The Lumbar Spine
Third Edition

*Official Publication of the International Society
for the Study of the Lumbar Spine*

The Lumbar Spine
Third Edition

*Official Publication of the International Society
for the Study of the Lumbar Spine*

Edited by

Harry N. Herkowitz, M.D.

*Chairman
Department of Orthopaedic Surgery
William Beaumont Hospital
Royal Oak, Michigan*

Jiri Dvorak, M.D.

*Professor
Department of Neurology
University of Zurich
Chief
Department of Neurology, Spine Unit
Schulthess Clinic
Zurich, Switzerland*

Gordon R. Bell, M.D.

*Vice-Chairman
Cleveland Clinic Spine Institute
Vice-Chairman
Department of Orthopaedic Surgery
Cleveland Clinic Foundation
Cleveland, Ohio*

Margareta Nordin, Dr.Sci., P.T., C.I.E.

*Research Professor and Director
Program of Ergonomics and Biomechanics
Departments of Orthopaedics and Environmental
Medicine
New York University School of Medicine
Director
Occupational and Industrial Orthopaedic Center
(OIOC)
Hospital for Joint Diseases
Mount Sinai-NYU Health
New York, New York*

Dieter Grob, M.D.

*Professor
Department of Orthopedics
University of Zurich
Chief
Department of Orthopedics, Spine Unit
Schulthess Hospital
Zurich, Switzerland*

LIPPINCOTT WILLIAMS & WILKINS
A **Wolters Kluwer** Company
Philadelphia · Baltimore · New York · London
Buenos Aires · Hong Kong · Sydney · Tokyo

2004

Acquisitions Editor: Robert Hurley
Developmental Editor: Kerry Barrett
Production Editor: Karina Mikhli
Manufacturing Manager: Benjamin Rivera
Cover Designer: Brian Crede
Compositor: Lippincott Williams & Wilkins Desktop Divison
Printer: Maple-Press

© 2004 by LIPPINCOTT WILLIAMS & WILKINS
530 Walnut Street
Philadelphia, PA 19106 USA
LWW.com

Printed in the USA

Library of Congress Cataloging-in-Publication Data

The lumbar spine / official publication of the International Society for the Study of the Lumbar Spine ;
    edited by Harry N. Herkowitz ... [et al.].—3rd ed.
        p. ; cm.
    Includes bibliographical references and index.
    ISBN 0-7817-4297-8
        1. Backache. 2. Lumbar vertebrae—Diseases. I. Herkowitz, Harry N. II. International Society for
the Study of the Lumbar Spine.
        [DNLM: 1. Lumbar Vertebrae. 2. Spinal diseases. WE 750 L95665 2004]
    RD771.B217L86 2004
    617.5′6—dc22
                                                                    2003065939

Care has been taken to confirm the accuracy of the information presented and to describe generally accepted practices. However, the authors, editors, and publisher are not responsible for errors or omissions or for any consequences from application of the information in this book and make no warranty, expressed or implied, with respect to the currency, completeness, or accuracy of the contents of the publication. Application of this information in a particular situation remains the professional responsibility of the practitioner.

The authors, editors, and publisher have exerted every effort to ensure that drug selection and dosage set forth in this text are in accordance with current recommendations and practice at the time of publication. However, in view of ongoing research, changes in government regulations, and the constant flow of information relating to drug therapy and drug reactions, the reader is urged to check the package insert for each drug for any change in indications and dosage and for added warnings and precautions. This is particularly important when the recommended agent is a new or infrequently employed drug.

Some drugs and medical devices presented in this publication have Food and Drug Administration (FDA) clearance for limited use in restricted research settings. It is the responsibility of the health care provider to ascertain the FDA status of each drug or device planned for use in their clinical practice.

10 9 8 7 6 5 4 3 2 1

Dedication

The International Society for the Study of the Lumbar Spine (ISSLS) is a unique organization. Its membership includes representatives from all the continents who come together yearly to discuss their unique perspectives on all facets of lumbar disease. It is an organization that thrives on discussion and whose members have dedicated their professional lives to advancing the knowledge of spine disease so that people may live active and productive lives. Many of the membership, past and present, were and are "household names" in the spine world who, through their research and teaching, have made significant contributions to our understanding of the spine. Many others who are not "household names" have also contributed to advancing our knowledge through their active participation in the society. This third edition of the ISSLS textbook is dedicated to the following members who have passed on; each of them has contributed through their research, teaching, and discussion that are reflected in the pages of this third edition: Alf Breig, Alexander Brodsky, John Bromley, Ralph Cloward, Stephan Dorhring, George Dommissee, Alan Dwyer, George Ehni, Harry Farfan, Harry Fahrni, William Fielding, Edward Froning, Jacob Graham, Beckett Howorth, Carlyle Hudson, Shunichi Inoue, Bernard Jacobs, Rae Jacobs, Henry LaRocca, Bruno Lassale, Ian MacNab, John McCulloch, James Morris, Philip Newmann, William Park, Homer Pheasant, Frank Raney, Lester Russin, Antonio Martino, David Selby, Lyman Smith, Arthur Thibodeau, Henk Verbiest, Henrik Weber, Thomas Whitecloud.

The Editorial Board on behalf of the ISSLS membership

Contents

SECTION I. BASIC SCIENCE

SECTION V. SPECIFIC CLINICAL ENTITIES

Contributing Authors

Todd J. Albert, M.D.
Professor and Vice Chairman
Department of Orthopaedic Surgery
Thomas Jefferson University Medical College
and The Rothman Institute
Philadelphia, Pennsylvania

Howard S. An, M.D.
The Morton International Professor
Director of Spine Surgery
Department of Orthopaedic Surgery
Rush University Medical Center
Chicago, Illinois

Gunnar B.J. Andersson, M.D., Ph.D.
Professor and Chairman
Senior Vice President, Medical Affairs
Department of Orthopedic Surgery
Rush University Medical Center
Chicago, Illinois

James A. Antinnes, M.D.
Department of Orthopaedic Surgery
University of California at San Francisco
San Francisco, California
Department of Orthopaedic Surgery
Hattiesburg Clinic Spine Center
Hattiesburg, Mississippi

Josef C. Assheuer, M.D.
Institute f. Kernspintomographie
Koln, Germany

Orin Atlas, M.D.
Spine Surgeon
Department of Orthopaedics
Virtua Memorial Hospital
Mt. Holly, New Jersey

Federico Balagué, M.D.
Adjunct Associate Professor
Department of Orthopedic Surgery
New York University School of Medicine
New York, New York
Médecin-chef Adjoint
Department of Rheumatology, Physical
Medicine and Rehabilitation
Cantonal Hospital
Fribourg, Switzerland

Michele C. Battié, Ph.D.
Professor and Canada Research Chair
Department of Physical Therapy
University of Alberta
Edmonton, Canada

Gordon R. Bell, M.D.
Vice-Chairman
Cleveland Clinic Spine Institute
Vice-Chairman
Department of Orthopaedic Surgery
Cleveland Clinic Foundation
Cleveland, Ohio

Tom Bendix, M.D., Dr.Med.Sci.
Professor
Institute of Sports and Biomechanics
University of Southern Denmark
Odense, Denmark
Bach Research Center
Fyen Hospital Ringe
University of Southern Denmark
Ringe, Denmark

Ashok Biyani, M.D.
Spine Fellow
Rush-Presbyterian-St. Luke's Medical Center
Chicago, Illinois

Scott L. Blumenthal, M.D.
Texas Back Institute
Musculoskeletal Research Foundation
Texas Health Research Institute
Plano, Texas

Scott D. Boden, M.D.
Professor
Department of Orthopaedic Surgery
Director
The Emory Spine Center
Emory University School of Medicine
Decatur, Georgia

Christopher M. Bono, M.D.
Chief of Spine Surgery
Department of Orthopaedic Surgery
Boston University School of Medicine
Boston, Massachusetts

David Borenstein, M.D., F.A.C.P., F.A.C.R.
Clinical Professor of Medicine
Arthritis and Rheumatism Associates
The George Washington University Medical
 Center
Washington, D.C.

Dahari D. Brooks, M.D.
State University of New York Health Science
 Center
Upstate Medical University
Syracuse, New York

Charles W. Cha, M.D.
Clinical Instructor
The Emory Spine Center
Department of Orthopaedic Surgery
Emory University School of Medicine
Atlanta, Georgia

Eric C. Chamberlin, M.D.
Pittsburgh Bone and Joint Surgeons
McKeesport, Pennsylvania

Kenneth M.C. Cheung, M.D., F.R.C.S.,
 F.H.K.C.O.S., F.H.K.A.M.(Orth.)
Associate Professor
Department of Orthopedic Surgery
The University of Hong Kong
Honorary Consultant and Deputy Chief
Division of Spine Surgery
Queen Mary Hospital and The Duchess of Kent
 Children's Hospital
Hong Kong, China

Gianluca Cinotti, M.D.
Associate Professor
Department of Orthopaedics and Traumatology
University La Sapienza
Rome, Italy

Scott D. Daffner, M.D.
Resident
Department of Orthopaedic Surgery
Thomas Jefferson University Hospital
Philadelphia, Pennsylvania

Rick Delamarter, M.D.
The Spine Institute at Saint John's Health
 Center
Santa Monica, California

Richard Derby, M.D.
Associate Clinical Professor
Department of Physical Medicine and
 Rehabilitation
Stanford University
Stanford, California
Medical Director
Spinal Diagnostic and Treatment Center
Daly City, California

Richard A. Deyo, M.D., M.P.H.
Professor
Departments of Medicine and Health Services
University of Washington
Staff Physician
Department of Medicine
University of Washington Medical Center
Seattle, Washington

Jean Dudler, M.D.
Maître d'Enseignement et de Recherche
Faculté de Biologie et de Médecine
Université de Lausanne
Médecin-associé
Servie de Rhumatologie
Médecine Physique et Rééducation
Centre Hospitalier Universitaire Vaudois
Lausanne, Switzerland

Jiri Dvorak, M.D.
Professor
Department of Neurology
University of Zurich
Chief
Department of Neurology, Spine Unit
Schulthess Clinic
Zurich, Switzerland

Anthony P. Dwyer, M.D.
Professor
Department of Orthopaedics
University of Colorado Health Science Center
Co-Director
Spine Service
Denver Health Medical Center
Denver, Colorado

Peter Dyck, M.D., F.A.C.S.
Clinical Professor
Department of Neurological Surgery
University of Southern California
Keck School of Medicine
Los Angeles, California

N. Ebraheim, M.D.
Spine Research Center
University of Toledo and Medical College
of Ohio
Toledo, Ohio

Stephen Eisenstein, Ph.D., F.R.C.S.
Director
Centre for Spinal Studies
The Robert Jones and Agnes Hunt Orthopaedic
Hospital
Oswestry, Shropshire
United Kingdom

Frank J. Eismont, M.D.
Vice-Chairman
University of Miami Department of Orthopedics
and Rehabilitation
University of Miami School of Medicine
Miami, Florida

Thomas J. Errico, M.D.
New York University Medical Center
New York, New York

Jeremy Fairbank, M.D., F.R.C.S.
Consultant Orthopaedic Surgeon
Nuffield Orthopaedic Centre
Senior Clinical Lecturer
Nuffield Department of Orthopaedic Surgery
Oxford, United Kingdom

Peter J. Fazey, M.D.
Centre for Musculoskeletal Studies
School of Surgery and Pathology
The University of Western Australia
Royal Perth Hospital
Perth, Western Australia

Yizhar Floman, M.D.
Professor (Emeritus)
Department of Orthopedic Surgery
Hadassah-Hebrew University Medical School
Jerusalem, Israel
Director
Israel Spine Center
Assuta Hospital
Tel Aviv, Israel

Robert D. Fraser, M.D.

Bruce E. Fredrickson, M.D.
Professor
Department of Orthopedic and Neurologic
Surgery
Upstate Medical University Hospital
Syracuse, New York

Brian J.C. Freeman, M.B., B.Ch., B.A.O.,
F.R.C.S. (Tr & Orth)
Clinical Tutor
Department of Orthopaedic and
Accident Surgery
University of Nottingham
Queens Medical Centre
Consultant Spinal Surgery
The Centre for Spinal Surgery
University Hospital
Queens Medical Centre
Nottingham, United Kingdom

Ioannis N. Gaitanis, M.D.
Department of Orthopaedic Surgery-
Traumatology
University of Crete at Heraklion
Crete, Greece

Steven R. Garfin, M.D.
Professor and Chair
Department of Orthopaedics
University of California at San Diego
San Diego, California

Robert J. Gatchel, M.D., Ph.D.
Elizabeth H. Penn Professor
Department of Clinical Psychology
Professor
Department of Psychiatry
The University of Texas Southwestern Medical
Center at Dallas
Dallas, Texas

Matthew J. Geck, M.D.
Spine Surgeon
Brain and Spine Center
Brackenridge Hospital
Texas Scoliosis and Spine, P.A.
Austin, Texas

Stanley D. Gertzbein, M.D., F.R.C.S.(C)
Clinical Professor
Department of Orthopedic Surgery
Baylor College of Medicine
Active Staff Consultant
Department of Orthopedic Surgery
Saint Joseph Hospital
Houston, Texas

Lars G. Gilbertson, Ph.D.
Associate Professor
Department of Orthopaedic Surgery
University of Pittsburgh Medical Center
Pittsburgh, Pennsylvania

**Wolfgang Gilliar, D.O., F.A.A.P.M.R.,
O.M.M.**
Assistant Clinical Professor
Department of Functional Restoration
Stanford University School of Medicine
Palo Alto, California

Vijay K. Goel, Ph.D.
Professor and Chair
Department of Bioengineering
University of Toledo
Professor and Co-Director
Department of Orthopedics
Medical College of Ohio
Toledo, Ohio

Philippe Goupille, M.D.
Professor
Department of Rheumatology
François Rabelais University
Department of Rheumatology
Trousseau Hospital
Tours, France

**Shunmugam Govender, M.D., M.M.B.S.,
F.R.C.S.**
Professor and Head
Department of Orthopaedics
University of Natal
Director
Department of Spinal Services
King George V Hospital
Durban, Natal

John N. Graber, M.D., F.A.C.S.
Clinical Instructor
Department of Surgery
University of Minnesota
Minneapolis, Minnesota

Jonathan N. Grauer, M.D.
Assistant Professor
*Department of Orthopaedics and
Rehabilitation*
Yale University School of Medicine
Yale New Haven Hospital
New Haven, Connecticut

**Charles G. Greenough, M.D., M.Chir.,
F.R.C.S.**
Professor
University of Durham
Durham, United Kingdom
Clinical Director
Spinal Injuries Centre
The James Cook University Hospital
Middlesbrough, United Kingdom

Dieter Grob, M.D.
Professor
Department of Orthopedics
University of Zurich
Chief
*Department of Orthopedics,
Spine Unit*
Schulthess Hospital
Zurich, Switzerland

Mats Grönblad, M.D., Ph.D.
Associate Professor
*Division of Physical Medicine and
Rehabilitation*
University of Helsinki
Chief
*Division of Physical Medicine and
Rehabilitation*
University Central Hospital
Helsinki, Finland

Robert Gunzburg, M.D., Ph.D.
Senior Consultant
Department of Orthopedics
Centenary Clinic
Antwerp, Belgium

Richard D. Guyer, M.D.
Associate Clinical Professor
Department of Orthopedic Surgery
Univeristy of Texas Southwestern Medical
* School*
Dallas, Texas
Director
Texas Back Institute Spine Fellowship
Texas Back Institute
Plano, Texas

Holger Haak, M.D.
Orthopaedic University Hospital
Duesseldorf, Germany

Alexander G. Hadjipavlou, M.D.
Professor and Chairman
Department of Orthopaedic Surgery
Traumatology
University of Crete Medical School
Crete, Greece

Yong Hai, M.D.
Professor and Chairman
Department of Orthopaedic Surgery
Spinal Surgery Center
306 Hospital
Beijing, China

Scott Haldeman, D.C., M.D., Ph.D.
Clinical Professor
Department of Neurology
University of California at Irvine
Irvine, California
Adjunct Professor
Department of Epidemiology
University of California at Los Angeles
* School of Public Health*
Los Angeles, California

David J. Hall, M.B.B.S., F.R.A.C.S.
Clinical Lecturer
Department of Orthopaedics and Trauma
University of Adelaide
Senior Visiting Medical Specialist,
* Spinal Unit*
Royal Adelaide Hospital
Adelaide, South Australia

Edward N. Hanley, Jr., M.D.
Chair
Department of Orthopaedic Surgery
Carolinas Medical Center
Charlotte, North Carolina

Kambiz Hannani, M.D.

Kenneth B. Heithoff, M.D.
Center for Diagnostic Imaging
Minneapolis, Minnesota

Joerg Herdmann, M.D.
Neurosurgical University Hospital
Duesseldorf, Germany

Harry N. Herkowitz, M.D.
Chairman
Department of Orthopaedic Surgery
William Beaumont Hospital
Royal Oak, Michigan

Arto Herno, M.D., Ph.D.
Senior Consultant
Department of Physical and Rehabilitation
* Medicine*
Kuopio University Hospital
Kuopio, Finland

Alan S. Hilibrand, M.D.
Assistant Professor
Department of Orthopaedic Surgery
Jefferson Medical College
The Rothman Institute
Thomas Jefferson University Hospital
Philadelphia, Pennsylvania

Sten H. Holm, Ph.D.
Professor and Chief
Department of Surgery
Sahlgrenska University Hospital
Göteborg, Sweden

Serena Shaw Hu, M.D.
Associate Professor
Department of Orthopaedic Surgery
University of California at San Francisco
Staff Surgeon
Department of Orthopedic Surgery
Moffitt-Long Hospitals, UCSF
San Francisco, California

Aage Indahl, M.D., Ph.D.
Associate Professor
Department of Physical Medicine and
* Rehabilitation*
University of Oslo
Kysthospitalet ved Stavern
Stavern, Norway

Hirokazu Ishihara, M.D., Ph.D.
Senior Lecturer
Department of Orthopaedic Surgery
Toyama Medical and Pharmaceutical University
Toyama, Japan

Manabu Ito, M.D., Ph.D.
Assistant Professor
Department of Orthopaedic Surgery
Hokkaido University Graduate School of
* Medicine*
Chief
Spine Section
Department of Orthopaedic Surgery
Hokkaido University Hospital
Sapporo, Japan

Ragnar Johnsson, M.D., Ph.D.
Associate Professor
Department of Orthopedics
Consultant, Spine Unit
Lund University Hospital
Lund, Sweden

Bo Jönsson, M.D., Ph.D.
Department of Orthopaedics
Lund University Hospital
Helsingborg Hospital
Helsingborg, Sweden

Allison M. Kaigle Holm, Ph.D.
Senior Research Engineer
Department of Orthopaedics
Sahlgrenska University Hospital
Göteborg, Sweden

Masahiko Kanamori, M.D., Ph.D.
Lecturer and Chief
Department of Orthopedics
Toyama Medical and Pharmaceutical University
Toyama, Japan

Kiyoshi Kaneda, M.D.
Professor Emeritus
Hokkaido University
Director General
Bibai Rosai Hospital
Bibai, Japan

James D. Kang, M.D.
Associate Professor
Department of Orthopaedic Surgery
University of Pittsburgh School of Medicine
Associate Professor
Department of Orthopaedic Surgery
University of Pittsburgh Medical Center
Pittsburgh, Pennsylvania

Babek Kateb, M.D.

P. Katonis, M.D.
Assistant Professor and Lecturer
Department of Orthopaedic Surgery-
* Traumatology*
University of Crete at Heraklion
Crete, Greece

Christopher P. Kauffman, M.D.
Assistant Clinical Professor
Department of Orthopaedic Surgery
Division of Spine Surgery
University of California at San Diego
San Diego, California

Yoshiharu Kawaguchi, M.D., Ph.D.
Assistant Professor
Department of Orthopaedic Surgery
Toyama Medical and Pharmaceutical
* University*
Toyama, Japan

Mamoru Kawakami, M.D., Ph.D.
Assistant Professor
Department of Orthopaedic Surgery
Wakayama Medical University
Wakayama, Japan

Tony S. Keller, Ph.D.
Department of Mechanical Engineering
Musculoskeletal Research Laboratory
The University of Vermont
Burlington, Vermont

K. Anthony Kim, M.D.

Shinichi Kikuchi, M.D., Ph.D.
Department of Orthopaedic Surgery
Fukushima Medical University
Fukushima City, Japan

Mark A. Knaub, M.D.
Fellow, Spinal Surgery
Department of Orthopaedic Surgery
William Beaumont Hospital
Royal Oak, Michigan

Kenneth J. Kopacz, M.D.
Assistant Clinical Professor
Department of Orthopaedics
New Jersey Medical School
Newark, New Jersey
Attending
Department of Orthopaedic Surgery
St. Barnabas Medical Center
Livingston, New Jersey

Victor Kosmopoulos, Ph.D.
Assistant Professor
Department of Engineering
The College of New Jersey
Ewing, New Jersey

Juergen Kraemer, M.D.
Orthopaedic University Hospital
Bochum, Germany

Robert Krämer, Dr. Med.
Associate Doctor
Cirugia Ortopedica y
   Traumatologia
Centro Medico Teknon
Co-Chief
Cirugia de la Columna
Consultorios Marquesa
Barcelona, Spain

Hiroshi Kuroki, M.D., D.M.Sc.
Instructor
Department of Orthopaedic Surgery
Faculty of Medicine
University of Miyazaki
Miyazaki, Japan

Christian Lattermann, M.D.
Resident
Department of Orthopaedic Surgery
University of Pittsburgh Medical Center
Pittsburgh, Pennsylvania

William C. Lauerman, M.D.
Professor and Chief
Division of Spine Surgery
Department of Orthopaedic Surgery
Georgetown University Hospital
Washington, DC

Casey K. Lee, M.D.
Clinical Professor
Department of Orthopaedic Surgery
New Jersey Medical School
Newark, New Jersey
Attending Surgeon
Department of Orthopaedic Surgery
St. Barnabas Medical Center
Livingston, New Jersey

**John C.Y. Leong, O.B.E., F.R.C.S.,
   F.R.C.S.E., F.R.A.C.S., F.H.K.A.M.
   (Orth), J.P.**
Chair, Professor, and Head
Department of Orthopaedic Surgery
The University of Hong Kong
Hong Kong

Simon Macklin, M.B.B.S., F.R.C.A.
Senior Staff Specialist
Department of Anaesthesia and Intensive Care
Royal Adelaide Hospital
Adelaide, South Australia

Marianne L. Magnusson, Dr.Med.Sc.
Liberty Worksafe Research Centre
Department of Environmental and
   Occupational Medicine
University of Aberdeen
Aberdeen, Scotland

Chris J. Main, M.D.
University of Manchester
School of Epidemiology
Manchester, United Kingdom

Joseph Y. Margulies, M.D., Ph.D.
Consultant Orthopaedic Surgeon
Maurice E. Mueller Institute
Berne, Switzerland
Associate Professor
Department of Surgery
Albert Einstein College of
   Medicine
New York, New York

William S. Marras, Ph.D., C.P.E.
Biodynamics Laboratory
The Ohio State University
Columbus, Ohio

Hisao Matsui, M.D., Ph.D.
Chief
Department of Orthopaedic Surgery
Takaoka City Hospital
Takaoka, Toyama, Japan

H. Michael Mayer, M.D., Ph.D.
Associate Professor, Head, and Medical
   Director
Spine Center Munich
Orthozentrum Meunchen
Meunchen, Germany

Geoffrey M. McCullen, M.D.
Spine Surgeon
Department of Orthopedics
Neurological and Spinal Surgery, LLC
Lincoln, Nebraska

Dennis P. McGowan, M.Sc., M.D.
Staff Surgeon
Department of Orthopedic Surgery
Good Samaritan Hospital
Kearney, Nebraska

Anis O. Mekhail, M.D., M.S.
Clinical Assistant Professor
Department of Orthopedic Surgery
University of Illinois at Chicago
Chicago, Illinois
Spine Surgeon
Department of Orthopedic Surgery
Palos Community Hospital
Palos Heights, Illinois

Akio Minami, M.D.
Professor and Chairman
Department of Orthopaedic Surgery
Hokkaido University Graduate School of
  Medicine
Sapporo, Japan

Robert J. Moore, Ph.D., B.App.Sc.,
  M.App.Sc.
Affiliate Senior Lecturer
Department of Pathology
The University of Adelaide
Head
The Adelaide Centre for Spinal
  Research
Institute of Medical and Veterinary
  Science
Adelaide, South Australia

Mohamed Mostafa Mossaad, M.D.,
  M.S.C., M.D., Orth.
Professor
Spine Unit, Department of
  Orthopaedics
Faculty of Medicine
Zagazig University
Chief
Spine Unit, Department of
  Orthopaedics
Zagazig University Hospital
Zagazig, Egypt

Robert R. Myers, Ph.D.
Department of Anesthesiology and Pathology
  (Neuropathology)
University of California at San Diego
VA Healthcare System
San Diego, California

Alf L. Nachemson, M.D., Ph.D.
Professor Emeritus
Department of Orthopaedics and Surgical
  Sciences
Göteborg University
Sahlgrenska Hospital
Göteborg, Sweden

Hiroaki Nakamura, M.D., Ph.D.
Associate Professor
Department of Orthopaedic Surgery
Osaka City University Medical School
Subchief
Department of Orthopaedic Surgery
Osaka City University Hospital
Osaka, Japan

Margareta Nordin, Dr.Sci., P.T., C.I.E.
Research Professor and Director
Program of Ergonomics and Biomechanics
Departments of Orthopaedics and
  Environmental Medicine
New York University School of Medicine
Director
Occupational and Industrial Orthopaedic
  Center (OIOC)
Hospital for Joint Diseases
Mount Sinai-NYU Health Center
New York, New York

Donna D. Ohnmeiss, Dr.Med.
Director of Research
Texas Back Institute Research Foundation
Plano, Texas

Juan Carlos Rodriguez Olaverri,
  M.D., Ph.D.
Attending Spine Section
Department of Orthopaedic Surgery
Hospital Universitario Miguel Servet
Zaragoza, Spain

Kjell Olmarker, M.D.
Department of Orthopaedics
Sahlgren Hospital
Gothenburg, Sweden

Conor O'Neill, M.D.
Assistant Clinical Professor
Department of Radiology
University of California at San Francisco
Private Practice
San Francisco Spine Diagnostics
San Francisco, California

Orso L. Osti, M.D., Ph.D., F.R.A.C.S.,
  F.A.Ortho.A.
Head
Spinal Service
The Queen Elizabeth Hospital
Woodville, South Australia
Clinical Senior Lecturer
Adelaide University
North Adelaide, South Australia

Paul Pagano, M.D.
Tulane University Health Sciences Center
New Orleans, Louisiana

Manohar M. Panjabi, Ph.D.
Professor and Director
Department of Orthopaedics and Rehabilitation
Biomechanics Research Laboratory
Yale University School of Medicine
New Haven, Connecticut

Frank M. Phillips, M.D.
Associate Professor and Co-Director Spine
*   Fellowship*
Department of Orthopaedic Surgery
Rush University Medical Center
Chicago, Illinois

Malcolm H. Pope, Dr.Med.Sc., Ph.D., D.Sc.
Department of Environmental and
*   Occupational Medicine*
Liberty Worksafe Research Centre
University of Aberdeen
Aberdeen, Scotland

Franco Postacchini, M.D.
Professor
Department of Orthopaedic Surgery
University La Sapienza
Chairman
Department of the Orthopaedics
Policlinico Umberto I
Rome, Italy

Christopher S. Raffo, M.D.
Instructor
Department of Orthopaedics
Georgetown University
Washington, D.C.

James Rainville, M.D.
Clinical Assistant Professor
Department of Physical Medicine and
*   Rehabilitation*
Harvard Medical School
Chief
Department of Physical Medicine and
*   Rehabilitation*
New England Baptist Hospital
Boston, Massachusetts

S. Rajasekaran, M.S., Ph.D.
Academic Director
Department of Orthopaedics
Ganga Institute of Orthopaedics
Department of Orthopaedics and Spine Surgery
Ganga Hospital
Coimbatore, India

Ralph F. Rashbaum, M.D.
Texas Health Research Institute
Texas Back Institute
Musculoskeletal Research
*   Foundation*
Plano, Texas

Donald L. Renfrew, M.D.
Musculoskeletal Radiologist
Department of Radiology
Center for Diagnostic Imaging
Winter Park, Florida

Setti S. Rengachary, M.D.
Professor and Associate Academic
*   Chairman*
Department of Neurosurgery
Wayne State University
Attending Neurological Surgeon
Department of Neurosurgery
Harper Hospital
Detroit, Michigan

Peter A. Robertson, M.D., F.R.A.C.S.
Orthopaedic and Spinal Surgeon
Department of Orthopaedic Surgery
Auckland City Hospital
Auckland, New Zealand

Stephen L. Gabriel Rothman, M.D.
Clinical Professor
Department of Radiology
University of Southern California School of
*   Medicine*
Los Angeles, California
Spinal Injury Service
Rancho Los Amigos Hospital
Downey, California

Björn L. Rydevik, M.D., Ph.D.
Professor and Chairman
Institute for Surgical Sciences
Göteborg University
Professor
Department of Orthopaedics
Sahlgrenska University Hospital
Göteborg, Sweden

Jeffrey A. Saal, M.D., F.A.C.P.
Associate Clinical Professor
Department of Functional Restoration
Stanford University School of
*   Medicine*
Stanford, California
SOAR, Physiatry Group
Redwood City, California

Joel S. Saal, M.D.
Associate Clinical Professor
Department of Functional Restoration
Stanford University School of Medicine
Stanford, California
SOAR, Physiatry Group
Redwood City, California

Srinath Samudrala, M.D.
Assistant Professor
Department of Neurological Surgery
Keck School of Medicine
University of Southern California
Los Angeles, California

Steven C. Scherping, Jr., M.D.
Assistant Professor
Department of Orthopaedic Surgery
Georgetown University Hospital
Washington, D.C.

Klaus-Peter Schulitz, M.D.
Professor Emeritus
Department of Orthopaedic Surgery
Heinrich-Heine Universitaet
Duesseldorf, Germany

Dilip K. Sengupta, M.B.B.S., M.S., Dip. N.B.E., M.Ch.
Staff Spine Surgeon
Department of Orthopaedics
William Beaumont Hospital
Royal Oak, Michigan

William O. Shaffer, M.D.
Associate Professor and Surgery Residency
  Program Director
Department of Surgery
Division of Orthopaedic Surgery
University of Kentucky Medical School
Attending Orthopaedic Surgeon
Department of Surgery
Division of Orthopaedic Surgery
Chandler Medical Center of the University
  of Kentucky
Lexington, Kentucky

Francis H. Shen, M.D., F.A.C.S.
Assistant Professor
Department of Orthopaedic Surgery
University of Virginia School of Medicine
Assistant Professor
Department of Orthopaedic Surgery
Health Sciences Center
University of Virginia
Charlottesville, Virginia

Osamu Shirado, M.D.
Associate Professor
Department of Orthopaedic Surgery
Saitama Medical School
Saitama, Japan
Vice President
Department of Orthopaedic Surgery
Sapporo Orthopaedic and Cardiovascular
  Hospital
Sapporo, Japan

Jeff Scott Silber, M.D.
Assistant Professor
Department of Orthopedic Surgery
Albert Einstein College of
  Medicine
Bronx, New York
Assistant Professor
Department of Orthopedics
Chief, Orthopedic Spine Surgery
Long Island Jewish Medical Center
New Hyde Park, New York

Edward D. Simmons, M.D., C.M., M.Sc., F.R.C.S.(C.)
Associate Clinical Professor
Department of Orthopaedic Surgery
State University of New York at
  Buffalo
Attending Orthopaedic Surgeon
Department of Orthopaedic Surgery
Buffalo General Hospital
Buffalo, New York

Edward H. Simmons, M.D., B.Sc.(Med.), F.R.C.S.(C.), M.S.(Tor.), F.A.C.S.
Emeritus Professor
Department of Orthopedic Surgery
State University of New York at
  Buffalo
Emeritus Chief
Department of Orthopaedic Surgery
State University of New York at Buffalo
Buffalo, New York

Kevin P. Singer, Ph.D., P.T.
Associate Professor and Director
The Centre for Musculoskeletal
  Studies
School of Surgery and Pathology
The University of Western Australia
Royal Perth Hospital
Perth, Western Australia

Kevin F. Spratt, Ph.D.
Adjunct Assistant Professor
Department of Psychological and Quantitative
 Foundations
College of Education
University of Iowa
Senior Project Leader
Department of Orthopaedic Surgery
University of Iowa Hospitals and
 Clinics
Iowa City, Iowa

Thomas Steffen, M.D., Ph.D., M.B.A.
Associate Professor and Research
 Director
Division of Orthopaedic Surgery
Orthopaedic Research Laboratory
McGill University
Montreal, Quebec, Canada

Björn Strömqvist, M.D., Ph.D.
Associate Professor
Department of Orthopedics
Head of Spine Unit
Lund University Hospital
Lund, Sweden

Marek Szpalski, M.D.
Associate Professor
School of Medicine
Free University of Brussels
Chairman
Department of Orthopedic and Trauma
 Surgery
IRIS South Teaching Hospitals
Brussels, Belgium

Tetsuya Tamaki, M.D., Ph.D.
Professor Emeritus
Department of Orthopaedic Surgery,
Wakayama Medical University
Medical Director
Aitoku Medical Welfare Center
Wakayama, Japan

Naoki Takeda, M.D.
Professor
Department of Health Sciences
Hokkaido University School of Medicine
Sapporo, Hokkaido, Japan

Ensor E. Transfeldt, M.D.
Associate Professor
University of Minnesota
Twin Cities Spine Center
Minneapolis, Minnesota

Jayesh M. Trivedi, F.R.C.S.(Orth.)
Consultant Spinal Surgeon
Department of Orthopaedics
Robert Jones and Agnes Hunt
 Hospital
Oswestry, United Kingdom

George M. Tsoukas, M.D.
Department of Endocrinology
McGill University
Montreal, Quebec, Canada

Michael N. Tzermiadianos, M.D.
Department of Orthopaedic Surgery and
 Traumatology
University of Crete at Heraklion
Crete, Greece

Alexander R. Vaccaro, M.D.
Professor and Co-Director
Delaware Valley Regional Spinal
Cord Injury Center
Co-Chief
Spine Service
Co-Director
Spine Fellowship Program
Thomas Jefferson University and the Rothman
 Institute
Philadelphia, Pennsylvania

Tapio Videman, M.D., Dr.Med.Sc.
Alberta Heritage Foundation for Medical
 Research Scientist and Professor
Faculty of Rehabilitation Medicine
University of Alberta
Edmonton, Canada

Robert G. Watkins IV, M.D.
Los Angeles Spine Surgery Institute
Los Angeles, California

Robert Watkins III, M.D.
Los Angeles Spine Surgery Institute
Los Angeles, California

Thomas S. Whitecloud III, M.D.
Ray J. Haddad Professor and Chairman
Tulane University of Health Sciences
 Center
New Orleans, Louisiana

Sam W. Wiesel, M.D.
Professor and Chair
Department of Orthopedics
Georgetown University
Washington, D.C.

Alexander Wild, M.D.
Orthopaedic University Hospital
Duesseldorf, Germany

Leon L. Wiltse, M.D.
Wiltse Spine Institute
Carmel Valley, California

Douglas S. Won, M.D.
Fellow, Spinal Surgery
Department of Orthopaedic Surgery
William Beaumont Hospital
Royal Oak, Michigan

Hansen A. Yuan, M.D.
Professor
Department of Orthopaedic and Neurological
  Surgery
State University of New York, Upstate Medical
  University
Syracuse, New York

Yinggang Zheng, M.D.
Research Fellow
Department of Orthopaedic Surgery
State University of New York at Buffalo
Research Fellow
Simmons Orthopaedic and Spine Associates
Buffalo, New York

Preface

This third edition of the International Society for the Study of the Lumbar Spine textbook represents a complete revision of the prior edition. A significant amount of new information is included— from the basic science of spine disease to surgical management of lumbar disorders. The members of this society who have contributed their excellent work are also the ones whose research has led to the many advances in the care and management of spinal disorders. This is an inclusive textbook emphasizing the basic science behind the clinical problems we face on a daily basis; it is comprehensive and covers all facets of the diseases that affect the lumbar spine. We are grateful to all the members of this society who have contributed chapters in order to make this the authoritative textbook on the lumbar spine.

This book is intended for all physicians and allied personnel who care for patients with low-back disorders. Hopefully, it will answer all the questions that the reader has to better understand the etiology, pathophysiology, clinical diagnosis, and management of lumbar disease.

Harry N. Herkowitz, M.D.
Jiri Dvorak, M.D.
Gordon R. Bell, M.D.
Margareta Nordin, Dr.Sci., P.T., C.I.E.
Dieter Grob, M.D.

Acknowledgments

No textbook makes it to press without the dedication of those behind the scenes. The International Society for the Study of the Lumbar Spine (ISSLS) textbook is no different.

First, I would like to acknowledge Shirley Fitzgerald, our administrator, friend, and the one person who keeps ISSLS on track making sure the business of the society is dealt with in a timely fashion. Many of us have "grown up with her" over the years and her dedication to the well-being of the society cannot be overstated. She is a unique individual who we are lucky to have in ISSLS.

Second, each Editorial Board member has his/her administrative assistant who helps organize the paperwork, correspondence, and chapter reviews. We would like to thank Christine Musich, Susana Kuster, Katrin Knecht, Elisabeth Weiss, and Katherine Habler.

Without their dedication and organization, the fruition of this textbook would have been significantly delayed. We wish to thank each of you for your outstanding effort.

Finally, we are grateful to Robert Hurley, Kerry Barrett, and Karina Mikhli at Lippincott Williams & Wilkins and Ted Huff, the illustrator, for supporting our organization, for being so professional in putting this textbook together, and for seeing it through to publication.

SECTION I

Basic Science

CHAPTER 1

Epidemiology and the Economics of Low Back Pain

Alf Nachemson

Epidemiology is critical to understanding the scope of a problem and gives information about its magnitude and the demand on medical and social resources. It is extremely important in our industrialized societies and gives information on the natural history, important for patient counseling about prognosis. It can also identify risk factors, both individual and external, which is beyond the scope of this chapter. It is also of importance to demonstrate both the societal burden of the ailment and its severe consequences for the individual quality of life (1).

Most studies in the literature talk about *prevalence* which is the percentage of people in a known population who have the symptom during a specified period. Point prevalence is the percentage who has pain on the day of the interview. One-month or one-year prevalence is the percentage who has pain at sometime within the past month or the past year. Lifetime prevalence is the percentage who can remember pain at sometime in their life. *Incidence* is the percentage of people in a known population who develop new symptoms during a specified period of time. It is commonly applied to those who report injuries or present for health care within a specified period.

Most recent surveys define low back pain as pain occurring between the costal margins and the gluteal folds. Some surveys use a diagram to show pain areas.

Back pain has often been defined differently. Epidemiologic rates for "back symptoms," "back disability," or "health care for back pain" respectively can all differ dependent of study sample.

Another major limitation of defining back pain is that surveys depend entirely on individual's own report of pain and disability, which is open to subjective bias, particularly when one is reporting from a disliked working environment. There may be recall bias: the longer ago the time of back pain is asked about, the more unreliable the answer. People with more severe trouble may be more likely to include earlier information within the period of the question (2–4) and present pain when questioned increases recall of earlier periods (5). Official statistics may overcome this problem to provide more accurate data about work loss, health care use, sickness verification and benefits, but these usually give lower rates for each of these than self-reports from population surveys (6). For example, a Danish study showed that only 25% of those reporting lower back pain in the past month ever visited a health care practitioner and less than 5% received sickness benefits; i.e., collecting unemployment (7).

There may also be sampling bias. Many surveys study selected group(s) of workers or patients, who may not be representative of the general population.

Raspe (8), Shekelle (9), and Andersson (2) reviewed altogether several hundred epidemiologic studies of low back pain from North America, Great Britain and Europe, in particular the Scandinavian countries. Because many of the surveys do not ask comparable questions, they give different results. Thus, the definition of morbidity chosen for the survey is of importance for the resulting frequency of pain.

The best available evidence on the epidemiology of low back pain is from large, representative, population surveys (2,10–19). Most recent surveys have used similar wording for their questions, and many have asked about pain lasting more than 24 hours, to exclude minor or passing symptoms.

Many international surveys of low back pain report a point prevalence of 15% to 30%, a 1-month prevalence between 19% and 43%, and a lifetime prevalence of about 60% to 80%. The exact figures in different studies appear to depend mainly on the wording of the question rather than any difference in the people studied (Table 1-1). What is clear, however, are the similarities of prevalence at any age, from 10 to 90 years of age.

TABLE 1-1. *One-month back pain prevalence at different ages and in different countries*

Age (yr)	Country	Yes (%)[a]
10–15	Sweden	40
12–15	France	50
15–18	Switzerland, Finland	32
25–35	Sweden, Denmark, Great Britain	35
40–50	Great Britain, Germany, Sweden, Finland, Tibet	40
40–60	Austria	68
55–65	Great Britain, Holland	30
70–85	Sweden	45
85+	Sweden	40

[a]Percentage of individuals who responded "yes" to the question, "Have you had any low back pain in the last month?"

The Nuprin Pain Report (17) found that 56% of American adults said they had at least one day of back pain in the last year. Fourteen percent had pain for more than 30 days in the year. Back pain was the second most common pain after headache. Most back pain was mild and short-lived and had very little effect on daily life, but recurrences were common. The most recent larger population study from Canada reported 8% with significant back pain in a 6-month period (20).

Von Korff et al. (18) found that 41% of American adults between the ages of 26 and 44 years had back pain in the last 6 months. Most people had occasional short attacks of pain, but they reported that they had had these attacks over a long period. Their pain was usually mild or moderate and did not limit their activities.

Some British surveys give comparable figures; Mason (21) found point prevalence around 15%, 1-month prevalence of 40%, and lifetime prevalence of 60%. Walsh et al. (19), Mason (21), and Papageorgiou et al. (13) found an almost identical lifetime prevalence of 60%, the same as reported in Belgium (16). In Tibet rural population the point prevalence was 34% and 12-month prevalence was 42% (22).

Population surveys suggest that the age of onset of back pain is spread fairly evenly from the teens to the early 40s. It is uncommon to develop nonspecific low back pain for the first time after the mid-50s. However, several recent studies of children show a higher prevalence of back pain than previously realized (Table 1-1). Brattberg (23,24) carried out a longitudinal study of 471 schoolchildren aged 10, 13, and 15 years in the county of Gävleborg in Sweden. In each year's survey, about 26% of children said they had back pain, but only 9% of the children reported back pain in both surveys in 1989 and 1991. Burton et al. (25) prospectively studied 216 adolescents from 11 through 15 years of age. Only 12% of 11-year-olds said they had ever had back pain, but by age 15 this number rose to 50%. The back pain these children describe was usually recurrent but did not deteriorate

with time. Adolescents appear to have about the same prevalence of back pain as adults, but it is rarely disabling and few seek health care. Burton et al. (25) suggest that most adolescent back trouble should be considered a normal life experience and should not have undue significance attached to it. There is no evidence on whether it predicts low back trouble in adult life. The study by Hellsing (26) of 19-year-old conscripts suggests the same finding when they were followed up to 10 years later.

The General Survey on Living Conditions in Sweden (27) found that neck and back problems are among the most common causes of "chronic sickness." About 3% to 5 % of the population between the ages of 16 and 44 years and 11% to 12% of those between the ages of 45 and 64 years report back problems as a "chronic sickness". For those between the ages of 65 and 84 years the frequency of back pain is somewhat reduced or 9% to 11%, although Brattberg (28,29) reported a higher prevalence of 45%. Back trouble is the most common cause of chronic sickness in both men and women under age 64 and the second most common cause of sickness for those between the ages of 65 and 74. Only circulatory system problems are more common among those in the 65+ age group. There is a slight increase over time of back pain in the general population according to the General Survey on Living Conditions (27). As an average for the population between 16 and 84 years (men and women), 6.5% reported back pain symptoms in 1985 compared to 8.0% in 1994. Linton et al. (30), in a study covering subjects living in the middle part of Sweden, but limited to subjects 35 to 45 years of age, found even higher prevalence figures, although these were probably dependent on how the questions were asked.

Other Scandinavian studies (3,31–33) have all described point prevalence of around 30%, 1-year prevalence of around 50%, and lifetime prevalence up to 80% or more.

The traditional clinical classification of back pain is acute, recurrent, and chronic, but recent epidemiologic studies show that back pain is usually a recurrent, intermittent, and episodic problem. Croft et al. (12,34) suggest that the most important epidemiologic concept, and also an important clinical concept, is the pattern of back pain over long periods of the individual's life, and that the experience of back pain may be better expressed as the total days of pain over 1 year. Von Korff et al. (18) also described this recurrent trait in back symptoms in the United States, as have others (35,36).

WORK LOSS DUE TO BACK PAIN

It is difficult to get accurate information on the amount of work loss attributed to back pain. In many countries, including Sweden since 1991, the first 2 weeks of sick pay are paid by employers who hold the data individually and do not return any statistics to any central authority.

Social security data contain claims and benefits paid, which depend on entitlement. The recent monograph by Waddell et al. (37) goes to unsurpassed length to describe this. The back pain absenteeism from no less than 13 countries was compared, demonstrating differences as well as similarities. There is little, if any evidence to suggest any physical basis to the overall level of reported back pain or disability in any of the examined industrialized societies. Instead, cultural, societal, and economic factors seem to play a more important role. According to the Waddell report, "There is now extensive evidence that psychosocial factors are more important than any physical changes in the back for development and maintenance of chronic pain and disability" (37).

In the 1970s, Valkenburg and Haanen (38) conducted a study in Zoetermeer, Netherlands of 6,500 men and women 20 years of age and older and provided data as seen in Table 1-2. These authors performed a physical and X-ray examination that demonstrated increasing "degenerative" changes with age that were not directly related to disability. Many others have since supported these findings.

Andersson (2) found that back problems were the most common cause of activity limitation in adults under age 45 and the fourth most common in those between the ages of 45 to 64. Seven percent of adults reported a disability due to their back or due to both their back and other joint problems that limited their activities for an average of about 23 days each year. These figures suggest that 7% to 14% of U.S. adults have some disability due to back pain for a least 1 day each year, and just over 1% of Americans are permanently disabled by back pain and another 1% are temporarily disabled by back pain at any one time. These figures have been confirmed by Murphy and Volinn (39), with little observable change over the years studied.

Walsh et al. (19) conducted a population survey using clinical measures of low back disability based on eight activities of daily living. The 1-year prevalence of a disability score of 50% or more was 5.4% for men and 4.5% for women, while the lifetime prevalence was 16% and 13%, respectively. The 1-year prevalence of time off work because of back pain was 11% for men and 7% for women, while the lifetime prevalence was 34% and 23%, respectively.

The South Manchester Study (14) found that 8% of adults said they had bed rest for back pain at some time in the past 12 months. However, these figures are again self-reports about what people said they did about back pain, not the treatment they received.

The Clinical Standards Advisory Group (40) estimated that work loss due to back pain in the United Kingdom in 1993 was about 52 million days, while 106 million days' sickness and invalidity benefits were paid for back pain. However, there was only overlap of 7 million days between these two groups. Most of the workers who lost short periods of work were paid by their employers, did not receive any state sickness benefits, and did not appear in the official statistics, while most of the benefits went to people who were not employed (41).

Guo et al. (42) provide the best estimate of work loss due to back pain in the United States, using data on 30,074 workers from the National Health Interview Survey. In 1988, about 22.4 million people, or 17.6% of all U.S. workers, lost an estimated 149 million days of work due to back pain. This can be compared to the very recent figures in Sweden that claim the world record of sickness absence in recent years. Short-term sickness of less than 1 year was registered for a total of 380,000 workers in a population of 4.4 million of working age; and 480,000 subjects were sick more than 1 year or permanently disabled in 2001 (43,44). According to Murphy and Volinn (39), the prevalence of back illness has not changed much in the U.S. since those 1988 rates. Comparison can be made to recent Swedish rates provided in the following paragraphs.

In most studies, about half the total days missed from work due to back pain are accounted for by the 85% of people who are off work for short periods, with a median of less than 7 days (45). The other half is accounted for by the 15% of people who are off work for more than 1 month. This is reflected in the total social costs of back pain. It is widely quoted that 80% to 90% of the health care costs of back pain are for the 10% of patients with chronic low back pain and disability (2,46–48). Watson et al. (49) showed that the same is true for the social costs. In 1994, back pain in the island of Jersey accounted for 11% of all sickness absence. Only 3% of those off work with back pain were off for more than 6 months, but they accounted for 33% of the benefits paid.

TABLE 1-2. *Low back complaints and work disability in the Dutch city of Zoetermeer (38) in the 1970s*

	Men (%)	Relative (%)	Women (%)	Relative (%)
Point-prevalence	22.2		30.2	
Lifetime incidence	51.4		57.8	
>3 months	14.3	28	19.6	34
Unfit for work	24.3	47	19.5	34
Work change	4.2	8	2.4	4

WORK LOSS DUE TO BACK PAIN IN SWEDEN

The city of Gothenburg, with its 450,000 inhabitants, has been a source of much Swedish epidemiologic data through the late 1990s (2,45,47,50–54).

In the studies just mentioned from the 1970s, Svensson and Andersson (50–52) indicated that between 2% and 6% of all people reporting illness in Gothenburg suffered work loss due to back pain. An interesting fact was that one-fourth of the men who said they never had had back pain actually had been off work 1 day or more with that diagnosis when insurance data were checked. This illustrates the difficulty in relying on memory in questionnaire surveys. Sweden's workforce of approximately 4.4 million people between the ages of 18 and 65 years of age lost approximately 58 workdays per year on an average due to sickness in 2001. As a comparison, it can be calculated that the annual amount of working days lost among the 125 million people of similar age in the U.S. amounts to 150 million per year (42). In Sweden with 4.4 million people of working age the same work loss due to low back pain was 50 million days (i.e., approximately 8 times higher).

There was a reduction in number of subjects on overall sick leave from 1993 to 1997 after which time sick-listing again increased considerably (55) (Fig. 1-1). In addition there has been a steep increase in new permanent disability claims granted, from 45,000 in 1997 to 70,000 in 2002; 20% of which are due to back pain (43,44,54) (Table 1-3). The total number of days lost because of back

TABLE 1-3. *New disability pensions granted in Sweden (1996–2002)*

Year	Total no.	No. for back pain
1996	39.245	8.464
1997	41.198	8.673
1998	34.487	5.951
1999	39.506	6.735
2000	49.237	8.458
2001	57.081	10.014
2002 (approx.)	63.000	13.000

disability in Sweden, including both short-term absenteeism and those on permanent disability exceeded 50 million in 2002 (43,44,55). This figure may be somewhat uncertain because the exact diagnosis is not always clear; it is known, however, that 49% of all sick subjects for more than 1 year have a musculoskeletal disorder, and

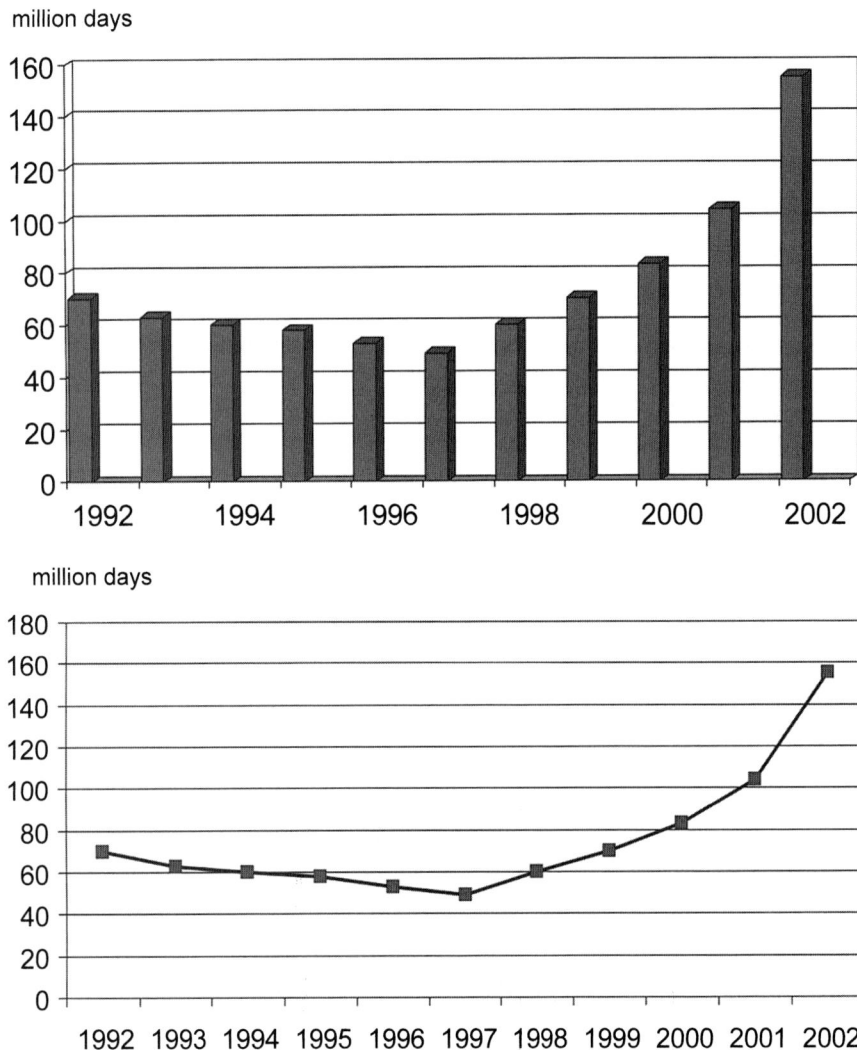

FIG. 1-1. Total number of sick days paid 1992 to 2002 in Sweden (excluding the first 14 days covered by employer), approximately 30% due to low back pain (43–45,54).

70% of this percentage according to the Gothenburg studies (45,54) is back pain, while 25% of permanent disability pensions are granted for back problems.

SCIATICA

Few surveys use strict criteria for "sciatica." Several reports give a lifetime prevalence of 14% to 40% for leg pain associated with back problems but they do not distinguish true radicular pain from the more common referred leg pain. Deyo and Tsui-Wu (56) estimated the lifetime prevalence of "surgically important disc herniation" to be about 2%. Lawrence (57) reported a prevalence of "sciatica suggesting a herniated lumbar disc" in 3.1% of men and 1.3% of women. Neither of these studies gave diagnostic criteria. Heliovaara et al. (58) in Finland reported the only large population survey with clinical criteria of radicular pain. That study had a lifetime prevalence of back pain of 77% in men and 74% in women, while the lifetime prevalence of any associated leg pain was 35% in men and 45% in women. Applying strict diagnostic criteria for radicular pain, however, the lifetime prevalence of actual "sciatica" was only 5% in men and 4% in women, also later confirmed (59). Svensson and Andersson (50–52) performed cross-sectional studies of two groups of subjects, one consisting of 940 men between the ages 40 and 46 years and 1,760 women between the ages of 38 and 64 years. They found prevalence rates for all back pain between 60% and 70% with a 1-month prevalence of 35%. Sciatica (or any leg pain) was described by around 30%. This is, however, a different symptom than true radiculopathy. In Belgium, such symptoms necessitating surgery amounted to a yearly incidence of 1 per 1,000 population (60).

WORK-RELATED BACK INJURIES

Back injuries make up almost one-third of all work-related injuries in the U.S., where there are now about 1 million worker compensation claims for back injuries per annum; the percentage in Sweden, with its general insurance system, is considerably less (5% to 6%) and actually not increasing (54). In Sweden, a steep decline by 80% was noted in 1995/1996 when the rules were changed and back pain was no longer regarded as clearly work-related (47,54).

In the U.K. in 1990/1991, the Health and Safety Executive recorded 34,720 nonfatal back injuries causing at least 3 days off work, which accounted for approximately 23% of all work-related injuries (61,62). Most back injuries were less serious "sprains or strains," but these minor back injuries led to longer time off work and to higher health and compensation costs than any other minor injuries. The issues of work-relatedness are dealt with in several recent reviews including those by the U.S. National Research Council (63) and the Sweden Institute for Working Life (64) as well as large prospective cohort studies (65). There is an association between reported low back pain and low back pain disability with certain taxing work postures, but there is an equally strong association between low back pain disability and psychosocial factors, especially those related to the workplace (37,66,67). The socioeconomic burden of back pain was recently very thoroughly described in a monograph by Waddell et al. (37). The authors describe how the whole problem of disabling low back pain must be looked upon from a wider psychological, social, and political perspective. When the different trends in low back pain disability are related to the ease of getting benefits, as well as the cultural views in different countries, the different percentages of wage replacements of sickness and permanent disability, and subsequently the absence rates are better understood. How a person is looked upon and accepted in society when declaring they are not fit for work is obviously also a factor.

IS BACK PAIN INCREASING?

An historical review by Allan and Waddell (68) concluded that human beings have had back pain all through history, and it is no more common or severe today than it has always been. Epidemiologic studies show no evidence of any convincing change in the prevalence of back pain. Leboeuf-Yde and Lauritsen (69) found no definite trend in 26 Nordic studies from 1954 through 1992, and apparent differences are probably mainly due to the wording of the questions. Leino et al. (66) in Finland found that the prevalence of back pain remained unchanged from 1978 to 1992 in annual surveys that have used identical questions each year. Murphy and Volinn (39) analyzed U.S. National Health Interview Survey data and found a 22% increase in chronic low back pain (continuous for more that 3 months) and a 35% increase in activity limitation due to back pain between 1987 and 1994, but a reduction thereafter.

Similarly, there is no clear evidence of any increase in the number of work-related back injuries. Data from the U.K. (11,40,62) show no definite trend. Data from the U.S. are conflicting (39,69). The National Council on Compensation Insurance (70) reported a gradual rise in the proportion of worker compensation claims due to back injuries from 1981 to 1990. However, Murphy and Volinn (39), also using data from the Washington State Department of Labor and Industries and a large worker compensation provider covering approximately 10% of the privately insured labor force, estimated that the annual low back pain claim rate actually decreased by 30% between 1987 and 1995. In Norway and the Netherlands, however, low back disability is increasing at a rate similar to Sweden (37,43,44).

Swedish data detailed until 1991 in the The Swedish State Health Technology Board (SBU) report (45) showed an increase in the incidence and duration of sickness absence due to back pain in the 1970s and 1980s, and a particular increase in the number of people going on long-term disability and early retirement between the mid-1980s and early 1990s; however, since the early 1990s until 1997 there was a definite decrease in sickness absence and early retirement due to back pain followed by a steep increase until 2002 (43). These changes can be partly explained by both increasing loss of jobs and increasing sickness benefits. Data from the U.K. suggest that the annual rate of new Department of Social Services (DSS) claims for invalidity benefit for back pain have changed very little over the past 20 years, but an increasing proportion of people receive benefit for much longer periods so that the total numbers on benefit and the amount and costs of benefit paid are increasing (37,62). Cross-cultural or international comparisons are, however, difficult to make (37,71).

Despite popular belief, there is no clear historical or epidemiologic evidence that the symptom of back pain has changed since the time any recording has been done. There is no evidence of any change in the pathology of the lower back throughout recorded history. The prevalence of low back pain has not changed, at least over the past 30 years. Instead, all the evidence is of an increase in chronic disability attributed to nonspecific low back pain.

HOW BACK PAIN BECOMES DISABLING

Pain and disability are subjective. Pain per se does not meet the definition of impairment (abnormality), but if activity aggravates pain and the individual avoids or reduces their activities, then pain may lead to disability. However, low back pain and disability depend more on psychosocial factors than on the physical condition of the back, and can best be understood and managed by a biopsychosocial model (37,61), which is more consistent with the latest evidence on the development of chronic pain and disability:

- The symptom of back pain arises from a physical process in the back and ensuing nociception. The key to chronic pain and disability may be failure to recover, rather than the development of a different syndrome.
- As pain becomes chronic (greater than 12 weeks) attitudes and beliefs, distress, and illness behavior play an increasing role in the development of chronicity and disability (34,37,66,67,72–76).

In an attempt to explain the transition from acute to chronic low back pain, Turk (77) stressed that demographic and psychosocial factors, including socioeconomic ones, are better predictors of chronicity than clinical, radiologic, or physical factors. This was reiterated in the same author's argument for more attention to the psychosocial dimension when treating patients with chronic back pain (78). This all occurs within the social context

(varying worldwide), and leads to social interactions with others, including in particular family, coworkers, and health care providers.

It is well known that there are close links between physiological and psychological events (37,54,76). Nonspecific low back pain seems to be mainly a matter of disturbed function or painful musculoskeletal dysfunction. Disability is reduced function (76). It is a matter of what the individual does (or does not do) and of altered performance. Pain behavior or illness behavior is also a matter of what the individual does (or does not do) (76).

Disability due to back pain involves both physical dysfunction and illness behavior, which in a sense are simply two sides of the same coin. Behavior always involves motor and physiologic activity; and physiologic processes always have behavioral expressions (72,73).

Low back pain and disability are clearly related, but they are not the same and the link between them may be much weaker than often assumed. One study (75) found that severity of pain only accounted for about 10% of the variance of low back disability. It is important to make a very clear distinction between pain and disability conceptually, in clinical practice, and as the basis for social security and sickness benefits (76,79). Another example of importance for ratings of disability is the fact that measured reduced mobility of the lower back is not related to pain or overall ability (80).

Pain is "an unpleasant sensory and emotional experience associated with actual or potential tissue damage, or described in terms of such damage" (81). Pain is a symptom, not a clinical sign, a diagnosis, or a disease. It is not possible to assess pain directly: assessment always depends on the individual's report of their subjective experience, so the report of pain always depends on how the individual thinks and feels about it and communicates it. A disability, on the other hand, is restricted activity. The most comprehensive definition of disability is by the World Health Organization (WHO) (82), which defines a disability as "any restriction or lack (resulting from an impairment) of ability to perform an activity in the manner or within the range considered normal for a human being." There are a number of assumptions in the WHO definition. It assumes that what is normal is to have no disability or restriction of any kind, which does not allow for the range that is normal by gender and age. It assumes that disability is "due to an impairment," which implies a physical basis and cause-and-effect relationship that may not be an accurate reflection of disability associated with pain. It is often taken to imply that disability is a health problem, which is not always true. Nevertheless, the core of all the definitions of disability is that it is restricted activity. For the purpose of sickness benefits or compensation, disability is often considered as incapacity for work, although the definition and degree of incapacity varies in different jurisdictions. Clinical assessment of disability usually relies on the patient's own report, so again the definition is subjective and open to the same influences as the report of pain (83–85).

Fordyce et al. (72) considered further the nature of impairment and disability associated with low back pain from a biopsychosocial perspective. The problem is that it is not possible to assess back pain, but only the person with the pain. Pain, suffering, and pain behavior all confound questions of impairment and disability. The term *disability* may mean either loss of capacity or simply reduced activity, but observation of performance cannot distinguish these. Reduced performance may reflect actual loss of capacity, or the individual may stop before they reach their physical limits, or they may not even attempt the activity. Fordyce (73) further defines a "state of disability as when the person prematurely terminates an activity, under-performs or declines to undertake it." The concept and measure of disability cannot be independent of performance. It is not possible to separate body and mind. Physical defects affect a person's beliefs and expectations about their situation. On the other hand, beliefs and expectations help to shape the impact of physical defects on activity. The extent to which psychological and social processes can influence physical activity should not be underestimated, and vice versa. Concepts of impairment and disability must allow for this dynamic interaction. Disability is not only a question of physical impairment, nor is it only functional capacity: it is a question of behavior and performance. Performance depends on anatomical and physiological abilities, but also on psychological and social resources. Performance depends on effort. Testing itself may cause pain and inhibit performance. Capacity may be set by physiological limits; but performance is set by psychological limits. (72,73).

ACKNOWLEDGMENT

Special thanks to Anders Norlund, PhD, and Gordon Waddell, MD, FRCS, for valuable help with important facts and figures.

REFERENCES

1. Sprangers MAG, de Regt EB, Andries F, et al. Which chronic conditions are associated with better or poorer quality of life? J Clin Epidemiol 2000;53:895–907.
2. Andersson GBJ. The epidemiology of spinal disorders. In: Frymoyer JW, ed. The adult spine: principles and practice, 2nd ed. New York: Raven Press, 1997;1:93–141.
3. Biering-Sørensen F, Hilden J. Reproducibility of the history of low back trouble. Spine 1984;9:280–286.
4. van Poppel M. The prevention of low back pain in industry [thesis]. Amsterdam: Amsterdam University; 1999.
5. Haas M, Nyiendo J, Aickin M. One-year trend in pain and disability relief recall in acute and chronic ambulatory low back pain patients. Pain 2002;95:83–91.
6. Smedley J, Egger P, Cooper C, et al. Manual handling activities and risk of low back pain in nurses. Occupation Environ Med 1995;52:160–163.
7. Lonnberg F. The management of back problems among the population II. Therapists' and patients' perception of the disease. Ugeskr Laeger 1997;159:215–221.
8. Raspe H. Back pain. In: Silman AJ, Hochberg MC, eds. Epidemiology of the rheumatic diseases. Oxford: Oxford University Press, 1993: 330–374.
9. Shekelle P. The epidemiology of low back pain. In: Giles LGF, Singer KP, eds. Clinical anatomy and management of low back pain. London: Butterworth Heinemann, 1997:18–31.
10. Cassidy JD, Carroll LJ, Côté P. The Saskatchewan Health and Back Pain Survey: the prevalence of low back pain and related disability in Saskatchewan adults. Spine 1998;23:1860–1867.
11. Consumer's Association 1985 Back Pain Survey. London: Research Surveys of Great Britain Ltd, 1985.
12. Croft P, Joseph S, Cosgrove S, et al. Low back pain in the community and in hospitals. A report to the Clinical Standards Advisory Group of the Department of Health. Prepared by the Arthritis & Rheumatism Council, Epidemiology Research Unit, University of Manchester, 1994.
13. Papageorgiou AC, Croft PR, Ferry S, et al. Estimating the prevalence of low back pain in the general population. Evidence from the South Manchester back pain survey. Spine 1995;20:1889–1894.
14. Papageorgiou AC, Croft PR, Thomas E, et al. Influence of previous pain experience on the episode incidence of low back pain: results from the South Manchester Back Pain Study. Pain 1996;66:181–185.
15. Shekelle PG, Markovich M, Louie R. An epidemiologic study of episodes of back pain care. Spine 1995;20:1668–1673.
16. Skovron ML, Szpalski M, Nordin M, et al. Sociocultural factors and back pain. A population-based study in Belgian adults. Spine 1994;19:129–137.
17. Taylor H, Curran NM. The Nuprin Pain Report. New York: Louis Harris and Associates 1985:1–233.
18. Von Korff M, Dworkin SF, Le Resche LA, et al. An epidemiologic comparison of pain complaints. Pain 1988;32:173–183.
19. Walsh K, Cruddas M, Coggon D. Low back pain in eight areas of Britain. J Epidemiol Community Health 1992;46:227–230.
20. George C. The six-month incidence of clinically significant low back pain in the Saskatchewan adult population. Spine 2002;27:1778–1782.
21. Mason V. The prevalence of back pain in Great Britain. Office of Population Censuses and Surveys, Social Survey Division (now Office of National Statistics.) London: Her Majesty's Stationary Office, 1994: 1–2.
22. Hoy D, Toole MJ, Morgan D, et al. Low back pain in rural Tibet. Lancet 2003;361:225–226.
23. Brattberg G. Back pain and headache in Swedish schoolchildren: a longitudinal study. Pain Clin 1993;6:157–162.
24. Brattberg G. The incidence of back pain and headache among Swedish schoolchildren. Qual Life Res 1994;3:S27–S31.
25. Burton KA, Clarke RD, McClune TD, et al. The natural history of low back pain in adolescents. Spine 1996;21:2323–2328.
26. Hellsing AL. Work absence in a cohort with benign back pain: prospective study with 10 year follow-up. J Occup Rehabil 1994;4(3):153.
27. SCB. Statistiska centralbyrån [Statistics Sweden]. Undersökningar av levnadsförhållanden, ULF [National household surveys]. Stockholm: SCB, 1996.
28. Brattberg G, Parker MG, Thorslund M. The prevalence of pain among the oldest old in Sweden. Pain 1996;67:29–34.
29. Brattberg G, Parker MG, Thorslund M. A longitudinal study of pain: reported pain from middle age to old age. Clin J Pain 1997;13:144–149.
30. Linton SJ, Hellsing AL, Halldén K. A population-based study of spinal pain among 35–45 year old individuals. Prevalence, sick leave, and health care use. Spine 1998;23:1457–1463.
31. Bergenudd H, Nilsson B. Back pain in middle age; occupational workload and psychologic factors: an epidemiologic survey. Spine 1988;13:58–60.
32. Bergenudd H. Talent, occupation and locomotor discomfort [thesis]. Lund: Lund University; 1989.
33. Hagberg M, Wegman D H. Prevalence rates and odds ratios of shoulder-neck diseases in different occupational groups. Br J Industr Med 1987;44:602–610.
34. Croft PR, Papageorgiou AC, Ferry S, et al. Psychological distress and low back pain: evidence from a prospective study in the general population. Spine 1995;20:2731–2737.
35. Carey TS, Garrett JM, Jackman A, et al. Recurrence and care seeking after acute back pain: results of a long-term follow-up study. North Carolina Back Pain Project. Med Care 1999;37:157–164.

36. Rossignol M, Lortie M, Ledoux E. Comparison of spinal health indicators in predicting spinal status in a 1-year longitudinal study. Spine 1993;18(1):54–60.
37. Waddell G, Aylward M, Sawney P. Back pain, incapacity for work and social security benefits: an international literature review and analysis. London: The Royal Society of Medicine Press, 2002.
38. Valkenburg HA, Haanen HCM. The epidemiology of low back pain. In: White AA, Gordon SL, eds. Symposium on idiopathic low back pain. St. Louis: Mosby, 1982:9–22.
39. Murphy PL, Volinn E. Is occupational low back pain on the rise? Spine 1999;24:691–697.
40. Clinical Standards Advisory Group Epidemiology Review: the epidemiology and cost of back pain. Annex to the CSAG Report on Back Pain. London: Her Majesty's Stationary Office, 1994:1–72.
41. Macfarlane GF, Thomas E, Papageorgiou AC, et al. Employment and work activities as predictors of future low back pain. Spine 1997;22:1143–1149.
42. Guo H-R, Tanaka S, Cameron LL, et al. Back pain among workers in the United States: national estimates and workers at high risk. Am J Industr Med 1995;28:591–602.
43. Nybeviljade förtidspensioner/sjukbidrag 2002. Statistikinformation Is-1 2003:1. Stockholm, Riksförsäkringsverket: 2002 [in Swedish].
44. Nybeviljade förtidspensioner och psykisk ohälsa—ålder, kön och diagnos. Redovisar 2003. Stockholm, Riksförsäkringsverket: 2003 [in Swedish].
45. Nachemson A. 1991 Ont i Ryggen. Back pain—causes, diagnosis, treatment. SBU Report. Swedish Council on Technology Assessment in Health Care. Stockholm: Workers Compensation Back Claim Study, 1992.
46. Johansson J Å, Rubenowitz S. Risk indicators in the psychosocial and physical work environment for work-related neck, shoulder and low back symptoms: a study among blue- and white-collar workers in eight companies. Scand J Rehabil Med 1994;26:131–142.
47. Nachemson A. Back pain in the workplace: a threat to our welfare states. In: Wolter D, Seide K, Hrsg. Berufsbedingte Erkrankungen der Lendenwirbelsäule. Springer Verlag 1998; Kapitel 15:191–206.
48. Weill C, Ghadi V, Nicoulet I, et al. Back pain in France. Epidemiology, present knowledge, current practice and costs. CD-Santé. Paris 1 July 1998.
49. Watson PJ, Main CJ, Waddell G, et al. Medically certified work loss, recurrence and costs of wage compensation for back pain: a follow-up study of the working population of Jersey. Br J Rheumatol 1998;37:82–86.
50. Svensson HO, Andersson GBJ. Low back pain in forty to forty-seven year old men: work history and work environment factors. Spine 1983;8:272–276.
51. Svensson HO, Andersson GBJ, Johansson S, et al. A retrospective study of low back pain in 38- to 64-year old women. Frequency and occurrence and impact on medical services. Spine 1988;13:548–552.
52. Svensson HO, Andersson GBJ. The relationship of low-back pain, work history, work environment, and stress: a retrospective cross-sectional study of 38- to 64-year-old women. Spine 1989;14:517–522.
53. Westrin CG. Low-back sick listing. A nosological and medical insurance investigation. Acta Soc Med Scand 1970;2–3:127–134.
54. Nachemson A, Jonsson E, eds. Neck and back pain. The scientific evidence of causes, diagnosis and treatment. Philadelphia: Lippincott Williams & Wilkins, 2000.
55. Statens Offentliga Utredningar SOU 2002 [in Swedish]. Available at: http://www.regeringen.se/propositioner/sou/sou2002.htm. Accessed October 23, 2003.
56. Deyo R A, Tsui-Wu Y-J Functional disability due to back pain. Arthritis Rheumat 1987;30:1247–1253.
57. Lawrence JS. Rheumatism in populations. London: Heinemann, 1977.
58. Heliovaara M, Impivaara O, et al. Lumbar disc syndrome in Finland. J Epidemiol Community Health 1987;41:251–258.
59. Manninen P, Riihimäki H, Heliövaara M. Incidence and risk factors of low-back pain in middle-aged farmers. Occupation Med (Oxf) 1995;45:141–146.
60. Du Bois M, Donceel P. Epidemiology, fitness for work, and costs. In:
Gunzburg R, Szpalski M, eds. Lumbar disc herniation. Philadelphia: Lippincott Williams & Wilkins, 2000.
61. Waddell G. The epidemiology of low back pain. In: Waddell G, ed. The back pain revolution. New York: Churchill Livingstone, 1998:69–84.
62. Erens B, Ghate D. Invalidity benefit: a longitudinal study of new recipients. Department of Social Security Research Report Number 20. London: Her Majesty's Stationary Office, 1993:1–127.
63. National Research Council and Institute of Medicine. Musculoskeletal disorders and the workplace. Low back and upper extremities. Washington DC: National Academy Press, 2001.
64. Hansson T, Westerholm P. Arbete och besvär i rörelseorganen. En vetenskaplig värdering av frågor om samband. Arbete och Hälsa 2001: 12. Arbetslivsinstitutet, Stockholm, 2001 [in Swedish].
65. Croft P, Papageorgiou A, McNally R. Low back pain. In: Stevens A, Rafferty J, eds. Health care needs assessment. Second Series. Oxford: Radcliffe Medical Press, 1997:129–182.
66. Leino PI, Hanninen V. Psychosocial factors at work in relation to back and limb disorders. Scand J Work Environ Health 1995;21:134–142.
67. Hoogendoorn WE, Bongers PM, de Vet HC, et al. Psychosocial work characteristics and psychological strain in relation to low-back pain. Scand J Work Environ Health 2001;27:258–267.
68. Allan DB, Waddell G. An historical perspective on low back pain and disability. Acta Orthop Scand 1989[Suppl];234(60):1–23.
69. Leboeuf-Yde C, Lauritsen JM. The prevalence of low back pain in the literature: a structured review of 26 Nordic studies from 1954 to 1993. Spine 1995;20:2112–2118.
70. National Council on Compensation Insurance, Florida. Report 1992; 1–25.
71. Sanders SH, Brena SF, Spier CJ et al. Chronic low back pain patients around the world: cross-cultural similarities and differences. Clin J Pain 1992;8:317–323.
72. Fordyce WE, ed. Back pain in the workplace: management of disability in non-specific conditions. Seattle: International Association for the Study of Pain (IASP) Press, 1995.
73. Fordyce WE. On the nature of illness and disability [Editorial]. Clin Orthop 1997;336:47–51.
74. Papageorgiou AC, Macfarlane GF, Thomas E, et al. Psychosocial factors in the workplace—do they predict new episodes of low back pain? Spine 1997;22:1137–1142.
75. Waddell G, Main CJ. Assessment of severity in low-back disorders. Spine 1984;9:204–208.
76. Waddell G, Main CJ, Morris EW, et al. Chronic low-back pain, psychologic distress, and illness behavior. Spine 1984;9:209–213.
77. Turk DC. The role of demographic and psychosocial factors in transition from acute to chronic pain. In: Jensen TS, Turner JA, Wiesenfeld-Hallin Z, eds. Proceedings of the 8th World Congress on Pain. Progress in pain research and management. Vol 8. Seattle: IASP Press, 1997.
78. Turk DC. Clinical effectiveness and cost-effectiveness of treatments for patients with chronic pain. Clin J Pain 2002;18:355–365.
79. Vowles KE, Gross RT. Work-related beliefs about injury and physical capacity for work in individuals with chronic pain. Pain 2003;101:291–298.
80. Parks KA, Chrichton KS, Goldford RJ, et al. A comparison of lumbar range of motion and functional ability scores in patients with low back pain: assessment for range of motion validity. Spine 2003;28:380–384.
81. International Association for the Study of Pain (Subcommittee on Taxonomy). 1979 pain terms: a list with definitions and notes on usage. Pain 1979;6:249–252.
82. World Health Organization. International Classification of Impairments, Disabilities and Handicaps. Geneva: World Health Organization, 1980.
83. Swales K, Craig P. Evaluation of the Incapacity Benefit medical test. In-house report 26. London: Social Research Branch, Department of Social Security, 1997.
84. Suter PB. Employment and litigation: improved by work, assisted by verdict. An adversarial situation also prolongs time off work due to occupational back pain. Pain 2002;100:249–257.
85. Atlas SJ, Chang Y, Kammann E, et al. Long-term disability and return to work among patients who have a herniated lumbar disc: the effect of disability compensation. J Bone Joint Surg Am 2000;82:4–15.

CHAPTER 2

Pathophysiology of Nerve Root Pain in Disc Herniation and Spinal Stenosis

Kjell Olmarker, Robert R. Myers, Shinichi Kikuchi, and Björn Rydevik

Lumbosacral nerve roots are known to be intimately involved in the pathophysiology of disc herniation and spinal stenosis (1). During the last decade there has been an increasing interest in this topic, and recent research has aimed at defining basic pathophysiologic events at the cellular or subcellular level responsible for the pathophysiology of nerve root pain. In this chapter, the current knowledge about these mechanisms is reviewed and discussed in relation to the clinical features of lumbar disc herniation and spinal stenosis.

SYMPTOMATOLOGY OF NERVE ROOT INVOLVEMENT

The symptoms of nerve root pathophysiology may be divided into two main categories: pain and nerve dysfunction (2). Nerve root pain is typically radiating in nature, and is usually related to a specific nerve root or roots innervating tissue below the knee. Nerve dysfunction may be present in both motor and sensory modalities, thus producing both motor weakness and sensory disturbances. One may assume that pain and nerve dysfunction result from different pathophysiologic events, but they usually coincide, indicating that nerve root pathophysiology is very complex.

PATHOPHYSIOLOGIC MECHANISMS

Two specific mechanisms at the "tissue level" may be defined: mechanical deformation of the nerve roots and biologic or biochemical activity of the disc tissue with effects on the roots. The mechanical deformation theory is the oldest concept of nerve root injury induced by herniated disc tissue and dates back to the turn of the last century with some clinical observations on injuries in the lumbosacral junction with subsequent leg pain, and more

recently to Mixter and Barr's seminal observations (1–5). The theory that biologic activity of the disc tissue may injure the nerve roots recently was confirmed experimentally (6). The experimental knowledge regarding these two mechanisms is discussed separately.

MECHANICAL EFFECTS

The spinal nerve roots are relatively well protected from external trauma because they are enclosed by the vertebral bones (Fig. 2-1). However, the nerve roots do not posses the same amounts and organization of protective connective tissue sheaths as do the peripheral nerves (Fig. 2-2). Therefore, the spinal nerve roots may be particularly sensitive to mechanical deformation resulting from intraspinal disorders such as disc herniations or protrusions, spinal stenosis, degenerative disorders, and tumors (7–9). There has been moderate interest in studying nerve root compression in experimental models. Gelfan and Tarlov in 1956 and Sharpless in 1975 performed initial experiments on the effects of compression on nerve impulse conduction (10,11). Although no calibration was performed of the compression devices used, both papers indicated that nerve roots were more susceptible to compression than peripheral nerves. During recent years, however, the interest in nerve root pathophysiology has increased considerably. A number of studies are reviewed in the following.

Experimental Nerve Root Compression

Some years ago, a model was presented for evaluation of the effects of compression of the cauda equina in pigs that allowed for experimental, graded compression of cauda equina nerve roots at known pressure levels for the first time (7,8). In this model, the cauda equina was

11

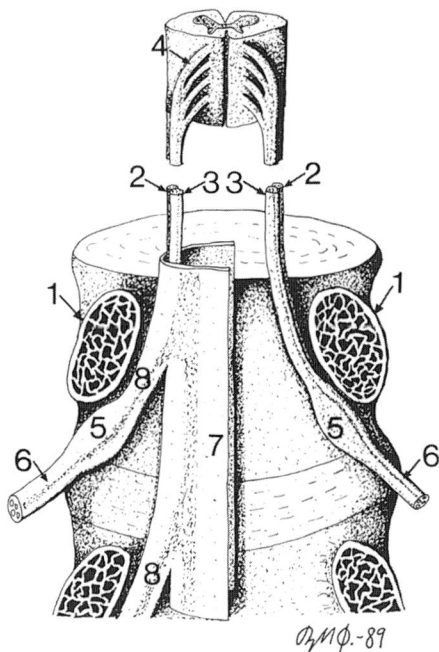

FIG. 2-1. Drawing of the intraspinal course of a human lumbar spinal nerve root segment. The vertebral arches have been removed by cutting the pedicles *(1)*, and the opened spinal canal can be viewed from behind. The ventral *(2)* and dorsal *(3)* nerve roots leave the spinal cord as small rootlets *(4)* that caudally converge into a common nerve root trunk. Just prior to leaving the spinal canal, there is a swelling of the dorsal nerve root called the dorsal root ganglion *(5)*. Caudal to the dorsal root ganglion, the ventral and dorsal nerve roots mix and form the spinal nerve *(6)*. The spinal dura encloses the nerve roots both as a central cylindrical sac *(7)*, and as separate extensions called root sleeves *(8)*. (From Olmarker K. Spinal nerve root compression. Thesis. Göteborg, Sweden: Göteborg University, 1990, with permission).

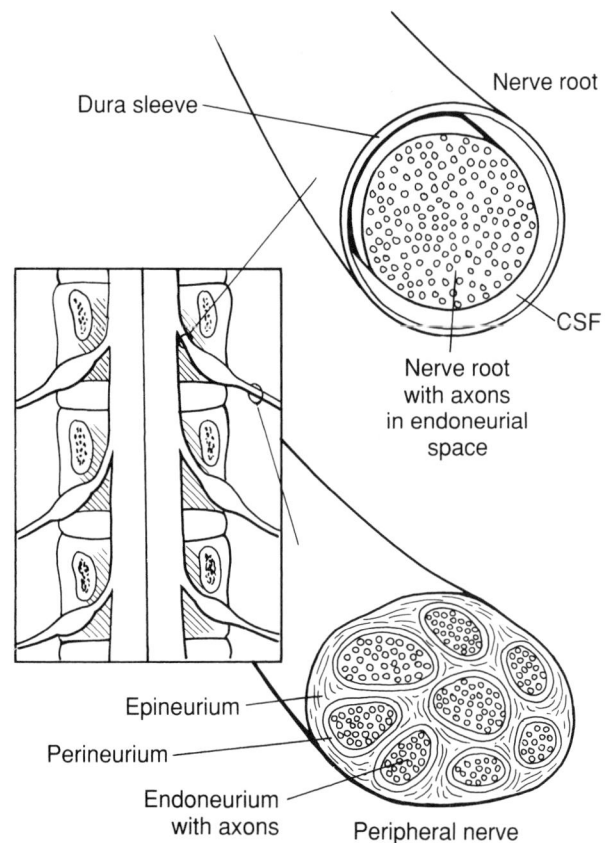

FIG. 2-2. The nerve root and the peripheral nerve differ in their microscopic anatomy. The axons of the nerve root are located in the endoneurial space and covered by cerebrospinal fluid and the dura sleeve. The axons of the peripheral nerves are located in the endoneurium of the fascicles that are enclosed by the perineurium. These fascicles are all enclosed by the epineurium that is formed by loose connective tissue. (From Weinstein JN, Rydevik BL, Sonntag VKH, eds. Essentials of the spine. New York: Raven Press, 1995, with permission.)

compressed by an inflatable balloon that was fixed to the spine (Fig. 2-3). The cauda equina could be observed through the translucent balloon also. This model made it possible to study the flow in the intrinsic nerve root blood vessels at various pressure levels (12). The experiment was designed in a way that the pressure in the compression balloon was increased by 5 mm Hg every 20 seconds. The blood flow and vessel diameters of the intrinsic vessels could be observed simultaneously through the balloon using a vital microscope. The average occlusion pressure for the arterioles was found to be slightly below and directly related to the systolic blood pressure. The blood flow in the capillary networks was intimately dependent on the blood flow of the adjacent venules. This corroborates the assumption that venular stasis may induce capillary stasis and thus changes in the microcirculation of the nerve tissue, which has been suggested as one mechanism in carpal tunnel syndrome (13). The mean occlusion pressures for the venules demonstrated large variations; however, a pressure of 5 to 10 mm Hg was sufficient to induce venular occlusion. It is assumed that the capillary blood flow also is affected in such situations because of retrograde stasis.

In the same experimental setup, the effects of gradual decompression were studied after initial acute compression for a short while (14). The average pressure for starting the blood flow was slightly lower at decompression than at compression for arterioles, capillaries, and venules. However, it was found that there was not a full restoration of the blood flow until the compression was lowered from 5 to 0 mm Hg. This observation further stressed the previous impression that vascular impairment is present even at low-pressure levels.

Compression-induced impairment of the vasculature may be one mechanism for nerve root dysfunction because the nutrition of the nerve root is affected. However, the nerve roots also have a considerable nutritional supply via diffusion from the cerebrospinal fluid (CSF) (15). To assess the compression-induced effects on the

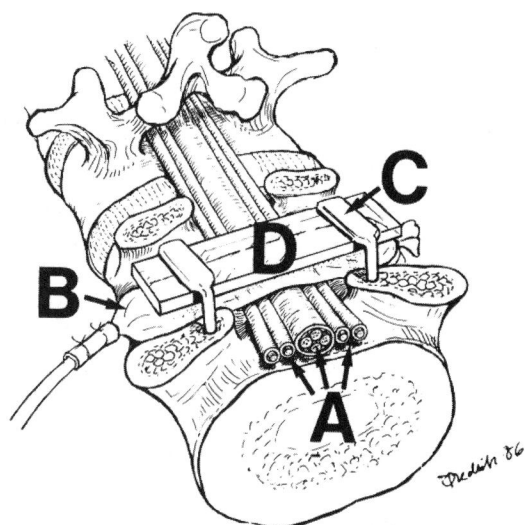

FIG. 2-3. Schematic drawing of experimental nerve root compression model. The cauda equina **(A)** is compressed by an inflatable balloon **(B)** that is fixed to the spine by two L-shaped pins **(C)** and a Plexiglas plate **(D)**. (From Olmarker K, Holm S, Rosenqvist AL, et al. Experimental nerve root compression. A model of acute, graded compression of the porcine cauda equina and an analysis of neural and vascular anatomy. Spine 1991;16(1):61–69, with permission.)

total contribution to the nerve roots, an experiment was designed where ^{3}H-labeled methylglucose was allowed to be transported to the nerve tissue in the compressed segment both via the blood vessels and via the CSF diffusion after systemic injection (16). The results showed that no compensatory mechanism from CSF diffusion could be expected at the low-pressure levels. On the contrary, 10 mm Hg compression was sufficient to induce a 20% to 30% reduction of the transport of methylglucose to the nerve roots as compared to control.

It is known from experimental studies on peripheral nerves that compression also may induce an increase in the vascular permeability, leading to intraneural edema formation (17). Such edema may increase the endoneurial fluid pressure, which in turn may impair the endoneurial capillary blood flow and in such a way jeopardize the nutrition of the nerve roots (18–21). Because the edema usually persists for some time after the removal of a compressive agent, edema may negatively affect the nerve root for a longer period than the compression itself. The presence of an intraneural edema is related also to subsequent formation of intraneural fibrosis (22), and may contribute to the slow recovery of some patients with nerve compression disorders. To determine if intraneural edema may form in nerve roots because of compression, the distribution of Evan's blue albumin (EBA) in the nerve tissue was analyzed after compression at various pressures and durations (23). The study showed that edema formed even at low-pressure levels, predominantly at the edges of the compression zone.

The function of the nerve roots has been studied by direct electrical stimulation and recordings either on the nerve itself or in the corresponding muscular segments (24–27). During a 2-hour compression period, a critical pressure level for inducing a reduction of Monophasic action potential (MAP) amplitude seems to be located between 50 and 75 mm Hg. Higher pressure levels (100 to 200 mm Hg) may induce a total conduction block with varying degrees of recovery after compression release. To study the effects of compression on sensory nerve fibers, the electrodes in the sacrum were used to record a compound nerve action potential after stimulating the sensory nerves in the tail (i.e., distal to the compression zone). The results showed that the sensory fibers are slightly more susceptible to compression than the motor fibers (26,27). Also, the nerve roots are more susceptible to compression injury if the blood pressure is lowered pharmacologically (25). This further implies the importance of the blood supply to maintain the functional properties of the nerve roots.

Onset Rate of Compression

One factor that has not been fully recognized in compression trauma of nerve tissue is the onset rate of the compression. The onset rate (i.e., the time from start to full compression) may vary clinically from fractions of seconds in traumatic conditions to months or years in degenerative processes. There may be a wide variation even in clinically rapid onset rates. With the presented model it was possible to vary the onset time of the applied compression. Two onset rates have been investigated. Either the pressure is preset and compression is started by flipping the switch of the compressed air system used to inflate the balloon, or the compression pressure is slowly increased over 20 seconds. The first onset rate was 0.05 to 0.1 seconds, which provided a rapid inflation of the balloon and a rapid compression onset.

Such a rapid onset rate has been found to induce more pronounced effects on edema formation (23), methylglucose transport (16), and impulse propagation (24) than the slow onset rate. Regarding methylglucose transport, the results show that the levels within the compression zone are more pronounced at the rapid than at the slow onset rate at corresponding pressure levels. There was also a striking difference between the two onset rates when considering the segments outside the compression zones. The levels approached baseline values closer to the compression zone in the slow rather than the rapid onset series. This may indicate the presence of a more pronounced edge zone edema in the rapid onset series, with a subsequent reduction of the nutritional transport also in the nerve tissue adjacent to the compression zone.

For the rapid onset compression, which is likely to be more closely related to spine trauma or disc herniation than to spinal stenosis, a pressure of 600 mm Hg maintained only for 1 second is sufficient to induce a gradual impairment of nerve conduction during the 2 hours studied after the compression was ended (28). Overall, the mechanisms for these pronounced differences between the different onset rates are not clear, but may be related to differences in displacement rates of the compressed nerve tissue toward the uncompressed parts because of the viscoelastic properties of the nerve tissue (9). Such phenomena may lead not only to structural damage of the nerve fibers, but also to structural changes in the blood vessels with subsequent edema formation. The gradual formation of intraneural edema also may be closely related to the described observations of a gradually increasing difference in nerve conduction impairment between the two onset rates (23,24).

Multiple Levels of Nerve Root Compression

Patients with double or multiple levels of spinal stenosis seem to have more pronounced symptoms than patients with stenosis only at one level (29). The presented model was modified to address this interesting clinical issue. Using two balloons at two adjacent disc levels, which resulted in a 10-mm uncompressed nerve segment between the balloons, induced a much more pronounced impairment of nerve impulse conduction than had been previously found at corresponding pressure levels (30). For instance, a pressure of 10 mm Hg in two balloons induced a 60% reduction of nerve impulse amplitude during 2 hours of compression, whereas 50 mm Hg in one balloon showed no reduction.

The mechanism for the difference between single and double compression may not simply be because the nerve impulses have to pass more than one compression zone at double level compression. There also may be a mechanism based on the local vascular anatomy of the nerve roots. Unlike for peripheral nerves, there are no regional nutritive arteries from surrounding structures to the intraneural vascular system in spinal nerve roots (7,31–34). Therefore, compression at two levels might induce a nutritionally impaired region between the two compression sites. In this way, the segment affected by the compression would be widened from one balloon diameter (10 mm) to two balloon diameters, including the interjacent nerve segment (30 mm). This hypothesis was partly confirmed in an experiment on continuous analyses of the total blood flow in the uncompressed nerve segment located between two compression balloons. The results showed that a 64% reduction of total blood flow in the uncompressed segment was induced when both balloons were inflated to 10 mm Hg (35). There was complete ischemia in the nerve segment at a pressure close to the systemic blood pressure. Data from a study on the nutritional transport to the nerve tissue at double level compression demonstrated that there is a reduction of this transport to the uncompressed nerve segment located

between the two compression balloons similar to that within the two compression sites (36). Thus, there is experimental evidence that the nutrition to the nerve segment located between two compression sites in nerve roots is severely impaired, although the nerve segment itself is uncompressed.

Also, it was evident that the effects of nerve conduction were enhanced if the distance between the compression balloons was increased from one to two vertebral segments (30). However, this was not the case in the nutritional transport study where the methylglucose levels in the compression zones and the uncompressed intermediate segment were similar between double compression over one and two vertebral segments (36). This indicates that the nutrition to the uncompressed nerve segment located between two compression sites is affected almost to the same extent as at the compression sites, regardless of the distance between the compression sites, but that functional impairment may be directly related to the distance between the two compression sites. The impairment of the nutrition to the nerve segment between the two compression balloons thus seems to be more important than the fact that the nerve impulses have to overcome two compression sites in double-level compression.

Double-level compression of pig cauda equina with electrical nerve root stimulation to simulate a walking situation showed that an initial short-term increase in cauda equina blood flow rapidly decreased (37). Such observations further support the pathophysiologic significance of double-level cauda equina compression in spinal stenosis.

Chronic Experimental Nerve Root Compression

The discussion of compression-induced effects on nerve roots has dealt with acute compression so far (i.e., compression that lasts for some hours and with no survival of the animal). To better mimic various clinical situations, compression must be applied over longer periods. Probably many changes in the nerve tissue, such as adaptation of axons and vasculature, occur in patients but cannot be studied in experimental models using only 1 to 6 hours of compression. Another important factor in this context is the onset rate, which was discussed in the preceding text. In clinical syndromes with nerve root compression, the onset time probably is quite slow. For instance, a gradual remodeling of the vertebrae to induce spinal stenosis leads to an onset time of many years. Of course, it is difficult to mimic such a situation in an experimental model. Also, it is impossible to have absolute control over the pressure acting on the nerve roots in chronic models because of the remodeling and adaptation of the nerve tissue to the applied pressure. However, knowledge of the exact pressures is probably less important in chronic than acute compression situations. Instead, chronic models should induce a controlled compression with a slow onset time that is easily reproducible. Such models may be well suited for studies on pathophysiologic events as well as intervention by surgery or drugs. Some attempts have been made to induce such compression.

Delamarter et al. presented a model on the dog cauda equina in which they applied a constricting plastic band (38). The band was tightened around the thecal sac to induce a 25%, 50%, or 75% reduction of the cross-sectional area. The band was left in place for various lengths of time. Analyses were performed and showed both structural and functional changes that were proportional to the degree of constriction.

To induce a slower onset and more controlled compression, Cornefjord and collaborators used a constrictor to compress the nerve roots in the pig (39). The constrictor initially was intended to induce vascular occlusion in experimental ischemic conditions in dogs. The constrictor consists of an outer metal shell that is covered on the inside with a material called amaroid that expands when in contact with fluids. Because of the metal shell, the amaroid expands inward with a maximum expansion after 2 weeks, resulting in compression of a nerve root placed in the central opening of the constrictor. Compression of the first sacral nerve root in the pig resulted in a significant reduction of nerve conduction velocity and axonal injuries using a constrictor with a defined original diameter (39). Also, it was found that there is an increase in substance P in the nerve root and dorsal root ganglion following such compression (40). Substance P is a neurotransmitter related to pain transmission. Thus, the study may provide experimental evidence that nerve root compression produces pain. The constrictor model also has been used to study blood flow changes in the nerve root vasculature (41). It could then be observed that the blood flow is not reduced just outside the compression zone, but significantly reduced in parts of the nerve roots located inside the constrictor.

One important aspect in clinical nerve root compression conditions is that the compression level is probably not stable but varies as the result of changes in posture and movements (42,43). Konno and collaborators recently introduced a model where the pressure could be changed after some time of initial chronic compression (44). An inflatable balloon was introduced under the lamina of the seventh lumbar vertebra in the dog. The normal anatomy and the effects of acute compression using compressed air were first evaluated in previous studies (45). By inflating the balloon at a known pressure slowly over 1 hour with a viscous substance that would harden in the balloon, a compression of the cauda equina could be induced with a known initial pressure level. The compression was verified by myelography. Because the balloon under the lamina comprised a twin set of balloons, the second balloon component could be connected to compressed air and could be used to add compression to the already chronically compressed cauda equina.

In conclusion, acute nerve root compression experiments have established critical pressure levels for interference with various physiologic parameters in the spinal nerve roots. However, studies on chronic compression may provide knowledge more applicable to the clinical situation.

Spinal Stenosis: Experimental–Clinical Correlation

There is substantial knowledge about critical levels of pressure for inducing changes in nerve root nutrition and function. These critical levels are of interest in understanding the basic pathophysiologic mechanisms of compression-induced changes in nerve roots. However, such absolute pressure levels may be of relatively less significance in chronic situations. When nerve tissue is compressed, there is a gradual displacement of the nerve tissue from the compressed to the uncompressed segments (46,47). If the pressure is of an extremely low onset rate (e.g., spinal stenosis), there may be an adaptation of the nerve tissue to the applied pressure. In cadaver experiments, Schönström et al. found that when a hose clamp was tightened around a human cadaver cauda equina specimen, there was a critical cross-sectional area of the dural sac when the first signs of pressure increase among nerve roots were recorded by a catheter placed in the compression zone (48). This cross-sectional area was approximately 75 mm^2, which was found also to correlate with a corresponding measurement on CT scans in spinal stenosis patients (49). The pressure increased when the hose clamp was further tightened. However, pressure dropped with time because of creep phenomena in the nerve tissue the. When the pressure did not normalize within 10 minutes, the "sustained size" was registered and was found to be in the range of 45 to 50 mm^2 (48). This indicates that even in acute compression, there is an adaptation of the nerve tissue to the applied pressure. In a longer perspective, this probably means that the nerve also may be reorganized in its microstructural elements, which results in a nerve with a smaller diameter. Under such circumstances, with gradually decreasing nerve diameter, the nerve pressure acting on the nerve is reduced to some degree.

Despite these important aspects regarding chronic changes in compressed spinal nerve roots, it is interesting to note the correlation between the animal experimental observations regarding critical pressures for functional and nutritional changes in nerve roots under compression on one side, and the measurements of pressure levels among nerve roots in human cadaver lumbar spines following experimental constriction of the dural sac. Acute pressure increase among cauda equina nerve roots to 50 mm Hg was induced when the cross-sectional area of the dural sac was reduced to 63 mm^2, and a pressure of 100 mm Hg was induced at a cross-sectional of 57 mm^2 (50). Such pressure levels correlate with *in vivo* observations regarding physiologic changes in cauda equina nerve roots following experimental compression (7,12,23).

Epidural pressure measurements have been performed, evaluating for example the relationship between epidural pressure and posture (43). It was found that the local epidural pressure at the stenotic level was low in lying and sitting postures, and high in standing postures. Pressure was increased with extension but decreased with flexion of the spine. The highest epidural pressure, 117 mm Hg, was found in standing with extension. Measurements also have been reported regarding changes in epidural pressure during walking in patients with lumbar spinal stenosis (51). It was found that the pressure changed during walking with a wave pattern of increase and decrease. Such observations correlate with the previously mentioned experimental observations regarding intermittent cauda equina compression (42).

Mechanical Deformation and Pain

There are some experimental observations that indicate that mechanical nerve deformation per se may induce impulses that could be interpreted as pain by the central nervous system. Howe and collaborators found that mechanical stimulation of nerve roots or peripheral nerves resulted in nerve impulses of short duration, and that these impulses were prolonged if the nerve tissue had been exposed to mechanical irritation by a chromic gut ligature for 2 to 4 weeks (52). The same results were obtained in an *in vitro* system using rabbit nerve roots (53). However, in this setup it was also evident that the dorsal root ganglion was more susceptible to mechanical stimulation than the nerve roots. The dorsal root ganglion has drawn a special interest in this regard, and an increase in the level of neurotransmitters related to pain transmission has been found in the dorsal root ganglion in response to whole body vibration of rabbits (54). A similar increase also has been seen in the dorsal root ganglion and nerve root after local constriction of the same nerve root (40). *In vivo* models of pain behavior have demonstrated that a severe mechanical deformation, such as ligation, of the nerve root generally is not painful (55–57). However, it seems that if chromic gut sutures are used, the additional irritation makes the mechanical compression painful. Recent studies have shown that disc incision with leakage of nucleus pulposus into the epidural space or a light mechanical deformation and slight medial displacement of the nerve root, does not produce pain behavior in a rat model, whereas the combination of the two factors produces pain (58–60). This is discussed in the following.

Interesting observations have been made regarding contact pressure between the nerve root and the disc in patients with lumbar disc herniation (61). Nerve root pressure before discectomy varied from 7 to 256 mm Hg (mean, 53 mm Hg). The magnitude of nerve root pressure correlates with the severity of neurologic deficits, but not with the degree of straight leg rising.

Neuropathology and Pain

There is a considerable body of work on the relationship of pain to neuropathologic changes that has been reviewed recently (62). In fact, much of what is known has been studied in relationship to mechanical and inflammatory injury of the sciatic nerve in the rat. Entrapment of a peripheral nerve produces pathologic change in proportion to the degree of compression and its duration (63), as is known to be the case for nerve root compression. In an electron microscopic study (63), minor degrees of nerve compression were associated with ischemic injury to Schwann cells, resulting in their necrosis and in demyelination. Severe nerve compression was associated with injury to the axon resulting in Wallerian degeneration. Subsequent experiments established the relationship of pain to these forms of neuropathologic change (64). These studies established that mild levels of ischemia producing demyelination generally were not painful, whereas severe ischemia producing Wallerian degeneration resulted in hyperalgesia. In fact, the pathology of the chronic constriction injury model of neuropathic pain is based on this relationship and the added insult of inflammation caused by the chromic gut ligatures used to compress the nerve (65). It is now recognized that the cytokine-driven processes of Wallerian degeneration are the dominant neuropathologic factors linking nerve injury and pain (64,66, 67) and that the degree and extent of wallerian degeneration relates directly to the magnitude and duration of hyperalgesia (68).

BIOLOGIC AND BIOCHEMICAL EFFECTS

The clinical picture of sciatica with a characteristic distribution of pain and nerve dysfunction, but in the absence of herniated disc material both at radiologic examination and at surgery, has indicated that the mechanical component is not the only factor that may be responsible for sciatic pain. Therefore, it has been suggested that the disc tissue per se may have injurious properties that may be of pathophysiologic significance (9). However, not until recently was it confirmed in an experimental setup that local, epidural application of autologous nucleus pulposus in the pig with no mechanical deformation, induces significant changes in both structure and function of the adjacent nerve roots (6). This finding has opened up a new field of research, which is reviewed in the following.

Biologic Effects of Disc Tissue (Nucleus Pulposus)

No changes in nerve function or structure were observed after placing autologous nucleus pulposus, obtained from a lumbar disc in the same animal, onto the tibial nerve in a rabbit (69). However, there are certain differences in microscopic anatomy and vascular permeability between peripheral nerves and nerve roots that make the extrapolation from peripheral nerve experiments to spinal conditions difficult. McCarron and collaborators applied autologous nucleus pulposus from discs of the dog's tail in the epidural space of the animal (70). They observed that an epidural inflammatory reaction did not occur when saline was injected as control. However, the nerve tissue was not assessed in this study.

Olmarker and collaborators presented a study that demonstrated that autologous nucleus pulposus might induce a reduction in nerve conduction velocity and light microscopic structural changes in a pig cauda equina model of nerve root injury (Fig. 2-4) (6). However, these axonal changes had a focal distribution and the quantity of injured axons was too low to be responsible for the significant neurophysiologic dysfunction observed. A follow-up study of areas of the nerve roots exposed to nucleus pulposus that appeared to be normal by light microscopy, revealed that there were significant injuries of the Schwann cells with vacuolization and disintegration of the Schmidt-Lanterman incisures (Fig. 2-5) (71). Schmidt-Lanterman incisures are essential for the normal exchange of ions between the axon and surrounding tissues. Therefore, an injury to this structure would be likely to interfere with the normal impulse conduction properties of the axons. However, the distribution of changes was too limited to fully explain the neurophysiologic dysfunction observed. For instance, a recent study that demonstrated that freezing of the nucleus pulposus prevented the reduction in nerve conduction velocity also demonstrated these characteristic changes histologically in spite of normal nerve conduction (72). However, the potency of the nucleus pulposus was further emphasized in an experiment using a dog model where it was seen

that a surgical incision of the annulus fibrosus, with minimal leakage of nucleus pulposus, was enough to induce significant changes in structure and function of the adjacent nerve root (73).

Because there is no structural correlate to the functional changes, continued studies have assessed the potential effects of nucleus pulposus on the nerve root nutrition. Epidural application of autologous nucleus pulposus within 2 hours induces an intraneural edema (74,75) that leads to a reduction of the intraneural blood flow (75). Histologic changes of the nerve roots are present after 3 hours (76), and a subsequent reduction of the nerve conduction velocity starts 3 to 24 hours after application (6,76).

From these initial experiments, it could be concluded that nucleus pulposus has significant properties to injure the nerve roots by its mere presence. However, the mechanisms for the nucleus pulposus–induced nerve root injury are not yet fully understood. These studies indicated that inflammatory reactions were present, at least epidurally. This initiated a study where a potent anti-inflammatory agent, methylprednisolone, was administered at different times intravenously after nucleus pulposus application (77). The results showed clearly that the nucleus pulposus–induced reduction in nerve conduction velocity was eliminated if methylprednisolone was administered within 24 hours of application. If methylprednisolone was administered within 48 hours the effect was not eliminated but significantly lower than if no drug was used. This observation indicates that the negative effect does not occur immediately but develops during the first 24 hours after application. However, if methylprednisolone is administered within 24 hours, some areas in the nerve roots demonstrate normal impulse conduction properties with light microscopic axonal changes in the same magnitude as in the previous study (6). This further corroborates the impression that the structural nerve

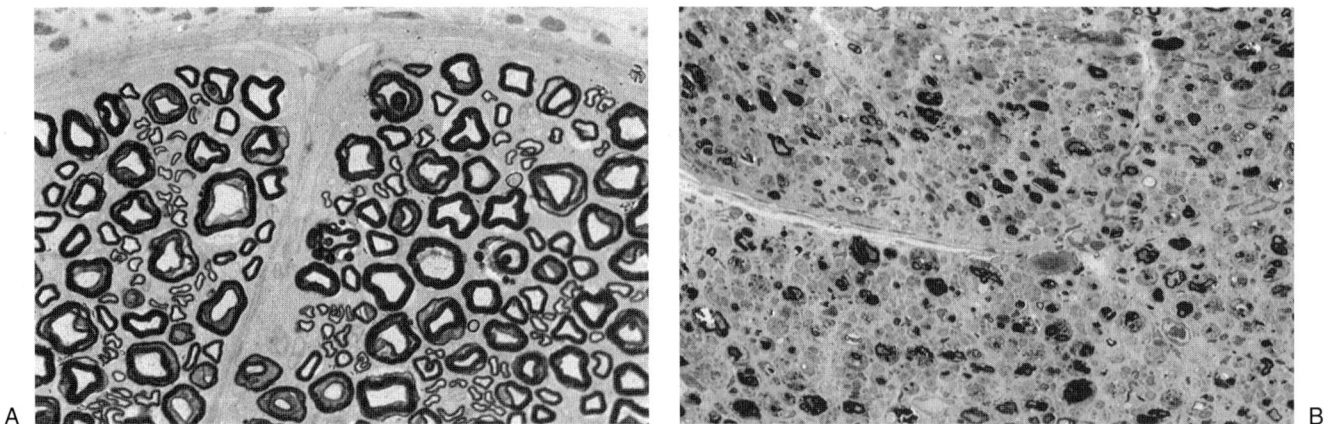

FIG. 2-4: **A:** A nerve root exposed to fat for seven days. There are no apparent changes. **B:** A nerve root exposed to autologous nucleus pulposus for seven days. There is pronounced axonal degeneration and the normal architecture of the endoneurial space has been markedly changed.

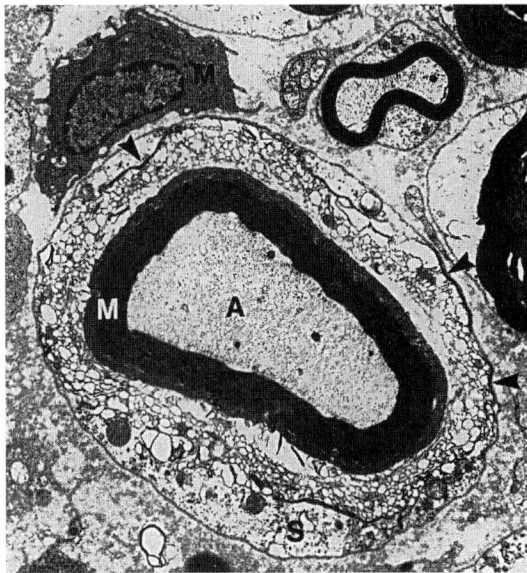

FIG. 2-5. Seven days after the application of nucleus pulposus. Myelinated nerve fiber with prominent vesicular swelling of a Schmidt-Lanterman incisure *(SL).* Note the mononuclear cell *(M)* in close contact with the nerve fiber. *A,* Well-preserved axon; *M,* myelin sheath; *S,* outer Schwann cell cytoplasm; *Arrowheads,* Myelin sheath layers outside the Schmidt-Lanterman incisure. (Bar: 2.5 mm) (From Olmarker K, Nordborg C, Larsson K, et al. Ultrastructural changes in spinal nerve roots induced by autologous nucleus pulposus. Spine 1996;21(4):411–414, with permission.)

injury inducing nerve dysfunction may not be found at the light microscopic level but must be sought for at the subcellular or molecular level.

Although methylprednisolone may intervene with the pathophysiologic events of the nucleus pulposus–induced nerve root injury, it was not clear if this resulted from the anti-inflammatory properties of the methylprednisolone or something else. To establish if the presence of autologous nucleus pulposus could initiate a leukotactic response from the surrounding tissues, a study was initiated that assessed the potential inflammatory properties of the nucleus pulposus (78). Autologous nucleus pulposus and autologous retroperitoneal fat were placed in separate perforated titanium chambers and placed subcutaneously with a sham chamber in the pig. Seven days later, the number of leukocytes was assessed for the chambers. The number of leukocytes was the same between the fat and the sham chambers. However, the nucleus pulposus–containing chambers had a number of leukocytes that exceeded the two others by 250%. In another experiment, autologous nucleus pulposus and muscle were placed in Gore-Tex (W. L. Gore & Associates, Inc., Flagstaff, AZ) tubes subcutaneously in rabbits (79). After 2 weeks, there was an accumulation of T-helper and T-suppresser cells in the tube with nucleus pulposus that persisted the full observation time of 4 weeks.

Nucleus pulposus may also interfere with the nutrition to the intraspinal nerve tissue. Following application to the dorsal root ganglion, the intraneural blood flow was dramatically decreased and there was a simultaneous increase of the tissue fluid pressure (75). The authors suggested that this might indicate that the nucleus pulposus induced intraneural edema because of the increased vascular permeability of the intraneural capillaries.

Kawakami et al. recently showed that neuropathic pain in an experimental setting seems to be mediated by infiltrating leukocytes (80), a finding consistent with the observations of neuroimmune inflammatory changes and pain (81). In rats made leukopenic by nitrogen mustard, the pain response was absent after application of nucleus pulposus, whereas normal rats with nucleus pulposus application displayed a pathologic response to stimulation. The same group also demonstrated that inhibition of cox-2 might reduce nucleus pulposus–induced pain behavior (82). Taken together, this further supports the idea that autologous nucleus pulposus may elicit inflammatory reactions when outside the intervertebral disc space and that such reactions may not necessarily be restricted to resorption of the herniated tissue but be intimately involved in the pathophysiology of sciatica.

Nucleus Pulposus and Sciatic Pain

Pain is much more difficult to assess that nerve conduction in controlled experimental studies for obvious reasons. The available literature indicates that pain may be induced by both mechanical and nucleus pulposus–mediated factors. The role of the nucleus pulposus in this context is interesting although uncommon in patients with obvious symptoms of disc herniation but no visible herniation at radiologic examination or surgery (19,83). The existing data suggest that communication between the intradiscal and epidural space is sufficient for inducing effects on the nerve roots, indicating that annular disruption with a discrete leakage of nucleus pulposus material into the spinal canal, with no visible herniation, could be enough to induce symptoms. The potential of nucleus pulposus material to induce pain was indicated in clinical studies that showed that noncontained herniations (where the nucleus pulposus is in contact with the epidural space) are much more painful and have a more pronounced straight leg-raising (SLR) than contained herniations (84–86).

Recent studies on rats, using pain behavior assessment, have indicated that nucleus pulposus may well be involved in pain production. Pain behavior in this context refers to response thresholds to thermal and mechanical stimulation. Kawakami et al. showed that a three-level laminectomy and an application of homologous nucleus pulposus or annulus fibrosus taken from three intervertebral discs in another rat, applied at three nerve roots, produced pain behavior (57); whereas Olmarker and Myers showed that facetectomy with incision of the disc and transfer of the autologous nucleus pulposus to the adjacent nerve root or dorsal root ganglion did not produce pain behavior (58). This indicates that there may be a dose-response curve between pain behavior and the amount of nucleus pulposus material in the epidural space. However, in Olmarker's model, pain behavior was present when the disc incision was combined with a slight medial displacement of the nerve root or dorsal root ganglion (DRG), and induced a mild mechanical deformation; whereas the displacement per se was found not to produce pain behavior (58). This observation is consistent with the neuropathologic understanding of pain and the consequences of combined mechanical and inflammatory injury to nerve fibers that are superimposed to increase the number of fibers injured and the corresponding increase in proinflammatory cytokines (67,68). The same pathophysiologic response was observed in a study assessing walking patterns, in which it was seen that the combination of displacement and disc incision produced detectable changes (60). A pain behavior study assessing changes in spontaneous behavior showed that the combined action of displacement and disc incision produced changes, whereas displacement or disc incision alone did not produce changes (87).

These experimental studies on pain behavior may indicate that the presence of nucleus pulposus has sensitized the nerve tissue to become sensitive to mechanical deformation. It is known that compression of peripheral nerves is not painful and that touching of a normal nerve root during local anesthesia is not painful (88). However, touching of a nerve root exposed to a disc herniation often reproduces sciatic pain (88). This clinical observation and the experimental finding that nucleus pulposus sensitizes the nerve root relates very well. It may be assumed that, in the pathophysiology of sciatica, except for inducing nerve dysfunction, nucleus pulposus can sensitize the nerve tissue to produce pain when exposed to mechanical stimulation.

Although the combination of a mechanical component and the presence of nucleus pulposus seems to be a prerequisite to produce changes in the *in vivo* situation, neurophysiologic studies have demonstrated that the mere application of nucleus pulposus may induce increased neuronal pain transmission (89). This may indicate that pain behavior assessment is a gross instrument to detect pain and that nucleus pulposus may induce pain in the absence of a mechanical component as well.

Theoretically, one may hypothesize two different mechanisms by which mechanical or biologic factors may induce pain; either by direct stimulation of nerves or innervated structures, or by neuroischemia. A vascular impairment of the nerve tissue with a nutritional deficit that results in ischemia of the nerve seems to be a likely pain mechanism, and could be induced by both mechanical and biologic factors. In studies where pain was suspected to result from direct stimulation of the nerve roots, the nucleus pulposus material primarily was in contact with the surrounding meninges, not the axons (56–58,60,84,

87,90). Also, in a study where locally anesthetized patients re-experienced their sciatic pain after local stimulation of the nerve root, the meninges might have been the actual tissue of stimulation (88). The spinal dura mater is known to contain nerve endings, and stimulation of the dura has been suggested as a mechanism for sciatic pain (9,91,92). Irritation or stimulation of the dura as an important factor for sciatica could explain many clinical features. The dura is segmentally innervated, as indicated in Figure 2-6; the sensory nerves travel in a caudal-lateral direction and are drained to the corresponding nerve root by the nerve of Luschka (93–96). Stimulation of the dura at a point where the dorsolateral herniations appear (Fig. 2-6I) should be recorded by the corresponding nerve root (97). However, the irritation may spread medially to the contralateral segment at this location, producing bilateral symptoms; or laterally, producing symptoms from levels above. Similarly, a lateral disc herniation (Fig. 2-6II) could produce symptoms in the lower level. If the pain of the straight leg raising test is the result of dura irritation caused by friction to the herniated mass, one may consider the phenomenon of "crossed SLR" to be based on simultaneous stimulation of the contralateral dura. Such a "radiculitis" or "local meningitis" could be regarded as similar to peritonitis. In peritonitis, a reflector muscle contraction usually is present

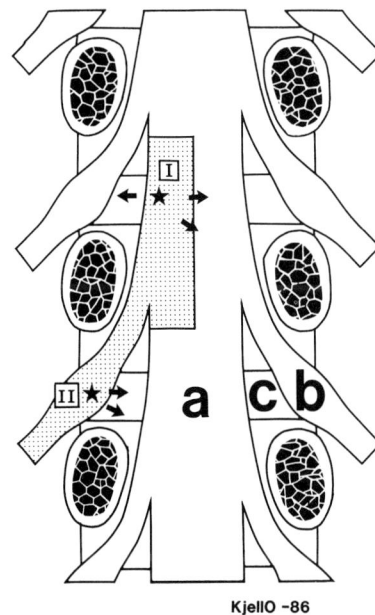

KjellO -86

FIG. 2-6. Suggested area of innervation by one recurrent sinuvertebral nerve (nerve of Luschka). Disc herniation at location *I* may be recorded by the same nerve and also by the nearby innervation areas, laterally and contralaterally, as indicated by the arrows. At location *II*, a lateral disc herniation of the disc one level below may affect the same nerve root but also the root one level below, located medial to this root, as indicated by the arrows. (From Olmarker K. The experimental basis of sciatica. J Orthop Sci 1996;1:230–242, with permission.)

over the affected area. An analog for this local meningitis could be the reflector ipsilateral contraction of the spinal muscles, producing "sciatic scoliosis," or lateral bending of the spine at the level of herniation.

To speculate further, one could elaborate that the deep visceral pain presented earlier as referred pain may be related to painful conditions in the nerve (e.g., neuroischemia), and that the sharp, distinct pain presented as radicular pain may be related to dura irritation. However, although these proposed mechanisms are subject to speculation, the view of spinal pain may change dramatically in coming years based on new ideas and concepts as well as rapidly increasing knowledge about the molecular events active in the pathophysiology of sciatica.

Mechanisms and Transport Routes

When considering various pathophysiologic mechanisms below the tissue level, three mechanisms seem reasonable: (a) a direct neurotoxic effect on the nerve tissue; (b) a vascular impairment; and (c) inflammatory or immunologic reactions.

It is difficult to relate the observed histologic changes of nerve tissue as induced by nucleus pulposus to direct neurotoxic effects or ischemia. There is always reason to assume that there are neurotoxic substances acting on the axons present in the nucleus pulposus. However, histologic observations indicate that the changes are focal and mainly found in the center of the nerve roots, resembling a mononeuritis simplex induced by nerve infarction caused by embolism of the intraneural vessels (6,71,98). Particularly in view of the work of Jayson et al. that indicate an impairment of the venous outflow from the nerve roots owing to periradicular vascular changes, one must consider vascular impairment as a highly interesting factor (99–102). Even relatively large molecules deposited in the epidural space may be found in the intraneural vessels of the adjacent nerve roots within seconds after application (103). Considering the possibility of epidurally placed substances to penetrate the relatively impermeable dura, cross over the CSF, and then diffuse through the root sheath and into the axons, this vascular route may seem more relevant. As mentioned, nucleus pulposus seems to have certain inflammatory properties (6,78–80,104). Because many inflammatory mediators are involved in vascular and rheologic phenomena such as coagulation, one may suspect that vascular impairment of the nerve root may result from vascular embolism. In fact, it was observed in a vital microscopic study that the presence of nucleus pulposus may induce thrombus formation in microvessels (78). Inflammatory mediators might also exert a direct effect on the myelin sheaths, as indicated by an electron microscopic study of nerve roots exposed to autologous nucleus pulposus in the pig (71). There were significant injuries of Schwann cells with vacuolization and disintegration of the Schmidt-Lanterman incisures, which closely resembles the

injury pattern of inflammatory nerve disease (105,106). As described, results from recent studies have indicated that epidural application of nucleus pulposus induces an increase of the vascular permeability and a subsequent reduction of the blood flow in the adjacent nerve roots, which suggests that vascular impairment is pathophysiologically important.

It has been suggested also that because the nucleus pulposus is avascular and thus "hidden" from the systemic circulation, presentation of the nucleus pulposus could result in an autoimmune reaction directed to antigens present in the nucleus pulposus, and that bioactive substances from this reaction could injure the nerve tissue (107–113). Also, there could be autoimmune reactions, not only in the disc, but also in components from the nerve tissue that are released as the result of injury, such as basic myelin protein. It is not clear if such immunologic reactions occur, but ongoing research has demonstrated immunoreactivity in some patients at the time of surgery. An interesting study assessed the possible presence of immune complexes in herniated disc tissue obtained at surgery as an indicator of immunoactivation (114). It was found that there was IgG in close relation to the disc cells in herniated disc material. However, no IgG was found in the residual disc evacuated at the time of surgery. Neither immune complex was found in control disc material obtained at spine surgery for causes other than pain. Although inconclusive, this study might indicate that immunologic activation may be present in some cases of sciatica.

Components of the Nucleus Pulposus of the Intervertebral Discs

The nucleus pulposus mainly comprises proteoglycans, collagen, and cells (115,116). Therefore, the observed effects as induced by the nucleus pulposus at local application probably should be contributed to one or more of these components. The proteoglycans have gained most attention; and are suggested to have a direct irritating effect on the nerve tissue (113,117,118). Neither the collagen nor the cells previously were suggested to be of pathophysiologic importance. However, recent studies of the cells of the nucleus pulposus showed that these cells are capable of producing metalloproteases such as collagenase or gelatinase, as well as interleukin-6 and prostaglandin E_2, and do so spontaneously in culture (104). Using the same pig model as described, the possible role of the nucleus pulposus cells for the nucleus pulposus–induced nerve injury has been assessed (72). In a blind fashion, autologous nucleus pulposus was subjected to 24 hours of freezing at -20°C and digestion by hyaluronidase or a heating box at 37°C for 24 hours. The treated nucleus pulposus was reapplied after 24 hours and analyses were performed 7 days later. It was evident that there were no changes in nerve conduction velocity in animals where the nucleus pulposus had been frozen and the cells killed, whereas in the other two series the results were similar to application of unaltered nucleus pulposus. Therefore, it seems reasonable that the cells are responsible in some way for inducing the nerve injury and that the structural molecules are of less importance. This assumption was further supported by a study using the same model, which showed that application of cultured pig disc cells to the cauda equina reproduced the reduction in nerve conduction velocity (119). However, application of disc cell membranes also reproduced this reduction, indicating that the responsible substances probably are membrane bound.

Substances such as IgG, hydrogen ions, NO, and PLA2 might be responsible for the pathophysiologic reactions (113,120–124). Another substance produced by the disc cells that has similar pathophysiologic effects as nucleus pulposus is tumor necrosis factor-a (TNF-a) (125). The possible involvement of TNF and other related cytokines in the pathophysiology of sciatica is discussed in the following.

Cytokines as Mediators of Nerve Dysfunction and Pain

Tumor necrosis factor is known to be a regulatory proinflammatory cytokine that has both specific biologic effects as well as the ability to up-regulate and act synergistically with other cytokines, such as IL-1B and IL-6 (126–131). Immediately after nerve injury, TNF is released and up-regulated by Schwann cells at the site of nerve injury (132). This is followed by the release and up-regulation of TNF in many other endoneurial cells, including endothelial cells, fibroblasts, and mast cells. Tumor necrosis factor also is produced by chondrocytes and disc cells (125, 133–136). The local production of TNF is the stimulus that results in macrophage attraction to the injury site (66), which then contributes massively to the concentration of proinflammatory cytokines in the injured tissue. Several studies have clearly shown that blocking TNF production or delaying the invasion of macrophages to the site of nerve injury results in reduced or delayed neuropathologic change and reduced hyperalgesia (81,137). When performing a meta-analysis on the biologic or pathophysiologic effects induced by TNF and nucleus pulposus, one may find that there is almost a perfect match. For instance, TNF is known to induce axonal and myelin injury similar to that observed after nucleus pulposus application (138–144), intravascular coagulation (145–147), and increased vascular permeability (147). Tumor necrosis factor is also known to be neurotoxic (141,143,148,149) and to induce painful behavioral changes (138,150) as well as ectopic nerve activity when applied locally (139,151). Interestingly, TNF is sequestered in a membrane-bound form and is activated after shedding by certain enzymes. Matrix metalloproteinases (MMP) are particularly important in this regard. MMP-9 and MMP-2 are up-regulated immediately after a nerve injury (152). Matrix metalloproteinases process the inactive, membrane-bound form of TNF and its receptors to the biologically active form. MMP-9 and TNF receptors are also retrogradely transported from the site of nerve injury to the corresponding dorsal root ganglion and spinal cord (153), where they may have a direct role in gene regulation. This may relate to the observation that cell membranes of disc cells are sufficient to mediate nucleus pulposus–induced effects (119).

Tumor necrosis factor was found in disc cells; when TNF was inhibited with a nonspecific cytokine inhibitor, the nucleus pulposus–induced reduction in nerve conduction velocity following experimental application of nucleus pulposus in a pig model was completely blocked (125). When using more specific TNF inhibitors, such as a monoclonal antibody to TNF (infliximab) and a soluble TNF-receptor (etanercept), the inhibition was equally effective (154). Application of selected cytokines in the pig model showed that TNF reduced the nerve conduction velocity per se (155). IL-1B and interferon-γ only induced a slight reduction of nerve conduction velocity.

Application of certain cytokines to intraspinal nerves may also increase the somatosensory neural response (156). Discharges from wide dynamic range neurons following stimulation of a receptor field of a dorsal root ganglion exposed to nucleus pulposus increased significantly following application (157). This may be related to the sensitization of the sensory system caused by proinflammatory cytokines and the production of low-grade spontaneous electrophysiologic activity in nociceptors by TNF (151), which by itself is an important factor that contributes to sensitization. The administration of an antibody specific for TNF efficiently inhibited this effect. An in vivo study assessing changes in spontaneous behavior clearly showed that changes induced by the combined action of mechanical deformation and disc incision was markedly inhibited by intraperitoneal injection of a monoclonal antibody specific for TNF (59). It seems that TNF is an important mediator both for the observed effects on nerve function and pain induced by local application of nucleus pulposus. Additional support for this hypothesis comes from previous work which showed that blockade of TNF up-regulation in macrophages by thalidomide (137) and down-regulation of TNF by IL-10 administration (158) reduced the magnitude and duration of hyperalgesia following nerve injury. Because cytokine interactions are complex, other cytokines, such as IL-1B and IL-6, may be involved as well (155,156,159,160). However, because these cytokines are induced by TNF, their exact role has not been completely evaluated.

Suggested Mechanism of Action of Tumor Necrosis Factor

It is known that even relatively large substances that are placed in the epidural space are found in the intraneural capillaries of the nerve root and dorsal ganglion (103). Therefore one may assume that TNF may reach the intraneural capillaries following release from disc cells in the herniated nucleus pulposus. Tumor necrosis factor induces an activation of endothelial adhesion molecules (e.g., ICAM and VCAM), thereby adhering circulating immune cells to the vessel walls (Fig. 2-7) (129,161,162). Because of the TNF-induced increased vascular permeability, these cells migrate into the endoneurial space where the axons are located (163–165). The cells then release their content of TNF and other cytokines, which may induce an accumulation of ion channels locally in the axonal membranes (166–168). The channels may allow for an increased passage of sodium and potassium, which may result in spontaneous discharges and discharges of ectopic impulses following mechanical stimulation. Tumor necrosis factor by itself can cause spontaneous electrical activity in A-delta and C-nociceptors (151). Such discharges, regardless of whether they come from a pain fiber or a nerve fiber transmitting other sensory information, are interpreted as pain by the brain (169–172). Such a mechanism may relate to the sensitization of the nerve roots seen in the mentioned experimental and clinical studies and may relate to motion-evoked sciatic pain, such as the straight-leg raising test.

Studies have also indicated that local application of nucleus pulposus may disintegrate the myelin sheath (71, 73). This is a known effect of TNF (138,163,173–175). In particular, this injury seems to affect the Schmidt-Lanterman incisures, which are responsible for the ion exchange between the axon and surrounding tissues (176–179). This could also contribute to the formation of ectopic impulses and the sensitization to mechanical stimuli.

Recent work regarding molecular events in the pathophysiology of neuropathic pain has suggested a potential role of TNF for inducing allodynia (139,180–185). Tumor necrosis factor may mediate the formation of allodynic states in both the dorsal root ganglion and spinal cord level because of its local up-regulation, which occurs via a positive feedback loop caused by TNF itself. Interestingly, this cycle seems to be broken by a direct effect of TNF on the up-regulation of anti-inflammatory cytokines such as IL-10, which eventually leads to a reduction of TNF and the physiologic balance of proinflammatory and anti-inflammatory cytokines. Such regulation seems to be induced both by mechanical injury to peripheral parts of the axons and also as a direct effect of TNF exposure, and thereby further enhances the impression that TNF may be an important mediator of neuropathic pain. Tumor necrosis factor is a potent activator of cells, and because it is

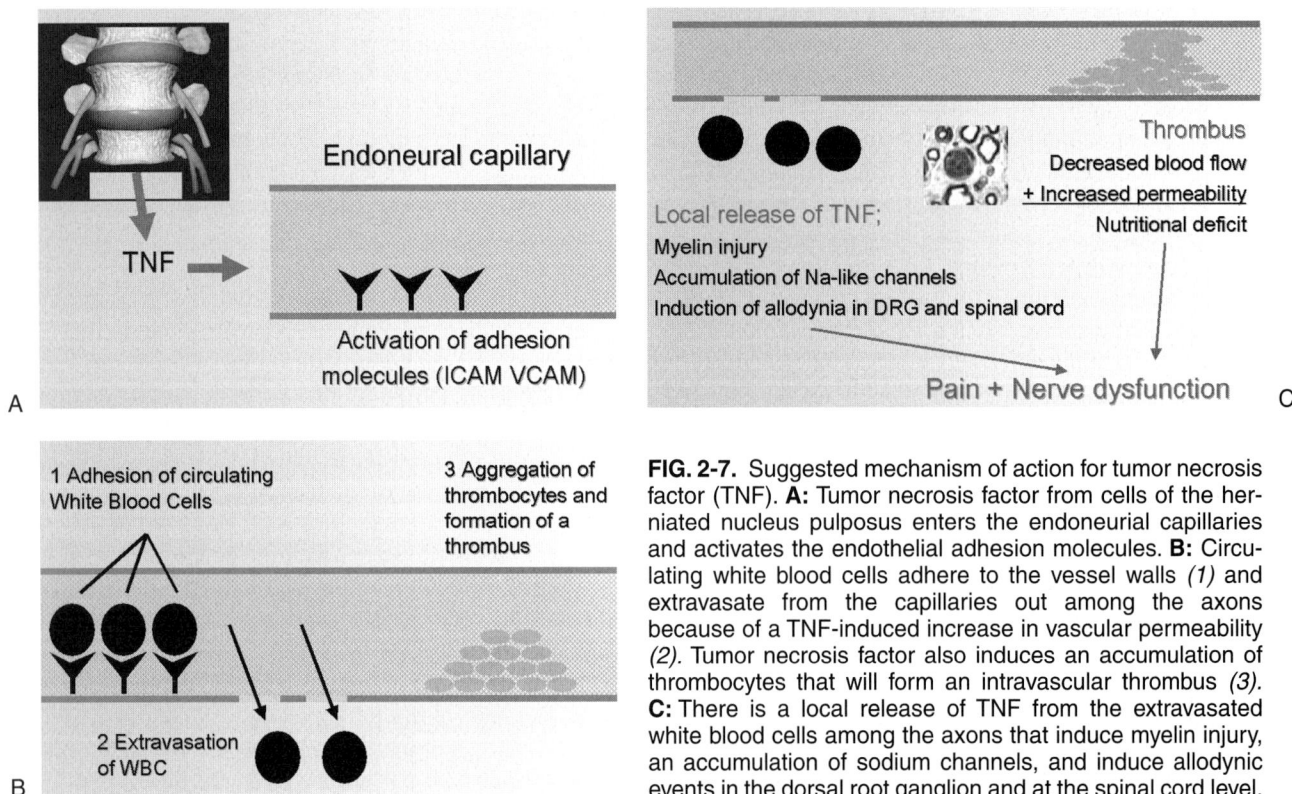

FIG. 2-7. Suggested mechanism of action for tumor necrosis factor (TNF). A: Tumor necrosis factor from cells of the herniated nucleus pulposus enters the endoneurial capillaries and activates the endothelial adhesion molecules. B: Circulating white blood cells adhere to the vessel walls (1) and extravasate from the capillaries out among the axons because of a TNF-induced increase in vascular permeability (2). Tumor necrosis factor also induces an accumulation of thrombocytes that will form an intravascular thrombus (3). C: There is a local release of TNF from the extravasated white blood cells among the axons that induce myelin injury, an accumulation of sodium channels, and induce allodynic events in the dorsal root ganglion and at the spinal cord level. The thrombus, together with the edema, induces a nutritional deficit in the nerve root because of increased permeability. Both the local effects of TNF and the nutritional deficit may induce pain and nerve dysfunction.

intraneural blood flow in the porcine cauda equina. J Orthop Res 1993;11(1):104–109.

36. Cornefjord M, Takahashi K, Matsui Y, et al. Impairment of nutritional transport at double-level cauda equina compression. An experimental study. Neuroorthopaedics 1992;13:107–112.

37. Baker AR, Collins TA, Porter RW, et al. Laser Doppler study of porcine cauda equina blood flow. The effect of electrical stimulation of the rootlets during single and double site, low pressure compression of the cauda equina. Spine 1995;20(6):660–664.

38. Delamarter RB, Bohlman HH, Dodge LD, et al. Experimental lumbar spinal stenosis. Analysis of the cortical evoked potentials, microvasculature, and histopathology. J Bone Joint Surg (Am) 1990;72(1):110–120.

39. Cornefjord M, Sato K, Olmarker K, et al. A model for chronic nerve root compression studies. Presentation of a porcine model for controlled, slow-onset compression with analyses of anatomic aspects, compression onset rate, and morphologic and neurophysiologic effects. Spine 1997;22(9):946–957.

40. Cornefjord M, Olmarker K, Farley DB, et al. Neuropeptide changes in compressed spinal nerve roots. Spine 1995;20(6):670–673.

41. Sato K, Olmarker K, Cornefjord M, et al. Changes of intraradicular blood flow in chronic nerve root compression. An experimental study on pigs. Neuroorthopaedics 1994;16:1–7.

42. Konno S, Olmarker K, Byrod G, et al. Intermittent cauda equina compression. An experimental study of the porcine cauda equina with analyses of nerve impulse conduction properties. Spine 1995;20(11):1223–1226.

43. Takahashi K, Miyazaki T, Takino T, et al. Epidural pressure measurements. Relationship between epidural pressure and posture in patients with lumbar spinal stenosis. Spine 1995;20(6):650–653.

44. Konno S, Yabuki S, Sato K, et al. A model for acute, chronic, and delayed graded compression of the dog cauda equina. Presentation of the gross, microscopic, and vascular anatomy of the dog cauda equina and accuracy in pressure transmission of the compression model. Spine 1995;20(24):2758–2764.

45. Sato K, Konno S, Yabuki S, et al. A model for acute, chronic, and delayed graded compression of the dog cauda equina. Neurophysiologic and histologic changes induced by acute, graded compression. Spine 1995;20(22):2386–2391.

46. Rydevik B, Lundborg G, Skalak R. Biomechanics of peripheral nerves. In: Nordin M, Frankel VH, eds. Basic biomechanics of the musculoskeletal system. Philadelphia: Lea & Febiger, 1989, 75–87.

47. Macgregor RJ, Sharpless SK, Luttges MW. A pressure vessel model for nerve compression. J Neurol Sci 1975;24(3):299–304.

48. Schonstrom N, Bolender NF, Spengler DM, et al. Pressure changes within the cauda equina following constriction of the dural sac. An in vitro experimental study. Spine 1984;9(6):604–607.

49. Schonstrom NS, Bolender NF, Spengler DM. The pathomorphology of spinal stenosis as seen on CT scans of the lumbar spine. Spine 1985;10(9):806–811.

50. Schonstrom N, Hansson T. Pressure changes following constriction of the cauda equina. An experimental study in situ. Spine 1988;13(4):385–388.

51. Takahashi K, Kagechika K, Takino T, et al. Changes in epidural pressure during walking in patients with lumbar spinal stenosis. Spine 1995;20(24):2746–2749.

52. Howe JF, Loeser JD, Calvin WH. Mechanosensitivity of dorsal root ganglia and chronically injured axons: a physiological basis for the radicular pain of nerve root compression. Pain 1977;3(1):25–41.

53. Cavanaugh JM, Ozaktay AC, Yamashita T, et al. Mechanisms of low back pain: a neurophysiologic and neuroanatomic study. Clin Orthop 1997(335):166–180.

54. Weinstein J, Pope M, Schmidt R, et al. Neuropharmacologic effects of vibration on the dorsal root ganglion. An animal model. Spine 1988;13(5):521–525.

55. Chatani K, Kawakami M, Weinstein JN, et al. Characterization of thermal hyperalgesia, c-fos expression, and alterations in neuropeptides after mechanical irritation of the dorsal root ganglion. Spine 1995;20(3):277–289; discussion 290.

56. Kawakami M, Weinstein JN, Spratt KF, et al. Experimental lumbar radiculopathy. Immunohistochemical and quantitative demonstrations of pain induced by lumbar nerve root irritation of the rat. Spine 1994;19(16):1780–1794.

57. Kawakami M, Weinstein JN, Chatani K, et al. Experimental lumbar radiculopathy. Behavioral and histologic changes in a model of radicular pain after spinal nerve root irritation with chromic gut ligatures in the rat. Spine 1994;19(16):1795–1802.

58. Olmarker K, Myers RR. Pathogenesis of sciatic pain: role of herniated nucleus pulposus and deformation of spinal nerve root and dorsal root ganglion. Pain 1998;78(2):99–105.

59. Olmarker K, Nutu M, Storkson R. Changes in spontaneous behavior in rats to experimental disc herniation are blocked by selective TNF-alpha inhibition. Spine 2003;28(15):1635–1641.

60. Olmarker K, Iwabuchi M, Larsson K, et al. Walking analysis of rats subjected to experimental disc herniation. Eur Spine J 1998;7(5):394–399.

61. Takahashi K, Shima I, Porter RW. Nerve root pressure in lumbar disc herniation. Spine 1999;24(19):2003–2006.

62. Myers R, Shubayev VI, Campana WM. Neuropathology of painful neuropathies. In: Sommer C, ed. Pain in peripheral nerve disease. Basel: Karger; 2001:8–30.

63. Powell HC, Myers RR. Pathology of experimental nerve compression. Lab Invest 1986;55(1):91–100.

64. Myers RR, Yamamoto T, Yaksh TL, et al. The role of focal nerve ischemia and Wallerian degeneration in peripheral nerve injury producing hyperesthesia. Anesthesiology 1993;78(2):308–316.

65. Sommer C, Galbraith JA, Heckman HM, et al. Pathology of experimental compression neuropathy producing hyperesthesia. J Neuropathol Exp Neurol 1993;52(3):223–233.

66. Stoll G, Jander S, Myers RR. Degeneration and regeneration of the peripheral nervous system: from Augustus Waller's observations to neuroinflammation. J Peripher Nerv Syst 2002;7(1):13–27.

67. Myers R, Wagner R, Sorkin LS. Hyperalgesic action of cytokines on peripheral nerves. In: Watkins LR, Maier SF, eds. Cytokines and pain. Basel: Birkhäuser Verlag, 1999:133–157.

68. Myers RR, Heckman HM, Powell HC. Axonal viability and the persistence of thermal hyperalgesia after partial freeze lesions of nerve. J Neurol Sci 1996;139(1):28–38.

69. Rydevik B, Brown MD, Ehira T, et al. Effects of graded compression and nucleus pulposus on nerve tissue: an experimental study in rabbits. Proceedings of the Swedish Orthopaedic Association, Göteborg, Sweden, August 7, 1982. Acta Orthopaedica Scand 1983;54:670–671.

70. McCarron RF, Wimpee MW, Hudkins PG, et al. The inflammatory effect of nucleus pulposus. A possible element in the pathogenesis of low-back pain. Spine 1987;12(8):760–764.

71. Olmarker K, Nordborg C, Larsson K, et al. Ultrastructural changes in spinal nerve roots induced by autologous nucleus pulposus. Spine 1996;21(4):411–414.

72. Olmarker K, Brisby H, Yabuki S, et al. The effects of normal, frozen, and hyaluronidase-digested nucleus pulposus on nerve root structure and function. Spine 1997;22(5):471–475.

73. Kayama S, Konno S, Olmarker K, et al. Incision of the anulus fibrosus induces nerve root morphologic, vascular, and functional changes. An experimental study. Spine 1996;21(22):2539–2543.

74. Byrod G, Otani K, Brisby H, et al. Methylprednisolone reduces the early vascular permeability increase in spinal nerve roots induced by epidural nucleus pulposus application. J Orthop Res 2000;18(6):983–987.

75. Yabuki S, Kikuchi S, Olmarker K, et al. Acute effects of nucleus pulposus on blood flow and endoneurial fluid pressure in rat dorsal root ganglia. Spine 1998;23(23):2517–2523.

76. Byrod G, Rydevik B, Nordborg C, et al. Early effects of nucleus pulposus application on spinal nerve root morphology and function (in process citation). Eur Spine J 1998;7(6):445–449.

77. Olmarker K, Byrod G, Cornefjord M, et al. Effects of methylprednisolone on nucleus pulposus–induced nerve root injury. Spine 1994;19(16):1803–1808.

78. Olmarker K, Blomquist J, Stromberg J, et al. Inflammatogenic properties of nucleus pulposus. Spine 1995;20(6):665–669.

79. Takino T, Takahashi K, Miyazaki T, et al. Immunoreactivity of nucleus pulposus. Trans. International Society for the Study of the Lumbar Spine. Helsinki, Finland, 1995.

80. Kawakami M, Tamaki T, Matsumoto T, et al. Role of leukocytes in radicular pain secondary to herniated nucleus pulposus. Clin Orthop 2000(376):268–277.

81. Myers RR, Heckman HM, Rodriguez M. Reduced hyperalgesia in nerve-injured WLD mice: relationship to nerve fiber phagocytosis, axonal degeneration, and regeneration in normal mice. Exp Neurol 1996;141(1):94–101.

82. Kawakami M, Matsumoto T, Hashizume H, et al. Epidural injection of cyclooxygenase-2 inhibitor attenuates pain-related behavior following application of nucleus pulposus to the nerve root in the rat. J Orthop Res 2002;20(2):376–381.

83. Crock HV. Observations on the management of failed spinal operations. J Bone Joint Surg Br 1976;58(2):193-199.

84. Jonsson B, Stromqvist B. Clinical appearance of contained and non-contained lumbar disc herniation. J Spinal Disord 1996;9(1):32–38.

85. Ito T, Takano Y, Yuasa N. Types of lumbar herniated disc and clinical course. Spine 2001;26(6):648–651.

86. Nygaard OP, Mellgren SI, Osterud B. The inflammatory properties of contained and noncontained lumbar disc herniation. Spine 1997;22 (21):2484–2488.

87. Olmarker K, Storkson R, Berge OG. Pathogenesis of sciatic pain: a study of spontaneous behavior in rats exposed to experimental disc herniation. Spine 2002;27(12):1312–1317.

88. Kuslich SD, Ulstrom CL, Michael CJ. The tissue origin of low back pain and sciatica: a report of pain response to tissue stimulation during operations on the lumbar spine using local anesthesia. Orthop Clin North Am 1991;22(2):181–187.

89. Anzai H, Hamba M, Onda A, et al. Epidural application of nucleus pulposus enhances nociresponses of rat dorsal horn neurons. Spine 2002;27(3):E50–E55.

90. Kawakami M, Tamaki T, Weinstein JN, et al. Pathomechanism of pain-related behavior produced by allografts of intervertebral disc in the rat. Spine 1996;21(18):2101–2107.

91. Olmarker K, Rydevik B. Pathophysiology of sciatica. Orthop Clin North Am 1991;22(2):223–234.

92. El-Mahdi MA, Abdel Latif FY, Janko M. The spinal nerve root "innervation," and a new concept of the clinicopathological interrelations in back pain and sciatica. Neurochirurgia (Stuttgart) 1981;24(4): 137–141.

93. Edgar MA, Nundy S. Innervation of the spinal dura. J Neurol Neurosurg Psychiatry 1966;29:530–534.

94. Kaplan EB. Recurrent meningeal branch of the spinal nerve. Bull Hospital Joint Dis 1947.

95. von Luschka H. Die Nerven des Menschen. 1850.

96. Rudinger N. Die Gelenkennerven des menschlichen Körpers. Erlangen: Ferdinand Enke, 1857.

97. Olmarker K. Experimental basis of sciatica. J Orthop Sci 1996;1: 230–242.

98. Dyck PJ, Karnes J, Lais A, et al. Pathologic alterations of the peripheral nervous system of humans. In: Dyck PJ, Thomas PK, Lambert EH, et al., eds. Peripheral neuropathy. Philadelphia: WB Saunders, 1984: 828–930.

99. Hoyland JA, Freemont AJ, Jayson MI. Intervertebral foramen venous obstruction. A cause of periradicular fibrosis? Spine 1989;14(6): 558–568.

100. Cooper RG, Freemont AJ, Hoyland JA, et al. Herniated intervertebral disc-associated periradicular fibrosis and vascular abnormalities occur without inflammatory cell infiltration. Spine 1995;20(5):591–598.

101. Jayson MI, Keegan A, Million R, et al. A fibrinolytic defect in chronic back pain syndromes. Lancet 1984;2(8413):1186–1187.

102. Klimiuk PS, Pountain GD, Keegan AL, et al. Serial measurements of fibrinolytic activity in acute low back pain and sciatica. Spine 1987; 12(9):925–928.

103. Byrod G, Olmarker K, Konno S, et al. A rapid transport route between the epidural space and the intraneural capillaries of the nerve roots. Spine 1995;20(2):138–143.

104. Kang JD, Georgescu HI, McIntyre-Larkin L, et al. Herniated lumbar intervertebral discs spontaneously produce matrix metalloproteinases, nitric oxide, interleukin-6, and prostaglandin E_2. Spine 1996;21(3): 271–277.

105. Dalcanto MC, Wisniewski HM, Johnson AB, et al. Vesicular disruption of myelin in autoimmune demyelination. J Neurol Sci 1975;24 (3):313–319.

106. Hahn AF, Gilbert JJ, Feasby TE. Passive transfer of demyelination by experimental allergic neuritis serum. Acta Neuropathol (Berlin) 1980; 49(3):169–176.

107. Bisla RS, Marchisello PJ, Lockshin MD, et al. Auto-immunological basis of disc degeneration. Clin Orthop 1976(121):205–211.

108. Bobechko WP, Hirsch C. Auto-immune response to nucleus pulposus in the rabbit. J Bone Joint Surg 1965;47B:574–580.

109. Gertzbein SD, Tile M, Gross A, et al. Autoimmunity in degenerative disc disease of the lumbar spine. Orthop Clin North Am 1975;6(1): 67–73.

110. Gertzbein SD. Degenerative disc disease of the lumbar spine: immunological implications. Clin Orthop 1977(129):68–71.

111. Gertzbein SD, Tait JH, Devlin SR. The stimulation of lymphocytes by nucleus pulposus in patients with degenerative disc disease of the lumbar spine. Clin Orthop 1977(123):149–154.

112. LaRocca H. New horizons in research on disc disease. Orthop Clin North Am 1971;2(2):521–531.

113. Naylor A. The biophysical and biochemical aspects of intervertebral disc herniation and degeneration. Ann Roy Col Surg (England) 1962; 31:91–114.

114. Satoh K, Konno S, Nishiyama K, et al. Presence and distribution of antigen-antibody complexes in the herniated nucleus pulposus (in process citation). Spine 1999;24(19):1980–1984.

115. Bayliss MT, Johnstone B. Biochemistry of the intervertebral disc. In: Jayson MIV, ed. The lumbar spine and back pain. New York: Churchill Livingstone, 1992:111–131.

116. Eyre D, Benya P, Buckwalter J. Intervertebral disc. In: Frymoyer JW, Gordon SL, eds. New perspectives on low back pain. Rosemont, IL: American Academy of Orthopaedic Surgeons, 1988:149–207.

117. Marshall LL, Trethewie ER. Chemical irritation of nerve-root in disc prolapse. Lancet 1973;2(7824):320.

118. Marshall LL, Trethewie ER, Curtain CC. Chemical radiculitis. A clinical, physiological and immunological study. Clin Orthop 1977(129): 61–6.

119. Kayama S, Olmarker K, Larsson K, et al. Cultured, autologous nucleus pulposus cells induce structural and functional changes in spinal nerve roots. Spine 1998;23(20):2155–2158.

120. Brisby H, Byrod G, Olmarker K, et al. Nitric oxide as a mediator of nucleus pulposus–induced effects on spinal nerve roots. J Orthop Res 2000;18(5):815–820.

121. Diamant B, Karlsson J, Nachemson A. Correlation between lactate levels and pH in discs of patients with lumbar rhizopathies. Experientia 1968;24:1195–1196.

122. Nachemson A. Intradiscal measurements of pH in patients with lumbar rhizopathies. Acta Orthop Scand 1969;40:23–42.

123. Pennington JB, McCarron RF, Laros GS. Identification of IgG in the canine intervertebral disc. Spine 1988;13(8):909–912.

124. Saal JS, Franson RC, Dobrow R, et al. High levels of inflammatory phospholipase A2 activity in lumbar disc herniations. Spine 1990;15 (7):674–678.

125. Olmarker K, Larsson K. Tumor necrosis factor alpha and nucleus-pulposus-induced nerve root injury. Spine 1998;23(23):2538–2544.

126. Chao CC, Hu S, Ehrlich L, et al. Interleukin-1 and tumor necrosis factor-alpha synergistically mediate neurotoxicity: involvement of nitric oxide and of N-methyl-D-aspartate receptors. Brain Behav Immun 1995;9(4):355–365.

127. Gadient RA, Cron KC, Otten U. Interleukin-1 beta and tumor necrosis factor-alpha synergistically stimulate nerve growth factor (NGF) release from cultured rat astrocytes. Neurosci Lett 1990;117(3): 335–340.

128. Bluthe RM, Dantzer R, Kelley KW. Interleukin-1 mediates behavioural but not metabolic effects of tumor necrosis factor alpha in mice. Eur J Pharmacol 1991;209(3):281–283.

129. McHale JF, Harari OA, Marshall D, et al. TNF-alpha and IL-1 sequentially induce endothelial ICAM-1 and VCAM-1 expression in MRL/lpr lupus-prone mice (in process citation). J Immunol 1999;163 (7):3993–4000.

130. Siwik DA, Chang DL, Colucci WS. Interleukin-1beta and tumor necrosis factor-alpha decrease collagen synthesis and increase matrix metalloproteinase activity in cardiac fibroblasts in vitro. Circ Res 2000;86(12):1259–1265.

131. McGee DW, Bamberg T, Vitkus SJ, et al. A synergistic relationship between TNF-alpha, IL-1 beta, and TGF-beta 1 on IL-6 secretion by the IEC-6 intestinal epithelial cell line. Immunology 1995;86(1):6–11.

132. Wagner R, Myers RR. Schwann cells produce tumor necrosis factor alpha: expression in injured and non-injured nerves. Neuroscience 1996;73(3):625–629.

133. Satomi N, Haranaka K, Kunii O. Research on the production site of tumor necrosis factor (TNF). Jpn J Exp Med 1981;51(6):317–322.

134. Bachwich PR, Lynch JP 3rd, Larrick J, et al. Tumor necrosis factor production by human sarcoid alveolar macrophages. Am J Pathol 1986;125(3):421–425.

135. Robbins DS, Shirazi Y, Drysdale BE, et al. Production of cytotoxic factor for oligodendrocytes by stimulated astrocytes. J Immunol 1987;139(8):2593–2597.

136. Sayers TJ, Macher I, Chung J, et al. The production of tumor necrosis factor by mouse bone marrow-derived macrophages in response to bacterial lipopolysaccharide and a chemically synthesized monosaccharide precursor. J Immunol 1987;138(9):2935–2940.

137. Sommer C, Marziniak M, Myers RR. The effect of thalidomide treatment on vascular pathology and hyperalgesia caused by chronic constriction injury of rat nerve. Pain 1998;74(1):83–91.

138. Wagner R, Myers RR. Endoneurial injection of TNF-alpha produces neuropathic pain behaviors. Neuroreport 1996;7(18):2897–2901.

139. Igarashi T, Kikuchi S, Shubayev V, et al. 2000 Volvo Award winner in basic science studies: Exogenous tumor necrosis factor-alpha mimics nucleus pulposus–induced neuropathology. Molecular, histologic, and behavioral comparisons in rats. Spine 2000;25(23):2975–2980.

140. Liberski PP, Yanagihara R, Nerurkar V, et al. Further ultrastructural studies of lesions produced in the optic nerve by tumor necrosis factor alpha (TNF-alpha): a comparison with experimental Creutzfeldt-Jakob disease. Acta Neurobiol Exp (Warsz) 1994;54(3):209–218.

141. Madigan MC, Sadun AA, Rao NS, et al. Tumor necrosis factor-alpha (TNF-alpha)-induced optic neuropathy in rabbits. Neurol Res 1996; 18(2):176–184.

142. Redford EJ, Hall SM, Smith KJ. Vascular changes and demyelination induced by the intraneural injection of tumour necrosis factor. Brain 1995;118(Pt 4):869–878.

143. Selmaj K, Raine CS. Tumor necrosis factor mediates myelin damage in organotypic cultures of nervous tissue. Ann NY Acad Sci 1988; 540:568–570.

144. Stoll G, Jung S, Jander S, et al. Tumor necrosis factor-alpha in immune-mediated demyelination and Wallerian degeneration of the rat peripheral nervous system. J Neuroimmunol 1993;45(1–2):175–182.

145. Nawroth P, Handley D, Matsueda G, De, et al. Tumor necrosis factor/cachectin-induced intravascular fibrin formation in meth A fibrosarcomas. J Exp Med 1988;168(2):637–647.

146. van der Poll T, Jansen PM, Van Zee KJ, et al. Tumor necrosis factor-alpha induces activation of coagulation and fibrinolysis in baboons through an exclusive effect on the p55 receptor. Blood 1996;88(3): 922–927.

147. Watts ME, Arnold S, Chaplin DJ. Changes in coagulation and permeability properties of human endothelial cells in vitro induced by TNF-alpha or 5,6 MeXAA. Br J Cancer 1996;74(suppl 27):S164–S167.

148. Viviani B, Corsini E, Galli CL, et al. Glia increase degeneration of hippocampal neurons through release of tumor necrosis factor-alpha. Toxicol Appl Pharmacol 1998;150(2):271–276.

149. Wuthrich RP, Jevnikar AM, Takei F, et al. Intercellular adhesion molecule-1(ICAM-1) expression is upregulated in autoimmune murine lupus nephritis. Am J Pathol 1990;136(2):441–450.

150. Sommer C, Schmidt C, George A, et al. A metalloprotease-inhibitor reduces pain associated behavior in mice with experimental neuropathy. Neurosci Lett 1997;237(1):45–48.

151. Sorkin LS, Xiao WH, Wagner R, et al. Tumour necrosis factor-alpha induces ectopic activity in nociceptive primary afferent fibres. Neuroscience 1997;81(1):255–262.

152. Shubayev VI, Myers RR. Upregulation and interaction of TNF alpha and gelatinases A and B in painful peripheral nerve injury. Brain Res 2000;855(1):83–89.

153. Shubayev VI, Myers RR. Axonal transport of TNF-alpha in painful neuropathy: distribution of ligand tracer and TNF receptors. J Neuroimmunol 2001;114(1–2):48–56.

154. Olmarker K, Rydevik B. Selective inhibition of tumor necrosis factor-alpha prevents nucleus pulposus–induced thrombus formation, intraneural edema, and reduction of nerve conduction velocity: possible implications for future pharmacologic treatment strategies of sciatica. Spine 2001;26(8):863–869.

155. Aoki Y, Rydevik B, Kikuchi S, et al. Local application of disc-related cytokines on spinal nerve roots. Spine 2002;27(15):1614–1617.

156. Ozaktay AC, Cavanaugh JM, Asik I, et al. Dorsal root sensitivity to interleukin-1 beta, interleukin-6 and tumor necrosis factor in rats. Eur Spine J 2002;11(5):467–475.

157. Onda A, Yabuki S, Kikuchi S. Effects of neutralizing antibodies to tumor necrosis factor-alpha on nucleus pulposus–induced abnormal nociresponses in rat dorsal horn neurons. Spine 2003;28(10):967–972.

158. Wagner R, Janjigian M, Myers RR. Anti-inflammatory interleukin-10 therapy in CCI neuropathy decreases thermal hyperalgesia, macrophage recruitment, and endoneurial TNF-alpha expression. Pain 1998;74(1):35–42.

159. Wehling P, Cleveland SJ, Heininger K, et al. Neurophysiologic changes in lumbar nerve root inflammation in the rat after treatment with cytokine inhibitors. Evidence for a role of interleukin-1. Spine 1996;21(8):931–935.

160. Brisby H, Olmarker K, Rosengren L, et al. Markers of nerve tissue injury in the cerebrospinal fluid in patients with lumbar disc herniation and sciatica. Spine 1999;24(8):742–746.

161. Mattila P, Majuri ML, Mattila PS, et al. TNF alpha-induced expression of endothelial adhesion molecules, ICAM-1 and VCAM-1, is linked to protein kinase C activation. Scand J Immunol 1992;36(2): 159–165.

162. Pober JS. Effects of tumour necrosis factor and related cytokines on vascular endothelial cells. Ciba Found Symp 1987;131:170–184.

163. Creange A, Barlovatz-Meimon G, Gherardi RK. Cytokines and peripheral nerve disorders. Eur Cytokine Network 1997;8(2):145–151.

164. Munro JM, Pober JS, Cotran RS. Tumor necrosis factor and interferon-gamma induce distinct patterns of endothelial activation and associated leukocyte accumulation in skin of Papio anubis. Am J Pathol 1989;135(1):121–133.

165. Oku N, Araki R, Araki H, et al. Tumor necrosis factor-induced permeability increase of negatively charged phospholipid vesicles. J Biochem (Tokyo) 1987;102(5):1303–1310.

166. Kagan BL, Baldwin RL, Munoz D, et al. Formation of ion-permeable channels by tumor necrosis factor-alpha. Science 1992;255(5050): 1427–1430.

167. Baldwin RL, Stolowitz ML, Hood L, et al. Structural changes of tumor necrosis factor alpha associated with membrane insertion and channel formation. Proc Natl Acad Sci USA 1996;93(3):1021–1026.

168. Wei Y, Babilonia E, Pedraza PL, et al. Acute application of TNF stimulates apical 70-pS K+ channels in the thick ascending limb of rat kidney. Am J Physiol Renal Physiol 2003;285(3):F491–F497.

169. Woolf CJ. The pathophysiology of peripheral neuropathic pain—abnormal peripheral input and abnormal central processing. Acta Neurochir Suppl (Wien) 1993;58:125–130.

170. Attal N, Bouhassira D. Mechanisms of pain in peripheral neuropathy. Acta Neurol Scand Suppl 1999;173:12–24; discussion 48–52.

171. Zimmermann M. Pathobiology of neuropathic pain. Eur J Pharmacol 2001;429(1–3):23–37.

172. Wall PD. Neuropathic pain and injured nerve: central mechanisms. Br Med Bull 1991;47(3):631–643.

173. Selmaj K, Raine CS, Cross AH. Anti-tumor necrosis factor therapy abrogates autoimmune demyelination. Ann Neurol 1991;30(5):694–700.

174. Selmaj KW, Raine CS. Tumor necrosis factor mediates myelin and oligodendrocyte damage in vitro. Ann Neurol 1988;23(4):339–346.

175. Villarroya H, Violleau K, Ben Younes-Chennoufi A, et al. Myelin-induced experimental allergic encephalomyelitis in Lewis rats: tumor necrosis factor alpha levels in serum and cerebrospinal fluid immunohistochemical expression in glial cells and macrophages of optic nerve and spinal cord. J Neuroimmunol 1996;64(1):55–61.

176. Ghabriel MN, Allt G. Schmidt-Lanterman incisures. I. A quantitative teased fibre study of remyelinating peripheral nerve fibres. Acta Neuropathol (Berlin) 1980;52(2):85–95

177. Shanklin WM, Azzam NA. Histological and histochemical studies on the incisures of Schmidt-Lanterman. J Comp Neurol 1964;123:5–10.

178. Robertson JD. The ultrastructure of Schmidt-Lanterman clefts and related shearing defects of the myelin sheath. J Biophys Biochem Cytol 1958;4(1):39–46.

179. Todd BA, Inman C, Sedgwick EM, et al. Ionic permeability of the frog sciatic nerve perineurium: parallel studies of potassium and lanthanum penetration using electrophysiological and electron microscopic techniques. J Neurocytol 2000;29(8):551–567.

180. Schafers M, Sorkin LS, Geis C, et al. Spinal nerve ligation induces transient upregulation of tumor necrosis factor receptors 1 and 2 in injured and adjacent uninjured dorsal root ganglia in the rat. Neurosci Lett 2003;347(3):179–182.

181. Schafers M, Lee DH, Brors D, et al. Increased sensitivity of injured and adjacent uninjured rat primary sensory neurons to exogenous tumor necrosis factor-alpha after spinal nerve ligation. J Neurosci 2003;23(7):3028–3038.

182. Schafers M, Svensson CI, Sommer C, et al. Tumor necrosis factor-alpha induces mechanical allodynia after spinal nerve ligation by acti-

vation of p38 MAPK in primary sensory neurons. J Neurosci 2003;23 (7):2517–2521.

183. Winkelstein BA, Rutkowski MD, Sweitzer SM, et al. Nerve injury proximal or distal to the DRG induces similar spinal glial activation and selective cytokine expression but differential behavioral responses to pharmacologic treatment. J Comp Neurol 2001;439(2):127–139.

184. Raghavendra V, Rutkowski MD, DeLeo JA. The role of spinal neuroimmune activation in morphine tolerance/hyperalgesia in neuropathic and sham-operated rats. J Neurosci 2002;22(22):9980–9989.

185. DeLeo JA, Rutkowski MD, Stalder AK, et al. Transgenic expression of TNF by astrocytes increases mechanical allodynia in a mouse neuropathy model. Neuroreport 2000;11(3):599–602.

186. Spillert CR, Sun S, Ponnudurai R, et al. Tumor necrosis factor-induced necrosis: a monocyte-mediated hypercoagulable effect. J Natl Med Assoc 1995;87(7):508–509.

187. Aderka D. Role of tumor necrosis factor in the pathogenesis of intravascular coagulopathy of sepsis: potential new therapeutic implications. Isr J Med Sci 1991;27(1):52–60.

188. Karppinen J, Korhonen T, Malmivaara A, et al. Tumor necrosis factor-alpha monoclonal antibody, infliximab, used to manage severe sciatica. Spine 2003;28(8):750–753.

189. Genevay S, Stingelin S, Gabay C. Efficacy of etanercept in the treatment of acute sciatica. In: European league against rheumatism. Rheumatology Sept. 16, 2003.

190. Cooper RG, Freemont AJ. TNF-alpha blockade for herniated inter-vertebral disc-induced sciatica: a way forward at last? Rheumatology Sept. 16, 2003.

191. Olmarker K, Størkson R, Berge O-G. Pathogenesis of sciatic pain: a study of spontaneous behavior in rats exposed to experimental disc herniation. Spine 2002;27(12):1312–1317.

192. Palmgren T, Gronblad M, Virri J, et al. An immunohistochemical study of nerve structures in the anulus fibrosus of human normal lumbar intervertebral discs. Spine 1999;24(20):2075–2079.

193. Cavanaugh JM, Kallakuri S, Ozaktay AC. Innervation of the rabbit lumbar intervertebral disc and posterior longitudinal ligament. Spine 1995;20(19):2080–2085.

194. Kojima Y, Maeda T, Arai R, et al. Nerve supply to the posterior longitudinal ligament and the intervertebral disc of the rat vertebral column as studied by acetylcholinesterase histochemistry. I. Distribution in the lumbar region. J Anat 1990;169:237–246.

195. McCarthy PW, Carruthers B, Martin D, et al. Immunohistochemical demonstration of sensory nerve fibers and endings in lumbar intervertebral discs of the rat. Spine 1991;16(6):653–655.

196. Takebayashi T, Cavanaugh JM, Yamashita T, et al. Characteristics of sympathetic afferent units from the lower lumbar disc. Edinburgh: Trans. International Society for the Study of the Lumbar Spine, 2001.

197. Andersson GBJ. Intervertebral disc herniation: Epidemiology and natural history. In: Weinstein JL, eds. Low back pain. A scientific and clinical overview. Rosemont, IL: American Academy of Orthopaedic Surgeons; 1995:7–21.

CHAPTER 3

Biomechanical Considerations of Disc Degeneration

Allison M. Kaigle Holm and Sten H. Holm

Mobility and stability of the spine are governed by a complex neuromusculoskeletal system. Panjabi (1) eloquently described the spinal stabilizing system as three subsystems (Fig. 3-1): *passive* (disc, ligament, bone, and passive muscle), *active* (tendons and active muscle), and *neural* (the nervous system and neural components within the passive and active structures). The biomechanical characteristics of the lumbar spine are dependent upon the integrity of all three subsystems. Under normal conditions, the musculoskeletal structures interact in a highly coordinated and optimized fashion via neural networks, to produce the desired movements and achieve the requirements for stability. However, injury or degenerative processes disrupt the intricate balance, and cause a transfer in unfavorable loads onto other spinal structures. This often leads to pain or dysfunction. With regard to the intervertebral disc, degenerative processes are believed to alter the disc's mechanical properties as well as the surrounding structures. This underlying belief has fueled an extensive amount of research aimed at elucidating the biomechanical consequences of disc degeneration.

STRUCTURE AND FUNCTION

It is important to have some basic knowledge of the individual structures of the lumbar spine, as well as their functions and interactive processes, in order to understand how disturbances to a single structure can adversely affect secondary structures, and ultimately the spinal system as a whole. Many examples of this can be found in the literature. Disc degeneration transmits unfavorable stresses onto other spinal structures, particularly the facet joints. A radiographic study by Butler et al. (2) found that disc degeneration caused secondary osteoarthritic changes in the facet joints, most likely due to a shift in the mechanical loading. Using a sheep model, facet joint arthrosis has been shown

to occur in response to experimentally induced disc degeneration (3). Substantial bone remodeling in vertebrae adjacent to intervertebral discs that sustained lesions of the annulus has also been observed (4). Changes in muscle fiber type of the multifidus and erector spinae muscles (5–7), and structural changes in the connective tissue of the multifidus (8) have been reported clinically in patients with lumbar disc herniation.

The intervertebral disc is a deformable connective structure, with a very low capacity for remodeling and repair due to its avascularity in the mature state. This makes it particularly vulnerable to fatigue failure. A turgescent central nucleus pulposus exists in the healthy state; it is designed to sustain and transmit pressure while surrounded by an annulus fibrosus, a highly organized arrangement of collagen fiber layers that can resist movements in all directions due to the fibers' alternating oblique orientation. Due to the arrangement of the annulus fibers and regardless of the type of loading, the disc annulus, partly or in whole, is subjected to tensile stresses. The three major constituents of the intervertebral disc are water, collagen, and proteoglycans. Their proportions vary radially within the disc, as well as with aging and degeneration (9,10). The outer annulus has the highest collagen content and the lowest water and proteoglycan contents, whereas the nucleus has high water and proteoglycan contents and low collagen content (11). The biomechanical properties of the intervertebral disc depend largely on the tissue's hydration. The collagen fibrils provide the tensile strength of the intervertebral disc. The turgid action of the water-binding proteoglycans surrounded by the collagenous framework provides the load-bearing capacity (12). The principal functions of the intervertebral disc are to allow joint mobility and transfer axial loads between the vertebrae. Together with the vertebrae, the disc resists approximately 80% of the compressive force acting on the spine in the upright standing

ACTIVE STRUCTURES : **PASSIVE STRUCTURES**

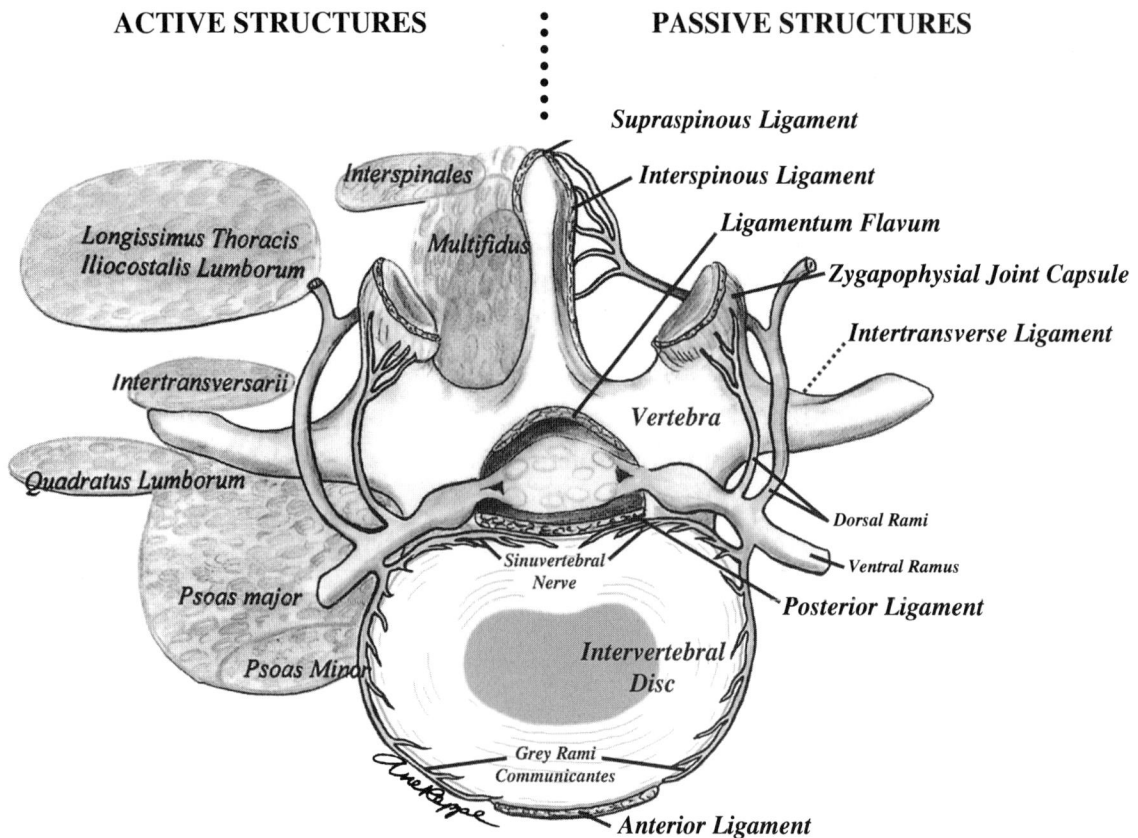

FIG. 3-1. Schematic of the bilateral active and passive structural arrangement and sensory innervation on the L3-L4 level.

posture (13). The intervertebral disc allows rotations (flexion-extension, lateral bending, and axial) between the vertebrae, as well as translational movements caused by compressive or shear forces.

A cartilaginous end plate, which joins the vertebral body and intervertebral disc, provides a nutritional pathway to the avascular intervertebral disc. The end plates deflect when sufficient axial loads are transferred between the intervertebral disc and vertebral body. Disruption in the nutritional pathways through the end plate is believed to be a key mechanism for disc degeneration (14).

The zygapophysial joints, or commonly called facet joints, are synovial joints formed between the superior and inferior articular processes of adjacent vertebrae. These cartilage-covered articulating processes or facets, along with the fibrous capsule that encloses the joint, provide a locking mechanism that can resist shear translation and axial rotation between the vertebrae. Bony impact, as well as tension of the joint capsule, play major roles in providing passive stability during bending of the lumbar spine. According to Adams and Hutton (15), the facet joints normally bear approximately 20% of the spinal compressive force, but if there is a loss in disc height due to degenerative changes, load bearing can be as high as 70%. In a lumbar motion segment, the intervertebral disc provides approximately 40% to 50% torque strength, while the

remaining strength is attributed to the posterior elements and the interspinous ligaments (16).

The ligaments of the lumbar spine provide passive tensile resistance to external loads. The amount of stability provided by a particular ligament depends not only on its strength, but also on its architectural arrangement and the loading circumstances. Ligaments are most effective in resisting loads along the same direction of their fibers. With disc degeneration, narrowing of the disc space can reduce the ligamentous tension, and thus decrease its effectiveness in providing passive translatory or rotatory stability.

Devoid of the muscles, the osseoligamentous spine is inherently unstable at low loads (approximately 90 N) (1,17). Therefore, the neuromuscular system must fulfill the supplementary and adaptive role of maintaining postural stability *in vivo*. Disturbances in the precise motor control strategies, particularly those of repetitive nature, may have detrimental effects on the lumbar spinal structures (e.g., cause pain or dysfunction). The lumbar spine is directly influenced by a number of bilateral muscles, both intersegmental and polysegmental, acting in a well-coordinated manner in order to balance the actions of gravity or execute controlled movements, as well as provide passive elastic tension. The muscles not only produce movements, but also generate compressive and shear forces that contribute to the high internal forces to which the lumbar spine is subjected. The complex recruitment patterns of the lumbar musculature are not well established. However, biomechanical and neurophysiologic evidence suggests that the deep intrinsic muscles are recruited to control motions at the intervertebral level, whereas the long multisegmental muscles may be involved in a more "global" control of the overall spinal orientation (18–20).

The innervation pattens of the active and passive structures of the lumbar spine have, for the most part, been determined. The load-sensitive nerve endings, or mechanoreceptors, found in muscle (muscle spindles) and tendon (Golgi tendon organs), provide proprioceptive information regarding tension levels, essential for controlling muscle tone. Although the presence of nerve endings in the passive structures has been well documented (21–28), their role has not been clearly established. Regarding the articular structures, the outer annulus of the intervertebral disc and the capsules of the facet joints contain both free nerve endings and mechanoreceptors. These structures act as proprioceptive transducers for monitoring the position and movements of the motion segment. The neurologic feedback from these passive structures provides sensory information needed to regulate muscle tension, and hence the mobility and stability of the lumbar spine. In addition to a regulatory function, the presence of a nerve supply in the articular structures makes these structures potential sources of pain (22).

BIOCHEMICAL AND STRUCTURAL CHANGES ASSOCIATED WITH DISC DEGENERATION

Disc degeneration is the deterioration and remodeling of the physical and chemical properties of the tissue—whole or in part—with retrogressive pathologic changes in the cells or macromolecules (14). The changes observed in degenerated discs are similar to those found in normal aging (29,30), but they are more pronounced with disc degeneration, may occur earlier in life and with more severe changes, and are often associated with clinical symptoms (31).

The principal biochemical sign of disc degeneration and aging is the loss in proteoglycans and hence loss of water, particularly in the nucleus (11,30,32,33). Cells in the nucleus change their shape and begin to synthesize collagen types not found in normal intervertebral discs (34). Structurally, the nucleus pulposus becomes progressively more fibrous and opaque, with increased pigmentation (34–37). The demarcation between the annulus-nucleus boundary becomes less distinct and delamination of the mid-to-outer annulus occurs, particularly in the anterior annulus (38,39) (Fig. 3-2). Delamination is believed to be a precursor stage for the development of concentric tears in the annulus fibrosus (40). Abnormalities can be found in the ultrastructural features of the collagen fibrils of the annulus fibrous (e.g., widened fibrils or irregular fibril cross-sectional diameters) (41). Radial fissures and cracks

in the annulus fibrosus can form cavities within the disc (42). There can be inward buckling of the inner annulus as well as increased radial bulging of the annulus (43,44). Radiographically identifiable pathology associated with disc degeneration includes disc space narrowing, osteophyte formation around the margins of the vertebral bodies, and sclerosis of the vertebral end plates (45,46).

For describing the degree of degeneration according to morphologically observed changes, Nachemson (47) created an integer grading scale ranging from 0 (no macroscopic signs of degeneration) to 4 (severely degenerated). This grading scheme or versions similar to it are commonly referred to when classifying the degeneration status of specimens used in biomechanical studies. Kirkaldy-Willis (48) described the process of degeneration as having three sequential phases: (a) an early phase of dysfunction, where the motion segment does not function normally but the pathologic changes are minimal (grade 1); (b) instability, an intermediate phase where there is increased joint laxity which may be exemplified as abnormal segmental motion (grade 2); and (c) the restabilization phase characterized by fibrosis in the posterior joints and osteophyte formations, which lead to decreased segmental motion (grades 3 and 4).

MECHANICAL FACTORS AS POSSIBLE PATHOMECHANISMS OF DISC DEGENERATION

There are several theories about the possible pathomechanisms of disc degeneration. Mechanical, chemical, age-related, autoimmune, hereditary, and genetic factors have all been implicated (49). Considerable attention has focused on trying to understand the etiologic role mechanical loading plays in disc degeneration. This partially stems from the fact that back pain is the leading cause of disability among the working population (50). There is an underlying belief that pathology leading to back symptoms can result from mechanical factors that damage spinal structures (51–53). Farfan et al. (16), for example, postulated that intervertebral disc degeneration results from imposed torsional strains that cause impairment in the function of the facet joints. Although there is no clear dose-response relation between occupational loading exposure and degenerative findings, physical workload has been found to predict spinal injury in truck drivers (54). Suspected occupational risk factors for back pain include the following physical demands: heavy physical loading; materials handling including lifting, bending, twisting, pulling or pushing; prolonged static postures; and whole body vibration (52,55–57). However, there are discrepancies in the literature regarding which physical factors are associated with an increased prevalence of low back pain. Marras et al. (58) assessed the contribution of dynamic trunk motions to the risk for low

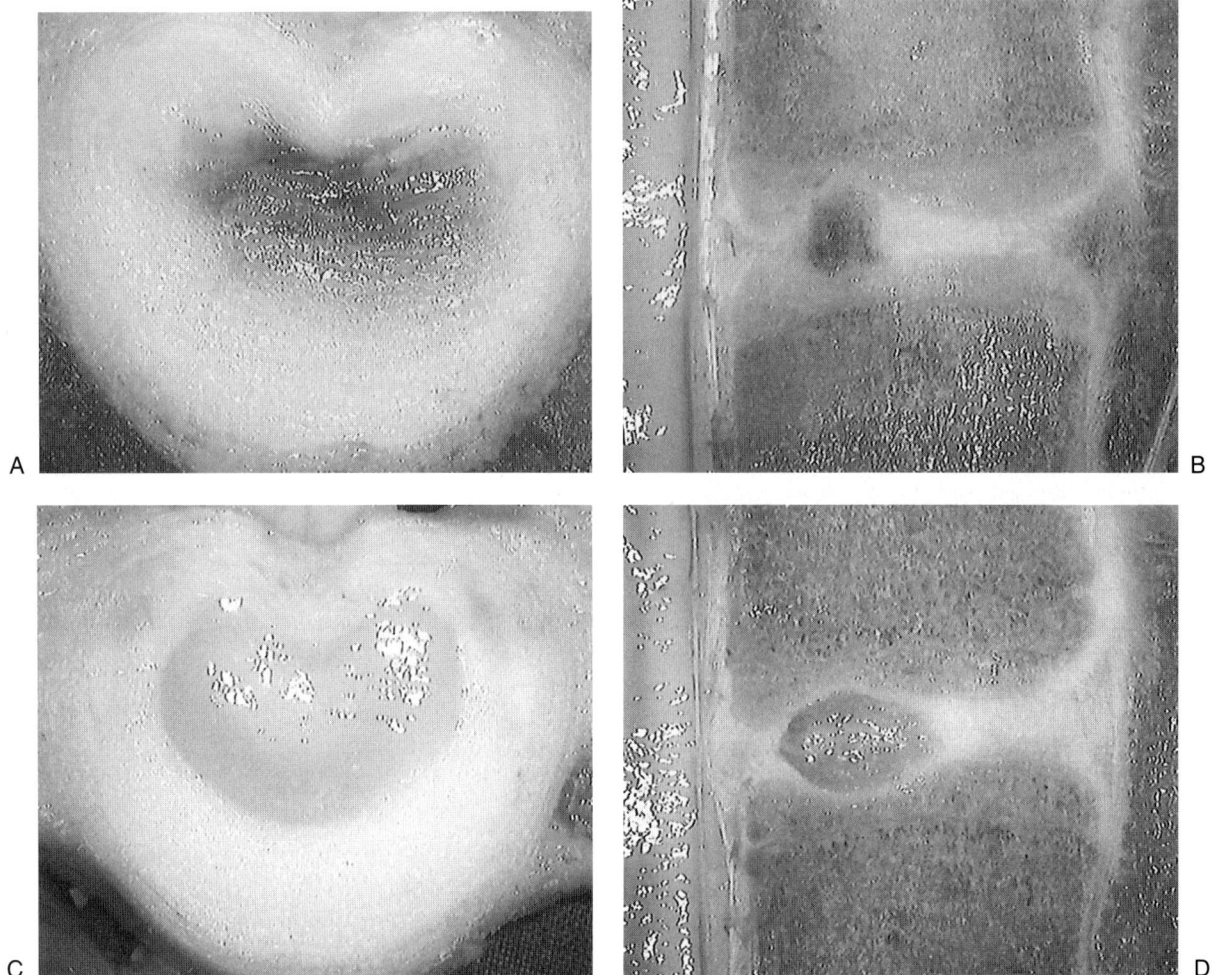

FIG. 3-2. Comparative photographs of cross-sectional and sagittal views of a degenerated disc **(A, B)** and the adjacent disc **(C, D)** from an experimental model (end-plate injury) of disc degeneration, showing gross morphologic changes in both the annulus and nucleus structures. (From Kawchuk GN, Kaigle AM, Holm SH, et al. The diagnostic performance of vertebral displacement measurements derived from ultrasonic indentation in an *in vivo* model of degenerative disc disease. Spine 2001;26:1348–1355, with permission.)

back disorders during occupational lifting in industry. An increase in the magnitude of the following workplace factors significantly increased the risk for low back disorders: lifting frequently, load movement, trunk lateral velocity, trunk twisting velocity, and trunk sagittal angle.

There is evidence to suggest that occupational exposures have an effect on disc degeneration, specifically with regard to lumbar disc degeneration; however, the contribution of such risk factors appears to be modest, particularly when compared to familial influences (52). A critical review of the literature was recently made by Hansson and Westerholm (59) to assess whether or not existing scientific evidence substantiates relationships between low back problems and the following different physical work exposures: patient handling and care, lifting of patients, materials handling, heavy physical work, heavy lifting, bent or twisted work positions, standing or walking, prolonged sitting, and exposure to whole body vibration. The review revealed that

there is strong evidence of an association between an increased occurrence of low back problems and frequent heavy lifting (greater than 15 kg) and twisted or bent working positions, whereas frequent lifting of less than 10 kg shows a strong negative association. Moderate evidence supports an association between whole body vibration and an increased occurrence of low back problems. Limited evidence yields an association between patient handling and care, patient lifting, and heavy physical work and an increased occurrence of low back problems. There is currently insufficient evidence for an association between low back pain and standing, walking, or prolonged sitting.

Loading effects on the lumbar spine during physically demanding tasks are not only dependent on the load magnitude, but also the loading rate and history (60,61). This is partly because the intervertebral disc and ligaments are viscoelastic structures. The viscoelastic behavior has been well documented for the intervertebral disc, both normal and degenerated (62–70). The outflow of tissue fluid and the stretching of the collagen fibers of the annulus fibrosus under loading cause approximately a 20% reduction in the height and volume of the disc (71). Intradiscal pressure has also been shown to decrease with creep loading (72). Such reductions make the tissue more elastic (73), less resistant to bending (60) and shear loading (74), and causes greater axial loading on the facet joints (75). When loading is removed, the disc imbibes fluid and recovers from the deformation, although complete recovery requires a considerable amount of time. With repetitive physical tasks, even at relatively low physiologic loads, the spinal structures may suffer from fatigue. Mechanical fatiguing can make the disc, as well as other viscoelastic spinal structures (e.g., ligaments, tendons, and fascia) more vulnerable to microdamage. Considering the very low repair capacity of the mature intervertebral disc, accumulative structural damage is believed to be an underlying cause of disc degeneration and low back pain (76).

Trying to establish cause and effect in disc degeneration is extremely difficult. In a degenerated disc, structural disruption is accompanied by cell-mediated changes in composition. It is not clear as to whether progressive biochemical changes in the disc alter its structural integrity, or whether mechanical disturbances precipitate biochemical changes in disc cell metabolism (77). Adams and Dolan (76) described how structural failure may cause biologic degeneration of tissues by a number of mechanisms: by altering the mechanical environment of the cells, by interfering with metabolite transport to and from the cells, or by breaking down barriers and allowing an inflammatory or even autoimmune reaction to occur. Biochemical observations by Pearce et al. (78) support the hypothesis that low proteoglycan concentrations in all the discs of a spine precede degeneration.

EXPERIMENTAL MODELS OF DISC DEGENERATION

In order to perform controlled investigations of the etiology and progression of disc degeneration, animal models are often used. Experimental models have the advantage of allowing standardized evaluations of biomechanical, histochemical, and morphologic phenomena of the degenerative process, directly from initiation of the process. There are several different ways in which experimental disc degeneration can be induced in vivo, either chemically or mechanically. Injection of a matrix-degrading enzyme (e.g., chymopapain), into the disc can produce degenerative changes (79). A number of investigators have mechanically produced degeneration in vivo in rat and mice tail discs chronically loaded with an external compression device (80–82). Disc degeneration as a result of torsional injuries has been demonstrated in vivo in rabbit models (83,84). A scalpel stab incision into the annulus fibrosus, with or without penetration into the nucleus pulposus (Fig. 3-3), is a technique that has frequently been used to mechanically induce disc degenera-

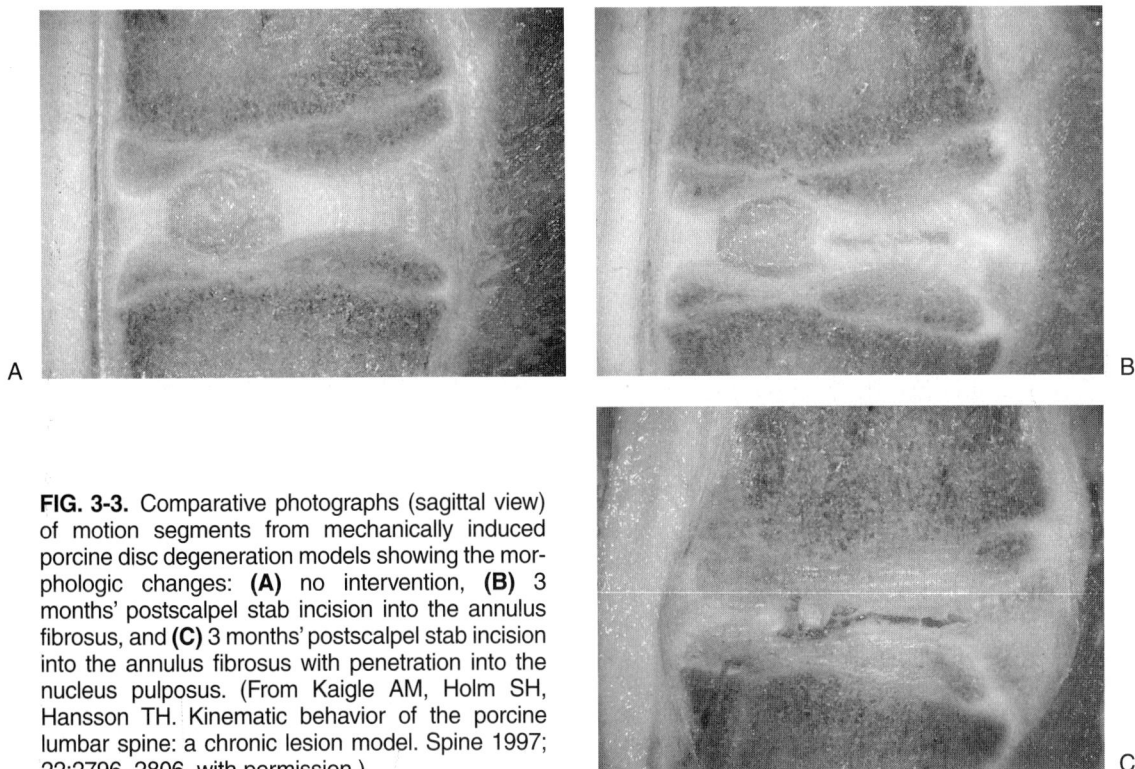

FIG. 3-3. Comparative photographs (sagittal view) of motion segments from mechanically induced porcine disc degeneration models showing the morphologic changes: (A) no intervention, (B) 3 months' postscalpel stab incision into the annulus fibrosus, and (C) 3 months' postscalpel stab incision into the annulus fibrosus with penetration into the nucleus pulposus. (From Kaigle AM, Holm SH, Hansson TH. Kinematic behavior of the porcine lumbar spine: a chronic lesion model. Spine 1997; 22:2796–2806, with permission.)

tion (85–94). In rabbit, sheep and pig, this model has been shown to cause progressive degeneration which biochemically and structurally resembles that in human disc degeneration. A new injury model, involving penetration of the end plate via the vertebral body, has been shown to produce symmetrically widespread degenerative changes in the disc that resemble human disc degeneration (i.e., declines in concentrations of water, cells, and proteoglycans as well as intradiscal pressure) (38). This is a model in which the severity of the degenerative changes can vary according to the penetration diameter or depth (38,95). Loss in hydrostatic pressure in the nucleus and disruption of nutritional pathways through the end plate are believed to be two key mechanisms behind this model of disc degeneration. Deficient metabolite transport has been linked with degenerative changes (96). This model mimics human degeneration caused by end-plate fractures or nucleus herniation through the end plate.

BIOMECHANICAL CONSEQUENCES OF DISC DEGENERATION

In everyday life, the structures of the lumbar spine are continuously subjected to pure as well as combined physiologic loads (e.g., compressive, tensile, shear, torsional, and combinations thereof). Disc degeneration affects both the geometry and material properties of the motion segment. While geometric changes can be expected to decrease flexibility, changes in material properties may cause the opposite response. The extent to which each of these factors affects the spinal behavior is also dependent on the direction of loading. For these reasons, along with the fact that the intervertebral disc is an anisotropic structure, it is necessary to perform biomechanical testing which includes both simple and complex loading modes.

For several decades, numerous studies have been performed in order to assess how the biomechanical properties of the lumbar spine are affected by intervertebral disc degeneration. Accurate knowledge of the intervertebral disc's biomechanical properties in healthy, injured, or diseased states is essential for performing valid mathematical analyses of the intervertebral disc, for refining injury (failure) criteria, and for developing artificial disc replacements, as a few examples. Studies have used various methodologies in order to quantify the physical properties—elastic and viscoelastic—as well as the kinematic behavior. Since the degenerative status can be determined, the majority of studies of intervertebral disc degeneration are conducted using cadaveric material (isolated discs, motion segments, or whole lumbar spines) or *in vivo* animal models. Methodologies for performing such analyses have primarily employed servohydraulic-type material testing devices or used similar techniques that can measure the load-displacement behavior.

Elastic Behavior

With regard to biomechanical testing, axial compression has been a popular test mode for studying the intervertebral disc, perhaps due to physiologic as well as practical considerations; namely that the disc is a major compression-carrying structure in the spine (97) and that compression testing is a relatively straightforward experimental test mode that can provide considerable information about the disc's physical properties. Early biomechanical studies from the 1950s by Brown et al. (98) and Hirsch et al. (99–101) described the nonlinear mechanical characteristics of *in vitro* lumbar motion segments under axial compression, as well as other test conditions. Studies such as these were motivated by the fact that disc degeneration was viewed as a possible pathologic anatomical explanation for low back pain, and although no pain mechanisms were identifiable at the time, the importance of mechanical factors was strongly recognized. Hirsch and Nachemson (101) demonstrated differences in the mechanical behavior between cadaveric motion segments with normal and degenerated discs, noting that for the same applied axial load, degenerated discs deformed more easily than healthy discs, particularly at higher loads. Nachemson et al. (102) reported differences in stiffness between less degenerated discs [grades 0 to 2 on a total 5-point scale of 0 (normal) to 4] and grossly degenerated discs (grades 3 and 4) that were dependent on the loading configuration. In axial compression, less degenerated discs were stiffer than grossly degenerated discs. However, in flexion and extension modes, more degenerated discs were found to be less flexible, while in lateral bending and torsion, there were no significant differences. Fibrosis in the posterior joints of the grossly degenerated discs may explain the observed increase in stiffness in the flexion and extension loading modes observed in the degenerated discs. Keller et al. (68) also reported a decrease in axial compressive stiffness with increasing grades of degeneration [1 to 3 on a total 4-point scale of 1 (normal) to 4]. In a recent *in vitro* study, Brown et al. (103) examined lumbar motion segment stiffness under flexion-traction loading. A nonlinear trend, which coincided with the degenerative process described by Kirkaldy-Willis (48), dysfunction-instability-restabilization, was observed between motion segment stiffness and degeneration grade; reduced stiffness was found in discs with early stages of degeneration whereas discs with more severe degenerative changes showed a tendency toward increased stiffness.

Viscoelastic Behavior

Using static and dynamic axial compression test modes, it has been shown that degeneration alters the viscoelastic (time-dependent) behavior of the intervertebral disc. Virgin (70) was the first to demonstrate that the hysteresis behavior was greater in discs that showed actual signs of degeneration than in middle-aged or older discs that did not show any degenerative signs. This means that, in the degenerate state, there is greater energy loss during loading-unloading cycles, which can be of considerable importance with regard to repetitive axial vibration. Koeller et al. (69) studied the effects of age and degeneration on the creep response of the intervertebral disc under dynamic axial compression. From the middle of the third to the beginning of the sixth decade, only slight alterations in the biomechanical properties were found, whereas later in life, where there was a greater occurrence of disc degeneration, increased creep was observed in the lumbar spine. Kazarian (65) performed static axial compression tests on older cadaveric lumbar motion segments with various degrees of degeneration. The creep behavior was found to correlate with the degree of degeneration; the degenerate discs exhibited greater initial deformation and approached equilibrium at a more rapid rate compared with the nondegenerate discs. Similar behavior has been confirmed by Keller et al. (68).

Internal Disc Mechanics

With the intervertebral disc being an inhomogeneous structure, there are regional material property differences, particularly in the annulus fibrosus, which reflect the variations in structural and biochemical composition. Such regional properties will affect the manner in which the intervertebral disc responds to loading and must be taken into consideration when performing analytical representations. Brown et al. (98) were perhaps the first group to map the regional tensile strengths of the intervertebral disc. Rectangular vertebra-disc-vertebra sections from different locations of the disc were axially stretched to failure. In this normal material, the strongest areas were found to be in the anterior and posterior portions of the disc, while the central portion was the weakest.

More recent studies of the radial and circumferential variations in the tensile properties of nondegenerate lumbar disc specimens have reported that, when loaded along the plane of the lamella, the anterior annulus is stiffer and stronger than the posterolateral regions, and the outer annulus is stiffer and stronger than the inner regions (10,104). Ebara et al. (104) speculated as to how load distribution would benefit from a lower tensile modulus in the inner annulus fibrosus. They stated that the lower values for the tensile modulus and the larger values for strain suggest that the inner annulus fibrosus is likely to be more deformable, and thus be more successful at distributing applied loads in a uniform manner across the inner annulus fibrosus, as compared to the more restrictive outer annulus. Therefore, the more deformable inner annulus fibrosus may provide for significant energy dissipation within the tissue. Acaroglu et al. (105), using

multiple-layer annulus specimens, evaluated the effects of aging and degeneration on the regional tensile properties when loaded along the plane of the lamellae. Degeneration was found to be accompanied by significant decreases in the failure properties (i.e., failure stress and strain energy density), indicating that degenerated annulus fibrosus will fail at lower stresses and require less energy to fail. Also, a significant decrease in the Poisson ratio, which is a ratio of the transverse and axial strains in the tissue, was found. This indicates structural changes in the annulus lamellae, which will affect the internal stresses in the disc and thus the overall manner in which the disc bears loads. Fujita et al. (106) studied *in vitro* the radial tensile properties of normal and degenerated lumbar annulus fibrosus, when loading perpendicular to the plane of the lamellae. The radial tensile behavior of the annulus was highly nonlinear and showed region-dependent behavior that was likely due to radial variations in interlaminar weaving. Compared to specimens from both the inner and outer annulus of normal discs, specimens from the middle layers were stiffer and failed at smaller strain magnitudes with radial tensile loading. Differences due to degeneration were noted; moderately degenerated discs showed a 30% decrease in yield and ultimate stress compared with normal discs.

Umehara et al. (107) studied variations in the disc's axial compressive properties as a function of location in the disc and degeneration. Using an indentation technique on whole disc specimens, the axial compressive elastic modulus was assessed in lumbar discs with various degrees of degeneration. In normal discs, the elastic moduli were lowest in the nucleus as well as the lateral portions of the annulus, whereas the values were significantly greater in the posterior and anterior annulus, being greatest in the anterior portion. This normal distribution pattern, which correlated with the distributions of tensile strengths reported in earlier studies, was affected by disc degeneration. In normal discs, the distribution was symmetrical about the midsagittal plane, whereas the more severely degenerated discs showed asymmetrical and irregular profiles and higher nucleus moduli. In the slightly degenerated discs, the lowest values of the elastic moduli were found in the posterolateral portions of the disc, which is also the region where disc disruption is clinically found to occur most frequently (108). Farfan et al. (16) found that the location of maximum stress under torsional loading was at the posterolateral angles of the intervertebral disc, again coinciding with the common site of clinical disc protrusion.

Annular lesions of the radial, circumferential, or rim-lesion type compromise the disc's internal mechanical integrity. Such lesions appear to evolve independent of age or each other (40), and may be the result of fatigue failure or part of a degeneration process. A study has examined how the type and severity of such lesions in lumbar intervertebral discs alter the biomechanical properties (109). Flexion-extension stiffness increased with greater tear severity, which was believed to be partly due to the accompanied loss in disc height. Increasing severity of circumferential tears and rim lesions correlated with decreasing joint axial torsional stiffness. With a circumferential tear, interlamellar bonding is absent in a portion of the annulus; thus the disc's ability to transfer shear forces induced by torsional loading is reduced. It has been suggested that interlaminar separation and matrix failure between the lamellae might be a more clinically relevant injury mechanism than tensile failure of the collagen fibers within a lamella (106). It is believed that with loss of cohesion between the annulus lamellae, other structures of the motion segment, particularly the facet joints, have to provide a greater portion of torsional resistance, and that this could play a major role in early degenerative changes (16). With a rim lesion, there is a defect in the annulus attachment close to the bone of the vertebral rim, which compromises the transferring of torsional loads across the motion segment. Thompson et al. (109) reported that radial tears showed little or no effect on the axial torsional stiffness. Schmidt et al. (110) compared the stiffness (flexion-extension, axial rotation, lateral bending) in cadaveric motion segments with and without high intensity zones (i.e., radial tears, in the annulus fibrosus viewed on magnetic resonance images). In this study, the presence of a radial tear was associated with a significant reduction in stiffness in the motion segment in axial rotation.

A direct means for measuring loading on the spine is with intradiscal pressure measurement techniques. In a healthy disc, the pressurized gelatinous nucleus pulposus acts as a hydraulic cushion that generates tensile stresses in the annulus, permitting applied loads and pressures to be evenly distributed over multiple spinal segments. The lamellae of the annulus fibrosus are believed to primarily bulge radially outward due to the hydrostatic pressure in the nucleus. However, with aging and degenerative processes, the reduction in water content and increased fibrosis in the nucleus result in reduced hydrostatic behavior, and there are structural disruptions in the annulus lamellae and end-plate regions. In degenerated discs, there have been reported observations of inward bulging of the inner lamellae (43,44,77), and that such bulging is associated with pressure loss in the nucleus (81). Under loading, such changes alter the internal disc mechanics, producing high stress concentrations that may cause pain or even further disc disruption. Since the nucleus of a severely degenerated disc does not always exhibit hydrostatic behavior, discometric studies of such material must be interpreted with caution.

In a number of pioneering *in vivo* human studies, Nachemson et al. (111–116) measured intradiscal pressure in lumbar intervertebral discs during various activities. From these and the later studies by Andersson et al. (117,118) and Schultz et al. (119), intradiscal pressure measurements, electromyographic data, and biomechanical modeling have altogether provided vital information that has been used to establish workplace recommendations as well as clinical treatment strategies for disc diseases. Recent *in vivo* investigation (120,121) using modern pressure transducer technology has substantiated the findings of the intradiscal pressure studies from the 1960s and 1970s. In a healthy male volunteer, Wilke et al. (121) measured the intradiscal pressure in the L4-L5 disc and found good correlation with Nachemson's data, with two exceptions. First, intradiscal pressure was found to be lower in relaxed sitting than in relaxed standing, and second, the pressures while lying supine and lying on the side were essentially the same, whereas Nachemson found a threefold pressure increase in side lying. However, in a larger group of subjects (8 healthy volunteers and 28 patients with low back pain), Sato et al. (120) measured L4-L5 intradiscal pressures during various postures that corroborated the earlier findings of Nachemson et al.

Several investigators have examined how the internal disc mechanics are altered by disc degeneration. In moderately degenerated human discs, the intradiscal pressure has been shown to be approximately 30% less than in nondegenerate discs (111,114). Using an *in vivo* porcine model, Ekström et al. (122,123) and Holm et al. (38) measured the intradiscal pressure in normal lumbar discs and discs with experimentally induced degeneration, as well as the disc adjacent to the degenerated level. The intradiscal pressure in the disc adjacent to the degenerated level, which did not show morphologic signs of degeneration, was found to be slightly higher than in normal discs. This increase can be expected due to the redistribution in mobility demands and alignment of the segments adjacent to those with increased stiffness (i.e., degenerated or fused) (124). Intradiscal pressure has been shown to be highly dependent on the angle of the motion segment (120). Similar to the *in vivo* human studies discussed previously, the intradiscal pressure in the degenerated disc was significantly lower (more than 50%) compared to the pressures in the adjacent and normal discs. Sato et al. (120) reported a progressive decline in intradiscal pressure with increasing disc degeneration grade. Using stress profilometry, age-related degenerative changes in cadaveric lumbar motion segments have been shown to reduce the sagittal diameter of the central hydrostatic region (nucleus and inner annulus) of the disc by approximately 50% and the pressure by 30%, and increase the width of the "functional" annulus by 80% (125) (Fig. 3-4). Structural disruptions, such as radial fissures or fractures in the end plate, increase the space available to nucleus material, thus reducing the central intradiscal pressure (77). Stress profilometry has shown that compressive stresses are transferred from the nucleus to the annulus, particularly the posterior region where increases in peak stresses by 160% have been reported (125). Similar effects in the stress redistribution (i.e., reduced nucleus pressure and increased peak compressive stresses in the posterior annulus) have been observed with sustained (creep) loading (72).

Spinal Kinematics

Several biomechanical investigations, both *in vitro* and *in vivo*, have looked at the effects of disc degeneration on spinal kinematics. Mimura et al. (126) performed a comprehensive investigation into the relationship between multidirectional flexibility of whole cadaveric lumbar spines and disc degeneration. Flexion-extension, lateral bending, and axial rotation pure movements were applied and the motion parameters used to describe the nonlinear spinal behavior were neutral zone, range of motion, and neutral zone ratio. The neutral zone is an absolute measure of the joint laxity around the neutral position, where little resistance is offered by the passive spinal column (127). In an *in vitro* study, the neutral zone has been shown to increase with disc degeneration, particularly in axial rotation and anteroposterior shear motions, and is considered to be a more sensitive parameter than range of motion in relating to disc degeneration (128). The neutral zone ratio, a quotient of the neutral zone and the range of motion, increases in value with greater joint laxity. In the presence of increasing disc degeneration, Mimura et al. (126) reported an increase in intervertebral joint laxity around the neutral position, believed to be due to lax collagenous tissues, as demonstrated by an increase in the neutral zone ratio for all three types of loading

modes. With regard to range of motion, a significant decrease in lateral bending was found, perhaps resulting from facet hypertrophy. Tendencies toward decreased flexion-extension and increased axial rotation ranges of motion were observed. In a clinical study, a reduction in disc height was found to be significantly associated with reduced flexion-extension range of motion (129). The finding of an increase in axial rotation with higher degrees of disc degeneration has been corroborated in other studies (128,130–132), presumably due to fissure formations in the annulus fibrosus and a reduction in disc height. While segmental motion has been shown to increase with increasing severity of degeneration, a decrease has been found at the highest grade of degeneration (126,131). This is in accordance with the final phase of degeneration, as reported by Kirkaldy-Willis (48), where there is a restabilization due to osteochondrotic changes.

Using an *in vivo* porcine model, Kaigle et al. (133) studied dynamically the alterations in segmental kinematics during flexion-extension as a result of acute interventions to the passive stabilizing components of the lumbar spine and to the musculature. Acute injury to the intervertebral disc resulted in greater axial joint laxity during flexion-extension maneuvers, while acute injury to the facet joints caused greater segmental sagittal plane rotation. A facetectomy resulted in considerable destabilization of the motion segment, particularly in the neutral region, where erratic behavior was exhibited during flexion-extension. Although increasing the flexion-extension range of motion, activation of the lumbar paraspinal muscles was shown to have a stabilizing effect on the segmental patterns of motion in the

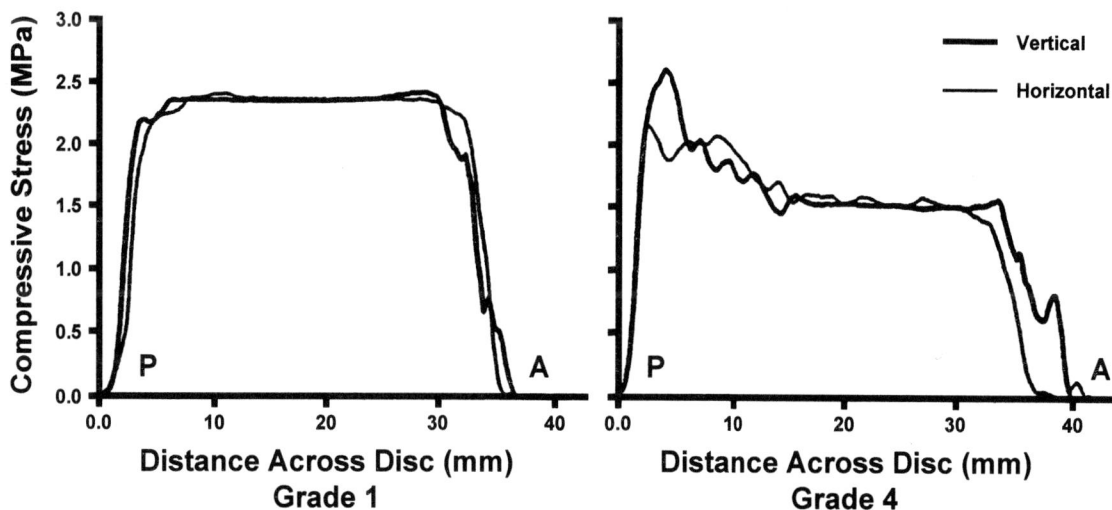

FIG. 3-4. Stress profiles (posterior-anterior). **Left:** Grade 1 disc, female, 27 years old, L1-L2. **Right:** Grade 4 disc, female, 82 years old, L4-L5. (Redrawn from Adams MA, McNally DS, Dolan P. Stress distributions inside intervertebral discs. The effects of age and degeneration. J Bone Joint Surg Br 1996;78:965–972, with permission.)

acutely injured porcine motion segment by reducing the abrupt kinematic behavior in the neutral region. Similar findings were reported in an *in vitro* study by Panjabi et al. (134), where it was demonstrated that the application of simulated intersegmental muscle forces maintained or decreased intervertebral motions (i.e., maintained or decreased neutral zone) for intact and injured motion segments, except the range of motion in flexion which increased with muscle force. In a chronic lesion model, however, the musculature was overall less efficient at providing stability when the intervertebral disc or facet joints were degenerated (87). This may have been due to altered mechanisms in the neuromuscular feedback system in the degenerated motion segments and consequently, the lumbar spine as a whole.

In the clinical situation, there are some important aspects to consider regarding increased joint laxity. Daily activities involve movements across the neutral position (e.g., right-to-left lateral bending, forward flexion to extension, etc.). This transition requires well-coordinated activation/deactivation of various different muscles. With increased joint laxity, there may be insufficient tension in the spinal ligaments and annulus fibers, both of which are known to contain nerve endings that allow them to act as proprioceptive transducers. Lack of sufficient tension may delay or even prevent the detection and delivery of sensory information needed to regulate muscle tension. Stability becomes compromised when the recruitment of the appropriate sequence of muscles needed to overcome the loading demands is too slow, too late, or insufficient.

In a clinical study, *in vivo* segmental motion, overall trunk bending, and myoelectric activity of the lumbar erector spinae muscles were continuously measured during flexion-extension maneuvers in patients with suspected degenerative instability and in healthy volunteers (135). Segmental motion as well as trunk mobility was significantly less in the patients during flexion-extension. Reduced range of motion on functional radiographs has previously been found in patients with low back pain and degenerative changes in the lumbar spine (136–138). The patterns of motion in flexion were also significantly different from the controls. Using videofluoroscopy, Okawa et al. (139) found that, compared to a control group, patients with lumbar degenerative spondylolisthesis showed disordered patterns of motion in forward flexion and a tendency toward smaller ranges of motion, however, the degree of disc degeneration alone did not correlate with the disordered motion patterns. In contrast, in patients with degenerative disorders in the lumbar spine, it has been reported that anterior translatory instability as measured on flexion-extension radiographs is positively associated with disc degeneration and facet joint osteoarthritis, while other forms of sagittal plane instability (rotatory, posterior) have shown no association (140).

In a clinical study, McGregor et al. (141) were unable to find a relationship between degenerative disc disease as seen on plain lateral radiographs and the overall lumbar range of motion. Altogether, the findings suggest that degenerative changes in the lumbar spine and the accompanying aberrant kinematic behavior are associated with alterations in the neuromuscular system. Analyzing the muscular behavior during flexion-extension, Kaigle et al. (135) found that flexion relaxation (i.e., decreased myoelectric activity with extreme trunk flexion) was demonstrated in healthy volunteers but not in the group of chronic low back pain patients with suspected degenerative instability (Fig. 3-5). The restricted segmental mobility found in these patients was believed to be due to the persistent activation of the musculature. It is conceivable that the activated muscles behaved more as stabilizers rather than mobilizers, compensating for the laxity in the diseased motion segment. Such activation would also allow loads to be transferred via the muscles instead of the diseased passive structures, perhaps as a means for avoiding pain. Pain is one factor that has been shown to inhibit flexion relaxation (142,143). Ahern et al. (144) showed that pain behavior, particularly guarded movement, was significantly related to flexion relaxation. Wolf et al. (145) suggested that chronic low back pain patients develop postural abnormalities, such as guarded movement and splinting, in order to compensate for actual or anticipated pain, and that over time, these postural adjustments could alter the normal neuromuscular function.

CONCLUDING REMARKS

The behavior of the lumbar spine is dependent upon the characteristics of its passive, active, and neural subsystems, any of which can become injured or diseased, and all of which undergo the aging process. The neuromuscular system controls the movements and stability in the lumbar spine and can compensate, to a certain degree, for loss in function of one or more of the structures. As conceptually described by Panjabi (1), dysfunction in any of the subsystems may lead to one or more of the following responses in the other subsystems: (a) an immediate, compensatory response, which would result in normal function; (b) a long-term adaptation response, which would result in normal function but with an altered spinal stabilizing system; and (c) an injury which would lead to overall system dysfunction, producing, for example, low back pain.

Numerous investigations have demonstrated that disc degeneration alters the biomechanical behavior of the lumbar spine in a number of ways. However, discrepancies in the literature exist regarding the exact manner in which a disc's biomechanical properties are affected by degeneration. Although grouping of *in vitro* disc specimens according to degeneration grade facilitates compar-

Control L4-L5

Patient L4-L5

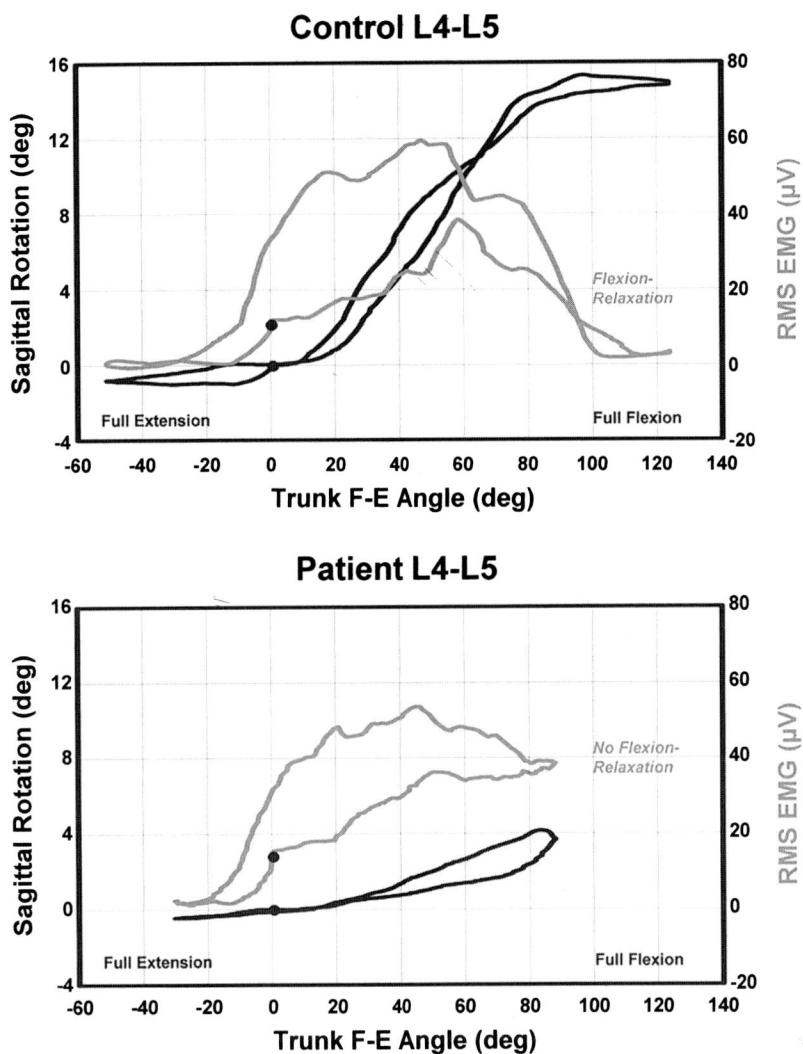

FIG. 3-5. Segmental kinematic (sagittal rotation) and myoelectric [right-side erector spinae surface Root Mean Square electromyography (RMS EMG)] experimental data as a function of the overall trunk flexion-extension angle during a flexion-extension cycle from the L4-L5 motion segment of a control subject **(top)** and a patient with degenerative instability **(bottom)**. Note the absence of flexion-relaxation in patient myoelectric data.

isons, averaging results in groups of motion segments with diverse degenerative changes may obscure the effects of degeneration on the biomechanical response. This may be a factor contributing to the disparities reported in the literature. Additionally, it has also been pointed out by Vernon-Roberts et al. (40) that to properly classify disc disease, it is essential to examine disc slices at multiple levels within a disc since abnormalities are three-dimensionally complex. However, very few studies have reported employing such procedures. It should also be noted that the majority of *in vitro* studies have been performed on lumbar motion segments obtained from cadaveric specimens beyond the sixth decade in age, suggesting that the degenerative changes were age-related. Although biochemical and biomechanical changes due to normal aging are similar to those found in degeneration,

it would be more appropriate to perform biomechanical studies on degenerate discs from specimens in the middle decades of life, which is the time in life where there is a maximal incidence of disc-related back problems (146).

Since disc degeneration is a process, the biomechanical properties will undergo changes throughout this process. An observed increase in flexion-extension stiffness, for example, during one stage of the degenerative process may not necessarily be present at a later point in time. Even at a similar point in time, while changes in the material properties may increase the flexibility of the motion segment, geometric changes may produce an opposite affect, thus producing no net effect on the overall behavior. Clinically, patients suspected of having degenerative segmental instability display vertebral misalignment on functional radiographs, accompanied by morphologic changes in the intervertebral disc, vertebrae, and possibly facet joints. However, clinical studies as a whole have been unable to demonstrate segmental hypermobility (i.e., greater range of motion), which correlates with the pathologic signs and symptoms. On the contrary, the majority of studies have found hypomobility in the suspected 'unstable' motion segment. This raises an important issue regarding the ability of the neuromuscular feedback system to compensate for joint laxity or abnormal movements in a lumbar motion segment. To better understand the mechanisms by which the passive, active, and neural structures interact, refer to Chapter 11.

In summary, the overall findings reported in the literature indicate that with disc degeneration, the biochemical and structural changes compromise the disc's structural integrity, regionally and subsequently as a whole. The effects of disc degeneration on the motion segment stiffness are a function of the loading mode. When loaded in axial compression or torsion, degenerated discs display a reduction in stiffness, whereas in flexion-extension and lateral bending, a stiffening effect has generally been found. Disc degeneration alters the normal stress distribution patterns. The failure properties of the annulus lamellae are reduced along with the intradiscal pressure in the nucleus. This produces high stress concentrations in the posterior annulus, the region where disc disruption is clinically found to occur most frequently. Such alterations in the internal disc mechanics may cause pain or precipitate further disc disruption. Degenerative changes in the lumbar spine cause aberrant kinematic behavior, particularly around the neutral position. Although increased intervertebral laxity around the neutral position has been associated with disc degeneration, the majority of in vivo studies have found reduced ranges of motion. Persistent muscle activation is believed to be a mechanism by which the neuromuscular system provides stabilization in order to guard diseased passive structures from abnormal motion, which may cause pain or further tissue damage.

REFERENCES

1. Panjabi MM. The stabilizing system of the spine. Part I. Function, dysfunction, adaptation, and enhancement. J Spinal Disord 1992;5:383–389.
2. Butler D, Trafimow JH, Andersson GB, et al. Discs degenerate before facets. Spine 1990;15:111–113.
3. Moore RJ, Crotti TN, Osti OL, et al. Osteoarthrosis of the facet joints resulting from anular rim lesions in sheep lumbar discs. Spine 1999;24:519–525.
4. Moore RJ, Vernon-Roberts B, Osti OL, et al. Remodeling of vertebral bone after outer anular injury in sheep. Spine 1996;21:936–940.
5. Mattila M, Hurme M, Alaranta H, et al. The multifidus muscle in patient with lumbar disc herniation. A histochemical and morphometric analysis of intraoperative biopsies. Spine 1986;11:732–738.
6. Zhao W-P, Kawaguchi Y, Matsui H, et al. Histochemistry and morphology of the multifidus muscle in lumbar disc herniation. Comparative study between diseased and normal sides. Spine 2000;25:2191–2199.
7. Zhu X-Z, Parnianpour M, Nordin M, et al. Histochemistry and morphology of erector spinae muscle in lumbar disc herniation. Spine 1989;14:391–397.
8. Lehto M, Hurme M, Alaranta H, et al. Connective tissue changes of the multifidus muscle in patients with lumbar disc herniation. An immunohistologic study of collagen types I and III and fibronectin. Spine 1989;14:302–309.
9. Eyre DR. Biochemistry of the intervertebral disc. Int Rev Conn Tiss Res 1979;8:227–291.
10. Skaggs DL, Weidenbaum M, Iatridis JC, et al. Regional variation in tensile properties and biomechanical composition of the human annulus fibrosus. Spine 1994;19:1310–1319.
11. Urban J. Biochemistry: disc biochemistry in relation to function. In: Wiesel SW, Weinstein JN, Herkowitz H, et al., eds. The lumbar spine, 2nd ed. Philadelphia: WB Saunders, 1996:271–281.
12. Holm S. Nutritional and pathophysiologic aspects of the lumbar intervertebral disc. In: Wiesel SW, Weinstein JN, Herkowitz H, et al., eds. The lumbar spine, 2nd ed. Philadelphia: WB Saunders, 1996:285–310.
13. Yoganandan N, Myklebust JB, Wilson CR, et al. Functional biomechanics of the thoracolumbar vertebral cortex. Clin Biomech 1988;3:11–18.
14. Holm S. Pathophysiology of disc degeneration. Acta Orthop Scand Suppl 1993;251:13–15.
15. Adams MA, Hutton WC. The effect of posture on the role of the apophyseal joints in resisting intervertebral compressive force. J Bone Joint Surg 1980;62B:358–362.
16. Farfan HF, Cossette JW, Robertson GH, et al. The effects of torsion on the lumbar intervertebral joints: the role of torsion in the production of disc degeneration. J Bone Joint Surg 1970;52A:468–497.
17. Crisco JJ. The biomechanical stability of the human lumbar spine. Experimental and theoretical investigations [dissertation]. New Haven, CT: Yale University; 1989.
18. Bergmark A. Stability of the lumbar spine. A study in mechanical engineering. Acta Orthop Scand 1989;60[Suppl]:230.
19. Hodges, P. The role of the motor system in spinal pain: implications for rehabilitation of the athlete following lower back pain. J Sci Med Sport 2000;3:243–253.
20. Moseley GH, Hodges PW, Gandevia SC. Deep and superficial fibers of the lumbar multifidus muscle are differentially active during voluntary arm movements. Spine 2002;27:E29–E36.
21. Bogduk N. Clinical anatomy of the lumbar spine and sacrum, 3rd ed. London: Churchill Livingstone, 1997.
22. Cavanaugh JM. Neural mechanisms of lumbar pain. Spine 1995;20:1804–1809.
23. Holm S, Indahl A, Kaigle A, et al. The neuromuscular role of mechanoreceptors in the porcine lumbar intervertebral disc. Adelaide, Australia: Proceedings from the ISSLS Annual Meeting, 2000.
24. Jackson HC, Winkelmann RK, Bickel WH. Nerve endings in human lumbar spinal column and related structures. J Bone Joint Surg 1966;48A:1272–1281.
25. Kääpä E, Grönblad M, Holm S, et al. Neural elements in the normal and experimentally injured porcine intervertebral disc. Eur Spine J 1994;3:137–142.
26. Roberts S, Eisenstein SM, Menage J, et al. Mechanoreceptors in intervertebral discs. Morphology, distribution and neuropeptides. Spine 1995;20:2645–2651.
27. Yamashita T, Cavanaugh JM, El-Bohy AA et al. Mechanosensitive afferent units in the lumbar facet joint. J Bone Joint Surg Am 1990;72:865–870.
28. Yamashita T, Minaki Y, Oota I, et al. Mechanosensitive afferent units in the lumbar intervertebral disc and adjacent muscle. Spine 1993;18:2252–2256.
29. Adams P, Muir H. Quantitative changes with age of proteoglycans of human lumbar discs. Ann Rheum Dis 1976;35:289–296.
30. Ayad S, Weiss JB. Biochemistry of the intervertebral disc. In: Jayson MIV, ed. The lumbar spine and back pain, 3rd ed. London: Churchill Livingstone, 1987:100–137.
31. Magara A, Schwartz A. Relation between low back pain syndrome and x-ray findings. I. Degenerative osteoarthritis. Scand J Rehab Med 1976;8:115–125.
32. Adams P, Eyre DR, Muir H. Biochemical aspects of development and ageing of human lumbar intervertebral discs. Rheum Rehab 1977;16:22–29.
33. Lyons G, Eisenstein SM, Sweet MBE. Biochemical changes in intervertebral disc degeneration. Biochim Biophys Acta 1981;673:443–453.

34. Kääpä E. Collagens, proteoglycans, and neural structures in a porcine model of intervertebral disc degeneration [dissertation]. Oulu, Finland: University of Oulu; 1993.

35. Buckwalter JA. Spine update. Aging and degeneration of the human intervertebral disc. Spine 1995;20:1307–1314.

36. Hickey DS, Hukins DWL. Aging changes in the macromolecular organization of the intervertebral disc: an x-ray diffraction and electron microscope study. Spine 1982;7:234–242.

37. Yasuma T, Arai K, Suzukk F. Age-related phenomena in the lumbar intervertebral discs. Lipofuscin and amyloid deposition. Spine 1992; 17:1194–1198.

38. Holm S, Kaigle AM, Ekström L, Hansson T. Degenerative properties of the porcine intervertebral disc due to endplate injury. Kona, Hawaii: Proceedings from the ISSLS Annual Meeting, 1999.

39. Marchand F, Ahmed AM. Investigation of the laminate structure of lumbar disc annulus fibrosus. Spine 1990;15:402–410.

40. Vernon-Roberts B, Fazzarli NL, Manthey BA. Pathogenesis of tears of the anulus investigated by multiple-level transaxial analysis of the T12-L1 disc. Spine 1997;22:2641–2646.

41. Gruber HE, Hanley EN. Ultrastructure of the human intervertebral disc during aging and degeneration. Spine 2002;27:798–805.

42. Farfan HF, Huberdeau RM, Dubow HI. Lumbar intervertebral disc degeneration: the influence of geometrical features on the pattern of disc degeneration—a post mortem study. J Bone Joint Surg Am 1972; 54:492–510.

43. Gunzburg R, Parkinson R, Moore R, et al. A cadaveric study comparing discography, MRI, histology, and mechanical behavior of the human lumbar disc. Spine 1992;17:417–423.

44. Tanaka M, Nakahara S, Inoue H. A pathologic study of discs in the elderly. Spine 1993;18:1456–1462.

45. Friberg S, Hirsch C. Anatomical studies on lumbar disc degeneration. Acta Orthop Scand 1948;17:224–230.

46. Harris RI, Macnab I. Structural changes in the lumbar intervertebral disc. J Bone Joint Surg 1954;36B:304.

47. Nachemson A. Lumbar intradiscal pressure. Experimental studies on post-mortem material. Acta Orthop Scand Suppl 1960;XLIII:1–104.

48. Kirkaldy-Willis WH. Presidential symposium on instability of the lumbar spine. Spine 1985;10:254.

49. Hadjipavlou AG, Simmons JW, Pope MH, et al. Pathomechanics and clinical relevance of disc degeneration and annular tear: a point-of-view review. Am J Orthop 1999;28:561–571.

50. Bernard BP. Musculoskeletal disorders and workplace factors: a critical review of epidemiologic evidence for work-related musculoskeletal disorders of the neck, upper extremity, and low back. Cincinnati: U.S. Department of Health and Human Services, National Institute for Occupational Safety and Health, 1997.

51. Magora A. Investigation of the relation between low back pain and occupation: III. Physical requirements: sitting, standing, and weight lifting. Ind Med 1972;41:5–9.

52. Videman T, Battié MC. Spine update. The influence of occupation on lumbar degeneration. Spine 1999;24:1164–1168.

53. Hartvigsen J, Bakketeig LS, Leboeurf-Yde C, et al. The association between physical workload and low back pain clouded by the "healthy worker" effect. Spine 2001;26:1788–1793.

54. Krause N, Ragland DR, Fisher JM, et al. Psychosocial job factors, physical workload, and incidence of work-related spinal injury: a 5-year prospective study of urban transit operators. Spine 1998;23:2507–2516.

55. Kelsey JL, Githens PB, White AA, et al. An epidemiologic study of lifting and twisting on the job and risk for acute prolapsed lumbar intervertebral disc. J Orthop Res 1984;2:61–66.

56. Pope MH, Andersson GBJ, Frymoyer JW, et al., eds. Occupational low back pain: assessment, treatment, and prevention. St. Louis: Mosby–Year Book, 1991.

57. Videman T, Nurminen M, Troup JDG. Lumbar spinal pathology in cadaveric material in relation to history of back pain, occupation, and physical loading. Spine 1990;15:728–740.

58. Marras WS, Lavender SA, Leurgans SE, et al. Biomechanical risk factors for occupationally related low back disorders. Ergonomics 1995;38:377–410.

59. Hansson T, Westerholm P, eds. Arbete och besvär i rörelseorganen. En vetenskaplig värdering av frågor om samband. Arbete och hälsa 2001;12.

60. Adams MA, Dolan P. Time-dependent changes in the lumbar spine's resistance to bending. Clin Biomech 1996;11:194–200.

61. Hutton WC, Adams MA. Can the lumbar spine be crushed in heavy lifting? Spine 1982;7:586–590.

62. Adams MA, Hutton WC. The effect of posture on the fluid content of lumbar intervertebral discs. Spine 1983;8:665–671.

63. Casper RA. The viscoelastic behavior of the human intervertebral disc [dissertation]. Durham, NC: Duke University; 1980.

64. Hirsch C. The reaction of intervertebral discs to compression forces. J Bone Joint Surg 1955;37A:1188–1196.

65. Kazarian L. Creep characteristics of the human spinal column. Orthop Clin North Am 1975;56A:675–687.

66. Kaigle AM, Magnusson M, Pope MH, et al. In vivo measurement of intervertebral creep: a preliminary report. Clin Biomech 1992;7: 59–62.

67. Keller TS, Hansson TH, Holm SH, et al. In vivo creep behavior of the normal and degenerated porcine intervertebral disc: a preliminary report. J Spinal Disord 1989;1:267–278.

68. Keller TS, Spengler DM, Hansson TH. Mechanical behavior of the human lumbar spine. I. Creep analysis during static compressive loading. J Orthop Res 1987;5:467–478.

69. Koeller W, Muehlhaus S, Meier W, et al. Biomechanical properties of human intervertebral discs subjected to axial dynamic compression—influence of age and degeneration. J Biomech 1986;19:807–816.

70. Virgin WJ. Experimental investigations into physical properties of intervertebral disc. J Bone Joint Surg 1951;33B:607–611.

71. Botsford DJ, Esses SI, Ogilvie-Harris DJ. In-vivo diurnal variation in intervertebral disc volume and morphology. Spine 1994;19: 935–940.

72. Adams MA, McMillan DW, Green TP, et al. Sustained loading generates stress concentrations in lumbar intervertebral discs. Spine 1996; 21:434–438.

73. Smeathers JE. Some time-dependent properties of the intervertebral joint when under compression. Eng Med 1984;13:83–87.

74. Cyron BM, Hutton WC. The behaviour of the lumbar intervertebral disc under repetitive forces. Int Orthop 1981;5:203–207.

75. Dunlop RB, Adams MA, Hutton WC. Disc space narrowing and the lumbar facet joints. J Bone Joint Surg 1984;66B:706–710.

76. Adams MA, Dolan P. Recent advances in lumbar spinal mechanics and their clinical significance. Clin Biomech 1995;10:3–19.

77. Adams MA, Freeman BJC, Morrison HP, et al. Mechanical initiation of intervertebral disc degeneration. Spine 2000;25:1625–1636.

78. Pearce RH, Grimmer BJ, Adams ME. Degeneration and the chemical composition of the human lumbar intervertebral disc. J Orthop Res 1987;5:198–205.

79. Bradford DS, Cooper KM, Oegema TR. Chymopapain, chemonucleolysis and nucleus pulposus regeneration. J Bone Joint Surg 1983; 65A:1220–1231.

80. Iatridis JC, Mente PL, Stokes IA, et al. Compression-induced changes in intervertebral disc properties in a rat tail model. Spine 1999;24: 996–1002.

81. Lotz JC, Colliou OK, Chin JR, et al. Compression-induced degeneration of the intervertebral disc: an in vivo mouse model and finite-element study. Spine 1998;23:2493–2506.

82. Walsh A, Bradford DS, Kleinstueck F, et al. In situ growth factor stimulation of degenerated intervertebral discs. Adelaide, Australia: Proceedings from the ISSLS Annual Meeting, 2000.

83. Hadjipavlou AG, Simmons JW, Yang JP, et al. Torsional injury resulting in disc degeneration: I. An in vivo rabbit model. J Spinal Dis 1998;11:312–317.

84. Sullivan JD, Farfan HF, Kahn DS. Pathologic changes with intervertebral joint rotational instability in the rabbit. Can J Surg 1971;4: 71–79.

85. Ahlgren BD, Vasavada A, Brower RS, et al. Anular incision technique on the strength and multidirectional flexibility of the healing intervertebral disc. Spine 1994;19:948–954.

86. Kaigle A, Ekström L, Holm S, et al. In vivo dynamic stiffness of the lumbar spine exposed to cyclic loading: influence of load and degeneration. J Spinal Dis 1998;11:65–70.

87. Kaigle AM, Holm SH, Hansson TH. Kinematic behavior of the porcine lumbar spine—a chronic lesion model. Spine 1997;22: 2796–2806.

88. Kääpä E, Grönblad M, Holm S, et al. Neural elements in the normal and experimentally injured porcine intervertebral disc. Eur Spine J 1994;3:137–142.

89. Kääpä E, Holm S, Inkinen R, et al. Proteoglycan chemistry in exper-

imentally injured porcine intervertebral disc. J Spinal Disord 1994;7: 296–306.

90. Latham JM, Pearcy MJ, Costi JJ, et al. Mechanical consequences of annular tears and subsequent intervertebral disc degeneration. Clin Biomech 1994;9:211–219.

91. Lipson SJ, Muir H. Proteoglycans in experimental intervertebral disc degeneration. Spine 1981;6:194–210.

92. Moore RJ, Osti OL, Vernon-Roberts B, et al. Changes in endplate vascularity after an outer anulus tear in the sheep. Spine 1992;17: 874–878.

93. Osti OL, Vernon-Roberts B, Fraser RD. Anulus tears and intervertebral disc degeneration. An experimental study using an animal model. Spine 1990;15:762–767.

94. Smith JW, Walmsley STA. Experimental incisions of the intervertebral disc. J Bone Joint Surg 1951;33B:612–625.

95. Cinotti G, Giannicola G, Della Rocca C, et al. Disc degeneration induced by injury of vertebral endplate. Adelaide, Australia: Proceedings from the ISSLS Annual Meeting, 2000.

96. Holm S, Nachemson A. Nutritional changes in the canine intervertebral disc after spinal fusion. Clin Orthop 1982;169:243–258.

97. Markolf KL, Morris JM. The structural components of the intervertebral disc. A study of their contributions to the ability of the disc to withstand compressive forces. J Bone Joint Surg 1974;56A:675–687.

98. Brown T, Hansen RJ, Yorra AJ. Some mechanical tests on the lumbosacral spine with particular reference to the intervertebral discs. J Bone Joint Surg 1957;39A:1135–1164.

99. Hirsch C. The mechanical response in normal and degenerated lumbar discs. Acta Orthop Scand 1956;38A:242–243.

100. Hirsch C. The reaction of intervertebral discs to compression forces. J Bone Joint Surg 1955;37A:1188–1196.

101. Hirsch C, Nachemson A. New observations of the mechanical behavior of lumbar discs. Acta Orthop Scand 1954;23:254–283.

102. Nachemson AL, Schultz AB, Berkson MH. Mechanical properties of human lumbar spine motion segments. Influence of age, sex, disc level, and degeneration. Spine 1979;4:1–8.

103. Brown MD, Holmes DC, Heiner AD. Measurement of cadaver lumbar spine motion segment stiffness. Spine 2002;27:918–922.

104. Ebara S, Iatridis JC, Setton LA, et al. Tensile properties of nondegenerate human lumbar anulus fibrosus. Spine 1996;21:452–461.

105. Acaroglu ER, Iatridis JC, Setton LA, et al. Degeneration and aging affect the tensile behavior of human lumbar anulus fibrosus. Spine 1995;20:2690–2701.

106. Fujita Y, Duncan NA, Lotz JC. Radial tensile properties of the lumbar annulus fibrosus are site and degeneration dependent. J Orthop Res 1997;15:814–819.

107. Umehara S, Tadano S, Abumi K, et al. Effects of degeneration on the elastic modulus distribution in the lumbar intervertebral disc. Spine 1996;21:811–819.

108. Schultz AB, Ashton-Miller JA. Biomechanics of the human spine. In: Mow VC, Hayes WC, eds. Basic orthopaedic biomechanics. New York: Raven Press, 1991:337–374.

109. Thompson RE, Pearcy MJ, Downing KJ, et al. Disc lesions and the mechanics of the intervertebral joint complex. Spine 2000;25: 3026–3035.

110. Schmidt TA, An HS, Lim T-H, et al. The stiffness of lumbar spinal motion segments with a high-intensity zone in the anulus fibrosus. Spine 1998;23:2167–2173.

111. Nachemson A. In vivo discometry in lumbar discs with irregular nucleograms: some differences in stress distribution between normal and moderately degenerated discs. Acta Orthop Scand 1965;36: 418–434.

112. Nachemson A. The effect of forward leaning on lumbar intradiscal pressure. Acta Orthop Scand 1965;35:314–328.

113. Nachemson A. The influence of spinal movements on the lumbar intradiscal pressure and on the tensile stresses in the annulus fibrosus. Acta Orthop Scand 1963;33:183–207.

114. Nachemson A. The load on lumbar discs in different position of the body. Clin Orthop 1966;45:107–122.

115. Nachemson A, Elfström G. Intravital dynamic pressure measurements in lumbar discs. A study of common movements, maneuvers and exercises. Scand J Rehabil Med Suppl 1970;1:1–40.

116. Nachemson A, Morris JM. In vivo measurements of intradiscal pressure. J Bone Joint Surg [Am] 1964;46:1077–1092.

117. Andersson GBJ, Örtengren R, Nachemson A. Intradiscal pressure, intra-abdominal pressure and myoelectric back muscle activity related to posture and loading. Clin Orthop 1977;129:156–164.

118. Andersson GBJ, Örtengren R, Nachemson AL, et al. The sitting posture: an electromyographic and discometric study. Orthop Clin North Am 1975;6:105–120.

119. Schultz A, Andersson GBJ, Örtengren R, et al. Loads on the lumbar spine. Validation of a biomechanical analysis by measurements of intradiscal pressures and myoelectric signals. J Bone Joint Surg Am 1982;64:713–720.

120. Sato K, Kikuchi S, Yonezawa T. In vivo intradiscal pressure measurement in healthy individuals and in patients with ongoing back problems. Spine 1999;24:2468–2474.

121. Wilke H-J, Neef P, Caimi M, et al. New in vivo measurements of pressures in the intervertebral disc in daily life. Spine 1999;24:755–762.

122. Ekström L, Holm S, Kaigle AM, et al. In-vivo porcine intervertebral disc pressure as a function of external loading. Brussels: Proceedings from the ISSLS Annual Meeting, June 1998.

123. Ekström L, Kaigle AM, Holm S, et al. In-vivo intradiscal pressure in the degenerated porcine spine. Kona, Hawaii: Proceedings from the ISSLS Annual Meeting, June 1999.

124. Cunningham BW, Kotani Y, McNulty PS, et al. The effect of spinal destabilization and instrumentation on lumbar intradiscal pressure. An in vitro biomechanical analysis. Spine 1997;22:2655–2663.

125. Adams MA, McNally DS, Dolan P. Stress distributions inside intervertebral discs. The effects of age and degeneration. J Bone Joint Surg Br 1996;78:965–972.

126. Mimura M, Panjabi MM, Oxland TR, et al. Disc degeneration affects the multidirectional flexibility of the lumbar spine. Spine 1994;19: 1371–1380.

127. Panjabi MM. The stabilizing system of the spine. Part II. Neutral zone and instability hypothesis. J Spinal Disord 1992;5:390–397.

128. Panjabi MM, Goel V, Summers D. Relationship between chronic instability and disc degeneration. Toronto: Proceedings from the ISSLS Annual Meeting, 1982.

129. Burton AK, Battie MC, Gibbons L, et al. Lumbar disc degeneration and sagittal flexibility. J Spinal Disord 1996;9:418–424.

130. Adams MA, Hutton WC. The relevance of torsion to the mechanical derangement of the lumbar spine. Spine 1981;6:241–248.

131. Fujiwara A, Lim T-H, An HS, et al. The effect of disc degeneration and facet joint osteoarthritis on the segmental flexibility of the lumbar spine. Spine 2000;25:3036–3044.

132. Krismer M, Haid C, Behensky H, et al. Motion in lumbar functional spine units during side bending and axial rotation moments depending on the degree of degeneration. Spine 2000;25:2020–2027.

133. Kaigle AM, Holm SH, Hansson, TH. Experimental instability in the lumbar spine. Spine 1995;20:421–430.

134. Panjabi M, Abumi K, Duranceau J, et al. Spinal stability and intersegmental muscle forces. A biomechanical model. Spine 1989;14: 194–200.

135. Kaigle AM, Wessberg P, Hansson TH. Muscular and kinematic behavior of the lumbar spine during flexion-extension. J Spinal Disord 1998;11:163–174.

136. Dvorák J, Panjabi MM, Novotny JR, et al. Clinical validation of functional flexion-extension roentgenograms of the lumbar spine. Spine 1991;16:943–950.

137. Murata M, Morio Y, Kuranobu K. Lumbar disc degeneration and segmental instability: a comparison of magnetic resonance images and plain radiographs of patients with low back pain. Arch Orthop Trauma Surg 1994;113:297–301.

138. Pearcy M, Portek I, Shepherd J. The effect of low-back pain on lumbar spinal movements measured by three-dimensional x-ray analysis. Spine 1985;10:150–153.

139. Okawa A, Shinomiya K, Komori H, et al. Dynamic motion study of the whole lumbar spine by videofluoroscopy. Spine 1998;23: 1743–1749.

140. Fujiwara A, Tamai K, An HS, et al. The relationship between disc degeneration, facet joint osteoarthritis, and stability of the degenerative lumbar spine. J Spinal Disord 2000;13:444–450.

141. McGregor AH, Cattermole HR, Hughes SPF. Spinal motion in lumbar degenerative disc disease. J Bone Joint Surg Br 1998;80B: 1009–1013.

142. Ahern DK, Follick MJ, Council JR, et al. Comparison of lumbar paravertebral EMG patterns in chronic low back pain patients and non-patient controls. Pain 1988;34:153–160.

143. Sihvonen T, Partanen J, Hänninen O, et al. Electric behavior of low
     back muscles during lumbar pelvic rhythm in low back pain patients
     and healthy controls. Arch Phys Med Rehabil 1991;72:1080–1087.
144. Ahern DK, Hannon DJ, Goreczny AJ, et al. Correlation of chronic
     low-back pain behavior and muscle function examination of the flex-
     ion-relaxation response. Spine 1990;15:92–95.
145. Wolf SL, Nacht M, Kelly JL. EMG biofeedback training during
     dynamic movement for low back pain patients. Behav Ther 1992;13:
     395–406.
146. Praemer A, Furner S, Rice DP. Musculoskeletal conditions in the
     United States. Park Ridge, IL: American Academy of Orthopaedic
     Surgeons, 1992:26–27.

CHAPTER 4

Morphologic Changes of End Plates in Degenerative Disc Disease

Robert J. Moore

The vertebral bodies of the axial skeleton are separated by intervertebral discs, which are highly specialized structures that enable a range of physiologic and mechanical functions associated with motion. The discs have three main structural components—a central nucleus pulposus surrounded by the annulus fibrosus and the end plates, which are located at the cranial and caudal interfaces with the vertebrae. While the structure and function of the annulus and nucleus are well characterized, much less is known about the end plates. Perhaps this is because their constitution has not yet been consistently defined, or because structural changes to the end plates are more subtle than changes to other disc components, and therefore easily overlooked.

In some early anatomical studies the end plates were described as the transitional zone between the vertebral body and the adjacent disc because they possessed both an osseous and a hyaline cartilage component (1,2). Other authors, however, proposed a more limited situation, and described the end plates as the thin layer of hyaline cartilage interposed between the vertebral body and the disc (3,4). For whatever reason, this latter concept has survived and they are now more commonly known as the "cartilage end plates" or simply the "end plates."

Volumes of literature have been devoted to the normal development of the end plates that are recognizable from an early embryologic stage and retain their cartilaginous nature during normal maturation while the adjacent vertebrae undergo ossification (5). The cartilaginous component of the mature end plate is essentially an aqueous gel containing large proteoglycan molecules within a dense mesh of collagen fibrils that are aligned along the longitudinal axis (horizontally in the human). Although it has been suggested that there is no direct physical connection between the end plates and the underlying bone (6), their juxtaposition almost certainly contributes to the strong bond that is essential for the normal function of the end plate (7). When the epiphyses fuse in the young adult spine, only the outer rim of the end plates is ossified, leaving a broad central cartilaginous plate. The lamellae of the outer annulus attach directly to the adjacent bone, while the fibers of the inner annulus connect the end plates directly with the disc.

The end plates are thin, particularly in the center of the disc, measuring no more than 1 mm at maturity (8), but there can be considerable variation from one side to the other (9). In the lower lumbar spine the end plates are roughly cardioid to elliptical in shape (10). While this fact in itself may seem to have little relevance, shape is the only one of several parameters investigated by computed tomography-myelography that is claimed to be significantly related to the development of disc herniation (11). The most abundant cell type in the end plate is the chondrocyte, distributed more uniformly than the clearly defined layers of cells within articular cartilage. Otherwise the end plate bears a close similarity to the articular cartilage of synovial joints.

The biochemical characteristics of the end plates, from normality through the spectrum of degenerative conditions, are well documented (12,13). The two most abundant families of molecules in the disc are the collagens and the proteoglycans that are found in varying proportions in the annulus, the nucleus, and the end plates. Of the several species of collagen, type X is probably the most important in the end plates because it is a marker of hypertrophic chondrocytes and is thought to be involved in cartilage calcification (14). It has been detected mainly in the central region (15).

Proteoglycan molecules are essential for the maintenance of the water content and overall integrity of the nucleus (16). It is known that altered tissue levels of proteoglycans can adversely influence disc function (17). The proteoglycans of the end plate have not been studied extensively, but suffice to say loss of proteoglycans from the end plate is implicated in loss of proteoglycans from the nucleus (18). It follows that disc degeneration invariably is preceded by widespread degradation of disc proteoglycans (19). It has long been suspected that alterations to the biochemical composition of the end plate, particularly during the growth phase, may be involved in the development of scoliosis (20–22).

Heterozygous inactivation of the Col2a1 gene allele in 1-month old mice has been shown to lead to lower glycosaminoglycan concentration in the end plates and thicker and more irregular end plates that become calcified prematurely (23).

The developing discs receive essential nourishment from two sources. From the embryonic stage, a network of blood vessels penetrates the annulus no deeper than about one-third of its total thickness (24). Most of these vessels do not persist beyond maturity and by adulthood they can be seen in only the outer two or three lamellae. Blood vessels also penetrate the end plates from the vertebral body margins (5) and arise from ramifications of a large primary nutrient artery on the dorsal surface of each vertebral body. With maturation however, these small vessels also disappear, leaving only a limited blood supply in the form of capillary buds that perforate the osseous component of the end plate (25). It is curious that mammalian discs have evolved in this way, since the central nucleus pulposus in the adult human can be up to 20 mm from the nearest blood vessels and is therefore totally reliant on diffusion of solutes across the end plates and the annulus for nutrition. No other tissue in the body is so distanced from a blood supply, and presumably therefore so susceptible to deterioration.

Extensive *in vitro* study of the transport of solutes, disc nutrition, and metabolism using small dye molecules has shown that the lateral end plate at the vertebral rim is relatively impermeable compared with the central portion, and even the entire annulus fibrosus (26). The contribution of the periannular blood supply was well accepted, but the permeability of the capillary network immediately beneath the end plate attracted new attention. Quantitative analysis of human autopsy specimens that had been injected with dye solution subsequently confirmed that there were significantly more marrow contacts along the central end plate adjacent to the nucleus than there were in the lateral margins (27,28).

While determining the significance of these vessels to disc nutrition and cell metabolism, diffusion was shown to be the principal mechanism for transporting small dissolved solutes into the disc (29). Further, the size and ionic charge of the molecules were also shown to govern the rate and extent of diffusion (29,30). As the high proteoglycan content in the nucleus confers a net negative charge to the normal disc, small, uncharged molecules such as glucose and oxygen and positively charged ions such as sodium and calcium diffuse into the disc with relative ease. Conversely, it is much more difficult for negatively charged molecules such as sulfate and chloride ions to enter the nucleus. Macromolecules such as immunoglobulins and enzymes are totally excluded.

The relative contribution and importance of the end plate and annular routes to disc nutrition were established independently using biochemical (31), histologic (25), and radiologic (32) methods. Each of these studies confirmed the importance of the central end plate in the metabolic processes of the disc.

Soon after maturity the cartilage of the end plate undergoes extensive mineralization and eventually this tissue is resorbed and replaced by true bone (33,34). It is likely that this remodeling, as well as the calcification of vascular channels in the end plate region both contribute substantially to a reduction in the normal exchange of nutrients across the end plate with increasing age (35).

Since the end plate is capable of remodeling after maturity it seems reasonable to expect the obliteration and loss of vascular channels could also be reversed. This does appear to be possible, and in fact has been demonstrated in an experimental ovine model of annular lesions (36). In the context of that study it was presumed that neovascularization was a basic survival mechanism for discs undergoing severe pathologic deterioration, although it was in vain, since they continued to degenerate. Although not specifically tested in that study it is likely that such new blood vessels are formed by activation of normally latent enzymes of the matrix metalloproteinase (MMP) family, which are regulated by tissue inhibitors (37–41). Increased levels of several MMP species have been detected in surgical and postmortem samples of human discs (40,42), and although the end plate itself was not analyzed in these studies, it is reasonable to assume that they would be no different.

As well as providing an axis for the diffusion of nutrients to the avascular disc, the end plates also are important for the mechanical function of the spine. In the course of normal physical activity, mechanical loading (especially axial compression) can alter the shape of the disc to the extent that the end plates and the subchondral trabecular bone become deformed (43). This deformation is reversible in young healthy end plates that are subjected to even moderate loading, but when the forces are higher and applied repeatedly, the end plates sustain irreversible damage. There is evidence that the integrity of the end plate and subchondral bone, rather than the degree of disc degeneration, influence how much damage occurs during axial compression (44). It was also noted that the radiographic appearance of the end plates in this study was similar to those of osteoporotic patients, in whom the end plates become more concave with age and progressive vertebral osteopenia (45,46).

Morphologic changes to the end plates occur with advancing age but also may be seen in association with pathology in either the nucleus or the annulus. Either way, the changes are essentially microscopic and become evident macroscopically only in the advanced stages of disease (47).

In the earliest changes after maturity fissures and clefts appear along the length of the end plate in the horizontal plane. Occasionally there is evidence of chondrocyte death. The cartilage may be invaded by microscopic blood vessels and there also may be ossification extending from the adjacent bony end plate. With time the cartilage becomes depleted progressively and undergoes further ossification. The nucleus fills the small voids created as more blood vessels perforate the end plate, but these defects do not breach the bony end plate.

The most dramatic changes occur after the fifth decade. It is not unusual to observe nuclear material protruding into the adjacent vertebral marrow with foci of bony sclerosis resulting from active remodeling at these sites. Often there is total loss of the cartilage end plate. In an experimental murine spondylosis model disc degeneration, including loss of the end plate, was accompanied by increased apoptosis in end plate chondrocytes relative to naturally aged mice, suggesting that programmed cell death plays a role in age-related changes of the disc (48).

Of all the structural elements that constitute the disc, the end plate appears to be most susceptible to mechanical failure. Theoretical modeling using finite element analysis has shown that mechanical failure always begins with separation of the end plate from the subchondral bone (49), in complete agreement with the microscopic observations of Vernon-Roberts (47). Autopsy studies also confirm that portions of the end plate become separated from the vertebral body and are herniated from the disc along with attached annular fibers (50,51). A significant weak point of the motion segment appears to be near the epiphyseal ring, where the annulus fibers insert directly into the vertebral bone. Not only is it a common site for fracture causing back pain and radiculopathy in adolescents and young adults (52) but it has been shown to be particularly susceptible to failure during experimental mechanical compression tests in the adolescent pig (53). This is a different injury pattern to that seen in adults, where the end plate and adjacent trabecular bone are affected (54,55).

Schmorl nodes are relatively common features of the end plate that have been characterized in considerable detail. These vertical protrusions of nucleus pulposus into either (and occasionally both) of the adjacent vertebrae were first described by Luschka in the late 19th century and subsequently named by Schmorl (2). They are found in more than 70% of autopsy spines with equal frequency above and below the age of 50 years, suggesting that they appear relatively early in life (56). Schmorl observed that they were twice as common in men up to the age of 59 years and attributed this to lifestyle factors, in particular a greater risk of occupational trauma. After the age of 60 years, however, they are twice as common in women, presumably at a stage when the disc is more liable to rupture

due to changes associated with advanced age, including vertebral osteopenia. In any case there is clear evidence that discs with Schmorl nodes are more degenerate than other discs at an early age (57).

Schmorl nodes are encountered less frequently on clinical radiographs than by autopsy examination (2,58). In general this is because they are small, but in other instances they can be so immature to have not yet caused any significant structural changes. Ultimately there is loss of disc height from nuclear prolapse or subsequent formation of a cartilaginous cap and eventually new bone around the prolapsed tissue.

Despite being relatively common, it is still not known how Schmorl nodes are formed. It seems obvious that nuclear protrusion can only occur through openings in the end plate, but under normal circumstances these defects do not exist. Schmorl himself suggested that these lesions could result from weaknesses in the end plate due to foci of degenerate cartilage (2). In the absence of significant destruction, such as direct trauma or neoplasm, it is assumed that scar tissue in the end plates is a legacy of the closure and repair of the nutrient vessels in the developing years (59), and this leaves congenitally weak spots through which protrusion is possible (60). The latter study also demonstrated a significantly higher proportion of marrow contacts in the end plates of specimens with Schmorl nodes, and suggested that these lesions could contribute to further pathology such as Scheuermann disease in which they feature prominently.

With the development of implantable devices aimed at augmenting spinal fusion, the end plate assumes a critical role. It was previously thought that mechanical stability, and therefore a good clinical outcome following interbody fusion, could be achieved only if the end plates were preserved, whether bone was used alone or in conjunction with these devices (61). The design of implants therefore appears to be critical for successful fusion. It is claimed, for instance, that threaded cages compromise end-plate integrity, but while nonthreaded cages address this problem, their design generally does not conform to the normal profile of the end plate, providing limited opportunity for bony incorporation (62). The inherent strength of titanium cages offers greater resistance to axial loading, which can be achieved by preservation of the end plates in thoracolumbar column reconstruction (63). More recent work in cadavers however, suggests that an implant with only peripheral support provides the same axial strength as an implant with full support, and that there is no mechanical advantage gained by maintaining a solid implant face (64). In fact, it has been claimed that removal of the central end plate actually promotes graft incorporation without affecting mechanical strength. In another study that has implications for interbody cage design, both the sacral and inferior end plates were shown to be stronger than the superior lumbar end plates, while the central region of both the lumbar and sacral end plates was also identified as being a structurally weak point (65). The importance of preserving the end plate to prevent graft subsidence was further emphasized in a report of compression testing conducted on cervical spine segments (66). As we move from "classical" fusion methods to the realm of spinal arthroplasty, where the aim is to maintain or even restore function as well as relieve pain, it is clear that these considerations will have major implications for the design of implantable devices in spinal surgery (67).

REFERENCES

1. Harris RI, MacNab I. Structural changes in the lower intervertebral discs. J Bone Joint Surg 1954;36B:304–322.
2. Schmorl G, Junghanns H. The human spine in health and disease, 2nd Am ed. New York: Grune and Stratton, 1971.
3. Peacock A. Observations on the prenatal development of the intervertebral disc in man. J Anat 1951;85:260–274.
4. Walmsley R. The development and growth of the intervertebral disc. Edinburgh Med J 1953;60:341–364.
5. Taylor JR, Twomey LT. Growth of human intervertebral discs and vertebral bodies. J Anat 1988;120:49–68.
6. Inoue H. Three-dimensional architecture of lumbar intervertebral discs. Spine 1981;6:139–146.
7. Aspden RM, Hickey DS, Hukins DWL. Determination of collagen fibril orientation in the cartilage of vertebral endplate. Connect Tiss Res 1981;9:83–87.
8. Edwards WT, Zheng Y, Ferrara LA, et al. Structural features and thickness of the vertebral cortex in the thoracolumbar spine. Spine 2001;26:218–225.
9. Roberts S, Menage J, Urban JPG. Biochemical and structural properties of the cartilage end-plate and its relation to the intervertebral disc. Spine 1989;14:166–174.
10. Hall LT, Esses SI, Noble PC, et al. Morphology of the lower vertebral endplates. Spine 1998;23:1517–1522.
11. Harrington J Jr, Sungarian A, Rogg J, et al. The relation between vertebral endplate shape and lumbar disc herniations. Spine 2001;26:2133–2138.
12. Antoniou J, Goudsouzian M, Heathfield TF, et al. The human lumbar endplate. Evidence of changes in biosynthesis and denaturation of the extracellular matrix with growth, maturation, aging, and degeneration. Spine 1996;21:1153–1161.
13. Bayliss MT, Johnstone B. Biochemistry of the intervertebral disc. In: Jayson MIV, ed. The lumbar spine and back pain, 4th ed. Edinburgh: Churchill Livingstone, 1992:111–131.
14. Aigner T, Gresk-Otter KR, Fairbank JC, et al. Variation with age in the pattern of type X collagen expression in normal and scoliotic human intervertebral discs. Calcif Tissue Int 1998;63:263–268.
15. Lammi P, Inkinen RI, von der Mark K, et al. Localization of type X collagen in the intervertebral disc of mature beagle dogs. Matrix Biol 1998;17:449–453.
16. McDevitt CA. Proteoglycans of the intervertebral disc. In: Ghosh P, ed. The biology of the intervertebral disc. Boca Raton, FL: CRC Press, 1988:151–170.
17. Urban JP, Maroudas A. Swelling of the intervertebral disc in vitro. Connect Tiss Res 1981;9:1–10.
18. Roberts S, Urban JP, Evans H, et al. Transport properties of the human cartilage endplate in relation to its composition and calcification. Spine 1996;21:415–420.
19. Pearce RH, Grimmer BJ, Adams ME. Degeneration and the chemical composition of the human intervertebral disc. J Orthop Res 1987;5:198–205.
20. Antoniou J, Arlet V, Goswami T, et al. Elevated synthetic activity in the convex side of scoliotic intervertebral discs and endplates compared with normal tissues. Spine 2001;26:E198–E206.
21. Pedrini-Mille A, Pedrini VA, Tudisio C, et al. Proteoglycans of human scoliotic intervertebral disc. J Bone Joint Surg 1983;65A:815–823.
22. Roberts S, Menage J, Eisenstein SM. The cartilage end-plate and intervertebral disc in scoliosis: calcification and other sequelae. J Orthop Res 1993;11:747–757.
23. Sahlman J, Inkinen R, Hirvonen T, et al. Premature vertebral endplate

ossification and mild disc degeneration in mice after inactivation of one allele belonging to the Col2a1 gene for type II collagen. Spine 2001;26:2558–2565.
24. Taylor JR. Growth and development of the human intervertebral disc [PhD thesis]. Edinburgh: University of Edinburgh; 1973.
25. Holm S, Maroudas A, Urban JPG, et al. Nutrition of the intervertebral disc. Solute transport and metabolism. Connect Tiss Res 1981;8:101–119.
26. Nachemson A, Lewin T, Maroudas A, et al. In vitro diffusion of dye through the endplate and the annulus fibrosus of human intervertebral discs. Acta Orthop Scand 1970;41:589–607.
27. Crock HV, Yoshizawa H. The blood supply of the lumbar vertebral column. Clin Orthop Rel Res 1976;115:6–21.
28. Maroudas A, Stockwell RA, Nachemson A, et al. Factors involved in the nutrition of the human lumbar intervertebral disc: cellularity and diffusion of glucose in vitro. J. Anat 1975;120:113–130.
29. Urban JPG, Holm S, Maroudas A, et al. Nutrition of the intervertebral disc. An in vivo study of solute transport. Clin Orthop Rel Res 1977;129:101–114.
30. Urban JPG, Holm S, Maroudas A. Diffusion of small solutes into the intervertebral disc. An in vivo study. Biorheology 1978;15:203–221.
31. Ogata K, Whiteside LA. Nutritional pathways in the intervertebral disc. An experimental study using hydrogen washout technique. Spine 1981;6:211–216.
32. Crock HV, Goldwasser M. Anatomic studies of the circulation in the region of the vertebral endplate in adult greyhound dogs. Spine 1984;9:702–706.
33. Bernick S, Caillet R. Vertebral end-plate changes with aging of human vertebrae. Spine 1982;7:97–102.
34. Oda J, Tanaka H, Tsuzuki N. Intervertebral disc changes with aging of human cervical vertebra from the neonate to the eighties. Spine 1988;13:1205–1211.
35. Roberts S, McCall IW, Menage J, et al. Does the thickness of the vertebral subchondral bone reflect the composition of the intervertebral disc? Eur Spine J 1997;6:385–389.
36. Moore RJ, Osti OL, Vernon-Roberts B, et al. Changes in endplate vascularity after an outer anulus tear in the sheep. Spine 1992;17:874–878.
37. Crean JK, Roberts S, Jaffray DC, et al. Matrix metalloproteinases in the human intervertebral disc: role in disc degeneration and scoliosis. Spine 1997;22:2877–2884.
38. Goupille P, Jayson MI, Valat JP, et al. Matrix metalloproteinases: the clue to intervertebral disc degeneration? Spine 1998;23:612–626.
39. Kang JD, Stefanovic-Racic M, McIntyre LA, et al. Toward a biochemical understanding of human intervertebral disc degeneration and herniation. Contributions of nitric oxide, interleukins, prostaglandin E2 and matrix metalloproteinases. Spine 1997;22:1065–1073.
40. Roberts S, Caterson B, Menage J, et al. Matrix metalloproteinases and aggrecanase: their role in disorders of the human intervertebral disc. Spine 2000;25:3005–3013.
41. Weiler C, Nerlich AG, Zipperer J, et al. SSE Award Competition in Basic Sciences: Expression of major matrix metalloproteinases is associated with intervertebral disc degeneration and resorption. Eur Spine J 2002;11:308–320.
42. Kanemoto M, Hukuda S, Komiya Y, et al. Immunohistochemical study of matrix metalloproteinase-3 and tissue inhibitor of metalloproteinase-1 in human intervertebral discs. Spine 1996;21:1–8.
43. Brinckmann P, Frobin W, Hierholzer E, et al. Deformation of the vertebral end-plate under axial loading of the spine. Spine 1983;8:851–856.
44. Holmes AD, Hukins DWL, Freemont AJ. End-plate displacement during compression of lumbar vertebra-disc-vertebra segments and the mechanism of failure. Spine 1993;18:128–135.
45. Twomey LT, Taylor JR. Age changes in lumbar vertebrae and intervertebral discs. Clin Orthop 1987;224:97–104.
46. Twomey LT, Taylor JR, Furniss B. Age changes in the bone density and structure of the lumbar vertebral column. J Anat 1983;136:15–25.
47. Vernon-Roberts B. Age-related and degenerative pathology of intervertebral discs and apophyseal joints. In: Jayson MIV, ed. The lumbar spine and back pain, 4th ed. Edinburgh: Churchill Livingstone, 1992:17–41.
48. Ariga K, Miyamoto S, Nakase T, et al. The relationship between apoptosis of endplate chondrocytes and aging and degeneration of the intervertebral disc. Spine 2001;26:2414–2420.
49. Natarajan RN, Ke JH, Andersson GB. A model to study the disc degeneration process. Spine 1994;19:259–265.
50. Moore RJ, Vernon-Roberts B, Fraser RD, et al. The origin and fate of herniated lumbar intervertebral disc tissue. Spine 1996;21:2149–2155.

51. Tanaka M, Nakahara S, Inoue H. A pathologic study of discs in the elderly. Separation between the cartilaginous endplate and the vertebral body. Spine 1993;18:1456–1462.
52. Beggs I, Addison J. Posterior vertebral rim fractures. Br J Radiol 1998; 71:567–572.
53. Lundin O, Ekstrom L, Hellstrom M, et al. Injuries in the adolescent porcine spine exposed to mechanical compression. Spine 1998;23: 2574–2579.
54. Lundin O, Ekstrom L, Hellstrom M, et al. Exposure of the porcine spine to mechanical compression: differences in injury pattern between adolescents and adults. Eur Spine J 2000;9:466–471.
55. Rolander SD, Blair WE. Deformation and fracture of the lumbar vertebral endplates. Orthop Clin North Am 1975;6:75–81.
56. Hilton RC, Ball J, Benn RT. Vertebral end-plate lesions (Schmorl's nodes) in the dorso-lumbar spine. Ann Rheum Dis 1976;35: 127–132.
57. Vernon-Roberts B, Pirie CJ. Degenerative changes in the intervertebral discs and their sequelae. Rheum Rehab 1977;16:13–21.
58. Pfirrmann CWA, Resnick D. Schmorl nodes of the thoracic and lumbar spine: radiographic-pathologic study of prevalence, characterization, and correlation with degenerative changes of 1,650 spinal levels in 100 cadavers. Radiol 2001;219:368–374.
59. Chandraraj S, Briggs CA, Opeskin K. Disc herniation in the young and end-plate vascularity. Clin Anat 1998;11:171–176.
60. McFadden KD, Taylor JR. End-plate lesions of the lumbar spine. Spine 1989;14:867–869.
61. Zindrick MR, Selby D. Lumbar spinal fusion: different types and indications. In: Wiesel SW, Weinstein JN, Herkowitz H, et al, eds. The lumbar spine, 2nd ed. Philadelphia: Saunders, 1996.
62. Steffen T, Tsantrizos A, Fruth I, et al. Cages: designs and concepts. Eur Spine J 2000;9[Suppl 1]:S89–S94.
63. Hollowell JP, Vollmer DG, Wilson CR, et al. Biomechanical analysis of thoracolumbar interbody constructs—how important is the endplate? Spine 1996;21:1032–1036.
64. Steffen T, Tsantrizos A, Aebi M. Effect of implant design and endplate preparation on the compressive strength of interbody fusion constructs. Spine 2000;25:1077–1084.
65. Grant JP, Oxland TR, Dvorak MF. Mapping the structural properties of the lumbosacral vertebral endplates. Spine 2001;26:889–896.
66. Lim TH, Kwon H, Jeon CH, et al. Effect of endplate conditions and bone mineral density on the compressive strength of the graft-endplate interface in anterior cervical spine fusion. Spine 2001;26:951–956.
67. Szpalski M, Gunzburg R, Mayer M. Spine arthroplasty: a historical review. Eur Spine J 2002; 11[Suppl 2]:S65–S84.

CHAPTER 5

Clinical Spinal Instability Resulting from Injury and Degeneration

Manohar M. Panjabi, Vijay K. Goel, Allison M. Kaigle Holm, Malcolm H. Pope

The origin of most cases of low back pain is unknown (1). Clinical spinal instability is considered as one of the most common causes (2). It is hypothesized that mechanical derangement by degeneration, injury, or muscle dysfunction produces spinal instability that results in pain or dysfunction. It is assumed that an underlying intervertebral motion abnormality exists, which is magnitude and direction dependent (3).

Although the phrase spinal instability is commonly used in a clinical setting, there is no single accepted definition (4). Thirty spine surgeons were asked to define clinical instability and its symptoms and signs, and 30 different answers were received! Clinical instability has two parts: mechanical derangement and clinical consequences. It has been concisely put in a definition with which many clinicians agree. It is the loss of the ability of the spine to maintain its physiologic patterns of displacement that cause no incapacitating pain or neurologic dysfunction (3).

Spinal stability is provided by three interrelated systems: the spinal column (passive system); spinal muscles (active system); and control system, which coordinates the muscles in response to the stability needs of the spine (Fig. 5-1). Instability results when single or multiple components of the systems fail or malfunction (5). This conceptual framework is useful in understanding the roles of various spinal system components in providing spinal stability.

Clinical spinal instability may be described by its causes, methods for its diagnosis, and treatments. Past research concerned with these aspects of spinal instability is described. At present, the causes are thought to be injury, degeneration, and muscle dysfunction or insufficiency, or a combination of all three. Diagnostic methods generally include flexion-extension roentgenograms, but other techniques such as magnetic resonance imaging (MRI) are now available. Treatment methods include exercises and surgery. Also presented are future directions for research.

CAUSES OF SPINAL INSTABILITY

The degenerative process of the functional spinal unit (FSU) is usually described by dysfunction, instability, and restabilization (6). (The FSU is the smallest unit of the spine, consisting of two adjacent vertebrae and the connecting ligaments, disc, and facet capsules.) The unstable phase is characterized by reduction in disc height, laxity of the ligaments and facet capsules, and degeneration of the facet joint, which result in abnormal spinal movement. A positive relationship with low back pain was found if the disc height decreased by 40% (7). Osteophytes have been proposed as indicators of instability (8). A traction spur is said to result from increased tensile stresses at the annulus, whereas the claw spur results from compressive loads.

Injury

Microtrauma occurring for long periods may lead to accelerated degeneration and spinal instability (9). This can include occupational exposures (e.g., whole-body vibrations) (10). A major overload may fracture facets and end plates, produce annular tears of the disc, or rupture ligaments, which also may lead to spinal instability. Surgical procedures (e.g., total facetectomies) may cause instability as well.

What roles do the ligaments, facets, and disc components play in providing stability? The contribution of the facet joints in the lumbar spine was experimentally determined to be 50% in resisting torsional loads (9). The other 50% is provided by the intervertebral disc. Using pure moments and measuring three-dimensional 6 degrees-of-freedom intervertebral motions, the effects of

51

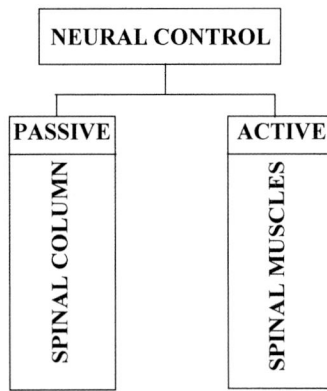

FIG. 5-1. The spinal stabilizing system. A conceptual framework in which the passive spinal column, active spinal muscles, and neuromuscular control subsystems together provide the spinal stability. (From Panjabi M. The stabilizing system of the spine. Part I. Function, dysfunction, adaptation, and enhancement. J Spinal Disord 1992;5(4):383–389.)

posterior ligamentous injury and partial and total facetectomies were recorded (11). With physiologic loads of 8 nm, the average ranges of motion (and neutral zones) for the intact lumbar spine were found to be as follows: flexion, 8.2 (0.93) degrees; extension, 4 (0.93) degrees; lateral bending, 6.2 (0.97) degrees; and axial rotation, 3.5 (1.1) degrees (Fig. 5-2). (The concept of neutral zone is indicated in Figure 5-5.) Cutting of the supraspinous and interspinous ligaments produced a 2-degree increase in flexion, but no change in other motions. Unilateral facetectomies produced increases of 4.2 degrees in flexion and 1.8 degrees in rotation, but no marked changes in other motions. Bilateral total facetectomy, compared with the case with the spine intact, produced increases of 63% in flexion, 78% in extension, 15% in lateral bend-

ing, and 126% in axial rotation. Thus, the facets play a significant mechanical role, especially in rotatory stability. The conclusion was made that the partial facetectomy of one or both facets at a single level does not cause spinal instability, whereas the loss of a complete facet joint on one or both sides makes the spine acutely unstable. These *in vitro* experimental results should be carefully interpreted for clinical use because they do not include the muscles and effects of healing. To understand the role played by all spinal column components in providing stability, fresh cadaveric functional spinal units were studied in response to either flexion or extension loads, while the various spinal components were transected from either a posterior-to-anterior direction or vice versa (12). Vertebral movements in response to transection of the components were monitored in the sagittal plane. This study formed the basis of the guidelines for determining thresholds of clinical instability in the lumbar (1).

Does an injury to the disc repair itself? The disc does not have the healing potential of most other structures in the body because it lacks a blood supply (13). Repair, however, involves a process of vascular ingrowth. The concept of a mechanical self-sealing phenomenon that would seal off the defect was advocated (14) but was later shown to be a fallacy, especially for multidirectional instabilities (15,16).

The process of repair and restabilization after injury, if it occurs, cannot be studied by *in vitro* biomechanical studies. Neither can the clinical studies provide useful information concerning the natural time course of an injury, because all significant injuries in humans are usually surgically or otherwise stabilized. Thus, there is limited information regarding the natural history of most spinal injuries. In a set of *in vivo* experiments using two

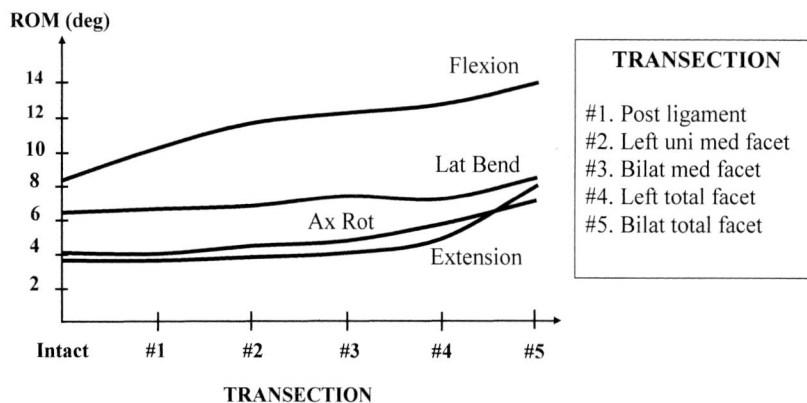

FIG. 5-2. Average multidirectional intervertebral ranges of motion of fresh cadaveric lumbar spine specimens as functions of injury. The motions were: flexion, extension, lateral bending, and axial rotation. The injuries sequential were: posterior ligaments (supraspinous and intraspinous), left unilateral medial facetectomy, bilateral medial facetectomy, left total facetectomy, and bilateral total facetectomy. (From Abumi K, Panjabi MM, Kramer KM, et al. Biomechanical evaluation of lumbar spinal stability after graded facetectomies. Spine 1990;15:1142–1147.)

different animals, three graded spinal injuries (interspinous and supraspinous ligament transections, laminectomy, and facetectomy) at the C4-5 level were studied by functional flexion-extension stereoradiographs for up to 24 weeks (17,18). In these *in vivo* animal experiments, contrary to expectations, the spine at the injury site became more stable (even compared with the intact spine) as measured by standardized functional X-ray studies during the healing period (Fig. 5-3). Although the facetectomy resulted in the largest increase in motion acutely, it also produced the largest decrease in motion *in vivo*. At 6 weeks after the injury, the range of motion (ROM) decreased from 23 degrees preoperatively to 5 degrees postoperatively. These findings are supported by studies using a canine (19) and a porcine model (20). In the later study, explanation was provided for the decreased motion. At 3 months post facetectomy, we found hypertrophy of the facet joints, which limited the range of motion.

Degeneration

For an in-depth description of degeneration, please see Chapter 3.

The spine degenerates with age; this is a normal process that results in altered mechanical characteristics. It also may lead to low back problems. Kirkaldy-Willis (6) provided a classification of degeneration of the spine based on three stages.

Stage 1. Dysfunction. This includes low back pain with nonspecific syndrome. The facet capsule may be lax and disc degeneration is of grade 1 to 2 on a scale of 1 to 4.

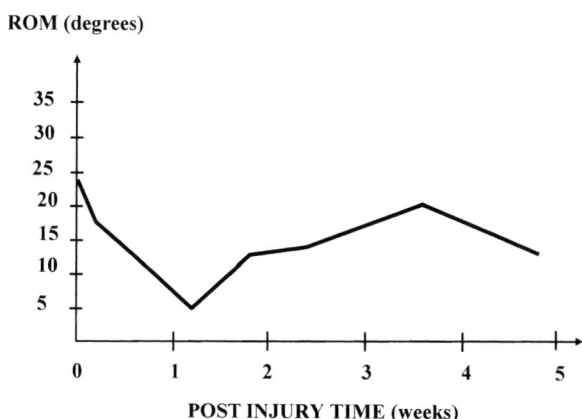

ROM (degrees)

POST INJURY TIME (weeks)

FIG. 5-3. Average intervertebral range of motion at the injury site as a function of healing time. The injury was bilateral facetectomy at C4-5 in a canine model. The injury was unprotected during the entire healing phase, and the motion measurements were made using functional flexion-extension stereoradiographs. (From Panjabi M, Pelker K, Crisco J, et al. Biomechanics of healing of posterior cervical spinal injuries in canine model. Spine 1988;13:803–807.)

Stage 2. Instability. This is marked by increased facet joint laxity and moderate disc degeneration (grades 2 to 3). Clinical syndrome can be identified, and the instability can be measured by functional X-ray studies.

Stage 3. Restabilization. This is characterized by fibrosis in posterior joints and osteophytic formations leading to decreased overall motion. Disc generation has reached the final stage (grades 3 to 4).

A recent study has confirmed the biomechanical aspects of the preceding hypothesis using an intraoperative instrumented lamina spreader (21). It consisted of an electric motor, which spread the adjacent laminae, and the strain gauges attached to the spreader legs, which measured the force applied. Based on a study of nearly 300 patients and 650 FSUs intraoperatively, we conclude the following. The average stiffness reaches its peak of 120 N/mm at about 25 years of age, decreases thereafter to less than 20 N/mm at about 55 years, and then increases once more to about 80 N/mm above the age of 60 (Fig. 5-4). The stiffness seems to have an inverse relationship to the disc degeneration and range of motion.

The degeneration effect on the mechanical properties of the spine is specific and direction dependent. Several parameters may be obtained from load-displacement curves of a lumbar spine specimen to quantify the mechanical properties. These are: the neutral zone (NZ), representing "looseness" of the specimen; the elastic zone (EZ), which may equate with elastic deformation; and the range of motion (Fig. 5-5). Another parameter is the neutral zone ratio (NZR), equal to NZ divided by ROM. In a study using fresh cadaveric lumbosacral spine specimens, intervertebral flexion-extension, lateral bending, and axial rotation were measured and plotted against disc degeneration grade (22). In flexion-extension, there was some tendency for ROM to decrease and NZ to increase. The lateral bending showed significant decrease in ROM and significant increase in NZR. In axial rotation there were significant changes in ROM, which decreased, and in NZ and NZR, both of which increased.

The preceding knowledge has been obtained mostly from *in vitro* experiments. The general degeneration of the spine, seen on X-ray films as decreased disc height, deformed end plates, and osteophyte formation, has not been found to be a reliable predictor of subsequent low back pain. On the other hand, evidence suggests that increased disc degeneration carries a significantly higher risk of low back problems (23). During discography, 23% of patients with nondegenerated discs reported pain, and 77% felt either pressure only or no pain at all. On the other hand, among patients with a severely degenerated annulus, 90% reported pain during discography, whereas only 10% felt no pain or simply some pressure. Thus, a significant relationship seems to exist between disc degeneration and low back pain, even though it may not

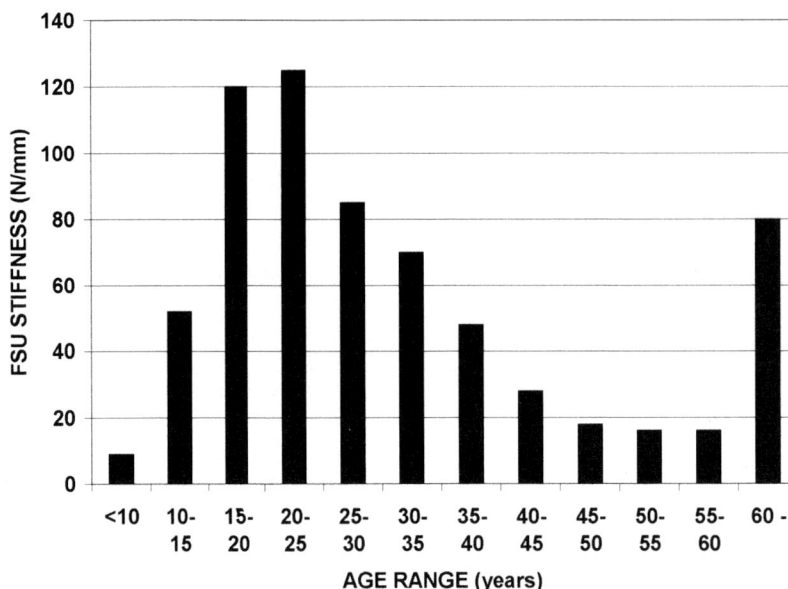

FIG. 5-4. Functional spinal unit (FSU) stiffness distribution with age. (From Brown MD, Holmes DC, Heiner AD, et al. Intraoperative measurement of lumbar spine motion segment stiffness. Spine 2002;27(9):954–958.)

be a one-to-one correspondence. This and similar *in vivo* studies provide a link to the *in vitro* biomechanical studies, by which the mechanical characteristics of the spine and the clinical symptoms of low back pain may be related.

Role of Spinal Muscles

The understanding of the primary role of musculature in providing spinal stability and the extent to which the

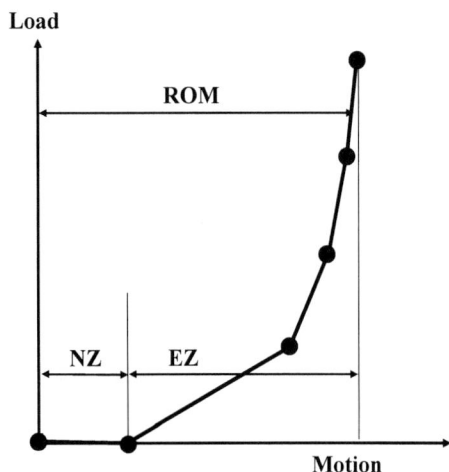

FIG. 5-5. Load-displacement curve of a spine specimen. The measurements for neutral zone *(NZ)*, elastic zone *(EZ)*, and range of motion *(ROM)* are obtained from the curve.

musculature contributes to pain production, modulation, and prevention is not well understood. Muscle dysfunction may result from muscle weakness, in the form of decreased strength or endurance, and possibly from a disturbance in the neuromuscular control system, in the form of altered recruitment patterns. Muscle spasm and pain may be indicators of muscular overload owing to the reduced efficiency in weakened passive structures of the spinal system. As described, muscles form an important subsystem of the overall spinal stabilizing system.

A lumbo-sacral (L1-sacrum) spinal column that is devoid of musculature is a mechanically unstable structure, with a load-carrying capacity of less than 90 N (or 20 pounds) (24). However, with properly coordinated muscle action, the spine can sustain large loads, which is exemplified by the action of weight lifters. In the past, the complexity of the muscular anatomy and physiology hindered the development of biomechanical models for studying the stabilizing role of muscle, as well as various passive components of the spine (e.g., ligaments, discs, vertebrae, and facet joints). Detailed morphologic and biomechanical analyses of the lumbar musculature are now available (25–27). The spinal muscles may be conceptualized as local (intersegmental) and global (multisegmental), which helps us to understand their functions of stabilizing the spine and producing motion (28,29). Advanced mathematical models are helping us to better understand the instability (30).

A modeling study based on radiographs from normal subjects was performed to determine the effects of flexion on the forces exerted by the lumbar muscles (27). The act of flexing caused substantial elongation of many muscle fascicles, which consequently reduced the maximum active tension they could exert. Consequently, it was found that the compressive forces and moments exerted by the back muscles in full flexion are not significantly different from those in the upright posture. However, major changes in shear forces were found, particularly at L5-S1, where there was a reversal from a net anterior to a net posterior force. These shear forces must be considered when prescribing therapeutic exercise, particularly in patients with translatory instability in the lower lumbar and lumbosacral region.

Using an anatomically detailed biomechanical model, the role of the lumbar erector spinae musculature in offsetting the anterior shear forces on L4-5 (58 to 324 N) and upper body mass during different dynamic lifts (squat and stoop) were studied (31,32). They found that, during the squat lift, the maximum peak forces supported by the facet joints and possibly the disc remained relatively constant at approximately 200 N, regardless of the load mass. When comparing the two different lifting styles, the stoop lift, which produced a more flexed lumbar spine than did the squat lift, and had greater contributions from the passive lumbar structures (e.g., ligamentous strain), although the peak moments provided by these tissues were less than 60 nm.

The effects of simulated intersegmental muscle forces on spinal instability in an in vitro experiment have been investigated (33). In flexion loading, range of motion increased and neutral zone decreased with the application of muscle forces, whereas both variables decreased in extension loading. Similar observations have been made in an in vivo investigation using a porcine model to study alterations in segmental kinematics as a result of injury to the passive stabilizing components and stimulation of the lumbar musculature (34). When compared with the unstimulated situation, stimulation of the paraspinal muscles produced significantly greater range of motion in sagittal rotation and shear translation in the L3-4 motion segment after injuries to the disc or facet joints. Although it increased the range of motion, the increased muscular activity also stabilized the injured motion segment. This stabilization was indicated by a reduction in the abrupt changes in the pattern of motion for sagittal rotation during the transitional phase between dynamic flexion and extension (neutral region).

Electromyographic signals of the paraspinal and abdominal muscles have been studied both in normal subjects and in patients with low back pain. Some studies have shown that the electromyographic patterns displayed some abnormalities in patients with low back pain compared with the normal group (35–37). Also, the flexion-relaxation phenomenon of the erector spinae muscle group is absent in some patients with acute low back pain but returns after the pain has gone. The flexion-relaxation phenomenon is the myoelectric silence at approximately

two thirds of maximum flexion angle, at which the load moment is carried by the soft tissues (e.g., ligaments, fascia, and passive elongated muscle) (38,39). It is now believed that intra-abdominal pressure stabilizes the spine (40).

However, studies show diverging results as to whether increased intra-abdominal pressure loads or unloads the spine (30,41,42). The muscles not only apply loads and provide stability, but also help control the posture and movement (5). In a study of low back patients and healthy controls, patients demonstrated poorer balance control while sitting on an unstable hemisphere and had longer reaction times to sudden horizontal loadings (43).

DIAGNOSTIC METHODS

Roentgenographic Motion Studies

Besides the grades of disc degeneration, which are related to a greater risk of low back pain, other motion and posture measures can be obtained from radiographs or computed tomography or MRI images. Functional radiographs (e.g., a pair of radiographs taken, generally, at the extremes of a motion in a certain plane) form the basis of most clinical studies of motion. Knutsson (44) was probably the first to indicate a relationship between excessive anteroposterior translation seen on flexion-extension radiographs and low back problems. In another study, patients with low back pain were examined in lateral bending, and centers of rotation were calculated for various positions of the lumbar spine. An increased area occupied by the locus of the centers of rotation at a particular level was found to be directly related to the pain at that level (45). In another study, motions were measured from lateral radiographs taken in three specified postures (46). Normal patients were found to be different from the patients with spondylosis in translation and rotation and in coupling between these motions.

The spinal movements of patients with low back pain who are suspected of having instability may not always be greater in magnitude. It is known clinically, quantified using stereoradiographic analysis, that patients with low back pain have restricted flexion-extension intervertebral motion. The total flexion (L1-S1) of about 50 degrees in normal individuals decreases to less than 20 degrees in patients with low back pain and nerve root tension signs (47). Associated with the restricted flexion-extension spinal motion are increased coupled motions (i.e., lateral bends and axial rotations). The coupled motion is defined as the associated motion produced during the main motion (e.g., lateral bending or axial rotation produced during flexion). Theoretically, there are up to five coupled motions for every main motion. Both observations may be explained by the fact that spinal instability resulted in activation of the muscular system. Increased muscle forces restricted the overall motion of the spine and at the same time, owing to muscle imbalance, resulted in asymmetric spinal movements (e.g., out-of-sagittal plane coupled motion during flexion-extension). Functional flexion-extension X-ray studies were performed passively on a patient population that was subdivided into different groups having similar pathologic conditions (48). When compared with a normal population, all patients exhibited less motion, except for high-performance athletes who showed more motion compared to the controls. Therefore, it was concluded that a kinematic analysis of the lumbar spine using passive flexion-extension was not a clinically useful method.

Inferior-superior loading using functional X-ray examinations also has been investigated as a measure of spinal instability (49,50). The motion was measured at two extremes of motion obtained by (a) spinal traction (suspending the individual from his or her hands); and (2) compression (using a weighted backpack during standing). Anteroposterior translation measurements were taken from lateral X-ray films of patients who had spondylolisthetic or retrospondylolisthetic displacement. In accordance with the severity of symptoms, the patients were divided into the following groups: (a) asymptomatic patients; (b) those with moderate symptoms and (c) patients with severe symptoms. The degree of primary anterior slip was almost equal in the three groups, but the translator movement differed significantly among them, as follows: 0.7, 5.2, and 7.5 mm, respectively.

Stereoradiographic techniques have been used to analyze three degrees-of-freedom sagittal plane motion (sagittal rotation, antero-posterior translation, and inferior-superior translation) in patients with low back pain and suspected segmental spinal instability (51). The average angular ROM in patients at the unaffected level (9.67 degrees) was not different from that at the affected level (8.45 degrees). The same was true for antero-posterior shear translation values, which were 1.54 and 0.92 mm, respectively. However, the ratio (i.e., coupled shear translation divided by the flexion angle) was significantly different (+0.18 versus −0.13 mm/degree) at the unaffected and affected levels, respectively. The retrodisplacement (anterior-to-posterior translation during flexion from extended position) was associated with the restricted motion, especially for sagittal plane rotations of less than 5 degrees, but was not correlated with the specific clinically unstable levels.

In a recent study, three-dimensional coupled motions were measured in low back pain patients (52). The patients were asked to move in three planes (sagittal, transverse, and frontal) while the intervertebral motions of pedicle screws inserted into the vertebrae above and below the suspected painful level were measured. During flexion-extension, there were small out of plane rotations. During axial rotation there was considerable variability in the coupled motions. The same was true for the lateral bending. The authors concluded that in contrast to well-defined *in vivo* and *in vitro* coupling patterns observed in the controls, the low back pain patients showed significantly greater variability. The inherent coupling pattern of the osseoligamentous spine was modified by the altered muscle pattern or pain.

Other Measures of Instability

Measurement of ROM, especially flexion-extension, is easy *in vivo*. For this reason, the ROM has been used often as an indicator of instability (4). Unfortunately, the ROM is not related to clinical instability, as exemplified by a young gymnast who may have extensive ROM but no clinical symptoms of instability (3). Further, the measurement of the ROM is affected by voluntary effort that the subject applies at the time of examination and motion limitation because of pain. Thus, investigating other measures of motion as possible indicators of instability has merit.

One such variable is the neutral zone, which represents looseness of the spinal column around the neutral position. Support for the coupled motions concept is provided by an *in vivo* study, which documented the presence of these motions in patients with suspected clinical instability (47). The neutral zone has been studied only *in vitro*. The increase in the neutral zone was found to be associated with disc degeneration and its decrease was related to simulated muscle force application (22,33). No direct clinical evidence is yet available. Because both measures are generally smaller in magnitude compared with the ROM, new and more accurate diagnostic methods are needed. In a recent study using ultrasound Doppler effect, the neutral zones of the sacroiliac joint have been measured in subjects without pain (53). Future studies with low back pain patients using this technique will be interesting to see if the neutral zone concept is clinically useful.

Using an intervertebral motion device for continuously measuring sagittal plane motion in the human lumbar spine, the intervertebral motion, along with the overall trunk angle, was measured dynamically during standing flexion-extension, both in normal subjects in patients suspected of having clinical instability in a lumbar motion segment (39). There exists a characteristic pattern of motion during flexion-extension for normal lumbar motion segments and patients (Fig. 5-6). The main findings were the following. Motion was significantly less, by at least 50%, in patients compared to the controls. A 78% reduction in muscle activity at full flexion (flexion relaxation) occurred in controls, whereas only a 13% reduction was found in patients. These observations were explained by hypothesizing that the neuromuscular control system provides active stabilization needed to protect the injured or diseased passive structures from movements that may cause pain, similar to the stabilization concepts proposed by Panjabi (5).

Control L4-L5

Patient L4-L5

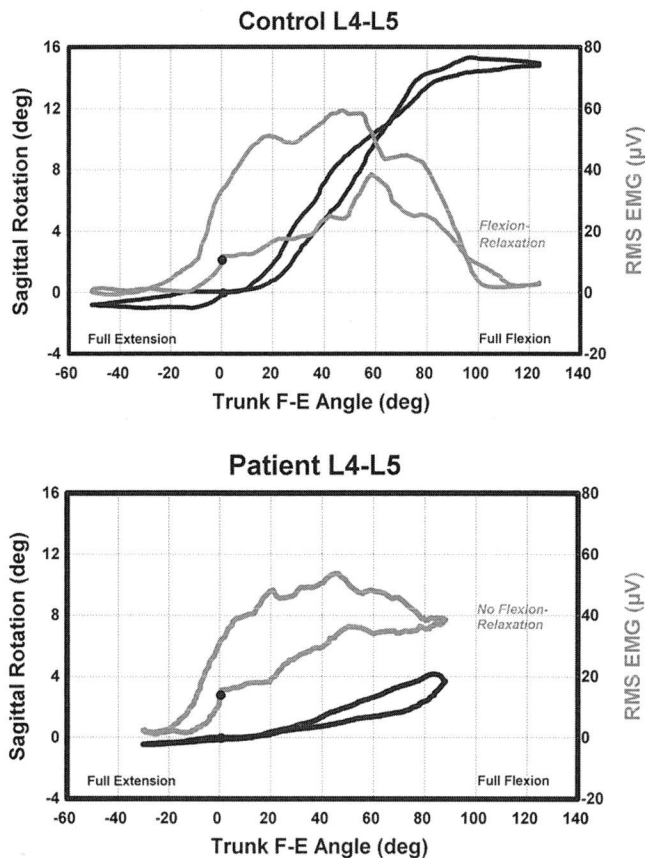

FIG. 5-6. Segmental kinematics (sagittal rotation) and myoelectric experimental data during a flexion-extension (F-E) cycle from the L4-5 motion segment plotted as a function of trunk F-E angle for a control and a patient. (Neutral standing position = trunk F-E angle = 0 degrees. Root mean square of the right-side erector spinae myoelectric activity (RMS EMG).) (From Kaigle AM, Wessberg P, Hansson T. Muscular and kinematic behavior of the lumbar spine during flexion-extension. J Spinal Disord 1998;11(2):163–174.)

TREATMENTS

Spinal instability is treated clinically by diverse conservative methods, some of which seem to be paradoxic. Both the flexion exercises, which strengthen abdominal muscles, and the extension exercises, which strengthen back muscles, have been effective (54). To increase spinal stability co-contraction of both the front and back muscles is needed (55). This may be the explanation for the effectiveness of both the flexion and extension exercises. Rotational exercises have been found to be effective in patients who did not respond to other treatments (56). In addition to strengthening the spinal muscles, improving muscle coordination is important in enhancing spinal stability (5). Muscle stabilization has been advocated and shown to be effective in treating back pain patients (57). Various fusion techniques are reported to have clinical success (3).

FUTURE RESEARCH

Several aspects of spinal instability need to be investigated from the biomechanical viewpoint. A short list is provided.

1. By means of *in vitro* simulations (using human cadaveric material), *in vivo* animal models, and mathematical models, investigate the role of intersegmental (deep) as well as multisegmental (superficial) muscles in providing spinal stability.
2. Develop techniques that measure the dynamic intervertebral motion continuously.
3. Using *in vivo* animal models, study the role of healing and adaptation after injury in altering the spinal stability.
4. Develop new and more accurate diagnostic methods for determining abnormalities of coupled motion, neutral zones, and other motion variables, which may help to provide more sensitive and specific measurements of spinal instability than are presently available.
5. Conduct clinical studies (prospective, double blind, and controlled) that correlate carefully obtained measures of instability of intervertebral motions (representing spinal column) and muscle function (representing neuromuscular control) with the clinical symptoms. These studies may help to bridge the gap between instability indicators and clinical symptoms.

REFERENCES

1. White A, Gordon S. Synopsis: workshop on idiopathic low-back pain. Spine 1982;7:141–149.
2. Moran FP, King T. Primary instability of lumbar vertebrae as a common cause of low back pain. J Bone Joint Surg 1957;39B:6–22.
3. White AA, Panjabi MM. The clinical biomechanics of the spine. Philadelphia: JB Lippincott, 1990.
4. Nachemson A. A critical update and symposium summary. Spine 1985; 10:290–291.
5. Panjabi MM. The stabilizing system of the spine. Part I. Function, dysfunction, adaptation, and enhancement. J Spinal Disord 1992;5(4): 383–389.
6. Kirkaldy-Willis WH. Managing low back pain. New York: Churchill Livingstone, 1983.
7. Nakana T, Nakano K, Nakano N. Does the disc narrowing of the lumbar spine cause symptoms? Proceedings of the International Society for the Study of the Lumbar Spine. Boston, 1990.
8. Macnab I. The traction spur: an indicator of segmental instability. J Bone Joint Am 1971;53(4):663–670.
9. Farfan HF, Cosette IW, Robertson GH, et al. The effects of torsion on the lumbar intervertebral joints: The role of torsion in the production of disc degeneration. J Bone Joint Surg 1970;52A:468–497.
10. Bongers P, Boshnizan H. Back disorders and whole body vibration at work. Amsterdam: Akademisch Proefschrift, University of Amsterdam. 1990.
11. Abumi K, Panjabi MM, Kramer KM, et al. Biomechanical evaluation of lumbar spine stability after graded facetectomies. Spine 1990;15: 1142–1147.
12. Posner I, White AA, Edwards WT, et al. A biomechanical analysis of the clinical stability of the lumbar and lumbosacral spine. Spine 1982; 374–388.
13. Hirsch C. The mechanical response in normal and degenerated lumbar discs. J Bone Joint Surg 1956;38A:242.
14. Markolf KI, Morris JM. The structural components of the intervertebral disc: J Bone Joint Surg 1974;56A:675.

15. Goel CK, Nishiyama K, Weinstein JN, et al. Mechanical properties of lumbar spinal motion segments as affected by partial disc removal. Spine 1986;11:1008–1012.
16. Panjabi MM, Krag MH, Chung TQ. Effects of disc injury on mechanical behavior of the human spine. Spine 1984;9(7):707–713.
17. Panjabi MM, Pelker K, Crisco J, et al. Biomechanics of healing of posterior cervical spinal injuries in a canine model. Spine 1988;13: 803–807.
18. Wetzel FT, Panjabi MM, Pelker RR. Biomechanics of the rabbit cervical spine as a function of component transection. J Orthop Res 1989;7: 723–727.
19. Whitehill R, Stowers SF, Fechner RE, et al. Posterior cervical fusions using cerclage wires, methylmethacrylate cement and autogenous bone graft. An experimental study of a canine model. Spine 1987;12:12–22.
20. Kaigle AM, Holm SH, Hansson TH. Kinematic behavior of the porcine lumbar spine: a chronic lesion model. Spine 1997;22(24):2796–2806.
21. Brown MD, Holmes DC, Heiner AD, et al. Intraoperative measurement of lumbar spine motion segment stiffness. Spine 2002;27(9):954–958.
22. Mimura M, Panjabi MM, Oxland TR, et al. Disc degeneration affects the multidirectional flexibility of the lumbar spine. Spine 1994;19(12): 1371–1380.
23. Vanharanta H, Sachs BL, Spivey MA, et al. The relationship of pain provocation to lumbar disc deterioration as seen by CT/discography. Spine 1987;12:295–298.
24. Crisco JJ, Panjabi MM, Yamamoto I, et al. Euler stability of the human ligamentous lumbar spine: Part II. Experiment. Clin Biomech 1992;7: 27–32.
25. Bogduk N, Macintosh JE, Pearcy MJ. A universal model of the lumbar back muscles in the upright position. Spine 1992;17:897–913.
26. Macintosh JE, Bogduk N. The biomechanics of the lumbar multifidus. Clin Biomech 1986;1:205–213.
27. Macintosh JE, Bogduk N, Pearcy M. The effects of flexion on the geometry and actions of the lumbar erector spinae. Spine 1993;18:884–893.
28. Bergmark A. Stability of the lumbar spine. A study in mechanical engineering. Acta Orthop Scand Suppl 1989;230:1–54.
29. Crisco JJ, Panjabi MM. The intersegmental and multisegmental muscles of the lumbar spine: a biomechanical model comparing lateral stabilizing potential. Spine 1991;16(7):793–799.
30. Cholewicki J, VanVleit JJ. Relative contribution of trunk muscles to the stability of the lumbar spine during isometric exertions. Clin Biomech 2002;17(2):99–105.
31. Potvin JR, McGill SM, Norman RW. Trunk muscle and lumbar ligament contributions to dynamic lifts with varying degrees of trunk flexion. Spine 1991;16:1099–1107.
32. Potvin JR, Norman RW, McGill SM. Reduction in anterior shear forces on the L4-L5 disc by the lumbar musculature. Clin Biomech 1991;6: 88–96.
33. Panjabi MM, Abumi K, Duranceau J, et al. Spinal stability and intersegmental forces—a biomechanical model. Spine 1989;14:194–199.
34. Kaigle AM, Holm SH, Hansson TH. Experimental instability in the lumbar spine. Spine 1995;(4):421–430.
35. Floyd WF, Silver PHS. The function of erector spinae muscles in certain movements and postures in man. J Physiol 1955;129:814–203.
36. Sihvonen T, Partanen J, Hänninen O, et al. Electric behavior of low back muscles during lumbar pelvic rhythm in low back patients and healthy controls. Arch Phys Med Rehabil 1991;72:1080–1087.
37. Triano JJ, Schulz AB. Correlation of objective measure of trunk motion and muscle function with low-back disability ratings. Spine 1987;12: 561–565.
38. Kippers V, Parker AW. Posture related to myoelectric silence of erectors spinae during trunk flexion. Spine 1984;9:740–745.
39. Kaigle AM, Wessberg P, Hansson T. Muscular and kinematic behavior of the lumbar spine during flexion-extension. J Spinal Disord 1998;11 (2):163–174.
40. Hodges PW, Cresswell AG, Daggfeldt K, et al. In vivo measurement of the effect of intra-abdominal pressure on the human spine. J Biomech 2001;34:347–353.
41. Daggfeldt K, Thorstensson A. The role of intra-abdominal pressure in spinal unloading. J Biomech 1997;30:1149–1155.
42. Gracovetsky S, Farfan H, Helleur C. The abdominal mechanism. Spine 1985;10:317–324.
43. Radebold A, Cholewicki J, Polzhofer GK, et al. Impaired postural control of the lumbar spine is associated with delayed muscle response times in patients with chronic idiopathic low back pain. Spine 2001;26 (7):724–730.
44. Knutsson F. The instability associated with disc degeneration in the lumbar spine. Acta Radiol 1944;25:593–609.
45. Dimnet J, Fischer LP, Gonon G, et al. Radiographic studies of lateral flexion in the lumbar spine. J Biomech 1978;11:143–150.
46. Keeson W, During J, Beeker TW, et al. Recordings of the movement at the intervertebral segment L5-S1: a technique for the determination of the movement in the L5-S1 spinal segment by using three specified postural postures. Spine 1984;9:83–90.
47. Pearcy M, Portek I, Shepherd J. The effect of low-back pain on lumbar spinal movements measured by three-dimensional x-ray analysis. Spine 1985;10:150–153.
48. Dvořák J, Panjabi MM, Novotny JE, et al. Clinical validation of functional flexion-extension roentgenograms of the lumbar spine. Spine 1991;16:943–950.
49. Friberg O. Lumber instability: a dynamic approach by traction-compression radiograph. Spine 1987;12:119–129.
50. Käleho P, Kadziolka R, Sward L, et al. Stress views in the comparative assessment of spondylolytic spondylolisthesis. Skel Radiol 1989;17: 570–575.
51. Stokes IAF, Wilder DG, Frymoyer JW, et al. Assessment of patients with low back pain by biplanar radiographic: measurement of intervertebral motion. Spine 1981;6:233–240.
52. Lund T, Nydegger T, Schlenzka D, et al. Three-dimensional motion patterns during active bending in patients with chronic low back pain. Spine 2002;27(17):1865–1874.
53. Buyruk HM, Snijders CJ, Vleeming A, et al. The measurements of sacroiliac joint stiffness with colour Doppler imaging: a study of healthy subjects. Eur J Radiol 1995;87(2):127–133.
54. Williams PC. Examination and conservation treatment for disc lesions of lower spine. Clin Orthop 1955;5:28–35.
55. Cholewicki J, Ivancic PC, Radebold A. Can increased intra-abdominal pressure in humans be decoupled from trunk muscle co-contraction during steady state isometric exertions? Eur J Appl Physiol 2002;21: 117–121.
56. Polermo K, Panjabi MM. Role of trunk rotation endurance exercise in failed back treatment. Arch Phys Med Rehabil 1986;67:620.
57. Hides JA, Jull GA, Richardson CA. Long-term effects of specific stabilizing exercises from first-episode low back pain. Spine 2001;26(11): E243–248.

CHAPTER 6

Spinal Instrumentation

Vijay K. Goel, Manohar M. Panjabi, Huroshi Kuroki, Setti S. Rengachary, D. McGowan, and N. Ebraheim

In recent years, surgeons have well-accepted surgical stabilization and fusion of the spine using instrumentation. Accordingly, the number of available devices for use by a surgeon has increased (1–4). The types and complexity of procedures (e.g., posterior, anterior, interbody) (3) have produced novel design challenges, requiring sophisticated testing protocols (3). In addition, most contemporary implant issues of stabilization and fusion of the spine are mostly mechanical in nature (4). [Biologic factors related to the adaptive nature of living tissue further complicate mechanical characterization (3,5,6).] Accordingly, researchers have designed various methods of testing to assess the mechanical nature of the spine and implants, both as separate and united entities. These evaluation regimens have produced valuable information and have led to the design and development of state-of-the-art systems. The most efficient way to describe the biomechanical issues relating to stabilization and fusion in the thoracolumbar region is to group the literature that concerns the major testing modalities. Results of specific studies are presented to show the type of information provided by the various testing methods.

CLINICAL SCOPE AND OBJECTIVE OF SPINAL FUSION

Low back pain is responsible for approximately 14% of visits to physicians that do not involve preexisting conditions (2). Others have estimated 70% of the population in the United States has experienced back pain in their lives, leading to surgical intervention of the lumbar spine in 4% of the population (2). Surgical treatments most often promote fusion of the painful segments, with an estimated 25% of the 280,000 operations involving the lumbar spine (4,7).

The objective of spinal fusion is to eliminate pain and allow the patient to resume normal activities. Elimination of relative motion between the affected joints often

reduces this type of segmental pain. Spinal fusion is also performed to prevent or correct deformity (3) and stabilize the spine after trauma. Pathologic degeneration of the bony elements, intervertebral disc, and soft tissues are also indicators for fusion (3). Although intervertebral disc conditions seem to account for a significant proportion of the lesions leading to fusion, other indications include segmental instability, both degenerative and iatrogenic, and failed previous surgery. Although the aforementioned indications are commonly cited in the literature as grossly appropriate, there is considerable debate as to the degree of the lesion that indicates fusion (8).

Properly applied, spinal instrumentation maintains alignment and shares spinal loads until a solid, consolidated fusion is achieved. As instrumentation procedures have become increasingly popular, the number of available fixation systems has grown. With few exceptions, these hardware systems are used in combination with bone grafting procedures, and may be augmented by external bracing systems.

BIOMECHANICAL EVALUATION OF INSTRUMENTATION PERFORMANCE

Spinal implants typically follow loosely standardized testing sequelae during the design and development stage and in preparation for clinical use. The design and development phase goal, from a biomechanical standpoint, seeks to characterize and define the geometric considerations and load-bearing environment to which the implant will be subjected. Various testing modalities exist that elucidate which components may need to be redesigned. Not including the testing protocols for individual components of a device, plastic vertebrae (corpectomy) models are one of the first-stage tests that involve placing the assembled device on plastic vertebral components in an attempt to pinpoint which component of the assembled device may be the weakest mechanical link in the worst case scenario, vertebrectomy. The *in vivo* effectiveness of the device may be limited by its attachment to the vertebrae (fixation). Thus, testing of the implant-bone interface is critical in determining the fixation of the device to biologic tissue. Construct testing on cadaveric specimens provides information about the effectiveness of the device in reducing intervertebral motion across the affected and adjacent segments during quasi-physiologic loading. Animal studies provide insight with respect to the long-term biologic effects of implantation. Analytic modeling, such as the finite element method, is an extremely valuable tool for determining how implants and osseous loading patterns change with varying parameters of the device design. This type of modeling may also provide information about temporal changes in the bone quality due to the changing loading patterns as bone adapts to the implant (e.g., stress shielding-induced bone remodeling). After a certain level of confidence in the implant's safety and effectiveness is established through all or some of the aforementioned tests, controlled clinical trials allow for the determination of an implant's suitability for widespread clinical use. The following sections discuss each of these testing modalities, with specific examples used to illustrate the type of information that different tests can provide.

Implant-Bone Interface

Device-Vertebra Interface

Depending upon the spinal instrumentation, the device-vertebra interface may deal with laminae, pedicles, the vertebral body itself, or the end plates.

Interlaminar Hooks

Interlaminar hooks are used as a means for fixing the device to the spine. Hook dislodgment, slippage, and incorrect placement have led to loss of fixation, however, resulting in nonfusion and pseudoarthrosis. Purcell et al. (9) investigated construct stiffness as a function of hook placement with respect to affected level in a thoracolumbar cadaver model. They created posterior ligamentous defects through sectioning and imposed bony fracture at T-12 and L-1 by flexion testing to failure. The unstable spines were instrumented with Harrington distraction instrumentation and interlaminar hooks placed initially on T-11 and L-2. The hooks were relocated to various levels about the affected area and the construct retested. The failure moment was found to be a function of the hook placement. The authors recommended hook placements three levels above and two levels below the affected area. This placement reduced vertebral tilting (analogous to intervertebral motion) across the stabilized area, where fusion is to be promoted.

Transpedicular Screws

Proper application of screw-based anterior or posterior spinal devices requires an understanding of screw biomechanics, including screw characteristics and insertion techniques, as well as an understanding of bone quality, pedicle and vertebral body morphometries, and salvage options (10–12). This is best illustrated by the fact that the pedicle, rather than the vertebral body, contributes approximately 80% of the stiffness and about 60% of the pullout strength across the screw-bone interface (10).

Carlson et al. (13) evaluated the effects of screw orientation, instrumentation, and bone mineral density (BMD) on screw translation, rotation at maximal load, and compliance of the screw-bone interface in human cadaveric bones. An inferiorly directed load was applied to each screw, inserted either anteromedially or anterolaterally, until failure of the fixation was perceived. Anteromedial screw placement with fully constrained loading linkages provided the stiffest fixation at low loads and sustained the highest maximal load. Larger rotation of the screws, an indication of screw-out failure, was found with the semi-constrained screws at maximal load. BMD directly correlated with maximal load, indicating that bone quality is a major predictor of bone-screw interfacial strength. Peiffer et al. and Ryken et al. also found a significant correlation between BMD and torque ($p < .0001$, r < 0.42), BMD and pullout force ($p < .0001$, r < 0.54), and torque and pullout force (14–16).

Since the specimens used for pullout strength studies primarily come from older adult subjects, Choi et al. used foams of varying densities to study the effect of BMD on the pullout strength of several screws (17). Pedicle screws (6.0 mm × 40 mm, 2 mm pitch, titanium alloy) of several geometric variations were used for the study. They included the buttress (B), square (S), and V-shape (V) screw tooth profiles. For each type of tooth profile, its core shape (i.e., minor diameter) also varied, either straight (i.e., cylindrical, core diameter < 4.0 mm) or tapered (i.e., conical, core diameter < 4.0 mm/2.0 mm). In addition, for the cylindrical screws the major diameter was kept straight or tapered. The conical screws had their major diameters tapered only. Therefore, screws with a total of nine different geometries were prepared and tested (Fig. 6-1A). Nomenclature used for identifying each screw type followed this sequence: tooth profile, the shape of the major diameter, and core type. For example, BST represents the screw with the *bu*ttress tooth profile and *s*traight major diameter on a *t*apered core. The screws were implanted in the rigid polyurethane foams (77 cm × 127 cm × 77 cm) (Sawbones, Pacific Research Laboratory, Vashon Island, WA) of three different grades (grades 10, 12, and 15). These grades "simulated" the variations in BMD (10 lbm/ft³, 12 lbm/ft³, and 15 lbm/ft³, respectively) of the cancellous bone of a vertebra. Screws were implanted according to the American Society for Testing and Materials (ASTM: F1839-97) protocol. The

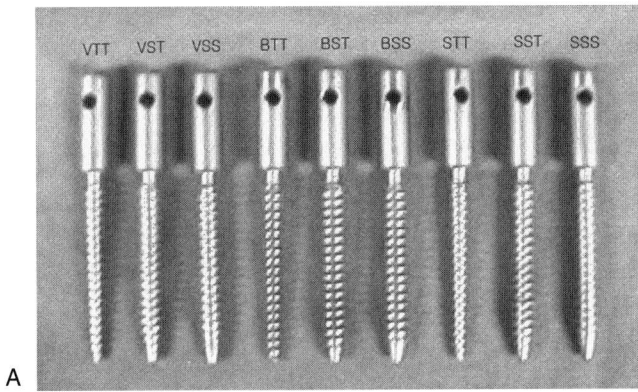

FIG. 6-1. A: Different types of screws used in the foam model to determine the pullout strengths of various designs. The nomenclature used is as follows: thread shape—square *(S)*, buttress *(B)*, V-shape *(V)*; screw diameters—straight major diameter on straight core *(SS)*, straight major diameter on tapered core *(ST)*, tapered major diameter on tapered core *(TT)*. **B:** Regression analysis. The maximum and minimum values from pullout test for each foam grade were used regardless of tooth or core profiles. (From Choi W, Lee S, Woo KJ, et al. Assessment of pullout strengths of various pedicle screw designs in relation to the changes in the bone mineral density. Paper presented at: 48th Annual Meeting of the Orthopedic Research Society; February 10–13, 2002; Dallas, TX.)

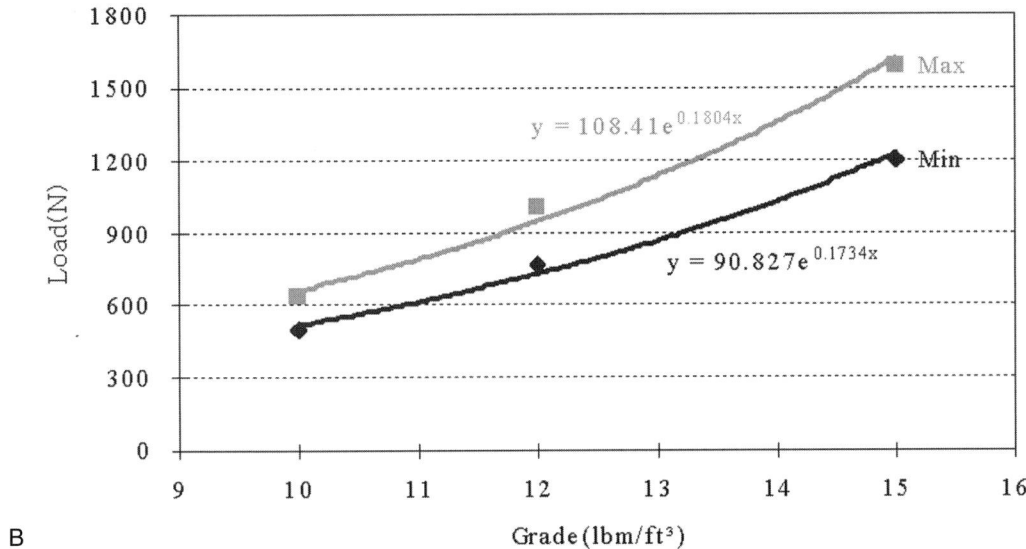

screws were pulled out at a loading rate of 5 mm per minute (ASTM: F1691-98) using MTS858 Bionix Machine (MTS Corp., Eden Prairie, MN). A one-way analysis of variance (ANOVA) test was done for the statistical analysis with SPSS 7.0 (SPSS, Inc., Chicago, IL). Comparison of the pullout strength between the screw types was assessed with the Tukey test and Scheffe test. P values less than 0.05 were regarded as statistically significant.

The maximum pullout strengths for various screw designs are shown in Table 6-1. The highest purchasing

TABLE 6-1. *Axial strength (N) data for different types of screws pulled out in foam of different densities*

Foam grade	Body profile	Tooth profile (mean ±SD)		
		Square	Buttress	V-shape
10	SS	591 ± 22	497 ± 80	615 ± 36
	ST	622 ± 43	598 ± 25	634 ± 19
	TT	525 ± 36	547 ± 30	568 ± 74
12	SS	864 ± 50	769 ± 56	987 ± 55
	ST	956 ± 30	825 ± 108	1,005 ± 92
	TT	811 ± 41	808 ± 25	944 ± 32
15	SS	1,397 ± 93	1,303 ± 126	1,516 ± 78
	ST	1,582 ± 82	1,438 ± 36	1,569 ± 79
	TT	1,197 ± 43	1,352 ± 88	1,396 ± 68

SD, standard deviation; SS, straight major diameter on straight core; ST, straight major diameter on tapered core; TT, tapered major diameter on tapered core.

Source: Choi W, Lee S, Woo KJ, et al. Assessment of pullout strengths of various pedicle screw designs in relation to the changes in the bone mineral density. Paper presented at: 48th Annual Meeting or the Orthopedic Research Society; February 10–13, 2002; Dallas, Texas.

power in any screw design was observed in foams with the highest density (grade 15). Exponential increase in pullout strength was seen when the foam density increased from grade 10 through 15 (Fig. 6-1B). The VST screws exhibited the highest strength while the BSS the lowest with grades 10 and 12. The SST type screws were strongest against pullout with grade 15 foam while the STT the weakest. Statistical analysis showed that regardless of the foam grades or tooth profiles, the conical screws with straight major diameter (i.e., ST types) were stronger than the other two designs (i.e., SS or TT, $p < .05$). Within the ST types, the buttress (B) tooth screws showed the lowest pullout strength among the three tooth profiles ($p < .05$), while there was no statistical difference between the square and V-shape tooth with grades 12 and 15. However, with grade 10 foam, no significant difference was observed statistically among the three. In a case for the SS type screws, the buttress (B) tooth was the weakest regardless of the foam grades. Between the square and V-shape tooth screws, no difference was found. As for the TT types, V-shape screws had higher pullout strength than the square with grades 12 and 15. No statistical differences were found between the V-shape and the buttress (B) screws with grades 12 and 15, nor were any found among the three tooth types with grade 10.

The use of foam for pullout tests afforded a control on the variability in the quality of bone that is prevalent in other studies. Thus, the foam allowed for characterization of the effects of screw variables on the pullout strength. Overall, results demonstrate that the conical screws are consistently more effective against the pullout than the cylindrical designs. This is especially evident when the major diameter of the screw is kept straight. In this case, the contact area between the screw thread and surrounding foam is large. Although no consistent statistical superiority was found with the tooth profiles, results did suggest that the V-shape tooth screws ranked highest in many statistical comparisons and the buttress types showed comparatively lower pullout strength than the other types. This finding may be somewhat different from the literature. This can be due to the absence of the cortical purchase in foam model used in this study. On the other hand, the square tooth screws faired well in terms of pullout strength when the major diameter was kept straight but did not do so when tapered. Results also suggest that as the density of the host site is decreased no clear choice of tooth profile could be found.

Likewise, McKinley et al. developed a synthetic model to study the role of variations in pedicle morphology on the loads in pedicle screws (18). Synthetic vertebral analogs were fabricated, varying in pedicle height, length, or width independently. Pedicle screws internally instrumented with strain gauges were used as load transducers to determine screw-bending moments within the pedicle and body of the analog. Analogs were loaded in compression to simulate loading of an unstable burst fracture.

Screw bending moments within the pedicle increased incrementally with increasing pedicle length, rising 30% as length increased from 8 mm to 12 mm. Screw moment increased 20% when pedicle height dropped below 15 mm, consistent with a threshold effect. Changes in pedicle width did not affect screw loads within the pedicle. Thus, *in situ* pedicle screw loads increased significantly as pedicle length increased and as pedicle height decreased.

Lim et al. investigated the relationship between the BMD of the vertebral body and the number of loading cycles to induce loosening of an anterior vertebral screw (19). (Screw loosening was defined as 1 mm displacement of the screw relative to bone.) There was a positive correlation between the number of loading cycles to induce screw loosening and BMD ($r < 0.8$, $p < .01$). The average number of loading cycles to induce screw loosening was significantly less for specimens with BMD less than 0.45 g/cm^2 compared to those with BMD greater than or equal to $0.45 g/cm^2$. These findings suggest that BMD may be a good predictor of anterior vertebral screw loosening as well, just like the pedicle screws.

These findings of increase in pullout strength, number of cycles to failure, and tightening torque with BMD, however, are not fully corroborated with the corresponding *in vivo* work. For example, moments and forces during pedicle screw insertion were measured *in vivo* and *in vitro* and correlated to BMD, pedicle size, and other screw parameters (material, diameter) (20). The mean *in vivo* insertion torque (1.29 Nm) was significantly greater than the *in vitro* value (0.67 Nm). The linear correlation between insertion torque and BMD was significant for the *in vitro* data but not for the *in vivo* data. No correlation was observed between insertion torque and pedicle diameter. However, another investigation that clinically evaluated 52 patients who underwent pedicle screw fixation augmenting posterior lumbar interbody fusion (PLIF) supports the *in vitro* findings. BMD was measured using dual energy X-ray absorptiometry (DEXA) and radiographs were assessed for detecting loosening and at the pedicle screw bone interface. BMD was found to have a close relationship with the stability of pedicle screw *in vivo*, and BMD values below 0.674 ± 0.104 g/cm^2 suggested a potential increased risk of "nonunion". Similar studies pertaining to screw vertebral body interface for the anterior instrumentation have yet to be undertaken.

The current literature is based on studies of cylindrical pedicle screw designs. Conical screws have been introduced that may provide better "fit and fill" of the dorsal pedicle as well as improved resistance to screw bending failure. However, there is concern about loss of fixation if conical screws must be backed out after insertion (21). Abshire et al. evaluated these issues by pulling out cylindrical and conical screws inserted in pedicles of porcine vertebrae (21). Pullout results were comparable to data from healthy human vertebrae. Conical screws provided a 17% increase in the pullout strength compared with cylindrical screws of the same size and thread design. The results also suggest that appropriately designed conical screws can be backed out 180° and 360° for intraoperative adjustments without loss of pullout strength, stiffness, and so forth. These findings are in agreement with the foam specimen work described earlier by Choi et al. (17).

Most recently, due to the experience gained with the use of pedicle screw-based fixation systems for the lumbar region, surgeons have extended the indications for such devices to the thoracic region. However, most of the basic science work and consequently our understanding of the biomechanics of thoracic pedicle screws is extrapolated from the work of various researchers on the lumbar spine. The specifics of how thoracic pedicle screw biomechanics may differ and hence any differences in use or application have not been elucidated (10).

Cages

Total disc removal alone or in combination with other surgical procedures invariably leads to a loss of disc height and an unstable segment. Both allologous and autologous bone grafts have been used as interbody spacers. Associated with the harvest and use of autogenous bone grafts are several complications: pain, dislodgment of the anterior bone graft, loss of alignment, and so forth. Recently, the use of inserts, fabricated from synthetic materials (metal or bone-biologic), has gained popularity. These may be implanted through an anterior or posterior approach. Interbody devices promote fusion by imparting immediate postoperative stability, by load bearing, while allowing long-term fusion incorporation of the bone chips packed inside and around the cage (22). Anterior procedures used to implant cages often involve extensive removal of the anterior portion of the annulus fibrosis and anterior longitudinal ligament. The strength of the construct relies in part on the tension capacity of the remaining annulus (22,23). The posterior interbody fusion procedures involve removal of various posterior elements. Iatrogenic or acquired (spondylolytic) posterior column instability frequently necessitates the application of posterior fusion hardware. Combined fusions of the lower lumbar spine (posterior arthrodesis with anterior or posterior interbody fusion) usually involve partial or complete facetectomy and removal of the pars interarticulars with the required partial or complete discectomy. These constructs require a significant amount of load bearing by the graft (or cage) construct and posterior hardware to resist external forces (22,23).

The cages of varying sizes, shapes, and materials have been made available to surgeons. Thus, like the screw-bone interface, one needs to understand the biomechanics of cage–end-plate interaction. The interface mechanics are affected by several factors: size, shape, and material

of the cage; end-plate properties such as BMD and preparation (contact area with cage and removal of the central bony region), and the approach used to place the cage. Both axial compressive strength and pullout resistance functions are important parameters to study (24).

Axial Compression Force

In axial compression, higher failure loads were observed with greater bone densities (25). Steffen et al. undertook a human cadaveric study with the objectives to assess the axial compressive strength of an implant with peripheral end-plate contact as opposed to full surface contact, and to assess whether removal of the central bony end plate affects the axial compressive strength (25). Neither end-plate contact region nor its preparation technique affected yield strength or ultimate compressive strength. Age, bone mineral content, and the normalized end-plate coverage were strong predictors of yield strength ($p < .0001$; $r^2 < 0.459$) and ultimate compressive strength ($p < .0001$; $r^2 < 0.510$). An implant with only peripheral support resting on the apophyseal ring offers axial mechanical strength similar to that of an implant with full support. Neither supplementary struts nor a solid implant face has any additional mechanical advantage, but reduces graft-host contact area. Removal of the central bony end plate is recommended because it does not affect the compressive strength and promotes graft incorporation.

Tsantrizos et al. compared compressive strength of PLIF implants using a new cortical bone spacer machined from allograft to that of titanium-threaded and non-threaded PLIF cages [Ray Threaded Fusion Cage (TFC), Contact Fusion Cage, and PLIF Allograft Spacer] (26). The Contact Fusion Cage and PLIF Allograft Spacer constructs had a higher ultimate compressive strength than the Ray TFC. The PLIF Allograft Spacer is biomechanically equivalent to titanium cages but is devoid of the deficiencies associated with other cage technologies.

There are drawbacks to using threaded cylindrical cages (e.g., limited area for bone ingrowth and metal precluding radiographic visualization of bone healing). To somewhat offset these drawbacks, several modifications have been proposed, including changes in shape and material (27–29). For example, the central core of the barbell-shaped cage can be wrapped with collagen sheets infiltrated with bone morphogenetic protein. The biomechanical properties of an anterior lumbar interbody reconstruction using 18 mm diameter threaded cylindrical cages, or barbell cages (18 mm diameter and 6 mm wide at both cylindrical ends, with a round 4 mm diameter bar joining the two ends) were compared. Following the axial compression tests to failure, the specimens with cage *in situ* were then radiographed and bisected through the disc, and the subsidence (or penetration) of the cage(s) into the cancellous bone of the vertebral bodies was measured. There was no difference in terms of stiffness between the motion segments with the threaded cylindrical cage(s) inserted and those with the barbell cage(s) inserted ($p > .15$). The average values of subsidence were 0.96 mm for the threaded cylindrical cage group and 0.80 mm for the barbell cage group (difference not significant: $p < .38$). The femoral ring allograft (FRA) and PLIF spacers have been developed as biological cages that permit restoration of the anterior column with a machined allograft bone (27). Test results demonstrate that the FRA and PLIF spacers have a compressive strength over 25,000 N. According to Bianchi, the average load-bearing capacity of allograft spacers ranged from 10,308 N to 31,015 N (30). Strength dropped by less than 2% per decade of age of the donors and did not depend on the sex of the donor. Thus, the load-carrying capacity of the allografts exceeded the applied compressive loads of the spine. These precision cortical grafts withstand much higher loads when compared to conventional allografts that are composed mostly of cancellous bone.

Pullout Strength

Dietl et al. pulled out cylindrical threaded cages (Ray TFC, Raymedica Inc, Bloomington, MN), bullet-shaped cages, and newly designed rectangular titanium cages with an end-plate anchorage device used as posterior interbody implants (31). The Stryker cages required a median pullout force of 130 N (minimum, 100 N; maximum, 220 N), as compared with the higher pullout force of the Marquardt cages (median, 605 N; minimum, 450 N; maximum, 680 N), and the Ray cages (median, 945 N; minimum, 125 N; maximum, 2230 N). Differences in pullout resistance were noted depending on the cage design. A cage design with threads or a hook device provided superior stability, as compared with ridges. The pyramid-shaped teeth on the surfaces and the geometry of the implant increased the resistance to expulsion at clinically relevant loads (1053 N and 1236 N, respectively) (31).

Construct Testing

Spinal instrumentation needs to be applied to a spine specimen to evaluate its effectiveness. As a highly simplified model, two plastic vertebrae serve as the spine model. Loads are applied to the plastic vertebrae and their motions are measured. This provides some idea of the rigidity of the instrumentation. However, a better picture can be obtained by attaching the device to the cadaveric spine specimen and by evaluating the assembly. One may choose a free level above and below the instru-

mented segment to choose the length of the specimen, as the specimen is anatomically identical to the *in vivo* situation, more clinically relevant results concerning the device performance are obtained.

Plastic Vertebra (Corpectomy) Models

Clinical reviews of failure modes of the devices indicate that most designs satisfactorily operate in the immediate postoperative period. Over time, however, these designs can fail because of the repeated loading environment to which they are subjected. Thus, fatigue testing of newer designs has become an extremely important indicator of long-term implant survivorship. Although cadaveric studies have proved extremely valuable in the evaluation of screw and hook fixation designs, the rapid deterioration of cadaveric material precludes this testing method for long-term fatigue evaluation in which testing may continue over periods of weeks. Protocols have been developed wherein the vertebrae are represented by plastic components, usually medical-grade ultra–high-molecular-weight polyethylene (UHMWPE) (32). A plastic vertebra protocol was developed by Goel et al. (33) for the evaluation of the Kaneda device (first-generation design [DePuy Spine, Inc., Raynham, MA]). The test design (Fig. 6-2) resulted in axial loading, producing a flexion-bending moment secondary to the offset of the hardware

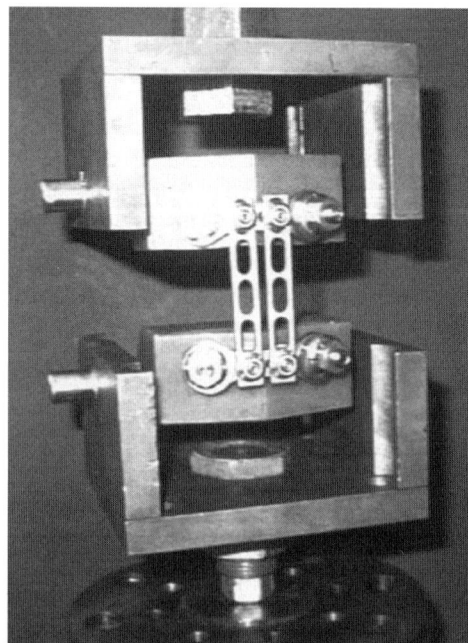

FIG. 6-2. Fixture used to determine the static and cyclic bending failure loads of a posterior device.

from the loading axis. Quasi-static bending loads to failure showed that the paraspinal rods permanently deformed at an axial load of 806.3 ± 6.0 N. This loading produced an associated bending moment on the paraspinal rods of 28.8 ± 0.2 Nm. Fatigue testing showed that the endurance limit of the construct was 380.0 N with a bending moment of 13.6 Nm. The preceding protocol was modified to accommodate evaluation of semirigid or flexible devices using a plastic vertebra approach (34). Because appreciable compression-bending support is not afforded by the flexible devices, the testing protocol was changed to include a steel fulcrum that bridged the UHMWPE block gap.

Cunningham et al. undertook testing of 12 anterior thoracolumbar instrumentation systems in static and fatigue modes using a plastic vertebra model (32). The static destructive and fatigue tests up to 2 million cycles at three-load levels were conducted, followed by the failure mode analysis. Twelve anterior instrumentation systems, consisting of five plate and seven rod systems were compared in stiffness, bending strength, and cycles to failure. Static and fatigue test parameters both demonstrated highly significant differences between devices. The stiffness ranged from 280.5 kN/m in the Synthes plate (Synthes, Paoli, PA) to 67.9 kN/m in the Z-plate (Sofamor-Danek, Memphis, TN). The Synthes plate and Kaneda SR (new design) titanium (AcroMed, Cleveland, OH) formed the highest subset in bending strength of 1516.1 N and 1209.9 N, respectively, whereas the Z-plate showed the lowest value of 407.3 N. There were no substantial differences between plate and rod devices. In fatigue, only three systems: the Synthes plate, the Kaneda SR titanium, and the Olerud plate (Nord Opedic AB, Sweden) withstood 2 million cycles at 600 N. The failure mode analysis demonstrated plate or bolt fractures in plate systems and rod fractures in rod systems.

Clearly, studies such as these involving missing vertebra (corpectomy) artificial models reveal the weakest components or linkages of a given system. Results must be viewed with caution since they do not shed light on the biomechanical performance of the device. Furthermore, we do not know the optimum strength of a fixation system. These protocols do not provide any information about the effects device implantation may have on individual spinal components found in vivo. For these data, osteoligamentous cadaveric models need to be incorporated in the testing sequelae and such studies are more clinically relevant

Osteoligamentous Cadaver Models

For applications, such as fusion and stabilization, initial reductions in intervertebral motion are the primary determinants of instrumentation success, although the optimal values for such reductions are not known and probably not needed to determine relative effectiveness. Thus, describing changes in motion of the injured and stabilized segments in response to physiologic loads is the goal of most cadaveric studies. Many times, these data are compared with the intact specimen, and the results are reported as the instrumentation's contribution to providing stability (35). To standardize, the flexibility testing protocol has been suggested (36). Here a load is applied and resulting motions are measured. Three loads, flexion/extension, lateral bending, and axial torsion, are applied one at a time. It is suggested that the loads be pure moments so that the entire length of the specimen is subjected to the same moment. This method standardizes the testing protocol and helps identify weakness in the construct (36). Additionally, most of these studies involve quasi-static loading; however, short-term fatigue characteristics have also been investigated. Both posterior and anterior instrumentation employed for the promotion of fusion have been evaluated using cadaveric specimens. Examples of both these types of devices, which are discussed within the context of this testing modality, follow.

The stability analysis of devices with varying stiffness is best exemplified in a study by Gwon et al. (37) who evaluated the stability characteristics of three different transpedicular screw devices: spinal rod-transpedicular screw system (RTS), the Steffee System (Variable Screw Plate System [VSP], DePuy Spine, Inc., Raynham, MA), and Crock device (CRK). All devices provided statistically significant ($p < .01$) motion reductions across the affected level (L4-L5). The differences among the three devices in reducing motion L4-L5, however, were not significant. Also, the changes in motion patterns of segments adjacent to the stabilized level compared with the intact case were not statistically significant. These findings have been confirmed by Rohlmann et al. who used a finite element model to address several implant-related issues, including this one (38).

In an in vitro study, Weinhoffer et al. (39) measured intradiscal pressure in lumbosacral cadaver specimens subjected to constant displacement before and after applying bilateral pedicle screw instrumentation across L4-S1. They noted that intradiscal pressure increased in the disc above the instrumented levels. Also, the adjacent level effect was confounded in two-level instrumentation compared with single-level instrumentation. Opposite results, however, are presented by several others (37,40). These authors tested intact and stabilized spines under constant loads. Results based on in vitro studies must be interpreted with caution, being dependent on the testing mode chosen (displacement or load control) for experiments. In the displacement control-type studies, in which applied displacement is kept constant during testing of intact and stabilized specimens, higher displacements and related parameters (e.g., intradiscal pressure) at the adjacent segments are reported. This is not true for the results based on the load control-type studies, in which the applied loads are kept constant.

Lim et al. assessed the biomechanical advantages of diagonal transfixation compared to horizontal transfixation (41). Diagonal cross-members yielded more rigid fixation in flexion and extension but less in lateral bending and axial rotational modes, as compared to horizontal cross- members. Furthermore, greater stresses in the pedicle screws were predicted for the system having diagonal cross-members. The use of diagonal configuration of the transverse members in the posterior fixation systems did not offer any specific advantages, quite contrary to the common belief.

Using an experimental approach in which pressure sensors were inserted into the disc space and strain gauges were mounted on the spinal rods, Cripton et al. determined the load sharing among the spinal components in response to external loads (42). A large majority of the applied moments were found to be supported by an equal and opposite force pair between the intervertebral disc and fixator rods in flexion, extension, and an equal and opposite force pair between the left and right fixator rods in lateral bending. Torsional moments were shared approximately equally between the posterior elements; intervertebral disc, an equal and opposite shear force pair in the transverse plane between the right and left fixators and internal fixator moments. The authors concluded that when posterior instrumentation devices are used to stabilize severe anterior column injuries, the implants may be at risk of fracture secondary to reversed bending moments.

Biomechanical cadaveric studies of anterior fusion-promoting and stabilizing devices have become increasingly more common in the literature, due to this procedure's rising popularity. For example, in vitro testing was performed using the T9-L3 segments of human cadaver spines (43). An L-1 corpectomy was performed, and stabilization was achieved using one of three anterior devices: the anterior thoracolumbar locking plate, (ATLP [Synthes, Paoli, PA]) in nine spines, the smooth rod Kaneda, (SRK [DePuy Spine, Inc. Raynham, MA]) in ten, and the Z-plate in ten. Specimens were load tested. Testing was performed in the intact state, in spines stabilized with one of the three aforementioned devices after the devices had been fatigued to 5,000 cycles at ±3 Nm, and after bilateral facetectomy. There were no differences between the SRK-instrumented and Z-plate–instrumented spines in any state. In extension testing, the mean angular rotation (± standard deviation) of spines instrumented with the SRK (4.7° ± 3.2°) and Z-plate devices (3.3° ± 2.3°) was more rigid than that observed in the ATLP-stabilized spines (9° ± 4.8°). In flexion testing after induction of fatigue, however, only the SRK (4.2° ± 3.2°) was stiffer than the ATLP (8.9° ± 4.9°). Also, in extension postfatigue, only the SRK (2.4° ± 3.4°) provided more rigid fixation than the ATLP (6.4° ± 2.9°). All three devices were equally unstable after bilateral facetectomy. The SRK and Z-plate anterior thoracolumbar implants were both more rigid than the ATLP, and of the former two, the SRK was stiffer. The results suggest that in cases in which profile and ease of application are not of paramount importance, the SRK has an advantage over the other two tested implants in achieving rigid fixation immediately postoperatively. Lee et al. also reached similar conclusions (44).

The biomechanical properties of several different spinal instrumentations have been studied in various spinal injury models. Only a few studies, however, investigate the stabilization methods in spinal tumor vertebral body replacement surgery (45). Thus, the biomechanical characteristics of short-segment anterior, posterior, and combined instrumentations in lumbar spine tumor vertebral body replacement surgery were investigated in a cadaver model. The L2 vertebral body was resected and replaced by a carbon-fiber cage. Different fixation methods were applied across the L1 and L3 vertebrae. One anterior, two posterior, and two combined instrumentations were tested. The anterior instrumentation, after vertebral body replacement, showed greater motion than the intact spine, especially in axial torsion (range of motion, 10.3° vs. 5.5°; neutral zone, 2.9° vs. 0.7°; p < .05). Posterior instrumentation provided greater rigidity than the anterior instrumentation, especially in flexion-extension (range of motion, 2.1° vs. 12.6°; neutral zone, 0.6° vs. 6.1°; p < .05). The combined instrumentation provided superior rigidity in all directions compared with all other instrumentations. Posterior and combined instrumentations provided greater rigidity than anterior instrumentation. Anterior instrumentation should not be used alone in vertebral body replacement.

Lim et al. undertook a study to test the biomechanical efficacy of using polymethylmethacrylate (PMMA) block, tricortical iliac crest bone graft, one large Harms cage, and two small Harms cages as spacers in a corpectomy model (46). The Harms cage, especially one large cage, improved the axial rotational stability significantly in both anterior and posterior fixation groups as compared with the iliac bone or polymethylmethacrylate. No significant difference in the stabilizing role was found among different grafting devices in lateral bending, flexion, and extension. These results suggest that a more rigid spinal construct can be obtained by using a metal cage with improved friction at the cage-bone interface.

Oda et al. nondestructively compared three types of anterior thoracolumbar multisegmental fixation to investigate the effects of rod diameter and rod number on construct stiffness and rod-screw strain (47). Three types of anterior fixation were then performed at L1-L4: (a) 4.75 mm diameter single-rod system, (b) 4.75 mm dual-rod system, and (c) 6.35 mm single-rod system. A carbon fiber cage was used for restoring intervertebral disc space. Single screws at each vertebra were used for single-rod fixation and two screws were used for dual-rod fixation. The 6.35 mm single-rod fixation significantly improved construct stiffness compared with the 4.75 mm single rod fixation only under torsion ($p < .05$). The 4.75 mm dual-rod construct resulted in significantly higher stiffness than did both single-rod fixations ($p < .05$), except under compression. For single-rod fixation, increased rod diameter neither markedly improved construct stiffness nor affected rod-screw strain, indicating the limitations of a single-rod system. In thoracolumbar anterior multisegmental instrumentation, the dual-rod fixation provided higher construct stiffness and less rod-screw strain compared with single-rod fixation.

Cage-Related Studies

Restoring stability to the anterior column is essential for achieving normal spinal biomechanics. A variety of mechanical spacers have been developed and advocated for both anterior and posterior approaches. These devices have been used to enhance the fusion process and reduce the complications associated with the traditional autografts. Due to widespread use of the cages as interbody spacers, we have decided to devote this entire section to dealing with construct evaluation using cages. These studies range from evaluations of cages as stand-alone devices to use of anterior or posterior instrumentation for additional stabilization. The orientation of the cage within the disc space can also be varied. Finally, radiodense cage materials impede radiographic assessment of the fusion, and may cause stress shielding of the graft. The following studies describe the biomechanics of the cage-based constructs from these perspectives.

Cage-Alone Studies

The changes in stiffness and disc height of porcine functional spinal units (FSUs) by installation of a threaded interbody cage and those by gradual resection of the annulus fibrosus were quantified (48). Flexion, extension, bending, and torsion testing of the FSUs were performed in four sequential stages:

- Stage I, intact FSU
- Stage II, the FSUs were fitted with a threaded fusion cage
- Stage III, the FSUs were fitted with a threaded fusion cage with the anterior one-third of the annulus fibrosus excised, including excision of the anterior longitudinal ligament
- Stage IV, in addition to stage III, the bilateral annulus fibrosus was excised.

Segmental stiffness in each loading in the four stages and a change of disc height induced by the instrumentation were measured. After instrumentation, stiffness in all loading modes ($p < .005$) and disc height ($p < .002$)

increased significantly. The stiffness of FSUs fixed by the cage decreased with gradual excision of the annulus fibrosus in flexion, extension, and bending. These results suggest that distraction of the annulus fibrosus and posterior ligamentous structures by installation of the cage increases the soft-tissue tension, resulting in compression to the cage and a stiffer motion segment. This study explains the basic mechanism through which the cages may provide the stability in various loading modes.

Three PLIF implant constructs (Ray TFC, Contact Fusion Cage, and PLIF Allograft Spacer) were tested for stability in a cadaver model (26). Changes in the neutral zone, and range of motion were analyzed. None of the stand-alone implant constructs reduced the neutral zone. The constructs decreased the range of motion in flexion and lateral bending. The data did not suggest any implant construct to behave superiorly. Specifically, the PLIF Allograft Spacer is biomechanically equivalent to titanium cages and is devoid of the deficiencies associated with metal cages. Therefore, the PLIF Allograft Spacer is a valid alternative to conventional cages. Lund et al. has confirmed these results in a similar study (23).

Murukami et al., in an *in vitro* model, compared the stability of a posterior interbody reconstruction using two standard threaded cages (18 mm diameter), a single mega-cage (24 mm diameter), or a reconstruction using dual-nested cages (22 mm diameter (29). After testing, each specimen was bisected through the disc and the surface area of the reamed (exposed) vascular bed was calculated. The dual-nested cages produced the stiffest reconstruction. However, there was no significant difference between the standard and nested cages, and compared with the mega-cage, the only difference was in flexion. The surface area of cancellous bone exposed by reaming for each of the three reconstructions showed the greatest value with the dual-nested cages. These findings, together with the improved safety afforded by the nested or mega-cage, suggest that they are appropriate alternatives to the standard dual-threaded cage reconstruction.

Nibu et al. (40) investigated the stability afforded by the BAK interbody fusion device (Spine Tech, Minneapolis, MN) in four human cadaveric specimens (L5-S1) with implants placed from the anterior approach. The BAK device increased the stiffness of the spinal unit for all motions except extension ($p < .05$) (Table 6-2). Finite element model analyses of the spinal segment with and without the cage have also revealed similar results (49,50) (Fig. 6-3).

The lateral orientation of the cage placement within the disc has been increasingly used for fusion, but a direct biomechanical comparison between cages implanted either anteriorly or transversely in human cadaveric spines has not been performed (51). Fourteen spines were randomized into the anterior group (anterior discectomy and dual anterior cage—TFC placement) and the lateral group (lateral discectomy and single transverse cage

TABLE 6-2. *Average stiffness (Nm/deg) calculated from the flexibility data between zero and 10 Nm load*

Stiffness (N/degree)	Intact	Flexion	Increase (%)
Flexion	1.15	2.12	84.3
Extension	1.25	1.09	−12.8
Axial rotation	8.30	13.90	67.5
Latral bending	1.90	5.54	191.6

Source: Nibu K, Panjabi MM, Oxland T, et al. Multidirectional stabilizing of BAK interbody spinal fusion system for anterior surgery. *J Spinal Disord* 1997;10:357.

placement) for load-displacement evaluations. Segmental ranges of motion were similar between spines undergoing either anterior or lateral cage implantation. Combined with a decreased risk of adjacent structure injury through a lateral approach, these data support a lateral approach for lumbar interbody fusion.

When used alone to restore stability, the orientation of the cage (oblique vs. posterior) affected the outcome (52). In flexion, both the OBAK (oblique placement of one cage) and CBAK (conventional posterior placement of two cages) orientations provided significant stability. In lateral bending, CBAK orientation was found to be better than OBAK. In axial mode, CBAK orientation was significantly effective in both directions while OBAK was effective only in right axial rotation. Owing to the differences in the surgical approach and the amount of dissection, the stability for the cages when used alone as a function of cage orientation was different.

The metallic cages being very stiff may lead to stress-shielded environments within the devices with potential adverse effect on growth of the cancellous bone within the

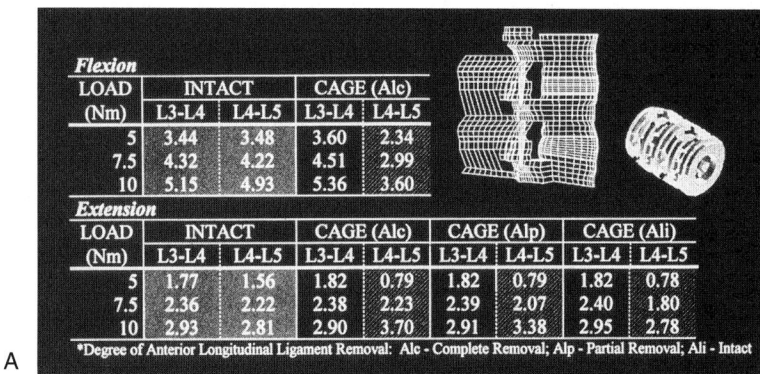

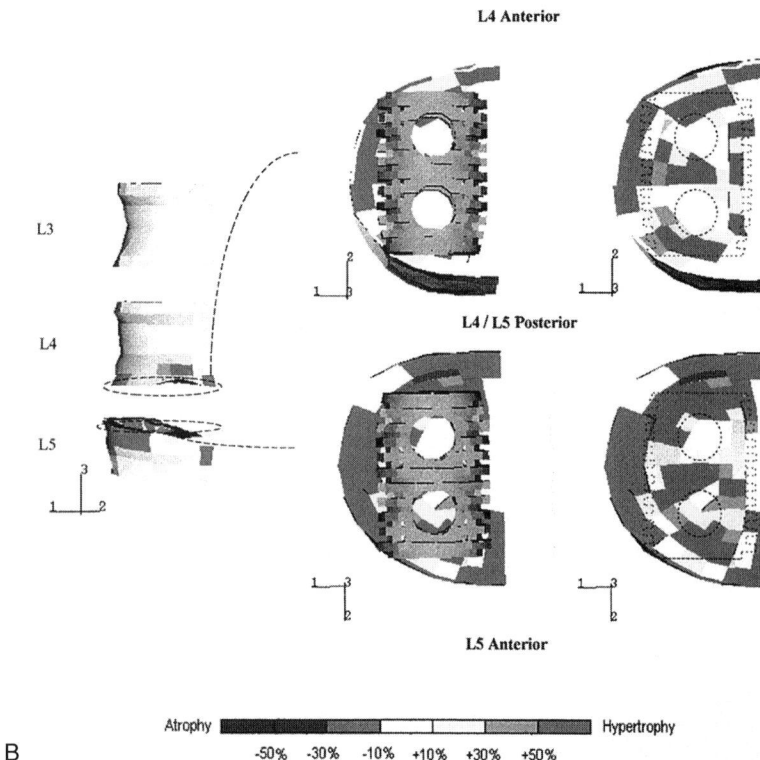

A:

Flexion				
LOAD (Nm)	INTACT		CAGE (Alc)	
	L3-L4	L4-L5	L3-L4	L4-L5
5	3.44	3.48	3.60	2.34
7.5	4.32	4.22	4.51	2.99
10	5.15	4.93	5.36	3.60

Extension								
LOAD (Nm)	INTACT		CAGE (Alc)		CAGE (Alp)		CAGE (Ali)	
	L3-L4	L4-L5	L3-L4	L4-L5	L3-L4	L4-L5	L3-L4	L4-L5
5	1.77	1.56	1.82	0.79	1.82	0.79	1.82	0.78
7.5	2.36	2.22	2.38	2.23	2.39	2.07	2.40	1.80
10	2.93	2.81	2.90	3.70	2.91	3.38	2.95	2.78

*Degree of Anterior Longitudinal Ligament Removal: Alc - Complete Removal; Alp - Partial Removal; Ali - Intact

FIG. 6-3. **A:** The finite element model of a ligamentous motion segment was used to predict load-displacement behavior of the segment following cage placement. *Alc,* anterior longitudinal ligament completely removed/cut; *Alp,* partially cut; *Ali,* intact. **B:** Percentage change in density of the bone surrounding the BAK cage. (From Goel VK, Grosland NM, Scifert JL. Biomechanics of the lumbar disc. J Musculoskeletal Res 1997;1:81 and Grosland NM, Goel VK, Grobler LJ, et al. Adaptive internal bone remodeling of the vertebral body following an anterior interbody fusion: a computer simulation. Paper presented at the 24th Meeting of the International Society for the Study of the Lumbar Spine; June 3–6, 1997; Singapore.)

cage itself (53). Using a calf spine model, a study was designed to compare the construct stiffness afforded by 11 differently designed anterior lumbar interbody fusion devices: four different threaded fusion cages (BAK device, BAK Proximity, Center Pulse, Minneapolis, MN; Ray TFC; and Danek TIBFD, Sofamor-Danek, Memphis, TN), five different nonthreaded fusion devices (oval and circular Harms cages, Brantigan PLIF and ALIF cages, and InFix device); two different types of allograft (femoral ring and bone dowel), and to quantify their stress-shielding effects by measuring pressure within the devices. Before testing, a silicon elastomer was injected into the cages and intra-cage pressures were measured using pressure needle transducers. No statistical differences were observed in construct stiffness among the threaded cages and non-threaded devices in most of the testing modalities. Threaded fusion cages demonstrated significantly lower intra-cage pressures compared with nonthreaded cages and structural allografts. Compared with nonthreaded cages and structural allografts, threaded fusion cages afforded equivalent reconstruction stiffness but provided a more stress-shielded environment within the devices. (This stress shielding effect may further increase in the presence of supplementary fixation devices.)

It is known that micromotion at the cage–end-plate interface can influence bone growth into its pores. Loading conditions, mechanical properties of the materials, friction coefficients at the interfaces, and geometry of spinal segments would affect relative micromotion and spinal stability. In particular, relative micromotion is related closely to friction at bone-implant interfaces after arthroplasty. A high rate of pseudarthrosis and a high overall rate of implant migration requiring surgical revision have been reported following PLIF using BAK threaded cages. A high rate of both pseudarthrosis and implant migration may be due to poor fixation of the implant, in addition to stress-shielding phenomena previously described. Thus, Kim developed an experimentally validated finite element model of an intact FSU and the FSU implanted with two threaded cages to analyze the motion of threaded cages in PLIF (54). The model responses were analyzed, without preload, under forces of axial compression (600 N), torsion (25 Nm), and shearing force (250 N). Motion of the implants was not seen in compression. In torsion, a rolling motion was noted, with a range of motion of 10.6° around the central axis of the implant when left/right torsion (25 Nm) was applied. The way the implants move within the segment may be due to their special shape: the thread of the implants cannot prevent the BAK cages rolling within the disc space. However, it must be noted that the author considered the torsional load value to high; such values may not be clinically relevant. Using a finite element approach, Kim also studied the effects of mechanical parameters at bone-implant interfaces of the lumbar spine segments on micromotion (54). Relative micromotion (slip distance

on the contact surfaces), posterior axial displacement, and stress were predicted as a function of coefficient of friction, loading conditions, and age-related material-geometric properties of the spinal segments. Relative micromotion (slip distance) at the interfaces was obvious at their edges under axial compression. The slip occurred primarily at the anterior edges under torsion with preload, whereas it occurred primarily at the edges of the left cage under lateral bending with preload. Relative micromotion at the interfaces increased significantly as the apparent density of cancellous bone or the friction coefficient of the interfaces decreased. A significant increase in slip distance at the anterior annulus occurred with an addition of torsion to the compressive preload. Relative micromotion was sensitive to the friction coefficient of the interfaces, the bone density, and the loading conditions. A reduction in age-related bone density was less likely to allow bone growth into surface pores of the cage. It was likely that the larger the disc area the more stable the interbody fusion of the spinal segments. However, the amount of micromotion may change in the presence of posterior fixation technique, an issue that was not reported by the author.

Almost every biomechanical study has shown that interbody cages alone, irrespective of their shapes, sizes, surface type, material, and approach used for implantation, do not stabilize the spine in all of the modes. It is suspected that this may be caused by the destruction of the appropriate spinal elements like the anterior longitudinal ligament and anterior annulus fibrosus or facets. Thus, use of additional instrumentation to augment cages seems to have become a standard procedure.

The three-dimensional flexibility in six human lumbar functional spinal units was measured after the anterior or anterolateral insertion of an interbody cage with transfacetal screws (55). The implant used was a central, porous, contoured implant with end-plate fit. The translaminar screw fixation masked the differences in stability due to cage orientation and construct became stable in all directions.

Wang et al. used a multisegmental cadaveric spine model to quantify the load-displacement behavior of intact spine specimens, injured and stabilized using BAK cages as lumbar interbody fusion devices with posterior instrumentation across two levels (L4-S1) (52). The obliquely inserted BAK cage has the advantages of reducing exposure and precise implantation. The biomechanical efficacy of this procedure is sparse, especially in comparison to the PLIF with posterior instrumentation. With the supplementary posterior fixation, the differences in stability due to the orientations were not noticeable at all, both before and after cyclic tests; underscoring the importance of using instrumentation when cages are used as PLIFs. However, the oblique insertion may be more favorable since it requires less exposure, enables precise implantation, and is less expensive.

Tsantrizos et al. undertook a human cadaveric study to compare the initial segmental stability of a PLIF construct tested with supplemental pedicle screw fixation (26). Three PLIF implant constructs (Ray TFC, Contact Fusion Cage, and PLIF Allograft Spacer) were tested nondestructively in axial rotation, flexion-extension, and lateral bending. Supplemental pedicle screw fixation decreased the neutral zone in flexion-extension and lateral bending. It significantly decreased the range of motion in all loading directions with no differences between implant constructs. The biomechanical data did not suggest any implant construct to behave superiorly with supplemental posterior fixation.

Lund et al. examined the effects of cross-bracing the posterior instrumentation in stabilizing the intervertebral disc implanted with one of the three cage designs from the posterior side (23). As compared to stabilization with posterior instrumentation, the addition of cross-bracing had a stabilizing effect in axial rotation.

Cyclic Loading

The function of interbody fusion cages is to stabilize the spinal segment primarily by distracting it as well as allowing bone ingrowth and fusion (22). An important condition for efficient formation of bone tissue is achieving adequate spinal stability. However, the initial stability may be reduced due to repeated movements of the spine during activities of daily living. Before and directly after implantation of a Zientek, Stryker, or Ray PLIF cage, 24 lumbar spine segments were evaluated for stability analyses (22). The specimens were then loaded cyclically for 40,000 cycles at 5 Hz with an axial compression load ranging from 200 N to 1,000 N. The specimens were tested again in the spine tester. Generally, a decrease in motion in all loading modes was noted after insertion of the Zietek and Ray cages and an increase after implantation of a Stryker cage. In all three groups, greater stability was demonstrated in lateral bending and flexion then in extension and axial rotation. Reduced stability during cyclic loading was observed in all three groups; however, loss of stability was most pronounced in the Ray cage group. The authors thought that this may be due to the damage of the cage—bone interface during cyclic loading which was not the case for the other two since they have flat brick-type interfaces.

Animal Models

An approximation of the *in vivo* performance of spinal implants in humans can be attained by evaluation in animal models (56,57). Specifically, animal models provide a dynamic biologic and mechanical environment in which the implant can be evaluated. Temporal changes in both the host biologic tissue and instrumentation can be assessed with selective incremental sacrificing of the ani-

mals. Common limitations of animal studies include the method of loading (quadruped vs. biped) and the size adjustment of devices needed so that proper fit is achieved in the animals.

Animal studies have revealed the fixation benefits of grouting materials in the preparation of the screw hole. Spivak et al. (58) undertook an investigation in which 16 dogs were subjected to bilateral drilling and placement of transpedicle screws from L1 to L6 and sacral alar screws. The lumbar screw population included both standard and plasma-sprayed hydroxyapatite (HA)-coated screws, both with and without HA grout added to over-drilled screw holes before screw insertion. The major findings showed that the HA grouting of the screw hole bed before insertion significantly increased fixation (pullout) of the screws. Scanning electron microscopy analysis revealed that HA plasma spraying had deleterious effects on the screw geometry, dulling the self-tapping portion of the screw and reducing available space for bony ingrowth.

An animal model of anterior and posterior column instability was developed by McAfee et al. (59) to allow *in vivo* observation of bone remodeling and arthrodesis after spinal instrumentation. An initial anterior and posterior destabilizing lesion was created at the L5-6 vertebral levels in 63 adult beagle dogs. Observations 6 months after surgery revealed a significantly improved probability of achieving a spinal fusion if spinal instrumentation had been used. Nondestructive mechanical testing after removal of all metal instrumentation in torsion, axial compression, and flexion revealed that the fusions performed in conjunction with spinal instrumentation were more rigid. Quantitative histomorphometry showed that the volumetric density of bone was significantly lower (i.e., device-related osteoporosis occurred) for fused versus unfused spines. In addition, a linear correlation occurred between decreasing volumetric density of bone and increasing rigidity of the spinal implant; device-related osteoporosis occurred secondary to Harrington, Cotrel-Dubousset, and Steffee pedicular instrumentation. These studies have several limitations, in addition to the ones already stated. In their model, the spinal implant spanned two vertebral bodies completely separated from each other, with the exceptions being the spinal cord and some perispinous ligaments. In patients, a degenerated disc or interbody bone graft (or a similar device) is always present between the two vertebral bodies. Thus, the implant was subjected to 100% load in McAfee's models as opposed to the load-sharing role the device plays in patients. The clinical follow-up studies also do not lend support to the animal model-based findings. Thus, the stress-induced changes in the bone quality found in the animal models are not likely to correlate well with the actual changes in the spinal segment of a patient. In fact, it is suggested that the degeneration in a patient may be determined more by individual characteristics than by the fusion itself (60).

In long bone fractures, internal fixation improves the union rate but does not accelerate the healing process. Spinal instrumentation also improves the fusion rate in spinal arthrodesis. However, it remains unclear whether the use of spinal instrumentation expedites the healing process of spinal fusion (61). Accordingly, an *in vivo* sheep model was used to investigate the effect of spinal instrumentation on the healing process of posterolateral spinal fusion (61). Sixteen sheep underwent posterolateral spinal arthrodeses at L2-L3 and L4-L5 using equal amounts of autologous bone. One of those segments was selected randomly for further augmentation with transpedicular screw fixation (Texas Scottish Rite Hospital spinal system; Sofamor Danek, Memphis, TN). The animals were euthanized at 8 weeks or 16 weeks after surgery. Fusion status was evaluated through biomechanical testing, manual palpation, plain radiography, computed tomography, and histology. Instrumented fusion segments demonstrated significantly higher stiffness than noninstrumented fusions at 8 weeks after surgery. Radiographic assessment and manual palpation showed that the use of spinal instrumentation improved the fusion rate at 8 weeks (47% vs. 38% in radiographs, 86% vs. 57% in manual palpation). Histologically, the instrumented fusions consisted of more woven bone than the noninstrumented fusions at 8 weeks after surgery. The 16-week-old fusion mass was diagnosed biomechanically, radiographically, and histologically as solid, regardless of pedicle screw augmentation. The results demonstrated that spinal instrumentation created a stable mechanical environment that enhanced the early bone healing of spinal fusion.

Strain-gauge instrumented interbody implants were placed into the L4-5 disc space of a motion segment in two baboons (62) to directly measure *in vivo* loads in the lumbar spine by telemetry transmitter. Radiographs were taken monthly to assess fusion. During extreme activity, highest measurable strain values were indicative of loads in excess of 2.8 times body weight. Measuring load on an intradiscal implant over the course of healing provides key information about the mechanics of this process and may assist with the implant design. More recently, Kanayama et al. (61) performed a study in 24 skeletally mature sheep in which they sought to characterize load sharing between the instrumentation and the fusion mass through the osseous union process. The authors destabilized the posterior elements (via bilateral facetectomy, excision of the spinous processes, and excision of the supraspinous and interspinous ligaments) between L3-4 and L5-6. The segments were stabilized with the Texas Scottish Rite Hospital instrumentation, which uses transpedicular screws and short segment rods. Bone graft from the spinous processes and iliac crest was applied to one of the stabilized levels, with the other stabilized level used as the control. Animals were euthanized at 0 (control data), 4, 8, 12, and 16 weeks; their spines were

removed and kept frozen until mechanical testing. The spine was divided into the two-instrumented functional spinal units, L3-4 and L5-6, and each was tested separately. Strain on the hardware was measured using uniaxial strain gauges and loads applied in axial compression (500 N), flexion-extension (±6 Nm), and lateral bending (±6 Nm). After the instrumented spines were tested, the device was removed and the fusion mass mechanically evaluated in the same manner. The data indicated that the posterolateral fusion masses were significantly stiffer ($p < .01$) beginning at 8 weeks compared with the 0-week controls. Also the fusion masses had higher stiffness beginning at 12 weeks ($p < .05$), compared with the instrumented controls. Strain recordings on the spinal rods indicated that deformation with the fusion mass during lateral bending, and axial compression was significantly decreased ($p < .05$) at 8 weeks. Flexion and extension strain recordings showed that this parameter became statistically significant at 16 weeks compared with 8 weeks. This study conclusively showed that the instrumentation became unloaded as the fusion mass developed. [However, as shown in the next section, the *in vivo* clinical investigation of Rohlmann et al. contradicts these findings and thus suggest that additional studies in this area are needed (38,63–66).] Histologic and radiographic evaluations did not indicate complete maturation of the fusion mass even though the mechanical data showed that the bony union had achieved sufficient biomechanical integrity. Studies such as these provide biomechanists and clinicians with observations about how bone adapts to the disrupted *in vivo* loading environment with the implantation of the device to the destabilized area, thus providing a window to clinical performance.

IN VIVO CLINICAL STUDIES

Loads in posterior implants were measured in 10 patients using telemeterized internal spinal fixation devices (63–66). The telemeterized internal spinal fixator allowed the measurement of three force components and three moments acting in the fixator. Implant loads were determined in up to 20 measuring sessions for different activities, including walking, standing, sitting, lying in the supine position, and lifting an extended leg while in the supine position. Implant loads often increased shortly after anterior interbody fusion was performed. Several patients retained the same high level even after fusion had taken place. This explains the reason why screw breakage sometimes occurs more than half a year after implantation. The time of fusion could not be pinpointed from the loading curves. The results showed that fixators may be highly loaded even after fusion has occurred. A flexion bending moment acted on the implant even when the body was in a relaxed lying position. This meant that shortly after the anterior procedure, the shape of the spine was not neutral and unloaded, but slightly deformed, which loaded the fixators. Pedicle screw breakage more than half a year after insertion does not prove that anterior interbody fusion had not occurred. In another study the same authors used the telemeterized internal spinal fixation devices to study the influence of muscle forces on the implant loads in three patients before and after anterior interbody fusion. Contracting abdominal or back muscles in a lying position was found to significantly increase implant loads. Hanging by the hands from wall bars as well as balancing with the hands on parallel bars reduced the implant loads compared with standing; however, hanging by the feet with the head upside down did not reduce implant loads, compared with lying in a supine position. When lying on an operating table with only the foot end lowered so that the hips were bent, the patient had different load measurements in the conscious and anesthetized state before anterior interbody fusion. The anesthetized patient evidenced predominately extension moments in both fixators, whereas flexion moments were observed in the right fixator of the conscious patient. After anterior interbody fusion had occurred, the differences in implant loads resulting from anesthesia were small. The muscles greatly influence implant loads. They prevent an axial tensile load on the spine when part of the body weight is pulling (e.g., when the patient is hanging by his or her hands or feet). The implant loads may be strongly altered when the patient is under anesthesia.

Fusion is currently determined using radiographic techniques. Discrepancies exist between radiographic evidence and more direct measurements of fusion such as operative exploration and biomechanical or histologic measurements (67). To facilitate the return of patients to full unrestricted activity, it would be useful to develop a technique for accurate *in vivo* determination of fusion. The technique developed by Rohlmann et al., as described earlier, is not only impractical for use in a larger patient population but also cannot provide an indication of the time when the fusion has taken place in a patient. Szivek et al. undertook a study to identify strain- gauge placement sites by testing cadaver spines *in vitro*, and to evaluate an implantable gauge bonding technique and subminiature radio transmitter for accurate strain monitoring *in vivo* (67). Three cadaver spines were tested during anteroposterior bending and torsional loading in the control, instrumented, and instrumented plus polymethylmethacrylate states. The spines were instrumented with an ISOLA (AcroMed Corporation, Cleveland, OH) construct, and a simulated fusion was achieved through the application of PMMA. Strain gauges were attached in uniaxial, biaxial, and rosette configurations. The principal strains were calculated. Calcium phosphate (CaP) ceramic-coated gauges were implanted in patients and recovered after up to 15 months *in vivo*. A radio transmitter was developed and tested for use in patients. The largest and most consistent strain changes after simulated fusion were recorded during torsional loading on the laminae of a vertebra directly underneath a hook. CaP ceramic-

coated strain gauges showed excellent bone bonding to the lamina when fusion occurred. Radiotelemetry accurately tracked strain magnitudes and strain rates expected in patients. The consistency obtained in torsional loading indicated that this type of loading will provide the most useful data from patients *in vivo*.

Finite Element Models

Investigations *in vitro* and animal studies *in vivo* contain numerous limitations, including that these are both time-consuming and monetarily expensive. The most important limitations of *in vitro* studies are that muscle contributions to loading are not usually incorporated and the highly variable quality of the cadaver specimens. As stated earlier, *in vivo* animal studies usually involve quadruped animals, and the implant sizes usually need to be scaled according to the animal size. In an attempt to complement those previously discussed protocols, several finite element (FE) models of the ligamentous spine have been developed.

Goel et al. (68) generated osteoligamentous FE models of intact lumbar one segment (L3-L4) and two segments (L3-L5). Using the L3-L4 model, they simulated fusion with numerous techniques in an attempt to describe the magnitude and position of internal stresses in both the biologic tissue (bone and ligament) and applied hardware. Specifically, the authors modeled bilateral fusion using unilateral and bilateral plating. Bilateral plating models showed that cancellous bone stresses were significantly reduced with the instrumentation simulated in the immediate postoperative period. Completely consolidated fusion mass load transmission led to unloading of the cancellous bone region, even after simulated removal of the device. Thus, this model predicted that removal of the device would not alleviate stress shielding–induced osteopenia of the bone and that this phenomenon may truly be a complication of the fusion itself. As would be expected, unilateral plating models revealed higher trabecular bone stresses than were seen in the bilateral plating cases. The degree of stability afforded to the affected segment, however, was less. Thus, a system that allows the bone to bear more load as fusion proceeds may be warranted. Several solutions have been proposed to address this question.

For example, a fixation system was developed that incorporated polymer washers in the load train (Steffee variable screw placement, VSP). The system afforded immediate postoperative stability and reduced stiffness with time as the washers undergo stress relaxation (a viscoelastic effect) (69). FE modeling of this system immediately after implantation showed that internal bony stresses were increased by about 20% over the same system without the polymeric material. In addition, mechanical property manipulation of the washers simulating their *in vivo* stress relaxation revealed these stresses were continuously increasing, promoting the likelihood that decreased resorption would occur. The other solution is the use of dynamized fixation devices, which will be discussed later in this chapter.

The ability of a hinged pedicle screw-rod fixation (dynamized) device to transmit more loads across the stabilized segment compared with its rigid equivalent system was predicted using the FE models (70). In general, the hinged screw device allowed for slightly larger axial displacements of L3, while it maintained flexion rotational stability similar to the rigid screw device (Table 6-3). Slightly larger axial displacements may be sufficient enough to increase the load through the graft since the stiffness of the disc was increased by replacing it (shown as the "nucleus" in the tables) with a cancellous, cortical, or titanium interbody device to simulate the fusion mass in the model (Table 6-4).

The work of Goel et al. described above neglects the effect of muscle forces on the construct mechanics. Rohlmann et al. developed a set of FE models of the lumbar segment to address such issues (66). The diameters of the longitudinal rod of the fixator were also varied to be 3, 5, 7, and 10 mm in the model, and the forces of the trunk muscles were simulated. The diameter of the longitudinal rod strongly affected the fixator loads but hardly influenced the stresses in the vertebral end plates. The stresses in the bridged discs were strongly reduced. However, the internal fixator had only a minor influence on the stresses in the annulus fibrosus and the pressure in the nucleus pulposus of the adjacent discs. These results support the cadaver-based motion data of Gwon et al. described in an earlier section (37).

FE modeling coupled with adaptive bone remodeling algorithms has been used to investigate temporal changes associated with interbody fusion devices. Grosland et al. (50) have predicted the change in bone density distribution after implantation of the BAK device (Fig. 6-3). The major findings include hypertrophy of bone directly in the load train (directly overlying and underlying the implant) and lateral atrophy secondary to the relatively high stiffness of the implant. The model also predicted that bone grows into and around the larger holes in the implant, resulting in sound fixation of the device. Further insight into the biomechanics of the cages using the FE models was provided in an earlier section of this chapter.

TABLE 6-4. *Loads transferred through the "nucleus" and the device for the 800 N axial compression*

Graft	Rigid		Hinged	
	"Nucleus"	Device	"Nucleus"	Device
Cancellous	712.4	87.6	767.9	32.1
Cortical	741.2	58.8	773.5	26.5
Titanium	742.5	57.5	774.3	25.7

Obviously the value of FE modeling is that mapping of the osseous, ligamentous, and instrumentation stresses and strains can be obtained in a relatively inexpensive and time-efficient manner. Predictions of temporal changes of bone in response to the implantation of a device have yielded important data. Also, design perturbations can be quickly assessed as to their relative advantages (and disadvantages).

MORE RECENT FUSION INITIATIVES

The preceding review clearly shows that a large number of fusion enhancement instrumentation is available to surgeons. However, none of the instrumentation is totally satisfactory in its performance and there is room to improve the rate of fusion success, if fusion is the goal. Naturally, alternative fusion approaches (mechanical, biological) are currently being pursued.

The rigidity of a spinal fixation device and its ability to share load with the fusion mass is considered essential for the fusion to occur. If the load transferred through the fusion mass, however, is increased without sacrificing the rigidity of the construct, a more favorable environment for fusion may be created. To achieve this objective, posterior as well as anterior "dynamized" systems have been designed (70–72). One such posterior system consists of rods and pedicle screws and has a hinged connection between the screw head and shaft compared with the rigid screws (73,74) (Fig. 6-4A). Another example of the dynamized antero-lateral compression device (ALC [DePuy Spine, Inc., Raynham, MA]) is shown in Figure 6-4B. Load-displacement tests were performed to assess the efficacy of these devices in stabilizing a severally destabilized spinal segment. The hinged and rigid posterior systems provided significant stability across the L2-L4 segment in flexion, extension, and lateral bending as compared with the intact case ($p < 0.05$). The stabilities imparted by the hinged-type and its alternative rigid devices were of similar magnitudes (Fig. 6-4A) (71). The ALC dynamized and rigid anterior systems also provided significant stability across the L3-L5 segment in flexion, extension, and lateral bending ($p <. 05$). The stability imparted by the Dynamized ALC and its alternate rigid system did not differ significantly (Fig. 6-4B) (72).

Anterior bone graft in combination with posterior instrumentation has been shown to provide superior sup-

TABLE 6-3. *Axial displacement and angular rotation of L3 with respect to L4 for the 800 N axial compression*

Graft	Axial displacement (mm)		Rotation (degrees)	
	Rigid	Hinged	Rigid	Hinged
Cancellous	−0.258	−0.274	0.407	0.335
Cortical	−0.134	−0.137	0.177	0.127
Titanium	−0.132	−0.135	0.174	0.126

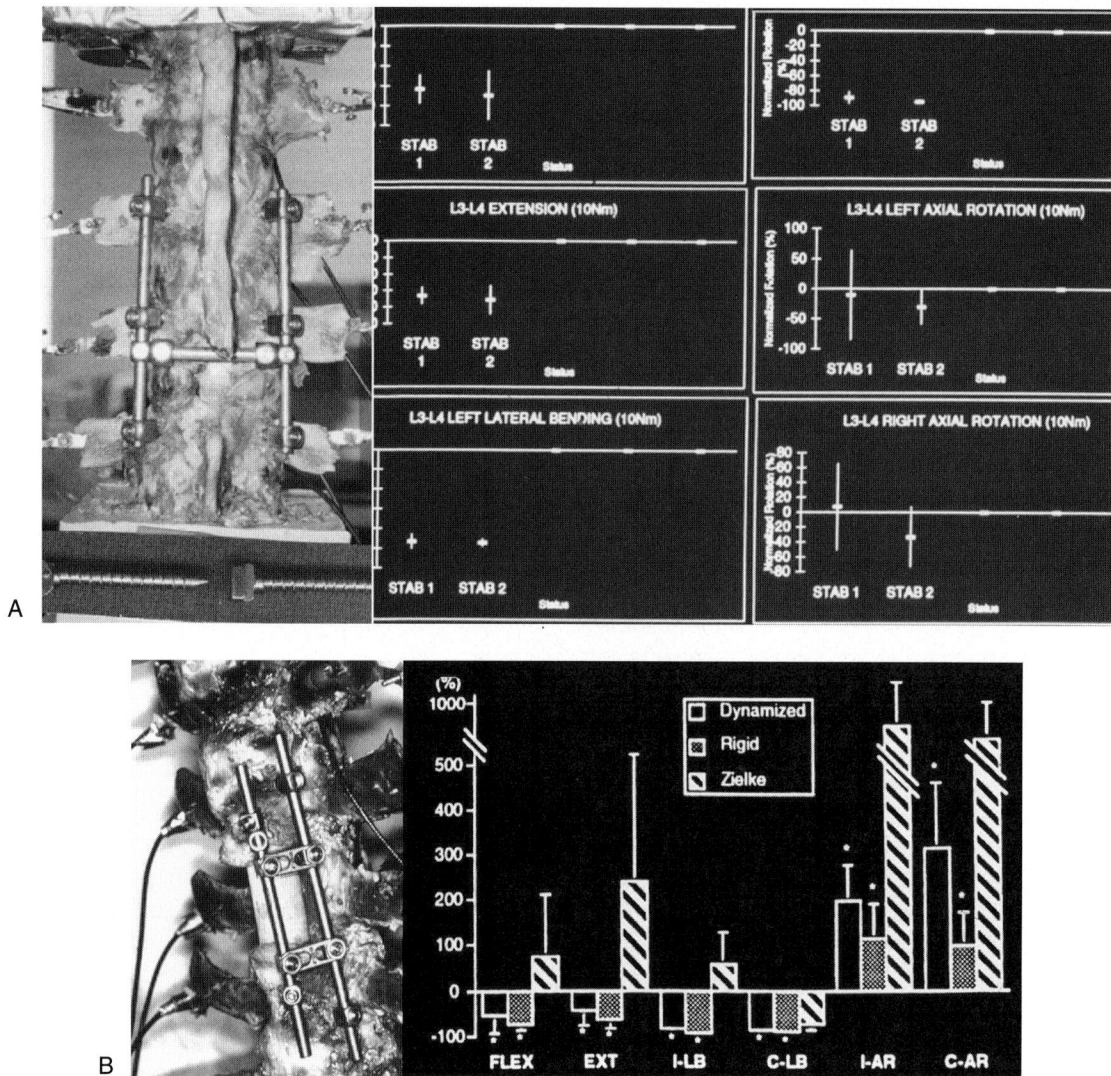

FIG. 6-4. The two different types of dynamized systems used in a cadaver model to assess their stability characteristics. The data were compared with the corresponding "rigid" systems. **A:** Posterior system. **B:** Anterior system. (From Scifert J, Sairyo K, Goel VK, et al. Stability analysis of an enhanced load sharing posterior fixation device and its equivalent conventional device in a calf spine model. *Spine* 1999;24:2206–2213 and Hitchon PW, Goel VK, Rogge T, et al. Biomechanical studies of a dynamized anterior thoracolumbar implant. Spine 2000;25(3):306–309.)

port because the graft is in line with axial loads and posterior elements are left intact. However, employing posterior instrumentation with anterior grafting requires execution of two surgical procedures. Furthermore, use of a posterior approach to place an interbody graft requires considerable compromise of the posterior elements, although it reduces the surgery time. It would be advantageous to minimize surgical labor and structural damage caused by graft insertion into the disc space through a posterior approach. This issue has been addressed by preparing an interbody bone graft using morselized bone (73,74). This device consists of a gauze bag of Dacron inserted into the disc space, filled with morselized bone,

and tied shut (Fig. 6-5). Testing *in vitro* measured the rotations of each vertebral level of mechanically loaded cadaver lumbar spines, both in intact and several experimental conditions. With the tension band alone, motion was restored to the intact case, except in extension where it was reduced (Fig. 6-5). With the graft implant, motion was restored to intact in all of the loading modes, except in flexion where it was reduced. With the tension band and graft, motion was again restored to intact except in flexion and extension where it was reduced. The *in vitro* results suggest that a tension band increases stability in extension, while the bag device alone seems to provide increased stability in flexion. The implanted bag filled

Selspot Testing

MTS Testing

Cavity Measurement

A

Mode	Band Alone	BAG Alone	Band + BAG
Flexion	↓	↓	↓
Extension	↓	↓	↓
Lateral Bending	—	↑	↓
Axial Rotation	—	—	—

B

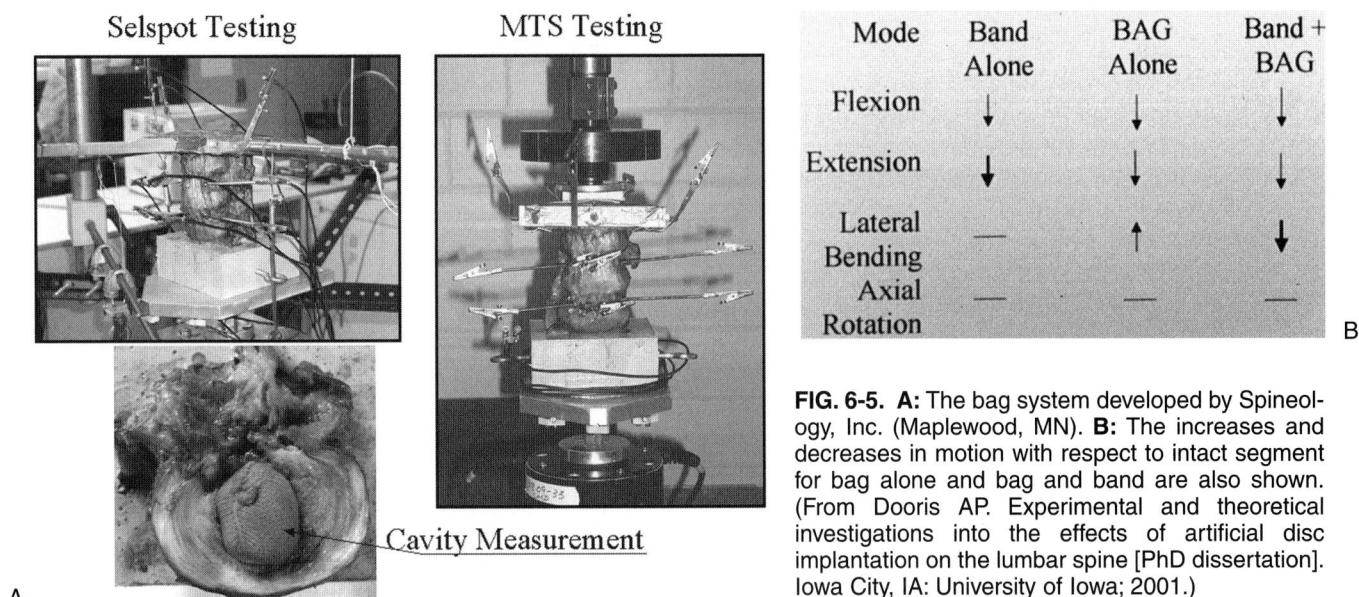

FIG. 6-5. A: The bag system developed by Spineology, Inc. (Maplewood, MN). B: The increases and decreases in motion with respect to intact segment for bag alone and bag and band are also shown. (From Dooris AP. Experimental and theoretical investigations into the effects of artificial disc implantation on the lumbar spine [PhD dissertation]. Iowa City, IA: University of Iowa; 2001.)

with morselized bone in combination with a posterior tension band, restores intact stiffness. Postcyclic results in axial compression suggest that the morselized bone in the bone-only specimens either consolidates or extrudes from the cavity despite confinement. Motion restoration or reduction as tested here is relevant both to graft incorporation and segment biomechanics. The posterior interbody grafting method using morselized bone is amenable to orthoscopy. It produces an interbody graft without an anterior surgical approach. In addition, this technique greatly reduces surgical exposure with minimal blood loss and no facet compromise. This technique would be a viable alternative to current 360° techniques pending animal tests and clinical trials.

Bone grafting is used to augment bone healing and provide stability after spinal surgery. Autologous bone graft is limited in quantity and unfortunately associated with increased surgical time and donor-site morbidity. Recent research has provided insight into methods that may modulate the bone healing process at the cellular level in addition to reversing the effects of symptomatic disc degeneration which is a potentially disabling condition, managed frequently with various fusion procedures. Alternatives to autologous bone graft include allograft bone, demineralized bone matrix, recombinant growth factors, and synthetic implants. Each of these alternatives could possibly be combined with autologous bone marrow or various growth factors. Although none of the presently available substitutes provides all three of the fundamental properties of autograft bone (osteogeneticity, osteoconductivity, and osteoinductivity), there are a number of situations in which they have proven clinically useful. A literature review indicates that alternatives to autogenous bone grafting find their greatest appeal when autograft bone is limited in supply or when acceptable

rates of fusion may be achieved with these substitutes (75). For example, bone morphogenetic proteins have been shown to induce bone formation and repair (75).

Relatively little research has been undertaken to investigate the efficacy of osteoconductive protein 1 (OP-1) in the aforementioned stated role (75,76). Grauer et al. performed single-level intertransverse process lumbar fusions at L5-L6 in 31 New Zealand White rabbits (76). These were divided into three study groups: autograft, carrier alone, and carrier with OP-1. The animals were euthanized 5 weeks after surgery. Five (63%) of the eight in the autograft group had fusion detected by manual palpation, none (0%) of the eight in the carrier-alone group had fusion, and all eight (100%) in the OP-1 group had fusion. Biomechanical testing results correlated well with those of manual palpation. Histologically, autograft specimens were predominantly fibrocartilage, OP-1 specimens were predominantly maturing bone, and carrier-alone specimens did not show significant bone formation. OP-1 was found to reliably induce solid intertransverse process fusion in a rabbit model at 5 weeks.

Smoking interferes with the success of posterolateral lumbar fusion and a group of authors from the aforementioned investigation extended their study to review the effect of using OP-1 to enhance the fusion process in patients who smoke (77). OP-1 was able to overcome the inhibitory effects of nicotine in a rabbit posterolateral spine fusion model, and to induce bony fusion reliably at 5 weeks.

Magin et al. undertook a study to determine whether the use of recombinant human (rh) OP-1 or HA would improve on the intercorporal fusion achieved by interbody autologous bone grafting in a sheep model (78). Vertebral fusion quality was examined by plain radiograph at 4-week intervals, by scintigraphy at 3 and 6 months, and by computed tomography scan, magnetic resonance imaging, biomechanical testing, and histologic evaluation. All examination methods demonstrated superior fusion after administration of rhOP-1, with radiologic fusion apparent at 4 months. Autologous bone grafts eventually produced bony healing in most cases, albeit of a lower quality than with rhOP-1. HA use led only to the formation of a tight pseudoarthrosis. The results indicated that rhOP-1 use was an appropriate method for improving interbody fusion in the sheep spine. In addition to offering the potential for improved bone healing, rhOP-1 use may permit less invasive surgery such as transpedicular fusion and the use of cages. In another similar study, Sandhu et al. investigated the efficacy of recombinant human bone morphogenetic protein 2 (rhBMP-2)-collagen composite in comparison with autograft to enhance spinal interbody fusion. Comparisons were drawn from temporal radiographic and end-point biomechanical and histologic data (79). Twelve sheep underwent single-level anterior lumbar interbody fusion performed with a cylindrical fenestrated titanium interbody fusion device (INTER FIX, Medtronic Sofamor Danek, Inc., Memphis, TN). The device was filled either with rhBMP-2-collagen (n < 6) or autogenous iliac crest bone graft (n < 6). Radiographs revealed a bony bridge anterior to the cage in five of six rhBMP-2-treated animals, whereas it was present only in one of five in the autogenous bone graft group. Segments treated with rhBMP-2 were 20% stiffer in flexion than autograft-treated segments at 6 months. All six in the rhBMP-2 group and two of six in the autograft group showed complete fusion. There was a significantly higher rate of bony continuity observed at the fenestrations of the rhBMP-2 group. Three times more cage fenestrations in the rhBMP-2 group demonstrated "all-bone" when compared with the autograft group ($p < .001$). Further, the scar tissue in and around the autograft-treated cages was 16-fold more ($p < .01$) than that seen for rhBMP-2-treated cages. The study demonstrated that rhBMP-2 can lead to earlier radiologic fusion and a more consistent increased stiffness of the segments when compared with autograft in sheep anterior lumbar interbody fusion. Furthermore, a three times higher histologic fusion rate was attainable with significantly reduced fibrous tissue around the implant when rhBMP-2 is used.

NONFUSION TREATMENT ALTERNATIVES

Various methods have been employed in the characterization of device effectiveness for which spinal fusion is indicated. Because of the nonphysiologic nature of fusing the spinal segments that are supposed to provide motion/flexibility, adjacent-level degeneration, and other complications associated with the fusion process, alternatives to fusion have been proposed.

Nucleus Replacements

Ray Nucleus

In 1988 Ray presented a prosthetic nuclear replacement consisting of flexible woven filaments (Dacron) surrounding an internal semipermeable polyethylene membranous sac filled with hyaluronic acid and a thixotropic agent (i.e., a hydrogel) (73,80). As a nucleus replacement, the implant can be inserted similar to a thoracolumbar interbody fusion device, either posteriorly or transversely. Two are inserted per disc level in a partly collapsed and dehydrated state, but would swell due to the strongly hygroscopic properties of the hyaluronic acid constituent. The designer expects the implant to swell enough to distract the segment while retain enough flexibility to allow a normal range of motion. An option is to include therapeutic agents in the gel that would be released by water flow in and out of the prosthesis according to external pressures.

Recent reports on biomechanical tests of the device show that it can produce some degree of stabilization and distraction (73,80). Loads of 7.5 Nm and 200 N axial were applied to six L4-L5 specimens. Nucleotomized spines increased rotations by 12% to 18% depending on load orientation, but implanted spines (implant placed transversely) showed a change of −12% to +2% from the intact with substantial reductions in neutral zone. Up to 2 mm of disc height was recovered by insertion. The implant, however, was implanted and tested in its nonhydrated form. The biomechanics of the hydrated prosthesis may vary considerably from its desiccated form.

In situ Curable Prosthetic Intervertebral Nucleus Device

The prosthetic intervertebral nucleus (PIN) device (Disc Dynamics, Inc., Minnetonka, MN) consists of a compliant balloon connected to a catheter (Fig. 6-6) (73,74). This is inserted and liquid polymer injected into the balloon under controlled pressure inflating the balloon, filling the cavity, and distracting the intervertebral disc. Within 5 minutes the polymer is cured. Five fresh-frozen osteoligamentous three-segment human lumbar spines, screened for abnormal radiograph and low bone density, were used for the biomechanical study. The spines were tested under four conditions: intact, denucleated, implanted, and fatigued. Fatiguing was produced by cyclic loading from 250 to 750 N at 2 Hz for at least 100,000 cycles. Nucleotomy was performed through a 5.5 mm trephine hole in the right middle lateral side of the annulus. The device was placed in the nuclear cavity as described earlier. Following biomechanical tests, these specimens were radiographed and dissected to determine any structural damage inflicted during testing. Middle segment rotations generally increased with discectomy

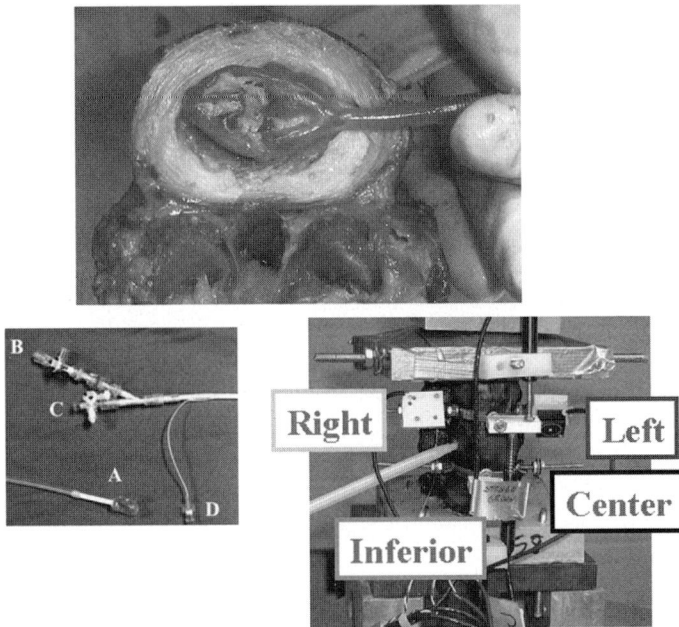

FIG. 6-6. *In situ* curable prosthetic intervertebral nucleus (PIN) device being developed by Disc Dynamics, Inc., Minnetonka, MN. (From Dooris AP. Experimental and theoretical investigations into the effects of artificial disc implantation on the lumbar spine [PhD dissertation]. Iowa City, IA: University of Iowa; 2001.)

but were restored to the normal intact range with implantation. After fatiguing, rotations across the implanted segment increased. However, these were not more than, and often less than the intact adjacent segments. During polymer injection under compressive load, the segment distracted as much as +1.8 mm (average) at the disc center as determined by the surrounding gauges. Over 1.6 mm was maintained during polymer cure with compression. The immediate goals of a disc replacement system are to restore disc height and provide segment mobility without causing instability. This study showed that the PIN device could reverse the destabilizing effects of a nucleotomy and restore normal segment stiffness. Significant increases in disc height can also be achieved. Implanting the majority of disc replacement systems requires significant annulus removal. This device requires minimal surgical compromise and has the potential to be performed arthroscopically.

Artificial Disc

One of the most recent developments for nonfusion treatment alternatives is replacement of the intervertebral disc. The goal of this treatment alternative is to restore the original mechanical function of the resected disc (81). One of the stipulations of artificial disc replacement is that the remaining osseous spinal and paraspinal soft tissue components are not compromised by pathologic changes. Bao et al. (82) have classified the designs of total disc replacements into four categories: (a) low-friction sliding surface; (b) spring and hinge systems; (c) contained fluid-filled chambers; and (d) discs of rubber and other elastomers. The former two designs seek to take advantage of the inherently high fatigue characteristics

that all-metal designs afford. The latter two designs attempt to incorporate some of the viscoelastic and compliant properties that are exhibited by the normal, healthy intervertebral disc. The disc must be able to maintain its mechanical integrity to approximately 85 million cycles; consist of biocompatible materials; exist entirely within the normal disc space and maintain physiologic disc height; restore normal kinematic motion wherein the axes of each motion, especially sagittal plane motion, are correctly replicated; duplicate the intact disc stiffness in all three planes of rotation and compression; provide immediate and long-term fixation to bone; and, finally, provide *fail-safe* mechanisms so that if an individual component of the design fails, catastrophic failure is not immediately imminent and does not lead to peri-implant soft tissue damage. This is certainly one of the greatest design challenges that bioengineers have encountered to date. In the following paragraphs, some of the methods are discussed that are being employed in an attempt to meet this rigorous challenge.

One of the available studies reviews iterative design of the artificial disc replacement based on measured biomechanical properties. Lee et al. (83,84) looked at incorporating three different polymers into their prosthetic intervertebral disc design and tried to represent the separate components (annulus fibrosis and nucleus) of the normal disc in varying proportion. They loaded their designs under 800 N axial compression and in compression-torsion out to 5°. The results indicated that discs fabricated from homogeneous materials exhibited isotropy that could not replicate the anisotropic behavior of the normal human disc. Thus, 12 layers of fiber reinforcement were incorporated in an attempt to mimic the actual annulus fibrosis. This method did result in more closely approxi-

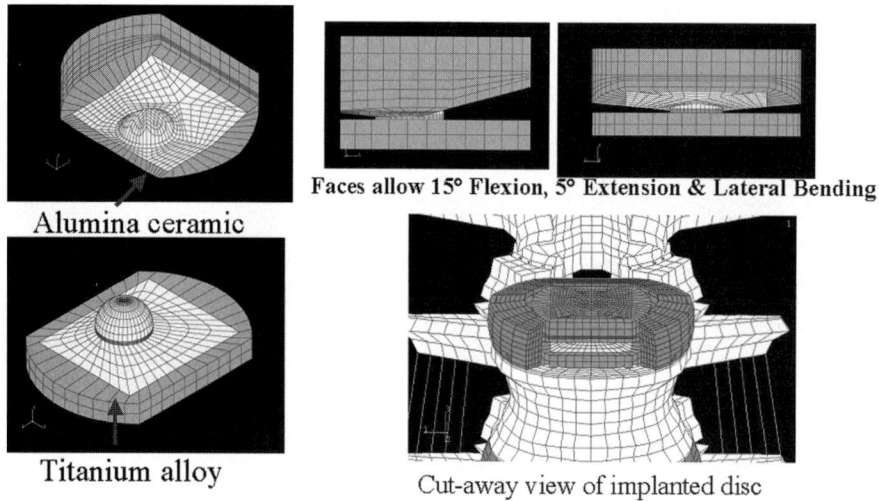

FIG. 6-7. The intact finite element model of a ligamentous segment was modified to simulate the ball-and-socket type artificial disc implant. (From Dooris AP. Experimental and theoretical investigations into the effects of artificial disc implantation on the lumbar spine [PhD dissertation]. Iowa City, IA: University of Iowa; 2001.)

mating the mechanical properties of the normal disc. Through this method of redesign and testing, the authors claim that eventually "a disc prosthesis that has mechanical properties comparable to the natural disc could be manufactured" (83, 84).

Another artificial intervertebral disc has been developed, and its intrinsic biomechanical properties, bioactivity, and effectiveness as a total disc replacement were evaluated *in vitro* and *in vivo* (85). The artificial intervertebral disc consists of a triaxial three-dimensional fabric (3-DF) woven with a UHMWPE fiber, and spray-coated with bioactive ceramics on the disc surface. The arrangement of weave properties was designed to produce mechanical behavior nearly equivalent to the natural intervertebral disc. Total intervertebral disc replacement at L2-L3 and L4-L5 was performed using a 3-DF disc with or without internal fixation in a sheep lumbar spine model. The segmental biomechanics and interface histology were evaluated after surgery at 4 and 6 months. The tensile-compressive and torsional properties of prototype

3-DF were nearly equivalent to those of human lumbar disc. The lumbar segments replaced with the 3-DF disc alone showed a significant decrease of flexion-extension range of motion to 28% of control values as well as partial bony fusion at 6 months. However, the use of temporary fixation provided a nearly physiologic mobility of the spinal segment after implant removal as well as excellent bone-disc fusion at 6 months. An artificial intervertebral disc using 3D-F demonstrated excellent *in vitro* and *in vivo* performance in both biomechanics and interface histology. There is a potential for future clinical application.

FE analyses have also been recruited in an effort to perturb design with an eye toward optimizing the mechanical behavior of artificial discs. Langrana et al. (83) generated an FE model that examined the effect of orientation of the synthetic disc fiber layers, number of fiber layers, and the order of the reinforcing layers. Dooris et al. modified a previously validated intact FE model to create models implanted with a ball-and-socket

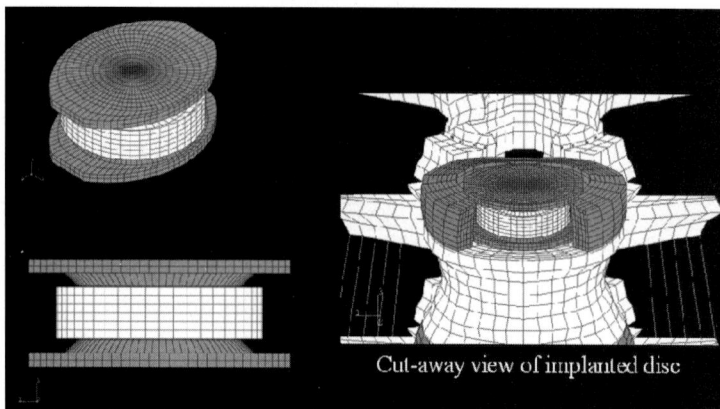

FIG. 6-8. The intact finite element model of a ligamentous segment was modified to simulate the slip-core–type artificial disc implant. (From Dooris AP. Experimental and theoretical investigations into the effects of artificial disc implantation on the lumbar spine [PhD dissertation]. Iowa City, IA: University of Iowa; 2001.)

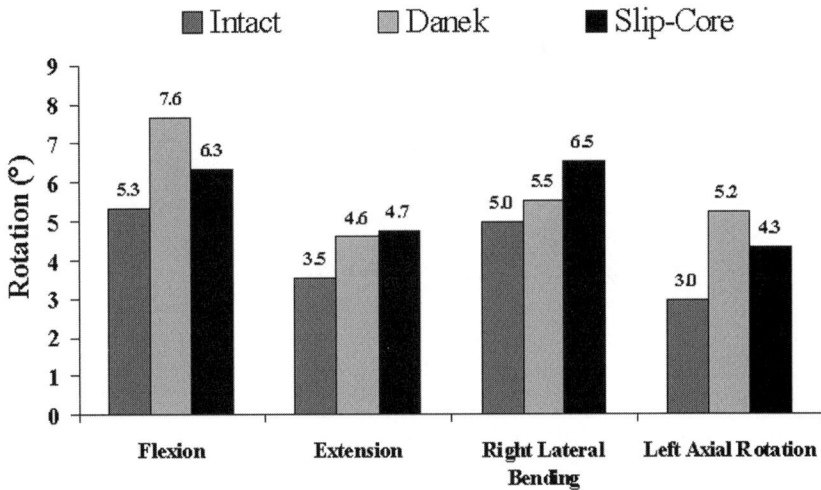

FIG. 6-9. Predicted rotations for the ball-and-socket and slip-core disc designs as compared to the intact case. (From Dooris AP. Experimental and theoretical investigations into the effects of artificial disc implantation on the lumbar spine [PhD dissertation]. Iowa City, IA: University of Iowa; 2001.)

and slip-core–type artificial disc models through an anterior approach (73,86) (Figs. 6-7, 6-8). To study surgical variables, small and large windows were cut into the annulus, and the implants were placed anteriorly and posteriorly within the disc space. The anterior longitudinal ligament was also restored. Models were subjected to either 800 N axial compression force alone or to a combination of 10 Nm flexion-extension moments and 400 N axial preload. Implanted model predictions were compared with those of the intact model. The predicted rotations for the two-disc implanted models were in agreement with the experimental data (73).

For the ball-and-socket design disc facet loads were more sensitive to the anteroposterior location of the artificial disc than to the amount of annulus removed. Under 800 N axial compression, implanted models with an anteriorly placed artificial disc exhibited facet loads 2.5 times

greater than loads observed with the intact model, whereas posteriorly implanted models predicted no facet loads in compression. Implanted models with a posteriorly placed disc exhibited greater flexibility than the intact and implanted models with anteriorly placed discs. Restoration of the anterior longitudinal ligament reduced pedicle stresses, facet loads, and extension rotation to nearly intact levels. The models suggest that, by altering placement of the artificial disc in the anteroposterior direction, a surgeon can modulate motion-segment flexural stiffness and posterior load sharing, even though the specific disc replacement design has no inherent rotational stiffness. The motion data, as expected, differed between the two disc designs (ball and socket, and slip core) and as compared to the intact disc as well (Fig. 6-9). Similar changes were observed for the loads on the facets (Fig. 6-10).

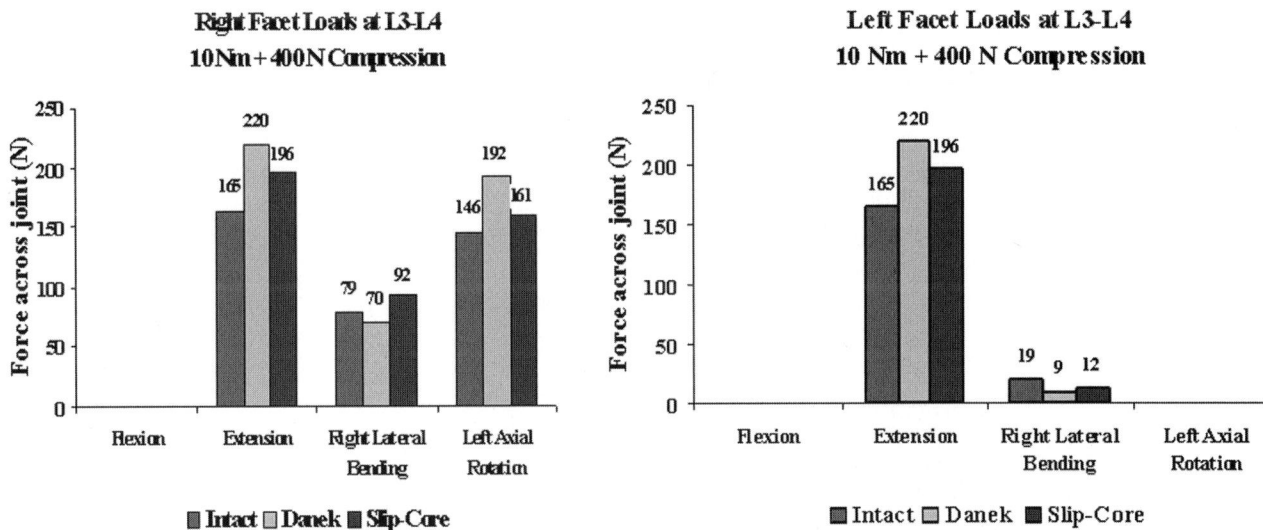

FIG. 6-10. Predicted facet loads for ball-and socket and slip-core disc designs as compared to the intact case. (From Dooris AP. Experimental and theoretical investigations into the effects of artificial disc implantation on the lumbar spine [PhD dissertation]. Iowa City, IA: University of Iowa; 2001.)

The experimentally validated FE models of the intact and disc-implanted L3-L5 segments revealed that both of these devices do not restore motion as well as loads across facets back to the intact case. (These designs restore the intact biomechanics in a limited sense.) These differences are not only due to the size of the implants but the inherent design differences. Ball-and-socket design has a more "fixed" center of rotation as compared to the slip-core design in which the center of rotation (COR) undergoes a wider variation. A further complicating factor is the location of the disc within the annular space itself, a parameter under the control of the surgeon. Thus, it will be difficult to restore biomechanics of the segment back to normal using such designs. Only clinical follow-up studies will provide the effects of such variations on the changes in spinal structures as a function of time (8).

MORE RECENT AND FUTURE INITIATIVES

Although many of the well-accepted investigation techniques and devices have been discussed herein, other techniques for the stabilization/fusion of the spine and nonfusion approaches are currently being investigated. These concepts are likely to play a significant role in the future and are discussed in the following sections.

Vertebroplasty

A citation of the review article by Garfin et al. is the most appropriate way to introduce this topic for further discussion. Painful vertebral osteoporotic compression fractures lead to significant morbidity and mortality (87). This relates to pulmonary dysfunction, eating disorders (nutritional deficits), pain, loss of independence, and mental status change (related to pain and medications). Medications to treat osteoporosis (primarily antiresorptive) do not effectively treat the pain or the fracture, and require over 1 year to reduce the degree of osteoporosis. Kyphoplasty and vertebroplasty are new techniques that help decrease the pain and improve function in fractured vertebrae.

Vertebroplasty is the percutaneous injection of PMMA cement into the vertebral body. While PMMA has high mechanical strength, it heals fast and thus requires only a short handling time. Other potential problems of using PMMA injection may include damage to surrounding tissues by a high polymerization temperature or by the non-reacted toxic monomer, and the lack of long-term biocompatibility. Bone mineral cements, such as calcium carbonate and CaP cements, have longer working time and low thermal effect. They are also biodegradable while having a good mechanical strength. However, the viscosity of injectable mineral cements is high, and the infiltration of these cements into vertebral body has been questioned. Recently, the infiltration properties of a CaP cement have been significantly improved, which is ideal

for the transpedicular injection to the vertebral bodies for vertebroplasty or augmentation of osteoporotic vertebral body strength. Little is known, however, about the biomechanics of this treatment. Various authors have evaluated the biomechanical efficacy of this procedure by comparing it with respect to the intact, the axial strength of the vertebral body following fracture and injection of the cement, and the corresponding load-displacement behavior of the constructs.

Lim et al. evaluated the compression strength of human vertebral bodies injected with new CaP cement with improved infiltration properties before compression fracture and also for vertebroplasty in comparison with PMMA injection (88). The bone mineral densities of 30 vertebral bodies (T2-L1) were measured using DEXA. Ten control specimens were compressed at a loading rate of 15 mm per minute to 50% of their original height. The other specimens had 6 mL of PMMA (n < 10) or the new CaP (n < 10) cement injected through the bilateral pedicle approach before being loaded in compression. Additionally, after the control specimens had been compressed, they were injected with either CaP (n < 5) or PMMA (n < 5) cement using the same technique, to simulate vertebroplasty. Loading experiments were repeated with the displacement control of 50% vertebral height. Load to failure was compared among groups and analyzed using analysis of variance. Mean bone mineral densities of all five groups were similar and ranged from 0.56 to 0.89 g/cm2. The size of the vertebral body and the amount of cement injected were similar in all groups. Load to failure values for PMMA, the new CaP, and vertebroplasty PMMA were significantly greater than that of controls. Load to failure of the vertebroplasty CaP group was higher than the control group but not statistically significant. The mean stiffness of the vertebroplasty CaP group was significantly smaller than control, PMMA, and the new CaP groups. The mean height gains after injection of the new CaP and PMMA cements for vertebroplasty were minimal (3.56% and 2.01%, respectively). Results of this study demonstrated that the new CaP cement can be injected and infiltrates easily into the vertebral body. It was also found that injection of the new CaP cement can improve the strength of a fractured vertebral body to at least the level of its intact strength. Thus, the new CaP cement may be a good alternative to PMMA cement for vertebroplasty, although further *in vitro*, *in vivo* animal, and clinical studies should be done. Furthermore, the new CaP may be more effective in augmenting the strength of osteoporotic vertebral bodies, and for preventing compression fractures considering our biomechanical testing data and the known potential for biodegradability of the new CaP cement. Belkof et al. found that the injection of either Orthocomp (Orthovita, Malvern, PA) or Simplex P (Howmedica, Inc., Allendale, NJ) resulted in vertebral body strengths that were significantly greater than initial strength values (89). Vertebral bodies augmented with Orthocomp recovered their initial stiffness; and, vertebral bodies augmented with Simplex P were significantly less stiff than they were in their initial condition. However, these biomechanical results have yet to be substantiated in clinical studies.

Previous biomechanical studies have shown that injections of 8 to 10 mL of cement during vertebroplasty restore or increase vertebral body strength and stiffness; however, the dose-response association between cement volume and restoration of strength and stiffness is unknown. Belkof et al. (89) investigated the association between the volume of cement injected during percutaneous vertebroplasty and the restoration of strength and stiffness in osteoporotic vertebral bodies. Two investigational cements were studied: Orthocomp and Simplex 20 (Simplex P with 20% by weight barium sulfate). Compression fractures were experimentally created in 144 vertebral bodies (T6-L5) obtained from 12 osteoporotic spines harvested from female cadavers. After initial strength and stiffness were determined, the vertebral bodies were stabilized using bipedicular injections of cement totaling 2, 4, 6, or 8 mL and recompressed, from which posttreatment strength and stiffness were measured. Strength and stiffness were considered restored when posttreatment values were not significantly different from initial values. Strength was restored for all regions when 2 mL of either cement was injected. To restore stiffness with Orthocomp, the thoracic and thoracolumbar regions required 4 mL, but the lumbar region required 6 mL. To restore stiffness with Simplex 20, the thoracic and lumbar regions required 4 mL, but the thoracolumbar region required 8 mL. These data provide guidance on the cement volumes needed to restore biomechanical integrity to compressed osteoporotic vertebral bodies.

Liebschner et al. undertook an FE-based biomechanical study to provide a theoretical framework for understanding and optimizing the biomechanics of vertebroplasty, especially the effects of volume and distribution of bone cement on stiffness recovery of the vertebral body, just like the preceding experimental study (90). An experimentally calibrated, anatomically accurate FE model of an older adult L1 vertebral body was developed. Damage was simulated in each element based on empirical measurements in response to a uniform compressive load. After virtual vertebroplasty (bone cement filling range of 1 to 7 cm3) on the damaged model, the resulting compressive stiffness of the vertebral body was computed for various spatial distributions of the filling material and different loading conditions. Vertebral stiffness recovery after vertebroplasty was strongly influenced by the volume fraction of the implanted cement. Only a small amount of bone cement (14% fill or 3.5 cm3) was necessary to restore stiffness of the damaged vertebral body to the pre-damaged value. Use of a 30% fill increased stiffness by more than 50% compared with the pre-damaged value. Whereas the unipedicular distributions exhibited a comparative stiffness to the

bipedicular or posterolateral cases, it showed a medial-lateral bending motion ("toggle") toward the untreated side when a uniform compressive pressure load was applied. Only a small amount of bone cement (15% volume fraction) is needed to restore stiffness to pre-damage levels, and greater filling can result in substantial increase in stiffness well beyond the intact level. Such overfilling also renders the system more sensitive to the placement of the cement because asymmetric distributions with large fills can promote single-sided load transfer and thus toggle. These results suggest that large fill volumes may not be the most biomechanically optimal configuration, and an improvement might be achieved by use of lower cement volume with symmetric placement. These theoretical findings support the experimental observations described in the preceding paragraph, except these authors did not analyze the relationship between cement type and volume needed to restore strength.

Hitchon et al. compared the stabilizing effects of the HA product with PMMA in an experimental compression fracture of L-1 (91). No significant difference between the HA- and PMMA-cemented-fixated spines was demonstrated in flexion, extension, left lateral bending, or right and left axial rotation. The only difference between the two cements was encountered before and after fatiguing in right lateral bending ($p < .05$). The results of this study suggest that the same angular rigidity can be achieved by using either HA or PMMA. This is of particular interest because HA is osteoconductive, undergoes remodeling, and is not exothermic.

According to Garfin et al. both vertebroplasty and kyphoplasty have had a very high acceptance and use rate (87,92). There is 95% improvement in pain and significant improvement in function following treatment by either of these percutaneous techniques. Kyphoplasty improves height of the fractured vertebra, and improves kyphosis by over 50%, if performed within 3 months from the onset of the fracture (onset of pain). There is some height improvement, though not as marked, along with 95% clinical improvement, if the procedure is performed after 3 months. Complications occur with both and relate to cement leakage in both, and cement emboli with vertebroplasty. Kyphoplasty and vertebroplasty are safe and effective, and have a useful role in the treatment of painful osteoporotic vertebral compression fractures that do not respond to conventional treatments. Kyphoplasty offers the additional advantage of realigning the spinal column and regaining height of the fractured vertebra, which may help decrease the pulmonary, gastrointestinal, and early morbidity consequences related to these fractures. Both procedures are technically demanding.

Bioartificial Disc

The rapidly advancing field of tissue engineering opens new possibilities to solving spine problems. By seeding and growing intervertebral disc cells, it could be possible to grow a new bioartificial disc to be implanted into the spine. Studies are in progress at a number of centers, including our own (93).

The FE model studies can be used to simulate even the smallest of systems. For example, Baer et al. have developed an FE model to study the cell micromechanical environment in the intervertebral disc (94). Hopefully, this approach can be used to investigate the effects of various spinal instrumentations at the cellular level.

CONCLUSION

The prevalence of spinal fusion and stabilization procedures is continuously increasing. This chapter has presented many of the contemporary biomechanical issues germane to stabilization and fusion of the spine. Because of the wide variety of devices available, various testing protocols have been developed in an attempt to describe the mechanical aspects of these devices. Many *in vitro* studies are performed during the earlier stages of implant development to characterize and optimize the mechanical behavior of the device. In addition, the investigations reveal comparative advantages (and disadvantages) of the newer designs to existing hardware. Subsequent *in vivo* testing, specifically animal models, provides data on the performance of the device in a dynamic physiologic environment. All of the testing, *in vitro* and *in vivo*, helps to build confidence that the instrumentation is safe for clinical trial. The biomechanical testing and evaluation of spinal fusion and stability has produced an extensive knowledge base that has allowed for the design, development, and implementation of various devices. Future biomechanical work is required to produce newer devices and optimize existing ones, with an eye toward reducing the rates of nonfusion and pseudarthrosis. In addition, novel devices and treatments that seek to restore normal spinal function and loading patterns without fusion continue to necessitate advances in biomechanical methods. These are the primary challenges that need to be incorporated in future biomechanical investigations. Finally, one has to gain understanding of the effects of devices at the cellular level and one must undertake outcome assessment studies to see if the use of instrumentation is warranted for the enhancement of the fusion process.

ACKNOWLEDGMENTS

This chapter is based on the work sponsored by various funding agencies over the last 20 years. Part of the literature review and writing of the actual manuscript was done while the senior author (Goel) was a Visiting Professor at the Department of Electronic and Computer Engineering, Tokyo Denki University, Ishizaka, Hatoyama-machi, Hiki-Gun, Saitama 350-0394, Japan.

REFERENCES

1. Davis H. Increasing rates of cervical and lumbar spine surgery in the United States 1979–1990. Spine 1994;19:1117.
2. Sonntag VKH, Marciano FF. Is fusion indicated for lumbar spinal disorders? Spine 1995;20:138S.
3. Goel VK, Weinstein JN. Clinical biomechanics of the lumbar spine. Boca Raton, FL: CRC Press, 1990.
4. Goel VK, Gilbertson LG. Basic science of spinal instrumentation. Clin Orthop 1987;335:10.
5. Goel VK, Pope MH. Biomechanics of fusion and stabilization. Spine 1995;20:35S.
6. White AAA, Panjabi MM. Clinical biomechanics of spine, 2nd ed. Philadelphia: Lippincott-Raven, 1990.
7. Katz JN. Lumbar spinal fusion—surgical rates, costs and complications. Spine 1995;20:78S.
8. Zdeblick TA. A prospective, randomized study of lumbar fusion—preliminary results. Spine 1993;18:983.
9. Purcell GA, Markolf KL, Dawson EG. Twelfth thoracic-first lumbar vertebral mechanical stability of fractures after Harrington-rod instrumentation. J Bone Joint Surg Am 1981;63:71.
10. Lehman RA, Kuklo TR, O'Brien MF. Biomechanics of thoracic pedicle screw fixation. Part I—Screw biomechanics. Semin Spine Surg 2002;14(1):8–15.
11. Okuyama K, Abe E, Suzuki T, et al. Influence of bone mineral density on pedicle screw fixation: a study of pedicle screw fixation augmenting posterior lumbar interbody fusion in elderly patients. Spine J 2002; 1:402–407.
12. Okuyama K, Sato K, Abe E, et al. Stability of transpedicle screwing for the osteoporotic spine. Spine 1993;18:2240.
13. Carlson GD, Abitbol JJ, Anderson DR, et al. Screw fixation in the human sacrum—an in vitro study of the biomechanics of fixation. Spine 1992;17:S196.
14. Pfeiffer M, Gilbertson LG, Goel VK, et al. Effect of specimen fixation method on pullout tests of pedicle screws. Spine 1996;21:1037.
15. Pfeiffer M, Hoffman H, Goel VK, et al. In vitro testing of a new transpedicular stabilization technique. Eur Spine J 1997;6:249.
16. Ryken TC, Clausen JD, Traynelis VC, et al. Biomechanical analysis of bone mineral density, insertion technique, screw torque, and holding strength of anterior cervical plate screws. J Neurosurg 1995;83: 324–329.
17. Choi W, Lee S, Woo KJ, et al. Assessment of pullout strengths of various pedicle screw designs in relation to the changes in the bone mineral density. Paper presented at the 48th Annual Meeting of the Orthopedic Research Society; February 10–13, 2002; Dallas, TX.
18. McKinley TO, McLain RF, Yerby SA, et al. The effect of pedicle morphometry on pedicle screw loading a synthetic model. Spine 1997;22 (3):246–252.
19. Lim TH, Kim JG, Fujiwara A, et al. Prediction of fatigue screw loosening in anterior spinal fixation using dual energy x-ray absorptiometry. Spine 1995;20(23):2565–2568; discussion 2569.
20. Bühler, DW, Berlemann U, Oxland, TR, et al. Moments and forces during pedicle screw insertion in vitro and in vivo measurements. Spine 1998;23(11):1220–1227.
21. Abshire BB, Mclain RF, Valdevitt A, et al. Characteristics of pull out failure in conical and cylindrical pedicle screws after full insertion and back out. TSJ 2001;1(6):408–414.
22. Ketller A, Wilke HJ, Dietl R, et al. Stabilizing effect of posterior lumbar interbody fusion cages before and after cyclic loading. J Neurosurg 2000;92(1):87–92[Suppl].
23. Lund T, Oxland TR, Jost B, et al. Interbody cage stabilisation in the lumbar spine: biomechanical evaluation of cage design, posterior instrumentation and bone density. J Bone Joint Surg Br 1998;80(2): 351–359.
24. Rapoff AJ, Ghanayem AJ, Zdeblick TA. Biomechanical comparison of posterior lumbar interbody fusion cages. Spine 1997;22:2375.
25. Steffen T, Tsantrizos A, Aebi M. Effect of implant design and endplate preparation on the compressive strength of interbody fusion construct. Spine 2000;25(9):1077–1084.
26. Tsantrizos A, Baramki HG, Zeidman S, et al. Segmental stability and compressive strength of posterior lumbar interbody fusion implants. Spine 2000;25(15):1899–1907.
27. Janssen ME, Nguyen C, Beckham R, et al. A biological cage. Eur Spine J 2000;9 [Suppl 1]:S102–S109.

28. Murakami H, Boden SD Hutton WC. Anterior lumbar interbody fusion using a barbell-shaped cage: a biomechanical comparison. J Spinal Disord 2001;14(5):385–392.

29. Murakami H, Horton WC, Kawahara N, et al. Anterior lumbar interbody fusion using two standard cylindrical threaded cages, a single mega-cage, or dual nested cages: a biomechanical comparison. J Orthop Sci 2001;6(4):343–348.

30. Bianchi JR. Design and mechanical behavior of the MD series of bone dowels [PhD dissertation]. Gainesville, FL: University of Florida; 1999.

31. Dietl R, Krammer HJ, Kettler M, et al. Pullout test with three lumbar interbody fusion cages. Spine 2002;27(10):1029–1036.

32. Cunningham BW, Sefter JC, Shono Y, et al. Static and cyclic biomechanical analysis of pedicle screw constructs. Spine 1993;18:1677.

33. Goel VK, Winterbottom JM, Weinstein JN. A method for the fatigue testing of pedicle screw fixation devices. J Biomech 1994;27:1383.

34. Clausen JD, Goel VK, Sairyo K, et al. A protocol to evaluate semi-rigid pedicle screw systems. J Biomech Eng 1997;119:364.

35. Chang KW, Dewei Z, McAfee PC, et al. A comparative biomechanical study of spinal fixation using the combination spinal rod plate and transpedicular screw fixation system. J Spinal Disord 1989;1:257.

36. Panjabi MM. Biomechanical evaluation of spinal fixation devices: Part I. A conceptual framework. Spine 1988;13(10):1129–1134.

37. Gwon JK, Chen J, Lim TH, et al. In vitro comparative biomechanical analysis of transpedicular screw instrumentations in the lumbar region of the human spine. J Spine Disord 1991;4:437.

38. Rohlmann A, Bergmann G, Graichen F, et al. Comparison of loads on internal spinal fixation devices measured in vitro and in vivo. Med Eng Phys 1997;19:539.

39. Weinhoffer SL, Guyer RD, Herbert M, et al. Intradiscal pressure measurements above an instrumented fusion—a cadaveric study. Spine 1995;20:526.

40. Nibu K, Panjabi MM, Oxland T, et al. Multidirectional stabilizing of BAK interbody spinal fusion system for anterior surgery. J Spinal Disord 1997;10:357.

41. Lim T-H,An HS, Hasegawa T, et al. Biomechanical evaluation of diagonal fixation in pedicle screw instrumentation. Spine 2001;26(22):2498–2503.

42. Cripton PA, Jain GM, Wittenberg RH, et al. Load-sharing characteristics of stabilized lumbar spine segments. Spine 2000;25(2):170.

43. Hitchon PW, Goel VK, Rogge TN, et al. In vitro biomechanical analysis of three anterior thoracolumbar implants. J Neurosurg (Spine 2) 2000;93:252–258.

44. Lee SW, Lim TH, You JW, et al. Biomechanical effect of anterior grafting devices on the rotational stability of spinal constructs. J Spinal Disord 2000;13(2):150–155.

45. Vahldeik MJ, Panjabi MM. Stability potential of spinal instrumentations in tumor vertebral body replacement surgery. Spine 1998;23(5):543–550.

46. Lim T-H, Kim JG, Fujiwara A, et al. Load-sharing characteristics of stabilized lumbar spine segments. Spine 2000;25(2):170.

47. Oda I, Cunningham BW, Lee GA, et al. Biomechanical properties of anterior thoracolumbar multisegmental fixation—an analysis of construct stiffness and screw-rod strain. Spine 2000;25(8):2303–2311.

48. Hasegawa K, Ikeda, M Washio, et al. An experimental study of porcine lumbar segmental stiffness by the distraction-compression principle using a threaded interbody cage. J Spinal Disord 2000;13(3):247–252.

49. Goel VK, Grosland NM, Scifert JL, et al. Biomechanics of the lumbar disc. J Musculoskeletal Res 1997;1:81.

50. Grosland NM, Goel VK, Grobler LJ, et al. Adaptive internal bone remodeling of the vertebral body following an anterior interbody fusion: a computer simulation. Paper presented at the 24th International Society for the Study of the Lumbar Spine; June 3–6, 1997; Singapore.

51. Heth JA, Hitchon PW, Goel VK, et al. A biomechanical comparison between anterior and transverse interbody fusion cages. Spine 2001;26:E261–E267.

52. Wang S-T, Goel VK, et al. Posterior instrumentation reduces differences in spine stability due to different cage orientations—an in vitro study. Spine (accepted).

53. Kanayama M, Cunningham BW, Haggerty CJ, et al. In vitro biomechanical investigation of the stability and stress-shielding effect of lumbar interbody fusion devices. J Neurosurg 2000;93:2[Suppl]:259–265.

54. Kim Y. Prediction of mechanical behaviors at interfaces between bone and two interbody cages of lumbar spine segments. Spine 2001 26(13):1437–1442.

55. Volkman T, Horton WC, Hutton WC. Transfacet screws with lumbar interbody reconstruction: biomechanical study of motion segment stiffness. J Spinal Disord 1996;9(5):425–432.

56. Shirado O, Zdeblick TA, McAfee PC, et al. Quantitative histologic study of the influence of anterior spinal instrumentation and biodegradable polymer on lumbar interbody fusion after corpectomy—a canine model. Spine 1992;17:795.

57. Smith KR, Hunt TR, Asher MA, et al. The effect of a stiff spinal implant on the bone mineral content of the lumbar spine in dogs, J Bone Joint Surg Am 1991;73:115.

58. Spivak JM, Neuwirth MG, Labiak JJ, et al. Hydroxyapatite enhancement of posterior spinal instrumentation fixation. Spine 1994;19:955.

59. McAfee PC, Farey ID, Sutterlin CE, et al. The effect of spinal implant rigidity on vertebral bone density: a canine model. Spine 1991;16:S190.

60. Penta M, Fraser RD. Anterior lumbar interbody fusion—a minimum 10 year follow-up. Spine 1997;22:2429.

61. Kanayama M, Cunningham BW, Sefter JC, et al. Does spinal instrumentation influence the healing process of posterolateral spinal fusion? An in vivo animal model. Spine 1999;24(11):1058–1065.

62. Eric H, Ledet MS, Sachs BL, et al. Real-time in vivo loading in the lumbar spine. Part 1. Interbody implant: load cell design and preliminary results. Spine 2000 25(20):2595–2600

63. Rohlmann A, Bergmann G, Graichen F. A spinal fixation device for in vivo load measurement. J Biomech 1994;27:961.

64. Rohlmann A, Graichen F, Weber U, et al. Biomechanical studies monitoring in vivo implant loads with a telemeterized internal spinal fixation device. Spine 2000;25(23):2981–2986.

65. Rohlmann A, Calisse J, Bergmann G, et al. Internal spinal fixator stiffness has only a minor influence on stresses in the adjacent discs. Spine 1999;24(12):1192.

66. Rohlmann A, Bergmann G, Graichen F, et al. Influence of muscle forces on loads in internal spinal fixation devices Spine 1998;23(5):537–542.

67. Szivek JA, Roberto RF, Slack JM, et al. An implantable strain measurement system designed to detect spine fusion preliminary results from a biomechanical in vivo study. Spine 2002;27(5):487–497.

68. Goel VK, Lim TH, Gilbertson LG, et al. Clinically relevant finite element models of a ligamentous lumbar motion segment. Semin Spine Surg;1993;5:29.

69. Goel VK, Lim TH, Gwon J, et al. Effects of rigidity of an internal fixation device—a comprehensive biomechanical investigation. Spine 1991;16:S155.

70. Goel V, Konz R, Chang H-T, et al. Hinged dynamic stability as compared to dynamic rigid device. Paper presented at the 45th Annual Meeting of the Orthopaedic Research Society; Feb. 1–4, 1999; Anaheim, CA.

71. Scifert J, Sairyo K, Goel VK, et al. Stability analysis of an enhanced load sharing posterior fixation device and its equivalent conventional device in a calf spine model. Spine 1999;24:2206–2213.

72. Hitchon PW, Goel VK, Rogge T, et al. Biomechanical studies of a dynamized anterior thoracolumbar implant. Spine 2000;25(3):306–309.

73. Dooris AP. Experimental and theoretical investigations into the effects of artificial disc implantation on the lumbar spine [PhD dissertation]. Iowa City, IA: University of Iowa; 2001.

74. Dooris A, Hudgin G, Goel V, et al. Restoration of normal multisegment biomechanics with prosthetic intervertebral disc. Paper presented at the 48th Annual Meeting of the Orthopedic Research Society; February 10–13, 2002; Dallas, TX.

75. Yamashita H, Dijke PT, Heldin CH, et al. Bone morphogenetic protein receptors. Bone 1996;19:569.

76. Grauer JN, Patel TC, Erulkar JS, et al. 2000 Young Investigator Research Award Winner: Evaluation of OP-1 as a graft substitute for intertransverse process lumbar fusion. Spine 2001;26(2):127–133.

77. Patel TC, Erulkar JS, Grauer JN, et al. Osteogenic protein-1 overcomes the inhibitory effect of nicotine on posterolateral lumbar fusion. Spine 2001;26(15):1661–1661.

78. Magin MN, Delling G. Improved lumbar vertebral interbody fusion using rhOP-1: a comparison of autogenous bone graft, bovine hydroxylapatite (Bio-Oss), and BMP-7 (rhOP-1) in sheep. Spine 2001;26(5):469–478.

79. Sandhu HS, Toth JM, Diwan AD, et al. Histologic evaluation of the efficacy of rhBMP-2 compared with autograft bone in sheep spinal anterior interbody fusion. Spine 2002;27(6):567–575.

80. Klara PM, Ray CD. Artificial nucleus replacement clinical experience. Spine 2002;27(12):1374–1377.

81. Kostuik JP. Intervertebral disc replacement—experimental study. Clin Orthop 1997;337:27.

82. Bao QB, McCullen GM, Higham PA, et al. The artificial disc: theory, design and materials. Biomaterials 1996;17:1157.

83. Langrana NA, Lee CK, Yang SW. Finite element modeling of the synthetic intervertebral disc. Spine 1991;16:S245.

84. Lee CK, Langrana NA, Parsons JR, et al. Development of a prosthetic intervertebral disc. Spine 1991;16:S253.

85. Kotani Y, Kuniyoshi A, Yasuo S, et al. Artificial intervertebral disc replacement using bioactive three-dimensional fabric design, development, and preliminary animal study. Spine 2002;27(9):929–935

86. Dooris AP, Goel VK, Grosland NM, et al. Load-sharing between anterior and posterior elements in a lumbar motion segment implanted with an artificial disc. Spine 2001;26(6):E122–E129.

87. Garfin SR, Yuan, HA, Reiley MA. New technologies in spine kyphoplasty and vertebroplasty for the treatment of painful osteoporotic compression fractures. Spine 2001; 26(14):1511–1515.

88. Lim T-H, Brebach T, Renner SM, et al. Biomechanical evaluation of an injectable calcium phosphate cement for vertebroplasty. Spine 2002;27 (12):1297–1302.

89. Belkof SM, Mathis JM, Erbe EM, et al. Biomechanical evaluation of a new bone cement for use in vertebroplasty. Spine 2000;25(9):1061–1064.

90. Liebschner MAK, Rosenberg WS, Keaveny TM. Effects of bone cement volume and distribution on vertebral stiffness after vertebroplasty. Spine 2001;26:1547–1554, .

91. Hitchon PW, Goel V, Drake J, et al. A biomechanical comparison of hydroxyapatite and polymethylmethacrylate vertebroplasty in a cadaveric spinal compression fracture model. J Neurosurg (Spine 2) 2001; 95:215–220.

92. Vaccaro AR, Kazuhiro Chiba, Heller JG, et al. Bone grafting alternatives in spinal surgery. Spine J 2002;2:206–215

93. Huntzinger J, Phares T, Goel V, et al. The effect of concentration on polymer scaffolds for bioartificial intervertebral discs. Paper presented at the 49th Annual Meeting of the Orthopaedic Research Society; Feb. 2–5, 2003; New Orleans, LA.

94. Baer AE, Setton LA. The mechanical environment of intervertebral disc cells: effect of matrix anisotropy and cell geometry predicted by a linear model. J Biomech Eng 2000;122, 245–251.

CHAPTER 7

Fracture and Repair of Lumbar Vertebrae

Tony S. Keller, Victor Kosmopoulos, and Thomas Steffen

The lumbar spine, located between the sacrum and thoracic regions of the vertebral column (the lower back), typically consists of five vertebrae. These five vertebrae generally increase in size from the superior to the inferior lumbar spine and are larger than both the cervical and thoracic vertebrae. Similar to size, the weight-bearing ability of lumbar vertebrae is often greater, resulting in a higher incidence of pain following injury. From a mechanical point of view, the weight-bearing or structural capacity (force at failure) of the vertebrae depends on both material properties (bone mineral content, trabecular bone tissue density, and apparent density) and geometric properties (size, orientation, and connectivity of bone elements). A close association between bone mineral loss due to osteoporosis and the risk of fracture has been clearly established. Skeletal structures such as the vertebral bodies, which are comprised primarily of trabecular bone, are particularly at risk. The purpose of this chapter is to discuss the mechanics of vertebral compression fractures and trabecular bone damage. An understanding of microdamage and microfracture of vertebrae is used to facilitate discussions of cement repair strategies.

STRUCTURAL AND MECHANICAL BEHAVIOR OF LUMBAR VERTEBRAE

Mechanical properties not only vary from vertebra to vertebra or level to level, but also can vary dramatically within a given vertebral body. Trabeculae tend to be denser, rodlike structures in the inferior and superior sections in contrast to the less dense, platelike trabeculae that are associated with the central region of the lumbar vertebral centrum (1). Studies that have examined the physical and mechanical properties of lumbar vertebral trabecular bone have also shown that trabecular bone underlying the normal intervertebral disc nucleus is significantly stronger, stiffer, and denser in comparison to trabecular bone underlying the disc annu-

lus (2–4). Such intravertebral variations in trabecular bone properties have been attributed, in part, to adaptation to the heterogeneous pressure distribution within the normal intervertebral disc (4). Namely, the pressurized disc nucleus exerts higher stresses on the underlying end plate and trabecular bone compared to pressure transmitted by the disc annulus. Keller et al. (2,4) also noted that disc degeneration reduces intravertebral variations in trabecular bone-apparent stiffness, strength, and density in regions adjacent to the end plate, which presumably reflects a more uniform or homogeneous distribution of pressure and stress within the degenerated disc.

The architectural design or structure of bone in human vertebrae and elsewhere in the body is very complex ranging from a very porous solid (trabecular bone) to a very dense solid (compact bone). The anterior column, or centrum, of human vertebrae is comprised of only a very thin cortical shell (less than 2 mm), which is virtually indistinguishable from the trabeculae that comprise the bulk of the vertebral centrum (Fig. 7-1). Silva et al. (5) performed a finite element analysis of an idealized lumbar vertebrae, and reported that the cortical shell's contribution was only 10% of the total vertebral strength, thus making the trabecular centrum the main load-bearing structure. Using anatomically accurate microstructural finite element simulations, the authors estimate that removal of the trabecular centrum, leaving only the vertebral shell, results in over an eightfold decrease in apparent stiffness compared to the intact vertebrae (having both the vertebral shell and centrum) (Fig. 7-2). Finite element analysis of vertebral mechanics is covered in more detail in later sections of this chapter.

Given the porous nature of bone, the relative amount of bone tissue is described histologically using apparent density (ρ_a). Apparent density is defined as the mass of bone tissue present within a given volume. Clinically, estimates of bone mass are most commonly obtained using dual energy X-ray absorptiometry (DEXA). This

85

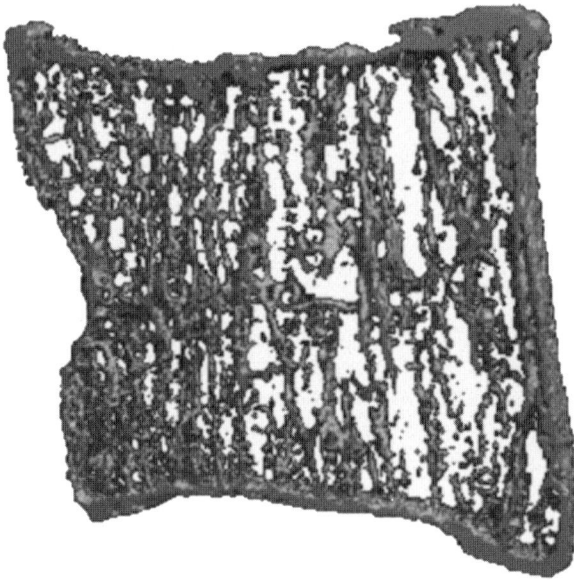

FIG. 7-1. Volume rendering of microcomputed tomography scan image of T10 osteopenic vertebral body (1.8-mm thick section). (From Keller TS, Kosmopoulos V, Liebschner MAK. Modeling of bone loss and fracture in osteoporosis. In: Gunzburg R, Szpalski M, eds. Vertebral osteoporotic compression fractures. Philadelphia: Lippincott Williams & Wilkins, 2002: 35–50.)

low-radiation method provides measures of the bone mineral content (BMC, g/cm) and bone mineral density (BMD, g/cm²) distributions within the body (6).

Although BMC and BMD are not true volumetric measures of tissue mass or apparent density, both have been shown to be useful predictors of bone fragility (2,7–9). Hansson (8) performed *in vitro* mechanical compression tests on 109 intact L1-L4 vertebral centrum specimens from subjects spanning five decades in age (31 to 79 years). In this test series, the BMC ranged from 1.44 g/cm to 6.39 g/cm (mean 3.33 g/cm), and the compressive force at failure F_{ult} ranged from 1,520 Newtons (N) to 10,987 N (mean 3,850 N). From this data the following linear correlations are obtained (10):

$$F_{ult} = 1,535 \text{ BMC} - 1,258 \ (R^2 = 0.74)$$

$$F_{ult} = -75 \text{ AGE} + 8,199 \ (R^2 = 0.30)$$

Examination of these relationships indicates that the compressive strength of the lumbar vertebral centrum is strongly and positively correlated to BMC, but is weakly and negatively correlated to subject age. After age 30, lumbar vertebral compressive strength is predicted to decrease 750 N per decade, declining to 1,500 N at 89 years of age. When the lumbar vertebral strength decreases to 1,500 N or lower, failure of the vertebral structures can occur under postural loads imposed by the weight of the body above the vertebrae (10,11).

From a mechanical point of view, ultimate force is a structural property that is dependent upon both the size

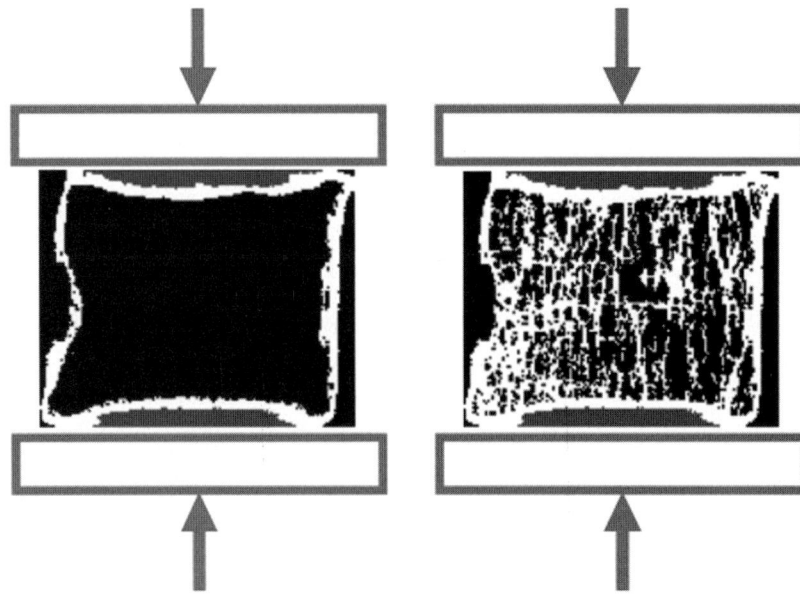

FIG. 7-2. Finite element microstructural models used to simulate experimental compression of **(A)** just the cortical shell (without the trabecular centrum) and **(B)** of the complete vertebral body (cortical shell and trabecular centrum).

(geometry) and composition (material) of the tissue. Thus, one cannot directly compare the ultimate force of vertebrae from different regions in the spine because the size of the cervical, thoracic, and lumbar vertebrae varies appreciably from each other and from one level to the next. For this reason, material property measurements, such as stress or force/area are often preferred, since they account for geometry variations of different size structures. An estimate of the apparent stress at failure (σ_{ult}, MPa or 10^6 N/m^2) can be obtained for Hansson's data by dividing the ultimate force (F_{ult}, N) by the cross-sectional area (mm^2) reported for the vertebral end plate. The apparent stress at failure of the lumbar vertebrae is found to range from 0.95 to 4.95 MPa (mean 2.29 MPa). Here apparent stress refers to the fact that we still have not accounted for the porosity of the vertebral centrum. Namely, two similar size vertebrae can have very different structural properties if their porosity or apparent density differs appreciably.

Keller (12) published empirical relationships from *in vitro* mechanical tests that can be used to calculate the compressive apparent strength (ρ_a, MPa) of vertebral bone:

$$\sigma_a = 97.8 \, \rho_a^{2.30}$$

where ρ_a is the apparent density ($0.05 < \rho_a < 0.30$ g/cm^3). Note that the approximately square exponent means that a relative reduction in apparent density of one half will produce a corresponding relative reduction in compressive apparent strength of one fourth. In older adults (more than 70 years), the apparent density of human vertebral trabecular bone can be as low as 0.05 g/cm^3, which corresponds to an ultimate compressive strength of only 0.05 MPa. Stresses much greater than 0.05 MPa are produced in vertebrae when subjected to compressive forces associated with weight bearing in upright postures (10).

OSTEOPOROSIS

Osteoporosis is a skeletal disorder distinguished by weakened skeletal architecture caused by suboptimal bone development or a reduction in bone mass. It is a disease that weakens the structural properties of bone in both men and women, and results in fracture when loads applied to bone exceed the bone's ability to support those loads. Thus, osteoporosis is a significant risk factor for fracture and its incidence increases with age. In the United States, 10 million individuals have been diagnosed with osteoporosis and another 18 million have low bone mass, which places them at increased risk for osteoporosis and fracture. Treatment of osteoporotic fracture is estimated to be as high as $15 billion annually (13).

Osteoporosis is accompanied by reduced bone strength, and has been clinically characterized using non-invasive radiographic measures such as BMD, BMC, and apparent density (ρ_a). The standard diagnosis for osteoporosis is 2.5 standard deviations or more below the mean BMD (or BMC) for an average 30-year-old adult of the same sex. Osteoporosis affects bone quality, which refers to bone architecture, rate of adaptation/remodeling, level of mineralization, and damage accumulation (13).

In osteoporosis perforations exist within the structure causing increased fragility (Fig. 7-3). One reason for this fragility increase is due to the replacement of the plate-like closed cell trabecular structures by open cell rodlike structures, resulting in an increasingly porous appearance. Mechanically, trabecular-buckling strength is dependent on the diameter, length, distance between cross-links, and the material properties of individual trabeculae. In osteoporosis the vertebral trabeculae become thinner and cross-linking continuity with horizontal trabeculae is reduced without compensation by the vertebral shell. Throughout the progression of this disease, deterioration of the trabecular structure induces the

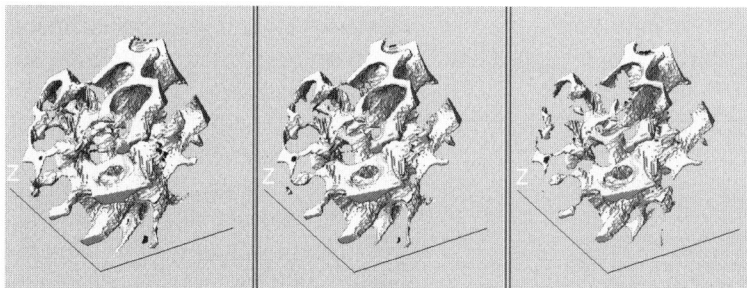

FIG. 7-3. Volumetric rendering of a 2.56 mm × 2.56 mm × 2.56 mm region of trabecular bone from the human lumbar vertebral centrum. The panels **(from left to right)** illustrate progressive and uniform bone loss resulting in a decrease of the bone volume fraction from 15.3% to 11.1% to 7.66%. Note that there is significant loss of trabecular connectivity following the simulated bone loss. The 20 μm voxel (volume pixel) images were reconstructed from a histologic specimen using a quantitative serial imaging and marching cubes algorithm. (From Saxena R, Keller TS. Computer modeling for evaluating trabecular bone mechanics. In: An YH, Draughn RA, eds. Mechanical testing of bone and the bone-implant interface. Boca Raton, FL: CRC Press, 1999:407–436.)

reduction in bone mass (and thus density) ensuring an increased rate of fracture.

VERTEBRAL FRACTURE

Approximately 700,000 osteoporotic vertebral fractures occur per year in the United States with 230,000 resulting in chronic disabling pain (13,14). Vertebral fractures alter force transmission to the vertebral body segments, lead to vertebral body collapse, increase fracture risk (fivefold) to neighboring vertebrae (15), and result in progressive spinal deformity (e.g., kyphosis) (16).

Vertebral fracture may occur as a result of a traumatic force exceeding the load-bearing capacity of the vertebral body, or by the accumulation of trabecular tissue-level damage (microdamage) from repeated (fatigue), uniform and nonuniform, everyday subfailure-type postural loading (no trauma) (10,11,17). A traumatic force can result from high-impact falls to normal lifting and bending (13).

Apparent density and its clinical counterpart BMD provide good estimates of bone mechanical properties but are not definitive in predicting vertebral strength (12). The load-bearing capacity of the lumbar vertebrae (structural characteristics) coupled with the applied loads (magnitude, duration, rate) determine fracture risk (Fig. 7-4). Vertebral

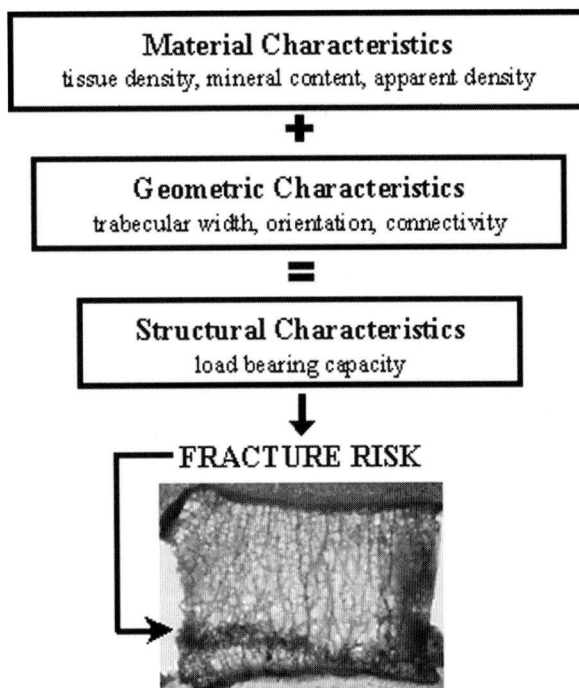

FIG. 7-4. Vertebral material, geometry, and structure are biomechanical determinants of fracture risk. Loading characteristics (magnitude, profile, duration, and rate) also influence fracture risk.

fracture is about four times more common in women than in men, and the risk for a vertebral fracture has been found to increase almost exponentially with age. The frequency of osteoporotic vertebral fracture also increases during menopause in women and continues to steadily increase in frequency throughout the remainder of life. Furthermore, depending on the age groups studied (40 years to more than 80 years), the prevalence of osteoporotic vertebral fractures varies from around 5% to somewhat over 50% (18–21).

Compression Fracture Classification

Vertebral compression fractures are primarily caused by excessive axial loads that may result in vertebral body height reductions, and in the more extreme cases, deformities. The axial failure loads for lumbar vertebrae have been estimated and classified by age. In general, a force of approximately 4,200 N produces fracture in individuals over the age of 60, whereas under the age of 40, an increased load of approximately 7,600 N causes fracture (22,23). As we noted earlier, however, the compressive strength of lumbar vertebrae is closely dependent on the size and quality of the segment, and, in the case of osteoporosis, can be substantially lower than 4,200 N.

Different postural loading conditions (e.g., uniform and nonuniform) endured by the vertebral body result in different vertebral fracture geometries at failure. In the most general case, postural loads are greatest on the anterior aspect of the vertebral body resulting in what is known as anterior wedge-type compression fractures. Anterior compression fractures have been classified into four subtypes (22): (a) both end plates are damaged; (b) only the superior end plate is damaged (most common); (c) only the inferior end plate is damaged; and (d) both end plates are intact but anterior cortical shell is damaged.

In the least severe case, hairline fractures to the cortical shell or the vertebral end plate may occur. These types of hairline fractures are difficult to diagnose and may plague the patient with pain. End-plate damage can occur in the central regions, periphery regions, or as transverse cracks across the end plate (22). End-plate damage has been proposed to be the initial stage of more severe vertebral compression fractures (1,24,25). Burst fractures are the most severe and can range from an end-plate fracture resulting in disc intrusion into the vertebral body (22) to complete shattering of the vertebral body. Burst fractures occur at axial loads ranging from 6,000 to 10,000 N (26).

Clinical Definition of Vertebral Fracture

Radiographic detection of vertebral compression fractures is often the confirmation of the presence of osteoporosis or bone fragility. Without any known pathomorphologic aberrations distinguishing osteoporotic bone from nonosteoporotic bone tissue, the fracture itself defines pathology. Since the occurrence of a fracture is not only the result of the mechanical properties of the bone, but is also a function of the fracturing trauma, both factors must be considered when defining osteoporosis. In the presence of a patient with a recent fracture, knowing nothing or very little about the patient's bone quality or the forces involved in the trauma, the most practical way for clarifying whether a fracture is osteoporotic or not is Harold Frost's criterion of the "everyday trauma." Frost stated that a fracture occurring because of an everyday trauma indicates that the patient has osteoporosis or bone fragility. Even if current technology allows us to determine, for example, the amount of bone mineral in different parts of the human skeleton, we still lack practical techniques for measuring the fracture-generating forces. Therefore the "everyday trauma" definition is still a practical measure for estimating bone fragility (27). Hence, development of models that can simulate both the loading and structural (trabecular) damage behavior of vertebral bodies are important for understanding clinical pathologies (e.g., osteoporosis) and for predicting bone fragility and its risk for fracture.

TRABECULAR BONE DAMAGE

Trabecular bone is a porous structure (Figs. 7-1 to 7-4), which behaves similarly to typical engineering materials (and cortical bone) in compression until the ultimate stress is reached. The mechanical behavior in trabecular bone shows a relatively linear or elastic response for deformations less than 1% (Fig. 7-5). The point at which the mechanical behavior becomes nonlinear (strain increasing at a greater rate than the stress) is defined as the yield strain and permanent or inelastic deformation and damage occurs beyond yield. The yield point of ver-

tebral trabecular bone is similar for both compression and tension: 0.84% and 0.78% indicate compressive and tensile yield strain, respectively, for vertebral trabecular bone specimens (28). However, beyond yield the compressive load capacity of trabecular bone does not go to zero as would be expected. Instead the load is maintained or may even show a slight increase compared to the previously recorded ultimate load (Fig. 7-5B.).

Physically this behavior can be explained by understanding the compressive mechanics of porous structures. As the pore spaces begin to collapse, the trabeculae collide and compress into each other increasing the trabecular bone-volume fraction (bone volume/combined bone and pore space volume) of the specimen. This reduction in pore space and consequent increase in volume fraction results in a temporary load tolerance by the trabecular structure. Thus, the load-carrying capacity of trabecular bone is still quite substantial following compression fracture, and results in a large post-yield stress-strain response (28). This behavior is similar to elastoplastic materials having large post-yield regions and therefore can be modeled as such. In contrast, during tensile loading the load-carrying capacity of trabecular bone is minimal resulting in a smaller post-yield region and abrupt failure. Note that in studying the mechanics of porous structures it is often useful to clarify between whole specimen properties (e.g., vertebral body) by referring to them as "apparent" and site-specific properties of the individual constituents (e.g., trabeculae) by referring to them as "tissue."

Stress-Strain Behavior

The inelastic stress-strain behavior of bone is mainly a result of cracks, plasticity, and viscous creep. Cracks degrade stiffness, strength, and other material properties

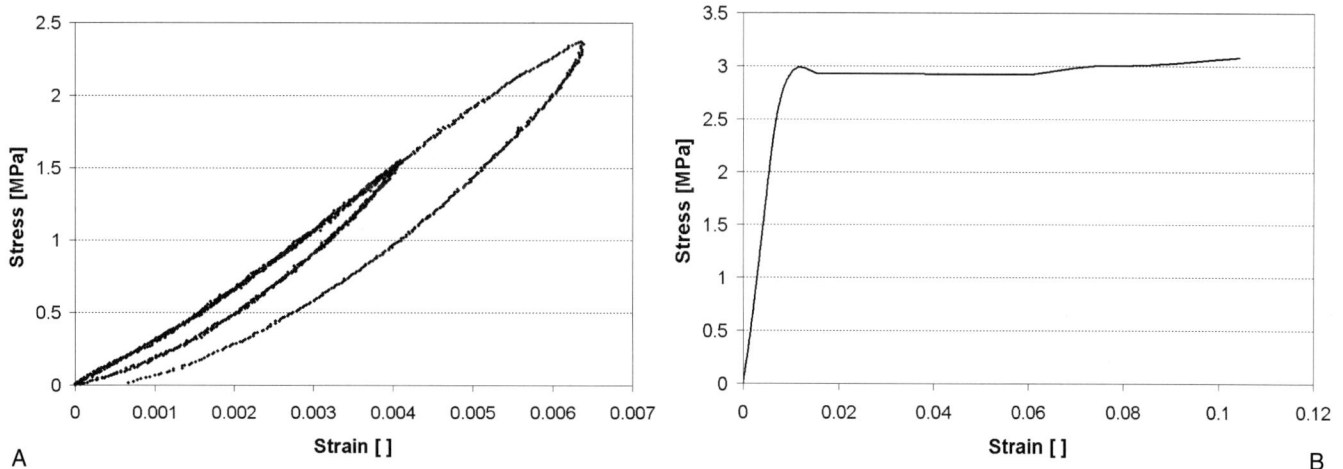

FIG. 7-5. Experimental stress-strain curve displaying the load-unload-reload mechanical behavior **(A)** and post-yield mechanical behavior **(B)** of an osteoporotic vertebral body.

because of the imposed material discontinuities. The complex strain behavior of vertebral trabecular bone and other porous materials is a result of the cumulative effects of the elastic strain, inelastic strain due to damage accumulation, plastic strain, and anelastic (viscous) strain (29). Such strain behavior can be differentiated using a load-unload-reload protocol. After unloading from a damaging event, the stress-strain behavior of bone (trabecular and compact) is similar to that of composites (30). Namely, bone recovers approximately three-fourths of the total inelastic strains (29). Damaged bone shows relatively small changes in its elastic modulus or stiffness during the initial onset (at low strain levels) of a reload. As loads are increased (relatively high strain levels) however, cracks propagate, and residual stresses are relieved resulting in a curvilinear stress-strain behavior (Fig. 7-5) (31). This cyclic load-unload-reload behavior in time produces bone fatigue, which in turn reduces bone strength and stiffness (32–36). Bone damage resulting from fatigue or creep can occur under elastic conditions (pre-yield loading) and has been accepted as a normal physiologic process (37–39).

Damage Mechanics

A microstructural reduction in tissue mechanical properties (e.g., strength, stiffness) is often referred to as microdamage. The accumulation of microdamage, microfracture, leads to local tissue discontinuities within a single trabecula and a decrease in apparent vertebral bone strength. Both microdamage and microfracture are load-dependent, although bone microdamage occurs at a higher incidence than microfracture (40). Microdamage or microfracture may act as a precursor for bone remodeling (41–44). The resorption phase of bone remodeling can in turn induce further microdamage (45,46) by increasing pore size. This increase in pore size (decrease in apparent density and volume fraction) consequentially reduces the apparent modulus, increases the tissue strain, and results in a temporary increase in bone fragility and osteoporotic fracture risk (39,47–50). Gross vertebral fracture can be a result of extensive microdamage or microfracture accumulation to the trabecular structure (47,51,52).

Continuum damage mechanics (CDM) is a rapidly developing area in the study of bone fracture. For a simple isotropic or axisymmetric material, the presence of cracks or damage (D) can be expressed as a simple scalar representing the loss of load-carrying area (Fig. 7-6) (53). An effective modulus (E_{EFF}) can then be determined by scaling the elastic modulus (E) by the damage parameter (D):

$$E_{EFF} = (E)(D)$$

where D is continuous between zero (fractured material) and 1 (undamaged material).

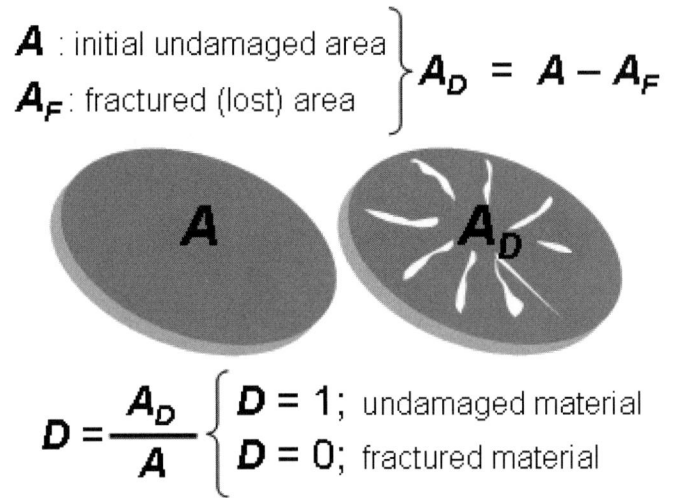

$$A_D = A - A_F$$

A : initial undamaged area
A_F : fractured (lost) area

$$D = \frac{A_D}{A} \quad \begin{cases} D = 1; \text{ undamaged material} \\ D = 0; \text{ fractured material} \end{cases}$$

FIG. 7-6. Schematic illustration of the isotropic damage concept defined by continuum damage mechanics.

To study vertebral trabecular bone damage a quasi-continuum CDM approach has been developed based on an empirical nonlinear stress-strain relationship (generalized tangent hyperbolic law) (54,55) and an elasto-plastic modulus reduction (EPMR) scheme (56,57). The latter assumes that the evolution of trabecular bone microdamage (D) can be modeled as a change in bone elastic modulus or stiffness, wherein the elastic modulus of bone is assumed to be proportional to the apparent density cubed (discussed earlier) (12,58). The EPMR scheme is easily implemented using the finite element method and can therefore be used to model the damage evolution behavior of complex material geometries. The following sections illustrate the use of CDM and the finite element method to study vertebral damage and cement repair.

Finite Element Damage Simulations

The finite element method is a numerical technique that provides approximations to theory. Finite element analysis is an efficient method used to solve differential equations over complex domains or structures. The structure is discretized and represented by finite elements formed by nodes. Finite element modeling is especially attractive in the analysis of heterogeneous and anisotropic structures, such as trabecular bone, for which a closed form solution using analytic methods will be impossible. In recent years, anatomically accurate models of trabecular bone can and have been investigated (59–61). These microstructural finite element models are usually constructed from micro-computed tomography raster arrays at spatial resolutions of 150 μm or less for large volumes and 50 μm or less for small volumes of bone (less than 50 mm³). Microstructural finite element models enable calculation and visualization of internal tissue stresses and strains.

Damage simulations of complex structures, such as that of trabecular bone in the vertebral body, can be studied using microstructural finite element models. Continuum damage and EPMR approaches have been integrated within the finite element numerical framework and used as a research tool to investigate existing or potential bone damage (56,57,62–65). Furthermore, finite element bone damage models can be used to study the mechanics of surgical repair. To date however, only a few studies have used finite element damage models to study the failure mechanisms (56,57,64–67) and surgical repair (vertebroplasty) efficacy (56,64,67) of the vertebral body. Simulation of vertebral body damage using the finite element approach is presented in the following section, and repair simulations will be discussed later in this chapter.

Kosmopoulos and Keller (64) coupled the EPMR damage approach with an anatomically accurate two-dimensional (2D) microstructural finite element model of a midsagittal vertebral body section. Two vertebral loading postures were simulated by using a uniform loading profile and a nonuniform (ramped) loading profile. Compressive loads were applied incrementally over a stress range of 0 to 3 MPa. The experimentally validated (65) EPMR scheme and iterative finite element analysis resulted in a nonlinear stress-strain response (Fig. 7-5A) and a decrease in the apparent modulus of the vertebral body. At the highest stress the uniformly loaded model resulted in a total vertebral body apparent modulus reduction of 32%, while the ramp-loaded model resulted in a 95% apparent modulus reduction, compared to the initial undamaged vertebral body apparent modulus (E_0 = 444 MPa). Microdamage initiation (modulus reduction of 5%) was first apparent at an applied stress level of 1.5 MPa for both the uniform-loaded and ramped-loaded cases. At the maximum applied stress there was a trabecular bone modulus reduction of 40% or more in 10.4% and 15.9% of the total bone elements for the uniform-loaded and ramped-loaded microdamage models, respectively (Fig. 7-7). For the uniform-loaded vertebral body the distribution of highly stressed elements followed a column-wise (superior-inferior) pattern within the cortical shell and more centrally located trabeculae, in contrast to the ramped-loaded case where the highly stressed elements were located on the posterior vertebral shell. The ramp-loaded model resulted in a substantially greater number of highly stressed bone elements (20.9% of bone elements with stress concentrations greater than 3) compared to the uniform-loaded model (4.2% of bone elements with stress concentrations greater than 3).

VERTEBRAL REPAIR

Most compressive fractures do not affect the spinal cord, are relatively stable, and are therefore asymptomatic in nature. These types of fractures rarely require surgical intervention (68,69) and are treated using conservative nonsurgical approaches. These treatments often involve a short period of postural reduction (bed rest) directly after incidence, followed by external immobilization, and finally by gradual ambulation (16,70). Bed rest is usually recommended for the first 4 to 6 weeks followed by 6 to 12 weeks of bracing using a rigid orthosis. In severe cases of burst fractures, tissue fragments may enter the spinal canal and cause myelopathy (71). Fractures may lead to progressive deformity and instability, spinal stenosis, neurologic deficit, and pain requiring surgical intervention. The probability of fracture healing without surgery decreases as the severity or amount of tissue involved in the fracture increases (72).

Bone Cement Augmentation

Vertebroplasty and kyphoplasty are two recently developed minimally invasive repair techniques for the treatment of vertebral compressive fractures. Unlike traditional treatments, these bone cement augmentation repair procedures help to restore spinal alignment and decrease chronic pain (73).

Vertebroplasty involves the forced injection, usually using either a parapedicular or transpedicular approach, of bone cement, usually polymethylmethacrylate (PMMA), through one (unipedicular) or two bone (bipedicular) biopsy needles into the closed space of a collapsed vertebral body (16,73). The injections are performed under continuous fluoroscopic guidance, and for high-risk cases, computed tomography is also used (74,75). This technique provides pain relief and stabilization, but typically does not restore the height of the collapsed vertebral body.

Kyphoplasty involves the insertion of a bone balloon into the vertebral body using biplanar fluoroscopic image guidance. The balloon is inflated causing the trabecular bone to compact, resulting in a suitable cavity to re-expand the vertebral body. In kyphoplasty, bone cement is injected with more control and with less pressure than during vertebroplasty. Another advantage of kyphoplasty is the restoration of vertebral body height and reduction of spinal deformity (16,73).

The main complication with each of these cement repair techniques is associated with the use of PMMA. In vertebroplasty cement, extravasation may occur since the PMMA is injected at much higher pressures. The rates of this occurrence have been reported to be as high as 40% when PMMA cement is used in the treatment of osteoporotic compression fractures (15), and is greater when using higher injection volumes or less viscous cement (76). Another concern with PMMA is its high polymerization temperature. Polymerization has been reported to produce average peak cement core temperatures of 87°C and 108°C for small (approximately 14.9 cm^3) and larger (approximately 27.6 cm^3) cement volume fills (77).

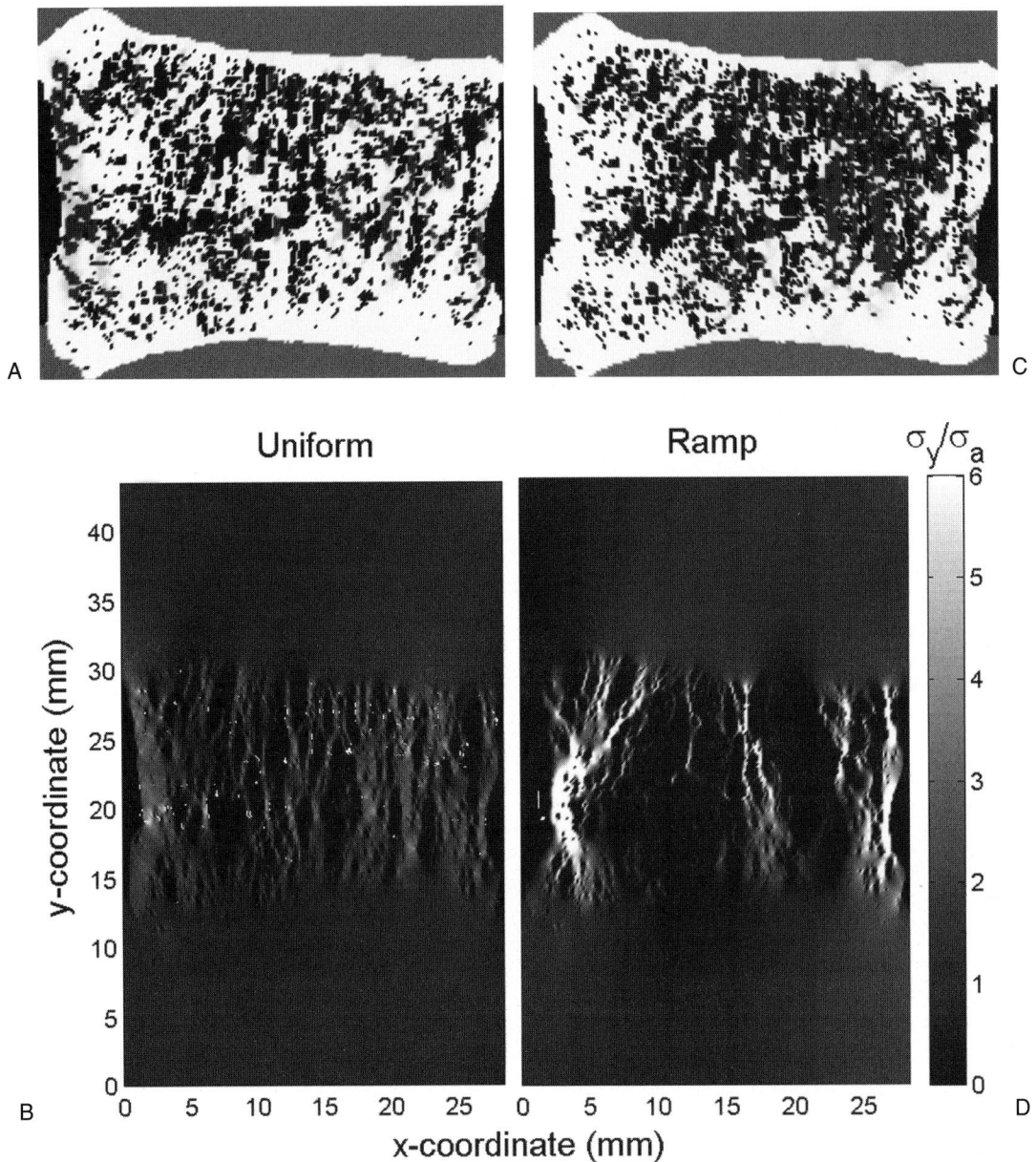

FIG. 7-7. Numerical simulation of vertebral trabecular bone microdamage using the elastoplastic modulus reduction finite element scheme. Four-node isoparametric elements were used to represent the vertebral body structure, which was assumed to have isotropic material properties. The applied compressive stress (3 MPa) corresponds to upright posture loads acting on the lumbar spine (10). Two vertebral loading postures were simulated by using a uniform **(A, B)** and a nonuniform or ramped **(C, D)** loading profile. In **(A)** and **(C)** the bone and marrow tissues are depicted as white and black elements, respectively, whereas bone tissue damage (modulus reduction of 40% or greater) is depicted by the dark gray elements. In **(B)** and **(D)**, the gray scale intensity plots show the resulting stress concentrations (element axial stress/apparent stress, σ_y/σ_a) following the uniform and ramp loading profiles, respectively. Highly stressed elements are depicted as lighter gray (max $\sigma_y/\sigma_a < 6$) and less severely stressed elements as darker gray to black (min $\sigma_y/\sigma_a > 0$).

Bone-forming cells (osteoblasts) have been shown to undergo thermal necrosis when exposed to relatively lower temperatures than cement polymerization (as low as 50°C for more than 1 minute) (78,79). Clinically the complication rate (between 1% to 3%) associated with PMMA-induced temperature elevation and PMMA extravasation is insignificant for treatment of vertebral fracture (74), but long-term effects are still being investigated. Another noteworthy complication from the resulting increased strength and stiffness of cement-augmented vertebrae is the modified load transfer to adjacent vertebral bodies. Recent findings suggest that the cement augmentation results in higher stresses and strains to adjacent vertebrae, thus facilitating their future collapse (80).

Biomechanical Studies of Cement Augmentation

Biomechanical studies of cement augmentation have demonstrated that vertebroplasty treatment of experimentally created compression fractures is an effective means to restore the strength, and to a lesser extent, the stiffness of the damaged vertebrae (81). These authors noted that 2 mL of PMMA cement restored the strength of thoracolumbar and lumbar vertebrae, but 8 mL and 4 mL of cement were necessary to restore the stiffness of the thoracolumbar and lumbar vertebrae, respectively, to predamage levels using a bipedicular approach. Furthermore, it has been shown that lumbar vertebral strength can be significantly restored using either a unipedicular (6 mL injection through one pedicle) or bipedicular (5 mL injections through each pedicle) approach (70).

The biomechanical aspects of kyphoplasty are less well understood. Reductions in risk of cement extravasation and vertebral height restoration have been suggested as the main advantages of kyphoplasty compared to vertebroplasty (16). Researchers have reported a 47% restoration in vertebral height in 70% of the collapsed vertebral bodies following kyphoplasty (16). Furthermore their findings support that lower pressure, higher viscosity cement injections reduced the rate of cement extravasation as compared to published findings for vertebroplasty.

Computer models and numerical tools to simulate and guide surgical repair are becoming more routine, and are rapidly advancing treatment of musculoskeletal disorders (82). One of the main advantages of computer models is that they can be used as their own repeated measure. Different cement repair strategies can be studied using a single bone specimen and can be evaluated in an unlimited manner using different loading modes and boundary conditions. The ability of microstructural finite element models to represent complex structures lends this technique to the study of trabecular bone microdamage and repair. Numerical examples of cement augmentation repair are discussed and presented in the following sections.

Numerical Simulations of Cement Augmentation

Validated finite element models can act as replacements to experimental testing (44). Liebschner et al. (67) used an experimentally validated apparent lumbar vertebral damage model to investigate vertebroplasty cement repair. In their study, cement repair was modeled by the introduction of PMMA cement elements within the vertebral centrum. Four PMMA cement bolus volumes (1.0, 3.5, 5.0, and 7.0 cm^3) were investigated with an assumed cylindric cement shape. Using this repair modeling approach, the authors reported that only small amounts of PMMA (approximately 14% fill or 3.5 cm^3) were required to restore apparent stiffness to intact levels, and that symmetric PMMA placement was preferential compared to asymmetric distributions.

The EPMR damage simulation scheme and finite element method was recently used to investigate damage-repair of human vertebrae (64). Microstructurally damaged finite element models were repaired using four different PMMA cement repair strategies:

- replacement of marrow elements by PMMA cement elements at each of the four interior corners of the midsagittal model (referred to as model A)
- central placement of cement consistent with a parapedicular surgical approach (model B)
- strategic placement of equivalent cement quantities at five damage initiation sites (model C), and
- complete vertebral cement fill (replacement of all marrow elements) (model D) (Table 7-1).

The first three repair strategies used equivalent amounts of cement elements (25% of the marrow elements were replaced by PMMA bone cement). For the third strategy, the five trabecular microdamage initiation sites were used as the central locus for repair (each

TABLE 7-1. *Summary of finite element simulations of several PMMA cement repair strategies[a]*

Loading regimen	Vertebroplasty repair regimen	Normalized apparent modulus (E_R/E_0)	Bone element stress concentrations (% >3)
Uniform	Undamaged	1.0	4.5
	Damaged	0.68	5.5
	Repair A	1.67	3.5
	Repair B	1.60	3.3
	Repair C	2.10	3.4
	Repair D	4.06	0.0
Ramped	Undamaged	1.0	4.6
	Damaged	0.05	20.1
	Repair A	1.26	14.4
	Repair B	0.38	17.5
	Repair C	1.52	11.6
	Repair D	3.53	0.4

PMMA, polymethylmethacrylate.
[a]See text for definitions of repair regimens.

site with PMMA comprising 5% of the marrow elements). The motivation for studying partial cement fill was the notion that reductions of cement volume during vertebroplasty may reduce the likelihood of cement leakage. Plane stress, static finite element analyses were performed on each of the damage-repair models (eight in total). Loading profiles used for the repair models were identical to the EPMR damage simulation (uniform and nonuniform). Stress-strain results (apparent modulus) were normalized to undamaged vertebral body results.

Examination of the eight-vertebroplasty repair models revealed that only the ramp-loaded central placement cement regimen (model B) did not restore the microstructurally damaged vertebral body apparent modulus to the initial undamaged apparent modulus ($E_0 = 444$ MPa). The repair strategy using a central placement, cement regimen (model B), was the least effective of all the partial fill repair strategies for both loading conditions in increasing vertebral body structural stiffness (Table 7-1). In the case of the uniform-loaded microdamage regimen, model B resulted in a repair modulus/initial modulus ratio $E_R/E_0 = 1.60$, which is still significantly (135%) above the damaged apparent modulus ($E_D = 302$ MPa). Of the strategic partial cement fill regimens, model C was most effective in increasing the apparent modulus above the initial undamaged apparent modulus for both the uniform ($E_R/E_0 = 2.10$) and ramped ($E_R/E_0 = 1.52$) microdamage models. Each of the partial cement repair strategies (models A through C) resulted in complete recovery of the apparent modulus above the undamaged levels except model B for the severely damaged ramp-loaded case.

In the case of the complete fill repair regimen (model D), the number of highly stressed elements (trabecular bone stress concentrations greater than 3) decreased to less than 0.4% (98% reduction) of the total bone elements for the ramp-loaded model and were completely removed (100% reduction) for the uniform-loaded microdamage model. The least effective cement repair strategy for reducing the number of highly stressed bone elements was model A for the uniform-load microdamage model (36% reduction with respect to the untreated damage model), and model B for the ramp-load microdamage model regimen (14% reduction with respect to the untreated damage model) (Table 7-1). Strategic placement of cement at damage initiation sites, model C, resulted in a 38% and 43% reduction in the number of highly stressed elements for the uniform-loaded and ramp-loaded microdamage models, respectively, compared to the untreated damaged model.

The previous analysis was limited to a single vertebral body. Keller et al. (10) studied the effects of spinal deformity and vertebral height loss associated with osteoporosis using an anatomically accurate sagittal plane postural loading model of the anterior spinal column (C2-S1) in conjunction with the EPMR scheme. This analytic model was found to reproduce the salient features of thoracic spinal deformities caused by osteoporotic wedge fractures (Fig. 7-8A). This model was used to simulate the effects of vertebral cement augmentation (vertebroplasty) on spinal deformity. Spine stiffness was parametrically varied over the range of 1× to 2× that of a normal healthy spine. An increase of 2× in vertebral body stiffness corresponds to complete cement fill of the normal vertebral body (64). Increases in thoracic kyphosis and decreases in vertebral body height resulted in a 34.9% overall decrease in spinal height (C2-S1), 12.0% decrease in body height, and a 22.8 cm anterior translation of C2. The resulting thoracic kyphotic deformity (86.4° T2-T10) qualitatively resembled deformities observed in elderly individuals with osteoporotic compression fractures.

To prevent severe thoracic deformity (greater than 70°) cement augmentation of three or more thoracic segments and a 60% increase in vertebral body stiffness was required. Doubling the vertebral body stiffness of one segment resulted in only a 10° reduction in thoracic kyphosis deformity, whereas stiffness doubling combined with augmentation of 11 segments (T2-T12) reduced the kyphotic deformity to 50° (height change = 2.4%, C2 translation = 10.9 cm) (Fig. 7-8B). The effects of cement augmentation on postural load-induced osteopenic thoracic kyphosis are summarized in Figure 7-8C. These analytic results suggest that cement augmentation of vertebrae can reduce the severity of osteoporotic spine deformities. Model data provide insight for surgical procedures (optimal cement material and volume, number of treatment levels) designed to prevent or treat vertebral fractures and deformity of the thoracolumbar skeleton. Ultimately, identification of subjects who are at risk for vertebral microdamage and fracture may facilitate early prophylactic treatments using cement augmentation. Clinical repair of fractures using small cement quantities at locations where damage is greatest or where damage initiates may become comparable to current cement-filling regimens used during vertebroplasty.

CONCLUSION

Lumbar vertebral compression fractures are primarily caused by overloading, but even postural loads may result in vertebral body height reduction, deformity, myelopathy, and pain. Restoration of vertebral geometry and mechanical properties to undamaged levels using cement repair strategies is dependent on a number of factors including bone density, damage, cement quantity, quality (modulus) and placement (within a single and at multiple vertebral segments), and surgical approaches and techniques. These factors, together with the complexity of vertebral bone geometry and material properties, suggest

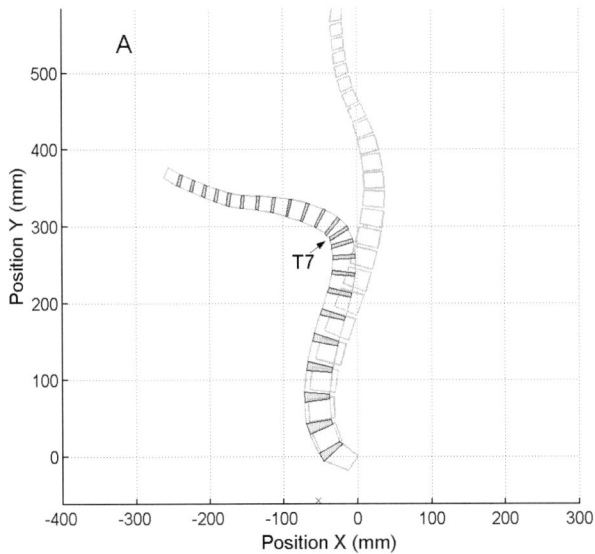

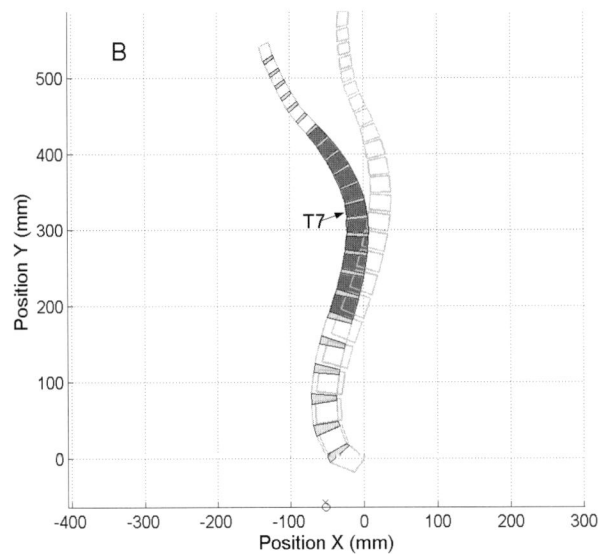

FIG. 7-8. Graphic depiction showing the resulting spinal deformity and anterior wedge-type fractures of the T7 and T8 vertebral bodies following osteoporosis simulations **(A)** and multisegment vertebroplasty repair **(B)**. The three-dimensional surface plot depicts thoracic angle changes (vertical axis) with respect to cement augmentation (represented by changes in segment stiffness from 1× to 2× normal) and the number of augmented segments (thoracic levels, T1-T12) **(C)**.

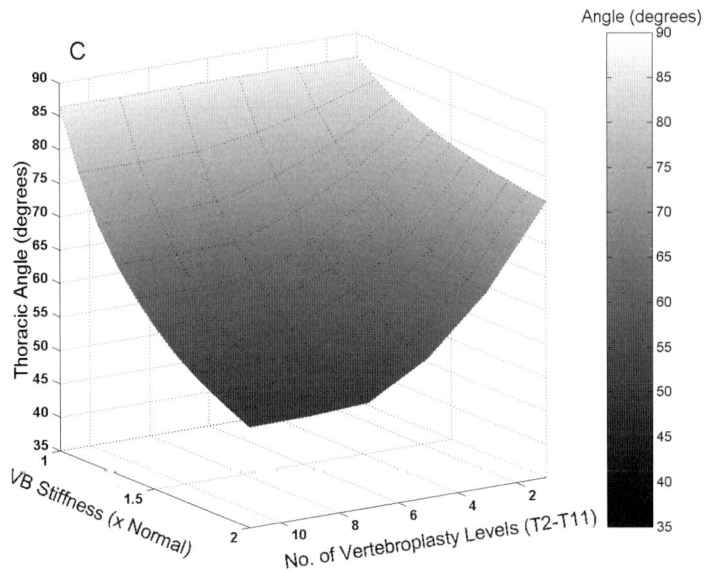

that computational tools and algorithms using anatomically precise two-dimensional and three-dimensional vertebral geometry derived from radiographic images may prove to be valuable for clinical management of vertebral osteoporotic compression fractures and tumors. In this regard, simple analytic models and more complex microstructural finite element models provide a framework for understanding microdamage and fracture of vertebrae, and investigating surgical treatment, including design and development of tissue-engineered fracture repair materials. Additional work is needed to identify the effects of cement augmentation on the load transfer and stress distributions of adjacent vertebrae. Whether or not altered load transfer is sufficient to facilitate collapse of adjacent (untreated) vertebral bodies, as has been recently suggested (80), remains to be determined.

ACKNOWLEDGMENTS

Research supported by Department of Energy Experimental Program to Stimulate Competitive Research (EPSCoR) and National Aeronautics and Space Administration (NASA) EPSCoR.

REFERENCES

1. Hansson TH, Keller TS, Panjabi MM. A study of the compressive properties of lumbar vertebral trabeculae: effects of tissue characteristics. Spine 1987;11:56–62.
2. Keller TS, Hansson TH, Abram AC, et al. Regional variations in the compressive properties of lumbar vertebral trabeculae. Spine 1989;14:1012–1019.
3. Keller TS, Moeljanto E, Main JA, et al. Distribution and orientation of bone in the human vertebral centrum. J Spinal Disord 1992;5:60–74.
4. Keller TS, Ziv I, Moeljanto E, et al. Interdependence of lumbar disc

and subdiscal bone properties: a report of the normal and degenerated spine. J Spinal Disord 1993;6:106–113.

5. Silva MJ, Keaveny TM, Hayes WC. Load sharing between the shell and centrum in the lumbar vertebral body. Spine 1997;22:140–150.

6. Dunn WL, Wahner HW, Riggs BL. Measurement of bone mineral content in human vertebrae and hip by dual photon absorptiometry. Radiology 1980;136:485–487.

7. Eriksson SA, Isberg BO, Lindgren JU. Prediction of vertebral strength by dual photon absorptiometry and quantitative computed tomography. Calc Tissue Int 1989;44:243–250.

8. Hansson T. The bone mineral content and biomechanical properties of lumbar vertebrae [PhD thesis]. Göteborg: University of Göteborg; 1977.

9. Hansson T, Roos B, Nachemson A. The bone mineral content and ultimate compressive strength in lumbar vertebrae. Spine 1980;1:46–55.

10. Keller TS, Harrison DE, Colloca CJ, et al. Prediction of osteoporotic spinal deformity. Spine 2003;28:455–462.

11. Keller TS, Nathan M. Height change due to creep in intervertebral discs: a sagittal plane model. J Spinal Disord 1999;12:313–324.

12. Keller TS. Predicting the compressive mechanical behavior of bone. J Biomech 1994;27:1159–1168.

13. Osteoporosis prevention, diagnosis, and therapy. NIH Consensus Statement 2000;17:1–36.

14. Cyteval C, Sarrabere M, Rouz JO, et al. Acute osteoporotic vertebral collapse: open study on percutaneous injection of acrylic surgical cement in 20 patients. AJR Am J Roentgenol 1999;173:1685–1690.

15. Jensen ME, Evans AJ, Mathis JM, et al. Percutaneous polymethylmethacrylate vertebroplasty in the treatment of osteoporotic vertebral compression fractures: technical aspects. Am J Neuroradiol 1997;18:1897–1904.

16. Lieberman IH, Dudeney S, Reinhardt M-K, et al. Initial outcome and efficacy of `kyphoplasty' in the treatment of painful osteoporotic vertebral compression fractures. Spine 2001;26:1631–1638.

17. Cooper C, Atkinson EJ, O'Fallon WM, et al. Incidence of clinical diagnosed vertebral fractures: a population based study in Rochester, Minnesota, 1985–1989. J Bone Miner Res 1992;7:221–227.

18. Jensen GF, Christiansen C, Boesen J, et al. Epidemiology of postmenopausal spinal and long bone fractures: a unifying approach to postmenopausal osteoporosis. Clin Orthop 1982;166:75–81.

19. Gershon-Cohen J, Rechtman AM, Schraer H. Asymptomatic fractures in osteoporotic spines of the aged. JAMA 1953;153:625–627.

20. Melton LJ. Epidemiology of vertebral fractures. Aalborg, Denmark: Proceedings of the Internal Symposium on Osteoporosis, Sept. 27–Oct. 2, 1987.

21. Zetterberg C, Mannius S, Mellstrom D, et al. Osteoporosis and back pain in the elderly. A controlled epidemiologic and radiographic study. Spine 1990;15:783–786.

22. Garfin SR, Gertzbein S, Eismont F. Fractures of the lumbar spine: evaluation, classification, and treatment. In Wiesel SW, Weinstein JN, Herkowitz H, et al., eds. The lumbar spine, 2nd ed. Vol 2. Philadelphia: Saunders, 1996:822–873.

23. Perey O. Fractures of the vertebral endplate in the lumbar spine. Acta Orthop Scand 1957;25[Suppl]:237–238.

24. Brinckmann P, Biggemann M, Hilweg D. Fatigue fracture of human lumbar vertebrae. Clin Biomech 1988;1[Suppl]:1–23.

25. Hansson T, Keller TS, Jonson R. Fatigue fracture morphology in human lumbar motion segments. J Spinal Disord 1988;1:33–38.

26. Willen J, Lindahl S, Irstram L, et al. Unstable thorocolumbar fractures: a study by CT and conventional roentgenology of the reduction effect of Harrington instrumentation. Spine 1984;9:214–219.

27. Frost HM. (1993). Suggested fundamental concepts in skeletal physiology. Calcif Tissue Int 1993;52:1–4.

28. Kopperdahl DL, Keaveny TM. Yield strain behavior of trabecular bone. J Biomech 1998;31:601–608.

29. Jepsen KJ, Davy DT, Akkus O. Observations of damage in bone, In: Cowin SC, ed. Bone mechanics handbook, 2nd ed. Boca Raton, FL: CRC Press, 2001:17.1–17.12.

30. LeMaitre J. A course on damage mechanics, 2nd ed. Berlin: Springer-Verlag, 1996.

31. Fondrk MT, Bahniuk E, Davy DT, et al. Some viscoplastic characteristics of bovine and human cortical bone. J Biomech 1988;21:623–630.

32. Carter DR, Hayes WC. Compact bone fatigue damage: residual strength and stiffness. J Biomech 1977;10:325–337.

33. Carter DR, Caler WE, Spengler DM, et al. Fatigue behavior of adult cortical bone: the influence of mean strain and strain range. Acta Orthop Scand 1981;52:481–490.

34. Pattin CA, Caler WE, Carter DR. Cyclic mechanical property degradation during fatigue loading of cortical bone. J Biomech 1996;29:69–79.

35. Zioupos P, Wang XT, Currey JD. Experimental and theoretical quantification of the development of damage in fatigue tests of bone and antler. J Biomech 1996;29:989–1002.

36. Zioupos P, Casinos A. Cumulative damage and the response of human bone in two-step loading fatigue. J Biomech 1998;31:825–833.

37. Frost HM. Presence of microscopic cracks in vivo in bone. Henry Ford Hospital Med Bull 1960;8:25–35.

38. Hansson T, Roos B. Microcalluses of the trabeculae in lumbar vertebrae and their relation to the bone mineral content. Spine 1981;6:375–380.

39. Burr DB, Forwood MR, Fyhrie DP, et al. Bone microdamage and skeletal fragility in osteoporotic and stress fractures. J Bone Miner Res 1997;12:6–15.

40. Yeh OC, Keaveny TM. Relative roles of microdamage and microfracture in the mechanical behavior of trabecular bone. J Orthop Res 2001;19:1001–1007.

41. Tschantz P, Ritishauser E. La surcharge mechanique de l'os vivant. Ann Anat Pathol 1967;12:223–248.

42. Pugh JW, Rose RM, Radin EL. A possible mechanism of Wolff's law: trabecular microfractures. Arch Int Physiol Biochim 1973;81:21–40.

43. Martin RB, Burr DB. A hypothetical mechanism for the simulation of osteonal remodeling by fatigue damage. J Biomech 1982;15:137–139.

44. Keaveny TM. Strength of trabecular bone. In: Cowin SC, ed. Bone mechanics handbook, 2nd ed. Boca Raton, FL: CRC Press, 2001:16.1–16.42.

45. Scully TJ, Besterman G. Stress fracture: a preventable training injury. Military Med 1982;147:285–287.

46. Martin RB. A mathematical model for fatigue damage repair and stress fracture in osteonal bone. J Orthop Res 1995;13:309–316.

47. Fyhrie DP, Schaffler MB. Failure mechanisms in human vertebral cancellous bone. Bone 1994;15:105–109.

48. Wachtel EF, Keaveny TM. Dependence of trabecular damage on the mechanical strain. J Orthop Res 1997;15:781–787.

49. Martin RB, Burr DB, Sharkey NA. Skeletal tissue mechanics. New York: Springer, 1998.

50. Keaveny TM, Wachtel EF, Kopperdahl DL. Mechanical behavior of human trabecular bone after overloading. J Orthop Res 1999;17:346–353.

51. Fazzalari NL, Forwood MR, Smith K, et al. Assessment of cancellous bone quality in severe osteoarthrosis: bone mineral density, mechanics, and microdamage. Bone 1998;22:381–388.

52. Kopperdahl DL, Pearman JL, Keaveny TM. Biomechanical consequences of an isolated overload on the human vertebral body. J Orthop Res 2000;18:685–690.

53. Kachanov LM. Introduction to continuum damage mechanics. Dordrecht: Martinus Nijhoff Publishers, 1986.

54. Betten J. Bemerkungen zum Versuch von Hohenemser. ZAMM 1975;55:149–158.

55. Betten J. Generalization of nonlinear material laws found in experiments to multi-axial states of stress. Eur J Mech, A/Solids 1989;8:325–339.

56. Keller TS, Kosmopoulos V, Liebschner MAK. Modeling of bone loss and fracture in osteoporosis. In: Gunzburg R, Szpalski M, eds. Vertebral osteoporotic compression fractures. Philadelphia: Lippincott Williams & Wilkins, 2002:35–50.

57. Kosmopoulos V, Keller TS. Finite element modeling of trabecular bone damage. Comp Meth Biomech Biomed Eng 2003;6:209–216.

58. Carter DR, Hayes WC. The compressive behavior of bone as a two-phase porous structure. J Bone Joint Surg 1977;59A:954–962.

59. van Rietbergen B, Weinans H, Huiskes R, et al. A new method to determine trabecular bone elastic properties and loading using micromechanical finite-element models. J Biomech 1995;28:69–81.

60. Saxena R, Keller TS, Sullivan JM. A three-dimensional finite element scheme to investigate the apparent mechanical properties of trabecular bone. Comp Meth Biomech Biomed Eng 1999a;2:285–294.

61. Saxena R, Keller TS. Computer modeling for evaluating trabecular bone mechanics. In: An YH, Draughn RA, eds. Mechanical testing of bone and the bone-implant interface. Boca Raton, FL: CRC Press, 1999:407–436.

62. Taylor M, Verdonschot N, Huiskes R, et al. A combined finite element method and continuum damage mechanics approach to simulate the in vitro fatigue behavior of human cortical bone. J Mat Sci Mat Med 1999;10:841–846.
63. Pidaparti RM, Liu Y. Bone stiffness changes due to microdamage under different loadings. Biomed Material Eng 1997;7:193–203.
64. Kosmopoulos V, Keller TS. Bone microdamage and repair simulations using an elastoplastic numerical scheme. Marbella, Spain: Proceedings from IASTED on Applied Simulation and Modelling, Sept. 3–5, 2003.
65. Kosmopoulos V, Keller TS, Baroud G, et al. Experimental and numerical simulation of microdamage and failure of thoracic vertebral trabecular bone. New Orleans: Transactions of the Orthopaedic Research Society. Feb. 2–5, 2003.
66. Kopperdahl DL, Roberts AD, Keaveny TM. Localized damage in vertebral bone is most detrimental in regions of high strain energy density. J Biomech Eng 1999;121:622–628.
67. Liebschner MAK, Rosenberg WS, Keaveny TM. Effects of bone cement volume and distribution on vertebral stiffness after vertebroplasty. Spine 2001;26:1547–1554.
68. Bostrom MP, Lane JM. Future directions: augmentation of osteoporotic vertebral bodies. Spine 1997;22[Suppl 24]:38S–42S.
69. Hu SS. Internal fixation in the osteoporotic spine. Spine 1997;22 [Suppl 24]:43S–48S.
70. Tohmeh AG, Mathis JM, Fento DC, et al. Biomechanical efficacy of unipedicular versus bipedicular vertebroplasty for the management of osteoporotic vertebral compression fractures. Spine 1999;24:1772–1776.
71. Lowery GL, Grobler LJ, Kulkarni SS. Challenges of internal fixation in osteoporotic spine. In: An YH, ed. Orthopaedic issues in osteoporosis. Boca Raton, FL: CRC Press, 2003:355–369.
72. Gertzbein SD, Court-Brown CM. Rationale for the management of flexion/distraction injuries of the thoracolumbar spine based on a new classification. Spine 1988;13:892–895.
73. Garfin SR, Yuan HA, Reiley MA. New technologies in spine: kyphoplasty and vertebroplasty for the treatment of painful osteoporotic compression fractures. Spine 2001;26:1511–1515.
74. Deramond H, Depriester C, Galibert P, et al. Percutaneous vertebroplasty with polymethylmethacrylate: technique, indications, and results. Radiol Clin North Am 1998;36:533–546.
75. Barr JD, Barr MS, Lemley TJ, et al. Percutaneous vertebroplasty for pain relief and spinal stabilization. Spine 2000;25:923–928.
76. Martin JB, Jean B, Sugiu K, et al. Vertebroplasty: clinical experience and follow-up results. Bone 1999;25[Suppl 2]:11S–15S.
77. Leeson MC, Lippitt SB. Thermal aspects of the use of polymethylmethacrylate in large metaphyseal defects in bone: a clinical and laboratory study. Clin Orthop 1993;295:239–245.
78. Eriksson RA, Albrektsson T, Magnusson B. Assessment of bone viability after heat trauma: a histological, histochemical and vital microscopic study in the rabbit. Scand J Plast Reconstr Surg 1984;18: 261–268.
79. Rouiller C, Majno G. Morphologische and chemische Untersuchung an Knochen nach Hitzeeinwirkung. Beitr Pathol Anat Allg Pathol 1953;113:100–120.
80. Polikeit A, Nolte LP, Ferguson J. The effect of cement augmentation on the load transfer in an osteoporotic functional spinal unit: finite element analysis. Spine 2003;28:991–996.
81. Belkoff SM, Mathis JM, Jasper LE, et al. The biomechanics of vertebroplasty: the effect of cement volume on mechanical behavior. Spine 2001;26:1537–1541.
82. Nolte LP, Visarius H, Arm E, et al. Computer-aided fixation of spinal implants. J Image Guid Surg 1995;1:88–93.

CHAPTER 8

Genetic Transmission of Common Spinal Disorders

Michele C. Battié and Tapio Videman

Spinal disorders such as disc degeneration and hernia-tion, sciatica, and back pain have commonly been attrib-uted to the accumulation of environmental effects, pri-marily mechanical insults and injuries, imposed on normal aging changes. Accordingly, environmental fac-tors received much attention as possible risk factors dur-ing the prior half-century, and only recently have studies on hereditary aspects of disc degeneration, disc failure, and back symptoms begun to accumulate (1).

A decade ago, in reviewing the epidemiology of degenerative disc disease, Frymoyer wrote: "Among the factors associated with its occurrence are age, gender, occupation, cigarette smoking, and exposure to vehicu-lar vibration. The contribution of other factors such as height, weight, and genetics is less certain" (2). Research since that time has dramatically changed views of genetic and environmental determinants of many common spinal disorders. When reviewing the same topic of "disc disease" in 2002, Ala-Kokko came to the following conclusion: "Even though several envi-ronmental and constitutional risk factors have been implicated in this disease, their effects are relatively minor, and recent family and twin studies have sug-gested that sciatica, disc herniation and disc degenera-tion may be explained to a large degree by genetic fac-tors" (3). We concur and will discuss the basis for this tentative conclusion in this chapter.

The role of genetics in common musculoskeletal dis-orders has been studied more in primary osteoarthritis than in spinal disorders. In a recent review article, Loughlin concluded that primary osteoarthritis has a major genetic component, but that osteoarthritis "is rarely transmitted as a Mendelian trait and that environ-mental factors play a significant role in disease expres-sion." He also classified osteoarthritis as a common, oli-gogenic, multifactorial genetic disease (4). These views are concordant with those on common spinal disorders,

which would be logical because joints and intervertebral discs are to a major part composed of the same proteins. To date more than a dozen gene loci associated with osteoarthritis have been identified, and a half dozen associated with disc degeneration, mainly from chromo-somes 2, 4, 6, 7, 11, 16, and X. Only a few loci have been associated with both joint and spine degeneration. However, it is likely that the genes representing the most significant genetic susceptibility to these common con-ditions have yet to be identified. (4).

We will briefly review the evidence suggesting genetic transmission, from case reports and more formal studies of familial aggregation to classic twin studies attempting to separate genetic and shared environmental influences, to the identification of gene forms. The primary focus of this chapter is on genetic influences on common spinal disorders, including disc degeneration and herniation, sciatica, and back pain.

IDENTIFYING AND CONFIRMING GENETIC INFLUENCES

Studies of the genetic epidemiology of common spinal disorders begin with determining whether familial aggre-gation of the disease or disorder is present. This is done by examining the frequency of disease in relatives of those affected as compared to the frequency of disease in the general population. If relatives are at increased risk, the pattern of familial aggregation can be further defined through various types of family studies (5). Most of the studies on common spinal disorders fall into this cate-gory. Once evidence for familial aggregation has been obtained, there is a need to distinguish between biologic (genetic) and social (cultural inheritance) sources of familial similarity (6). One method of accomplishing this is through classic twin studies of monozygotic and dizy-gotic twin pairs.

The genetic architecture of a trait includes information on how many gene loci are involved and which of the loci are polymorphic, with at least two common forms of the genes or alleles. The number of alleles and their frequencies are then determined for each gene locus. Allele frequencies and average effects associated with the alleles determine the contribution of allelic variation to the overall genetic variation. These can be further partitioned into additive genetic variance, due to gene "dosage," and variance due to dominance (7).

A growing number of monogenic diseases have been successfully analyzed down to the molecular level and have shown how a biochemical defect evolves from a single mutation, which parts of a gene are indispensable for normal function, and how phenotypes develop from different mutations. Based on these insights, molecular genetics can yield information on normal traits and common diseases. Normal traits and common diseases generally have a genetic contribution from more than one gene locus.

Genes suspected of involvement in the etiology of disease are called candidate genes. Candidate genes may be used as targets, with potential genetic variation leading to differences in the proteins encoded by the genes. These proteins are part of the physiologic system that, when disturbed, gives rise to the disease being studied. Also, for specific genes and some environmental factors, gene-gene interactions and gene-environment interactions may exist. For example, Solovieva et al. presented evidence suggesting that the effect of weight on lumbar disc degeneration is modified by COL9A3 gene polymorphisms in Finnish men (8). Simple linear models may, therefore, fail to grasp the complexity of the real world, and unraveling the contribution of genes and environment in diseases of multifactorial etiology is a challenging proposition (9).

DISC HERNIATION AND SCIATICA

The clearest association between back-related symptoms and the disc is for severe sciatica, often leading to surgery to remove an offending herniated disc. This condition also has been the focus of several investigations into genetic influences on common spinal disorders. As is typically the case, observations of familial aggregation lead to hypotheses of genetic susceptibility for sciatica and disc herniation.

It should be noted, however, that in juveniles and adults, persons identified as having disc herniations are those who access and receive spine surgery for pain with the diagnosis of disc herniation. Although discectomy may appear to be a clear indicator of the presence of a symptomatic disc herniation, the significant regional variations in rates of spine surgery demonstrate that this outcome is likely to be significantly influenced by other factors as well (10). Thus, some degree of classification error is involved when studying the occurrence of severe symptomatic disc herniation using the surrogate of discectomy.

Familial Aggregation of Juvenile Lumbar Disc Herniation

Two reports in 1990 documented cases of identical twins with similar histories of radicular symptoms and lumbar disc herniation. Matsui et al. documented a case of a 16-year-old girl who was admitted to a hospital for low back and left leg pain (11). Myelography and subsequent laminotomy revealed a protruded mass at the L4-5 level with left L5 root compression. Two years later, the patient's identical twin was admitted complaining of back pain of 2 years' duration and right leg symptoms of approximately 8 months. Results from myelography and discography prompted the surgeon to perform laminotomy and discectomy at the L4-5 and L5-S1 levels. The observation that herniated lumbar discs in young patients are relatively rare and the absence of a history of trauma, suggested that the similarity of the local disc pathology in the twins was not a chance occurrence. Matsui et al. thus concluded that their findings suggest that genetic factors are involved in the development of juvenile herniated nucleus pulposus (11).

Gunzburg et al. documented a similar case of identical twin girls who experienced radicular pain within 1 year of one another when they were approximately 13 years of age (12). Computed tomography scans revealed posterior bulging at the L4-5 level and herniation at the L5-S1 level in both. As in the case presented by Matsui et al., the onset of symptoms was similar and neither twin cited an injury or trauma (11). The twins experienced progressive symptoms that led to surgery in one case and chemonucleolysis in the other, with subsequent pain relief and return to normal activities.

These case reports demonstrate that familial aggregation occurs, but clarifying whether or not it occurs more often than would be expected through random occurrence requires comparison to controls or a reference group. The generally low incidence of juvenile disc herniation would suggest that such aggregation as seen in the cases just described would be extremely unlikely chance events. A rare population-based study of the incidence of surgeries for juvenile disc herniation was conducted among more than 75,000 Japanese elementary, junior high, and high school students. It revealed incidence rates of 1.69 per 100,000 person-years for 10- to 12-year-olds, 3.2 for 13- to 15-year-olds, and 9.4 for 16- to 18-year-olds. The mean incidence rate for all the schoolchildren was 5.4 per 100,000 person-years (13).

Two subsequent papers reported on the degree of familial aggregation in cases versus control groups. Varlotta et al. investigated the incidence of severe low back pain, sciatica, and surgically treated herniated discs among the parents of 63 patients under 21 years of age who had herniated lumbar discs and the parents of a control group of nonback patients (14). They also tried to eliminate reporting bias by family members by requiring confirmation from medical records. The estimated risk of developing a herniated disc before the age of 21 was four to five times greater for patients who had a positive family history, as compared to those who did not.

A year later Matsui et al. reported on the occurrence of lumbar disc herniation in the siblings and parents of 40 patients under 18 years of age who had undergone surgery for lumbar disc herniation and a referent group composed of the families of 120 controls (patients treated in the same department who had "normal spines") (13). The odds ratio of a patient with juvenile disc herniation to have a family history of disc surgery was 5.61 times that of a patient without disc herniation. The authors concluded that their results "strongly suggest that lumbar disc herniation in patients aged 18 years or younger shows familial predisposition and clustering."

Because family members can become affected even though the disease is not familially transmitted, the risk in family members ideally should be compared with the population risk. The finding by Matsui et al. of a higher incidence of a positive family history in juveniles with disc herniation, yielding an odds ratio of 5.61, is directly useful clinical information when combined with the incidence of 5.4 per 100,000 children and adolescents (13). Varlotta et al. used matched patient-control pairs in their series of 63 disc herniations in patients under 21 years of age (14). The age-adjusted relative risk of herniation in family members of patients compared to family members of controls was 4.5, which was quite similar to that found by Matsui et al. despite differences in methods and sample populations (13).

Younger patients who had undergone discectomy also were found to be significantly more likely to have a family history of back disorders by Nelson et al. in a study comparing three age groups, those 9 through 15, 16 through 19, and 20 through 25 years of age (15). Such a finding would be consistent with genetic epidemiologic literature, indicating that stronger genetic effects are associated with earlier onset.

Familial Aggregation of Lumbar Disc Herniation in Adults

There also have been over a half-dozen reported observations of familial aggregation of lumbar disc herniation in adults, raising interest in the possibility of genetic susceptibility (16–19). Scapinelli described a striking family history of a 44-year-old patient who had undergone surgery for lumbosacral disc herniation (17). Six of the patient's 14 siblings (five brothers and one sister) also had undergone surgery for lumbar disc herniation, with unusually large volumes of herniated disc material noted. In addition, two other siblings, one brother and one sister,

had been diagnosed as having lumbar disc herniation and were treated conservatively. The author noted an early onset of symptoms, usually in the third decade, which was not precipitated by trauma. He concluded that the high proportion of members of this generation affected could be due to transmission by both branches of the family of a genetic predisposition to premature degeneration or soft tissue weakness. He also hypothesized that a defective autosomal-dominant major gene with low penetrance may be responsible for increasing risk among some persons.

Similarly, Varughese and Quartey reported on the case histories of four brothers who had spinal surgery between 27 and 39 years of age for severe leg pain associated with disc herniation and concomitant spinal stenosis (18). Both parents reported similar histories of symptoms and spine surgery. The authors concluded that the familial aggregation, along with the relatively young ages of the brothers at the time of their acute radicular symptoms, suggest that developmental or hereditary factors may have been responsible for the pathogenesis of spinal problems in this family.

These observations were followed by several case-control studies of familial aggregation of disc herniation or "discogenic" low back pain. For example, Postacchini et al. studied the occurrence of "discogenic" low back pain in the relatives of patients attending a low back pain clinic for persistent and recurrent symptoms, patients who had undergone discectomy for lumbar disc herniation, and individuals with no history of low back pain (20). They identified familial aggregation in families of discogenic low back pain and surgery for herniated discs. Of the patients with discogenic low back pain and discectomy, 35% and 37%, respectively, had first-degree relatives with a history of discogenic low back pain. Five percent of patients with discogenic pain and 10% of those with discectomy had first-degree relatives who had undergone disc surgery. In comparison, only 12% of subjects without a history of back pain problems had relatives with discogenic low back pain and 1% had relatives with discectomy (20).

In one other case-control study, Simmons et al. investigated the family histories of back problems in first- and second-degree relatives of 65 patients who underwent surgery for "degenerative disc disease," as compared to 67 controls who had undergone orthopedic surgery for nonspine-related problems (21). Patients who had undergone spine surgery were 2.4 times more likely to have a positive family history of recurrent, incapacitating low back pain as those in the control group. In the spine surgery group, 18.5% of the relatives had a history of having spinal surgery, as compared with only 4.5% of the control group, yielding an odds ratio of 4.8 (21).

Richardson et al. noted methodologic limitations in earlier investigations of familial aggregation of disc-related low back problems, including unknown reliability of questionnaires to identify "discogenic" low back pain, overly exclusive control group criteria, and failure to control for potentially confounding extrinsic factors (22). They attempted to address these methodologic issues in a study of symptoms of lumbar disc herniation in the immediate relatives of 38 patients with disc herniation confirmed at surgery and 50 control subjects with upper extremity disorders. Although the numbers of subjects were relatively small and response rates limited, subjects with disc herniation confirmed at surgery were 16.5 times more likely to have a family history of symptoms of disc herniation as compared to the control subjects.

Matsui et al. assessed disc degeneration and herniation in 24 subjects with a history of disabling low back pain or unilateral leg pain who sought medical care and who also had immediate relatives who had undergone surgery for disc herniation (23). The frequency and extent of degenerative changes were then compared to those of 72 age- and sex-matched controls with a similar symptom history, but without a family history of disc surgery. The grade of disc degeneration according to magnetic resonance imaging (MRI) signal intensity was significantly more severe, and the incidence of lower lumbar herniation/bulging was higher in cases with a family history of disc surgery compared to controls. These findings led the authors to speculate that a familial predisposition for disc herniation may be an expression of disc degeneration (23).

Collectively, the observations and studies of familial aggregation make a convincing case that intervertebral disc herniations for which care is sought in juveniles and adults are indeed influenced by familial factors. The studies do not, however, provide data on the relative contributions of genetic and shared environmental factors and their complex interactions.

Classic Twin Studies of Disc Herniation and Sciatica

Classic twin studies comparing concordance of findings within monozygotic and dizygotic twin pairs provide a methodologic strategy for disentangling genetic and shared environmental influences. Heikkilä et al. conducted such a study of sciatica and hospitalization for disc herniation by comparing pair-wise concordance of monozygotic and dizygotic twins (24). The data from this Finnish study are valuable in that both self-report and hospital data are available, covering mild cases, which are less reliably reported, and generally more severe cases, which are more reliably categorized but more selected. In addition, the series was large (more than 9,000 same-sex twin pairs) and representative. Heritability estimates were 21% for sciatica and 11% for associated hospitalizations. The difference in the observed versus expected incidence of sciatica between monozygotic and dizygotic pairs decreased with increasing age. Thus, genetic influences were more significant in persons under 40 years of age. This finding is consistent with the literature, which indi-

cates that stronger genetic effects are associated with an earlier onset of disease (5). The apparently greater genetic influence in younger subjects may be due, in part, however, to a higher rate of misclassification caused by forgetfulness that occurs with advancing age.

Direct Genetic Evidence for Disc Herniation and Sciatica

Two collagen IX alleles have been recently identified to be associated with sciatica and lumbar disc herniation, confirming the role of genetics in spinal disorders. A study from 1999 reported that a tryptophan allele (Trp2) in the human COL9A2 gene was associated with sciatica, although it was present only in about 4% of the patients (25). There was also a trend for increased prevalence of radial tears in nonherniated discs among the Trp2 allele–positive subjects (3 of 6 patients with sciatica and 3 of 11 family members) (26). More recently it was discovered that 12.2% of patients with sciatica had a Trp3 allele in the COL9A3 compared with 4.7% among controls (27). Ala-Kokko has concluded from these findings that disc disease is not one entity, but instead is likely to consist of several related phenotypes (3).

LUMBAR DISC DEGENERATION

It is of little surprise that the size and shape of spinal structures in family members are more similar than in unrelated individuals. The reports of twin pairs that demonstrate similarities in spinal and other skeletal morphology simply provide confirmatory evidence (11, 28–31). Such similarities have been amply demonstrated for other anthropometrics, such as height and dental structure (16,32). Of greater interest is the possibility that degenerative changes commonly attributed primarily to environmental factors may be, in part, a function of genetic predisposition, and that this influence may be substantial. Disc degeneration is of interest because it is believed to be a factor in the pathogenesis of disc herniation and may play a contributory role in back symptoms.

Familial Aggregation of Disc Degeneration

We presented evidence of substantial familial aggregation of disc degeneration in terms of extent and location of changes in two earlier studies of monozygotic twins published in 1995 (33,34). The first study assessed the degree of similarities in degenerative findings by spinal level in the lumbar discs of 20 pairs of monozygotic twins from 36 to 60 years of age, relative to what would be expected by chance based on the prevalence of the findings by level among all 40 subjects (33). The MRI assessments were conducted blinded to twinship and revealed a higher degree of twin similarities than would be expected by chance. Only 15% of the variance in disc bulging/herniation was explained by age and smoking, but the variance explained rose to 54% with the addition of a variable representing familial aggregation in the L1-L4 discs. Approximately 26% of the variance was explained by familial aggregation in the L4-5 and L5-S1 levels. These results suggested a substantial familial influence on lumbar disc degeneration and warranted further investigation.

In a later study spine MR images of 115 pairs of male identical twins were assessed blinded to twinship and exposure history to estimate the effects of commonly suspected risk factors on disc degeneration, as determined from signal intensity, bulging, and height narrowing, relative to the effects of age and familial aggregation (34). In the multivariable analysis of the T12-L4 region, occupational physical loading conditions explained 7% of the variance in disc degeneration scores among the 230 subjects; this rose to 16% with the addition of age and to 77% with the addition of a variable representing familial

aggregation. In the L4-5 and L5-S1 region, leisure-time physical loading was the only behavioral or environmental factor investigated that entered the multivariate model and it explained only 2% of the variance in disc degeneration summary scores. The portion of the variance in lower lumbar disc degeneration scores explained rose to 9% with the addition of age and to 43% with the addition of familial aggregation. Examples of spine MR images from three pairs of twin siblings from this study cohort are provided in Figure 8-1.

Significantly more of the variance in degeneration remained unexplained in the lower lumbar region, as compared to the upper lumbar region. This discrepancy could be due to environmental conditions, which are likely mechanical in nature, and interact with spinal anthropometrics in such a way as to have a disproportional effect on the lower lumbar levels. However, the factors involved are not simply a function of the magnitude

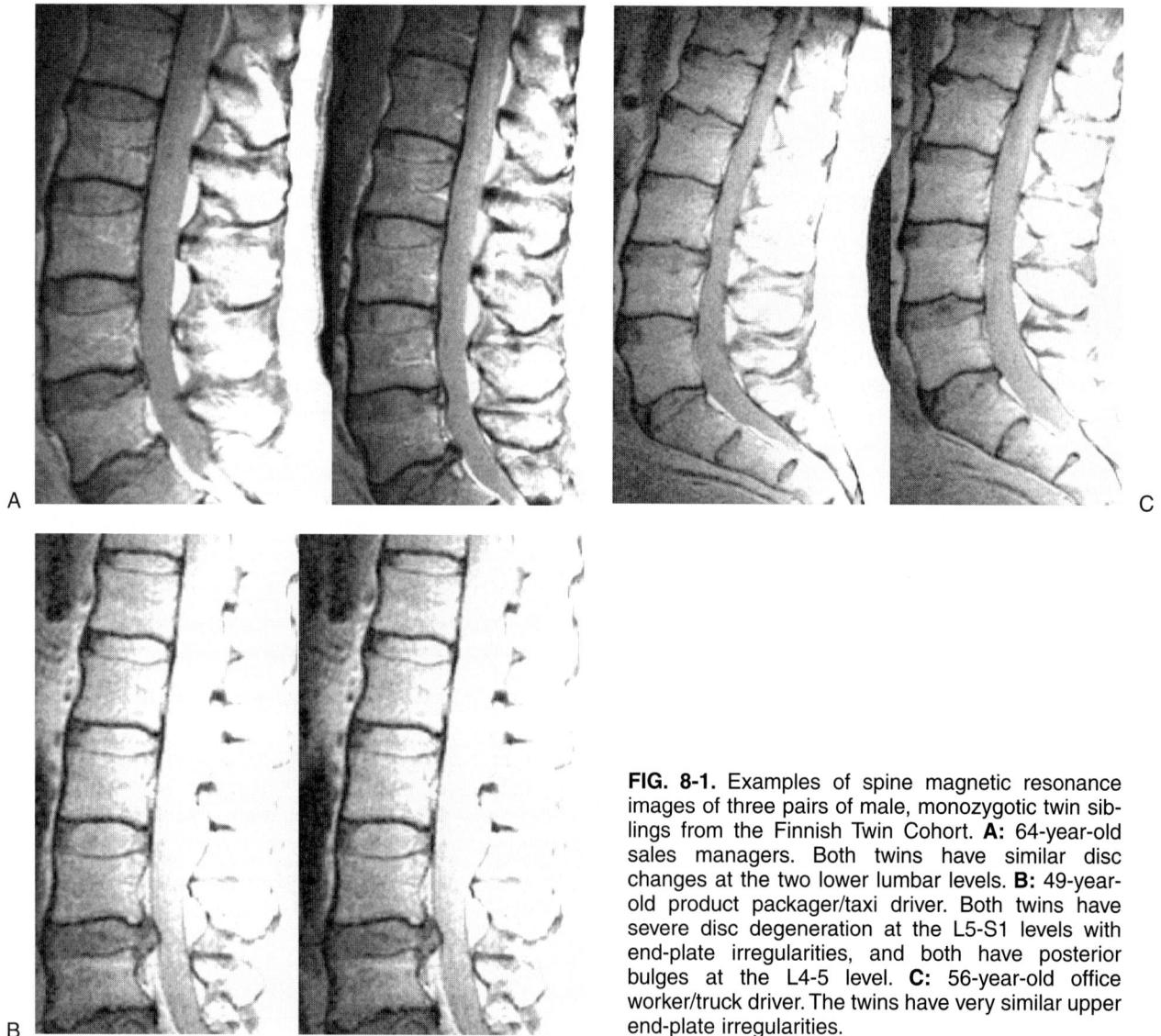

FIG. 8-1. Examples of spine magnetic resonance images of three pairs of male, monozygotic twin siblings from the Finnish Twin Cohort. **A:** 64-year-old sales managers. Both twins have similar disc changes at the two lower lumbar levels. **B:** 49-year-old product packager/taxi driver. Both twins have severe disc degeneration at the L5-S1 levels with end-plate irregularities, and both have posterior bulges at the L4-5 level. **C:** 56-year-old office worker/truck driver. The twins have very similar upper end-plate irregularities.

of occupational physical loading from materials handling and work postures. The study findings indicated that disc degeneration may be explained primarily by familial influences, which are most likely genetic, and as yet unidentified factors, which may include complex interactions. This study provides a first estimate of the relative importance of specific environmental agents and overall familial influences, including genetic factors (34). The remaining variance that is unaccounted for by the specific environmental and familial sources of variation is due to measurement error and yet unknown environmental effects.

Classic Twin Studies of Disc Degeneration

Following the earlier studies suggesting the possibility of a substantial genetic influence, Sambrook et al. conducted a classic twin study to examine the hypothesis that disc degeneration has a major genetic component (35). Spine MR images were obtained for 86 pairs of monozygotic twins and 154 dizygotic twins, 80% of who were female, from Australian and British twin registries. A substantial genetic influence on disc degeneration was found. For an overall score of disc degeneration, comprised of disc height, signal intensity, bulging, and anterior osteophyte formation, heritability estimates were 74% [95% confidence interval (CI), 64% to 81%] for the lumbar spine and 73% (95% CI, 64% to 80%) for the cervical spine. Heritability estimates were adjusted for age, weight, smoking, occupation, and physical activity. An analysis of individual MRI findings suggested that disc bulging and height were the primary contributors to the genetic determination of the disc degeneration summary score. Interestingly, a genetic influence was not apparent for signal intensity (35).

The findings of Sambrook et al. indicate a substantial genetic influence. What is not known is whether specific gene effects of relatively large magnitude exist or if the genetic contribution is due to small effects of many genes (35).

Direct Evidence of a Genetic Influence on Disc Degeneration

Genetic influences on intervertebral disc degeneration in humans were confirmed in 1998. In a study, using spine MRI it was shown that low-signal intensity of thoracic and lumbar discs was associated with TaqI tt-genotypes of the vitamin D receptor gene. A similar pattern was found between the summary scores of signal intensity, bulging, and disc height for both TaqI and FokI genotypes (36). TaqI and FokI each accounted for a substantial portion (6% to 7%), of the inter-individual variance in disc degeneration as measured through signal intensity. Another study using spine X-ray found an association between Taq polymorphisms and the severity of

osteophytosis and presence of disc narrowing, and more weakly, with the presence of osteophytosis (37).

A later investigation of the associations of vitamin D receptor TaqI polymorphisms and spine degeneration demonstrated that those with the tt genotype also had more anular tears but less bulges and osteophytes than those with the TT genotype (38). These findings emphasized the need for caution in combining specific suspected degenerative phenomena into summary scores. Also, the finding of the association between anular tears and genetics could be of importance because anular tears may be related to the pathophysiology of back pain. In another study, multilevel and severe lumbar disc degeneration was observed among 64 women with shorter variable numbers of tandem repeat length of the aggregate gene (39). In addition, the 5A5A and 5A6A genotypes of metalloproteinase-3 gene were associated with more degenerative findings in elderly individuals than those with the 6A6A genotype (40).

In animal studies, accelerated joint and intervertebral disc degeneration were observed in transgenic mice (COL9A1) based on X-rays and histologic methods. The spinal changes included shrinkage of the nucleus pulposus, anular fissures and herniations, and slight osteophyte formation (41). However, none of the known mutations in COL9A1 have been associated with disc degeneration in humans.

Although several gene forms associated with various aspects of disc degeneration have already been identified, it is likely that new gene forms associated with lumbar degeneration, pathology, and symptoms will be found over the coming years with the rapid growth in genetic research.

Several mechanisms have been suggested through which hereditary factors could influence disc degeneration and herniation. Genetic effects on the size and shape of spinal structures could affect the spine's mechanical properties, and thus its vulnerability to external forces (42). Biologic processes associated with the synthesis and breakdown of the disc's structural and biochemical constituents could be genetically predetermined, in part, leading to accelerated degenerative changes in some persons relative to others. The latter hypothesis has received some support from the recent findings of Annunen et al. and Paassilta et al. who found mutations in two collagen IX genes, COL9A2 and COL9A3, to be associated with disc pathology and symptoms (25,27).

BACK PAIN

Much more than just structural variations need to be considered in genetic and other determinants of back pain. For example, genetic influences could affect pain through a variety of mechanisms dealing with structural, neurologic, inflammatory, other physiologic and behavioral characteristics.

The relative importance of genes versus experience in human pain perception remains unclear; in animal studies there are significant individual differences in both nociceptive and analgesic sensitivity. Yet such differences are not necessarily attributable to genetics. Most often the familial aggregation of pain has been attributed to shared environmental influences and familial modeling (43–46). MacGregor et al., in a classic twin study of sensitivity to forehead pressure pain threshold, found heritability estimates of only 10%, indicating that shared family environmental factors may be significant in pain thresholds (47).

Classic Twin Studies Suggesting Genetic Susceptibility

Little is known about the role of genes in common low back pain problems or the pathways or mechanisms through which they may influence these problems. There have, however, been a of couple classic twin studies suggesting a genetic component. Bengtsson and Thorson investigated possible genetic influences on back pain in a cohort of 5,029 monozygotic and 7,876 dizygotic Swedish twin pairs (48). Back pain was defined as an affirmative answer to the question, "Have you had so much back pain during the last few years that you found it difficult to work?" Such pain was reported by about 15% of this cohort of twins ranging from 15 to 47 years of age. Pain concordance among twins with similar physical work environments was higher among monozygotic (25%) than dizygotc (15%) twin pairs (except in men performing light work), leading the authors to conclude that there is a relationship between genetic factors and back pain (48). The Swedish data are reported by gender, workload, and zygosity, but not by age, which is unfortunate given the findings of Heikkilä et al. of a differential effect of heredity by age on sciatica and associated hospitalizations (24).

Another classic twin study using over 700 twin pairs was presented by MacGregor et al. at an American College of Rheumatology meeting in 1999 (49). They found a substantial genetic contribution to the occurrence of severe back pain, with genetic factors accounting for 73% of the variance in population liability. They also reported on a subset of 97 monozygotic and 234 dizygotic pairs that had MR images available for analyses and found that more than 50% of the total genetic variance in back pain remained unexplained by genes involved in MRI changes. This suggests that there are other mechanisms through which genes may influence back pain than simply through structural changes in the disc. Mogil has noted that pain is considered both a sensation and an emotion, with considerable complexity and subjectivity. Yet, pain is also being studied at the level of the gene (50). The aforementioned studies should motivate more studies of the roles and relative contributions of cultural and genetic inheritance of back pain.

OTHER SPINAL DISORDERS WITH GENETIC CONTRIBUTIONS

Genetic contributions have been suggested or identified for a number of other spinal disorders, such as scoliosis, Scheuermann disease, spondylolysis, spina bifida, and spinal stenosis. Several family studies indicate that heredity has a role in scoliosis. Nearly identical "mirror images" of congenital lumbar scoliosis for a brother and sister, and two sets of identical twins with concordant scoliotic curves have been reported (51). In one family study from 1975, scoliosis appeared in 15 members of a family in 3 generations (52).

Segregation analysis was applied to 101 pedigrees from Russia with idiopathic scoliosis (more than 10°) and to 90 pedigrees with Scheuermann disease. Using transmission probability models, a significant contribution of one major causal gene was established and inheritance could be described according to a dominant major gene diallele model for both diseases. The authors concluded that only the carriers of the mutant allele develop pronounced forms of the disease. For scoliosis, only 30% of males and 50% of females with the mutant gene should manifest the disease (53). All male carriers of the mutant allele develop Scheuermann disease, while only half of female carriers manifest the disease. The frequency of scoliosis in the families with Scheuermann disease was 8%. The authors concluded that the "familial aggregation of these two spinal pathologies in the present sample may indicate a genetic unity of Scheuermann disease and idiopathic scoliosis" (53,54).

Scoliosis can also be a consequence of other severe diseases such as Marfan syndrome, familial dysautonomia, spondylocostal dysostosis, congenital lordoscoliosis due to lumbar segmentation defects and incomplete formation of lumbar vertebrae, diastrophic dwarfism, and familial Rett syndrome (55–57). The occurrence of scoliosis in the presence of other hereditary connective tissue syndromes raises the possibility that idiopathic scoliosis and congenital scoliosis are in fact a heterogeneous group of disorders with varied pathogenetic mechanisms (58).

From a systematic review using different genome databases, there were three candidate loci for human scoliosis (58). Genome-wide linkage surveys in large multiplex families indicate concordantly a limited number of genetic loci predisposing to idiopathic scoliosis: three loci on chromosomes 6p, distal 10q, and 18q in one family and distal chromosome 10q on another (59). The role of genetic factors in the development of scoliosis has been well documented; however, reports of the specific mode of genetic inheritance are inconclusive. These facts, combined with the phenotypic variability of this disorder, suggest that the genetic expression of idiopathic scoliosis may be dependent upon multiple factors and genetic interactions (60).

Spondylolysis also is suspected of having a genetic component. Spondylolysis was found in 13% of young Eskimos and in 74% of older Eskimos, a rate that is higher in the older age group than in other ethnic groups, leading Simper et al. to suspect a genetic influence (61). Several family studies support that there is an inheritance component in spondylolysis: 21% of descendants of a male ancestor with spondylolysis also had the condition, 4% had also spina bifida occulta. This pedigree was consistent with autosomal-dominant inheritance and incomplete (about 75%) penetrance for spondylolysis (56). One other survey identified 19% of relatives with spondylolysis (57). In addition, the reported cases of multiple lumbar spondylolysis could indicate the hereditary component (62–64). Spondylolysis can also be part of other syndromes, such as osteopetrosis, where other findings usually are clinically more important (65).

There are several reports about small case series indicating familial aggregation of spinal stenosis, commonly associated with a narrow cervical canal and disc herniations and sometimes with other congenital anomalies (66–69). Familial spinal canal stenosis has also been associated with autosomal-dominant osteosclerosis, and acrodysostosis (70). In addition, there are also case reports about hypophosphatemic vitamin D–resistant rickets as a cause of spinal canal stenosis (71).

SUMMARY

The study of genetic influences on common spinal disorders is rapidly progressing. Studies of familial aggregation were an initial step along this line of inquiry. Familial aggregation, well beyond what would be expected by chance occurrence, has been found for outcomes such as hospitalizations for disc herniation in juveniles and adults, sciatica, back pain, and disc degeneration. Familial aggregation also has been found to be greater in younger than older subjects in the case of hospitalizations for disc herniation, which would be congruent with a genetic component to this condition. The classic twin studies reported to date also suggest a genetic component to common spinal disorders and in some cases, such as for disc degeneration, a substantial one that overshadows the role of suspected environmental risk factors. Specific gene forms associated with these conditions also have been identified, which may eventually provide key insights into the mechanisms underlying back disorders. Although the complex contributions and interactions of genetic and environmental factors are currently unknown, these are fertile areas for future research.

REFERENCES

1. Riihimäki H. Low-back pain, its origin and risk indicators. Scand J Work Environ Health 1991;17:81–90.
2. Frymoyer JW. Lumbar disk disease: epidemiology. Instr Course Lect 1992;41:217–223.
3. Ala-Kokko L. Genetic risk factors for lumbar disc disease. Ann Med 2002;34:42–47.
4. Loughlin J. Genetic epidemiology of primary osteoarthritis. Curr Opin Rheumatol 2001;13:111–116.
5. Khoury MJ, Beaty TH, Cohen BH. Fundamentals of genetic epidemiology. New York: Oxford University Press, 1993.
6. Cavalli-Sforza LL, Feldman MW. Cultural transmissions and evolution: a quantitative approach. Princeton, NJ: Princeton University Press, 1981.
7. Sing CF, Moll PP. Genetics of atherosclerosis. Annu Rev Genet 1990;24:171–187.
8. Solovieva S, Lohiniva J, Leino-Arjas P, et al. COL9A3 gene polymorphism and obesity in intervertebral disc degeneration of the lumbar spine: evidence of gene-environment interaction. Spine 2002;27(23):2691–2696.
9. Zebra KE, Sing CF. The role of genome type-environment interaction and time in understanding the impact of genetic polymorphisms on lipid metabolism. Curr Opin Lipidol 1993;4:152–162.
10. Cherkin DC, Deyo RA, Loeser JD, et al. An international comparison of back surgery rates. Spine 1994;19:1201–1206.
11. Matsui H, Tsuji H, Terahata N. Juvenile lumbar herniated nucleus pulposus in monozygotic twins. Spine 1990;15:1228–1230.
12. Gunzburg R, Fraser RD, Fraser GA. Lumbar intervertebral disc prolapse in teenage twins. A case report and review of the literature. J Bone Joint Surg Br 1990;72:914–916.
13. Matsui H, Terahata N, Tsuji H, et al. Familial predisposition and clustering for juvenile lumbar disc herniation. Spine 1992;17:1323–1328.
14. Varlotta GP, Brown MD, Kelsey JL, et al. Familial predisposition for herniation of a lumbar disc in patients who are less than twenty-one years old. J Bone Joint Surg Am 1991;73:124–128.
15. Nelson CL, Janecki CJ, Gildenberg PL, et al. Disk protrusions in the young. Clin Orthop 1972;88:142–150.
16. Porter RW, Thorp L. Familial Aspects of disc protrusion. Orthop Trans 1986;10:524.
17. Scapinelli R. Lumbar disc herniation in eight siblings with a positive family history for disc disease. Acta Orthop Belg 1993;59:371–376.
18. Varughese G, Quartey GR. Familial lumbar spinal stenosis with acute disc herniations. Case reports of four brothers. J Neurosurg 1979;51:234–236.
19. Wilde GP, Narth AD, Kerslake R. The familial incidence of disc degeneration. In: Proceedings of the Annual Meeting of the Society for Back Pain Research, Oswestry, England. Hastings, England: Society for Back Pain Research, 1990.
20. Postacchini F, Lami R, Pugliese O. Familial predisposition to discogenic low-back pain. An epidemiologic and immunogenetic study. Spine 1988;13:1403–1406.
21. Simmons ED Jr, Guntupalli M, Kowalski JM, et al. Familial predisposition for degenerative disc disease. A case-control study. Spine 1996;21:1527–1529.
22. Richardson JK, Chung T, Schultz JS, et al. A familial predisposition toward lumbar disc injury. Spine 1997;22:1487–1492; discussion 1493.
23. Matsui H, Kanamori M, Ishihara H, et al. Familial predisposition for lumbar degenerative disc disease. A case-control study. Spine 1998;23:1029–1034.
24. Heikkilä JK, Koskenvuo M, Heliövaara M, et al. Genetic and environmental factors in sciatica. Evidence from a nationwide panel of 9365 adult twin pairs. Ann Med 1989;21:393–398.
25. Annunen S, Paassilta P, Lohiniva J, et al. An allele of COL9A2 associated with intervertebral disc disease. Science 1999;285:409–412.
26. Karppinen J, Pääkkä E, Raina S, et al. Magnetic resonance imaging findings in relation to the COL9A2 tryptophan allele among patients with sciatica. Spine 2002;27:78–83.
27. Paassilta P, Lohiniva J, Goring HH, et al. Identification of a novel common genetic risk factor for lumbar disk disease. JAMA 2001;285:1843–1849.
28. Bull J, el Gammal T, Popham M. A possible genetic factor in cervical spondylosis. Br J Radiol 1969;42:9–16.
29. King JB. A radiographic survey of 9 pairs of elderly identical twins. Clin Radiol 1968;19:315–317.
30. King JB. A radiographic survey of nine pairs of elderly identical twins. Clin Radiol 1971;22:375–378.
31. Hurxthal LM. Schmorl's nodes in identical twins: their probable genetic origin. Lahey Clin Foundation 1966;15:89–92.

32. Langinvainio H, Koskenvuo M, Kaprio J, et al. Finnish twins reared apart. II: Validation of zygosity, environmental dissimilarity and weight and height. Acta Genet Med Gemellol (Roma) 1984;33: 251–258.

33. Battie MC, Videman T, Gibbons LE, et al. 1995 Volvo Award in clinical sciences. Determinants of lumbar disc degeneration. A study relating lifetime exposures and magnetic resonance imaging findings in identical twins. Spine 1995;20:2601–2612.

34. Battie MC, Haynor DR, Fisher LD, et al. Similarities in degenerative findings on magnetic resonance images of the lumbar spines of identical twins. J Bone Joint Surg Am 1995;77:1662–1670.

35. Sambrook PN, MacGregor AJ, Spector TD. Genetic influences on cervical and lumbar disc degeneration: a magnetic resonance imaging study in twins. Arthritis Rheum 1999;42:366–372.

36. Videman T, Leppävuori J, Kaprio J, et al. Intragenic polymorphisms of the vitamin D receptor gene associated with intervertebral disc degeneration. Spine 1998;23:2477–2485.

37. Jones G, White C, Sambrook P, et al. Allelic variation in the vitamin D receptor, lifestyle factors and lumbar spinal degenerative disease. Ann Rheum Dis 1998;57:94–99.

38. Videman T, Gibbons LE, Battie MC, et al. The relative roles of intragenic polymorphisms of the vitamin D receptor gene in lumbar spine degeneration and bone density. Spine 2001;26:E7–E12.

39. Kawaguchi Y, Osada R, Kanamori M, et al. Association between an aggrecan gene polymorphism and lumbar disc degeneration. Spine 1999;24:2456–2460.

40. Takahashi M, Haro H, Wakabayashi Y, et al. The association of degeneration of the intervertebral disc with 5a/6a polymorphism in the promoter of the human matrix metalloproteinase-3 gene. J Bone Joint Surg Br 2001;83:491–495.

41. Kimura T, Nakata K, Tsumaki N, et al. Progressive degeneration of articular cartilage and intervertebral discs. An experimental study in transgenic mice bearing a type IX collagen mutation. Int Orthop 1996; 20:177–181.

42. Palmer PE, Stadalnick R, Arnon S. The genetic factor in cervical spondylosis. Skeletal Radiol 1984;11:178–182.

43. Bachiocco V, Scesi M, Morselli AM, et al. Individual pain history and familial pain tolerance models: relationships to post-surgical pain. Clin J Pain 1993;9:266–271.

44. Edwards PW, Zeichner A, Kuczmierczyk AR, et al. Familial pain models: the relationship between family history of pain and current pain experience. Pain 1985;21:379–384.

45. Lester N, Lefebvre JC, Keefe FJ. Pain in young adults: I. Relationship to gender and family pain history. Clin J Pain 1994;10:282–289.

46. Violon A, Giurgea D. Familial models for chronic pain. Pain 1984;18: 199–203.

47. MacGregor AJ, Griffiths GO, Baker J, et al. Determinants of pressure pain threshold in adult twins: evidence that shared environmental influences predominate. Pain 1997;73:253–257.

48. Bengtsson B, Thorson J. Back pain: a study of twins. Acta Genet Med Gemellol (Roma) 1991;40:83–90.

49. MacGregor AJ, Andrew T, Snieder H, et al. A genetic model for lower back pain: a population-based MRI study of twins. Presented at the annual meeting of the American College of Rheumatology, Session B: poster 452,1999.

50. Mogil JS. The genetic mediation of individual differences in sensitivity to pain and its inhibition. Proc Natl Acad Sci U S A 1999;96:7744–7751.

51. Gaertner RL. Idiopathic scoliosis in identical (monozygotic) twins. South Med J 1979;72:231–234.

52. Robin GC, Cohen T. Familial scoliosis. A clinical report. J Bone Joint Surg Br 1975;57:146–148.

53. Axenovich TI, Zaidman AM, Zorkoltseva IV, et al. Segregation analysis of idiopathic scoliosis: demonstration of a major gene effect. Am J Med Genet 1999;86:389–394.

54. Axenovich TI, Zaidman AM, Zorkoltseva IV, et al. Segregation analysis of Scheuermann disease in ninety families from Siberia. Am J Med Genet 2001;100:275–279.

55. Hayek S, Laplaza FJ, Axelrod FB, et al. Spinal deformity in familial dysautonomia. Prevalence, and results of bracing. J Bone Joint Surg Am 2000;82-A:1558–1562.

56. Haukipuro K, Keränen N, Koivisto E, et al. Familial occurrence of lumbar spondylolysis and spondylolisthesis. Clin Genet 1978;13: 471–476.

57. Wynne-Davies R, Scott JH. Inheritance and spondylolisthesis: a radiographic family survey. J Bone Joint Surg Br 1979;61-B:301–305.

58. Giampietro PF, Raggio CL, Blank RD. Synteny-defined candidate genes for congenital and idiopathic scoliosis. Am J Med Genet 1999; 83:164–177.

59. Wise CA, Barnes R, Gillum J, et al. Localization of susceptibility to familial idiopathic scoliosis. Spine 2000;25:2372–2380.

60. Miller NH. Spine update. Genetics of familial idiopathic scoliosis. Spine 2000;25:2416–2418.

61. Simper LB. Spondylolysis in Eskimo skeletons. Acta Orthop Scand 1986;57:78–80.

62. Mathiesen F, Simper LB, Seerup A. Multiple spondylolyses and spondylolistheses. Br J Radiol 1984;57:338–340.

63. Al-Sebai MW, Al-Khawashki H. Spondyloptosis and multiple-level spondylolysis. Eur Spine J 1999;8:75–77.

64. Ravichandran G. Multiple lumbar spondylolyses. Spine 1980;5:552–557.

65. Martin RP, Deane RH, Collett V. Spondylolysis in children who have osteopetrosis. J Bone Joint Surg Am 1997;79:1685–1689.

66. Igarashi S, Koyama T, Shimosaka S, et al. [Familial narrow spinal canal (lumbar canal stenosis with narrow cervical canal): case reports of three brothers]. No Shinkei Gekakei Geka 1982;10:961–966.

67. Postacchini F, Massobrio M, Ferro L. Familial lumbar stenosis. Case report of three siblings. J Bone Joint Surg Am 1985;67:321–323.

68. Iida H, Shikata J, Yamamuro T, et al. A pedigree of cervical stenosis, brachydactyly, syndactyly, and hyperopia. Clin Orthop 1989;80–86.

69. Hughes PJ, Edwards JM, Ridler MA, et al. A balanced autosomal translocation (3;9) associated with primary hypogonadism and dorsal spine stenosis. Clin Genet 1993;43:44–45.

70. Hamanishi C, Nagata Y, Nagao Y, et al. Acrodysostosis associated with spinal canal stenosis. Spine 1993;18:1922–1925.

71. Adams JE, Davies M. Intra-spinal new bone formation and spinal cord compression in familial hypophosphataemic vitamin D resistant osteomalacia. Q J Med 1986;61:1117–1129.

CHAPTER 9

Genetic Applications to Lumbar Disc Disease

Christian Lattermann, Lars G. Gilbertson, and James D. Kang

The etiology and pathophysiology of degenerative disc disease (DDD) are still unknown. However, it is believed, that it is the result of a complex interaction between biologic and mechanical factors.

New biologic techniques may allow for addressing intervertebral disc degeneration on a molecular level. Recent advancements in recombinant DNA technology have led to the decoding of many human genes that appear to be attractive for the scientific and clinical use in musculoskeletal disorders (1,2). Growth factors and embryogenic differentiation factors have been isolated and studied for many musculoskeletal conditions. Bone morphogenetic proteins (BMPs), for example, are successfully being used to enhance bone healing and fusion in humans (3). Other growth factors such as transforming growth factor β (TGF-β), or insulin-derived growth factor 1 (IGF-1) have been shown to be able to influence the proliferation and extracellular matrix production of various different musculoskeletal tissues (4–6).

After this brief overview we will introduce several novel approaches involving molecular genetic techniques and how their use can be advantageous for the treatment of DDD in the lumbar spine.

IDENTIFICATION OF GENES FOR TARGETED GENE MANIPULATION

Intervertebral disc disease occurs because of a complex interaction of cells, cell products, inflammatory cytokines, and degradative processes occurring in the intervertebral disc. All of these to-date identified mechanisms are naturally occurring processes that are designed to maintain the intervertebral disc homeostasis. One or multiple unknown triggers mark the beginning of disc degeneration by causing a shift of the anabolic/catabolic equilibrium. The goal of any biologic therapy for DDD therefore must be to reinstate the equilibrium or slow down the shift of the anabolic/catabolic equilibrium.

In order to be able to identify the different pathways in which a gene therapy protocol would be able to intervene toward a slowing of the degenerative process one has to understand the process of disc degeneration. While there are still many secrets to be solved in the complex process of disc degeneration it seems that there is a fundamental concept of homeostasis that is gradually disrupted during the degeneration of the intervertebral disc. To facilitate the understanding of the complex process of intervertebral disc degeneration and the possible ways of therapeutic intervention one can group the different mechanisms responsible for maintenance of disc homeostasis into two major categories: nutritional and catabolic.

Nutritional

One of the first steps in disc degeneration may be the increase in fibrochondrocytes along the annulus fibrosus. This increased fibrosis has been observed parallel to a decrease in diffusion of substances throughout the intervertebral disc. This in turn may be responsible for the declining oxygen tension within the intervertebral disc. A decrease in oxygen tension most likely will result in impairment of cellular function within the nucleus and thus may lead to a decrease in matrix synthesis. Decreased matrix synthesis will lead to a favored production of the smaller, less complex keratan sulfate shifting the equilibrium toward a higher concentration of nonaggregated proteoglycans that bind fewer water molecules (7–9). As a result, the overall capacity of the nucleus pulposus to imbibe water decreases. In addition there seems to be an abundance of smaller proteoglycan fragments that appear in early disc degeneration secondary to the collapse of adequate matrix proteoglycan production. These smaller, nonaggregate proteoglycans and breakdown products decrease the fluid flow throughout the disc and thus, even further inhibit the diffusion capacity of nutrients throughout the disc. This again limits the oxygen tension and nutrient supply to and from the intervertebral disc cells.

A further cascade involved in disruption of normal disc homeostasis is the constant maintenance of different collagen types within the intervertebral discs. The intervertebral disc is predominantly composed of type I and II collagen. The annulus is predominantly composed of type I collagen fibers. Type II collagen is mainly found in the nucleus pulposus. The distribution shows a small gradient toward the periphery, with the concentration of collagen type II decreasing and type I collagen fibers increasing toward the annulus. Despite the fact that this collagen scaffold does not seem to change significantly during the aging process, DDD shows significant alteration of the collagen composition early on. In early degeneration more type I and II collagen is expressed, however, in tandem with an increase in minor collagen types (III, V, VI). During the course of further degeneration collagen type II will disappear in the nucleus and be replaced by collagen type I. The minor collagen types of fibrosis (III, IV, and X) become more abundant within the nucleus pulposus and gradually lead to a loss of elasticity.

Catabolic

An inflammatory component has been discussed as a major entity in degeneration of the intervertebral disc. Nitric oxide (NO), interleukin-1 (IL-1) and 6 (IL-6), and prostaglandin E_2 (PGE_2) are powerful inflammatory mediators which have been shown to be elevated in degenerated human intervertebral discs. Although the mechanisms are not fully understood to date NO, IL-6, and PGE_2 appear to be up-regulated in response to the main inflammatory cytokine IL-1. It is likely that these inflammatory mediators have multiple functions but one of their functions is to support the breakdown of proteoglycans mediated by degradative enzymes called matrix metalloproteinases (MMPs). These MMPs are a family of enzymes responsible for the breakdown of collagens and extracellular matrix. The MMPs include well-known enzymes such as, collagenase 1-3, gelatinases, stromelysin, or aggrecanase. These powerful catabolic enzymes are able to breakdown different sizes of matrix proteoglycans and collagens and show a significantly higher activity in degenerated intervertebral disc cells than in normal discs. It is surprising, however, that the actual amount of MMPs is not increased in the degenerated intervertebral disc. In fact, the increase in proteoglycan breakdown may be more likely a result of the lack of inhibition of the MMPs.

In a normal intervertebral disc MMPs are inhibited by molecules called tissue inhibitors of metalloproteinases (TIMPs). The concentration of these TIMPs is greatly decreased in degenerated intervertebral discs. This mechanism, therefore, suggests a breakdown of the anti-catabolic system within the intervertebral disc during degeneration.

Strategies that result in a net increase in proteoglycans may have therapeutic potential in altering the natural history of disc degeneration. These strategies could involve increasing the production of proteoglycans, blocking their catabolic degradation, or a combination of both.

Possible Targets for Gene or Protein Transfer

One common way to increase the productivity of cells in the presence of impaired function uses small proteins called *growth factors*. These growth factors have the ability to override and steer cellular protein synthesis in less than optimal surroundings. Naturally occurring, these growth factors offer a way in which intervertebral disc cells can be influenced and guided to produce extracellular matrix and collagen when disc degeneration occurs and thus counteract the degradation of the intervertebral disc.

Several promising growth factors have been isolated which have the ability to increase extracellular matrix production and collagen production in intervertebral disc cells. Transforming growth factor-β (TGF-β1) and bone morphogenetic proteins (BMPs) are two examples of growth factors (out of many) with strong potential for altering intervertebral disc (IVD) biology. Thompson et al. studied the *in vitro* response of canine IVD tissue to the following growth factors: human recombinant IGF-1, epidermal growth factor (EGF), fibroblast growth factor (FGF), and TGF-β1. Incorporation rates by the tissue regions of up to five times the control rate were reported, with the nucleus and transition zone responding more than the annulus. TGF-β1 and EGF elicited greater response than FGF, while IGF-1 produced only a marginally significant response in the nucleus and no response in the annulus and transition zone (10). Our group showed that the use of TGF-β1 and BMP-2 lead to higher levels of proteoglycan production in degenerative human and rabbit nucleus pulposus cells (6). Takegami et al. studied the effect of human recombinant osteogenic protein (hrOP-1) on cell proliferation as well as on proteoglycan production and collagen synthesis. They showed that there is a dose-dependent increase in proliferation rate as well as collagen and proteoglycan production of rabbit intervertebral disc cells treated with hrOP-1. They were also able to show the restoration of proteoglycan in previously proteoglycan-depleted cultures of intervertebral disc cells if they were treated with hrOP-1 (11). Our laboratory has just recently shown that the treatment of degenerative intervertebral disc cells with TIMP-1 will increase proteoglycan production and the rate of proteoglycan synthesis by a factor of 5.

However, the critically important issue for the delivery of growth factors is the length of therapeutic effect of these exogenous growth factors to targeted cells in the IVD. The normal half-life for most of these growth factors *in vivo* is approximately 20 minutes. Therefore, the therapeutic effect of injecting growth factors directly into the IVD may be too transient to have a major long-lasting effect on a chronic disorder such as DDD, and repeated injections may not be practical or well tolerated by patients.

THE CONCEPT OF GENE TRANSFER

A sophisticated way to deliver sustained levels of growth factors to musculoskeletal tissues has been shown to be gene transfer technology. Particularly, the use of viral vectors appears to be highly efficient in the delivery of the desired transgene to most mesenchymal tissues.

Gene transfer is a novel technique in which genes of interest are inserted into target cells, causing them to synthesize the protein encoded by the inserted gene. This technique can be used as an approach for treating genetic diseases by compensating for mutant genes or as a means of delivering a therapeutic substance to the area of interest.

Protein synthesis within a mammalian cell involves several steps. At first a gene, consisting of specific DNA sequence is transcribed into a complementary chain heterogeneous to nuclear RNA. This is then processed into messenger RNA (mRNA) by a series of modifications that include capping, splicing, and the addition of a polyadenosine tail. The mature mRNA leaves the nucleus of the cell and is translated by ribosomes into a sequence of amino acids that form the protein. When an exogenous gene is introduced into the nucleus of a cell, it is also transcribed into mRNA and thus produces the protein encoded by the gene. The cell may normally not make this protein of interest, or it may be made in insufficient amounts. There are different techniques available that aid the insertion of a foreign gene into the genome of a mammalian cell. Gene transfer to cells normally requires the assistance of a vehicle or vector, which may be viral or nonviral in nature. The nonviral techniques typically use small particles like liposomes or spheroblasts carrying the gene of interest. These particles have the ability to fuse with the target cell or to enter the cell by endocytosis. Other techniques like elec-

troporation and microparticle bombardment use physical strain or electric shock in order to break small temporary defects into the cell wall without severely damaging the cell, allowing the DNA strand to travel into the cell. Another approach uses a direct microinjection of the gene into the cell. These methods tend to be inefficient (5).

Viral-based vectors generally use the inherent capacity of a virus to attach to the surface of a cell, through specific receptors, and insert its genome into the cell (Fig. 9-1). For safety reasons the viral vector must be altered to render the virus incapable of replicating. Hence viral vectors are engineered such that endogenous gene sequences required for replication and pathology are removed. The ideal viral vector therefore carries the genes of interest into cells with high efficiency, but does not replicate or cause pathology.

By far the most commonly used vectors are retroviral and most are based upon the Molony murine leukemia virus. Retroviral vectors specifically infect dividing cells with a very high efficiency. They insert their genes into the chromosomes of the target cell. This leads to reproduction of the inserted gene each time the infected cell divides. Clinical trials have already been successfully initiated using retroviral vectors. Although retroviral vectors are the most commonly used vectors in human clinical trials at present, there are certain disadvantages in their use. For example, retroviruses do not infect nondividing cells. Furthermore, there is a theoretical risk of mutagenesis due to the random integration of the viral DNA into the chromosome of the target cell. If chromosomal integration occurs near a site of an oncogene, activation may occur causing the cell to transform. Because of this potential risk, most investigators have used the retroviral vectors in an *ex vivo* approach (discussed later in the chapter). Presently, however, there are no reports of malignancy caused by gene therapy using retroviral vectors.

The second most commonly used viral vector is derived from the adenovirus. This is a DNA virus that is highly infectious to a number of different cell types. The

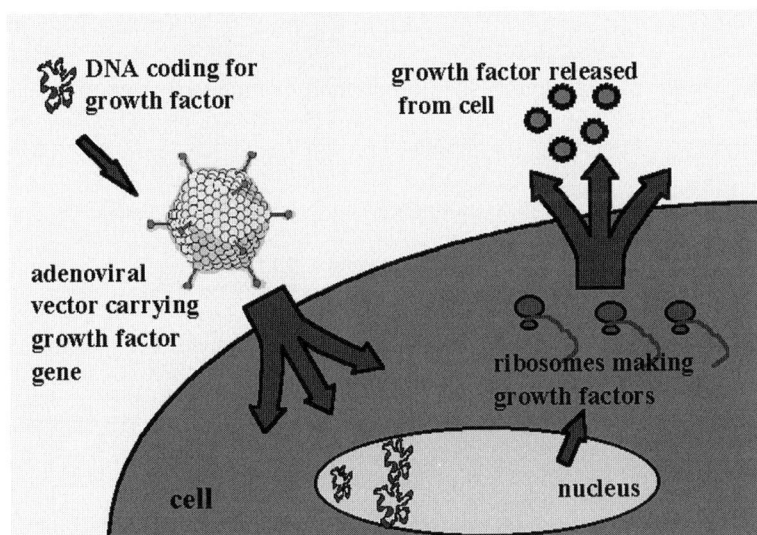

FIG. 9-1. The DNA coding for a growth factor is engineered into a vector (i.e., adenoviral vector capsid). The vector is applied to the tissue or cell culture and attaches to the cell membrane. The DNA is inserted into the cell and travels to the nucleus where it integrates episomally or integrates into the chromosome. The inserted DNA then uses the regular transcription and translation process of the host cell and is translated into the protein of interest. The treated cell now begins to produce the protein of interest in high amounts.

adenoviral vector infects dividing as well as nondividing cells and can be prepared in high titers. In contrast to the retroviral vectors, the genome of the adenoviral vector is not integrated into the chromosome of the target cell. The adenoviral vector inserts its genome as an episome within the nucleus of the target cell. Thus, the inserted genes will not be automatically passed on during cell division. As a result the percentage of infected daughter cells will rapidly decrease as a result of dilution with every cell generation. However, adenoviral vectors are highly antigenic and initiate strong immune responses. Likewise, herpes viral vectors, which have the capability of including multiple transgenes, are also antigenic and often cytotoxic to the host cell or tissues. Currently, new generations of viral-based vectors are under development. These will increase the efficiency of transduction of both dividing and nondividing cells. The most promising of these are based upon adeno-associated virus (AAV), the herpes simplex virus (HSV), and the lenti-retrovirus. These vectors show a high infectivity and may provide a long-term expression. The goal is to generate new viral vectors which can escape the surveillance of the host immune system and which can express the desired gene product in a tissue-specific manner.

Gene transfer can be accomplished by two main approaches, *ex vivo* or *in vivo*, in order to transduce target cells.

The *ex vivo* approach transduces target cells after harvest and culture *in vitro* under sterile conditions. The cells are transduced and selected in culture and then prepared for injection into the recipient tissue. Because no viral particles enter the human body, *ex vivo* gene therapy provides a measure of safety that is not found with *in vivo* gene delivery.

In vivo transduction is a more straightforward procedure. The vector is directly applied into the tissue of interest by catheter or needle injection. This approach however, does not allow control over the rate of target cell transduction. Due to the direct introduction of viral particles into the body, safety concerns are higher. The choice of the approach to achieve target cell transduction is dependent upon the desired longevity of gene expression, the viral vector chosen, the anatomy and physiology of the target organ, safety considerations, and the underlying cause of the disease to be treated. Generally, the *ex vivo* approach is usually employed when using retroviral vectors because of the necessity for high rates of cell division and safety concerns surrounding the injection of retrovirus into the body. Due to their high infectivity and ability to infect nondividing cells, adenoviral vectors are often used experimentally in the *in vivo* approach (5).

Gene Transfer to the Intervertebral Disc

Several authors have previously shown successful transfer of exogenous genes to musculoskeletal tissues. In our laboratory we have pioneered the viral gene transfer to the intervertebral disc using adenoviral and retroviral gene transfer protocols.

Wehling et al. reported the successful gene transfer of the LacZ marker gene as well as the interleukin receptor antagonist gene (IRAP) to bovine intervertebral disc cells (12). Subsequently, Nishida et al. performed a study which showed that the adenoviral transfer of the LacZ marker gene to the rabbit intervertebral disc is feasible and will lead to long-term expression of the marker gene (13). This has since been proved to be the case with different viral vectors including AAV (Figs. 9-2 and 9-3A,B). Surprisingly the intervertebral disc allowed for long-term gene expression after use of an adenoviral vector, suggesting that the intervertebral disc may be an immune-privileged site within the human body. This observation has since been underlined by Park et al. He found an unusually high expression of FAS ligand, a suppressor of cellular immunity, within the intervertebral disc (14). In a follow-up study Nishida et al. transferred the gene for TGF-β to rabbit intervertebral discs *in vivo* and could show that the overall proteoglycan production of the intervertebral disc cells increased (15). Moon et al.

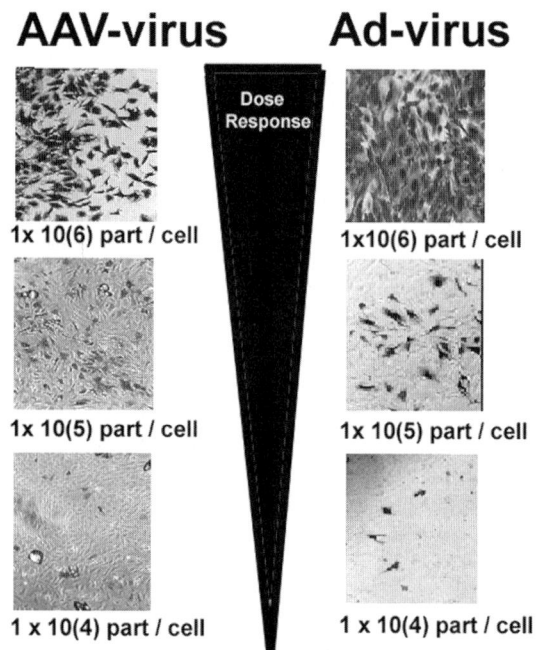

FIG. 9-2. *In vitro* transduction of human intervertebral disc cells with two different viral vectors. The adeno-associated virus vector *(AAV)* and the adenoviral vector *(ad)* both transfer the LacZ marker gene to human intervertebral disc cells. Both viruses show a clearly dose-dependent transduction efficacy. The adenoviral vector is overall more efficient. Adenoviral vectors have the advantage of efficient transduction of nondividing cells. The AAV shares this advantage but in addition is much less immunogenic and is not associated with any known disease in humans. Thus, the AAV vectors may be potentially safer than adenoviral or retroviral vectors.

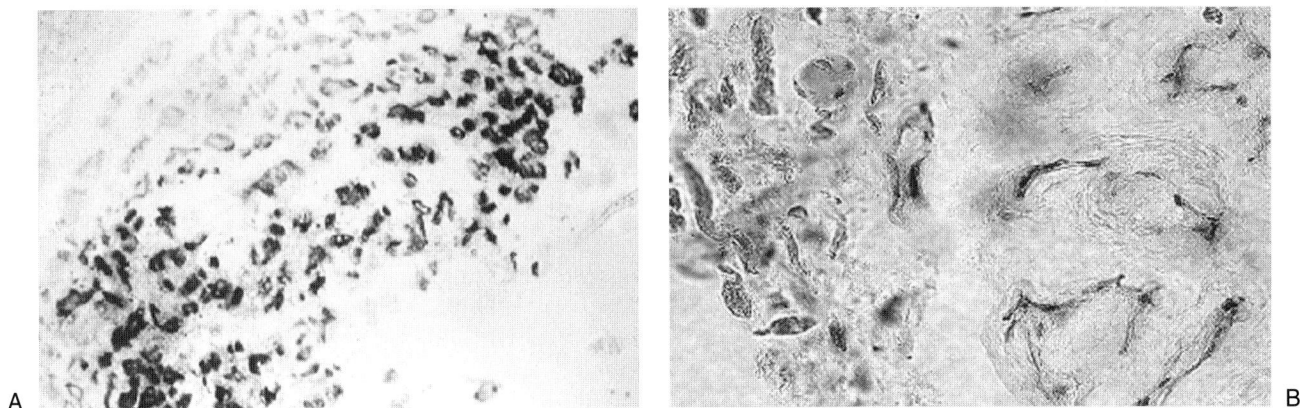

FIG. 9-3. *In vivo* transduction of intervertebral disc cells in rabbits can be achieved using a simple injection technique. Adenoviral gene transfer of the LacZ marker gene **(A)** at 6 weeks can be traced as long as 1 year post-injection. The *in vivo* delivery of the LacZ marker gene using the novel AAV vector **(B)** can be detected for at least 6 weeks post-injection.

investigated the effect of different growth factors transferred to human intervertebral disc cells using an adenoviral vector. He showed synergism between the expression of TGF-β, BMP-2, and IGF-1 with respect to the overall proteoglycan production in culture (6). In a recently published study Yung et al. applied a pellet culture technique in order to grow intervertebral disc cells in a three-dimensional matrix. Transduction of these pellet cultures with an adenoviral vector coding for the BMP-2 gene led to an increase in proteoglycan synthesis and total proteoglycan content (16).

FUTURE PERSPECTIVES

Clearly there are still many obstacles to overcome before a viral or nonviral gene transfer protocol can be used as a viable treatment option in DDD. Molecular biologists and surgeons, however, are feverishly working to develop safer methods of gene transfer in order to be able to influence the biologic environment within soft tissues such as the intervertebral disc. We know from animal experimental data that the approach is feasible *in vivo*. Safety studies are currently underway to determine if these technologies may be applicable to humans.

In addition to the development of novel and safe vectors researchers are developing new models to mimic intervertebral discs *in vitro* and *in vivo*.

Finally, it is important to understand the goal of any therapeutic approach to disc degeneration. The major issue to overcome at this time is still the early detection of disc degeneration. Questions that need to be answered, address the time course of degeneration. When is a disc too degenerated for therapy? How much regeneration potential does a degenerated disc have? How well does the magnetic resonance image signal change correlate with the biologic activity of the intervertebral disc? All these questions will have to be addressed before a broad-

based attempt to treat this disease using gene therapy can be made. As of now, we still do not know the exact cause of disc degeneration. It is certainly not feasible to prophylactically treat all degenerated discs at all levels with a gene therapy approach. It is therefore important to focus treatment using this new technology to very limited and clearly defined problems. One of these problems, for example, is disc degeneration occurring above and below fusions in the lumbar or cervical spine. At the time of fusion an injection into the adjacent discs could be performed without any problems.

In conclusion, gene transfer technology offers a sophisticated way to influence the biochemical environment inside the degenerated intervertebral disc and may be a useful tool to treat this highly prevalent disease in the future. The transfer of growth factors to the intervertebral disc may be able to limit disc degeneration or it may be able to prevent disc degeneration if the gene transfer is done prophylactically at a junctional level at the time of posterior spinal fusion. Viral or nonviral gene transfer is an emerging technology that will be able to offer exciting new perspectives in research and treatment of intervertebral disc disease.

REFERENCES

1. Evans CH, Scully SP. Orthopaedic gene therapy. Clin Orthop 2000;379 [Suppl]:S2
2. Jaffurs D, Evans CH. The Human Genome Project: implications for the treatment of musculoskeletal disease. J Am Acad Orthop Surg 1998;6 (1):1–14.
3. Boden SD, Zdeblick TA, Sandhu HS, et al. The use of rhBMP-2 in interbody fusion cages. Definitive evidence of osteoinduction in humans: a preliminary report. Spine 2000;25(3):376–381.
4. Puolakkainen PA, Twardzik DR, Ranchalis JE, et al. The enhancement in wound healing by transforming growth factor-beta 1 (TGF-beta 1) depends on the topical delivery system. J Surg Res 1995;58(3):321–329.
5. Gruber HE, Hanley EN Jr. Human disc cells in monolayer vs 3D culture: cell shape, division and matrix formation. BMC Musculoskeletal Disord 2000;1(1):1.
6. Moon SH, Gilbertson LG, Nishida K, et al. Human intervertebral disc

cells are genetically modifiable by adenovirus-mediated gene transfer: implications for the clinical management of intervertebral disc disorders. Spine 2000;15;25 (20):2573–2579.

7. Lipson SJ, Muir H. 1980 Volvo award in basic science. Proteoglycans in experimental intervertebral disc degeneration. Spine 1981;6(3):194–210.

8. Pearce RH, Grimmer BJ, Adams ME. Degeneration and the chemical composition of the human lumbar intervertebral disc. J Orthop Res 1987;5(2):198–205.

9. Stevens RL, Ryvar R, Robertson WR, et al. Biological changes in the annulus fibrosus in patients with low-back pain. Spine 1982;7(3):223–233.

10. Thompson JP, Oegema TR Jr, Bradford DS. Stimulation of mature canine intervertebral disc by growth factors. Spine 1991;16(3):253–260.

11. Takegami K, Thonar EJ, An HS, et al. Osteogenic protein-1 enhances matrix replenishment by intervertebral disc cells previously exposed to interleukin-1. Spine 2002;15;27 (12):1318–1325.

12. Wehling P, Schulitz KP, Robbins PD, et al. Transfer of genes to chondrocytic cells of the lumbar spine. Proposal for a treatment strategy of spinal disorders by local gene therapy. Spine 1997;15;22 (10):1092–1097.

13. Nishida K, Kang JD, Suh JK, et al. Adenovirus-mediated gene transfer to nucleus pulposus cells. Implications for the treatment of intervertebral disc degeneration. Spine 1998;15;23 (22):2437–2442.

14. Park JB, Chang H, Kim KW. Expression of Fas ligand and apoptosis of disc cells in herniated lumbar disc tissue. Spine 2001;15;26 (6):618–621.

15. Nishida K, Kang JD, Gilbertson LG, et al. Modulation of the biologic activity of the rabbit intervertebral disc by gene therapy: an in vivo study of adenovirus-mediated transfer of the human transforming growth factor beta 1 encoding gene. Spine 1999;1;24 (23):2419–2425.

16. Yung Lee J, Hall R, Pelinkovic D, et al. New use of a three-dimensional pellet culture system for human intervertebral disc cells: initial characterization and potential use for tissue engineering. Spine 2001;1;26 (21):2316–2322.

CHAPTER 10

Clinical Neurophysiologic and Electrodiagnostic Testing in Disorders of the Lumbar Spine

Jiri Dvorak and Scott Haldeman

Patients with symptoms related to the lumbar spine can be differentiated into two groups: those with neurologic deficits and those with more benign pathology causing pain. This differentiation carries significant clinical importance when considering prognosis as well as the necessity for nonsurgical or surgical intervention. The patient presenting with neurologic findings suggestive of a spinal cord or cauda equina lesion may represent a medical or surgical emergency. Patients with acute or progressive radiculopathy may respond to nonsurgical care but require more intense investigation than the patient without radiculopathy and may benefit from surgical decompression.

Patients with chronic neurologic lesions carry a poorer prognosis than appropriately treated patients with acute neurologic deficits. For this reason the documentation of neurologic deficits is one of the primary goals of the diagnostic process when evaluating patients with disorders of the lumbar spine.

When neurologic deficits are noted on examination of patients with lumbar radicular pain syndromes due to disc herniation or stenosis there may be a discrepancy between clinical and neuroradiologic imaging (magnetic resonance imaging, computed tomography, myelogram) findings. Furthermore, virtually all forms of nondestructive pathology noted on an imaging test can exist in the absence of symptoms. This can make it difficult to identify the particular nerve root or spinal cord level responsible for the patient's complaints. In other patients the clinical examination may be equivocal and there may be considerable doubt regarding the presence of neurologic deficits when patients present with vague nonspecific sensory or motor symptoms in the lower extremities.

Neurologic deficits in the lower extremities, even in patients with low back pain, may represent disorders that are not related to the lumbar spine. There are a number of compression lesions such as peroneal neuropathy and tarsal tunnel syndrome that can mimic radicular clinical pictures, especially if the symptoms are diffuse or the clinical examination is superficial. Surgery to the lumbar spine in these patients is unlikely to be of any benefit in reducing such deficits.

A surgeon contemplating surgery often has to answer two questions. The first is the determination of the presence and degree of neurologic loss. The second is the level of a spinal cord lesion or the nerve root that that may respond to decompressive surgery. If there is close concordance between clinical and imaging findings there is no need to consider further testing. However, in cases where imaging and clinical findings are not in complete agreement, the surgeon may require additional testing in order to make the correct decision on whether to operate and at what level surgery should be contemplated. It is in these cases, where there is doubt as to the presence of neurologic deficits or the level of such deficits, that neurophysiologic and electrophysiologic tests can become important in the diagnostic process.

There still remain some questions related to the sensitivity, specificity, and positive predictive value of certain electrophysiologic tests that often raise unreasonable expectations for these tests. There has also been a trend toward the indiscriminate ordering of batteries of tests in patients with sciatica. This has often led to confusing results that may not be of much help to the treating physician. Despite these shortcomings, the use of electrodiagnostic testing has become routine in most clinical settings that treat patients with disorders of the lumbar spine. This chapter will attempt to outline the most common electrophysiologic tests and to describe how they can be of the most value to both surgical and nonsurgical treating physicians.

ELECTRODIAGNOSTIC TESTING

Electrodiagnostic testing can be divided into three distinct areas of interest.

1. *The investigation of a suspected radiculopathy.* This is often the primary goal of electrodiagnostic testing. In this setting the testing is used to document the presence of and the level of a radiculopathy as well as to give some indication of the chronicity of the neurologic loss. The mainstay of this testing is electromyography (EMG). Electromyography, however, can be supplemented by the use of H-reflexes and possibly F-responses in order to make the testing more meaningful.

2. *The investigation of myelopathy.* The presence of symptoms suggestive of a myelopathy may represent a medical emergency and may have to be confirmed in a confusing clinical setting. Somatosensory evoked potentials (SEPs) and motor evoked potentials (MEPs) are most commonly used to investigate conduction within the spinal cord. SEP-techniques can be used to evaluate the sensory pathways within the spinal cord whereas MEPs allow for assessment of lesions that affect motor neuron pathways. Both SEPs and MEPs, however, are impacted by lesions that affect nerve roots as well as the lumbosacral plexus and depend on the integrity of peripheral nerves for accurate recording. This can make it difficult to interpret these tests if more than one lesion is present in a patient.

3. *The differentiation of proximal nerve root lesions from other peripheral or entrapment neuropathies.* The primary tool for this process is peripheral motor and sensory nerve conduction studies or conventional neurography (electronystagmogram, or ENG). It is often necessary to supplement these studies or at least correlate findings from ENG studies with F-wave, H-reflex, and EMG findings. Electromyography of limb and paraspinal muscles, for example, may allow a distinction to be made between lesions affecting motor roots and more peripheral nerve elements. Electroneurography, F-wave, and H-reflex studies may be the only manner to distinguish between proximal root and peripheral nerve disease with a high degree of confidence.

SEPS

SEPs can be recorded over the scalp adjacent to the sensory cortex on electric stimulation of the large mixed motor-sensory nerves, small sensory peripheral nerves, or the skin over specific dermatomes. Responses can also be recorded on magnetic stimulation of paraspinal and peripheral muscles. The recording of these potentials, due to their small amplitude in comparison with the background electrical noise, requires the computer averaging of multiple responses. Most laboratories will record simultaneously the sensory action potential within the peripheral nerve and, where possible, a response over the lower lumbar spine. The latter, however can be difficult in older patients and especially in overweight patients.

The nerves most commonly used for the diagnosis of spinal cord lesions are the large mixed sensory-motor posterior tibial and common peroneal nerves of the lower limbs usually at the level of the ankle. The absolute latency of scalp response and the difference in latency of the responses from the two legs can be used as an indication of reduced conduction within the spinal cord. By recording the peripheral sensory nerve conduction and measuring the height of the patient, it is possible to calculate the expected normal latency. If a spinal response is obtained, a central conduction time can be calculated by subtracting the latency of the spinal response from the latency of the cortical response.

Attempts to diagnose radiculopathy by stimulating dermatomes and small sensory nerves have led to disappointing results and suggest that the sensitivity, specificity, and reliability of SEPs in radiculopathy is not sufficient for general use. These tests are also very time-consuming and technically challenging as the responses have much smaller amplitude than those obtained from larger nerves. The use of mixed nerve responses is very insensitive in the diagnosis of radiculopathy because both the posterior tibial and peroneal nerves contain fibers from multiple nerve roots. However, in patients with multilevel radiculopathy or plexopathy marked abnormalities can be seen on stimulation of these large nerves.

SEPs have, however, been shown to be of value in documenting cauda equina and spinal cord lesions that affect bowel, bladder, and sexual function. In these patients cortical evoked potentials and bulbocavernosus reflex responses on stimulation of the pudendal nerve may give some indication whether the bowel, bladder, or sexual dysfunction is due to a lesion within the spinal cord or more peripherally within the nerve root and pudendal nerve.

MEPS

Barker et al. first introduced the method of painless magnetoelectric transcranial stimulation of the cerebral cortex in 1985 (1,2). They applied short magnetic pulses to the scalp produced by a device designed to stimulate peripheral nerves, and recorded muscle action potentials from upper and lower limb muscles. The magnetic field produced by this instrument passes through scalp and skull to stimulate the cerebral cortex. Magnetoelectric stimulation can also be used to stimulate deep-lying proximal segments of peripheral nerves and nerve roots (3), thus allowing for evaluation of central and proximal peripheral pathways. This equipment has also been used to stimulate paraspinal muscles and record cortical evoked potentials that can be influenced by muscle spasm.

The muscles most commonly used for recording cortically evoked MEPs in the lower extremities are the quadriceps, tibialis anterior, gastrocnemius, extensor hallucis, and abductor hallucis muscles (4). Surface recording electrodes are placed over the motor end plate. The segmental innervation of these muscles is used to determine the level of the lesion.

When recording MEPs on stimulation of motor roots at the lumbar spine, the intensity of the stimulator must be adjusted so that a potential with a steep negative rise can be recorded. In this situation the onset latency is not critically dependent on the positioning of the coil or the stimulation strength (3). The site of excitation of the nerve root is most probably the nerve root as it exits from the intervertebral foramen (3).

In order to interpret the MEP waveform it is necessary to obtain an M-wave recording by means of conventional neurography. The M-wave is the electric potential recorded from the muscle in response to a supramaximal stimulus of the peripheral nerve. This provides a measure of muscle electric response "size" (5) and is used as a reference signal with which transcranial stimulation MEP amplitude and duration are compared (i.e., MEP amplitude and duration are expressed as ratios of M-wave amplitude and duration).

F-WAVES

F-waves are long latency responses recorded over distal muscles on stimulation of motor nerves innervating the muscle. This is achieved through the stimulation of a Renshaw cell in the anterior horn of the spinal cord through antidromic stimulation of the motor nerve. Distinct left-right latency differences that exceed normal values or a reduced number of F-waves after a given number of supramaximal peripheral stimuli in the presence of normal distal motor conduction can be a sign of a proximal neuronal lesion in the sciatic plexus or nerve root. F-waves, however, must be interpreted with caution. The F-wave is often normal in mild cases of radiculopathy, especially if only one nerve root is involved.

In conjunction with MEPs, however, F-wave recordings may give information about conduction times in motor fibers within the proximal segments of spinal nerves that may be compressed by a disc herniation. F-wave recordings allow for the determination of peripheral nerve conduction time or peripheral latency (PL), the time it takes for impulses to travel from the anterior horn cell to the muscle. This latency includes conduction over the motor root from the spinal cord through its exit from the intervertebral foramen to the muscle where it is recorded. Calculation of PL is especially important in lumbar spine disorders where motor roots measure 10 to 20 cm (6) and contribute considerably to peripheral latency. F-wave recordings can therefore help localize the site of a lesion (7).

H-REFLEX

The H-reflex was first described by Hoffmann in 1918 (8). It is a reflex motor response within a muscle elicited on electric stimulation of large, low-threshold sensory nerve fibers within the nerve from that muscle. The response on stimulation of this nerve results in excitation of the motor neuron pool that innervates the muscle (from which the H-wave is recorded) through the same nerve. It is a monosynaptic reflex response that has a strong correlation with the tendon jerk but bypasses the muscle spindles.

In adults the H-reflex is recordable in a limited group of extensor muscles, especially the soleus/gastrocnemius muscles in the calf innervated by the S1 nerve root. Low-amplitude voluntary muscle contraction may facilitate the H-response (9). Stimulation of the tibial nerve at the knee with slowly increasing intensity from subthreshold to submaximal levels allows for recording of H-responses with increasing amplitude from the soleus muscle. Further increase in stimulus intensity elicits M-waves of increasing size, while the H-reflex diminishes progressively and is eventually replaced by the F-wave on supramaximal stimulus intensity. H-reflexes and F-waves have similar latencies when stimulus and recording sights are at the same location. S1 sensory or motor root deficits reduce H-responses and increase their latency. Right/left latency differences can be a sensitive indicator of unilateral S1-radiculopathy. Braddom et al. and Aiello et al. noted a 90% to 100% true-positive rate and 0% true-negative rate in S1 radiculopathies using the H-reflex from the soleus/gastrocnemius muscles (10,11).

EMG

EMG performed with concentric or monopolar needle electrodes is the oldest and the most widely used neurophysiologic test for the diagnosis of nerve root compression syndromes (12). It is often used as an extension of the physical and neurologic examination and the muscles selected for testing are usually selected based on the clinical findings (Fig. 10-1).

Needle EMG requires the physician to study the muscle under different conditions of muscle contraction. Four specific forms of electric muscle activity are recorded and noted for each muscle tested:

1. *Insertional activity* is evaluated at the time of insertion of the needle into the bulk of the muscle and at each repositioning of the needle electrode within the muscle. It is common practice to sample muscle electric activity at 10 to 20 locations within the muscle.

2. *Spontaneous activity* is studied with the muscle at rest. At each location within the muscle, the needle electrode is maintained in a stationary and stable positioning and muscle electric activity is recorded with the muscle at rest. This allows for the detection of abnormal electric activity such as fibrillation potentials and positive sharp

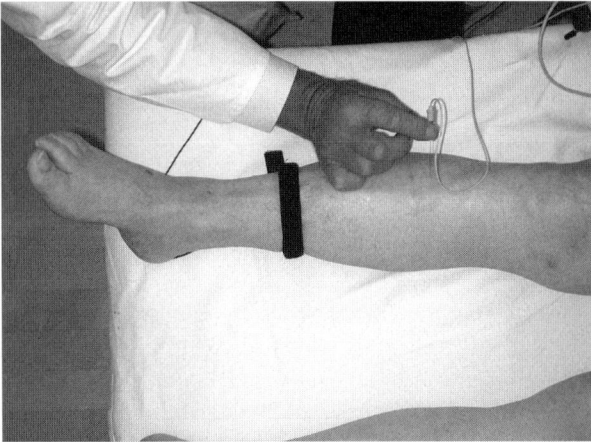

FIG. 10-1. Electromyogram with concentric needle electrode from tibialis anterior muscle

waves that are indication of acute denervation of the muscle (Fig. 10-2).

3. *Single motor unit action potentials* (MUAPs) are recorded during light voluntary contraction of the muscle and examined with respect to amplitude, duration, and number of phases of the electric potentials. An average of 20 MUAPs are commonly evaluated and can vary slightly from muscle to muscle.

4. *Motor unit recruitment* and the *interference pattern* are recorded during a gradual increase of voluntary muscle contraction and during maximal voluntary contraction to obtain a crude indication of the degree of muscle loss following denervation (Fig. 10-3).

In normal muscles, MUAPs are only seen during voluntary muscle contraction. The membranes of denervated muscle fibers become unstable and sensitive to mechanical or chemical irritation. This results in increased insertional activity and spontaneous activity that can be recorded in the absence of muscle contraction. These signs of denervation noted on EMG testing become evident at about 14 to 21 days after the nerve lesion. As the nerves to paraspinal muscles are shorter than those traveling to distal muscles, the spontaneous activity is first seen in paravertebral muscles followed by proximal and then distal muscles of the leg. These potentials represent signs of *acute* denervation of the muscle.

The analysis of single MUAPs may reveal characteristics that are typical but not specific for lower motor neuron injury that can occur in radiculopathy. The finding of increased amplitude, increased number of phases, and increased duration of the motor unit potentials are classically seen only after reinnervation of denervated muscle fibers as the result of sprouting from adjacent unaffected fibers. These changes are therefore termed signs of *chronic* denervation or reinnervation. Decreased motor unit recruitment and discharge are crude signs of the degree of neuronal loss as the result of radiculopathy.

SENSITIVITY AND SPECIFICITY OF NEUROPHYSIOLOGIC TESTING

There are numerous problems in the interpretation of published research studies that have looked at the sensitivity and specificity of the different electrodiagnostic tests. The primary difficulty is the determination of a gold standard for comparison. The studies that have been published have attempted to correlate the tests with either clinical examination findings, imaging studies such as computed tomography (CT), magnetic resonance imaging (MRI) or myelography, or the observation of nerve root compression noted during surgery. The difficulty in attempting to correlate electrodiagnostic testing with the clinical examination is that many clinical findings such as motor and sensory changes can be equivocal and influenced by pain that the patient may be experiencing. There may also be a fair degree of interobserver differences noted in neurologic clinical findings, especially among nonneurologists, that can make it difficult to interpret these results. The difficulty in using imaging studies such as CT, MRI, or myelography as a gold standard is that virtually all findings considered abnormal on these studies, including some of the most severe lesions that appear to be causing neuronal compression, can be seen in the asymptomatic population with a normal examination. One of the primary reasons for conducting the electrodiagnostic testing is to document the significance of a suspected compressive lesion. It therefore does not make sense to use imaging studies as the gold standard. The problem with surgical observation is that there is considerable subjectivity on the part of the surgeon in documenting the presence of root compression and the sur-

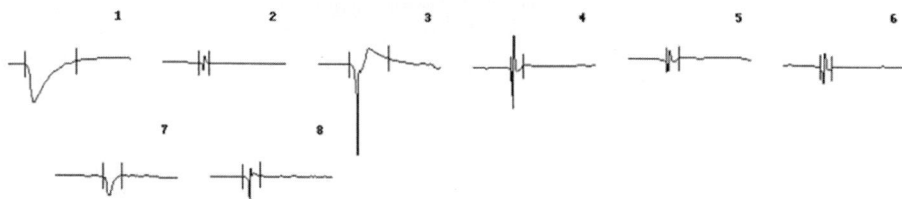

FIG. 10-2. Summary of different typical spontaneous activity from denervated tibialis anterior muscle as shown in Figure 10-1 (*1,* sharp positive wave; *2,* fibrillation; *3* and *4,* fasciculation).

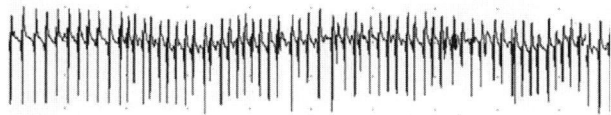

FIG. 10-3. Motor unit recruitment (interference pattern) during voluntary reduced contraction from denervated tibialis anterior muscle.

geon often does not have full visualization of the root or explore all potential nerve roots, especially in the newer minimally invasive procedures.

A number of studies however have attempted to address the issue of sensitivity and specificity of the neurophysiologic assessment of nerve root compression syndromes when compared to clinical, imaging, and surgical findings (13–15). The results of these studies have varied greatly from as little as 20% to as much as 90% or better correlation. The often markedly different results reported in other studies is due, in part, to the different electrodiagnostic tests used, the number of electrodiagnostic tests studied, and the basis of documenting the lesion (clinical, imaging, or surgical). The greater the number of electrodiagnostic tests used and the greater the number of tests the more sensitive the study is likely to be, but at the same time the results are likely to be less specific as each test has its own unique level of accuracy. The less precise the imaging or clinical finding the less likely that a correlation will be found.

These studies have been reviewed in detail by a number of authors and we will simply discuss a few of these papers to illustrate this point. Tullberg et al. (16), for example, looked at a series of electrodiagnostic tests in 20 patients who had undergone lumbar surgery for CT-documented disc herniations. They used a wide variety of tests including standard-needle EMG, F-wave responses on stimulation of the peroneal nerve (L5 root), and tibial nerve (S1 root) and dermatomal SEPs. They compared these studies with clinical neurologic findings such as motor, sensory, or reflex changes, CT scan results, and surgical observation of root compression. Using multiple diagnostic tools and multiple points for correlation, it is not surprising that these authors found poor reliability to predict results using electrodiagnostic testing. They noted that clinically only 4 patients with documented root compression on CT scan had motor loss and only 10 had sensory loss with very little correlation between the different findings on clinical examination. They noted that 13 of the 20 patients had abnormal electrodiagnostic test results but the correlation between tests and between tests and CT findings was low. As expected EMG was the most sensitive of these three testing methods for determining the presence of radiculopathy (45%) but it was less sensitive in determining the level of the disc protrusion (20%). The sensitivity of the F-wave to document the

presence of a root lesion noted on CT or surgery was 35%, which is in agreement with other investigations (17–20). However, the results were again unreliable in predicting the exact level. These authors concluded that there was no correlation between electrodiagnostic studies and the outcome of surgery.

The lack of correlation between electrodiagnostic studies, clinical findings, and imaging was studied by Haldeman et al. in 100 patients with chronic low back and leg pain who were undergoing disability evaluations for work-related injuries (21). The most revealing part of this study was the lack of correlation between clinical findings and imaging studies. The conclusion was that, in patients with chronic persistent back pain, there is a breakdown in the correlation between the clinical presentation and pathology. This makes it difficult to use patients with chronic pain complaints as a means of determining the reliability of any test in documenting disability.

Most studies, however, that have looked at the correlation of a single electrodiagnostic test and a specific clinical or imaging finding have found a correlation of between 75% and 85% in the documentation of radiculopathy (22,23). The results of Toyokura et al. (24), who looked at patients with a well-defined lesion rather than conduct a global study, conflict markedly with the results of Tullberg et al (16). Tokoyura et al. found that there was a significant improvement in F-responses after surgery that correlated with the improvement of muscle weakness after surgery.

There has also been a fairly high correlation between electrodiagnosis and the evaluation of muscle or motor function. Carter and Fritz compared EMG findings of acute denervation in patients with MRI findings of root compression (25). They compared the findings on EMG with the findings on short-time inversion recovery (STIR) MRI of the muscles affected by the nerve roots. STIR MRI has been noted to have a strong correlation with peripheral nerve injury that causes denervation and associated muscle edema. They noted a 92% correlation between denervated muscle on EMG and that was noted on STIR MRI. Zsu et al. provided more evidence of a close correlation been different electrodiagnostic tests and gave some indication how they could be used (26). They noted that in 227 patients with signs of acute denervation on EMG due to radiculopathy 47% of patients with L5 radiculopathies had an abnormal peroneal nerve F-wave. There was an abnormal H-reflex in 73% of cases with a S1 radiculopathy. The posterior tibial F-response was less sensitive showing only a 23% abnormal rate in patients with an S1 radiculopathy. They found no false-positive results. These authors believe that the use of long latency responses is primarily to confirm the findings on EMG and more accurately define the level of the lesion, but they also believe that these tests should not be performed without EMG because of the large false-negative results of using F-waves as a freestanding test.

Tullberg et al. (16) found that dermatomal SEP showed only 15% reliability in documenting the level of a root lesion, a finding that has been observed in a number of other studies. The studies of Dermatomal Sensory Evolved Potentials (DSERs), however, have given conflicting results that have fueled considerable controversy over the use of these tests. Yazicioglu et al. found that these tests were misleading in 27% of patients and predicted the presence and level of the lesion in only 7.2% of patients (27). This has led many authorities, including the American Academy of Neurology, to issue statements that DSERs do not add anything significant to the electrodiagnostic evaluation of radiculopathy (19). This has not, however, eliminated the controversy. Pape et al. recently reported a strong correlation between SERs and subsets of patients with sciatica (28). They found a strong correlation in patients with sciatica due to facet joint hypertrophy causing nerve root compression with or without disc pathology.

Studies on combining motor and sensory evoked responses that theoretically would increase reliability have also been disappointing. For example, Vohanka and Dvorak (29) correlated the neurophysiologic findings with CT or MRI findings of the lumbar spine. The quantitative analysis of motor unit potentials showed 30% sensitivity in patients with radiculopathy, but without motor deficit. The MEPs and SEPs combined reached sensitivities of 55%, but the MEPs had 75% false- negative findings.

One of the difficulties in electrodiagnostic studies has been the lack of lower extremity muscles and easily accessed peripheral nerves that can be tested for high lumbar disc herniations. Haig et al. (30, 31) has been studying the sensitivity of needle EMG of paraspinal muscles using a very precise mapping technique in fairly large samples of patients with and without low back pain and radiculopathy. They found that patients who are clinically normal have few if any EMG abnormalities in the paraspinal musculature despite a high incidence of abnormalities found on CT and MRI (32) in asymptomatic subjects. However, patients with radiculopathy as documented on pain drawings had a high degree of correlation with denervation in needle EMG of paraspinal muscles. The authors recommend EMG mapping of paraspinal muscles to rule out false-positive imaging studies. They found that the combination of paraspinal EMG mapping and lower extremity EMG showed a very strong correlation with imaging of root compression with a false-positive rate of only 8% and a false-negative rate of only 5%. In the small subset of patients with lack of correlation between imaging studies and electrodiagnostic testing it is still not possible to indicate the more reliable test for determining the presence of clinically significant radiculopathy.

Correlation between axial CT imaging and narrow spinal canal and electrophysiologic conduction studies has been prospectively evaluated in 132 patients by Vohanka et al. (33). Neurogenic claudication was initially declared by 59% of the patients. Twenty-six patients had one level, 68 had two levels, and 37 had three levels of central stenosis. No statistically significant relationship was found among the number of levels of the stenosis and the nerve conduction studies. However a significant relationship was found between minimum sagittal spinal canal diameter and the delay of central conduction time by transcranial magnetic stimulation. A similar correlation was detected in amplitude of the H-reflex and minimum transversal diameter.

Adamova et al. (34) introduced an exercise treadmill test in patients with mild lumbar spinal stenosis. It is a simple examination that can verify walking capacity and confirm neurogenic claudication described by the patient. Unfortunately an extensive electrophysiologic testing (H-reflex, F-response, MEP) and the analysis of obtained data before and after the treadmill test did not show significant changes in comparison with control groups.

CONCLUSIONS

There are ongoing studies that will hopefully clarify some of the difficulties clinicians have in interpreting imaging and electrodiagnostic testing. At this time, however, it is clear that it is not possible to take any one clinical finding, imaging study finding, or electrodiagnostic test out of context with other studies or findings. The most accurate method of determining the presence of a neurologic lesion is to conduct the electrodiagnostic test in conjunction with the other tests and clinical findings.

It is increasingly being recommended that the ideal approach to the study of radiculopathy is the electrodiagnostic consult by a specialist rather than the electrodiagnostic test by a technician. In this situation the electrodiagnostic specialist performs a history and examination of the patient and reviews all imaging studies. The determination of which electrodiagnostic test should be performed is based on the questions that arise from the examination of the patient.

If the clinical picture is clear, it may not be necessary to perform any testing. If there is concern as to whether an obvious radiculopathy is acute or chronic it may be sufficient to perform only needle EMG to look for signs of acute denervation or chronic reinnervation patterns. If there is concern as to whether a specific lesion on imaging is causing a radiculopathy then it may be important to include H-reflex or peroneal F-wave studies for the documentation of an S1 lesion or F-responses if polyradiculopathy is being considered. Paraspinal EMG mapping may be most appropriate when an upper lumbar radiculopathy is being considered. If there is confusion as to whether a neurologic deficit is due to a peripheral metabolic or entrapment neuropathy then it becomes necessary to consider nerve conduction studies. If there is consideration of a myelopathy or cauda equina lesion then somatosensory evoked responses, bulbocavernosus reflex responses, or cortical motor evoked responses may be necessary. It may be necessary to consider other neurophysiologic tests such as cystometry, nocturnal penile tumescence, or specific tests of the autonomic nervous system not mentioned in this chapter in order to obtain a clear picture of the nature of the neurologic lesion causing a patient's symptoms.

It is the tailoring of the clinical neurophysiologic test to the patient and, in particular, the clinical question being asked that gives these tests their greatest value. The more qualified the specialist performing the test and the manner in which the tests are correlated with the clinical findings the more reliable the testing can be considered. The indiscriminate use of electrodiagnostic testing by technicians (even when a physician is acting as a technician) appears to be the primary reason for the variation in the results in the different studies. It is hoped that the evolution of the ordering of electrodiagnostic testing into the requesting of a consult with a clinician with the capability to examine a patient, review the imaging studies, and determine the testing approach most likely to answer specific questions will lead to the answers to questions commonly asked by surgeons and other clinicians attempting to determine whether a patient with low back symptoms has a radiculopathy, myelopathy, or other neurologic lesion.

REFERENCES

1. Barker AT, Freeston IL, Jalinous R, et al. Magnetic stimulation of the human brain. J Physiol 1985;369:3P.
2. Barker AT, Jalinous R, Freeston IL. Non-invasive magnetic stimulation of the human motor cortex. Lancet 1985;1:1106–1107.
3. Britton TC, Meyer BU, Herdmann J, et al. Clinical use of the magnetic stimulator in the investigation of peripheral conduction time. Muscle Nerve 1990;13:396–406.
4. Chomiak J, Dvorak J, Antinnes J, et al. Motor evoked potentials: appropriate positioning of recording electrodes for diagnosis of spinal disorders. Eur Spine J 1995;4:180–185.
5. Reiners K, Herdmann J, Freund H-J. Altered mechanisms of muscular force generation in lower motor neuron disease. Muscle Nerve 1989;12:647–659.
6. Herdmann J, Dvorak J, Rathmer L, et al. Conduction velocities of pyramidal tract fibres and lumbar motor nerve roots: normal values. Zent Neurochir 1991;52:197–199.
7. Dvorak J, Herdmann J, Theiler R, et al. Magnetic stimulation of motor cortex and motor roots for painless evaluation of central and proximal peripheral motor pathways. Normal values and clinical application in disorders of the lumbar spine. Spine 1991;16(8):955–960.
8. Hoffmann P. Ueber die Beziehung der Sehnenreflexe zur willkuerlichen Bewegung und zum Tonus. Zschr Biologie 1918;68(1111): 351–370.
9. Stanley EF. Reflexes evoked in human thenar muscles during voluntary activity and their conduction pathways. J Neurol Neurosurg Psychiatry 1978;41:1016.
10. Braddom R, Joynson E. Standardization of H reflex and diagnostic use in S1 radiculopathy. Arch Phys Med Rehabil 1974;55:1661–1666.
11. Aiello I, Serra G, Migliore A. Electrophysiological findings in patients with lumbar disc prolapse. Clin Neurophysiol 1984. 24(4): p. 3313–3320.
12. Shea P, Woods W, Werden D. Electromyography in diagnosis of nerve root compression syndrome. Arch Neurol Psychiatry 1950;64:93–104.
13. Knuttsson B. Comparative value of electromyographic, myelographic and clinical-neurological examinations in diagnosis of lumbar root compression syndrome. Arch Orthop Scand Suppl 1961;49:1–135.
14. Kimura J. Electrodiagnosis in diseases of nerve and muscle: principles and practice, 2nd ed. Philadelphia: F.A. Davis, 1989.
15. Wilbourn AJ, Aminoff MJ. The electrodiagnostic examination in patients with radiculopathies. Muscle Nerve 1998;21:1612–1631.
16. Tullberg T, Svanborg E, Isacsson J, et al. A preoperative and postoperative study of the accuracy and value of electrodiagnosis in patients with lumbosacral disc herniation. Spine 1993;18(7):837–842.
17. Aminoff M, Goodin D, Parry G. Electrophysiologic evaluation of lumbosacral radiculopathies: electromyography, late response, and somatosensory evoked potentials. Neurology 1985;35:1514–1518.
18. Eisen A, Hoirch M. The electrodiagnostic evaluation of spinal root lesions. Spine 1983; 8:1(459):98–106.
19. Fisher M, Shivde A, Texeira C, et al. Clinical and electrophysiological appraisal of the significance of radicular injury in back pain. J Neurol Neurosurg Psychiatry 1978;41:303–306.
20. Tonzola R, Ackil A, Shahani B, et al. Usefulness of electrophysiological studies in the diagnosis of lumbosacral root disease. Ann Neurol 1981;9:305–308.
21. Haldeman S, Shouka M, Robboy S. Computed tomography, electrodiagnostic and clinical findings in chronic worker's compensation patients with back and leg pain. Spine 1988;13:345–350.
22. LaJoie W. Nerve root compression: correlation of electromyographic, myelographic and surgical findings. Arch Phys Med Rehab 1972;53: 390–392.
23. Lane M, Tamhankar M, Demopoulos J. Discogenic radiculopathy: Use of electromyography in multidisciplinary management. NY State J Med 1978;78:32–36.
24. Toyokura M, Ishida A, Murakami K. Follow-up study on F-wave in patients with lumbosacral radiculopathy. Comparison between before and after surgery. Electromyogr Clin Neurophysiol 1996;36:207–214.
25. Carter GT, Fritz RC. Electromyography and lower extremity short time to inversion recovery magnetic resonance imaging findings in lumbar radiculopathy. Muscle Nerve 1997;20:1191–1193.
26. Zsu Y, Weber R, Li J, et al. F-waves of peroneal and tibial nerve provide unique information in ongoing L5 and S1 radiculopathies. Paper presented at: Proceedings of the International Society for the Study of the Lumbar Spine; Cleveland; 2002; No. 158.
27. Yazicioglu K, Ozgul A, Kalyon TA, et al. The diagnostic value of dermatomal somatosensory evoked potentials in lumbosacral disc herniations: a critical approach. Electromyogr Clin Neurophysiol 1999;39: 175–181.
28. Pape E, Eldevik P, Vanvik B. Diagnostic validity of somatosensory evoked potentials in subgroups of patients with sciatica. Eur Spine J 2002;11:38–46.
29. Vohanka S, Dvorak J. Motor and somatosensory evoked potentials in lumbar spinal stenosis. Paper presented at 40th Congress of the Czech and Slovak Neurophysiology. Brno; 1993.
30. Haig AJ, LeBreck DB, Powly SG. Paraspinal mapping. Quantified needle electromyography of paraspinal muscles in persons without low back pain. Spine 1995;20:715–721.
31. Haig AJ, Vamakawa K, Hudson DM. Paraspinal electromyography in high lumbar and thoracic lesions. Am J Phys Med Rehabil 2000;79: 336–342.
32. Boden S, McCowin P, Davis D, et al. Abnormal magnetic resonance scans of the cervical spine in asymptomatic subjects. J Bone Joint Surg 1990;72-A(8):1178–1184.
33. Vohanka S, Adamova B, Dusek L. Correlation between axial CT imaging of the narrow lumbar spinal canal and electrophysiological conduction studies. Eur Spine J 2002;11S:11–12.
34. Adamova B, Vohanka S, Dusek L. The contribution of an exercise treadmill test to diagnosis in patients with mild lumbar spinal stenosis. Eur Spine J 2002;11S:54.

CHAPTER 11

Sensorimotor Control of the Lumbar Spine

Sten H. Holm and Aage Indahl

ETIOLOGY OF LOW BACK PAIN

Low back pain has probably been an integral part of most human lives through the ages. Tattoos on the back of the "Iceman" recently found in the Swiss Alps have been interpreted as a possible treatment for low back pain. At the beginning of the 20th century, the sacroiliac joint was thought of as the main pain generator of the back, and sacroiliac dysfunction was described (1). With the passing of time, other structures have come into focus. The term "facet syndrome" was coined in 1933 by Ghormley, although the meaning was different from that of today (2). It is still an undefined entity as is the "sacroiliac syndrome" (3). The major breakthrough came in 1934 when Mixter and Barr described how herniated nucleus material from the intervertebral disc, pressing on the nerve root, was the cause of sciatic pain (4). Although many details are now known about what Mixter and Barr described, it is still not fully understood why disc herniations occur. The mechanisms behind spinal disorders can either act as single variables or in combination. Derangement in the lumbar intervertebral disc and zygapophysial joints can contribute at the same segmental level or at different levels and be independently painful causing direct and referred pain. A similar situation can arise when the sacroiliac joint system itself is disturbed, or indirectly affected through derangement in the lumbar spine or its supporting structures (5–10). The relationship between pain and structural derangement is still not fully understood.

Low back pain is one of the most common medical problems of the middle-aged population, and from society's point of view, it is the most costly musculoskeletal disease in industrialized countries today (11–13). In the majority of cases, the origin of the pain remains obscure. Much of low back pain is thought to arise from damage to the intervertebral disc or the zygapophysial joints, either directly through traumatic injuries or disc prolapse, or indirectly through degenerative processes that transmit unfavorable loading patterns onto other spinal structures

(e.g., ligaments, tendons, and supporting musculature) as well as to the sacroiliac joint (8,14–20).

In the clinical situation, the surgery rate for chronic back pain is still growing, thus indicating strong beliefs in pathoanatomic derangements. *Stability* and *instability* are terms that are fundamental in describing the function of the different back structures. Despite the lack of a working clinical definition for these terms in a biomechanical system, they are widely used. Instability of one or more spinal segments is accepted as one cause for low back pain and the growing number of spinal fusion operations supports this belief. The need for strong trunk muscles and ergonomic advice to preserve the stability and integrity of the spine have dominated conservative treatments (e.g., stabilizing exercises) for many decades. Even if there is no clear definition of instability, there seems to be a common understanding that instability is a situation where a pathologic motion occurs within the motion segment. Attempts to measure such pathologic motions using advanced techniques have not been able to demonstrate instability (i.e., hypermobility) (21). However, this appears not to have had any impact on the clinical belief regarding the existence of instability. Terms that cannot be defined, processes that cannot be measured, or exercises that have no clear criteria for being a stabilizing exercise are of little value as scientific tools. For biomechanical systems, it might be more useful to use the terms such as *motion, balance* or *postural control*, and *transfer of loading* with regard to the function of the spine and its motion segments. An increased insight and understanding of the sensorimotor control system that takes care of these functions may lead us closer to the nature of low back pain.

In order to understand sensorimotor control, it is necessary to have knowledge of the different structures that are involved. All clinical entities for the treatment of low back pain are unfortunately lacking a physiologic backup and verification from adequate experimentally controlled trials. Injuries and structural degeneration cannot be

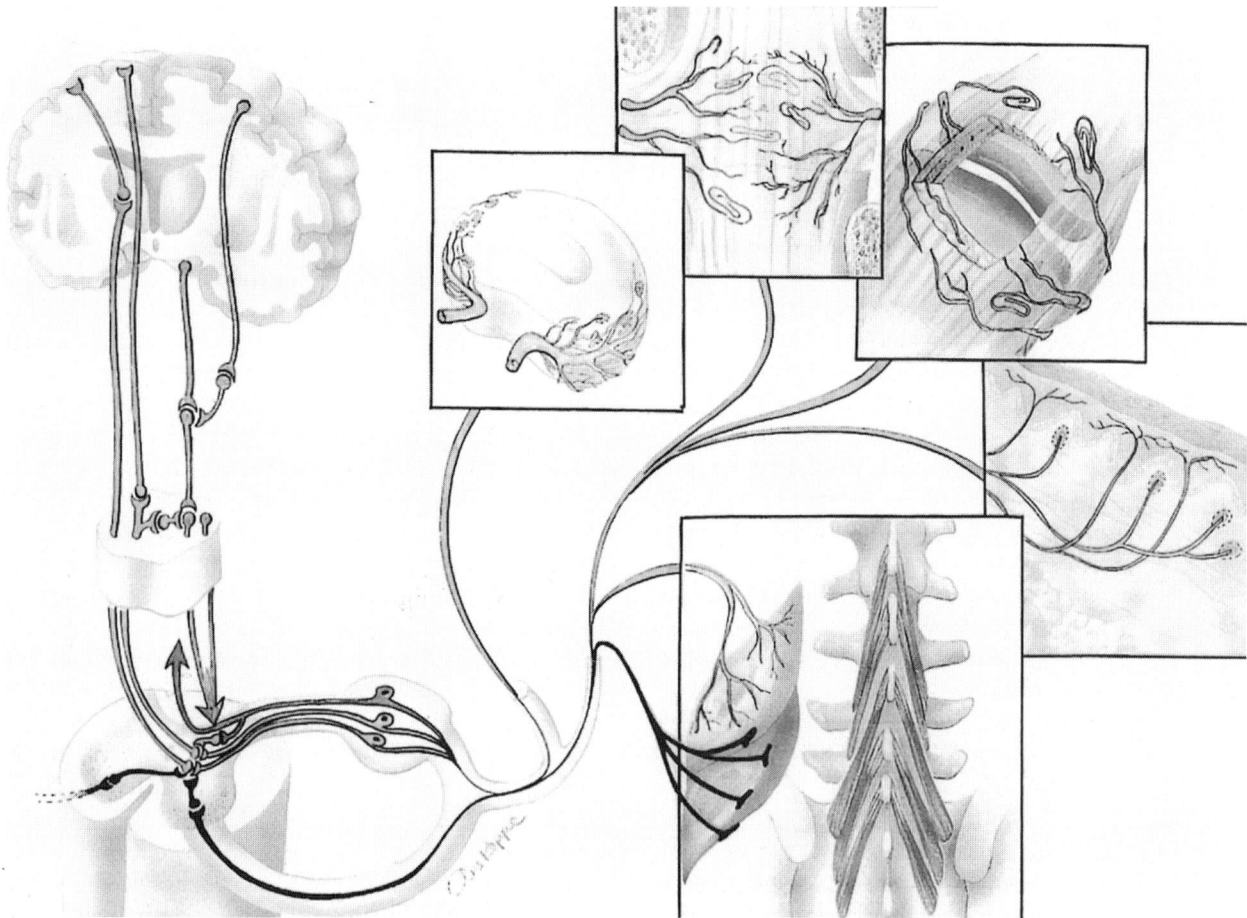

FIG. 11-1. Neuromuscular network connecting the central nervous system to peripheral structures **(shown in boxes)**: intervertebral disc, zygapophysial joint, skin, and spinal muscles. (Reprinted with permission from Holm S, Indahl A, Solomonow M. Sensorimotor control of the spine. *J EMG & Kinesiol* 2002;12:219-34.)

properly studied in the human situation because of the ongoing aging process. There remains an absolute need for interdisciplinary studies and experimental models in order to evaluate the neuromuscular interaction and the muscular control in the spine (22,23).

The peripheral part of the intervertebral disc, as well as the zygapophysial joint capsules, are richly innervated by different nerves that serve the function of pain and mechanical reception (20,24–26) (Fig. 11-1). Both injury as well as noxious stimulation of the spinal structures have been shown to cause spasm of the lumbar muscles and hamstrings (10,27), and may induce perturbations in the proprioceptive function (14). Such observations indicate possible mechanisms for long-term activation of the musculature as an important factor in low back problems.

LUMBAR AND SACRAL STRUCTURES AND INNERVATION PATTERNS

This section contains a brief summary of important structures and mechanisms involved in control and move-

ments of the back. Also discussed is how lesions in the avascular supporting structures, depending on location, size, and degree of inflammation, can cause perturbations to the proprioceptive function of the different receptors and result in increased or prolonged muscle activation that may cause pain. Irritation of low threshold nerve endings in the sacroiliac joint, intervertebral disc, or the zygapophysial joint tissue may trigger a reflex activation of the gluteal and paraspinal muscles that may become painful over time. To come closer to a solution to many low back problems, a better understanding of muscle function and their interactions with the passive structures through the neural structures is needed.

The Lumbar Intervertebral Disc

The intervertebral disc is a deformable connective structure that allows mobility and transfer loads between the vertebrae. A normal intervertebral disc consists of a gel-like central nucleus pulposus designed to sustain pressure. Surrounding the nucleus pulposus is a special arrangement of layers of collagen fibers, known as the annulus fibrosus, which can resist movements in all directions due to their alternating oblique orientation. A cartilaginous end plate joins the vertebral body and the intervertebral disc, and provides a nutritional pathway to the disc, which is an avascular structure (28).

In the superficial layers of the disc, nerves form simple free endings in the fetal stage, which increase in number as the fetus matures. During the postnatal period, various types of receptors develop, and in adult material, five types of nerve terminations can be found. The complexity of the receptors on the surface of the annulus increases with age. Within a given disc, the receptors are not uniformly distributed (Fig. 11-2). After postnatal development, there is a relative decrease in the number of receptors in the anterior region. In adults the greatest number of endings are found in the lateral regions of the disc, a smaller number occur in the posterior region, and the least number occur in the anterior region. The source of the nerve endings in the lumbar disc is the lumbar sinuvertebral nerves and branches of the lumbar ventral rami and the gray rami communicantes. Each lumbar sinuvertebral nerve supplies the disc at its level of entry into the vertebral canal and the disc above. The posterolateral corner of each lumbar disc receives branches from the lumbar ventral rami that originate just outside the intervertebral foramina. This region of the disc receives a branch from the gray ramus communicantes before its connection with the ventral ramus. Branches of the gray rami communicantes innervate discs at various levels. Even though the lumbar intervertebral discs are innervated by branches of the sympathetic nervous system, it does not necessarily mean that afferent fibers from these structures return to the nervous system through the sympathetic trunk. It has been suggested that somatic afferent fibers from the discs simply use the course of the rami communicantes to return to the ventral rami (20).

The presence of nerve endings in the lumbar intervertebral disc raises the question as to their function. Malinsky (29) proposed a proprioceptive function based on its morphology; however Kumar and Davis (30) did not find any evidence to support this theory. Two studies have demonstrated that mechanoreceptors are present in the outer annulus fibrosus of the intervertebral disc (20,31). Furthermore, it has been shown that in the rat the dorsal portions of intervertebral discs from L1-L2 to L4-L5 are multisegmentally innervated by the T11-L5 dorsal root ganglions (32).

For acute pain to occur, nerves must be involved. The disc itself may be an intrinsic source of pain originating from mechanical or chemical disturbances (33) (Fig. 11-3). As previously described, it has been established that the intervertebral disc receives innervation and that there are pain potentials in the outer part of the annulus fibrosus. It is possible that discogenic pain from a single level may involve more than one recurrent branch of the spinal nerves. Free nerve ending associated with blood vessels in the disc may be considered as having a vasomotor or vasosensory function, but because the annulus fibrosus contains so few blood vessels, this is less likely to be the function for the majority of the nerve fibers in the disc. Although there is no absolute explicit evidence that disc pain can be ascribed to a particular type of nerve ending in the disc, there is abundant evidence suggesting that the disc can be painful (33,34).

The Zygapophysial Joints

Together with the intervertebral disc, the lumbar zygapophysial joints, or more commonly called facet

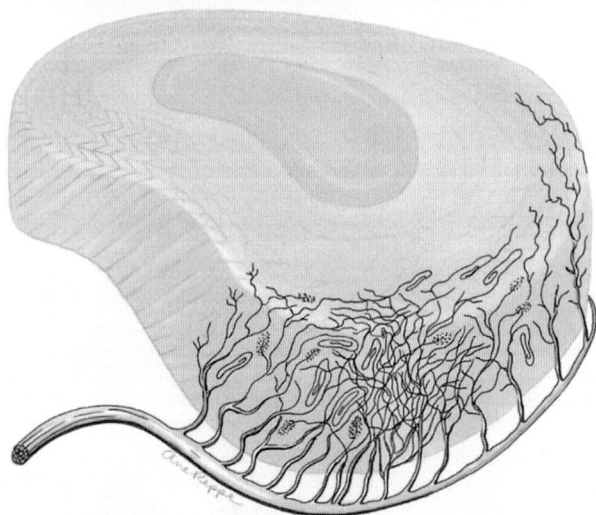

FIG. 11-2. Schematic of the lumbar intervertebral disc showing nonuniform innervation in the peripheral part.

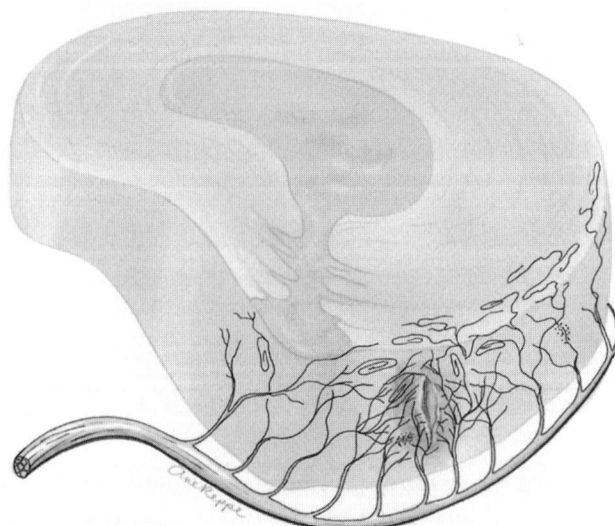

FIG. 11-3. Schematic of a lumbar intervertebral disc showing lesions that may or may not cause pain.

joints, are responsible for mechanical guidance of the motion segment (35). The inferior articular processes of one lumbar vertebra with the superior articular processes of the lower adjacent vertebra form the lumbar facet joints. The joints exhibit features typical of synovial joints and the articulating surfaces are covered by articular cartilage. The amount of weight bearing has been difficult to calculate, but is estimated to range from 0 to 20% (36,37).

Sensory innervation of the facet joints is derived from the posterior ramus of the spinal nerves, with each joint receiving branches from the level above, the same level, and the level below. These branches supply filaments to the capsule surrounding the facet joint, which is attached to the articular cartilage. Anteriorly, the fibrous capsule of the joint is replaced entirely by the ligamentum flavum, which attaches close to the articular margin. The enclosing joint capsule is thick dorsally and is reinforced by some of the deep fibers of the multifidus muscle. The consensus is that the facet joint is a possible source of low back pain (38). Marked degenerative changes can often be demonstrated on imaging. Attempts have been made to establish the "facet joint syndrome" as a clinical entity, but this remains questionable (10).

The Ligaments

The different ligaments provide substantial stability of the spine. The anterior and posterior longitudinal ligaments resist separation between adjacent as well as multiple vertebral bodies. Posteriorly, ligamentous structures provide resistance to flexion or axial separation between adjacent laminae (ligamentum flavum) and spinous processes (interspinous and supraspinous ligaments). The iliolumbar ligament provides a strong resistance to forward displacement between the L5 vertebra and the ilium. The intertransverse ligament, which spans between consecutive transverse processes, is considered part of the fascial system, which separates different muscular compartments within the spine (24).

Apart from ligamentum flavum, all ligaments seem to be innervated (39). The ligaments around the disc receive their innervation from the same nerves as the disc. The dorsal longitudinal ligament is more densely innervated than the anterior longitudinal ligament, receiving nerve endings from both sides. The more lateral and posteriorly located ligaments receive their innervation mainly from the posterior branch of the spinal nerve (24).

The Sacroiliac Joint

The sacroiliac joint (SIJ) is a true synovial joint with an auricular shape and a very limited amount of motion. The joint is relatively small, considering the large forces transmitted across it. The SIJ does, however, have an extensive network of strong ligaments that helps maintain stability and is constructed in such a way that the liga-

ments are self-tightening with increasing load. Roentgen stereophotogrammetric analysis has shown the amount of SIJ motion to range from 0.5 to 1.6 mm for translation and up to 4° for rotation (40).

The SIJ appears to be richly innervated, although there seems to be some uncertainty as to the exact innervation patterns (Fig. 11-4). Solonen found the SIJ to be predominantly innervated by the L4-S1 nerve roots, with some contribution from the superior gluteal nerve, but with a lesser contribution from S2, and rarely from L3 nerve roots (41). Grob et al. (42), in a study on adult human cadavers, found the SIJ to be innervated by fine nerve branches derived exclusively from dorsal rami of the S1-S4 spinal nerves. Ikeda reported that the upper ventral portion of the SIJ was mainly supplied by the ventral ramus of the fifth lumbar nerve, while the lower ventral portion was mainly supplied by the ramus of the S2 nerve (43). Thick, thin, and unmyelinated nerve fibers have been reported, which are compatible with a broad repertoire of sensory receptors, including encapsulated mechanoreceptors (42,43).

In search of causes of low back pain, the SIJ has gained renewed interest as a possible pain generator (44,45). There is a special awareness of the SIJ as a source of pain in pregnant and postpartum women, and although the mechanism is not understood, relaxation of the SIJ before childbirth is believed to play a role (9). Instability or subluxation has most often been suggested as mechanisms behind sacroiliac dysfunction (7,46). Despite any proven clinical findings or clearly defined function of the joint,

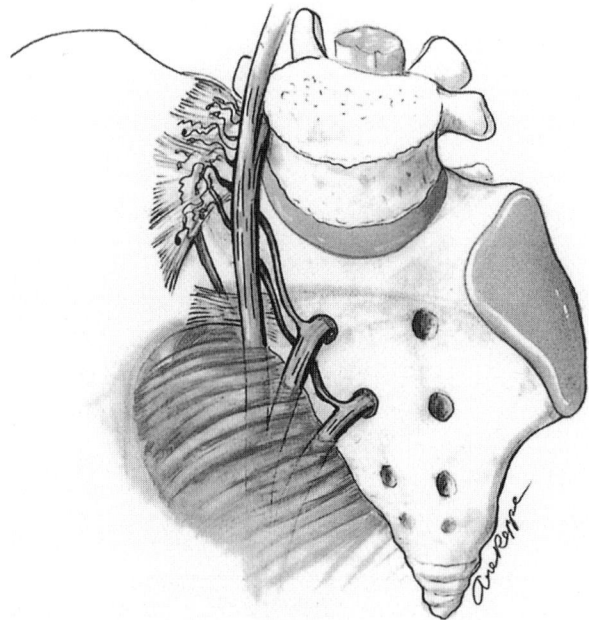

FIG. 11-4. Representation showing the sacroiliac joint, stabilizing ligaments, and innervation.

"sacroiliac dysfunction" has been established as a clinical entity (5,7,46,47).

The Supporting Musculature

The system responsible for muscle coordination around a joint is called the "myotactic unit." Muscle spindle afferents make direct connections to motor neurons responsible for activation of synergist muscles and to interneurons inhibiting motor neurons of antagonist muscles. Through these divergent connections to the different muscles around a joint, a strong neural network is established so that muscles do not act independently of each other. Such arrangements are responsible for joint stiffness.

Neural control on multiple levels is required to maintain normal locomotion. In order to support the body against gravity, maintain posture, and to propel it forward, muscle contractions must be well coordinated for several joints. At the same time, the nervous system must exert active control to maintain balance of the moving body, and it must adapt the locomotion patterns to the environment and to the overall behavioral goals. The spinal circuits activated by descending signals from higher centers accomplish this. Neural circuits in the spinal cord play an essential role in motor coordination. Spinal reflexes, where the "myotactic units" are the building blocks, provide the nervous system with a set of elementary patterns of coordination that can be activated, either by sensory stimuli or by descending signals from the brainstem and cerebral cortex.

The lumbar musculature exerts various forces on the spinal motion segments. Each muscle not only acts as a moment-producer, but also generates compressive and shear forces. The functions of these muscles are to stabilize the spine while providing mobility (21,48,49). The recruitment patterns for these muscles are not well established. The multifidus muscles are the longest and most medial of the lumbar back muscles. They consist of repeating series of fascicles that originate from the laminae and the spinous processes of the lumbar vertebrae and display consistent patterns of attachments caudally (24). The key feature of the morphology of the lumbar multifidus is that its fascicles are arranged polysegmentally (Fig. 11-5). Each lumbar vertebra is supplied with a group of fascicles that radiate from its spinous process, anchoring it below to mammillary processes. The fibers of the multifidus are designed to act together on a single spinous process of two to four levels. All the fascicles originating from the spinous processes of a given vertebra are innervated by the medial branch of the dorsal ramus that originates from below that vertebra. The muscles that act directly on a particular vertebral segment are innervated by the nerve of that segment (50–52). Although the paraspinal musculature has been studied quite extensively, its role in the formation of low back pain is far from clear (53). Electromyographic evaluations of various back lesions have contributed to the current understanding of low back pain (54–58). The clinical picture often seen is one of tense and painful paraspinal muscles and reduced flexibility in the lumbar spine. This

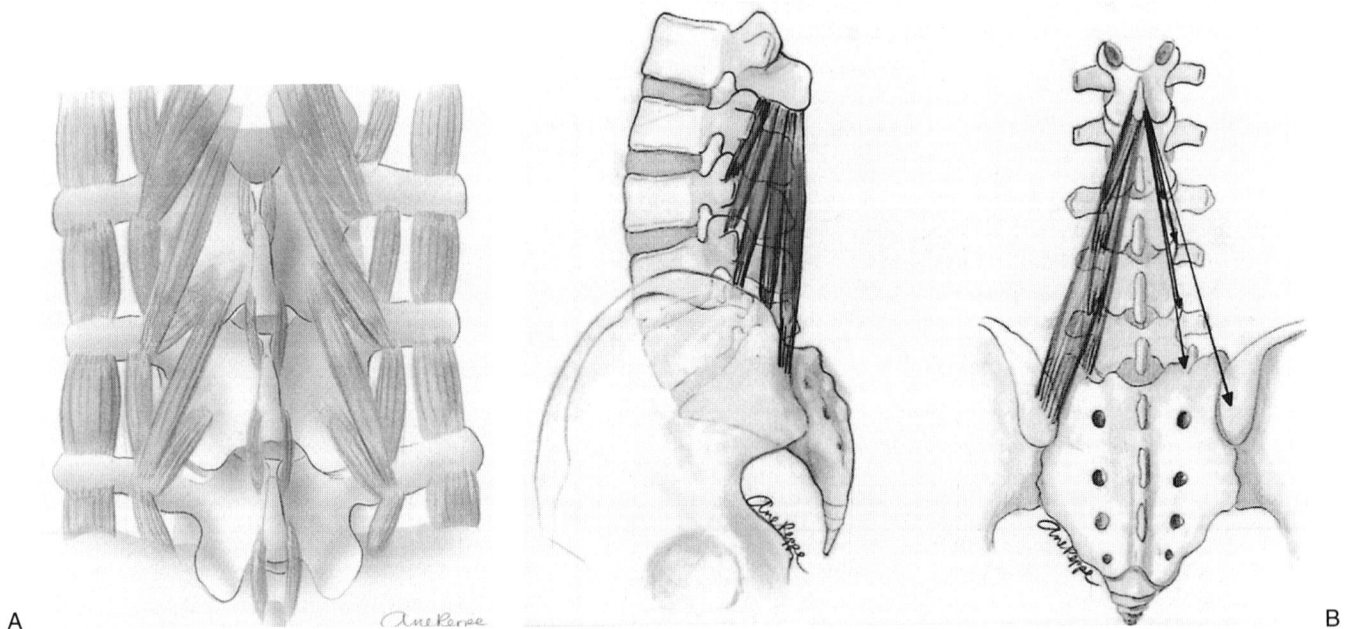

A

B

FIG. 11-5. A: Schematic of the interspinales, intertransversarii mediales and laterales, and parts of the multifidus muscles. **B:** Schematic showing the polysegmental attachments of the multifidus fascicles originating from L1 vertebra. (From Holm S, Indahl A, Solomonow M. Sensorimotor control of the spine. J EMG Kinesiol 2002;12:219–234, with permission.)

is thought to be caused by reflex stabilization by the paraspinal muscles.

SENSORIMOTOR CONTROL

The innervation patterns of the active and passive structures of the lumbar spine have, for the most part, been experimentally determined. The spinal nerve roots (dorsal and ventral), which exit from the spinal canal, connect the central nervous system and the peripheral nerves. The dorsal nerve root contains sensory fibers and the ventral root contains motor and some sensory fibers. The nerve roots join to form a spinal nerve. For each lumbar vertebra, there is an associated lumbar spinal nerve. Peripherally, each lumbar spinal nerve divides into a dorsal and ventral ramus, which branch further to provide innervation to the various passive and active structures (Fig. 11-6). Three branches stem from the dorsal ramus: lateral, intermediate, and medial. The lateral and intermediate branches innervate iliocostalis lumborum and the longissimus thoracis muscles, respectively. The medial branch provides innervation to a number of structures which lie posteriorly: muscles (interspinales, intertransversarii mediales, and multifidus), ligaments (interspinous and perhaps the supraspinous), and

the zygapophysial joint capsules. The ventral ramus provides innervation to structures that lie anteriorly: muscles (intertransversarii laterales, psoas major), the intertransverse ligament, and the lateral aspects of the intervertebral disc. The gray ramus communicans, which is an autonomic root from the sympathetic trunk, also provides innervation to the lateral aspects of the intervertebral disc and to the intervening anterior longitudinal ligament.

The control of movement depends on the sensory system working together with the motor system. Sensory information influences motor output in many ways and at all levels of the motor system. Sensory input to the spinal cord directly triggers reflex responses. The reflexes are involuntary and relatively stereotyped responses to certain sensory stimuli. Reflexes in which the sensory stimuli arise from receptors in muscles, joints, and skin, and in which the neural circuitry is entirely contained within the spinal cord are called spinal reflexes (Fig. 11-1).

In muscle and tendon, the motor and sensory functions of the neural structures for controlling posture and movements are well established. The load-sensitive nerve endings, or mechanoreceptors, found in muscle (muscle spindles) and tendon (Golgi tendon organs), provide proprioceptive information regarding tension levels, essen-

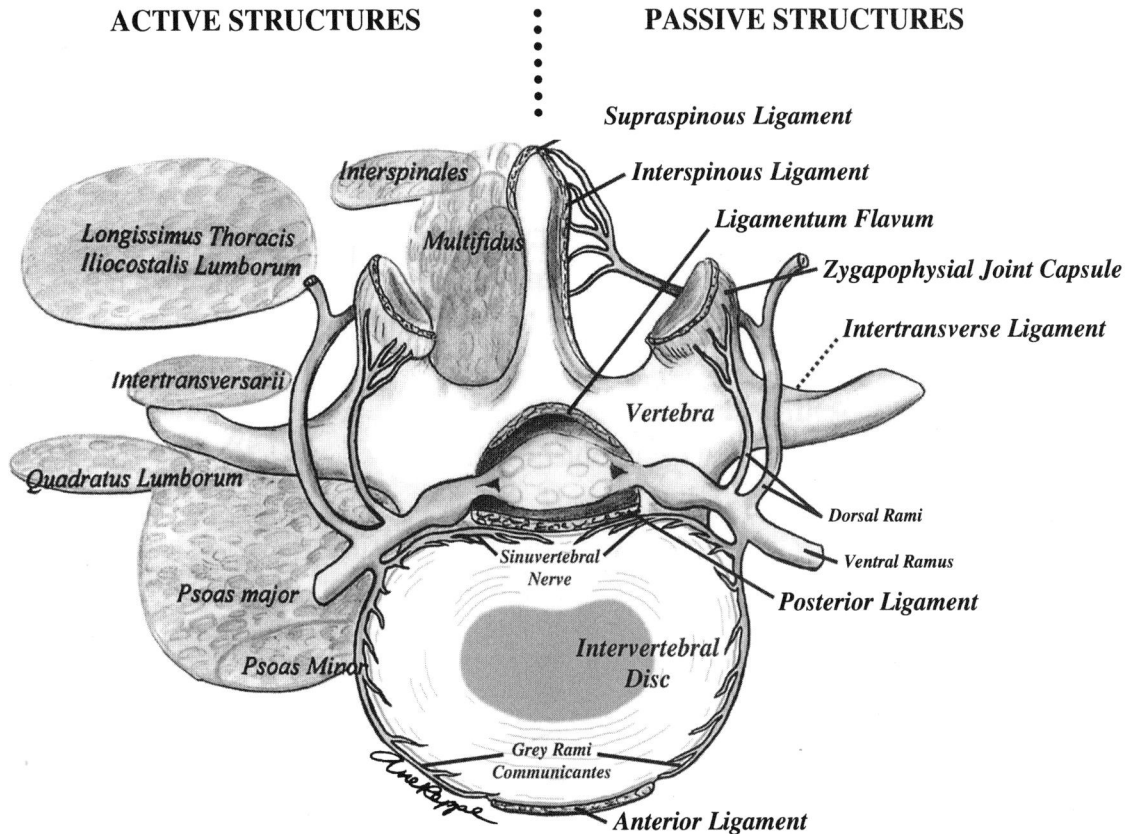

FIG. 11-6. Schematic drawing of the bilateral active and passive structural arrangement and sensory innervation on the L3-L4 level. (From Holm S, Indahl A, Solomonow M. Sensorimotor control of the spine. J EMG Kinesiol 2002;12:219–234, with permission.)

tial for controlling muscle tone, and therefore joint stability (Fig. 11-7). Although the presence of nerve endings in passive structures (ligaments, intervertebral disc, zygapophysial joint capsule) in the spinal column has been documented, their role is not clearly defined. Regarding the articular structures, the outer annulus of the intervertebral disc and the capsules of the zygapophysial joint contain both free nerve endings and mechanoreceptors. In addition to being potential sources of pain, these structures may act as transducers for monitoring the position and movements in the motion segment. The neurologic feedback from passive structures provides sensory information needed to regulate muscle tension, and hence, the stability in the lumbar spine.

Normal locomotion requires multiple levels of neural control. To support the body against gravity, maintain posture and to transport it forward, the nervous system must coordinate muscle contractions. At the same time, the nervous system must exert active control to maintain balance of the moving body and adapt the locomotion patterns.

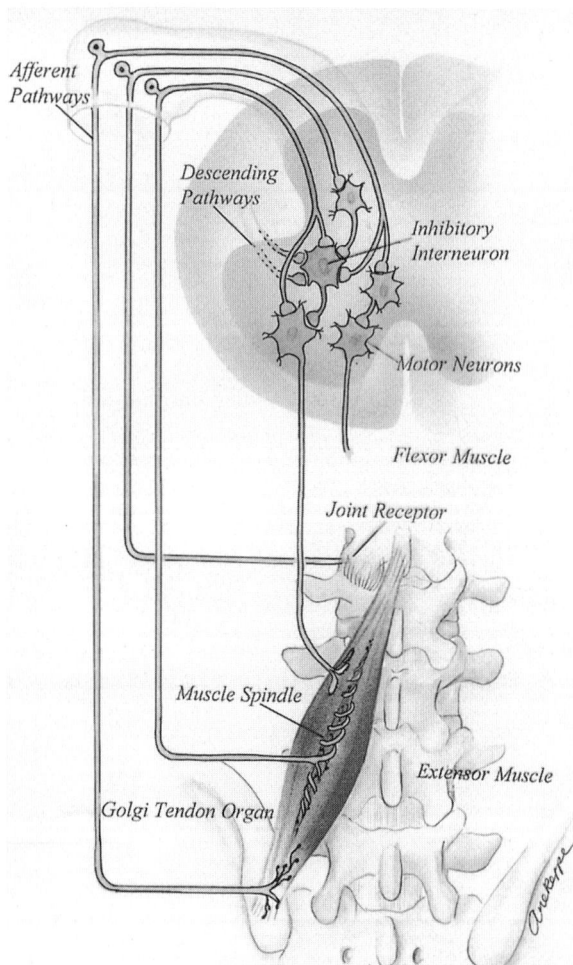

FIG. 11-7. Neuromuscular feedback system depicting the afferent sensory information from joint receptors, muscles spindles, and Golgi tendon organs for regulating muscle tension.

Neural circuits in the spinal cord play an essential role in motor coordination. Spinal reflexes provide the nervous system with a set of basic patterns of coordination that can be activated, either by sensory stimuli or by descending signals from the brainstem and cerebral cortex.

Functioning of the motor system is strongly related to that of the sensory system. Proper functioning of the motor system depends on a continuous inflow of sensory information. Sensory input to the spinal cord directly triggers reflexes. It is also essential for determining the parameters of programmed voluntary responses. Finally, both feedback and feed-forward mechanisms provide flexibility in the control of motor output (Fig. 11-8). Although the same sensors may provide information for both feedback and feed-forward control, the manner in which the information is processed varies. Biologic feedback processes generally operate continuously but slowly and are therefore used to maintain posture and regulate slow movements, while feed-forward systems, with an intermittent mode, operate more quickly.

FUNCTION AND DYSFUNCTION

In low back pain, where no pathoanatomic findings can be demonstrated, the cause of the pain may mainly be a functional disturbance. In order to be able to describe possible functional disturbances, the normal function must first be described. However, this is not always the case in medicine. For example, sacroiliac dysfunction was described 90 years ago, but the function of this joint has not yet been established. The hypothesis laid out below takes into account the muscular, ligamentous, and nervous networks, and their various interactive processes (Fig. 11-1). It builds upon what is known about neural control of other joints, and it is reasonable to believe that the same mechanisms apply to the spinal motion segments.

To understand the nature of a functional disturbance and how this can occur, it is necessary to first describe normal function. The nerve endings in the outer annulus fibrosus of the disc, in the capsule of the facet joints, and in the ligaments are most likely part of a proprioceptive system responsible for optimal recruitment of the paraspinal muscles (29,31). Mechanoreceptors are thought to play an important role in monitoring position and joint movement by regulating and modifying muscle tension. These different nerve endings can record the loading on the different spinal structures. The descending signals that initiate muscle action are modified by the sensory input from the proprioceptive nerve endings. Recruitment of the paraspinal muscles may thus be coordinated in such a manner that the forces applied to the various structures are properly distributed regardless of position. In such a system, the action of the muscles can provide the different spinal structures with the support needed in order to counteract detrimental forces and avoid injury. Overload of specific structures can be detected by high threshold nerve endings, and in due

Feed-forward control

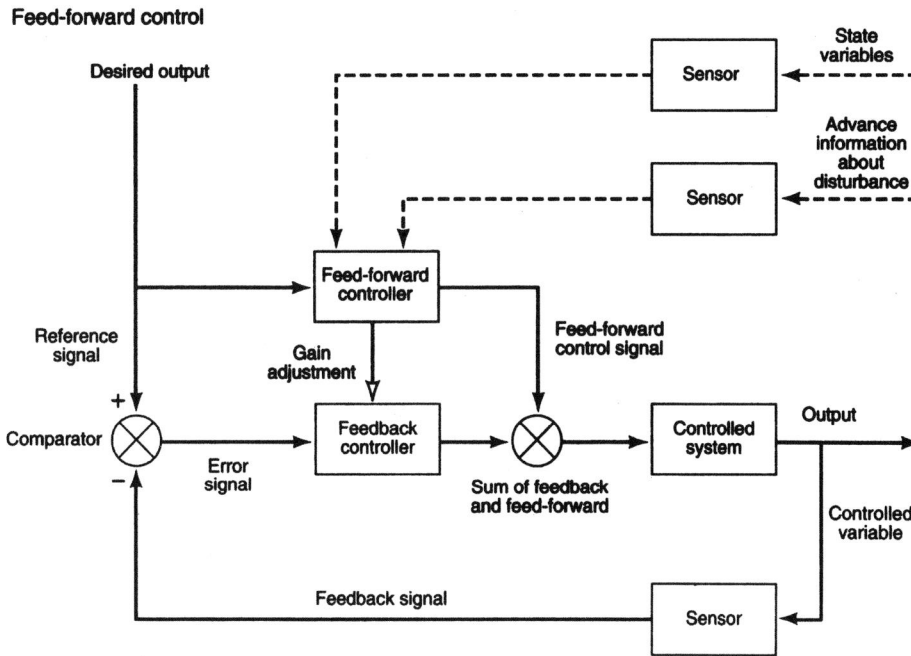

FIG. 11-8. Flowchart showing the functioning of the motor system involving feed-forward control in relation to feedback compensatory corrections. (From Ghez C. The control of movement. In: Kandel ER, Schwartz JH, Jessel TM, eds. Principles of neural science, 3rd ed. Norwalk, CT: Appleton & Lange, 1991:536, with permission.)

process inhibit muscle actions responsible for increasing the loading, and thereby prevent injury. This may be a reason why heavy physical loading does not seem to have the impact on degeneration of the spine as earlier assumed (59–61).

The common clinical finding of decreased range of motion of the spine in patients with low back pain points to increased muscle activity presumably caused by alterations in the recruitment system. The origin of such a change in paraspinal muscle recruitment is thought to be a lesion of some kind in one or more spinal structures. The intervertebral disc is the spinal structure where lesions are most readily detected. Even if it is not yet known exactly why disc lesions occur, since the time when Mixter and Barr demonstrated herniation of the nucleus pulposus and its effect on the nerve root as a mechanism behind sciatic pain, there has been mounting evidence for disc pathology and disc changes (4). Some of these changes can be seen on imaging, but others may only be demonstrated through histologic methods. In most cases, the likely site of the lesion is probably the annulus fibrosus of a lumbar disc. Such a lesion must occur in an innervated region of the annulus fibrosus (Fig. 11-3). Depending on the size of the lesion, the density of the neural structures, and the damage done to them, the firing patterns from these nerve endings may be altered in such a manner to cause increased activation of the paraspinal muscles. This muscle activation may occur in a "bracing" fashion and subject the muscles to static work, which is believed to be responsible for muscle pain (62).

Toward the latter part of trunk flexion, there is a spontaneous reduction in the muscle electric activity in certain paraspinal muscles. This behavior is known as flexion-relaxation and was first recognized by Floyd and Silver in 1951 (63). Paquet et al. (64) have demonstrated altered muscle activation patterns in patients with a former history of back pain compared to similar back patients without previous back pain experience. Haig et al. (65) have shown changes in the flexion-relaxation phenomenon in a patient with acute disc herniation, and Sihvonen et al. (17) have demonstrated increased muscle activation and lack of flexion-relaxation in patients with chronic low back pain. Pain, for whatever reason, lasting for some time may lead to the establishment of a more "bracing" pattern as the dominating strategy for muscle activation.

Even though it is not known which processes are responsible for muscle pain, it is a common human experience that muscles can be painful (66). There is no suitable experimental evidence supporting the hypothesis that a "pain-spasm-pain" cycle can exist in the back. Studies have shown that experimental pain in muscles does not increase the firing of γ-motor units, but it does increase the stretch reflex (67). Increase in such reflexes may result in inappropriate muscle activation.

NEUROMUSCULAR REFLEX SYSTEM

A thorough description of reflex systems essential for sensorimotor control has been provided by Gordon (68).

A summary, in part, is provided in this section. The stretch reflex is the only known monosynaptic reflex in the mammalian nervous system. Because the participating afferent and efferent axons have large diameters and are among the most rapidly conducting neurons in the nervous system, the stretch reflex pathway is adapted for speed of operation. The economy of the neural circuit for the stretch reflex allows muscle tone to be regulated quickly and efficiently without direct intervention by higher centers. Descending control signals adjust the gain of the reflex loops, adapting them to the requirements of specific motor acts.

A characteristic aspect of muscle tone is that the tension produced by the muscle increases approximately in proportion to the amount of stretch. Moreover, when muscle is released from a stretch, the tension decreases progressively to its resting level. This symmetric response is present whether the muscle is stretched slowly or abruptly and is due to a combination of the mechanical properties of muscle and the neural components provided by the stretch reflex. In slowly imposed stretches, this springlike behavior occurs because of the intrinsic length-tension properties of muscle. In rapid stretches, however, the intrinsic mechanical response is an initial increase in tension followed by a transient collapse even as the muscle continues to be stretched.

The increased focus on the innervation of different spinal structures has led to a new understanding and awareness that they may play an important role in a complex regulating system (20,24–26,42). Reflexes from ligaments in many of the joints of the extremities have previously been established (69–71). Spasms and elevated activity of the lumbar paraspinal muscles are common in patients with low back pain. In the spine, several ligaments are associated with each motion segment, thus comprising a complex proprioceptive measurement system, particularly when combined with the sensory inputs from nearby discs and capsules. The existence of sensory receptors in the various spinal ligaments has been established (51,72–75). Solomonow et al. have experimentally investigated whether or not a ligament-muscular reflex exists from the spinal ligaments to related muscles (76). Furthermore, it has been demonstrated that static constant load applied to the lumbar spine through the supraspinous ligament results in spasm of the multifidus muscles, although the stretching was below the physiologic range limit and spasms were evident regardless of the loading magnitude (22). A conclusion drawn from these studies is that there exists a clear chain of events consisting of viscoelastic tissue damage, pain, and muscular spasm. The spasms are most likely triggered by nerve endings, which are found in the spinal ligamentous tissues. These receptors monitor tissue injury and trigger responses such as pain and probably its associated spasms. The finding that the viscoelastic structures were stretched, although the applied load was constant was

very interesting as this indicates that the tension developed may be a stimulus that elicits reflexive activity in the muscles (22). These two separate sensory feedback mechanisms are probably in synergy with each other to protect the spinal structures from instability and injury.

Possible muscle activation because of damage to passive viscoelastic spinal structures is difficult to detect. Painful stimuli seem to have an inhibitory effect on muscle activation. But damage done to ligaments and perhaps other passive structures does not necessarily have to result in a lot of pain. Depending on the size of the lesion, the density of the neural structures, and damage done to them, and the degree of irritation to the surrounding nerve endings, the firing pattern from these nerve endings may be altered in such a manner so as to cause increased activation of the paraspinal muscles. Studies have shown that experimental pain in muscles does not increase the firing of γ-motor units, but it does increase the stretch reflex (67). Increase in such reflexes may result in inappropriate muscle activation.

In muscle and tendon, the motor and sensory functions of the neural structures for controlling posture and movements are well established (77); however, until recently, this has not been the case for the spinal structures. Stimulation of the outer annulus of the disc or zygapophysial joint, both of which have been shown to contain nerve endings, causes activation of paraspinal musculature. This not only occurs on the same segmental level but also on different levels, indicating a complex interaction (15). Such an interaction is necessary in order to stabilize different segments, not only in relation to each other, but also in the process of maintaining posture. However, a lesion at one location may cause alterations in muscle activation at a location other than the actual segment and even on the contralateral side. Avramov et al. (78) have shown that loading excites three patterns of nerve discharges from the zygapophysial joints: short duration bursts during changes in loading, prolonged discharges at low levels, and prolonged discharges at high load levels. These results indicate that different units in the joint capsule have different levels of stress threshold.

The range of motion and innervation of the SIJ seems well suited for detecting various loading patterns during locomotion. In humans, the slanted position of the L5-S1 motion segment and the relative position of the SIJ appear to have physiologic importance for load detection. The afferent input from SIJ receptors, as well as mechanoreceptors in the intervertebral disc and zygapophysial joints, will contribute to different degrees of muscle activation and may constitute an integral regulatory system (79). Changes in loading on the SIJ may result in altered activation of the stabilizing muscles, and thus play an important regulatory function in stabilization and movement of the upper body during postural changes.

Instability of a spinal motion segment, as a result of degeneration of the disc or zygapophysial joints, is believed to be manifested as "slipping" because of laxity in the motion segment. Kaigle et al. (21) have shown that this kind of hypermobility does not seem to occur, but that the segmental motion pattern is greatly altered. The change in length and loading of the spinal ligaments may cause alterations in the firing patterns and consequently, coordination of the muscle activity. With decreased disc height as a result of degeneration, adaptation of the surrounding nerve endings may be less efficient and thus result in less optimal neuromuscular reflexes. Better knowledge of the sensory function of the passive spinal structures should influence the manner in which these structures are treated clinically.

In healthy persons, the paraspinal muscles display the flexion-relaxation phenomenon (i.e., muscle activity decreases as flexion of the trunk increases), and the muscles become silent in the fully bent posture (15,63,79). In a patient with a herniated nucleus pulposus, Haig et al. found that the flexion-relaxation phenomenon was absent (65). It may be assumed that in patients in whom the phenomenon is absent, there is an imbalance between nerve discharges to the muscles from a pathologic structure and inhibitory discharges from the zygapophysial joint capsule in forward bending. Conversely, inhibitory discharges from the joint capsule can explain why manipulative treatment and mobilization of the zygapophysial joint provide relief in some cases.

Using an experimental model, it has been demonstrated by Indahl et al. (15) that stimulation of nerve endings in the intervertebral disc and zygapophysial joint capsule elicited responses in the paraspinal muscles, thereby demonstrating neuromuscular interaction exists between these structures. Stretching on the zygapophysial joint capsule inhibited the muscular response, thus suggesting the existence of a complex reflex system that is responsible for the motion and stabilization of the lumbar spine.

Stretching of more than one joint can increase inhibition and make the treatment more effective. Muscle spasm is a common clinical feature in patients with back problems, and manipulation of the zygapophysial joints may elicit a stretch reflex from the capsule, contributing to an inhibitory action on muscle spasm, thereby relieving pain (Fig. 11-9). Thus, it appears that there is a delicate interaction between the different parts of the spinal motion segments, and proprioceptive nerve endings may play a vital part in load distribution during movements.

In addition to the lumbar motion segments, the SIJ is of great importance in stabilization of the lumbosacral area. Despite this, there have been surprisingly few experimental studies investigating SIJ function. The results of mapping studies (80), the innervation of the SIJ (41–43), its position and range of motion (81), altogether give reason to believe that the SIJ also plays a regulatory

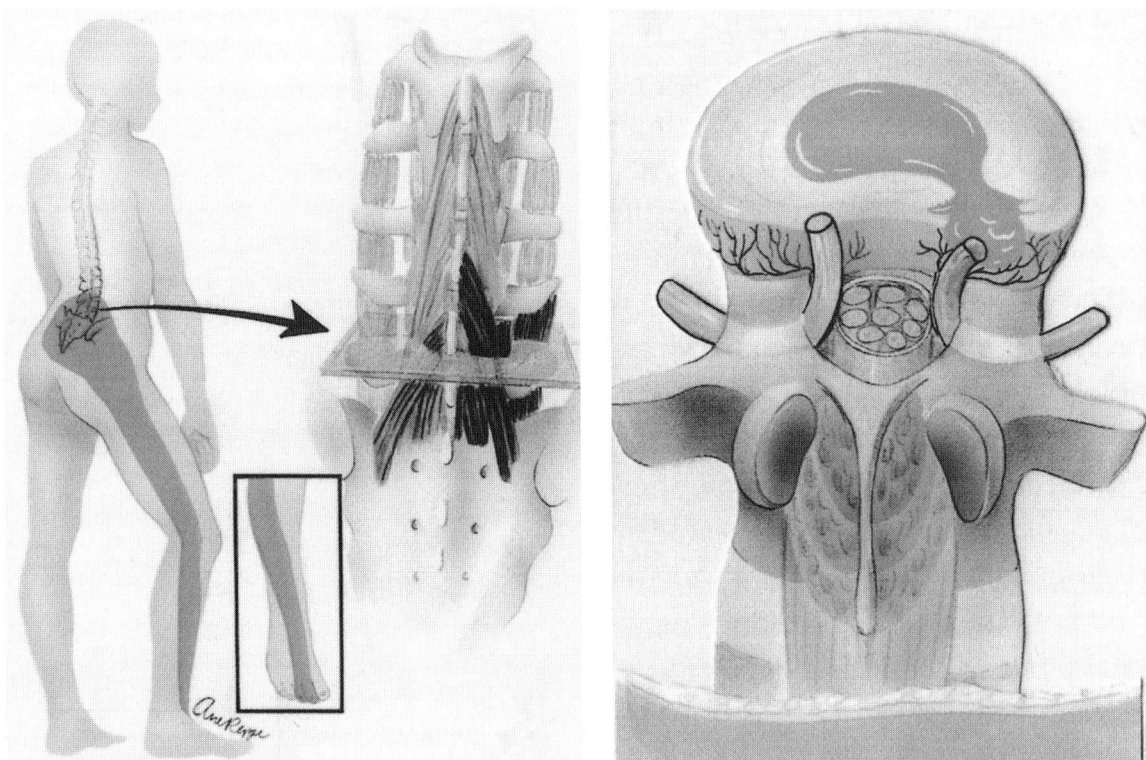

FIG. 11-9. Schematic representation of patient pain and how it relates to muscle activation (left) and disc herniation (right).

function involving reflex muscle activation responsible for stabilization and movement of the upper body during locomotion. Furthermore, it was shown by Indahl et al. (15) that stimulation of nerve and nerve endings in the deep part of the ventral SIJ, as well as in the superficial part of the dorsal capsule, elicits motor action potentials in different muscles. Interesting patterns were revealed. Stimulation of nerve elements in the ventral area of the SIJ produced predominant contractions in the gluteus medius and quadratus lumborum muscles. However, stimulation of the superficial dorsal layer of the SIJ capsule elicited responses predominantly in the medially located multifidus fascicles. It is possible that the different areas of the SIJ play different roles in regulating the locomotion system and the response may therefore vary depending on the stimulation site.

SUMMARY

Despite a pathophysiologic understanding of the involved structures, no single group of patients can, with certainty, be identified at an early stage and be given a specific treatment. This seems to support the basic notion that low back pain is multicausal, and that the prognosis depends on a variety of factors. Furthermore, this suggests that movement-related pain should be considered as a complex behavior, and not solely as a psychiatric or a neurologic problem, but rather as a problem related to the integration of nervous and biomechanical mechanisms. This involves the sensorimotor control, with feedback from muscles, discs, and joints, all in a complex interaction with the central nervous system, as well as the traditional peripheral pain mechanisms.

REFERENCES

1. Albee FH. A study of the anatomy and the clinical importance of the sacroiliac joint. JAMA 1909;53:1273–1276.
2. Ghormley RK. Low back pain with special reference to the articular facets, with presentation of an operative procedure. JAMA 1933;101:1773–1777.
3. Mooney V. Facet syndrome. In: Wiesel SW, Weinstein JN, Herkowitz HN, et al., eds. The lumbar spine. Philadelphia: WB Saunders, 1996:538–558.
4. Mixter WJ, Barr JS. Rupture of the intervertebral disc with involvement of the spinal canal. N Engl J Med, 1934;2A:210–215.
5. Bernard PN, Cassidy JD. Sacroiliac joint syndrome: pathophysiology, diagnosis and management. In: Frymoyer JW, ed. The adult spine: principles and practice. New York: Raven Press, 1991:2107–2131.
6. Daum WJ. The sacroiliac joint: an underappreciated pain generator. Am J Orthop 1995;24:475–478.
7. DonTigny RL. Dysfunction of the sacroiliac joint and its treatment. J Orthop Sports Phys Ther 1979;1:23–35.
8. Wiberg G. Back pain in relation to the nerve supply of the intervertebral discs. Acta Orthop Scand 1947;19:211–221.
9. MacLennan AH, Green RC, Nicolson R, et al. Serum relaxin and pelvic pain of pregnancy. Lancet 1986;2:243–245.
10. Mooney V. Evaluation and treatment of sacroiliac dysfunction. In: Wiesel SW, Weinstein JN, Herkowitz HN, et al., eds. The lumbar spine. Philadelphia: WB Saunders, 1996:559–569.
11. Anderson J. Pathogenesis of back pain. In: Grahame R, Andersson JAD, eds. Low back pain. Vol 2. Westmount, Montreal, Canada: Eden Press, 1980:23–32.
12. Nachemson A. The lumbar spine: an orthopaedic challenge. Spine 1976;1:59–71.
13. Swezey RL, Clements PJ. Conservative treatment of back pain. In: Jayson MIV, ed. The lumbar spine and back pain, 3rd ed. Edinburgh: Churchill Livingstone, 1987:299–314.
14. Indahl A, Kaigle A, Reikerås O, et al. Electromyographic response of the porcine multifidus musculature after nerve stimulation. Spine 1995;20:2652–2658.
15. Indahl A, Kaigle A, Reikerås O, et al. Interaction between the porcine lumbar intervertebral disc, zygapophysial joints, and paraspinal muscles. Spine 1997;22:2834–2840.
16. Lamb DW. The neurology of spinal pain. Phys Ther 1979;59:971–973.
17. Sihvonen T, Partanen J, Hanninen O, et al. Electric behavior of low back muscles during lumbar pelvic rhythm in low back pain patients and healthy controls. Arch Phys Med Rehabil 1991;72:1080–1087.
18. Taylor JR, Twomey LT. Innervation of lumbar intervertebral discs. Med J Aust 1979;2:701–702.
19. Wyke B. The neurology of low back pain. In: Jayson MIV, ed. The lumbar spine and back pain, London: Longman, 1987:58–99.
20. Yamashita T, Minaki Y, Oota I, et al. Mechanosensitive afferent units in the lumbar intervertebral disc and adjacent muscle. Spine 1993;18:2252–2256.
21. Kaigle AM, Holm S, Hansson T. Experimental instability in the lumbar spine. Spine 1995;20:421–430.
22. Solomonow M, Zhou B, Baratta RV, et al. Neuromuscular disorders associated with static lumbar flexion: a feline model. J EMG Kinesiol 2002;12:81–90.
23. Kaigle AM, Holm SH, Hansson TH. Kinematic behavior of the porcine lumbar spine—a chronic lesion model. Spine 1997;22:2796–2806.
24. Bogduk N, Tynan W, Wilson AS. The nerve supply to the human lumbar intervertebral discs. J Anat 1981;132:39–56.
25. Cavanaugh JM, El-Bohy AA, Hardy WH, et al. Sensory innervation of soft tissues of lumbar spine in the rat. J Orthop Res 1989;7:389–397.
26. Kojima Y, Maeda T, Arai R, et al. Nerve supply to the posterior longitudinal ligament and the intervertebral disc of the rat vertebral column as studied by acetylcholinesterase histochemistry. J Anat 1990;169:237–255.
27. Basmajian JV. Acute back pain and spasm. A controlled multicenter trial of combined analgesic and antispasm agents. Spine 1989;14:438–439.
28. Holm S. Pathophysiology of disc degeneration. Acta Orthop Scand Suppl 1993;251:13–15.
29. Malinsky J. The ontogenetic development of nerve terminations in the intervertebral disc of man. Acta Anat 1959;38:96–113.
30. Kumar S, Davis PR. Lumbar intervertebral innervation and intra-abdominal pressure. J Anat 1973;114:47–53.
31. Roberts S, Eisenstein SM, Menage J, et al. Mechanoreceptors in intervertebral discs. Spine 1995;20:2645–2651.
32. Ohtori S, Takahashi K, Chiba T, et al. Sensory innervation of the dorsal portion of the lumbar intervertebral discs in rats. Spine 2001;26 (8):946–950.
33. Kuslich SD, Ulstrom CL, Michael CJ. The tissue origin of low back pain and sciatica: a report of pain response to tissue stimulation during operations on the lumbar spine using local anesthesia. Orthop Clin North Am 1991;22:181–189.
34. Wyke B. The neurology of low back pain. In: Jayson MIV, ed. The lumbar spine and back pain. London: Longman, 1987:58–99.
35. Stokes IAF. Mechanical function of facet joints in the lumbar spine. Clin Biomech 1988;3:101–105.
36. Adams MA, Hutton WC, Stott JRR. The resistance to flexion of the lumbar intervertebral joint. Spine 1980;5:245–253.
37. Lorentz M, Patwardhan A, Vanderby R. Load-bearing characteristics of lumbar facets in normal and surgically altered spinal segments. Spine 1983;8:122–130.
38. Ashton IK, Ashton BA, Gibson SJ, et al. Morphological basis for back pain: the demonstration of nerve fibers and neuropeptides in the lumbar zygapophysial joint capsule, but not in the ligamentum flavum. J Orthop Res 1992;10:72–78.
39. Buckmill A T, Covard K, Plumton C, et al. Nerve fibers in lumbar spine structures, and injured spinal roots express the sensory neuron specific sodium channels SNS/PN3 and NaN/SNS2. Spine 2002;27:135–140.

40. Sturesson B, Selvik G, Uden A. Movements of the sacroiliac joints: a roentgen stereophotogrammetric analysis. Spine 1989;14:162–165.
41. Solonen KA. The sacroiliac joint in the light of anatomical, roentgenological and clinical studies. Acta Orthop Scand Suppl 1957;27:1–27.
42. Grob KR, Neuberger WL, Kisslig RO. Die innervation des sacroiliacgelenkes beim menschen. Zeitschrift fur Rheumatologie 1995;54:117–122.
43. Ikeda R. Innervation of the sacroiliac joint. Macroscopical and histological studies [in Japanese]. J Nippon Med Sch 1991;58:587–596.
44. Daum WJ. The sacroiliac joint: an underappreciated pain generator. Am J Orthop 1995;24:475–478.
45. Schwarzer AC, Aprill CN, Bogduk N. The sacroiliac joint in chronic low back pain. Spine 1995;20:31–37.
46. Mooney V. Understanding, examining for, and treating sacroiliac pain. J Musculoskel Med 1993;37–49.
47. Dreyfuss P, Michalsen M, Pauza K, et al. The value of medical history and physical examination in diagnosing sacroiliac joint pain. Spine 1996;21:2594–2602.
48. Bogduk N, Macintosh JE, Pearcy MJ. A universal model of the lumbar back muscles in the upright position. Spine 1992;17:897–913.
49. Bogduk N, Twomey L. Clinical anatomy of the lumbar spine. New York: Churchill Livingstone, 1987.
50. Bogduk N. The myotomes of the human multifidus. J Anat 1983;136:148–149.
51. Bogduk N, Wilson A, Tynan W. The human lumbar dorsal rami. J Anat 1982;134:383–397.
52. Macintosh JE, Valencia F, Bogduk N, et al. The morphology of the lumbar multifidus muscles. Clin Biomech 1986;1:196–204.
53. Cailliet R. Low back pain syndrome, 4th ed. Philadelphia: FA Davis, 1988:63–75.
54. Eisen A, Hoirch M. The electrodiagnostic evaluation of spinal root lesion. Spine 1983;8:98–116.
55. Haldeman S. The electrodiagnostic evaluation of nerve root function. Spine 1984;9:42–48.
56. Jacobsen RE. Lumbar stenosis. An electromyographic evaluation. Clin Orthop 1976;115:68–71.
57. Johnson EW, Melvin JL. Value of electromyography in lumbar radiculopathy. Arch Phys Med Rehabil 1971;52:239–243.
58. Wise CS, Ardizzone I. Electromyography in intervertebral disc protrusions. Arch Phys Med Rehabil 1954;35:442–446.
59. Battie MC, Videman T, Gibbons LE, et al. Determinants of lumbar disc degeneration: a study relating lifetime exposures and magnetic resonance imaging findings in identical twins. Spine 1995;20:2601–2612.
60. Lundberg U, Mardberg B, Frankenhauser M. The total work load of male and female white collar workers as related to age, occupational level, and number of children. Scand J Psychol 1994;35:315–337.
61. Nachemson AL. The load on lumbar discs in different positions of the body. Clin Orthop 1966;45:107–122.
62. Edwards RHT. Hypotheses of peripheral and central mechanisms underlying occupational muscle pain and injury. Eur J Appl Physiol 1988;57:275–281.
63. Floyd WF, Silver PHS. Function of the erectors spinae muscles in flexion of the trunk. Lancet 1951;15:133–143.
64. Paquet N, Malouin F, Richards C. Hip-spine movement interaction and muscle activation patterns during sagittal trunk movements in low back pain patients. Spine 1994;19:596–603.
65. Haig AJ, Weismann G, Haugh LD, et al. Prospective evidence for change in paraspinal muscle activity after herniated nucleus pulposus. Spine 1993;18:926–930.
66. Ursin H, Endresen I, Ursin G. Psychological factors and self-reports of muscle pain. Eur J Appl Physiol 1988;57:282–290.
67. Matre DA, Sinkjr T, Svensson P, et al. Experimental muscle pain increases the human stretch reflex. Pain 1998;75:331–339.
68. Gordon G. Spinal mechanisms of motor coordination. In: Kandel ER, Schwartz JH, Jessel TM, eds. Principles of neural science, 3rd ed. Norwalk, CT: Appleton & Lange, 1991:581–595.
69. Knatt T, Guanche C, Solomonow M, et al. The glenohumeral-biceps reflex in the feline. Clin Orthop 1995;314:247–252.
70. Phillips D, Petrie S, Solomonow M, et al. Ligamento-muscular protective reflex in the elbow. J Hand Surg 1997;22:473–478.
71. Solomonow M, Baratta RV, Zhou B, et al. The synergistic action of the ACL and thigh muscles in maintaining knee stability. Am J Sports Med 1987;15:207–213.
72. Hirsch C, Inglemark B, Miller M. The anatomical basis for low back pain: study on presence of sensory nerve endings in ligaments, capsular and disc structures in human lumbar spine. Acta Orthop Scand 1963;33:1–17.
73. Jackson H, Winkleman R, Bickel W. Nerve endings in the human lumbar spinal column and related structures. J Bone Joint Surg Am 1966;48:1272–1281.
74. Rhalmi W, Yahia H, Newman N, et al. Immunohistochemical study of nerves in lumbar spine ligaments. Spine 1993;18:264–267.
75. Yahia H, Newman N. Innervation of spinal ligaments of patients with disc herniation. Pathol Res Pract 1991;187:936–938.
76. Solomonow M, Zhou B, Harris M, et al. The ligamento-muscular stabilizing system of the spine. Spine 1998;23:2552–2562.
77. Ghez C, Gordon J. The control of movement. In: Kandel ER, Schwartz JH, Jessel TM, eds. Principles of neural science, 3rd ed. Norwalk, CT: Appleton & Lange, 1991:533–547.
78. Avramov AI, Cavanaugh JM, Ozaktay CA, et al. The effects of controlled mechanical loading on group II, III, and IV afferent units from the lumbar zygapophysial joint and surrounding tissue. An in vitro study. J Bone Joint Surg Am 1992;74:1464–1471.
79. Indahl A, Kaigle A, Reikerås O, et al. Sacroiliac joint involvement in activation of the porcine spinal and gluteal musculature. J Spinal Disord 1999;12:325–330.
80. Fortin JD, Dwyer AP, West S, Pier J. Sacroiliac joint: pain referral maps upon applying a new injection—arthrography technique. Part I: asymptomatic volunteers. Spine 1994;19:1475–1482.
81. Vleeming A, Volkers ACW, Snijders CJ, et al. Relation between form and function in the sacroiliac joint. Part II: biomechanical aspects. Spine 1990;15:133–135.

CHAPTER 12

Outcomes Assessment: Overview and Specific Tools

Kevin F. Spratt

Clinical outcomes were often what clinicians said they were in the days before 1982. "My doctor says I'm doing very well." Since the early 1980s, in spine care and many other disciplines where pain and suffering are major symptoms associated with the complaints that bring the patient to health care providers, outcomes have become more strongly associated with patient self-report. The argument is clear: Who but the patient is in a position to accurately recount symptom magnitude and quality?

In spine care, the 1982 *Spine* publications of the Million et al. pain interference scale (1) (popularly called the Million Visual Analogue Scale) and the 1983 Roland and Morris Disability Questionnaire (2) signaled the beginning of legitimizing patient self-report for spine-related disease outcomes.

THE NOTION OF CLINICAL OUTCOMES

The universe of outcome instruments potentially applicable to the spine care professional is reasonably large. Gattchel (3) edited a compendium of outcome instruments for assessment and research of spinal disorders, where he categorized such biopsychosocial measures as the following:

1. Physical or "hard" measures
   a. Range of motion: using inclinometers or Isostation B-200 equipment (Isotechnologies, Hillsborough, NC)
   b. Spine strength: using Cybex (a division of Lumex Corporation, Ronkonkoma, NY) or Isostation B-200 equipment
   c. Lifting capacity functional measures: using Cybex and MedX (MedX Corporation, Altamonte Springs, FL) equipment
   d. Other tests of human performance capacity: aerobic capacity and treadmill tolerance
2. Psychological or "soft" measures

   a. Psychological tests: depression, MMPI-2, Symptom Checklist 90-Revised (4–7)
   b. Self-report measures of pain and disability: the SF-36, Chronic Pain Coping Inventory, Coping Strategies Questionnaire, McGill Pain Questionnaire, Oswestry Disability Index, Roland and Morris Disability Questionnaire, Multidimensional Pain Inventory (MPI), Quebec Back Pain Disability Scale, Sickness Impact Profile, and Activities of Daily Living (ADL) scales (8–24)
   c. Clinical interview: the structured clinician interview for the DSM-IV (SCID) (25)
   d. Clinical ratings of overt pain behavior: the Waddell Non-Organic Signs Test (26)

The clinical outcomes chapter by Spratt and Weinstein (27) in *The Lumbar Spine*, vol. 2, provides greater detail regarding the types of outcomes as well as classification schemes for a wide variety of outcomes measures.

RELIABILITY AND VALIDITY

For any outcome measure, whether based on patient self-report or a laboratory test, the psychometric properties of primary interest are the same: reliability or precision and validity or accuracy. Methods for evaluating reliability and validity are major topics in measurement theory and are beyond the scope of this chapter. Impressive overviews of the concepts of reliability are provided by Feldt and Brennan (28), and for validity by Cronbach (29).

As a brief primer of reliability in the clinical setting, reliability considerations are usually evaluated in two ways, internal consistence of items, and test-retest reliability. Typically internal consistency is of primary importance when considering scale construction and test-retest or stability of the score is of primary importance when considering clinical value. With test-retest reliability the object of measurement (a patient) is assessed on multiple (usually two) occasions under the assumptions that the first assessment does not affect, or is independent of, the second or subsequent assessments. In many cases, including clinical settings, this can be problematic because: (a) a second assessment shortly after the first assessment is not likely to be independent because the patient is likely to remember what he or she said and try for consistency rather than an accurate estimate of the current state, or (b) a second assessment a few days after the first assessment may be influenced by treatments that resulted from the initial visit. Thus, the most accurate method for establishing test-retest reliability for an instrument is to have the patient respond to the instrument on separate occasions with nothing but a short natural history intervening between the events. In this situation, which is rarely evaluated in the clinical setting, low reliabilities, meaning large discrepancies within a patient across time, could reflect: (a) an instrument that does not have adequate psychometric properties, or (b) a construct under assessment (e.g., pain, function, or attitudes) that are more state-like than trait-like, meaning that the construct may not be stable. The consequence of this result is that the instrument is not useful in evaluating treatment progress because the score might vary independently of treatment effectiveness on any given day. Thus, the single most important aspect of the reliability of an instrument used in the clinical setting is that it demonstrates stability, meaning that the score measures a condition or construct that is not amenable to quick and unpredictable changes across short time increments. In practice, internal consistency reliability estimates often are used as proxies for test-retest reliability. Because instrument construction often is guided by internal consistency estimates, the general sense is that internal consistency reliabilities are positively biased estimates of test-retest reliability; therefore, the amount of error expected in a score that is most relevant to the clinical setting is often underestimated.

This notion of stability, of course, begs the issue of validity because it suggests that the specific constructs chosen to be of interest need to be reasonably stable in the short run. Strictly speaking, instruments do not have validity, but the scores they generate have validity to the extent that those scores provide information that aids in making appropriate decisions. If a test produces a score that is likely to be interpreted as high today but low tomorrow, then the lack of stability in that score indicates that it does not provide information useful in making appropriate decisions.

Measures of reliability include Cronbach's alpha for internal consistency, kappa for categorical outcomes, and intraclass correlations or generalizability coefficients (30) when outcomes are reasonably continuous. It has been argued that generalizability coefficients are preferable to kappa coefficients under circumstances when kappa struggles, such as when the number of categories becomes large (e.g., more than four levels); when the number of raters scores being compared are greater than two (although generalized kappa statistics can be computed); and when the prevalence of one of the categories is low or the sample size is small.

The value of generalizability coefficients is that they can be developed in ways that isolate potential culprits or candidates for lack of reliability, and that they allow estimation of what some consider the most relevant form of reliability in the clinical setting: the estimate of the reliability for a single rater on a single occasion; in other words, the reliability in the classical clinical situation where one clinician is evaluating a score based on a single reading. A problem with reliability coefficients, including generalizability coefficients, always has been that the meaning of the magnitude of the coefficient is not set. A reliability of .7 in some fields is considered good to excellent, whereas .8 is considered dismal in other fields.

To better understand the relationship between the reliability coefficient and the consequent differences in assessments between raters, 100,000 pairs of random normal scores were generated, transformed to have exact reliabilities of .30, .40, .50, .60, .70, .80, .90, .95, and .99, again transformed to have the mean and standard deviation associated with selected SF-36 scores and then broken down into six mutually exclusive and exhaustive categories based on the tenth, 25th, 50th, 75th, and 90th percentiles, as summarized in Table 12-1. These six cate-

TABLE 12-1. *Descriptive statistics amd cut points for selected SF-36 scales*

Statistics	PCS	MCS	SF	PF	Example: PCS
Mean	30.6	45.9	39.1	40.8	
SD	7.2	14.5	25.0	22.4	
Min	13.0	16.0	0	0	
P10	22.0	21.5	12.5	15.0	Category 1:(13–21.9) Min–P10;10% of scores
P25	26.0	35.0	25.0	25.0	Category 2:(22–25.9) P10–P25;15% of scores
P50	30.0	52.5	37.5	40.0	Category 3:(26–29.9) P25–P50;25% of scores
P75	35.0	58.0	50.0	55.0	Category 4:(30–34.9) P50–P75;25% of scores
P90	39.0	60.0	75.0	75.0	Category 5:(35–38.9) P75–P90;15% of scores
Max	58.0	63.0	100	100	Category 6:(39–58) P90–Max;10% of scores

MCS, mental component summary; PCS, physical component summary; PF, physical functioning; SD, standard deviation; SF, social functioning.

Description statistics are based on the initial visit for 376 University of Iowa patients presenting with low back troubles.

gories for each pair of ratings with the specified reliability were then crossed and the level of agreement and disagreement determined based on differences in classification group. The percentage of same and different categorization is summarized in Table 12-2 for each reliability level. This pattern is consistent for all outcome measures under the assumption of normality; therefore, separate tables for each outcome were unnecessary.

By way of interpreting the information provided in Tables 12-1 and 12-2, suppose a test-retest reliability of .8. In this situation, 42.63% of scores from that instrument are expected to remain in the score category; 45.56% are expected to be in adjacent categories; and 1.87% to differ by two categories, .915% to differ by three categories, and .026% to differ by four categories. With a test-retest reliability of .8, a miss by two or more categories is expected 11.81% of the time. Across 400 patients, just considering two category differences, this means that approximately 44 patients might have a score:

In category 1 (13 to 21.9), but a true score in category 3 (26 to 29.9); worst case difference 16.9, best case 4.1
In category 2 (22 to 25.9), but a true score in category 4 (30 to 34.9); worst case difference 13.9, best case 4.1
In category 3 (26 to 29.9), but a true score in category 5 (35 to 38.9); worst case difference 12.9, best case 5.1
In category 4 (30 to 34.9), but a true score in category 6 (39 to 58); worst case difference 28, best case 4.1

Of course, the reverse pattern is equally likely: An observed score in category 3 (26 to 29.9) might reflect a true score in category 1 (13 to 21.9). Thus, overtreatment or undertreatment might result if the observed score overestimates or underestimates severity. To the extent that overestimates of symptom severity result in a differential diagnosis suggesting a more aggressive treatment path (e.g., surgery), or underestimates of symptom severity result in a differential diagnosis suggesting a less aggressive or immediate treatment path (e.g., watchful waiting), the lack of reliability of the diagnostic tool clearly affects quality of care.

It should be noted that a test-retest reliability estimated based on the clinically relevant generalizability coefficient of one clinician making one rating is likely to be lower than the .8 estimate used in this example. Further note that if dropping to a reliability of .7, only 36.18% of scores are expected to be in the same category if a second independent evaluation is done at the same time. Thus, the stability of many outcome measures employed at initial visits, which are often used as ancillary diagnostic tools in clinical research, may have marginal value when applied to clinical practice.

In sum, the reliability of many outcome tools used to evaluate patients presenting with low back pain have limited test-retest reliability evidence. The proxy internal consistency reliability estimates used are likely to be positively biased, suggesting that the differences between the observed and true scores are likely to be larger than expected; therefore, clinical decisions based on these scores are likely to be based on unreliable information. This may be one explanation for the often repeated, generally accepted, but not necessarily well-documented cliché that if you do not like the opinion of your clinician, get a second opinion because it will probably be different.

GENERIC VERSUS CONDITION-SPECIFIC INSTRUMENTS

Outcomes associated with evaluating patients with low back pain employ two broad types of measures: (a) generic outcomes typically assessing general health that were developed with the general population in mind, and (b) condition-specific outcomes typically constructed by

TABLE 12-2. *Magnitudes of disagreement for selected reliabilities*

Reliability	Number of categories of disagreement					
	Match	1	2	3	4	5
0.30	23.40	37.99	24.34	10.63	3.06	0.586
0.40	25.65	39.55	23.41	8.966	2.079	0.348
0.50	28.24	41.35	22.00	6.957	1.293	0.158
0.60	31.62	42.99	19.79	4.890	0.663	0.052
0.70	36.18	44.73	16.12	2.765	0.201	0.010
0.80	42.63	45.56	10.87	0.915	0.026	—
0.90	54.15	42.14	3.665	0.046	—	—
0.95	65.79	33.58	0.630	—	—	—
0.99	84.45	15.55	—	—	—	—

For categories of disagreement:
Match indicates no disagreement (i.e., 1-1, 2-2, 3-3, 4-4, 5-5, 6-6)
1 indicates disagreement by 1 category (i.e., 1-2, 2-3, 3-4, 4-5, 5-6)
2 indicated disagreement by 2 categories (i.e., 1-3, 2-4, 3-5, 4-6)
3 indicated disagreement by 3 categories (i.e., 1-4, 2-5, 3-6)
4 indicated disagreement by 4 categories (i.e., 1-5, 2-6)
5 indicates disagreement by 5 categories (i.e, 1-6)

practitioners in a particular field to more carefully assess the outcomes thought to be relevant to the specific condition under consideration. The SF-36 is a well-known example of a generic health outcome tool. The Roland and Morris Disability Questionnaire and the Oswestry Disability Index are well-known examples of condition-specific instruments. In practice, the title of condition-specific instrument is a misnomer because these instruments are not meant to be linked to a particular condition or diagnosis, but rather to a particular region of the body. The Roland and Morris Disability Questionnaire, for example, is a list of 24 statements associated with actions or activities, such as, "Because of my back or leg I stay at home," and, "Because of my back or leg I sit down for most of the day."

In practice, the differences between generic and condition-specific instruments are more in name than anything else. The intent of using both types of instruments may be to differentiate between non–back/leg and back/leg-specific symptoms. In practice, judging by the correlations in the .7 to .9 range between generic and condition-specific outcome instruments, respondents either can not or do not differentiate between the sources or causes of their pain and symptoms. These high correlations can be worse news for the researcher when considering the notion of correlational attenuation. In short, this concept of attenuation allows the researcher to estimate the true correlation between two scores adjusting for the unreliability in each measure. The logic is that the unreliability in a measure reflects random error, and random error is uncorrelated. Thus, when one correlates two scores that are not perfectly reliable, the resultant correlation is an underestimate of the true correlation because of the error in each of the two measures. The formula for correcting for attenuation is given by:

$$R_{12} = \frac{r_{12}}{\sqrt{r_{11}r_{22}}}$$

where R_{12} is the disattenuated correlation between 1 and 2; r_{12} is the attenuated correlation between 1 and 2; r_{11} is the reliability associated with instrument 1; and r_{22} is the reliability associated with instrument 2.

From this formula, as shown in Table 12-3, a consequence of a high correlation between two instruments with moderate reliabilities is a disattenuated correlation that approaches or even exceeds 1.0. This makes logical sense when one considers, for example, that two instruments with reliabilities of .7 that correlate with each other at .8, in essence, are correlated higher with each other than they are with themselves, because reliability can be thought of as the extent that a score correlates with itself. Thus, from Table 12-3, if instruments 1 and 2 both have reliabilities of .7, and the observed correlation between instruments 1 and 2 (r_{12}) = .8, then the disattenuated correlation between instruments 1 and 2 (R_{12}) is 1.14, indicating the unlikely event that two distinct instruments correlate higher with each other than with themselves. This situation suggests that the two instruments are not distinct. In a more common example, consider the situation were two instruments both have test-retest reliabilities of .8 and the intercorrelation between the two instruments is .7. In this case the disattenuated correlation is .88, which is higher than the reliabilities for either of the two instruments and suggests that they should not be considered distinct.

Perhaps the worst consequence of labeling instruments as condition specific when, in fact, they are region specific (i.e., the back or leg areas) is that clinicians have not tried to establish stronger links between outcome measures and specific conditions. Spratt (31), in discussing the clinical model for health care, argues that the classic Diagnosis-Treatment model should be expanded to an Assessment-Diagnosis-Treatment-Outcome (ADTO) model, which should be viewed as an iterative cycle where: (a) Assessment leads to diagnosis; (b) diagnosis leads to treatment; (c) treatment goals suggest relevant outcomes; and (d) out-

TABLE 12-3. *The relationship between instrument reliability and disattenuated correlations among instruments*

r_{11}	r_{22}	r_{12}	R_{12}	r_{12}	R_{12}	r_{12}	R_{12}	r_{12}	R_{12}	r_{12}	R_{12}	r_{12}	R_{12}	r_{12}	R_{12}
0.30	0.30	0.30	1.00	0.50	1.67	0.70	2.33	0.80	2.67	0.85	2.83	0.90	3.00	0.95	3.17
0.50	0.50	0.30	0.60	0.50	1.00	0.70	1.40	0.80	1.60	0.85	1.70	0.90	1.80	0.95	1.90
0.70	0.70	0.30	0.43	0.50	0.71	0.70	1.00	0.80	1.14	0.85	1.21	0.90	1.29	0.95	1.36
0.75	0.75	0.30	0.40	0.50	0.67	0.70	0.93	0.80	1.07	0.85	1.13	0.90	1.20	0.95	1.27
0.80	0.80	0.30	0.38	0.50	0.63	0.70	0.88	0.80	1.00	0.85	1.06	0.90	1.13	0.95	1.19
0.85	0.85	0.30	0.35	0.50	0.59	0.70	0.82	0.80	0.94	0.85	1.00	0.90	1.06	0.95	1.12
0.90	0.90	0.30	0.33	0.50	0.56	0.70	0.78	0.80	0.89	0.85	0.94	0.90	1.00	0.95	1.06
0.95	0.95	0.30	0.32	0.50	0.53	0.70	0.74	0.80	0.84	0.85	0.89	0.90	0.95	0.95	1.00
0.30	0.50	0.30	0.77	0.50	1.29	0.70	1.81	0.80	2.07	0.85	2.19	0.90	2.32	0.95	2.45
0.50	0.70	0.30	0.51	0.50	.085	0.70	1.18	0.80	1.35	0.85	1.44	0.90	1.52	0.95	1.61
0.70	0.80	0.30	0.40	0.50	0.67	0.70	0.94	0.80	1.07	0.85	1.14	0.90	1.20	0.95	1.27
0.75	0.90	0.30	0.37	0.50	0.61	0.70	0.85	0.80	0.97	0.85	1.03	0.90	1.10	0.95	1.16
0.80	0.95	0.30	0.34	0.50	0.57	0.70	0.80	0.80	0.92	0.85	0.98	0.90	1.03	0.95	1.09
0.85	0.50	0.30	0.46	0.50	0.77	0.70	1.07	0.80	1.23	0.85	1.30	0.90	1.38	0.95	1.46
0.90	0.50	0.30	0.45	0.50	0.75	0.70	1.04	0.80	1.19	0.85	1.27	0.90	1.34	0.95	1.42
0.95	0.50	0.30	0.44	0.50	0.73	0.70	1.02	0.80	1.16	0.85	1.23	0.90	1.31	0.95	1.38

comes lead to reassessment of the patient's condition, which suggests a potential shift in diagnosis. In this framework, an outcome might reasonably be considered an extension of the assessment conducted to determine diagnosis. In this way, outcomes of interest are in fact condition specific because these aspects of the patient's health status are evaluated, presumably, because the patient's states and traits (e.g., pain or symptom location, magnitude, stability, progression, radiographic evidence of degeneration or lesions, etc.) are fundamental to determining what is wrong with the patient. Logically, effective treatment results in changes in these conditions; therefore, the very assessments and diagnostic tests done to establish a specific diagnosis seem to provide the basis for determining the condition- or diagnosis-specific outcomes of interest for evaluating a patient's health status. Within this framework, a clinically relevant change in outcome could be defined as a change in diagnosis based on changes in the assessments of the patient's health status originally used to inform the diagnosis.

CLINICALLY RELEVANT DIFFERENCES

Currently, a concern among clinicians wishing to use outcome instruments to help understand a patient's progress is determining the minimum clinically significant difference; that is, the smallest change in a patient's score from time 1 to time 2 than can be considered a clinically relevant change. Unfortunately, a *real* change need not be synonymous with one that is greater than can be expected by chance, is clinically relevant, and reflects a meaningful amount of movement in terms of resulting clinical decisions. A real change at the group level is a simple statistical procedure. One compares the two groups' distribution of scores, determines the appropriate statistical test based on those distributions, performs the test, and obtains the probability that such a difference is likely to have occurred by chance. If the likelihood is low (<1/20 or .05), the decision is typically that the difference is too large to expect under the assumption that there was no change and the decision is to reject the notion that there was no change. If the change is for the better, the conclusion is that the patient improved over time, or if there were two treatment groups, that one group did better than the other.

However, at the clinical level, where the sample size is 1 (i.e., the individual patient), inferential statistical procedures are not of much practical value. In this case, however, the notion of a reliable difference is still quantifiable within measurement theory by estimating the standard error of measurement defined as:

$$SEM = S_x \sqrt{1 - r_{xx}}$$

where *SEM* is the standard error of measurement; S_X is the standard deviation of instrument X; and r_{xx} is the reliability associated with instrument X.

From this equation, it should be clear that the standard error of measurement (SEM) for an instrument X is smaller as the standard deviation of the scores decreases and the reliability (range, 0 to 1) increases.

Under small sample probability theory ($n = 1$ surely qualifies as small), multiplying the obtained standard error of measurement by two and adding it to a patient's score would approximate a 95% confidence interval around that score. From Table 12-1, consider the SF-36 for the PCS outcome: Mean = 30.6, SD = 7.2, and assume test-retest reliability of .85. In this situation the SEM computes to be 2.79. Thus, a follow-up score of 30.6 + 2 × 2.79 ≥36.18 or a score ≤25.03 (30.6 − 2 × 2.79) indicates a reliable change in the score; that is, a score different from the initial one by more than could be expected because of unreliability. In other words, the approximate 95% confidence interval around the initial score of 30.6 is (25.03 − 36.18). If the reliability of this score was lower, say .75, this 95% confidence interval would become (23.4 − 37.8), indicating a change of around 7.2 points for the difference to be considered greater than might be expected because of lack of reliability. This analysis assumes that the underlying scores are continuous, unimodal, and reasonably symmetrical, all fairly reasonable for the SF-36 PCS and MCS scales.

However, consider the SF-36 Social Functioning (SF) scale: a two-item scale with each item effectively scored as 0, 25, 50, 75, and 100 so that possible averaged scores are 0, 12.5, 25, 37.5, 50, 62.5, 75.0, 87.5, and 100. In this case, the assumption of continuous data clearly does not hold. If one ignores the volition of assumptions and applies the SEM formula to these data, assuming a generous test-retest reliability of .7, one obtains a SEM of 13.7 and a 95% confidence interval around the mean of 39.1 of (11.7 − 66.5). However, these calculations mean virtually nothings because the changes that can occur on the SF scale are such that a single change of one level on one item will move the score 12.5 points, which is close to 1 SEM. Thus, a "reliable" difference can be obtained by consistent changes on one or more units on each of the two items making up the scale. This example should highlight the need to have a large enough number of items to allow a reasonable assumption of continuous data and range of responses to an item to allow adequate discrimination among responses.

In sum, the notion of SEM provides a coherent theoretical framework for establishing how much change in an outcome is required to be comfortable that the observed change is more than could be expected because of an inherent error in the assessment. This represents a necessary condition for establishing whether or not an observed change in outcome is clinically relevant. A second necessary condition, based on the logic provided in the previous section regarding the true concept of condition-specific outcomes guided by the ATDO clinical model is to demonstrate that the changes observed in the outcome(s) of interest are sufficient to change the diagnostic status of the patient. It seems that these two necessary conditions for establishing the clinical relevance of changes in outcome represent a sufficient condition for establishing the clinical relevance of an observed difference.

THE FUTURE OF OUTCOMES

In the early 1980s, when clinicians interested in studying and treating low back pain began to embrace patient self-report as an important tool in evaluating patients' health status, and by proxy treatment efficacy, I felt that clinicians had found the path to righteousness (i.e., finding the truth about treatment efficacy). More than 20 years later the path remains a long a winding road and the potential is unfulfilled.

Einstein defined insanity as doing the same thing over and over again and expecting different outcomes. Over the course of the last 20 years three common themes recur that seem to support Einstein's notion of insanity as it applies to the use of outcomes by clinicians treating patients with back troubles.

Shorter is better. If a set of 10 items have been identified as providing a reasonably reliable and valid score, then shortening this instrument to five items will make it twice as good. Hopefully, the potential consequences of shorting a scale on the SEM, as illustrated with the social functioning subscale on the SF-36, provide compelling reasons why shorter is not always better.

The best way to implement an outcomes program is to start with a core set of items and expand this core as needed. The thinking is that, in theory, it is relatively easy to establish a reasonably small information system, get the technology up and running, and train the clinician users in the system. Once this system is in operation, clinicians will demand improvements in reporting, which will expand the core. In practice, the changes in technology (e.g., additional programming and reconciling reports) required to expand questionnaires usually are perceived by those who administer the system to outweigh the potential gains to the clinician users that would result from adding to the core set. Conversely, but consistent with the aforementioned short is better bias, it is generally perceived to be easy to remove items from a core, even though this act also requires changes in programming and reconciling reports.

The clinical community is unable to appreciate and the measurement community to clarify the distinction between outcomes as applied to groups of patients as opposed to a given patient. In general, the current state of clinical outcomes measures is adequate in many ways when used to evaluate treatment efficacy within a randomized controlled trial. However, these tools typically are not sufficiently reliable and valid for use in clinical practice, nor does reporting at the patient level typically provide clinicians with adequate warnings about the potential magnitude of error in the score they are using to inform their decision making. Efforts to improve the accuracy and precision of outcome instruments and the score reporting to the point that these scores would be appropriate in clinical situations would make these tools better in the aggregate sense as well, thus indicating a win-win situation. The catch? Clinically relevant outcomes require more rather than fewer items to achieve the accuracy and precision demanded at the individual patient level.

REFERENCES

1. Million R, Hall W, Haavik Nilsen K, et al. Assessment of the progress of the back-pain patient. Spine 1982;7:204–212.
2. Roland M, Morris R. A study of the natural history of back pain. Part I: Development of a reliable and sensitive measure of disability in low-back pain. Spine 1983;8:141–144.
3. Gatchel RJ. Compendium of outcome instruments for assessment and research of spinal disorders. La Grange, IL: North American Spine Society, 2001.
4. Beck A, Ward C, Mendelson M, et al. An inventory for measuring depression. Arch Gen Psychiatry 1961;4:561–571.
5. Zung WWK. A self-rating depression scale. Arch Gen Psychiatry 1965;12:63–70.
6. Keller L, Butcher J. Assessment of chronic pain patients with the MMPI-2. Minneapolis: University of Minnesota Press, 1991.
7. Derogatis L. Symptom checklist-90-R: administration, scoring and procedures manual. Minneapolis: National Computer Systems, 1994.
8. Ware JE Jr, Sherbourne CD. The MOS 36-item short-form health survey (SF-36): I. conceptual framework and item selection. Med Care 1992;30:473–483.
9. Ware JEJ, Kosinski M, Keller SD. SF-36 Physical and mental health summary scales: a user's manual. Boston: The Health Institute, New England Medical Center, 1994.
10. Ware JEJ, Snow KK, Kosinski M, et al. SF-36 Health survey manual and interpretation guide. Boston: The Health Institute, New England Medical Center, 1993.
11. Jensen M, Turner J, Romano J, et al. The Chronic Pain Inventory: development and preliminary validation. Pain 1995;60:203–216.
12. Rosenstiel A, Keefe F. The use of coping strategies in low back pain patients: relationship to patient characteristics and current adjustment. Pain 1983;17:33–40.
13. Melzack R. The McGill Pain Questionnaire: major properties and scoring methods. Pain 1975;1:277–299.
14. Fairbank J. Revised Oswestry Disability Questionnaire (comment). Spine 2000;25(19):2552.
15. Fairbank J. Use of Oswestry Disability Index (comment). Spine 1995;20(13):1535–1537.
16. Fairbank JC, Cooper J, Davies JB, et al. The Oswestry low back pain disability questionnaire. Physiotherapy 1980;66(8):271–273.
17. Kerns RD, Turk DC, Rudy TE. The West Haven-Yale Multidimensional Pain Inventory. Pain 1985;23:345–356.
18. Kopec J, Esdaile J, Abrahamowicz M, et al. The Quebec Back Pain Disability Scale: conceptualization and development. J Clin Epidemiol 1996;49:151–161.
19. Kopec J, Esdaile J, Abrahamowicz M, et al. The Quebec Back Pain Disability Scale: measurement properties. Spine 1995;20:341–352.
20. Bergner M, Bobbitt RA, Carter WB, et al. The Sickness Impact Profile: development and final revision of a health status measure. Med Care 1981;19(8):787–805.
21. Bergner M, Bobbitt RA, Pollard WE, et al. The sickness impact profile: validation of a health status measure. Med Care 1976;14(1):57–67.
22. Katz S. Index of Independence in Activities of Daily Living. In: Ward MJ, Lindeman CA, eds. Instruments for measuring nursing practice and other health care variables. Washington, DC: US Government Printing Office, 1979:275–228; 275–280.
23. Katz S, Akpom CA. Index of ADL. Med Care 1976;14:116–118.
24. Katz S, Ford AB, Moskowitz RW, et al. Studies of illness in the aged.

The Index of ADL: a standardized measure of biological and psychosocial function. JAMA 1963;185:914–919.

25. First M, Spitzer R, Gibbon M, et al. Structured clinical interview for DSM-IV axis I disorders: nonpatient version 2. New York: New York State Psychiatric Institute, 1995.

26. Waddell G, McCulloch JA, Kummell E, et al. Nonorganic physical signs in low-back pain. Spine 1980;5:117–125.

27. Spratt KF, Weinstein JN. Measuring clinical outcomes. In: Weisel S, ed. The lumbar spine. Philadelphia: WB Saunders, 1996:1313–1338.

28. Feldt LS, Brennan RL. Reliability. In: Linn RL, ed. Educational measurement. New York: Macmillan, 1989:105–146.

29. Cronbach LJ. Test validation. In: Thorndike RL, ed. Educational measurement. Washington, DC: American Council on Education, 1971: 443–507.

30. Brennan RL. Generalizability theory. New York: Springer, 2001.

31. Spratt KF. Statistical relevance. In: Fardon DF, Garfin SR, Abitbol J-J, et al, eds. Orthopaedic knowledge update: spine 2. Rosemont, IL: The American Academy of Orthopaedic Surgeons, 2002:497–505.

CHAPTER 13

The Role of Outcomes and How to Integrate Them into Your Practice

Richard A. Deyo

Outcomes research became a buzzword in the 1990s, although it seems to mean different things to different people. In general, it refers to a strategy of assessing clinical practices according to patient outcomes, rather than to some prespecified, often arbitrary, set of criteria for the process of care. For example, we might judge the quality of care for a patient with metastatic cancer to the lumbar spine by his neurologic function, activities of daily living, and survival, rather than by whether the patient received a particular surgical implant or a particular diagnostic test.

Several important trends have led to the increasing interest in outcome assessment. First, medical care costs are rising much more rapidly than inflation, and the employers and government agencies who pay the bills are asking if they are getting their money's worth. This seems to be an important question, because per capita costs for medical care in the United States are well above any other country in the world, and yet measures of population health, such as morbidity and mortality, are substantially worse in the U.S. than in many other developed countries (1).

A second trend has been the observation that medical practices vary widely from place to place, even among very small geographic areas (2). At an international level, the United States appears to perform roughly twice as much back surgery as most developed countries, and five times more back surgery than the United Kingdom (3). No one knows which rate is optimal, but it seems unlikely that differences in surgical rates reflect any significant differences in the prevalence of back pain or disc disease. Thus, explanations often invoke differences in training, surgeons' beliefs, public attitudes, financial incentives, imaging strategies, and professional uncertainty. Unfortunately, the differences do not seem to be based on evidence about which style of practice produces the best patient outcomes.

One implication of these findings is that some medical services may be unnecessary. Without information on patient outcomes, however, it is impossible to know whether, and when, this is the case. Recent data from the Maine Lumbar Spine Study (MLSS) suggest that outcomes do vary from one geographic area to the next. In fact, within the state of Maine, the best surgical outcomes—in terms of pain relief, functional status, disability compensation, and patient satisfaction—all occur in the areas with the lowest surgical rates. In contrast, the region of the state with the highest surgical rates reports the worst surgical outcomes. The area of the state with intermediate surgical rates has intermediate outcomes by every measure (4). Thus, it seems clear that more is not necessarily better. Such observations have led to greater calls for accountability by the medical profession.

TYPES OF OUTCOME MEASURES

The Problem of Surrogate Outcomes

Traditionally, many research studies have focused on physiologic outcomes or anatomic outcomes as indicators of success. Examples would be whether a solid fusion is achieved in a patient who undergoes lumbar spine fusion. Other examples would be spinal range of motion as a measure of improvement, spinal fluid endorphins as a measure of possible pain relief, or surface electromyography as an indicator of "muscle spasm." Unfortunately, as suggested in Table 13-1, these are all intermediate or "surrogate" outcomes, that may or may not reflect the end results in which we—and our patients—are most interested. That is, these outcomes do not necessarily correlate well with pain relief, return to work, or improvement in daily function. The implication is that if we are interested in the outcomes of pain relief, return to work, and daily functioning, we must measure them directly rather than try to infer them from these physiologic or anatomic surrogates (5).

139

TABLE 13-1. *Contrasting results for "surrogate" outcomes versus end results*

Treatment (reference)	Surrogate outcome	End result
Lumbar fusion for degenerative discs	Solid fusion achieved	Many patients with solid fusion continue to have pain; many patients without solid fusion have good pain relief
Biofeedback (28)	Reduced paraspinal EMG activity	No change in pain
Antidepressant drugs (29)	No change in spinal fluid endorphins	Better pain relief than placebo
Surgical discectomy (20)	Recovery of motor deficits equal, with or without surgery	Better pain relief with surgery

EMG, electomyogram.

Dissociations among Outcomes

Another problem has been that, in the past, much of the research on back problems focused only on measuring pain, to the exclusion of other dimensions of outcome. However, in a modern understanding of chronic pain management, it has become apparent that both clinical and research work may need to focus more on patient functioning than on pain reports. Some clinical trials have shown that it is possible to improve pain reports without improving functional status scores, suggesting that even though pain reports diminish, behavior may not change in any significant way. This highlights the fact that even among the results most important to us, there are often dissociations among outcomes.

As one example, in the MLSS, patients treated surgically for herniated discs were compared to others treated nonsurgically. Even after statistically adjusting for many baseline characteristics to produce more nearly equivalent groups, surgical outcomes were substantially better than nonsurgical outcomes regarding pain and daily functioning. However, return to work was equivalent between the two arms (6). If one focused only on return to work, one might erroneously conclude that surgery was not helpful for herniated discs. If one focused on pain and function, however, a large advantage of surgery would be apparent.

In another example, we studied long-term outcomes in a longitudinal cohort of primary care patients seen in a managed care organization. After 2 years of follow-up, even among those with the worst pain ratings (6 to 10 on a 10-point scale), the vast majority of patients were still working. Only 11.3% were unemployed despite their high levels of pain (Table 13-2). Conversely, among those who reported no pain at all, 6.5% remained unemployed. In other words, those with the least pain had a higher employment rate, but even there, a substantial fraction remained unemployed (7). Thus, even among the outcomes that may be most relevant to doctors and patients, there are often dissociations, and these different dimensions of outcome must be measured independently.

This is one reason why the traditional outcome scale of "excellent/good/fair/poor" is often inadequate. Howe and Frymoyer noted that different definitions of these terms result in dramatically different conclusions about the

efficacy of surgical procedures, even with the same data in hand (8). Furthermore, as the examples given earlier suggest, any attempt to combine pain, function, and employment status into a single scale may be misleading, because the different outcomes can move in different directions, or one may improve while others do not.

In studying patients with degenerative spinal disorders, death and cure are generally not relevant measures of outcome. Very few patients die from back pain or disc disease. Thus, unlike the study of heart disease or cancer, death rate is a poor outcome measure for spinal degenerative conditions. Furthermore, patients are rarely cured of these degenerative conditions, because the degenerative process continues even after successful surgical intervention. In most studies of both surgical and nonsurgical treatments, a substantial proportion of patients continue to have pain symptoms, although the symptoms may be improved by the treatments under study. Unlike infectious diseases or the surgical treatment of appendicitis, it is generally inappropriate to talk about "cure."

Modern Outcome Questionnaires

All of these factors help to explain the growing interest in questionnaire-based measures of a patient's pain, back-specific functioning, general health status, and work disability. Indeed, these are the dimensions of outcome recommended for routine measurement by an international working group (9) and in an update, by the participants in

TABLE 13-2. *Dissociations among outcomes at 2-year follow-up of patients in primary care[a]*

Worst pain rating (6–10): 11.3% unemployed
Best pain rating (0): 6.5% unemployed
Worst modified Roland score (37.6–100%): 11.4% unemployed
Best modified Roland score (0): 4.3% unemployed

[a]Excludes subjects keeping house, retired, or otherwise outside the work force.
From Dionne CE, Von Korf M, Koepsell TD, et al. A comparison of pain, functional limitations, and work status indices as outcome measures in back pain research. *Spine* 1999;24:2339–2345, with permission.

TABLE 13-3. *Reproducibility of patient self-reports and physician observations[a]*

Test-retest reliability of patient self-reports over several weeks	Kappa[b]	Interobserver agreement by expert clinicians	Kappa[b]
Health history questionnaire	0.79	Ankle reflexes normal	0.50
Daily function: sickness impact profile	0.87	Soft tissue tenderness	0.24
Physical function: SF-36	0.89	Lumbar spine x-ray, normal or abnormal	0.51
Pain: visual analog scale	0.94	Presence of osteophytes on x-ray	0.64

[a]Data are from Deyo (5), Deyo, et al. (12), Deyo, et al. (13), Patrick (14), Pecoraro (15), McCombe (16), with permission.

[b]Kappa quantifies agreement on two measures after adjusting for chance agreements.

a "focus" issue of Spine (10). Reliable and valid measures of each of these dimensions are available because of fusing clinical expertise with social science methodology.

A common concern about questionnaire measures is that they are "soft data." Physiologic measures are attractive in part because they seem "harder." However, the boundary between hard and soft data is indistinct at best. Feinstein pointed out that we might judge the hardness of data by their objectivity (physician finding versus patient report); preservability (e.g., radiologic or histologic specimen); or by the ability to quantify (e.g., a hematocrit versus the observation that a patient is pale). However, he concluded that the essence of "hardness" was the reproducibility of data when measured repeatedly under the same circumstances (11). By this measure, many modern questionnaires are at least as hard as the clinical observations with which we are more familiar. For example, Table 13-3 shows the test-retest reliability of several self-report questionnaires, and contrasts these with interobserver agreement on several clinical measures (12–16). In many cases, the reproducibility of the questionnaire measures substantially exceeds that of the clinical measures.

In addition to reproducibility, these measures have demonstrable validity, as judged by comparison with other more objective measures of health. For example, in a national survey, middle-aged men responded to a single question about whether their health was excellent, very

good, good, fair, or poor. The responses to this single question predicted 10-year mortality. In fact, the survival rates fell in perfect order according to the initial self-evaluation of health, and ranged from about 60% survival among those who indicated poor health to 95% survival among those who indicated excellent health (17). Although we know little about how subjects made their self-evaluations at baseline, this simple self-rating obviously had important prognostic ability.

Questionnaires for studying back-related dysfunction have been validated against a variety of clinical measures, with reassuring results. Table 13-4 provides an example that compares the Roland Disability Questionnaire, the Short Form 36 (SF-36), and some "disability day" measures from U.S. population surveys (14). While some association is expected between a valid questionnaire and other measures of health status (e.g., opioid use, or physical examination findings), such an association would not necessarily be expected to be a strong association. In the absence of a "gold standard" for daily functioning, this sort of cumulative "construct validation" is generally the best we can do.

Performance Measures

Tests of patient performance have sometimes been used to evaluate physical capacity. Such tests may include, for example, computerized dynamometry, or

TABLE 13-4. *Construct validation of several patient self-report measures by comparison with other clinical phenomena[a]*

Outcome questionnaire	Opioids in past mo		Workers' comp		Abnormal straight leg raising	
	Yes	No	Yes	No	Yes	No
Modified Roland scale[a]	17.5	14.2	17.6	14.9	16.8	13.9
SF-36 physical function[b]	7.6	16.8	3.1	16.8	9.4	18.4
SF-36 pain[b]	19.2	33.0	21.4	28.7	23.4	32.3
Days of reduced activity[c]	21.3	18.1	24.3	17.4	20.2	18.7

[a]Mean scores at baseline for sciatica patients seen in surgical practices. All differences are significant at p ≤ .005. Higher scores on the Roland scale represent worse function; range 0–2.4.

[b]All differences are significant at $p \leq .005$. Higher scores on the SF-36 represent better function, range 0–100.

[c]All differences are significant at $p \leq .005$ except for those with and without abnormal SLR.

From Patrick DL, Deyo RA, Atlas SJ, et al. Assessing health related quality of life in patients with sciatica. Spine 1995;20:1899–1909, with permission.

timed or measured performance on a standardized set of tasks. While this approach has the attraction of seeming objective, patient mood, motivation, and other factors affect performance. Further, they require in-person evaluation (rather than by mail or telephone) and may require special equipment, making them less practical and affordable than questionnaire measures. How these performance measures may compare with self-report measures in terms of validity and responsiveness remains unclear and is an area for further investigation.

OUTCOME ASSESSMENT FOR QUALITY IMPROVEMENT

One application of outcome measurement is for improving clinical practices. In this circumstance, patients would use outcome questionnaires in the course of routine clinical care. The results might be used to evaluate changes in clinical practice, surgical technique, staffing patterns, or other aspects of care.

As one example, Zucherman et al. reported their experience of measuring patient outcomes with different surgical implants for performing spinal fusions. Unfortunately, they found that with successive waves of new surgical implants, their outcomes became worse rather than better (18). Only with the most recent implants at the time did their results finally improve, though they remained worse than their results using bone grafts without surgical implants. It seems unlikely that these surgeons were less technically skilled than other surgeons. Instead, they seemed to identify an important trend in their own practice that might otherwise have gone unnoticed. Even though their report did not make use of some of the newer outcome instruments, their data were sufficient for monitoring and improving their own clinical practice.

Such quality improvement efforts may have been part of the motivation for developing the Musculoskeletal Outcomes Data Evaluation and Management System (MODEMS) program by the American Academy of Orthopaedic Surgeons (AAOS). That program was designed to have surgeons implement outcome measures routinely in their own practices, with data submitted to a central database. Unfortunately, the effort was not highly successful, and this experience may point to some of the problems with outcome assessment in routine practice.

Measuring outcomes in routine care requires real resources. In addition to identifying and duplicating questionnaires, one must have some means of entering the data into a computerized database, calculating scores, and reporting the results. Some practices have succeeded in doing this at baseline for most new patients, but have found it difficult to obtain uniform follow-up. Some patients do not return to clinic, some return at unexpected intervals, and some simply do not respond to mail or telephone surveys. Obtaining a high rate of follow-up at consistent time intervals is likely to require dedicated personnel who are able to conduct multiple mailings or phone calls, and this adds to the expense. These activities are not a part of routine care as it is currently conceived, and therefore are not reimbursed by patients or insurance companies. Thus, many practices find it difficult to collect uniform outcome data.

In part for this reason, we have proposed a simple set of outcome questions that might be used in routine care and would require minimal resources (9). This is a set of just six questions, all derived from well-validated outcome questionnaires, and covering several important dimensions of outcome: pain, back-related functioning, general health status, work disability, and satisfaction with care (Table 13-5). Even this short set of measures appears to be a substantial improvement compared with measuring pain severity alone, or by "excellent/good/fair/poor" standards. The questions were intended to be examined individually, without generating an overall score, in part to avoid obscuring the situation in which one dimension improves while others do not. A 1-week period for measuring symptoms was suggested because it allows the patient to integrate recent experience for a long enough interval to be meaningful, but short enough to avoid important problems with recall and to identify relatively short-term improvements. Many of these items are included in the lumbar cluster of the AAOS outcome instruments used for the MODEMS program.

While these outcome measures may be useful for monitoring quality improvement over time, they should be used with caution to compare individual physicians, clinics, or hospitals. Such cross-system comparisons may be misleading because of important demographic or clinical differences in the patient populations served. Thus, for example, a hospital serving low-income patients with low levels of literacy, language barriers, high levels of comorbidity, poor health insurance, and menial if any work, is likely to have worse outcomes than a health care system serving well-insured, affluent, and well-educated patients. Similarly, a physician with a reputation for excellence may have the most difficult cases referred to him or her, while a less-skilled physician may see patients with less severe problems. The patients of the more skilled physician might have worse outcomes despite higher quality care simply because of a worse initial prognosis. Comparing outcomes under these circumstances could lead to an erroneous conclusion about the quality of care. Having measures of baseline demographic and clinical characteristics for patients would help to avoid such mistaken conclusions, but may not completely adjust for all the differences in patient populations.

Furthermore, if financial incentives are tied to outcome measures, there is a substantial risk of "gaming" the results. This could occur if a health care system made only nominal efforts to collect data from patients with low literacy, limited English fluency, the most severe illness, or simply removed "outliers" from calculations or adjusted inclusion and exclusion criteria to optimize their apparent outcomes. The gaming that has been well

TABLE 13-5. *Parsimonious routine care*

Patient outcomes[a]

1. During the past week, how bothersome have each of the following symptoms been? (circle one number in each row)

	Not at all bothersome	Slightly bothersome	Moderately bothersome	Very bothersome	Extremely bothersome
a. Low back pain	1	2	3	4	5
b. Leg pain (sciatica)	1	2	3	4	5

2. During the past week, how much did pain interfere with your normal work (including both work outside the home and housework)?

☐ Not at all ☐ A little bit ☐ Moderately ☐ Quite a bit ☐ Extremely

3. If you had to spend the rest of your life with the symptoms you have right now, how would you feel about it?

☐ Very dissatisfied ☐ Somewhat dissatisfied ☐ Neither satisfied nor dissatisfied ☐ Somewhat satisfied ☐ Very satisfied

4. During the past 4 weeks, about how many days did you cut down on the things you usually do for more than half the day because of back pain or leg pain (sciatica)? _____ Number of days

5. During the past 4 weeks, how many days did low back pain or leg pain (sciatica) keep you from going to work or school? _____ Number of days

6. Over the course of treatment for your low back pain or leg pain (sciatica), how satisfied were you with your overall medical care?

☐ Very dissatisfied ☐ Somewhat dissatisfied ☐ Neither satisfied nor dissatisfied ☐ Somewhat satisfied ☐ Very satisfied

[a]Note: most of these items are included in the AAOS Lumbar Cluster, the Low Back Pain TyPE, and the NASS low back outcome instrument.
From Deyo RA, Battie M, Beurskens AJ, et al. Outcome measures for low back pain research. A proposal for standardized use. Spine 1998;23:2003–2013, with permission.

demonstrated in diagnosis coding for reimbursement suggests that this is a real concern.

Aside from quality improvement, some practices have adopted routine measurement of health outcomes for helping to inform clinical care. Thus, for example, some practices have routinely had patients complete the SF-36 or the Oswestry Disability Questionnaire, and made the results available to clinicians as they see the patients. In many cases, these have been academic practices where extramural resources, including grants, could help to support these activities. Nonetheless, some private practitioners have also adopted the strategy and find the information useful to inform their own care of individual patients.

OUTCOME MEASUREMENT FOR RESEARCH PURPOSES

Aside from their use in quality improvement, outcome measures might be used for comparing the effectiveness of different clinical approaches to a particular problem. In some circumstances, this might be done in the form of a randomized controlled trial. However, randomized trials are probably less common in routine practice settings than observational studies, such as cohort studies. In cohort studies, patients may receive different treatments for the same condition, but with the treatments determined by the course

of usual care rather than the dictates of a randomization schedule. Although such studies do not yield information as definitive as randomized trials with regard to treatment efficacy, outcome studies using cohort designs have sometimes added greatly to our understanding of patient experience of various outcomes, unexpected consequences of therapy, and important gaps in clinical knowledge.

An example of such work can be found in the MLSS, where we followed patients with either herniated lumbar discs or lumbar spinal stenosis with pretreatment measures, and follow-up data collected at 3 months, 6 months, 1 year, and annually thereafter. Table 13-6 provides selected data from that study, using several state-of-the art outcome questionnaires (19).

The MLSS collected data from the offices of orthopedic surgeons, neurosurgeons, and occupational medicine physicians. The study provided much greater detail regarding patient outcomes than was previously available from the one randomized trial of surgical versus nonsurgical treatment for sciatica (20). Like that study, the MLSS suggested that surgery offered an advantage in outcomes for several years, although the differences in outcome between surgical and nonsurgical treatment gradually narrowed over several years. The MLSS also found that return to work after 1 year and 3 years was virtually the same with or without surgery (6).

TABLE 13-6. *Outcomes data for patients with sciatica, comparing surgical and nonsurgical therapy in a cohort study*

| Outcome variable[a] | Treatment group | | P value |
	Surgical (n = 219)	Nonsurgical (n = 170)	
Symptoms			
Low back pain compared to baseline[b]			<0.001
Better	75.0	54.5	
Same	16.8	29.9	
Worse	8.2	15.6	
Leg pain compared to baseline[b]			<0.001
Better	81.3	55.8	
Same	13.4	33.3	
Worse	5.3	10.9	
Change in predominant symptom[c]			<0.001
Completely gone	30.6	11.4	
Much better	40.2	31.7	
Better	9.1	13.2	
About the same or a little better	14.3	29.9	
A little worse to much worse	5.8	13.8	
Sciatica Frequency Index, mean change	−11.2	−3.4	<0.001
Functional status			
Roland score, mean change (1-yr baseline)	−11.1	−4.7	<0.001
SF-36 score, mean change (1-yr baseline)			
Physical function	40.3	17.5	<0.001
Bodily pain	44.0	20.4	<0.001
Disability days in past month, mean changes[d]			
In bed	−10.1	−3.3	<0.001
Decreased activity	−16.0	−12.5	0.04
Absent from work	−10.2	−8.0	0.06
Quality of life, ≥ moderate improvement	79.7	57.6	<0.001
Patient satisfaction			
Overall results of treatment, ≥ very good	61.1	46.0	0.005
Spend rest of life like now, satisfied	60.1	39.6	<0.001
If surgery, still choose back operation, yes	86.5		
Employment and WC status			
If receiving WC at entry	(n = 60)	(n = 63)	
Unemployed at 1-yr evaluation	30.5	44.1	0.13
Receiving WC at 1-yr evaluation	45.6	55.2	0.30
If employed at entry	(n = 113)	(n = 78)	
Unemployed at 1-yr evaluation	5.4	6.9	0.68
Receiving WC at 1-yr evaluation	4.6	7.1	0.47

SF-36, Short Form 36; WC, workers' compensation.
[a]All variables expressed in percentages, except where noted.
[b]Symptom severity was reported to be "better" if the response was "better" to "completely gone," the same if the response was "about the same" or "a little better," and worse if the response was "a little worse" or "much worse."
[c]Predominant symptom, either leg or back pain, at entry.
[d]Comparing difference of two distributions using the Kolmogorow-Smirnov statistic.
From Atlas SJ, Deyo RA, Kellar RB, et al. The Maine Lumbar Spine Study, Part II.
One year outcomes of surgical and non-surgical management of sciatica. Spine 1996;21:1777–1786, with permission.

An example of a randomized trial using similar outcome measures is the Spine Outcome Research Trial (SPORT) currently underway in the United States. This study is randomizing patients to surgical or nonsurgical treatment for herniated discs, spinal stenosis, or degenerative spondylolisthesis. The trial involves data collected from numerous clinical practices around the country. In this trial, patients usually complete questionnaires using electronic "tablets," allowing instant data entry and analysis. Outcome measures in this study include the Oswestry Disability Questionnaire, the SF-36, and symptom measures, as well as a

measure of patient satisfaction (21). For projects such as these, which enjoy extramural research funding, it is feasible to use a larger set of questionnaires than the simple measures proposed for quality improvement purposes

RECOMMENDED QUESTIONNAIRES FOR STUDYING OUTCOMES OF LUMBAR SPINE DISORDERS

As a result of an international low back pain forum, and a subsequent focus workshop on outcome research, a core

TABLE 13-7. *A proposed set of patient-based outcome measures for use in spinal disorders*

Domain	Instrument	No. of items (response options)	Score (best to worse)	Time to complete	Dimensions
Back specific function	Roland-Morris	24 (yes/no)	0–24	5 min	Physical activities, housework, mobility, dressing, getting help, appetite, irritability, pain
	or Oswestry	10 (6 levels)	0–100	5 min	Pain intensity, personal care, lifting, walking, sitting, standing, sleeping, sex life, social life, traveling
Generic health status	SF-36 version 2.0	36 (variable)	8 dimensions: 100–0 each or norm-based: mean: 50; SD: 10	10 min	Eight dimensions: physical function, role physical, bodily pain, general health, vitality, social function, role emotional, and mental health Can be aggregated into two components: Physical and mental health
Pain	Bodily pain scale of SF-36	2 (variable)	100–0 or norm-based: mean: 50; SD: 10	2 min	Pain intensity, pain interference with work and housework
	(optional) Chronic pain grade	7 (11-point NRS) + no. of days in pain		5 min	Current, worse, and average pain, disability days, interference with usual activities, recreational, social and family activities, and work (including housework)
Work disability[a]	Work status	10 categories	Nominal scale	1 min	Employed at usual job, on light duty, or some restricted work assignment, paid leave/sick leave, unpaid leave, unemployed because of health problems, unemployed because of other reason, student, keeping house/homemaker, retired, on disability
	Days off work and days of reduced work[b]	No. of days		2 min	
	Time to return to work	No. of days		2 min	
Satisfaction: back specific	*Satisfaction with care:* Patient Satisfaction Scale	17 (5 levels)			Information, caring, effectiveness of treatment, and others
	Satisfaction with treatment outcome: Global question	1 (7 levels)	1–7	1 min	Extremely, very, somewhat satisfied, mixed, somewhat, very, extremely dissatisfied

NRS, Numerical Rating Scale.

[a]The SF-36 physical and mental role scales refer to all roles (work as well as housework). The reader specifically interested in work-related disability would need to modify these scales to refer to work roles only.

[b]The U.S. National Health Interview Survey asks about days off work and reduced activity both from usual work and other role activities. The reader specifically interested in work-relatedness would need to modify these questions to refer to work roles only.

From Bombardier C. Outcome assessments in the evaluation in the treatment of spinal disorders; summary and general recommendations. Spine 2000;25:3100–3103, with permission.

set of patient-based outcome measures for research purposes has been proposed (9,10). As shown in Table 13-7, these include measures of back-specific functioning, generic health status, pain, work disability, and patient satisfaction. Each of the instruments in Table 13-7 has been well validated, and the characteristics of the questionnaires are indicated in the table. This set of measurement instruments corresponds closely to the lumbar spine cluster proposed by the AAOS and to the North American Spine Society (NASS) spine questionnaires. The special focus issue of Spine contains a summary of the data relating to these questionnaires, including information about their reliability, reproducibility, and responsiveness to changes over time (10,22,23). For key elements of this recommended set, such as the Roland and Morris disability questionnaires and the SF-36, well-validated versions are available in many languages, especially European languages.

This set of instruments was intended to be a core set that might be used by most investigators studying low back problems, to help improve comparability among studies and also to facilitate formal meta-analysis of multiple studies. However, the intent was to make this core set sufficiently brief so that investigators could add additional instruments for purposes specific to the conditions and treatments they are studying. Thus, investigators may wish to add more psychological measures or disease-specific modules such as measures for spinal stenosis or scoliosis.

This is certainly not an exhaustive list of validated instruments for studying low back pain. However, it does represent a set that appears to be well validated, widely used, and at least equivalent in performance characteristics to other available instruments.

HAZARDS IN OUTCOME MEASUREMENT

The difficulties in making fair comparisons among physicians or hospitals have previously been addressed. In general, valid comparisons of outcomes would require at least adjustment for disease severity, comorbid conditions, baseline health status, and several important demographic variables. Even with such adjustment, comparisons should be made with caution, because we do not yet know all the relevant variables for predicting patient prognosis or outcome.

Those who assess spine outcomes must be aware that many factors other than medical care can affect the results of a particular disease. Patients with multiple comorbid diseases (e.g., heart disease or diabetes) are likely to have worse outcomes than patients without comorbid illnesses. Low income or homeless patients are likely to have worse outcomes than more affluent patients. Patient compliance, genetic endowment, psychological characteristics, and environmental factors (such as workplace characteristics) may also have a major influence on patient outcomes. Thus, in comparing qual-

ity of care between providers or in comparing the effectiveness of different treatments, caution is warranted if outcomes are used. In most situations, random allocation to alternative treatments is the best way to assure that one is truly comparing equivalent groups, but this is rarely feasible in comparing health care providers or workplaces.

The optimal timing and duration of follow-up for outcome assessment may vary according to the condition or treatment under study. For example, studies of spinal manipulation have suggested that any benefits occur within a few days or weeks of treatment, and do not have long-lasting effects. In contrast, surgical intervention may result in a temporary decline in patient functioning during the postoperative recovery period, with benefits only becoming apparent in long-term follow-up. Similarly, the timing of outcome measures may vary according to whether one is studying patients with acute pain or chronic pain.

Patients' literacy and language fluency are additional potential barriers to the use of questionnaire measures such as those presented here, though these barriers can sometimes be overcome (24). Standards for developing equivalent questionnaires in different languages have been proposed (25), and oral interviews can sometimes replace self-administration.

An important caveat is that financial incentives may affect a patient's self-report. If financial gain may result from high levels of disability (e.g., disability compensation), patients may report worse functioning on standardized questionnaires. This is not being dishonest as much as it is a natural tendency to maximize symptoms and dysfunction under such circumstances. Conversely, some patients have reported fear of losing their insurance coverage if they admit to any functional problems that might be seen as "preexisting conditions" in any new insurance application. Such patients would perceive a financial incentive to report excellent functioning and no symptoms, skewing results in the opposite direction. The magnitude of such effects has not been well-quantified or studied, although it seems clear that outcomes are generally worse among patients who receive disability compensation than among those who do not, even with apparently similar levels of anatomic or physiologic disruption. Such incentives may also influence performance on standardized physical tasks.

FUTURE DEVELOPMENTS

Item response theory has been well known among those who do psychological testing for many years, but its application to health status measures is relatively recent. Item response theory allows one to rate the "difficulty" of a question in comparison to other similar questions. Thus, for example, "walking one block" would be rated easier than "walking one mile". Although the ranking of these two items is obvious, the relative rankings of other functional items may be less clear. Item response theory allows a diverse range of items to be ranked by their difficulty. Such techniques can allow the construction of a large bank of individual questions that measure the same underlying construct (such as physical function or emotional function) and calibration of every item within that bank (26).

With computer technology, adaptive testing would then become possible. The idea is that if a patient indicates he or she is able to walk a mile, then questions about less demanding activities would be avoided. Instead, a series of more difficult questions would be posed, allowing the investigator to reach a very precise estimate of a patient's physical functional ability with just a few items. Thus, after the first question, the computer selects each subsequent item from the pool of calibrated items according to the subject's responses to the initial and each subsequent item. The goal is to achieve a high level of accuracy with as few items as possible.

Item response theory models have been used for some scale validation, and the Quebec Back Pain Disability Scale was developed using this technique (27). An effort to calibrate all the items found in major scales for back pain should be encouraged, because this could lead to construction of a relevant item bank, and in turn toward computerized adaptive testing (26).

Adaptive testing aside, the Internet offers enticing prospects for the future of studying patient outcomes. If Internet access was widely available in patients' homes, patients would be able to complete questionnaires and transmit data to a central database without using pencil and paper, stamps, or envelopes. In settings where computer access is widely available, this may already be feasible.

CONCLUSION

Variations in care and rising health care costs have led to growing calls for accountability by those who pay the bills. In many cases, studying patient outcomes in a rigorous fashion is likely to be the best way to identify effective treatments and to assess the quality of care. For low back disorders, traditional measures such as death, cure, and physiologic outcomes have only limited applicability. In many cases, patients' symptoms, function, and work status are the most important outcomes to measure. While these are subjective, modern instruments can assess these dimensions of outcome with demonstrable reliability and validity. A standard battery of instruments can be recommended for measuring several dimensions of patient outcome, generally obviating any need to "reinvent the wheel." However, improvements in such measures will inevitably be developed, and comparisons among potential outcome measures should be encouraged. Such comparisons should quantify the construct validity, reproducibility, and responsiveness of these instruments.

When comparing providers with regard to quality of care, or when comparing treatment effectiveness, extreme care is warranted to assure that the comparisons are fair, considering potential baseline differences in disease severity, health status, and demographic characteristics. A variety of logistic barriers must be overcome before these instruments are widely used in routine practice, including the resource requirements for collection, automation, analysis, and reporting of the data. Nonetheless, such efforts offer the promise of substantial improvements in quality of care and in the effectiveness of treatment approaches.

ACKNOWLEDGMENTS

Supported in part by grant no. 1 P60 AR 48093 from the National Institute of Arthritis, Musculoskeletal and Skin Diseases.

REFERENCES

1. Geyman JP. Evidence-based medicine in primary care: an overview. J Am Board Fam Pract 1998;11:46–56.
2. Center for the Evaluative Clinical Sciences at Dartmouth Medical School. The Dartmouth Atlas of Musculoskeletal Health Care. Am. Academy of Orthopedic Surgeons, 2000.
3. Checkin DC, Deyo RA, Loeser JD, et al. An international comparison of back surgery rates. Spine 1994;19:1201–1206.
4. Keller RB, Atlas SJ, Soule DN, et al. Relationships between rates and outcomes of operative treatment for lumbar disc herniation and spinal stenosis. J Bone Joint Surg 1999;81-A:752–762.
5. Deyo RA. Measuring the functional status of patients with low back pain. Arch Phys Med Rehabil 1988;69:1044–1053.
6. Atlas SJ, Chang YC, Kammann E, et al. Long term disability and return to work among patients who have a herniated lumbar disc: the effect of disability compensation. J Bone Joint Surg 2000;82-A:4–15.
7. Dionne CE, Von Korf M, Koepsell TD, et al. A comparison of pain, functional limitations, and work status indices as outcome measures in back pain research. Spine 1999;24:2339–2345.
8. Howe J, Frymoyer JW. The effects of questionnaire design on the determination of end results in lumbar spine surgery. Spine 1985;10:804–805.
9. Deyo RA, Battie M, Beurskens AJ, et al. Outcome measures for low back pain research. A proposal for standardized use. Spine 1998;23:2003–2013.
10. Bombardier C. Outcome assessments in the evaluation in the treatment of spinal disorders; summary and general recommendations. Spine 2000;25:3100–3103.
11. Feinstein AR. Clinical biostatistics. XLI. Hard science, soft data, and challenges of choosing clinical variables in research. Clin Pharmacol Ther 1977;22:485–498.
12. Deyo RA, Rainville J, Kent DL. What can the history and physical examination tell us about low back pain? JAMA 1992;268:760–765.
13. Deyo RA, McNiesh LM, Cone RO. Observer variability in the interpretation of lumbar spine radiographs. Arthritis Rheum 1985;28:1066–1070.
14. Patrick DL, Deyo RA, Atlas SJ, et al. Assessing health related quality-of-life in patients with sciatica. Spine 1995;20:1899–1909.
15. Pecoraro RE, Inui TS, Chen MF, et al. Validity and reliability of a self-administered health history questionnaire. Public Health Rep 1979;94:231–238.
16. McCombe PS, Fairbanks JCT, Cockersole DC, et al. Reproducibility of physical signs of low back pain. Spine 1989;14:908–919.
17. Idler EL, Angel RJ. Self-rated health and mortality in the NHANES-I Epidemiologic Follow-Up Study. Am J Public Health 1990; 80:446–452.
18. Zucherman J, Hsu K, Piccetti G, et al. Clinical efficacy of spinal instrumentation in lumbar degenerative disc disease. Spine 1992;17:834–837.

19. Atlas SJ, Deyo RA, Keller RB, et al. The Maine Lumbar Spine Study, Part II. One year outcomes of surgical and non-surgical management of sciatica. Spine 1996;21:1777–1786.
20. Weber H. Lumbar disc herniation: a controlled prospective study with ten years of observation. Spine 1983;8:131–140.
21. Weinstein JN, Deyo RA. Clinical research: issues and data collection. Spine 2000;25:3104–3109.
22. Roland M, Fairbank J. The Roland-Morris disability questionnaire and the Oswestry disability questionnaire. Spine 2000;25:3115–3124.
23. Ware JE. SF-36 Health Survey update. Spine 2000;25:3130–3139.
24. Deyo RA, Patrick DL. Barriers to the use of health status measures in clinical investigation, patient care, and policy research. Med Care 1989;27[3 Suppl]:S254–S268.
25. Beaton DE, Bombardier C, Guillemin F, et al. Guidelines for the process of cross-cultural adaptation of self-report measures. Spine 2000;25:3186–191.
26. Kopec JA. Measuring functional outcomes in persons with back pain: a review of back specific questionnaires. Spine 2000;25:3110–3114.
27. Kopec JA, Esdaile JM, Abrahamowicz M, et al. The Quebec Back Pain Disability Scale: conceptualization and development. J Clin Epidemiol 1996;49:151–161.
28. Nouwen A. EMG biofeedback used to reduce standing levels of paraspinal muscle tension in chronic low back pain. Pain 1983;17:353–360.
29. Ward NG. Tricyclic antidepressants for chronic low-back pain: mechanisms of action and predictors of response. Spine 1986;11:661–665.

SECTION II

Alternatives to Traditional Nonoperative Treatment

CHAPTER 14

Manual Therapy in Patients with Low Back Pain

Jiri Dvorak, Scott Haldeman, and Wolfgang Gilliar

The hands are one of the oldest tools available to clinicians for healing. References to manual treatment methods can be found in the writings of virtually all ancient and modern civilizations. This discipline, in its broadest definition and as it relates to low back pain, includes all procedures where practitioners apply their hands for diagnostic and therapeutic purposes in the hope of relieving symptoms and restoring function. Since the 1950s, and in particular since the 1970s, manual medicine has experienced unprecedented growth and acceptance, not only by the general population, but also by traditionally orthodox branches of medicine. This growing interest is due to a number of social and political forces. One of the strongest of these forces has been the failure of traditional medicine practitioners to develop treatment methods that control low back pain to the satisfaction of patients.

Despite the marked increase in diagnostic technology and improvements in both medications and surgical procedures, there is no evidence that the amount of suffering and related disability due to back pain has improved, and if anything, it appears to be increasing. There has also been a marked resurgence in interest by the public in so-called alternative and complementary medicine, or CAM approaches to health care. This may, in part, be a response to the more aggressive use of medications, injection therapies, and surgery along with the growing realization that these procedures rarely cure back pain, at least in the long term, and have significant complication rates and expenses. A recent series of publications has shown that more patients use CAM therapies to treat their low back pain than conventional medical therapies, and that satisfaction with CAM providers is markedly higher than for traditional medical providers. The most popular CAM treatment for low back pain is spinal manipulation and massage, both of which fall into the category of manual therapies, although particularly in Europe, manual medicine is integrated within the classic education of physicians. In several countries (e.g., Switzerland, Germany, Czech Republic, France) a subspecialization in manual

medicine has been established within the normal medical associations.

The initial response by the mainstream medical community to the popularity of manual therapy through the first 75 years of the 20th century was an attempt to ostracize practitioners, especially chiropractors and osteopathic physicians, and to isolate those medical practitioners who recommended and taught manual therapy. There was, however, a small group of pioneering allopathic physicians such as James Cyriax, Robert Maigne, Karl Lewit, and John Mennell, particularly in Europe, and later within North America and the rest of the world, who maintained an interest in the manual therapies throughout the 20th century. The "modern" era of manual therapy has often been attributed to the Swiss physician O. Nägeli (1843–1922), who described a series of "handgriffe" (hand applications) for cervical manipulations in 1894. It was during the same period, at the end of the 19th century and early 20th century, that Andrew Taylor Still, M.D., formulated the concepts of osteopathy and chiropractics was established as a practice devoted to spinal manipulation by Daniel David Palmer. There was a parallel growth of the three groups of practitioners of manual therapy (medical physicians, chiropractors, and osteopaths) through the 20th century that gradually resulted in communication of ideas and the teaching of techniques between these different groups of practitioners. At the same time massage and manual mobilization, which have always been part of rehabilitation and the practice of physical therapy, became more formalized within this medical profession. There is a growing body of academic physical therapists that have become very active in research in the manual therapies and are responsible for the publication of a number of clinical trials on the topic. Components of the manual medicine armamentarium are increasingly being adopted and integrated in general medical practice and are being included within the teachings of many medical specialties including neurology, orthopedics, physical medicine, rehabilitation, and rheumatology (1). In some settings the manual therapies are practiced by a medical physician but in many interdisciplinary centers these therapies are performed by chiropractors, osteopathic physicians, and sometimes by physical therapists.

DEFINITIONS

Terminology used by practitioners can be difficult to understand for many physicians who do not have formal training in the manual medicine field. The German term "manuelle medizin", or manual medicine has become the standard term used for the manipulative therapies practiced by medical physicians in most of Europe. On the other hand, in North America 90% of the manipulative treatments are performed by chiropractors who use the term "chiropractic adjustment" to describe their procedures. Osteopathic physicians refer to specific "osteopathic manipulative therapy (OMT)." Many of the mobilization and massage techniques are generally offered by physical therapists and a growing number of massage therapists. Each of these professions, in turn, has numerous techniques or named methods of providing their form of manual therapy.

It is possible to divide the manual therapies into three major subdivisions with a fourth category representing a combination of some of the techniques. The most common procedure, and that which also requires the greatest amount of skill and training, is the classic "thrust technique." The thrust technique is also described as "mobilization-with-impulse" technique, or "high velocity, low amplitude (HVLA) thrust" (Fig. 14-1). The second gen-eral treatment category is represented by the nonthrust mobilization techniques, which are also known as "mobilization-without-impulse" techniques. They are easier to perform and do not take the joint beyond the normal range of motion. The third category includes the so-called soft tissue techniques, consisting of various methods of mobilization and massage applied to the soft tissues of the spine without movement of a joint.

The fourth manual technique, the "neuromuscular therapy (NMT)" is a hybrid of the classic manual techniques and includes treatment procedures that attempt to mobilize and stretch the muscles by engaging specific muscle action or invoking associated neuromuscular reflex mechanisms. These techniques rely on direct muscle force (NMT 1) in order to move the spine and stretch muscles or they include a postisometric relaxation phase (NMT 2) (Fig. 14-2). Another variation attempts to take advantage of the reciprocal innervation for inhibition of specific muscle groups (NMT 3). This form of manual therapy is based, in part, on the observation that rotation of the spine to one side is caused by the contralateral transversospinal muscular system but may be typically limited by shortened ipsilateral transversospinal muscles. Rotational motion of the superior partner of the vertebral spinal segment is initiated to one side by the rotator and multifidi muscles on the contralateral side. Thus, the right rotator and multifidi muscles function as agonists for rotation to the left side (Fig. 14-3). When the rotatores and multifidi muscles are shortened in the same spinal segment it is assumed that they diminish rotation to the

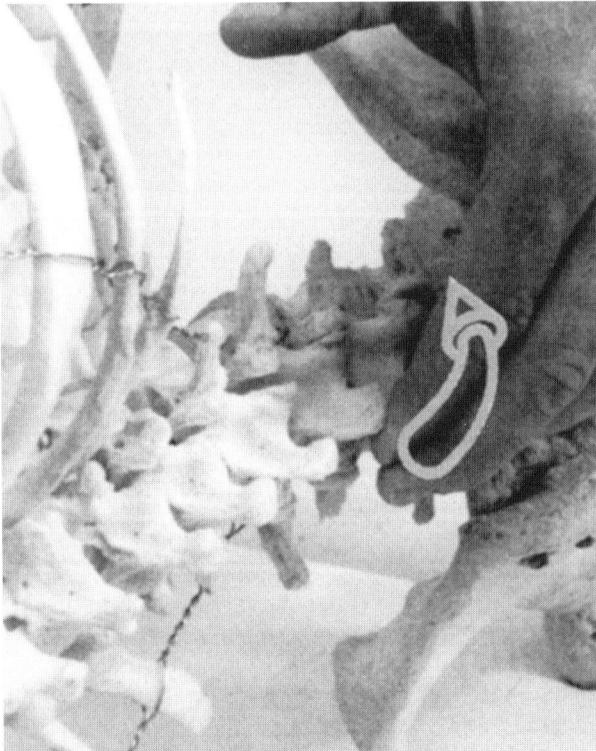

FIG. 14-1. Manipulation of lumbar spine in side position (mobilization with impulse). (From Dvorak J, Dvorak V, Schneider W, et al. Musculoskeletal medicine (manual therapy), 3rd English ed. Stuttgart/New York: G. Thieme Verlag, 2004, with permission.)

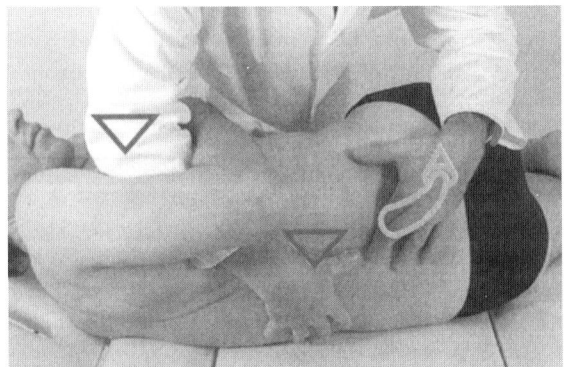

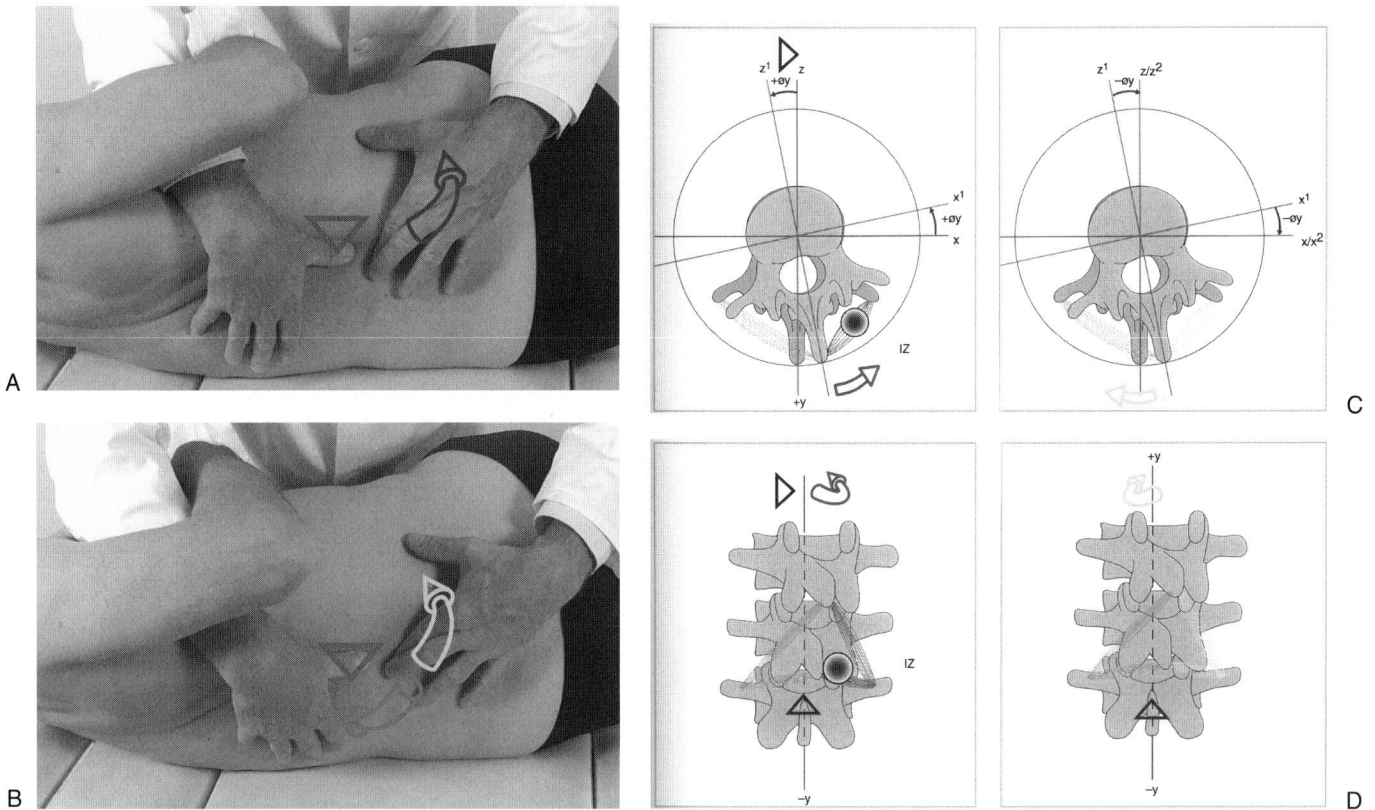

FIG. 14-2. Mobilization without impulse of the lumbar spine **(A)** and mobilization without impulse using the postisometric relaxation of the antagonistic muscle groups **(B)** also described as neuromuscular therapy (NMT). **C:** *Arrow* indicates the direction of isometric muscle contraction. **D:** *Arrow* indicates the direction of mobilization. (From Dvorak J, Dvorak V, Schneider W, et al. Musculoskeletal medicine (manual therapy), 3rd English ed. Stuttgart/New York: G. Thieme Verlag, 2004, with permission.)

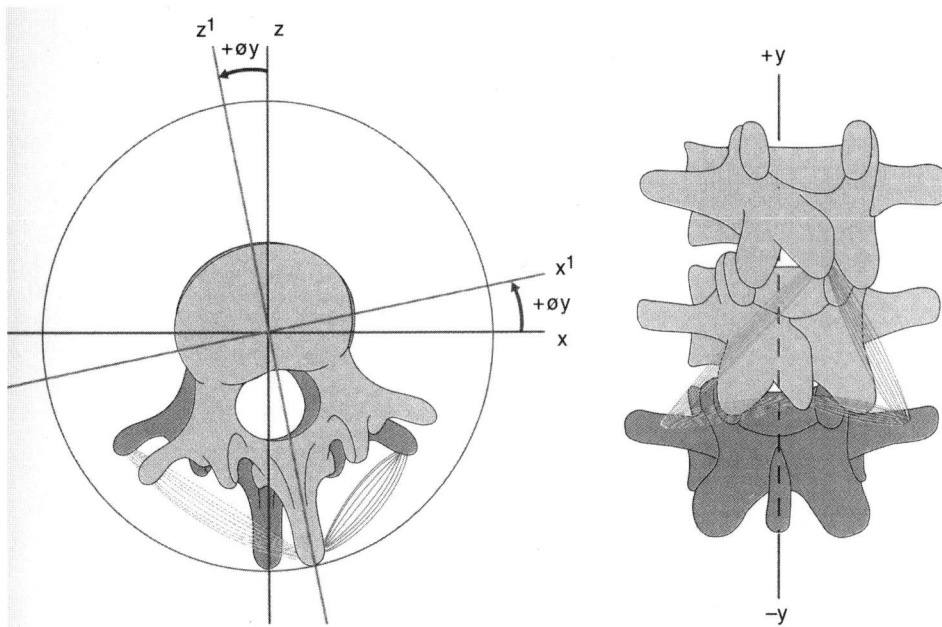

FIG. 14-3. Schematic drawing of the function of intersegmental rotatory muscles. (From Dvorak J, Dvorak V, Schneider W, et al. Musculoskeletal medicine (manual therapy), 3rd English ed. Stuttgart/New York: G. Thieme Verlag, 2004, with permission.)

right. These techniques then attempt to increase spinal motion by stretching the incriminated shortened muscles and restoring mobility (Tables 14-1, 14-2).

CLINICAL MODEL FOR USE OF MANUAL THERAPY

Rehabilitative efforts for low back pain, especially when chronic, often present both a diagnostic and therapeutic challenge. Many practitioners of manual therapy have found it useful to approach to this complex clinical presentation by addressing specific clinical parameters first. They then attempt to integrate the findings (or lack thereof) within the greater clinical context. Three major domains of decision making have been identified as important when considering manual therapy for patients with low back pain or sciatica. These domains of diagnosis, in turn, are often further subdivided into specific subcategories.

According to this diagnostic approach there are three separate but interrelated thought processes involved when formulating a diagnosis for a patient where manual therapy is being considered. The first domain, the "structural diagnosis," refers to specific organic pathology and relies on the ability to define an objective veri-fiable pathologic lesion (e.g., disc herniation), osteoporosis, spondylosis, spinal stenosis, spondylolisthesis, and others. The second domain refers to a "functional diagnosis" that is based on both manual and functional performance tests including such findings as muscle spasm or muscular contraction, gross range of motion, focal intersegmental restrictions in motion, spinal biomechanics, posture, and gait. The third level of information in the diagnostic process is the domain of the patient's "pain perception" including those that exacerbate or decrease the pain and the psychosocial issues that affect pain.

This model infers that the resolution or diminution of a patient's pain can only occur when there is improvement on all three domains. The practitioner of manual therapy, using this model, will often include specific and individually tailored rehabilitation exercises along with carefully chosen passive physical therapeutic modalities all the while being cognizant of the patient's psychosocial situation. The unique clinical setting of the manual medicine practitioner, where there is physical contact with the patient and often multiple office visits, allows for a closer doctor-patient interaction than is commonly noted in conventional medical practices.

TABLE 14-1. *Overview of some of the most commonly used manual therapy techniques*[a]

Manual therapies			
Manual medicine techniques			Therapeutic massage
Mobilization with impulse	Mobilization without impulse	Soft tissue techniques	Common massage techniques
Thrust techniques 1. Chiropractic adjustment 2. Osteopathic Thrust Terminology *Thrust* is also known as: 1. High-velocity/low impulse technique or 2. Manipulation (nonspecific, general term)	Counterstrain technique Craniosacral technique Functional technique Muscle energy technique Myofascial release technique Ligamentous release technique Myofascial trigger point technique Visual techniques	Articulatory technique Deep pressure technique Diaphragmatic release Lymphatic pump technique Mesenteric release Pectoral release Stretch techniques: Lateral, linear, diagonal, etc. Traction	Swedish-type massage Effleurage (stroking) Pétrissage (kneading) Friction (rubbing) Tapotement (percussion) Acupressure Bindegewebsmassage Deep tissue massage Lymphatic massage Reflexology Shiatsu Sports massage (variation of Swedish massage)
Combined techniques			
		Neuromuscular treatment I Neuromuscular treatment II Neuromuscular treatment III	Integrating/movement approaches 1. Alexander technique 2. Feldenkrais method 3. Rolfing 4. Many others
	Remarks: The nonthrusting techniques typically take into account articular and/or soft tissue motion restrictions.	Remarks: Soft tissue techniques are used for preparation or can be used independently.	Remarks: There are numerous types of massage approaches with even more variations

[a]As with any classification, this table should be used as a general guide rather than a definitive one, since there is a considerable amount of overlap among the various manual medicine techniques, as well as with some of the massage techniques.

TABLE 14-2. *Comparison of the terms "manipulation" and "mobilization" showing continental differences*

	Europe	USA	Comments
Manipulation	Refers usually to the *thrusting* techniques, which are also known as high-velocity/low-amplitude techniques or the "mobilization-with-impulse" techniques.	A rather general term, which may refer to any therapeutic procedure in which the hands are used to treat the patient, including thrust techniques. *Chiropractic adjustment* is a generic term with over 100 sub-techniques, including the high-velocity/low-amplitude (HVLA) thrust and the low-force techniques. *Osteopathic manipulative treatment (OMT)* encompasses the entire spectrum of manual therapies from thrust to nonthrust, including the soft tissue techniques.	When possible, and in order to avoid confusion, the newer terminology of "mobilization-with-impulse" (= thrust = high-velocity/low-amplitude [HVLA] technique) *or* "mobilization-without-impulse" (= nonthrust techniques) should be used.
Mobilization	Refers essentially to any type of induced tissue or joint movement which is then qualified by describing the presence or absence of impulse forces (thrust vs. nonthrust techniques, respectively).	Usually refers to the various nonthrusting and soft tissue techniques.	It is best to qualify the type of mobilization used.

From Dvorak J, Dvorak V, Schneider W. (eds). Manual medicine 1984. Heidelberg: Springer Verlag, 1984, and Dvorak J., et al. Manual medicine: diagnostics and therapy, 3rd English ed. Stuttgart: Thieme Publisher, 2004, with permission.

INDICATIONS AND CONTRAINDICATIONS FOR SPINAL MANIPULATION

The appropriate application of manual medicine procedures, as with any other treatment approach, requires not only theoretical knowledge and training about the indications and contraindications of a particular technique, but also a high level of technical skill and experience by the practitioner (1–3). Unfortunately the identification of the patient likely to respond to manual therapy is not yet clear. This lack of information has, as in the case of many medical procedures, led to reliance on consensus conferences to determine the indications for manual medicine.

In 1990, the RAND Corporation, which has produced appropriateness guidelines for several health care provider groups, convened two expert panels to help establish indications for spinal manipulation for back pain conditions (4). These indications, when appropriately applied, would include by far the majority of patients with low back problems (4). These panels stated that, in the absence of contraindications, a short trial of therapy using spinal manipulation for patients with lower back pain with or without sciatica was appropriate.

The absolute or relative contraindications to manual therapy identified by these panels included progressive neurologic deficits from any cause, the most common of which are disc herniation, space-occupying lesions, and progressive spinal stenosis. Other contraindications include segmental hypermobility due to pathologic and traumatic fractures, acute rheumatoid inflammatory joint disease, destructive bone lesions secondary to tumor or infection, and bleeding disorders due to metabolic, congenital, or medication causes. Some of these conditions may show some symptomatic relief because of manual therapy as long as the mobilizations and the therapeutic massage techniques are carefully chosen and cautiously applied.

Major complications from manual therapy applied to the lumbar spine appear to be extremely rare. There have been a few case reports of cauda equina syndrome following lumbar manipulation (5) but it is not yet evident whether the cases would have progressed in the natural course of the disc herniation or were directly affected by a manipulation. Thus far there are no good data indicating spinal manipulation can adversely affect lumbar discs. The risk of irreversible cauda equina syndrome was estimated by Shekelle et al. (6) to be as low as 1 in 100 million lumbar spine manipulations, but this estimate was based only on reported cases and presumably there are a number of additional cases where a temporal relationship exists.

One point that is evident from both clinical practice and the scientific literature is that manual therapy is not a panacea and not all patients with low back pain respond with reduction of symptoms. Explanations for this variation in patient responses include three possibilities (7): (a) an inadequate workup of the patient's symptoms leading to a wrong diagnosis; (b) the unnecessary or inappropriate application of manual therapy (the diagnosis may have been correct but treatment was "wrong"); and (c) the probability that, for many patients with low back pain, there may be no current adequate treatment.

EFFECTIVENESS OF MANUAL THERAPY IN THE TREATMENT OF BACK PAIN SYNDROMES

One of the difficulties in performing randomized clinical trials to determine the effectiveness of manual therapy is the ability to perform a double-blind study and the inability to establish a placebo treatment. This is not unique to the manual therapies, but is true of all active treatment approaches including the physical therapies and exercise. The comparison of manual medicine treatment approaches with other treatment interventions and the development of placebos based on touching the patient or performing massage, however, have allowed certain conclusions to be drawn regarding effectiveness of the manual therapies relative to no treatment and to many of the common approaches to patients with low back pain. Currently there are more than 45 randomized clinical trials, more than almost any other treatment approach to low back pain, that have attempted to evaluate the effectiveness of the manual and manipulative therapies. There are also over 50 reviews of the studies that have been published in peer-reviewed journals. It is only possible to list a few of these in a short chapter on the topic and to discuss some of the key findings and conclusions from these papers.

An example of the type of study that has been attempted to look at the effectiveness of manual therapy is a prospective randomized clinical study by Koes et al., published in 1992 (8), where 256 patients with chronic low back pain were referred for one of four categories of treatment (manipulation, physical therapy, placebo, or treatment by a general practitioner). The patients in the manipulation group and those in the active physical therapy group showed a more favorable outcome at the 3- and 6-week follow-up than those who had been assigned to either the placebo group or treatment by the general practitioner. However, by 12 weeks the differences had almost entirely disappeared. Yet, patients in the manual medicine group had received less treatment (5.4 treatment sessions versus 14.7 treatments) than those in the physical therapy group, and the authors thought that this might be regarded as a considerable advantage. The acceptance of the treatment was greater by the patients in the manual medicine group than in the other treatment groups. In a follow-up paper, the authors noted that improvement in the main complaint was larger with manipulative therapy (4.5 times) than with physiotherapy (3.8 times) after 12 months' follow-up (difference 0.9; 95% confidence interval 0.1 to 1.7). Manipulative therapy also resulted in larger improvements in physical functioning (difference 0.6; −0.1 to 1.3). The authors concluded that manual therapy and physiotherapy are better than general practitioner and placebo treatments, and that manipulative therapy is slightly better than physiotherapy after 12 months. These observations are similar to those presented in the retrospective study by Patijn (9).

Triano et al. (10) elected to use a sham manipulation as a control group in an attempt to create a placebo. These authors reported on a prospective clinical trial of 145 patients who had experienced chronic back pain who were randomized into three groups according to specific manipulation, sham manipulation, and a group who received instruction materials. Two-week follow-up revealed that the group that had received specific manipulation showed a significantly lower visual analog pain scale value and a greater willingness to participate in rehabilitation, that is there was a greater trust in actively participating in their program. The recent study by Aure et al. (11), on the other hand, looked at the issue as to whether manual therapy was, as effective as well-established treatment approaches such as exercise. They evaluated patients with chronic low back pain randomized to either exercise or manipulation with 1-year follow-up to compare the effect of manual therapy to exercise therapy in work-disabled patients. Although improvement was observed in both groups, the manual therapy group showed significantly greater improvement than the exercise therapy group in all outcome variables. Immediately after the 2-month treatment period, 67% in the manual therapy group and 27% in the exercise therapy group had returned to work.

Reviews of the literature on the manual therapies have included meta-analyses, reviews grading the methodologic quality of the clinical trials, and the use of evidence tables and best evidence synthesis such as that done through the Cochrane Collaboration. Koes et al. have published a series of reviews of the scientific literature over the past 12 years using a described method of ranking the quality of the clinical trials. This group performed one of the earliest meta-analyses of the manipulation literature in 1991. Unfortunately 36 of the randomized clinical studies that they reviewed were thought to have low methodologic quality scores. They noted that approximately half of the studies indicated a positive result for manual medicine approaches on patients suffering from various disorders although the most favorable results were often in the studies with low methodologic scores. Similar observations were made when evaluating studies that looked at the evidence in favor of other treatments such as physical therapy and training therapy (12), and the evidence for these common treatment approaches was often less than that for the manual therapies. In 1991, Shekelle et al. (4), in a very detailed and critical evaluation of the randomized clinical trials, came to a similar conclusion with a slightly different emphasis. These authors thought that spinal manipulation had been demonstrated to be of short-term benefit in certain patients, particularly those with uncomplicated acute lower back pain. They based this conclusion on a meta-analysis of a subset of seven clinical trials in which recovery at 3 weeks could be compared with that of other therapies. The pooled estimate showed a 17% higher likelihood of recovery in favor of spinal manipulation. Again, a substantial number of trials were excluded from the meta-analysis by these investigators because most of the published randomized clinical trials at the time had used outcomes measured on a quantitative scale, such as pain and disability, rather than dichotomous outcomes.

The most comprehensive systematic reviews involving an array of different treatments for low back pain have been performed by van Tulder et al. (13,14) on a regular basis over the past few years with regular re-analysis of the newer trials. These authors have assessed the methodologic quality of the trials and used specific evidence-based rules to determine the presence and strength of evidence of efficacy. They concluded that for acute low back pain there was evidence to suggest that spinal manipulation is better than placebo, physical therapy, exercise, and short-wave diathermy. For chronic lower back pain, they found strong evidence that spinal manipulation was better than placebo, and moderate evidence that it was better than the treatment offered by a general practitioner, massage, bed rest, and analgesics. Bronfort et al. (15) published a systematic review of the efficacy of spinal manipulation emphasizing the magnitude of treatment effects compared to other treatments in determining the strength of evidence. These authors elected to set aside the conclusions by the investigators of the individual randomized clinical trials and to focus on the data only. Their analysis reached a conclusion similar to that of van Tulder et al. in that there is evidence of short-term efficacy for spinal manipulation in patients with both acute and chronic lower back pain.

SUMMARY

Although manual therapy is one of the oldest and most widely practiced treatments for low back pain, there has been a rapid growth over the past 20 years in its acceptance and use on an international basis. This is primarily due to the publication of a large number of clinical trials, most of which suggest that this therapeutic approach is at least as efficacious as other established treatment approaches and is more efficacious than placebo and usual medical care.

There remain, however, numerous unanswered questions concerning manual therapy. The exact physiologic effects and mechanisms of manual therapy are not known. The relative effectiveness of the choice of manual therapy approach depends primarily on the training and experience of the clinician. Current experimental and clinical research is beginning to look at these issues and hopefully, within the near future, it will be possible to identify the patient who would most likely benefit from manual therapy and to explain the mechanism through which the treatment effect is achieved.

REFERENCES

1. Dvorak J, Dvorak V, Schneider W, et al. Musculoskeletal medicine (manual therapy), 3rd English ed. Stuttgart/New York: G. Thieme Verlag, 2004.
2. Lewit K. Nebenwirkungen und kontraindikationen der manuellen therapie im bereich der halswirbelsaeule. Manuelle Medizin, 1987;25 (2092):42–43.
3. Schneider W. Muskulaere dysbalance. Der informierte Arzt, Gazette Medicale, 1988;2(1077):66–70.
4. Shekelle PG, Adams AH, Chassin M. The appropriateness of spinal manipulation for low-back pain: indications and ratings by a multidisciplinary expert panel. Santa Monica, CA: RAND Corporation, 1991.
5. Haldeman S, Rubinstein SM. Cauda equina syndrome in patients undergoing manipulation of the lumbar spine. Spine 1992;17(12): 1469–1473.
6. Shekelle PG, Adams AH, Chassin MR, et al. Spinal manipulation for low-back pain. Ann Intern Med 1992;117(7):590–598.
7. Kraft GH. The physiatric approach to upper limb pain syndromes. In: Physical medicine and rehabilitation clinics of North America. Philadelphia: WB Saunders, 1996.
8. Koes BW, Bouter LM, van Mameren H, et al. The effectiveness of manual therapy, physiotherapy, and treatment by the general practitioner for nonspecific back and neck complaints: a randomized clinical trial. Spine 1992;17:1:28–35.
9. Patijn J, Durinck JR. Effects of manual medicine on absenteeism. J Manual Med 1991;6(2):49–53.
10. Triano JJ, McGregor M, Hondras MA, et al. Manipulative therapy versus education programs in chronic low back pain. Spine 1995;20:948–955.
11. Aure OF, Nilsen JH, Vasseljen O. Manual therapy and exercise therapy in patients with chronic low back pain: a randomized, controlled trial with 1-year follow-up. Spine 2003;28(6):525–531; discussion 531–532.
12. Koes BW, Assendelft WJ, Van der Heijden GJ, et al. Spinal manipulation and mobilisation for back and neck pain: a blinded review. Br Med J 1991;303:1298–1303.
13. van Tulder MW, Koes BW, Bouter LM. Conservative treatment of acute and chronic nonspecific low back pain. A systematic review of randomized controlled trials of the most common interventions. Spine 1997;22(18):2128–2156.
14. van Tulder MW, Koes BW, Metsemakers JF, et al. Chronic low back pain in primary care: a prospective study on the management and course. Fam Pract 1998;15(2):126–132.
15. Bronfort G, Haldeaman S. Spinal manipulation in patients with lumbar disc disease. Spine Surg 1999;11(2):97–103.

CHAPTER 15

Acupuncture and Reflexology

Marianne L. Magnusson and Malcolm H. Pope

COMPLEMENTARY AND ALTERNATIVE MEDICINE IN TREATMENT OF LOW BACK PAIN

Despite the increased use and acceptance of complementary and alternative medicine (CAM), there is relatively little information available concerning efficacy. A survey of 542 patients attending 16 family practice clinics was conducted to determine patients' reasons for using CAM and the impact of CAM on health and well-being (1). Approximately 21% of the patients used one or more forms of CAM, of which the most common were chiropractic (34.5%), herbal remedies (26.7%), and massage therapy (17.2%). In spite of poor evidence for efficacy, CAM is used for low back pain (LBP) more frequently than for any other indication. Expert opinions on the use of CAM for LBP could therefore be helpful until more randomized controlled trials (RCTs) are available. Ernst and Pitller (2) sent a questionnaire to 50 clinical experts on LBP to assess the perceived clinical effectiveness of CAM for four categories of LBP. The conclusions were that expert opinion is in favor of the effectiveness of acupuncture for acute uncomplicated LBP, whereas homeopathy was perceived ineffective for LBP.

REFLEXOLOGY

Furlan et al. (3) conducted a Cochrane Review on massage therapy. Four randomized controlled trials met the inclusion criteria. Two trials were of high and two were of low methodologic quality. None evaluated massage as the main intervention. Rather, it was the control intervention in studies evaluating manipulation, electric stimulation, and a lumbar corset. There was limited evidence showing that massage is less effective than manipulation immediately after the first session and moderate evidence showing it is less effective than transcutaneous electric nerve stimulation (TENS) during the course of sessions in relieving pain and improving activity. At the completion of treatment and at 3 weeks after discharge there was no difference among massage and manipulation, electric stimulation, or corsets, but this evidence is limited. The reviewers concluded that there is insufficient evidence to recommend massage as a stand-alone treatment for nonspecific LBP.

Reflexology has been in existence for many thousands of years and can be considered a type of massage. It was first practiced in India, China, and Egypt and then introduced to the West at the beginning of the 20th century as zone therapy (4). It was suggested that pressure on specific parts of the body could have an anesthetizing effect on a related area. The body is divided into 10 equal vertical zones, and pressure on one part of a zone is said to affect all structures within that zone. It was taught that "bioelectric energy" flowed through these zones to "reflex points" in the hands and feet. In the 1930s, the zone therapy was refined into what was termed "foot reflexology," which suggests that "congestion" or tension in any part of the foot mirrors "congestion" or tension in a corresponding part of the body (5).

Charts with organs superimposed on the foot, hand, or ear are used to map these points. The reflexologist looking for constrictions or painful areas probes the theoretical reflex points by using the charts to determine what body part corresponds to that area of the foot (or hand or ear, etc.). There are areas that are said to correspond with the lumbar spine. Several products (e.g., sandals, shoe inserts, foot massage devices) are sold based on this theory.

Jarvis (6) concluded, because of a carefully conducted trial, that reflexology could not reliably find conditions known to be present and thus was not predictive or therapeutic. Jarvis concludes that reflexology has little potential for direct harm, but can mislead people into believing that it can be used for screening or having real therapeutic value. No scientific trials were found that showed any value of reflexology for lumbar spine problems. Jarvis advises us to be skeptical of therapeutic claims beyond the ability of foot massage for relaxation.

ACUPUNCTURE

Acupuncture, a form of Eastern medicine that has been practiced for many centuries, is the stimulation of special "points" on the body, usually by the insertion of fine needles. Originally there were 365 such points, corresponding to the days of the year, but the number identified by proponents during the past 2,000 years has increased gradually to over 2,000 (7). Acupuncture uses the meridian systems of the body (Chinese system of energy flow in the body) to promote healing and treat injury and disease. Through the insertion of needles into well-defined acupuncture sites, the nervous system is stimulated to release chemicals in the muscles, spinal cord, and brain. These chemicals will either change the experience of pain, or they will trigger the release of other chemicals and hormones that influence the body's own internal regulating system. The improved energy and biochemical balance produced by acupuncture results in stimulating the body's natural healing abilities, and in promoting physical and emotional well-being. The use of heat and electric stimulation at the acupuncture sites is thought to augment the therapeutic effect of needling and is used particularly in treating chronic pain (8).

The following mechanisms have been proposed to explain acupuncture's presumed action on pain: The effects of acupuncture, particularly on pain, are partially explicable within a conventional physiologic model, which suggests that acupuncture stimulates A_δ fibers entering the dorsal horn of the spinal cord. This mediates segmental inhibition of pain impulses carried in the slower, unmyelinated C fibers and, through connections in the midbrain enhances descending inhibition of C fiber pain impulses at other levels of the spinal cord. This helps explain why acupuncture needles in one part of the body can affect pain sensation in another region. Acupuncture is also said to stimulate release of endorphins and other neurotransmitters such as serotonin. This is likely to be another mechanism for the effects of acupuncture, such as in acute pain (8). Another explanation is the "gate theory", which suggests that if pain fibers carry impulses from an acupuncture site, impulses from a painful body organ will be unable to reach the brain. Attention can be diverted from a symptom by stimulating or irritating another part of the body. Psychological mechanisms—including suggestion, operant conditioning, and other psychological mechanisms—may be involved in the placebo effect.

Theory and Practice

Acupuncture is based on ancient Chinese medical philosophy, which views illness quite differently than contemporary science (9). In ancient China, diseases were not systematically described or classified (10). Internal organs, which were felt to be intermediaries between the body and nature, were assigned qualities representing emotional states, colors, and seasons. Some organs, such as the "triple warmer," were imaginary. There were no concepts of modern physiology, biochemistry, nutrition, or mechanisms of healing. There was no knowledge of the existence of cells, the circulation of the blood, the function of nerves, or the existence of hormones. Knowledge of anatomy was incomplete.

Diagnosis

Traditional Chinese diagnosis does not correlate with modern scientific concepts. An ill person was considered out of balance with nature and its two opposing forces, yin and yang. Yin represented the feminine, passive, or accepting qualities and yang the masculine, aggressive, or forceful ones. Diseases were not described or named. Diagnoses were made from examining the pulse (of which there were supposedly six variations) and the tongue, which was said to vary in appearance with certain disease states.

Treatment

Although the details of practice differ between schools, all traditional acupuncture theory is based on the concept of yin and yang. Illness is seen as excess or deficiency in various exogenous and endogenous pathogenic factors, and treatment is aimed at restoring balance. This reestablishing of "balance" and "harmony" supposedly occurs as symptoms improve. Since there was no formal study of diseases or description of their natural history, the ancient Chinese could rarely determine how an illness actually improved. Treatments were chosen by trial and error, and perpetuated by personal experience. Since there were no scientific criteria for success or failure, the judgment that "healing" had taken place was based on the word of the therapist or the patient.

Acupuncture points were assigned to "meridians" on the surface of the body. These supposedly represent channels through which flows the life force, "Ch'i" (or "Qi"). Insertion of needles at the designated points was said to increase or decrease the flow of Ch'i to achieve a more normal and harmonious state (7).

The life force, Ch'i, has no basis in human physiology. The meridians are imaginary; their locations do not relate to internal organs, and therefore do not relate to human anatomy. Acupuncture points are also imaginary. (Various acupuncture charts give different locations for the points.) These concepts continue to form the basis of modern acupuncture therapy even though extremely sophisticated methods are used to measure its reputed biochemical effects. Although scientific methods may be applied to biochemical studies, many published reports are based solely and uncritically on clinical anecdotes and tradition (11). In conclusion, the existence of "meridians," "acupuncture points," or Ch'i has never been scientifically validated.

VARIATIONS AND OFFSHOOTS OF ACUPUNCTURE

Acupressure

Acupressure uses firm digital pressure on trigger or acupuncture points. Shiatsu, a modified form of acupressure, is a form of Japanese traditional medicine (12).

Auriculotherapy

Auriculotherapy is based on the notion that the body and organs are represented on the ear (13). Needles are placed in the imaginary points representing the diseased organs. There is no scientific evidence that these points exist or that auriculotherapy has any therapeutic value (14).

Staplepuncture

In staplepuncture, staples are placed at acupuncture points on the ear, typically to aid smoking cessation or drug withdrawal.

PROS AND CONS OF ACUPUNCTURE

The World Health Organization recognizes the use of acupuncture in the treatment of a wide range of medical problems including neurologic and muscular disorders:

1. Digestive disorders: gastritis and hyperacidity, spastic colon, constipation, diarrhea.
2. Respiratory disorders: sinusitis, sore throat, bronchitis, asthma, and recurrent chest infections.
3. Neurologic and muscular disorders: headaches, facial tics, neck pain, rib neuritis, frozen shoulder, tennis elbow, and various forms of tendonitis, LBP, sciatica, and osteoarthritis.
4. Urinary, menstrual, and reproductive problems.
5. Smoking cessation.

The National Council Against Health Fraud (NCAHF) believes:

1. Acupuncture is an unproved modality of treatment.
2. Its theory and practice are based on primitive and fanciful concepts of health and disease that bear no relationship to present scientific knowledge.
3. Research during the past 20 years has failed to demonstrate that acupuncture is effective against any disease.
4. Perceived effects of acupuncture are probably due to a combination of expectation, suggestion, counterirritation, operant conditioning, and other psychological mechanisms.
5. The use of acupuncture should be restricted to appropriate research settings.

6. Insurance companies should not be required by law to cover acupuncture treatment.
7. Licensure of lay acupuncturists should be phased out (15).

EVIDENCE OF ACUPUNCTURE EFFICACY

Symptom relief with acupuncture is difficult to assess because there is no objective standard of measurement. Double-blind studies comparing the insertion of needles at acupuncture points and at other points ("sham acupuncture") are difficult to design. If an experienced acupuncturist locates the points, the practitioner's expectations may be transmitted to the patient. If an inexperienced person inserts the points, misplaced needles may undermine the results. Moreover, practitioners may differ about the location of the points, so it may be difficult to find a patch of skin that has not been labeled an "acupuncture point." Chronic pain is often cyclic, with periods of relief. Since people often request help when their pain is most severe, spontaneous improvement may occur, independent of the treatment (16). The natural history of most acute pain is that it improves with time and no intervention. Thus, there may be reports of improvement of symptoms from any intervention. There is general agreement that 30% to 35% of subjects' pain improves from suggestion or placebo effect alone. Thus, measuring a small difference between placebo and acupuncture requires a large number of subjects to show as little difference as 25%. People who volunteer for acupuncture may have a conscious or unconscious bias toward the procedure and thus may be more prone to suggestion.

RESEARCH EVIDENCE

Richardson and Vincent analyzed 28 studies on the effect of acupuncture on pain. All were published between 1973 and 1986 in English language peer-reviewed journals. Fifteen showed no difference in effectiveness between acupuncture and control groups. Thirteen showed some effectiveness for acupuncture over control groups, but not all controls were the same. (Some were compared to sham acupuncture, some to medical therapy, etc.) Overall, the differences were small (17,18). The NCAHF Task Force on Acupuncture evaluated the above studies, as well as more recent ones, and found that reported benefits varied inversely with quality of the experimental design. The greater the benefit claimed the worse the experimental design. Most studies that showed positive effects used too few subjects to be statistically significant. The best designed experiments—those with the highest number of controls on variables—found no difference between acupuncture and control groups (15). In 1989 Dutch epidemiologists reported similar conclusions in 91 separate clinical trials of acupuncture for various disorders. They also found that the stricter the controls, the smaller the difference between acupuncture and control groups (19).

Research evidence also shows that acupuncture has greater effects than placebo. Randomized trials have found that true acupuncture is more effective in relieving pain than a "sham" technique, such as inserting needles away from true points (however, the aforementioned disagreement about the localization of points should be considered). Of the numerous studies on nausea, a condition that readily lends itself to placebo controlled trials, almost all show that stimulating true acupuncture points is more effective than stimulating false points. Studies showing that acupuncture can affect anesthetized animals provide further evidence that its effects probably cannot be explained purely in psychological terms (7).

It is less clear whether acupuncture has clinically important benefits in the conditions for which it is typically used. Much of the research evidence comes from hospital-based studies of acute conditions such as postoperative pain rather than studies of chronic conditions in primary care. Moreover, most trials have had small numbers of patients and only short-term follow-up. Overall, evidence from several randomized controlled trials supports the use of acupuncture in pain conditions, particularly migraine, headache, and postoperative pain. Such trials also provide evidence of an effect of acupuncture in substance misuse, nausea, and stroke. Trials of acupuncture in asthma and hay fever have produced conflicting results. Systematic reviews and randomized controlled trials suggest that acupuncture is probably not of benefit for stopping smoking, tinnitus, or obesity.

ACUPUNCTURE AND LBP

The use of acupuncture to treat LBP has increased dramatically in the past few decades. In spite of this, there is very sparse scientific documentation of outcomes from these treatments. In one study, 12 patients suffering chronic LBP were treated with both acupuncture and TENS. The order of treatments was balanced, and changes in the intensity and quality of pain were measured with the McGill Pain Questionnaire. Pain relief was produced in both groups and lasted between 23 hours for TENS and 40 hours for acupuncture. The difference between the treatments was not statistically significant. According to the authors, both methods could be equally effective, and probably have the same underlying mechanism of action (20). However, as there was no pure control treatment group the pain relief could be a Hawthorne effect or the two treatments were equally effective or ineffective.

Carlsson and Sjölund (21) randomly assigned 50 patients who had been suffering chronic LBP for a minimum of 6 months and had tried a variety of other therapies to a manual acupuncture group, an electroacupuncture group, or a placebo group. Treatment was delivered once per week for 8 weeks and follow-up treatments after 6 months or longer. The placebo group was given mock stimulation. An independent and blinded-to-treatment assessment (clinical interview, physical examination) at baseline and at follow-ups at 1, 3, and 6 months classified the patient's pain as improved, unchanged, or worse. Subjectively, patients reported pain intensity at the follow-ups. At the 1-month independent assessment, 16 of 34 patients in the acupuncture group and 2 of 16 in the placebo group improved ($p < .05$). There was also a significant decrease of pain intensity at 1 and 3 months in the acupuncture group. Sleep pattern was less disturbed and total intake of analgesics dropped dramatically after the treatment period in the acupuncture group, but not in the placebo patients. After 6 months, 14 acupuncture patients and two placebo patients were still improved ($p < .05$). There was no difference between types of acupuncture.

Kalauokalani et al. (22) analyzed 135 patients with chronic LBP who received acupuncture or massage in a randomized trial. Before randomization, study participants were asked to describe their expectations regarding the helpfulness of each treatment on a scale of 0 to 10. The primary outcome was level of function at 10 weeks as measured by the modified Roland Disability Scale. Improved function was observed for 86% of the participants with higher expectations for the treatment they received as compared with 68% of those with lower expectations ($p < .01$). Furthermore, patients who expected greater benefit from massage than from acupuncture were more likely to experience better outcomes with massage than with acupuncture, and vice versa ($p < .03$). The study suggests that patient expectations may influence clinical outcome independently of the treatment itself. In contrast, general optimism about treatment, divorced from a specific treatment, is not strongly associated with outcome.

Cherkin et al. (23) randomized 262 patients with persistent LBP to receive traditional Chinese medical acupuncture ($n < 94$), therapeutic massage ($n < 78$), or self-care educational materials ($n < 90$). Telephone interviewers masked to treatment group assessed symptoms and dysfunction. Follow-up was available for 95% of patients after 4, 10, and 52 weeks, and none withdrew for adverse effects. Treatment groups were compared after adjustment for pre-randomization covariates using an intent-to-treat analysis. At 10 weeks, massage was significantly superior to self-care on the symptom ($p < .01$) and the disability scale ($p < .001$). Massage was significantly superior to acupuncture on the disability scale ($p < .01$). After 1 year, massage was not better than self-care but was better than acupuncture on the symptom and dysfunction scales ($p < .002$ and $p < .05$, respectively). The massage group used the least medications and had the lowest costs of subsequent care ($p < .05$). Therapeutic massage was effective for persistent LBP, providing long-lasting benefits. Traditional Chinese medical acupuncture was relatively ineffective.

A systematic review to assess the effects of acupuncture as treatment of nonspecific LBP was conducted by van Tulder et al. (24). Eleven studies were included, of which only two were of high quality. In the review, van Tulder et al. disagree with the original authors' conclusions in 7 of the 11 studies. According to van Tulder et al., there was no difference between acupuncture and control in seven trials. Acupuncture was superior in only two studies, whereas the results were unclear in the remaining two trials. Thus, 9 of the 11 studies could not show that acupuncture was more effective than placebo or sham acupuncture, nor with trigger-point injection or TENS. The reviewers' conclusions were that this systematic review did not indicate that acupuncture is effective for the treatment of back pain.

A meta-analysis by Ernst et al. (25), of randomized controlled trials on acupuncture for back pain involving data from nine studies, showed improvement with acupuncture compared with control intervention with an odds ratio of 2.30 (95% confidence interval 1.28 to 4.13). It was concluded that collectively, the data implied that acupuncture is superior to various control interventions, although there was insufficient evidence to prove whether it is superior to placebo.

Although both studies, which virtually used the same RCTs, conclude that there is not enough evidence to prove acupuncture more effective than any other treatment, they present contradicting results. This is due to the different methods of assessing methodologic quality and of summarizing the results that were chosen. Because of the low quality, methodologic problems, and in some trials, the use of an invalid acupuncture treatment, van Tulder et al. used a qualitative analysis, which took into account the levels of evidence rather than a statistical pooling across trials. Ernst et al. used a meta-analysis and quantitatively pooled the results from the trials.

SAFETY OF ACUPUNCTURE

As with all CAM, the absence of a formal system for reporting adverse effects means that acupuncture's safety is difficult to assess. The definition of adverse effect varies and both under- and over-reporting occur. Most adverse effects are relatively minor events such as bruising and dizziness but more serious events have been reported such as hepatitis and pneumothorax (26,27). A prospective study of over 55,000 acupuncture treatments given in a college for medically trained acupuncturists confirms that acupuncture is probably safe in qualified hands (28). Only 63, mostly minor, adverse events were identified, and no cases of serious adverse events such as pneumothorax, infection, or spinal lesions were reported, although these have been described in the literature (27).

The adverse effects of acupuncture are probably related to the nature of the practitioner's training. A sur-

vey of 1,135 Norwegian physicians revealed 66 cases of infection, 25 cases of punctured lung, 31 cases of increased pain, and 80 other cases with complications (29). A parallel survey of 197 acupuncturists, who are more apt to see immediate complications, yielded 132 cases of fainting, 26 cases of increased pain, 8 cases of pneumothorax, and 45 other adverse results (29).

In summary, because the quality of the RCTs that evaluated acupuncture was generally poor, the effectiveness of acupuncture for treating acute or chronic back pain is unclear. However, acupuncture seems to be relatively safe (30).

REFERENCES

1. Palinkas LA, Kabongo ML. The use of complementary and alternative medicine by primary care patients. A SURF*NET study. J Fam Pract 2000;49(12):1121–1130.
2. Ernst E, Pittler MH. Experts' opinions on complementary/alternative therapies for low back pain. J Manipulative Physiol Ther 1999;22(2):87–90.
3. Furlan AD, Brosseau L, Welch V, et al. Massage for low back pain (Cochrane Review). In: The Cochrane Library, 1. Oxford: Update Software, 2002.
4. Raso J."Alternative" healthcare: a comprehensive guide. Buffalo, NY: Prometheus Books, 1994:126.
5. Ingham ED. The development of foot reflexology in the U.S., part I. Massage Therapy J 1989;28:127.
6. Jarvis WT. NCAHF Position Paper on Reflexology. Loma Linda, CA: The National Council Against Health Fraud, 1996.
7. Skrabanek P. Acupuncture: past, present, and future. In: Stalker D, Glymore C, eds. Examining holistic medicine. Buffalo, NY: Prometheus Books, 1985.
8. Vickers A, Zollman C. Clinical review ABC of complementary medicine: acupuncture. BMJ 1999;319:973–976.
9. Motokawa T. Sushi science and hamburger medicine. Perspect Biol Med 1989;32:489–504.
10. Kaptchuk TJ. The web that has no weaver, understanding Chinese medicine. New York: Congden & Weed, 1983.
11. Patel MS. Problems in the evaluation of alternative medicine. Soc Sci Med 1987;25:669–678.
12. Brady LH, Henry K, Luth JF 2nd, et al. The effects of shiatsu on lower back pain. J Holist Nurs 2001;19(1):57–70.
13. Oleson TD, Kroenig RI, Breisier DE. An experimental evaluation of auricular diagnosis: the somatic mapping of musculoskeletal pain at ear acupuncture points. Pain 1980;8:217–229.
14. Melzack R, Katz K. Auriculotherapy fails to relief chronic pain: a controlled crossover study. JAMA 1974;228:1544–1551.
15. NCAHF Position Paper on Acupuncture. Washington, DC: National Council Against Health Fraud, 1990.
16. Malone RD, Strube MJ. Meta-analysis of non-medical treatments for chronic pain. Pain 1988;34:231–244.
17. Richardson PH, Vincent CA. The evaluation of therapeutic acupuncture: concepts and methods. Pain 1986;24:1–13.
18. Richardson PH, Vincent CA. Acupuncture for treatment of pain. Pain 1986;24:1540.
19. Ter Riet G, et al. The effectiveness of acupuncture. Huisarts Wet 1989;32:170–181, 308–312.
20. Fox EJ, Melzock R. Transcutaneous electrical stimulation and acupuncture comparison treatment for low back pain. Pain 1976;2(2):141–148.
21. Carlsson C, Sjölund B. Acupuncture for chronic low back pain: a randomized placebo-controlled study with long-term follow-up. Clin J Pain 2001;17(4): 296–305.
22. Kalauokalani D, Cherkin DC, Sherman KJ, et al. Lessons from a trial of acupuncture and massage for low back pain: patient expectations and treatment effects. Spine 2001;26(13):1418–1424.
23. Cherkin DC, Eisenberg D, Sherman KJ, et al. Randomized trial comparing traditional Chinese medical acupuncture, therapeutic massage,

and self-care education for chronic low back pain. Arch Intern Med 2001;161(8):1081–1088.

24. van Tulder MW, Cherkin DC, Berman B, et al. Acupuncture for low back pain (Cochrane Review). Spine 1999;24(11):1113–1123.

25. Ernst E, White AR, Wider B. Acupuncture for back pain: meta-analysis of randomised controlled trials and an update with data from the most recent studies. Schmerz 2002;16(2):129–139.

26. Yamashita H, et al. Adverse events related to acupuncture. JAMA 280: 1563–1564, 1998.

27. Cantan R, Milesi-Defrance N, Hardenberg K, et al. Bilateral pneumothorax and tamponade after acupuncture [in French]. Departement d'anesthesie-reanimation, Hopital General, Dijon. Presse Med 2003;32 (7):311–312.

28. Shin HR, Kim JY, Kim JI, et al. Hepatitis B and C virus prevalence in a rural area of South Korea: the role of acupuncture. Br J Cancer 2002; 87:314–318.

29. Norheim JA, Fennebe V. Adverse effects of acupuncture. Lancet 1995; 345:1576.

30. Cherkin DC, Sherman KJ, Deyo RA, et al. A review of the evidence for the effectiveness, safety, and cost of acupuncture, massage therapy, and spinal manipulation for back pain. Ann Intern Med 2003;138(11): 898–906.

SECTION III

The Injured Worker

CHAPTER 16

Returning Workers to Gainful Employment

Margareta Nordin

Returning workers to gainful employment after work absence due to low back pain has become a public health policy problem. Being unemployed or disabled from work due to low back pain of benign nature is a societal problem in industrialized and industrializing parts of the world. Compounding this problem is the fact that the reputation of low back pain and its potential incapacitating symptoms has worsened. In industrialized countries, the public still believes that low back pain is crippling, leading to serious disability and the loss of gainful employment and a satisfying lifestyle. Without great fanfare, back pain became the leading 20th century medical disaster (1), with an estimated cost of 1% to 2% of gross national product (GNP) in Organisation for Economic Co-operation and Development (OECD) countries (2) and a cost of about $50 billion in the United States (or 0.5% to 0.6% of GNP based on data from 2001) (3). Cats-Baril and Frymoyer (4) estimated that costs for back pain in the United States were equivalent to 0.5% to 2.0% of GNP in 1991. In these and other industrialized countries, the cost structure for low back ailments is the same, with approximately 10% to 30% of being spent for direct costs and 70% to 90% on indirect costs.

It is technically difficult to estimate work loss due to back pain, however work loss due to back pain has been reported in several studies. For example, Guo et al. (5) reported in 1988 that 17.6% of the respondents (n < 30,074) to the National Health Interview Survey lost an estimated 149 million workdays in the United States. The Office of National Statistics in the United Kingdom reports from 1993 to 1998 approximately 5% of employed individuals said they had taken time off from work for back pain over a 4-week period being questioned (6).

In Sweden about 2% to 6% of the working population experiences work loss from back pain (7). The differences in reported work loss may be due to different reporting systems, national versus non-national health systems, and various compensation systems, among others. There are indications that sickness absence is increasing (8) and early retirement resulting from back pain is decreasing (7), however there are also indications that an increasing proportion of people receive benefits for much longer time and that the amount of benefits paid are increasing (7). This would make a strong argument to intensify the prevention of disability and encourage work ability for individuals experiencing low back pain.

COMMONALITY OF BACK PAIN EPISODES

Prevalence of low back pain is high. International studies reveal a point prevalence (about 1 week) of 15% to 30%, a 1-month prevalence of 10% to 43%, and a lifetime prevalence of low back pain of 51% to 81% (1,7). It is important to note that study design and cultural differences in self-reporting, more so than actual differences of the populations studied, may cause the variation of these estimates (7,8). Therefore, one can reasonably state that it is more common during life to have experienced back pain than not to have experienced back pain. In fact, when conducting a study, it is actually quite difficult to find individuals who have never experienced or been out of work for back pain (9,10).

BACK PAIN CLASSIFICATION

Pain in the lumbar spine can be classified as specific or nonspecific pain. These terms are convenience terms created to establish some sort of triage mechanism. Specific low back pain means that the pain originates from a known structure, abnormality, tumor, trauma, or systemic or established disease. All other conditions are classified and diagnosed as nonspecific low back pain (NSLBP), a diagnosis that stems from the fact that science has not yet revealed which structure in the spine generates the pain.

This classification system has been very helpful for researchers and clinicians.

One point of encouragement is that large working population cohorts using the classification of NSLBP have a good prognosis for 90% of affected individuals to return to work. Studies show that 75% of compensable back pain resolved within 4 weeks, 90% within 3 months, and 95% within 6 months (1,11,12). The probability of an NSLBP diagnosis developing into "chronic back pain syndrome" (often defined as disabling pain of more than 3 to 6 months) is approximately 5% to 6%, compared to patients presenting with a specific diagnosis of low back pain for whom about 35% to 40% will develop a chronic and disabling condition (13–15).

Although chronicity as defined by continuous pain or permanent work disability affects about 3% to 5% of patients seeking care for low back pain, recurrence of low back pain is more frequent. For example: in Canada the frequency of recurrent episodes after compensable back injury was 36% over 3 years (11). In a survey of approximately 3,800 Belgian adults, 85% of those reporting back pain at the time of interview had experienced prior episodes (16). Some authors claim that low back pain should be regarded as a persistent problem with intermittent exacerbation (Fig. 16-1) (1,17,18) that may seriously affect work ability (19).

This chapter will focus on the prevention of work-related disability in the working population with NSLBP. It will discuss the return of workers to gainful employment and the subsequent retention of that gainful employment.

MISUNDERSTANDINGS AND A PHILOSOPHICAL SHIFT REGARDING BACK PAIN

The Paris Task Force (20) best describes the philosophical and evidence-based shift from passive to active treatment. The treatment of low back pain has not advanced beyond the outdated prescription for bed rest, because the role of activity in its treatment has been the object of three misunderstandings:

1. The first misunderstanding is related to the fact that certain activities (mainly occupational) are undeniably risk factors for low back pain and there is a natural tendency to avoid activity once an episode of back pain has begun. Although reexposure to the conditions that triggered the episode often causes pain, which may sometimes be intolerable (reinforcing the idea that it is better to avoid the conditions altogether), conditions that cause back pain are not necessarily risk factors for chronicity.

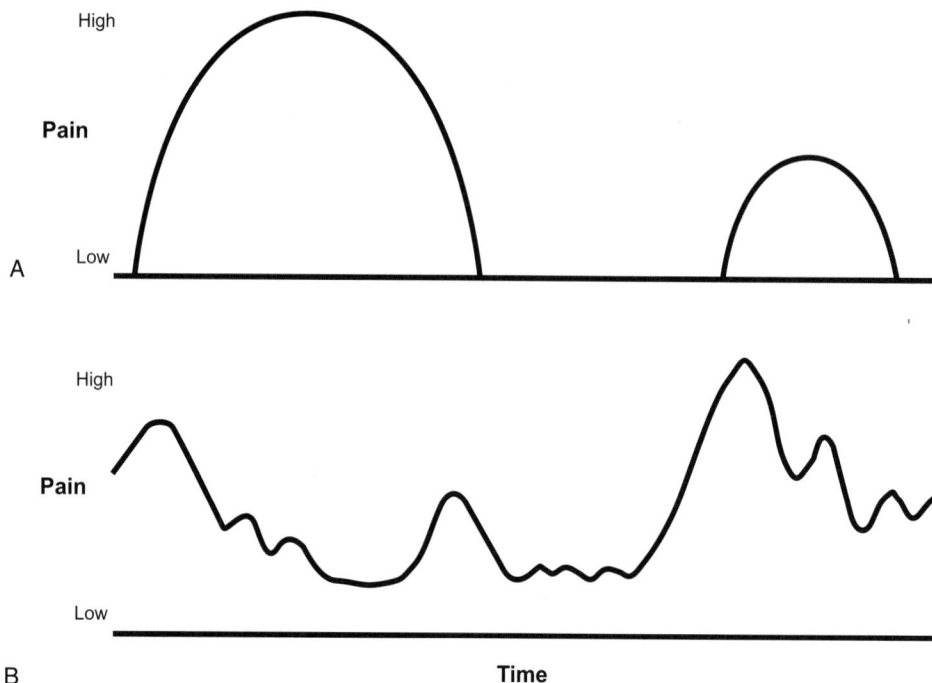

FIG. 16-1. Examples of concepts in studies including duration and pain in the lumbar spine. A: More traditional concepts where the bouts of pain are represented with a pain-free period in between. B: More current and debated concept in subgroups of patients where the pain over time may vary and not subside completely. (Adapted from Croft P, Papageorgiou A, McNally R. Low back pain. In: Stevens A, Raftery J, eds. Health care needs assessment. Second series: The epidemiologically based needs assessment reviews. Oxford: Radcliffe Medical Press, 1996:129–182.)

2. The second misunderstanding stems from the association many people make between "sciatica" (i.e., low back pain accompanied by spinal symptoms and signs) and low back pain unaccompanied by neurologic sequelae. However, low back pain accompanied by spinal damage only accounts for a very low percentage (approximately 5%) of all cases of low back pain, and there is no longer any consensus on the existence of a continuum linking the two types of conditions.

3. The third misunderstanding arises from current approaches to pain management. While it is common to neglect, if not disparage, specific and effective pain relief, it is nevertheless considered important to avoid anything that might trigger pain. In the absence of specific pain relief, rest becomes the only possible choice, with unfortunate results.

APPROACH TO TREATMENT FOR NSLBP

Despite the time and effort spent preventing and treating NSLBP, the costs associated with NSLBP continue to rise (1,2,8). This may, in part, be attributed to the current management of NSLBP in which the patient is either over- or under-treated. It is often assumed that pain is due to either a specific underlying cause or that it is of a nonmedical origin. Both conclusions do a disservice to the patient with NSLBP.

In the first scenario, attempting to provide a specific diagnosis to a patient with NSLBP can have deleterious consequences. For example, Abenhaim et al. (11) observed that patients given a specific spine diagnosis faired worse than patients given a diagnosis of NSLBP. The authors further discussed the possibility that medically "labeling" a condition of NSLBP with specific diagnoses may convince the patient that the pain is of a purely physical origin, suggesting that pain requires medical interventions such as medication, injections, manipulations, and even surgery. In order to relieve pain, the patient may then engage, to no avail, in negative health behaviors such as "doctor shopping," avoidance of movement and activities, and an over-reliance on medication or other passive treatments.

In the second scenario, attributing pain to nonmedical factors such as psychological conditions alone invalidates the true nature of pain, causing serious psychological distress to the patient. Furthermore, this attribution of NSLBP to nonphysical conditions may backfire as the patient seeks validation of the physical pain by over-focusing on the pain in an effort to convince others that it is "real." The health care provider may also grow frustrated and give up on the patient prematurely.

In the best scenario, however, the successful treatment of NSLBP requires a unique approach where the true nature and prognosis of NSLBP are shared with the patient. This is best accomplished proactively through an evaluation and treatment program derived from the application of the biopsychosocial model (1,8,21).

A Proactive Approach to NSLBP

A proactive approach to NSLBP includes the following:

1. The health care provider forms a partnership with the patient. Together they follow evidence-based medical practices and timelines for evaluation and treatment.
2. The health care provider must also be able to identify risk factors for chronicity as they emerge and make timely referrals when appropriate (19,22).
3. The patient is monitored on a regular basis so that changes in treatment needs may be assessed and implemented in a timely manner. For example, NSLBP may sometimes become specific as when true sciatica or a discitis develop. This can only be detected if the patient is monitored properly.

A proactive approach to NSLPB works best in the context of a biopsychosocial paradigm (8). A biopsychosocial perspective takes into consideration psychological and social factors related to pain, as well as physical factors and has been proven successful for the treatment of NSLBP. By definition, NSLBP has no identifiable known medical cause and therefore traditional medical approaches often fail. In the context of failed medical treatment approaches, as time goes on, psychological and social factors become increasingly important in determining pain and its subsequent disability. These factors must be acknowledged for successful outcomes in treating NSLBP (19,22–25).

WORKER'S CHOICE: TO SEEK OR NOT TO SEEK TREATMENT

Pain developing in the lumbar spine may be or may not be attributed to work functions; however, the pain may still affect the work capacity and be aggravated during working hours. An individual may or may not seek help for the condition (26). The difference in action taken transpires in the predicament of the worker/employee and the system in which that individual works. Hadler described the process of predicament (27). The individual considers the pain, the restriction in function, and the options for action. There may or may not be an event that ignited the pain. All these factors influence the idiosyncratic decision to seek help based on prior experience, education, environment, and possible fear for the seriousness of the condition. Three obvious choices are relevant at this point:

1. Endure the pain and continue to work, which is not uncommon. However, few studies have focused on the individual who continues to work with low back pain.

2. Seek professional medical advice and be considered a person with an illness (i.e., a patient under medical or other care). Most studies of low back pain have focused on this group of individuals.
3. Report an occupational injury or illness and file a claim. The individual who reports a claim becomes a claimant with an injury or illness. Fewer studies have focused on treatment of work-related low back pain and claimants.

The choice an individual makes may affect the outcome of the condition. Because the environment in which the condition is treated or left untreated varies, the health care and reimbursement provided may be different. As well, the external perception of the individual with low back pain differs. For example, a person who chooses to continue to work with moderate NSLBP will probably do fine except in very physically demanding jobs such a construction, firefighting or rescue work, nursing, or jobs with exposure to whole body vibration (i.e., driving a truck) (28). An individual who seeks medical care for acute or subacute NSLBP should be advised by their health care provider to keep active and to return to work as soon as possible based on the international scientific guidelines for low back pain (19,23,29,30). The outcome for these patients, which is measured as return to work and well-being, will be far more successful than those undergoing a long-term bed rest or passive modality treatment. Finally, a claimant experiencing NSLBP who is told by the employer's physician to return to work as soon as possible will usually start to negotiate about the date to return to work. The outcome is usually very favorable if the health care provider takes the time to explain the condition and establishes trust with the claimant, and recommends continued activity, short course of active treatment, and light work duty during the next 1 to 4 weeks. The recommendation to return to the regular work is usually negotiated based on type of work, exposures to hazardous or unsafe working conditions, and tasks to be performed.

Health care providers must acknowledge and understand the options and predicaments of choice for the individual with back pain. None of the choices are wrong or right, however, they are personal and choices that are not always well understood in the scientific and medical environment. The health care provider who chooses to manage the working/employed patient should reinforce the distinction between impairment and disability, hurt and harm (1,23), and should recognize that work disability is a multidimensional problem of which clinicians and researchers have only just begun to unravel the complexity (8).

RULING OUT RED FLAGS

The evaluation of low back pain should involve ruling out specific signs, referred to as "red flags" (23) and identifying risk factors for chronicity, referred to as "yellow flags" (22). A diagnostic triage has been suggested by the Clinical Guidelines for the Management of Acute Low Back Pain from the Royal College of General Practitioners (19). Diagnostic imaging tests are not routinely indicated (31).

Red flags are signs and symptoms detected by the clinician that may indicate possible serious spinal pathology and require referral to a specialist (23). A standardized physical examination is necessary to exclude possible specific conditions. The examination must consist of a patient history that includes trauma, systemic diseases, cancer, infection, or major neurologic compromise (red flags). The patient history is followed by a physical evaluation that includes posture, gait, toe and heel walk, palpation, range of motion, the effect of trunk sagittal flexion/extension and lateral flexion on low back pain and leg pain, and a neurologic examination of the lower extremities to test motor, sensory, and reflexes (32,33). The presence of red flags or neurologic signs and symptoms (such as back pain with radiation to a leg below the knee level or sensory-motor dysfunction) will classify low back pain as specific and may require a referral to a specialist for treatment (19,23). All other patients can be classified as having NSLBP.

PHYSICAL AND PSYCHOSOCIAL RISK FACTORS ASSOCIATED WITH DELAYED RECOVERY

A number of physical, personal, psychosocial, and environmental factors have been associated with the outcome of NSLBP. Physical signs that have been found to be predictors of delayed return to work in patients with acute (up to 4 weeks of duration of pain) NSLBP are altered gait and pain below the knee in a nondermatomic topography (32,34–37). Since these signs are present in both specific LBP and NSLBP, their meaning for NSLBP is still unclear. It is possible that they may reflect aspects of fear of pain and behaviors intended to communicate suffering to the health care provider rather than actual physical abnormality (38). Personal factors, such as age, affect recovery and therefore work ability (39–41). For example, it takes a person about twice as long to return to work at age 50 compared to age 30. Clinical factors such as the duration of back pain have also been associated with poor prognosis in that the likelihood of recovery diminishes steadily after as early as 4 weeks (39).

Most significantly, studies have revealed a number of psychological risk factors. For example, strong associations between delayed recovery in acute NSLBP and psychological distress have been found (38,42–44); depressive mood and somatization are consistently observed in the transition from acute to chronic low back pain (21); and high self-perceived disability and short-term changes in perceived disability have been associated with return to work outcomes such that higher perceptions of disability are related to poorer outcome (19,38,39,41,42,44,45). Other factors have been associated with poor outcome, including the belief that back pain is harmful or potentially severely disabling; fear avoidance beliefs (the belief that certain movements or activities will exacerbate pain); perceived inability to return to work; and the belief that passive treatment is preferable to active participation in care (19,22).

These psychosocial factors can be summarized as negative beliefs about low back pain and its consequences and negative emotional states. They may be considered "yellow flags" (22) or "early predictors" (38,36) because, while they do not indicate the same urgency of treatment as red flags, there is enough evidence to recommend that they receive attention when present. Guidelines from New Zealand stress the importance of assessing psychological and psychosocial risk factors as early as 2 weeks after the onset of NSLBP (22).

In an occupational health setting, psychosocial factors such as work-related perceptions constitute additional risk factors (46). Job dissatisfaction, monotony, poor social support, high perceived stress, and high perceived job demands have all shown a strong association with NSLBP (47). Therefore, it is reasonable to evaluate these perceptions in patients with NSLBP and discuss with the patient how these factors may influence the perceived back pain.

Physical characteristics of the job (such as excessive overtime or heavy workload) may also contribute to stress (28,43,48–50). Physical characteristics may be assessed subjectively and objectively. It is less understood what impact reducing perceived or actual physical stressors at work may have on psychological distress, NSLBP, and disability.

THE IMPACT OF COMORBIDITY ON DISABILITY IN NSLBP

There is recent information in the literature about the relationship between comorbidity and work disability from back pain. In a prospective, randomized case-controlled study Seferlis et al. (41) compared somatic and personality characteristics of acute LBP patients with healthy matched controls and found a fourfold increase in sick leave episodes in LBP patients for reasons other than spine morbidity. Fanuele et al. (51), in their prospective observational study on spine center patients, demonstrated that comorbidity affects the physical function, showing that the more comorbidities a patient has, the lower the physical functional status.

Nordin et al. (12) examined the relationship between comorbidity and the initial return to work following first episodes of work-disabling NSLBP. An inception cohort of workers with new episodes of NSLBP was identified from administratively maintained occupational health

records. A comparison of 6-month return to work rates between workers with one or more comorbid conditions to those without documented comorbidity was conducted. Workers with comorbidity were 1.3 times more likely to remain work-disabled than those with uncomplicated NSLBP, after adjusting for age, gender, lifting demands, and type of work (adjusted hazard ratio 1.31, 95% confidence interval 1.12 to 1.52). Concurrent injury (i.e., sprains or strains of the neck, upper and lower extremity, and contusions and lacerations) had the strongest association with delayed return to work (adjusted hazard ratio 1.49, 95% confidence interval 1.21 to 1.83). The authors concluded that occupational health professionals should routinely evaluate comorbidities at the first, as well as subsequent visits to better manage disability associated with NSLBP.

ESTABLISHING AN EVIDENCE-BASED TREATMENT PLAN

Researchers and clinicians have used an additional categorization of NSLBP based on the onset and duration of pain in the lumbar spine to develop evidence-based guidelines of treatment (20). Clinical and accepted categorizations for duration of NSLBP are:

1. *Acute:* Pain with a duration ≤ 4 weeks.
2. *Subacute:* Pain with a duration ≥ 4 weeks but ≤ 12 weeks.
3. *Chronic:* Unremitting pain with a duration ≥ 12 weeks

For many individuals, however, NSLBP is not a one-time event but tends to recur (18,52). Therefore, an additional classification, *recurrent NSLBP,* signifies intermittent pain with a pain-free period in between in which the individual could resume work (7,20). Recurrent NSLBP may be acute or subacute, but since chronic pain signifies unremitting pain of more than 12 weeks, by definition, it cannot be chronic (53).

Considering the socioeconomic impact of NSLBP there is an obvious need for effective interventions, especially in occupational health care. The ultimate goal of such interventions for workers is return to work, either to a preinjury or modified work capacity. Given the favorable natural course in the acute phase of NSLBP of return to work, the challenge becomes returning an employee to work who is in the subacute or chronic phase.

A variety of treatment interventions are typically used for individuals presenting with NSLBP (54,55). Several authors have published systematic reviews of the efficacy of these interventions (19,20,53,56–58). Studies show that for subacute NSLBP exercise therapy, behavioral therapy, and intensive multidisciplinary rehabilitation with functional restoration all reduce pain and improve function in workers (20,32,59,60). Graded activity leads to earlier return to work and reduced long-term sick leave in workers with subacute low back pain. Lindström et al. (60) described the goal of the graded activity approach as being return of an individual to the previous nonmodified workplace. Positive reinforcement to return to work is an important aspect of graded activity as well as continuous encouragement to resume work. Multidisciplinary treatment consisting of a combination of exercises, education, and a behavioral approach seems the most effective intervention in the subacute phase of NSLBP. Lindström et al. (60) conducted a randomized control trial aimed at restoring occupational function in workers in an automobile plant. The multidisciplinary intervention team included a physician, a physical therapist, and a social worker. All workers (n < 103) participating in the study had been out of work for more than 8 weeks for NSLBP. Half of the participants were randomized to an intervention including an operant-behavioral conditioning program and the other half received what is considered "usual care." The intervention program consisted of four parts: measurements of functional physical capacity, a workplace visit, "back-to-school" education, and an individual, submaximal, gradually increased exercise program. The individually tailored exercise program was based on an operant-conditioning behavioral approach and the result of the

tests and the demands of the patient's work. No ergonomic or other changes in the work situation were needed in the study. The results were significant and positive.

The rate of return to work was significantly faster in the intervention group than in the control group ($\kappa 2 < 4.7$, $p < .03$) (Fig. 16-2). The intervention group had 7 weeks' less sick leave in the follow-up period of 1 year than the control group receiving "usual care." Four patients in the control group went on permanent disability versus one patient in the intervention group. The study did not have an independent evaluator, causing a methodologic weakness, however it was the first randomized control trial in the industry that emphasized the importance of activity and exercise, a behavioral approach, and an individual tailored program to resume work demands. It was also a program that demonstrated the importance of full support from the employer.

One approach to augment return to work for chronic NSLBP patients is functional restoration (61–63), the goal being to restore a patient's function. This approach leads to the decrease of and control of pain through the combination of exercise with functional work simulation and behavioral support. The exercise program uses a

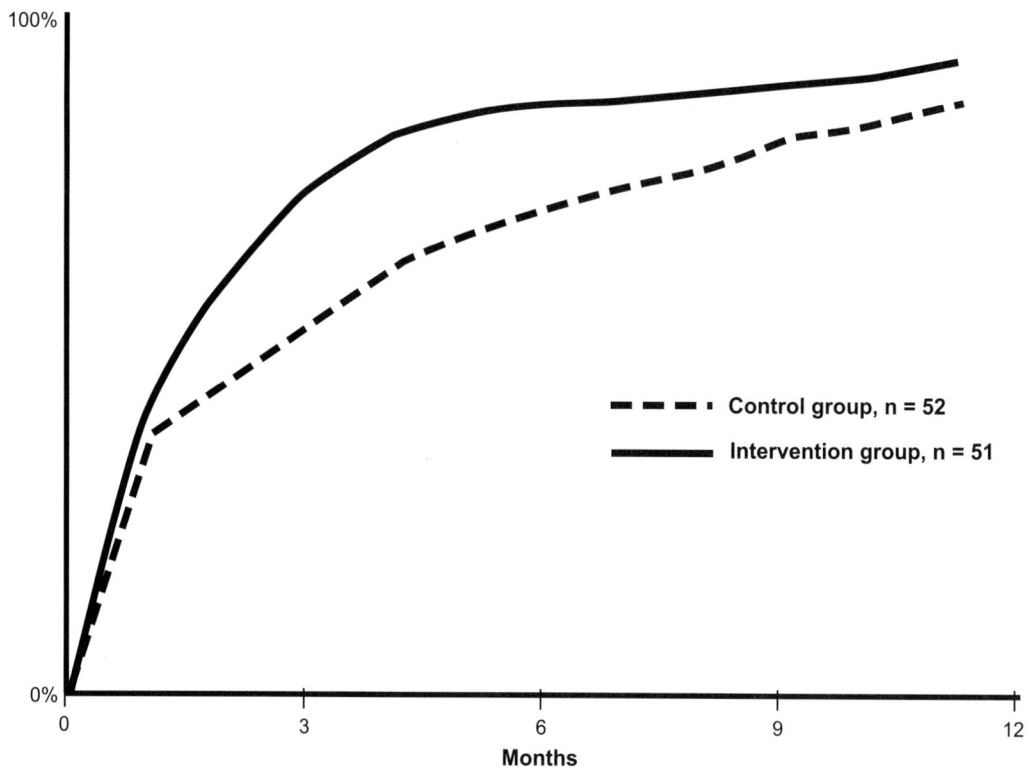

FIG. 16-2. Proportion returning to regular work. Randomized control trial from Sweden showing results from active intervention including exercise, behavioral approach and workplace visit versus usual care. (Adapted from Lindström I, Öhlund C, Eek C, et al. The effect of graded activity on patients with subacute low back pain: a randomized prospective clinical study with an operant-conditioning behavioral approach. Phys Ther 1992;72:279–290.)

sports exercise approach, and emphasizes mobility, strengthening, endurance, and flexibility. The functional simulation program is conducted in a specially developed occupational gymnasium and includes tasks that are commonly required in the workplace. The behavioral support consists of cognitive-behavioral treatment, relaxation, education, biofeedback, and individual and group counseling. The workers are treated in groups of up to 10 to 12 individuals (61,64).

In summary, multifactorial and multidisciplinary treatment consisting of a combination of exercises, education, and a behavioral approach seems the most effective intervention. This is especially true of graded activity (32,60) for workers with subacute low back pain and functional restoration (64) for workers with chronic low back pain. Both of these approaches offer the most promising results.

Multidisciplinary treatment is still somewhat of a gray area. It is unclear what the most effective contribution is of each of the program components. Studies are lacking and are needed to clarify the efficacy, cost utility, and cost-effectiveness of such programs. Nevertheless, literature reviews by Scheer et al. (63) and Rivier et al. (65) and one systematic review by van Tulder et al. (53) indicate favorable results for the outcome of multidisciplinary active intervention programs related to occupational subacute and chronic NSLBP, clinical improvement and well-being. The results are less explicit on return to work, work retention, and cost.

In moving forward, health care providers must simultaneously rely on and challenge evidence-based practices. Scientific evidence from clinical trials, systematic reviews, and meta-analyses on the effectiveness of interventions form a sound basis for clinical guidelines. Guidelines are efficient means to close the gap between research and practice. Good clinical guidelines, however, also consider other aspects such as side effects, costs, availability, and preferences of injured workers and clinicians (66). At present, several guidelines have been published addressing the specific issues of management of low back pain in an occupational health care setting. This includes: (a) Quebec Task Force, Canada (30); (b) Victoria Workcover Authority, Australia (67); (c) American College of Occupational and Environmental Medicine (68); (d) Dutch Association of Occupational Medicine, The Netherlands (69); (e) Accident Compensation Corporation and National Health Committee, New Zealand, 1997(22); and (f) Faculty of Occupational Medicine, United Kingdom (70). The guidelines show general agreement on numerous issues fundamental to occupational management of low back pain. The assessment recommendations consist of diagnostic triage, screening for "red flags" and neurologic problems, and the identification of potential psychosocial and workplace barriers for recovery. The recommendations for treatment of workers with low back pain include:

1. Reassuring the worker and providing adequate information about the self-limiting nature and good prognosis of low back pain.
2. Advising the worker to continue ordinary activities and working, or to return to normal activity and work as soon as possible, even if there is still some pain.
3. Most workers with low back pain manage to return to more or less normal duties quite rapidly. Consider temporary adaptations of work duties (hours/tasks) only when necessary.
4. When a worker fails to return to work within 2 to 12 weeks (there is considerable variation in the time scale in different guidelines), refer the worker/employee to a gradually increasing exercise program or multidisciplinary rehabilitation program (exercises, education about condition and prognosis, reassurance, and pain management following behavioral principles). These rehabilitation programs should be embedded in an occupational setting or occupational-related care setting.

The guidelines also recommend, on advice from health care provider, that low back pain is a self-limiting condition and, importantly, that remaining at work or an early (gradual) return to work, if necessary with modified duties, should be encouraged and supported.

RETURN TO WORK AS A THERAPEUTIC MODALITY

The therapeutic value of return to work is a novel concept and some studies have looked at efficacy of restricted duty (71) and workplace modifications (72). Loisel et al. (72) states that a return to "usual" work is the only worthwhile therapeutic objective. Returning workers to modified workstations allows them to resume their work after a back injury but does not lead to therapeutic success. In fact, some companies have used a return to modified workstations to hide cases from official occupational accident statistics. The same study also clearly demonstrated that therapeutic success, measured by return to usual work, is dependent on the efficacy of workplace interventions, with medical interventions (both diagnostic and therapeutic) and graded activity programs significantly less effective. In this study, the workplace interventions consisted of workplace meetings with supervisors to discuss modifications to the organization of the patient's work. Attempts to modify workstations were relatively uncommon, but if made, they were simple (72).

Restricted work or light duty is popular among some employers and health care provider, while other organizations do not use it. It is believed to reduce indirect cost, augment work retention, and expedite the transfer of the individual from the restricted work position to full preinjury capacity duty in a more time-efficient manner. However, few studies have looked at restricted work procedures that are commonly used in industry. Hiebert et al. (71) carried out a retrospective cohort study (n < 240). The objectives were to evaluate the associations of prescribed work restrictions with work absenteeism and recurrence in cases of NSLBP. Employees absent from work because of back pain were identified from medical records of a utility company, and were placed into two groups: those who received a work restriction for back pain and those who did not. After 1 year of follow-up, the duration of sickness-related absence was compared between the two groups. Employees who returned to work within the follow-up period were followed for one additional year to determine rates of recurrence between the two groups. The Cox proportional hazards model was used to generate hazard ratios adjusted for age, gender, and job category.

Work restrictions were given to 43% of the workers reporting disabling NSLBP. Sickness-absence duration did not differ between those who received restrictions as compared to those who did not (adjusted hazard ratio < 1.12, $p < .41$). The median duration of restricted duty was 32.5 days; for 22% of workers restricted duty was never lifted. Injury recurrence appeared less likely for those who had work restrictions in their initial episode; however, it was not statistically significant (adjusted hazard ratio < 0.77, $p < .48$). The conclusion of the study was that work restriction was not associated with early return to work and thus to returning to full preinjury duty. The authors concluded that the findings of this study should be interpreted cautiously; a recommendation to discontinue the practice of prescribing work restrictions should not be made on the basis of the findings from this paper alone. This study should be interpreted as a first critical attempt to evaluate a common clinical practice and to highlight the need for further research.

"SAFE" RETURN TO WORK

The management of low back pain in an occupational health setting should be aimed at a "safe" return to work. Current occupational guidelines are consistent regarding their recommendations to reassure the worker with low back pain, and to encourage and support return to work even with some persisting symptoms. Evidence on the effectiveness of ergonomic and workplace adaptations are lacking and guidelines do not specifically recommend this type of intervention. "Participatory ergonomics" interventions which propose consultations with the worker, the employer and an ergonomist, might be effective as the potential value of "getting all the players on one side" has been stressed (55).

The Paris Task Force (20) favors workers returning to their usual workstations or regular duty with the following conditions in place. One, several or all conditions may be used to return the employee to regular duty:

1. Management of the process by occupational physicians and the human resources department
2. Workstation assessment

3. Evaluation of workers' physical capacity
4. Identification of workstations that are congruent with workers' physical capacities
5. Communication between workers and supervisors
6. Regular clinical follow-up during the adaptation period.

If all of the above has failed a reclassification of the employee/worker to other type of work/duty, retraining to other type of work, or permanent disability may be considered. The most important message in this instance is to use a systematic approach to reclassify the ability or possible disability for work. The focus of this chapter is to discuss successful reintegration of the worker with low back pain episode(s) into the workplace; the reader is referred to a text by Waddell et al. (8) for further discussion of the incapacity for work and back pain in a social context, from an international point of view. Waddell et al. stress that "from a social perspective, trends of incapacity for work attributed from low back pain and social security benefits paid back for back pain form a social phenomenon which is related to the economic and labor market situation." Most important, the text emphasizes that back pain is not simply a health problem but often raises more fundamental psychosocial issues which health care providers and social security systems are often ill-equipped to handle (73). Being ill-equipped to handle these problems or worse, refusal to recognize the problems leads to slow intervention and promotes disability.

WORK RETENTION AFTER NSLBP

Few studies have been conducted verifying the relationship between work retention and NSLBP. Work retention is an important outcome of NSLBP as it contains information about symptom control over a period of time, medical utilization, and loss of productivity. Amick et al. (74) suggested that there are many reasons to measure work outcomes, such as evaluation of effectiveness of health services, assessment of productivity loss, and targeting injury prevention programs. Additionally, reports in the literature have shown that people who are out of work because of either disability or unemployment are more likely to develop other diseases, and ultimately their life span is reduced when compared to people who are employed (75). Work retention is therefore an important outcome of a successful intervention and workers' well-being as a health improvement measurement.

Campello (76) studied physical and psychosocial associations and work retention. Sixty-seven patients (mean age 40, SD 12 years) with NSLBP participated in a 4-week multidisciplinary rehabilitation program. Patients returning to work were followed for 2 years. Physical and psychosocial baseline measures were collected, including performance and functional capacity tests. Psychosocial baseline measures were somatization scales, pain beliefs, and perceived disability. Physical parameters included trunk flexibility, lifting capacity, and aerobic capacity, among others. The dependent variable, work retention, was defined as the number of days that the subject worked during the 2-year follow-up period. Survival analysis was used to establish a predictive model. The average time out of work before treatment was 9 months (SD 12). Average work retention was 362 days (range 47 to 682 days) for 18 patients that relapsed with NSLBP. Results showed that posttest trunk flexion and somatization were the strongest predictors for work retention [final trunk flexion hazard ratio 2.5 (95% confidence interval 1.26 to 4.79, $p < .01$), somatization scale hazard ratio 2.5 (95% confidence interval 1.25 to 4.93, $p < .01$)]. The author concluded that psychosocial and physical factors are associated with work retention for NSLBP patients.

Beliefs and perceptions have also been found to be associated with work retention. Linton and Hallden (77) observed a significant difference in beliefs that one should not work with current pain levels between groups of acute and subacute NSLBP patients seeking primary care. There was a significant difference between individuals who retained work and groups that have missed work because of NSLBP problems subsequent to their return to work. Individuals who believed they should not work because of the level of pain experienced were less likely to retain work in a 6-month follow-up period. High levels of perceived disability were found to be negatively associated with work retention in a study conducted in a group of subacute and chronic NSLBP patients undergoing rehabilitation in outpatient clinics. Individuals who perceived high levels of disability were more likely to experience an interruption of work because of NSLBP in a 6-month follow-up period following completion of a treatment program and return to work (78).

High levels of anxiety were found to be negatively associated with work retention. Individuals who reported feeling tense and anxious at the time of intervention were less likely to retain work after they returned to work (77). Changes in depression and anxiety were also found to be predictive for work retention in a study conducted of patients with chronic NSLBP enrolled in an intensive rehabilitation program (79). Individuals who showed a decrease in anxiety and depression levels (from high to low levels) were more likely to retain work than individuals who did not show a decrease in levels of distress after multidisciplinary intervention. In conclusion, physical and psychosocial factors affect work retention after an episode of disabling low back pain.

CONCLUSIONS

The probability of returning to work decreases very rapidly with increasing duration of work absence in every study reviewed by the Paris Task Force (20). The risk of chronicity and work incapacity increased very rapidly in the first weeks of the episode of back pain, and the prognosis is greatly compromised well before the third month of disability. This chapter has focused on the prevention of work disability and the different possibilities a worker might undergo to return to gainful employment after an episode of NSLBP. Perhaps the most important message to the health care provider is to accept that the diagnosis of NSLBP is an accurate and a "good" diagnosis with a good prognosis. Scientific studies may change this concept in the future when scientists discover the cause(s) of NSLBP.

A working person is at great risk for delayed recovery and long-term disability from 6 to 12 weeks following the onset of symptoms of NSLBP and work incapacity. At this time there are successful interventions to return a person to gainful employment. Based on scientific evidence these interventions must be active, include exercises, and take into account psychosocial and workplace interventions after a careful multidisciplinary evaluation of the work-disabled patient.

ACKNOWLEDGMENTS

A special thanks to Katherine Hahler and Rudi Hiebert for preparing this manuscript and checking references.

REFERENCES

1. Waddell G, Nachemson AL, Phillips RB. The back pain revolution. Edinburgh: Churchill Livingstone, 1998.
2. Norlund A, Waddell G. Cost of back pain in some OECD countries. In: Nachemson A, Jonsson E, eds. Neck and back pain: the scientific evidence of causes and treatment. Philadelphia: Lippincott Williams & Wilkins, 2000:421–426.
3. Bureau of Economic Analysis. Gross National Product, Seasonally Adjusted 1959–2002. Washington, DC: U.S. Department of Commerce, 2003.
4. Cats-Baril WL, Frymoyer JW. The economics of spine disorders. In: Frymoyer JW, Ducker TB, Hadler NM, et al., eds. The adult spine: principles and practice. New York: Raven Press, 1991:85–105.
5. Guo HR, Tanaka S, Cameron LL, et al. Back pain among workers in the United States: national estimates and workers at high risk. Am J Industr Med 1995;28:591–602.
6. Office of National Statistics. The prevalence of back pain in Great Britain in 1998. 1998/18. London: Department of Health Statistics Division 3, 1999.
7. Nachemson A, Waddell G, Norlund A. Epidemiology of neck and back pain. In: Nachemson A, Jonsson E, eds. Neck and back pain: the scientific evidence of causes and treatment. Philadelphia: Lippincott Williams & Wilkins, 2000:165–188.
8. Wadell G, Aylward M, Sawney P. Back pain, incapacity for work and social security benefits: An international literature review and analysis. London: The Royal Society of Medicine Press Limited, 2002.
9. Hultman G, Nordin M, Saraste H. Physical and psychological workload in men with and without low back pain. Scand J Rehabil Med 1995;27:11–17.
10. Hultman G, Nordin M, Saraste H, et al. Body composition, endurance, strength, cross-sectional area, and density of MM erector spinae in men with and without low back pain. J Spinal Disord 1993;6:114–123.
11. Abenhaim L, Rossignol M, Gobeille D, et al. The prognostic consequences in the making of the initial medical diagnosis of work-related back injuries. Spine 1995;20:791–795.
12. Nordin M, Hiebert R, Pietrek M, et al. The association of comorbidity and outcome in episodes of non-specific low back pain in occupational populations. J Occupation Environ Med 2002;44:1–8.
13. Hashemi L, Webster BS, Clancy EA, et al. Length of disability and cost

of workers' compensation low back pain claims. J Occupation Environ Med 1997;39:937–945.

14. Murphy PL, Courtney TK. Low back pain disability: relative costs by antecedent and industry group. Am J Industr Med 2000;37:558–571.
15. Volinn E, Van Koevering D, Loeser JD. Back sprain in industry. The role of socioeconomic factors in chronicity. Spine 1991;16:542–548.
16. Skovron ML, Szpalski M, Nordin M, et al. Sociocultural factors and back pain. A population-based study in Belgian adults. Spine 1994;19:129–137.
17. Croft P, Papageorgiou A, McNally R. Low back pain. In: Stevens A, Raftery J, eds. Health care needs assessment. Second series: The epidemiologically based needs assessment reviews. Oxford: Radcliffe Medical Press, 1996:129–182.
18. Deyo RA, Weinstein JN. Low back pain. N Engl J Med 2001;344:363–70.
19. Waddell G, McIntosh A, Hutchinson A, et al. Low back pain evidence review. London: Royal College of General Practitioners, 1999.
20. Abenhaim L, Rossignol M, Valat JP, et al. The role of activity in the therapeutic management of back pain. Report of the International Paris Task Force on Back Pain. Spine 2000;25:1S–33S.
21. Weiser S, Cedraschi C. Psychosocial issues in the prevention of chronic low back pain—a literature review. In: Nordin M, Vischer TL, eds. Common low back pain: prevention of chronicity. Baillière's clinical rheumatology: international practice and research. London: Harcourt Brace Jovanovich Ltd, 1992:657–684.
22. Kendall NAS, Linton SJ, Main CJ. Guide to assessing psychosocial yellow flags in acute low back pain: risk factors for long term disability and work loss. Wellington: Accident Rehabilitation and Compensation Insurance Corporation of New Zealand and the National Health Committee, 1997.
23. Bigos SJ, Bowyer O, Braen G. Acute low back problems in adults. Clinical Practice Guideline, No. 14. Rockville, MD: U.S. Department of Health and Human Services, Public Health Service, Agency for Health Care Policy and Research, 1994.
24. Fransen M, Woodward M, Norton R, et al. Risk factors associated with the transition from acute to chronic occupational back pain. Spine 2002;27:92–98.
25. Nordin M, Weiser S, Van Doorn JW, et al. Nonspecific low back pain. In: Rom W, ed. Environmental and occupational medicine. Philadelphia: Lippincott-Raven Publishers, 1998:947–957.
26. Carey TS, Evans AT, Hadler NM, et al. Acute severe low back pain. A population-based study of prevalence and care-seeking. Spine 1996;21:339–344.
27. Hadler MN. Occupational musculoskeletal disorders. New York: Raven Press, 1993;1–14.
28. Vingard E, Nachemson A. Work related influences on neck and low back pain. In: Nachemson A, Jonsson E, eds. Neck and back pain: the scientific evidence of causes and treatment. Philadelphia: Lippincott Williams & Wilkins, 2000:997–1126.
29. Koes BW, van Tulder MW, Ostelo R, et al. Clinical guidelines for the management of low back pain in primary care: an international comparison. Spine 2001;26:2504–2513.
30. Spitzer WO, LeBlanc FE, DuPuis M. Scientific approach to the assessment and management of activity-related spinal disorders. A monograph for clinicians. Report of the Quebec Task Force on Spinal Disorders. Spine 1987;12:1S–59S.
31. van Tulder MW. Spinal radiographic findings and nonspecific low back pain. A systematic review of observational studies. Spine 1997;22:427–434.
32. Campello M, Weiser S, van Doorn JW, et al. Approaches to improve the outcome of patients with delayed recovery. In: Nordin M, Cedraschi C, Vischer TL, eds. New approaches to the low back pain patient. Baillière's clinical rheumatology: international practice and research. London: Harcourt Brace Jovanovich Ltd, 1998:93–113.
33. Spengler DM. Clinical evaluation of the low back region. In: Nordin M, Andersson GBJ, Pope MH, eds. Musculoskeletal disorders in the workplace. principles and practice. Philadelphia, PA: Mosby–Year Book, Inc., 1997:278–287.
34. Cherkin DC, Deyo RA, Street JH, et al. Predicting poor outcomes for back pain seen in primary care using patients' own criteria. Spine 1996;21:2900–2907.
35. Hazard RG, Haugh LD, Reid S, et al. Early prediction of chronic disability after occupational low back injury. Spine 1996;21:945–951.
36. Klenerman L, Slade PD, Stanley IM, et al. The prediction of chronic-

ity in patients with an acute attack of low back pain in a general practice setting. Spine 1995;20:478–484.
37. Balagué F, Nordin M, Sheikhzadeh A, et al. Recovery of severe sciatica. Spine 1999;24:2516–2524.
38. Nordin M, Skovron ML, Hiebert R, et al. Early predictors of delayed return to work in patients with low back pain. J Musculoskel Disord 1997;5:5–27.
39. Dionne CE, Koepsell TD, Von Korff M, et al. Predicting long-term functional limitations among back pain patients in primary care settings. J Clin Epidemiol 1997;50:31–43.
40. Lehmann TR, Spratt KF, Lehmann KK. Predicting long-term disability in low back injured workers presenting to a spine consultant. Spine 1993;18:1103–1112.
41. Seferlis T, Nemeth G, Carlsson AM. Prediction of functional disability, recurrences, and chronicity after 1 year in 180 patients who required sick leave for acute low-back pain. J Spinal Disord 2000;13:470–477.
42. Burton KA, Waddell G. Clinical guidelines in the management of low back pain. In: Nordin M, Cedraschi C, Vischer TL, eds. New approaches to the low back pain patient. Baillière's clinical rheumatology: international practice and research. London: Harcourt Brace Jovanovich Ltd, 1998:17–36.
43. Ferguson SA, Marras WS. A literature review of low back disorder surveillance measures and risk factors. Clin Biomech 1997;12:211–226.
44. Waddell G. Biopsychosocial analysis of low back pain. In: Nordin M, Vischer TL, eds. Common low back pain: prevention of chronicity. Baillière's clinical rheumatology: international practice and research. London: Harcourt Brace Jovanovich Ltd, 1992:523–557.
45. Burton AK, Tillotson KM, Main CJ, et al. Psychosocial predictors of outcome in acute and subchronic low back trouble. Spine 1995;20:722–728.
46. Truchon M. Determinants of chronic disability related to low back pain: towards an integrative biopsychosocial model. Disabil Rehabil 2001;23:758–767.
47. Hurrel JJ, Murphy RM. Psychological job stress. In: Rom WM, ed. Environmental and occupational medicine. Philadelphia: Lippincott-Raven Publishers, 1998:905–914.
48. Burton AK, Erg E. Back injury and work loss. Biomechanical and psychosocial influences. Spine 1997;22:2575–2580.
49. Garg A, Moore JS. Epidemiology of low-back pain in industry. Occupation Med 1992;7:593–608.
50. Papageorgiou AC, Macfarlane GJ, Thomas E, et al. Psychosocial factors in the workplace—do they predict new episodes of low back pain? Evidence from the South Manchester Back Pain Study. Spine 1997;22:1137–1142.
51. Fanuele JC, Birkmeyer NJ, Abdu WA, et al. The impact of spinal problems on the health status of patients: have we underestimated the effect? Spine 2000;25:1509–1514.
52. Von Korff M, Saunders K. The course of back pain in primary care. Spine 1996;21:2833–2837.
53. van Tulder MW, Ostelo R, Vlaeyen JW, et al. Behavioral treatment for chronic low back pain: a systematic review within the framework of the Cochrane Back Review Group. Spine 2000;25:2688–2699.
54. Atlas SJ, Nardin RA. Evaluation and treatment of low back pain: An evidence-based approach to clinical care. Muscle Nerve 2003;27:265–284.
55. Frank J, Sinclair S, Hogg-Johnson S, et al. Preventing disability from work-related low-back pain. New evidence gives new hope—if we can just get all the players onside. Can Med Assoc J 1998;158:1625–1631.
56. Guzman J, Esmail R, Karjalainen K, et al. Multidisciplinary rehabilitation for chronic low back pain: systematic review. Br Med J 2001;322:1511–1516.
57. Karjalainen K, Malmivaara A, van Tulder M, et al. Multidisciplinary biopsychosocial rehabilitation for subacute low back pain in working-age adults: a systematic review within the framework of the Cochrane Collaboration Back Review Group. Spine 2001;26:262–269.
58. Panel P. Philadelphia panel evidence-based clinical practice guidelines on selected rehabilitation interventions for low back pain. Phys Ther 2001;81:1641–1674.
59. Hansen FR, Bendix T, Skov P, et al. Intensive, dynamic back-muscle exercises, conventional physiotherapy, or placebo-control treatment of low-back pain. A randomized, observer-blind trial. Spine 1993;18:98–108.
60. Lindström I, Öhlund C, Eek C, et al. The effect of graded activity on patients with subacute low back pain: a randomized prospective clinical study with an operant-conditioning behavioral approach. Phys Ther 1992;72:279–290.

61. Bendix AF, Bendix T, Labriola M, et al. Functional restoration for chronic low back pain. Two-year follow-up of two randomized clinical trials. Spine 1998;23:717–725.

62. Härkäpää K, Mellin G, Järvikoski A, et al. A controlled study on the outcome of inpatient and outpatient treatment of low back pain. Part III. Long-term follow-up of pain, disability, and compliance. Scand J Rehabil Med 1990;22:181–188.

63. Scheer SJ, Watanabe TK, Radack KL. Randomized controlled trials in industrial low back pain. Part 3. Subacute/chronic pain interventions. Arch Phys Med Rehabil 1997;78:414–423.

64. Mitchell RI, Carmen GM. The functional restoration approach to the treatment of chronic pain in patients with soft tissue and back injuries. Spine 1994;19:633–642.

65. Rivier G, Nordin M, Rossignol M. Impact socioprofessionnel des programmes de prise en harge des dorso-lombalgies. In: Deburge A, Benoist M, Morvan G, et al., eds. Degénérescence du Rachis Lombaire et Lombalgies. Monographie des journées de l'hôpital Beaujon. Montpellier: Sauramps Médical, 1999:181–212.

66. Shekelle PG, Woolf SH, Eccles M, et al. Clinical guidelines: developing guidelines. Br Med J 1999;318:593–596.

67. Victorian Workcover Authority. Guidelines for the management of employees with compensable low back pain. Melbourne: Workcover Authority, 1996.

68. Harris JS. The ACOEM occupational medicine guidelines. In: Harris JS, Loeppke RR, eds. Integrated health management: the key role of occupational medicine in managed care disability management and integrated delivery systems. Boston: OEM Press, 1998.

69. Dutch Association of Occupational Medicine. Dutch guideline for the management of occupational physicians of employees with low back pain. (Nederlandse Vereniging voor Arbeids-en Bedrijfsgeneeskunde (NVAB). Handelen van de bedrijfsarts bij werknemers met lage-rugklachten. Richtlijnen voor Bedrijfsartsen). Brussels, 1999.

70. Carter JT, Birrell LN. Occupational health guidelines for the management of low back pain at work—principal recommendations. London: Faculty of Occupational Medicine, 2000.

71. Hiebert R, Skovron ML, Nordin M, et al. Work restrictions and outcome of nonspecific low back pain. Spine 2003;28: (in press).

72. Loisel P, Abenhaim L, Durand P, et al. A population-based, randomized clinical trial on back pain management. Spine 1997;22:2911–2918.

73. Nordin M. 2000 International Society for the Study of the Lumbar Spine Presidential Address: Backs-to-Work: some reflections. Spine 2001;26:851–856.

74. Amick BC, Lerner D, Rogers WH, et al. A review of health-related work outcome measures and their uses, and recommended measures. Spine 2000;25:3152–3160.

75. Janlert U. Unemployment as a disease and diseases of the unemployed. Scand J Work Environ Health 1997;23:79–83.

76. Campello M. Physical and psychosocial predictors of work retention after a multidisciplinary rehabilitation program for non-specific low back pain patients [doctoral thesis]. New York: New York University. Ann Arbor, MI: UMI Dissertation Services, UMI Number: 3062794, Proquest Information and Learning Co, 2002:1–116.

77. Linton SJ, Hallden K. Can we screen for problematic back pain? A screening questionnaire for predicting outcome in acute and subacute back pain. Clin J Pain 1998;14:209–215.

78. Infante-Rivard C, Lortie M. Relapse and short sickness absence for back pain in the six months after return to work. Occupation Environ Med 1997;54:328–334.

79. Garcy P, Mayer T, Gatchel RJ. Recurrent or new injury outcomes after return to work in chronic disabling spinal disorders. Tertiary prevention efficacy of functional restoration treatment. Spine 1996;21:952–959.

CHAPTER 17

Occupational Ergonomics

William S. Marras

Ergonomics has been defined as "a multidisciplinary activity dealing with the interactions between man and his *total* working environment" (1). Ergonomic design attempts to create workplaces to accommodate or "fit" the workers. The goal of ergonomics is to create a work environment that is efficient, productive, and optimizes worker health. Inherent in this definition is the idea that ergonomics deals with not only the physical components of the workplace, but addresses the mental or cognitive components as well. Among the scientific disciplines employed to achieve these goals are biomechanics, biochemistry, psychology, cognitive science, physiology, physical anthropometry, organizational design, and medicine.

The science of ergonomics is primarily concerned with the *prevention* of problems in the workplace. Over the past several decades, ergonomics has been employed with increasing frequency by organizations of all sizes. Many large as well as small companies have permanent ergonomic programs in place that have derived significant benefits from these efforts (2). There are several motivations for the incorporation of ergonomic principles in the design of the workplace. These motivations are associated with the direct and indirect costs associated with musculoskeletal disorders in the workplace. Direct costs are associated with the rapidly increasing health care costs associated with a work-related musculoskeletal disorder. Indirect costs associated with work-related musculoskeletal disorders include the training of new workers that replace the injured worker, employee turnover costs including administrative costs, loss of productivity, lower product quality, and the cost of the injury investigation. Many businesses have discovered that the prevention of injuries is much more economically advantageous than rehabilitating a musculoskeletal disorder that has already occurred.

Ergonomic approaches alter the work environment to control risk exposure and optimize efficiency and productivity. Two types of risk controls or ergonomic interventions are used in the design of the workplace. First, engineering controls are used to physically change the orientation of the work environment relative to the person. Engineering controls ideally alter the workplace and create a work environment where the risk has been minimized so that the work-person interface is optimal. Second, administrative controls are often employed when it is not possible to provide engineering controls. Administrative controls do not eliminate the risk. Instead they attempt to control risk by managing the time of worker exposure to the risks in the workplace. This is often accomplished through rotation of workers exposed to a risk or ensuring that workers have adequate time to recover from exposure to workplace risks through appropriate scheduling of days off work.

While ergonomics typically addresses all aspects of musculoskeletal disorders as well as performance issues, the discussion of ergonomics in this chapter will be limited in scope to issues and principles associated with the prevention of low back disorders (LBDs) due to physical work activities (not related to whole-body vibration).

MAGNITUDE OF THE LOW BACK PAIN PROBLEM AT WORK

It should be acknowledged that since most people work, workplace risk factors and individual risk factors are difficult to separate (3). However, potential patterns can be identified through surveys of working populations. In the United States back disorders are associated with more days away from work than those related to any other part of the body (4). Recent studies of 17,000 men and women of working age population in Sweden (5) indicated that 5% of workers sought care for a new low back pain episode over a 3-year period. They also found that many of these cases became chronic. Evaluations of data from a large sample of U.S. households collected by the National Health Injury Survey (NHIS) found that back pain accounts for about one-fourth of the workers'

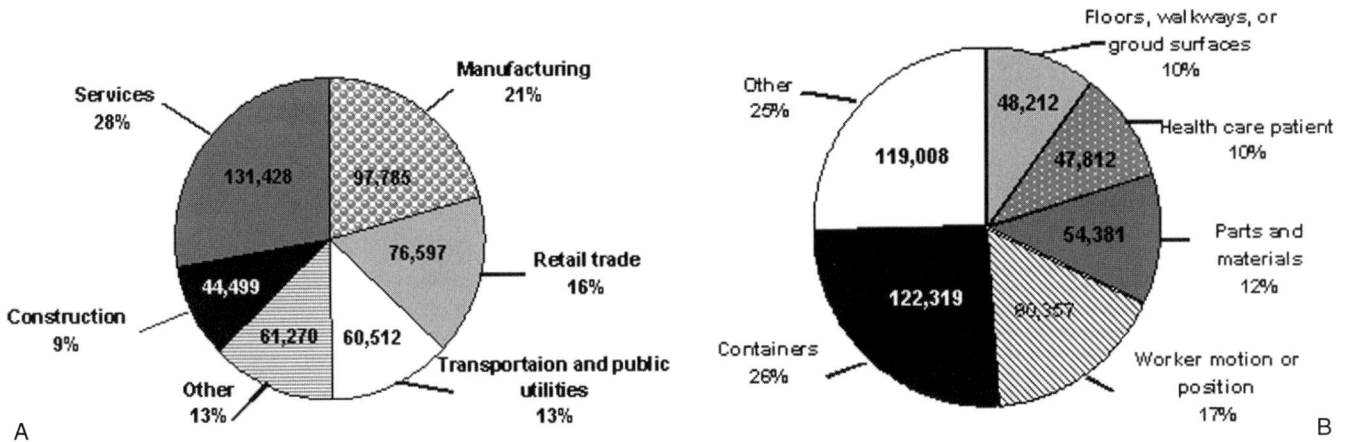

FIG. 17-1. A: Number and distribution of back cases with days away from work in private industry by industry division during 1997. **B:** Number and distribution of back cases with days away from work in private industry by source of the disorder during 1997. (Data for both **A** and **B** from National Institute for Occupational Safety and Health. Worker health chartbook. Cincinnati, 2000.)

compensation claims in the United States (6). Two-thirds of the low back pain cases were attributed to occupational activities. Prevalence of lost workdays due to back pain was found to be 4.6% (7). Certain occupations were also found to be significantly linked to greater rates of low back pain reporting. Risk appeared to be highest for construction laborers (prevalence 22.6%) and nursing aides (19.8%) (6). Figure 17-1 summarizes the findings of a National Institute for Occupational Safety and Health (NIOSH) analysis of work-related LBDs (4). This figure indicates that, in terms of prevalence, the service industry followed by manufacturing account for nearly half of all occupationally related LBDs. The analysis also indicates that handling of containers and worker motions and position assumed during work are most often associated with LBDs in U.S. industry. Hence, these data strongly suggest that occupational factors appear to be related to risk of LBDs.

EPIDEMIOLOGY OF WORK RISK FACTORS

Several reviews have identified specific risk factors that increase the risk of LBDs in the workplace. The NIOSH performed a critical review of the epidemiologic evidence associated with musculoskeletal disorders (8). Five categories of risk factors were evaluated. The critique concluded that strong evidence existed for an association between LBDs and lifting/forceful movements and LBDs and whole-body vibration. Significant evidence was found for the associations between heavy physical work and awkward postures and back problems. The review concluded that insufficient evidence was available to make any conclusions between static work postures and LBD risk. In a methodologically rigorous review Hoogendoorn et al. (9) were generally able to support these conclusions. They found that manual materials

handling, bending, twisting, and whole-body vibration were risk factors for back pain.

Several studies have been in search of a dose-response relationship among work risk factors and low back pain. Two studies (10,11) suggest that cumulative loading of the spine might be associated with risk of LBD at work. However, Videman et al. (12) suggested that the relationship might not be as straightforward as the linear relationships suggested. When examining the relationship between back pain, history of physical loading, and occupation in cadaveric specimens, Videman et al. concluded that the risk relationship between LBD risk and loading was "J-shaped" with sedentary jobs being associated with moderate levels of risk, heavy work being associated with the greatest degree of risk, and moderate exposure to loading being associated with the lowest level of risk. Seidler et al. (13) have recently suggested that the combination of occupational lifting and trunk flexion, and duration of the activities significantly increased risk.

Over the past decade, studies have also assessed the impact of psychosocial factors in the workplace in relation to the risk of LBDs (14–17). Studies often show that monotonous work, high perceived workload, time pressure, low job satisfaction, and lack of social support are related to LBD risk. However, Davis and Heaney (18) found that the impact of psychosocial factors was diminished, yet still significant, once biomechanical factors were accounted for in the study designs.

Secondary prevention studies of LBD have begun to explore the interaction between LBDs, physical factors, and psychosocial factors. Frank et al. (19) as well as Waddell (20,21) have pointed out that much of low back pain treatment is multidimensional. Epidemiologic studies of the role of variables in primary prevention of work-related low back pain have suggested that

TABLE 17-1. *Summary of epidemiologic evidence with risk estimates (null, positive, and attributable fraction) of associations with work-related factors associated with low back disorders*

Work-related risk factor	Risk estimate					
	Null association[a]		Positive association		Attributable fraction (%)	
	n	Range	n	Range	n	Range
Manual material handling	4	0.90–1.45	24	1.12–3.54	17	11–66
Frequent bending and twisting	2	1.08–1.30	15	1.29–8.09	8	19–57
Heavy physical load	0		8	1.54–3.71	5	31–58
Static work posture	3	0.80–0.97	3	1.30–3.29	3	14–32
Repetitive movements	2	0.98–1.20	1	1.97	1	41
Whole-body vibration	1	1.10	16	1.26–9.00	11	18–80

n, Number of associations presented in epidemiologic studies.
[a]Confidence intervals of the risk estimates included the null estimate (1.0). In only 12 of 16 null associations was the magnitude of the risk estimate presented.
From NRC. Musculoskeletal disorders and the workplace: low back and upper extremity. Washington DC: National Academy Press, 2001, with permission.

multiple dimensions, such as physical stressors and psychosocial factors, play a role in low back pain risk (22). Tubach et al. have recently shown that low social support at the workplace and bending at work are strongly associated with extended work absence due to low back pain (23).

Recent rigorous epidemiologic reviews of the literature performed by the National Research Council (3) have concluded that there is a clear relationship between back disorders and physical load imposed by manual material handling, frequent bending and twisting, physically heavy work, and whole-body vibration. The risk attributable to these risk factors is summarized in Table 17-1. This analysis indicates that the vast majority of high quality epidemiologic studies have associated LBDs with these risk factors and up to two-thirds of risk can be attributed to materials handling activities. As a result of these epidemiologic analyses, it was concluded that preventive measures may reduce the exposure to risk factors and reduce the occurrence of back problems.

OCCUPATIONAL BIOMECHANICS LOGIC

The epidemiologic literature helps to understand what factors might be associated with work-related LBDs but the body of literature is problematic in that it has great difficulty prescribing an optimal level of exposure in order to minimize risk. The National Research Council's review of epidemiologic evidence and LBDs concluded that "epidemiologic evidence itself is not specific enough to provide detailed, quantitative guidelines for design of the workplace, job, or task. This lack of specificity results from the absence of exposure measurements on a continuous scale, as opposed to the more commonly used dichotomous (yes/no) approach. Without continuous measures, it is

not possible to state the 'levels' of exposure associated with increased risk of low back pain" (3). In order to more fully understand "how much exposure is too much exposure" to risk factors, we must develop an understanding of how work-related factors might lead to LBDs. This causality pathway is typically addressed through biomechanical and ergonomic analyses. If one views the biomechanical literature as a whole, it is clear that these analyses represent a promising approach to controlling low back injury risk in the workplace.

Biomechanical logic presents a format to help us understand the mechanisms that might effect the development of a LBD. At the heart of this logic is the idea that risk is associated with a load-tolerance relationship. Figure 17-2 shows this relationship graphically. As explained by McGill (24), when work is performed the structures and tissues of the spine undergo a loading pattern with each repeated job cycle. If the magnitude of the load imposed upon a structure or tissue exceeds the structural tolerance of this tissue, damage occurs and this damage might be capable of setting off the sequence of events that could lead to LBD. If the magnitude of the imposed load is below the structural tolerance, the task is safe. The magnitude of the distance between the structure loading and the tolerance is considered the safety margin (Fig. 17-2A). If the load exceeds the tolerance then risk is present (Fig. 17-2B).

Biomechanics can also be used to describe the processes believed to be at work during exposure to cumulative trauma disorders. As shown in Fig. 17- 2C, when exposed to repetitive exertions, one would expect the tolerance to be subject to degradation over time. As the work is performed repeatedly, we would expect that the loading pattern would remain relatively constant, however, with overuse we would expect the tolerance limit to decrease over time. This makes it more probable

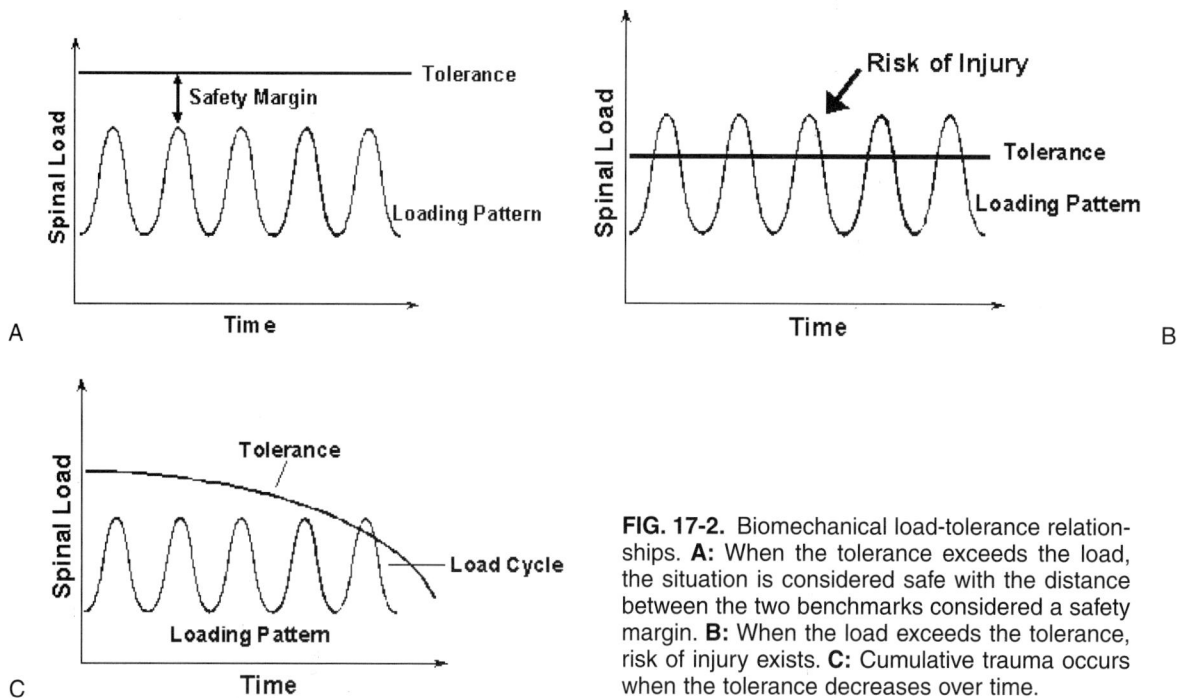

FIG. 17-2. Biomechanical load-tolerance relationships. **A:** When the tolerance exceeds the load, the situation is considered safe with the distance between the two benchmarks considered a safety margin. **B:** When the load exceeds the tolerance, risk of injury exists. **C:** Cumulative trauma occurs when the tolerance decreases over time.

for the load to exceed the tolerance and thus trigger a potential disorder.

PAIN AND BIOMECHANICAL TOLERANCE

It is believed that there are numerous pathways to pain perception associated with LBDs. It is important to understand these pathways since they are the basis for the structure and tissue limits employed in ergonomic logic. One can consider the quantitative limits above which a pain pathway is initiated as a tolerance limit for ergonomic purposes. While none of these pathways have been defined definitively, these pathways are appealing since they represent biologically plausible mechanisms that complement the view of injury association derived from the epidemiologic literature.

In general, three broad categories of pain pathways are believed to exist that may affect the design of the workplace. These categories are associated with: (a) structural and tissue stimulation, (b) physiologic limits, and (c) psychophysical acceptance. Each of these pathways is expected to have different tolerance limits to mechanical loading of the tissue. Thus, in order to properly design a workplace one must design tasks so the ultimate limit within each of these categories is not exceeded.

Pathways between Tissue Stimulation and Pain

The literature suggests that there are several structures in the back that when stimulated are capable of pain perception. Both cellular and neural mechanisms can lead to pain and both laboratory and anatomic investigations have indi-

cated neurophysiologic and neuroanatomic origins of back pain (25–29). These pathways often involve pressure on a structure that can directly stimulate pain receptors or trigger the release of pain-stimulating chemicals.

Pain pathways have been identified for joint pain, pain of disc origin, longitudinal ligaments, and mechanisms for sciatica. Facet pain mechanisms are associated with an extensive distribution of small nerve fibers and endings in the lumbar facet joint, nerves containing substance P, high-threshold mechanoreceptors in the facet joint capsule, and sensitization and excitation of nerves in the facet joint and surrounding muscle when the nerves are exposed to inflammatory or algesic chemicals (30–32). The pathway for disc pain has been suggested through an extensive distribution of small nerve fibers and free nerve endings in the superficial annulus of the disc and small fibers and free nerve endings in the adjacent longitudinal ligaments (25,28,33,34). Sciatic pain can be associated with mechanical stimulation of spine structures. Even moderate pressure on the dorsal root ganglia results in vigorous and long-lasting excitatory discharges that might explain sciatica. Additionally, sciatica might be explained by excitation of dorsal root fibers when the ganglia were exposed to the nucleus pulposus. Stimulation and nerve function loss in nerve roots exposed to phospholipase A_2 might also explain sciatica (27,35,36). Recent work is showing the importance of proinflammatory agents such as tumor necrosis factor-α (TNF-α) and interleukin-1 (IL-1) (37). These agents upregulate under certain conditions and set the stage for pain perception. It is possible that mechanical stimulation of tissues can initiate this sequence of events and thus become the initiator of pain. Thus, it may be possible to consider the role of these agents in a load-tolerance model where tolerance may be considered the point at which these agents are upregulated.

These studies provide the framework for an established and logical link between the mechanical stimulation of spinal tissues and structures and the sensation of low back pain that is the foundation of occupational biomechanics and ergonomics.

Functional Lumbar Spinal Unit Tolerance Limits

The tolerances of the individual structures of the functional lumbar spinal unit are often considered collectively as part of the structural support system. The vertebral body can typically withstand large loads when compressed. The tolerance limits are often considered along with those of the end plate. A review by Jager (38) indicated the compressive tolerance reported in the literature could be large (over 8 kN) especially in an upright posture, but highly variable with some specimens indicating failure at 2 kN. Damage to human vertebral cancellous bone is typically a result of shear stress and the ultimate strength is correlated with tissue stiffness when exposed to compressive loading (39). Bone failure often occurs along with disc herniation and annular delamination (40). Thus, damage to the bone itself appears to be part of the cascading series of events associated with low back pain (29,41,42).

There is a debate in the literature as to the pain pathway associated with vertebral end-plate microfracture. One line of thinking maintains that health of the vertebral body end plate is essential for proper mechanical functioning of the spine. Damage to the end-plate nutrient supply can result in damage to the disc and disruption of spinal function (43). Traditionally, the literature has supported the idea that the disruption of nutrient flow is capable of initiating a cascading series of events that can lead to low back pain (29,41,42,44). Tolerances of the vertebral end plate have been studied in several investigations. These studies suggest that the end plate is the first structure to be damaged when the spine is loaded, especially at lower load rates (43,45–47). End-plate failure commonly occurs with compressive loads of 5.5 kN (47). End-plate tolerances have been observed to decrease by 30% to 50% with exposure to repetitive loading (45) which suggests the disc is affected by cumulative trauma. Integrity also appears to be influenced by anterior-posterior shear loading. Shear limits tolerances of 1290 to 1770 N for soft tissue and 2000 to 2800 N for the hard tissue have been reported for the spine (48,49).

Activity-related damage might also be indicated by the presence of Schmorl nodes. Some have suggested that Schmorl nodes might be remnants of healed end-plate fractures (50,51) and might be linked to trauma (51,52). Position or posture of the spine appears to strongly influence end-plate tolerance during loading. Flexed

spine postures can greatly reduce loading tolerance (40,53). Hence, trunk posture is an important consideration for occupational risk assessment. Industrial surveillance studies by Punnett et al., Marras et al., and Norman et al. (10,54–56) all suggest that LBD increases as trunk postures during work deviate from an upright posture.

Individual factors can also influence end-plate integrity. Age and gender have been found to greatly influence the biomechanical tolerance of the end plate (57). Brinkmann (45) has shown that bone mineral content and end-plate cross-sectional area can explain much of the variance in tolerance (within 1 kN).

The disc can be subject to damage with sufficient loading. Disc herniation can occur when the spine is subject to compression and positioned in an excessively flexed posture (53). Repeated flexion under moderate compressive loading can also produce disc herniations (46). Excessive anterior-posterior shear may produce avulsion of the lateral annulus (58,59). The torsion tolerance limit of the disc can occur at loads as low as 88 Nm in an intact disc and 54 Nm in the damaged disc (60,61). The literature indicates that when the spine assumes complex spinal postures such as hyperflexion with lateral bending and twisting, disc herniation is likely to occur (62,63).

The biomechanical tolerance of the disc may also be associated with the time of day when the lifting is performed. Snook et al. (64) found that flexion early in the morning was associated with greater risk of pain. Fathallah et al. (65) reported similar results and concluded that risk of injury was greater early in the day when disc hydration was at a high level. Thus, the temporal component of risk associated with biomechanical exposure must be considered when assessing risk.

This discussion has indicated that the tolerance limits of the functional lumbar spinal unit may vary considerably. Adams et al. (66) has described how repeated microfractures of the vertebrae and scarring of the end plate can lead to an interruption of nutrient flow to the disc. This event can result in weakening of the annulus which may permit protrusion into the surrounding structures or spinal instability. The end plate and much of the annulus are not capable of sensing pain. However, once protrusion occurs or instability results in the application of loads of surrounding tissues, inflammatory responses can occur and nociceptors of surrounding tissues can be stimulated, thus initiating a sequence of events associated with pain. Quantitative ergonomics attempts to design work tasks so that these tolerance limits are not exceeded. Thus, although a wide range of tolerance limits are reported for the functional lumbar spinal unit, most authorities have adopted the NIOSH lower limit of 3400 N for compression as the protective limit for most male workers and 75% of that limit for female workers (67). This is the limit at which end-plate microfracture is believed to begin for some workers. Similarly, a limit of 6400 N represents the limit at which 50% of workers would be at risk (68). Contemporary quantitative assessments are recognizing the complex interaction of spine position, frequency, and complex spine forces (compression, shear, and torsion) as more realistic assessments of risk. However, these contemporary ergonomic assessments have not resulted in best practices or standards by governmental agencies to date.

Ligament Tolerance Limits

The literature suggests that ligament tolerances are affected by the load rate (69). Avulsion occurs at low load rates and tearing occurs at high load rates. Hence load rate may explain the increased risk associated with bending motions (velocity) that have been observed in surveillance studies (70) as well as injuries from slips or falls that may be a result of injuries at greater load rates (24). Posture can also play a role in tolerance. Under load, the architecture of the interspinous ligaments can result in significant anterior shear forces on the spine when flexed in a forward bending posture (71). This result is consistent with the recent field observations of risk (10,54–56, 72,73). Studies have identified 60 Nm as the point at which damage begins to occur (74). This finding is consistent with the field observations (55,56) that have found exposures to external load movements of at least 73.6 Nm as associated with high risk of occupationally related low back pain reporting. Similarly, Norman et al. (10) reported nearly 30% greater load movement exposure in those jobs associated with risk of LBP. Mean movement exposure associated with the LBP cases in this study was 182 Nm of total load movement (due to the load lifted plus body segment weights).

Lordic spine curvature may also affect the loading and tolerance of the spinal structures. The research team at the University of Waterloo has shown that when lumbar spinal curvature is maintained during bending the extensor muscles support the shear forces of the torso. If the spine is flexed during bending and posterior ligaments are flexed, then significant shear can be imposed on the ligaments (75–77). Other studies have indicated that shear tolerance (2000 to 2800 N) of the spine can be easily exceeded when the spine is in full flexion (49).

A strong temporal component to ligament recovery appears to exist. Solomonow has found that ligaments require long periods to regain structural integrity and compensatory muscle activities are recruited (78–84). Recovery time has been found to be several-fold the loading duration and can easily exceed the typical work-rest cycles observed in industry.

Facet Joint Tolerance

Failure of the facet joints can occur in response to shear loading. Investigations by McGill have concluded that much of the tissues that load the facets have signif-

icant horizontal loading components and thus place these structures at risk from occupational tasks (85). Cripton et al. have estimated a shear tolerance for the facet joints of 2000 N (86). These findings are consistent with industrial observations that have shown that exposure to lateral motions and shears is associated with increased risk of LBD reporting (10,55,56). Laboratory assessments have confirmed that exposure to high lateral velocities can result in significant lateral shear forces (87).

Torsional forces can also cause the facet joints to fail (60). Exposure to high torsional movements, especially when combined with high velocity, have been associated with increased loading (88–91). Field studies have also shown that these movements are associated with high-risk jobs (10,55,56). Loading when exposed to torsional moments also depends upon the posture of the torso, with greater load observed with more deviated postures from neutral (89). Specific structure loading depends upon specific posture and curvature of the spine since load sharing occurs between the apophyseal joints and the disc (74). Therefore, spine posture dictates both the nature of spine loading and whether damage might occur to the facet joints or the disc.

Adaptation

An important consideration in the load-tolerance relationship is that of adaptation. Wolff's law dictates that tissues adapt and remodel in response to load. In the case of the spine, adaptation in response to load has been acknowledged for bone (92), the ligaments (93), the disc (94), and the vertebrae (95). Adaptation may explain the observation that the greatest risk has been associated with jobs involving both high loading and very low levels of spinal loading, whereas job demands associated with moderate spine loading have the lowest levels of risk (96,97). Hence, there appears to be an ideal zone of loading that minimizes risk of exceeding the tolerance limit.

Psychophysical Tolerance Limits

The tolerance limits of tissue are typically derived from cadaveric studies. While these mechanical limits of performance may be adequate for the analysis of tasks that may lead to an acute trauma event, their application to tasks that may lead to cumulative trauma disorder may be less clear. Since adaptation may play a role, such quantitative analyses of the load-tolerance relationship becomes difficult. In addition, some dynamic tasks such as pushing and pulling may be difficult to characterize through quantitative biomechanical analyses and their injury pathway may be poorly understood.

When mechanical tolerances are not known such as in these circumstances, one approach used to establish tolerance limits has been the psychophysical approach. The psychophysical approach is a means of strength testing where subjects are asked to progressively adjust the amount of load they can push, pull, lift, or carry until they subjectively feel the load is of a magnitude that would be acceptable to them over an 8-hour work shift. Task variables such as lift origin, height, load dimensions, frequency of exertion, push/pull heights, carrying distance, and so forth are all systematically altered so that a database of conditions and the acceptable exertion range is cataloged for a spectrum of male and female subjects. These data are typically presented in tables that indicate the percentage of subjects who would find a particular load acceptable for a given task. Snook et al. have produced extensive description of these tolerances (98–103). An example of this information for pushing activities is shown in Table 17-2.

Few investigations have explored whether the design of work tasks through psychophysical tolerance limits is protective and minimizes low back pain at work. However, Snook (99) has observed that low back-related injury claims were three times more prevalent in jobs exceeding the psychophysically determined strength tolerance of 75% of men compared with jobs demanding less strength.

Physiologic Tolerance Limits

Work tasks requiring high energy expenditure are thought to limit the ability of the body to deliver oxygen to the muscles. When oxygen debt occurs, insufficient release of adenosine triphosphate (ATP) occurs within the muscle and prolonged muscle contractions cannot be sustained. Hence, under high-energy expenditure work conditions, aerobic capacity may be considered as a physiologic tolerance limit for low back pain.

Physiologic criteria for limiting low back pain due to heavy physical work requiring high levels of energy

TABLE 17-2. *Example of psychophysical table used to determine the acceptable load an individual is willing to accept. The table indicates the maximum amount of push force acceptable for males and females under various conditions.*

From Snook SH. The design of manual handling tasks. Ergonomics 1978;21:963–985, with permission.

expenditure have been defined by the NIOSH (104). This document considers an energy expenditure rate of 9.5 kcal per minute as a baseline measure for maximum aerobic lifting capacity. Seventy percent of this baseline is considered the aerobic tolerance limit for work that is defined primarily as "arm work". Of the baseline energy expenditure, 50%, 40%, and 33% are considered the tolerance limits for lifting task durations of 1 hour, 1 to 2 hours, and 2 to 8 hours, respectively.

Minimal epidemiologic evidence is available to support these limits, although Cady et al. have demonstrated the importance of aerobic capacity in back injury for a large sample of firefighters (105,106).

PSYCHOSOCIAL PATHWAYS

A body of literature exists that has attempted to explain how psychosocial factors might relate to the risk of suffering an LBD. Reviews have implicated psychosocial factors as associated with risk (14,107) and some have dismissed the role of biomechanical factors. However, few studies have properly evaluated biomechanical exposure along with psychosocial exposure in these assessments. A recent study by Davis and Heaney (18) has shown that no studies have been able to adequately assess both risk dimensions concurrently.

Recent biomechanical studies (108,109) have indicated that psychosocial stress does have the capacity to influence biomechanical loading. These laboratory studies have demonstrated how individual factors such as personality can interact with perception of psychosocial stress to increase trunk muscle coactivation and subsequent spine loading. Hence, these studies provide evidence that psychosocial stress may influence risk through a biomechanical pathway.

SPINE LOAD ASSESSMENT

An important component of evaluating the load-tolerance relationship, and the potential risk associated with work is an accurate assessment of the loading experienced by a tissue. The review of the tolerance literature suggests that it is important to understand the specific nature of the tissue loading including factors such as compression force, shear force in multiple dimensions, load rates, positions of the spine structures during loading, frequency of loading, and so forth. Thus, accurate and specific information about loading is essential if one is to use this information to assess potential risk associated with occupational tasks.

Presently it is not feasible to directly monitor the loads imposed upon the spine structures and tissues while workers are performing an occupationally related task in the workplace. Instead, indirect means such as biomechanical models are typically used to estimate loading. All biome-

chanical models attempt to understand how exposure to external loads results in internal forces that may exceed a tolerance limit. External forces reside outside the body (e.g., gravity or inertia) and must be overcome by the worker to do work. Internal forces are the structures inside the body (e.g., muscles, ligaments, etc.) that must supply counterforces to support the external load. However, since the internal forces are typically at a biomechanical disadvantage, these internal forces can be very large and result in large force applications on spine tissues. Several approaches to biomechanical modeling have been used for these purposes resulting in different trade-offs between their ability to realistically assess spine loading associated with a task and ease of model use.

The first models used to assess spine loading during occupational tasks were reported in the 1970s. Early models of spine loading made assumptions about which trunk muscles supported the external load held in the hands during a lifting task (110,111). These models assumed that a single muscle vector within the trunk could summarize the internal supporting force (and spine loading) required to counteract an external load lifted by a worker. The model assumes that a lift could be represented by a static equilibrium-lifting situation and that no muscle coactivation occurs among the trunk musculature during lifting. The model employs anthropometric regression relationships to estimate body segment lengths representative of the general population. Two output variables are predicted that can be used in a load-tolerance assessment of work exposure. The first model output is spine compression that is typically compared to the NIOSH compression limits of 3400 N and 6400 N. The second model output is population static strength of six joints. L5/S1 joint strength is used to assess overexertion risk to the back. The model has evolved into a computer-based model (3-dimensional static-strength prediction program [3DSSPP]) and is typically used for general assessments of materials handling tasks involving slow movements where excessive compression loads are suspected of contributing to risk. An example of the computer program is shown in Fig. 17-3. The model can be linked to field observations by videotaping a lifting task and recording the weight of the object lifted. Early risk assessments of the workplace have used this method to assess spine loads on the job (112).

During the 1980s, biomechanical models were expanded to account for the contribution of multiple internal muscles' reactions in response to the lifting of an external load. Much of the spine tolerance literature was beginning to recognize the significance of three-dimensional spine loads as compared to only compression loads in defining potential risk. Thus, biomechanical models were developed that predicted compression forces as well as shear forces imposed upon the spine. The first functional multiple muscle system model proposed for mate-

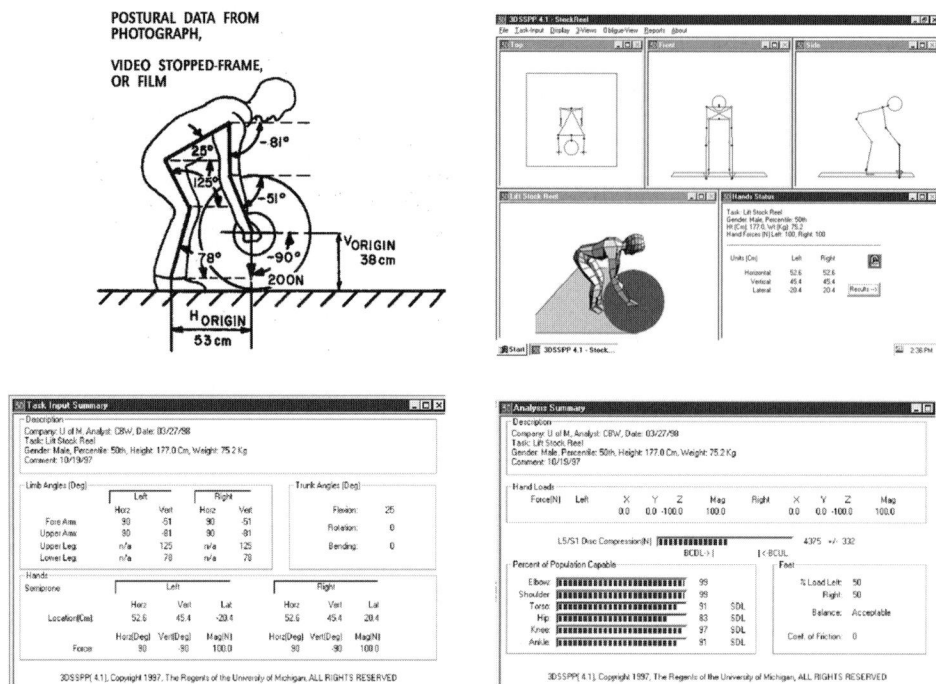

FIG. 17-3. Example of three-dimensional static strength prediction program. (Courtesy of D. Chaffin.)

rial handling assessments was developed by Schultz and Andersson (113). This model demonstrated how loads manipulated outside the body could impose large spinal loads due primarily to the coactivation of trunk muscles necessary to counteract this external load. The modeling approach represented much more realism than previous models, however, the approach resulted in indeterminate solutions (since there were more muscles' forces represented in the model than functional constraints unique solutions became difficult). In order to overcome this problem, modeling efforts attempted to determine which muscles would be active (114–116). These efforts resulted in models that worked well for static representations of a lift but not necessarily for dynamic lifting situations (117).

In order to better account for spine loads under dynamic, complex lifting situations, later efforts attempted to directly monitor muscle activity using electromyography (EMG) as an input to multiple muscle models. EMG eliminated the problem of indeterminacy since specific muscle activities were uniquely defined through the neural activation of each muscle. These biologically assisted models were not only able to accurately assess compression and shear spine loads for specific occupationally related movements (88,89,118–129) but are also able to predict differences among individuals so that variations in loading among a population

could be assessed (87,108,130–133) (Fig. 17-4). Validation measures suggest that these models have excellent external as well as internal validity (133,134). Granata and Marras (135) demonstrated the importance of accounting for trunk muscle coactivation when assessing spine loading and found that not accounting for coactivation could result in miscalculations of spinal loading by up to 70%.

The disadvantage of biologically assisted models is that they require EMG recordings that are often not tolerated well in the workplace. Therefore many of the studies of loadings associated with the spine during work have been performed under laboratory conditions and have attempted to assess specific aspects of the work that may be common to many work conditions. Several efforts used EMG-assisted models to assess three-dimensional spine loading during materials handling activities (87,118,123,136–138). There are many examples of information provided from these in-depth analyses using biologically assisted models. Figure 17-5 shows the difference in spine compression as subjects lift with one hand versus two hands as a function of lift asymmetry (118). This figure indicates that compressive loading of the spine is not simply a matter of load-weight lifted. Significant trade-offs occur as a function of asymmetry and the number of hands involved with the lift. The concept of trade-offs among workplace factors was reinforced in a study that evaluated order-selecting activi-

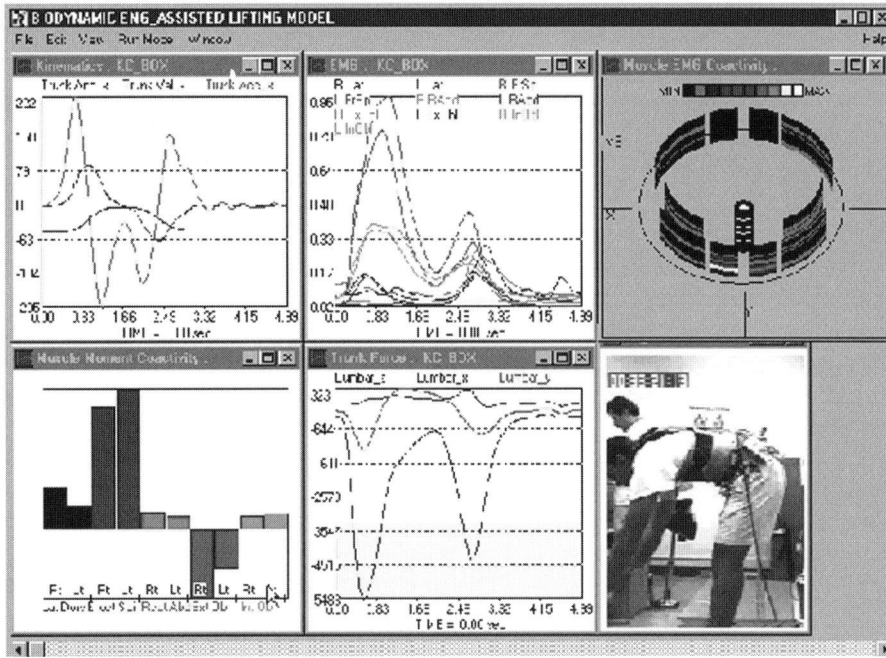

FIG. 17-4. Electromyography (EMG)-assisted model used to evaluate spine loading during simulated work activities. Sample window panels clockwise from upper left: spine position, velocity, and acceleration during task, EMG activities of 10 trunk muscles, muscle coactivation representation, movements imposed on the spine by each muscle, and video of task activity.

ties in a laboratory setting (139). Some of the results from this study are displayed in Table 17-3. This table shows the interaction between load weight, location of the lift (region on the pallet), and presence of handles on spine compression (benchmark). This analysis indicates that all three factors significantly affected the loading on the spine. Another study indicated the trade-offs between spine compression and shear loads as a function of how many hands were involved in the lift, whether both feet were in contact with

the ground, lift origin, and height of a bin from which subjects were lifted (140) (Table 17-4). Similar studies have also helped to understand spine loading trade-offs associated with team lifting (141), patient lifting (Table 17-5) (142), the assessment of lifting belts (77,143–146), and while using lifting assistance devices (147). Efforts have also been made to apply the in-depth knowledge obtained from these biologically assisted models through regression models of workplace characteristics (148,149). Recently,

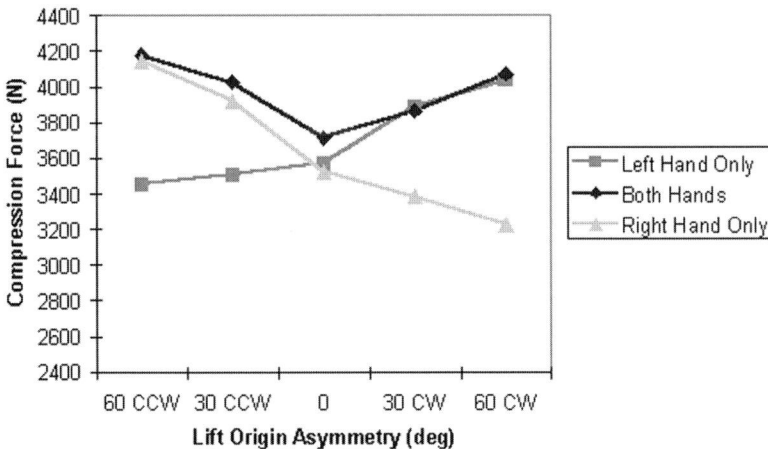

FIG. 17-5. Mean peak compression force as a function of lift asymmetry [clockwise *(CW)* versus counterclockwise *(CCW)*] and hand(s) used to lift load. Results derived from electromyography-assisted model simulation of tasks (118).

TABLE 17-3. *Percentage of lifts during order selection tasks within various spine compression benchmark zones as a function of the interaction between load weight, location of the lift (region on the pallet), and presence of handles. Spine loads estimated by an EMG-assisted model (139).*

Region on the pallet	Spine compression benchmarks	Box weight					
		18.2 kg		22.7 kg		27.3 kg	
		Handles	No handles	Handles	No handles	Handles	No handles
Front-top	<3,400 N	100.0	100.0	100.0	99.2	99.2	100.0
	3,400–6,400 N	0.0	0.0	0.0	0.8	0.8	0.0
	>6,400 N	0.0	0.0	0.0	0.0	0.0	0.0
Back-top	<3,400 N	98.2	89.1	84.5	76.4	83.6	67.3
	3,400–6,400 N	1.8	10.9	15.5	23.6	16.4	32.7
	>6,400 N	0.0	0.0	0.0	0.0	0.0	0.0
Front-middle	<3,400 N	98.7	91.3	94.7	82.7	92.6	76.0
	3,400–6,400 N	1.3	8.7	5.3	17.3	7.4	23.3
	>6,400 N	0.0	0.0	0.0	0.0	0.0	0.7
Back-middle	<3,400 N	88.7	82.0	80.7	75.3	76.7	64.7
	3,400–6,400 N	11.3	18.0	19.3	24.7	23.3	34.6
	>6,400 N	0.0	0.0	0.0	0.0	0.0	0.7
Front-bottom	<3,400 N	45.3	30.0	29.3	14.0	16.0	3.3
	3,400–6,400 N	52.0	62.0	62.7	65.3	72.0	66.0
	>6,400 N	2.7	8.0	8.0	20.7	12.0	30.7
Back-bottom	<3,400 N	35.3	24.0	30.0	10.7	9.3	2.0
	3,400–6,400 N	60.7	67.3	56.7	65.3	71.3	62.0
	>6,400 N	4.0	8.7	13.3	24.0	19.3	36.0

EMG, electromyogram; N, Newton.

efforts have also employed these models to assess the role of psychosocial factors, personality, and mental processing on spine loading (108,109).

Efforts have also attempted to use stability as criteria to govern detailed biologically assisted biomechanical models of the torso (84,150–157). One potential injury pathway for LBDs suggests that the unnatural rotation of a single spine segment that may create loads on passive tissue or other muscle tissue can result in irritation or injury (85). Much of the work performed in this area

to date has been directed toward static response of the trunk as well as sudden loading responses (151,152,154, 155,158,159).

ASSESSMENT METHODS AND THE IDENTIFICATION OF LBD RISK AT WORK

Previous sections have introduced methods used in studies of the assessment of spine loads in response to various work-related factors that are common to many

TABLE 17-4. *Spine forces (means and standard deviations for lateral shear, anterior-posterior shear, and compression) as a function of the number of hands used, the number of feet supporting the body during the lift, the region of a pallet and the height of a bin when lifting items from an industrial bin (140)*

Independent measures	Condition	Lateral shear force (N)	Anterior-posterior shear force (N)	Compression force (N)
Hand	One-hand	472.2 (350.5)[a]	1093.3 (854.7)	6033.6 (2981.2)
	Two-hand	233.8 (216.9)[a]	1136.9 (964.1)	5742.3 (1712.3)
Feet	One-foot	401.7 (335.1)[a]	1109.4 (856.1)	6138.6 (2957.5)[a]
	Two-feet	304.3 (285.1)[a]	1120.8 (963.3)	5637.3 (2717.9)
Region	Upper front	260.2 (271.7)[b]	616.6 (311.1)[b]	3765.7 (1452.8)[b]
	Upper back	317 (290.8)[b]	738.0 (500.0)[b]	5418.1 (2364.2)[c]
	Lower front	414.4 (335.0)[c]	1498.3 (1037.8)[c]	6839.8 (2765.4)[d]
	Lower back	420.4 (329.0)[c]	1607.5 (1058.4)[c]	7528.2 (2978.4)[e]
Bin height	94 cm	361.9 (328)	1089.9 (800.8)	5795.8 (2660.4)
	61 cm	344.1 (301)	1140.3 (1009.1)	5980.2 (3027.4)

[a]Indicates significant difference at $\alpha = 0.05$.

[b-e]Region has four experimental conditions, therefore letters b–e are used to indicate which regions are significantly different from one another. Regions with different letters were significantly different at $\alpha = 0.05$.

N, Newton.

TABLE 17-5. *Spine loads estimated during patient transfer as a function of the number of lifters and the transfer technique (142)*

		Spinal loads		
Transfer technique		Maximum lateral shear force (N)	Maximum A-P shear force (N)	Maximum compression force (N)
Lifting phase				
One-person				
	Hug	1060.7 (697.6)[B]	908.5 (555.9)[B]	6336.3 (2044)[C]
Two-person				
Left-side lifter	Hook	731.7 (442.6)[A]	955.6 (436.5)[B]	4948.2 (1598.6)[B]
	Gait belt	702.6 (495.1)[A]	916.7 (549.1)[B]	4895.5 (1633.1)[B]
Right-side lifter	Hook	697.1 (435.8)[A]	892.8 (495.6)[A]	4455.8 (1539.9)[A]
	Gait belt	664.2 (461.5)[A]	985.7 (567.6)[B]	4600.9 (1437.6)[AB]
Lowering phase				
One-person				
	Hug	1127.9 (621.6)[B]	1111.69 (614.6)[C]	6007.9 (1859.2)[C]
Two-person				
Left-side lifter	Hook	845.2 (489.0)[A]	1020.8 (503.0)[C]	4713.4 (1640.1)[B]
	Gait belt	781.4 (506.1)[A]	1005.4 (523.8)[C]	4597.5 (1454.9)[AB]
Right-side lifter	Hook	830.4 (463.9)[A]	935.6 (478.9)[A]	4314.1 (1694.4)[A]
	Gait belt	815.5 (469.8)[A]	1097.4 (487.6)[B]	4571.8 (1529.7)[AB]

*Different Alpha Characters Indicate Significant Difference at $p = .05$.
N, Newton.

workplaces (e.g., one-hand versus two-hand lifting). These studies have resulted in a rich body of literature that can be used as a guide for the proper design of many work situations. However, a need still exists for assessing unique work situations that may not have been explored in these laboratory studies. The more robust methods for assessing spine loads (e.g., EMG-assisted models) may not be usable for assessment on the job since they require extensive instrumentation. This section reviews the methods and tools available for the assessment of LBD risk at the work site along with a review of the literature that supports their usage.

Three-Dimensional Static Strength Prediction Program

The three-dimensional static strength prediction program (3DSSPP) has been described previously. This program considers the load-tolerance relationship from two aspects. An estimate of spine compression is generated and compared to the generally accepted tolerance limits of 3400 N. In addition, the load imposed by the task on six joints is compared to the static strength of the muscle groups. This last relationship has been defined as a lifting strength rating (LSR) and was used to prospectively assess low back injuries in an industrial environment (97). The LSR is defined as the weight of the maximum load lifted on the job divided by the lifting strength measured in the same lifting posture for a large, strong man. The study concluded that "the incidence rate of low back pain [was] correlated [monotonically] with higher lifting strength requirements as determined by assessment of

both the location and magnitude of the load lifted." This was one of the first quantitative ergonomic studies to conclude that not only was load lifting potentially hazardous, but it was also important to consider the load location when assessing risk. The study also suggested that exposure to moderate lifting frequencies appeared to be protective, whereas, high or low rates of lifting were common in jobs with greater reports of back injury.

An industrial study using both the LSR and estimates of back compression forces observed jobs over 3 years in 5 large industrial plants where 2,934 material handling tasks were evaluated (112). The results suggested a positive correlation between the lifting strength ratio and back incidence rates. The study also reported that musculoskeletal injuries were twice as likely for predicted spine compression forces that exceeded 6800 N. However, this was not true for back incidents specifically. The study also suggested that prediction of risk was best associated with the most stressful tasks (as opposed to indices that represent risk aggregation).

Job Demand Index

A similar concept to the LSR was reported by Ayoub et al. (160) in terms of a job severity index (JSI). This index considers the ratio of the job demands relative to the lifting capacities of the worker. Job demands include factors such as the weight of the object lifted, the frequency of lifting, exposure time, and lifting task origins and destinations. A comprehensive task analysis is required to assess job demands. The worker capacity includes the strength and body size of the worker. Strength is determined through psychophysical testing. A prospective study using the JSI was performed by Liles et al. (161). Results suggested a threshold of a job demand relative to worker strength above which the risk of low back injury increased. The authors suggest that this method could identify the more costly injuries.

NIOSH Lifting Guide and Revised Lifting Equation

The NIOSH has developed two tools to help industry assess the risk associated with materials handling jobs. The objective of both tools was to "prevent or reduce the occurrence of lifting-related low back pain among workers" (162). Both tools considered biomechanical, physiologic, and psychophysical limits in their development.

The first tool was a guide based upon biomechanical, physiologic, and psychophysical information (68). This method assessed job characteristics and assessed the magnitude of the load that must be lifted for spine compression to reach 3400 N (the action limit, or AL) or 6400 N (the maximum permissible limit, or MPL). The AL was defined as the tissue tolerance where damage begins to occur in the spine. In theory, to be protective, work tasks should be designed so that the load lifted by the worker was below the calculated AL limit. The AL was determined through a functional equation that considered four discounting factors multiplied by a constant. The constant (90 lbs or 40 kg) was assumed to be the magnitude of the weight lifted under ideal lifting conditions that would result in a spine compression of 3400 N. The four discounting factors consist of: (a) horizontal distance of the load from the spine, (b) the vertical height of the load off the floor, (c) the vertical travel distance of the load, and (d) the frequency of lifting. These discounting factors were governed by functional relationships that reduced the magnitude of the allowable load (constant). An MPL was determined by multiplying the AL by 3. It was assumed that if the load lifted by the worker exceeded the MPL, more than 50% of the workers were at risk and engineering controls were needed. If the load lifted by the worker was between the AL and the MPL then the task placed less than 50% of the workforce at risk and either engineering or administrative controls were required. The guide was designed to be used for primarily sagittally symmetric lifts that were slow and smooth. Only one evaluation of the guide's effectiveness could be found in the literature (73). Comparing the predictions with historical data of back injury reporting in industry, this evaluation indicated an odds ratio (OR) of 3.5 with good specificity but low sensitivity.

A revision of this method was published in 1993 and has become known as the "revised NIOSH lifting equation" (162). The revision was intended to consider asymmetric lifting situations as well as tasks with various types of coupling (handles). The revised equation was similar in form to the 1981 guide in that it included a load

constant that was mediated by several work characteristic "multipliers." However, several components of the equation were different. First, the value calculated was a recommended weight limit (RWL). If the load lifted by the worker was below this value the load was considered safe. Second, the load constant was reduced to 23 kg or 51 lbs (from the 40 kg or 90 lbs in the 1981 guide). Third, the form of the multipliers was changed and the functional relationship between discounting and the workplace measure was slightly more liberal for the four factors originally contained in the 1981 guide (horizontal distance, vertical distance, vertical travel distance, and frequency). This was done to compensate for a lower load constant. Fourth, two new multipliers (task asymmetry and coupling) were added to the equation. Once the RWL is calculated for a given work situation, it is compared (as a denominator) to the load lifted by the worker to form a lifting index (LI). If the LI is less than the value 1, the job is considered safe. If the LI is greater than 1, then risk is present. LI values above 3 are thought to place nearly all workers at increased risk (104).

Two assessments of the revised equation to injury reporting have been performed. One assessment compared the ability of the tool to identify high- and low-risk jobs based upon a historical database (73). This assessment yielded an OR of 3.1. Further analyses indicated higher sensitivity than the 1981 guide but lower specificity. A second analysis using a different data set assessed ORs as a function of the LI. For LIs between 1 and 3 the ORs ranged from 1.54 to 2.45, indicating an increasing OR with increasing low back pain reporting. However, the OR for LIs over 3 was lower (OR of 1.63) indicating a nonmonotonic relationship between the LI and risk.

Video-Based Biomechanical Models

Norman et al. (10) used a quasi-dynamic two-dimensional biomechanical model to assess cumulative biomechanical loading of the spine in 234 automotive assembly workers. This study identified four independent factors for LBD reporting consisting of integrated load movement (over a work shift), hand forces, peak shear force on the spine, and peak trunk velocity. They concluded that workers in the top 25% of loading exposure on all risk factors were at about six times the risk of reporting back pain than those in the bottom 25% of loading.

Lumbar Motion Monitor Risk Assessment

In an attempt to consider the contribution of trunk dynamics as well as the traditional biomechanical factors in workplace assessment of risk, Marras et al. (55,56) biomechanically evaluated over 400 industrial jobs (with documented LBD risk history) by observing 114 workplace and worker-related variables. Of the variables explored, exposure to load movement (load magnitude × distance of load from spine) was found to be the single most powerful predictor of LBD reporting. This study also identified 16 trunk kinematic variables that resulted in statistically significant ORs associated with risk of LBD reporting in the workplace. None of the single kinematic variables were as strong a predictor as load moment, however, when load moment was combined with three kinematic variables (relating to the three dimensions of trunk motion) along with an exposure frequency measure, a strong multiple logistic regression model resulted that described reporting of back disorder well (OR of 10.7). The analysis indicated that risk was multivariate in nature and that exposure to the combination of the five variables described reporting well. This information was incorporated into a functional risk model (Fig. 17-6) that accounted for trade-offs between risk variables. For example, a job task that exposes a worker to low magnitude of load moment can represent a high-risk situation if the other four variables in the model were of sufficient magnitude. The model has been validated in a prospective workplace intervention study (72). The risk model has been linked with a lumbar motion monitor (LMM) (Fig. 17-7) in a computer program to document trunk motion exposure on the job.

When the findings from these studies are considered in conjunction with previous epidemiologic studies in the workplace (54), it is clear that work associated with activity performed in nonneutral postures increases the risk to the back. Collectively these studies indicate that as trunk posture becomes more extreme or the trunk motion becomes more rapid, reporting of back disorder is greater.

These results suggest that occupational risk of LBD is associated with mechanical loading of the spine and suggest that when tasks involve greater three-dimensional loading, the association with risk becomes much stronger.

A database of 126 jobs including LMM information was evaluated by Fathallah et al. (70) to precisely quantify and assess the complex trunk motions of groups with varying degrees of LBD reporting. They determined that groups with greater reporting rates exhibited complex trunk motion patterns involving high magnitudes of combined trunk velocities, especially at extreme sagittal flexion, whereas the low-risk groups did not exhibit these patterns. This study suggested that elevated levels of complex simultaneous velocity patterns along with key workplace factors (load moment and frequency) were unique to those with increased LBD risk.

Workplace Assessment Summary

The findings of recent quantitative studies used to assess workplace LBD risk using available workplace assessment tools are summarized in Table 17-6. The studies are consistent in that even though these studies have not evaluated spinal loading directly, the exposure measures included were indirect indicators of spinal load and suggest that as these risk factors increase in magnitude the risk increases. Load location or strength ratings both appear to be indicators of the magnitude of the load imposed upon the spine. The exposure metrics (load location, kinematics, and three-dimensional analyses) are important from a biomechanical standpoint because they

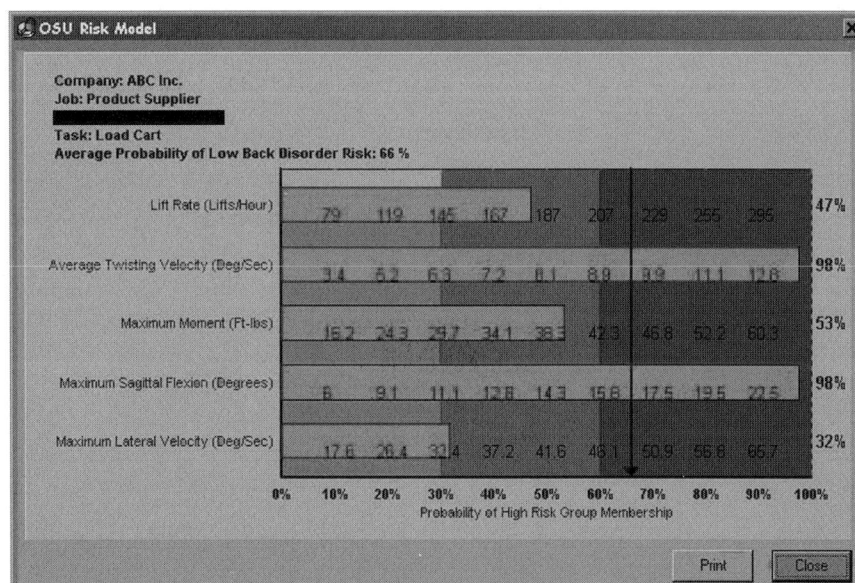

FIG. 17-6. Lumbar motion monitor risk model. The probability risk of high risk (of low back pain) group membership is quantitatively indicated for a particular task for each of five risk factors indicating how much exposure is too much exposure for a particular risk factor. The *vertical arrow* indicates the overall probability of high-risk group membership due to the combination of risk factors.

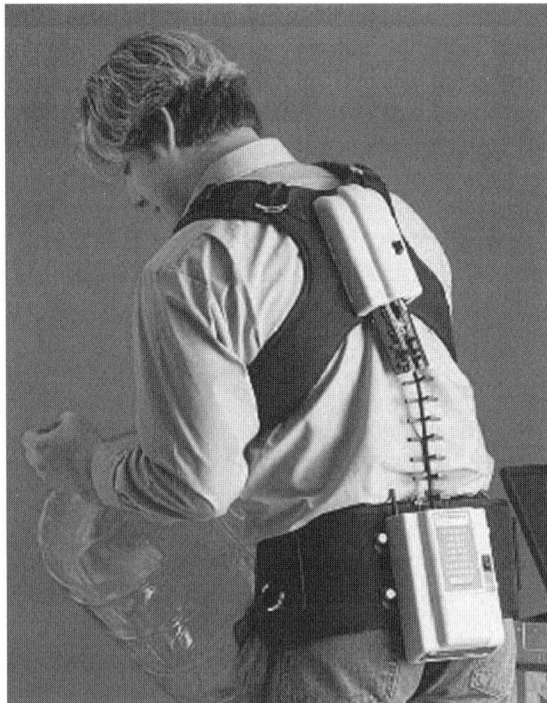

FIG. 17-7. The lumbar motion monitor used to track trunk kinematics during occupational activities.

at the workplace, associations between biomechanical factors and risk of LBD reporting are evident. Several common components of biomechanical risk assessment can be derived from these studies. First, increased LBD reporting is associated with work primarily when the specific load location relative to the body (load moment or load location) is quantified in some way. Most studies have shown that these factors are closely associated with increased low back pain reports. Second, many studies have shown that increased reporting of low back pain can be well characterized when the three-dimensional kinematic demands of the work are described. Finally, nearly all of these assessments have demonstrated that risk is multidimensional in that there is a synergy among risk factors that is often associated with increased reporting of low back pain. Several studies have also suggested that some of these relationships are nonmonotonic. In summary, these efforts have suggested that the better the lift characteristics can be characterized in terms of biomechanical demand the better the association with risk.

mediate the ability of the trunk's internal structures to support the external load. As these metrics change they can change the nature of the loading on the back's internal structures.

Collectively, these studies demonstrate that when meaningful biomechanical assessments are performed

THE PROCESS OF IMPLEMENTING ERGONOMIC CHANGE

Recent findings have shown that there are substantial links between biomechanical loading of the spine and psychosocial factors (108,109). Hence, ergonomic changes to the work environment must consider biomechanical loading as well as the psychosocial environment. A review of ergonomic interventions (163) has shown that such interventions can reduce workers'

TABLE 17-6. *Summary of recent field evaluations of low back disorder risk factors and strength of association with risk (odds ratio). The more precisely the lifting requirements (e.g., load location, moment, etc.) are specified the better the association with risk*

		Risk factors identified								
Authors	No. of jobs	Capacity/demand ratio	Load location	Load moment	Frequency	Kinematics	2-D	3-D	Multiple factors	Odds ratio (CI)
Punnett et al., 1991	95 case 124 refferant					x		x	x	Max flex 5.7 (1.6–20.4) Twist/lat 5.9 (1.6–21.4)
Marras et al., 1993/1995	403		x	x	x	x		x	x	5 var = 10.7 (4.9–23.6)
Norman et al., 1998	104 cases 130 refferant			x		x	x		x	4 var = 5.7 (1–31.2)
Waters et al., 1999	36	x	x	x	x			x	x	Max OR = 2.45 (1.29–4.85)

CI, confidence interval; OR, odds ratio.

compensation costs if they are implemented correctly. However, experience has also shown that unless workers are accepting of workplace redesign, the interventions will not be effective.

A proven method to maximize the effectiveness of workplace interventions is through the implementation of an ergonomics process. These processes are designed to address occupational health issues in a timely manner and create an environment that fosters worker acceptance of engineering interventions. Ergonomics processes grew out of efforts to control musculoskeletal disorders in meat packing facilities (164). The logic behind this approach is to develop a system or process to identify and correct musculoskeletal problems associated with work. It is considered a process instead of a program since it is intended to become an ongoing surveillance and correction component of the business operation instead of a one-time effort.

The process is intended to encourage management and labor to communicate and work as a team to accomplish a common goal of worker health. In order to address the psychosocial issues in the workplace, a key component of an ergonomics process is worker empowerment. Workers are encouraged to take an active role in the process and take control and ownership of work design suggestions and changes. Thus, the process encourages a participatory approach. Benefits of such an approach include increased worker motivation, job satisfaction, and greater acceptance of change. The goal is to create an environment where the success of the operation is the objective as opposed to the interests of any given individual.

There are several functions of a successful ergonomics process. These functions include: management leadership and commitment, employee participation, job analysis leading to injury prevention and control, training, medical management, program evaluation, and documentation. A successful process begins with the creation of an ergonomics committee. The committee composition should be balanced between management and labor to encourage a balanced effort to work toward the common goal. Committee members should include those involved with the design of work layout as well as those empowered to dictate scheduling. In addition, labor representatives to the committee should include those employees who have broad experience with many of the jobs in the facility as well as those employees who can communicate well with the majority of the other workers. This committee then becomes the center of all ergonomic-related activities within the facility.

The ergonomics process is actually a system where the different components of the system interact to produce the desired effect. The interactions within this system are shown in Fig. 17-8. This figure indicates that the ergonomics committee is at the heart of the interactions with all the components of the process. The process begins with management involvement. Ergonomics processes must be driven from the top down. Thus, management

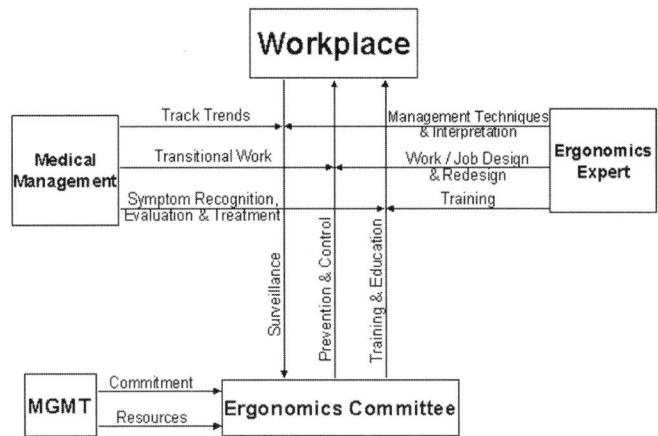

FIG. 17-8. The interaction of elements within an ergonomics process.

must initiate the process and visibly demonstrate commitment to the process. In addition, management must provide resources to the committee. These resources should include financial resources so that physical interventions can be implemented as well as access to information such as injury records, production schedules, and so forth.

As indicated in Figure 17-8, the fundamental responsibilities of the ergonomics committee are threefold. First, the committee must monitor the workplace to determine where clusters of work-related musculoskeletal injuries are located. Techniques for surveillance include injury reports as well as surveying workers for symptom recording. In order that ergonomic efforts become preventive rather than reactive it is important to solicit the cooperation of all workers in this effort. Medical personnel can help facilitate this effort by helping the committee interpret the trends in an objective fashion. The second responsibility of the committee is the prevention and control of occupationally related musculoskeletal disorders. For the purposes of LBD, the techniques discussed earlier can be employed to help isolate the nature of any potential problems associated with the design of work. The issue of interest here is often "how much exposure to risk factors is too much exposure?" Thus, quantitative methods can be used to help determine which changes are needed and their likely impact. As indicated in the figure, ergonomic experts can be useful in assisting the committee in performing these assessments. The third responsibility of the committee is the training and education of the workers. Several levels of training are typically necessary. All workers should receive short duration awareness training to inform them that an ergonomics process is in place, familiarize them with risk factors, and explain to them how to interact with the process. In addition, workers should receive training as to the types of symptoms that need to be reported to the committee for prevention to be successful. Higher level training should also be provided to engineers and supervisors. In general, training should be of sufficient detail so that management understands the functioning of the process and so that they do not become an impediment to the process success. Both medical professionals and ergonomic specialists can facilitate these activities.

Medical management and the ergonomic experts serve as resources to the committee for the process responsibilities. The goal of a process is not to make the ergonomics committee into ergonomics experts, but to encourage them to actively involve experts to accomplish the goals of the process. These experts can be valuable in terms of advising the committee as to how and when to perform surveillance activities as well as suggesting appropriate interventions for a given situation.

It is imperative that the program be evaluated regularly to justify its continuation. Issues such as the achievement of program goals, reductions of musculoskeletal disorders, hazard reduction, and employee feedback should be considered. Corrective actions should be taken in response to the evaluation. Finally, documentation is an important part of a successful program. Records should be kept that document the changes made to the workplace and that can serve as justification of expenditures. These records can also be used to transfer knowledge to new team members.

Ergonomics processes can have a significant impact on musculoskeletal risk, but only if the process is performed correctly and maintained. Keys to process maintenance include strong direction, realistic goals, establishment of a system to address employee concerns, early intervention success, and publicity for the intervention.

CONCLUSIONS

This review has shown that LBDs are common in the workplace and associated with occupational tasks when the risk factors of manual materials handling, bending and twisting, and whole-body vibration are present. The load-tolerance relationship represents a sound biomechanically plausible avenue to support the epidemiologic findings. Sophisticated biologically assisted biomechanical models have been developed that have been used to quantitatively assess many situations (in the laboratory) that are common to workplaces. There are also a host of quantitative workplace assessment tools available to assess risk directly at the work site. These tools appear to be most sensitive if they are multifactorial in nature and assess the load movement exposure and torso kinematic responses to work situations in three-dimensional space. The more precisely these job requirements are documented the better the association with risk. Finally, the implementation of ergonomic change in the workplace must consider psychosocial issues in the workplace in order to foster worker acceptance of change. The imple-

mentation of an ergonomics process can be useful for these purposes.

REFERENCES

1. Tichauer ER. The biomechanical basis of ergonomics. New York: John Wiley and Sons, 1978.
2. Government Accounting Office. Worker protection: private sector ergonomics programs yield positive results. Washington, DC: Government Accounting Office, 1997.
3. National Research Council. Musculoskeletal disorders and the workplace: low back and upper extremity. Washington DC, National Academy Press, 2001.
4. National Institute for Occupational Safety and Health. Worker health chartbook. Cincinnati, 2000.
5. Vingard E, Mortimer M, Wiktorin C, et al. Seeking care for low back pain in the general population: a two-year follow-up study: results from the MUSIC-Norrtalje study. Spine 2002;27:2159–2165.
6. Guo HR, Tanaka S, Cameron LL, et al. Back pain among workers in the United States: national estimates and workers at high risk. Am J Ind Med 1995;28:591–602.
7. Guo HR, Tanaka S, Halperin WE, et al. Back pain prevalence in US industry and estimates of lost workdays. Am J Public Health 1999;89:1029–1035.
8. National Institute for Occupational Safety and Health. Musculoskeletal disorders and workplace factors. Washington, DC: Department of Health and Human Services, 1997.
9. Hoogendoorn WE, van Poppel MN, Bongers PM, et al. Physical load during work and leisure time as risk factors for back pain [see Comments]. Scand J Work Environ Health 1999;25:387–403.
10. Norman R, Wells R, Neumann P, et al. A comparison of peak vs cumulative physical work exposure risk factors for the reporting of low back pain in the automotive industry. Clin Biomech (Bristol, Avon) 1998;13:561–573.
11. Kumar S. Cumulative load as a risk factor for back pain. Spine 1990;15:1311–1316.
12. Videman T, Nurminen M, Troup JD. 1990 Volvo Award in clinical sciences. Lumbar spinal pathology in cadaveric material in relation to history of back pain, occupation, and physical loading. Spine 1990;15:728–740.
13. Seidler A, Bolm-Audorff U, Heiskel H, et al. The role of cumulative physical work load in lumbar spine disease: risk factors for lumbar osteochondrosis and spondylosis associated with chronic complaints. Occup Environ Med 2001;58:735–746.
14. Bongers PM, de Winter CR, Kompier MA, et al. Psychosocial factors at work and musculoskeletal disease. Scand J Work Environ Health 1993;19:297–312.
15. Karasek R, Brisson C, Kawakami N, et al. The Job Content Questionnaire (JCQ): an instrument for internationally comparative assessments of psychosocial job characteristics. J Occup Health Psychol 1998;3:322–355.
16. van Poppel MN, Koes BW, Deville W, et al. Risk factors for back pain incidence in industry: a prospective study. Pain 1998;77:81–86.
17. Hoogendoorn WE, van Poppel MN, Bongers PM, et al. Systematic review of psychosocial factors at work and private life as risk factors for back pain. Spine 2000;25:2114–2125.
18. Davis KG, Heaney CA. The relationship between psychosocial work characteristics and low back pain: underlying methodological issues. Clin Biomech (Bristol, Avon) 2000;15:389–406.
19. Frank JW, Kerr MS, Brooker AS, et al. Disability resulting from occupational low back pain. Part I: What do we know about primary prevention? A review of the scientific evidence on prevention before disability begins. Spine 1996;21:2908–2917.
20. Waddell G. The back pain revolution. Edinburgh: Churchill Livingstone, 1999.
21. Waddell G. Biopsychosocial analysis of low back pain. Baillieres Clin Rheumatol 1992;6:523–557.
22. Krause N, Ragland DR, Fisher JM, et al. Psychosocial job factors, physical workload, and incidence of work-related spinal injury: a 5-year prospective study of urban transit operators. Spine 1998;23:2507–2516.
23. Tubach F, Leclerc A, Landre MF, et al. Risk factors for sick leave due

to low back pain: a prospective study. J Occup Environ Med 2002;44:451–458.

24. McGill SM. The biomechanics of low back injury: implications on current practice in industry and the clinic. J Biomech 1997;30:4 65–475.

25. Bogduk N. The anatomical basis for spinal pain syndromes. J Manipulative Physiol Ther 1995;18:603–605.

26. Cavanaugh JM. Neural mechanisms of lumbar pain. Spine 1995;20:1804–1909.

27. Cavanaugh JM, Ozaktay AC, Yamashita T, et al. Mechanisms of low back pain: a neurophysiologic and neuroanatomic study. Clin Orthop 1997;166–180.

28. Kallakuri S, Cavanaugh JM, Blagoev DC. An immunohistochemical study of innervation of lumbar spinal dura and longitudinal ligaments. Spine 1998;23:403–411.

29. Siddall PJ, Cousins MJ. Spinal pain mechanisms. Spine 1997;22:98–104.

30. Dwyer A, Aprill C, Bogduk N. Cervical zygapophyseal joint pain patterns. I: A study in normal volunteers. Spine 1990;15:453–457.

31. Ozaktay AC, Cavanaugh JM, Blagoev DC, et al. Phospholipase A2-induced electrophysiologic and histologic changes in rabbit dorsal lumbar spine tissues. Spine 1995;20:2659–2668.

32. Yamashita T, Minaki Y, Ozaktay AC, et al. A morphological study of the fibrous capsule of the human lumbar facet joint. Spine 1996;21:538–543.

33. Bogduk N. The lumbar disc and low back pain. Neurosurg Clin N Am 1991;2:791–806.

34. Cavanaugh JM, Kallakuri S, Ozaktay AC. Innervation of the rabbit lumbar intervertebral disc and posterior longitudinal ligament. Spine 1995;20:2080–2085.

35. Chen C, Cavanaugh JM, Ozaktay AC, et al. Effects of phospholipase A2 on lumbar nerve root structure and function. Spine 1997;22:1057–1064.

36. Ozaktay AC, Kallakuri S, Cavanaugh JM. Phospholipase A2 sensitivity of the dorsal root and dorsal root ganglion. Spine 1998;23:1297–1306.

37. Dinarello CA. Proinflammatory cytokines. Chest 2000;118:503–508.

38. Jager M. Biomechanisches Modell des Menschen zu Analyse und Beureilung der Belastung der Wirbelsaule bie der Handhabung von Lasten in VDI Berlage, Vol. 33, Reihe 17 Boeechnik Nr. 1987.

39. Fyhrie DP, Schaffler MB. Failure mechanisms in human vertebral cancellous bone. Bone 1994;15:105–109.

40. Gunning JL, Callaghan JP, McGill SM. Spinal posture and prior loading history modulate compressive strength and type of failure in the spine: a biomechanical study using a porcine cervical spine model. Clin Biomech (Bristol, Avon) 2001;16:471–480.

41. Kirkaldy-Willis WH. The three phases of the spectrum of degenerative diseases. In: Kirkaldy-Willis WH, ed. Managing low back pain. New York: Churchill-Livingstone, 1998.

42. Brinkmann P. Pathology of the vertebral column. Ergonomics 1985;28:77–80.

43. Moore RJ. The vertebral end-plate: what do we know? European Spine J 2000;9:92–96.

44. Siddall PJ, Cousins MJ. Neurobiology of pain. Int Anesthesiol Clin 1997;35:1–26.

45. Brinkmann P, Biggermann M, Hilweg D. Fatigue fracture of human lumbar vertebrae. Clin Biomech (Bristol, Avon) 1988;3:S1–S23.

46. Callaghan JP, McGill SM. Intervertebral disc herniation: studies on a porcine model exposed to highly repetitive flexion/extension motion with compressive force. Clin Biomech (Bristol, Avon) 2001;16:28–37.

47. Holmes AD, Hukins DW, Freemont AJ. End-plate displacement during compression of lumbar vertebra-disc-vertebra segments and the mechanism of failure. Spine 1993;18:128–135.

48. Begeman PC, Visarius H, Nolte LP, et al. Viscoelastic shear responses of the cadaver and hybrid III lumbar response. In: Proceedings of the 38th Stapp Car Crash Conference; Ft. Lauderdale, FL; 1994.

49. Krypton P, Berlemen U, Visarino H, et al. Response of the lumbar spine due to shear loading. In: Kang KH, ed. Injury prevention through biomechanics. Wayne State University, Detroit, Michigan, May 4–5

50. Vernon-Roberts B, Pirie CJ. Degenerative changes in the intervertebral discs of the lumbar spine and their sequelae. Rheumatol Rehabil 1977;16:13–21.

51. Vernon-Roberts B, Pirie CJ. Healing trabecular microfractures in the bodies of lumbar vertebrae. Ann Rheum Dis 1973;32:406–412.

52. Kornberg M. MRI diagnosis of traumatic Schmorl's node. A case report. Spine 1988;13:934–935.

53. Adams MA, Hutton WC. Prolapsed intervertebral disc. A hyperflexion injury 1981 Volvo Award in Basic Science. Spine 1982;7:184–191.

54. Punnett L, Fine LJ, Keyserling WM, et al. Back disorders and nonneutral trunk postures of automobile assembly workers. Scand J Work Environ Health 1991;17:337–346.

55. Marras WS, Lavender SA, Leurgans SE, et al. Biomechanical risk factors for occupationally related low back disorders. Ergonomics 1995;38:377–410.

56. Marras WS, Lavender SA, Leurgans SE, et al. The role of dynamic three-dimensional trunk motion in occupationally-related low back disorders. The effects of workplace factors, trunk position, and trunk motion characteristics on risk of injury. Spine 1993;18:617–628.

57. Jager M, Luttmann A, Laurig W. Lumbar load during one-hand bricklaying. Int J Industr Ergo 1991;8:261–277.

58. Yingling VR, McGill SM. Anterior shear of spinal motion segments. Kinematics, kinetics, and resultant injuries observed in a porcine model. Spine 1999;24:1882–1889.

59. Yingling VR, McGill SM. Mechanical properties and failure mechanics of the spine under posterior shear load: observations from a porcine model. J Spinal Disord 1999;12:501–508.

60. Adams MA, Hutton WC. The relevance of torsion to the mechanical derangement of the lumbar spine. Spine 1981;6:241–248.

61. Farfan HF, Cossette JW, Robertson GH, et al. The effects of torsion on the lumbar intervertebral joints: the role of torsion in the production of disc degeneration. J Bone Joint Surg [Am] 1970;52:468–497.

62. Adams MA, Hutton WC. Gradual disc prolapse. Spine 1985;10:524–531.

63. Gordon SJ, Yang KH, Mayer PJ, et al. Mechanism of disc rupture. A preliminary report. Spine 1991;16:450–456.

64. Snook SH, Webster BS, McGorry RW, et al. The reduction of chronic nonspecific low back pain through the control of early morning lumbar flexion. A randomized controlled trial. Spine 1998;23:2601–2607.

65. Fathallah FA, Marras WS, Wright PL. Diurnal variation in trunk kinematics during a typical work shift. J Spinal Disord 1995;8:20–25.

66. Adams M, McNally D, Wagstaff J, et al. Abdominal stress concentrations in lumbar intervertebral discs following damage to the vertebral bodies: a cause of disc failure. Eur Spine J 1993;1:214–221.

67. Chaffin DB, Andersson GBJ, Martin BJ. Occupational biomechanics. New York: John Wiley and Sons, 1999.

68. National Institute for Occupational Safety and Health. Work practices guide for manual lifting. Washington, DC: Department of Health and Human Services, 1981.

69. Noyes FR, De Lucas JL, Torvik PJ. Biomechanics of ligament failure: an analysis of strain-rate sensitivity and mechanisms of failure in primates. J. Bone Joint Surgery 1994;56A:236–253.

70. Fathallah FA, Marras WS, Parnianpour M. The role of complex, simultaneous trunk motions in the risk of occupation-related low back disorders. Spine 1998;23:1035–1042.

71. Heylings DJ. Supraspinous and interspinous ligaments of the human lumbar spine. J Anat 1978;125:127–131.

72. Marras WS, Allread WG, Burr DL, et al. Prospective validation of a low-back disorder risk model and assessment of ergonomic interventions associated with manual materials handling tasks [In Process Citation]. Ergonomics 2000;43:1866–1886.

73. Marras WS, Fine LJ, Ferguson SA, et al. The effectiveness of commonly used lifting assessment methods to identify industrial jobs associated with elevated risk of low-back disorders. Ergonomics 1999;42:229–245.

74. Adams M, Dolan P. Recent advances in lumbar spinal mechanics and their clinical significance. Clin Biomech (Bristol, Avon) 1995;10:3–19.

75. McGill SM, Norman RW. Effects of an anatomically detailed erector spinae model on L4/L5 disc compression and shear. J Biomech 1987;20:591–600.

76. Potvin JR, McGill SM, Norman RW. Trunk muscle and lumbar ligament contributions to dynamic lifts with varying degrees of trunk flexion [see Comments]. Spine 1991;16:1099–1107.

77. McGill S, Seguin J, Bennett G. Passive stiffness of the lumbar torso in flexion, extension, lateral bending, and axial rotation. Effect of belt wearing and breath holding. Spine 1994;19:696–704.

78. Solomonow M, He Zhou B, Baratta RV, et al. Biexponential recovery model of lumbar viscoelastic laxity and reflexive muscular activity after prolonged cyclic loading. Clin Biomech (Bristol, Avon) 2000; 15:167–175.

79. Solomonow M, Zhou BH, Harris M, et al. The ligamento-muscular stabilizing system of the spine. Spine 1998;23:2552–2562.

80. Stubbs M, Harris M, Solomonow M, et al. Ligamento-muscular protective reflex in the lumbar spine of the feline. J Electromyogr Kinesiol 1998;8:197–204.

81. Wang JL, Parnianpour M, Shirazi-Adl A, et al. Viscoelastic finite-element analysis of a lumbar motion segment in combined compression and sagittal flexion. Effect of loading rate. Spine 2000;25:310–18.

82. Gedalia U, Solomonow M, Zhou BH, et al. Biomechanics of increased exposure to lumbar injury caused by cyclic loading. Part 2. Recovery of reflexive muscular stability with rest. Spine 1999;24: 2461–2467.

83. Solomonow M, Zhou B, Baratta RV, et al. Neuromuscular disorders associated with static lumbar flexion: a feline model. J Electromyogr Kinesiol 2002;12:81–90.

84. Solomonow M, Zhou BH, Baratta RV, et al. Biomechanics of increased exposure to lumbar injury caused by cyclic loading: Part 1. Loss of reflexive muscular stabilization. Spine 1999;24:2426–2434.

85. McGill S. Low back disorder. Champaign, Illinois: Human Kinetics, 2002.

86. Cripton P, Berlemen U, Visarino H, et al. Response of the lumbar spine due to shear loading in injury prevention through biomechanics. Yang KH, ed. At the proceedings of Injury Prevention through Biomechanics, Wayne State University, Detroit, Michigan, May 4–5, 1995.

87. Marras WS, Granata KP. Changes in trunk dynamics and spine loading during repeated trunk exertions. Spine 1997;22:2564–2570.

88. McGill SM. Electromyographic activity of the abdominal and low back musculature during the generation of isometric and dynamic axial trunk torque: implications for lumbar mechanics. J Orthop Res 1991;9:91–103.

89. Marras WS, Granata KP. A biomechanical assessment and model of axial twisting in the thoracolumbar spine. Spine 1995;20:1440–1451.

90. Pope MH, Andersson GB, Broman H, et al. Electromyographic studies of the lumbar trunk musculature during the development of axial torques. J Orthop Res 1986;4:288–297.

91. Pope MH, Svensson M, Andersson GB, et al. The role of prerotation of the trunk in axial twisting efforts. Spine 1987;12:1041–1045.

92. Carter DR. Biomechanics of bone. In: Nahum HM, Melvin J, eds. Biomechanics of trauma. Norwalk, CT: Appleton Century Crofts, 1985.

93. Woo SL-Y, Gomez MA, Akeson WH. Mechanical behaviors of soft tissues: measurements, modifications, injuries, and treatment. In: Nahum HM, Melvin J, eds. Biomechanics of trauma. Norwalk, CT: Appleton Century Crofts, 1985.

94. Porter RW, Adams MA, Hutton WC. Physical activity and the strength of the lumbar spine. Spine 1989;14:201–203.

95. Brinkmann P, Biggermann M, Hilweg D. Prediction of the compressive strength of human lumbar vertebrae. Clin Biomech (Bristol, Avon) 1989;4:S1–S27.

96. Videman T, Nurminen M, Troup JD. 1990 Volvo Award in clinical sciences. Lumbar spinal pathology in cadaveric material in relation to history of back pain, occupation, and physical loading. Spine 1990; 15:728–740.

97. Chaffin DB, Park KS. A longitudinal study of low-back pain as associated with occupational weight lifting factors. Am Ind Hyg Assoc J 1973;34:513–525.

98. Ciriello VM, Snook SH, Blick AC, et al. The effects of task duration on psychophysically-determined maximum acceptable weights and forces. Ergonomics 1990;33:187–200.

99. Snook SH. The design of manual handling tasks. Ergonomics 1978; 21:963–985.

100. Snook SH. Psychophysical considerations in permissible loads. Ergonomics 1985;28:327–330.

101. Snook SH. Psychophysical acceptability as a constraint in manual working capacity. Ergonomics 1985;28:331–335.

102. Snook SH. Approaches to preplacement testing and selection of workers. Ergonomics 1987;30:241–247.

103. Snook SH, Ciriello VM. The design of manual handling tasks: revised tables of maximum acceptable weights and forces. Ergonomics 1991; 34:1197–1213.

104. Waters TR, Putz-Anderson V, Garg A. Applications manual for the revised NIOSH lifting equation. Cincinnati: National Institute for Occupational Safety and Health, 1994.

105. Cady LD, Bischoff DP, O'Connell ER, et al. Strength and fitness and subsequent back injuries in firefighters. J Occup Med 1979;21: 269–272.

106. Cady LD, Jr., Thomas PC, Karwasky RJ. Program for increasing health and physical fitness of fire fighters. J Occup Med 1985;27: 110–114.

107. Burton AK, Tillotson KM, Main CJ, et al. Psychosocial predictors of outcome in acute and subchronic low back trouble. Spine 1995;20: 722–728.

108. Marras WS, Davis KG, Heaney CA, et al. The influence of psychosocial stress, gender, and personality on mechanical loading of the lumbar spine. Spine 2000;25:3045–3054.

109. Davis K, Marras WS, Heaney CA, et al. The impact of mental processing and pacing on spine loading. Spine 2002 (in press).

110. Chaffin DB, Herrin GD, Keyserling WM, et al. A method for evaluating the biomechanical stresses resulting from manual materials handling jobs. Am Ind Hyg Assoc J 1977;38:662–675.

111. Chaffin DB, Baker WH. A biomechanical model for analysis of symmetric sagittal plane lifting. AIIE Transactions 1970;2:16–27.

112. Herrin GD, Jaraiedi M, Anderson CK. Prediction of overexertion injuries using biomechanical and psychophysical models. Am Ind Hyg Assoc J 1986;47:322–330.

113. Schultz AB, Andersson GB. Analysis of loads on the lumbar spine. Spine 1981;6:76–82.

114. Hughes RE, Chaffin DB. The effect of strict muscle stress limits on abdominal muscle force predictions for combined torsion and extension loadings. J Biomech 1995;28:527–533.

115. Schultz A, Andersson GB, Ortengren R, et al. Analysis and quantitative myoelectric measurements of loads on the lumbar spine when holding weights in standing postures. Spine 1982;7:390–397.

116. Bean JC, Chaffin DB, Schultz AB. Biomechanical model calculation of muscle contraction forces: a double linear programming method. J Biomech 1988;21:59–66.

117. Marras WS, King AI, Joynt RL. Measurement of loads on the lumbar spine under isometric and isokinetic conditions. Spine 1984;9:176–187.

118. Marras WS, Davis KG. Spine loading during asymmetric lifting using one versus two hands. Ergonomics 1998;41:817–834.

119. Granata KP, Marras WS. An EMG-assisted model of trunk loading during free-dynamic lifting. J Biomech 1995;28:1309–1317.

120. Granata KP, Marras WS. An EMG-assisted model of loads on the lumbar spine during asymmetric trunk extensions. J Biomech 1993; 26:1429–1438.

121. Granata KP, Marras WS. Relation between spinal load factors and the high-risk probability of occupational low-back disorder. Ergonomics 1999;42:1187–1199.

122. Marras WS, Davis KG, Granata KP. Trunk muscle activities during asymmetric twisting motions. J Electromyogr Kinesiol 1998;8:247–256.

123. Marras WS, Davis KG, Splittstoesser RE. Spine loading during whole body free dynamic lifting. Columbus, Ohio: The Ohio State University Press, 2001.

124. Marras WS, Granata KP. Spine loading during trunk lateral bending motions. J Biomech 1997;30:697–703.

125. Marras WS, Granata KP. The development of an EMG-assisted model to assess spine loading during whole-body free-dynamic lifting. J Electromyogr Kinesiol 1997;7:259–268.

126. Marras WS, Sommerich CM. A three-dimensional motion model of loads on the lumbar spine: I. Model structure. Hum Factors 1991;33: 123–137.

127. Marras WS, Sommerich CM. A three-dimensional motion model of loads on the lumbar spine: II. Model validation. Hum Factors 1991; 33:139–149.

128. McGill SM. The influence of lordosis on axial trunk torque and trunk muscle myoelectric activity. Spine 1992;17:1187–1193.

129. McGill SM. A myoelectrically based dynamic three-dimensional model to predict loads on lumbar spine tissues during lateral bending. J Biomech 1992;25:395–414.

130. Marras WS, Davis KG, Jorgensen MJ. Spine loading and gender. Spine 2002 (in press).

131. Marras WS, Davis KG, Ferguson SA, et al. Spine loading characteristics of patients with low back pain compared with asymptomatic individuals. Spine 2001;26:2566–2574.

132. Mirka GA, Marras WS. A stochastic model of trunk muscle coactivation during trunk bending. Spine 1993;18:1396–1409.
133. Granata KP, Marras WS, Davis KG. Variation in spinal load and trunk dynamics during repeated lifting exertions. Clin Biomech (Bristol, Avon) 1999;14:367–375.
134. Marras WS, Granata KP, Davis KG. Variability in spine loading model performance. Clin Biomech (Bristol, Avon) 1999;14:505–514.
135. Granata KP, Marras WS. The influence of trunk muscle coactivity on dynamic spinal loads. Spine 1995;20:913–919.
136. Davis KG, Marras WS. Assessment of the relationship between box weight and trunk kinematics: does a reduction in box weight necessarily correspond to a decrease in spinal loading? [In Process Citation]. Hum Factors 2000;42:195–208.
137. Davis KG, Marras WS, Waters TR. Reduction of spinal loading through the use of handles. Ergonomics 1998;41:1155–1168.
138. Davis KG, Marras WS, Waters TR. The evaluation of spinal loads during lowering and lifting. Clin Biomech (Bristol, Avon) 1998;13:141–152.
139. Marras WS, Granata KP, Davis KG, et al. Effects of box features on spine loading during warehouse order selecting. Ergonomics 1999;42:980–996.
140. Ferguson SA, Gaudes-MacLaren LL, Marras WS, et al. Spinal loading when lifting from industrial storage bins. Ergonomics 2002;45:399–414.
141. Marras WS, Davis KG, Kirking BC, et al. Spine loading and trunk kinematics during team lifting. Ergonomics 1999;42:1258–1273.
142. Marras WS, Davis KG, Kirking BC, et al. A comprehensive analysis of low-back disorder risk and spinal loading during the transferring and repositioning of patients using different techniques. Ergonomics 1999;42:904–926.
143. McGill SM, Norman RW, Sharratt MT. The effect of an abdominal belt on trunk muscle activity and intra-abdominal pressure during squat lifts. Ergonomics 1990;33:147–160.
144. Marras WS, Jorgensen MJ, Davis KG. Effect of foot movement and an elastic lumbar back support on spinal loading during free-dynamic symmetric and asymmetric lifting exertions. Ergonomics 2000;43:653–668.
145. Jorgensen MJ, Marras WS. The effect of lumbar back support tension on trunk muscle activity. Clin Biomech (Bristol, Avon) 2000;15:292–294.
146. Granata KP, Marras WS, Davis KG. Biomechanical assessment of lifting dynamics, muscle activity and spinal loads while using three different styles of lifting belt. Clin Biomech (Bristol, Avon) 1997;12:107–115.
147. Marras WS, Granata KP, Davis KG, et al. Low back disorder risk and spine loading during the use of lifting assistance devices (LADs). Columbus, Ohio: The Ohio State University, 1996.
148. McGill SM, Norman RW, Cholewicki J. A simple polynomial that predicts low-back compression during complex 3-D tasks. Ergonomics 1996;39:1107–1118.
149. Fathallah FA, Marras WS, Parnianpour M. Regression models for predicting peak and continuous three-dimensional spinal loads during symmetric and asymmetric lifting tasks. Hum Factors 1999;41:373–388.
150. Cholewicki J, McGill S. Mechanical stability of the in vivo lumbar spine: implications of injury and chronic low back pain. Clin Biomech (Bristol, Avon) 1996;11:1–15.
151. Cholewicki J, VanVliet IJ. Relative contribution of trunk muscles to the stability of the lumbar spine during isometric exertions. Clin Biomech (Bristol, Avon) 2002;17:99–105.
152. Cholewicki J, Simons AP, Radebold A. Effects of external trunk loads on lumbar spine stability. J Biomech 2000;33:1377–1385.
153. Granata KP, Marras WS. Cost-benefit of muscle cocontraction in protecting against spinal instability [In Process Citation]. Spine 2000;25:1398–1404.
154. Granata KP, Orishimo KF. Response of trunk muscle coactivation to changes in spinal stability. J Biomech 2001;34:1117–1123.
155. Granata KP, Wilson SE. Trunk posture and spinal stability. Clin Biomech (Bristol, Avon) 2001;16:650–659.
156. Panjabi MM. The stabilizing system of the spine. Part II. Neutral zone and instability hypothesis. J Spinal Disord 1992;5:390–396; discussion 397.
157. Panjabi MM. The stabilizing system of the spine. Part I. Function, dysfunction, adaptation, and enhancement. J Spinal Disord 1992;5:383–389; discussion 397.
158. Cholewicki J, Polzhofer GK, Radebold A. Postural control of trunk during unstable sitting. J Biomech 2000;33:1733–1737.
159. Granata KP, Orishimo KF, Sanford AH. Trunk muscle coactivation in preparation for sudden load. J Electromyogr Kinesiol 2001;11:247–254.
160. Ayoub MM, Bethea NJ, Deivanayagam S, et al. Determination and modeling of lifting capacity. Lubbock, TX: Texas Tech University, 1978.
161. Liles DH, Deivanayagam S, Ayoub MM, et al. A job severity index for the evaluation and control of lifting injury. Hum Factors 1984;26:683–693.
162. Waters TR, Putz-Anderson V, Garg A, et al. Revised NIOSH equation for the design and evaluation of manual lifting tasks. Ergonomics 1993;36:749–776.
163. Government Accounting Office. Worker protection: private sector ergonomics programs yield positive results. Washington DC, 1997.
164. Occupational Safety and Health Administration. Ergonomics program management guidelines for meatpacking plants. Washington DC, U.S. Department of Labor, 1993.

SECTION IV

Surgery

CHAPTER 18

Preparation for Surgery

Orso L. Osti, Simon Macklin, and Hiroaki Nakamura

PREOPERATIVE ASSESSMENT

Significant changes have occurred over the last 30 years in the way patients are counseled before surgery. It is paramount that plainly written information on the relevant surgical procedure, containing appropriate illustrations, be available to patients before surgery. Audiovisual equipment can be used; however, in view of the emotional implications of surgical intervention for pain, a face-to-face preoperative discussion between the surgeon and patient is advised. The surgeon needs to ensure that all appropriate imaging is available at the time of the surgery and that a recent body pain drawing is available to confirm the site and pattern of distribution of preoperative symptoms. Obtaining informed written consent, which should include financial details of the surgery, is mandatory before the operation. The consent form should be signed by the surgeon and patient at the same time and, preferably, within days of the operation. Consent should be obtained immediately before scheduling the patient for surgery and one should reappraise the consent form with the patient on the day of the operation.

PREANESTHETIC ASSESSMENT

A detailed preanesthetic assessment is an essential prerequisite to safe anesthetic practice. It offers the anesthetist the opportunity to identify the presence of comorbid medical conditions, arrange for optimization of those conditions if required, identify other confounding factors (e.g., difficult venous access or airway), discuss options for preoperative medication and postoperative analgesia, and obtain informed consent for the anesthetic. It is important to discuss the possible requirement for blood transfusion at this point and explore potential strategies for blood conservation. This may be particularly relevant in those with a religious objection to the use of homologous blood products.

A number of specific questions should be considered: Is there a previous anesthetic history? If so, were there any complications? Are there cardiac, respiratory, or endocrine comorbidities? Is airway management expected to be difficult?

Most institutions have guidelines for appropriate preoperative investigations based on the patient's age and comorbidities. Table 18-1 shows the guidelines currently in use at the Royal Adelaide Hospital.

PREOPERATIVE MEDICATIONS

With few exceptions, therapeutic drugs taken for concurrent diseases should be continued up to the time of surgery (1). The notable exceptions to this rule are: aspirin and other nonselective nonsteroidal antiinflammatory drugs (NSAIDS), hypoglycemic agents, and monoamine oxidase inhibitors. Aspirin and nonselective NSAIDS (which act on both cyclooxygenase 1 and 2 enzymes) should be discontinued for 7 to 10 days before surgery to allow recovery of platelet aggregation. The newer cyclooxygenase 2 inhibitors (e.g., rofecoxib and celecoxib) are free from platelet aggregation inhibition and can be continued up to the time of surgery without a risk of increased bleeding because of platelet dysfunction.

A range of new specific platelet aggregation inhibitors, clopidogrel (Iscover [Bristol-Myers Squibb Pharmaceuticals, Australia] and Plavix [Sanovi-Synthelabs, Australia]) or ticlopidine (Ticlid [Roche Products, Australia]), recently have been introduced for use in patients with acute coronary syndrome or for use in thromboembolic prophylaxis. These should be stopped at least 5 days prior to surgery to prevent excess bleeding owing to platelet dysfunction.

Monoamine oxidase inhibitors are associated with a high incidence of CNS side effects if piperidine-based opioids are used for analgesia. These side effects may be

TABLE 18-1. *The current guidelines for preoperative investigations in use at the Royal Adelaide Hospital*

Investigations	Clinical Indications	Investigations	Clinical Indications
Electrocardiogram (ECG)[a]	Men aged 45 years and over Women aged 50 years and over Hypertension Current or past significant cardiac disease Current or past significant circulatory disease Current or past significant pulmonary disease Diabetes mellitus; person aged 35 years and over Renal disease Thyroid or other metabolic disease Morbid obesity Sleep apnea History of alcoholism Cardiac drug therapy Radiation or chemotherapy Other clinical indications	CBE, *continued* Biochemistry (Urea and electrolytes)[e]	History of alcoholism Severe chronic disease History of current infection Other clinical indications (e.g., platelet count for regional anesthesia) Aged 65 years or over and when clinically indicated Renal disease Diabetes mellitus Cardiovascular disease Hypertension Adrenal and other endocrine disease Liver disease Cardiac drugs Diuretics Steroids Chemotherapy Fluid and electrolyte abnormality (e.g., diarrhea, malabsorption, or bowel preparation) Other clinical indications

Chest x-ray (CXR)[b]	Current or past significant pulmonary disease
	Asthma or COAD that is debilitating or with a change of symptoms
	Ongoing pulmonary infection (productive cough with colored sputum or a change in nature of sputum)
	Cardiovascular disease
	  Current or past significant disease, *or*
	  A change in symptoms
	Cardiothoracic procedure since last CXR
	Cardiac pacemaker or implanted defibrillator
	Thyroidectomy for information on trachea
	Malignancy
	Sleep apnea
	Radiation or chemotherapy
	Other clinical indications
		Liver function tests[f]
		
		Lung function tests[g,h]
			Hepatobiliary disease
			Pancreatic disease
			Bleeding disorder
			History of or exposure to hepatitis
			Human immunodeficiency virus or acquired immunodeficiency syndrome
			History of alcoholism
			Chemotherapy
			Other clinical indications
			History of lung disease, dyspnea, or orthopnea *and*
			  Need to determine degree of reversibility *or*
			  Determine baseline condition, in anticipation of postoperative ventilation
			Cardiothoracic procedure
			Significant skeletal abnormality (e.g., kyphoscoliosis)
			Morbid obesity
			Other clinical indications

Compete blood examination (CBE)[c,d]	Aged 65 years or over and when clinically indicated Surgery with a potential for significant blood loss Recent history of blood loss or donation Known anemias Bleeding disorders Anticoagulation therapy Malignancy, including hematologic Radiation or chemotherapy Renal disease	Echocardiogram (ECHO)[i]	Previously uninvestigated or undocumented heart murmur Severe cardiac disease *or* symptoms of severe dyspnea *or* unstable angina where an assessment of left ventricular function is valuable

(continued)

[a]An ECG is valid for 6 months unless there has been a change in symptoms or clinically indicated.

[b]If a CXR is clinically indicated, obtain a CXR if none was obtained in the last year or if symptoms have changed since the last CXR.

[c]A hemoglobin level +/− platelet count my suffice in the majority of cases.

[d]A CBE is valid 6 months unless clinically indicated.

[e]Valid for 6 months if last set of results is normal unless clinically indicated.

[f]Valid for 6 months unless clinically indicated.

[g]Specify tests required (i.e., spirometry, blood gases, or carbon monoxide diffusion factor)

[h]Valid for 1 year unless clinically indicated.

[i]Valid for 1 year unless symptoms have changed or clinically indicated.

either excitatory or depressive and are most commonly seen when meperidine (pethidine) is coadministered (2). Other opioids with a piperidine base (e.g., fentanyl) have been used without complications. The assumption is that alfentanil and sufentanil are probably safe (3,4). No literature addresses the safety of remifentanil.

The current recommendations are that the newer reversible monoamine oxidase inhibitors (MAOIs) should be discontinued 24 hours before anesthesia. The older irreversible MAOIs should be continued because of the high risk of uncontrolled depression in the weeks leading up to surgery. Under these circumstances, all opioids may display an exaggerated depressant effect and smaller doses should be used in the first instance. Meperidine (pethidine) should be avoided.

Most institutions, and all anesthetists, should have a management plan for the diabetic patient. Ideally the diabetic should appear as early as possible on the theater list (operating schedule). Management should be directed to avoid dangerous hypoglycemia and excessive hyperglycemia. An intravenous dextrose infusion, combined with a sliding scale of actrapid insulin, is often used to facilitate perioperative glycemic control.

The use of specific analgesic or anxiolytic medication in the immediate preoperative period is a matter of personal choice and can be tailored to the individual patient's requirements.

CONSENT FOR ANESTHESIA

In the current climate with the drive for increased day of surgery admissions, a strong argument can be made for the anesthetic assessment and consent to be performed before admission to the hospital for surgery. This allows time for appropriate investigations to be organized and the results to be reviewed before admission to the hospital. This is particularly pertinent for those with cardiorespiratory disease, in whom modification of therapy may be required for optimization of the medical condition before anesthesia. It also enables the risks and complications to be explained to the patient in a nonthreatening environment.

POSITIONING

Enough emphasis cannot be placed on the care that must be taken in positioning the patient under anesthesia to minimize the risk of pressure injury. Surgery on the lumbar spine may be undertaken in the lateral or prone position. For combined anterior and posterior stabilization, the patient needs to be rotated part way through the procedure.

The patient in the prone position is at particular risk. Appropriate padding and supports should be used to prevent pressure injury to soft-tissue structures (e.g., breast

and penis) and bony prominences (e.g., iliac crest, knees, and elbows). Special attention should be given to protecting the orbital structures from trauma. The eyes should be taped closed to prevent corneal abrasions and the head should be supported to prevent pressure on the supraorbital nerves. There is little evidence to suggest that use of ophthalmic lubrication confers any benefit. Pressure on the globe must be avoided at all costs because of the danger of retinal vein occlusion or retinal ischemia. The latter is of particular concern if hypotensive anesthesia is employed. Both of these complications may lead to blindness.

Before positioning in the prone position, it is worth identifying limitations in cervical spine movement and assessing the range of shoulder movement. The arms may be positioned with the arms flexed at the elbow, externally rotated and abducted at the shoulder and placed on a support. This has the advantage of allowing easy access to peripheral veins, arterial monitoring, pulse oximetry, and neuromuscular monitoring. However, the ulnar nerve and brachial plexus must be protected to avoid pressure or overextension leading to neuropraxia. An alternative is to place the arms alongside the torso if there are physical limitations that prevent the former position. Access to monitoring devices is limited in this position.

Regardless of the position, the ulnar nerve is at high risk of damage, which may occur in spite of one's best efforts to protect it. The mechanisms behind the damage are not altogether clear, and preventative measures cannot be implemented without definitive causation. Nevertheless, it is imperative to avoid pressure or excessive stretching of the ulnar nerve at the elbow (5).

A number of devices are commercially available for surgery in the prone position. These range from the simple (e.g., firm blocks to be placed under the hips and chest) to the sophisticated (e.g., the Andrew's table). These devices are designed to avoid pressure on the abdomen and thereby avoid splinting of the diaphragm and minimal epidural bleeding from abdominal compression. As intra-abdominal pressure increases, the vertebral venous pressure raises in parallel with raising pressure of the inferior vena cava (IVC) (6–8). Appropriately designed surgical frames have been proved to reduce the pressure within the IVC compared with more conventional chest rests (9). Reduction of intra-abdominal and IVC pressure lower blood loss (10). The spinal frame used in our institution is shown in Figure 18-1. The iliac crest padded supports are modifiable to accommodate different patient sizes. The frame is radiolucent to allow biplanar fluoroscopy.

Approximately 20% of patients operated in the prone position using iliac crest support frames complain postoperatively of symptoms linked to neuropraxia of the lateral cutaneous nerve of the thigh. This is more common in obese individuals and where the surgery is prolonged

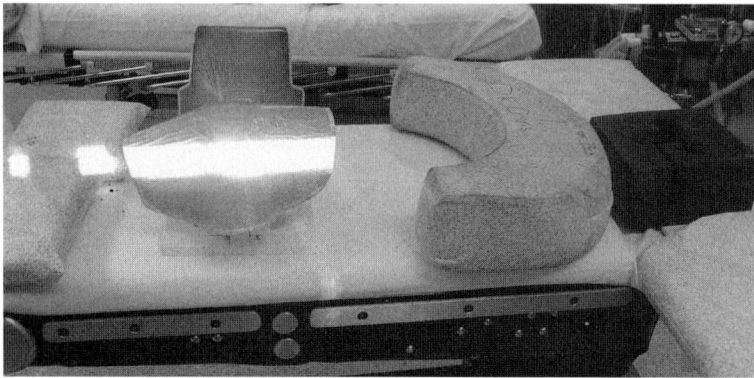

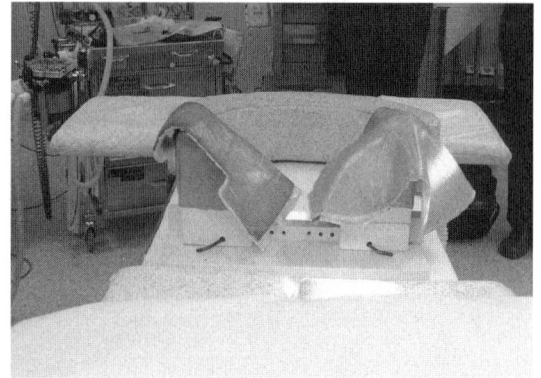

FIG. 18-1. Spinal frame. The iliac crest padded supports are modifiable to accommodate for different patients' sizes. The frame is radiolucent to allow biplanar fluoroscopy.

(over 2 hours). In most cases, the neurapraxia fully resolves within 6 weeks.

KNEE-CHEST POSITION

One of the potential advantages of the knee-chest position over iliac crest support frames for lumbar spine surgery is the greater opening of the interlaminar space compared to the iliac crest support frame. However, it is possible that the dural sac and individual nerve roots may be under increased tension in this position; therefore, safe retraction of the neural tissue may be more difficult to achieve. Potential circulatory disturbance in the legs should be carefully monitored in view of the significant bend at the knees. It is common for older individuals to complain after the surgery of increased knee pain, especially if patello-femoral osteoarthritis is present preoperatively.

Intraoperative preservation of the physiologic lumbar lordosis may become critical when stabilization procedures are performed. A decrease in the lordosis angle has been correlated with increased symptoms and gait abnormality following lumbar fusion (11–13). The hip flexion angle relates to lumbar lordosis (14–16), and it appears that iliac crest support–type frames may lead to better maintenance of physiologic lumbar lordosis compared with knee-chest devices because they involve less flexion of the hip joint.

LATERAL DECUBITUS

This position may be used when the upper lumbar spine is approached retroperitoneally. In most cases, the approach is carried out through the left side with the patient lying onto his or her right side. The right (bottom) knee is flexed to approximately 90° with the left (upper) knee extended. An axial pad is placed just underneath the waistline, and the pelvis and head of the fibula are protected with adequate padding. The patient's right upper extremity is placed on the operating table with the left

side in a padded gutter arm support. An axillary roll may be used to take pressure off the brachial plexus to avoid disabling postoperative neurapraxia.

BLOOD CONSERVATION

The requirement for blood transfusion depends on a multitude of factors, not the least of which is an agreement on the threshold hemoglobin before transfusion. Most departments of transfusion medicine have guidelines for transfusion that have reduced the threshold level from a previously accepted level of 100 g/L (10 g/dL). In the absence of confounding comorbid disease, there is little indication for transfusion unless the hemoglobin concentration has fallen below 80 g/L (8 g/dL) in the absence of ongoing blood loss.

A number of strategies have been proposed to reduce the incidence of homologous transfusion. These include autologous predonation, isovolemic hemodilution and perioperative cell salvage. Autologous predonation can be logistically difficult and costly to institute; it may result in a relaxation of the transfusion trigger and result in inappropriate transfusion; it does not remove the risk of clerical error; and it does not remove the risk of transmission of bacterial infection. If the blood is harvested but not reinfused, it is not suitable to be used in the general blood pool and therefore becomes an expensive and useless commodity.

Isovolemic hemodilution refers to the practice of harvesting a quantity of blood at the beginning of a procedure and replacing it with a crystalloid or colloid solution to prevent a fall in circulating volume. This has the effect of immediately reducing the hemoglobin concentration and therefore reducing the amount of hemoglobin lost per volume of shed blood. Providing the blood has been harvested correctly, it will contain fresh platelets and coagulation factors not usually present in stored blood. In addition, the harvested blood can be processed to extract a platelet concentration rich in growth factors, which may be of benefit to osteogenesis at the surgical site. The harvested blood can then be reinfused during the later stages of the operation.

Perioperative cell salvage has been extensively used as a blood conservation technique. Despite the equipment becoming increasingly sophisticated, its application is still limited to those procedures where blood loss is anticipated to be excessive, such as more extensive and lengthy spinal procedures.

BLOOD LOSS AND THE SURGICAL FIELD

It is important to realize that the second arm of blood conservation techniques are directed at reducing blood loss to optimize the surgical field. A number of basic strategies should be employed; these are summarized in Table 18-2. Remember that bleeding can be venous or arterial.

Venous bleeding occurs predominantly from the epidural veins, which are in communication with the IVC. Therefore, strategies to reduce IVC pressure reduce epidural venous pressure. Positive pressure ventilation tends to reduce venous return and increase IVC pressure. Consequently, efforts to limit the positive inspiratory pressure while maintaining appropriate gas exchange should be made. This can be achieved by maintaining an adequate level of neuromuscular blockade, together with adjustments of inspiratory time, pressure, and flow rate. Appropriate use of bronchodilating drugs may help in the bronchospastic patient. Positive end expiratory pressure (PEEP) should be avoided (17). Careful positioning on a suitable support system avoids abdominal compression. This has been shown to reduce IVC pressure with reduction in epidural venous pressure. This position also avoids diaphragmatic splinting from abdominal compression, which would otherwise cause a rise in ventilatory inflation pressure and increase IVC pressure (18).

Avoiding vasodilatation and reducing the perfusion pressure can reduce arterial bleeding. Vasodilatation can be minimized by controlled hyperventilation to produce hypocapnia. The perfusion pressure can be reduced by a number of pharmacologic interventions that come under the broad heading of hypotensive anesthesia. A wide range of drugs has been used to induce hypotension under anesthesia; a full discussion on the relative merits can be found elsewhere (19). However, hypotensive anesthesia is

TABLE 18-2. *Strategies for minimizing blood loss*

Prevent venous bleeding	Reduce arterial bleeding
Avoid abdominal compression	Control heart rate
Avoid diaphragmatic splinting	Hyperventilate to hypocapnia
Minimize peak inspiratory pressure	Induce hypotension
Avoid positive end expiratory pressure	

not without its complications and consideration must be given to the risk-benefit assessment for each individual patient. The risks of hypotensive anesthesia are hypoperfusion of vital organs, principally those organs whose function is not conventionally monitored. The CNS is of prime concern. Cerebral hypoperfusion may lead to a range of postoperative complications from short-term confusion and disorientation to massive cerebral infarction. Although cerebral autoregulation maintains cerebral blood flow through a range of blood pressure variations, blood flow is pressure dependent beyond the extremes of these variations. Volatile anesthetic agents may offer some cerebral protection by reducing cerebral metabolic oxygen consumption. A more scientific method of determining adequacy of cerebral blood flow is to monitor jugular bulb oxygenation or cerebral blood flow by means of transcranial Doppler. These techniques are becoming recognized as having a role to play in carotid vascular surgery and neurosurgery, but their role in hypotensive anesthesia outside of these domains has yet to be determined. In addition, spinal cord ischemia may occur if blood flow through the anterior spinal artery is compromised. The effects of hypoperfusion of the CNS may be exacerbated by hyperventilation and consequent hypocarbia leading to vasoconstriction deliberately induced to reduce bleeding.

Modern volatile anesthetic agents are an attractive option to induce hypotension. Agents, such as isoflurane and sevoflurane, with relatively low blood-gas solubility coefficients cause depression of medullary cardiac centres while depressing myocardial contractility directly. This leads to a reduction in cardiac output and a fall in blood pressure. Because of their low solubility, changes in inspired volatile agent concentration lead to rapid changes in blood concentration. This offers a level of titratability that makes them useful agents for inducing hypotension without a prolonged recovery time.

A special mention should be made regarding perioperative β-blockade. In addition to its advantageous effects on slowing heart rate and reducing force of contractility and thereby reducing blood pressure, evidence is becoming available that the use of perioperative β-blockade may reduce the all-cause mortality in high risk surgical patients undergoing noncardiac surgery (20–22). Their potential benefit to patients who are not considered high risk is yet to be determined (23).

A conservative approach to hypotensive anesthesia for surgery on the lumbar spine would be to use β-adrenergic blockade with atenolol for a target heart rate of 60 to 70 beats per minute and a volatile anesthetic agent 0.5 to 1.5 μg/kg clonidine to provide a modest fall in blood pressure but maintain a mean arterial pressure above 70 mm Hg. By using a drug such as clonidine with a long half-life (compared to agents such as sodium nitroprusside), the problems of rebound hypertension or rapid return to normotension are avoided.

Finally, two additional concerns must be addressed. First, the negative impact of perioperative hypothermia on the incidence of wound infection has been investigated (24,25). Hypothermia leads to increased shivering in the immediate postoperative period, which increases the basal metabolic rate. This increases respiratory and myocardial work and can be relevant in patients with impaired cardiorespiratory function to the point of precipitating cardiorespiratory failure. In addition, hypothermia has an adverse effect on normal hemostatic function. Although major blood loss is uncommon in most surgery on the lumbar spine, the impact of moderate hypothermia, below 35°C, on platelet function and the coagulation cascade must be considered (26,27). If efforts to create a bloodless surgical field are to be successful, meticulous attention to detail is required. This should include the avoidance of hypothermia by the use of appropriate warming devices. The introduction of forced air warming devices, which direct warmed air through an inflatable blanket to provide body surface heating, has been a huge advance in this field (28). Most of the work on the effects of hypothermia and coagulation has been done on either trauma or cardiopulmonary bypass patients. Further work needs to be done on patients undergoing elective noncardiac surgery. Nevertheless, it seems prudent to minimize hypothermia for the reasons mentioned in the preceding.

Finally, what is the role of the serine protease inhibitor, aprotinin, and the lysine analogs, tranexamic acid and aminocaproic acid? Both of these groups of agents have been shown to be beneficial in cardiac surgery or knee arthroplasty (29–31). Tranexamic acid has been shown to be beneficial in pediatric scoliosis surgery (32). The emphasis has been on the reduction in blood transfusion. The role of these agents in reducing bleeding to improve the surgical field has yet to be determined.

ANTIBIOTICS

Infection rates with spinal surgery vary widely among published series and according to the type of surgery performed. Wimmer et al. reported on 22 cases out of 850 clean spinal procedures with an overall infection rate of 2.6% (33). In that study, it was suggested that extended preoperative hospitalization, large intraoperative blood loss, and prolonged operating time were correlated with increased risk of postoperative infection. The authors also suggested that routine prophylactic antibiotics may not be necessary, although parenteral postoperative antibiotic should be administered when segmental instrumentation is used.

The overall risk of infection is higher in acute trauma than in elective surgery. Patients with significant preoperative neurologic deficit are also at higher risk. It has been shown that penetration of antibiotics into the disc is poor and that a critical relationship exists between serous antibiotic concentration and disc antibiotic levels that may have a prophylactic effect on infection. It has been suggested that antibiotic concentration within the disc is highest between 15 and 80 minutes following intravenous administration (34).

Prophylactic administration of antibiotics should be considered mandatory for all procedures that may violate the intervertebral disc. In experimental studies where lumbar intervertebral discs were inoculated with staphylococcus epidermidis cultures, no discitis developed with prophylactic intravenous or intradiscal administration of cephalosporins, whereas large doses of antibiotics administered following the inoculation of bacteria into the disc did not prevent disc infection (35,36).

Different classes of antibiotics have been demonstrated to penetrate the intervertebral disc at different rates. Aminoglycosides and glycopeptides appear to penetrate into the nucleus pulposus well, whereas penicillins and cephalosporins have been proven to enter the disc at much lower concentrations. Prophylactic antibiotics are even more critical when percutaneous disc procedures are performed. The administration of antibiotics should be planned so that the highest intradiscal concentration may be achieved when the surgical insult to the disc is likely to occur. Maximal antibiotic concentration in the disc, as indicated, occurs 15 to 80 minutes following parenteral antibiotic administration; the likely average time for broad-spectrum antibiotics is 30 to 45 minutes.

POSTOPERATIVE PAIN MANAGEMENT

The mainstay of acute pain management is opioid analgesia. Postoperative analgesia should be administered by a route that offers rapid onset and the ability to titrate the dose to achieve optimal effect. The intravenous route is the most suitable in the recovery unit, where the patient can be closely monitored for the adverse effects of opioids. Central nervous system depression is initially manifest and may then present with more serious effects, such as respiratory depression. A simple sedation score can be used as an early warning sign for the clinician before more significant CNS depression occurs. Figure 18-2 gives the protocol for intravenous opioid loading used at the Royal Adelaide Hospital. Once therapeutic plasma concentrations of opioid analgesics have been achieved, it is appropriate to convert to a patient controlled analgesia (PCA) system. Most institutions have a protocol for drug concentration, bolus dose, and lockout time to be used for PCA. A simple protocol for the fit patient under 65years of age is the following:

- Morphine: 1 mg/mL
- Bolus dose: 1 mg
- Lockout time: 5 minutes

The bolus dose can be increased if analgesia is inadequate and decreased if excessive sedation occurs. It is

Sedation Score

0	**None**
1	**Mild:** occasionally drowsy, easy to rouse
2	**Moderate:** constantly drowsy, easy to rouse
3	**Severe:** somnolent, difficult to rouse
S	**Normally Asleep**

BEGIN

Pain? — NO → Routine observations

YES

"Pain Protocol" and opioid ordered? — NO → Get order

YES

Prepare in Saline **morphine** 1mg/ml, or **fentanyl** 20 micrograms/ml

10ml syringe
Draw up **10mg morphine** or **200 micrograms fentanyl** and make up to 10ml with saline

20ml syringe
Draw up **20mg morphine** or **400 micrograms fentanyl** and make up to 20ml with saline

Routine observations

Pain? — YES → ... NO → Is sedation score less than 2? — NO → Seek medical advice

YES

Is respiratory rate greater than 8/min? — NO → Seek medical advice

Hold further doses until sedation score less than 2 and respiratory rate greater than 8/min. Consider use of naloxone 100 microgram increments IV.

WAIT 3 min

YES

B.P. OK? — NO → Seek medical advice

YES

Under 70 years old? — NO →

YES

Give 1ml IV ← NO — **Severe pain?** — YES → 1st or 2nd dose? — YES → Give 2ml IV

Severe pain? — YES → 1st or 2nd dose? — YES → Give 1ml IV — NO → Give 0.5ml IV

NO — Some relief with last 2 doses? — NO → Give 4ml IV / YES → Give 2ml IV

NO — Some relief with last 2 doses? — NO → Give 1ml IV / YES → Give 1ml IV

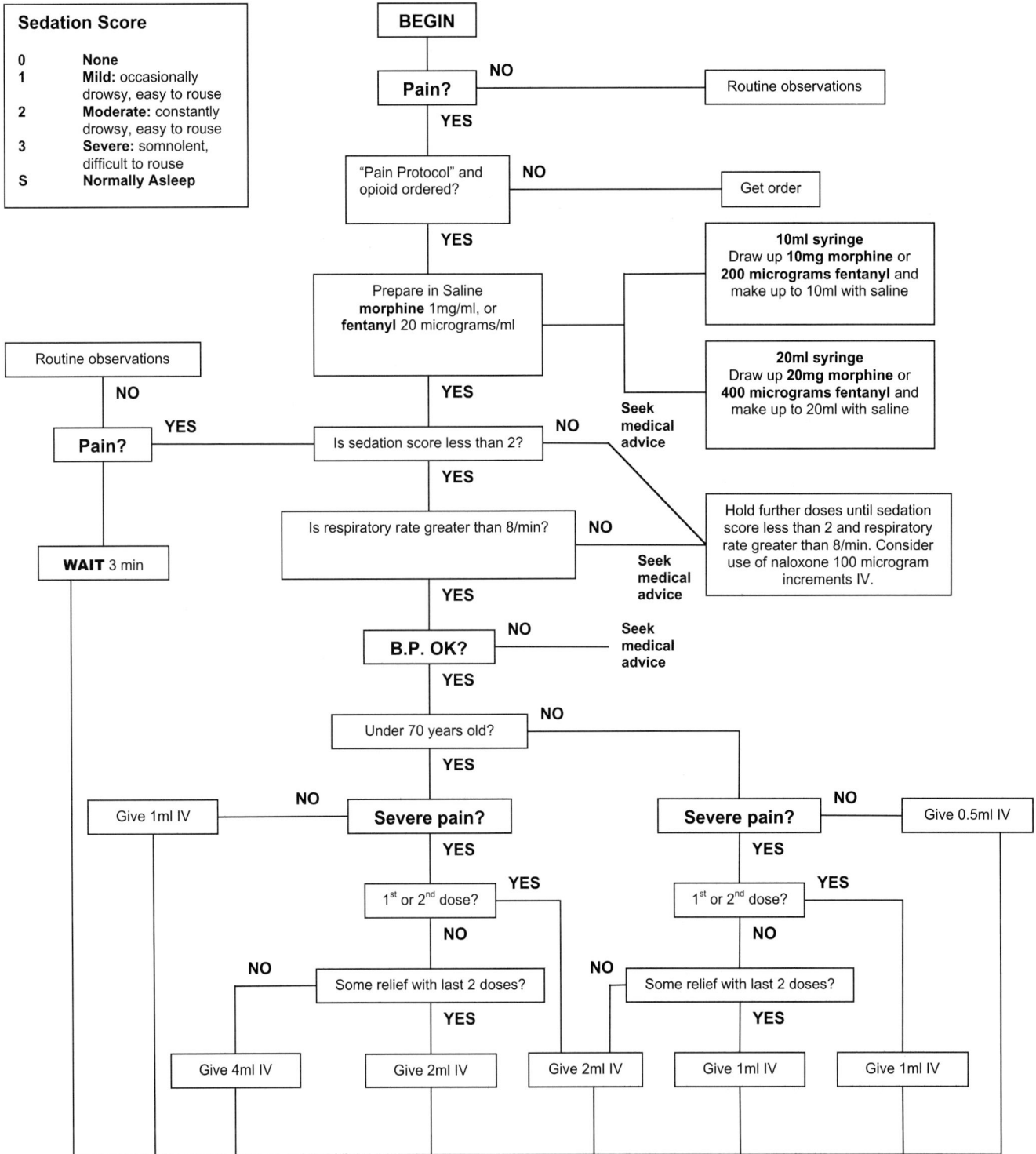

FIG. 18-2. Guidelines for intravenous opioid administration. These guidelines are/should: (1) Only to be used by staff in recovery wards who have been instructed in this technique; (2) NOT appropriate for routine maintenance of analgesia in general wards; (3) Note that the peak effect of an intravenous dose may not occur for over 15 minutes, therefore all patients should be observed closely during this time; (4) All patients receiving repeated doses of IV opioids should be ordered oxygen; and (5) "Pain Protocol" should cease when the patient is comfortable (they will not necessarily be pain free). From The Acute Pain Service, Royal Adelaide Hospital, with permission.

generally accepted that a background infusion ordinarily should not be prescribed because it appears not to improve the analgesia but may increase the incidence of side effects (38).

Morphine should be the first line agent of choice, but fentanyl can be used as an alternative. Meperidine (pethidine) should be avoided if feasible because of the possibility of CNS toxicity associated with its metabolite, normeperidine (norpethidine). Normeperidine plasma concentrations can be achieved with PCA pethidine and can lead to CNS excitability, and manifest as agitation and even convulsions (39,40).

It is worth considering the use of adjuvant analgesic agents that do not specifically target opioid receptors. Use of nonspecific cyclooxygenase inhibitors may increase intra and post-operative bleeding and should be avoided. However, the more recently released selective cox-2 inhibitors (celecoxib and parecoxib) may have a role to play and further investigation of these drugs is warranted. Similarly, centrally acting drugs that are α-adrenergic agonists stimulate the descending spinal inhibitory pathways. These pathways originate in the periaqueductal gray matter and reticular formation, to run in the dorsolateral fasciculus. They synapse in the substantia gelatinosa of the dorsal horn where norepinephrine and serotonin are released. They are involved in the highly complex system of interneurons, which modify nociceptive input to the spinal cord. Clinical data do not support the use of clonidine by the epidural or intrathecal route with conflicting data on its analgesic efficacy. However, its sedative effects may be beneficial in patients with a high preoperative opioid intake. Similarly, tramadol may be beneficial by preventing reuptake of noradrenaline and serotonin at the spinal cord level. It has only weak intrinsic opioid activity and is thought to exert its effects at a supraspinal or spinal cord level.

Finally, if pain control in the immediate postoperative period is difficult, ketamine by intravenous infusion of 2 to 8 mg/hour (depending on age and comorbid disease) can be used. Ketamine is the only clinically available NMDA (N-methyl-D-aspartate) receptor antagonist and provides analgesia at the spinal cord level where NMDA is an excitatory neurotransmitter.

ACKNOWLEDGMENT

Hiroaki Nakamura's contribution was supported by a grant from Medtronic-Sofamor Danek International.

REFERENCES

1. Noble DW, Kehlet H. Risks of interrupting drug treatment before surgery. BMJ 2000; 321:719–20
2. Stack CG, Rogers P, Linter SP. Monoamine oxidase inhibitors and anaesthesia. Br J Anaesthesiol 1988;60:222.
3. Fobe F, Kestens-Servaye Y, Baele P, et al. Heart transplant and monoamine oxidase inhibitors. Acta Anaesthesiol (Belgium) 1989;40 (2):131–138.
4. Ure DS, Gillies MA, James KS. Safe use of remifentanil in a patient treated with the monoamine oxidase inhibitor phenelzine. Br J Anaesthesiol 2000;84(3): 414–416.
5. Practice advisory for the prevention of perioperative peripheral neuropathies. Anesthesiology 2000;92(4):1168–1182.
6. Distefano VJ, Klein KS, Nixon JE, et al. Intraoperative analysis of the effects of position and body habitus on surgery of the low back. A preliminary report. Clin Orthop 1974;99:51–56.
7. McNulty SE, Weiss J, Azad SS, et al. The effect of the prone position on venous pressure and blood loss during lumbar laminectomy. J Clin Anesthesiol 1992;l4:220–225.
8. Wayne SJ. The trunk position for lumbar-disc surgery. J Bone Joint Surg 1967;49:1195–1198.
9. Lee TC, Yang LC, Chen HJ. Effect of patient position and hypotensive anaesthesia on inferior vena caval pressure. Spine 1998;23:941–948.
10. Sivarajan M, Amory DW, Everett GB, et al. Blood pressure not cardiac output, determines blood loss during induced hypotension. Anesthesiol Analg 1980;59:203.
11. Grobler Lj, Moe JH, Winter RB, et al. Loss of lumbar lordosis following surgical correction of thoracolumbar deformity. Orthop Trans 1978;2:239–244.
12. Hasty CA, Passoff TL, Perry J. Gait abnormalities arising from iatrogenic loss of lumbar lordosis secondary to Harrington instrumentation in lumbar fractures. Spine 1983;8:501–511.
13. Wasylenko MJ, Skinner S, Perry J. Analysis of posture and gait following spinal fusion with Harrington instrumentation. Orthop Trans 1981;5:21–25.
14. Tan SB, Kozak JK, Dickson JH, et al. Effect of operative position on sagittal alignment of the lumbar spine. Spine 1994;19:314–318.
15. Steohens CG, Yoo JU, Wilbur G. Comparison of lumbar sagittal alignment produced by different operative positions. Spine 1996;21:1802–1807.
16. Benfanti PL, Geissele AE. The effect of intraoperative hip position on maintenance of lumbar lordosis. Spine 1997;22:2299–2303.
17. Mitaka C, Nagura T, Tsunoda Y, et al. Two-dimensional echocardiographic evaluation of inferior vena cava, right ventricle and left ventricle during positive pressure ventilation with varying levels of positive end-expiratory pressure. Crit Care Med 1989;17(3):205–210.
18. Lee TC, Yang LC, Chen HJ. Effect of patient position and hypotensive anaesthesia on inferior vena caval pressure. Spine 23(8):941–947.
19. Miller RD. Anaesthesia, 4th ed. New York: Churchill Livingstone, 1994.
20. Auerbach AD, Goldman L. β-Blockers and reduction of cardiac events in noncardiac surgery: scientific review. JAMA 2002;287(11): 1435–1444.
21. Mangano DT, Layug EL, Wallace A, et al. Effect of atenolol on mortality and cardiovascular morbidity after noncardiac surgery. Multicenter Study of Perioperative Ischemia Research Group. N Engl J Med 1996;335(23):1713–1720.
22. Jones KG, Powell JT. Slowing the heart saves lives: advantages of perioperative beta-blockade. Br J Surg 2000;87(6):689–690.
23. Howell SJ, Sear JW, Foex P. Peri-operative beta-blockade: a useful treatment that should be greeted with cautious enthusiasm. Br J Anaesthesiol 2001;86(2):161–164.
24. Kurz A, Sessler DI, Lenhardt R. Perioperative normothermia to reduce the incidence of surgical-wound infection and shorten hospitalization. Study of Wound Infection and Temperature Group. N Engl J Med 1996;334(19):1209–1215.
25. Beilin B, Shavit Y, Razumovsky J, et al. Effects of mild perioperative hypothermia on cellular immune responses. Anesthesiology 1998;89 (5):1133-1140.
26. Watts DD, Trask A, Soeken K, et al. Hypothermic coagulopathy in trauma: effect of varying levels of hypothermia on enzyme speed, platelet function, and fibrinolytic activity. J Trauma 1998;44(5):846–854.
27. Reed RL 2nd, Bracey AW Jr, Hudson JD, et al. Hypothermia and blood coagulation: dissociation between enzyme activity and clotting factor levels. Circ Shock 1990;32(2):141–152.
28. Giesbrecht GG, Ducharme MB, McGuire JP. Comparison of forced-air patient warming systems for perioperative use. Anesthesiology 1994; 80(3):671–679.
29. Hiippala S, Strid L, Wennerstrand M, et al. Tranexamic acid (Cyklokapron) reduces perioperative blood loss associated with total knee arthroplasty. Br J Anaesthesiol 1995;74(5):534–537.
30. Casati V, Sandrelli L, Speziali G, et al. Hemostatic effects of tranexamic acid in elective thoracic aortic surgery: a prospective, randomized, double-blind, placebo-controlled study. J Thorac Cardiovasc Surg 2002;123(6):1084–1091.
31. Benoni G, Fredin H. Fibrinolytic inhibition with tranexamic acid

reduces blood loss and blood transfusion after knee arthroplasty: a prospective, randomised, double-blind study of 86 patients. J Bone Joint Surg Br 1996;78(3):434–440.

32. Neilipovitz DT, Murto K, Hall L, et al. A randomized trial of tranexamic acid to reduce blood transfusion for scoliosis surgery. Anesthesiol Analg 2001;93(1):82–87.

33. Wimmer C, Gluch H, Franzreb M, et al. Predisposing factors for injections in spine surgery: a survey of 850 spinal procedures. J Spinal Disord 1998;11:124–128.

34. Guiboux J-P, Cantor JB, Small SD, et al. The effect of prophylactic anti-biotics on iatrogenic intervertebral disc infection: rabbit model. Spine 1995;20:685–688.

35. Fraser RD, Osti OL, Vernon-Roberts B. Discitis after discography. J Bone Joint Surg 1987;69B:26–35.

36. Osti OL, Fraser RD, Vernon-Roberts B. Discitis after discography. The role of prophylactic anti-biotics. J Bone Joint Surg 1990;72B:271–274.

37. Owen H, et al. Variables of patient controlled analgesia 2 Concurrent infusion. Anaesthesia 1989;44:11–13.

38. McHugh GJ Norpethidine accumulation and generalized seizure during pethidine patient-controlled analgesia. Anaesthesiol Int Care 1999;27(3):289–291.

39. Stone PA, Macintyre PE, Jarvis DA. Norpethidine toxicity and patient controlled analgesia. Br J Anaesthesiol 1993;71(5):738–740.

CHAPTER 19

Surgical Approaches to the Thoracolumbar Spine

Scott D. Daffner and Todd J. Albert

The thoracolumbar spine offers numerous challenges in treatment, particularly with regard to anterior surgical approaches. The unique biomechanics of this region, particularly the transition from thoracic kyphosis to lumbar lordosis, put it at increased risk for degeneration. In addition, a wide variety of traumatic and neoplastic conditions may also affect the thoracolumbar spine.

Two basic surgical approaches exist for surgery in this region—anterior and posterior. Posterior approaches are most frequently used for procedures involving the posterior elements, although modifications of the posterior exposure may allow access to the anterior portion of the spine. Anterior approaches are generally required for access to the vertebral body itself. In addition, combined anterior and posterior approaches are occasionally used, depending on the type of pathology, the extent of the injury, and the judgment of the physician.

BONY ANATOMY OF THE THORACOLUMBAR SPINE

The thoracolumbar region represents the transition from one type of vertebral body to another. Thoracic vertebrae are generally smaller than those of the lumbar region. Their facet joints are oriented more frontally, the spinous process is longer and angled more distally, the pedicles are narrower and shorter, and the articulations with the ribs distinguish the thoracic vertebrae. The short transverse processes are angled posterolaterally, articulating with the ribs (1,2).

The lower thoracic vertebrae begin to resemble lumbar vertebrae. Their facet joints change from a frontal orientation to one that more closely resembles those of the lumbar vertebrae in which the superior articular facets are anterolateral to the inferior articular facets of the vertebra above and are directed dorsomedially. From L1 to L5, the pedicles become larger in diameter and become more medially oriented (1,2).

Several ligamentous structures stabilize the bony elements of the vertebrae (Fig. 19-1). The supraspinous and interspinous ligaments connect the spinous processes, while the intertransverse ligaments segmentally connect the transverse processes. The ligamentum flavum passes between the ventral side of the lamina to the superior lip of the next caudal lamina. The ligamentum flavum has a midline raphe, providing a convenient plane through which the canal may be entered. The broad anterior longitudinal ligament runs the length of the spinal column, intimately integrated with the periosteum of the anterior vertebral body, while the posterior longitudinal ligament lies along the posterior aspect of the vertebral body, adhering strongly to the intervertebral discs.

POSTERIOR APPROACH

The most commonly used approach to the spine is the posterior approach (3). This approach differs little along the entire length of the spine, and is used for laminectomy and posterior, transpedicular, or posterolateral fusion.

Posterior Anatomy

To fully appreciate this approach, one must understand the anatomy (Fig. 19-2). The muscular layers of the back can be divided into three distinct layers (Fig. 19-3). The *superficial layer* consists of the trapezius, which inserts on the T12 spinous process most caudally, and the latissimus dorsi which arises from the spinous processes and inserts onto the humerus. The *intermediate layer* is composed of the serratus posterior inferior, while the *deep layer* includes the erector spinae group (spinalis, longissimus, and iliocostalis) lying superficial and lateral to the

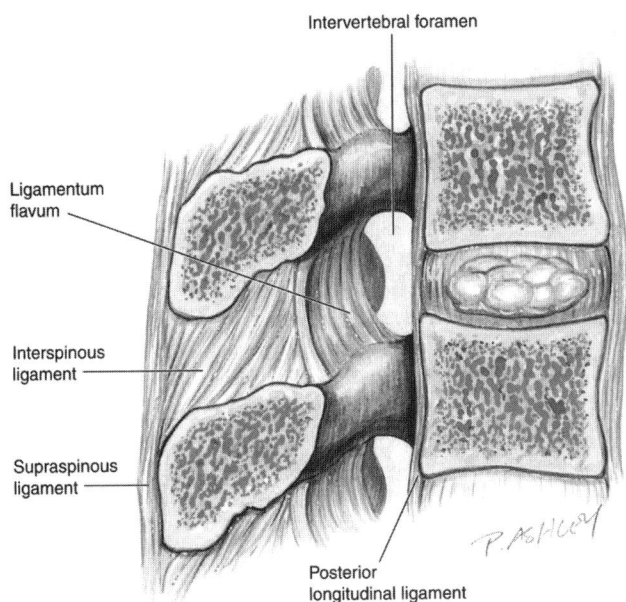

FIG. 19-1. Ligamentous stabilization of the vertebra and ribs. (From Albert TJ, Balderston RA, Northrup BE, eds. Surgical approaches to the spine. Philadelphia: WB Saunders, 1997, with permission.)

transversospinalis group (rotatores, multifidus, and semispinalis). These latter muscle groups are often detached as a single mass during this approach. The bony structures revealed during this approach include the spinous processes, laminae, and transverse processes. The facet joint capsules are also visualized from this approach.

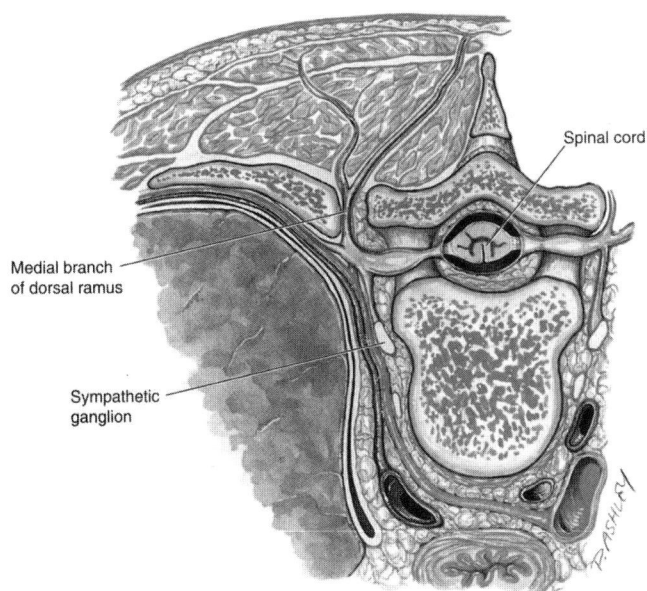

FIG. 19-2. Axial view demonstrating posterior exposure of the thoracolumbar spine. (From Albert TJ, Balderston RA, Northrup BE, eds. Surgical approaches to the spine. Philadelphia: WB Saunders, 1997, with permission.)

Surgical Technique

The patient is placed in either the prone or kneeling position with the abdomen hanging free to reduce pressure on the abdomen and thereby reduce epidural venous pressure and decrease intraoperative bleeding (Fig. 19-4). It is important to pad all bony prominences (2,3).

The skin incision is made in the midline over the spinous processes at the appropriate level. The incision is carried down through the subcutaneous tissue to the deep fascia. By dissecting the deep fascia subperiosteally from the spinous processes, one can preserve the attachments of fascia and can avoid bleeding from intramuscular blood vessels. The erector spinae muscles should be gently retracted with a Cobb elevator, helping to avoid straying into the musculature (Fig. 19-2). Subperiosteal dissection should be carried out in a caudal to cephalad direction. The dissection may be extended laterally to facilitate posterolateral fusion or pedicular instrumentation. Unless a facet fusion is planned, care should be taken to avoid subperiosteal dissection into the facet joint (2). Transverse processes may be palpated inferolateral to the facet joint by following the base of the superior articular process out laterally. After defining the superior and inferior borders of the transverse process, electrocautery may be used to continue the subperiosteal dissection of the segmental musculature, taking care to preserve the intertransverse ligament.

This approach may be extended to allow exposure of the posterior and anterior spinal elements. The extended posterior approach is primarily used for tumor resection and for osteotomies. The extensive nature of this approach may increase the risk for neurovascular damage, including spinal ischemia. The skin incision is extended three or four levels proximal and distal to the desired level of resection. The contents of the spinal canal may be visualized by performing a complete laminectomy. In the low thoracic region, ribs may be divided lateral to the costotransverse joints. If the pleura is entered, a chest tube may need to be inserted. Mobilizing the vascular structures may require ligation of the segmental vessels. The vertebral bodies may then be excised through the disc space above and below the pathology. Posterior stabilization should be performed before the anterior vertebral body resection to avoid neurologic compromise resulting from a completely destabilized spine (1).

Complications associated with the posterior approach may be minimized by careful planning and meticulous surgical technique. Identification of the appropriate level should be verified by taking an intraoperative radiograph. Neural elements, including nerve roots, must be clearly identified and protected. Excessive bleeding may be minimized by performing a subperiosteal dissection. Identification and cauterization of the segmental facetal artery lateral to the pars will minimize bleeding as the dissec-

FIG. 19-3. Superficial, intermediate, and deep muscular layers of the back. (From Albert TJ, Balderston RA, Northrup BE, eds. Surgical approaches to the spine. Philadelphia: WB Saunders, 1997, with permission.)

tion is carried out laterally. Epidural bleeding may be controlled by using Gelfoam or thrombin-soaked pledgets and bipolar cautery (2).

ANTERIOR APPROACHES

Two basic anterolateral approaches to the thoracolumbar spine may be used. These are the transpleural retroperitoneal and the retropleural retroperitoneal approaches. While the transpleural approach provides excellent exposure of the anterior vertebral column over a number of segments, it involves extensive soft-tissue dissection and the rib head may impair visualization. In addition, bleeding from the epidural veins may be difficult to control. The retropleural approach is more lateral than the transpleural approach. Because the rib head and

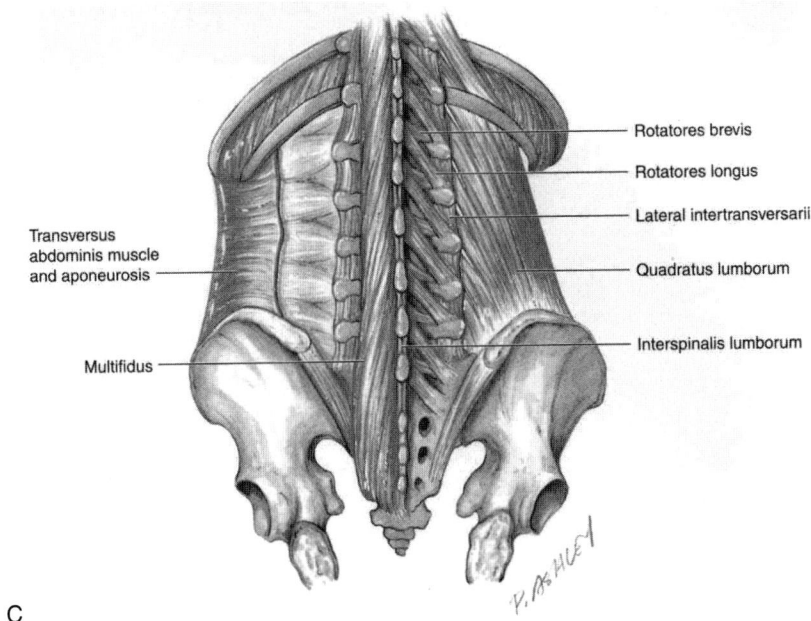

Transversus abdominis muscle and aponeurosis

Multifidus

Rotatores brevis

Rotatores longus

Lateral intertransversarii

Quadratus lumborum

Interspinalis lumborum

C

FIG. 19-3. *(continued).*

pedicle are resected, this approach offers better visualization of the anterolateral spinal canal during decompression, although it may be associated with a great deal of bleeding (1,4,5).

Anterior Anatomy

Anterior approaches to the thoracolumbar junction require a solid understanding of the associated anatomy of the chest and abdominal walls, the diaphragm, and the retroperitoneal contents. Within the chest wall, the ribs articulate with the spine at the level of the disc space above (e.g., the 9th rib articulates at the level of the T8-9 disc space) and the transverse process of the same level. Caudally, the 11th and 12th ribs lack costotransverse articulations. The ribs are stabilized by a number of strong ligamentous attachments, particularly the costovertebral and costotransverse ligaments (Fig. 19-5). The superior costotransverse ligament runs from the inferior aspect of the transverse process to the superior aspect of the rib below. The medial (capsular) ligament attaches the posterior neck of the rib to the anterior border of the

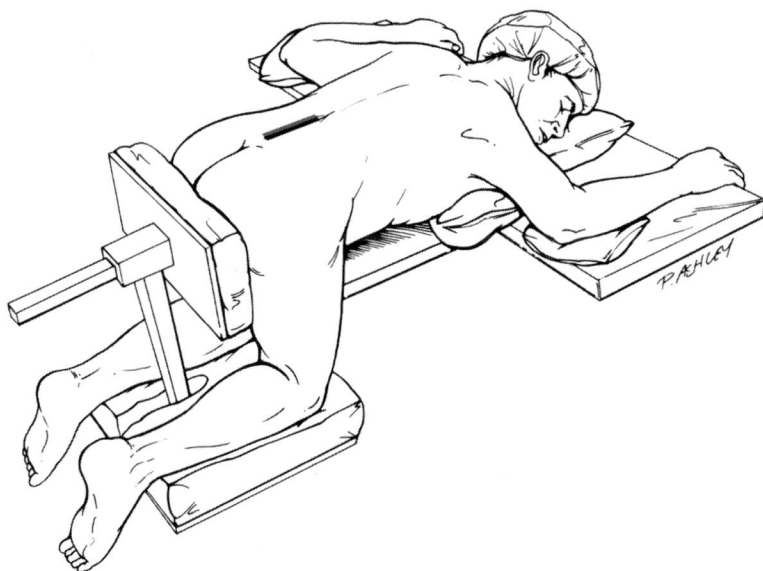

FIG. 19-4. Patient positioning in the kneeling posture on an Andrews table. Note the rolls allowing for decompression of the abdominal contents, which decreases intraoperative blood loss. Alternatively, the patient may be placed on a posted frame. (From Albert TJ, Balderston RA, Northrup BE, eds. Surgical approaches to the spine. Philadelphia: WB Saunders, 1997, with permission.)

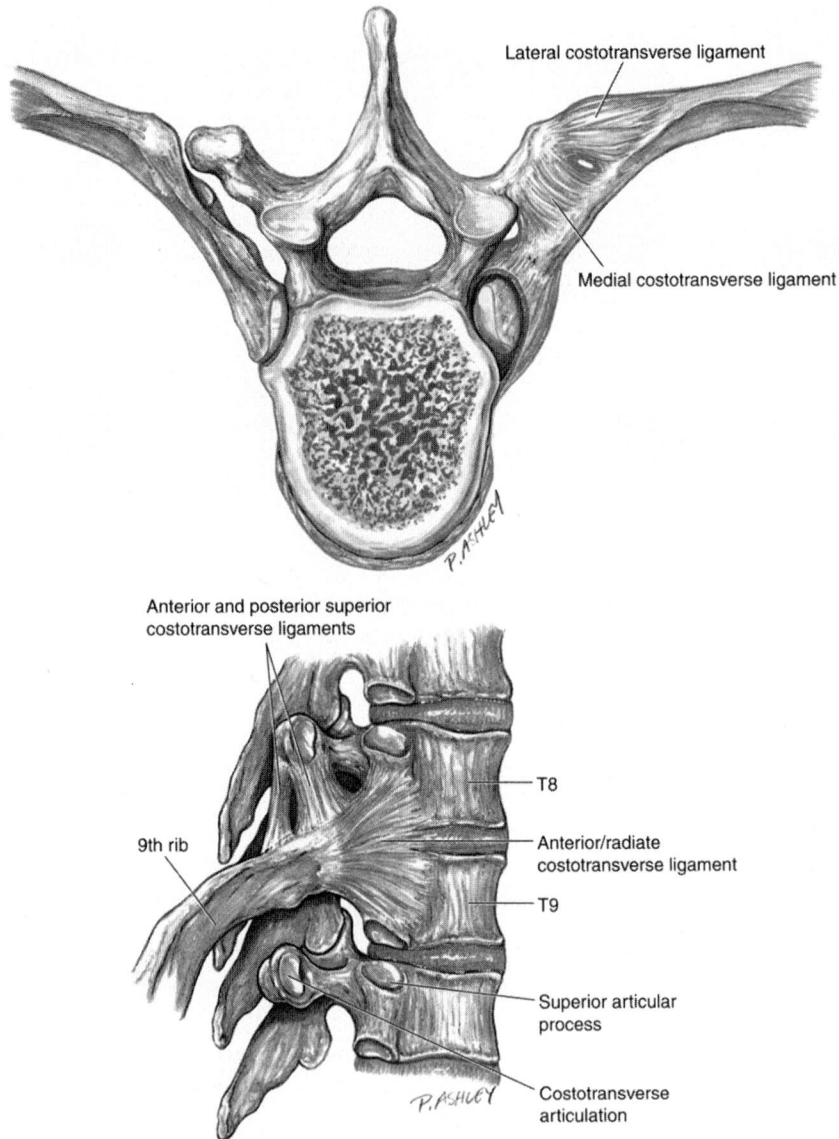

FIG. 19-5. Ligaments stabilizing the ribs. **A:** Axial view. **B:** Sagittal view. (From Albert TJ, Balderston RA, Northrup BE, eds. Surgical approaches to the spine. Philadelphia: WB Saunders, 1997, with permission.)

transverse process. The lateral costotransverse ligament connects the posterior tubercle of the rib to the tip of the transverse process. The anterior costotransverse (radiate) ligament connects the head of the rib to its respective vertebral body. The intercostal neurovascular bundle runs along the inferior surface of the rib in the costal groove. The endothoracic fascia lies deep to the intercostal muscles. Beneath this lies the pleura, which extends to the 10th rib in the midaxillary line and to T12 or L1 in the midline posteriorly (6).

The muscles of the anterior abdominal wall represent a continuation of the layers of the intercostal muscles, with the external, internal, and innermost intercostals muscles continuing as the external oblique, internal oblique, and transversus abdominus muscles, respectively. The transversalis fascia, which lies deep to the transversus aponeurosis, represents the abdominal equivalent of the endothoracic fascia and adheres loosely to the parietal peritoneum.

The diaphragm attaches anterolaterally to the lower six costal cartilages, lower four ribs, xiphoid process, and the thoracolumbar vertebral bodies posteriorly. The crura of the diaphragm insert on the lumbar spine between L1 and L3, and the aorta passes through the crura at the T12 level. The medial arcuate ligament spans the psoas muscle at L1 or L2, and the lateral arcuate ligament bridges the quadratus lumborum from the transverse process of L1 to the 12th rib (Fig. 19-6) (6).

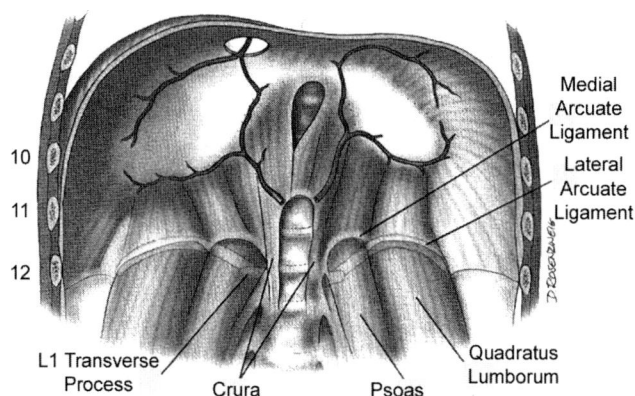

FIG. 19-6. The crura and arcuate ligaments of the diaphragm's insertion on the posterior abdominal wall. (Modified from Birch BD, Desai RD, McCormick PC. Surgical approaches to the thoracolumbar spine. Neurosurg Clin 1997;8 (4):471–485.)

Vascular structures encountered in the anterior approach include the aorta, diaphragmatic arteries, celiac trunk, superior renal artery, and the left renal artery on the left and the inferior vena cava on the right. The aorta is essentially tethered to the spine by the segmental arteries, which run toward their respective foramina. The artery of Adamkiewicz usually arises from the aorta in the lower thoracic or upper lumbar level along the left side (3).

The ilioinguinal and iliohypogastric nerves course inferolaterally over the quadratus. The genitofemoral nerve emerges from the body of the psoas, lying on its anterior surface in the lower lumbar region. The sympathetic trunk lies anterior to the psoas along its junction with the spinal column and may need to be divided (unilaterally) during an anterior approach.

The retroperitoneal space contains the kidneys, adrenal glands, and the ureters, which course inferomedially along the ventral aspect of the psoas toward the bladder between the peritoneum and the psoas fascia. Because the ureters adhere loosely to the peritoneum, they are usually safely retracted with the peritoneum and its contents during anterior surgical approaches.

Surgical Technique

The spine is usually approached from the left side, since it is much easier to mobilize the aorta than the vena cava. The patient should be positioned in the lateral position with the area of interest over the break in the table. An axillary roll and sufficient padding should be used to prevent neurovascular compression injuries (Fig. 19-7). The patient may be rolled slightly posteriorly by 45° to 60° (1,3,5).

At our institution, we prefer the transpleural retroperitoneal approach. The incision is made over the rib one or two levels proximal to the level of spinal pathology. The incision extends anteroinferiorly from just lateral to the paravertebral musculature over the rib (10th, 11th or 12th), toward the anterior superior iliac spine. The subcutaneous tissue and musculature are divided with electrocautery to help control bleeding. The periosteum of the rib is then dissected free, taking care to preserve the intercostal neurovascular bundle inferior to the rib. After stripping the periosteum from the rib to within 1 or 2 cm of the costotransverse joint, the rib is resected using rib cut-

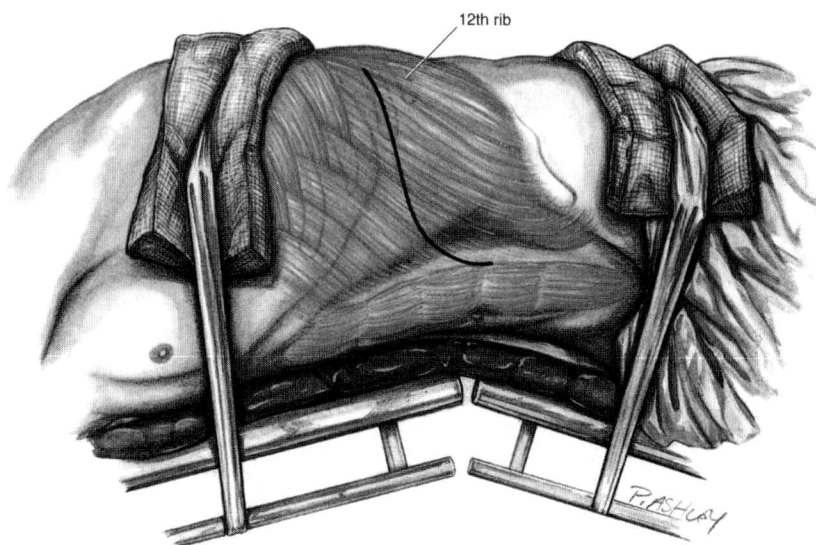

FIG. 19-7. Patient positioning for the anterior approach to the thoracolumbar spine. The level of interest should be placed over the break in the table and the incision should be made over the rib two levels above the level of interest in the midaxillary line. (From Albert TJ, Balderston RA, Northrup BE, eds. Surgical approaches to the spine. Philadelphia: WB Saunders, 1997, with permission.)

ters and is saved for possible future bone grafting (Fig. 19-8). The pleura is then incised (3–5).

The diaphragm may be released from its lateral insertions in the thoracoabdominal wall (Fig. 19-9). The peritoneum is then gently mobilized away from the posterior abdominal wall with blunt dissection. Dissection of the diaphragm then proceeds medially, elevating the medial and lateral arcuate ligaments from the underlying musculature. The medial attachment of the lateral arcuate ligament and the lateral attachment of the medial arcuate ligament are divided at their insertion on the L1 transverse process, taking care to retain sufficient tissue to permit reattachment of the diaphragm. Finally, the left crus of the diaphragm is divided approximately 2 cm from the vertebral body, allowing communication between the thoracic and abdominal cavities (1,4–6).

The lung is then retracted medially along with the diaphragm and peritoneum. The intercostal and lumbar vessels should be ligated close to the aorta to mobilize the great vessels (3). Elevation of the psoas muscle laterally to the pedicles allows for adequate exposure of lumbar segments. Occasionally, the sympathetic chain, which lies along the anterior spine, may need to be transected during this approach. If this is done, the patient should be told that the foot on the side of the sympathetectomy will become warmer (5). The periosteum of the vertebral body is incised and dissected away. Care is taken not to cauter-

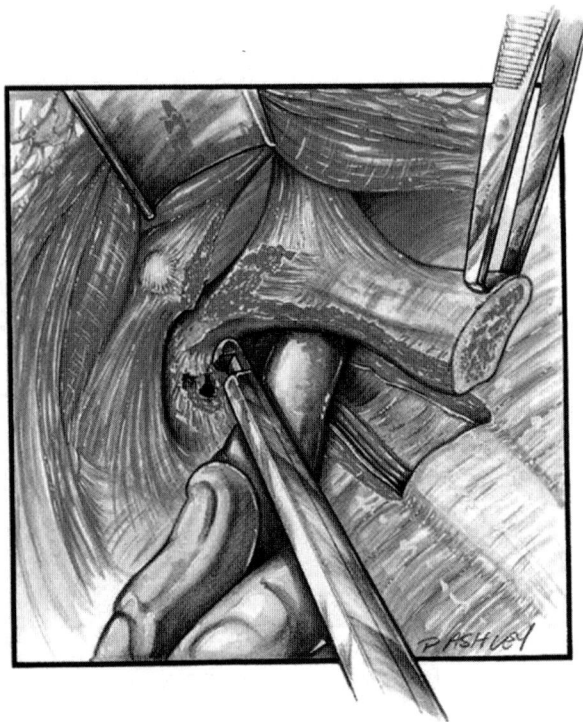

FIG. 19-9. Line of incision to detach the diaphragm from the posterior and lateral abdominal wall. One should leave a cuff of approximately 1 cm for reattachment. (From Albert TJ, Balderston RA, Northrup BE, eds. Surgical approaches to the spine. Philadelphia: WB Saunders, 1997, with permission.)

ize blood vessels around the intervertebral foramen. Once exposed, decompression and stabilization may be performed (Fig. 19-10).

Closure begins with reattachment of the diaphragm to the psoas, L1 transverse process, quadratus, and the cuff of tissue remaining along the anterior and lateral chest wall from which it was initially dissected. A chest tube and retroperitoneal drain are inserted, and the abdominal and chest walls are then closed in layers.

A retropleural retroperitoneal approach may also be used to expose the thoracolumbar spine (1,5,6). This approach is similar to the one described previously, with the incision made along the rib, two levels above the spinal pathology, from the paraspinal muscles to the midaxillary line. The rib that crosses the midaxillary line on the lateral chest radiograph should be resected. The rib is dissected subperiosteally and removed, taking care not to damage the underlying pleura. The endothoracic fascia, which lies deep to the rib periosteum, may then be incised with scissors in line with the incision. The parietal pleura is then carefully freed from this fascial layer by blunt dissection with either a finger or a sponge on forceps beginning anteriorly and progressing posteriorly.

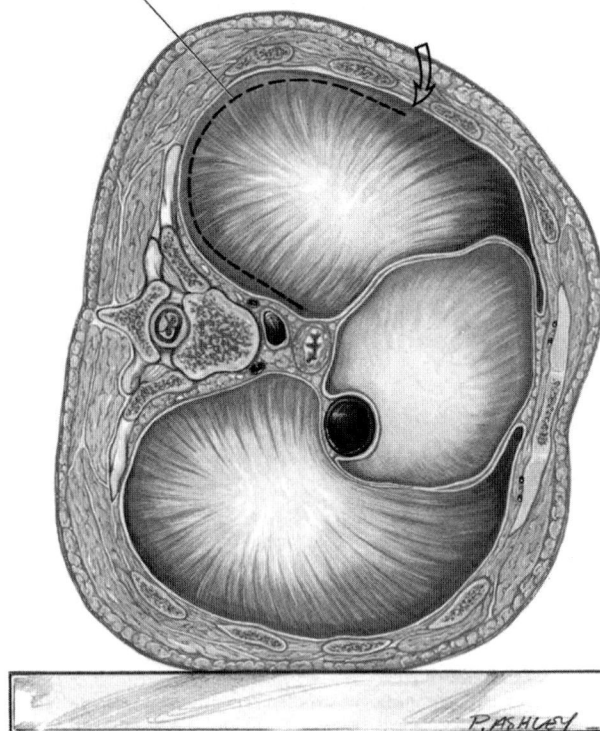

FIG. 19-8. Removal of the rib 1 to 2 cm distal to the costotransverse joint. (From Albert TJ, Balderston RA, Northrup BE, eds. Surgical approaches to the spine. Philadelphia: WB Saunders, 1997, with permission.)

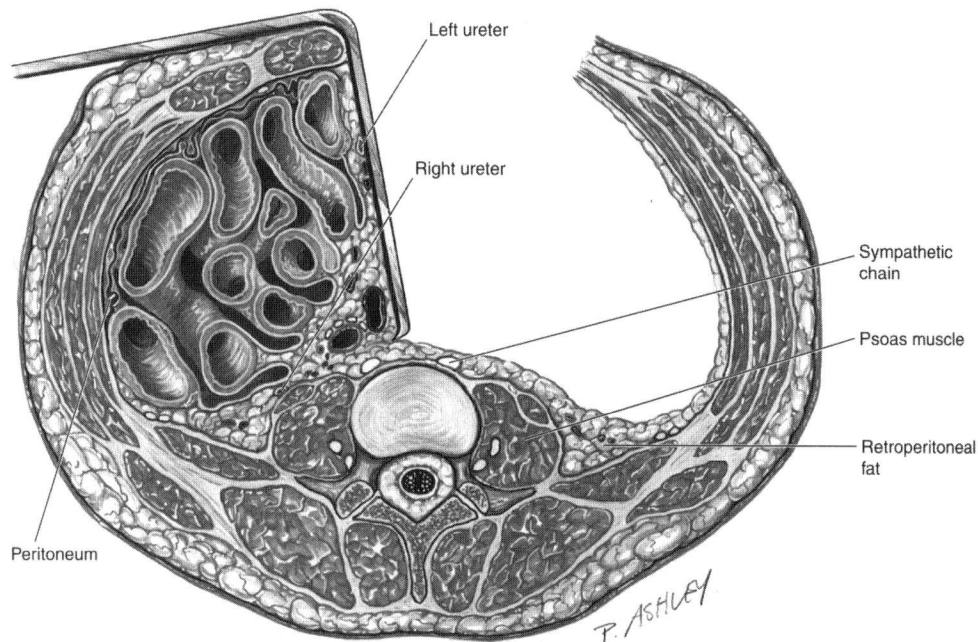

FIG. 19-10. Axial section demonstrating the anterior retroperitoneal exposure of the thoracolumbar spine. The lungs and abdominal contents are retracted medially, providing excellent exposure. (From Albert TJ, Balderston RA, Northrup BE, eds. Surgical approaches to the spine. Philadelphia: WB Saunders, 1997, with permission.)

The abdominal muscles are divided and the peritoneum is carefully mobilized. The costal cartilage may then be divided allowing the peritoneum and abdominal contents to be swept laterally from the undersurface of the diaphragm. The diaphragm is then incised, leaving a 1 cm cuff of tissue for reattachment. The vertebral column is then approached as described earlier. The diaphragm is reattached, and if the pleura was violated during the approach, a chest tube should be placed at the time of closure.

Complications associated with the anterior approach include vascular and visceral injuries, chyle leak, dural tears, neurologic injury, and hernias (1,5). At our institution, somatosensory evoked potentials (SEP) and motor evoked potentials (MEP) are routinely used. Blood loss is best controlled by carefully cauterizing or ligating small bleeding vessels during the approach. Bone wax or Gelfoam pledgets may be used for dissection adjacent to the neural elements; as monopolar electrocautery should be avoided here, only bipolar cautery should be used. A thorough knowledge of anatomy is the key to identifying and ligating blood vessels (especially veins) during this approach.

A dural tear may occur during decompression. Anterior dural tears are difficult to repair, and may be treated alternatively by application of Gelfoam. Direct suturing of the tear or application of fat or muscle patches may also be tried. Additionally, placement of a subarachnoid drain may be considered if closure cannot be obtained.

As mentioned previously, the sympathetic chain is often sacrificed or injured during the anterior approach with no long-term effects. Patients must be forewarned, however, that a temperature difference between the limbs may be experienced, with the leg on the sympathectomized side feeling warmer.

Finally, because the diaphragm is incised for this approach, care must be taken to securely reattach it to the chest wall to avoid herniation of abdominal contents into the thoracic cavity. Postoperative pulmonary toilet must be employed, and close attention should be paid to chest tube protocol if one is used.

COMBINED ANTERIOR AND POSTERIOR APPROACH

Occasionally, the degree and complexity of pathology is best treated with a combined anterior and posterior approach. This is most often used for tumorous or traumatic injuries resulting in three-column instability and neural compression. The sequence of the surgical approach—anterior followed by posterior, posterior followed by anterior, or simultaneous—depends upon the pathology and the patient, and should therefore be determined on a case-by-case basis (7).

An anterior, followed by a posterior, procedure is useful in situations where the use of anterior instrumentation is contraindicated, or when anterior instrumentation alone may not adequately stabilize the spine, but the coronal alignment of the spine is satisfactory. In these instances, an anterior decompression and fusion is followed by a posterior stabilization procedure. For deformity surgery, the anterior approach is generally done to decompress and release a kyphotic deformity with the use of structural graft for fusion. Additional correction may be attempted by the posterior procedure.

A posterior, followed by an anterior, procedure may be indicated in patients with significantly displaced fracture dislocations. The initial posterior procedure restores realignment of the spine in the coronal and sagittal planes. In patients with loss of anterior column support, an anterior procedure may be necessary. Finally, the posterior reduction and decompression may not adequately decompress the spinal canal, in which case an anterior procedure should also be performed.

The inherent instability of injuries requiring combined anterior and posterior procedures increases the risk of complications. Careful electrophysiological monitoring can help avoid intraoperative neurologic injuries. Blood loss is increased in these combined procedures due to the extended operative time needed. An operating table which allows axial rotation of the patient's body without the need for repositioning can help decrease the potential for complications by reducing procedure time as well as avoiding any potential injuries which may occur from patient movement (7).

REFERENCES

1. Kostuik JP. Surgical approaches to the thoracic and thoracolumbar spine. In: Frymoyer JW, Ducker TB, Hadler NM, et al., eds. The adult spine: principles and practice, 2nd ed. Philadelphia: Lippincott-Raven, 1997:1437–1470.
2. Kramer DL, Booth RE, Albert TJ, et al. Posterior lumbar approach. In: Albert TJ, Balderston RA, Northrup BE, eds. Surgical approaches to the spine. Philadelphia: WB Saunders, 1997:173–192.
3. Hoppenfeld S, de Boer P. The spine. In: Hoppenfeld S, de Boer P, eds. Surgical exposures in orthopaedics: the anatomic approach, 2nd ed. Philadelphia: JB Lippincott Co, 1994: 215–301.
4. Adams PR, Cotler HB. Alternative anterior lumbar exposures. In: Albert TJ, Balderston RA, Northrup BE, eds. Surgical approaches to the spine. Philadelphia: WB Saunders, 1997:157–172.
5. Emery SE. Anterior retroperitoneal lumbar exposures. In: Albert TJ, Balderston RA, Northrup BE, eds. Surgical approaches to the spine. Philadelphia: WB Saunders, 1997:145–156.
6. Birch BD, Desai RD, McCormack PC. Surgical approaches to the thoracolumbar spine. Neurosurg Clin North Am 1997;8:471–485.
7. Vaccaro AR. Combined anterior and posterior surgery for fractures of the thoracolumbar spine. Instr Course Lect 1999;48:443–449.

CHAPTER 20

Surgical Approaches to the Lumbar Spine: Anterior and Posterior

Anthony P. Dwyer

This chapter discusses the surgical anatomy of the anterior and posterior approaches to the lumbar spine, including the advantages, disadvantages, risks, and complications of each approach. It does not discuss specific anatomic detail, which can be reviewed in many excellent surgical anatomy textbooks (1–5).

Surgical anatomy consists of surface anatomy, radiologic anatomy, and the surgical approach anatomy (4,6). There must be an understanding of the principle of the internervous plane and the steps to expand the approach of surgical dissection (7). Such anatomic knowledge helps the surgeon anticipate the complications of each approach and assists in potential disaster planning, such as injury to a major vessel, the spinal cord, nerves, or viscera.

Finally, it is important to remember the principles of all surgical approaches (4).

1. Each surgical layer must expose the margins of the wound.
2. Exposure of each surgical layer must be completed before the next layer is exposed.

These principles avoid a conical exposure, whereby the exposure is narrow with deeper dissection.

The decision to use the anterior or posterior approach to the lumbar spine is based on the site of the pathology and the best approach to that pathology afforded by each. It is also important to know and understand the vital structures that are encountered with each approach. Each pathology must be considered, as well as its location. Such pathologies include: coronal or sagittal deformity, neurologic compression, infection, primary and metastatic tumors, nonunion, and instability of the spinal column.

The surgical management of these pathologies must be easily and safely attainable with the selective surgical approach.

There are general indications, contraindications, and specific risks for each approach. Ideally the lumbar spine should be approached from the left side because the arterial structures are more resistant to surgical trauma than are venous structures, but a right-sided retroperitoneal approach can be used if it there has been a previous left-sided approach, which may produce significant scarring and fibrosis. Other examples of conditions that might alter the choice of surgical approach include: excessive subcutaneous fibrosis following burns or radiation therapy that prevent a safe posterior approach to the lumbar spine, or the potential for an anterior approach to the lumbar spine to cause retrograde ejaculation from damage to the hypogastric plexus (8).

Each surgical approach has its own advantages and disadvantages, and at times both must be used in a single stage (9). For example, the anterior approach may require the presence of a general or vascular surgeon, but the reduced surgical trauma associated with the minimized muscular cutting of the new approaches may result in a shorter hospital stay and quicker rehabilitation. On the other hand, the posterior approach is more common and routine, but is associated with more surgical trauma from ischemia and denervation of the muscles. In addition, the prone position may be associated with cardiopulmonary problems in the older patient, injury to the peripheral nerves, and ophthalmic complications.

ANTERIOR SURGICAL APPROACH TO THE LUMBAR SPINE

This discussion covers the retroperitoneal approach to the lumbar spine, as popularized by Hodgson and others (10–12). Both the antero-lateral approach (with the patient in the lateral or semilateral position), and the direct anterior midline approach (via the rectus abdominus muscle and the transversalis fascia muscle, with the patient in the supine position) are discussed. This section does not cover the transperitoneal approach to the lumbar spine, because this is generally used only for exposure of the lumbosacral junction and is discussed in a separate section.

The retroperitoneal approach to the lumbar spine has the advantage of being readily expanded to provide access to the anterior and middle columns of the lumbar spine. Also, it allows ready access to the vertebral bodies, the annulus and intervertebral disc, the anterior aspects of the transverse process and lateral pedicle, the neural foramen, and the anterial epidural space.

It is useful for surgical access for vertebral body and disc space infection, primary and secondary tumors, decompression of the vertebral canal from anterior pathology, correction of lumbar deformity, reconstruction of the anterior column, and stabilization and fusion of a symptomatic unstable segment.

DIRECT ANTERIOR APPROACH

Surface and Radiologic Anatomy

The surface landmarks for the anterior approach to the lumbar spine consist of the iliac crest, anterior superior iliac spine, pubic symphysis, the coastal margin and the umbilicus (6).

In a thin patient the lumbar sacral junction and the aorta can be readily palpable through the midline.

The surface anatomic landmarks need to be compared with a careful study of the antero-posterior (AP) and lateral views of the lumbar spine, noting the relationship between anatomic landmarks and X-ray anatomy in order to properly plan the skin incision and surgical approach.

Usually the intercristal line on top of the iliac crest passes through the L4-5 disc, but this varies among individuals and may be altered with lumbosacral anomalies such as sacralization of the fifth lumbar vertebrae or lumbarization of the sacrum.

Inadvertent operating at the wrong level of the lumbar spine may be prevented by "signing your site" and confirming the specific level with intraoperative X-rays.

Patient Position

For the direct anterior approach to the lumbar spine, the patient is positioned in the supine position with a padded support under the prominence of the sacrum and the lumbar spine centered over the break in a radiolucent operating table to allow for adjustment in the degree of extension of the lumbar spine. The direct anterior approach is ideal for an average-sized patient but a large patient may require the antero-lateral approach to allow the abdominal contents to conveniently fall away from the lumbar spine. The head and neck are in the neutral posi-

tion with the upper extremities partially abducted. Compression stockings to the lower extremities should be used and an indwelling urinary catheter inserted.

Incision

There are four choices for the skin incision:

1. Horizontal paramedian
2. Vertical paramedian (Fig. 20-1)
3. Pfannenstiel or horizontal incision above the pubic symphysis
4. Oblique

The horizontal and vertical paramedian incisions are most commonly used. The Pfannenstiel incision may be used for cosmetic reasons and the oblique incision is rarely used for the direct anterior approach because the anatomy is the same as in the antero-lateral approach.

The level of a transverse incision depends on the specific level of pathology. As mentioned, the surface and radiologic anatomy need to be correlated with each other to make sure that the intercristal line does indeed go through the L4-5 disc. With that determined, the L3-4 disc generally is at the level of the umbilicus, and the L5-S1 disc is usually halfway between the umbilicus and pubic symphysis.

Access to more than two lumbar levels usually requires the use of a vertical paramedian decision, with the length determined by the specific number of levels required. Access is through the rectus-abdominus muscle to the posterior rectus sheath above the arcuate line, or by mobilization of the rectus laterally. Incision of the anterior rectus sheath in line with the skin incision or it can be enlarged by making a vertical incision at both its medial and lateral margins as described by Henderson (8) and Fraser (13,14). The specifics of this are described in the following.

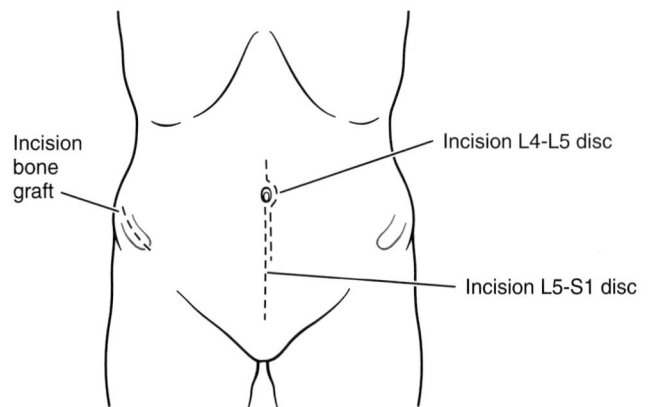

FIG. 20-1. Vertical paramedian incisions. (Modified from Henderson, RJ. Anterior approach for lumbar fusions and associated morbidity. In: Spine care. St. Louis: Mosby, 1995:1112–1134, with permission.)

Surgical Anatomy

The key muscle in the direct anterior approach is the rectus abdominus with its anterior and posterior sheaths above the arcuate line. Division of the anterior rectus sheath exposes the rectus muscle (Fig. 20-2). The underlying transversalis fascia is defined and carefully incised to gain entry into the retroperitoneal space. The peritoneal fat is gently freed with a finger from the transversalis fascia. The freed peritoneum, with its contents, is retracted medially (Fig. 20-3). The psoas is encountered posteriorly and medially with the genitofemoral nerve located on its surface and the sympathetic trunk located medially.

The ureter is identified by its peristaltic movements and accompanying blood vessels. The ureter usually stays with the posterior peritoneum as it is moved forward. The major blood vessels are identified: the aorta and common iliac and iliac arteries anteriorly and to the left of the corresponding veins.

The left iliolumbar vein may have several different configurations and should be doubly ligated before it is incised and mobilized (Fig. 20-4) (2).

The presence of the hypogastric plexus coming off the aorta can be at risk of damage as it courses over the anterior aspect of the lumbosacral disc (Fig. 20-5). Electrocautery should not be used in this area in males in order to avoid damage to the hypogastric plexus, which could result in retrograde ejaculation.

Contraindications and Disadvantages of the Anterior Approach

Contraindications to the direct anterior approach to the lower lumbar spine include the presence of pathology in the posterior column, and situations where the anatomy does not allow safe access to the anterior and middle columns. This includes low bifurcation of the aorta that may prevent safe access to the L5-S1 or L4-5 disc or the presence of significant retroperitoneal scarring from previous surgeries.

Disadvantages include the technical challenges of dissecting and manipulating major arteries and veins; namely, the iliolumbar vein, vena cava, common iliac vein, and accompanying arteries.

As indicated, the arterial structures are more resistant to manipulation than veins, so the approach to and the

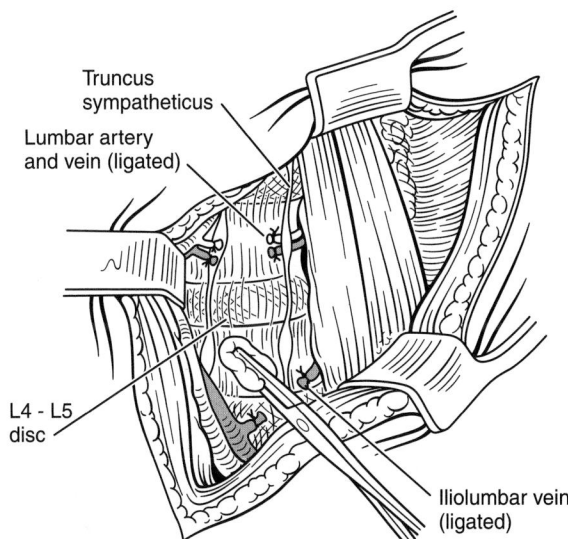

FIG. 20-3. Direct retroperitoneal approach. (Modified from Nakano N, Nakano T. Anterior extraperitoneal lumbar discectomy without fusion. In: The lumbar spine. Philadelphia: WB Saunders, 1990:987–989, with permission.)

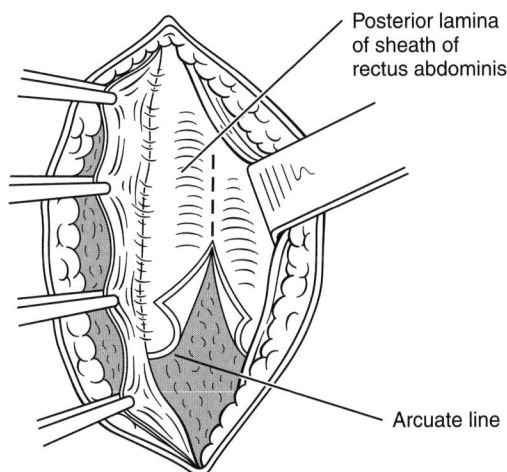

FIG. 20-2. Rectus abdominis. (Modified from Nakano N, Nakano T. Anterior extraperitoneal lumbar discectomy without fusion. In: The lumbar spine. Philadelphia: WB Saunders, 1990:987–989, with permission.)

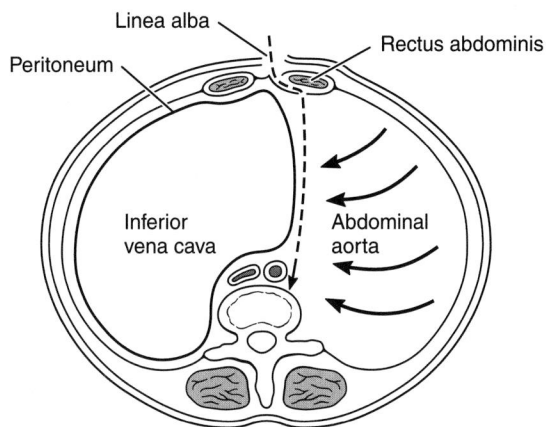

FIG. 20-4. Retroperitoneal structures at the L4-5 disc level. (Modified from Henderson, RJ. Anterior approach for lumbar fusions and associated morbidity. In: Spine care. St. Louis: Mosby, 1995:1112–1134, with permission.)

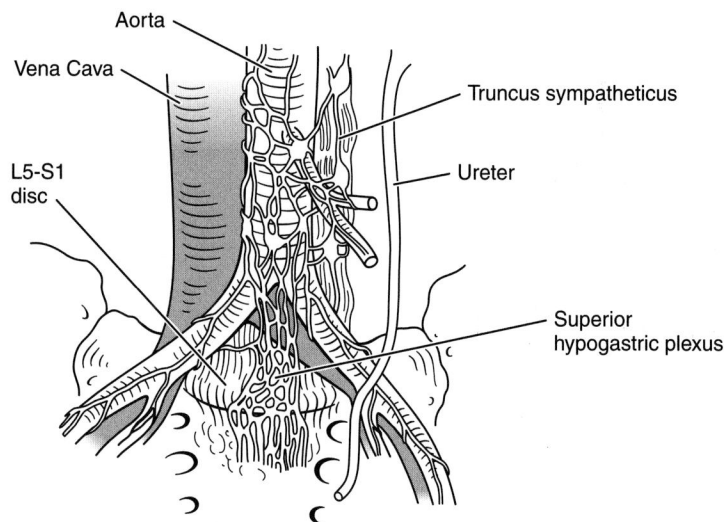

FIG. 20-5. Hypogastric plexus, vessels, and ureter. (Modified from Henderson, RJ. Anterior approach for lumbar fusions and associated morbidity. In: Spine care. St. Louis: Mosby, 1995:1112–1134, with permission.)

dissection of the lower lumbar spine should be done from the left. This approach also minimizes the potential damage to hypogastric plexus over the lumbosacral disc, minimizes the risk of injury to the ureter and the genitofemoral nerve and other nerves that lie within and on the psoas muscle.

The surgeon should be aware that anterior and lateral vertebral osteophytes can cause adherence of venous structures to the spine and make their dissection and manipulation difficult and dangerous because of the potential of injuring one of the veins. The assistance of an experienced vascular surgeon is invaluable to minimize this occurrence and help manage it if it occurs.

ANTEROLATERAL APPROACH

Indications for the anterolateral approach are similar to those for the direct anterior approach. It is particularly helpful in the obese patient, where the lateral decubitus position permits the viscera and abdominal wall to fall out of the way.

Patient Position

The patient is positioned in the decubitus position with the left side up over a beanbag on a radiolucent operating table. The patient must be positioned over the break in the table so that flexion of the table will permit lateral flexion of the patient. This lateral flexion increases the interval among the costal margin, iliac crest, and pubic symphysis to facilitate exposure. An auxiliary role is placed under the dependent axilla and the upper arm is placed in a relaxed neutral position over a pillow or armboard. The hips and knees are flexed and padded to protect the peripheral nerves, particularly the lateral popliteal nerve at the knee. Flexion of the hips relaxes the psoas muscle, which aids in its dissection from the lateral aspect of the lumbar bodies and the transverse process.

Once the patient is properly positioned, a beanbag is inflated to provide support. The bean bag must not come higher than the umbilicus anteriorly and the spinous process posteriorly in order to avoid limitation of the surgical exposure. The patient is secured with strapping around the shoulders and over the greater trochanter, to stabilize the patient when the table is rotated.

It is very important to keep the posterior cortex on the vertebra in a direct vertical alignment when decompressing the spine anteriorly in order to avoid disorientation and potential neural injury by penetration through the posterior cortical wall into the anterior epidural space of the vertebral canal.

Incision

As with the direct anterior approach to the lumbar spine, the incisions for the antero-lateral approach to the lower lumbar spine depend on which levels require exposure (Fig. 20-6). Usually the lateral edge of the incision is

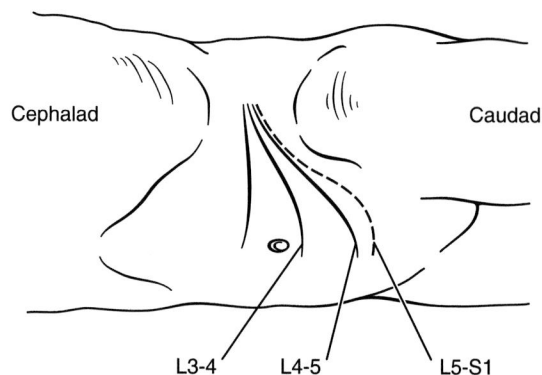

FIG. 20-6. Variation in oblique incision for specific lumbar level. (Modified from Watkins RG. Surgical approaches to the spine. In: The lumbar spine. Philadelphia: WB Saunders, 1996:1263–1271, with permission.)

in the midauxiliary line proceeding medially and curving inferiorly to the midline anteriorly. The surface and radiologic anatomy must be checked to be sure that the intercristal line passes through the L4-5 disc and appropriate adjustments in the incision should be made if necessary. For exposure of the L3-4 level the medial aspect of the incision should be in the midline at or below the umbilicus. For access to the L4-5 disc, the medial aspects of the incision should be in the mid- to upper third of the way between the umbilicus and pubic symphysis. Access to the L5-S1 disc should be midway between the umbilicus and pubic symphysis.

Surgical Anatomy

Knowledge of the muscles of the lateral abdominal wall is the key to this approach. The fascia and fibers of the external oblique usually run along the line of the incision, and the fibers of the internal oblique run at nearly 90 degrees to the external oblique fibers. The transversus abdominus muscle runs nearly horizontally above the transversalis fascia. After blunt dissection between the fibers of the external and internal obliques, the transversalis fascia is defined and reflected laterally to gain access to the retroperitoneal space. The peritoneum is carefully swept off the transversalis fascia and the retroperitoneal fat is encountered in the retroperitoneal space. The dissection is bluntly carried down to the psoas muscle. The mobilization, dissection, and manipulation of the psoas laterally are important to obtain access to the lateral aspect of the lower lumbar spine. Care must be taken to avoid injury to the sympathetic trunk lying along its medial aspect, the nerves of the lumbar plexus in its substance, and the genitofemoral nerve along the surface of the psoas. The ureter is identified by its peristaltic movement and usually moves with the posterior peritoneum as the peritoneum and its contents are reflected anteriorly.

The relationship of the major blood vessels, iliolumbar vein, and hypogastric plexus are the same as with the direct anterior approach.

POSTERIOR APPROACH

This discussion covers the posterior approach to the lumbar spine through the following incisions and dissections: direct midline, paramedian muscle splitting, and far lateral or oblique.

The posterior approach provides access to the posterior column, including the pedicle, transverse process, facet joint lamina, and spinous process; the vertebral canal; the middle column, including the disc, posterior longitudinal ligament, and posterior vertebral body; and limited access to the anterior column.

The posterior approach is commonly used for the following surgical procedures: decompression of the verte-

bral canal, nerve root canal and foramen; posterior fusion and instrumentation for management of deformity and instability; excision of primary and secondary spinal tumors; and débridement of spinal infections.

Surgical and Radiologic Anatomy

The surface anatomic landmarks include the midline lumbar spinous processes, intercristal line, and posterior superior and inferior iliac spines. Usually the sacral dimple area is at the level of the lumbosacral disc.

The radiologic anatomy must be checked on the AP and lateral X-rays, taking care to ensure that there are no lumbosacral anomalies such as lumbarization of the sacrum, or sacralization of L5, spina bifida occult, or prior laminectomy defect. The intercristal line must be checked on both the AP and lateral views to see its exact location with respect to the 4-5 intervertebral disc. Care must be taken to assure the appropriate level and confirm this with cross-table lateral X-rays if necessary. The key to orientation within the spinal canal is the pedicle: medial to the pedicle is the nerve root and superior to it is the intervertebral disc.

Patient Position

The patient is placed prone on a suitably padded spinal frame that provides the required position and posture of the lumbar spine. This may be in lumbar flexion for a simple laminotomy and disc prolapse or in extension and lordosis for decompression of spinal stenosis. The lordotic position is mandatory if instrumentation and fusion is required to assure that lumbar lordosis is achieved. This minimizes the risk of developing a "flat back" position.

The spinal frame must allow the abdomen to hang free to avoid compression of the abdominal contents, which can cause excessive epidural bleeding by shunting of blood from the vena cava through Batson's plexus into the epidural veins. Epidural bleeding also can be minimized by having the anesthesiologists avoid overinflation of the lungs and overdistention of the diaphragm, which can increase abdominal pressure and shunt blood from the vena cava into the epidural veins.

The patient also can be placed in the kneeling position, which also avoids abdominal compression. Care must be taken to avoid pressure on the knees and other bony prominences.

Incisions

Midline

The midline incision is centered over the appropriate level and is the most commonly used incision in gaining access to the posterior lumbar spine. It provides ready access to unilateral or bilateral pathologies. The length of the incision can be minimized by taking a cross-table X-ray beforehand to accurately identify the level or levels in question.

The incision is taken directly down through the superficial and deep subcutaneous fascia to the middle of the posterior tip of the spinous process and the lumbo dorsal fascia. Stripping and dissection of the subcutaneous tissue from the lumbar dorsal fascia avoids producing a dead space that can fill with serous fluid and blood.

Paramedian Incision

The paramedian incision is used for the paraspinal approach popularized by Wiltse that involves splitting of the sacrospinous muscle in the sagittal plane, two or three fingerbreadths from the midline (15,16). Wiltse recommended bilateral skin incisions, whereas others have advocated a midline skin incision with bilateral incision of the thoracolumbar fascia and splitting of the sacrospinalis muscle (Fig. 20-7). This provides access to the facet joint and transverse processes, and for lateral pathology such as a far lateral disc prolapse.

A midline incision for the bilateral paramedian approach has the advantage of a single skin incision but requires a longer cut than a bilateral skin incision. A bilateral incision also provides adequate access for pedicle screw and instrumentation insertion.

Far Lateral Incision

This incision is placed over the lateral edge of the erector spinae muscle, usually between the junction of the medial spinalis muscle and the intermediate longissimus muscle portion of the erector spinae muscle. This approach provides access to the transverse process and is the least used incision or approach to the posterior lumbar spine.

Surgical Anatomy

The lumbar dorsal fascia is detached from the tips of the spinous process and is followed by subperiosteal dissection of the paraspinal muscles from the spinous process, lamina, and posterior facet joint. If necessary, this can be carried out all the way to the transverse processes.

Posterior Lumbar Muscles

The lumbar musculature can be grouped into the following types:

- short intersegmental muscles, which include interspinales and intertransversarii mediales;
- short polysegmental muscles, which include multifidus and the lumbar portions of longissimus and iliocostalis (the lumbar erector spinae); and

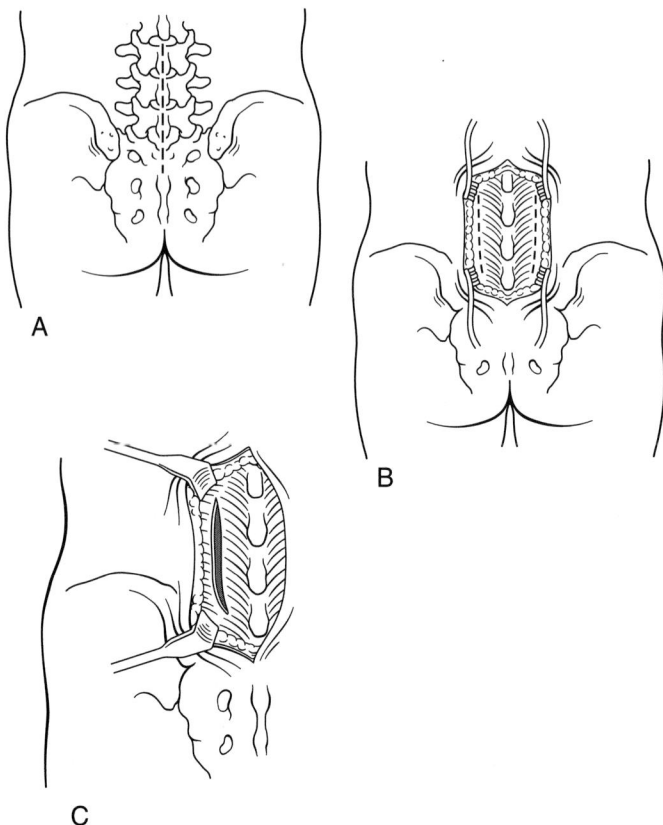

FIG. 20-7. Midline incision for paraspinal approach. (Modified from Wiltse LL, Bateman GI, Hutchinson RH, et al. The paraspinal sacra spinalis splitting approach to the lumbar spine. J Bone Joint Surg 1968;50A:919; Wiltse LL. The paraspinal sacra spinalis splitting approach to the lumbar spine. Clin Orthop 1973;91:48, with permission.)

- long polysegmental muscles, which include thoracic portions of longissimus and iliocostalis(1).

Short Intersegmental

Interspinalis. There are four pairs of lumbar interspinalis, each pair lying lateral to the interspinous ligament and connecting the adjacent spinous processes.

Intertransversarii Medialis. These arise from the accessory and mamillary processes and from the mamillo-acessory ligament between the processes, and are innervated at each level by the lumbar dorsal rami.

Short Polysegmental

Multifidus. Multifidus is invariably encountered in posterior midline approaches to the lumbar spine, as it is the most medial and the largest of the posterior lumbar musculature.

There is a constant pattern of fascicles, either short thin fascicles arising from the caudal portion of the dorsal aspect of each lumbar and inserted into the mamillary process of the vertebra two levels caudal, or larger longer fascicles arising from the spinous process radiating out in five overlapping groups that form the bulk of the multifidus. The fascicles arise either from the base of the spinous process or from the common tendon at the caudal tip of the spinous process and are inserted three levels caudal into the mamillary process—the posterior superior iliac spine, the posterior iliac crest, or the sacrum.

Lumbar Erector Spinae. The lumbar erector spinae is made up of two named muscles—the longissimus thoracis and iliocostalis lumborum—that are separated by the lumbar intermuscular aponeurosis. Each has two named portions: *lumbar* fascicles arising from the lumbar vertebrae and *thoracic* fascicles arising from the thoracic vertebrae.

The longissimus thoracis pars lumborum has five fascicles, each arising from the mamillary process and the adjacent transverse process of each vertebra and inserted into the medial aspect of the posterior superior iliac spine.

The iliocostalis lumborum pars lumborum has four overlapping fascicles arising from the tip of the transverse process of L1, L2, L3, and L4 vertebrae as well as the adjacent middle layer of the thoracolumbar fascia, and insert into the iliac crest lateral to the posterior superior iliac crest.

The thoracic portions of these muscles make up the long polysegmental muscles, arising from the ribs and transverse processes, and attach to the sacrum and iliac crest, as well as the tendinous portions forming the erector spinae aponeurosis that are attached to the ilium, the sacrum, and the sacral and lumbar spinous processes.

The thoracolumbar fascia is made up of three layers—anterior, middle, and posterior—that separate the posterior lumbar and trunk muscles into separate compartments and has significant biomechanical functions.

The posterior layer is the most significant surgically and consists of superficial and deep laminae forming a retinaculum over the lumbar muscles. The posterior layer is attached medially to the midline and laterally to the lateral raphe, arising vertically from the iliac crest.

Other anatomical works list these lumbar muscles into layers:

Superficial: the thoracic portions of longissimus thoracis and iliocostalis lumborum.
Intermediate: the multifidus and the lumbar portions of longissimus thoracis and iliocostalis lumborum.
Deep: the interspinales and intertransversarii.

Ligamentum Flavum

Knowledge of the ligamentum flavum, and understanding its attachment at each level, aids in its safe dissection and removal. The ligamentum flavum runs in a vertical direction attaching to the cephalic tip of the distal lamina and halfway up the ventral surface of the proximal lamina (Fig. 20-8) (18). The ligamentum flavum also attaches laterally to the undersurface of the facet joint, and its fibers blend with those of the anterior capsule of the facet joint.

The facet joints are innervated by the posterior rami of the spinal nerves, which gain access to the posterior compartment at the lateral edge of the pars interarticularis and are accompanied by the intertransverse artery, which supplies the muscles of the deep layer. These vessels frequently are breached during posterior exposures and bleed during routine dissection of the pars, particularly during dissection out to the lateral tip of the transverse process at each level.

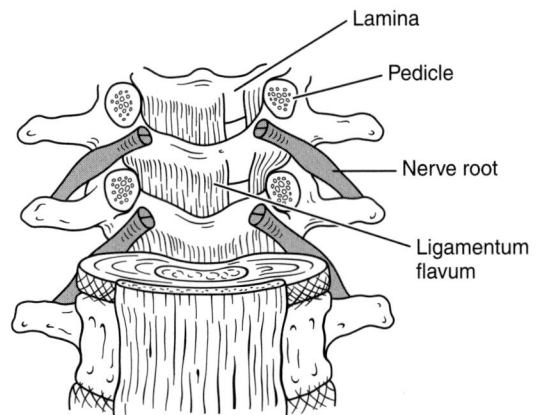

FIG. 20-8. Ligamentum flavum, nerve root, and pedicle. (Modified from Watkins RG. Surgical approaches to the spine. In: The lumbar spine. Philadelphia: WB Saunders, 1996:1263–1271, with permission.)

The Pedicle

The superficial landmarks, entry point, length, breadth, and direction of each lumbar pedicle are important. The pedicle is the key landmark to safely find the lateral edge of the nerve root and the intervertebral disc immediately above it. Pedicle fixation requires thorough knowledge of the pedicle entry point, which usually is located at the junction of the lateral edge of the facet and the midpoint of the transverse process.

Usually the pars of L5 is in line with the lateral portion of the L5 pedicle. Proceeding proximally, the lateral portion of the pars moves medially, so in the upper lumbar spine the medial edge of the pars is in line with the medial border of the pedicle.

Erector Spinae Muscle

The paravertebral approach of Wiltse exposes the spine in the interval between the multifidus and lateral muscles (longissimus and iliocostalis) (Fig. 20-9). The posterior and lateral aspect of the facet joint is palpated and the lateral muscles are retracted and dissected off the transverse process. The transverse process is identified and followed medially to pedicle, which can be palpated and used to identify the exiting nerve root. This approach provides access to a far lateral disc.

Indications and Advantages

The direct posterior approach to the lumbar spine provides safe access to posterior pathology and limited access to anterior column pathology through the pedicle or by gentle cauda equina retraction.

Contraindications

Potential contraindications to the posterior approach include anterior column pathology and significant skin or post-subcutaneous scarring and fibrosis related to previous radiation therapy or significant burns.

Disadvantages

One disadvantage to the posterior approach is the stripping of the paraspinal musculature, which can be associated with impairment of its nerve and blood supply and the formation of thick scar tissue, which can contribute to development of the postlaminectomy syndrome. Long and wide muscle stripping can be associated with prolonged recovery and postoperative pain and disability that can persist despite extensive postoperative rehabilitation.

Postlaminectomy scarring can occur as the muscle grows back into the laminectomy site and into the exposed dura and nerve roots. This also can produce difficulty in obtaining safe exposure for a redo posterior decompression. The scarring is often associated with dural tear and nerve root damage during repeat decompression.

There have been reports of injury to the aorta, vena cava, and retroperitoneal viscera with inadvertent placement of the instruments through the anterior longitudinal ligament. Therefore, it is imperative to know the length of the instruments being used and the depth to which it can be safely inserted into the disc space. It is also recommended that the pituitary rongeur be placed through the annulotomy with the jaws closed and then opened to avoid inadvertent grabbing of neural structures.

Intraoperative ophthalmic complications are uncommon but catastrophic. These include postoperative blindness and visual field defects. Contributing etiologies include an underlying vascular diathesis, diabetes, and direct pressure to the globe.

Prolonged positioning in the prone position also can result in cardiopulmonary shunting, which can be problematic in the elderly population undergoing multilevel decompression and fusion.

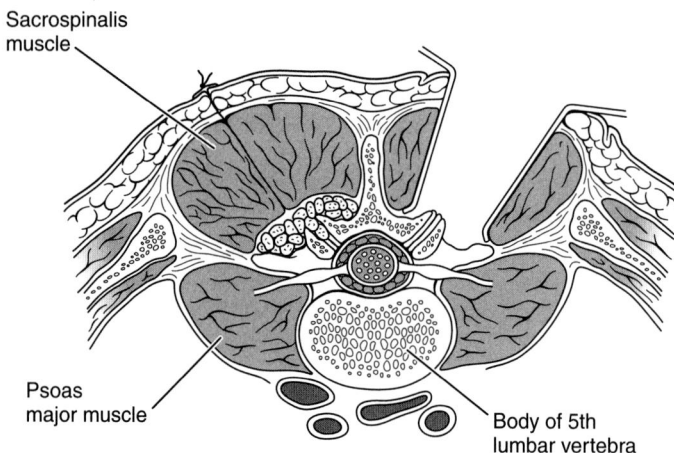

FIG. 20-9. Paramedian muscle splitting approach. (Modified from Wiltse LL, Bateman GI, Hutchinson RH, et al. The paraspinal sacra spinalis splitting approach to the lumbar spine. J Bone Joint Surg 1968;50A:919; Wiltse LL. The paraspinal sacra spinalis splitting approach to the lumbar spine. Clin Orthop 1973;91:48, with permission.)

REFERENCES

1. Bogduk NE, Twomey LT. Clinical anatomy of the lumbar spine. Edinburgh: Churchill Livingstone, 1991.
2. Crock HV. A short practice of spinal surgery. New York: Springer-Verlag Wien, 1993.
3. Hodgson AR, Yau ACMC. Anterior approaches to the spinal column. In: Apley AG, ed. Recent advances in orthopedics. Baltimore: Williams & Wilkins, 1964:289–323.
4. Hollingshead WH. Anatomy for surgeons, 3rd ed. Philadelphia: Harper & Row, 1982.
5. Selby DK, Henderson RJ, et al. Anterior lumbar fusion. In: White AH, Rothman R, eds. Lumbar spine surgery. St. Louis: CV Mosby, 1987:383.
6. Dwyer AP. Clinically relevant anatomy. In: Wiesel, Weinstein, Herkowitz, et al., eds. The lumbar spine. 2nd ed. Philadelphia: WB Saunders, 1996:57–73.
7. Hoppenfeld S, DeBoer P. Surgical exposure in orthopedics: the anatomical approach. Philadelphia: JB Lippincott, 1984.
8. Henderson RJ. Anterior approach for lumbar fusions and associated morbidity. In: Spine care. St. Louis: Mosby, 1995:1112–1134.
9. Fountain SS. A single stage combined surgical approach for vertebral resection. J Bone Joint Surg 1979;61A:1011.
10. Hanley ED, Delamater RB, McCulloch JA, et al. Surgical indications and techniques. In: Wiesel, Weinstein, Herkowitz, et al., eds. The lumbar spine. Philadelphia: WB Saunders, 1996:492–524.
11. Hodgson AR, Stock FE. Anterior spine fusion, a preliminary communication on the radical treatment of Pott's disease and Pott's paraplegia. Br J Surg 1956;44–266.
12. Hodgson AR, Stock FE. Anterior spinal fusion for the treatment of tuberculosis of the spine. J Bone Joint Surg 1960;42A:295.
13. Fraser RD, Gogan NJ. A modified muscle splitting approach to the lumbar sacral spine. Spine 1992;17:943.
14. Fraser RD. A wide muscle splitting approach to the lumbar sacral spine. J Bone Joint Surg 1982;64B:44–46.
15. Watkins RG. Surgical approaches to the spine. In: Wiesel, Weinstein, Herkowitz, et al., eds. The lumbar spine. Philadelphia: WB Saunders, 1996:1263–1271.
16. Wiltse LL, Bateman GI, Hutchinson RH, et al. The paraspinal sacra spinalis splitting approach to the lumbar spine. J Bone Joint Surg 1968;50A:919.
17. Nakano N, Nakano T. Anterior extraperitoneal lumbar discectomy without fusion. In: Wiesel, Weinstein, Herkowitz, et al., eds. The lumbar spine. Philadelphia: WB Saunders, 1990:987–989.
18. Watkins RG. Surgical approaches to the spine. New York: Springer-Verlag, 1983.
19. Nakano N, Nakano T. Anterior extraperitoneal lumbar discectomy without fusion. In: Wiesel, Weinstein, Herkowitz, et al., eds. The lumbar spine. Philadelphia: WB Saunders, 1990:1273–1274.
20. Wiltse LL. The paraspinal sacra spinalis splitting approach to the lumbar spine. Clin Orthop 1973;91:48.

CHAPTER 21

Posterior and Anterior Surgical Approaches to the Lumbosacral Junction

Peter A. Robertson

SEGMENTATION

Normal segmentation at the lumbosacral junction is frequently assumed, yet abnormal segmentation has been described in 33% of a cohort of patients (1). The presence of a transitional vertebra at the lumbosacral junction confuses nomenclature. Failure to recognize abnormal segmentation may cause incorrect interpretation of pathology, incorrect recognition of anatomic features at surgery, and increased risk of operating at an incorrect level.

Segmentation variations include extra or missing vertebrae within the spinal column (2); supernumerary or absent ribs; transitional lumbosacral segmentation with L5 transverse process articulation with the sacral ala; and incomplete coalescence of S1 and S2 with a well-formed S1-2 intervertebral disc. A wide variety of combinations may make it difficult to define levels with certainty. Options include classification of the whole spinal segmentation from proximal to distal, or counting from the sacrum up, to define levels. The former gives accurate labeling of the whole spine yet requires cumbersome total spinal X-rays and unwarranted exposure to radiation. The latter is more practical when dealing with the lumbosacral spine.

A practical approach to the nomenclature of atypical lumbosacral segmentation is to identify the transitional vertebra and describe it based on its most salient characteristics. A transitional vertebra that has all the appearances of an L5 vertebra, apart from a unilateral articulation between a transverse process and the sacral ala, is described as a sacralized L5. Conversely, if the upper sacral segment has all the hallmarks of an S1 segment, yet there is a significant rudimentary disc between S1 and S2, it is regarded as a lumbarized S1 (Fig. 21-1).Clear identification of a transitional lumbosacral segment requires lateral and special antero-posterior (AP) radiographs. The lateral allows definition of the vertebral body and sacral shape and the degree of formation of the abnormal disc. The AP views must include a view so that the X-ray beam is parallel to the lumbosacral disc. The beam should be centered on the disc. The lordosis thus requires the beam to be angled cephalad by approximately 20°, although this angulation varies dependent on the lordosis and should be judged from the lateral view. This is to accurately define the anatomic relationship between the transverse processes of L5 and the ala of the sacrum.

Once the transitional vertebra characteristics are defined and clarified, the adjacent segments can be numbered. When the number of lumbar vertebrae differs from normal (as defined by the absence of articulating ribs), some refer to the lumbosacral segment as the L4-S1 level or the L6-S1 level. Alternatively, the lumbar vertebrae may be numbered above an L5 segment to maintain familiarity with traditional segment numbering.

Because of the potential for confusion, it is essential that the treating doctors recognize any segmentation abnormalities and label the segments consistently. Consistent vertebral numbering and close correlation between preoperative and intraoperative lateral radiographs offer the best chance of avoiding incorrect levels.

POSTERIOR SURGICAL APPROACHES TO THE LUMBOSACRAL JUNCTION

The midline posterior approach to the lumbosacral junction, through a longitudinal incision, is an extensile approach that allows access to the posterior elements, the canal and the foramina, the posterolateral gutters, and the intervertebral disc space. It is the most frequently used approach and obviously can be extended to link with proximal dissection.

Identification of the level of incision is by relationship to the iliac crests (approximately L4 body level), palpa-

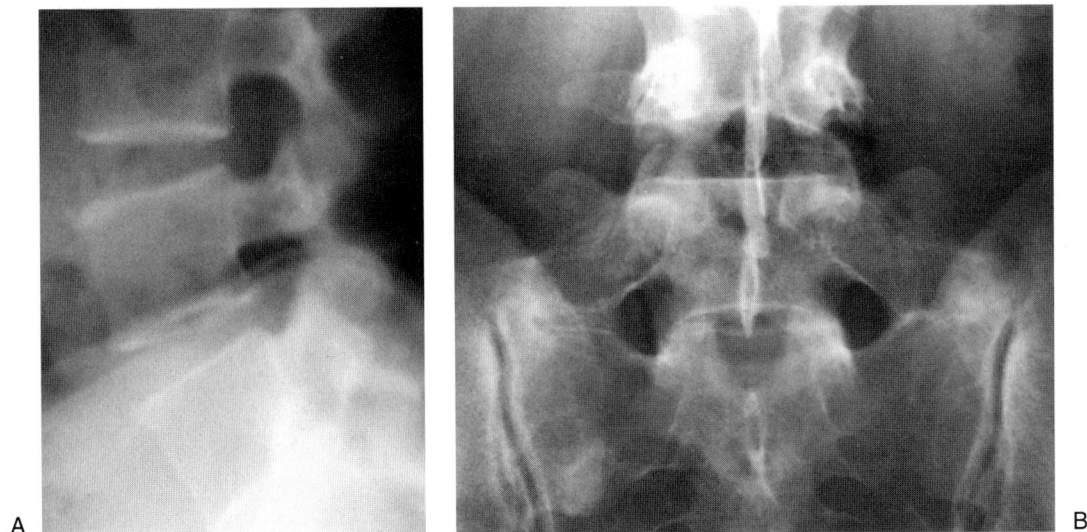

FIG. 21-1. A: A lateral X-ray of a transitional lumbosacral junction. The rudimentary disc space is between the upper sacral segment and the remainder of the sacrum. **B:** The anteroposterior radiograph angled parallel with the disc demonstrates the transitional vertebra with lateral articulation between the vertebra transverse processes and the sacral ala.

tion of the lumbosacral spinous process gaps, or use of skin markers and radiology.

Longitudinal division of the skin and subcutaneous tissue displays the deep fascia. This is a double-layered sheet that attaches to the spinous processes medially, and encloses the multifidus, the most medial of the paraspinal muscles. Although subperiosteal dissection is possible in children and adolescents, adults require division of the deep fascial attachment to the spinous process. The multifidus muscle attachment to the spinous processes and laminae of L5 and S1 is easily swept aside with a Cobb or Harrington periosteal elevator. The tendinous attachment of the multifidus is to the midline structures at the level of the supraspinous and interspinous ligaments. This attachment requires sharp division. Preoperative identification of any spina bifida is mandatory to allow cautious dissection of the upper sacrum—preventing inadvertent canal entry. Self-retaining retractors hold the multifidus muscle laterally and allow midline access to the canal by midline laminectomy or unilateral laminotomy. The parasagittal muscles can be swept further laterally, to display the glistening white lumbosacral facet joint capsule. The Taylor pointed retractor can then be placed lateral to the facet joint and levered laterally to retract the paraspinal muscles. This retraction technique is ideal for unilateral posterior lumbosacral approaches. Dissection proximal to the lumbosacral facet joint displays the pars interarticularis of L5. Definition of the lateral aspect of the pars is necessary to allow sufficient pars preservation when performing L5 laminectomy (Fig. 21-2).

More lateral development of this approach allows exposure to the posterolateral gutters, where bone grafting is performed in a posterolateral fusion. The multi-

fidus muscle has a further attachment to the posterolateral facet capsule and superior articular facet, which, when divided in a longitudinal direction, reveals loose fatty tissue that can be swept laterally to reveal the superior ala of the sacrum. Display of the transverse process of L5 requires detachment of multifidus from the posterolateral facet capsule of L4-5. Again, loose fatty tissue covers the transverse process of L5 and is easily swept laterally.

Troublesome bleeding may occur with exposure of the posterolateral gutters. The segmental vessels that accompany the nerve roots as they enter the foramen also give branches that course lateral to the pars interarticularis and supply the paraspinal muscle complex. These posterior vessels give off small, but occasionally troublesome, vascular branches that pass distally, lateral to the facet joint capsule and superior articular facet of the joint below (3). They frequently bleed as the transverse process or ala of the sacrum is displayed. Direct visualization can be difficult because of the paraspinal muscle mass that prevents retraction, so that it is difficult to see lateral to the facet joint capsule and superior articular facet. Useful tricks to prevent troublesome bleeding lateral to the facet joints include preemptive use of bipolar coagulation forceps in the loose fatty tissue lateral to the facet joint capsule (before sweeping the fatty tissue aside to display the transverse process or sacral ala), or bending the tip of the unipolar diathermy and sweeping that diathermy tip up the lateral aspect to the superior articular facet superior to the sacral ala or the lumbar transverse process. Troublesome bleeding is controllable with lateral gutter packing. More constant vascular ooze from the lateral gutter occurs after the transverse process and the lateral aspect of

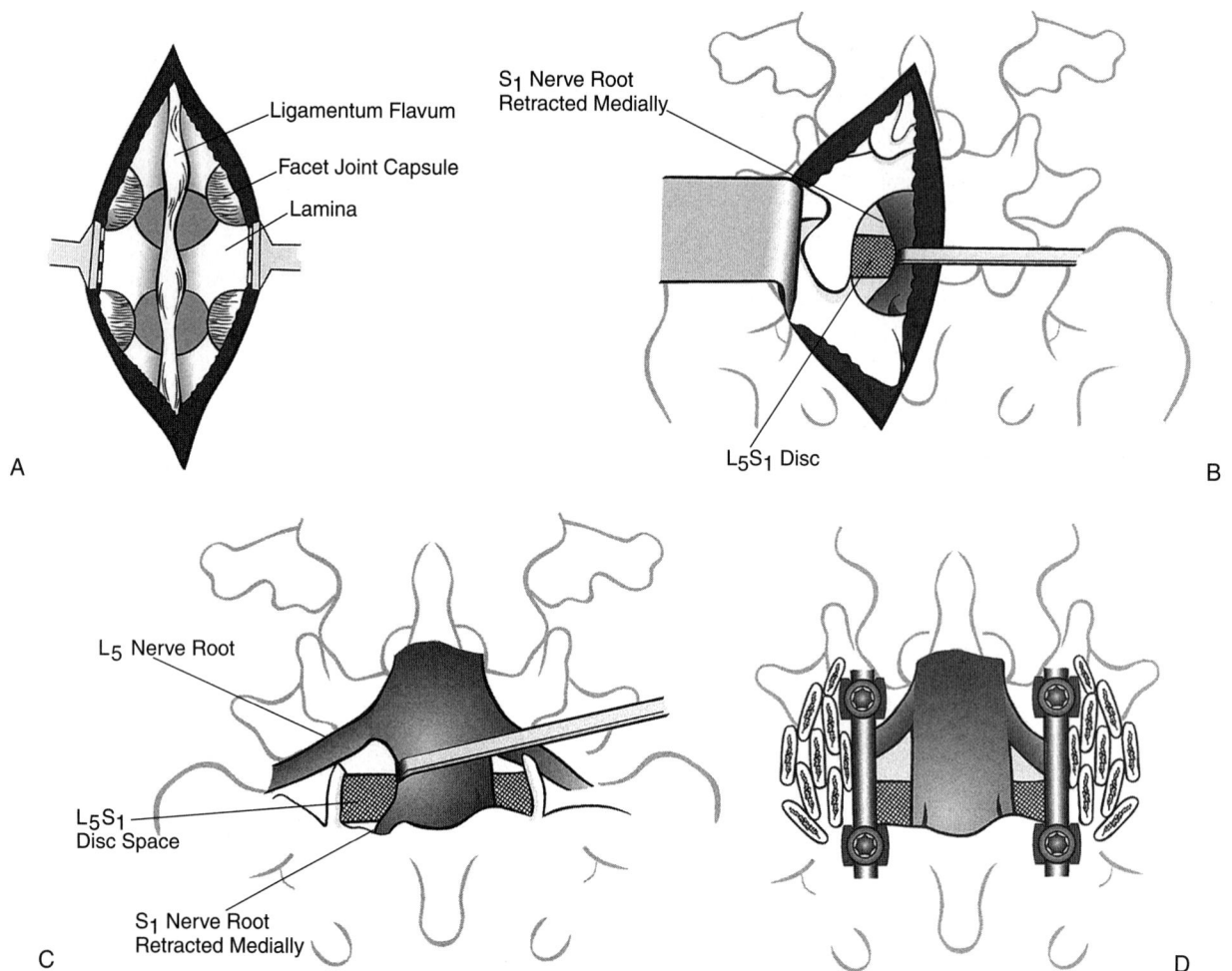

FIG. 21-2. Diagrammatic representation of the posterior approach to the lumbosacral junction. **A:** Posterior approach to the lumbosacral junction demonstrating laminae, ligamentum flavum, and facet joint capsules. **B:** Unilateral flavectomy, laminotomy, and approach for discectomy after retraction of the S1 nerve root. **C:** Extensive facetectomy to demonstrate the transforaminal "window" for access to the disc space. **D:** Posterolateral fusion with pedicle screws and rods after wide destabilizing facetectomy at the lumbosacral junction.

the superior articular facet are decorticated, before bone grafting and fusion procedures. For this reason decortication should be deferred until as late as possible in the procedure. Minor degrees of initial bleeding can occur with dissection around the S1 posterior foramen. This is best controlled with bipolar diathermy.

Attempts to coagulate the posterior branch of the segmental vessels, lateral to the pars interarticularis, threaten the posterior primary rami that accompany these vessels. At L4 and L5 these nerves do not have cutaneous sensory function (4), but the damage has implications for muscle function.

In unilateral posterior lumbosacral approaches effective retraction can be obtained with a Taylor pointed retractor, placed lateral to the facet joint, and retained by a weight and chain.

Bilateral approaches obtain best visualization with Travers (straight) or Adson (curved) self-retainers. Difficulty

with retraction is alleviated by proximal and distal release of the erector spinae from the midline structures. Careful use of self-retaining retractors and hand-held retractors gives adequate exposure to all posterior structures. Powerful crank type retractors can give wide exposure to the posterior structures, but can damage the paraspinal muscles, particularly if the retractor blades are forced hard up against the posterior iliac crest laterally. Muscle atrophy, weakness, and electromyographic changes occur following surgery, and these changes should be minimized (5–7). The crank retractor bulk can also limit access to the correct oblique pathway for pedicle screw placement at L5 and S1 (Fig. 21-3).

As an alternative to bilateral multifidus dissection off the spinous process and laminae for decompressive procedures, a unilateral multifidus strip combined with a spinous process osteotomy (at the base) allows midline access for decompression. This approach may limit mus-

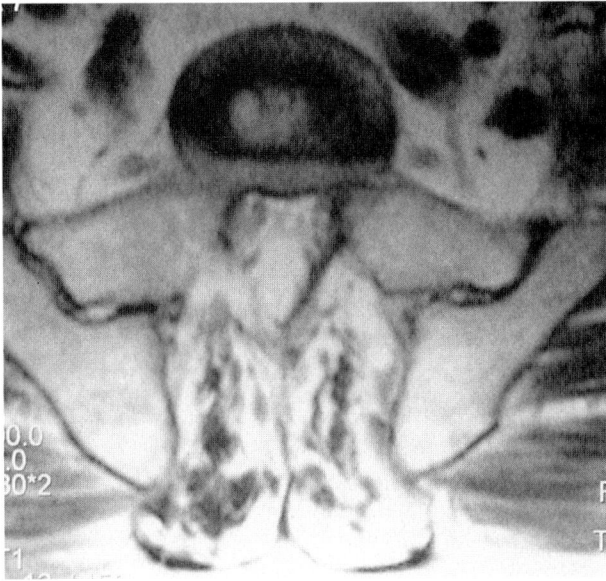

FIG. 21-3. Magnetic resonance imaging scan (axial) of the lumbosacral junction of an achondroplastic dwarf presenting for decompression of spinal stenosis. Note that the posterior iliac crests are very medial, causing herniation of the paraspinal muscle mass posteriorly. A posterior approach to this level is technically difficult because of muscle bulk and difficulty with retraction owing to the iliac crests. A limited amount of muscle excision may be required to access the spinal canal.

cle damage, preserve midline structures, and improve cosmesis, yet risks problems from spinous process nonunion, and cannot be applied if bilateral wider posterolateral exposure is needed (8).

SPINAL CANAL DISSECTION AT THE LUMBOSACRAL JUNCTION

Entry to the spinal canal at the lumbosacral junction requires removal of the ligamentum flavum on one or both sides of the midline. This can be achieved with either cautious sharp dissection in the midline or detachment of the ligamentum flavum at its periphery (easiest distally) using a small curved sharp curette. Once the epidural space is opened, it is explored and expanded with a dissector. A Kerrison up-cutting rongeur can be used to remove the ligamentum flavum and display the epidural space from the midline out to the facet joint.

The extent of dissection within the canal is determined by the pathology. Flavectomy alone gives adequate access to most posterolateral disc herniations. Partial laminectomy of either L5 proximally or S1 distally may be required for migrated disc fragments. Medial facetectomy is required where facet hypertrophy causes lateral recess stenosis at the entrance to the nerve root canal. Facetectomy can be performed with either rongeurs or osteotomes. Occasionally, more radical or complete facetectomy is required to decompress the L5-S1 foramen

and to allow access to the L5-S1 disc space to provide a working channel for interbody dissection and surgery. More proximal and lateral dissection is required if the L5 root needs decompression under the pars interarticularis, such as when there is a pars defect filled with hypertrophic fibrocartilage in association with a spondylolysis or spondylolisthesis (Fig. 21-2).

Once inside the canal it is essential to appreciate the position of the roots and dura at all times. A small layer of fat may cover the dura dorsally. The dural sac and traversing S1 root are medial to any working zone for discectomy or interbody work. The exiting L5 root has passed superiorly and laterally to the lumbosacral disc. If pathology about the exiting L5 root requires treatment at the lumbosacral junction, it is both superior and lateral to the flavectomy site for entry to the lumbosacral canal.

Epidural veins may be bountiful to the lateral and anterior regions of the canal, adjacent to the medial wall of the pedicle, and also to the posterior intervertebral body of L5 and S1. The vertebral body venous plexus communicates with the epidural veins anterior to the dural sac. The most effective way to prevent troublesome venous bleeding is to carefully position the patient before surgery, leaving the abdomen free from pressure, thereby avoiding engorgement of the epidural plexus.

If epidural venous bleeding is troublesome during canal dissection, careful packing with Gelfoam soaked in thrombin or with neurosurgical patties is useful. Larger veins may be cauterized with bipolar diathermy after careful retraction of neural structures. Occasional venous ooze from a cut bone at the edge of a laminectomy field may require the use of bone wax.

PARASAGITTAL APPROACH TO THE LUMBOSACRAL JUNCTION

Wiltse described the parasagittal approach to the lumbar spine (9), primarily for intertransverse fusion. It is particularly advantageous if surgery involves only posterolateral fusion without canal exploration. At the lumbosacral junction, in the presence of a high-grade spondylolisthesis, it can be very difficult to find and display the L5 transverse process in its forward slipped position. The Wiltse approach allows direct dissection on to the posterolateral structures with the minimum of muscle dissection (Fig. 21-4). Pedicle screws can be placed without excessive muscle retraction, a particularly helpful step at L5 where the pedicle is obliquely directed (10). This approach is also useful to treat the relatively uncommon far lateral disc herniation at L5-S1 and for excision of anomalous transverse processes that articulate with the sacrum and cause pain (Fig. 21-5) (11,12).

The approach is longitudinal and parasagittal between the multifidus muscle group medially and sacrospinalis laterally. Skin incision options include a midline longitudinal skin incision approach with bilateral parasagittal

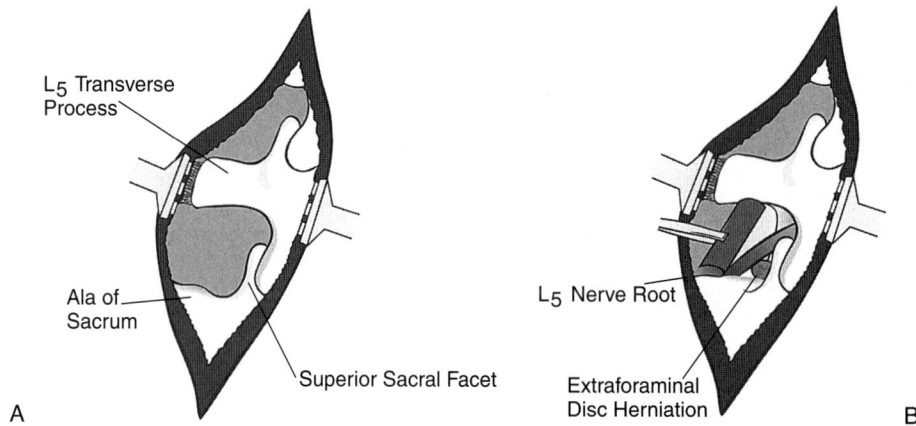

FIG. 21-4. Diagrammatic approach of the Wiltse parasagittal approach to the spine. **A:** The Wiltse parasagittal approach demonstrating the lateral aspects of the superior articular facets and the L5 transverse process and ala of the sacrum. **B:** Removal of the intertransverse membrane demonstrates the nerve root and the site of a far lateral (extraforaminal) disc prolapse.

fascial incisions two fingers breadth lateral to the midline; bilateral skin parasagittal incisions over the intermuscular interval; and a transverse skin incision at the lumbosacral junction with vertical fascial incisions over the parasagittal muscle interval. Bone graft may be harvested through any of the skin incisions by subcutaneous dissection. The latter incision may be cosmetic, avoiding a longitudinal lower lumbar incision.

The intermuscular interval is 2 to 3 centimeters lateral to the midline, and allows a direct approach to the lateral aspect of the superior articular facets of L5 and S1 and the transverse process of L5 and the ala of the sacrum. The lateral border of the L5 pars interarticularis is tra-

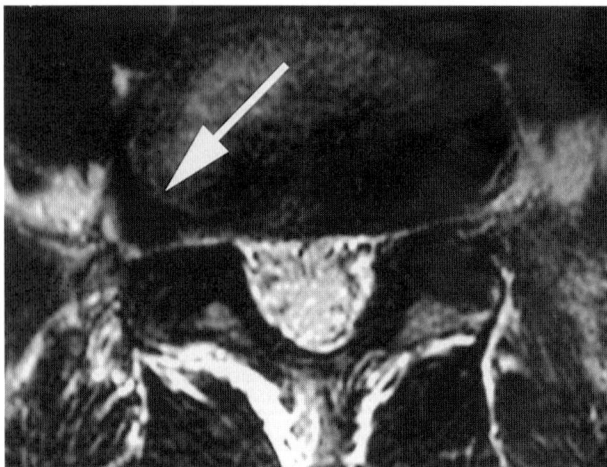

FIG. 21-5. Axial magnetic resonance imaging scan of a right far lateral disc prolapse (arrow) at the lumbosacral junction causing L5 root symptoms. This herniation can be approached surgically via a Wiltse parasagittal approach with minimal bone resection. Attempts to approach this from within the canal require destabilizing facet joint excision.

versed by the posterior primary ramus of L5 and the posterior branch of the segmental vessels. The latter frequently require coagulation.

The parasagittal approach gives excellent visualization of the posterolateral fusion bed and the lateral superior articular facet and the transverse process. Far lateral disc herniations may be resected after the intertransverse membrane is removed from its attachment to the adjacent transverse processes. The L5 nerve root traverses obliquely over the posterolateral aspect of the disc before forming a lumbosacral trunk.

This parasagittal approach can be used to access the spinal canal with multifidus retraction, hemilaminectomy on the surgical side, and then dissection beneath the lamina on the contralateral side so as to perform medial facetectomy and root decompression on that contralateral side (13).

A posterolateral approach lateral to iliocostalis has been described as an alternative approach to the far lateral disc prolapse (14). This approach develops a plane between iliocostalis and the flank muscles, and then follows the most lateral branch of the posterior primary rami down to the nerve root in the foramen. It is an approach perhaps more useful in the proximal lumbar spine, above the posterior iliac crest, yet has been used at L5-S1.

ANTERIOR APPROACHES TO THE LUMBOSACRAL JUNCTION

Anterior approaches to the lumbosacral junction require an approach between the great vessels to the lumbosacral disc. Retraction of the iliac arteries and veins laterally gives the broad expanse of the lumbosacral disc, with only the median sacral artery and the presacral autonomic nerves coursing inferiorly across the lumbosacral disc. Decisions as to the approach to this disc depend on a preference for a transperitoneal or retroperitoneal approach to the disc, and any requirement for dissection to include more proximal discs.

If only the lumbosacral disc requires surgery, then the transperitoneal approach offers a very direct approach and straightforward route to this disc. Division of the posterior parietal peritoneum allows direct display of the bifurcation of the great vessels, and the fine vessels and nerves that cross the disc (15). Obvious contraindications to this approach include acquired conditions resulting in extensive peritoneal adhesions.

The bifurcation of the aorta and inferior vena cava usually lie at the level of the L5 vertebral body, so the lumbosacral disc is approached between the bifurcations. Because the vena cava bifurcation is below and to the right of the aortic bifurcation, the vascular structure most at risk for injury is the left common iliac vein (16). Considerable variation exists in the relationship between the bifurcations and the body of L5 (17). When the bifurcation is proximal in relation to the spine there are occasions when the lower two lumbar discs can be approached through the bifurcation. At the other extreme, a low position of the vessels may result in a need to approach the lumbosacral disc lateral to the iliac vessels. In this latter situation, the iliolumbar vein should be divided to assist mobilization of the vessels.

The median sacral artery must be divided. Most surgeons advocate avoiding the use of diathermy about the presacral plexus over the front of the lumbosacral disc, for fear of the complication of retrograde ejaculation in male patients (15). Review has suggested that this complication is rare (18,19), yet it is prudent to cautiously isolate the presacral plexus and mobilize it to the side before approaching the lumbosacral disc (Fig. 21-6).

The lumbosacral junction also can be approached by a retroperitoneal method, with development of the retroperitoneal space, usually on the left side, allowing retraction of the viscera and display of the great vessels and spine. This is the approach required if the lumbosacral disc surgery is part of a combined procedure that involves surgery to the proximal discs.

The transperitoneal approach is best made through a vertical incision between the recti, with the incision located between the umbilicus and the symphysis. The parietal peritoneum is divided longitudinally, and with the patient in the Trendelenburg position, the abdominal contents are packed out of the way. This approach presents the posterior wall of the abdomen. Division of the posterior parietal peritoneum reveals the bifurcation of the aorta and inferior vena cava, and the lumbosacral disc between these structures. If the anterolateral disc region is to be exposed, the vessels must be carefully retracted to each side. The surgeon should make the incision low in the abdomen so that any instrumentation required for access to the lumbosacral disc can be performed with a direct view of the inferiorly directed L5-S1 disc space.

Approaches to the lumbosacral disc through a retroperitoneal route generally require a more lateral entry to the abdominal cavity. Approaches are either muscle-cutting or -splitting (19). Multiple descriptions of approach options exist, aiming to preserve abdominal wall muscle function (19–22). Incisions are horizontal or oblique along the line of the external oblique muscle, and placed at levels appropriate to allow access to the relevant discs. The deeper layers are either split or divided lateral to the recti. Most authors advocate avoidance of extensive longitudinal dissection lateral to the rectus abdominus, because of the risk of denervation of this muscle, yet this approach may yield a useful extensile approach that incorporates access to the lumbosacral disc along with several more proximal discs when extensive procedures are performed (20). In order to prevent possible denervation of the rectus, we have combined a paramedian longitudinal skin incision with a midline vertical incision between the recti, and a left-sided retroperitoneal dissection giving access to the lumbosacral junction, and combining this with access to the lumbar discs as high as L1.

Careful vascular retraction allows display of the lumbosacral disc. The adherent relationship between the great vessels and the lower lumbar vertebrae mean that

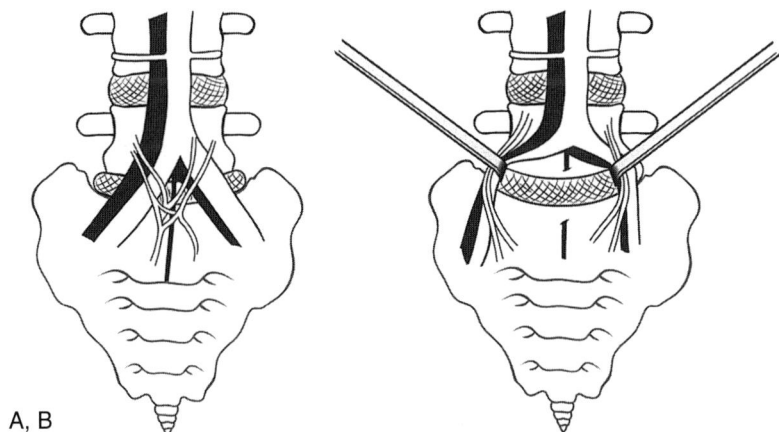

A, B

FIG. 21-6. Diagrammatic representation of the great vessel bifurcations overlying the lumbosacral disc, and the access to the disc with vessel retraction. **A:** Great vessels and presacral plexus overlying the lumbosacral disc. **B:** The lumbosacral disc after retraction of the presacral plexus and the great vessel bifurcations, and division of the median sacral artery.

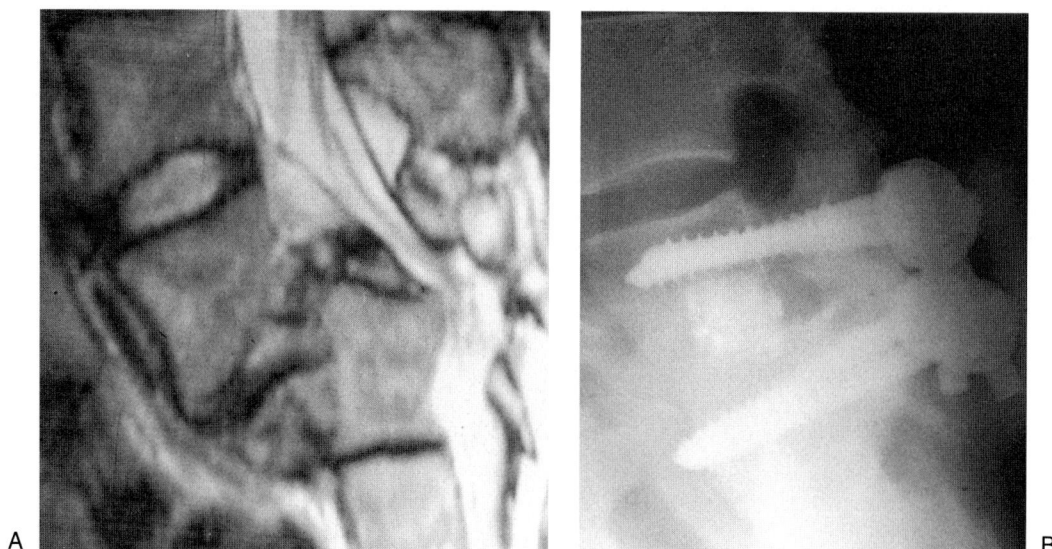

FIG. 21-7. A: Lateral radiograph of a 20-year-old woman with a delayed diagnosis and presentation (because of pregnancy) of a posttraumatic lumbosacral dislocation. **B:** Postoperative lateral radiograph after anterior transperitoneal approach, extensive mobilization of the great vessels, resection of anterior sacral callus, discectomy, inferior L5 hemicorpectomy (to avoid distraction during vertebral reduction), and subsequent posterior approach with transforaminal interbody fusion with titanium mesh cages and posterior pedicle screw instrumentation. The anterior approach was transperitoneal, with extensive mobilization of the great vessels to allow display of the L5 and S1 vertebral bodies.

greater anterior displays of the L5 body or upper sacrum require much greater mobilization of the vascular structures. Although this is infrequently required, a vascular surgeon can provide a very good working area for more extensive anterior surgery (Fig. 21-7).

REFERENCES

1. Wigh RE. Phylogeny and the herniated disc. South Med J 1979;72:1138–1143.
2. Wigh RE. The thoracolumbar and lumbosacral transitional junctions. Spine 1980;5:215–221.
3. Macnab I, Dall D. The blood supply of the lumar spine and its application to the technique of intertransverse lumbar fusion. J Bone Joint Surg (Britain) 1971;53B:628–637.
4. Last RJ. Anatomy: regional and applied. In: The nervous system. Edinburgh: Churchill Livingstone, 1978:20–31.
5. Mayer TG, Vanharnata H, Gatchel RJ, et al. Comparison of CT scan muscle measurements and isokinetic trunk strength in postoperative patients. Spine 1989;14:33–36.
6. See DH, Kraft GH. Electromyography in paraspinal muscles following surgery for root decompression. Arch Phys Med Rehab 1975;56:80–83.
7. Sihvonen T, Herno A, Paljava L, et al. Local denervation atrophy of paraspinal muscles in postoperative failed back syndrome. Spine 1993;18:575–578.
8. Weiner BK, Fraser RD, Peterson M. Spinous process osteotomies to facilitate lumbar decompressive surgery. Spine 1999;24:62–66.
9. Wiltse LL. The paraspinal sacrospinalis-splitting approach to the lumbar spine. Clin Orthop Rel Res 1973;91:48–57.
10. Fraser RD, Hall DJ. Laminectomy combined with posterolateral stabilisation: a muscle-sparing approach to the lumbosacral spine. Eur Spine J 1993;1:249–253
11. Jonsson B, Stromqvist B, Egund N. Anomalous lumbosacral articulations and low-back pain. Evaluation and treatment. Spine 1989;14(8):831–834.
12. Santavirta S, Tallroth K, Ylinen P, et al. Surgical treatment of Bertolotti's syndrome. Follow-up of 16 patients. Arch Orthop Trauma Surg 1993;112(2):82–87.
13. Wiltse LL, Spencer CW. New uses and refinements of the paraspinal approach to the lumbar spine. Spine 1988;13:696–706.
14. O'Brien MF, Peterson D, Crockard HA. A posterolateral microsurgical approach to extreme-lateral lumbar disc herniation. J Neurosurg 1995;83:636–640.
15. Freebody D, Bendall R, Taylor RD. Anterior transperitoneal lumbar fusion. J Bone Joint Surg 1971;53-B:617–627.
16. McAfee PC, Regan JR, Zdeblick T, et al. The incidence of complications in endoscopic anterior thoracolumbar spinal reconstructive surgery: a prospective multicenter study comprising the first 100 consecutive cases. Spine 1995;20:1624–1632.
17. Capellades J, Pellise F, Rovira A, et al. Magnetic resonance anatomic study of iliocava junction and left iliac vein positions related to L5-S1 disc. Spine 2000;25:1695–1700.
18. Flynn JC, Price CT. Sexual complications of anterior fusion of the lumbar spine. Spine 1984;9:489–492.
19. Hodgson AR, Wong SK. A description of a technic and evaluation of results in anterior spina fusion for deranged intervertebral disk and spondylolisthesis. Clin Orthop 1968;56:133–162.
20. Fraser RD, Gogan WJ. A modified muscle-splitting approach to the lumbosacral spine. Spine 1992;17(8):943–948.
21. Fraser RD. A wide muscle-splitting approach to the lumbosacral spine. J Bone Joint Surg Br 1982;64(1):44–46.
22. Allen BT, Bridwell KH. Paramedian retroperitoneal approach to the anterior lumbar spine. In: Bridwell KH, DeWald RL, eds. The textbook of spinal surgery. Philadelphia: JB Lippincott, 1991.

CHAPTER 22

Endoscopic Anterior Lumbar Procedures

Ensor E. Transfeldt and John N. Graber

Contemporary surgery of the lumbar spine is evolving into less invasive methods in an effort to decrease morbidity and hospital stay and speed up recovery and return to activity and work. The spine is enveloped by a variety of organs and muscles and traditional exposures alone have been frequently associated with a greater morbidity than many of the surgical procedures on the spine itself. Endoscopic techniques and image-guided surgery provide an exciting opportunity to provide minimal access to the spine. It is not intended to change the surgery, although many of the instruments and techniques have been modified to accommodate the endoscopic access. The indications for endoscopic access include surgery for trauma, tumor, infections, deformity, and degenerative conditions.

Laparoscopic- or endoscopic-assisted surgery is an alternative surgical approach to the spine rather than the development of a new operation. The development of this technique grew out of an interest in minimally invasive surgery. Initially, the approach was used for single-level anterior interbody fusions that evolved for use of interbody cage fixation and now has application for decompression, including corpectomies, débridement, and complex multilevel fusions and fixation. The indications for endoscopic procedures and the operation itself are the same as for any open procedure.

The laparoscopic technique requires an anatomic approach and the same attention to detail of the surgical technique and biology of fusion and healing as is needed with open approaches. Laparoscopic techniques are technically more demanding and present a different view of the anatomy than the conventional open approach. If the surgeon is unable to perform the operation through a conventional open technique, it is unlikely that he or she will be able to do it using an endoscope. The procedure requires a team approach with skill and experience, as well as a steep learning curve. Benefits include minimally invasive dissection of tissues, preservation of paraspinal musculature, decreased blood loss, shorter hospital stay, and faster recovery. This needs to be weighed against potential disadvantages, including the need for different instrumentation with unfamiliar tactile sensations and indirect visualization.

The endoscopic exposure can be done with either gas insufflation or "gasless" technique. Each has its proponents. Gas insufflation techniques require gas seals and special trocars as well as special instruments to maintain intra-abdominal pressure. This changes many aspects of the surgical procedure. The gasless technique allows standard instruments, but has other limitations. Once access is achieved, specialized equipment may be required to perform the surgery and insert implants. These instruments frequently are expensive. They have longer shafts and less tactile feedback and are more difficult to control; thus, the procedure takes longer. As newer equipment, including motorized equipment is being developed this will be improved. Gasless approaches allow the use of conventional instrumentation. Anatomic considerations are different, too. Experience helps to determine where to retract and where pressure can cause injury.

Visualization is made possible by fiberoptics, allowing illumination and magnification through a camera. Display is usually on a flat two-dimensional screen, thus losing some three-dimensional perception. The technology does offer the advantage of magnification.

Minimally invasive open techniques, such as the mini anterior lumbar interbody fusion (ALIF), have been described and developed and offer an attractive alternative to endoscopic techniques. They have the advantage of being able to perform the procedure with standard instruments, more rapid exposure of the spine, and with comparable morbidity and benefit to laparoscopic access. Stand-alone anterior fusion and instrumentation, especially with cages has waned in popularity. Laparoscopic surgical approaches appear to offer less advantage if a more expensive posterior operation is also required. All of these factors need to be considered when planning one's approach to spine fusion.

CLASSIFICATION OF ENDOSCOPIC ANTERIOR PROCEDURES

The major categories of laparoscopic surgery are:

I. Transperitoneal
   Gas insufflation
   Without insufflation
II. Retroperitoneal
   Gas insufflation
   Without insufflation
   Endoscopic-assisted mini open

Anterior lumbar endoscopic surgery developed originally as an extension of the techniques of laparoscopic surgery for the abdomen by general surgeons. The two methods of endoscopic access used more widely for anterior lumbar surgery are transperitoneal with insufflation and retroperitoneal gasless approaches.

TRANSPERITONEAL APPROACH

History

Obenchain (1) described a laparoscopic approach for anterior L5-S1 fusion without instrumentation. Zuckerman et al. first described instrumented anterior lumbar fusions through a transperitoneal approach with insufflation in 1995 (2). Matthews et al. (3) and Regan et al. (4) reported the technique and preliminary results.

Subsequently, the clinical effectiveness of laparoscopic ALIF has been reported extensively (3–13).

Regan et al. (14) described 249 patients undergoing laparoscopic ALIF and compared these to a cohort of 591 consecutive anterior fusions, using the same device. It basically showed that there was a decreased hospital stay, decreased blood loss, increased operative time, but operative time improved with time and experience.

Lieberman (15) did a prospective study and found that the laparoscopic technique resulted in decreased operative time with experience. Mean blood loss was 105 cc and the operative time was 2 hours, but was reduced to 1.5 hours with experience. The postoperative stay was 4 days. Postoperative functional outcomes assessment clearly needs to be done in these types of studies.

Kleeman and Hiscoe (16) described a prospective study comparing laparoscopic ALIFs to traditional posterolateral fusions with pedicle screws. He found that the fusion and complication rates were similar. In the laparoscopic group, blood loss was reduced by 90%, the hospital stay reduced by 50%, and the patients had an earlier return to work with a faster functional recovery. All the studies do show that there is a steep learning curve.

The transperitoneal approach with insufflation does provide direct anterior midline access to the L4-5 and L5-S1 levels and occasionally to the C3-4 level. It becomes increasingly more difficult to employ transperitoneal endoscopic techniques for more superior levels because

of the sigmoid colon and inferior mesenteric artery. The major advantage of air insufflation is that it allows fairly rapid exposure of the lumbar spine, as well as assistance in "organ retraction" by the increased intra-abdominal pressure, which helps keep the loops of the bowel out of the working field. Visual interference by loops of bowel still occurs and must be dealt with by use of retractors. The working field is also larger and there is less bleeding with this technique than that of the gasless transperitoneal approach. This approach requires trocars with specialized diaphragms to prevent air leaks. Specialized instruments and implants are needed to adapt to the use of the trocars.

Instruments for the insertion of interbody cages were easily adapted to this technique. Trephine discectomies are use for removal of a cylindric core of disc and a bone fold cage replaces the space. The disadvantage of this technique is that it results in a smaller surface area for exposure for bone fusion. Complete discectomy and preparation of the end plate is more tedious and difficult through trocars under conditions of insufflation. This approach has possible benefits for anterior-only surgery (e.g., stand-alone anterior cages). The addition of a more invasive posterior approach (e.g., for posterior fixation) eclipses the minimal invasiveness of the laparoscopic technique.

TECHNIQUE OF TRANSPERITONEAL APPROACH WITH INSUFFLATION

Positioning and Pneumoperitoneum

The patient is placed in the supine position with the arms by the side. The operating table is then placed in the steep Trendelenburg position. A lumbar roll under the patient's pelvis and lumbar spine is also placed in order to maintain lumbar lordosis, but also to facilitate use of a C-arm fluoroscope. The standard laparoscopic equipment used for this procedure includes a 0°, 10 mm telescope, camera lightsource, and insufflator. However, the use of angled viewing scopes offers advantage for more experienced surgeons. A 5 mm, 30° viewing scope has been our choice. The Trendelenburg position allows the bowels and the abdominal contents to fall in a cephalad direction.

A Veress needle is introduced supraumbilically into the abdomen in order to create a pneumoperitoneum. Pneumoperitoneum is created with carbon dioxide (CO_2) gas insufflation. Alternatively, a supraumbilical or infraumbilical incision is made with the introduction of a Hasson trocar for use of the endoscope. In this technique, all trocars have special valves to seal the escape of gas from the peritoneum. Through the umbilical trocars, the pneumoperitoneum can also be created. The other portals are then made under direct vision. The location of the working portal, which is usually through an 18 mm trocar, is dependent upon the trajectory of the intervertebral space being fused, and this assessment is made from preoperative X-rays (Fig. 22-1).

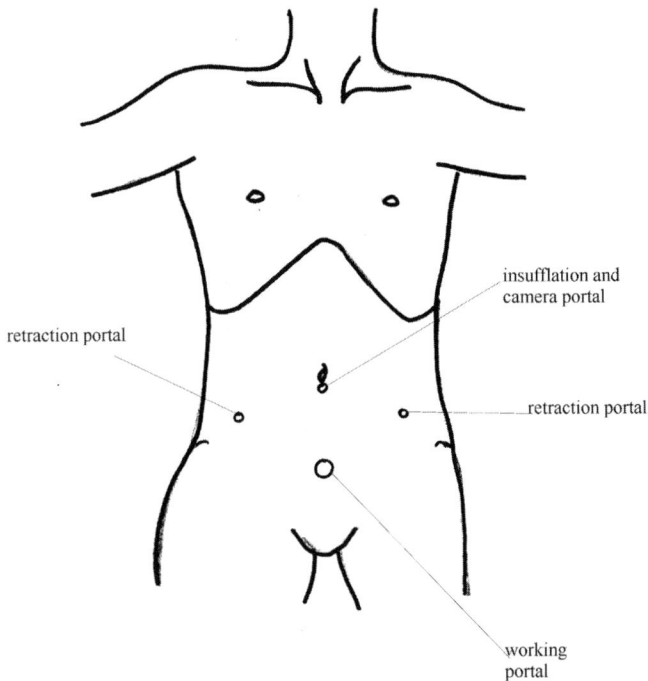

FIG. 22-1. Typical port placements for transperitoneal access to the lumbar spine. Camera access through this site is typical and a working portal is made on the midline lower abdominal wall in the trajectory of the desired interspace. The lateral portals are used for dissection and retraction.

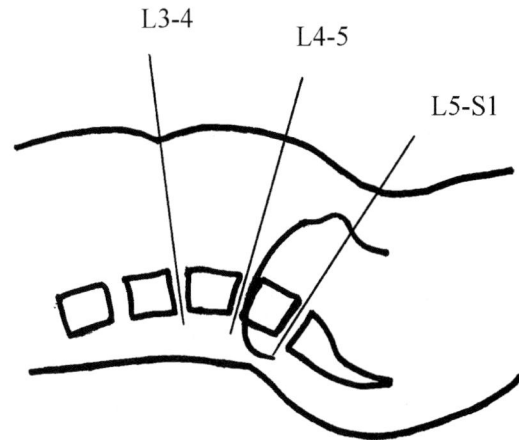

FIG. 22-2. The location of the working portal on the abdominal wall is determined by the trajectory of the interspace as seen on lateral spine films.

A 5 mm trocar is then inserted on each side, midway between the umbilicus and the pubis and lateral to the epigastric vessels. During the procedure, additional portals can be introduced if needed. The loops of small bowel are then placed into the epigastrium using special graspers. The location of the bifurcation of the great vessels is identified. The working portal is placed at a site on the abdominal wall in the interspace to be fused (Fig. 22-2).

Exposure of L5-S1 Disc Space

Having identified the bifurcation of the great vessels, the posterior peritoneum is incised longitudinally below the bifurcation and blunt dissection is used to visualize the L5-S1 disc space and median sacral vessels. The median sacral artery and vein are then clipped and divided. The iliac vein and artery must be swept off the lateral aspect of the interspace with laparoscopic Kittner dissectors. Ongoing retraction of these vessels can be done through trocars or by passing Steinmann pins though the abdominal wall. Dissection should generally be done without the use of monopolar cautery to avoid retrograde ejaculation in males. The approach for discectomy will then depend upon the individual preference of the surgeon. Special instruments for doing discectomies, as well as special metallic working portals with reamers

for insertion of cages and bone material have also been designed (Figs. 22-3, 22-4A, B).

Fluoroscopy is used at this point to visualize depth of the discectomy and reaming, as well as insertion of implants. The laparoscope allows simultaneous visualization to ensure that vascular and other structures are not damaged and remain out of the working site.

Technique for L4-5 Approach

The L4-5 disc space uses a similar approach, but the exact location of the dissection does depend on preoperative magnetic resonance (MR) images and computed tomography (CT) scans, which will help determine the location of the bifurcation. In the unlikely setting where the bifurcation of the great vessels is located above the L4-5 interspace, then the same dissection as already described will be used.

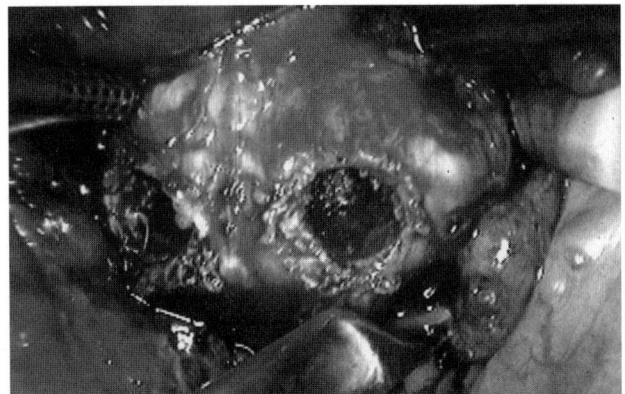

FIG. 22-3. Two sites of trephine partial discectomy are done on each side of midline on the L5-S1 disc space.

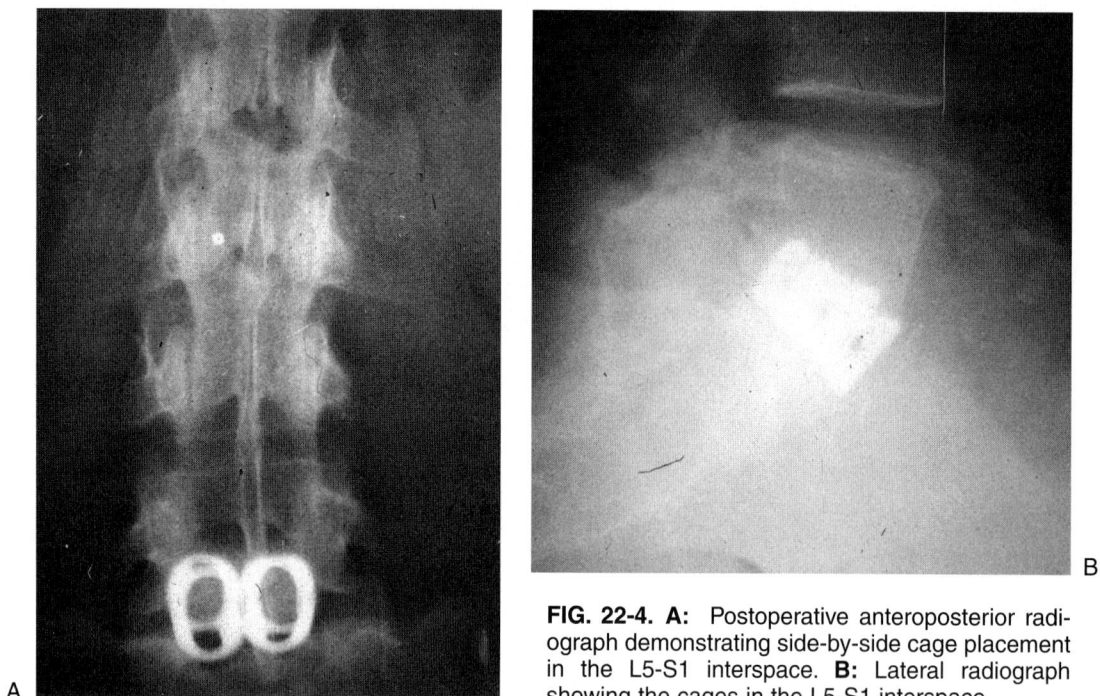

FIG. 22-4. A: Postoperative anteroposterior radiograph demonstrating side-by-side cage placement in the L5-S1 interspace. B: Lateral radiograph showing the cages in the L5-S1 interspace.

In most cases, the bifurcation is below or at the L4-5. The iliac artery and vein are first identified. Segmental vessels will also be identified, clipped, and divided and it is strongly recommended that the ascending iliolumbar vein be identified, clipped, and divided. These steps are important in mobilizing the aorta and the vena cava across the right side of the spine for adequate exposure of the L4-5 interspace. Percutaneous Steinmann pins can be placed to the vertebral bodies in order to assist with retraction or specialized retractors can be used through one of the working portals. Imaging with the C-arm of fluoroscope in two planes is necessary to ensure that implants are inserted centrally in the disc and to the correct depth.

TECHNIQUE OF TRANSPERITONEAL APPROACH WITHOUT INSUFFLATION

Maintaining a pneumoperitoneum requires the use of expensive special gas-sealing ports, as well as special instruments. The instruments need round shafts in order to accommodate the diaphragms. Albert Chin introduced the concept of a mechanical retraction device, the Laparolift (Origin Medsystems, Menlo Park, CA), which displaces the anterior abdominal wall and holds it up like a tent (17).

As a substitute for pneumoperitoneum, this system has a fan retractor that is inserted into the abdomen in a closed configuration through a 15 mm minilaparotomy incision and is then opened up. This fan retractor is attached to a powered hydraulic table-mounted device that provides the vertical lift and creates a working space.

The remainder of the portals, including the working portals and lateral portals, are similar to those described in the transperitoneal approach with insufflation. No gas seal however, is required. This allows use of conventional instrumentation and implants.

Before deploying the fan and applying lift, a finger should be introduced through the infraumbilical incision into the abdominal cavity and swept around to ensure no intra-abdominal adhesions are present. The fan retractor is then inserted and advanced in a plain parallel to the anterior abdominal wall. The fan blades are then opened and locked. Next, the retractor is attached to a sterile-draped lifting arm, which has previously been attached to the side rail of the operating room table. The retractor is then elevated using the hydraulic system of the lever arm, creating a "tent effect" by elevating the abdominal wall (Fig. 22-5A, B).

The endoscope is then inserted into the abdominal cavity through the fan insertion incision between the fan arms. This provides also provides an opportunity to visualize the arms of the fans to ensure that they have not entrapped any bowel or omentum. A force-limiting device is incorporated into the motor of the lifting arm to avoid excessive forces. The ancillary portals are then placed under direct visualization of the endoscope. The working portal is again strategically placed based on the trajectory of the interspace to be fused and gauged from preoperative X-rays. The ancillary ports are simple, rigid or flexible valveless sleeves, which are used simply to guide the insertion of instruments. It is possible with the flexible sleeves to introduce conventional curved and odd-shaped instruments into the abdominal cavity (Fig. 22-6A, B, C).

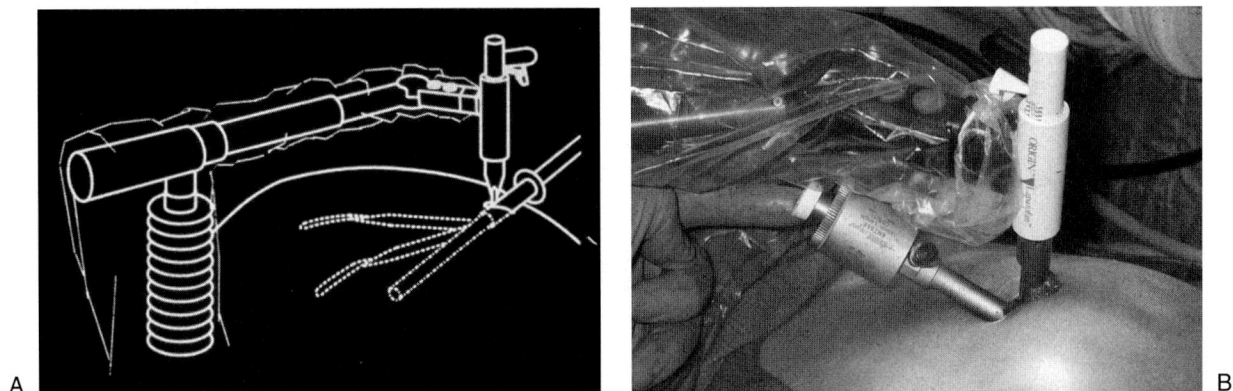

FIG. 22-5. A: Schematic drawing showing Laparolift (Origin Medsystems, Menlo Park, CA) with hydraulic arm, which is table-mounted and made to apply variable pressure to the anterior abdominal wall in a lifting fashion so as to create a space for visualization. **B:** Clinical photograph showing Laparolift (Origin Medsystems, Menlo Park, CA) in place with laparoscopic cannula placed through same portal as the Laparolift device. This is typically used for passage of the laparoscope.

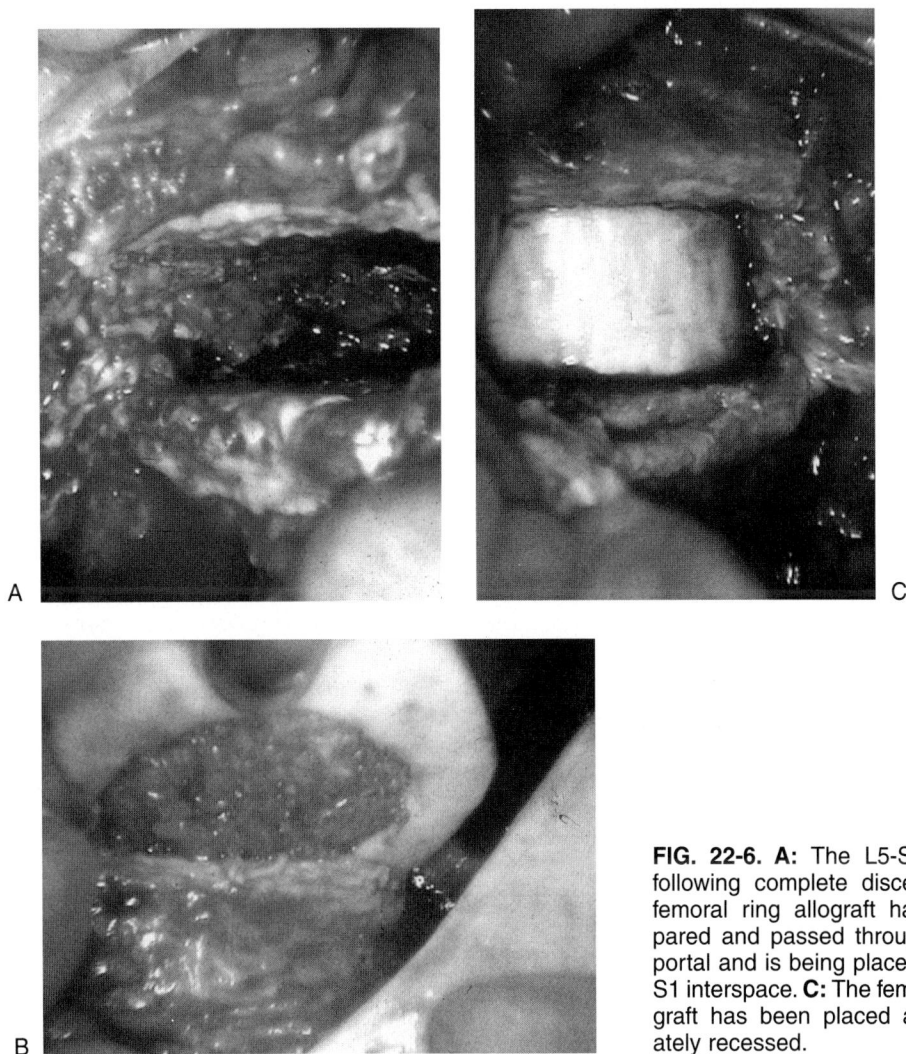

FIG. 22-6. A: The L5-S1 interspace following complete discectomy. **B:** A femoral ring allograft has been prepared and passed through a working portal and is being placed into the L5-S1 interspace. **C:** The femoral ring allograft has been placed and appropriately recessed.

RETROPERITONEAL APPROACH

History

The retroperitoneal is a potential space that can be created by dissection in natural anatomic and fascial planes. Retroperitoneoscopy was first described in the literature for straightforward smaller urologic and gynecologic procedures (18).

Introduction of CO_2 insufflators improved visualization and working space in the retroperitoneum. Fibrous bands limited the usefulness of CO_2 dissection. Balloons were introduced in the 1990s as an alternative for retroperitoneal dissection (19–22). The retroperitoneal approach is more versatile (1,23). McAfee has used a combination of video-assisted thorascopic and laparoscopic methods.

TECHNIQUE FOR RETROPERITONEAL APPROACH WITHOUT INSUFFLATION

The spine lies in the retroperitoneal space, which is only a potential space that can be created by retracting organs. This potential space is created by manual dissection and by the use of the balloon dissection of tissue planes. The cavity is then maintained with a mechanical lifting arm, as well as a specialized retractor. The dissecting balloon has a core cannula for placement of the endoscope so that the balloon dissection is performed under direct vision. The abdominal peritoneum is dissected off the abdominal wall and acts as an envelope containing the abdominal organs out of the view of the spine. A strategically placed working portal allows access for standard open surgical instruments, thus simplifying the endoscopic access (Fig. 22-7).

The patient is placed in the supine position with a sandbag under the left flank. Two incisions are made. The left flank incision for the balloon dissector and endoscope is placed halfway between the 11th rib and the iliac crest in the anterior auxiliary line. The second incision for the working portal is strategically placed, depending on the level and trajectory of the interspace that is to be fused. This approach allows fusion of any of the interspaces from T12-S1.

The flank incision is approximately 15 mm in length and dissection is carried out to the lateral abdominal musculature. The external oblique, internal oblique, and transverses muscles are bluntly separated to expose the extraperitoneal pararenal fatty tissue. A finger is again introduced into this space as a blunt dissector.

The elliptical-shaped preperitoneal dissecting balloon cannula (PDB) (Medsystems, Inc., Menlo Park, CA) is then introduced into the retroperitoneal space and once the balloon is within the incision, the endoscope is introduced into the core of the dissection cannula. The balloon is then deployed and expanded using an inflation bulb. Through the inflated balloon it is possible to identify the line of the peritoneum and observe its dissection on the

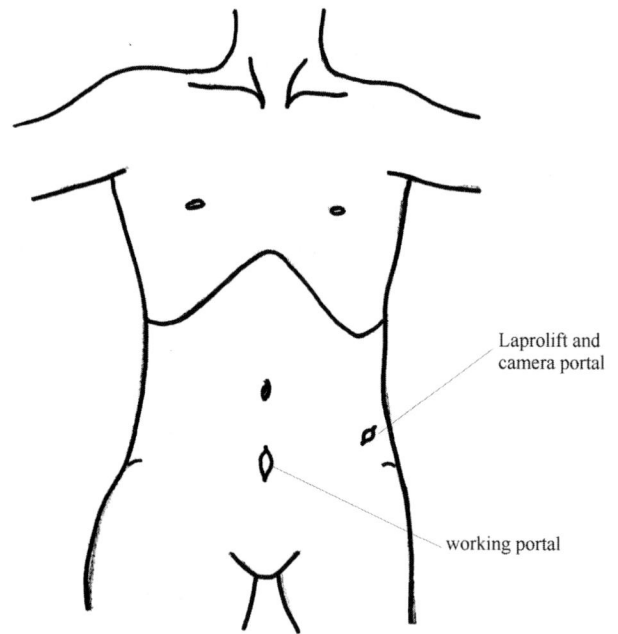

FIG. 22-7. Typical port placements for retroperitoneal access to the anterior lumbar spine. There are two portal sites. A midline site for access provides the working portal and a lateral site for a camera, Laparolift (Origin Medsystems, Menlo Park, CA), and retractors.

anterior abdominal wall. This line should be extended as close to the midline as possible to allow placement of the anterior working portal (Fig. 22-8A, B).

Once the retroperitoneal space has been developed and the peritoneum has been reflected from the undersurface of the anterior abdominal wall, the Laparolift retractor is inserted and a 10 cm long fan retractor (Laparofan, Medsystems, Inc., Menlo Park, CA) is inserted through the left flank incision and the arms of the fan are deployed under direct endoscopic visualization. The fan retractor is then attached to the mechanical lifting arm, which is then elevated again increasing the cavity. A flexible nonvalve trocar is then inserted behind the arms of the fan retractor, through which the endoscope is passed. A specialized balloon retractor can also be inserted through the same port or through the working port in the anterior abdominal wall. This retractor is only inflated once it has been introduced into the retroperitoneal space and is helpful in providing retraction of the peritoneum with its gastrointestinal contents.

The working portal is made through a 12 mm paramedian incision on the anterior abdominal wall, approximately 2 cm lateral to the midline. The level of the incision and the exact location may again depend on the level and trajectory of the interspace to be exposed. Through the para-midline skin incision, the anterior rectus sheath is identified and incised. The rectus muscle is retracted laterally, and the posterior rectus sheath is then incised and the peritoneum with its contents should have been

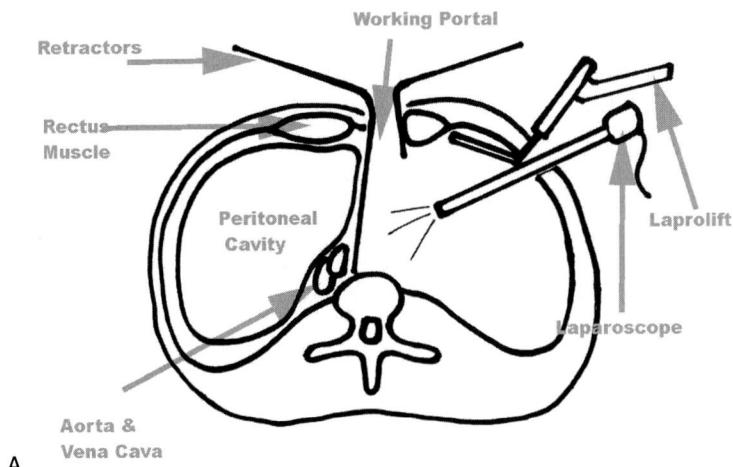

A

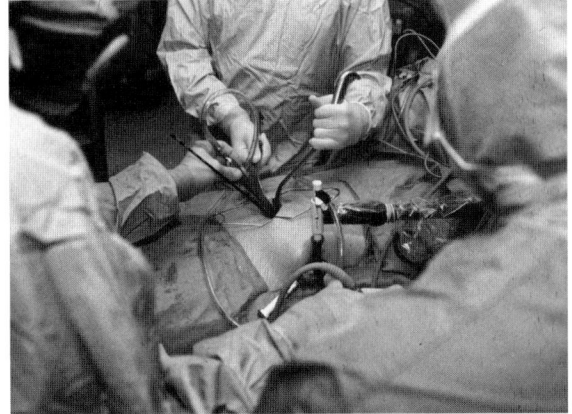

B

FIG. 22-8. A: Diagram demonstrating the concept of the retroperitoneal endoscopic approach with exposure of the anterior lumbar spine. A small skin incision is made anteriorly and the rectus muscle retracted laterally and after exposure of the preperitoneal space, the peritoneum bluntly dissected laterally and posteriorly and retracted to the right side. A Laparolift (Origin Medsystems, Menlo Park, CA) is placed anterolaterally through a small incision and a laparoscope is inserted through the same portal. The aorta and vena cava are identified and mobilized by clipping and diving the segmental vessels and then bluntly retracting them to the far side as well. B: Operating room photograph during retroperitoneal gasless exposure.

reflected across the midline, but this can additionally be assisted through this direct approach. Blunt dissection with the finger can again be used to sweep the peritoneum further off the abdominal wall if balloon dissection has not provided sufficient exposure.

The peritoneum contains the bowel, which can be retracted with inflatable or fan retractors. A supplemental balloon retractor may be introduced through the working portal as well, if necessary. The remainder of the procedure is then similar to that described in the transperitoneal technique. Exposure of the great vessels is necessary, and again isolation and retraction of these vessels will depend on the level of the interspace to be exposed. The L5-S1 interspace is again exposed below the bifurcation of the great vessels and the L4-5 and more proximal levels will require a retraction of the aorta and inferior vena cava to the right of the spine. Percutaneous Steinmann pins may then be used to maintain retraction of the great vessels (Fig. 22-9). Flexible endoscopic ports are introduced through the working portal. It is important to identify all the great vessels as well as the ureter to prevent injury. The sympathetic and parasympathetic presacral plexus are frequently approached from the side and elevated anteriorly with the great vessels. Lumbar segmental vessels should be clipped for more proximal lumbar spine dissection and at the L4-5 level the recurrent iliolumbar vein should also be identified and clipped. Conventional techniques for lumbar discectomy and preparation of the end plates can then be performed through this working portal.

Osteotomies and curettes of any shape or size can generally be used as well. In addition, a variety of intervertebral implants can be used, including screw-in cages, tap-in cages, cortical allografts, and prosthetic implants.

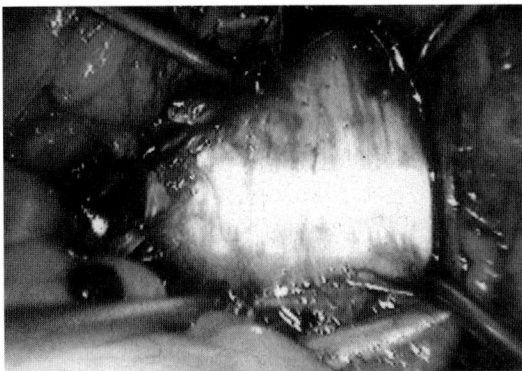

FIG. 22-9. Demonstrating the use of Steinmann pins to hold vessels and organs retracted. This technique can be employed in any of the endoscopic procedures discussed in this chapter. It could also be used for a mini anterior lumbar interbody fusion.

TECHNIQUE FOR RETROPERITONEAL WITH INSUFFLATION

There have been a few reports of a retroperitoneal exposure with insufflation dissection, but these were generally not widely embraced. In the anterior abdominal wall in the midline after exposure of the anterior abdominal wall, the section is carried down through the anterior and posterior sheath of the rectus muscle after retraction of the muscle itself. The posterior rectus sheath is then divided, exposing the extraperitoneal layer at the level of

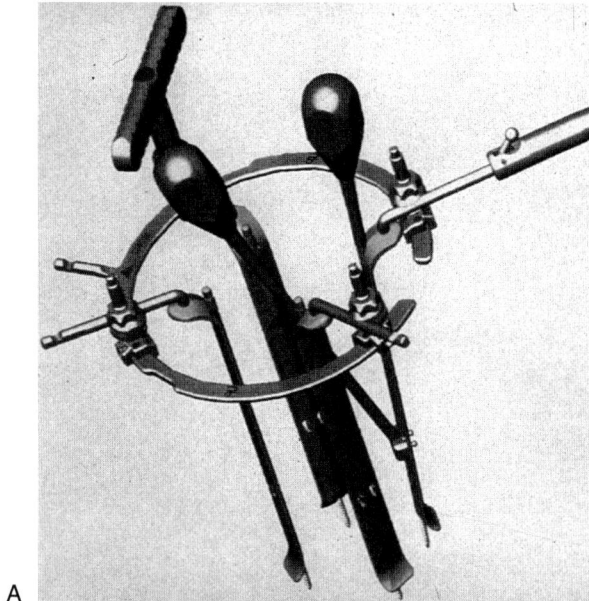

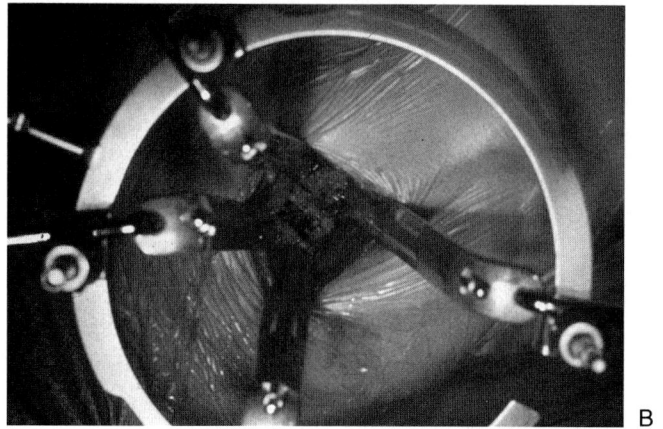

FIG. 22-10. A: Endo-Ring (Medtronic Sofamor Danek, Memphis, TN) in which Steinmann pins and retractors are used. The Endo-Ring is stabilized to the table. **B:** Clinical use of an Endo-Ring.

the arcuate ligament. Dissection with a finger is used to free up the peritoneum from the abdominal muscle wall. An inflatable balloon may be used for dissection and a 10 mm scope introduced bilaterally.

ENDOSCOPIC-ASSISTED MINI-OPEN APPROACH

Videoscopic-assisted open surgery with an enlarged working portal is an option. Essentially, this opening could employ a mini ALIF exposure, which is enhanced with an endoscope (Fig. 22-10A, B). An endoscope may be used through a separate portal. The newer technology of flexible fiberoptics allows the use of a camera and light source through a thin, flexible scope passed through the mini ALIF approach itself. The working portal may be small so that the only person having direct visualization of the surgical field is the operating surgeon. The addition of a videoscope allows the assistant to provide assistance or retraction.

COMPLICATIONS OF ENDOSCOPIC SPINE SURGERY

Complications can be divided into those caused by the technique of laparoscopy and those caused by the dissection necessary to expose the spine. Typical laparoscopic injuries include intestinal or other organ puncture caused by port placement, port site bleeding or hernia, cardiovascular dysfunction due to the increased intra-abdominal pressure, and CO_2 subcutaneous emphysema (23).

Intraoperative complications include major vessel injuries, distal arterial embolus, bowel injuries, and bladder and ureter injuries. Postoperative complications include deep vein thrombosis, ejaculatory dysfunction, and ileus.

The safest way to decrease complications in endoscopic spine surgery is to use an experienced laparoscopic general surgeon and to do careful preoperative planning. It is important to maintain good visualization, orientation, a maximum working space, and appropriate instrumentation.

It is vitally important to have an "emergency set" in the operating room for conversion to open procedures to minimize blood loss when vessel injuries occur (24). Conversion should not be considered a failure of the operation.

Specific complications are primarily related to exposure of the anterior lumbar spine, and usually include damage to vascular structures and the sympathetic plexus. Regan et al. (24) compared 249 laparoscopic patients to 591 open patients undergoing the same operation. Complications were comparable in both groups: 4.2% complications in the open group, 4.9% complications in the laparoscopic group. Device-related complications were increased in the laparoscopic group and these included disc herniations and no root irritation. Laparoscopic-related complications occurred in 4.7% of patients in the laparoscopic group and 2.3% in the open group. The authors point out that the laparoscopic procedures associated with a learning curve, but once mastered they believe this is an effective and safe procedure.

In Regan's series (25), there was a reoperation for nerve root compression or irritation in four patients, retrograde ejaculation occurred in 4.8% of males, and conversion to open procedure for excessive bleeding occurred in two patients. Major complications occurred in 13.4% of the first 40 cases.

VASCULAR INJURIES

The occurrence of vascular injuries should definitely be a primary concern for the use of the endoscopic approach. The literature seems to show a higher incidence of vascular injuries with endoscopic surgery than with the open approach. With the transperitoneal video-assisted approach the following vascular injury rates have been reported: McAfee (26) (1/22; 4.5%), Mathews et al. (3) (1/6; 17%), Zuckerman et al. (2) (2/17; 12%), Mahvi and Zdeblick (9) (2/20; 10%), Regan et al. (14) (5/58; 9.5%), Lieberman et al. (15) (1/47; 2.1%), Regan et al. (4) (6/24; 25%), and Escobar et al. (23) (2/34; 5.9%). In the video-assisted retroperitoneal gasless approach, reported vascular injury rates were as follows: Escobar (23) (0/30 patients), Onimus et al. (24) (0/20), and Thalgott et al. (27) (8/98; 8.1%).

Mini-laparotomy, an alternative minimal access approach has also been associated with vascular injuries. Escobar et al. (23) report two vascular injuries in 51 patients (4%), Mayer (28) reported none in 25 patients, Baker et al. (29) reported 18.4% in 19 patients. Vascular injuries have also been reported in traditional open approaches; however, the incidence appears to be much lower. Faciszewski et al. (30) reported only one major vessel injury in 350 anterior lumbar procedures (0.08%); Baker et al. (29) reported a 7.7% rate in 26 patients for this approach.

Vascular injuries may involve bleeding from small vessels or injury to the major vessels. It is important to ligate all bleeding vessels. Specialized equipment has been made for clipping vessels in surgeries where transperitoneal with insufflation approach is used. In the gasless approach, the conventional hemo-clips can be used. Injury to the major vessels requires immediate control of bleeding and if any difficulty is encountered, it is recommended to proceed with conversion to a conventional open approach as quickly as possible.

Anatomic variations increase incidence of vascular injuries and these occur most frequently at the L4-5 level. Zdeblick has described the incidence of vessel injuries and retrograde ejaculations at the L4-5 level. It is thought to be related to the vascular anatomy, especially the bifurcation of the aorta and the inferior vena cava (9,10,29, 31–34). Most often, the aorta and vena cava divide on the L5 vertebral body and exposure of the L4-5 disc is made above. However, at times the bifurcation is high and the L4-5 exposure more difficult. Sometimes it is easier to expose from below the bifurcation, but tears to the left common iliac vein are more common. We use the tenet that "it is easier to avoid bleeding than it is to stop it." In this case bleeding is best avoided by gently retracting the vein and observing sites of fixation by large branches that will tear with further retraction. Preemptive clipping and dividing of the L4 segmental lumbar artery and vein and the ascending iliolumbar vein is prudent if not necessary.

Retrograde Ejaculation

In Regan's series (35) in which he compared open techniques with laparoscopic techniques, the authors report that retrograde ejaculation occurred in 9.4% of laparoscopic cases compared to 4.7% of open cases. Complications of retrograde ejaculation vary between 0.42% and 45% of cases (12,34,36,37).

Retrograde ejaculation results from injury to the superior hypogastric plexus, which controls bladder-neck closure during ejaculation. The incidence reported varies between 0.42% and 45% of cases (13,14,34,38). The majority of these are thought to be transient. Retrograde ejaculation has been reported with open ALIF in 0.42% to 22% of cases (13,14,34,39,40). In Flynn's series (4,500 cases), 25% of patients reported retrograde ejaculation and had spontaneous resolution (39).

The superior hypogastric plexus lies in the retroperitoneal connective tissue anterior to the distal aorta and aortic bifurcation. It lies slightly to the left of the midline before dividing into the left and right hypogastric plexus. It is therefore most vulnerable with direct dissection from anterior and left-sided dissection. The retroperitoneal approach is usually done from the left side and is usually more posterior to the hypogastric plexus. This would explain why they are fewer patients with retrograde ejaculation (41).

Kleeman (16) recommends careful analysis of the vascular anatomy, especially at the L4-5 level and has classified the vascular anatomy at this area so that appropriate surgical approaches can be planned. This would reduce exposure on the side of the aorta and thus the hypogastric plexus. It is also recommended that bipolar cauterization be used.

Loss of Orientation

Loss of orientation regarding the center of the disc and the midline has been described in laparoscopic transperitoneal techniques and it is more difficult to identify during the procedure under visualization of a scope due to limitation of the exposure and orientation of the camera.

Loss of orientation can lead to asymmetric graft/cage placement. If placement is too lateral, then foraminal encroachment or vessel injury is a risk. It is therefore important to use X-rays in two planes.

Pseudoarthrosis

The most common cause for reoperation of interbody fusion cages is pseudoarthrosis. Salvage includes instrumented posterolateral fusions and frequent removal of the interbody device and replacement with autograft or allograft (42). This complication of pseudoarthrosis is seen more commonly in procedures where a trephine cylindric core of disc was removed and it is recommended that a complete discectomy would decrease the chances of nonunion. Studies using bone morphogenic protein (BMP) have shown remarkably high fusion rates.

Iatrogenic Nerve Root Impingement

This complication occurs due to disc herniation or retropulsed bone although it is not unique to endoscopic techniques, as described (23, 26). Neurologic problems including the radicular type of pain appeared to be unique to the transperitoneal insufflation technique. Regan et al. (14) reported six such cases in among 215 patients (2.8%), and a reoperation rate of 2.3% for nerve root decompression. Escobar et al. (23) reported six patients, all with transperitoneal insufflation approach for an incidence of 18% (6/34). All of these had undergone cylindric trephine discectomies and insertion of a screw-in cage device. One of the six patients had an acute cauda equina syndrome secondary to an acute disc herniation requiring emergent posterior decompression, which resulted in full neurologic recovery. Four of the six patients with new onset radicular symptoms had spontaneous resolution of the symptoms within 6 months after the index procedure.

Postoperative Ileus

Some degree of postoperative ileus is normal and to be expected after any surgery and anesthetic, even nonabdominal procedures (43). The degree of ileus is generally proportional to the extent of surgery, the amount of intestinal manipulation, the quantity of residual intraperitoneal blood or hematoma, the severity of physiologic disruption or infection, and the specific sensitivity of the individual patient. Paying strict attention to all these matters is important in avoiding extensive ileus. It has been shown that typical laparoscopic surgery is associated with less postoperative ileus than with comparable open procedures. The difference in ileus between mini-open spine access and the endoscopic exposure has not been specifically investigated. Unless the length of laparoscopic procedures can be decreased to that it compares with open procedures, it is unlikely to be much different.

Hernias

Hernias at the trocar site are a rare complication and occur more commonly in transperitoneal than in retroperitoneal endoscopy (26). This can be avoided by placing a stitch in the fascia of all ports greater than 10 mm in size.

Ureteral Injuries

The ureter is at risk for injury during anterior exposure of the lumbar spine and this may be higher with minimal access approaches. Escobar et al. (23) reported two (2/135; 1.5%) injuries: one with video-assisted extraperitoneal approach and one with a mini-laparotomy approach. There have been numerous single case reports regarding ureteral injuries with anterior lumbar surgery. Faciszewski et al. (30) has reported one case in a series of 350 traditional open approaches for an instance of 0.3%.

Laparoscopic Conversion

Conversion to an open approach may be due to vascular injury, abdominal adhesions, organ injury, or technical difficulties. Conversion should not be considered a failure.

COMPARISON OF MINI OPEN TECHNIQUE TO ENDOSCOPIC OPEN ALIF

The advantages of minimally invasive techniques are intended to reduce postoperative morbidity and decrease hospital stay. There should be no increase in complications of the approach and the outcomes should be comparable to traditional open approaches. The mini open technique offers many of the same advantages as the laparoscopic techniques. Mayer (28) has been credited for describing this approach. In contrast to standard laparotomy, this technique uses a muscle-splitting approach, separating muscles in the direction of the fiber orientation.

Another technique or approach is a vertical midline incision and division of the left rectus sheath in a vertical direction. The rectus muscle is retracted laterally and the posterior sheath is incised vertically as well. The preperitoneal plane is developed bluntly, first laterally and then posteriorly. Thereafter, the operation continues as with standard lateral open approaches.

Zdeblick and David reported a comparison of 25 anterior laparoscopic approaches with 25 mini open techniques for L4-5 fusion. Paired threaded cages were used in both cases. Operating time, blood loss, and length of hospital stay showed no statistical difference. There was a lower rate of complications in the mini open group (4%) versus a higher rate (20%) in the laparoscopic group. This study shows that even in technically competent hands laparoscopy has no advantage to a mini approach (34). There was significant increase in surgical time in the laparoscopic group when two-level procedures were evaluated (180 minutes versus 160 minutes).

Escobar et al. (23) reported on a retrospective review comparing 135 patients undergoing four different approaches: transperitoneal video-assisted surgery with insufflation, retroperitoneal endoscopic video-assisted surgery, mini laparotomy, retroperitoneal approach, and traditional oblique retroperitoneal surgery. There was onset of new radicular pain or numbness not experienced by the patient prior to surgery in six patients (18%); all with transperitoneal video-assisted surgery using insufflation. Vascular problems occurred in five patients (3%

overall); two in the transperitoneal video-assisted group (5.9%) and three in the mini-laparotomy group (8.7% of the group). Retrograde ejaculation occurred in four of 50 male patients (8%); three in the transperitoneal video-assisted group (25%) and one in the mini-laparotomy group (2%). Two patients had ureteral injuries (1.5% overall); one each in the retroperitoneal endoscopic and mini- laparotomy groups. Conversion to open procedures was performed in seven patients (11% of the video-assisted procedures).

The reasons for conversion included two major vessel lacerations and five peritoneal tears in the retroperitoneal video-assisted group. Overall, the incidence of complications in the endoscopic group was consistent with the literature for video-assisted techniques; it was thought to be higher than for open techniques. Reports in the literature do not show any advantage of laparoscopic versus mini-open for anterior lumbar surgery (34, 40).

In reviewing the literature, it would appear that the laparoscopic insufflation technique is associated with a higher rate of vascular injuries. These injuries usually require conversion to an open procedure, thus prolonging surgical time. However, vascular injuries occur with all approaches and successful vascular repair was the standard outcome for the aforementioned cited literature.

CONCLUSION

Minimizing access to the spine will remain a goal in spine surgery. Current techniques have some drawbacks, but should be regarded as a stepping stone to the future. There are good studies using prospective randomized controls, but no good outcome studies are described for fusion outcomes. These studies are necessary to establish superiority of any technique. The need for more minimally invasive techniques will always be there. The use of BMP and other materials to substitute for the patient's own bone have already reduced the need for harvesting of bone graft and lend themselves to easy implantation, thus making endoscopic techniques more attractive.

Evaluation of fusion by standard radiographs is unreliable. Thin section CTs with three-dimensional reconstruction are more reliable. CTs are usually performed when there is a suspicion of pseudoarthrosis or nonunion, or for evaluation of pain. There are few studies reporting CT evaluation of all patients in a laparoscopic cohort. Pellise et al. described a 16.6% fusion rate in patients fused with carbon fiber cages using laparoscopic techniques with complete discectomy (44). There was significant improvement in clinical outcomes however at a minimum follow-up of 2 years.

Fusion surgery comprises a large volume of spine surgery, and interbody fusions have become widely popular. The access for interbody fusions can be performed anteriorly or posteriorly. Interbody fusions through a posterior approach include a conventional posterolateral interbody fusion (PLIF) or the recently popularized translumbar interforaminal fusion (TLIF) and should be considered less invasive if they save the need for additional anterior access. Dural injury and epidural scarring however are a high risk. Image-guided interbody fusions and instrumentation have been a further development of the minimally invasive posterior approach.

Malberg et al. (45) have described a direct lateral approach to the spine employing minimal access. A small incision is used and a working channel is docked on the disc space after a series of dilators have prepared access through a psoas muscle–splitting approach. A guide frame coupled with X-rays provides image guidance to accurate placement of the dilators and working channel. An electromyogram neuromonitoring system is used to provide increased safety from nerve injury to the lumbar plexus. However, there have been no extensive reports on the clinical experience with this approach.

We have found many of the techniques and limitations of endoscopic approaches to be cumbersome and most often use mini open procedures. This has been especially true in multilevel fusions. The balance of benefits and drawbacks will continue to tip in favor of endoscopic approaches as technological advances continue to eliminate the problems.

REFERENCES

1. Obenchain T. Laparoscopic lumbar discectomy: case report. J Laparoendosc Surg 1991;1:145–149.
2. Zuckerman J, Zdeblick T, Bailey S, et al. Instrumented laparoscopic spinal fusion: preliminary results. Spine 1995;2:2029–2035.
3. Matthews H, Evans M, Molligan H, et al. Laparoscopic discectomy with anterior lumbar interbody fusion. Spine 1995;20:1797–1802.
4. Regan J, McAfee P, Guyer R, et al. Laparoscopic fusion of the lumbar spine in a multicenter series of the first 34 consecutive patients. Surg Laparosc Endosc 1996;6:458–468.
5. Boden S, Martin GJ, Horton W, et al. Laparoscopic anterior spinal arthrodesis with rhBMP-2 in a titanium interbody threaded cage. J Spinal Disord 1998;11:95–101.
6. Dickman C, Sonntag V, Russell J. The laparoscopic approach for instrumentation and fusion of the lumbar spine. BNI Q 1997;13:26–36.
7. Henry L, Cattey R, Stoll J, et al. Laparoscopically assisted spinal surgery. JSLS 1997;1:341–344.
8. Husson J, Le Huec J, Polard J, et al. Interbody arthrodesis of the lumbar vertebrae using retroperitoneal videoendoscopy: a preliminary study of 38 cases [in French]. Chirurgie 1998;123:491–499.
9. Mahvi D, Zdeblick T. A Prospective study of laparoscopic spinal fusion: technique and operative complications. Ann Surg 1998;224: 85–90.
10. McAfee P, Regan J, Zdeblick T, et al. The incidence of complications in endoscopic anterior thoracolumbar spinal reconstructive surgery. Spine 1995;20:1624–1632.
11. McLaughlin M, Comey C, Haid R. Laparoscopic anterior lumbar interbody fusion. Contemp Neurosurg 1998;20.
12. Silcox D. Laparoscopic bone dowel fusions of the lumbar spine. Orthop Clin North Am 1998;29:655–663.
13. Zdeblick T. Laparoscopic spinal fusion. Orthop Clin North Am 1998; 29:635–45.
14. Regan J, Yuan H, McAfee P. Laparoscopic fusion of the lumbar spine: minimally invasive spine surgery. Spine 1999;24:402–411.
15. Lieberman I, Willsher P, Litwin D, et al. Transperitoneal laparoscopic exposure for lumbar interbody fusion. Spine 2000;25:509–514.
16. Kleeman T, Hiscoe A. Critical Analysis of laparoscopic ALIF vs. posterolateral fusion with instrumentation. Paper presented at: 14th Annual North American Spine Society Meeting; 1999; Chicago.

17. Chin AK, Moll FH, McColl MB, et al. Mechanical peritoneal retraction as a replacement for carbon dioxide pneumoperitoneum. Journal Am Assoc Gynecol Laparoscopists 1993;1:62–66.

18. Bartel M. Retroperitoneoscopy. An endoscopic method for inspection and bioptic examination of the retroperitoneal space. Zentralbl Chir 1969;94(12):377–383.

19. Gaur DD. Retroperitoneoscopy: the balloon technique. Ann R Coll Surg Engl 1994;76(4):259–263.

20. Webb D. An aid to laparoscopic hernioplasty-balloon dissection. Med J Aust 1993;158(8):578.

21. Keizure JJ, Tashima M, Das S. Retroperitoneal laparoscopic renal biopsy. Surg Laparosc Endosc 1993;3(1):60–62.

22. Hirsch IH, Moreno JG, Lotfi MA, Gomella LG. Controlled dilatation of the extraperitoneal space for laparoscopic urologic surgery. J Laparoendosc Surg 1994;4(4):247–251.

23. Escobar E, Transfeldt E, Garvey T, et al. Video-assisted versus open anterior lumbar spine fusion surgery: a comparison of four techniques and complications in 135 patients. Spine 2003;28:729–732.

24. Onimus M, Papin P, Gangloff S. Extraperitoneal approach to the lumbar spine with video assistance. Spine 1996;21:2491–2494.

25. Regan J. Laparoscopic lumbar fusion: single surgeon experience in 127 consecutive cases. Proceedings of the 68th Annual Meeting of the American Academy of Orthopaedic Surgeons; San Francisco; 2001.

26. McAfee P, Regan J, Geis P, et al. Minimally invasive anterior retroperitoneal approach to the lumbar spine. Spine 1998;23:1476–1484.

27. Thalgott J. Balloon-assisted endoscopic retroperitoneal gasless approach to lumbar interbody fusion. Paper presented at: Third Annual Research Institute International Symposium; 1997; Scottsdale, AZ.

28. Mayer H. A new microsurgical technique for minimally invasive anterior lumbar interbody fusion. Spine 1997;22:691–700.

29. Baker J, Reardon P, Reardon M, et al. Vascular injury in anterior lumbar surgery. Spine 1993;18:2227–2230.

30. Faciszewski T, Winter R, Lonstein J, et al. The surgical and medical perioperative complications of anterior spinal fusion in the thoracic and lumbar spine in adults: a review of 1223 procedures. Spine 1995;20:1592–1599.

31. Dewald R. Roundtable discussion: minimally invasive and endoscopic anterior lumbar spine surgery. Orthop Today 2000;20:34–43.

32. Katkkhouda N, Guilherme M, Campos M, et al. Is laparoscopic approach to lumbar spine fusion worthwhile? Am J Surg 1999;178:458–461.

28. Lieberman I, Willsher P, Litwin D, et al. Transperitoneal laparoscopic exposure for lumbar interbody fusion. Spine 2000;25:509–514.

33. Rajaraman V, Vingan R, Roth P, et al. Visceral and vascular complications resulting from anterior lumbar interbody fusion. J Neurosurg 1999;91:60–64.

34. Zdeblick T, David S. A prospective comparison of surgical approach for anterior L4-L5 fusion: laparoscopic versus mini anterior lumbar interbody fusion. Spine 2000;25:2682–2687.

35. Regan J, McAfee P, Mack M. Atlas of endoscopic spine surgery. St. Louis, MO: Quality Medical Publishing, Inc., 1995.

36. Shaffrey C. Indications for threaded interbody devices. Proceedings of the 16th Annual Meeting of the Federation of Spine Associations; San Francisco; 2001.

37. Silber J, Anderson D, Hayes V, et al. Advances in surgical management of lumbar degenerative disease. Orthopaedics 2002;25:767–771.

38. McLaughlin M, Zhang J, Subach B, et al. Laparoscopic anterior lumbar fusion: technical note. Neurosurg Focus 1999;7:1–6.

39. Flynn J, Price C. Sexual complications of anterior fusion of the lumbar spine. Spine 1984;9:489–492.

40. Inoue S, Watanabe T, Hirose A, et al. Anterior discectomy and interbody fusion for lumbar disc herniation. Clin Orthop 1984;183:22–31.

41. Tiusanen H, Seitsalo S, Osterman K, et al. Retrograde ejaculation after anterior interbody lumbar fusion. Eur Spine J 1995;4:339–342.

42. Sylvain G, Raizadeh K, Macuire C, et al. Failure of lumbar interbody implants. Proceedings of the 68th Annual Meeting of the American Academy of Orthopaedic Surgeons; San Francisco; 2001.

43. Graber J, et al. Relationship of duration of postoperative ileus to extent and site of operative dissection. Surgery 1982;92:87–92.

44. Pellise F, Puig O, Rivas A, et al. Low fusion rate after L5-S1 laparoscopic anterior lumbar interbody fusion using twin stand-alone carbon fiber cages. Spine 2002;27:1665–1669.

45. Malberg MI. Extreme Lateral interbody fusion (XLIF): a new minimally invasive approach to the lumbar spine. In: Lieberman JR, et al., eds. Minimal access spine surgery. St. Louis: Quality Medical Publishing, 2002.

CHAPTER 23

Biology of Bone Grafting: Autograft and Allograft

Robert Gunzburg and Marek Szpalski

Spinal fusion is a well-accepted procedure for the treatment of disorders such as trauma, deformity, tumor, inflammation or infection, and common degenerative pathology. The aim of a spinal fusion is to eliminate the instability of the spine caused by these pathologies. By definition, spinal fusion means the achievement of a bony union between the involved vertebrae. In this chapter, the two types of bone grafts that are derived from natural bone (i.e., autograft and allograft) and are commonly used to achieve this goal will be discussed.

Far from being an inert structure, bone tissue can modify its mass and morphology in response to local and hormonal factors, thereby meeting the functional demands posed by various stimuli. Bone tissue also has the capacity for repairing itself without scarring. Bone grafting makes use of these core characteristics. In order to make optimal use of the clinically available graft options, the biology of bone, including its capacity for remodeling and self-repair, must be understood.

BONE STRUCTURE AND PHYSIOLOGY

Bone Cells

Osteoprogenitor cells are derived from mesenchymal cells and line the internal and external surfaces of bone. These cells have the capacity for differentiation into osteoblasts and related cells (e.g., fibroblasts) that comprise connective tissue.

Osteoblasts are active secretory cells derived from osteoprogenitor cells. Osteoblasts form the extracellular bone matrix by secreting osteoid (unmineralized matrix) and regulate its mineralization through the exocytosis of alkaline phosphatase-containing vesicles. Osteoblasts form a tight cell layer at the bone surface and have a life span of up to 8 weeks. The production of matrix proteins by osteoblasts decreases considerably with time, yet osteoblasts remain in communication with each other and

with related cells (e.g., osteocytes) by elaborating cytoplasmic processes that penetrate surrounding osteoid and terminate in gap junctions, creating an extensive intercellular communication network.

Osteocytes are derived from osteoblasts and comprise 90% of all cells in the mature skeleton; however, these mature cells differ significantly from osteoblasts in their biochemical, morphologic, and functional characteristics. Osteocytes are smaller, contain fewer organelles and have a higher ratio of nucleus to cytoplasm. They elaborate numerous filopodia, enabling interconnections and cellular communication. Occasionally, osteoblasts become trapped in the extracellular matrix, resulting in stimuli sufficient for their transformation into mature bone cells. Ongoing studies of the mechanosensory properties of osteocytes suggest that they are the primary regulators of bone remodeling, orchestrating the formation and resorption of bone in response to mechanical demands (1).

Osteoclasts are multinucleated, highly migratory, phagocytic cells derived from monocyte/macrophage precursors. Osteoclasts are responsible for the resorption of fully mineralized bone through acidic decalcification of bone matrix, followed by lysosomally mediated hydrolysis of its organic components. An activated osteoclast can resorb bone matrix at the rate of 200,000 μm^3 per day. Interestingly, 7 to 10 generations of osteoblasts are required to form this same amount of bone matrix (2).

Molecular Basis of Bone Remodeling

The regulation of osteoblastic and osteoclastic activities is dependent on a complex network of signaling molecules, including steroid hormones, prostaglandins, and cytokines; the molecular basis of osteoblast-osteoclast interactions is the subject of intensive research. The differentiation of osteoclast precursors into osteoclasts requires the expression of osteoclast differentiation factor

(ODF; also known as RANKL, TRANCE, and OPGL), a membrane-associated cytokine produced by osteoblasts in response to osteotropic factors such as parathyroid hormone, vitamin D, and cytokines such as tumor necrosis factor (TNF) and interleukins (3–5). Osteoclast precursors express the cell-surface receptor RANK, which binds ODF through cellular interaction with osteoblasts, in turn leading to osteoclast differentiation. ODF also plays a key role in the activation of osteoclasts into mature bone-resorbing cells (3). On the other hand, a number of cell types have been shown to secrete a soluble decoy receptor, known as osteoclastogenesis inhibitory factor (OCIF, also known as osteoprotegerin, or OPG) that competes for binding with RANK, thereby inhibiting osteoclast formation and subsequent bone resorption (5,3,6). The balance of molecular-signaling events, such as those touched upon in this chapter, most likely determine the outcome of stimuli leading to either net bone formation or net bone resorption.

Extracellular Matrix

Mineralization of osteoid, which consists primarily of collagen and ground substance, begins 10 to 15 days after its formation (7). Initially, mineral content rises rapidly to approximately 70% of its final amount; the remaining 30% being deposited over a period of several months. Even after mineralization is complete, bone still contains 25% organic matrix, including cells. Hydroxyapatite [$Ca_{10}(PO_4)_6(OH)_3$], the bone mineral, accounts for 70% of the final weight, while water accounts for the remaining 5%. Proteins, such as bone morphogenic proteins (BMP), growth factors, and cytokines, are embedded in the remaining extracellular matrix and play an important role in the mineralization process.

Bone Architecture

The matrix of mature cortical and cancellous bone has a lamellated structure. The lamellae run parallel to the trabeculae of cancellous bone or concentrically surround the Haversian canal in cortical bone, forming the so-called osteon, or functional unit of cortical bone. Typically, the long axis of the osteon runs parallel to the long axis of the bone. Osteons evolve into secondary osteons or haversian systems by resorption of preexisting bone. Modeling is the process whereby bone is laid down onto a surface without necessarily being preceded by resorption. Osteoblastic activity that fills voids following osteoclastic activity is referred to as remodeling. In the adult skeleton, remodeling is the more active process and gives bone the capacity to adapt to changes in loading and metabolic stimuli. Indeed, bone tissue adapts to mechanical stimuli (compression and bending movements) according to Wolff's law, which states, bone is laid down where stresses require its presence, and bone is absorbed where stresses do not require it.

Osteoinduction

In addition to differentiated bone cells such as osteoblasts, osteoclasts, and osteocytes, bone and adjacent tissue contain a number of less differentiated cells. Osteoinduction is the process by which these less differentiated, yet pluripotent cells are stimulated to develop into the bone-forming cell lineage (8). A great deal of research has focused on BMPs as inducing agents. BMPs are soluble glycoproteins (9) released in response to trauma, such as a fracture, or physical stimuli, such as mechanical, electrical, or magnetic alterations. Although osteoblasts present at the site of injury participate in the healing of a fracture, bone and soft tissue injuries are the primary trigger for the transformation of undifferentiated cells into osteoblasts. The response to injury involves the coordinated involvement of vascular and nervous tissue, as well as the sensitization of precursor cells, leading to the production of growth factors by these cells and their differentiation into actively remodeling cell types (8,10). Insofar as bone formation necessitates an adequate blood supply, bone growth factors are also angiogenic (11).

Osteoconduction

Osteoconduction is the appositional growth of bone on the three-dimensional surface of a suitable scaffold (12). This includes the ingrowth of capillaries, perivascular tissue, and osteoprogenitor cells and follows a highly organized, predictable spatial pattern (13).

Osteogenesis

Osteogenesis is the process of bone formation through cellular osteoblastic activity. Osteogenesis is dependent upon osteoconduction as a matrix for the delivery of the osteoinductive factors needed for the differentiation of osteoprogenitor stem cells.

SPINAL FUSION

Osseous spinal fusion remains the ultimate goal in the treatment of numerous spinal conditions. In spite of improvements in surgical techniques and instrumentation, failure (nonunion) has been estimated to occur in 5% to 35% of patients undergoing single-level fusions, and more frequently in patients undergoing multilevel fusions (14). The rate of clinical success does not necessarily parallel the rate of fusion. Numerous factors, such as mechanical stability, type of instrumentation, type of bone graft material, and individual biological factors, influence fusion rates.

Spinal arthrodesis can be achieved anteriorly by the fusion of vertebral bodies. This became a standard procedure in the cervical spine soon after Cloward first advocated this approach as a treatment for ruptured discs (15). At the levels of the thoracic and upper-lumbar spine, the approach is more difficult due to the presence of the rib cage and diaphragm; nonetheless, spinal interbody fusion can still be accomplished at these levels. Below the level of the conus, interbody fusion can be achieved either through an anterior or posterior approach.

Spinal arthrodesis can also be achieved posteriorly by bone bridging between the transverse processes and facet joints of the vertebrae involved in the fusion. All these fusion techniques are often combined with a variety of internal fixation devices. The choice of approach and technique depends on the type and location of the pathology and the surgeon's experience and knowledge.

BONE GRAFTS

Bone is a commonly transplanted tissue. Bone grafts have to promote osteogenesis and, in some applications, may need to provide mechanical support. The morphology of the required graft depends on the type of fusion being sought. Cortical bone is typically used for fixation and support, whereas cancellous bone provides osteogenic potential (16). For cervical interbody fusion or reconstruction or for thoracic and lumbar interbody fusions and reconstructions, corticocancellous grafts are required to provide structural support. However, when stabilizing devices such as cages are being used, cancellous bone chips (particulate grafts) may be preferred. Particulate graft materials may also be preferred for posterior and posterolateral intervertebral fusions. Cancellous bone grafts have been used to stimulate bone regeneration under a variety of pathologic circumstances, including trauma, infection, congenital defects, tumor invasion, and degenerative diseases. For optimal remodeling of bony tissue, these grafts need to mimic the properties of cancellous bone, providing the interrelated characteristics of osteoconduction, osteoinduction, and osteogenesis.

Revascularization occurs more rapidly with particulate grafts than with structural grafts. Particulate bone grafts tend to remodel entirely with time, whereas structural (cortical) grafts have a tendency to retain their shape and contain a mixture of necrotic and viable bone (17). The process of creeping substitution, "the temporal and spatial repair activities whereby viable new bone replaces necrotic old bone" (18), is also thought to differ between cancellous and cortical allograft (17). Whereas creeping substitution of cancellous bone involves appositional bone formation followed by resorption, this order of events is reversed for cortical bone, with osteoclastic activity initiating the repair process (17,18). Such differences in the biology of remodeling between different types of grafts may lead to significant differences in their clinical applications (17).

Autograft

Autografts are grafts harvested from the patient at the time of surgery. The autograft is the "gold standard" by which the success of other grafting techniques is assessed. Spinal fusion is the most common reason for the harvest of autogenous bone (19). The main source of autograft is the iliac crest, yet other sources, such as the proximal tibia, the fibula, or a rib, can be used if the iliac crest is not an option. Iliac crest bone can be harvested in the form of cancellous bone chips, respecting the inner and outer tables of the crista, or as tricortical strut grafts, providing bone capable of structural support (Fig. 23-1).

Cancellous bone autografts offer a number of positive features including histocompatibility, which precludes the risk of graft encapsulation and associated inflammation. Moreover, autografts maintain viable osteoblasts and osteoprogenitor cells, and also confer osteoconductive and osteoinductive potential (19,20). The calcified matrix of mature bone and its organic components (e.g., collagen and ground substance) supply the graft with biocompatible, osteoconductive properties (19). Noncollagenous growth factors, the most thoroughly investigated of which are the BMPs, are primarily responsible for the osteoinductive capacity of autograft (21). The highly porous, trabecular structure of autogenous cancellous bone permits the ingrowth of blood vessels needed for bone growth and reduces the risk of complications from hypoxia. Finally, autograft does not pose a risk of disease transmission. Autograft procedures show a high rate of success for certain spinal fusions, such as posterior-cervical arthrodesis.

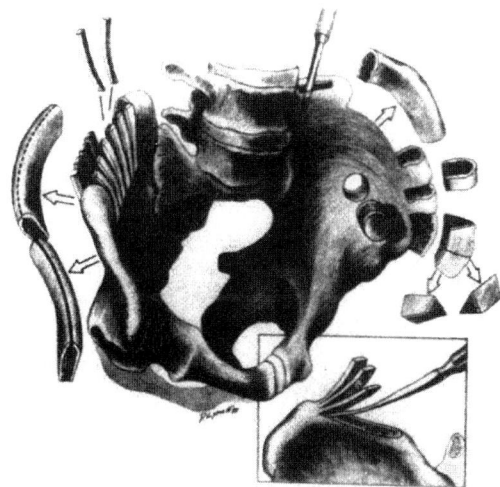

FIG. 23-1. Common types of iliac crest bone grafts. (From Sandhu HS, Grewal HS, Parvataneni H. Bone grafting for spinal fusion. Orthop Clin North Am 1999;30:686, with permission.)

Autograft, however, has several drawbacks, including both surgical complications and its limited supply. Although transplanted donor cells most likely contribute to new bone growth, most of the osteogenic cells that repopulate the graft are thought to migrate from the fusion bed (12,19). Although transplanted cells are initially alive, graft viability is diminished when the graft tissue is separated from its blood supply (19), leading to ischemic or apoptotic cell death (12) and leaving behind only a bone mineral scaffold (22). Although morselization may increase bone graft surface area, leading to increased accessibility of osteoinductive and osteogenic factors (19), additional processing of autogenous bone may contribute to further decreases in cell viability. The surviving cells receive their oxygen and nutrients by diffusion only; thus, cells are likely to die from ischemia before the graft is vascularized. Rapid vascularization of the graft site may be impeded by fibrin formation in the autograft and by the packing procedure used to place the graft into the surgical site; this is particularly of concern within the innermost region of the graft. Autogenous bone viability is further complicated by donor variables such as the age, gender, genetic makeup, and physical health of the patient.

Harvest of autogenous tissue is associated with high donor-site morbidity and is estimated to occur in 10% to 39% of patients (23). Donor-site morbidity is dependent upon the surgical approach; for example, sacroiliac sub-luxation and dislocation occur more frequently with the posterior approach, while infection occurs more frequently following the anterior approach (24). Minor complications are common and include superficial infections, temporary sensory impairment, and mild or transient pain. Acute and chronic pain at the donor site is commonly reported, but chronic pain may occur in over 25% of patients who undergo autograft procedures for spinal fusion (25,26). Although the precise cause of pain following iliac crest harvest is unknown, such pain is probably muscular or periosteal in origin and is often resistant to conventional treatment (26).

Major complications associated with the harvest of tissue from the iliac crest have been reported at rates of 0.7% to 25% (19). These include severe bleeding, herniation, serious infection, scarring, hematoma formation, injury to nervous or vascular tissue, pelvic fracture, and chronic pain at the procurement site (20,26–30). Skaggs et al. reported that after autogenous bone harvest, 15% of pediatric patients had complications that affected daily living activities (31).

Skillful surgical technique is essential to avoid injury to neurologic or vascular tissue during the harvest of iliac crest bone. Structures that often lie in the dissection path include the sciatic, iliohypogastric, lateral femoral cutaneous, and cluneal nerves, as well as the superior gluteal vessels (32) (Fig. 23-2). Damage to nervous and vascular

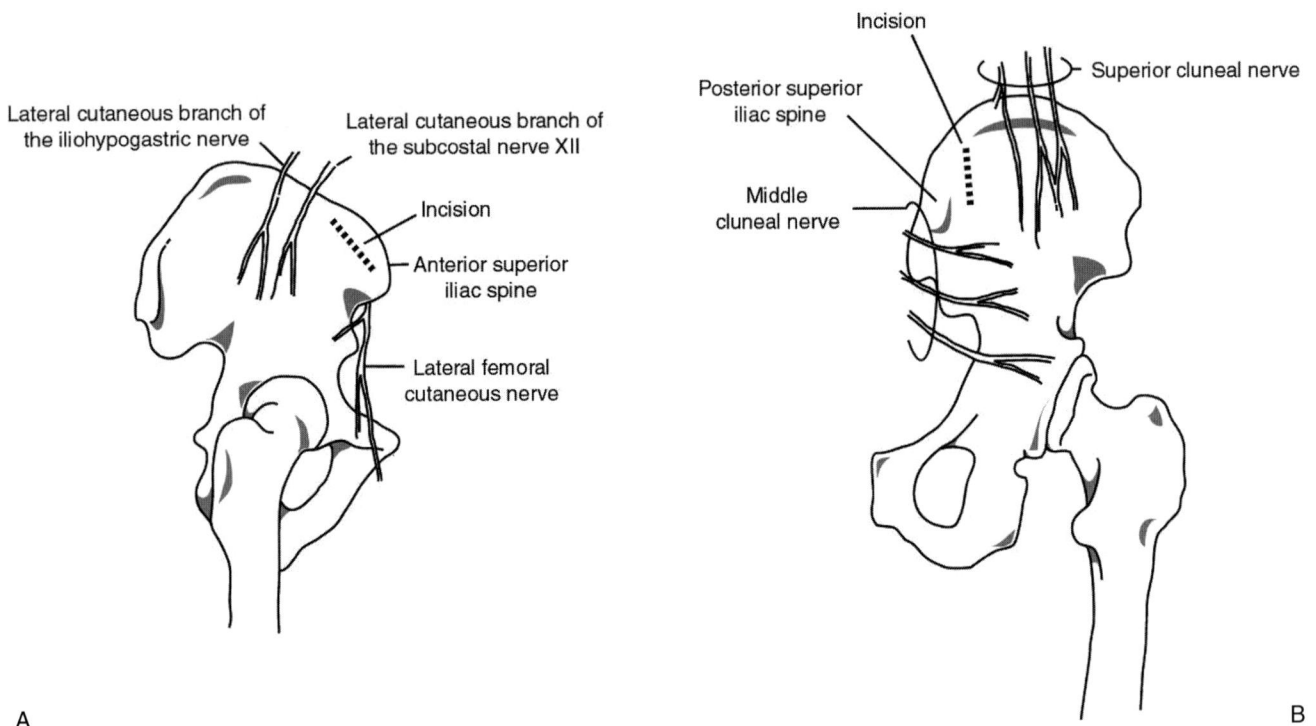

FIG. 23-2. Nervous tissue that can be damaged during harvest of bone from the iliac crest. **A:** Proximity of anterior incision (*dotted line*) relative to critical neurologic structures. **B:** Proximity of posterior incision (*dotted line*) to cluneal nerves.

tissue has been correlated with the amount of soft tissue dissected during the procedure (23). The superior gluteal vessels or the sciatic nerve may be damaged by dissection too close to the sciatic notch (33). In addition, chronic procurement-site pain may result from removal of bone in the sacroiliac region due to disruption of the sacroiliac joint (32). Since these iatrogenic complications may prolong recovery and increase disability, the surgeon should be thoroughly familiar with all anatomic structures that can be damaged during the harvest procedure (32).

Certain conditions require a relatively large amount of autogenous bone, limiting the applicability of autograft procedures. For example, obtaining adequate bone stock for multilevel spinal fusions may not be possible. Conversely, harvesting sufficient autogenous bone may be impractical in certain patient populations (i.e., older adults, children, or patients with metastatic carcinoma). Alternatives to autograft (e.g., allograft or composite materials) should be considered in these patients as well as in severely osteopenic patients (30). In patients with paralytic scoliosis and pelvic obliquity, posterior spinal fusion typically requires additional instrumentation to the pelvis, precluding harvest from the posterior ilium (34,35). An inadequate quantity of autogenous bone in a graft procedure may result in failure to fuse (36); supplementation of autograft with alternative graft materials should therefore be considered in cases that may lack sufficient autogenous bone stock.

ALLOGRAFT

Allografts are grafts previously harvested from another patient, or from the patient undergoing surgery at the time of surgery. Allografts were originally used only when the amount of bone-graft material required for a procedure exceeded the amount of autogenous bone that could be harvested. Recent improvements in the quality, safety, and availability of allogeneic materials have resulted in substantial increases in the use of allograft; in the mid-1990s, allograft comprised nearly 35% of all bone grafts performed in the United States (37). The advantages of allograft include avoidance of donor-site morbidity, the potential for providing immediate mechanical support, and availability in a variety of forms and shapes for customized applications. Allograft can be used as a particulate or structural material. As mentioned, the histology of bony incorporation differs significantly between these two preparations.

Although the rate of success for anterior spinal-lumbar arthrodesis with allograft has been reported to be similar to that of autograft, the two methods do not produce equivalent results (38). Allografts can have variability in bone quality and pose a small, but definite risk of disease transmission and immunogenic reactions (39). Processing techniques to reduce these risks result in a loss of osteogenic potential due to the lack of donor cells (40)

and reduced osteoinductive potential (19), presumably due to the inactivation or removal of osteotropic factors such as BMPs. The risk of disease transmission is related to the rigor with which allograft tissue is processed. For example, transmission of human immunodeficiency virus (HIV) has been documented in fresh-frozen allograft, but not in freeze-dried allograft (38,41). Transmission of HIV and hepatitis are also dependent on how carefully donors are screened. For orthopedic applications, freezing, freeze-drying, and irradiation, sometimes followed by demineralization, are commonly employed methods for processing and preserving allograft materials (17,40). Although freeze-drying reduces immunogenicity and lengthens shelf life relative to fresh-frozen allograft, freeze-drying also reduces mechanical strength by up to 50% (19,38,42). In addition, freeze-dried grafts are incorporated into host tissue less completely and retain BMPs less efficiently than fresh-frozen grafts. In summary, graft strength, immunogenicity, risk for transmission of disease, and capacity for incorporation into the host site can vary widely with the technique used for allograft preparation. One additional disadvantage of allograft is its expense.

Demineralized Bone Matrix

Brief mention should be made of demineralized bone matrix (DBM), a cortical allograft that is further processed by decalcification, leaving collagen, noncollagenous proteins, and growth factors (43). The resultant matrix lacks weight-bearing capacity (44) but has improved osteoinductive potential due to the presence of low-molecular-weight glycoproteins including BMPs (45). Decalcification of cortical bone increases the accessibility of these growth factors sequestered within the bone matrix (1,19,39). In addition, DBM is less immunogenic than conventionally processed allograft (43). Although DBM has been used clinically with proven success, the osteoinductive potential of DBM can vary, depending on the method of processing (46). Moreover, the effectiveness of DBM in promoting new bone formation is also related to the particle size of the matrix and to the method used for its sterilization (37).

Autograft and Allograft in Combination

As mentioned earlier, allograft may be needed to supplement autograft when the volume of the latter is not sufficient for a given procedure. Munting et al. used freeze-dried, cortical allograft for the repair of large, anterior segmental defects of the spine involving at least one vertebral body and its two adjacent discs (47). In 41 of 67 cases, autogenous bone, obtained from either the resected vertebral bodies or the ribs, was used to fill the medullary cavity. None of the patients experienced infection, transmission of disease, or long-term mechanical graft failure over the follow-up period, which averaged 31 months. Fusion was reported to have been obtained reliably. The authors noted that the use of autograft in the medullary cavity promoted successful fusion by providing a large surface area for load transmission at the graft-host interface.

Comparison of Autograft and Allograft

Successful incorporation of bone graft depends on the quality and quantity of graft material as well as host physiological responses. The graft material requires osteoconductive, osteoinductive, and osteogenic elements in order for successful new bone growth to occur. Since autogenous bone supplies all three of these items, it is generally considered superior to that of allograft. Moreover, autograft has produced less variability in clinical results. As observed by Ehrler and Vaccaro, two primary indications exist for the use of allograft bone: insufficient autograft and the requirement for immediate structural support (38).

In addition to being only weakly osteoinductive and devoid of osteogenic cells, allograft typically induces an inflammatory reaction in the host, thus producing an inflammatory response that may be an important contributor to graft failure (38,48,49). Indeed, allograft may induce a robust inflammatory reaction immediately after transplant, resulting in capillary thrombosis, thus further slowing revascularization and osteoinduction (38). This leads to tissue necrosis, comprising up to 50% or more of the graft (38). Animal studies suggest that the host immune response is specific to donor antigen and consists of killer/suppressor T cells, which are likely mediators of graft rejection (48). The human immune reaction to allograft bears resemblance to the immune reaction in animals (50), resulting in a rate of sensitization (67%) that is higher than that seen after blood transfusion (12% to 50%) (51). Immunologic factors that mediate rejection of foreign material share common bone-marrow–derived precursors and cytokines with the factors responsible for remodeling of bone; this may help explain the deleterious interaction between the two systems (48). In a study of 29 patients who received allograft, those who lacked sensitization to class II antigens achieved a more satisfactory clinical outcome compared with patients who exhibited such sensitization (50). This result provides evidence for a causal relationship between immunogenicity and less satisfactory outcome.

The rate of incorporation of graft material is determined by several factors, including anatomic site, size of the graft area, and size of the graft (12,22). Incorporation of allograft is qualitatively similar to that of autograft but occurs at a slower rate and with more variable results. The variable amount of inflammation arising from allograft procedures may be largely responsible for these differences. However, the weak osteoinductivity of allograft

may also be a contributing factor to its slower rate of incorporation relative to autograft. Demineralization of allograft material improves osteoinductivity. Pals and Wilkins have reported excellent functional outcomes with DBM in treating giant bony tumors (52); other authors, however, have reported variable efficacy in promoting bone induction (43).

Autograft has been used successfully in posterior cervical, thoracic, and intervertebral fusion procedures (e.g., achieving adequate fusion in over 90% of patients receiving posterior cervical fusions) (19), but less successfully in posterolateral lumbar fusion procedures, with some studies reporting adequate fusion in less than 60% of such surgeries (19). The success rate for posterolateral lumbar fusion is even lower when allograft is used alone or in combination with autograft (38). Success rates for anterior spinal lumbar fusions with allograft are comparable to autograft (38). High rates of success have also been reported for allograft posterior lumbar interbody fusion procedures (38).

Allograft has been shown to be useful as bone-void filler since it provides early structural support without donor-site morbidity (50). Perhaps the best indication for allograft is in adolescent patients undergoing scoliosis correction and fusion (19). In one study, 40 patients with idiopathic scoliosis who underwent corrective surgery were treated with either femoral head allograft or autograft from the iliac crest. Successful unions were obtained for all patients in both groups. Interestingly, the group treated with allograft experienced reduced postoperative pain relative to the group treated with autograft (53).

CONCLUSION

Spinal fusion is a common procedure for treating trauma, infection, congenital malformations, tumor growth, or degenerative diseases that threaten bone integrity. The vast majority of spinal fusion procedures rely on bone grafting techniques that support bone remodeling by providing osteogenic potential and, in some cases, mechanical support. Autogenous cancellous bone is the "gold standard" for bone graft materials, providing a matrix for osteoconduction, growth factors for osteoinduction, and osteoprogenitor cells for new bone formation. Autograft has several disadvantages, however, including limitations in the quality and quantity of bone available, and, most significantly, morbidity associated with the procurement site, usually the iliac crest. Complications of iliac crest harvest can occur in up to 25% of patients and may lead to prolonged recovery time and long-term morbidity.

The popularity of allograft has increased over the past few years due to improved safety, availability, and the potential for customizing allograft materials to specific applications. However, allograft has several drawbacks. Like autograft, allograft exhibits variations in the quality of tissue used for transplantation. Allograft also has a finite risk of transmitting disease and producing an immunogenic response in the host. In order to avoid these risks, allograft is extensively processed, resulting in reduced mechanical strength and osteoinductive potential. These characteristics probably affect clinical results obtained with allograft, resulting in less consistent surgical outcomes than are obtained with autograft. In spite of improvements in modern technology and instrumentation, the rate of failure (nonunion) of spinal arthrodesis remains relatively high, particularly in cases involving multilevel fusions. Insofar as fusion rates are related to factors such as mechanical stability and type of bone graft material, improvements in fusion rates may depend on further innovations in bone graft technology, including the use of autograft/allograft combinations and the development of composite materials that provide the scaffold and biologic stimuli necessary for successful bone remodeling.

REFERENCES

1. Burger EH, Klein-Nulend J. Mechanotransduction in bone—role of the lacuno-canalicular network. FASEB J 1999;13[Suppl[:S101–S112.
2. Albright JA, Skinner HCW. Bone: structural organization and remodeling dynamics. In: Albright JA, Brand RA, eds. The scientific basis of orthopaedics. East Norwalk, CT: Appleton & Lange, 1987:161–198.
3. Suda T, Kobayashi K, Jimi E, et al. The molecular basis of osteoclast differentiation and activation. Novartis Found Symp 2001;232: 235–250.
4. Lacey DL, Timms E, Tan H-L, et al. Osteoprotegerin ligand is a cytokine that regulates osteoclast differentiation and activation. Cell 1998;93:165–176.
5. Gravallese EM, Goldring SR. Cellular mechanisms and the role of cytokines in bone erosions in rheumatoid arthritis. Arthritis Rheum 2000;43:2143–2151.
6. Yasuda H, Shima N, Nakagawa N, et al. Identity of osteoclastogenesis inhibitory factor (OCIF) and osteoprotegerin (OPG): a mechanism by which OPG/OCIF inhibits osteoclastogenesis in vitro. Endocrinology 1998;139:1329–1337.
7. Sommerfeldt DW, Rubin CT. Biology of bone and how it orchestrates the form and function of the skeleton. Eur Spine J 2001;10[Suppl 2]: S86–S95.
8. Albrektsson T, Johansson C. Osteoinduction, osteoconduction and osseointegration. Eur Spine J 2001;10[Suppl 2]:S96–S101.
9. Urist MR, Mikulski A, Lietze A. Solubilized and insolubilized bone morphogenetic protein. Proc Natl Acad Sci U S A 1979;76:1828–1832.
10. Frost HM. The biology of fracture healing. An overview for clinicians. Part I. Clin Orthop 1989;(248):283–293.
11. Trippel SB. Growth factors as therapeutic agents. Instr Course Lect 1997;46:473–476.
12. Bauer TW, Muschler GF. Bone graft materials: an overview of the basic science. Clin Orthop 2000;(371):10–27.
13. Stevenson S. Biology of bone grafts. Orthop Clin North Am 1999;30: 543–552.
14. Marchesi DG. Spinal fusions: bone and bone substitutes. Eur Spine J 2000;9:372–378.
15. Cloward RB. The anterior approach for removal of ruptured cervical disks. J Neurosurg 1958;15:602–617.
16. Surgical techniques. In: Crenshaw AH, Daugherty K, eds. Campbell's operative orthopaedics. St. Louis: Mosby-Year Book, Inc., 1992:1–20.
17. Berven S, Tay BK, Kleinstueck FS, Bradford DS. Clinical applications of bone graft substitutes in spine surgery: consideration of mineralized and demineralized preparations and growth factor supplementation. Eur Spine J 2001;10[Suppl 2]:S169–S177.
18. Burchardt H. The biology of bone graft repair. Clin Orthop Rel Res 1983; (174):28–42.
19. Sandhu HS, Grewal HS, Parvataneni H. Bone grafting for spinal fusion. Orthop Clin North Am 1999;30:685–698.
20. Arrington ED, Smith WJ, Chambers HG, et al. Complications of iliac crest bone graft harvesting. Clin Orthop 1996;(329):300–309.
21. Boden SD. The biology of posterolateral lumbar spinal fusion. Orthop Clin North Am 1998;29:603–619.
22. Tägil M, Johnsson R, Strömqvist B, et al. Incomplete incorporation of morselized and impacted autologous bone graft. A histological study in 4 intracorporeally grafted lumbar fractures. Acta Orthop Scand 1999;70:555–558.
23. Banwart JC, Asher MA, Hassanein RS. Iliac crest bone graft harvest donor site morbidity: a statistical evaluation. Spine 1995;20:1055–1060.
24. Kurz LT, Garfin SR, Booth RE Jr. Harvesting autogenous iliac bone grafts: a review of complications and techniques. Spine 1989;14:1324–1331.
25. Fernyhough JC, Schimandle JJ, Weigel MC, et al. Chronic donor site pain complicating bone graft harvesting from the posterior iliac crest for spinal fusion. Spine 1992;17:1474–1480.
26. Summers BN, Eisenstein SM. Donor site pain from the ilium: a complication of lumbar spine fusion. J Bone Joint Surg Br 1989;71-B: 677–680.
27. Seiler JG, Johnson J. Iliac crest autogenous bone grafting: donor site complications. J South Orthop Assoc 2000;9:91–97.
28. Dösoglu M, Orakdögen M, Tevrüz M, et al. Enterocutaneous fistula: a complication of posterior iliac bone graft harvesting not previously described. Acta Neurochir (Wien) 1998;140:1089–1092.
29. Connolly JF, Guse R, Tiedeman J, et al. Autologous marrow injection as a substitute for operative grafting of tibial nonunions. Clin Orthop Rel Res 1991;(266):259–270.
30. Fernando TL, Kim SS, Mohler DG. Complete pelvic ring failure after posterior iliac bone graft harvesting. Spine 1999;24:2101–2104.
31. Skaggs DL, Samuelson MA, Hale JM, et al. Complications of posterior iliac crest bone grafting in spine surgery in children. Spine 2000;25: 2400–2402.
32. Hu RW, Bohlman HH. Fracture at the iliac bone graft harvest site after fusion of the spine. Clin Orthop 1994;(309):208–213.
33. Balderston RA, An HS. Complications in scoliosis, kyphosis, and spondylolisthesis surgery. In: Wickland E, ed. Complications in spinal surgery. Philadelphia: WB Saunders, 1991:20–22.
34. Gau YL, Lonstein JE, Winter RB, et al. Luque-Galveston procedure for correction and stabilization of neuromuscular scoliosis and pelvic obliquity: a review of 68 patients. J Spinal Disord 1991;4:399–410.
35. Bridwell KH, O'Brien MF, Lenke LG, et al. Posterior spinal fusion supplemented with only allograft bone in paralytic scoliosis. Does it work? Spine 1994;19:2658–2666.
36. McCarthy RE, Peek RD, Morrissy RT, et al. Allograft bone in spinal fusion for paralytic scoliosis. J Bone Joint Surg Am 1986;68-A: 370–375.
37. Boyce T, Edwards J, Scarborough N. Allograft bone: the influence of processing on safety and performance. Orthop Clin North Am 1999;30:571–581.
38. Ehrler DM, Vaccaro AR. The use of allograft bone in lumbar spine surgery. Clin Orthop 2000;(371):38–45.
39. Fleming JE Jr, Cornell CN, Muschler GF. Bone cells and matrices in orthopedic tissue engineering. Orthop Clin North Am 2000;31: 357–374.
40. Kerry RM, Masri BA, Garbuz DS, et al. The biology of bone grafting. AAOS Instr Course Lect 1999;48:645–652.
41. Tomford WW. Transmission of disease through transplantation of musculoskeletal allografts. J Bone Joint Surg Am 1995;77-A:1742–1754.
42. Pelker RR, Friedlaender GE. Biomechanical aspects of bone autografts and allografts. Orthop Clin North Am 1987;18:235–239.
43. Truumees E, Herkowitz HN. Alternatives to autologous bone harvest in spine surgery. Univ Penn Orthop J 1999;12:77–88.
44. Ludwig SC, Boden SD. Osteoinductive bone graft substitutes for spinal fusion: a basic science summary. Orthop Clin North Am 1999;30: 635–645.
45. Sandhu HS, Khan SN, Suh DY, et al. Demineralized bone matrix, bone morphogenetic proteins, and animal models of spine fusion: an overview. Eur Spine J, 2001;10[Suppl 2]:S122–S131.
46. Khan SN, Tomin E, Lane JM. Clinical applications of bone graft substitutes. Orthop Clin North Am 2000;31:389–398.
47. Munting E, Faundez A, Manche E. Vertebral reconstruction with cortical allograft: long-term evaluation. Eur Spine J 2001;10[Suppl 2]: S153–S157.

48. Friedlaender GE. Bone allografts: the biological consequences of immunological events. J Bone Joint Surg Am 1991;73-A:1119–1122.

49. Goldberg VM, Powell A, Shaffer JW, et al. Bone grafting: role of histocompatibility in transplantation. J Orthop Res 1985;3:389–404.

50. Friedlaender GE, Strong DM, Tomford WW, et al. Long-term follow-up of patients with osteochondral allografts. A correlation between immunologic responses and clinical outcome. Orthop Clin North Am 1999;30:583–588.

51. Strong DM, Friedlaender GE, Tomford WW, et al. Immunologic responses in human recipients of osseous and osteochondral allografts. Clin Orthop 1996;(326):107–114.

52. Pals SD, Wilkins RM. Giant cell tumor of bone treated by curettage, cementation, and bone grafting. Orthopedics 1992;15:703–708.

53. Dodd CAF, Fergusson CM, Freedman L, et al. Allograft versus autograft bone in scoliosis surgery. J Bone Joint Surg Br 1988;70-B: 431–434.

CHAPTER 24

Bone Graft Substitutes in Spinal Surgery

Anis O. Mekhail and Gordon R. Bell

Bone grafting is a prerequisite to obtaining a solid spinal fusion. Bone grafting can also be used for reconstruction of spinal defects caused by infection, trauma, or tumors. Autogenous bone graft is still the gold standard for augmenting spinal fusion. However, autogenous bone graft has significant limitations, including donor site morbidity and limited supply (1–5). The limitation in providing functional shapes, the increased operative time, the blood loss, and the possible need for transfusion are additional problems to be considered.

Although allograft is sometimes an attractive alternative to autograft, it has its own limitations and problems. These include loss of biologic and mechanical properties during its processing (6–8), the risk of disease transmission (9–13), immunogenicity (14,15), cost, and religious concerns. In general, allograft is associated with slower fusion rate, greater graft resorption, and increased infection rate when compared to autograft. This is especially true in lumbar intertransverse fusions and multiple-level anterior cervical fusions (16,17).

Despite the advances in spinal instrumentation, the incidence of nonunion has remained unacceptably high (10% to 40% without instrumentation, 10% to 15% with instrumentation) (18–25). Because of the limitations of autografts and allografts, scientists have sought to develop bone graft substitutes. In order to understand the value of the different bone graft substitutes, it is important to appreciate the different properties of graft materials that contribute to fusion (26,27). The ideal bone graft substitute should possess all the properties of autogenous bone graft, which include osteogenicity (the ability to directly produce bone by viable osteogenic cells), osteoinductivity (the ability to stimulate undetermined osteoprogenitor stem cells to differentiate into osteogenic cells and to induce the osteoblastic pathway even in a nonbony location), and osteoconductivity (the ability to provide a passive porous scaffold to support and direct new bone formation by allowing ingrowth of neovasculature and the infiltration of osteogenic precursor cells) (28). Bone graft substitutes should also be biocompatible,

bioabsorbable, be easy to use clinically, be cost-effective, provide the appropriate structural support required depending on the clinical situation (block form as well as granular), and be without risk of disease transmission. A composite graft (a mix of two or more graft materials) combines an osteoconductive matrix with bioactive agents that provide osteoinductive or osteogenic properties in order to closely replicate or supersede autograft properties. The bone graft substitute can be used as an extender if less bone graft is co-mixed and it can be used as an expander if the total volume of the mixture is increased, in an effort to increase the likelihood of bone healing. The bone graft substitute can replace bone graft if it can affect bone healing without adding bone.

Attaining spinal fusion does not only depend on the type of graft material used but also on several local and systemic factors, which include biomechanical stability and loading, blood supply, graft recipient site preparation, recipient bone pathology, nutrition, radiation, drugs, smoking, and several systemic diseases. These factors are discussed, for the most part, in Chapter 23. With all these factors taken into consideration, the basis of spinal fusion is simply bone formation, in an osteoconductive medium, by osteoprogenitor cells, which are induced by osteoinductive agents. However, for this scenario to occur, optimal local and systemic factors need to be present. The success of spinal fusion also varies depending on the location of the arthrodesis itself along the spine, and the biomechanical environment influencing the spinal fusion (posterolateral intertransverse process, anterior interbody, anteroposterior combined, presence or absence of internal fixation).

Differences in species used may also play a role, as they may heal differently and their spines are subjected to different loads. Animal models of spinal fusion should be evaluated with great caution. Structural grafts used for obtaining interbody fusion are located between two flat bones and are subjected to compressive loads, whereas graft materials used for posterior and posterolateral fusions are not structural, are surrounded mostly by soft tissue, and heal under tension loads. Also, the addition of instrumentation plays an important role in the success of fusion. Instrumentation adds to biomechanical stability and can affect the type of load applied, such as allowing a facet joint fusion to occur under compression rather than tension (29).

OSTEOCONDUCTIVE MATERIALS

Ceramics

The mineral phase of bone comprises approximately 60% to 70% of its dry weight (28). This carbonated calcium phosphate apatite mineral, termed *dahllite*, contains 4% to 6% carbonate by weight and small amounts of sodium, magnesium, and other trace elements (30). The structural integrity of bone, especially its compressive strength, directly depends on the state of the mineral phase. It has been demonstrated that the chemical structure of the substrate is vital to its observed osteoconductive properties. Ideally, a bone graft substitute would have a similar mineral composition and structure.

Because ceramics do not normally exhibit osteogenic or osteoinductive properties, when used alone they are dependent on local host tissues for osteoprogenitor cells and osteoinductive factors. When loaded with a source of osteogenic cells, such as autogenous bone or bone marrow, ceramic scaffolds facilitate cellular adhesion, support vascular ingrowth, and promote new bone formation (31).

The advantages of biodegradable osteoconductive ceramic bone graft substitutes include the availability in unlimited quantity and no donor site complications or infection risks. For synthetic materials to be useful *in vivo*, they must be compatible with surrounding tissues, be chemically stable in body fluids, have compatible mechanical and physical properties, be able to be produced in functional shapes, be able to withstand the sterilization process, have reasonable cost, and have a reliable quality control (32). Calcium phosphate, for the most part, possesses these properties (33–36). Although some inert metals, such as titanium and cobalt chrome, and some ceramics, such as aluminum oxide, can provide passageways for bone incorporation, bone does not directly bond to and proliferate along their surfaces. On the other hand, bone forms directly on the surface and chemically binds to bioactive osteoconductive ceramics. Moreover, the bone grows three-dimensionally along the ceramic's surface.

The most commonly used ceramics in bone surgery are calcium phosphates, which include coral-based or synthetic hydroxyapatite (HA) and tricalcium phosphate (TCP). They have a high degree of biocompatibility with host tissue (33,37) and they are brittle materials with low fracture resistance and variability in their chemical and structural (crystalline) composition (27). Optimal interconnection between pores (connective porosity

greater than 100 μm) and a pore size of 100 to 500 μm have been demonstrated to be essential for osteoconductivity (38,39). This is based on the three-dimensional interconnection between the lacunae in the bone that provide intercellular communication. Different preparative methods of ceramic bone graft substitutes lead to either a compact or a porous material. Greater crystalline formation and material density result in greater mechanical strength and resistance to dissolution with long-lasting stability. The poorly interconnected porosity created in artificially created ceramics retards normal rate of bone healing and remodeling required to obtain optimal mechanical strength. In contrast, an amorphous ultrastructure and greater porosity enhance interface activity and bone ingrowth, but they also enhance biodegradation of the implant (33).

Commercially available HA is relatively inert and biodegrades poorly (33,40,41). Nonresorbing materials may interfere with remodeling, create a stress riser, and impede the accretion of strength of the fusion mass (33). Conversely, ceramic TCP undergoes biodegradation within the first 4 to 8 weeks of implantation, which may be too early for optimal fusion mass healing (33,42). Biphasic ceramics, with an optimized ratio between HA and TCP may increase the mechanical strength or the degree and speed of resorption (43–47).

Natural ceramics derived from sea coral were first recognized by Chiroff et al. to have morphologically better interconnective porosity than artificially created HA, and with a structure similar to bone (48). Because the implant material is not coral but is derived from the mineral content of coral, the implants are called coralline. Coral is composed of 97% calcium carbonate in the form of aragonite. Coralline implants can be manufactured using one of two processes. The first is using natural coral in the calcium carbonate form (Biocoral; Inoteb, Saint-Gonnery, France) after removing the organics and sterilizing with radiation. Biocoral is available as blocks and in granular form. The other process is replamineform (involving a hydrothermal exchange reaction), which converts delicate coral calcium carbonate into mechanically superior HA (39,49). Because this is a solid-state reaction, the interconnected porosity is perfectly preserved (50). Two genera of stony corals are used: *Porites* and *Goniopora*. The exoskeleton of genus *Porites* is similar to cortical bone while that of *Goniopora* is similar to cancellous bone. Pro Osteon or Interpore porous HA (Interpore Cross International, Inc., Irvine, CA) are trade names for coralline HA. The number following the trade name designates the nominal pore diameter. Pro Osteon 200 HA is derived from *Porites* and has a pore diameter of 200 μm, while Pro Osteon 500 HA is derived from *Goniopora* and has a pore diameter of 500 μm (50).

Coralline implants are extremely biocompatible with promising results as a bone graft substitute to augment or replace autogenous bone graft (33,51–54) or as a part of a composite with an osteoinductive bone protein (55). However, the poor bioabsorbability of the HA can still effect poor bone remodeling. The alteration of the coral processing with a partial thermoreaction, where only 20% of the calcium carbonate is converted into HA, has been found to improve its bioresorbability (18,56). The HA layer delays the resorption of the underlying calcium carbonate to achieve a controlled rate of graft resorption. Bucholz et al. have noted that for invasion to occur, the coralline implants must be rigidly stabilized and in close apposition to the host bone (51).

Endobon (Merck, Darmstadt, Germany) and Pyrost (Stryker Howmedica Osteonics, Rutherford, NJ) are macroporous HA products derived from exposure of cancellous bovine bone to high temperatures. OsSatura porous-coated HA (IsoTis NV, Bilthoven, The Netherlands) is a porous calcium phosphate scaffold with a biomimetic coating: a first generation tissue-engineered product (57). Its surface structure resembles that of natural bone, which makes it osteoconductive. It is in the form of small granules with favorable handling characteristics.

Generally, TCP has inadequate porosity with a small grain size, and rapid dissolution that makes it a poor bone graft substitute. However, Vitoss (Orthovita, Malvern, PA) is an ultraporous formulation of β-TCP, with a broad range of pore size (1 μm to 1 mm) and interconnected porosity. The pore structure wicks blood, marrow, and cells. The material mimics human cancellous bone and is supplied as morsels or dowels that can be used as graft extenders in spinal surgery (58–60).

Emery et al. studied anterior interbody fusion in the thoracic spine of dogs, using autologous tricortical iliac crest bone graft, HA ceramics, calcium carbonate and a mixture of HA and TCP (45). All fusions were performed using anterior spinal instrumentation. Autologous bone graft was the most effective biomechanically and histologically. The same authors, in another study, found that autologous bone graft was also significantly better than calcium carbonate ceramics when combined with internal fixation (29). Although fixation did not statistically improve the biomechanical properties of ceramic fusion segments, it had a profound beneficial effect on the ability of the ceramic to be revascularized and remodeled.

Toth et al. assessed the effect of porosity of ceramic in a goat anterior cervical spine fusion model (61). Autograft was compared to 30%, 50%, and 70% porosity implants of 50:50 HA:β-TCP. All of the tested ceramic implants performed equal to or better than autograft iliac crest bone at 3 and 6 months. The more porous implants had a higher union rate early on, but also had a higher incidence of graft fracture. Overall fusion rates were 67% for the ceramic implants and 50% for autograft. The relatively low fusion rates in all groups were likely due to excessive neck motion in the goat; however, these low fusion rates put into question the ability of this model to be validly extrapolated to human anterior cervical fusions.

Posterolateral intertransverse lumbar fusion has been studied mainly in sheep (62). Some authors demonstrated better results with autologous bone when compared with different ceramics (43,56), others found similar results in terms of fusion rate when using coral *Porites* (calcium carbonate), a combination of HA and TCP, or resorbable coralline HA (46,63).

Baramki et al. evaluated the efficacy of porous HA granules in achieving posterolateral lumbar fusion in a sheep spine fusion model (56). Bisegmental instrumentation was performed using either no graft material, autologous bone, HA alone, or an HA/autograft composite in a 1:1 ratio. The radiographic images were difficult to interpret because of the radiodense interconnected porous HA granules. According to mechanical stability criteria, the fusion rate for the different groups was as follows: 100% (14/14) for the autologous bone group, 72% (10/14) for the bone/interconnected porous HA group, 50% (7/14) for the pure interconnected porous HA group, and 15% (2/14) for the sham group.

Delecrin et al. showed the influence of the fusion site microenvironment on incorporation of ceramic and new bone formation in a canine posterior lumbar fusion model (64). They evaluated bone growth into a macroporous ceramic implant in an interlaminar fusion site and a posterolateral intertransverse fusion site, using block HA/TCP (60%/40%) composite as a graft material. The percentage of newly formed fusion bone was significantly higher at the interlaminar fusion site compared to the intertransverse site, where decorticated bone in the fusion bed was scarce. For both locations, the highest amount of newly formed bone was observed in the area of close contact between ceramic and decorticated bone, and the lowest was observed in central areas. These results demonstrated the deficiency of osteoinduction properties of the graft, and a consequent reliance on bone growth induction, with the decorticated bleeding bone in the fusion bed serving as a source of stem cells and osteogenic factors.

Zdeblick et al. evaluated the efficacy of porous coralline HA as a substitute for autogenous or allogenic bone graft following multilevel anterior cervical discectomy in a goat cervical spine fusion model (65). They noted significant rates of implant collapse with bone graft substitute at 12 weeks but there was excellent biologic compatibility with good early creeping substitution of the graft by host bone. The concomitant use of an anterior cervical plate with the graft prevented extrusion and led to graft incorporation rates comparable to the autogenous bone group and superior to the allograft bone results. Mechanically, however, while the HA and allograft groups were comparable, they were significantly inferior to the autogenous graft group, leading to the early collapse of the fusion mass.

Clinically, ceramics have been mainly used as bone graft extenders with autologous bone, especially in fusion with long instrumentations (66–68). Ceramics are regulated by the Food and Drug Administration (FDA) as devices. Passati et al. used a combination of HA and TCP with autologous bone in 12 adolescent patients. All patients fused clinically and radiologically (68). Histologic analysis performed on specimens from two of these patients showed *de novo* bone ingrowth into ceramic pores. However, because these cases were instrumented posterior thoracic spines for adolescent deformities, the healing environment might have been less challenging than posterior lumbar intertransverse fusions in adults. Similarly, Ransford et al. compared 170 cases of posterior spinal fusion to treat idiopathic scoliosis using a synthetic porous ceramic (Triosite [Zimmer S.A.S., Cedex, France]) with 171 cases of autogenous bone graft in a prospective randomized study (69). Their results indicated no significant differences between the groups. In a prospective study of 32 patients treated with single-level posterolateral fusion using a biphasic calcium phosphate ceramic implant mixed with locally harvested bone, the overall rates of solid construct were 97% with clinical improvement in all but one case (70). However, there was a high rate of graft resorption, and poor fusion mass was evident on radiographs. The authors believed that the reason for a small fusion mass could be attributed to the tensile forces placed across the graft and the inferior supply of osteogenic factors as compared with massive autologous graft.

In patients undergoing anterior cervical interbody fusion using cages filled with coral HA, Thalgott et al. demonstrated a high fusion rate (71). McConnell et al. compared tricortical iliac crest bone graft to Pro Osteon 200 (coralline HA) in a prospective randomized study, of 29 patients, for anterior cervical interbody fusion with plating (72). There was no significant difference in clinical outcome and fusion rate. However, significant graft settling occurred in 50% of the HA grafts and 11% of the autografts ($p < .009$).

Other potential applications for ceramics is their use as mineral bone cement to augment osteoporotic vertebral compression fractures or pedicle screw fixation (73). The Norion Skeletal Repair System (Norion Core, Cupertino, CA) is a resorbable calcium phosphate cement that is composed of a combination of monocalcium phosphate, calcium carbonate, and β-TCP in a powder form and a solution of sodium phosphate, mixed into an injectable paste. Under physiologic conditions, the material hardens within 10 minutes, through precipitation, into dahllite (carbonated HA) in a nonexothermic reaction. The chemical composition and crystallinity of the material are similar to that of the mineral phase of bone. It also undergoes the same *in vivo* remodeling as normal bone.

Alpha-Bone Substitute Material (ETEX Corp, Cambridge, MA) is a poorly crystalline (mimics mineral phase of bone) calcium phosphate cement with favorable absorption and osseointegration characteristics and easy intraoperative handling characteristics (74–76). It is hydrated with saline to form a workable paste that hardens within 20 minutes at physiologic body temperature and can be prepared to harden to a variety of compressive strengths (5 to 40 milli-Pascals [mPA]). The setting reaction is endothermic, avoiding thermal damage. This substance appears to be suited to incorporation of antibiotics or other proteins, such as bone morphogenetic proteins (BMPs).

Calcium Sulfate

The first internal use of calcium sulfate as gypsum (plaster of Paris), to fill bony defects was reported in 1892 by Dressmann (77). Calcium sulfate is biocompatible and when it dissolutes it produces an acidic microenvironment (pH 5.6) that may help limit bacterial activity. Despite this local dissolution, on a systemic level, the breakdown of the graft material does not lead to any appreciable increase in serum calcium levels (78). Sidqui et al. found that osteoblasts can attach to calcium sulfate (79). In addition, osteoclasts can actively resorb the calcium sulfate, forming lacunae in a manner similar to natural bone. When mixed with water, calcium sulfate initiates an exothermic reaction that leads to recrystallization of the calcium sulfate into the solid form. Recrystallization occurs randomly and thus produces crystals of varying size and shape as well as multiple defects within the structure. This variability in the crystalline structure causes significant variability in solubility, mechanical properties, and porosity. In addition, it may resorb too rapidly, leading to fibrous ingrowth instead of bony substitution.

Medical grade calcium sulfate is in the form of regularly shaped crystals of similar size and shape. It possesses a slower, more predictable solubility and resorption. Medical grade calcium sulfate has been shown to possess an osteoconductivity equal to that of autogenous iliac crest marrow/bone with a rate of absorption that is equal to the rate at which new bone is formed (80–82). OsteoSet (Wright Medical Technology, Arlington, TN) is available in 3- and 4.8-mm pellets that dissolve *in vivo* within 30 to 60 days. The pellets are packaged in vials and are sterilized by gamma irradiation. Cunningham et al. showed that OsteoSet was comparable to autograft in a sheep posterolateral spinal fusion mode (83). OsteoSet is also available in a powdered form, thus maximizing the surgical options for adding antibiotics and filling defects with custom-molded beads or shapes. The chief advantage is that it can be used in the presence of infection (84–86).

Hadjipavlou et al. compared the effectiveness of calcium sulfate to other graft materials (autogenous iliac crest, frozen allogeneic bone, Pro Osteon 500 coralline graft, osteoinductive demineralized sheep bone preparation, and admixtures of autogenous iliac crest bone with calcium sulfate and coralline graft) in achieving lumbar interbody fusion in mature sheep (87). The substrates were placed into titanium mesh cages, which were implanted intervertebrally and recovered after 4 months. The histomorphometry suggested that the different graft types were equally effective at producing bone and were not different from the outcome of the empty control cages. Biomechanically, however, the behavior of the control fusion masses (with no graft material) was inferior to that of the fusion masses with other graft materials. The demineralized sheep bone preparations proved the least effective of the different substrates in achieving a solid interbody fusion. In terms of torsional strain, tensile failure, and volume of bone formed within the titanium cages, the effects of calcium sulfate and autogenous bone were indistinguishable from each other and similarly, that of calcium sulfate was indistinguishable from Pro Osteon and 1:1 admixtures of those substrates with autogenous bone. Elkins and Jones also noted no difference in the degree of bone healing between autogenous cancellous bone, calcium sulfate, and a composite of calcium sulfate and autogenous cancellous bone (88).

Calcium sulfate can also be used as a carrier for the local delivery of antibiotics. The elution of calcium sulfate is 17% at 24 hours; at 3 weeks, trace amounts are still detected. This profile compares favorably to polymethylmethacrylate, which releases 7% of its load by 24 hours, with trace amounts detected at 14 days (89).

Allergy to calcium sulfate, although rare and related to minor additives, should be considered when assessing the risk/benefit of using it as bone graft substitute. In a series of 15 implantations of calcium sulfate pellets (OsteoSet) used for bone reconstruction after resection of bone tumors, three cases of inflammatory reactions were noted (90). However, other investigators have noted that calcium sulfate is innocuous in terms of producing a local soft tissue chemical or pyogenic inflammatory reaction (80,81,88,91).

Collagen

Type I collagen, which is the most abundant protein in the extracellular matrix of bone, has a structure that is conductive for mineral deposition, vascular ingrowth, and growth-factor binding, and provides both a favorable physical and chemical milieu for bone regeneration (92). It binds the noncollagenous matrix proteins, which initiate and control mineralization. By itself, collagen functions poorly as a graft material, but when combined with bone morphogenetic proteins, osteoprogenitor precursors, or HA, it may enhance the incorporation of the grafts (57). Although it has potential immunogenicity, no significant adverse reactions have been shown with bovine collagen implanted in skeletal sites (93).

Collagraft (Zimmer, Warsaw, IN) is a composite of suspended fibrillar collagen (from bovine dermis) and a porous calcium phosphate ceramic (65% HA and 35%

TCP), in a ratio of 1:1 (93–96). It can be used as a paste or in strips and does not provide any structural support by itself. It is usually mixed with autologous bone as a bone graft extender or with autologous bone marrow aspirate. Collagen serves as a carrier for the ceramic and the autogenous marrow. Appositional new bone is formed directly on the calcium phosphate surfaces. The results of using this composite in spinal fusion in animal studies are mixed. The results from a study by Walsh et al., evaluating the use of the composite in a posterolateral intertransverse lumbar fusion in a sheep model, support the use of Collagraft (95). Zerwekh et al. showed that the use of Collagraft and autogenous bone mixture (3:1) for lumbar interbody fusion in a canine model provides a suitable osteoconductive alternative to the use of autogenous bone and results in the formation of a mechanically competent fusion mass not significantly different form that obtained with autogenous bone alone (97). On the other hand, Muschler et al. found collagraft to be inferior in union score when compared to autograft in a posterior segmental canine spinal fusion model (96). However, the material was applied in onlay fashion, which inhibits its incorporation.

Healos (Orquest, Mountain View, CA) is a mineralized collagen sponge, launched in Europe for clinical use in spine surgery in 2000. Each microscopic type I collagen fiber is coated with HA. By itself it is osteoconductive, but it can be mixed with bone marrow aspirate to provide osteogenic and osteoinductive potential. In a study of posterolateral intertransverse lumbar spine fusion in a New Zealand white rabbit model, Tay et al. concluded that Healos could be used in combination with an osteoinductive or osteogenic agent to ensure reliable fusion rates (98).

Nonbiologic Osteoconductive Materials

Degradable polymers, bioactive glasses, and various metals have been studied. The advantages of nonbiologic materials include the ability to control all aspects of the matrix, avoidance of immunologic reaction, and excellent biocompatibility. They provide structural support and can be used as spacers.

Polylactic and polyglycolic acid polymers slowly degrade by hydrolysis. Although well tolerated, these polymers may incite an inflammatory response in the surrounding tissues, especially with bulk implants. The materials can be assembled in various forms and can be integrated with growth factors or other compounds to create multiphase delivery systems. Porous foams of these polymers can be produced with optimum pore sizes for bone ingrowth. However, these materials by themselves have little osteoconductive potential, and bone ingrowth into them is not optimal (99). They are mainly used as growth factor delivery vehicles. Degradation of the polymer releases the factor locally.

Immix (Osteobiologics Inc., San Antonio, TX) is a synthetic bone graft scaffold, tissue engineered from amorphous D, L-polylactide–co-glycolide, and is designed to resorb within 12 to 20 weeks following implantation. It has been developed as granular particles, resembling allograft bone chips. It provides a porous architecture for the ingrowth of new bone and then fully degrades.

OSTEOINDUCTIVE MATERIALS

Demineralized bone matrix, which was first shown by Marshal Urist to induce ingrowth of connective tissue cells and differentiation of cartilage and bone, has been a great breakthrough in the advancement of biologic bone graft substitute technology (100,101). Advances in protein isolation technology yielded evidence of a series of osteoinductive glycoproteins, including BMP, transforming growth factor-β (TGF-β), platelet-derived growth factor (PDGF), epidermal growth factor (EGF), and others. Extracts of bone containing these growth factors produce new bone in ectopic sites in animal trials (102,103). The interaction of these factors with cytokines involves the regulation of chemotaxis and proliferation and differentiation of osteoprogenitor cells culminating in new bone formation. Of all these osteoinductive proteins, the most critical to bone formation are the BMPs, which have been shown to stimulate osteoblastic differentiation of pluripotent stem cells *in vitro* and are the only bioactive molecules capable of inducing ectopic bone production *in vivo* (104).

Demineralized Bone Matrix

Demineralized bone matrix (DBM) is an osteoconductive scaffold that is produced by acid extraction of banked allograft bone. It provides no structural support and contains noncollagenous proteins, osteoinductive growth factors, and type I collagen (105). DBM is a mixture of BMPs and immunogenic, noninductive proteins. It has greater osteoinductive potential than allograft due to enhanced bioavailability of growth factors secondary to the demineralization (106,107).

A great deal of variability in the osteoinductive potential of DBM products depends on a number of factors, such as processing solution, demineralization time, temperature extremes, DBM particle size, and method of terminal sterilization (108,109). Since the method of sterilization can reduce the activity of DBM, many suppliers prefer sterile procurement and processing. The variability in the DBM osteoinductive potential may reflect differences in the BMP content (110), although the absolute concentration of BMP within a particular DBM preparation does not necessarily correlate with its clinical efficacy. Another factor that may influence the efficacy of DBM is age. DBM acquired from young donors has been shown to have greater osteoinductive properties than those taken from older donors (111).

DBMs are usually suspended within a distinct carrier to modify their consistency and facilitate their use. A number of DBMs are associated with a glycerol carrier, and large amounts of these preparations have proven to be toxic when administered to athymic rats, eventually leading to death in a dose-dependent manner (112,113). However, there have been no reported cases of glycerol toxicity related to the implantation of these DBM products after years of use in humans. DBMs are currently available in a variety of configurations, and it appears that different configurations of the same DBM may perform differently, which can be the result of their different osteoconductive properties. A putty and flexible sheet form of a particular DBM was found to enhance spinal fusion to a greater extent than the gel form of the same DBM, most likely because these fiber-based preparations were thought to possess increased osteoconductivity compared to the particle form (114).

Because of the lack of an osteogenic potential of DBMs, they are most effective when implanted in environments that offer sufficient vascularity and an adequate supply of osteoprogenitor cells. DBMs have been found to promote successful arthrodesis of the spine when used alone or in conjunction with autograft, bone marrow, or ceramics (115–121). In humans, DBMs are mainly indicated as bone graft extenders when used in spinal fusion and are not thought to be sufficient for complete substitution for autogenous bone graft in the more challenging healing environments.

Several DBMs are now available commercially. Grafton (Osteotech, Inc., Eatontown, NJ) consists of DBM combined with a glycerol carrier and is available in the form of gel, malleable putty, or flexible sheets. Opteform (Medtronic Sofamor Danek, Memphis, TN), a moldable bone paste, contains cortical bone chips. Osteofil (Medtronic Sofamor Danek) is an injectable bone paste that combines DBM with thermoplastic, collagen-based hydrogel carrier matrix. This nonwater- soluble composite is easily extruded through a syringe when warmed to 46° to 50° but becomes firm when cooled to body temperature. Dynagraft (Regeneration Sciences, Inc., Irvine, CA) combines DBM with a pleuronic reverse-phase copolymer carrier that becomes firmer as it warms to body temperature. Both Dynagraft and Osteofil were reported to contain greater amounts of DBM per unit volume than the glycerol-containing composites (106).

Bone Morphogenetic Proteins

The BMPs are soluble, low-molecular-weight noncollagenous glycoproteins that belong to an expanding TGF-β superfamily of growth and differentiation factors. Unlike DBM, pure BMPs are nonimmunogenic and non-species-specific. BMPs are multifunctional; they regulate growth, differentiation, chemotaxis, and apoptosis, and play a pivotal role in the morphogenesis of a variety of tissues and organs (122). Different BMPs have different functions including extracellular and skeletal organogenesis and bone regeneration. Osteogenic BMPs act locally by binding to specific receptors present on the surface of mesenchymal stem cells. These receptors then transduce the signal through a group of proteins called Smads, which in turn activate particular genes. BMPs *in vivo* cause mesenchymal cells to differentiate into chondrocytes, which create a cartilage matrix that mineralizes and then is replaced by bone (endochondral ossification) which ultimately remodels. In higher concentrations, BMPs can result in direct (intramembranous) ossification. The relative amounts of endochondral and intramembranous ossification induced appear to be associated with the concentration of BMP implanted, the site of implantation, and the nature of the carrier and matrix material (123). The bone formed, as a result of the BMP induction, appears to be physiologically normal in all the species tested. The bone induction is observed only locally at the site of BMP and matrix implantation and is limited temporally only to the time when the BMP is present. The activity of BMPs is tightly controlled at many levels. Outside the cell, soluble inhibitory proteins such as nogin, chordin, and follistatin can bind certain of the BMPs and inhibit their binding to cell surface receptors. Inside the cell, the activity of BMPs is controlled through the combination of signal-transducing and inhibitory Smad proteins.

Human BMP is a rare and very expensive product. It comprises only 0.1% by weight of all bone protein, and is most abundant in diaphyseal cortical bone. It exists in the extracellular matrix, and is not accessible until the bone matrix has been demineralized (101,124). Mixtures of BMPs are available as purified bone extracts for clinical studies. Although these preparations may have the advantage of containing many potent osteogenic factors, including BMP heterodimers, they have lower BMP concentrations, contain other biologically inactive or inhibitory proteins, and may elicit a host immune response. A highly purified extract from a mixture of bovine bone morphogenetic proteins (bovine BMP extract or bBMPx) has demonstrated promising preclinical efficacy results (125). Using molecular cloning technology, it has been possible to produce recombinant human BMP (rhBMP) as a singular molecular species in unlimited quantities and without immunogenetic properties (126,127). In summary, this process involves inserting the human BMP DNA coding sequence (gene) for each protein into an expression vector. This vector is transfected into a mammalian cell host in order to produce a stable cell line that expresses that particular BMP. The rhBMPs extensively studied are rhBMP-2 (128) and rhBMP-7 (osteogenic protein-1, or OP-1) (129), which have similar osteoinductive activities *in vivo*.

Recombinant human BMPs are soluble factors and tend to diffuse away from the fusion site when used alone. Therefore, in larger animal models and human clinical trials, these factors are combined with a carrier matrix that serves to contain the BMPs and release them gradually. These carriers may also act as osteoconductive scaffolds (130). The ideal carrier system will retain and release the BMP in a controlled fashion, be biocompatible, not interfere with normal bony healing, be porous to promote osteoconductivity, be biomechanically suited for the site of implantation, be easy to apply, and be easy to manufacture. Once these BMPs are released, appropriately responding osteogenic cells must be present in the area for any significant bone formation to occur. In animal models, such as rabbit, dog, sheep, goat, and nonhuman primate, researchers have performed posterolateral intertransverse spinal arthrodesis or interbody arthrodesis with cages containing rhBMP-loaded carriers (collagen sponges, autogenous bone graft, DBM, ceramics, degradable polymers) (131–138). Uniformly, these studies have reported a dose-dependent increase in bone formation, consolidation, and remodeling with the rhBMP-loaded scaffolds compared to unloaded controls. Multiple animal studies have shown that rhBMP-mediated fusions rates were equivalent or superior to those obtained with autogenous bone graft and may generate fusion masses that are biomechanically stronger and stiffer (43,131, 138–141). The use of BMPs has been shown to obviate the need for decortication of the posterior elements that is usually required to provide endogenous osteoinductive growth factors that are necessary for obtaining posterolateral fusion (142). The osteoinductive activity of BMPs may even compensate for the inhibitory effects of nicotine and nonsteroidal antiinflammatory medications on spinal fusions (143–145).

Boden et al. conducted a multicenter trial to test the efficacy of rhBMP-2–mediated spinal arthrodesis (146). Fourteen patients were randomly treated with tapered titanium fusion cages containing either rhBMP-2 (1.5 mg/mL) soaked bovine collagen sponges or morselized autogenous iliac crest bone graft. The authors showed that this concentration of rhBMP-2 consistently resulted in spinal fusion. All of the 11 patients who received rhBMP-2 had solid fusions by 6 months compared with 2 out of 3 control patients. The Oswestry Disability Questionnaire scores of the rhBMP-2 group improved sooner (after 3 months) than those of the autograft group, with both groups demonstrating similar improvement at 6 months. There were no adverse events related to the rhBMP-2 treatment. The patients who received rhBMP-2 collagen sponges had shorter operative times, less blood loss, and shorter hospital stays.

Before embarking on the use of BMPs in humans on a big scale, certain issues have to be addressed. These issues include the cost-effectiveness, the optimal carrier systems, appropriate dose for the different spinal applications, and safety. It is important to realize that certain carrier materials that prove successful in one location may not be efficacious in another. Both rhBMP-2 and OP-1 appear to be safe, provided they are used appropriately, placed accurately, not allowed to come into contact with decompressed areas, and remain contained in the region of fusion (147). In some patients, transient antibody responses to the BMPs or carrier materials have been observed without clinical untoward effects. New bone formation may occur if rhBMP-2 or OP-1 comes in contact with laminectomy sites or decompressed neuroforamina, and may lead to restenosis. In a canine lumbar spine fusion model, the placement of OP-1 over a dural tear stimulated new bone formation in the subarachnoid space, resulting in mild spinal stenosis at the site of dural decompression (148). Adequate hemostasis should be performed to avoid the absorption of BMP by a hematoma at the decompression site. It is not advisable to leave collagen-based hemostatic agents in contact with the BMP implant where decompression has been performed, because BMP may elute from its collagen carrier into the collagenous hemostatic agent and thus enter the region of decompression. Leakage of rhBMP-2 or OP-1 outside the fusion area may lead to adjacent-level fusion. Appropriate carriers should adequately retain the BMP within the fusion area. Irrigation of the surgical site should not be performed after implantation of the BMP. Suction drains should not be placed directly in contact with BMP implants.

In a study by Ackerman et al., an economic analysis was performed comparing the total direct medical costs of BMP with autogenous iliac crest bone graft in single-level anterior lumbar fusion (149). Their preliminary results suggest that from a payer perspective, the upfront price of BMP is likely to be entirely offset by reductions in the use of other medical resources. That is, BMP appears to be cost neutral. The reason for these cost offsets was largely due to the prevention of pain and complications associated with iliac crest bone graft and reduction of costs associated with fusion failures. When considering the costs associated with an unsuccessful fusion as well as the cost offsets associated with obviating the need for autogenous iliac crest bone graft (e.g., iliac crest backfill, autograft extenders, and autograft harvesters), elimination, the associated donor site pain, and morbidity (e.g., infection, hematoma, neuroma, and vascular injury), a 9.3% increase in fusion success rate was required to achieve cost neutrality at a BMP price of $4,000. These analyses did not consider the health-related quality-of-life impact of eliminating donor site pain and complications. Since, at the present time, there are no large prospective randomized trials comparing the use of BMP to autologous bone graft, it is difficult to conclude that either graft material is more cost-effective.

Autologous Platelet Concentrate

Platelet α-granules contain several locally active factors, including PDGF, TGF-β, insulin-like growth factor, and epidermal growth factor, as well as important osteogenic substances like osteocalcin, all of which play specific roles in stimulating bone formation by promoting mesenchymal stem cell chemotaxis, proliferation, and other cellular processes (150,151). The clinical use of PDGFs to enhance bone healing involves extracting autologous growth factors (AGFs) from the patient's blood and mixing the AGF concentrate with a bone graft or a bone graft substitute. The AGF gel is obtained from the platelet-rich plasma (buffy coat) of the blood collected in the cell saver during surgery through centrifugation. The buffy coat is ultraconcentrated to a density of 1 million platelets/μL. This platelet-rich plasma, which is concentrated in a fibrinogen matrix, is combined with thrombin to form a fibrin clot (AGF gel). Approximately 20 mL of AGF is derived from 500 mL of blood in 10 minutes. The AGF gel also acts as a constraining gel, thus minimizing bone graft migration. In a retrospective study, 39 patients undergoing anterior or posterior fusion of the lumbar spine were treated with AGF concentrate, autogenous bone graft, and coralline HA in conjunction with stable internal fixation (152). After an average follow-up of 13 months, no pseudoarthroses were noted clinically or radiographically. Like DBMs, platelet gels are classified as minimally manipulated tissues and are therefore not closely regulated or subjected to rigorous testing.

BONE MARROW ASPIRATE

Autologous bone marrow contains both osteoprogenitor cells as well as growth factors that may enhance bone formation. Compared to autogenous bone graft harvesting, bone marrow aspiration is a much less aggressive technique with almost no donor site morbidity. Bone marrow is usually aspirated from the iliac crest but can be aspirated from any cancellous bone rich in bone marrow including vertebral bodies (through pedicles, before pedicle-screw placement). Bone marrow aspirates are usually combined to a carrier before application to the arthrodesis site in order to avoid its diffusion away from the area in need of repair.

Because the extent of osseous regeneration is dependent on the number of osteoprogenitor cells able to produce new bone, unfractionated bone marrow exhibits only moderate osteogenic potential, because it possesses only a limited quantity of mesenchymal stem cells. The bone marrow of healthy adults contains only one mesenchymal stem cell for every 50,000 nucleated cells, and this population is even further diminished in older patients and in those with metabolic diseases such as osteoporosis (153,154). Moreover, as bone marrow is aspirated from the iliac crest, it undergoes dilution with peripheral blood. Consequently, it has been recommended that no more than 2 mL of bone marrow should be aspirated from any single site (153). Centrifugation of the aspirated bone marrow separates the marrow cells from plasma and preserves the osteogenic potential of the cells, decreasing the volume of material injected (155). The proliferation and rate of differentiation of stem cells can be enhanced by the addition of growth factors (156) or by combining them with collagen (94)

Using special purification and subcultivation techniques, mesenchymal stem cells may be separated from other bone marrow elements and expanded *in vitro* without any loss in their multilineage potential (157). When supplied with the appropriate regulatory molecules in cell culture, these mesenchymal stem cells have the capacity to develop into mature osteoblasts (157,158). The amplification of osteoprogenitor cells that occurs after culture expansion of mesenchymal stem cells results in greater bone formation than with the unfractionated bone marrow (153,154). Mesenchymal stem cell therapy may be particularly valuable in older patients and those patients with reduced osteoprogenitor cell stores. This approach, however, carries the risk of *in vitro* contamination.

VivescOs (IsoTis, Bilthoven, The Netherlands) is a tissue-engineered bone developed for application in revision surgery, spinal fusion, and dental implants. The bone marrow cells are harvested from the patient and then expanded in tissue culture. The cells on the scaffold are then made into the desired shape and reimplanted into the patient. This process takes about 4 weeks (57).

GENE THERAPY

Several studies have shown that gene therapy is a safe and effective way of effecting new bone formation in animals (159,160). Gene therapy entails the transfer of genetic information to cells. When the gene (DNA encoding the protein) is transferred to a target cell, the cell synthesizes the protein encoded by the gene. Unlike gene therapy used for the treatment of genetic diseases, gene therapy used for bone induction is short-term, regional therapy.

The *in vivo* technique involves introduction of the gene directly to a specific anatomic site. This process is relatively simple and convenient, but limited by inefficient gene delivery, nonspecific targeting of cells, and the possibility of a vigorous host inflammatory response. In one study using the *in vivo* technique, the gene encoding for BMP-2 carried on an adenovirus vector was percutaneously injected in the paraspinal muscles of rats (160). Expression of BMP-2 by transfected muscle cells was shown to stimulate significant new bone formation.

The *ex vivo* technique involves harvesting cells from the patient, expanding the cells in tissue culture, and

genetically manipulating these cells which are subsequently reimplanted. Although this technique is more complex and expensive than the *in vivo* technique, it is considered to be safer after thorough screening of the genetically altered cells before their reimplantation. *Ex vivo* approaches are generally associated with high transduction rates and allow for preferential selection of certain target cells.

The vector (vehicle) for gene delivery can be viral (retrovirus, adenovirus, adeno-associated viruses) or nonviral. The gene can be selectively transferred to a targeted cell (osteoblast, fibroblast) at the bone induction site. Nonviral vectors are easier to produce, are more stable, and are less antigenic and theoretically safer than viral vectors. Nonviral vectors include liposomes, which are DNA suspended in lipid vesicles that are able to bind to cell membranes, and gene-activated matrices, which are osteoconductive scaffolds loaded with genetic material. Viral vectors possess superior transduction efficiencies and may be favored over nonviral vectors.

Gene therapy may provide a more potent osteoinductive signal than recombinant growth factors, because these methods result in the sustained local release of osteogenic proteins at levels that are more physiologic than the administration of a single large dose.

Using *ex vivo* gene therapy, Wang et al. implanted rat bone marrow cells, transduced with the BMP-2 gene, combined with a guanidine-extracted DBM in the posterolateral spine of rats (161). The BMP-2–producing cells resulted in solid fusion masses comparable to those produced from the use of recombinant BMP-2 protein. Boden et al. used a posterior spinal fusion model in athymic rats and grafted demineralized bone matrix with bone marrow cells (162). In each rat, one site received marrow cells transfected with the gene encoding the LIM mineralization protein-1 (LMP-1), a signaling intracellular protein (not a secreted factor) that acts by stimulating the synthesis and secretion of other osteoinductive factors and thus initiating bone formation *in vitro* and *in vivo*. At the other site for a control, the marrow cells were transfected with the reverse copy of the complimentary DNA (cDNA) that did not express any protein. Consistent fusions were obtained in all of the animals receiving bone marrow cells containing the LMP-1 DNA sequence, whereas no bone formation was observed in those implanted with cells carrying the inactive copy of the gene.

SUMMARY AND FUTURE DIRECTIONS

The mere formation of bone does not indicate fusion. For spinal fusion to occur, bone has to be formed and has to bridge vertebrae with incorporation of the graft material into the recipient site. Thus, there has to be an optimal local and systemic milieu for spinal fusion to occur; and that includes decortication of bone, optimal stability, optimal blood supply, normal bone physiology, and absence of systemic diseases and toxic materials that may suppress osteogenesis.

The newer forms of calcium sulfate and calcium phosphate materials possess a resorption profile that closely matches the rate at which new bone is deposited. They facilitate cellular adhesion, support vascular ingrowth, and promote new bone formation. They are purely osteoconductive materials and can be used as bone graft extenders or carriers for osteoinductive agents.

The advantages of nonbiologic materials such as degradable polymers, bioactive glasses, and various metals include the ability to control all aspects of the matrix, avoidance of immunologic reaction, and excellent biocompatibility. They provide structural support and can be used as spacers. However, these materials by themselves have little osteoconductive potential, and bone ingrowth into them is not optimal. They are mainly used as growth factor delivery vehicles.

Because of the lack of reliable noninvasive techniques to assess the success or failure of an arthrodesis, several investigators have found that an animal model would be a practical solution for studying the efficacy of the different bone graft substitutes. However, one should be cautious when interpreting the results of animal studies. The efficacy of osteoinductive agents largely depends on the amount of protein implanted. The threshold concentration of an osteoinductive agent, below which no significant bone is induced, may be different for different osteoinductive factors, different carrier matrices, different anatomic locations, and even different animal species. In addition, this threshold may need to be raised in the face of systemic healing challenges such as smoking, corticosteroids, chemotherapeutic agents, and diabetes mellitus.

The BMPs are differentiation factors, causing mesenchymal cells to differentiate into bone- and cartilage-forming cells. On the other hand, factors such as platelet-derived growth factor and TGF-β are growth factors. These growth factors cause cells to multiply and may cause cells to augment production of cellular products such as extracellular matrix proteins.

Platelets contain several locally active factors, which play specific roles in stimulating bone formation by promoting mesenchymal stem cell chemotaxis, proliferation, and other cellular processes. Several clinical studies to evaluate the use of PDGFs in enhancing spinal fusion are underway. It is still too early to identify the optimal method of obtaining PDGFs and applying the technology in spinal fusions.

Autologous bone marrow contains both osteoprogenitor cells as well as growth factors that may enhance bone formation. The procedure of obtaining bone marrow involves minimal morbidity. Bone marrow aspirates are usually combined to a carrier before application to the arthrodesis site in order to avoid its diffusion away from the area in need for repair.

Gene therapy may provide a more potent osteoinductive signal than recombinant growth factors, because of the sustained local release of osteogenic proteins obtained with gene therapy at levels that are more physiologic than the administration of a single large dose, as is the case with BMPs.

Ceramics, degradable polymers, bioactive glasses and metals, rhBMPs, PDGFs, autologous bone marrow aspirate, and *ex vivo* gene therapy can be used when there is concern about immune reactions and transferred infections, as in immunocompromised patients.

When considering the choice of bone graft substitute in order to attain bone formation, one has to think of the necessary triad for bone formation: osteogenesis, osteoinduction, and osteoconduction. Depending on the anatomic location and the biomechanical loading at the site of arthrodesis, one or more of the three elements has to be supplied. For an anterior cervical interbody fusion, an osteoconductive structural block may suffice in achieving fusion. The compressive loads, along with the contact to a bleeding end plate (provides bone marrow loaded with osteogenic and osteoinductive elements), with the intercession of the vertebral periosteum and surrounding muscle pericytes (osteoprogenitor cells), can provide all three necessary components for bone formation. On the other hand, posterolateral lumbar fusion usually requires at least an osteoconductive nonstructural bone graft substitute in addition to a strong osteoinductive agent provided there is good bridging to viable decorticated bone (primary source of blood supply, bone marrow, and osteoprogenitor cells to the fusion mass) (163).

Although only 10% of bone graft procedures worldwide have relied on synthetic materials (164), including ceramic and polymers, synthetic composite bone substitutes that combine an osteoconductive matrix with osteoinductive growth factors and osteogenic cells, rhBMPs, and gene therapy may ultimately surpass the use of bone grafts. Combined strategies of biologic and mechanical manipulation of spinal arthrodesis should be continuously prudently evaluated with sound scientific methods and well-designed, well-controlled, and rational clinical studies.

REFERENCES

1. Banwart JC, Asher MA, Hassanein RS. Iliac crest bone graft harvest donor site morbidity. A statistical evaluation. Spine 1995;20:1055–1060.
2. Betz RR. Limitations of autograft and allograft: new synthetic solutions. Orthopedics 2002;25[Suppl]:561–570.
3. Robertson PA, Wray AC. Natural history of posterior iliac crest bone graft donation for spinal surgery: a prospective analysis of morbidity. Spine 2001;26:1473–1476.
4. Summers BN, Eisenstein SM. Donor site pain from the ilium. A complication of lumbar spine fusion. J Bone Joint Surg 1989;71B:677–680.
5. Younger EM, Chapman MW. Morbidity of bone graft donor sites. J Orthop Trauma 1989;3:192–195.
6. Boyce T, Edwards J, Scarborough N. Allograft bone. The influence of

processing on safety and performance. Orthop Clin North Am 1999; 30:571–581.

7. Herron L, Newman M. The failure of ethylene oxide gas sterilized freeze-dried bone graft for thoracic and lumbar spine fusion. Spine 1989;14:496–500.

8. Pelker R, Friedlaender G. Biomechanical aspects of bone autografts and allografts. Orthop Clin North Am 1987;18:235–239.

9. Tomford WW. Transmission of disease through transplantation of musculoskeletal allografts. J Bone Joint Surg 1995;77A:1742–1754.

10. Conrad EU, Gretch DR, Obermeyer KR, et al. Transmission of the hepatitis-C virus by tissue transplantation. J Bone Joint Surg 1995; 77A:214–224.

11. Simonds RJ, Holmberg SD, Hurwitz RL, et al. Transmission of human immunodeficiency virus type 1 from a seronegative organ and tissue donor. N Engl J Med 1992;326:726–732.

12. Buck B, Malinin T, Brown M. Bone transplantation and human immunodeficiency virus. Clin Orthop 1989;240:129–136.

13. Centers for Disease Control. Transmission of HIV through bone transplantation: case report and public health recommendations. JAMA 1988;260:2487–2488.

14. Friedlaender GE. Bone allografts: the biological consequences of immunological events. J Bone Joint Surg 1991;73A:1119–1122.

15. Strong DM, Friedlaender GE, Tomford WW, et al. Immunologic responses in human recipients of osseous and osteochondral allografts. Clin Orthop 1996;326:107–114.

16. Jorgenson S, Lowe T, France J, et al. A prospective analysis of autograft versus allograft in posterolateral lumbar fusion in the same patient. Spine 1994;19:2048–2053.

17. Zdeblick T, Ducker T. The use of freeze-dried bone for anterior cervical fusions. Spine 1991;16:726–732.

18. Steinmann J, Herkowitz H. Pseudoarthrosis of the spine. Clin Orthop 1992;284:80–90.

19. Cleveland M, Bosworth D, Thomson F. Pseudoarthrosis in the lumbosacral spine. J Bone Joint Surg 1948;30A:302–311.

20. Stauffer R, Coventry M. Posterolateral lumbar spine fusion. J Bone Joint Surg 1972;54A:1195–1204.

21. DePalma AF, Rothman RH. The nature of pseudoarthrosis. Clin Orthop 1968;59:113–118.

22. West III JL, Bradford DS, Oglivie JW. Results of spinal arthrodesis with pedicle screw plate fixation. J Bone Joint Surg 1996;73A: 1179–1184.

23. Bridwell KH, Sedgewick TA, O'Brien MF, et al. The role of fusion and instrumentation in the treatment of degenerative spondylolisthesis with spinal stenosis. J Spinal Disord 1993;6:461–472.

24. McGuire RA, Amundson GM. The use of primary internal fixation in spondylolisthesis. Spine 1993;18:1662–1672.

25. Zdeblick TA. A prospective, randomized study of lumbar fusion: preliminary results. Spine 1993;18:983–991.

26. Lane JM, Sandhu HS. Current approaches to experimental bone grafting. Orthop Clin North Am 1987.;18:213–225.

27. Prolo DJ, Rodrigo JJ. Contemporary bone graft physiology and surgery. Clin Orthop 1985;200:322–342.

28. Posner AS. The mineral of bone. Clin Orthop 1985;200:87–99.

29. Fuller D, Stevenson S, Emery S. The effects of internal fixation on calcium carbonate. Ceramic anterior spinal fusion in dogs. Spine 1996;21:2131–2136.

30. Roufosse AH, Aue WP, Roberts JE, et al. Investigation of the mineral phases of bone by solid-state phosphorus-31 magic angle sample spinning nuclear magnetic resonance. Biochemistry 1984;23:6115–6120.

31. Ohgushi H, Goldberg VM, Caplan AI. Heterotopic osteogenesis in porous ceramics induced by marrow cells. J Orthop Res 1989;7:5 68–578.

32. Boden S, Schimandle J. Biologic enhancement of spinal fusion. Spine 1995;20:113S–123S.

33. Jarcho M. Calcium phosphate ceramics as hard tissue prosthetics. Clin Orthop 1981;157:259–278.

34. Flatley TJ, Lynch KL, Benson M. Tissue response to implants of calcium phosphate ceramic in the rabbit spine. Clin Orthop 1983; 179:246–252.

35. Osborn JF, Newesely H. The material science of calcium phosphate ceramics. Biomaterials 1980;1:108–111.

36. Spivak JM, Hasharoni A. Use of hydroxyapatite in spine surgery. Eur Spine J 2001;10[Suppl]:197–204.

37. Flattley T, Lynch K, Benson M. Tissue response to implants of cal-

cium phosphate ceramic in the rabbit spine. Clin Orthop 1983;179: 246–252.

38. Hulbert SF, Young FA, Mathews RS, et al. Potential of ceramic materials as permanently implantable skeletal prostheses. J Biomed Mater Res 1970;4:433–456.

39. White E, Shors EC. Biomaterial aspects of Interpore 200 porous hydroxyapatite. Dent Clin North Am 1986;30:49–67.

40. Holmes RE, Bucholz RW, Mooney V. Porous hydroxyapatite as a bone graft substitute in diaphyseal defects: a histometric study. J Orthop Res 1987;5:114–121.

41. Hoogendoorn HA, Renoooij W, Akkermans LMA, et al. Long-term study of large ceramic implants (porous hydroxyapatite) in dog femora. Clin Orthop 1984;187:281–288.

42. Ferraro J. Experimental evaluation of ceramic calcium phosphate as a substitute for bone grafts. Plast Reconstr Surg 1979;63:634–640.

43. Boden S, Martin G, Morone M, et al. Posterolateral lumbar intertransverse process spine arthrodesis with recombinant human bone morphogenetic protein-2/hydroxyapatite-tricalcium phosphate after laminectomy in the nonhuman primate. Spine 1999;24:1179–1185.

44. Daculsi G, LeGeros R, Nery E, et al. Transformation of biphasic calcium phosphate ceramics in vivo: ultrastructural and physico-chemical characterization. J Biomed Mater Res 1989;23:883–894.

45. Emery S, Fuller D, Stevenson S. Ceramic anterior spinal fusion. Biologic and biomechanical comparison in a canine model. Spine 1996; 21:2713–2719.

46. Guigui P, Plais P, Flautre B. Experimental model of posterolateral spinal arthrodesis in sheep. 2. Application of the model: evaluation of vertebral fusion obtained with coral (Porites) or with a biphasic ceramic (Triosite). Spine 1994;19:2798–2803.

47. Zerwekh J, Kourosh S, Scheinberg R. Fibrillar collagen-biphasic calcium phosphate composite as a bone graft substitute for spinal fusion. J Orthop Res 1992;10:562–572.

48. Chiroff RT, White EW, Weber KN, et al. Tissue ingrowth of replamineform implants. J Biomed Mater Res 1975;9:29–45.

49. White E, Shors EC. Biomaterial aspects of Interpore-200 porous hydroxyapatite. Dent Clin North Am 1986;30:49–67.

50. Shors EC. Coralline bone graft substitutes. Orthop Clin North Am 1999;30:599–613.

51. Bucholz R, Carlton A, Holmes R. Hydroxyapatite and tricalcium phosphate bone graft substitutes. Orthop Clin North Am 1987;18: 323–334.

52. Guillemin G, Meunier A, Dallant P. Comparison of coral resorption and bone apposition with two natural corals of different porosities. J Biomed Mater Res 1989;23:765–779.

53. Holmes R. Bone regeneration within a coralline hydroxyapatite implant. Plast Reconstr Surg 1979;63:626–633.

54. Holmes R, Bucholz R, Mooney V. Porous hydroxyapatite as a bone graft substitute in metaphyseal defects. J Bone Joint Surg 1986;68A: 904–911.

55. Damien C, Christel P, Benedict J, et al. A composite of natural coral, collagen, bone protein, and basic fibroblast growth factor tested in a rat subcutaneous model. Ann Chir Gynecol 1993;82:117–128.

56. Baramki H, Steffen T, Lander P, et al. The efficacy of interconnected porous hydroxyapatite in achieving posterior lumbar fusion in sheep. Spine 2000;25:1053–1060.

57. Parikh SN. Bone graft substitutes in modern orthopaedics. Orthopedics 2002;25:1301–1309.

58. Meadows GR. Adjunctive use of ultraporous beta-tricalcium phosphate bone void filler in spinal arthrodesis. Orthopedics 2002;25 [Suppl]:579–584.

59. Linovitz RJ, Peppers TA. Use of an advanced formulation of beta-tricalcium phosphate as a bone extender in interbody lumbar fusion. Orthopedics 2002;25[Suppl]:485–589.

60. Gunzburg R, Szpalski M. Use of a novel beta-tricalcium phosphate-based bone void filler as a graft extender in spinal fusion surgeries. Orthopedics 2002;25[Suppl]:591–595.

61. Toth JM, An HS, Lim TH, et al. Evaluation of porous biphasic calcium phosphate ceramics for anterior cervical interbody fusion in a caprine model. Spine 1995;20:2203–2210.

62. Guigui P, Plais P, Flautre B. Experimental model of posterolateral spinal arthrodesis in sheep. 1. Experimental procedures and results with autologous bone graft. Spine 1994;19:2791–2797.

63. Steffen T, Marchesi D, Aebi M. Posterolateral and anterior interbody spinal fusion models in the sheep. Clin Orthop 2000;371:28–37.

64. Delecrin J, Aguado E, Nguyen JM, et al. Influence of local environment on incorporation of ceramic for lumbar fusion. Comparison of laminar and intertransverse sites in a canine model. Spine 1997;22: 1683 1689.

65. Zdeblick TA, Cooke ME, Kunz DN, et al. Anterior cervical discectomy and fusion using a porous hydroxyapatite bone graft substitute. Spine 1994;19:2348–2357.

66. Heise U, Osborn J, Duwe F. Hydroxyapatite ceramic as a bone substitute. Int Orthop 1990;14:329–338.

67. Le Huec JC, Lesprit E, Delavigne C, et al. Tricalcium phosphate ceramics and allografts as bone substitutes for spinal fusion in idiopathic scoliosis: comparative clinical results at four years. Acta Orthop Belg 1997;63:202–211.

68. Passati N, Daculsi G, Rogez J, et al. Macroporous calcium phosphate ceramic performance in human spine fusion. Clin Orthop 1989;248: 169–176.

69. Ransford AO, Morley T, Edgar MA, et al. Synthetic porous ceramic compared with autograft in scoliosis surgery. A prospective, randomized study of 341 patients. J Bone Joint Surg 1998;80B:13–18.

70. Fujibayashi S, Shikata J, Tanaka C, et al. Lumbar posterolateral fusion with biphasic calcium phosphate ceramic. J Spinal Disord 2001;14: 214–21.

71. Thalgott J, Fritts K, Ginffre J, et al. Anterior interbody fusion of the cervical spine with coralline hydroxyapatite. Spine 1999;24: 1295–1299.

72. McConnell JR, Freeman BJC, Debnath UK, et al. A prospective randomized comparison of coralline hydroxyapatite with autograft in cervical interbody fusion. Spine 2003;28:317–323.

73. Bostrom MP, Lane JM. Future directions. Augmentation of osteoporotic vertebral bodies. Spine 1997;22[Suppl]:38–42. Erratum in: Spine 1998;23:1922.

74. Driessens FC, Planell JA, Boltong MG, et al. Osteotransductive bone cements. Proc Inst Mech Eng [H] 1998;212:427–435.

75. Fukase Y, Wada S, Uehara H, et al. Basic studies on hydroxy apatite cement: I. Setting reaction. J Oral Sci 1998;40:71–76.

76. Knaack D, Goad ME, Aiolova M, et al. Resorbable calcium phosphate bone substitute. J Biomed Mater Res 1998;43:399–409.

77. Dressmann H. Ueber knochenplombierungbei hohlebformigen defeckten des knochens. Beitr Klin Chirurgischen 1892;9:804–810.

78. Peltier L. The use of plaster of Paris to fill large defects in bone. Am J Surg 1959;97:311–315.

79. Sidqui M, Collin P, Vitte C, et al. Osteoblast adherence and resorption activity of isolated osteoclasts on calcium sulphate hemihydrate. Biomaterials 1995;16:1327–1332.

80. Hadjipavlou AG, Simmons JW, Yang J, et al. Plaster of Paris as an osteoconductive material for interbody vertebral fusion in mature sheep. Spine 2000;25:10–16.

81. Peltier LF. The use of plaster of Paris to fill defects in bone. Clin Orthop 1961;21:1–31.

82. Peltier LR, Bickel EY, Lillo R, et al. The use of plaster of Paris to fill defects in bone. Ann Surg 1957;146:61–69.

83. Cunningham BWO, Sefter JC, Buckley R, et al. An investigational study of calcium sulfate for posterolateral spinal arthrodesis—an invivo animal model. Paper presented at: Scoliosis Research Society Meeting; September 16–19, 1998; New York.

85. McKee MSE, Wild L, Waddell JP. The use of antibiotic impregnated, bioabsorbable bone substitute in the treatment of infected long bone defects: results of a prospective trial. J Orthop Trauma 2000;14: 137–138.

86. Armstrong DG, Findlow AH, Oyibo SO, et al. The use of absorbable antibiotic impregnated calcium sulphate pellets in the management of diabetic foot infections. Diabetes Med 2001;18:942–943.

75. Turner TM, Urban RM, Gitelis S, et al. Radiographic and histologic assessment of calcium sulfate in experimental animal models and clinical use as a resorbable bone-graft substitute, a bone-graft expander, and a method for local antibiotic delivery. One institution's experience. J Bone Joint Surg 2001;83A[Suppl]:8–18.

87. Hadjipavlou AG, Simmons JW, Tzermiadianos MN, et al. Plaster of Paris as bone substitute in spinal surgery. Eur Spine J 2001;10[Suppl 2]:189–196.

88. Edkins AD, Jones LP. The effects of plaster of Paris and autogenous cancellous bone on the healing of cortical defects in femur of dogs. Vet Surg 1988;17:71–76.

89. Miclau T, Dahners LE, Lindesey RW. In vitro pharmacokinetics of antibiotic release from locally implantable materials. J Orthop Res 1993;11:627–632.

90. Robinson D, Alk D, Sandbank J, et al. Inflammatory reactions associated with a calcium sulfate bone substitute. Ann Transplant 1999;4: 91–97.

91. Wilkins RM, Kelly CM, Giusti DE. Bioassayed demineralized bone matrix and calcium sulphate: use in bone-grafting procedures. Ann Chir Gynaecol 1999;88:180–185.

92. Cornell CN. Osteoconductive materials and their role as substitutes for autogenous bone grafts. Orthop Clin North Am 1999;30:591–598.

93. Chapman MW, Bucholz R, Cornell C. Treatment of acute fractures with a collagen-calcium phosphate graft material. A randomized clinical trial. J Bone Joint Surg 1997;79A:495–502.

94. Cornell CN, Lane JM, Chapman M, et al. Multicenter trial of Collagraft as bone graft substitute J Orthop Trauma 1991;5:1–8.

95. Walsh WR, Harrison J, Loefler A, et al. Mechanical and histologic evaluation of Collagraft in an ovine lumbar fusion model. Clin Orthop 2000;375:258–266;

96. Muschler GF, Negami S, Hyodo A, et al. Evaluation of collagen ceramic composite graft materials in a spinal fusion model. Clin Orthop 1996;328:250–260.

97. Zerwekh JE, Kourosh S, Scheinberg R, et al. Fibrillar collagen-biphasic calcium phosphate composite as a bone graft substitute for spinal fusion. J Orthop Res 1992;10:562–572.

98. Tay BK, Le AX, Heilman M, et al. Use of a collagen-hydroxyapatite matrix in spinal fusion. A rabbit model. Spine 1998;23:2276–2281.

99. Kadiyala S, Lo H, Leong KW. Biodegradable polymers and synthetic bone graft in bone formation and repair. Park Ridge, IL: American Academy of Orthopaedic Surgeons, 1994:317–324.

100. Urist M. Bone: formation by autoinduction. Science 1965;150: 839–899.

101. Urist M, Silverman B, Buring K, et al. The bone induction principle. Clin Orthop 1967;53:243–283.

102. Chalmers J, Gray D, Rush J. Observations on the induction of bone in soft tissues. J Bone Joint Surg 1975;57B:29–45.

103. Van Der Putte K, Urist M. Osteogenesis of the interior of intramuscular implants of decalcified bone matrix. Clin Orthop 1965;43: 257–270.

104. Wang EA, Israel D, Kelly S, et al. Bone morphogenetic protein-2 causes commitment and differentiation in C3H10T1/2 and 3T3 cells. Growth Factors 1993;9:57–71.

105. Ludwig SC, Boden SD. Osteoinductive bone graft substitutes for spinal fusion: a basic science summary. Orthop Clin North Am 1999; 30:635–645.

106. Sandhu HS, Grewal HS, Parvataneni H. Bone grafting for spinal fusion. Orthop Clin North Am 1999;30:685–698.

107. Fleming JE Jr, Cornell CN, Muschler GF. Bone cells and matrices in orthopedic tissue engineering. Orthop Clin North Am 2000;31: 357–374.

108. Buring K, Urist MR. Effects of ionizing radiation on the bone induction principle in the matrix of bone implants. Clin Orthop 1967;55: 225–234.

109. Aspenberg P, Johnson E, Thorngren KG. Dose-dependent reduction of bone inductive properties by ethylene oxide. J Bone Joint Surg 1990;72B:1036–1037.

110. Schwartz Z, Mellonin JT, Carnes DL Jr, et al. Ability of commercial demineralized freeze-dried bone allograft to induce new bone formation. J Periodontol 1996;67:918–926.

111. Schwartz Z, Somers A, Mellonig JT, et al. Ability of commercial demineralized freeze-dried bone allograft to induce new bone formation is dependent upon donor age but not gender. J Periodontol 1998;69: 470–478.

112. Bostrom MP, Yang X, Kennan M, et al. An unexpected outcome during testing of commercially available demineralized bone graft materials: how safe are the nonallograft components? Spine 2001;26: 1425–1428.

113. Wang JC, Kanim LE, Nagakawa IS, et al. Dose-dependent toxicity of a commercially available demineralized bone matrix. Spine 2001;26: 1429–1436.

114. Martin GJ, Boden SD, Titus L, et al. New formulations of demineralized bone matrix as a more effective graft alternative in experimental posterolateral lumbar spine arthrodesis. Spine 1999;24:637–645.

115. Edwards JT, Diegmann MH, Scarborough NL. Osteoinduction of human demineralized bone: characterization in a rat model. Clin Orthop 1998;357:219–228.
116. Frenkel SR, Moskovich R, Spivak J, et al. Demineralized bone matrix: enhancement of spinal fusion. Spine 1993;18:1634–1639.
117. Morone MA, Boden SD. Experimental posterolateral lumbar spinal fusion with demineralized bone matrix gel. Spine 1998;23:159–167.
118. Guizzardi S, Di Silvestre M, Scandroglio R, et al. Implants of heterologous demineralized bone matrix for induction of posterior spinal fusion in rats. Spine 1992;17:701–707.
119. Lindholm TS, Ragni P, Lindholm TC. Response of bone marrow stroma cells to demineralized cortical bone matrix in experimental spinal fusion in rabbits. Clin Orthop 1988;230:296–302.
120. Lindholm TS, Nilsson OS, Lindholm TC. Extraskeletal and intraskeletal new bone formation induced by demineralized bone matrix combined with bone marrow cells. Clin Orthop 1982;171: 251–255.
121. Ragni P, Lindholm TS. Interaction of allogeneic demineralized bone matrix and porous hydroxyapatite bioceramics in lumbar interbody fusion in rabbits. Clin Orthop 1991;272:292–2999.
122. Hogan BL. Bone morphogenetic proteins: Multifunctional regulators of vertebrate development. Genes Dev 1996;10:158–1594.
123. Wozney JM. Overview of bone morphogenetic proteins. Spine 2002; 27[Suppl]:2–8.
124. Urist M, Strates B. Bone formation in implants of partially and wholly demineralized bone matrix. Clin Orthop 1870;71:271–278.
125. Damien CJ, Grob D, Boden SD, et al. Purified bovine BMP extract and collagen for spine arthrodesis. Preclinical safety and efficacy. Spine 2002;27[Suppl]:50–58.
126. Wozney JM, Rosen V, Celeste AJ, et al. Novel regulators of bone formation: molecular clones and activities. Science 1988;242: 1528–1534.
127. Wozney J. The bone morphogenetic protein family and osteogenesis. Mol Reprod Dev 1992;32:160–167.
128. McKay B, Sandhu HS. Use of recombinant human bone morphogenetic protein-2 in spinal fusion application. Spine 2002;27[Suppl]: 66–85.
129. Vaccaro AR, Anderson DG, Toth CA. Recombinant human osteogenic protein-1 (Bone morphogenetic protein-7) as an osteoinductive agent in spinal fusion. Spine 2002;27[Suppl]:59–65.
130. Seeherman H, Wozney J, Li R. Bone morphogenetic protein delivery systems. Spine 2002;27[Suppl]:16–23.
131. Schimandle JH, Boden SD, Hutton WC. Experimental spinal fusion with recombinant human bone morphogenetic protein-2. Spine 1995; 20:1326–1337.
132. Martin GJ Jr, Boden SD, Marone MA, et al. Posterolateral intertransverse process spinal arthrodesis with rhBMP-2 in a nonhuman primate: important lessons learned regarding dose, carrier, and safety. J Spinal Disord 1999;12:179–186.
133. Boden SD, Martin GJ Jr, Horton WC, et al. Laparoscopic anterior spinal arthrodesis with rhBMP-2 in a titanium interbody threaded cage. J Spinal Disord 1998;11:95–101.
134. Boden SD, Schimandle JH, Hutton WC, et al. Volvo Award in basic sciences. The use of an osteoinductive growth factor for lumbar spinal fusion. Part I: Biology of spinal fusion. Spine 1995;20:2626–2632.
135. Boden SD, Schimandle JH, Hutton WC. Volvo Award in basic sciences. The use of osteoinductive growth factor for lumbar spinal fusion. II: Study of dose, carrier, and species. Spine 1995;20:2633–2644.
136. Sandhu HS, Kanim LE, Kabo JM, et al. Effective doses of recombinant human bone morphogenetic protein-2 in experimental spinal fusion. Spine 1996;21:2115–2122.
137. Sandhu HS, Kanim LE, Toth JM, et al. Experimental spinal fusion with recombinant human bone morphogenetic protein-2 without decortication of osseous elements. Spine 1997;22:1171–1180.
138. Cook SD, Dalton JE, Tan EH, et al. In vivo evaluation of recombinant human osteogenic protein (rhOP-1) implant as a bone graft substitute for spinal fusions. Spine 1994;19:1655–1663.
139. Muschler GF, Hyodo A, Manning T, et al. Evaluation of human bone morphogenetic protein 2 in a canine spinal fusion model. Clin Orthop 1994;308:229–240.
140. Holliger EH, Trawick RH, Boden SD, et al. Morphology of the lumbar intertransverse process fusion mass in rabbit model: a comparison between two bone graft materials—rhBMP-2 and autograft. J Spinal Disord 1996;9:125–128.
141. Grauer JN, Patel TC, Erulkar JS, et al. Evaluation of OP-1 as a graft substitute for intertransverse process lumbar fusion. Spine 2001;26: 127–133.
142. Sandhu HS, Kanim LE, Kabo JM, et al. Evaluation of rhBMP-2 with an OPLA carrier in a canine posterolateral (transverse process) spinal fusion model. Spine 1995;20:2669–2682.
143. Silcox DH, Boden SD, Schimandle JH, et al. Reversing the inhibitory effect of nicotine on spinal fusion using an osteoinductive protein extract. Spine 1998;23:291–296.
144. Martin GJ, Boden SD, Titus L. Recombinant human bone morphogenetic protein-2 overcomes the inhibitory effect of ketorolac, a nonsteroidal anti-inflammatory drug (NSAID), on posterolateral lumbar intertransverse process spine fusion. Spine 1999;24:2188–2193.
145. Patel TC, Erulkar JS, Grauer JN, et al. Osteogenic protein-1 overcomes the inhibitory effect of nicotine on posterolateral lumbar fusion. Spine 2001;26:1656–1661.
146. Boden SD, Zdeblick TA, Sandhu HS, et al. The use of rhBMP-2 in interbody fusion cages. Definitive evidence of osteoinduction in humans: a preliminary report. Spine 2000;25:376–381.
147. Poynton AR, Lane JM. Safety profile for the clinical use of bone morphogenetic proteins in the spine. Spine 2002;27[Suppl]:40–48.
148. Paramore CG, Lauryssen C, Rauzzino MJ, et al. The safety of OP-1 for lumbar fusion with decompression—a canine study. Neurosurgery 1999;44:1151–1155.
149. Ackerman SJ, Mafilios MS, Polly DW. Economic evaluation of bone morphogenetic protein versus autogenous iliac crest bone graft in single-level anterior lumbar fusion. Spine 2002;27[Suppl]:94–99.
150. Baylink DJ, Finkelman RD, Mohan S. Growth factors to stimulate bone formation. J Bone Miner Res 1993;8[Suppl]:565–572.
151. Slater M, Patava J, Kingham K, et al. Involvement of platelets in stimulating osteogenic activity. J Orthop Res 1995;13:655–663.
152. Lowery GL, Kulkarni S, Pennisi AE. Use of autologous growth factors in lumbar spinal fusion. Bone 1999;25[Suppl]:47–50.
153. Muschler GF, Boehm C, Easley KA. Aspiration to obtain osteoblast progenitor cells from human bone marrow: the influence of aspiration volume. J Bone Joint Surg 1997;79A:1699–1709.
154. Muschler GF, Nitto H, Boehm, et al. Age- and gender-related changes in the cellularity of human bone marrow and the prevalence of osteoblastic progenitors. J Orthop Res 2001;19:117–125.
155. Connolly J, Guse R, Lippiello L, et al. Development of an osteogenic bone marrow preparation. J Bone Joint Surg 1989;71A:684–691.
156. Lane JM, Yasko AW, Tomin E, et al. Bone marrow and recombinant human bone morphogenetic protein-2 in osseous repair. Clin Orthop 1999;361:216–227.
157. Jaiswal N, Haynesworth SE, Caplan AI, et al. Osteogenic differentiation of purified, culture-expanded human mesenchymal stem cells in vitro. J Cell Biochem 1997;64:295–312.
158. Kadiyala S, Young RG, Thiede MA, et al. Culture expanded canine mesenchymal stem cells possess osteochondrogenic potential in vivo and in vitro. Cell Transplant 1997;6:125–134.
159. Lieberman JR, Daluiski A, Stevenson S, et al. The effect of regional gene therapy with bone morphogenetic protein-2-producing bone-marrow cells on the repair of segmental femoral defects in rats. J Bone Joint Surg 1999;81A:905–917.
160. Alden TD, Pittman DD, Beres EJ, et al. Percutaneous spinal fusion using bone morphogenetic protein-2 gene therapy. J Neurosurg 1999;90[Suppl]:109–114.
161. Wang JC, Kanim LE, Yoo S, et al. Effect of regional gene therapy with bone morphogenetic protein-2-producing bone marrow cells on spinal fusion in rats. J Bone Joint Surg 2003;85A:905–901.
162. Boden SD, Titus L, Hair G, et al. Lumbar spine fusion by local gene therapy with a cDNA encoding a novel osteoinductive protein (LMP-1). Spine 1998;23:2486–2492.
163. Toribatake Y, Hutton C, Boden SD, et al. Revascularization of the fusion mass in a posterolateral intertransverse process fusion. Spine 1998;23:1149–1154.
164. Lewandrowski K, Gresser JD, Wise DL, et al. Bioresorbable bone graft substitutes of different osteoconductivities: a histologic evaluation of osteointegration of poly(propylene glycol-co-fumaric acid)-based cement implants in rats. Biomaterials 2000;21:757–764.

CHAPTER 25

Principles of Spinal Instrumentation in Degenerative Disorders of the Lumbar Spine

Ashok Biyani and Howard S. An

Approximately 72,000 lumbar fusion procedures were performed in 1993 in the United States for degenerative disorders of the lumbar spine (1), and the frequency of lumbar fusion has been on the rise at an annual rate of 8% for last two decades (2). The use of instrumentation to augment fusion in the lumbar spine has become quite popular over the last several years. Although it has been well established that posterior instrumentation enhances fusion rate, it is not clear whether it improves the functional outcome. Although transpedicular fixation has now become widely accepted as the posterior instrumentation system of choice for lumbar degenerative disorders, its indications are not well defined and are not universally accepted. Although several studies have focused on this subject over the last decade, many are retrospective in nature, contain a heterogeneous group of patients with different underlying disorders, and a variety of instrumentation systems have been used. Although there is a relative lack of prospective controlled data in the literature, a better understanding of the indications of transpedicular instrumentation and their outcome seems to be emerging. An increased emphasis is also being placed on the functional outcome and cost-effectiveness analysis of instrumentation.

HISTORICAL PERSPECTIVE

Internal fixation of the spine with wiring techniques has been known for over a century. Screw fixation was attempted by King (3) in the spine in 1940s even before hook-based systems were popularized by Harrington (4) in the 1960s. Harrington rods were used successfully in the surgical management of idiopathic scoliosis, but their applicability in the degenerative conditions of the lumbar spine was limited. Cotrel and Dubousset modified the hook-based systems and introduced the concept of seg-

mental fixation (5). The advent of Luque segmental sublaminar wiring technique brought forth the next major advance in the spinal instrumentation (6). This technique requires an intact lamina for a multilevel fusion construct and provides poor resistance to axial compression or distraction. Although sublaminar wiring is still widely used in the management of neuromuscular scoliosis, its role in management of degenerative spinal disorders is currently limited to correction of degenerative lumbar scoliosis by providing a posteriorly directed force and lateral translation of the apex of the deformity.

Pedicular fixation was first attempted in 1959 by Boucher, who tried inserting the pedicle screws through the facet joints (7). Roy-Camille (8,9) pioneered the technique of pedicle screw placement in the 1960s with further refinement in subsequent years. Transpedicular instrumentation was introduced in the United States by Steffee in 1983 (10). Numerous pedicle screw fixation systems have since been developed. Pedicle screws initially were attached to the plates, but rod-based systems have become more popular in the last decade.

INDICATIONS FOR THE USE OF INSTRUMENTATION IN LUMBAR DEGENERATIVE DISORDERS

The role of instrumentation as an adjunct to lumbar fusion in patients with lumbar degenerative disorders is not well defined. Although the literature is replete with reports on instrumented fusion for a variety of underlying disorders, there is a clear lack of consensus among spine surgeons on the indications for instrumented posterolateral fusion. Some of the more commonly accepted indications, although not without controversy or universal agreement, include degenerative spondylolisthesis and lumbar instability, multilevel fusion, revision surgery for pseudarthrosis, and spinal deformity including degenerative scoliosis and flat back syndrome. Posterior instrumented fusion for discogenic back pain remains the most controversial of all indications.

Degenerative Spondylolisthesis

Although untreated degenerative spondylolisthesis may progress over time in 30% of patients (11), the majority of patients respond well to conservative treatment, and only 10% to 15% of patients require operative intervention (12). Posterior decompression and fusion is the surgical treatment of choice for degenerative spondylolisthesis, because laminectomy alone is likely to further destabilize the spine. Herkowitz and Kurz (13) have demonstrated in a randomized, prospective study of patients with degenerative spondylolisthesis that superior results are obtained with decompression and concomitant fusion than with decompression alone. McCulloch (14) recently reported favorable results with microdecompression and uninstrumented single level fusion for degenerative spondylolisthesis in 21 patients. Several authors also have evaluated the role of instrumentation in degenerative spondylolisthesis. Fischgrund et al. (15) performed a prospective randomized study of 76 patients with degenerative spondylolisthesis and spinal stenosis. They reported a higher fusion rate (82%) in the instrumented group versus 45% in the noninstrumented group, but improved fusion rate with instrumentation did not translate into improved clinical outcome in patients undergoing single-level posterolateral fusion with transpedicular instrumentation. At a longer-term follow-up of the same group of patients, these authors reported worse outcome in patients with pseudarthrosis compared with patients who had solid fusion (16).

Yuan et al. (17) performed a large historical cohort study of patients, who underwent posterior spinal fusion with (2,177 patients) or without (456 patients) transpedicular instrumentation for degenerative spondylolisthesis. The fusion rate was 89.1% for the instrumented group and 70.4% for the uninstrumented group. Despite fewer reoperations, less number of spinal levels fused, less use of allograft and lower worker's compensation cases in the uninstrumented group, overall functional results were superior in the instrumented group. Shorter time to fusion, better neurologic recovery, and greater relief of back pain were noted in the instrumented group. The rate of complications, reoperation, and mortality was similar in the two groups.

Booth et al. (18) reviewed 49 consecutive patients with degenerative spondylolisthesis, who were treated with decompression, intertransverse process fusion, and segmental pedicle screw instrumentation. Eighty-three percent patients had satisfactory results with the procedure at a mean follow up of 6.5 years, and 86% reported last-ing improvement in their back and leg pain. Steffee and Brantigan (19) reported a fusion rate of 91.5% in a prospective study of 250 patients with spondylolisthesis who were treated with variable screw-plate system. Bridwell et al. (20) also reported significant improvement in radiographic fusion rate in patients with instrumented fusion for degenerative spondylolisthesis. Noninstrumented patients had significantly increased progression of spondylolisthesis compared with the instrumented group.

In a retrospective study of 30 patients with degenerative spondylolisthesis treated with decompression and instrumented posterior fusion, Nork et al. (21) reported improved functional outcome using standardized SF-36 questionnaire. Ninety-three percent of patients had successful radiographic fusion. Ninety-three percent of patients were satisfied with their outcome, and their SF-36 scores were superior to a previously published cohort of patients with low back pain. Eighty-three percent of patients had severe back pain preoperatively compared with 3% of patients having severe pain postoperatively. Poor outcome correlated with greater preoperative stenosis or occurrence of complications. The authors acknowledged that preoperative SF-36 scores were not available, and there was no control group of uninstrumented fusion in their study.

However, some studies have failed to find any significant advantages of instrumentation over no instrumentation. In a prospective randomized clinical study of primary or degenerative spondylolisthesis, Thomsen et al. (22) did not observe any significant difference in the fusion rate or functional outcome when decompression and posterolateral lumbar fusion was performed with or without Cotrel-Dubousset instrumentation. A few other authors have reported similar lack of improvement in outcome with instrumentation (23–25). It is obvious from the mixed results of these studies that there is no unanimity among spine surgeons on the role of instrumentation in patients with degenerative spondylolisthesis. Nevertheless, a clear trend seems to be emerging in management of degenerative spondylolisthesis with increasing usage of instrumentation. It is worth noting, however, that solid fusion does not necessarily translate in to a successful functional outcome.

The presence of L4-5 degenerative spondylolisthesis without obvious motion on preoperative flexion-extension lateral radiographs and narrow disc space with end plate-to-end plate contact is a relative indication for an uninstrumented posterolateral fusion following decompression. However, instrumented fusion is recommended in presence of documented instability or relatively preserved disc space height to prevent further postoperative olisthesis secondary to the destabilizing effect of the decompressive laminectomy (Fig. 25-1). The usage of instrumentation is also appropriate when there is a sig-

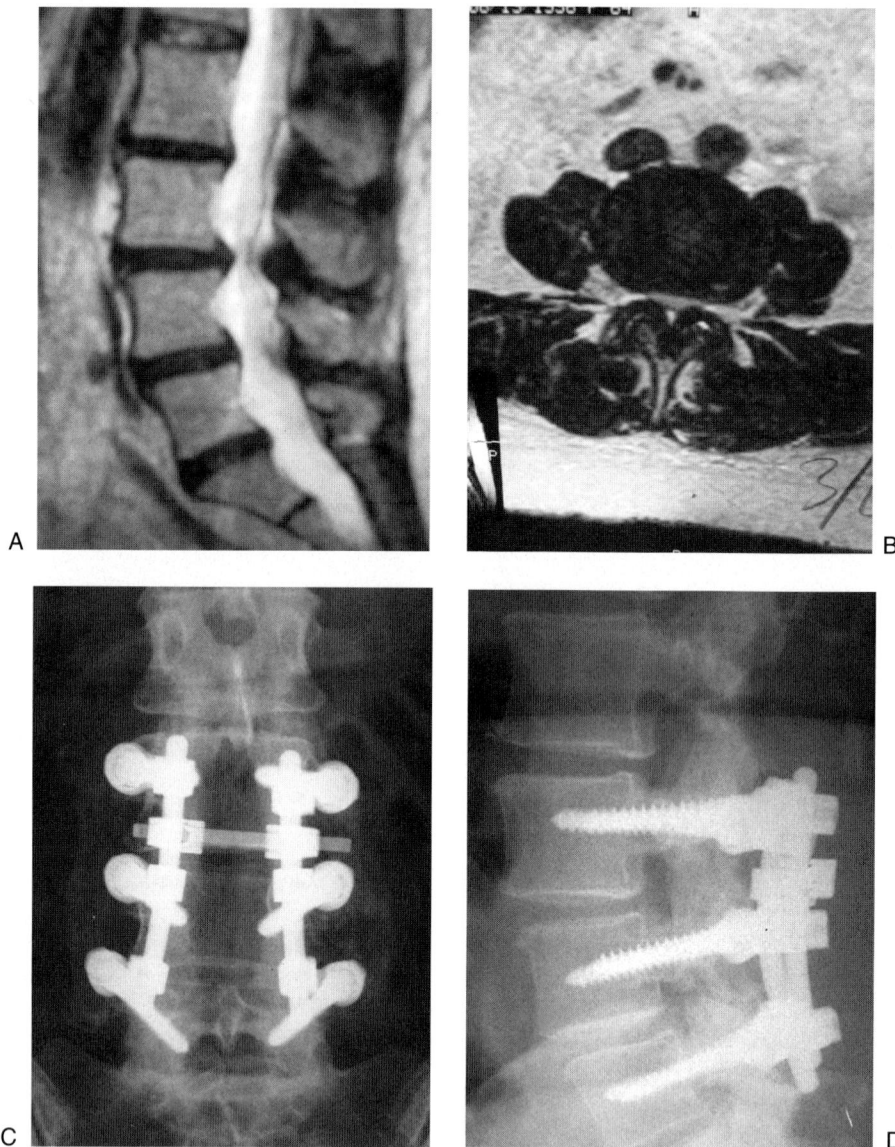

FIG. 25-1. Preoperative sagittal magnetic resonance image **(A)**, and axial image at L3-4 level **(B)** in a patient with degenerative spondylolisthesis at L4-5 and spinal stenosis at L3-4 and L4-5. Postoperative anteroposterior and lateral radiographs show decompression and instrumented fusion **(C,D)**.

nificant slippage with associated kyphosis. The instrumented posterolateral fusion should be performed either concomitantly with a posterior lumbar interbody fusion or extended to the sacrum for correction of the kyphotic deformity and to gain greater control of L4. Correction of kyphosis associated with spondylolisthesis and restoration of sagittal alignment is made possible by the usage of instrumentation, which not only improves the fusion rate, but may also delay the onset of adjacent segment breakdown (26).

Degenerative Scoliosis

Degenerative scoliosis may appear *de novo* or degenerative changes may develop in patients with preexisting idiopathic scoliosis. Degenerative scoliosis is most often accompanied by spinal stenosis. Progression of the deformity may occur because of destabilization if posterior decompression is performed without concomitant fusion, and several factors need to be considered when deciding whether concomitant arthrodesis is indicated. The scoliotic curve is likely to progress with decompression alone, if it is partially correctable on side bending films. Arthrodesis also is indicated when there has been a documented curve progression and in the presence of lateral spondylolisthesis, which is inherently unstable. Other risk factors for curve progression include a Cobb angle of 30 degrees or greater, and grade 3 apical vertebral body rotation. Lateral translation of greater than 6 mm and the presence of L5 seated above the intercrestal line are also indicative of instability (27). Finally, Loss of sagittal alignment renders the spine more vulnerable to developing progressive kyphosis after laminectomy alone (28).

Patients presenting with radiculopathy that coincides with the concavity of the curve may need wide lateral and foraminal decompression, including partial facetectomy. Fusion is indicated along with central and lateral canal decompression in the presence of degenerative scoliosis, particularly when the laminectomy is performed at the apex of the curve. If the spine is considered unstable intraoperatively after decompression, fusion should be performed. Resection of more than 50% of bilateral facet joints or a whole facet joint is considered to create spinal instability (29).

Fractional curve at the lumbosacral level is most often associated with foraminal stenosis. Adequate foraminotomy may require removal of a substantial part of the facet joints, which may lead to further destabilization. In addition to providing immediate stability, transpedicular instrumentation also facilitates reduction in pedicular kinking and indirect decompression of the foramina by segmental pedicular distraction (30,31). In a cadaveric study, Inufusa et al. (32) were able to increase the foraminal dimensions by 22.6% at L4-5 and by 39.6% at L5-S1 with 6 mm of rod distraction with transpedicular instrumentation.

Simmons and Simmons (34) retrospectively reviewed the results of decompression and instrumented fusion in patients with significant lumbar scoliosis and stenosis. Eighty-three percent of patients had severe pain preoperatively. Ninety-three percent of patients reported mild or no pain at follow-up. Overall fusion rate was 100%, and mean Cobb angle correction was 19 degrees. In another retrospective of 27 patients with adult onset scoliosis, Marchesi and Aebi (35) reported 86% satisfactory results and 4% rate of pseudarthrosis.

The degenerative lumbar curves often extend from the lower thoracic spine to the sacrum. Instrumentation decreases the rate of pseudarthrosis after multilevel arthrodesis, and facilitates correction of deformity and restoration of sagittal alignment. However, the extent of instrumented posterior fusion and concomitant anterior release and fusion are controversial issues in the surgical management of degenerative lumbar curves (33). Long instrumented fusion is associated with significant morbidity, and should be cautiously approached in the elderly population.

Degenerative Spinal Stenosis

Most patients with degenerative spinal stenosis can be treated with decompression alone in the absence of instability or significant kyphoscoliosis. A laminectomy with lateral recess decompression by undercutting the articular facets and adequate foraminotomy allows neural decompression and often can be performed without causing sig-

nificant iatrogenic instability (36). Mullin et al. (37) reported a 54% incidence of instability after decompressive laminectomy for stenosis, emphasizing the need for careful selection of patients with certain risk factors who may need a spinal fusion in addition to laminectomy. Presence of bridging osteophytes, narrowed disc spaces, calcified annulus, capsule or ligamentum flavum, and a high intercrestal line are considered to be preoperative indicators of spinal stability; such patients should be treated with decompression alone in the absence of other risk factors (38).

Garfin et al. (39) have summarized the predictors of postoperative instability after decompressive laminectomy alone for lumbar stenosis. These risk factors include a large preoperative slip, decompression across normal disc height, greater than 50% facet excision at a single level, increased numbers of levels decompressed, penetration of disc space at the decompressed level, and female sex. Presence of traction spurs and asymmetric narrowed disc space also are indicative of postoperative instability (38). All patients with aforementioned risk factors for postoperative progression of instability should be considered for a concomitant fusion.

Disc herniation is infrequently present in patients with spinal stenosis. A free fragment or a foraminal disc herniation is the most common presentations in this subset of patients. Decompressive discectomy is necessary in these instances to relieve the radicular symptoms. However, vigorous attempts at removing the disc material and radical disruption of the disc may produce iatrogenic instability, particularly in younger individuals with maintained disc height (40). A fusion procedure may be necessary when a radical discectomy is performed in conjunction with a decompressive laminectomy (28).

The criteria for addition of instrumentation to fusion have not been well established in surgical treatment of lumbar stenosis. In general, indications for adding instrumentation to posterolateral arthrodesis include the need for correction of kyphosis or scoliosis, decompression of the foramen, translational motion of more than 4 mm, and angulatory motion of more than 10 degrees in flexion extension lateral radiographs, and in presence of iatrogenic instability (28). By providing immediate stability, instrumentation halts further progression of olisthesis and increases the fusion rate. The presence of significant facet joint arthritis in patients with lumbar stenosis is a relative indication for concomitant instrumented fusion.

Hansraj et al. (41) noted that decompression and instrumented fusion was efficacious in management of complex spinal stenosis with a 96% patient satisfaction rate. Complex spinal stenosis was defined as the presence of radiographic instability in addition to stenosis, degenerative spondylolisthesis greater than grade 1 with instability, degenerative scoliosis with the curve greater than 20 degrees, and history of prior surgery with radiographic evidence of instability or junctional stenosis.

Recurrent stenosis is frequently seen in patients undergoing laminectomy without fusion, and occurs because of bone regrowth and formation of scar tissue. Postacchini and Cinotti (42,43) reported that recurrent stenosis was significantly less common in patients who underwent decompression and concomitant fusion compared with patients undergoing decompression alone. The reoperation rate for recurrent lumbar stenosis is estimated to be 5% to 23% (44). The management of adjacent segment stenosis usually is straightforward and involves simple decompressive laminectomy. However, management of recurrent stenosis of the previously operated levels is challenging. Significant bone regrowth, hypertrophic facets, and epidural scarring are frequently encountered in patients with recurrent spinal stenosis at the previously operated level, which necessitates more extensive facetectomies that may endanger the stability of the spine. Therefore, an arthrodesis with or without instrumentation may be recommended for patients undergoing decompression for recurrent lumbar stenosis. Because instrumentation improves the fusion rate, adding instrumented fusion to laminectomy is appropriate in these circumstances. However, these patients are often older and therefore are subject to a higher risk of overall complications. Consequently, instrumented arthrodesis should be performed sparingly, and usually is reserved for patients with spondylolisthesis and recurrent stenosis (28).

Pseudarthrosis and Flat Back Syndrome

The overall reported incidence of nonunion is approximately 5% to 7% for single-level uninstrumented fusion and 25% to 35% for uninstrumented degenerative spondylolisthesis (45). There is a significantly higher incidence of pseudarthrosis following multilevel uninstrumented fusion (46). Pseudarthrosis poses complex diagnostic and treatment dilemmas. Established pseudarthrosis can be detected on Ferguson views, AP, and flexion-extension lateral radiographs or reformatted computed tomography (CT) images. However, Kant et al. (47) reported 68% sensitivity of radiographs in correlating with intraoperative confirmation of pseudarthrosis.

The presence of pseudarthrosis does not necessarily correlate with the patient's symptoms. Once a diagnosis of pseudarthrosis has been established, the clinical picture should be carefully reviewed to assure that pseudarthrosis is indeed the underlying cause of persistent pain. The treatment of lumbosacral pseudarthrosis is complicated and challenging at best. Surgical treatment is dictated by a variety of factors, including prior history of instrumentation, associated spinal deformity, and patient factors such as history of smoking. A noninstrumented posterolateral lumbar pseudarthrosis is an indication for revision fusion with rigid transpedicular instrumentation. Rigid segmental fixation also is indicated when a posterolateral fusion is performed for treatment of a failed

posterior or anterior lumbar interbody fusion (48). A combined posterior instrumented revision fusion and anterior interbody fusion may be necessary in selected cases.

The outcome of surgical repair of pseudarthrosis is variable. The rate of successful fusion and improvement in functional outcome is less than primary fusions. Lauerman et al. (49) reported an overall fusion rate of 49% with use of a combination of sublaminar wires, Harrington compression rods, and variable pedicle screw-plate constructs and uninstrumented fusion in patient with pre-existing pseudarthrosis. Eighty-six percent of patients continued to experience low back pain, and 49% patients had poor clinical outcome. West et al. (50) reported 65% fusion rate after lumbar pseudoarthrosis repair with pedicle screw constructs, in contrast with 90% fusion rate in patients who underwent primary instrumented fusion for degenerative disc disease or spondylolisthesis. Horowitch et al. (51) reported a 68% fusion rate after instrumented fusion in a mixed group of patients, two thirds of whom had pseudarthrosis. Zdeblick reported on the results of a large cohort of patients undergoing lumbar fusion, some of who underwent repair of pseudarthrosis with and without instrumentation (52). The group treated with regrafting without instrumentation had a 20% fusion rate, whereas both semirigid and rigid instrumentation yielded 100% union. Despite an acceptable fusion rate, the functional outcome of instrumented repair of pseudarthrosis is more unpredictable.

Carpenter et al. (53) reported a 26% good or excellent outcome after pseudarthrosis repair despite a 94% fusion rate. Kim and Michelsen (54) retrospectively reviewed the results of surgical treatment in 50 failed back surgery patients. They noted an overall significant improvement in pain and function in 66% of the patients. Eighty-one percent of patients with a solid fusion had a satisfactory outcome compared with 23% in patients with failed pseudarthrosis repair. Stewart et al. (55) reported a 72% successful outcome following attempted pseudarthrosis repair, as determined by the ability of patients to return to work, the lack of a need for narcotic analgesics, and overall satisfaction.

Patients with a prior decompressive laminectomy may develop fixed sagittal imbalance owing to loss of posterior stabilizing structures. Fixed sagittal imbalance also may occur owing to breakdown through pseudarthrosis instability at a level above or below previous fusion, or because of multisegmental degenerative disc disease. Many patients with a flat back syndrome suffer from persistent back pain with erect posture owing to loss of lumbar posterior tension band and early fatigue of extensor muscles.

Approximately 15% to 20% of patients who have had a prior lumbar fusion for degenerative disease require revision lumbar surgery over the ensuing 3 to 5 years. Pseudarthrosis, flat back syndrome, and postlaminectomy instability are some of the common causes of persistent pain that require additional surgery. Correction of flat back syndrome and postlaminectomy kyphosis is best achieved with appropriate osteotomies, restoration of global sagittal alignment, and stabilization with transpedicular instrumentation (56). Although there is a higher risk of complications associated with the technically demanding revision surgery, high rate of osseous union, improved spinal alignment, and functional outcome can be achieved in carefully selected patients.

Degenerative Disc Disease

The role of posterior spinal fusion and instrumentation in degenerative disc disease without instability is highly controversial. The decision to perform an arthrodesis is based on the assumption that the pain generator can be localized to the degenerative disc space. Improvement in pain presumably occurs because of elimination of motion at a degenerated and painful segment. Posterolateral fusion may be considered for the treatment of intractable discogenic back pain. The fusion rate for single-level noninstrumented posterolateral fusion for degenerative disc disease is approximately 85% to 90% (46).

Several authors have reported improved fusion rate, less back pain, and higher return-to-work rates with instrumented than with noninstrumented fusion for degenerative disc disease (57–60). Lorenz et al. (57) prospectively evaluated 68 patients who underwent one level fusion with or without instrumentation for disabling back pain for 6 months or more, inability to work, and failed conservative care. None of the patients with instrumented fusion had pseudarthrosis and three fourths of patients reported improvement in pain and return to work. In contrast, 58% of patients in the uninstrumented group had nonunion and only one third of patients experienced pain relief and were able to return to work. Louise (58) reported a 97% fusion rate with pedicle screw-plate fixation in patients with intractable low back pain. Eighty-five percent of patients with sedentary work and 56.5% of heavy laborers were able to return to work in that study.

Dawson et al. (61) reported a 92% fusion rate and 70% to 80% clinical success rate in a retrospective study of 58 patients treated with posterolateral fusion for discogenic low back pain. These authors also reported a failure rate of 50% for patients undergoing revision surgery and 45% rate of pseudarthrosis for noninstrumented floating fusion. Hellstadius et al. (62) and Shaw and Taylor (63) also reported a 26% and 27% rate of pseudarthrosis, respectively, for posterolateral fusion without instrumentation. In another study, patients who underwent uninstrumented fusion for lumbar degenerative disc disease were 24 times more likely to have pseudarthrosis than comparable patients treated with transpedicular instrumented fusion (64).

Arthrodesis may be indicated for discogenic low back pain in certain circumstances. These include unremitting back pain and disability for 1 year, failure of conservative management including physical therapy for 6 months, magnetic resonance imaging (MRI) and discographic findings consistent with advanced degenerative disc disease and concordant symptom production at one or two levels. All patients with discogenic back pain who are being considered for spinal fusion also should have a normal psychological evaluation.

Patients with recurrent disc herniation at the same level usually are treated with repeat discectomy without fusion, unless preoperative instability is present or there is significant back pain associated with radicular pain. Routine use of instrumentation is not necessary in the absence of radiographically demonstrable instability. Patients with a second recurrence of disc herniation and those with preoperative or iatrogenically induced instability after their initial recurrence are candidates for arthrodesis (65), preferably with instrumentation. Smokers should have instrumented arthrodesis to enhance fusion rate.

Disc degeneration at a segment adjacent to prior fusion occurs because of increased stress concentration. Whitecloud et al. (66) treated 14 patients with adjacent segment degeneration with decompression and extension of fusion encompassing the degenerated motion segments. Ten of 12 patients treated with instrumented fusion had successful fusion. They recommended instrumented fusion for symptomatic adjacent degenerated segments, because instrumentation provides better control of the high stresses and improves the rate of fusion, compared with uninstrumented fusion.

Discogenic pain may persist despite a solid posterolateral fusion, presumably because of the presence of painful micromotion in the involved segment. Additionally, the disc itself may be a source of pain (67,68) that may benefit from interbody fusion, either with or without instrumentation. The role of interbody fusion is also a controversial subject that is beyond the scope of this chapter. Circumferential arthrodesis may reduce the rate of pseudarthrosis to less than 5%, but the morbidity associated with such an extensive procedure precludes its routine use in the management of lumbar degenerative disc disease. A circumferential fusion should be reserved for patients who are considered to be at high risk for pseudarthrosis, and is best reserved for revision cases and heavy smokers. Gertzbein et al. (69) reported 97% fusion rate and 77% good clinical outcome with circumferential fusion in a difficult group of patients, 62% of whom had previous surgery, 25% with prior pseudarthrosis, 55% with two or more levels fused, and 43% of whom were heavy smokers.

SPINAL INSTRUMENTATION SYSTEMS

Although a variety of spinal instrumentation systems are available, the role of hooks and sublaminar wires in the lumbar degenerative disorders is limited. Pedicle screws are available for use with plates or rods as the longitudinal members of the construct. However, rod based pedicle screw systems currently are more commonly used in management of degenerative conditions of the lumbar spine.

Pedicle Screws versus Hooks and Sublaminar Wires

Mardjetko et al. (70) concluded from their metaanalysis that adjunctive instrumentation leads to higher fusion rate, which, in turn, significantly improves patient satisfaction. However, these authors were not able to find any statistically significant difference in outcome between transpedicular systems and earlier instrumentation techniques such as hooks and rod construct and Luque wiring techniques. This metaanalysis had several design flaws, including a relatively small number of published articles, data from a wide variety of treatments over two decades, and variability in design and quality of many of the studies. Gurr et al. (71) biomechanically evaluated the strength of transpedicular fixation in a corpectomy model using calf spine. They compared posterior hook-based systems and pedicle screw constructs and found that the latter were more rigid, achieved greater fixation, and restored stability better than hook systems.

The use of sublaminar wiring and hook-based systems is outdated in the surgical management of degenerative lumbar spine disorders because of versatility and superior biomechanical characteristics of transpedicular fixation systems. Sublaminar wires are primarily used in the concavity of a degenerative scoliotic curve, whereas the terminal fixation is achieved with pedicle screws distally and either screws, hooks, or both proximally. The sublaminar wires provide a posteriorly directed force with torsional displacement of the vertebral body and lateral translation of the apex of a deformity. Hooks are used in the lumbar spine primarily as infralaminar hooks at the end of the construct or in patients with osteoporosis. Supralaminar or infralaminar hooks adjacent to pedicle screw instrumentation reduce the bending moments at the screw–rod junction (30).

The pedicle has been shown to be the strongest region within the vertebra and has been described as the "force nucleus" where the posterior elements meet the anterior column (10). Transpedicular fixation facilitates application of a rigid shorter length construct, thereby preserving more lumbar motion segment. Pedicle screws facilitate three-column control of the spine from the posterior approach, and permit restoration and maintenance of overall physiologic spinal alignment. An added advantage of a transpedicular system is that greater correction of deformity is feasible because of stronger points of fixation. In addition, concomitant laminectomy may be performed without adversely affecting the quality of fixation. Transpedicular systems avoid insertion of hardware

within the narrowed spinal canal. Solid fixation at the lumbosacral junction is also possible with pedicle screw placement (36,70).

Screw-Rod versus Screw-Plate Constructs

Several plate screw designs were introduced in the early stages of development of transpedicular instrumentation (8–10,24,72). The plate systems are low profile, and have the ability to resist torsion against large loads. The plates also provide large surface area under which the bone graft can be compressed against the spine. Although plate-based transpedicular fixation has some of the aforementioned advantages, screw-rod constructs are more popular because of several drawbacks of screw-plate constructs. It is difficult to place the plate on multiple screws if multilevel fusion is being performed. Although the plate may be bent in a sagittal plane, correction of a multiplane lumbar deformity is difficult to achieve with a screw-plate assembly. Attachment of sublaminar wires to correct degenerative scoliosis or its use with lamina hooks in patients with osteoporosis is not possible with plate systems. Impingement of adjacent facet joints by the plates is common, and cross connection of plates is difficult. Moreover, there is less space available for bone graft placement, and it is more difficult to visualize the fusion mass in postoperative radiographs in the presence of plates. Finally, the plate screw systems may be associated with a higher incidence of screw breakage because of angulation between the screws and the plate, which may lead to screw-plate malalignment. The reported rate of breakage of the early designs of pedicle screws inserted with plates varied from 4.3% to 23% of patients (73,74).

Screw-rod constructs, on the other hand, are very versatile and overcome many of the disadvantages of the plate systems. Rods also facilitate extension of the instrumentation to the pelvis. Rod systems are assembled either by lateral connectors to the screws or the rods are dropped directly in to the top-loading groove of the pedicle screws. In either case, the construct can be difficult to assemble at times. The overall assembly also tends to be bulkier than plate-based systems.

There are few clinical studies comparing the results of plate-screw and rod-screw constructs. Zdeblick reported on the results of fusion in lumbar degenerative disorders in a prospective clinical series of 124 patients (52). Patients were randomized into three groups; posterolateral fusion without instrumentation, posterolateral fusion with semirigid plate-screw instrumentation, and posterolateral fusion with rigid rod-screw constructs. The overall 1-year fusion rate determined by radiographic analysis showed fusion rates of 65%, 77%, and 95%, respectively. The fusion rate among those procedures augmented with rigid transpedicular fixation was significantly increased as compared with the other groups. In addition, the overall good to excellent clinical results were greater in the rigid instrumentation group (95%) as compared with the semirigid (89%) and uninstrumented groups (71%).

Biomechanical Considerations of Transpedicular Fixation

Transpedicular fixation permits rigid stabilization of the spine, which improves the fusion rate. Goel et al. (75) demonstrated a 70% reduction in flexion-extension and 65% decrease in lateral bending and axial motion with transpedicular fixation in a cadaver model. Kanayama et al. (76) observed significantly higher stiffness, more woven bone, and earlier fusion following instrumentation compared with uninstrumented fusion in a sheep model and concluded that spinal instrumentation creates a stable mechanical environment to enhance the early bone healing of spinal fusion. Kotani et al. (77) demonstrated that transpedicular fixation significantly contributed to anterior and middle column load sharing even after successful posterolateral fusion, when eccentric loading was applied *in vivo* in sheep. McAfee et al. (78) demonstrated an increased rate and cross-sectional area of fusion when posterior instrumentation was performed following anterior and posterior destabilization of the L5-6 motion segment in a beagle model. Although increased fusion rate was observed with a more rigid instrumentation, stiffer constructs also were associated with more severe device-related osteoporosis, although the clinical significance of this was unclear.

Several patient- and implant-related variables may affect the rigidity of transpedicular constructs. Inner diameter of the pedicle is the critical surgical diameter, and is directly related to the height of the patient, but not the gender (79). Several studies also have demonstrated that there are no significant racial differences in the morphology of the pedicle (80–83). Increasing the minor diameter of the pedicle screw decreases the risk of rate of screw fracture, whereas the major diameter, with greater depth of threads, determines the pullout strength of pedicle screws. Pedicle cortical disruption is unlikely if screw diameter is less than the endosteal diameter or is less than 80% of the cortical diameter (84). Consequently, determination of pedicular dimensions is important in preoperative planning.

Pedicle screws are available in conical and cylindrical designs. The potential advantages of conical pedicle screw design include less plastic deformation of the pedicle and improved thread purchase by compacting the cancellous bone at the cancellous–cortical bone interface throughout the pedicle. However, conical screws must be inserted to a correct depth, and loss of pullout strength may occur if the screw is backed out. In a calf model, Lill et al. (85) demonstrated that pullout strength of conical screws that had been backed out half a turn (180 degrees) was diminished by 50% even without cyclic loading. In

contrast, the pullout strength of cylindrical screws was that had been similarly backed out diminished only after cyclic loading.

Pintar et al. (86) performed a biomechanical study with the rods placed medial or lateral to the pedicle screws, and noted up to a 20% decrease in stiffness of transpedicular configuration with medial placement of longitudinal rods without cross connectors, compared with laterally placed rods without cross connectors. However, there was no significant difference in flexibility of the constructs with medially or laterally placed rods when one or more cross connectors were placed. They concluded that transverse connectors are necessary for constructs with medially placed rods to achieve rotational stiffness.

Although a few biomechanical studies have failed to show any biomechanical advantage of cross-linking of left and right longitudinal members (87,88), cross connectors are generally believed to significantly improve the torsional rigidity of the construct (89,90). Dick et al. (89) reported 44% increase in the torsional stiffness of pedicular constructs when one cross connector was used, and an additional 26% increase was noted with two cross-links. Cross sectional area of the cross-link correlated well with increase in torsional stiffness of a cross-linked construct. However, cross-links do not increase stiffness in the lateral flexion mode.

Several authors have recommended convergent placement of the pedicle screws (36,91,92), which decreases the likelihood of injury to the adjacent facet joints and allows insertion of a longer pedicle screw. Angled entry of the pedicle screws also provides an interlocking effect, which, in combination with longer screws, improves the pullout strength of the construct. In a biomechanical study, paired pedicle screws inserted at 30 degrees of convergence provided 28.6% higher resistance to axial pullout than paired pedicle screws placed in parallel (93). The pullout strength is also increased if the screw is placed into the end plate.

Biomechanical studies also have evaluated the optimal depth of insertion of the pedicle screw (91,94). The pedicles offer approximately 60% of fixation strength in the lumbar spine. An increase in the depth of insertion from 50% to 80% of the vertebral body improves the fixation strength by 30% (91). However, pedicle screws inserted to 80% of the anteroposterior depth of the vertebral body on lateral radiographs may penetrate the anterior cortex 10% to 30% of the time (95). The risk of potentially catastrophic vascular complications far outweighs the minor biomechanical advantages of bicortical fixation in lumbar spine (Fig. 25-2). However, bicortical fixation can be achieved safely in the sacrum by directing the screw medially, which increases the fixation strength by as much as 60%.

The bone–screw interface remains the most critical factor in determining the rigidity of transpedicular construct. Several authors (96,97) have shown that a higher

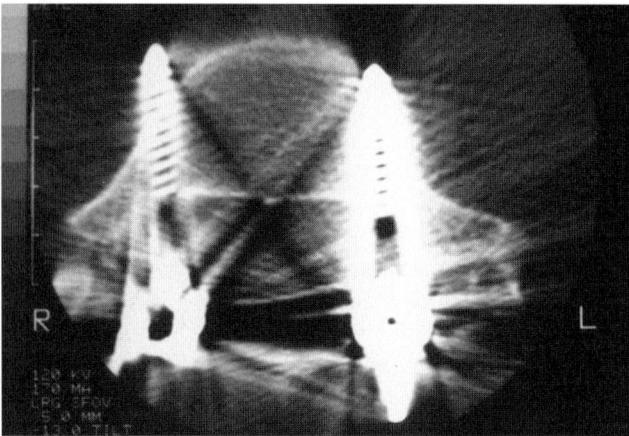

FIG. 25-2. Long screws may cause catastrophic vascular complications.

torque of insertion correlates with a higher screw pullout force. Halvorson et al. (98) showed that the pedicle screw pullout strength correlated highly with bone mineral density. Therefore, insertional torque aids the surgeon in determining overall quality of bone mineral density and gauges the rigidity of the pedicular construct intraoperatively. However, intraoperative insertional torque of pedicle screws is a poor predictor of postoperative screw loosening (99).

Poor fixation, intraoperative pedicle fracture, or postoperative screw migration with consequent risk of neurologic injury are major concerns in the presence of osteoporosis (Fig. 25-3). Biomechanical studies have shown that either untapping or undertapping the pedicle hole may improve the pullout force of pedicle screw in the osteoporotic spine (94,98). The bone mineral density of the lamina is affected less severely than that of the pedicles. Coe et al. (100) showed that the mean tensile

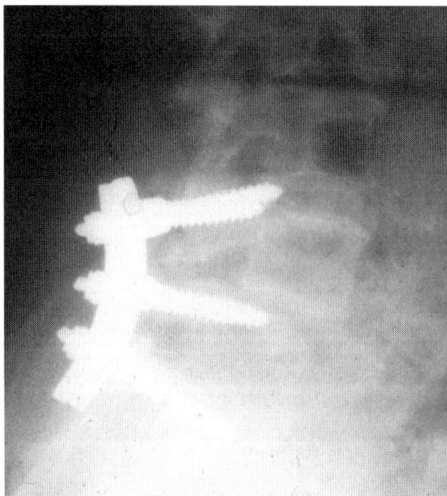

FIG. 25-3. Hardware migration in a patient with osteoporosis.

strength of lamina hook is 646 N lamina, and lamina hooks provide better fixation than pedicle screws in patients with severe osteoporosis. Other authors have also reported significant improvement in the stiffness of the construct when the pedicle screws are inserted in conjunction with laminar hooks (98,101–103).

Biomechanical and animal studies also have been performed to evaluate the efficacy of cement augmentation in improving the stiffness of pedicle screw based constructs. Pfeifer et al. (104) reported that low-pressure injection of polymethylmethacrylate (PMMA) into the pedicles increased the original pullout strength by 149% compared with 70% increase with milled bone and 56% increase with matchstick graft. Other investigators (105,106) have also reported improvement in pedicle screw pullout strength by PMMA injection into the pedicle. However, injection of PMMA into the pedicles may cause neurologic damage from extrusion of the cement into the spinal canal, and may complicate revision of the pedicle screw.

In one biomechanical study, revision of a 6-mm pedicle screw with a 7-mm screw decreased the pullout strength to 73% of the original pullout strength, but a 325% improvement was noted when a 7-mm screw was augmented with hydroxyapatite (107). In another study on human cadaveric lumbar vertebrae, Lotz et al. (108) demonstrated that augmentation of pedicle screws with injectable carbonated apatite cancellous bone cement improved the pullout strength of pedicle screws by 68%, and improved overall biomechanical performance by 30% to 63% on cyclic loading. Calcium phosphate cement augmentation increases the pullout strength of the pedicle screws by 10% compared with 147% increase by use of PMMA (105). The advantage of these newer bone cement materials is that they are bioabsorbable and are replaced during healing and normal bone remodeling.

Stainless Steel versus Titanium Implants

Titanium alloy implants have several potential advantages over stainless steel implants. Titanium implants offer superior MRI resolution (109–111), making it easier to interpret postoperative MRI scans. High bioactivity and more flexibility of titanium implants also may improve bone ingrowth and mechanical fixation. In an animal model, Christensen et al. (112) demonstrated 33% more bone growth with higher mechanical binding at the bone–screw interface with use of titanium implant. Generation of particulate debris, however, may occur with the use of titanium implant in the presence of pseudarthrosis. Histopathologic evaluation of periimplant tissue samples obtained during revision surgery in patients with failed lumbar fusion and titanium instrumentation revealed that the wear particles generated by titanium implants are present both in a free state within the fibrous tissue and intracellularly within the macrophages. The latter evokes a macrophage cellular response in tissues similar to that seen in total joint replacements. Patients with a solid spinal fusion have negligible levels of particulate debris (113,114).

TRANSPEDICULAR INSTRUMENTATION

The goals of adding instrumentation to a posterior lumbar fusion procedure are enhancement of the fusion rate, maintenance of correction of deformity while the fusion incorporates, preservation of maximum possible segments, and shortening of the time required for rehabilitation of the patient. The immediate rigidity provided by pedicle screw instrumentation permits earlier, more aggressive rehabilitation without the requirement for an external brace. Important principles of transpedicular instrumentation are careful patient selection, safe and reliable method of insertion of pedicle screws, restoration of spinal alignment, meticulous preparation of the fusion bed, and sound fusion technique. The instrumentation also should be easy to use, and surgeon familiarity with instrumentation system is paramount.

Preoperative Evaluation

Appropriate conservative management should be implemented before surgical treatment. Physical therapy or home exercises and nonsteroidal antiinflammatory drugs (NSAIDs) are recommended. Nonsteroidal antiinflammatory drugs should be used sparingly in the elderly population because of potential complications. If conservative treatment fails, it should be followed by a more detailed evaluation with additional imaging studies such as MRI or CT myelogram. In addition, provocative testing including discography, facet block, or selective nerve root injections may be necessary to determine the pain generator. Overall sagittal alignment should be evaluated on standing lateral radiographs, and the presence or absence of segmental instability should be determined on flexion-extension lateral radiographs. All this information helps the spine surgeon to formulate an appropriate surgical treatment plan that is tailored individually to each patient.

Specific anatomy of the lumbar spine should be carefully reviewed in each patient. Typically, the sagittal diameter of pedicle is greatest at the thoracolumbar level and decreases caudally, whereas transverse diameter of the pedicle is widest at L5 and gradually decreases at more proximal levels. The transverse diameter is the primary factor that determines the size of the pedicle screw. Plain radiographs reveal the relationship of the pedicle to each articular facet and transverse process. Preoperative knowledge of the mediolateral inclination of the pedicle in the presence of rotation is particularly helpful in patients with degenerative scoliosis. Preoperative and intraoperative lateral radiographs provide information on the cranial–caudal inclination of the pedicles at each level. The presence of identifiable transverse processes on AP radiographs also facilitates intraoperative estimation of the location of the pedicle in revision cases complicated by failed fusion. Computed tomographic or MRI axial images at the level of the pedicle also allow determination of appropriate medial-lateral angulation along with the dimensions of each pedicle.

Determination of bone quality also should be made, and a dual energy X-ray absorptiometry scan may be indicated in certain patients. Instrumentation is best avoided in elderly patients with osteoporosis because of relatively poor fixation afforded by transpedicular instrumentation and higher risk of intraoperative complications, including pedicle fracture, longer operating time, increased blood loss, and potentially higher infection rate. The risk of secondary neurologic complications from hardware migration and loss of fixation is significant as well.

All patients on chronic narcotic medications should be considered for detoxification prior to surgery, and a smoking cessation program should be advised. Smokers have a significantly higher nonunion rate than nonsmokers (115,116). Brown and associates (116) retrospectively reviewed 100 patients who had undergone one or two level laminectomy and fusion. Forty percent of the smokers developed pseudarthrosis compared with only 8% of nonsmokers. History of smoking is a relative indication for the use of instrumentation to improve fusion rate. Finally, preoperative donation of autologous blood should be recommended for all lumbar fusion procedures. Although preoperative administration of Procrit (epoetin alfa) has been advocated by some total joint surgeons to minimize the need for blood transfusion, its role in spine surgery has not been investigated.

Intraoperative Considerations

Although the choice of an operating table is surgeon dependent, it is critical that attention is paid to restoration of lumbar lordosis during positioning. Proper positioning of the upper extremities and placement of sequential compression stockings are necessary. Intravenous antibiotics are routinely administered and repeated throughout the procedure. Preoperative antibiotics have been demonstrated to diminish the incidence of deep postoperative infection in patients undergoing instrumented fusion (117). Intraoperative blood loss is minimized by use of appropriate hypotensive anesthesia, proper positioning without any pressure on the abdomen, meticulous hemostasis, and use of cell saver, particularly in multilevel fusion cases and revision procedures. Autograft iliac bone is preferred by most spine surgeons and remains the gold standard. Cancellous chip allograft and demineralized bone matrix also are frequently used as graft expanders. Bone morphogenic proteins such as RhBMP-

2 (Infuse), BMP-7 (OP-1), and BMP-14 (MP 52) are currently available for investigational use only. Bone morphogenic proteins may eliminate the need for autograft harvesting in the future if their effectiveness in achieving successful fusion is demonstrated in prospective controlled randomized studies.

The need for safe and accurate placement of pedicle screws cannot be overemphasized. Malpositioning of pedicle screws may cause dural laceration or neural injury (Fig. 25-4). Proper screw placement can be particularly difficult in revision lumbar surgery and in patients with significant degenerative scoliosis. In one of the earliest reported series on transpedicular instrumentation, Roy-Camille (8) reported a 10% incidence of incorrect placement of lumbar pedicle screws. Up to 40% of pedicle screws were placed incorrectly, and medial placement was noted in 29% in a recent study. A medial placement of 6 mm or more was significantly associated a neurologic injury (118). Schulze et al. (119) obtained CT scans in 50 patients after routine removal of 244 pedicle screws to eliminate any artifact from the hardware. Fifty-nine percent of screw tracks were located centrally within the pedicles, and 20% had violated the medial cortex by 2 mm or less. One patient had a neurologic injury because of pedicle screw malposition.

Roy-Camille (8,9) originally described use of a drill to create a pathway for the pedicle screw. However, creation of a burr hole at the screw entry point, followed by free hand development of screw tract with either a stiff probe (gearshift) or a curet, has currently become the most popular method of hole preparation. Boachie-Adjei et al. (120) found the free hand placement of pedicle screws to be safe, reliable, and cost effective in a prospective study of 50 patients with adult spinal deformity. Only 3% of screws were misplaced and 1% violated the medial wall, none with any clinical sequelae, in that study.

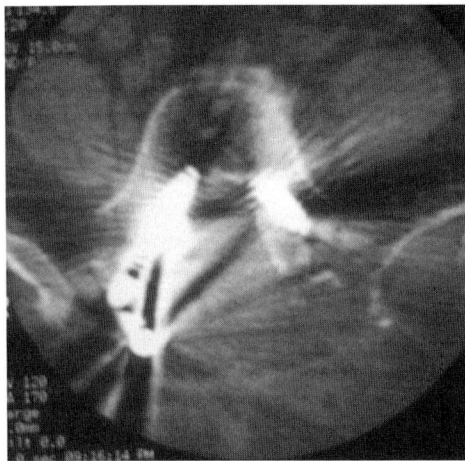

FIG. 25-4. Medial placement of pedicle screw may cause neurologic deficit and dural laceration.

Meter et al. (121) demonstrated that a true lateral or AP radiographic view of the vertebra provides a high degree of certainty that the screw has not crossed the end plate when a safe zone of 3 mm remains cephalad to the screw tip. Although intraoperative radiography can reduce concern about violation of the superior vertebral end plate, excessive use of intraoperative fluoroscopy should be avoided for fear of cumulative exposure to radiation (122). Biplanar roentgenography is only 73% to 83% accurate in determining position of the screw within the pedicle (123). Odgers et al. (124) prospectively inserted 238 screws from the T11 to L5 vertebral levels with the assistance of lateral plain radiographs. Eighteen screws had penetrated the pedicle wall medially and six laterally. Two screws penetrated the anterior vertebral body cortex. The overall success rate was 89.1%, and only two patients (0.84%) had neurologic complications. They concluded that pedicle screw insertion with the aid of lateral radiographs is safe and effective, and minimizes the operative time and expense arising from biplanar fluoroscopy.

Screw stimulation monitoring is a valuable adjunct to lumbar pedicle screw instrumentation. Several authors have demonstrated the usefulness of intraoperative screw testing by electrical stimulation to determine appropriate placement of pedicle screws (125–127). In general, electromyographic activity at a stimulation threshold of 8 to 10 mA is associated with breach in pedicle cortex, and activity at 4 to 6 mA or less is indicative of screw contact with nerve root or the dura. A stimulation threshold of 15 mA provides a 98% confidence in accuracy of pedicle screw placement.

Tactile sensory skills, anatomic knowledge, judicious usage of intraoperative radiography, and additional modalities such as electromyography monitoring are important in correct placement of pedicle screws. Several authors have reported favorable early experience with computer-assisted frameless stereotactic image guidance (128–131) and robot-assisted insertion techniques (132) in placement of pedicle screws in the lumbar spine. Frank et al. (133) reported the use of a malleable endoscope to visualize the pedicle cortex. However, these techniques are still evolving, and have not been fully evaluated. Moreover, these newer techniques are expensive, and their usefulness remains questionable at this time, given a high degree of accuracy with freehand placement of pedicle screws in all but certain revision cases and in patients with significant spinal deformity.

Percutaneous placement of pedicle screws is being developed also (134), but lack of adequate preparation of the intertransverse fusion bed as well as potentially higher risk of neurologic injury remain major points of concern. Most minimally invasive systems are designed to allow percutaneous screw insertion, and interbody fusion through a small tubular retractor. Some of the purported advantages of these minimally invasive approaches are reduced morbidity, less blood loss, cosmetically appealing smaller incisions, and reduced scarring. Such procedures, however, are technically highly demanding, have a high learning curve and limited application, and their usefulness has not yet been clearly documented in prospective studies.

Operative Technique

Important surgical principles of transpedicular instrumentation are strong biomechanical characteristics at the bone–implant interface, safe insertion of screws without neurovascular complications, avoidance of damage to the adjacent facet joints, and restoration of the sagittal balance. Wide surgical exposure of bony landmarks including the transverse processes, pars, and the mamillary processes is the first important step in accurate placement of lumbar pedicle screws. The facet joints at levels not included in the fusion must be preserved. When the sacrum is included in the fusion, lumbosacral facet joints and the ala are exposed, and the location of the first dorsal sacral foramen is determined. When decompression is performed as an integral part of the procedure, palpation of the pedicles from within the canal with the help of a Woodson also helps in determining the location of the pedicle. The accessory process is located in line with the lateral border of the pedicle, whereas the lateral border of pars interarticularis usually coincides with the center of L5 pedicle and medial border of the remaining lumbar pedicles (135).

Several methods of insertion of pedicle screws have been described. Roy-Camille (8,9) described a "straight-ahead" technique where the entrance point is chosen at the intersection of the middle third of the transverse process and a vertical line bisecting the center of the facet joint. A drill is then used to create the pathway for the screw, which is inserted parallel to the end plates in the sagittal plane. The Magerl technique (136) differs from that of Roy-Camille in that the entrance point is chosen at the intersection of the mid portion of the transverse process and the inferolateral aspect of the superior articular process, which allows more medial insertion of the screw parallel with the end plates. This course allows a longer-length screw to be inserted. A superomedially directed pedicle screw at the cranial end of the construct also has been recommended. The entry point for this superiorly directed screw tends to be at the intersection of the inferior one third of the transverse process and the vertical line along the lateral aspect of the superior articular facet (91). The advantage of this technique is that the prominent screw head is less likely to cause impingement at the adjacent intact facet joint at the cranial extent of the fusion. Gaines (137) recommends a direct funnel technique to identify and tap the pedicle isthmus, thereby obtaining a cortical purchase within the pedicle.

The sacral screws may be directed laterally into the ala, or more commonly, medially into the promontory (138,139). Insertion of sacral pedicle screws requires knowledge of the unique anatomy in this region. The entry point for S1 pedicle screws is located at a point inferolateral to the superior facet, and the screw is inserted caudally parallel with the superior surface of the sacrum. The screw is also angled medially to avoid neurovascular and visceral injury. Mirkovic et al. (139) studied the neurovascular and visceral anatomy anterior to the sacrum and noted that the lumbosacral trunk, internal iliac vein, and sacroiliac joint were most commonly at risk during insertion of the S1 pedicle screw. The sigmoid colon and internal iliac vein were most vulnerable to injury during S2 pedicle screw insertion.

Typically, a pilot hole is created with a burr at the entry point of the pedicle, and the pathway into the pedicle and vertebral body is developed either with a pedicle curette or a gearshift. A blunt probe is used to determine if the cortex has been violated. Radiopaque markers are placed in the pedicle holes and intraoperative lateral radiographs or fluoroscopy are used to determine accuracy and inclination of marker placement. Each screw hole is tapped beyond the pedicle into the vertebral body. Probing after the pedicle hole has been tapped provides an unmistakable tactile feedback of the threads within the pedicle. Tapping is optional in patients with osteoporosis. We prefer to perform decortication and preparation of the fusion bed and bone graft placement prior to screw insertion. Electromyographic stimulation of the pedicle screws may be done to further ensure proper screw placement. As the construct is put together with rods and connectors, care must be taken to avoid impingement on the facet joint at the cranial end of the fusion. The instruments must be handled very carefully while inserting the rod or tightening the set screws because inadvertent slippage of instruments into the spinal canal can cause dural laceration and neurologic damage.

Postoperative Care

Instrumentation obviates the absolute necessity of postoperative brace wear after lumbar fusion. However, most patients are typically immobilized in a lumbosacral orthosis or a thoracolumbosacral orthosis, depending on the length of the construct. Duration of brace wear varies depending on surgeon preference, length, and rigidity of the construct, and patient's body habitus and compliance. Transpedicular fixation appears to shorten the duration of postoperative rehabilitation.

Electrical stimulation devices are also sometimes recommended in the postoperative period to enhance fusion. In a controlled prospective study of patients undergoing posterior spinal instrumentation, Kucharzyk (140) reported a slightly improved fusion rate of 95.6% with the use of implantable electrical stimulation compared with 87% in the control group. Fifty-seven percent of patients in the stimulated group had clinical success compared with 46% in the nonstimulated group. Jenis et al. (141) performed a prospective study of 61 patients undergoing instrumented fusion who were randomized to receive no electrical stimulation and implantable device or an external stimulator. They did not find any significant difference in fusion rates in any group. Although there is a scarcity of additional prospective, controlled data on external electrical stimulation in patients with instrumented fusion, the use of external bone stimulation devices may be considered for high-risk patients.

Assessment of bony union is not always straightforward, particularly in the presence of bulky instrumentation. Oblique radiographs may help prevent the hardware from overshadowing the fusion mass and facilitate better assessment of the fusion status. Ferguson view radiographs are necessary for evaluation of lumbosacral fusion. Radiographic demonstration of trabeculation across the intertransverse area is necessary to assess union (142). We routinely also obtain flexion-extension lateral radiographs to document union and detect any instability 6 months postoperatively.

Prolonged stress shielding from retained instrumentation may be of concern. However, Craven et al. (143) reported that initial stress shielding of the bypassed vertebral column that occurs with the use of rigid internal fixation tends to lessen with time in a canine model. They attributed this rebound in the bone mineral density of the fused vertebral segments to several factors, most notably to a shift in load distribution from implant to the spine secondary to screw migration or loosening because of bone remodeling. Additional factors, such as implant–implant interface changes (e.g., loosening and corrosion) also may play a role. However, these authors had used human-sized bicortical pedicle screws in their canine experiment, and the longitudinal loads on the canine spine are typically one tenth of those observed in the human spine.

Retained hardware also may cause irritation from prominent hardware, late hematogenous infection, accelerated degeneration of the adjacent segment, long-term metal toxicity, and increased risk of neurologic injury in the event of future trauma (91). Previous studies (17,144,145) have reported a 12% to 23% incidence of hardware removal owing to local irritation caused by the pedicle screws. However, no data have been reported in the literature to support routine removal of pedicle screws, which in fact, may be dangerous because of significant risk of neurovascular injury. Consequently, routine removal of instrumentation should be avoided.

Complications

The complication rate with the usage of pedicle screw fixation is low if the surgeon is experienced and attention is paid to principles and details of the operative technique. Several authors have reported an acceptable complication rate and risk of neurologic injury during transpedicular instrumentation (17,145–147). In a historical cohort study, Yuan et al. (17) reported a 5% incidence of intraoperative events associated with the use of screws. Loss of purchase (1.7%) and pedicle fracture and screw breakout occurred in 1%. Neurologic injury, dural tear, and screw breakage were rare complications. In a series of 4,790 pedicle screw insertions, Lonstein (145) noted that 5.1% screws were inserted outside the pedicle, and the incidence of permanent nerve root injury owing to pedicle screw insertion was 0.3%.

When neurologic deficit is noted postoperatively, thin-cut CT scan is the imaging study of choice. Sapkas et al. (148) assessed the position of 220 pedicle screws with CT scan and lateral radiographs postoperatively in a prospective manner in 35 consecutive patients. They concluded that although the accuracy of CT imaging is better than that of plain radiographs, the difference is not statistically significant, and postoperative use of plain radiographs is a reliable method for evaluation of pedicle screw insertion in the absence of neurologic deficit. However, when neurologic deficit is present postoperatively, placement of questionable pedicle screws is best evaluated with thin section CT scan. Farber et al. (149) demonstrated that thin-cut CT scan is 10 times more sensitive than plain radiographs in determining violation of the medial cortex.

Postoperative infection in presence of instrumentation is worrisome. Pedicle screw fixation requires longer operative time with concerns of increased infection rates. Wimmer et al. (150) retrospectively reviewed a large series consisting of 574 posterior instrumented fusions and 274 anterior procedures. They identified an infection rate of 21/574 with posterior procedures and 1/274 with anterior surgery. Increased blood loss and prolonged operative time correlated with postoperative infection. Weinstein et al. (151) reviewed a series of 2,391 spinal operations with an overall infection rate of 1.9%. They observed increased infection rate in the presence of instrumentation and in patients with prior history of surgery. However, no significant difference was noted in the rate of infection between uninstrumented and instrumented spinal fusion in a large historic cohort study (17).

Glassman et al. (152) retrospectively reviewed 858 instrumented spinal fusion procedures and noted an overall infection rate of 4.2% and deep wound infection rate of 2.6%. Cigarette smoking and previous back surgery did not predispose to infection in that study. Staphylococcus aureus was the most common offending organism. All patients with deep infection were treated with serial wound irrigation and débridement and antibiotic mixed cement was placed in the lateral gutters. An 80% rate of improvement was noted after an average of 4.7 débridements. These authors concluded that postoperative infection does not adversely affect the rate of fusion. Weinstein et al. (151) also recommend an aggressive surgical approach consisting of repeated débridement followed by delayed wound closure. Viable bone graft and instrumentation may be left *in situ* to provide stability for achieving fusion.

There is a potential for increased blood loss owing to wider surgical exposure that is necessary for visualization of anatomic landmarks for pedicle screw insertion. Bulky pedicle screw based constructs also create a dead space by elevating the paraspinal musculature off the posterior elements, which may increase the risk of postoperative hematoma and infection secondary to a lack of tamponade effect (36).

Screw loosening at the bone–cement interface is the most common mechanism of failure in most pedicle screw instrumentation systems. However, some radiolucency may be present during the time preceding the union (36). Postoperative fracture of the instrumented pedicle is rare and its reported incidence is 0.2% to 2.7% of patients (143,144,146). Macdessi et al. (153) reported development of bilateral pedicle stress fractures at the uppermost level of the fusion mass in a patient 2 years after pedicle screw removal from an L4-S1 instrumented posterolateral lumbar spine fusion. They concluded that the pedicle is the weakest point in the neural arch after posterolateral fusion. Although movement continues at the level of the disc space anteriorly, the pedicle is susceptible to fracture.

Breakage of pedicle screws is uncommon with newer designs. Breakage of pedicle screws occurred in 0.5% of all screws in 2.2% patients in one study, in which most broken screws were of earlier designs (144). Screw breakage occurred more commonly with greater intervertebral motion, less anterior column loading, and presence of tall discs. Broken screws are not necessarily associated with pseudarthrosis (50), and breakage of hardware does not always require surgical management (Fig. 25-5).

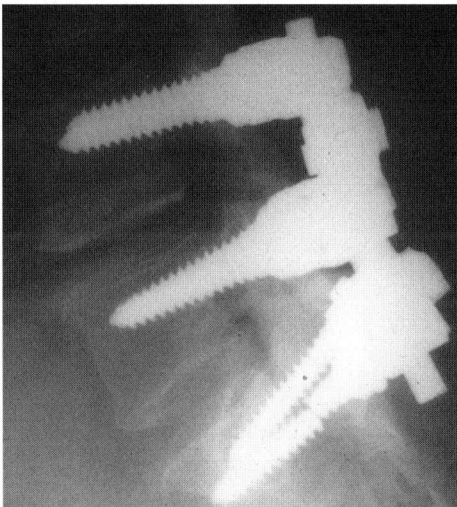

FIG. 25-5. Patients with broken hardware may have pseudarthrosis.

However, fusion status must be thoroughly evaluated in symptomatic patients, because up to two thirds of patients with broken screws may have pseudarthrosis (144).

Adjacent Segment Degeneration

Adjacent segment degeneration has been known to occur in patients with spinal fusion even before the use of instrumentation became widespread. Whether adjacent segment degeneration is a continuing degenerative process or a late complication of fusion is debatable. A solid fusion alters the biomechanics at the adjacent level, resulting in increased mechanical demands. Increased biomechanical forces, mobility, and intradiscal pressure in adjacent segments after fusion have been hypothesized to accelerate the pathologic changes (154–156). Lee (157) suggested that increased adjacent level changes after fusion occur because of stress concentration and posterior displacement of the center of rotation at the adjacent segment.

Whether instrumented fusion leads to acceleration in the degenerative process of the adjacent segments is not clear. Static kinematic testing has shown increased motion at adjacent segments in pedicle screw-based constructs (158). Stress transfer to the adjacent joints increases with increasing number of levels included in the fused segments (159). Wimmer et al. reported that adjacent segment degeneration was more common with multilevel than single-level instrumented circumferential fusion (160). Additionally, part of the facet joint cephalad to the fusion may be resected during insertion of the pedicle screws, or the hardware itself may abut against the facet joint, causing damage to it (91).

Degeneration most commonly occurs in the segment immediately cephalad to the fused segment. However, the next segment adjacent to that segment also has been reported to break down in 58% patients in one study (161). Aota et al. (162) reviewed 65 patients who underwent wide laminectomy, Cotrel-Dubousset instrumentation, and fusion for lumbar degenerative disorders. They used the Roy-Camille technique for insertion of pedicle screw, which involved resection of the tip of the inferior facet. They reported 24.6% incidence of postfusion instability, with a vast majority involving the adjacent segment above the fusion level. Seventy-eight percent instability occurred in sagittal plane and retrolisthesis was the most common instability pattern (nine of 15 patients). Age of the patient appeared to be the most significant factor, with a 36.7% incidence in patients older than 55 years compared with 12% incidence in younger patients.

Etebar and Cahill (163) reported adjacent segment degeneration in 18 of 125 consecutive patients who underwent instrumented posterior lumbar fusion for degenerative instability of the lumbar spine. The mean follow-up was 44.8 months. Twenty percent of all patients with next-segment failure were cigarette smokers. Adjacent segment involvement included spondylolisthesis (39%), stenosis (33%), stress fracture of the adjacent vertebral body (28%), and scoliosis (17%) in their study. The risk of adjacent-segment failure was particularly high in postmenopausal women with nearly 50% incidence. In a retrospective review of 49 patients who underwent instrumented lumbar fusion, Rahm and Hall (164) noted 35% incidence of adjacent-segment degeneration, and its occurrence was associated with increasing patient age, the use of interbody fusion, and a worsening of clinical results with time. An average of 2.5 levels were fused in their patient population with a mean age of 53.8 years. Based on their retrospective analysis of 83 patients, Kumar et al. (165) recommended restoration of sagittal alignment and normality of sacral inclination as paramount in minimizing the incidence of adjacent segment breakdown.

In contrast, Wiltse (166) concluded from a comparative study of 52 patients with instrumented fusion and a control group of 31 of uninstrumented fusion that the addition of pedicle screw fixation does not increase the incidence or severity of adjacent segment degeneration in the first 7 years after surgery.

It is clear that adjacent segment degeneration following instrumented lumbar fusion is a topic of major concern among spine surgeons. A thorough understanding of the patient- and surgeon-related factors may aid the surgeon in reducing the incidence of the degenerative process of adjacent unfused segments. Some of the surgeon-related factors include meticulous surgical techniques with preservation of the facet joint capsule, avoidance of facet damage during pedicle screw insertion or abutment of the facet joints against the hardware, and restoration of sagittal balance. Finally, careful consideration should be given to the health of adjacent discs and facet joints for possible inclusion in the proposed levels of fusion and prevention of early breakdown of an adjacent disc.

COST ANALYSIS

There has been significant increase in the number of instrumented fusion procedures performed in last several years. The economic implications of widening use of instrumentation in lumbar fusion procedures, their cost effectiveness, and potential value to the society are now receiving increased scrutiny. Katz et al. (167) performed a prospective observational study of 272 patients and concluded that uninstrumented fusion provided superior pain relief at 6 and 24 months postoperatively. They also noted that concomitant uninstrumented fusion procedure increased the hospital cost of decompressive laminectomy by 50% and instrumented fusion increased the cost by 100%, compared with patients who underwent uninstrumented fusion. Kuntz et al. (168) calculated the 10-year costs, quality-adjusted life years, and incremental cost effectiveness ratio of fusion lumbar fusion proce-

dures with and without instrumentation, and found instrumented fusion to be significantly more expensive in terms of incremental gain in health outcome. Gibson et al. (169) conducted meta-analysis of instrumented versus uninstrumented fusion and noted improved fusion rate with instrumentation, but no difference in the clinical outcome of the two groups. Whether the added cost of instrumentation is worth the benefit in overall health outcome remains a controversial and unresolved issue.

CONCLUSIONS

Pedicle screw fixation is a safe and reliable method of achieving rigid internal fixation of the lumbar spine in the hands of experienced surgeons. Instrumentation improves the rate of fusion and clinical outcome in certain degenerative disorders of the lumbar spine. However, more clinical data are needed for establishing the role of transpedicular fixation in patients with discogenic back pain. Although pedicle screw fixation offers several advantages, it should be used judiciously in carefully selected patients to minimize the risk of untoward complications. The risk-benefit ratio of adding instrumentation must be analyzed carefully, particularly in elderly patients. Finally, sound surgical principles of fusion must be practiced.

REFERENCES

1. Graves EJ. Detailed diagnoses and procedures, National Hospital Discharge Survey, 1993. Vital Health Stat 1995;122:1–288.
2. Davis H. Increasing rates of cervical and lumbar spine surgery in the United States, 1979–1990. Spine 1994;19:1117–1123.
3. King, D. Internal fixation for lumbosacral fusion. J Bone Joint Surg 1948;30A:560–565.
4. Harrington PR. Treatment of scoliosis: correction and internal fixation by spinal instrumentation. J Bone Joint Surg 1962;44A:591–610.
5. Sidhu K, Herkowitz H. Spinal instrumentation in the management of degenerative disorders of the lumbar spine. Clin Orthop Rel Res 1997;335:39–53.
6. Luque E. The anatomic basis and development of segmental spinal instrumentation. Spine 1982;7:256–259.
7. Boucher H. A method of spinal fusion. J Bone Joint Surg 1959;41B:248–259.
8. Roy-Camille R, Saillant G, Mazel C. Internal fixation of the lumbar spine with pedicle screw plating. Clin Orthop Rel Res 1986;203:7–17.
9. Roy-Camille R, Saillant G, Mazel C. Plating of thoracic, thoracolumbar, and lumbar injuries with pedicle screw-plates. Orthop Clin North Am 1986;17:147–159.
10. Steffee AD, Biscup RS, Sitkowski DJ. Segmental spine plates with pedicle screw fixation. A new internal fixation device for disorders of the lumbar and thoracolumbar spine. Clin Orthop Rel Res 1986;203:45–53.
11. Matsunaga S, Sakou T, Morizono Y, et al. Natural history of degenerative spondylolisthesis. Pathogenesis and natural course of the slippage. Spine 1990;15:1204–1210.
12. Postacchini F, Cinotti G, Perugia D. Degenerative lumbar spondylolisthesis. II. Surgical treatment. Ital J Orthop Traumatol 1991;17:467–477.
13. Herkowitz H, Kurz L. Degenerative lumbar spondylolisthesis with spinal stenosis. J Bone Joint Surg 1991;73A:802–808.
14. MuCulloch JA. Microdecompression and uninstrumented single level fusion for spinal canal stenosis with degenerative spondylolisthesis. Spine 1998;23:2243–2252.

15. Fischgrund JS, Mackay M, Herkowitz HN, et al. 1997 Volvo Award winner in clinical studies. Degenerative lumbar spondylolisthesis with spinal stenosis: a prospective, randomized study comparing decompressive laminectomy and arthrodesis with and without spinal instrumentation. Spine 1997;22:2807–2812.

16. Kornblum MB, Fishgrund JS, Herkowitz HN, et al. Degenerative lumbar spondylolisthesis with spinal stenosis: a prospective long-term study comparing fusion and pseudarthrosis. In: Proceedings of North American Spine Society, October 25–28, 2000. 15th Annual Meeting, New Orleans.

17. Yuan HA, Garfin SR, Dickman CA, et al. A historical cohort study of pedicle screw fixation in thoracic, lumbar, and sacral spinal fusions. Spine 1994;20S:2279S–2296S.

18. Booth KC, Bridwell KH, Eisenberg BA, et al. Minimum 5-year results of degenerative spondylolisthesis treated with decompression and instrumented posterior fusion. Spine 1999;24(16):1721–1727.

19. Steffee AD, Brantigan JW. The variable screw placement spinal fixation system. Report of a prospective study of 250 patients enrolled in Food and Drug administration clinical trials. Spine 1993;18:1160–1172.

20. Bridwell K, Sedgewick T, O'Brien M, et al. The role of fusion and instrumentation in the treatment of degenerative spondylolisthesis with spinal stenosis. J Spinal Disord 1993;6:461–472.

21. Nork SE, Hu SS, Workman KL, et al. Patient outcomes after decompression and instrumented posterior spinal fusion for degenerative spondylolisthesis. Spine 1999;24:561–569.

22. Thomsen K, Christensen FB, Eiskjaer SP, et al. 1997 Volvo Award winner in clinical studies. The effect of pedicle screw instrumentation on functional outcome and fusion rates in posterolateral lumbar spinal fusion: a prospective, randomized clinical study. Spine 1997;22:2813–2822.

23. McGuire R, Amundson G. The use of primary internal fixation in spondylolisthesis. Spine 1993;18:1662–1672.

24. Bernhardt M, Swartz DE, Clothiaux PL, et al. Posterolateral lumbar and lumbosacral fusion with and without pedicle screw internal fixation. Clin Orthop Rel Res 1992;284:109–115.

25. France JC, Yaszemski MJ, Lauerman WC, et al. A randomized prospective study of posterolateral lumbar fusion. Outcomes with and without pedicle screw instrumentation. Spine 1999;24:553–560.

26. Bridwell K. Acquired degenerative spondylolisthesis without lysis. In: Bridwell K, ed. The textbook of spinal surgery. Philadelphia: Lippincott-Raven, 1997:1299–1316.

27. Pritchett J, Bortel D. Degenerative symptomatic lumbar scoliosis. Spine 1993;18:700–703.

28. Garfin SR, Herkowitz HN, Mirkovic S. Spinal stenosis. J Bone Joint Surg 1999;81A:572–586.

29. Abumi K, Panjabi MM, Kramer KM, et al. Biomechanical evaluation of lumbar spine stability after graded facetectomies. Spine 1990;15:1142–1147.

30. Southern EP, An HS. Principles of spinal instrumentation in adult deformities. In: An HS, Cotler JM. Spinal instrumentation, 2nd ed. Philadelphia: Lippincott Williams & Wilkins, 1999:131–147.

31. Simmons ED. Surgical treatment of patients with lumbar spinal stenosis with associated scoliosis. Clin Orthop Rel Res 2001;384:45–53.

32. Inufusa A, An HS, Glover JM, et al. The ideal amount of lumbar foraminal distraction for pedicle screw instrumentation. Spine 1996;21:2218–2223.

33. McPhee IB, Swanson CE. The surgical management of degenerative lumbar scoliosis. Posterior instrumentation alone versus two stage surgery. Bull Hosp Jt Dis 1998;57(1):16–22.

34. Simmons E Jr, Simmons E. Spinal stenosis with scoliosis. Spine 1992;17:117S–120S.

35. Marchesi D, Aebi M. Pedicle fixation devices in the treatment of adult lumbar scoliosis. Spine 1992;17:S304–S309.

36. Jenis LG, An HS. Principles of spinal instrumentation in adult deformities. In: An HS, Cotler JM. Spinal instrumentation, 2nd ed. Philadelphia: Lippincott Williams & Wilkins, 1999:121–130.

37. Mullin BB, Rea GL, Irsik R, et al. The effect of post laminectomy spinal instability on the outcome of lumbar spinal stenosis patients. J Spinal Disord 1996;9:107–116.

38. Hopp E, Tsou P. Postdecompression lumbar instability. Clin Orthop Rel Res 1988;227:143–151.

39. Garfin S, Herkowitz H, Mirkovic S, et al. Nonoperative and operative treatment. In: Rothman R, Simeone F, eds. The spine, 3rd ed. Philadelphia: WB Saunders, 1992:857–875.

40. Waddell G, Kummell EG, Lotto WN, et al. Failed lumbar disc surgery and repeat surgery following industrial injuries. J Bone Joint Surg 1979;61A:201–207.

41. Hansraj KK, O'Leary PF, Cammisa FP Jr, et al. Decompression, fusion, and instrumentation surgery for complex lumbar spinal stenosis. Clin Orthop Rel Res 2001;384:18–25.

42. Postacchini F. Surgical management of lumbar spinal stenosis. Spine 1999;24:1043–1047.

43. Postacchini F, Cinotti G. Bone regrowth after surgical decompression for lumbar spinal stenosis. J Bone Joint Surg 1992;74:862–869.

44. Herno A, Airakisinen O, Saari T. Long term results of surgical treatment of lumbar spinal stenosis. Spine 1993;18:1471–1474.

45. Stauffer R, Coventry M. Posterior lateral lumbar spine fusion. J Bone Joint Surg 1972;54A:1195–1204.

46. Steinmann JC, Herkowitz HN. Pseudarthrosis of the spine. Clin Orthop Rel Res 1992;284:80–90.

47. Kant AP, Daum WJ, Dean SM, et al. Evaluation of lumbar spine fusion. Plain radiographs versus direct surgical exploration and observation. Spine 1995;20:2313–2317.

48. Larsen JM, Capen DA. Pseudarthrosis of the lumbar spine. JAAOS 1197;5:153–162.

49. Lauerman WC, Bradford DS, Ogilvie JW, et al. Results of lumbar pseudoarthrosis repair. J Spinal Disord 1992;5:149–157.

50. West JL 3rd, Bradford DS, Ogilvie JW, et al. Results of spinal arthrodesis with pedicle screw-plate fixation. J Bone Joint Surg (Am) 1991;73:1179–1184.

51. Horowitch A, Peek RD, Thomas JC, et al. The Wiltse pedicle screw fixation system. Early clinical results. Spine 1989;14:461–467.

52. Zdeblick TA. A prospective, randomized study of lumbar fusion. Preliminary results. Spine 1993;18:983–991.

53. Carpenter CT, Dietz JW, Leung KY, et al. Repair of a pseudarthrosis of the lumbar spine. A functional outcome study. J Bone Joint Surg Am 1996;78:712–720.

54. Kim SS, Michelsen CB. Revision surgery for failed back surgery syndrome. Spine 1992;17:957–960.

55. Stewart G, Sachs BL. Patient outcomes after reoperation on the lumbar spine. J Bone Joint Surg Am 1996;78:706–711.

56. Bridwell KH, Lenke LG, Lewis SJ. Treatment of spinal stenosis and fixed sagittal imbalance. Clin Orthop Rel Res 2001;384:35–44.

57. Lorenz M, Zindrik M, Schwaegler P, et al. A comparison of single-level fusions with and without hardware. Spine 1991;16S:455S–458S.

58. Louis R. Fusion of the lumbar and sacral spine by internal fixation with screw-plates. Clin Orthop Rel Res 1986;203:18–33.

59. Grubb S, Lipscomb H. Results of lumbosacral fusion for degenerative disc disease with and without instrumentation. Spine 1992;17:349–355.

60. Schwab FJ, Nazarian DG, Mahmud F, et al. Effects of spinal instrumentation on fusion of the lumbosacral spine. Spine 1995;20:2023–2028.

61. Dawson EG, Lotysch M 3rd, Urist MR. Intertransverse process lumbar arthrodesis with autogenous bone graft. Clin Orthop Rel Res 1981;154:90–96.

62. Hellstadius A. Experiences gained from spondylo-syndesis operations with H shaped bone transplantations in the case of degeneration of discs in the lumbar back. Acta Orthop Scand 1955;24:207–215.

63. Shaw EG, Taylor JG. The results of lumbosacral fusion for low back pain. J Bone Joint Surg 1956;38B:485–497.

64. Wood GW, Boyd RJ, Carothers TA, et al. The effect of pedicle screw/plate fixation on lumbar/lumbosacral autogenous bone graft fusions in patients with degenerative disc disease. Spine 1995;20:819–830.

65. Spengler DM. Perspectives on the indications and surgical management of patients with selected degenerative disorders of the lumbar spine. In: Bridwell KH, DeWald RL, eds. Philadelphia: Lippincott-Raven, 1997:1533–1545.

66. Whitecloud TS III, Wolfe MW. Indications for internal fixation and fusion in the degenerative lumbar spine. In: Bridwell KH, DeWald RL, eds. Philadelphia: Lippincott-Raven, 1997:1581–1600.

67. Weatherley CR, Prickett CF, O'Brien JP. Discogenic pain persisting despite solid posterior fusion. J Bone Joint Surg 1986;68B:142–143.

68. Kozak JA, O'Brien JP. Simultaneous combined anterior and posterior fusion. An independent analysis of a treatment for the disabled low back pain patient. Spine 1990;15:322–328.

69. Gertzbein SD, Betz R, Clements D, et al. Semi rigid instrumentation

in the management of lumbar spinal conditions combined with circumferential fusion. A multicenter study. Spine 1996;21:1918–1925.

70. Mardjetko S, Connolly P, Shott S. Degenerative lumbar spondylolisthesis: a meta-analysis of literature 1970–1993. Spine 1994;19:2256S–2265S.

71. Gurr K, McAfee P, Shih C. Biomechanical analysis of posterior instrumentation systems after decompressive laminectomy. An unstable calf-spine model. J Bone Joint Surg 1988;70A:680–691.

72. Thalgott JS, LaRocca H, Aebi M, et al. Reconstruction of the lumbar spine using AO DCP plate internal fixation. Spine 1989;14:91–95.

73. Zucherman J, Hsu K, White A, et al. Early results of spinal fusion using variable spine plating system. Spine 1988;13:570–579.

74. Davne SH, Myers DL. Complications of lumbar spine fusion with transpedicular instrumentation. Spine 1992;17:S184–S189.

75. Goel VK, Lim TH, Gwon J, et al. Effects of rigidity of an internal fixation device: a comprehensive biomechanical investigation. Spine 1991;16S:155.

76. Kanayama M, Cunningham BW, Sefter JC, et al. Does spinal instrumentation influence the healing process of posterolateral spinal fusion? An in vivo animal model. Spine 1999;24:1058–1065.

77. Kotani Y, Cunningham B, Cappuccino A, et al. The role of spinal instrumentation in augmenting posterolateral fusion. Spine 1996;21:278–287.

78. McAfee P, Farey I, Sutterling C, et al. 1989 Volvo Award in Basic Science. Device-related osteoporosis with spinal instrumentation. Spine 1989;14:919–926.

79. Skinner R, Maybee J, Transfeldt E, et al. Experimental pullout testing and comparison of variables in transpedicular fixation. A biomechanical study. Spine 1990;15:195–201.

80. Hou S, Hu R, Shi Y, et al. Pedicle morphology of the lower thoracic and lumbar spine in a chinese population. Spine 1993;18:1850–1855.

81. Kim NH, Lee HM, Chung IH, et al. Morphometric study of the pedicles of the thoracic and lumbar vertebrae in Koreans. Spine 1994;19:1390–1394.

82. Cheung KM, Ruan D, Chan FL, et al. Computed tomographic osteometry of the Asian lumbar pedicles. Spine 1994;19:1495–1498.

83. Anand N, Tanna DD. Unconventional pedicle spinal instrumentation. The Bombay experience. Spine 1994;19:2150–2158.

84. Misenhimer GR, Peek RD, Wiltse LL, et al. Anatomic analysis of pedicle cortical and cancellous diameter as related to screw size. Spine 1989;14:367–372.

85. Lill CA, Schlegel U, Wahl D, et al. Comparison of the in vitro holding strength of conical and cylindrical pedicle screws in a fully inserted setting and backed out 180°. J Spinal Disord 2000;13:259–266.

86. Pintar FA, Maiman DJ, Yoganandan N, et al. Rotational stability of a spinal pedicle screw/rod system. J Spinal Disord 1995;8:49–55.

87. Carson W, Duffield RC, Arendt M, et al. Internal forces and moments of transpedicular spine instrumentation. The effect of pedicle screw angle and transfixation: the 4R-4bar linkage concept. Spine 1990;15:893–901.

88. Ruland CM, McAfee PC, Warden KE, et al. Triangulation of pedicular instrumentation: a biomechanical analysis. Spine 1991;16:S270–S276.

89. Dick JC, Zdeblick TA, Bartel BD, et al. Mechanical evaluation of cross-link designs in rigid pedicle screw systems. Spine 1997;22:370–375.

90. Lynn G, Mukherjee DP, Kruse RN, et al. Mechanical stability of thoracolumbar pedicle screw fixation: The effect of cross-links. Spine 1997;22:1568–1573.

91. Krag M. Spinal instrumentation. Biomechanics of transpedicular spine fixation. In: Wiesel SW, Weinstein JN, Herkowitz HN, et al, eds. The lumbar spine, 2nd ed. Philadelphia: WB Saunders, 1996:1177–1203.

92. Zindrik MR, Lorenz MA. Posterior lumbar fusion. An overview of options and internal fixation devices. In: Frymoyer JW, ed. The adult spine. Principles and practice, 2nd ed. Philadelphia: Lippincott-Raven, 1997:2175–2203.

93. Barber JW, Boden SD, Ganey T, et al. Biomechanical study of lumbar pedicle screws: does convergence affect axial pullout strength? J Spinal Disord 1998;11:215–220.

94. Zindrik MR, Wiltse LL, Widell EH, et al. A biomechanical study of intrapedicular screw fixation in the lumbosacral spine. Clin Orthop Rel Res 1986;203:99–112.

95. Whitecloud TS, Skalley T, Cook SD, et al. Roentgenographic measurement of pedicle screw penetration. Clin Orthop Rel Res 1989;245:57–68.

96. Daftari TK, Horton WC, Hutton WC. Correlations between screw hole preparation, torque of insertion, and pullout strength for spinal screws. J Spinal Disord 1994;7:139–145.

97. Zdeblik TA, Kunz DN, Cooke ME, et al. Pedicle screw pull out strength. Correlation with insertional torque. Spine 1993;18:1673–1676.

98. Halvorson TL, Kelley LA, Thomas KA, et al. Effects of bone mineral density on pedicle screw fixation. Spine 1994;19:2415–2420.

99. Okuyama K, Abe E, Suzuki T, et al. Can insertional torque predict screw loosening and related failures? An in vivo study of pedicle screw fixation augmenting posterior lumbar interbody fusion. Spine 2000;25:858–864.

100. Coe JD, Warden KE, Herzig MA, et al. Influence of bone mineral density on the fixation of thoracolumbar implants. A comparative study of transpedicular screws, laminar hooks, and spinous process wires. Spine 1990;15:902–907.

101. Hasegawa K, Takahashi HE, Uchiyama S, et al. An experimental study of a combination method using a pedicle screw and laminar hook for the osteoporotic spine. Spine 1997;22:958–962.

102. Yerby SA, Ehteshami JR, Mclain RF. Offset laminar hooks decrease bending moments of pedicle screw during in situ contouring. Spine 1997;22:376–381.

103. Pfeifer BA, Krag MH, Johnson C. Repair of failed transpedicle screw fixation. A biomechanical study comparing polymethylmethacrylate, milled bone, and matchstick bone reconstruction. Spine 1994;19:350–353.

104. Margulies JY, Casar RS, Caruso SA, et al. The mechanical role of lamina hook protection of pedicle screws at the caudal end vertebra. Eur Spine J 1997;6:245–248.

105. Moore DC, Maitra RS, Farjo LA, et al. Restoration of pedicle screw fixation with an in situ setting calcium phosphate cement. Spine 1997;22:1696–1705.

106. Wittenberg RH, Lee KS, Shea M, et al. Effect of screw diameter, insertion technique, and bone cement augmentation of pedicular screw fixation strength. Clin Orthop Rel Res 1993;296:278–287.

107. Yerby SA, Toh E, McLain RF. Revision of failed pedicle screws using hydroxyapatite cement: a biomechanical analysis. Spine 1998;23:1657–1661.

108. Lotz JC, Hu SS, Chiu DF, et al. Carbonated apatite cement augmentation of pedicle screw fixation in the lumbar spine. Spine 1997;22:2716–2723.

109. Ebraheim NA, Rupp RE, Savolaine ER, et al. Use of titanium implants in pedicular screw fixation. J Spinal Disord 1994;7:478–486.

110. Wang JC, Sandhu HS, Yu WD, et al. MR parameters for imaging titanium spinal instrumentation. J Spinal Disord 1997;10:27–32.

111. Rudisch A, Kremser C, Peer S, et al. Metallic artifacts in magnetic resonance imaging of patients with spinal fusion. A comparison of implant materials and imaging sequences. Spine 1998;23:692–699.

112. Christensen FB, Dalstra M, Sejling F, et al. Titanium-alloy enhances bone-pedicle screw fixation: mechanical and histomorphometrical results of titanium-alloy versus stainless steel. Eur Spine J 2000;9:97–103.

113. Xu R, Ebraheim NA, Nadaud MC, et al. Local tissue of the lumbar spine response to titanium plate—screw system. Case reports. Spine 1996;21:871–873.

114. Wang JC, Yu WD, Sandhu HS, et al. Metal debris from titanium spinal implants. Spine 1999;24:899–903.

115. Boden SD, Sumner DR. Biologic factors affecting spinal fusion and bone regeneration. Spine 1995;23S:102–112.

116. Brown CW, Orme TJ, Richardson HD. The rate of pseudarthrosis (surgical nonunion) in patients who are smokers and patients who are nonsmokers: a comparison study. Spine 1986;11:942–943.

117. Wimmer C, Nogler M, Frischhut B. Influence of antibiotics on infection in spinal surgery: a prospective study of 110 patients. J Spinal Disord 1998;11:498–500.

118. Castro WH, Halm H, Jerosch J, et al. Accuracy of pedicle screw placement in lumbar vertebrae. Spine 1996;21:1320–1324.

119. Schulze CJ, Munzinger E, Weber U. Clinical relevance of accuracy of pedicle screw placement: a computed tomographic-supported analysis. Spine 1998;23:2215–2221.

120. Boachie-Adjei O, Girardi FP, Bansal M, et al. Safety and efficacy of pedicle screw placement for adult spinal deformity with a pedicle-

probing conventional anatomic technique. J Spinal Disord 2000;
13:496–500.
121. Meter JJ, Polly DW Jr, Miller DW, et al. A method for radiographic
evaluation of pedicle screw violation of the vertebral end plate. Spine
1996;21:1587–1592.
122. Rampersaud YR, Foley KT, Shen AC, et al. Radiation exposure to the
spine surgeon during fluoroscopically assisted pedicle screw insertion. Spine 2000;25:2637–2645.
123. Ferrick MR, Kowalski JM, Simmons ED Jr. Reliability of roentgenogram evaluation of pedicle screw position. Spine 1997;22:1249–1252.
124. Odgers CJ, Vaccaro AR, Pollack ME, et al. Accuracy of pedicle screw
placement with the assistance of lateral plain radiography. J Spinal
Disord 1996;9:334–338.
125. Lenke LG., Padberg AM, Russo MH, et al. Triggered electromyographic threshold for accuracy of pedicle screw placement. An animal
model and clinical correlation. Spine 1995;20:1585–1591.
126. Clements DH, Morledge DE, Martin WH, et al. Evoked and spontaneous electromyography to evaluate lumbosacral pedicle screw placement. Spine 1996;21:600–604.
127. Glassman SD, Dimar JR, Puno RM, et al. A prospective analysis of
intraoperative electromyographic monitoring of pedicle screw placement with computed tomographic scan confirmation. Spine 1995;
20:1375–1379.
128. Glossop ND, Hu RW, Randle JA. Computer-aided pedicle screw
placement using frameless stereotaxis. Spine 1996;21:2026–2034.
129. Girardi FP, Cammisa FP Jr, Sandhu HS, et al. The placement of lumbar pedicle screws using computerised stereotactic guidance. J Bone
Joint Surg (Br) 1999;81:825–829.
130. Carl AL, Khanuja HS, Gatto CA, et al. In vivo pedicle screw placement: image-guided virtual vision. J Spinal Disord 2000;13:225–229.
131. Amiot LP, Lang K, Putzier M, et al. Comparative results between conventional and computer-assisted pedicle screw installation in the thoracic, lumbar, and sacral spine. Spine 2000;25:606–614.
132. Abdel-Malek, K, McGowan DP, Goel VK, et al. Bone registration
method for robot assisted surgery: pedicle screw insertion. Proceedings of the Institute of Mechanical Engineers, Part H. J Eng Med
1997;211:221–233.
133. Frank EH. The use of small malleable endoscopes to assess pedicle
screw placement: technical note. Min Invas Neurosurg 1998;41:10–12.
134. Muller A, Gall C, Reulen HJ. A key hole approach for endoscopically
assisted pedicle screw fixation in lumbar spine instability. Neurosurgery 2000;47:85–95.
135. McCulloch JA. Microdecompression and uninstrumented single-level
fusion for spinal canal stenosis with degenerative spondylolisthesis.
Spine 1998;23:2243–2252.
136. Magerl F. Stabilization of the lower thoracic and lumbar spine with
external skeletal fixation. Clin Orthop Rel Res 1984;189:125.
137. Gaines RW Jr. Current concepts review. The use of pedicle-screw
internal fixation for the operative treatment of spinal disorders. J
Bone Joint Surg 2000;82A:1458–1476.
138. Xu R, Ebraheim NA, Yeasting RA, et al. Morphometric evaluation of
the first sacral vertebra and the projection of its pedicle on the posterior aspect of the sacrum. Spine 1995;20:936–940.
139. Mirkovic S, Abitbol JJ, Steinman J, et al. Anatomic considerations of
sacral screw placement. Spine 1991;16:289S,294S.
140. Kucharzyk DW. A controlled prospective outcome study of
implantable electrical stimulation with spinal fusion in a high-risk
spinal fusion population. Spine 1999;24:465–468.
141. Jenis LG, An HS, Stein R, et al. Prospective comparison of the effect
of direct current electrical stimulation and pulsed electromagnetic
fields on instrumented posterolateral lumbar arthrodesis. J Spinal
Disord 2000;13:290–296.
142. Blumenthal SL, Gill K. Can lumbar spine radiographs accurately
determine fusion in postoperative patients. Correlation of routine
radiographs with a second surgical look at lumbar fusions. Spine
1993;18:1186–1189.
143. Craven TG, Carson WL, Asher MA, et al. The effects of implant stiffness on the bypassed bone mineral density and facet fusion stiffness
of the canine spine. Spine 1994;19:1664–1673.
144. Blumenthal S, Gill K. Complications of Wiltse pedicle screw fixation
system. Spine 1993;18:1867–1871.
145. Lonstein JE, Denis F, Perra JH, et al. Complications associated with
pedicle screws. J Bone Joint Surg 1999;81A:1519–1528.

146. Faraj AA, Webb JK. Early complications of spinal pedicle screw. Eur
Spine J 1997;6:324–326.
147. Esses SI, Sachs BL, Dreyzin V. Complications associated with the
technique of pedicle screw fixation. A selected survey of ABS members. Spine 1993;18:2231–2238.
148. Sapkas GS, Papadakis SA, Stathakopoulos DP, et al. Evaluation of
pedicle screw position in thoracic and lumbar spine fixation using
plain radiographs and computed tomography. A prospective study of
35 patients. Spine 1999;24:1926–1929.
149. Farber GL, Place HM, Mazur RA, et al. Accuracy of pedicle screw
placement in lumbar fusions by plain radiographs and computed
tomography. Spine 1995;20(13):1494–1499.
150. Wimmer C, Gluch H, Frazreb M, et al. Predisposing factors for infection on spine surgery: a survey of 850 spinal procedures. J Spinal Disord 1998;11:124–128.
151. Weinstein MA, McCabe JP, Cammisa FP Jr. Postoperative spinal
wound infection: a review of 2,391 consecutive index procedures. J
Spinal Disord 2000;13:422–426.
152. Glassman SD, Dimar JR, Puno RM, et al. Salvage of instrumented
lumbar fusions complicated by surgical wound infection. Spine
1996;21:2163–2169.
153. Macdessi SJ, Leong AK, Bentivoglio JE. Pedicle fracture after instrumented posterolateral lumbar fusion: a case report. Spine 2001;26:
580–582.
154. Eck JC, Humphreys SC, Hodges SD. Adjacent-segment degeneration
after lumbar fusion: a review of clinical, biomechanical, and radiologic studies. Am J Orthop 1999;28:336–340.
155. Weinhoffer SL, Guyer RD, Herbert M, et al. Intradiscal pressure measurements above an instrumented fusion. A cadaveric study. Spine
1995;20:526–531.
156. Cunningham BW, Kotani Y, McNulty PS, et al. The effects of spinal
destabilization and instrumentation on lumbar intradiscal pressure: an
in vitro biomechanical analysis. Spine 1997;22:2655–2663.
157. Lee CK. Accelerated degeneration of the segment adjacent to a lumbar fusion. Spine 1988;13:375–377.
158. Yoganandan N, Pintar F, Maiman DJ, et al. Kinematics of the lumbar
spine following pedicle screw-plate fixation. Spine 1993;18:504–512.
159. Nagata A, Schendel MJ, Transfeldt EE, et al. The effects of immobilization of long segments of the spine on the adjacent and distal facet
force and lumbosacral motion. Spine 1993;18:2471–2479.
160. Wimmer C, Gluch H, Krismer M, et al. AP-translation in the proximal disc adjacent to lumbar spine fusion: a retrospective comparison
of mono- and polysegmental fusion in 120 patients. Acta Orthop
Scand 1997;68:269–272.
161. Schlegel JD, Smith JA, Schleusener RL. Lumbar motion segment
pathology adjacent to thoracolumbar, lumbar, and lumbosacral
fusions. Spine 1996;21:970–981.
162. Aota Y, Kumano K, Hirabayashi S. Postfusion instability at the adjacent segments after rigid pedicle screw fixation for degenerative lumbar spinal disorders. J Spinal Disord 1995;8:464–473.
163. Etebar S. Cahill DW. Risk factors for adjacent-segment failure following lumbar fixation with rigid instrumentation for degenerative
instability. J Neurosurg 1999;90(4 Suppl):163–169.
164. Rahm MD, Hall BB. Adjacent-segment degeneration after lumbar
fusion with instrumentation: a retrospective study. J Spinal Disord
1996;9:392–400.
165. Kumar MN, Baklanov A, Chopin D. Correlation between sagittal
plane changes and adjacent segment degeneration following lumbar
spine fusion. Eur Spine J 2001;10:314–319.
166. Wiltse LL, Radecki SE, Biel HM, et al. Comparative study of the incidence and severity of degenerative change in the transition zones after
instrumented versus noninstrumented fusions of the lumbar spine. J
Spinal Disord 1999;12:27–33.
167. Katz JN, Lipson SJ, Lew RA, et al. Lumbar laminectomy alone or
with instrumented or noninstrumented arthrodesis in degenerative
lumbar spinal stenosis. Patient selection, costs, and surgical outcomes. Spine 1997;22:1123–1131.
168. Kuntz KM, Snider RK, Weinstein JN, et al. Cost-effectiveness of
fusion with and without instrumentation for patients with degenerative spondylolisthesis and spinal stenosis. Spine 2000;25:1132–1139.
169. Gibson JNA, Grant IC, Waddell G. The Cochrane review of surgery
for lumbar disc prolapse and degenerative lumbar spondylosis. Spine
1999;24:1820–1832.

CHAPTER 26

Spinal Instrumentation Overview in Lumbar Degenerative Disorders: Cages

Kenneth M.C. Cheung and John C.Y. Leong

ROLE OF CAGES IN THE LUMBAR SPINE

Cages are interbody spacers used to bridge or reconstruct the interval between two vertebral bodies (1–4). There are many different designs, but in general, they all provide a mechanically strong scaffold inside of which osteoinductive or osteoconductive materials can be placed. Such material maybe autogenous bone graft, allograft, or more recently bone morphogenetic proteins (5–10).

Cages are used in either degenerative conditions of the spine requiring fusion, or as a form of anterior column reconstruction after destruction by tumor, infection, or trauma. This overview concentrates on its application in degenerative spinal conditions, in which cages are either used as an anterior load-sharing device after posterior spinal instrumentation and fusion (1,4,7,11,12); or as a replacement for bone graft after anterior lumbar interbody fusion (ALIF) (13), sometimes referred to as a "stand-alone" cage.

TYPES OF CAGES

There are no universally accepted classifications for the cages available today. However, they can be broadly divided into different types by their design or material (1).

Three general designs are used, as follows.

Horizontal Cylinders

One example is the Bagby and Kuslich lumbar (BAK/L) interbody fusion cage (Sulzer Spine-Tech, Minneapolis, MN) (Fig. 26-1). These devices generally are made from titanium. Usually a pair is inserted together by either the anterior or posterior approach, and by use of either open or minimally invasive techniques (11,13–19).

Vertical Rings

An example is the titanium mesh cage manufactured by DePuy AcroMed (Johnson & Johnson, Raynham, MA), sometimes referred to as the Harms cage (Fig. 26-2). They are designed to allow the length to be cut as desired; therefore, they can be used to span either a single disc space or multiple segments of the lumbar spine. Because of the presence of sharp edges, they are usually and more safely inserted via an open technique (20,21).

Open Boxes

An example is the Brantigan carbon cage (Fig. 26-3) (22–24). The boxes are designed either with conical superior and inferior surfaces for an anatomic fit into the disc space, or as wedges to recreate lumbar lordosis. Some are designed as a single large cage, which requires an open technique for insertion; whereas others involve two smaller rectangular cages, which can be inserted posteriorly using minimally invasive techniques.

Cage Materials

In general, these are usually made from titanium, carbon, or a carbon composite (polyetheretherketone [PEEK]). Titanium is a mechanically strong and bio-inert material that is magnetic resonance imaging (MRI) compatible. Therefore, cages made using this material can have relatively thin struts that allow more room for bone graft in its interior. The presence of a metallic shadow on radiographs makes the assessment of bony fusion within the cage difficult. Some surgeons attempt to overcome this by placing bone graft anterior to the cage as well as within it (5). Carbon and PEEK cages are radiolucent and allow for an easier assessment of bone fusion. Addition-

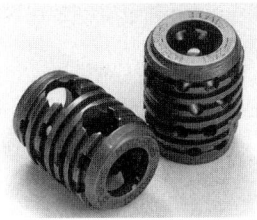

FIG. 26-1. Bagby and Kuslich lumbar interbody fusion cage, an example of a threaded horizontal cylinder.

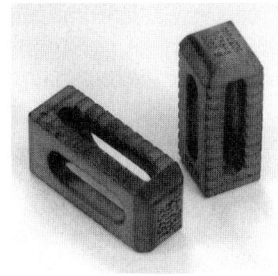

FIG. 26-3. Brantigan carbon cage, an example of an open box design.

ally, they have a Young's modulus that nearly matches that of cortical bone. This allows the compressive load on the cage to be shared by the bone graft inside the cage and may facilitate a more consistent and rapid bone fusion. Both carbon and PEEK cages are also MRI compatible.

INDICATIONS FOR CAGES

Before the advent of cages, bone grafts such as tricortical iliac crest grafts and fibula strut grafts were used very successfully as a form of anterior column support and to promote spinal fusion (25,26). Thus, there are no absolute indications for the use of cages, and the value of cages as an alternative to autogenous bone graft should be judged with the latter as a gold standard. Accordingly, the indication for use of a cage is the same as that for bone graft, namely, anterior column reconstruction and fusion.

Proponents of cages suggest that they may have a number of advantages over conventional bone graft material alone. Such advantages mainly stem from the separation of their mechanical and biological roles and may include:

1. Enhanced mechanical stability
2. Maintenance of intervertebral disc height
3. Avoidance of bone graft donor site morbidity by using alternative osteoconductive and osteoinductive materials inside the cage.

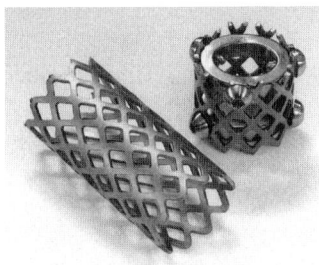

FIG. 26-2. Titanium mesh cage (Harms), an example of a vertical cylinder. End-rings **(right side)** can be added to the reduce stress concentration at the ends of the cage, and therefore reduce the chance of sinking into the end plate.

Cages are designed to have better mechanical stability than bone graft by virtue of their material and design. Cylindrical cages have a threaded design (Fig. 26-1) and use a screw-in technique for insertion (14,27), whereas box cages have a serrated surface (Fig. 26-3) (13,28). Both help to increase motion segment stiffness and resistance to pull-out. It is claimed that this may improve the chance of a successful fusion, although this point remains to be proved scientifically.

Cages may be better at maintaining disc height than bone graft alone. In our long-term follow-up study (mean duration of 14 years) of 67 patients that underwent anterior lumbar interbody fusion at L4-5 with autologous iliac crest graft (29), we demonstrated that there was an initial distraction of the disc space by 34% (4.1 mm) followed by an eventual partial loss of this distraction in 86% of cases despite a successful fusion. The mean preoperative disc space height was 12.1 mm, increased immediately after surgery to 16.2 mm, but settled to 12.6 mm at the latest follow-up. The reduction in distraction occurred within the first 3 months after surgery and was correlated with age, but not with recurrence of symptoms, the amount of initial distraction or sex of the individual. L4-5 segmental angulation followed a similar trend. The early loss of disc space distraction likely resulted from moulding of the bone graft into the created space, and bone graft softening and resorption during remodeling. Studies have shown that restoration of disc space height tightens the posterior ligaments and opens up the intervertebral foramina, thereby indirectly decompressing the neural foramina exiting nerve roots (30). Although this has been used as a justification for using cages, it should be borne in mind that our study showed that the loss of disc space distraction did not correlate with return of the patients' symptoms, and no long-term clinical study is available to demonstrate that disc space height is maintained with cages. Indeed, there is some evidence in both animal and human studies that disc space reduction and loss of lordosis also occur with threaded cylindrical cages (31,32). Special considerations should be given to patients with reduced bone density because there is a risk of end-plate fracture by the implanted cage, which may result in loss of distraction (29,33).

Avoidance of donor site morbidity (34,35) is often cited as another reason for using a cage. However, until recently only osteoconductive materials, such as allograft bone and hydroxyapatite blocks, were available as replacements for autogenous bone. We caution that the use of such materials as the ultimate aim is still to achieve a fusion and autogenous bone graft is still currently the best material for this purpose. There have been several studies examining the use of bone morphogenetic proteins placed inside cages in human patients (8,10). Both studies concluded that recombinant bone morphogenetic protein-2 (rhBMP-2), can effectively achieve a spinal fusion, although the number of patients involved were small, and the follow-up short. Large-scale randomized controlled trials with long-term follow-up are required to prove this definitively.

CHOICE OF CAGES

The ideal cage should rigidly immobilize the spine in all directions, be strong enough to withstand repeated loading, and have a modulus of elasticity close to that of cortical bone. It should also be easy to insert by either an open or minimally invasive approach, and should be clinically effective by randomized controlled trials and long-term follow-up.

It is difficult to advise readers on the optimal choice of cage because of the wide variety of cages currently available, with more likely to come on the market in the future. However, users should be aware of some biomechanical and clinical considerations with the currently available designs.

Biomechanical Considerations

In general, studies comparing the stiffness of the spine segment after cage insertion have shown no significant differences among the various designs (13,36–38). All are effective at stabilizing the spine, compared with its intact condition, in flexion, axial rotation, and lateral bending. This effectiveness is dependent on their ability to distract the surrounding soft tissues and their contact with the host bone. Hence, the cage needs to be appropriately sized for height as well as fit (13,39). Differences within a particular category of cage design may have an effect on mechanical stability. For instance, cages with sharp teeth have higher "pull-out" forces (13), whereas Harms cages without the addition of the end-rings impart only marginally better stability in rotation when compared to bone graft (40). All stand-alone cages, however, are less effective in stabilizing the spine in extension, and motion between the cage–bone junction is present unless supplemental fixation is used (41). Addition of fixation, whether anterior or posterior, and by translaminar or pedicle screws, will significantly improve the fusion segment stiffness (3,36,38,42).

One area of concern with the use of cages compared to bone graft is that the stiff struts of the cage stress shield the bone graft placed inside the cage. Because bone heals best under compression, this could result in reduced fusion rates. In a study by Kanayama et al. (37), a calf spine model was used to quantify the stress-shielding effects of 11 lumbar interbody fusion cages by measuring pressure within the cages. This was achieved by injecting the cages with a silicon elastomer before insertion, and intracage pressures were measured using pressure needle transducers. The authors concluded that threaded fusion cages demonstrated significantly lower intracage pressures compared with nonthreaded cages and structural allografts. Whether this is clinically relevant is not known, because there are no comparative studies examining fusion rates among the various types of cages.

The possibility of stress shielding and the presence of motion within the spine segment despite the use of cages raise the question of whether they can be used as stand-alone devices, without supplemental fixation. Because of a lack of clinical studies with long-term follow-up, this question cannot be currently answered. There are certainly advocates who recommend supplemental posterior fixation to improve the chance of fusion (38,42–46). It should be borne in mind that iliac crest bone grafting without instrumentation has been used successfully to perform anterior lumbar interbody fusion with fusion rates for a single level fusion of up to 96% (26,29,47,48). This should be the benchmark against which fusions with cages are compared.

Clinical Considerations

Interbody fusion in degenerative disc disease serves a number of purposes. First, by removing the disc it removes a potential source of pain, and by removing herniated fragments it decompresses the nerve roots. Second, fusion stabilizes the segment and augments the anterior column. Third, restoration of disc space height tightens up the posterior ligaments and opens up the intervertebral foramina, thus indirectly decompressing the nerve roots (30,31). The first two aims can be adequately achieved by anterior interbody fusion with tricortical iliac crest bone graft, whereas a cage may be required for the third aim. However, before a rational choice of fusion devices can be made, surgeons should be aware of the clinical track record of cages.

There are very few reports of long-term results of cages. One of the longest and earliest experiences in the use of interbody spacer was by the senior author in 1994 (49). A titanium mesh interbody spacer was inserted as a stand-alone device without bone grafting in 23 patients with an average follow-up period of 8 years (range, 5 to 12 years). This study demonstrated that bony ingrowth into the titanium mesh occurred in 18 of 23 patients, as shown by lack of a radiolucent line at the bone–implant junction, and was subsequently confirmed in retrieval studies. However, six of these 18 implants failed by a mid-substance disruption of the mesh, with three implants developing a crack, and three becoming deformed. In all six patients, movement could be demonstrated between the adjacent vertebral bodies, despite the lack of a radiolucent line. The authors postulated that with the solid metal–bone interface, the mesh became subjected to more stress during flexion and extension, such that if solid bone fusion did not occur, the implant failed in its mid-substance. One of the best ways to demonstrate bone fusion is the presence of anterior bridging bone (Fig. 26-4). This occurred in four of the 23 cases, and when this was seen, no further movement between the adjacent vertebral bodies could be demonstrated on flexion and extension, and no mesh failures occurred.

Based on this experience, the authors feel that one should make the distinction between *bone ingrowth* into the periphery of the cage, and *bone fusion,* which extends from one end plate to the other. If the latter does not occur, then the cage may fail in the long term. Thus, in reading the literature on the results of cages, the reader should make this distinction and note the duration of follow-up. Any study with less than 5 years of follow-up is very unlikely to see cage failure because of bone ingrowth only and the lack of a solid bone fusion.

One study examined needle biopsies from tissue within radiographically successful intervertebral body fusion cages filled with autograft (6). Five cages were implanted anteriorly, one with additional fixation, and four cages were implanted as part of a posterior lumbar interbody fusion. Five were carbon cages (Brantigan cage), whereas four were titanium mesh (Harms Cage), with a mean postimplantation biopsy duration of 28 months (range, 8 to 72 months). Biopsies were obtained from within the center of the cages and showed small fragments of

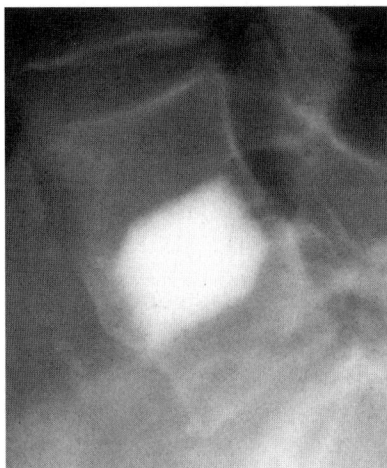

FIG. 26-4. Implanted titanium mesh block showing anterior bone bridging and solid fusion.

necrotic bone associated with viable bone and restoration of hematopoietic bone marrow. Numerous cement lines demarcated the edges of previous cycles of remodeling, and the ratio of necrotic to viable bone varied greatly among cases. Small particles of debris were found in four of the five carbon-fiber cages and in one of the four specimens from titanium cages, but there was no visible bone resorption or inflammation. It could be interpreted that, despite stress-shielding by the cage, solid bone fusion eventually may occur, although bone grafts contained within these cages are still undergoing remodeling beyond the 3 to 6 months that autograft is normally expected to fuse and remodel.

In 1997, Ray (50) reported his initial results of using a stand-alone threaded cage packed with autogenous bone graft and inserted via a posterior approach. Fusion, as assessed by plain lateral radiographs and lack of movement on flexion-extension radiographs, was said to occur in 91%. Lack of movement may result only from bony ingrowth into the superior and inferior faces of the cage for a limited distance. The word "fusion" should be used only if there is evidence of continuous bony ingrowth through the entire extent of the cage. To date, this has not been definitively demonstrated in any study.

Kuslich et al. reported on the 4-year follow-up results of the BAK cage in 25.6% of the original study population (18). Their overall "fusion rate" was 91.7% and 95.1% at 2 and 4 years, respectively. This was from a combination of anterior and posterior approaches. Whether or not additional instrumentation was used is unknown. The late-occurring complication rate was 13.8%. Complications necessitating a second operation occurred in 8.7%, and reoperations directly related to the device occurred in 3.1%. This study has been criticized for the small number of patients available for follow-up assessment (51,52).

Studies examining the use of other cages have tended to be combined with posterior fixation, and they all report "fusion rates" in the range of 90% to 100% (7,12,20,23,24,53). However, it should be noted that no movement would be detectable on flexion-extension radiographs with solid posterior fixation, thereby hampering fusion assessment. It requires long-term follow-up to demonstrate nonunion from loosening or implant failure (54).

One additional criterion in the choice of cages is the surgeon's familiarity with the techniques of insertion. Although the majority of the box cages are used in a similar manner to bone graft, the threaded cylindrical cages require a specialized technique of insertion. Attention to detail is important, because complications arising from inadequate distraction of the anulus fibrosus, under sizing of the cages, and dural tears from a posterior approach all have been described (55). Additionally, some cages are designed for anterior minimally invasive insertion (15–17,56–58), whereas others are designed for use as a PLIF only. These are all important issues to consider, and any surgeon intending to use such cages should be thoroughly familiar with their indications and design considerations.

SUMMARY

Lumbar interbody fusion cages may have some advantages over conventional autogenous bone grafting techniques. They have the theoretical potential to maintain vertebral distraction, and separate the structural and biological functions of an interbody spacer. With the development of osteoinductive compounds delivered as a recombinant protein or via gene therapy (59), bone graft harvesting and donor site morbidity theoretically could be avoided altogether. However, techniques of insertion may be demanding and surgeons should be familiar with the design before using a cage of their choice. Finally, one should balance the use of such expensive implants with the low cost and proven effectiveness of autogenous bone graft, which is the gold standard in anterior interbody reconstruction and fusion to date.

REFERENCES

1. Weiner BK, Fraser RD. Spine update lumbar interbody cages. Spine 1998;23(5):634–640.
2. Vaccaro AR, Cirello J. The use of allograft bone and cages in fractures of the cervical, thoracic, and lumbar spine. Clin Orthop Rel Res 2002;1(394):19–26.
3. Cunningham BW, Polly DW Jr. The use of interbody cage devices for spinal deformity: a biomechanical perspective. Clin Orthop Rel Res 2002;1(394):73–83.
4. McAfee PC. Interbody fusion cages in reconstructive operations on the spine. J Bone Joint Surg 1999;81(6):859–880.
5. Eck KR, Lenke LG, Bridwell KH, et al. Radiographic assessment of anterior titanium mesh cages. J Spinal Disord 2000;13(6):501–509.
6. Togawa D, Bauer TW, Brantigan JW, et al. Bone graft incorporation in radiographically successful human intervertebral body fusion cages. Spine 2001;26(24):2744–2750.
7. Whitecloud TS 3rd, Castro FP Jr, Brinker MR, et al. Degenerative conditions of the lumbar spine treated with intervertebral titanium cages and posterior instrumentation for circumferential fusion. J Spinal Disord 1998;11(6):479–486.
8. Boden SD, Zdeblick TA, Sandhu HS, et al. The use of rhBMP-2 in interbody fusion cages. Definitive evidence of osteoinduction in humans: a preliminary report. Spine 2000;25(3):376–381.
9. Kandziora F, Bail H, Schmidmaier G, et al. Bone morphogenetic protein-2 application by a poly(D,L-lactide)-coated interbody cage: in vivo results of a new carrier for growth factors. J Neurosurg 2002;97(1 Suppl):40–48.
10. Kleeman TJ, Ahn UM, Talbot-Kleeman A. Laparoscopic anterior lumbar interbody fusion with rhBMP-2: a prospective study of clinical and radiographic outcomes. Spine 2001;26(24):2751–2756.
11. Hacker RJ. Comparison of interbody fusion approaches for disabling low back pain. Spine 1997;22(6):660–665.
12. Schofferman J, Slosar P, Reynolds J, et al. A prospective randomized comparison of 270 degrees fusions to 360 degrees fusions (circumferential fusions). Spine 2001;26(10):E207–E212.
13. Tsantrizos A, Andreou A, Aebi M, et al. Biomechanical stability of five stand-alone anterior lumbar interbody fusion constructs. Eur Spine J 2000;9(1):14–22.
14. Brodke DS, Dick JC, Kunz DN, et al. Posterior lumbar interbody fusion. A biomechanical comparison, including a new threaded cage. Spine 1997;22(1):26–31.

15. Zucherman JF, Zdeblick TA, Bailey SA, et al. Instrumented laparoscopic spinal fusion. Preliminary Results. Spine 1995;20(18):2029–2034;discussion 2034-2035.
16. McAfee PC, Regan JJ, Geis WP, et al. Minimally invasive anterior retroperitoneal approach to the lumbar spine. Emphasis on the lateral BAK. Spine 1998;23(13):1476–1484.
17. Regan JJ, Aronoff RJ, Ohnmeiss DD, et al. Laparoscopic approach to L4-L5 for interbody fusion using BAK cages: experience in the first 58 cases. Spine 1999;24(20):2171–2174.
18. Kuslich SD, Danielson G, Dowdle JD, et al. Four-year follow-up results of lumbar spine arthrodesis using the Bagby and Kuslich lumbar fusion cage. Spine 2000;25(20):2656–2662.
19. Wong HK, Goh JC, Goh PS. Paired cylindrical interbody cage fit and facetectomy in posterior lumbar interbody fusion in an Asian population. Spine 2001;26(5):572–577.
20. Lenke LG, Bridwell KH. Mesh cages in idiopathic scoliosis in adolescents. Clin Orthop Rel Res 2002;1(394):98–108.
21. Eck KR, Bridwell KH, Ungacta FF, et al. Analysis of titanium mesh cages in adults with minimum two-year follow-up. Spine 2000;25(18):2407–2415.
22. Brantigan JW, McAfee PC, Cunningham BW, et al. Interbody lumbar fusion using a carbon fiber cage implant versus allograft bone. An investigational study in the Spanish goat. Spine 1994;19(13):1436–1444.
23. Brantigan JW, Steffee AD, Lewis ML, et al. Lumbar interbody fusion using the Brantigan I/F cage for posterior lumbar interbody fusion and the variable pedicle screw placement system: two-year results from a Food and Drug Administration investigational device exemption clinical trial. Spine 2000;25(11):1437–1446.
24. Hashimoto T, Shigenobu K, Kanayama M, et al. Clinical results of single-level posterior lumbar interbody fusion using the Brantigan I/F carbon cage filled with a mixture of local morselized bone and bioactive ceramic granules. Spine 2002;27(3):258–262.
25. Leong JC, Chun SY, Grange WJ, et al. Long-term results of lumbar intervertebral disc prolapse. Spine 1983;8(7):793–799.
26. Luk KD, Chow DH, Evans JH, et al. Lumbar spinal mobility after short anterior interbody fusion. Spine 1995;20(7):813–818.
27. Tencer AF, Hampton D, Eddy S. Biomechanical properties of threaded inserts for lumbar interbody spinal fusion. Spine 1995;20(22):2408–2414.
28. Dietl RH, Krammer M, Kettler A, et al. Pullout test with three lumbar interbody fusion cages. Spine 2002;27(10):1029–1036.
29. Cheung KMC, Zhang YG, Lu DS, et al. Reduction of disc space distraction after anterior lumbar interbody fusion with autologous iliac crest graft. Spine 2003;28(13):1385–1389.
30. Chen D, Fay LA, Lok J, et al. Increasing neuroforaminal volume by anterior interbody distraction in degenerative lumbar spine. Spine 1995;20(1):74–79.
31. Sandhu HS, Turner S, Kabo JM, et al. Distractive properties of a threaded interbody fusion device. An in vivo model. Spine 1996;21(10):1201–1210.
32. Goldstein JA, Macenski MJ, Griffith SL, et al. Lumbar sagittal alignment after fusion with a threaded interbody cage. Spine 2001;26(10):1137–1142.
33. Jost B, Cripton PA, Lund T, et al. Compressive strength of interbody cages in the lumbar spine: the effect of cage shape, posterior instrumentation and bone density. Eur Spine J 1998;7(2):132-141.
34. Cunningham BW, Kanayama M, Parker LM, et al. Osteogenic protein versus autologous interbody arthrodesis in the sheep thoracic spine. A comparative endoscopic study using the Bagby and Kuslich interbody fusion device. Spine 1999;24(6):509–518.
35. Younger EM, Chapman MW. Morbidity at bone graft donor sites. J Orthop Trauma 1989;3(3):192–195.
36. Oxland TR, Hoffer Z, Nydegger T, et al. A comparative biomechanical investigation of anterior lumbar interbody cages: central and bilateral approaches. J Bone Joint Surg 2000;82(3):383–393.
37. Kanayama M, Cunningham BW, Haggerty CJ, et al. In vitro biomechanical investigation of the stability and stress-shielding effect of lumbar interbody fusion devices. J Neurosurg 2000;93(2 Suppl):259–265.
38. Lund T, Oxland TR, Jost B, et al. Interbody cage stabilisation in the lumbar spine: biomechanical evaluation of cage design, posterior instrumentation and bone density. J Bone Joint Surg Br 1998;80(2):351–359.

39. Goh JC, Wong HK, Thambyah A, et al. Influence of PLIF cage size on lumbar spine stability. Spine 2000;25(1):35–39.
40. Lee SW, Lim TH, You JW, et al. Biomechanical effect of anterior grafting devices on the rotational stability of spinal constructs. J Spinal Disord 2000;13(2):150–155.
41. Kim Y. Prediction of mechanical behaviors at interfaces between bone and two interbody cages of lumbar spine segments. Spine 2001;26(13):1437–1442.
42. Le Huec JC, Liu M, Skalli W, et al. Lumbar lateral interbody cage with plate augmentation: in vitro biomechanical analysis. Eur Spine J 2002;11(2):130–136.
43. Hitchon PW, Goel V, Rogge T, et al. Spinal stability with anterior or posterior ray threaded fusion cages. J Neurosurg 2000;93(1 Suppl):102–108.
44. Nydegger T, Oxland TR, Hoffer Z, et al. Does anterolateral cage insertion enhance immediate stabilization of the functional spinal unit? A biomechanical investigation. Spine 2001;26(22):2491–2497.
45. Oxland TR, Lund T. Biomechanics of stand-alone cages and cages in combination with posterior fixation: a literature review. Eur Spine J 2000;9(Suppl 1):S95–S101.
46. Rathonyi GC, Oxland TR, Gerich U, et al. The role of supplemental translaminar screws in anterior lumbar interbody fixation: a biomechanical study. Eur Spine J 1998;7(5):400–407.
47. Inoue S, Watanabe T, Hirose A, et al. Anterior discectomy and interbody fusion for lumbar disc herniation. A review of 350 cases. Clin Orthop 1984;(183):22–31.
48. Fujimaki A, Crock HV, Bedbrook GM. The results of 150 anterior lumbar interbody fusion operations performed by two surgeons in Australia. Clin Orthop 1982;(165):164–167.
49. Leong JC, Chow SP, Yau AC. Titanium-mesh block replacement of the intervertebral disk. Clin Orthop Rel Res 1994;(300):52–63.
50. Ray CD. Threaded titanium cages for lumbar interbody fusions. Spine 1997;22(6):667–679.
51. Lonstein JE. Re: four-year follow-up results of lumbar spine arthrodesis using Bagby and Kuslich lumbar fusion cage. Spine 2001;26(13):1506–1508.
52. Winter RB. Re: four-year follow-up results of lumbar spine arthrodesis using Bagby and Kuslich lumbar fusion cage. Spine 2001;26(13):1507–1508.
53. Janssen ME, Lam C, Beckham R. Outcomes of allogenic cages in anterior and posterior lumbar interbody fusion. Eur Spine J 2001;10(Suppl 2):S158–S168.
54. Tullberg T. Failure of a carbon fiber implant. A case report. Spine 1998;23(16):1804–1806.
55. McAfee PC, Cunningham BW, Lee GA, et al. Revision strategies for salvaging or improving failed cylindrical cages. Spine 1999;24(20):2147–2153.
56. Mathews HH, Evans MT, Molligan HJ, et al. Laparoscopic discectomy with anterior lumbar interbody fusion. A preliminary review. Spine 1995;20(16):1797–1802.
57. Thalgott JS, Chin AK, Ameriks JA, et al. Minimally invasive 360 degrees instrumented lumbar fusion. Eur Spine J 2000;9(Suppl 1):S51–S16.
58. Heniford BT, Matthews BD, Lieberman IH. Laparoscopic lumbar interbody spinal fusion. Surg Clin North Am 2000;80(5):1487–1500.
59. Chen Y, Cheung KM, Kung HF, et al. In vivo new bone formation by direct transfer of adenoviral-mediated bone morphogenetic protein-4 gene. Biochem Biophys Res Commun 2002;298(1):121–127.

CHAPTER 27

Translaminar Screw Fixation

Dieter Grob

One of the surgical concepts to reduce pain originating from the lumbar spine is to immobilize the involved vertebrae. The most natural way to achieve this is to take advantage of the process of bone healing. By preparing the parts to be fixed with decortication and additional placement of bone graft, fusion may be enhanced. The mechanical situation of the spine, with considerable lever arms and multiple segmental centers of motion, implies a relatively low success rate of solid bony bridging.

To improve the fusion rate and reduce the need for rigid and cumbersome external fixation postoperatively, internal fixation has been introduced to temporarily immobilize the spine and thus enhance bony calcification. For this purpose Hadra (1) introduced first metallic wires in 1891. Before the era of pedicular screw fixation was introduced in Europe in the early 1960s (2), attempts to stabilize vertebrae posteriorly with screws only were attempted. The use of facet screws was first reported by King (3), whose technique was to immobilize the lumbosacral joints with short screws traversing the facets. With this technique he achieved a fusion rate of 91% without prolonged postoperative external fixation. Boucher (4) adopted this idea and improved the technique. He achieved a 100% fusion rate in single level fusions by penetrating the ipsilateral pedicle with the tip of the screw, thus improving the bony purchase. This method of screw insertion implied that the tip of the screw had to be placed near the foramen and the nerve root and carried the risk of nerve injury. In addition, there was a risk of decreased stability of this construct if the screw broke through the cortex of the posterior aspect of the facet. These complications of screw fixation in the lumbar spine made them unpopular despite the simplicity of the technique. It was Magerl 1984 (5) who modified and improved the technique of screw fixation and popularized revival of this type of immobilization. By inserting the screws from the contralateral side through the lamina, through the facet and ending in the base of the transverse process, most of the disadvantages of the former techniques were eliminated without losing their advantages.

Bony purchase was increased by the passage of the screw through the lamina, and the procedure was less risky because: (a) the insertion of the screw was clearly posterior to the neural elements; (b) the technique could be performed under direct visualization; and (c) the direction of screw insertion was parallel to the exiting nerve root, thereby minimizing the risk of injury to the nerve.

BIOMECHANICAL CONSIDERATIONS

A simplified but practical biomechanical concept of the lumbar spine with a three-column model was conceived by Louis (6). The anterior column is represented by the disc, the vertebral body, and the two posterior columns by the facets. In the course of evolution, anatomy adapted to the physiologic requirements of the spine; therefore, it seems reasonable to assume that the facets developed in response to mechanical necessity.

The importance of the facets has been demonstrated by several *in vitro* experiments in which partial or total resection of the facets led to dysfunction of the functional spinal motion unit (7,8). Together with the intervertebral disc, the facets share and support the axial load of the spine. Although the disc appears to be the primary load-bearing structure (8), the facets function as an indispensable part of the three-column concept to transmit part of the axial load, which varies according the position of the individual (9,10). Structural and morphologic changes that occur with destruction of cartilage and osteophyte formation underscore the important mechanical properties of the facets. Because the load passes partially through the facets, the lever arm acting on an internal fixation device through the facets remains small. A low-profile fixation device is sufficient to block segmental motion efficiently enough to enhance solid bony fusion (11,12).

Despite the fact that translaminar screw fixation represents the lowest profile implant for the lumbar spine, the stability in flexion achieved with this technique *in vitro* is similar to that provided by pedicle screw fixation (13,14).

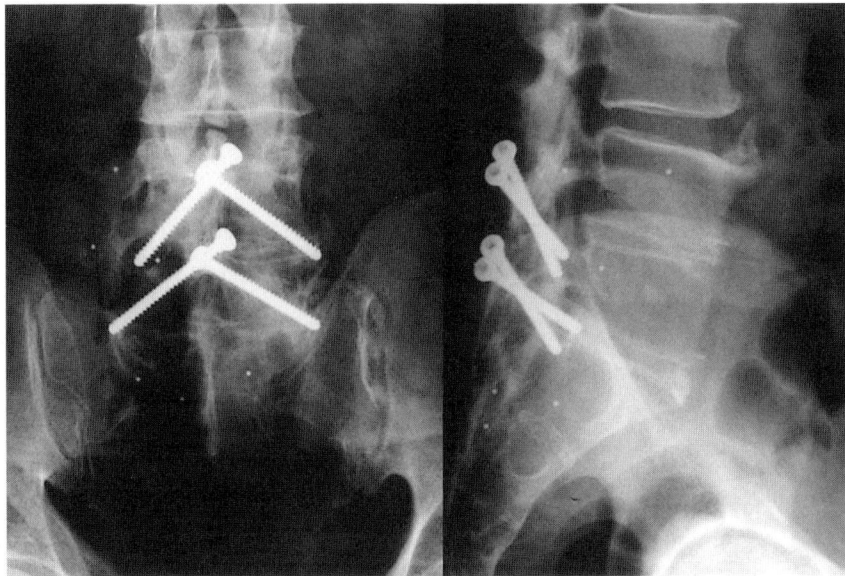

FIG. 27-1. Ten years postoperative: In addition to the solid fusion posteriorly, spontaneous calcification of the immobilized disc occurred. Axial loads are shared equally in the anterior and posterior columns.

The mechanical stiffness of a segment instrumented with translaminar screws is 2.4 times that of an uninstrumented segment; the stiffness was maintained for 5,000 cycles in static and cyclic loading tests (13,14).

The fact that the transfacet screw fixation *in vivo* might be less rigid than pedicle fixation may be an advantage rather than a disadvantage by promoting bone formation because rigid fixation results in stress shielding of the fusion and impedes bone remodeling (Fig. 27-1).

INDICATIONS

Translaminar screw fixation might be indicated in cases where segmental motion in the lumbar spine must be eliminated. It can be used as a primary fixation or as a supplemental procedure to protect and augment an existing fixation.

Translaminar Screws as Primary Procedure

Segmental Dysfunction

Motion between two or more anatomic structures causes wear and tear and a gradual change in their microstructure and macrostructure that may or may not lead to altered function and possibly pain (15). Given the complexity of the spine, diagnosis and localization of the pain source remains a challenging problem. In addition to clinical and radiologic examination (16), facet blocks and discography may be helpful to determine the painful segment. Temporary fixation with an external fixator also may be used as an invasive diagnostic method to identify a painful segment (17).

Once the diagnosis and localization of the painful segmental motion is established, posterior immobilization with translaminar screw fixation provides a simple and effective means of selective fusion of the involved segment (18). Dysfunction of a segment before the development of significant macroscopic structural changes represents an ideal indication for translaminar screw fixation.

Lumbar Spinal Stenosis

Degenerative lumbar spinal stenosis can be effectively treated with surgical decompression. If the compressive structures are removed, reduced leg pain and increased walking distance may be expected (19). It is reasonable to assume that the decompression may adversely affect the stability of the involved segment (7). Complete laminectomy with removal of a major portion of the facets, as may be required for lateral spinal stenosis, may jeopardize the segmental stability (8,20,21,22). Fusion also should be considered in these circumstances. Once the posterior elements have been removed, only transpedicular fixation systems are feasible. By using the more anatomic, atraumatic, and physiologic technique of "undercutting laminectomy," an effective decompression of the spinal canal can be performed leaving the posterior elements essentially intact (23–28). If fusion is considered necessary under these circumstances, the translaminar screws can provide fixation without considerable risk or lengthening of the operative time.

Revision Surgery

Persistent or recurrent pain after decompressive procedures might be associated with mechanical problems. Scar formation or persistent bony stenosis might irritate neurologic structures during motion. Therefore, immobilization of a previously operated segment may be indicated. If there is foraminal narrowing as a result of disc space narrowing following prior discectomy, additional distraction will open the foramen (29). Resection of one facet joint or bilateral resection of more than 50% of both facets may produce segmental instability (30). Because translaminar screws rely on the integrity of the posterior elements, this technique is only possible where the lamina and facet joint are sufficiently intact to receive a 4.5-mm cortical screw. Because the posterior bone stock is reduced, careful posterolateral intertransverse dissection must be done.

Disc-Related Syndromes

Lumbar Disc Herniation

Excision of a protruding disc fragment through a limited exposure is the accepted surgical treatment for herniated lumbar discs (31). A 5% to 10% incidence of recurrent disc herniation and a 10% to 15% incidence of postoperative low back pain is to be expected with this technique (32). Routine concomitant fusion after disc excision is not justified. However, in the presence of long-standing back pain and degenerative changes in the involved segment, fusion may help to improve outcome.

Disc Resorption and Internal Disc Disruption

When the underlying pathology is the degenerated disc itself (23,33), posterior fusion may help to relieve pain by immobilizing the segment. Posterior translaminar screw fixation is indicated if anterior surgery is not advised or indicated for other medical reasons or when posterior bony decompression is to be performed simultaneously.

Translaminar Screws as a Supplemental Procedure

Augmentation of Anterior Fusion

Translaminar screws efficiently immobilize the posterior columns in the presence of an intact anterior column. If there is a structural deficiency anteriorly, anterior reconstruction with a compression-resistant device must be performed. Biomechanically, anterior struts are ideal in resisting compressive forces but inadequate in neutralizing axial rotational forces. Therefore, supplemental translaminar screws are ideal in augmenting anterior procedures by immobilizing the facets and thereby eliminating axial rotation.

Augmentation of Pedicle Systems

The weak point in long lumbosacral pedicle constructs is sacral fixation. Different from the anatomy of the lumbar pedicles, the sacral pedicles are wider and provide less solid bone for screw fixation. The additional stability

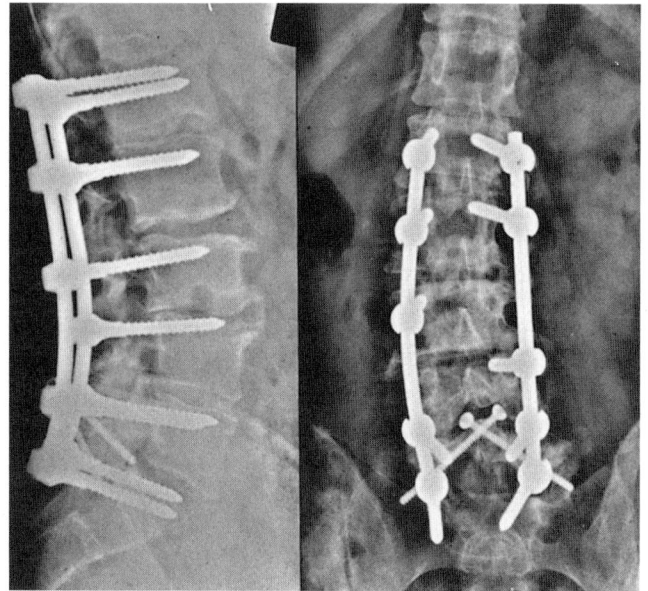

FIG. 27-2. Transarticular screw fixation as a supplement to increase stability at the lumbosacral junction.

achieved by supplementary transarticular screws fixation in the lumbosacral joint may help to overcome this anatomic disadvantage (Fig. 27-2).

Repair of Anterior Pseudarthrosis

In cases of anterior pseudarthrosis, posterior supplemental fusion is preferred to a repeat anterior procedure. Scar formation around the aorta, iliac vein, and vena cava may increase the operative risk of revision anterior surgery considerably. Translaminar screw fixation with additional posterior bone grafting offers a simple and effective method to stabilize the back.

CONTRAINDICATIONS AND LIMITATIONS

Translaminar screws rely on bony purchase to the posterior elements of the vertebrae (lamina, facets, and transverse process). Therefore, the posterior elements must be substantial enough to hold a screw. Severe osteopenia might jeopardize the screw purchase. Screw loosening and pseudarthrosis are more likely to occur in these cases. Because transfixed facets eliminate rotation in the y and z axis, but are less effective in the x axis, an intact anterior column is mandatory for this technique. The translaminar screws provide segmental fixation at each level fused, but avoids intersegmental connections between each fused segment. In our series, there were no statistical differences in solid bony union between monosegmental and bisegmental fixations; the number of three segmental fixations was too few to allow valid statistical analysis. However, for mechanical reasons, we do not advocate translaminar fixation of more than two adjacent segments.

For the same reason, translaminar screws should not be used to extend an existing fusion.

OPERATIVE TECHNIQUE

The surgical exposure is performed through a standard midline incision. The spinous processes, lamina, facet joints, and transverse processes are visualized and decorticated to receive the bone graft. The facet joints are opened by excision of the capsule, and osteophytes are removed. The cartilage of the dorsal aspect of the joint is removed, taking care not to injure the underlying subchondral bone in order to avoid loss of screw fixation.

The insertion of the screws by the Magerl technique is performed from the contralateral side of the spinous process of the segment to be fused, using a 50- to 54-mm long 4.5-mm screw. Fixation in slight flexion can be achieved if desired by applying interspinal distraction. Using a 3.2-mm drill bit, a hole is bored from the contralateral side of the spinous process into the opposite lamina. From there, the drill crosses the facet joint through its center and ends at the base of the transverse process (Fig. 27-3). This technique allows a nearly perpendicular screw direction in relation to the plane of the joint to be fused. In obese patients, percutaneous insertion of the drill through a separate stab incision may be necessary to obtain the proper direction of the screw. A dissector may be introduced between the attachment of the ligamentum flavum and the lamina, to minimize the risk of penetrating the spinal canal during the drilling procedure. An iliac bone graft must be placed posteriorly along the bony structures previously decorticated.

The postoperative management is straightforward and simple. Mobilization is begun on the first or second postoperative day. A soft corset brace is worn while out of bed for 3 months to restrict gross motions. Patients are encouraged to walk, and no physical therapy is performed during the first 2 months.

PATIENTS AND RESULTS

One hundred seventy-three consecutive patients underwent translaminar screw fixation of the lumbar spine, of which 145 (83%) were reassessed after an average follow-up of 58 months (34). Fifty-seven percent had a single-level fusion, 40% a two-level fusion, and 3% a three-level fusion. As a simultaneous procedure, 30% had a nucleotomy and 52% had a decompression of the spinal canal for clinically relevant symptoms of spinal stenosis.

A solid bony fusion, with a radiologically solid fusion mass and no apparent motion on the digitized flexion-extension radiographs in the fused segments, was documented in 163 patients (94%) and 241 segments (96%). Radiolucency around the screws was detected in five patients (3%). Two screws were broken; however, no motion could be detected on the flexion-extension radiographs.

Preoperatively the subjective pain rating was 7.6, which decreased to a pain rating of 2.9 at follow-up. Thirty-three patients (19%) were taking analgesics because of lumbar back pain. One hundred sixty (92%) of the patients stated that they would undergo the same treatment again if in the same situation as prior to surgery.

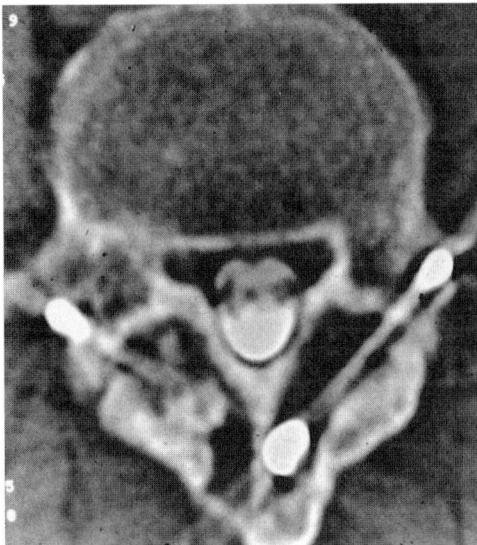

FIG. 27-3. Correct position of the screws in axial computed tomography scan: through the lamina and the facet joint into the base of the transverse process. Permanent stability is achieved with a proper grafting technique.

REFERENCES

1. Hadra BE. Wiring of the spinous processes in Pott's disease. Trans Am Orthop Assoc 1891;4:206–211.
2. Roy Camille R, Demeulenaere C. Osteosynthèse du rachis dorsal, lombaire et lombo-sacré par plaque métallique vissée dans les pédicules vertébraux et les apophyses articulaires. Presse Méd 1970;78:1447–1448.
3. King D. Internal fixation of lumbosacral fusion. J Bone Joint Surg 1948;30A:560–565.
4. Boucher HH. A method of spinal fusion. J Bone Joint Surg (British) 1959;41:248–259.
5. Magerl F. Stabilization of the lower thoracic and lumbar spine with external skeletal fixation. Clin Orthop 1984;189:125–141.
6. Louis R. Fusion of the lumbar and sacral spine by internal fixation with screw plates. Clin Orthop 1986;203:18–33.
7. Abumi K, Panjabi MM, Kramer KM. Biomechanical evaluation of lumbar spinal stability after graded facetectomies. Spine 1990;15:1142–1147.
8. Haher TR, O'Brien M, Dryer JW, et al. The role of the lumbar facet joints in spinal stability. Spine 1994;19:2667–2671.
9. Goel VK, Weinstein JN, Found EM. Biomechanics of lumbar and thoracolumbar spine surgery. In: Goel VK, Weinstein JN, eds. Biomechanics of the spine: clinical and surgical perspective. Boca Raton, FL: CRC Press, 1990:181–232.
10. Tencer A, Ahmed A, Burke D. Some static mechanical properties of the lumbar intervertebral joint, intact and injured. J Biomech Eng 1982;104:193–201.
11. Heggeness MH, Esses SI. Translaminar facet joint screw fixation for lumbar and lumbosacral fusion. A clinical and biomechanical study. Spine 1991;16S:266–269.

12. Kornblatt M, Casey MP, Jacobs RR. Internal fixation in lumbosacral spine fusion. A biomechanical and clinical study. Clin Orthop 1986; 203:141–150.

13. Deguchi M, Cheng, BC, Sato K, et al. Biomechanical evaluation of translaminar facet joint fixation. Spine 1998;23(12):1307–1313.

14. Vanden Berghe L, Mehdian H, Lee AJ, et al. Stability of the lumbar spine and method of instrumentation. Acta Orthop Belgica 1993;59: 175–180.

15. Eisenstein SM, Parry CR. The lumbar facet arthrosis syndrome. Clinical presentation and articular surface changes. J Bone Joint Surg 1987;69B:3–7.

16. Penning L, Blickman JR. Instability in lumbar spondylolisthesis: A radiologic study of several concepts. Am J Roentgenol 1980;134:293–301.

17. Olerud S, Sjöström L, Karlström G, et al. Spontaneous effect of increased stability of the lower lumbar spine in cases of severe chronic back pain. Clin Orthop 1986;203:67–74.

18. Stokes IA, Frymoyer JW. Segmental motion and instability. Spine 1987;12:688–691.

19. Grob D, Jeanneret B, Aebi M, et al. Atlantoaxial fusion with transarticular screw fixation. J Bone Joint Surg 1991;73B:972–976.

20. Hopp E, Tsou PM. Postdecompression lumbar instability. Clin Orthop 1988;227:143–151.

21. Katz J, Lipson S, Larson M, et al. The outcome of decompressive laminectomy for degenerative lumbar stenosis. J Bone Joint Surg 1991;73A:809–816.

22. Passuti N, Allioux JJ, Cistac C, et al. Sténoses lombaires dégénératives: interêt de l'instrumentation de Cotrel-Dubousset associé à la lamino-arthréctomie. Rev Chir Orthop 1990;76:23–29

23. Crock H. A short practice of spinal surgery. New York: Springer-Verlag, 1993.

24. De la Caffiniere JY. Evaluation du risque de glissement vertebral après traitement chirurgical d'une stenose lombaire. Rev Chir Orthop 1986; 72:73–80.

25. Getty CJ, Johnsson JR, Kirwan EO, et al. Partial undercutting facetectomy for bony entrapment of the lumbar nerve root. J Bone Joint Surg Br 1981;63-B(3) 330–335.

26. Grob D, Panjabi M, Dvorak J, et al. Die instabile Wirbelsäule-eine "In-vitro-" und "In-vivo-Studie" zum besseren Verständnis der klinischen Instabilität. Orthopäde 1994;23:291–298.

27. Nakai O, Okawa A, Yamaura I. Long term roentgenographic and functional changes in patients who were treated with wide fenestration for central lumbar stenosis. J Bone Joint Surg 1991;73A:1184–1191.

28. Senegas J, Etchevers JP, Vital JM, et al. Widening of the lumbar canal as an alternative to laminectomy in the treatment of lumbar stenosis. French J Orthop Surg 1988;2:93–99.

29. Humke T, Grob D, Dvorak J, et al. Foraminal changes with distraction and compression of the L4/5 and L5/S1 segments. Eur Spine J 1996;5: 183–186.

30. White AA, Panjabi MM, Posner I, et al. Spinal stability: evaluation and treatment. In: American Academy of Orthopedic Surgeons. Instructional Course Lectures. St. Louis: CV Mosby, 1981:457–483.

31. Benini A, Magerl F. Selective decompression and translaminar facet screw fixation for lumbar canal stenosis and disc protrusion. Br J Neurosurg 1993;7:413–418.

32. Hanley EN, Shapiro DE. The development of low back pain after excision of a lumbar disc. J Bone Joint Surg 1989;71A:719–721.

33. Weinstein J, Rydevik B. The pain of spondylolisthesis. Semin Sin Surg 1989;2:100–105

34. Grob D, Humke T. Translaminar screw fixation in the lumbar spine: indications, technique, results. Eur Spine J 1998;7:178–186.

Specific Clinical Entities

CHAPTER 28

Lumbar Disc Disorders

Mats Grönblad

Medicine, to produce health,
has to examine disease,
and music, to create harmony,
must investigate discord.
—Plutarch, c.e. 46–120

Low back pain, including that resulting from lumbar disc disorders, is multifactorial, as is the disability caused by it (1,2). Perhaps the most common causes of low back pain are musculoligamentous injuries and age-related degenerative processes of spinal structures (1). Degenerative processes are partly age-related and partly genetically determined (3–5). Spine problems and spinal degeneration are not problems of modern society, they have been reported in ancient times as well (6).

SOFT TISSUE

Definitions

Any muscle in the body may be strained or sprained, including low back muscles. Verifying such sprains as the cause of low back pain is, however, difficult. Often, however, either the term *low back strain* (7,8) or *sprain* (9) is used for any acute low back pain symptoms that commence suddenly (e.g., at the workplace). Of note, however, it has been suggested that sudden increases in physical activity will mainly affect the intervertebral disc, which is the most vulnerable spinal structure, due to its avascular nature and low metabolic rate. Thus, adaptive remodeling changes in the disc could lag behind those in other spinal tissues (10).

History and Physical Examination

Whenever a patient visits for low back pain, the most important thing is to first exclude any serious underlying disease or disorder that may warrant specific treatment. The so-called *red flags* (Table 28-1) are of great help when trying to exclude serious underlying disorder. When one or more of the red flags has been determined to be present, there is up to a 10% probability that the patient has a serious underlying disease causing the low back pain symptoms (13). A report of nighttime pain may also suggest underlying systemic disease (1) (e.g., malignant disease or inflammatory spondyloarthropathy). This is particularly the case if the pain shows progressive worsening with time. The combined history and erythrocyte sedimentation rate have been reported to have relatively high diagnostic accuracy in vertebral cancer (14). Moderately accurate items for diagnosing ankylosing spondylitis are a need to get out of bed at night and to move around a bit as well as reduced lateral mobility of the spine (14).

Pain radiating below the level of the knee may be suggestive of sciatica, and should warrant a thorough neurologic examination. While in the waiting room the patient may complete a pain drawing, depicting areas of pain and pain radiation, possibly with separate markings or colors for pain, numbness, and "pins and needles". Viewing such a precompleted chart will give the examining physician a quick notion of the presence or absence of sciatic pain radiation. Pain drawings may be an important adjunct in the assessment of chronic low back pain (15–18) and have been shown to have acceptable repeatability (18).

One should be alert to signs of systemic disease (e.g., fever). Following low back strain or sprains, possibly suggesting a muscular source for the pain, palpating vertebral muscles for tenderness can be done, but unfortunately, such palpation of tenderness is not reproducible between examiners (1). Interpreting limited spinal motion is also problematic, because the correlation with disability assessments or visual analog scale pain intensity is reportedly quite low (19). As well, in a normal busy clinical environment the reliability of such measurement of spinal motion is apparently quite low (20). With thoroughly trained examiners, however, the inter-tester reliability for physical examination findings may be somewhat better (21,22). Measures of spinal flexibility have been reported to be poor predictors of future back pain in an industrial setting (23). Borge et al. (24) recently con-

TABLE 28-1. Red flags *(somatic risk factors) for excluding serious underlying disorder in patients presenting with low back pain*

Age: >50 years
History of cancer
Unexplained weight loss
Pain: >1 month's duration
Absence of response to therapy
Pain becomes worse at rest
History of intravenous drug use
Presence of an infection, particularly urinary tract infection

From Bigos S, Bowyer O, Braen G, et al. Acute low back problems in adults. Clinical practice guideline no. 14. Rockville, MD: Agency for Health Care Policy and Research, 1994:iii, 1–26 (AHCPR publication no. 95-0642) and Lurie JD, Gerber PD, Sox HC. A pain in the back. *New Engl J Med* 2000;343:723–726, with permission.

cluded, based on a systematic literature review, that there is presently no satisfactory answer whether or not physical examination tests have any prognostic value in the nonoperative treatment of patients with low back pain. An exclusively medical approach for the measurement of physical disability following low back strain or sprains should probably be abandoned in favor of a multifactorial biopsychosocial approach to low back disability assessment (19,20).

Treatment

Following lumbar strain or sprains, the mainstay of any treatment should be to try to keep the patient active, not use bed rest as a treatment modality, and to support the patient in attempts to return to work as quickly as possible (25–27). The choice of treatments should be based upon published guidelines for treating patients with low back pain (11,28–32). It may also be helpful, when attempting to predict further chronicity of the low back problem, to consider so-called *yellow flags*, which are suggested psychological risk factors for delayed recovery (Table 28-2).

TABLE 28-2. Yellow flags *(psychological risk factors) that may help predict prolonged recovery*

Attitudes and beliefs: The experienced pain is harmful to the spine
Inadequate illness behavior (e.g., extended rest)
Compensation
Diagnosis and treatment: Causes confusion or fear about outcome
Emotions: fear, irritation, low mood
Work issues: Belief that work is harmful; absence of interest of employer; no possibilities for gradual return to work; high biomechanical demands

From Kendall NAS, Linton SJ, Main CJ. Guide to assessing psychosocial yellow flags in acute low back pain: risk factors for long-term disability and work loss. Wellington (NZ): Accident Rehabilitation & Compensation Insurance Corporation of New Zealand and the National Health Committee, 1997, with permission.

DISC DEGENERATION

Definition

A study by computed tomography (CT) discography on 300 patients with various prediscography diagnoses indicated a major role for intradiscal pathology in nonspecific low back pain syndromes (33). Also by CT discography, Schwarzer et al. (34) determined internal disc disruption to be present in 39% of 92 subjects studied. Such internal disc disruption was most commonly present at the L5-S1 and L4-L5 levels (34). Distinguishing pathologic disc degeneration from disc alterations due to normal aging is, however, problematic. In a clinical setting, it has only recently been possible to radiologically evaluate the extent and distribution of disc degeneration. Radiologic findings that have been interpreted as suggestive of disc degeneration are, however, also commonly observed in asymptomatic subjects (35,36). In a large-scale magnetic resonance imaging (MRI) study on asymptomatic women between the ages of 16 to 80 years, Powell et al. (35) noted a linearly increased prevalence of one or more degenerate disc with age. Disc degeneration on MRI was, however, already present in more than one-third of the women between the ages of 21 to 40 years (35). A more recent study by Goupille et al. (37) compared spinal cadavers of subjects who had suffered from chronic low back pain, in the absence of radicular pain, with subjects who had been free of back complaints. No individual type of degenerative abnormality was found to relate specifically to low back pain, but the extent of pathologic change did show such a relationship with prior chronic low back pain (37).

Natural History

There is now moderate evidence indicating that physical demands of work play only a minor role in the development of disc degeneration (3,38,39). In a recent large-scale longitudinal study on 1,165 nurses, low back pain at baseline was highly predictive of future low back pain, and the longer back pain was consistently reported (in a total of 8 follow-up questionnaires completed 3 months apart), the greater the likelihood that it would also be present at the next follow-up. Furthermore, the investigators showed that disabling low back pain carried a worse prognosis, as did back pain associated with sciatica (40). Thus, low back pain should not be regarded as an acute event that can be cured but as a persistent problem with intermittent exacerbations (1). As the observations by Smedley et al. (40) suggest, determining a presence or absence of disability, already at an early stage, is of paramount importance.

Follow-up by MRI of asymptomatic individuals with lumbar disc abnormalities, for an average of 5 years, showed progression of disc degeneration findings in 41.5% of the subjects (41). Medical consultation at follow-up was, however, not predicted by MRI findings at baseline, but by job-related variables (41). Another similar 7-year follow-up study on asymptomatic subjects showed that MRI findings were not predictive of either the development or the duration of low back pain (42). The individuals with the longest duration of low back pain did not have the greatest degree of abnormality on the baseline MRI scans (42). Interestingly, in schoolchildren degenerative abnormalities on MRI have been shown to predict future recurrent bouts of low back pain (43). It was suggested that disc degeneration present soon after the phase of rapid physical growth predicted recurrent pain up to early adulthood (43). At the other end of the age scale, a study by CT discography on 291 subjects with an age range of 17 to 79 years noted that the proportion of severely degenerated but painless discs increased with age, as did discs producing dissimilar pain (44). According to the investigators, such degenerated but asymptomatic discs, particularly in older subjects, may at least in part explain the well-recognized poor correlation between low back pain symptoms and radiographic images (44).

History and Physical Examination

In a study on male cadavers, examined radiographically and osteologically, history of back injury showed a relationship with the presence of symmetric disc degeneration, anular ruptures, and vertebral osteophytosis (45). In another study, lumbar disc degeneration, as observed by plain radiography, showed an age-independent association with both a history of lumbago and a history of sciatica (46).

The same basic principles presented previously for muscular strain and sprain also apply to patients with disc degeneration. Thus, it is of paramount importance to first exclude serious underlying disorder (Table 28-1). Unfortunately, there are no clinical tests that are specific for internal disc disruption that can be diagnosed by CT discography (34). Recent studies suggest that for measurements of spinal range of motion, there is both poor intra- and inter-rater reliability (47). Furthermore, range of motion measurements show poor validity with respect to relationships with physical and functional impairment (19,48). There is currently also strong evidence that back function testing machines producing isometric, isokinetic, or isoinertial measurements have no predictive value for either future low back pain or disability (39). Waddell et al. (49) have presented a validated battery of measures of physical impairment that can be recommended. Whichever symptom characteristics or clinical signs are used, they should show acceptable intra- and interexaminer repeatability and predictive validity with respect to major outcome measures of interest (50). Clinical observation of overt pain behavior may also be helpful, even if there may be a problem of standardization (51).

Imaging

Plain Radiography

The main indication of imaging is to exclude serious underlying disorder, when red flags are present (Table 28-1) or otherwise. In older patients the possibility of osteoporotic fracture should also be kept in mind (1). For the evaluation of disc degeneration, plain radiography produces far too many nonspecific findings, with doubtful clinical relevance (Figs. 28-1, 28-2). It is almost impossible to reliably relate such findings to clinical symptoms of low back pain. Overinterpretation is much too common, and may have an adverse effect on the outcome by labeling the patient and increasing the sick role. This will have an effect opposite to the mainstay of the treatment protocol, namely to keep the patient active, functional, and to decrease perceived disability (52). Reliability of measurement may pose a problem (53).

CT and MRI

As is the case with plain radiography, these imaging modalities should be used mainly to exclude serious underlying disorder (Table 28-1) or when the patient has progressive or persistent neurologic deficit. Of note, there is now strong evidence that plain radiography and MRI findings have no predictive value for future low back pain or disability (39). They also do not correlate well with clinical symptoms in patients with nonspecific low back pain, or with work capacity (39).

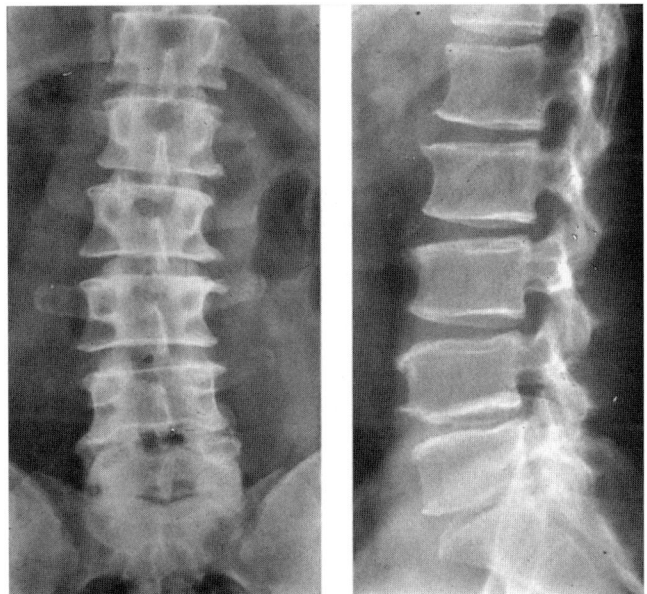

FIG. 28-1. Plain radiograph anteroposterior and sagittal views of the lumbar spine of an asymptomatic 61-year-old woman. Note general disc narrowing and minor osteophytes both anteriorly and laterally. There is also slight scoliosis. (Courtesy of Dr. Kaj Tallroth, Orton Hospital, Helsinki, Finland.)

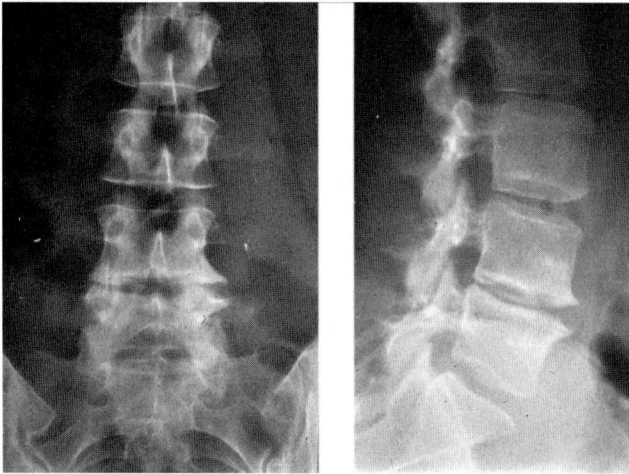

FIG. 28-2. Plain radiograph anteroposterior and sagittal views of a 46-year-old woman with low back pain. Disc narrowing, osteophytes, and end-plate changes appear only at the L4-L5 level. (Courtesy of Dr. Kaj Tallroth, Orton Hospital, Helsinki, Finland.)

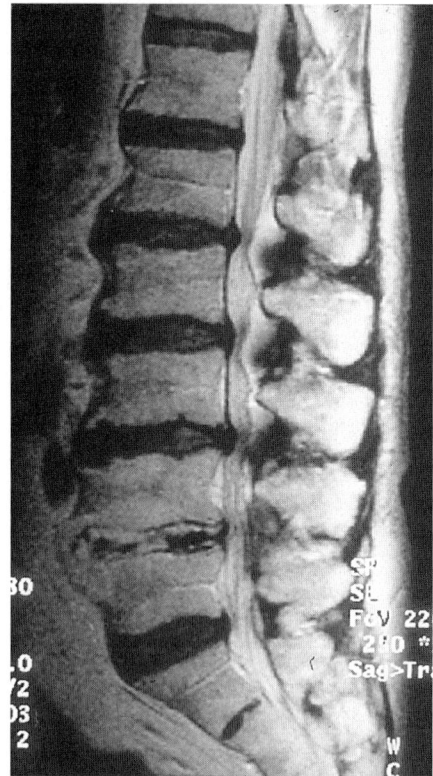

FIG. 28-3. T2-weighted sagittal magnetic resonance imaging scan (1.5 Tesla unit) of the lumbar spine of a 45-year-old man with low back pain. Note severe multiple level disc degeneration with end-plate abnormalities. The L4-L5 disc is almost totally obliterated, suggesting severe disc degeneration. (Courtesy of Dr. Kaj Tallroth, Orton Hospital, Helsinki, Finland.)

CT should be combined with discography for imaging disc degeneration. With respect to MRI, it should be kept in mind that particularly disc bulges and protrusions are commonly observed in asymptomatic subjects, whereas disc extrusions are not (Table 28-3). But even when extrusions are observed, they should be interpreted within the entire clinical context to determine whether neural compromise is present or not. Bulges and protrusions are particularly prevalent at the two lowest lumbar levels and the prevalence of disc bulges increases with age (36). There are now several studies that show MRI abnormalities in asymptomatic adults (1).

In a study on cadavers that used in parallel MRI, biochemical, and histologic analysis, decreased total proteoglycan content and chondroitin-keratan sulfate ratio in subjects with low signal intensity on T2-weighted MRI could be observed, supporting the validity of MRI for diagnosing disc degeneration (54). Signal intensity on T2-weighted MRI has been considered the most sensitive available measure of disc degeneration (Fig. 28-3),

whereas the assessment of disc height has less validity (55). In a large scale study, significant dehydration and degeneration on MRI was present in less than 5% at the two uppermost lumbar levels, whereas marked changes were observed at the two lowest lumbar levels in more than 20% of the patients (56).

Discography

When MRI and discography have been used in parallel for the assessment of disc degeneration, a high correlation has usually been observed (57–59). It is considered that MRI can be used for detecting early disc degeneration (58). Also quantitative disc manometry has been suggested to show good correlation with MRI for assessing disc degeneration (60). Disc manometry may be suitable for evaluating early stages of disc degeneration and may detect tears of annular fibers that go nondetected on MRI (60). Results are not entirely consistent, however (61).

Of all imaging modalities currently available, discography is the only one that can locate a degenerated and symptomatic disc and which visualizes internal disc disruption (Figs. 28-4, 28-5) (33,34,62–65) (Table 28-4).

TABLE 28-3. *Presence of disc abnormalities on magnetic resonance imaging in 98 asymptomatic subjects*

	%
Normal discs at all levels	36
Bulge (1 level)	52
Protrusion	27
Extrusion	1
Annular defects[a]	14
Abnormal finding in >1 disc	38

[a]Disruption of the outer annulus fibrosus ring of the disc.
Modified from Jensen MC, Brant-Zawadzki MN, Obuchowski N, et al. Magnetic resonance imaging of the lumbar spine in people without back pain. *N Engl J Med* 1994;331: 69–73, with permission.

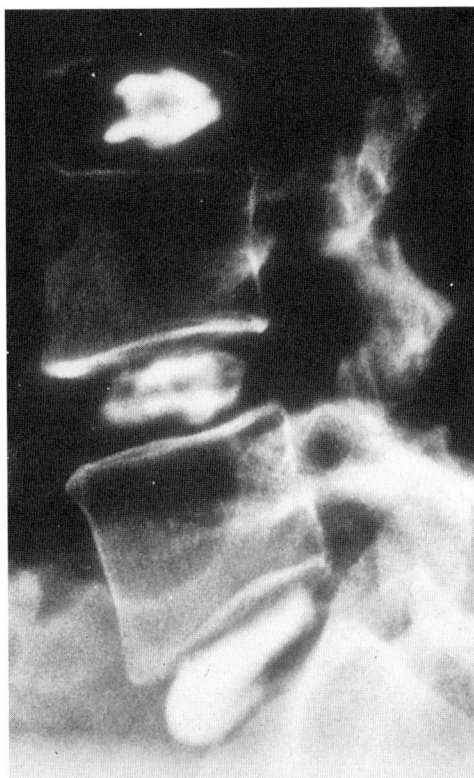

FIG. 28-4. Sagittal view discography in a 46-year-old man with low back pain. Note normal cotton ball–type images at L3-L4 and L4-L5, whereas there is abnormal spread of contrast in the L5-S1 disc. (Courtesy of Dr. Kaj Tallroth, Orton Hospital, Helsinki, Finland.)

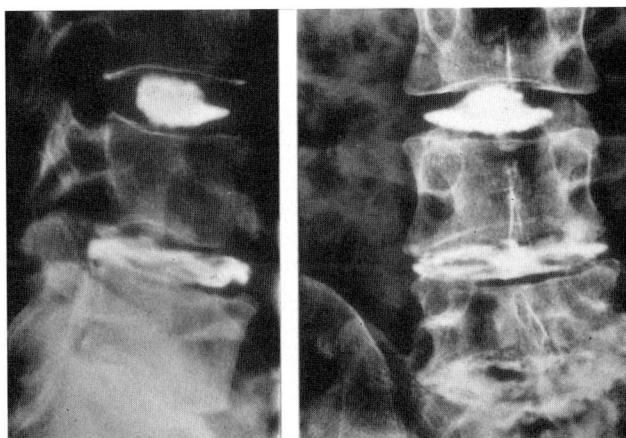

FIG. 28-5. Sagittal and anteroposterior discography views in a 36-year-old woman with low back pain. There is slight abnormal spread of contrast at the L3-L4 level, with more severe degeneration in the two lowermost discs, as seen by the widespread distribution of contrast. (Courtesy of Dr. Kaj Tallroth, Orton Hospital, Helsinki, Finland.)

TABLE 28-4. *Summary of position statement of North American Spine Society Diagnostic and Therapeutic Committee on lumbar discography*

Lumbar discography can be used in select cases such as:
- When there is persistent pain with suspicion of disc abnormality, and noninvasive tests have not provided sufficient diagnostic information.
- To determine whether discs within a proposed fusion segment are symptomatic, and whether adjacent discs are asymptomatic.
- In patients who have undergone previous spine surgery, but with nonremitting significant pain, to differentiate between postoperative scar and recurrent disc herniation.
- To investigate the condition of a disc within, or adjacent to, a fused spinal segment, to better delineate the source of symptoms.
- To confirm a contained disc herniation, possibly requiring minimally invasive discectomy.

Modified from Guyer RD, Ohnmeiss DD. Lumbar discography position statement from the North American Spine Society Diagnostic and Therapeutic Committee. Spine 1995;20:2048–2059, with permission.

Internal disc disruption has been postulated to be an important cause of low back pain, and a taxonomy has been established by the International Association for the Study of Pain (Table 28-5) (34). The clinical usefulness and interpretation of discography is, however, controversial (33,62–69). In particular, it has been observed that discographic pain reports are not only related to anatomic abnormalities within the disc, but also to scores on the Minnesota Multiphasic Personality Inventory (MMPI) (70), somatization disorder, compensation issues, and abnormal results on psychological testing (69). Thus, it would seem mandatory to perform psychological testing on any patient undergoing discography with interpretation of pain provocation, particularly if the discography procedure is used for preoperative evaluation. Even though discography may be problematic for clinical decision making, studies performed with discography have considerably widened the horizons for understanding mechanisms of low back pain and the locations of pain generators within the spine (62,64), including intricate mechanisms of pain radiation (65).

TABLE 28-5. *International Association for the Study of Pain (IASP) taxonomy for internal disc disruption*

The pain should be reproduced on provocation discography
Computed tomography/discography should reveal internal disc disruption
As a control, stimulation of at least one other disc should fail to reproduce the pain

From Schwarzer AC, Aprill CN, Derby R, et al. The prevalence and clinical features of internal disc disruption in patients with chronic low back pain. Spine 1995;20:1878–1883, with permission.

NONOPERATIVE TREATMENT

Types and Results

For treating lumbar disc disorders, a profusion of alternative therapies are available to the clinician, as is often the case when there is a lack of more precise knowledge regarding etiology and pathophysiology. The clinician may, however, obtain support in the choice of therapies from several recently published guidelines, and the mainstay of any treatment protocol should be to try to adhere to such guidelines whenever possible (11,28–32,39).

With an increasing shift to self-management strategies that empower patients to participate in decisions in their care (27,71,72), all patients should be provided with basic information regarding course and prognosis (Table 28-6). However, the mainstay of any treatment protocol should be to try to keep the patient active and to try to influence an often wide array of perceived functional limitations in daily activities and at work. The principal goal is to continue normal daily activities (27). Table 28-7 presents some main principles that will guide the clinician in the treatment of patients with lumbar disc disorders and nonspecific low back pain. Prolonged low back pain and disability will usually require a well-organized multidisciplinary rehabilitation program (82), even if there is presently a lack of knowledge regarding the optimal content of such programs (83) (e.g., whether any specific type of exercise has any specific physical effect or not) (84). In one study on multidisciplinary rehabilitation of patients with chronic low back pain, the most important variable for determining a successful treatment outcome was the reduction of subjective feelings of disability, whereas treatment outcome was not predicted by variables such as medical background, medical diagnosis, physical impairment, or physical variables such as mobil-

TABLE 28-6. *Some clinically relevant facts regarding the course and prognosis of nonspecific low back pain*

It is very common, in fact, it may be considered abnormal to live a single year *without* a backache (73).
Recovery from an acute spell of low back pain is generally rapid (74).
It is not an acute disease that can be cured, but once established, a chronic problem with intermittent exacerbations (1).
After 1 year 10%–45% still suffer from low back pain (75,76). In about one third the pain may still be disabling at 1 year (77).
Only about 2% remain on sick leave after 1 year (76).
Recurrences are common and have been reported in about 40% within 6 months (78) and about 75% within 1 year (75).
Even though recurrences are common, both pain and disability are usually less severe during such recurrences (75).
Once low back pain has become chronic, pain intensity and physical functioning improve only little after 1 year (79).

TABLE 28-7. *Main principles for managing lumbar disc disorders*

Neither sick leave nor inactivity will benefit recovery from low back pain (27).
To prevent adverse effects of fear avoidance beliefs, a principal goal should be the continuation of normal daily activities (27,80,81). Advice to stay active often leads to shorter periods of work loss and fewer recurrences, in comparison with traditional medical treatment (39).
Chronic cases will benefit from multidisciplinary rehabilitation programs (27).
Traditional biomedical education, based on an injury model, will not reduce future low back pain, nor work loss (39).
Lumbar belts or supports do not reduce work-related low back pain, nor work loss (39).
With respect to persistent symptoms and disability, and the response to treatment and rehabilitation, individual and work-related psychosocial factors play a key role (39).
Workers' own beliefs that their low back pain was caused by work, and their own expectations about inability to return to work, should be monitored, because they are important prognostic factors (39).
Most workers will be able to continue working, or can return to their ordinary work, within a few days or weeks, and do not need to wait until they are completely pain free (39).
The longer a worker is away from work, the lesser the chance of returning to work. For example, it has been shown that if a worker is off work for 4–12 weeks, the estimated risk of still being off work at 1 year is 10%–40%. With work absence of 1–2 years chances to return to any type of work are near nil (39).
With protracted work absence, treatments become ineffective for returning people to work, even though the treatments may still produce some clinical improvement (39).

ity, strength, endurance, or physical performance (82). There are several available validated condition-specific (19,85–93) and generic (94–97) functional disability scales that may be used for assessing outcome. It is important to remember, however, that disability is multifactorial (52,98).

With respect to the choice of treatment program, there is presently insufficient evidence to justify intensive and expensive programs, which are likely to be less cost-effective (39). In the treatment protocol, the role of the workplace and work-related factors should not be overlooked, since recent studies suggest that a close association between clinical care and occupational intervention may produce superior results to other treatment protocols, particularly in patients with subacute work-related low back pain (99). However, there is a need for more detailed information on the role of various risk factors for the various phases of work-related disability (100).

REFERENCES

1. Deyo RA, Weinstein JN. Low back pain. N Engl J Med 2001;344: 363–370.
2. Frank JW, Kerr MS, Brooker A-S, et al. Disability resulting from

occupational low back pain. Part I: What do we know about primary prevention? A review of the scientific evidence on prevention before disability begins. Spine 1996;21:2908–2917.

3. Battié MC, Videman T, Gibbons LE, et al. Determinants of lumbar disc degeneration. Spine 1995;20:2601–2612.

4. Annunen S, Paassilta P, Lohiniva J, et al. An allele of COL9A2 associated with intervertebral disc disease. Science 1999;285:409–412.

5. Paassilta P, Lohiniva J, Göring HHH, et al. Identification of a novel common genetic risk factor for lumbar disk disease. JAMA 2001;285:1843–1849.

6. Gerszten PC, Gerszten E, Allison MJ. Diseases of the spine in South American mummies. Neurosurgery 2001;48:208–213.

7. Aghababian RV, Voltur GA, Heifetz IN. Comparison of diflunisal and naproxen in the management of acute low back strain. Clin Ther 1986;9[Suppl C]:47–51.

8. Brown FL, Bodison S, Dixon J, et al. Comparison of diflunisal and acetaminophen with codeine in the treatment of initial or recurrent acute low back strain. Clin Ther 1986;9[Suppl C]:52–58.

9. Gunn CC, Milbrandt WE. Early and subtle signs in low-back sprain. Spine 1978;3:267–281.

10. Adams MA, Dolan P. Could sudden increases in physical activity cause degeneration of intervertebral discs? Lancet 1997;350:734–735.

11. Bigos S, Bowyer O, Braen G, et al. Acute low back problems in adults. Clinical practice guideline, no. 14. Rockville, MD: Agency for Health Care Policy and Research, 1994:iii, 1–26 (AHCPR publication no. 95–0642).

12. Lurie JD, Gerber PD, Sox HC. A pain in the back. New Engl J Med 2000;343:723–726.

13. Wipf JE, Deyo RA. Low back pain. Med Clin North Am 1995;79:231–246.

14. van den Hoogen HM, Koes BW, van Eijk JT, et al. On the accuracy of history, physical examination, and erythrocyte sedimentation rate in diagnosing low back pain in general practice. A criteria-based review of the literature. Spine 1995;20:318–327.

15. Chan CW, Goldman S, Ilstrup DM, et al. The pain drawing and Waddell's nonorganic physical signs in chronic low-back pain. Spine 1993;18:1717–1722.

16. Ohnmeiss DD, Vanharanta H, Ekholm J. Relation between pain location and disc pathology: a study of pain drawings and CT/discography. Clin J Pain 1999;15:210–217.

17. Ohnmeiss DD, Vanharanta H, Ekholm J. Relationship of pain drawings to invasive tests assessing intervertebral disc pathology. Eur Spine J 1999;8:126–131.

18. Ohnmeiss DD. Repeatability of pain drawings in a low back pain population. Spine 2000;25:980–988.

19. Grönblad M, Hurri H, Kouri JP. Relationships between spinal mobility, physical performance tests, pain intensity and disability assessments in chronic low back pain patients. Scand J Rehabil Med 1997;29:17–24.

20. Hunt DG, Zuberbier OA, Kozlowski AJ, et al. Reliability of lumbar flexion, lumbar extension, and passive straight leg raise test in normal populations embedded within a complete physical examination. Spine 2001;26:2714–2718.

21. Strender LE, Sjoblom A, Sundell K, et al. Interexaminer reliability in physical examination of patients with low back pain. Spine 1997;22:814–820.

22. Van Dillen LR, Sahrmann SA, Norton BJ, et al. Reliability of physical examination items used for classification of patients with low back pain. Phys Ther 1998;78:979–988.

23. Battié MC, Bigos SJ, Fisher LD, et al. The role of spinal flexibility in back pain complaints within industry. A prospective study. Spine 1990;15:768–773.

24. Borge JA, Leboeuf-Yde C, Lothe J. Prognostic values of physical examination findings in patients with chronic low back pain treated conservatively: a systematic literature review. J Manip Physiol Ther 2001;24:292–295.

25. Indahl A, Velund L, Reikeraas O. Good prognosis for low back pain when left untampered. A randomized clinical trial. Spine 1995;20:473–477.

26. Abenhaim L, Rossignol M, Valat J-P, et al. The role of activity in the therapeutic management of back pain. Report of the International Paris Task Force on Back Pain. Spine 2000;25:1S–33S.

27. Biering-Sorensen F, Bendix AF. Working off low back pain. Lancet 2000;355:1929–1930.

28. Accident Rehabilitation and Compensation Insurance Corporation (ACC) and the National Health Committee. New Zealand acute low back pain guide. Wellington, NZ: ACC, 1997.

29. Royal College of General Practitioners (RCGP). Clinical guidelines for the management of acute low back pain. London: RCGP, 1999.

30. Faas A, Chavannes AW, Koes BW, et al. Dutch college of general practitioners practice guideline for low back pain. Huisarts Wet 1996;39:18–31.

31. Kendall NAS, Linton SJ, Main CJ. Guide to assessing psychosocial yellow flags in acute low back pain: risk factors for long-term disability and work loss. Wellington, NZ: Accident Rehabilitation & Compensation Insurance Corporation of New Zealand and the National Health Committee, 1997.

32. Smeele IJM, van den Hoogen JMM, Mens JMA, et al. Dutch college of general practitioners practice guideline sciatica. Huisarts Wet 1996;39:78–89.

33. Vanharanta H, Guyer RD, Ohnmeiss DD, et al. Disc deterioration in low-back syndromes. A prospective, multi-center CT/discography study. Spine 1988;13:1349–1351.

34. Schwarzer AC, Aprill CN, Derby R, et al. The prevalence and clinical features of internal disc disruption in patients with chronic low back pain. Spine 1995;20:1878–1883.

35. Powell MC, Wilson M, Szypryt P, et al. Prevalence of lumbar disc degeneration observed by magnetic resonance in symptomless women. Lancet 1986;2(8520):1366–1367.

36. Jensen MC, Brant-Zawadzki MN, Obuchowski N, et al. Magnetic resonance imaging of the lumbar spine in people without back pain. N Engl J Med 1994;331:69–73.

37. Goupille P, Jayson MIV, Hoyland JA, et al. Association between increased extent and multilevel disc lesions with low back pain: a cadaveric study. Paper originally presented at: American College of Rheumatology, National Scientific Meeting; November 8–12, 1998; San Diego. Arthritis Rheum 1998;41[Suppl]:S90.

38. Videman T, Battié MC. The influence of occupation on lumbar degeneration. Spine 1999;24:1164–1168.

39. Waddell G, Burton AK. Occupational health guidelines for the management of low back pain at work: evidence review. Occupation Med 2001;51:124–135.

40. Smedley J, Inskip H, Cooper C, et al. Natural history of low back pain. A longitudinal study in nurses. Spine 1998;23:2422–2426.

41. Boos N, Semmer N, Elfering A, et al. Natural history of individuals with asymptomatic disc abnormalities in magnetic resonance imaging: predictors of low back pain-related medical consultation and work incapacity. Spine 2000;25:1484–1492.

42. Borenstein DG, O'Mara JW Jr, Boden SD, et al. The value of magnetic resonance imaging of the lumbar spine to predict low-back pain in asymptomatic subjects: a seven-year follow-up study. J Bone Joint Surg Am 2001;83-A:1306–1311.

43. Salminen JJ, Erkintalo MO, Pentti J, et al. Recurrent low back pain and early disc degeneration in the young. Spine 1999;24:1316–1321.

44. Vanharanta H, Sachs BL, Ohnmeiss DD, et al. Pain provocation and disc deterioration by age. A CT/discography study in a low-back pain population. Spine 1989;14:420–423.

45. Videman T, Nurminen M, Troup JD. Lumbar spinal pathology in cadaveric material in relation to history of back pain, occupation, and physical loading. Spine 1990;15:728–740.

46. Wiikeri M, Nummi J, Riihimäki H, et al. Radiologically detectable lumbar disc degeneration in concrete reinforcement workers. Scand J Work Environ Health, 1978;4[Suppl 1]:47–53.

47. Nitschke JE, Nattrass CL, Disler PB, et al. Reliability of the American Medical Association guides' model for measuring spinal range of motion. Its implication for whole-person impairment rating. Spine 1999;24:262–268.

48. Nattrass CL, Nitschke JE, Disler PB, et al. Lumbar spine range of motion as a measure of physical and functional impairment: an investigation of validity. Clin Rehabil 1999;13:211–218.

49. Waddell G, Somerville D, Henderson I, et al. Objective clinical evaluation of physical impairment in chronic low back pain. Spine 1993;17:617–628.

50. Viikari-Juntura E, Takala E-P, Riihimäki H, et al. Standardized physical examination protocol for low back disorders: feasibility of use and validity of symptoms and signs. J Clin Epidemiol 1998;51:245–255.

51. Waddell G, Richardson J. Observation of overt pain behaviour by

physicians during routine clinical examination of patients with low back pain. J Psychosom Res 1992;36:77–87.

52. Waddell G. Biopsychosocial analysis of low back pain. Baillieres Clin Rheumatol 1992;6:523–557.

53. Shao Z, Rompe G, Schiltenwolf M. Radiographic changes in the lumbar intervertebral discs and lumbar vertebrae with age. Spine 2002; 27:263–268.

54. Tertti M, Paajanen H, Laato M, et al. Disc degeneration in magnetic resonance imaging. A comparative biochemical, histologic, and radiologic study in cadaver spines. Spine 1991;16:629–634.

55. Luoma K, Vehmas T, Riihimäki H, et al. Disc height and signal intensity of the nucleus pulposus on magnetic resonance imaging as indicators of lumbar disc degeneration. Spine 2001;26:680–686.

56. DeCandido P, Reinig JW, Dwyer AJ, et al. Magnetic resonance assessment of the distribution of lumbar spine disc degenerative changes. J Spinal Disord 1988;1:9–15.

57. Gibson MJ, Buckley J, Mawhinney R, et al. Magnetic resonance imaging and discography in the diagnosis of disc degeneration. A comparative study of 50 discs. J Bone Joint Surg Br 1986;68:369–373.

58. Schneiderman G, Flannigan B, Kingston S, et al. Magnetic resonance imaging in the diagnosis of disc degeneration: correlation with discography. Spine 1987;12:276–281.

59. Linson MA, Crowe CH. Comparison of magnetic resonance imaging and lumbar discography in the diagnosis of disc degeneration. Clin Orthop, 1990;250:160–163.

60. Southern EP, Fye MA, Panjabi MM, et al. Disc degeneration: a human cadaveric study correlating magnetic resonance imaging and quantitative discomanometry. Spine 2000;25:2171–2175.

61. Castagnera L, Grenier N, Lavignolle B, et al. Study of correlation between intradiscal pressure and magnetic resonance imaging data in evaluation of disc degeneration. Therapeutic issue with percutaneous nucleotomy. Spine 1991;16:348–352.

62. Bernard TN Jr. Lumbar discography followed by computed tomography. Refining the diagnosis of low-back pain. Spine 1990;15:690–707.

63. Engelmann L, Hahnel H, Pfeiffer U. The status of discography in determining indications for therapy of intervertebral disk-induced diseases. Beitrage zur Orthop Traumatol 1990;37:85–92.

64. Guyer RD, Ohnmeiss DD. Lumbar discography position statement from the North American Spine Society Diagnostic and Therapeutic Committee. Spine 1995;20:2048–2059.

65. Ohnmeiss DD, Vanharanta H, Ekholm J. Degree of disc disruption and lower extremity pain. Spine 1997;22:1600–1605.

66. Nachemson A. Lumbar discography—where are we today? Spine 1989;14:555–557.

67. Carragee EJ. Is lumbar discography a determinate of discogenic low back pain: provocative discography reconsidered. Curr Review Pain 2000;4:301–308.

68. Carragee EJ, Chen Y, Tanner CM, et al. Can discography cause long-term back symptoms in previously asymptomatic subjects? Spine 2000;25:1803–1808.

69. Carragee EJ, Tanner CM, Khurana S, et al. The rates of false-positive lumbar discography in select patients without low back symptoms. Spine 2000;25:1373–1380.

70. Block AR, Vanharanta H, Ohnmeiss DD, et al. Discographic pain report. Influence of psychological factors. Spine 1996;21:334–338.

71. The Bone and Joint Decade 2000–2010 for prevention and treatment of musculo-skeletal disorders. Consensus document. Acta Orthop Scand 1998;69[Suppl 281]:1–86.

72. Carter JT, Birrell LN, eds. Occupational health guidelines for the management of low back pain at work—principal recommendations. London: Faculty of Occupational Medicine, 2000.

73. Hadler NM, Carey TS. Low back pain: an intermittent and remittent predicament of life. Ann Rheum Dis 1998;57:1–2.

74. Coste J, Delecoeuillerie G, Cohen de Lara A, et al. Clinical course and prognostic factors in acute low back pain: an inception cohort study in primary care practice. BMJ 1994;308:577–580.

75. van den Hoogen HJM, Koes BW, van Eijk JThM, et al. On the course of low back pain in general practice: a one year follow up study. Ann Rheum Dis 1998;57:13–19.

76. Schiottz-Christensen B, Nielsen GL, Hansen VK, et al. Long-term prognosis of acute low back pain in patients seen in general practice: a 1-year prospective follow-up study. Family Pract 1999;16:223–232.

77. Thomas E, Silman AJ, Croft PR, et al. Predicting who develops chronic low back pain in primary care: a prospective study. BMJ 1999;318:1662–1667.

78. Carey TS, Garrett JM, Jackman A, et al. Recurrence and care seeking after acute back pain: results of a long-term follow-up study. Med Care 1999;37:157–164.

79. van Tulder MW, Koes BW, Metsemakers JF, et al. Chronic low back pain in primary care: a prospective study on the management and course. Family Pract 1998;15:126–132.

80. Waddell G, Newton M, Henderson I, et al. A Fear-Avoidance Beliefs Questionnaire (FABQ) and the role of fear-avoidance beliefs in chronic low back pain and disability. Pain 1993;52:157–168.

81. Al-Obaidi SM, Nelson RM, Al-Awadhi S, et al. The role of anticipation and fear of pain in the persistence of avoidance behavior in patients with chronic low back pain. Spine 2000;25:1126–1131.

82. Hildebrandt J, Pfingsten M, Saur P, et al. Prediction of success from a multidisciplinary treatment program for chronic low back pain. Spine 1997;22:990–1001.

83. Kuukkanen T, Mälkiä E. Muscular performance after a 3 month progressive physical exercise program and 9 month follow-up in subjects with low back pain. A controlled study. Scand J Med Sci Sports 1996; 6:112–121.

84. van Tulder MW, Malmivaara A, Esmail R, et al. Exercise therapy for low back pain. The Cochrane Library, Issue 2. Oxford: Update Software, 2000.

85. Fairbank J, Couper J, Davies J, et al. The Oswestry low back pain questionnaire. Physiotherapy 1980;66:271–273.

86. Roland M, Morris R. A study of the natural history of low back pain: Part I. Development of a reliable and sensitive measure of disability in low-back pain. Spine 1983;8:141–144.

87. Grönblad M, Hupli M, Wennerstrand P, et al. Intercorrelation and test-retest reliability of the Pain Disability Index (PDI) and the Oswestry Disability Questionnaire (ODQ) and their correlation with pain intensity in low back pain patients. Clin J Pain 1993;9:189–195.

88. Grönblad M, Järvinen E, Hurri H, et al. Relationship of the Pain Disability Index (PDI) and the Oswestry Disability Questionnaire (ODQ) with three dynamic physical tests in a group of patients with chronic low-back and leg pain. Clin J Pain 1994;10:197–203.

89. Grönblad M, Järvinen E, Airaksinen O, et al. Relationship of subjective disability with pain intensity, pain duration, pain location, and work-related factors in nonoperated patients with chronic low back pain. Clin J Pain 1996;12:194–200.

90. Kopec JA, Esdaile JM. Spine update. Functional disability scales for back pain. Spine 1995;20:1943–1949.

91. Beurskens JA, de Vet HC, Köke JA, et al. A patient-specific approach for measuring functional status in low back pain. J Manip Physiol Ther 1999;22:144–148.

92. Kopec JA. Measuring functional outcomes in persons with back pain. A review of back-specific questionnaires. Spine 2000;25:3110–3114.

93. Roland M, Fairbank J. The Roland-Morris disability questionnaire and the Oswestry disability questionnaire. Spine 2000;25:3115–3124.

94. Dijkers M. Measuring quality of life. Methodological issues. Am J Phys Med Rehabil 1999;78:286–300.

95. Lurie J. A review of generic health status measures in patients with low back pain. Spine 2000;25:3125–3129.

96. Ware JE Jr. SF-36 health survey update. Spine 2000;25:3130–3139.

97. Tosteson ANA. Preference-based health outcome measures in low back pain. Spine 2000;25:3161–3166.

98. Turk DC, Rudy TE, Stieg RL. The disability determination dilemma: toward a multiaxial solution. Pain 1988;34:217–229.

99. Loisel P, Abenhaim L, Durand P, et al. A population-based, randomized clinical trial on back pain management. Spine 1997;22: 2911–2918.

100. Krause N, Dasinger LK, Deegan LJ, et al. Psychosocial job factor and return-to-work after compensated low back injury: a disability phase-specific analysis. Am J Industr Med 2001;40:374–392.

CHAPTER 29

Facet Joint Denervation:
A Minimally Invasive Treatment for
Low Back Pain in Selected Patients

David J. Hall

It is accepted that the lumbar zygapophyseal joints (facet joints) are a potential source of low back and referred leg pain. However, as a clinical entity, facet syndrome remains ill-defined and hence the extent and significance of its contribution in disabling low back pain is a subject of ongoing debate. Nevertheless, it is possible to identify, through diagnostic testing, a very select group of patients that can be successfully treated by percutaneous radiofrequency facet joint denervation.

BACKGROUND

Although Goldthwait (1), in 1911, is credited as the first to recognize the lumbar facet joint as a potential source of back and leg pain, it was Ghormley (2), in 1933, who first coined the term "facet syndrome." However, their theories focused more on the facet joint exerting mechanical pressure on nerves as the origin of symptoms.

Later, in 1971, Rees (3,4) published his work on multiple bilateral subcutaneous rhizolysis, where he reported a technique of denervation of the posterior spinal structures, including the facet joints, merely by the sweep of a Beaver blade and claimed apparently successful treatment in 998 out of 1,000 consecutively treated patients.

Following up on Rees' work, Shealy (5) initially experimented with Rees' technique but encountered problems with hematomata in several patients that led him to the use of a radiofrequency lesioning device under fluoroscopy guidance. Mooney (6) was impressed by his observations of Shealy's technique and was stimulated, along with Robertson (7), to undertake their important work in an attempt to provide more scientific evidence of the facet joint as a source of back pain. In their study, injection of the zygapophyseal joints in normal volunteers induced both back and referred leg pain and, moreover, they found that the pain could be obliterated by injection of local anesthetic into the same joints.

Accordingly, the concept of the facet joint block as a diagnostic test was born. Since then there have been numerous studies exploring the utility of facet joint injections as both a diagnostic and therapeutic tool in the treatment of low back pain; it is fair to say that there have been widely varying results (8–16). Nevertheless, injection of local anesthetic into lumbar facet joints or at their nerve supply is accepted as a diagnostic test of facet joint pain and it was a natural progression to explore facet joint denervation procedures in the hope of providing longer-lasting and perhaps permanent relief of facet joint pain (6,17–26). In order to refine techniques of facet joint denervation there was a renewed interest in anatomic studies to improve the understanding of innervation of lumbar spine structures and, in particular, to precisely map the afferent nerve supply of the facet joint (18, 26–30).

ANATOMY

The major afferent nerve supply to the facet joint is provided by the medial branch of the posterior primary ramus. The medial branch descends from the posterior primary ramus over the base of the transverse process in a groove at the root of the superior articular process, which is bridged by the mamillo-accessory ligament (Fig. 29-1). The mamillo-accessory ligament is formed by a condensation of the intertransverse ligament fibers passing from the mamillary body to the transverse process and occasionally it is ossified. After passing under the bridge of the mamillo-accessory ligament, the medial branch courses across the lamina deep to multifidus and

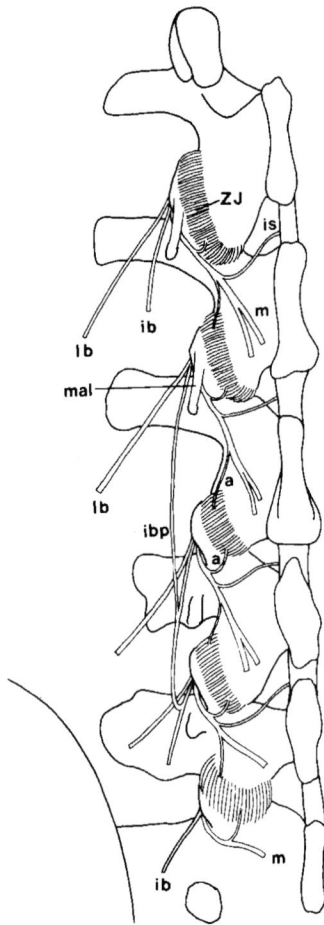

FIG. 29-1. A sketch of a dorsal view of the branches of the left lumbar dorsal rami. Mamillo-accessory ligaments (mal) have been left *in situ* covering the L1 and L2 medial branches. *A,* articular branches; *ib,* intermediate branch; *ibp,* intermediate branch plexus; *lb,* lateral branch; *m,* medial branch; *is,* interspinous branch, *zj,* zygapophyseal joint. (From Bogduk N. The innervation of the lumbar spine. Spine 1983;8(3):289.)

finally enters the muscle. Deep to the muscle it sends fibers innervating the caudal portion of the facet joint immediately above before sending fibers to the facet joint below.

Paris (29) proposed a greater multiplicity in afferent supply to the facet joint. In particular, he described an ascending facet branch that passed to the posterior aspect of the facet joint one level above, and throughout its course was entirely intramuscular and did not lie on any bony structures. He also suggested a more proximal origin of branches to multifidus and theorized that they would contain accessory afferent supply to the facet joints. However, this description of the anatomy, and in particular the ascending facet branch, could not be verified by Bogduk in his anatomical dissections (18,26–30). The existence of an intramuscular ascending facet joint branch infers a "triple innervation" of the facet joints

where a single medial branch supplies the adjacent facet joint and the joints above and below. However, there is broader acceptance of the "dual innervation" as proposed by Bogduk where the medial branch supplies its adjacent facet joint and the joint immediately below. There is agreement throughout the literature that the medial branch of the posterior primary ramus is constant and is fixed adjacent to the bone in the region of the mamillo-accessory ligament. There is no evidence of nerve fibers crossing the midline so that facet joints on each side have a unilateral innervation.

PATHOLOGY

In the majority of cases the cause of lumbar facet joint pain is not known. Although facet joint osteoarthritis is a relatively common occurrence, it is rare to find other definite recognizable pathology affecting the zygapophyseal joint such as systemic inflammatory arthropathy, facet joint fracture, or infection (6,7,15,31–34). Exclusion of such disorders is important, leaving osteoarthritis, which has been proposed as a cause of facet joint pain. Interestingly, it has been demonstrated that facet joint degeneration almost invariably follows disc degeneration at the same level and, accordingly, degenerative changes within the facet joint rarely, if ever, exist in isolation (32–34). In spite of this, a study by Schwarzer (12), evaluating patients by provocative discography and facet joint blocks, concluded that it was rare to suffer symptomatic disc degeneration in combination with symptomatic facet joints.

DIAGNOSIS

Although most clinicians recognize a clinical presentation, which is presumed attributable to facet joint pain, there is no literature to support any pathognomonic historical, physical examination or imaging findings associated with lumbar facet joint syndrome (6,9,11,14,15,16,19,31). Typically, it is thought that facet joint pain is aggravated by rest in any posture and is relieved by movement. The pain may be unilateral or bilateral in the lower back, with or without radiation to the lower limbs. Radiculopathy is absent and the pain should not radiate below the knee. Morning stiffness may be associated with a stooped posture on rising; lumbar extension is the movement most likely to aggravate symptoms. Despite the consistency of this description throughout the literature, clinical features have not proved to be predictive of the response to diagnostic facet joint blockade (13–16).

Facet joint injections form part of the investigative armamentarium when evaluating patients with nonradicular low back pain who have failed to respond to appropriate nonoperative management, including an exercise program, and in whom there are no sinister features of alternative underlying pathology. Lumbar facet joint injections, combined with the use of intra-articular corti-costeroids, have been used as both a diagnostic and therapeutic modality. However, their use remains controversial (7,8,10,11,15). As a therapeutic option, some authors have found facet joint injections to be of no use, whereas at best the injections may provide temporary relief of sufficient duration to allow resolution of symptoms by natural processes or through an appropriate rehabilitation program.

A series of studies undertaken by Bogduk and associates have shown that targeted medial branch blockade is a valid diagnostic test in the evaluation of facet joint pain (12,13,16). Indeed, from a technical viewpoint, medial branch block is more easily performed than facet joint injections and there is less prospect of diffusion of the local anesthetic to involve surrounding structures, which may confound the response.

In addition, differential blocks undertaken on separate occasions using local anesthetic agents with different pharmacologic properties and durations of action have been able to exclude false-positive results (13). Based on these studies and others where the placebo response is controlled, facet joint pain is thought to have a prevalence of up to 40% in chronic nonradicular low back pain (14,15).

If facet joint pain is accepted as a significant contributor in disabling low back pain, then it follows that facet joint denervation may provide long-term or even permanent relief of symptoms attributable to the facet joints. Facet joint denervation is appealing given the accessibility of the facet joint and, more particularly, the medial branch of the posterior primary ramus, which has a constant course adjacent to an easily identifiable bony landmark.

Bearing this in mind, when investigating a patient for consideration of radiofrequency denervation, it is logical that a medial branch block is a more appropriate diagnostic tool than facet joint block because it directly evaluates the structure scheduled for ablation.

TECHNIQUE

The original technique described by Shealy (5) targeted the electrode lateral to the midpoint of the facet joint and then swept the electrode in a cephalad and caudad direction so that there were three electrode positions for each joint covering the lateral aspect of the facet joint. The following modified technique is recommended in view of improved anatomic knowledge.

Under sterile conditions with the patient lying prone over a pillow to reduce the lumbar lordosis, on a radiolucent operating table, the levels to be denervated are located by antero-posterior (AP) fluoroscopy. The target point (i.e., the base of the transverse process where it meets the root of the superior articular process) is marked on the skin (Fig. 29-2). A puncture site is marked a cen-

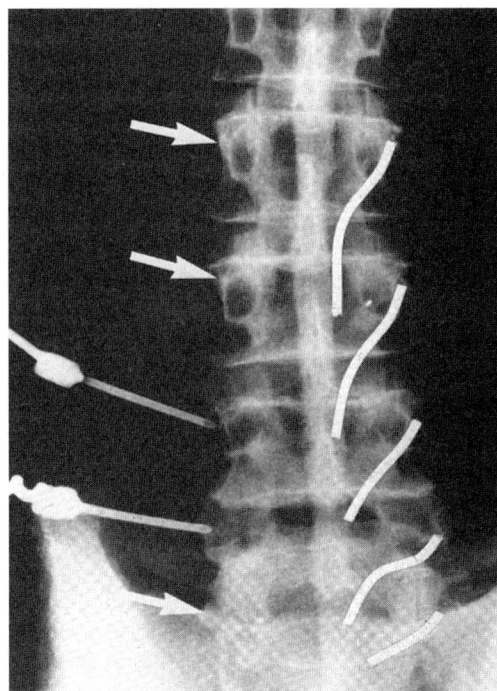

FIG. 29-2. Antero-posterior radiograph of lumbar spine illustrating target points for medial branch neurotomy. The target points lie exactly at the tip of either the *arrows* at L1, L2, and L5, or the guide needles at L3 and L4. Note, at the L3 and L4 levels, how the silhouette of the superior articular process overlaps the target point, demonstrating why electrodes should be introduced obliquely. The overhanging superior articular process protects the target point in a dorsoventral approach. The guide needles are indicating the target points; however, a more caudal entry point is now recommended in order to allow introduction of the electrode more or less parallel to the respective medial branches at L4 and above. On the **right side** of the figure the courses of the medial branches of the dorsal rami have been superimposed. (From Bogduk N, Long DM. Percutaneous lumbar medial branch neurotomy: a modification of facet denervation. Spine 1980; 5:196.)

timeter or two lateral and caudal to the target point for the L1 to L4 levels. (The L5 level is treated differently owing to the different anatomy, and is described in the following.) The lateral and caudal entry point is chosen to prevent deflection of the probe from the target at the base of the transverse process by the overhanging superior articular process and the bulging mamillary process. Because it has been shown that the uninsulated portion of the probe produces a radial spread of the lesion that does not extend beyond the tip of the electrode, a more caudal approach is chosen to allow the introduced probe to lie nearly parallel to the target nerve so that the nerve is more likely to be encompassed by the radial spread of the lesion (35). The L5 dorsal ramus courses in the groove between the ala and the superior articular facet of S1 and can be approached in a more sagittal direction with the probe laying parallel to the dorsal primary ramus proper as it hooks over the sacrum. The intended puncture sites are anesthetized using Lignocaine 1% down to the level of the deep fascia, being careful not to anesthetize deep around the facet joint, which may interfere with nerve conduction and patient response.

An 11 blade is used to puncture the skin before insertion of 3½-inch, 14-gauge Shiley needles with trocars under AP fluoroscopy. The Shiley needle is advanced until it is blocked by the base of the transverse process, which obviates the need for lateral fluoroscopy to check the depth of placement. The trocar is removed and the blunt-tipped electrode is introduced via the Shiley needle, which can be used to steer the electrode. The transverse process is palpated easily and the electrode is then directed in a cephalad and medial direction so that it slips off the transverse process into the intertransverse space. The probe is then gradually withdrawn so that the uninsulated portion lies at the root of the superior articular process, more or less parallel to the course of the medial branch. At L5, as mentioned, the probe comes to lie in a more sagittal direction in the groove on the superior aspect of the ala, adjacent to the superior articular facet and is parallel to the posterior primary ramus proper. Antero-posterior fluoroscopy is used to confirm the position of the tip of the electrode.

A stimulation mode can be used to confirm that the electrode tip is properly positioned adjacent to the medial branch of the posterior primary ramus and away from the anterior primary ramus. At 2 Hz, motor stimulation may occur and if twitching of the lower limb muscles is observed, the probe should be withdrawn to a more posterior position. At 100 Hz, a sensory response is elicited in the posterior primary ramus, which may produce pain or tingling similar to the presenting symptoms. However, the sensory response is not diagnostic and this step should not be necessary because the symptomatic levels should have been identified by prior medial branch blockade.

After satisfactory placement of the electrodes, lesions are made with a radiofrequency generator; the electrode tip temperature is raised to 80°C for 90 seconds. During the production of the lesion, the patient should be awake and cooperative in order to alert the surgeon as to the development of any radicular symptoms that would necessitate repositioning the lesioning electrode. Usually the patient experiences an exacerbation of back pain that reaches a crescendo and then settles as the lesion is completed. The neurologic status is checked immediately postoperatively. The procedure is undertaken on an outpatient basis with minimal or no sedation and the patient is allowed to return to normal activity as symptoms permit.

RESULTS

Since the introduction of radiofrequency denervation of the facet joint by Shealy (5), the technique has been modified and used with varying results (6,17,18–26).

To date only three randomized controlled trials (20,22,24) have been published evaluating the effect of radiofrequency lumbar facet joint denervation in chronic low back pain. However, the studies are not directly comparable because they each used either different diagnostic criteria or different surgical technique.

In 1994, Gallagher (20) included 60 patients who were judged on clinical grounds to have symptoms of low back pain suggestive of facet joint origin. Forty-one patients reported improvement or were equivocal in their response following injection of local anesthetic into and around the facet joints that were thought to be appropriate. Those patients were randomized to undergo either radiofrequency facet joint denervation or a sham procedure using the invalidated technique of Shealy. Nevertheless, relief of symptoms was noted in patients who had a clear improvement following facet joint injections compared to patients who were equivocal in their response to the injections. The results were evaluated at 1 and 6 months and were statistically significant.

Van Kleef (22), in 1999, reported results in 31 patients with chronic low back pain selected on the basis of pain relief following diagnostic blockade of the medial branch of the posterior primary rami. The technique of lesion production was similar to the modified technique as described in the preceding text, although the approach was more from a posterolateral oblique direction than the more caudal oblique approach, as promoted by Bogduk (35). At least 50% pain relief following medial branch blockade was required to be eligible to enter the study and then patients were randomized to undergo radiofrequency lesioning or a sham procedure. Interestingly, in the final analysis, the results were superior in patients who reported complete relief of pain with diagnostic nerve blocks compared to those with only partial relief of pain. Statistical analysis at 3, 6, and 12 months following treatment showed significant improvement in pain and functional disability in the treatment group.

In 2001, Leclaire (24) published results examining a larger sample size of 70 patients but a shorter follow-up of only 3 months and reported no significant improvement in the treatment group compared to the sham group. However, it is noteworthy that patients were included in the study based on their response to intra-articular facet joint injections rather than diagnostic medial branch blockade.

COMPLICATIONS

There have been no serious complications associated with the procedure apart from transient radiculopathy and the report of a skin burn through poor earthing (5,19–25).

CONCLUSION

It is apparent that there exists a very select group of patients with disabling low back pain that can be attributed to the facet joints and may be successfully treated by facet joint denervation.

The careful use of diagnostic medial branch blockade is the critical factor in patient selection for facet joint denervation. Meticulous attention to detail through the use of differential medial branch blockade is required to accurately identify a highly selected group of patients who may respond to radiofrequency denervation. Following recommended protocols is a tedious process that may test the patience of the clinician (not to mention the patient) and may explain the paucity of high-quality studies and the widely varying results published in the literature. Despite a plethora of literature dealing with anatomy and experimental studies, evaluating the facet joints as a potential source of pain, there is an extremely narrow evidence base of high-quality clinical studies examining the utility of radiofrequency denervation of the facet joints. In particular, there is a single study (22) that employed the theoretical best practice methods of patient selection, accurate lesioning technique, and rigorous scientific methodology that showed significant alleviation of pain and functional disability in a select group of patients both on a short- and long-term basis following radiofrequency denervation.

There are many factors that may lead to failure of the technique, including the technical adequacy of diagnosis by medial branch block and the adequacy of subsequent radiofrequency medial branch neurotomy. Additionally, there is always the question of alternate symptomatic pathology and, in particular, symptomatic disc degeneration because disc degeneration has been shown to always coexist with facet joint degeneration. It has been postulated that late resurgence of symptoms may be associated with nerve regeneration, in which case repeat procedures may be indicated after re-evaluation. Nevertheless, the minimally invasive technique of radiofrequency facet joint denervation is appealing given the accessibility of the medial branch of the posterior primary ramus and the reassurance that the reporting of complications from the procedure is virtually nonexistent.

REFERENCES

1. Goldthwait JE. The Lumbosacral Articulation. An explanation of many cases of "lumbago, sciatica and paraplegia." Boston Med Surg J 1911;164:365–372.
2. Ghormley K. Low back pain with special reference to the articular facets, with presentation of an operative procedure. JAMA 1933;101: 1773–1777.
3. Rees WES. Multiple bilateral subcutaneous rhizolysis of segmental nerves in the treatment of the intervertebral disc syndrome. Ann Gen Pract 1971;16:126–127.
4. Rees WS. Multiple bilateral subcutaneous rhizolysis. Med J Aus 1975; 1:536–537.
5. Shealy CN. Facet denervation in the management of back and sciatic pain. Clin Orthop 1976;115:157–164.
6. Mooney V. Facet syndrome. In: Weinstein JN, Wiesel SW, ed. The lumbar spine: the international society for the study of the lumbar spine. Philadelphia: WB Saunders, 1990:422–441.
7. Mooney V, Robertson J. The facet syndrome. Clin Orthop 1976;115: 149–156.
8. Fairbank JCT, Park WM, McCall IW, et al. Apophyseal injection of local anaesthetic as a diagnostic aid in primary low-back pain syndromes. Spine 1981;6:598–605.
9. Lewinnek GE, Warfield CA. Facet joint degeneration as a cause of low back pain. Clin Orthop 1986;213:216–222.
10. Lilius G, Laasonen EM, Myllynen P, et al. Lumbar facet joint syndrome. J Bone Joint Surg (Britain) 1998;71-B:681–684.
11. Jackson RP. The facet syndrome: myth or reality? Clin Orthop 1992; 279:110–121.
12. Schwarzer A, Aprill CN, Derby R, et al. The relative contributions of the disc and the zygapophyseal joint in chronic low back pain. Spine 1994;19:801–806.
13. Schwarzer AC, Aprill CN, Derby R, et al. The false-positive rate of uncontrolled diagnostic blocks of the lumbar zygapophyseal joints. Pain 1994;58:195–200.
14. Schwarzer A, Wang S, Bogduk N, et al. Prevalence and clinical features of lumbar zygapophyseal joint pain: a study in an Australian population with chronic low back pain. Ann Rheum Dis 1995;54:100–106.
15. Dreyfuss PH, Dreyer SJ, Herring SA. Contemporary concepts in spine care: lumbar zygapophysial (facet) joint injections. Spine 1995;20: 2040–2047.
16. Kaplan M, Dreyfuss P, Halbrook B, et al. The ability of lumbar medial branch blocks to anesthetize the zygapophysial joint: a physiologic challenge. Spine 1998;23:1847–1852.
17. McCulloch JA, Organ LW. Percutaneous radiofrequency lumbar rhizolysis (rhizotomy). Can Med Assoc J 1977;116:30–32.
18. Bogduk N, Long DM. The anatomy of the so-called "articular nerves" and their relationship to facet denervation in the treatment of low back pain. J Neurosurg 1979;51:172–177.
19. Rashbaum RF. Radiofrequency facet denervation: a treatment alternative in refractory low back pain with or without leg pain. Orthop Clin North Am 1983;14:569–575.
20. Gallagher J, Di Vadi PLP, Wedley JR, et al. Radiofrequency facet joint denervation in the treatment of low back pain: a prospective controlled double-blind study to assess its efficacy. Pain Clin 1994;7:193–198.
21. North RB, Han M, Zahurak M, et al. Radiofrequency lumbar facet denervation: analysis of prognostic factors. Pain 1994;57:77–83.
22. van Kleef M, Barendse GAM, Kessels A, et al. Randomized trial of radiofrequency lumbar facet denervation for chronic low back pain. Spine 1999;24:1937–1942.
23. Tzaan WC, Tasker RR. Percutaneous radiofrequency facet rhizotomy: experience with 118 procedures and reappraisal of its value. Can J Neurol Sci 2000;27:125–130.
24. Leclaire MD, Fortin L, Lambert R, et al. Radiofrequency facet joint denervation in the treatment of low back pain. Spine 2001;26: 1411–1417.
25. Geurts JW, van Wijk, RM, Stolker RJ, et al. Efficacy of radiofrequency procedures for the treatment of spinal pain: a systematic review of randomized clinical trials. Reg Anesth Pain Med 2001;26:394–400.
26. Bogduk N, Long DM. Percutaneous lumbar medial branch neurotomy: a modification of facet denervation. Spine 1980;5:193–200.
27. Bogduk N, Wilson AS, Tynan W. The human lumbar dorsal rami. J Anat 1982;134:383—397.
28. Bogduk N. The innervation of the lumbar spine. Spine 1983;8:286–293.
29. Paris SV. Anatomy as related to function and pain. Orthop Clin North Am 1983;14:475–489.
30. Bogduk N, Twomey LT. Clinical anatomy of the lumbar spine. London: Churchill Livingstone, 1997.
31. Eisenstein SM, Parry CR. The lumbar facet arthrosis syndrome: clinical presentation and articular surface changes. J Bone Joint Surg (Br) 1987;69:3–7.
32. Fujiwara A, Tamai K, Yamato N, et al. The relationship between facet joint osteoarthritis and disc degeneration of the lumbar spine: an MRI study. Eur Spine J 1999;8:396–401.
33. Butler D, Trafinow JH, Andersson GBJ, et al. Disc degenerate before facets. Spine 1990;15:111–113.
34. Vernon-Roberts B, Pirie CJ. Degenerative changes in the intervertebral discs of the lumbar spine and their sequelae. Rheum Rehab 1977;16: 13–21.
35. Bogduk N, Macintosh J, Marsland A. Technical limitations to the efficacy of radiofrequency neurotomy for spinal pain. Neurosurgery 1987; 20:529–535.

CHAPTER 30

Intradiscal Electrothermal Therapy

Jeffrey A. Saal and Joel S. Saal

The treatment of chronic discogenic low back pain presents one of the most difficult challenges to the spine specialist. Nonoperative measures are frequently unable to reduce pain and improve function in this patient subgroup (1, 2). Interbody fusion for these patients has yielded mixed and often poor results (3–5). An alternative therapy to address this problem is therefore desirable. The SpineCATH system (Smith & Nephew, Inc., Largo, FL) to perform intradiscal electrothermal therapy (IDET) was developed to address this difficult clinical dilemma.

Patients with chronic lumbar pain fall into two clinical categories: chronic recurrent and chronic persistent. Chronic recurrent patients have multiple pain flares with varying durations of 2 weeks to 3 months. Many patients within this group will begin to have more frequent recurrences with fewer pain-free intervals as time passes. Chronic persistent patients have persisting symptoms that do not abate and last longer than 3 months. The disc has been shown to be the pain source in the majority of patients with chronic symptoms (6). Carey et al. recently reported that patients who do not experience a resolution of their back pain within 3 months of onset had a poor prognosis for further recovery. When the patients were assessed at 22 months they continued to have persisting complaints of low back pain and were dissatisfied with their outcomes (1). Von Korff reported that although 80% of patients had resolution of their acute low back pain in 12 weeks, 60% of the patients experienced recurrent symptoms (2). These recent studies underline the fact that chronic low back pain does not necessarily have a favorable prognosis and that the long held truth that 90% of patients will experience resolution of their back pain within 6 to 12 weeks is incorrect and misleading.

PATHOPHYSIOLOGY OF INTERNAL DISC DERANGEMENT

The natural history of the degenerating disc includes loss of nuclear hydrostatic pressure, which leads to buckling of the annular lamellae. This phenomenon leads to increased focal segment mobility and increased shear stress to the annular wall. The process progresses to delamination and fissuring of the annular wall. Annular delamination has been shown to occur as a separate and distinct event from annular fissures (7). Fissures can be radial or concentric. In addition, electron microscopy has demonstrated micro "fractures" of collagen fibrils with disc degeneration. The progressive degeneration of the disc, manifested by any of these morphologic changes, has been shown to alter disc mechanics (8).

Tearing and delamination of the annulus can cause chronic pain. Mechanoreceptors in the disc have been shown to discharge with disc mobilization (9). Nociceptive tissue has been shown to be sensitized resulting in a decrease in their firing threshold after treatment with inflammatory enzymes and mediators (10–12).

A scenario for chronic discogenic pain is created when any combination of annular fissures, delamination, or microfractures of collagen fibrils leads to mechanical distortion of annular lamellae and subsequent sensitization of nociceptors that may have also been presensitized by PLA2 (13), nitrous oxide (14, 15), interleukin 1 (15), and metalloproteinase enzyme activity (15), or other chemical mediators. Afferent stimuli produce substance P release and nociception. Repetitive stimulation of the dorsal root ganglion (DRG) has been shown to create prolonged neural activity from the dorsal horn receptor fields (10,16,17). As the patient continues to load the disc, the neuronal activity continues. Clinically, the disrupted disc will often cause referral pain into the buttocks and leg due to DRG stimulation or from direct chemical irritation of the nerve roots.

A combination of mechanical and neural properties creates an interplay that leads to chronic discogenic pain. A high-intensity zone (HIZ) on the T2 of the magnetic resonance (MR) image has been shown to correlate with a pain-producing fissured disc 65% to 95% of the time (18–20). However, MRI predicts the presence of annular fissures less than 50% of the time and asymptomatic patients may have an HIZ (19–22). Therefore, a patient may have a painful annular tear without concomitant MRI findings. Disc bulging is due to, and directly associated with, annular degeneration and fissures; however, this phenomenon does not always create clinically significant low back pain (21).

Certainly not all chronic lumbar pain is discogenic. It is estimated that more than 50% of patients with chronic low back pain may have the disc as the primary source of pain (6), however, an accurate diagnosis can be elusive. Screening for patients with facet problems, sacroiliac joint dysfunction, psychosocial problems, systemic disease, neoplasm, and infection should be undertaken when appropriate. A chronic pain syndrome with primarily soft tissue pain and somatization often occurs in the low back pain population. Practitioners must be aware of the potential existence of these phenomena.

THERMAL IMPACT ON TISSUE

Innervation of the intervertebral disc has been well documented by researchers since the 1930s. More recently, Bogduk's work illustrated the sources of lumbar disc innervation (23). Coppes et al. found nociceptive properties in nerves of the outer annular wall. In fact, they observed nerve fibers "deeper than the outer third of the annulus fibrosus" (24). Freemont et al. also discovered significant neovascularization with neural expression of substance P, and linked that growth to disc degeneration and back pain. They identified nerve fibers as deep as the inner third of the annulus fibrosus and into the nucleus pulposus in several disc samples (25).

Letcher et al. established that irreversible nerve blocks due to neural thermocoagulation occur at 45°C in the brain (26), and Cosman et al. (27) used radiofrequency lesioning to produce 45°C isotherms for neural tissue lesioning. The intradiscal temperatures generated by the SpineCATH (48° to 75°C) are in the range necessary to create thermocoagulation of neural tissue in the target zone accessed (28, 29).

Collagen contraction, or shrinkage, has been well documented in the use of nonablative laser energy on joint capsular tissue and more recently in radiofrequency application in the glenohumeral joint capsule (30,31). Research has shown that there is a direct correlation between the amount of heat and duration of the heating applied to tissue and the resulting collagen contraction (32–36).

The breaking apart of the heat-sensitive bonds of the collagen fibrils causes tissue shrinkage. The framework of the intervertebral disc is composed primarily of types I and II collagen, which have a similar molecular structure. The tensile strength of these collagen fibers is derived from the extended conformation of the triple helix molecule, which is cross-linked with hydrogen

bonds. A portion of these bonds is heat sensitive, breaking apart when exposed to a range of temperatures over time. The disruption of these stabilizing hydrogen bonds releases the molecular strands, which collapse. This collapse, like the release of a spring-held taut, results in a new contracted state called the denatured or random coil conformation of the collagen fiber.

The optimal temperature for collagen contraction is reported to be 65°C. The lowest practical temperature at which heat-sensitive hydrogen bonds will start to break is 60° C. As the temperature increases, more bonds break. It is unclear whether there is an additional shrinkage effect over 75°C.

Kleinstueck et al. attempted to study intradiscal temperature dispersion from the SpineCATH (37). They placed the device in the nucleus rather than in the annulus and were able to measure temperatures of great than 42°C (temperature sufficient to thermocoagulate unmyelinated nerve fibers) at distances greater than 10 mm from the probe. However, their use of previously frozen cadaveric discs, and the placement of the heating element in the nuclear cavity rather than in the annulus as is done in clinical practice may have limited the peak temperatures. Freeman et al. presented temperature maps *in vivo* on sheep demonstrating higher peak temperatures (38). They found temperatures of greater than 65°C adjacent to the catheter. In a recent report Shah et al. found microscopic evidence of acute collagen modulation in cadaveric discs heated with a SpineCATH (29).

Recently Barensde et al. reported on a randomized controlled trial evaluating the efficacy of a radiofrequency probe placed into the center of the nucleus and then heated (39). The treated group fared no better than placebo. Houpt et al. (40) has previously demonstrated the inability of temperature dispersion for a radiofrequency device to raise intradiscal and annular temperatures. For these reasons the IDET technology (i.e., SpineCATH) does not use radiofrequency as a heating element but rather uses a thermal resistive coil, which produces conductive heat. Additionally, contrary to the radiofreqency device studied by Barendse (39), the IDET device is deployed into the annulus and is not deployed in the center of the nucleus (28,41).

CLINICAL RESEARCH REVIEW

The first published series of patients treated with IDET reported the 6-month (range 6 to 9 months, mean 7 months) outcome results for 25 patients with chronic low back pain of documented discogenic origin with mean duration of preoperative symptoms of 58.5 months. These were patients who failed to adequately improve with a comprehensively applied nonoperative care program and who elected IDET instead of chronic pain management or spinal fusion (41). The results demonstrated a statistically significant improvement in functional outcome as measured by Visual Analogue Scale (VAS) scores, Social Functioning (SF)-36 scores, sitting tolerance times, and narcotic analgesic medication. Sixty-two patients treated with IDET and followed for a minimum of 1-year (mean 16 months, range 12 to 23 months) postprocedure demonstrated outcome evaluation scores that did not statistically vary from the 6-month group. The mean group change for the SF-36 bodily pain was 17 and physical function was 20. These scores are consistent with significant clinical improvement (42).

A 2-year follow-up study noted continued improvement of SF-36 scores and sitting tolerance times (43).

Karasek and Bogduk (44) reported on the 1-year outcome of patients treated with IDET (35) and compared them to a control group of patients (17) similarly diagnosed but denied insurance authorization for IDET. The researchers used a 50% reduction of VAS scores as an indicator of success. On this basis, 60% were considered successes. Additionally, they noted that 23% of the patients had total relief of symptoms. They reported that only one patient in the control group improved and the remainder continued to have similar pain intensity.

Derby et al. (45) reported that 62.5% of patients treated with IDET had a favorable outcome based upon the Roland Morris Scale, VAS, North American

Spine Society (NASS) outcome instrument, and a general activity scale. If patients had preserved disc height and had not undergone previous surgery at the index level, the success rate was 76%.

Wetzel et al. presented the 2-year results of a multicenter prospective cohort study and found statistically significant improvement in pain reduction and physical function in their study group (46). To date, there are no published randomized controlled trials of IDET. Cleary, such trials will be extremely valuable in determining the validated efficacy of IDET and other spine therapies. Until those data are available, physicians and surgeons should proceed with caution prior to determining the path of care for their patients with chronic discogenic pain.

MECHANISMS OF ACTION

The precise mechanism of action of the observed positive clinical effect is currently under investigation. Moore et al. attempted to create annular in-growth of nerve fibers after surgically induced injury. They followed this with IDET in an attempt to determine if IDET reduced the population of nerve fibers in treated versus untreated control specimens. Unfortunately, neither the control nor the treated specimens had enough neural ingrowth to determine a differential effect (47). Pollintine et al. presented a cadaveric disc study demonstrating an equalization of stress across the IDET treated disc (48). This may lend useful insight into the mechanism of

action of IDET. Clearly, further work on the mechanism of action is required.

DIAGNOSTIC WORKUP AND PATIENT SELECTION FOR IDET

The following 12 criteria represent our present criteria for IDET candidacy. To date, these criteria have not been validated by controlled studies. They represent our experience, and are a work in progress.

1. Severe, function-limiting, chronic low back pain for more than 3 months.
2. Failure to adequately improve with a comprehensively applied aggressive nonoperative treatment program consisting of stabilization exercise training, back education, activity modification, and when appropriate, fluoroscopically guided selective epidural cortisone injections and, in some circumstances, facet injections.
3. A duration of 3 months for the nonoperative care program is recommended (this would bring the total duration of symptoms to an approximate minimum of 6 months prior to IDET).
4. Normal neurologic examination.
5. Negative straight leg raise (SLR)--no reproduction of "true sciatica".
6. MRI that does not demonstrate neural compressive disease.
7. Preservation of disc height at the symptomatic level (less than 30% disc space collapse).
8. No measurable segmental instability.
9. No lytic or degenerative spondylolisthesis.
10. Discogram that demonstrates an annular fissure and reproduces concordant pain at one or more levels at an injection volume of less than 2 cc, with a documented negative control level.
11. No irreversible psychosocial barriers to recovery.
12. Motivation to improve with realistic expectations of outcome.

In summary, IDET is intended for psychologically stable and motivated patients with chronic function limiting low back pain with a documented discogenic source of pain who have failed to improve with an aggressive exercise-based rehabilitation program. Discography criteria for low-volume concordant pain provocation attempts to separate appropriate patients with focal annular lesions who will experience pain reproduction at low volumes from patients who are questionable candidates with global annular degeneration who will often experience pain reproduction only at larger volumes of injectate (i.e., greater than or equal to 2 cc volumes). We have noted that patients with severe disc space collapse (greater than 50%) may have a lower likelihood of success than patients with preserved disc height. This theorem however has not been vigorously tested. In addition, the effectiveness of IDET on the previously operated segment remains an open question.

PROCEDURAL TECHNIQUE

Overview

Local anesthesia and conscious, monitored sedation is applied to the patient in an outpatient surgical or radiologic setting. A 17-gauge procedure needle is introduced into the symptomatic disc under multiplane fluoroscopic guidance. The SpineCATH is introduced through the procedure needle and navigated to the offending portion of the annulus. The SpineCATH position is documented in at least the anteroposterior and lateral radiologic view. Care must be undertaken to avoid catheter kinking, which may lead to catheter breakage. Treatment may be achieved with unilateral catheter deployment, but roughly 40% of the time, due to multiple annular fissures, bilateral deployment is necessary to cover the entire posterior annular wall. The ORA-50 (Smith & Nephew, Andover, MA) autotemperature heat generator controls the catheter heat delivery system. Typically a maximum catheter temperature of 90°C is attained (corresponding to tissue temperature adjacent to the catheter of approximately 72°C). There are occasions when the temperature profile must be modified to a maximum catheter temperature of 85° to 89°C to achieve patient comfort. The patient must be alert enough to be observed for the development of radicular pain during the procedure. If this occurs, the catheter is repositioned or removed. Most patients will experience their typical back pain and referral leg pain during the procedure. However, this must be differentiated from radicular pain, especially if the patient experiences it early in the heating cycle (i.e., catheter temperature 65° to 90°C). If this occurs, it is usually indicative of an extremely attenuated posterolateral annulus or a catheter that is extradiscal. It is our preference to inject 2 to 5 mg of cefazolin into the disc after treatment and removal of the SpineCATH.

A survey of complications was presented noting a 6 per 1,750 incidence of reversible nerve injury due to needle puncture and a 1 per 1,750 incidence of discitis. There is one published report of cauda equina injury due to IDET (49). IDET when performed by a skilled practitioner is relatively safe, but certainly not entirely without risk.

Course of Recovery and Postoperative Rehabilitation

Most patients will experience an increase in their typical pain (back, back and leg) in the early postoperative period. The postoperative pain gradually subsides over the first 1 to 7 days. Typically most patients will return to

at least their preprocedure pain level between the 7th and 14th postoperative day. We have noted that patients often have resolution of their preoperative leg pain symptoms in the first 4 weeks, whereas the improvement in back pain requires 6 to 12 weeks to occur. Initial study patients have been noted to progressively improve between 2 and 9 months. The 2-year data documented that the patient group demonstrated substantial improvement between 1- and 2-year follow-up points (43). The clinical course in the first 4 to 6 months is often variable. However, many of these patients will stabilize, and at 1-year follow-up demonstrate significant improvement. Patients who have not improved above their preoperative baseline by 6 months should be considered unsuccessful.

The most important postoperative principle appears to be allowing time for a healing reaction. This requires delaying aggressive exercise training for at least 3 months postprocedure. It is our practice to place patients in a semirigid lumbar corset for 8 weeks postprocedure. During this period, patients are encouraged to walk. At 8 weeks a progressive stabilization exercise program is begun and the corset is discontinued. Patients should be able to return to office work or light duty assignment by 2 weeks and light lifting duties at 6 weeks postprocedure, although return to heavy work may require 4 to 6 months. Optimization of return to work timing and postoperative management deserves further study.

CONCLUSION

IDET may offer a group of carefully selected patients with chronic discogenic low back pain an option other than chronic pain management or spinal fusion. Randomized control trials are necessary to validate the efficacy of IDET as well as spinal fusion for the treatment of patients with chronic discogenic low back pain.

ACKNOWLEDGMENTS

No funds were received in support of this chapter, and no benefits in any form have been received from a commercial party related directly or indirectly to the subject of this manuscript.

REFERENCES

1. Carey T, Garrett J, Jackman A. Beyond good prognosis: examination of an inception cohort of patients with chronic low back pain. Spine 2000;25(1):115.
2. Von Korff M. Studying the natural history of back pain. Spine 1994;19(18S):2041S–2046S.
3. Slosar PJ, Reynolds JB, Schofferman J, et al. Patient satisfaction after circumferential lumbar fusion. Spine 2000;25(6):722–726.
4. Wetzel FT, LaRocca SH, Lowery GL, et al. The treatment of lumbar spinal pain syndromes diagnosed by discography: lumbar arthrodesis. Spine 1994;19:792–800.

5. Zdeblick TA. A prospective, randomized study of lumbar fusions: preliminary results. Spine 1993;18:983–991.
6. Schwarzer A, Aprill C, Derby R, et al. The prevalence and clinical features of internal disc disruption in patients with chronic low back pain. Spine 1995;20(17):1878–2883.
7. Moore RJ, Vernon-Roberts B, Fraser RD, et al. The origin and fate of herniated lumbar intervertebral disc tissue. Spine 1996;21:2149–2155.
8. Schmidt TA, An HS, Lim T, et al. The stiffness of lumbar spinal motion segments with a high intensity zone in the anulus fibrosus. Spine 1998;23(20):2167–2173.
9. Robert S, Eisenstein SM, Menage J, et al. Mechanoreceptors in intervertebral discs. Spine 1995;20:2645–2651.
10. Ozaktay AC, Kallakuri S, Cavanaugh JM. Phospholipase A2 sensitivity of the dorsal root and dorsal root ganglion. Spine 1998;23(12):1296–1306.
11. Pateromichelakis S, Rood JP. Prostaglandin E increases mechanically evoked potentials in the peripheral nerve. Experientia 1981;27:282–284.
12. Wall PD, Gutnick M. Ongoing activity in peripheral nerves: the physiology and pharmacology of impulses originating in a neuroma. Exp Neurol 1974;43:580–593.
13. Franson R, Saal JS, Saal JA. Human disc phospholipase A2 is inflammatory. Spine 1992;17[Suppl]:S190–S192.
14. Kang JD, Georgescu HI, McIntyre L, et al. Herniated lumbar intervertebral discs spontaneously produce matrix metalloproteinases, nitric oxide, interleukin-6, and prostaglandin E2. Spine 1996;21(3):271–277.
15. Kawakami M, Tamaki T, Weinstein J, et al. Pathomechanism of pain related behavior produced by allografts of intervertebral disc in the rat. Spine 1996;21:2101–2107.
16. Devor M. Neuropathic pain and injured nerve: peripheral mechanisms. Br Med J 1991;47(3):619–630.
17. Utzschneider D, Kocsis J, Devor M. Mutual excitation among dorsal root ganglion neurons in the rat. Neurosci Letters 1992;146:53–56.
18. Aprill C, Bogduk N. High intensity zones in the disc anulus: a sign of painful disc on magnetic resonance imaging. Br J Radiol 1992;65:361–369.
19. Ito M, Incorvaia K, Yu S, et al. Predictive signs of discogenic lumbar pain on magnetic resonance imaging with discography correlation. Spine 1998;23(11):1252–1260.
20. Smith N, Hurwitz E, Solsberg D, et al. Interobserver reliability of detecting lumbar intervertebral disc high intensity zone on magnetic resonance imaging and association of high intensity zone with pain and anular disruption. Spine 1998;23(19):2074–2080.
21. Milette P, Fontaine S, Lepanto L, et al. Differentiating lumbar protrusions, disc bulges, and discs with normal contour but abnormal signal intensity: magnetic resonance imaging with discographic correlations. Spine 1999;24(1):44–53.
22. Osti OL, Vernon-Roberts B, Fraser RD. Anulus tears and intervertebral disc degeneration: an experimental study using an animal model. Spine 1990;15:762–767.
23. Bogduk N, Tynan W, Wilson AS. The nerve supply to the human lumbar intervertebral disc. J Anat 1981;132:39–56.
24. Coppes MH, Marani E, Thomeer RT, et al. Innervation of "painful" lumbar discs. Spine 1997;22(20):2342–2350.
25. Freemont AJ, Peacock TE, Goupille P, et al. Nerve ingrowth into diseased intervertebral disc in chronic back pain. Lancet 1997;350:178–181.
26. Letcher F, Goldring S. The effect of radiofrequency current and heat on peripheral nerve action potential in the cat. J Neurosurg 1968;29:42–47.
27. Cosman ER, Nashold BS, Ovelman-Levitt J. Theoretical aspects of radiofrequency lesions in the dorsal root entry zone. Neurosurgery 1984;15(6):945–950.
28. Saal JA, Saal JS. Thermal characteristics of lumbar disc: evaluation of a novel approach to targeted intradiscal thermal therapy. Paper presented at: 13th Annual Meeting of the North American Spine Society; 1998; San Francisco, California.
29. Shah R, Lutz GE, Lee J, et al. Intradiscal electrothermal therapy: a preliminary histologic study. Arch Phys Med Rehab 2001;82:1230–1237.
30. Fanton GS, Wall MS, Markel MD. Electrothermally assisted capsule shift (ETAC) procedure for shoulder instability. Am J Sports Med (in press).
31. Hecht P, Hayashi K, Cooley AJ, et al. The thermal effect of radiofrequency on joint capsular properties: an in vivo histological study using a sheep model. Am J Sports Med 1998;26(6):808-14.
32. Hayashi K, Markel M, Thabit G, et al. The effect of nonablative laser energy on joint capsular properties: an in vitro mechanical study using a rabbit model. Am J Sports Med 1995;23(4):482–487.
33. Hayashi K, Thabit G, Bogdanske GJJ, et al. The effect of nonablative laser energy on the ultrastructure of joint capsular collagen. Arthroscopy 1996;12(4):474–481.
34. Hayashi K, Thabit G, Vailas AC. The effect of nonablative laser energy on joint capsular properties: an in vitro histologic and biochemical study using a rabbit model. Am J Sports Med 1996;24(5):640–646.
35. Lopez M, Hayashi K, Fanton G, et al, The effect of radiofrequency energy on the ultrastructure of joint capsular collagen. Arthroscopy 1998;14:495–501.
36. Obrzut L, Hecht P, Hayashi K, et al. The effect of radiofrequency energy on the length and temperature properties of the glenohumeral joint capsule. Arthroscopy 1998;14:395–400.
37. Kleinstueck F, Diederich C, Nau W, et al. Acute biomechanical and histological effects of intradiscal electrothermal therapy on human lumbar discs. Spine 2001;26:2198–2207.
38. Freeman BJ, Walters R, Moore RJ, et al. In vivo measurement of peak posterior annular and nuclear temperatures obtained during intradiscal electrothermal therapy (IDET) in sheep. Paper presented at: 28th Annual Meeting of the International Society for the Study of the Lumbar Spine; 2001; Edinburgh, Scotland.
39. Barendse GA, van den Berg S, Kessels A, et al. Randomized controlled trial of percutaneous intradiscal radiofrequency thermocoagulation for chronic discogenic back pain: lack of effect from a 90 second 70°C lesion. Spine 2001;25(3):287–292.
40. Houpt J, Conner E, McFarland E. Experimental study of temperature distributions and thermal transport during radiofrequency current therapy of the intervertebral disc. Spine 1996;21(15):1808–1813.
41. Saal JS, Saal JA. Management of chronic discogenic low back pain with a thermal intradiscal catheter: a preliminary report. Spine 2000;25(3):382–388.
42. Saal JA, Saal JS. Intradiscal electrothermal treatment for chronic discogenic low back pain: a prospective outcome study with minimum one year follow-up. Spine 2000;25(20):2622–2627.
43. Saal JA, Saal JS. Intradiscal electrothermal treatment for chronic discogenic low back pain: a prospective outcome study with minimum two year follow-up. Spine 2002;27(9):966–974.
44. Karasek M, Bogduk N. Twelve-month follow-up of a controlled trial of intradiscal thermal annuloplasty for back pain due to internal disc disruption. Spine 2000;25(20):2601–2607.
45. Derby R, Eck B, Chen Y, et al. Intradiscal electrothermal annuloplasty (IDET): a novel approach for treating chronic discogenic back pain. Neuromodulation 2000;3(2):69–75.
46. Wetzel FT, Andersson GB, Peloza JH, et al. Intradiscal electrothermal therapy (IDET) to treat discogenic low back pain: two year results of a multi-center prospective cohort study. Paper presented at: 16th Annual Meeting of the North American Spine Society; 2001; Seattle, Washington.
47. Moore RJ, Walters R, Freeman BJ, et al. An assessment of the potential for IDET to denervate annular lesions. Paper presented at: Annual Meeting of the International Society for the Study of the Lumbar Spine; 2002; Cleveland, Ohio.
48. Pollintine P, Adams MA, Findlay G. IDET can equalize stress distributions inside intervertebral discs. Paper presented at: Annual Meeting of the International Society for the Study of the Lumbar Spine; 2002; Cleveland, Ohio.
49. Hsiu A, Isaac K, Katz J. Cauda equina syndrome from intradiscal electrothermal therapy. Neurology 2000;55(2):320.

CHAPTER 31

Operative Management of the Degenerative Disc: Posterior and Posterolateral Procedures

Gunnar B.J. Andersson and Francis H. Shen

In medicine, a successful outcome from a specific intervention is intimately associated with making an accurate diagnosis. In the case of degenerative disc disease making an accurate diagnosis can be challenging (1–3). Patients with degenerative disc disease may present with a variety of symptoms ranging from predominantly low back pain at one end of the spectrum, to leg pain at the other end (3–5). As a result, the management of degenerative disc disease has been controversial (4–8).

In patients with predominantly leg pain the source of the pain may be a degenerative herniated disc or associated lateral recess or foraminal stenosis resulting in lumbar radiculopathy. However, there is a subset of patients with axial back pain (low back pain without radiculopathy) where the history, physical findings, and confirmatory tests attempting to identify the source of pain have not been as clear. Pain generators in these patients may arise directly from the annulus of the degenerative disc (9,10), from arthritic facets (11,12), or from pathologic segmental instability and micromotion (13). It is this subset of patients that may benefit the most from a lumbar fusion.

In this section we review the operative indications, surgical options, techniques for posterolateral lumbar fusion, and role of instrumentation for axial back pain from disc degeneration. Management of the patient with radiculopathy from a herniated disc or stenosis is addressed in later chapters.

ETIOLOGY

Studies have focused on the annulus as a source of pain in the degenerative disc (9,10). Innervation of the annulus has been well characterized, with the outer third being innervated by pain transmitting free nerve endings (Figs. 31-1,31-2) (14). The sinuvertebral nerve, arising from the ventral root and gray rami communicans, provides innervation to structures within the spinal canal, the posterior longitudinal ligament, ventral dural sac, and posterior portion of the annulus (15). The ventral primary rami and the sympathetic nervous system innervate the lateral and anterior aspects of the annulus fibrosus, whereas branches of the gray rami communicans or the sympathetic trunk innervate the anterior longitudinal ligament (Figs. 31-1,31-2) (14,16). Furthermore, in a degenerative disc, the annulus fibrosus, as well as the cartilage end plates and underlying cancellous bone of the adjacent vertebra have been shown to be more extensively innervated than normal healthy discs and vertebra (17). In a study of 193 patients by Kuslich and colleagues, direct mechanical stimulation of the central and lateral portions of the annulus and vertebral end plates produced typical back pain symptoms in approximately two thirds of the patients (10).

Many of these same nerve endings are also involved with the production of pain-related neuropeptides (18). The number of neuropeptides known to be present in primary afferent neurons has been steadily increasing (19). These neuropeptides are produced within the dorsal root ganglion cell body and are delivered by axonal transport to the central and peripheral processes of the neurons. Their release has been demonstrated in response to intense electric stimulation of peripheral nerves; however, their exact role in pain modulation from degenerative disc disease has not yet been fully elucidated.

Because of the three-joint concept of the lumbar spine (20), axial back pain is likely the result of several factors (13). It is possible that with increasing ligamentous and capsular laxity there is progressive mechanical overload of the degenerative disc and facets resulting in segmental instability and pathologic motion potentially causing additional pain (13,21,22). The associated loss of disc height can increase stress across facet joints resulting in facet arthrosis. Although controversial, facet arthrosis has

317

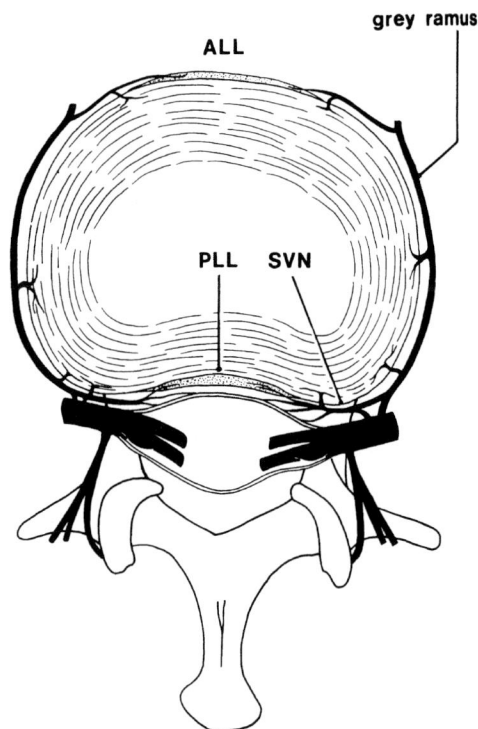

FIG. 31-1. The nerve supply of a lumbar intervertebral disc is depicted in a transverse view of the lumbar spine. Branches of the gray rami communicantes and the sinuvertebral nerves (SVN) are shown entering the disc and the anterior and posterior longitudinal ligaments (ALL and FLU). Branches from the sinuvertebral nerves also supply the anterior aspect of the dural sac and dural sleeve. (From Bogduk N, Twomey LT. Clinical anatomy of the lumbar spine, 2nd ed. Edinburgh: Churchill Livingstone, 1991:117.)

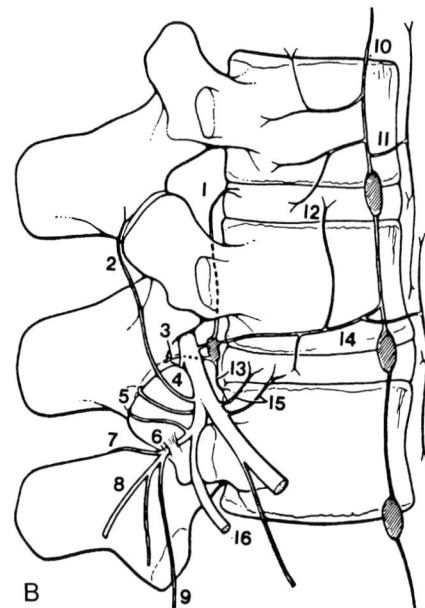

FIG. 31-2. Neuroanatomic definition of the lumbar motion segment. 1, Ascending branch of sinuvertebral nerve; 2, ascending facet branch; 3, sinuvertebral to facet; 4, direct branch to facet; 5, branches to multifidus; 6, medial branch of posterior primary ramus; 7, local facet branch; 8, descending facet branch; 9, branch to sacroiliac; 10, sympathetic chain; 11, branch under anterior longitudinal ligament; 12, branches from gray ramus to disc; 13, sinuvertebral to disc; 14, gray ramus communicans; 15, branches from anterior primary ramus to disc; 16, lateral branch of posterior primary ramus. (From Oudenhoven RC. The role of laminectomy, facet rhizotomy and epidural steroids. Spine 1979;4:145–147.)

also been implicated as a possible source of back pain (11,12,23). However, the clinical picture is variable. Although nociceptive nerve fibers have been clearly identified in facet joint capsules and pericapsular tissue, facet joint injections as a diagnostic and therapeutic modality are not always effective (23). Randomized studies have not demonstrated a difference between the efficacy of placebo and that of steroids and local anesthetics during facet injections (24,25).

OPERATIVE INDICATIONS

Before the diagnosis of degenerative disc disease can be made, a careful history, physical examination, and appropriate confirmatory studies should be performed. Once the diagnosis has been made, nonsurgical options should be exhausted before operative treatment is considered. The authors agree and stress that most individuals with chronic disc degeneration and axial back pain can be managed effectively with nonoperative treatment (2,4, 8,26). The natural history of axial back pain is continued improvement with resolution over time. In cases where

pain persists, it often becomes a diffuse process throughout the entire lumbar spine, and it becomes difficult to determine with certainty which of the several levels are the source of the pain.

Although the majority of patients improve with nonoperative measures, surgical intervention has a valuable role in selected cases. In a recent multicenter study, the Swedish Lumbar Spine Study Group randomized 294 patients with severe chronic low back pain into either surgical or nonsurgical treatment groups. The investigators concluded that in carefully selected patients with severe chronic low back pain without symptoms of leg pain or signs of nerve root compression, the improvement in pain and disability after surgical fusion was significantly superior to that of nonsurgical treatment (7). Current indications for fusion include the patient with (a) unremitting pain and disability for greater than 1 year; (b) failure of aggressive physical conditioning and conservative treatment for at least 3 to 4 months; (c) magnetic resonance imaging consistent with advanced disc degeneration limited to one or two disc levels; and (d) a negative psychiatric evaluation and lack of secondary gain (27,28).

TABLE 31-1. *Fusion techniques for degenerative disc disease*

Lumbar fusion techniques
Posterolateral intertransverse fusion
Posterior lumbar interbody fusion
Transforaminal lumbar interbody fusion
Anterior lumbar interbody fusion
Combined antero-posterior lumbar interbody fusion

Although some agreement has been reached concerning operative indications, the ideal surgical procedure for the management of the symptomatic degenerative disc has not yet been answered. Because the pain is believed to originate from either mechanical degeneration of the intervertebral disc or pathologic motion between vertebrae segments, the majority of surgical interventions focus on lumbar arthrodesis (Table 31-1). Fusion of the pathologic and painful lumbar segments would theoretically stabilize the progression of mechanical disc degeneration and eliminate pathologic motion and pain (2,4).

SURGICAL OPTIONS

Once the decision for operative intervention is decided on, then the options for arthrodesis include posterior-posterolateral fusions, posterior lumbar interbody fusions, anterior lumbar interbody fusions, and combined anterior-posterior fusions (4,5,27). There are few comparative studies that analyze the various techniques (29); the decision of whether or not to fuse the intervertebral disc is still under debate.

Some authors believe that a posterolateral fusion alone may be insufficient to address anterior pathology at the level of the intervertebral disc (30–32). They argue that if the annulus fibrosus has been identified as a potential pain generator, then treatment should address the pathology directly by complete elimination of the disc. Some studies have demonstrated anterior motion and concordant pain on discography of levels that lie beneath a solid posterior fusion (33). Proponents of posterolateral fusion argue that the posterior fusion alone is sufficient to provide relief of axial back pain symptoms in the majority of patients and that the associated morbidity from an interbody fusion cannot be justified (2,5,34).

Reported fusion rates vary among surgical techniques. Because of decreased vascularity of the vertebral endplates, pseudoarthrosis rates have been reported to be higher with interbody techniques (3,29). MacNab and Dall compared anterior interbody, posterior, and intertransverse fusions and found that the incidence of pseudoarthrosis after intertransverse fusions was significantly lower than with the other two methods. The investigators felt that the larger bone surface available from the transverse processes, lateral articular processes, and intervening isthmic region, combined with local vascu-

larity, enhanced the rate of neovascularization of the bone graft (29). Furthermore, interbody fusions often partially collapse and may potentially extrude during graft incorporation. Newer instrumentation and surgical techniques may improve fusion rates and decrease graft settling; however, long-term follow-up is still unavailable.

Biomechanically, the closer the fusion is to the centrode of the motion segment, the greater the stiffness achieved (3). Theoretically, interbody fusion techniques should have the highest rigidity, and the posterior and posterolateral fusions should have the least. However, the relatively larger fusion masses created posterolaterally during intertransverse process arthrodeses increases considerably the area moment of inertia, thus improving stability, particularly in axial rotation and lateral bending.

Historically, techniques that extend the fusion mass posteriorly to include the laminae, facet joints, and spinous processes have increased the rigidity of posterior fusions proportionally. However, this technique can lead to iatrogenic spinal and foraminal stenosis from bony overgrowth (4) and has been associated with a high rate of pseudarthrosis (35). In McBride's original description of the posterior fusion, he stressed the importance of the facet joint and used a morselized transfacet bone block for lumbosacral arthrodesis (36). Cadaveric studies performed by Boden et al. analyzed the axial and torsional stiffness of various techniques and questioned that method (37). Those authors concluded that disruption of the facet joint capsule required for placement of the transfacet bone blocks resulted in loss of spinal stability as compared with posterior intertransverse process arthrodesis alone. One significant advantage of the posterolateral technique over posterior fusions is that it can be performed in the absence of posterior elements. Posterior fusions are rarely performed today, and posterior and posterolateral techniques most commonly refer to intertransverse process arthrodeses (38).

POSTEROLATERAL INTERTRANSVERSE LUMBAR ARTHRODESIS

Historical Perspective

Spinal fusions were first reported in 1911 for the treatment of Pott disease by providing mechanical stability to inhibit progressive deformity and the spread of the tuberculous infections (39). Also in 1911, Hibbs described his experience with spinal fusion for tuberculosis and suggested that this technique could be used in the treatment of scoliosis (40). He performed his first fusion for scoliosis in 1914, and reported on his first 59 cases in 1924 (40). Eventually this led to the use of spinal fusions for the treatment of a variety of spinal deformities and diseases, including fractures, spondylolisthesis, scoliosis, kyphosis, and intervertebral disc disease.

Since that time, the techniques and surgical approaches for posterior-posterolateral lumbar fusions have changed significantly. There has been a significant increase in the basic science behind lumbar fusions and the understanding of the role of instrumentation. All fusion techniques involve surgical preparation of the site of intended fusion and an attempt to stimulate the formation of bone (41). Traditionally, graft materials were either autologous or allograft bone. However, an increasing number of synthetic and bioactive substances are currently in use or under investigation. Three basic requirements are necessary for a successful fusion: (a) graft material with adequate osteogenic, osteoinductive, and osteoconductive properties; (b) adequate local vascularity to produce and support the bone healing; and (c) an acceptable local environment for bone formation (41). A fusion is considered fused when the newly synthesized bone is mechanically contiguous with the local host bone and can sufficiently bear physiologic loads without failure of the fusion mass. A pseudarthrosis is said to take place if this does not occur.

Technique

This operation usually is performed under general anesthesia with the patient in the prone position. Chest and iliac crest rolls are placed with the chest and abdomen hanging free to allow pulmonary excursion, minimize abdominal compression, and minimize distention of the epidural veins. The use of prophylactic antibiotics is recommended.

A midline incision is centered slightly superior to the spinous processes of the involved levels, and the incision is extended proximally and distally to include the levels above and below to ensure adequate exposure. Electrocautery is used to divide the subcutaneous tissue down to the fascia in line with the skin incision. The fascia is incised in the midline and the paraspinous muscles are stripped subperiosteally from the spine with electrocautery and a Cobb periosteal elevator. Radiographs should be scrutinized for evidence of previous surgical or congenital bony defects to minimize inadvertent entry into the spinal canal. As the dissection progresses, sponges are packed tightly within the wound to help control bleeding. The facet joints are preserved until the appropriate levels have been identified. An intraoperative radiograph should be obtained if any question exists.

Once the level is confirmed, the dissection should progress laterally out to the transverse processes. This is performed by incising the fascia directly lateral to the facet joints and following the superior articular facet of the inferior vertebra out inferolaterally onto the transverse process. Deep retractors are repositioned as needed throughout the dissection. The muscle and soft tissue are carefully cleared off the transverse process, making sure not to fracture it. The dissection is carried superiorly and inferiorly as needed to include the appropriate levels. The spinous processes at the involved levels are connected by dissecting the muscle off the intertransverse ligament, thus creating space for the graft.

If the fusion is to extend to the sacrum, the ala should be prepared in a similar manner. The ala is exposed by dissecting lateral to the superior articular facet of the sacrum. It is important to note that in this area there are dense ligaments that must be dissected from the sacrum in order to obtain a clear exposure of the ala. At the end of the dissection, a continuous trough should exist laterally between the transverse processes and the ala. Bilateral decortication of the transverse processes, lateral portion of the pedicle, lateral portion of the articular facets, and ala is performed with a burr or sharp curettes (Fig. 31-3).

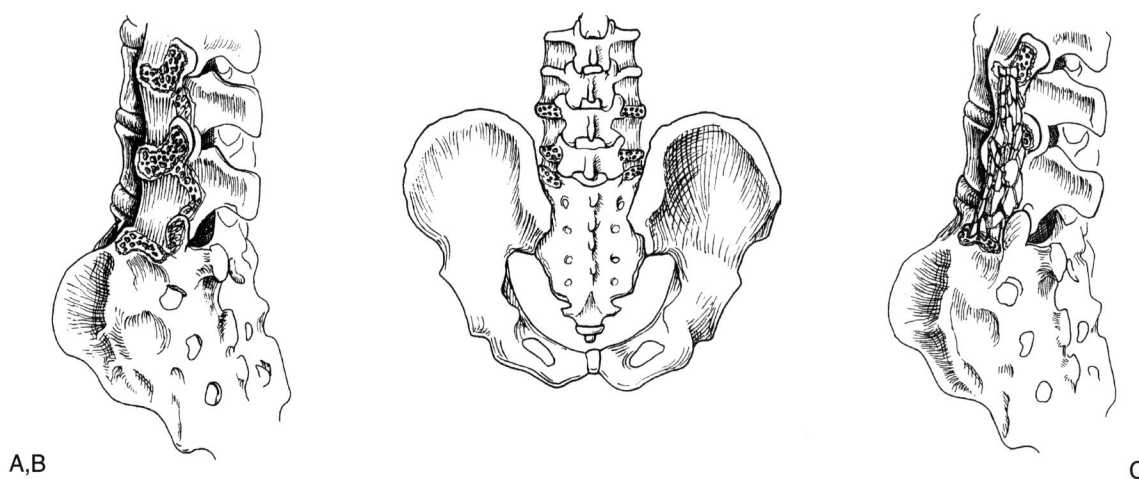

FIG. 31-3. Preparation of the fusion bed. **A:** Oblique view of meticulous decortication of the outer face of the facet joint, transverse process, pars, and alar cortical surfaces. **B:** Posterior view of decorticated bilateral lateral graft bed. **C:** Oblique view of fusion bed packed with cancellous and corticocancellous bone graft. (Zindrick MR, Selby D. Lumbar spine fusion: different types and indications. In: Wiesel SW, Weinstein JN, Herkowitz H, et al., eds. The lumbar spine, 2nd ed. New York: Lippincott Williams & Wilkins, 2004:600.)

At this point a preliminary sponge count should be performed and the wound checked both visually and with manual palpation to look for retained sponges. The wound is then irrigated and the posterolateral trough is packed ideally with autologous bone graft (see the following). The graft should not be harvested until the transverse processes, ala, and lateral structures have been exposed and decorticated to minimize the period when the bone is not in contact with tissue. At the end of the case hemostasis is obtained, any devitalized tissue is débrided, and a suction drain inserted into the wound if necessary. The fascia and subcutaneous tissue are closed in the standard manner.

Bone Graft Harvesting: Posterior Iliac Crest

Despite rapid advances in bone graft substitutes, the use of autologous iliac crest bone remains the gold standard at this time. Iliac crest is still the most common source of autologous bone harvest for posterolateral lumbar fusions because of its superior osteogenic, osteoconductive, and osteoinductive properties combined with easy accessibility.

If amenable, the same midline incision used during the exposure of the posterior spinal elements can be used to obtain access to the posterior ilium. Maintaining a full thickness flap, dissect just superficial to the fascia out laterally to the posterior superior iliac spine. If using the same incision results in excessive dissection or inadequate exposure, a second separate incision can be used. The second incision can be oriented either vertically or obliquely, with the posterior superior iliac spine at approximately the inferior or medial margin of the incision. Regardless of the approach, care should be taken, if possible, not to expose beyond 8 cm lateral to the posterior superior iliac spine, because this may result in injury to the superior cluneal nerves and cause numbness in the skin overlying the gluteal region (42).

Dissect down to the posterior superior iliac spine and expose the iliac crest. Incise the iliac crest periosteum and subperiosteally dissect the muscle and periosteum off the outer table of the posterior ilium. This is performed with a combination of electrocautery and a Cobb elevator. After the muscles and periosteum are stripped, a Taylor or similar retractor is placed deeply into the wound, taking care not to inadvertently enter into the greater sciatic notch distally.

Once the graft donor site is exposed, begin harvesting corticocancellous strips using a half-inch osteotome. Make sure to score the outer table only by creating several vertical strips approximately 7 mm in width. The distal extend of the vertical cuts are then connected horizontally with a curved osteotome to prevent distal propagation of the strips during harvest. Start at the top of the iliac crest, and use a curved osteotome wedged between the inner and outer tables of the ilium to remove

the precut corticocancellous strips. Once they are removed, the intramedullary cavity is available for cancellous bone removal with gouges or curettes. When an appropriate amount of bone graft has been obtained hemostasis is achieved, the wound irrigated, and a drain inserted if necessary. The incision is closed in the standard fashion.

Postoperative Management

Antibiotics are continued until the drains are removed, usually on the first or second postoperative day. Typically the diet is advanced as tolerated unless an ileus develops. The patient is encouraged to be out of bed and is allowed to ambulate the day of or day after surgery. An external orthosis or brace is recommended for support and comfort, particularly if multiple level fusions were performed. Early mobilization has not been shown to lower the rate of successful fusion and may actually improve muscle tone, decrease edema, promote hematoma resolution, and improve patient function and psychologic outlook.

After discharge from the hospital, the initial visit is often scheduled at 2 to 3 weeks postoperatively. The patient is then reevaluated at 6-week intervals for the first 3 months, and then every 3 months for the first year. The patient can usually return to light duty or part-time work by 4 to 6 weeks, although heavy lifting and vigorous athletics should be avoided for 6 months. As the patient's recovery improves, a more vigorous exercise program is gradually instituted with focus on proper back care and mechanics.

INSTRUMENTED VERSUS NONINSTRUMENTED POSTEROLATERAL FUSIONS

Significant interest and debate exists over the use of instrumentation in posterolateral lumbar fusions. Various constructs have been investigated and include wires, hooks, and pedicle-screw based segmental fixation techniques. Currently, segmental instrumentation with pedicle-screw fixation is the construct of choice because of the ability to control all three columns of the spine from a posterior approach, the ability to limit the fusion to involved motion segments, the ability to obtain spinal fixation in the absence of posterior elements, and the capability to avoid placement of instrumentation within the spinal canal (27,43,44).

From a theoretical standpoint, spinal instrumentation provides immediate stability to the spinal segments being fused and therefore increases fusion rates. Multiple studies support this hypothesis (4,44–47). For a single level posterolateral fusion without instrumentation pseudoarthrosis rates are reported to be between 10% and 15%. The addition of pedicle instrumentation may lower this to

5%. In a prospective, randomized trial of 49 patients, Zdeblick demonstrated a statistically significant difference in fusion rates between instrumented and noninstrumented posterior fusions for degenerative disc disease. The fusion rate for the group with pedicle instrumentation was 93% compared to 45% without instrumentation (47).

The use of instrumentation has been shown to reduce the pseudoarthrosis rate in patients undergoing multiple level fusions. In a prospective study by Grubb and Lipscomb (45) that looked at one- and two-level fusions, the authors found higher fusion rates in patients having instrumentation. Similar results from a prospective, multicenter trial were reported by Wood and colleagues (44), who examined the use of instrumentation in one- to four-level fusions, with the majority of them being two levels or greater. Compared to historic controls, the authors found that patients who underwent fusion without instrumentation were over 24 times more likely to develop a pseudoarthrosis when compared to patients with instrumented fusions.

Other reported advantages of instrumentation include decreased rehabilitation time, reduced need for postoperative bracing (47), and possible reduced requirement for postoperative use of pain medication (43,47,48). However, these findings should not mandate the routine use of instrumentation during lumbar arthrodesis. Compared to fusion *in situ,* the use of instrumentation has been associated with higher morbidity and mortality (Table 31-2). A cohort study sponsored by the North American Spine Society for the use of pedicle instrumentation reported an overall instrument related complication rate of 5% (48). The risks and benefits of instrumentation should be considered in each individual case, particularly in the elderly patient, where the advantages must be balanced carefully with the potential risks associated from the use of instrumentation. Furthermore, the use of instrumentation should be performed only by experienced surgeons, who are knowledgeable and comfortable with the specific techniques. The occasional use of instrumentation by the inexperienced surgeon is associated with an unacceptably high complication rate and should be avoided.

We believe that in cases where an increased risk of pseudoarthrosis is present, the use of adjuvant instrumentation is beneficial for posterolateral intertransverse lumbar fusions. In particular, this includes patients with risk factors such as diabetes and smoking, in multilevel fusions and in revision cases for failed back or surgical treatment of established pseudoarthrosis.

CONCLUSION

Significant debate exists over the role of surgery in the management of degenerative disc disease. The lack of randomized, prospective studies makes the comparison and evaluation of outcomes difficult to assess. Furthermore, studies on the role of posterolateral arthrodesis for the treatment of disc degeneration often includes patients with multiple pathologies, including herniated discs, spondylolisthesis, and spinal stenosis, some of whom may have undergone prior decompressive procedures or arthrodesis. Despite these shortcomings, posterolateral arthrodesis in properly selected patients is a viable option for the treatment of axial back pain from degenerative disc disease. Currently autologous iliac crest remains the gold standard for bone graft material during posterolateral lumbar fusions. The adjuvant judicious use of instrumentation improves fusion rates by providing immediate stability; however, its routine use should be avoided and decisions about its use should be made on an individual basis.

TABLE 31-2. *Complications of spinal instrumentation*

Complication	Reported rates
Neurologic injury	1%–5%
Infections	3%–6%
Instrumentation failure	6%–10%
Reoperation	20%

Source: Adapted from Yuan H, Garfin S, Dickman C, et al. A historical cohort study of pedicle screw fixation in thoracic, lumbar, and sacral spinal fusions. Spine, 1994;19(suppl 20):S2279–S2296, with permission.

REFERENCES

1. Andersson GBJ. The epidemiology of spinal disorders. In: Frymoyer J, ed. The adult spine: principles and practice, 2nd ed. Philadelphia: Lippincott-Raven, 1997:93–141.
2. Truumees E, Herkowitz HN. Degenerative disc disease. In: Chapman MW, Szabo RM, Marder R, eds. Chapman's orthopaedic surgery, 3rd ed. Philadelphia: Lippincott Williams & Wilkins, 2001:3775–3805.
3. Wisneski RJ, Garfin SR, Rothman RH, et al. Lumbar disc disease. In: Herkowitz H, Garfin S, Balderston R, et al., eds. Rothman Simeone the spine, 4th ed. Philadelphia: WB Saunders, 1999:613–679.
4. Hanley Jr EN, David SM. Lumbar arthrodesis for the treatment of back pain. J Bone Joint Surg 1999;81A(5):716–730.
5. Herkowitz HN, Sidhu KS. Lumbar spine fusion in the treatment of degenerative conditions: current indications and recommendations. J Am Assoc Orthop Surg 1995;3:123.
6. Bigos SJ. A literature-based review as a guide for generating recommendations to patients acutely limited by low back symptoms. In: Surg AAO, ed. Orthopaedic knowledge update: spine. Rosemont, IL: American Association of Orthopedic Surgeons, 1997:A15.
7. Fritzell P, Hagg O, Wessberg P, et al. Lumbar fusion versus nonsurgical treatment for chronic low back pain: a multicenter randomized controlled trial from the Swedish Lumbar Spine Study Group. Spine 2001;26(23):2521–2532.
8. Wilson-MacDonald J. Controversies in management: should backache be treated with spinal fusion? The case for spinal fusion is unproved. Br Med J 1996;312(7022):39–40.
9. Freemont AJ. Nerve ingrowth into diseased intervertebral disc in chronic back pain. Lancet 1997;350:178.
10. Kuslich SD, Ulstrom CL, Michael CJ. The tissue origin of low back pain and sciatica: a report of pain response to tissue stimulation during operations on the lumbar spine using local anesthesia. Orthop Clin N Am 1991;22:181–187.
11. Carrera GF. Lumbar facet joint injection in low back pain and sciatica: preliminary results. Radiology1980;137:665–667.
12. Lewinneck GE, Warfield CA. Facet joint degeneration as a cause of low back pain. Clin Orthop 1986;213:216–222.
13. Lanzino G, Shaffery CI, Ray CD. Posterior lumbar interbody fusion.

In: Benzel E, ed. Spine surgery: techniques, complications, avoidance, and management. Philadelphia: Churchill-Livingstone, 1999.

14. Bogduk N. The innervation of the lumbar spine. Spine 1983;8:286–293.
15. Hayashi N, Lee HM, Weinstein JN. The source of pain in the lumbar spine. In: Bridwell KH, DeWald RL, eds. The textbook of spinal surgery, 2nd ed. Philadelphia: Lippincott-Raven, 1997:1503–1514.
16. Bodguk N, Tynan W, Wilson AS. The nerve supply to the human lumbar intervertebral discs. J Anat 1981;132:39.
17. Brown MF, Hukkanen MVJ, McCarthy ID, et al. Sensory and sympathetic innervation of the vertebral endplate in patients with degenerative disc disease. J Bone Joint Surg 1997;79B(1):147–153.
18. Coppes MH, Marani E, Thomeer RT, et al. Innervation of "painful" lumbar discs. Spine 1997;22:2342–2349.
19. Ahmed M, Bjurholm A, Kreicbergs A, et al. Neuropeptide Y, tryosine hydroxylase and vasoactive intestinal peptide-immunoreactive nerve fibers in the vertebral bodies, discs, dura mater, and spinal ligaments of the rat lumbar spine. Spine 1993;18:268.
20. Yong-Hing K, Kirkaldy-Willis WH. The pathophysiology of disc degeneration of the lumbar spine. Orthop Clin N Am 1983;14:59.
21. Frymoyer JW, Selby DK. Segmental instability. Rationale for treatment. Spine 1985;10:280–286.
22. Stokes IA, Frymoyer JW. Segmental motion and instability. Spine 1987;12:688–691.
23. Carette S, Marcoux S, Truchon R, et al. A controlled trial of corticosteroid injections into facet joints for chronic low back pain. N Engl J Med 1991;325:1002–1007.
24. Jackson RP. The facet syndrome: myth or reality? Clin Orthop 1992;279:110.
25. Lilius G, Laasonen EM, Myllynen P, et al. The facet syndrome. J Bone Joint Surg 1989;71B:681.
26. Nachemson A. Lumbar disc disease with discogenic pain: what surgical treatment is most effective? Spine 1996;21(15):1835–1836.
27. Sidhu KS, Herkowitz HN. Spinal instrumentation in the management of degenerative disorders of the lumbar spine. Clin Orthop Rel Res 1997;335:39–53.
28. Srdjan M. The role of surgery for non radicular low back pain. Curr Opin Orthop 1994;5:37–42.
29. MacNab I, Dall D. The blood supply of the spine and its application tot the technique of intertransverse fusion. J Bone Joint Surg 1972;54B:1195.
30. Kozak JA, O'Brien JP. Simultaneous combined anterior and posterior fusion. An independent analysis of a treatment for the disabled low back pain patient. Spine 1990;115:322–328.
31. Newman MH, Grinstead GL. Anterior lumbar interbody fusion for internal disc disruption. Spine 1992;17:831–833.
32. Steffee AD, Sitkowski DJ. Posterior lumbar interbody fusion and plates. Clin Orthop 1988;227:99–102.
33. Weatherley CR, Prickett CF, O'Brien JP. Discogenic pain persisting despite solid posterior fusion. J Bone Joint Surg 1986;68B:142–143.
34. Zdeblick T. The treatment of degenerative lumbar disorders. A critical review of the literature. Spine 1995;20(suppl 24):S126–S137.
35. Fraser RD. Interbody, posterior, and combined lumbar fusions. Spine 1995;20(suppl 24):S167–S177.
36. McBride ED. A mortised transfacet bone block for lumbosacral fusion. J Bone Joint Surg 1949;31A:385–393.
37. Boden SD, Martin C, Rudolph R, et al. Increase of motion between lumbar vertebrae after excision of the capsule and cartilage of the facets. A cadaver study. J Bone Joint Surg 1994;76A:1847–1853.
38. Dawson EG, Lotysch M, Urist MR. Intertransverse process lumbar arthrodesis with autogenous bone graft. Clin Orthop 1981;154:90–96.
39. Albee FH. Transplantation of a portion of the tibia into the spine for Pott's disease. JAMA 1911;57:885–886.
40. Hibbs RA. An operation for progressive spinal deformities. NY Med J 1911;93:1013–1016.
41. Muschler GF, Lane JM. Spine fusion. In: Herkowitz H, Garfin S, Balderston R, et al., eds. Rothman Simeone the spine, 4th ed. Philadelphia: WB Saunders, 1999:1573–1629.
42. Hoppenfeld S, deBoer P. The pelvis: posterior approach to the iliac crest for bone graft. In: Hoppenfeld S, deBoer P, eds. Surgical exposures in orthopaedics: the anatomic approach. Philadelphia: JB Lippincott, 1994:307–309.
43. Kanwaldeep SS, Herkowitz HN. Spinal instrumentation in the management of degenerative disorders of the lumbar spine. Clin Orthop Rel Res 1997;335:39–53.
44. Wood II GW, Boyd RJ, Carothers TA, et al. The effect of pedicle screw/plate fixation on lumbar/lumbosacral autogenous bone graft fusions in patients with degenerative disc disease. Spine 1995;20:819–830.
45. Grubb SA, Lipscomb HJ. Results of lumbosacral fusion for degenerative disc disease with and without instrumentation: two to five year follow-up. Spine 1992;17:349–355.
46. Lorenz M, Zindrick M, Schwaegler P, et al. A comparison of single-level fusions with and without hardware. Spine 1991;16(suppl 8):S455–S458.
47. Zdeblick TA. A prospective, randomized study of lumbar fusion: preliminary results. Spine 1993;18:983–991.
48. Yuan HA, Garfin SR, Dickman CA, et al. A historical cohort study of pedicle screw fixation in thoracic, lumbar, and sacral spinal fusions. Spine 1994;19(suppl 20):S2279–S2296.

CHAPTER 32

Posterior Lumbar Interbody Fusion

Casey K. Lee and Kenneth J. Kopacz

Degenerative disc disorders are probably the most common cause of acute or chronic low back pain, but the natural history and the mechanism of pain production of degenerative disc disorders are poorly understood. Many different phases of degenerative disc disease (i.e., "degenerative cascade") are described well by Kirkaldy-Willis et al. (1). The acute onset of low back pain, the first time or very occasional recurrences, usually becomes symptom-free after a short duration. Some pathologic conditions of degenerative disc disease (DDD) are, however, responsible for recurrent or chronic persistent low back pain that significantly affects a patient's lifestyle. These include *internal disc derangement* which is defined as a derangement of the internal disc structure (nucleus and annulus) or biochemical alterations without having any external disc pathology such as disc bulge, herniation, disc height narrowing, or abnormal displacement. Another subtype of DDD is classified as stable DDD. This is described as degenerative disc changes without having gross abnormal displacement such as degenerative spondylolisthesis.

Spinal fusion for DDD has been a most controversial subject for many decades. The effectiveness of spinal fusion for DDD was difficult to prove without knowledge of the natural history of various degenerative conditions. Yet, DDD has been the most common pathologic condition for which spinal fusion is indicated. Davis reported that 51% of spinal fusions performed in the United States during a 10-year period (1980 to 1990) were for DDD (2). In a review of English-language literature by Bono and Lee (3) for spinal fusion for DDD between 1980 and 2000, spinal fusion was indicated for various conditions of DDD. The most common indication was for stable DDD (67%) which included internal disc derangement, DDD without instability, and postdisc excision for disc herniation. The second most common indication was for DDD with spondylolisthesis (25%).

Indication for spinal fusion for certain conditions of DDD such as degenerative spondylolisthesis, progressive degenerative scoliosis, or hypolordosis ("flat back syndrome") is well accepted while indication for others such as stable DDD and internal disc derangement (IDD) is still controversial. Spinal fusion for chronic low back pain caused by DDD has been proven more effective than nonoperative treatments in a recent controlled clinical study (4). For IDD, there is no controlled clinical study that conclusively proves the effectiveness of spinal fusion over the natural history or nonoperative treatments, and it remains a most controversial subject. There is, however, some indirect clinical information suggesting that spinal fusion for IDD may be a more effective treatment than the natural history or nonoperative treatments. In a 5-year follow-up study of patients with chronic low back pain caused by IDD (discography-positive) who were treated with nonoperative treatments, none of the patients became symptom-free and approximately 50% were experiencing the same or worse pain (5). In another study, patients who were candidates for spinal fusion with the diagnosis of IDD but were denied fusion by insurance payors were followed for one-and-a-half years. Two-thirds of patients were experiencing the same or worse symptoms at follow-up (6). The published results of spinal fusion for IDD indicate a high rate of symptom relief and return to work. In a report on a properly selected group of patients with IDD, spinal fusion provided better clinical success rates of pain relief (89%) and return to work (82%) (7).

CHOICE OF SPINAL FUSION TECHNIQUES

Posterolateral Fusion versus Interbody Fusion

Lumbar interbody fusion is preferred to posterior or posterolateral fusion in patients with discogenic pain (stable DDD and IDD) and in patients with anterior column weight-bearing deficiency, especially with angular instability in the sagittal or coronal plane. It is also preferred in patients with failed previous posterior or posterolateral fusion.

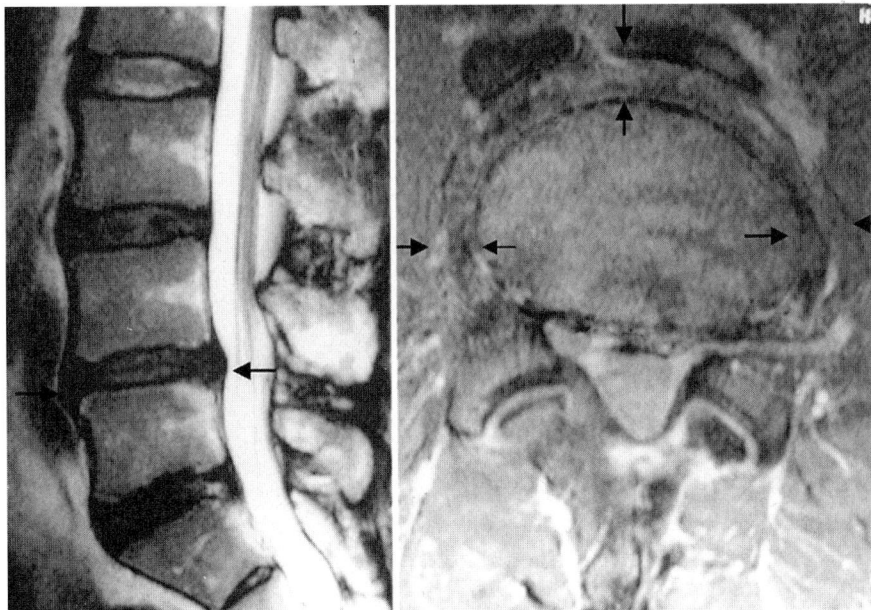

FIG. 32-1. Disc degeneration with anterior column weight-bearing function ("flat-tire syndrome"). Magnetic resonance imaging of the lumbosacral spine of a patient with chronic disabling low back pain shows the L4-5 disc with diffuse circumferential bulge *(arrows)* and with minimally decreased disc height. The disc has deficient anterior column weight-bearing function.

Various types of spinal fusion produce different biomechanical effects on the fused segment and on adjacent segments (8,9). In a biochemical study, Rolander reported that posterior fusion did not eliminate motion across the disc within the fused segment and suggested that this retained motion across the disc may be the source of chronic persistent pain after successful posterior fusion. Clinical studies by others further support this concept (10,11). In these clinical studies, some patients with discogenic pain had persistent pain after successful posterior or posterolateral fusion, and their pain symptom was successfully relieved after subsequent lumbar interbody fusion.

Effects of different types of lumbar fusion on adjacent segments are primarily caused by changes in stiffness and changes in the center of rotation of segmental motion of adjacent levels to fusion (9). Degeneration of the disc results in changes in biomechanics of the motion segment. In certain cases, the motion segment may become unstable in sagittal, coronal, axial or combination motions due to mechanical incompetence of the disc (anterior column weight-bearing deficiency) (Fig. 32-1). Interbody fusion is more effective in correcting the anterior column deficiency than is posterior or posterolateral fusion. Posterior or posterolateral fusion for DDD with anterior column deficiency, especially for angular instability (segmental hypolordosis or disc space wedging), may produce significant adverse effects on the adjacent segments (12,13).

Posterior Lumbar Interbody Fusion versus Anterior Lumbar Interbody Fusion

Indications for, and the fusion rate of posterior lumbar interbody fusion (PLIF) are very similar to those of anterior lumbar interbody fusion (ALIF). The clinical success rate is comparable for the two, but the "surgeon factor" (skills and experience) is an important factor (14). Each procedure has advantages and disadvantages. ALIF has a wider and easier surgical exposure, but often requires a second surgeon (vascular or general). It is associated with inherently more significant and serious complications than PLIF, such as vascular or visceral injuries, impotence, or retrograde ejaculation. When rigid fixation is required for ALIF, an additional posterior approach is required for pedicle screw fixation. PLIF is primarily indicated for the lower lumbar and lumbosacral spine (L3-5 and S1). In the upper lumbar spine above the L2 level, the surgical exposure for PLIF is limited by the presence of conus medullaris and by the short interpedicular distance. The surgical exposure of PLIF is more limited and more difficult to master than ALIF. However, PLIF has definite advantages over ALIF in other aspects: all three columns of the motion segment can be addressed through one exposure—posterior decompression, restoration of anterior column weight-bearing function, correction of degenerative deformities and instability, and rigid posterior fixation. It has different complications from ALIF: excessive epidural bleeding, dural tear, or neural injury. PLIF is preferred to ALIF for patients who require addressing all three columns at the same time: posterior decompression, restoration of anterior column weight-bearing function, and rigid posterior fixation.

PLIF Indications

Indications for PLIF are as follows:

1. The *preferred* indication for PLIF is DDD with anterior column weight-bearing deficiency (Fig. 32-2).

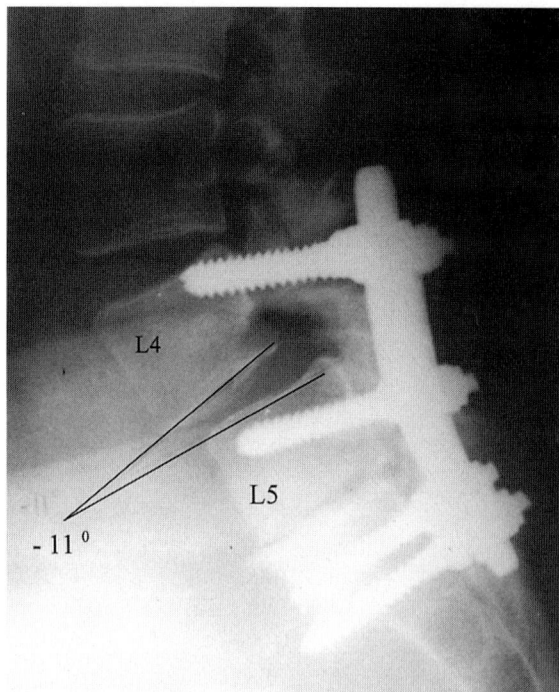

FIG. 32-2. Disc degeneration with disc space wedging and loss of lordosis. A lateral view of the lumbosacral spine of a female patient shows persistent segmental kyphosis at L4-5 after posterolateral fusion. She has severe persistent low back pain and was unable to stand up straight. Posterolateral spinal fusion failed to correct segmental kyphosis and failed to relieve her symptoms.

   a. DDD with diffuse circumferential disc bulge with or without disc space collapse ("flat-tire syndrome") (12) (Fig. 32-1)
   b. DDD with segmental instability such as degenerative spondylolisthesis
   c. DDD with segmental deformity—hypolordosis or disc space wedging (Fig. 32-2)
2. PLIF is a good choice for chronic disabling low back caused by:
   a. IDD
   b. Stable DDD
   c. Post-disc excision DDD
3. Other indications for PLIF are:
   a. Failed posterolateral fusion
   b. The rare indication of a disc space infection with epidural abscess resistant to nonoperative treatment that requires surgical intervention for débridement and stabilization
   c. Degenerative scoliosis where posterior decompression, correction of deformity, and rigid internal fixation are combined with fusion

PLIF Contraindications

PLIF is contraindicated where the neural elements cannot be retracted in such conditions as conjoined nerve roots or severe epidural scarring following previous surgery. PLIF is not recommended above L2 because of the very narrow interpedicular distance, narrow spinal canal, and proximity of the conus medullaris.

PLIF Surgical Techniques

Successful results of PLIF depend on proper patient selection, indications, and good surgical techniques. The PLIF procedure requires: (a) adequate exposure; (b) adequate mobilization, retraction, and protection of neural elements; (c) proper preparation of the vertebral end plates (graft bed); and (d) placement of an adequate amount of appropriate bone graft. Basic surgical techniques are described well by others (15–19). Some selected important points are described here.

Exposure

Bilateral large laminotomies and medial one-half facetectomies provide a sufficiently large enough exposure for the basic PLIF technique (Fig. 32-3). Proper control of epidural bleeding is essential for mobilization and retraction of the dura and nerve roots. Bipolar coagula-

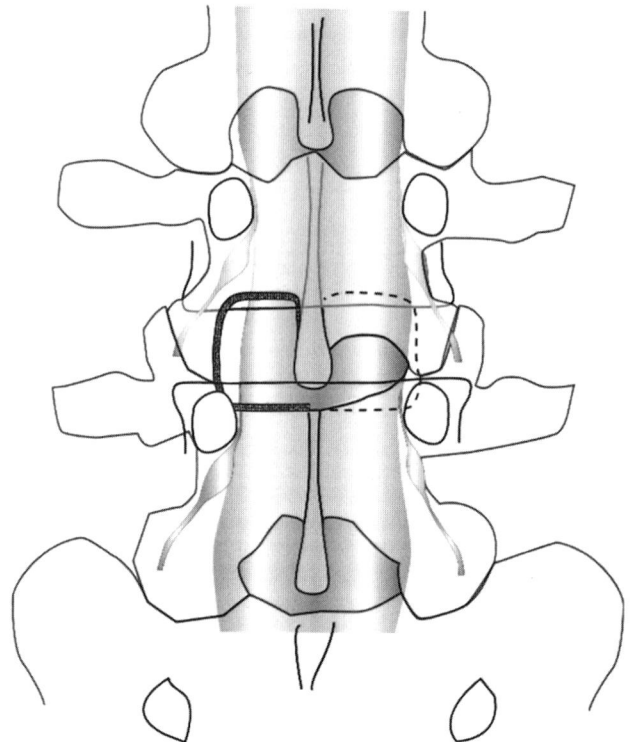

FIG. 32-3. The surgical exposure for the basic posterior lumbar interbody fusion (PLIF). Bilateral laminotomies and medial one-half facetectomies *(dotted line)* will provide sufficient exposure for the basic PLIF. Most of the lamina, spinous processes, interspinous and supraspinous ligaments, and lateral one-half of facet joints are saved for stability of the fusion construct.

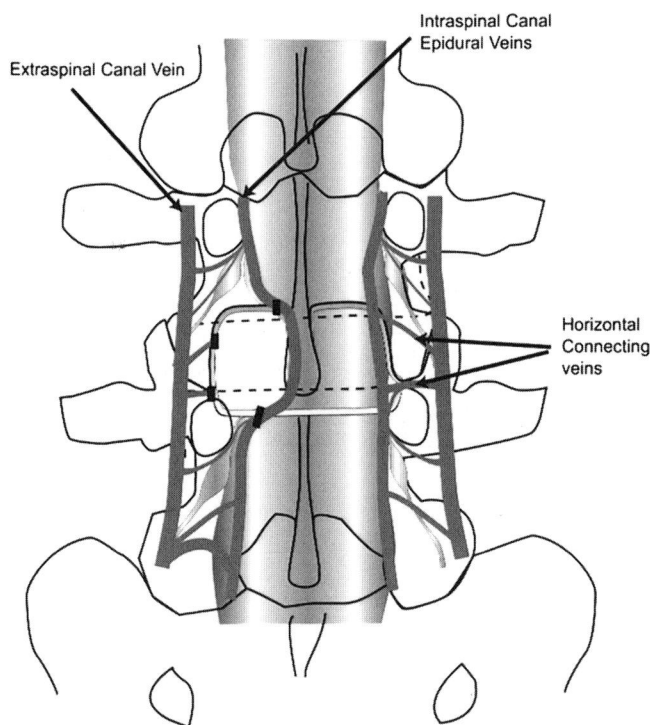

FIG. 32-4. Control of epidural bleeding and retraction of neural elements. Epidural vessels have regular anatomic arrangements, vertically running intraspinal canal vessels and horizontally running connecting vessels between intraspinal and extraspinal canal systems. Horizontally running vessels are coagulated with a bipolar cautery and divided immediately above the pedicles and near the lower vertebral end plate. The traversing nerve root, dura, and intraspinal vertical epidural vessels are retracted to the midline.

tion and division of cross-linking epidural veins between the extraspinal canal and intraspinal canal venous system superior to the pedicles provides a dry surgical field and allows easier mobilization of the dura and nerve roots medially to the midline (Fig. 32-4).

Mobilization, Retraction, and Protection of Neural Elements

The dura and the traversing nerve root may be retracted to the midline (Figs. 32-4, 32-5). A prolonged continuous retraction of the nerve root should be avoided, especially for patients who had previous posterior surgery. The exiting nerve root above the disc may occasionally be in the way at the superior lateral corner of the surgical field under the facet joint. All of these neural elements should be retracted and protected all the time during the procedure, especially during insertion of bone graft or any fusion device into the disc space.

Preparation of the Vertebral End Plates (Graft Bed)

Contact surface area between graft bed and bone graft is the most important factor for bone healing and subsi-

dence. Exposure of sub–end-plate cancellous bone promotes bone healing. Biomechanical tests indicate that decortication of the vertebral end plates does not have any significant effect on the compressive strength at the interface between bone grafts and vertebral bone (20). The three most important factors for subsidence of bone grafts or interbody fusion devices are bone mineral density of the vertebral bone, applied compressive load, and contact surface area at the interface. To prevent subsidence, a PLIF construct requires a minimum contact surface area of 6.25 cm^2 for stability at the interface for a patient with normal bone mineral density under normal postoperative physiologic conditions (21). This amount of contact surface area can be obtained by preparing the end plates for 2.5 cm × 2.5 cm for bone grafts. For the average-size adult Caucasian, laminotomies and medial one-half facetectomies with retraction of neural elements medially to the midline provide adequate exposure (1.3 to 1.5 cm on each side) for decortication of vertebral end plates between pedicles (1.25 cm from each side) and to the depth of 2.8 cm anteriorly. This contact surface area of 6.25 cm^2 is approximately equal to the total contact surface area of two tricortical iliac crest bone grafts.

Bone Graft Insertion

Stand-alone PLIF construct (PLIF construct without internal fixation systems such as pedicle screw fixation or facet screw fixation) requires bone grafts that provide sufficient compressive strength to prevent graft collapse, that provide a sufficiently large contact surface area to prevent subsidence, and that have good bone healing potential. Two autologous tricortical iliac crest bone grafts meet all of the requirements. Each tricortical iliac crest bone graft may be harvested and split in half and inserted in four blocks of split grafts (Fig. 32-5). An alternative graft is to remove the outer wall of the iliac crest, obtaining four corticocancellous blocks. These modifications allow easy placement of graft into the disc space without excessive retraction of neural elements, and save the inner cortical table of the iliac crest. Patients treated with stand-alone PLIF with four blocks of autologous one-half iliac crest bone grafts show no significant graft subsidence or graft collapse. Furthermore, there is no significant difference in graft subsidence or fusion rate between stand-alone PLIF and PLIF with pedicle screw fixation. This strongly suggests that stand-alone PLIF provides a high rate of fusion without subsidence or graft collapse when the basic principles of PLIF techniques are diligently followed. These include: (a) saving posterior structures of interspinous and supraspinous ligaments and lateral one-half facet joints; (b) adequate size of vertebral end-plate preparation for contact surface area with bone graft; and (c) proper choice of bone graft in quantity and quality.

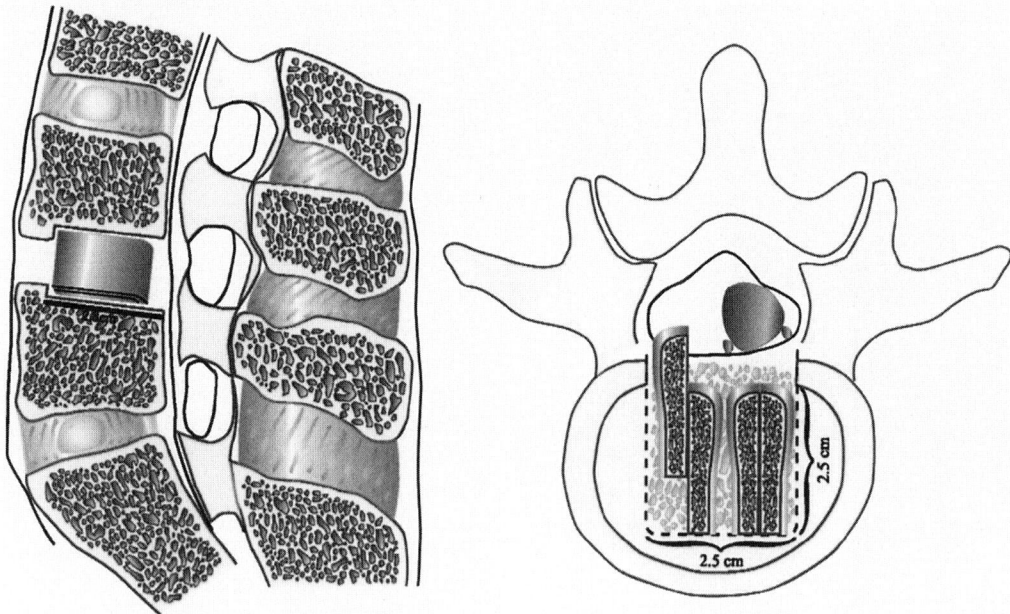

FIG. 32-5. Preparation of the vertebral end plates and insertion of bone grafts. The vertebral end plates are decorticated between the pedicles (about 2.5 cm) and to the depth of approximately 2.8 cm toward the anterior aspect of the spinal column. Four blocks of bicortical corticocancellous graft (each with 0.7 cm width, 2.5 cm depth, and with an appropriate height) are impacted into the disc space. The space available for bone graft insertion is limited to approximately 1.25 to 1.3 cm when the neural elements are retracted to the midline. A bone graft wider than 1.3 cm is very difficult and requires further retraction of neural elements or total facetectomy.

Modifications of the Basic PLIF Technique

Many different types of modification of PLIF surgical techniques have been described in the literature (22–31). Some advocate bilateral total facetectomies and laminotomies for a larger surgical exposure and for easier insertion of bone grafts or interbody fusion devices. This surgical exposure, however, produces an unstable PLIF construct and requires additional rigid internal fixation systems such as pedicle screw fixation or facet screw fixation. One other similar variation is unilateral approach: laminotomy and facetectomy, insertion of bone graft or interbody fusion devices and pedicle screw fixation are performed on one side only. Little information is available in the literature about the success rate of the unilateral PLIF.

Facet screw fixation or other posterior tension band devices have been used with PLIF for additional stability of the fusion construct. PLIF with pedicle screw fixation provides a marginally better fusion rate than stand-alone PLIF. A good stand-alone PLIF construct provides sufficient enough stability for prevention of subsidence or bone graft collapse. A clinical comparison study of stand-alone PLIF versus PLIF with pedicle screw fixation demonstrated no significant difference in subsidence and graft failure (32). Patients with stand-alone PLIF do not require any external brace postoperatively. Patients with PLIF and pedicle screw fixation appear to have easier and faster mobilization during the immediate postoperative period.

Although autologous iliac crest corticocancellous bone graft has been the standard for basic PLIF procedure, many other alternatives have been used. These include local bone graft from spinous process or lamina removed during the operation, cortical or corticocancellous allograft, graft substitutes, or various types of interbody fusion devices. In recent years, the use of ready made cortical or corticocancellous interbody fusion grafts or interbody fusion cages have become popular. Most of these products require facetectomies to provide a large exposure for insertion, and therefore require supplemental pedicle screw fixation. Some of these devices are poorly designed and do not satisfy the basic principles of interbody fusion techniques (Fig. 32-6).

The average interpedicular (right to left) distance of the lower lumbar spine of an adult Caucasian is about 2.5 cm, and the average disc height in the lower lumbar spine is 1.2 to 1.3 cm. In order to have a cylindric cage sufficiently contact the vertebral end plates, the diameter of the cage has to be greater than 1.6 cm. A smaller cage will result in gradual subsidence or failure of bony union. A cage with a 1.5 cm diameter or greater will be very difficult to insert posteriorly because of the anatomic limitations described herein. It requires total facetectomy or

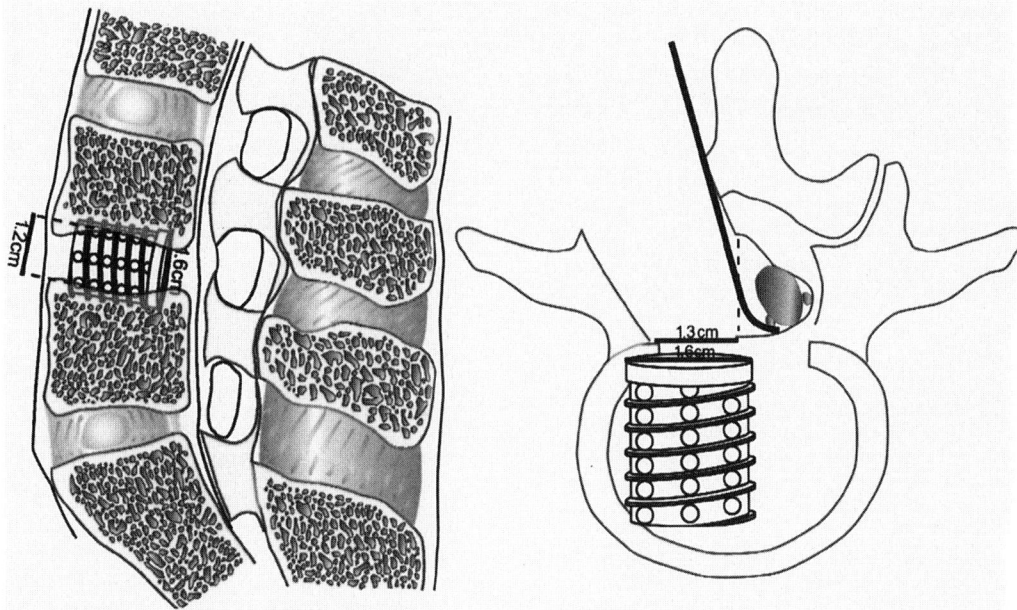

FIG. 32-6. Interbody fusion devises. For a lower lumbar disc with disc space height of 1.2 cm, the diameter of a cylindric cage should be more than 1.6 cm for adequate contact surface area. To insert this through the posterior approach, the surgical exposure requires total laminectomies and facetectomies and requires retraction of the neural elements far beyond the midline.

excessive retraction of the dura and the nerve root beyond the midline for insertion of such a large cage. The interpedicular distance in the Asian population is smaller than that of Caucasians, and the procedure becomes even more difficult and riskier for excessive bleeding and neural injury (33). Any interbody device or prepared bone graft in excess of 1 cm wide is difficult to insert posteriorly into the disc space, and it requires an excessive amount of retraction even with total facetectomies. The design of interbody fusion devices for PLIF should be different from that for ALIF because of these anatomic limitations. Surgeons must be familiar with these limitations and choose a proper device to avoid serious complications.

Complications of PLIF

PLIF has a steep learning curve and it carries the risk of various complications (34–41). Most complications during PLIF are related to inadequate exposure, excessive epidural bleeding, and poor understanding of anatomic and biomechanical principles of the procedure.

Excessive epidural bleeding can be a problem during the PLIF procedure. This may cause not only an excessive amount of blood loss but also poor visualization of the surgical field leading to dural tear or neural injury. Adequate bleeding control with a dry surgical field must be obtained before mobilization of neural elements and work within the disc space.

The incidence of neuropraxia is reported in the range of 1.5% to 4% (34,41). Okuyama et al. reported a high rate (8%) of neuropraxia, but all had transient neuropraxia with no permanent neural palsy (40). This is primarily due to excessive and prolonged retraction of the nerve root. To avoid this complication, one must have constant visualization and adequate mobilization of the dura and nerve roots, and must avoid prolonged retraction of neural elements. When PLIF procedure is performed on a patient who had previous posterior disc surgery with perineural scar, one must pay extra attention to mobilize the neural elements and release them more frequently from retraction. The incidence of dural laceration is reported in 1.5% (34). This is primarily due to poor visualization of the dura either by an inadequate size of exposure or by excessive bleeding. Over-sized bone graft or interbody fusion device is another cause for dural laceration during insertion.

The incidence of bone graft migration into the spinal canal is reported in the range of 0.3% to 2.4% (34,35, 41). The common causes for this complication are misfit of bone graft or interbody fusion device in the disc space or an unstable fusion construct. Proper preparation of the vertebral end plates and adequate size of bone graft are essential for a stable fusion construct. When posterior spinal structures are removed during the PLIF procedure, especially the facet joints, the fusion construct must be adequately stabilized with a rigid internal fixation system.

Excessive epidural fibrosis has been blamed to be a cause of failed PLIF procedure, although it has not been proven by any credible study. Excessive epidural bleeding and rough handling of the neural elements during the procedure may result in excessive scarring that may adversely affect the outcome. Adequate control of epidural bleeding, as described earlier, will minimize any significant epidural fibrosis.

REFERENCES

1. Kirkaldy-Willis WH, Wedge JH, Yong-Hing K, et al. Pathology and pathogenesis of lumbar spondylosis and stenosis. Spine 1978;3:319–328.
2. Davis H. Increasing rate of cervical and lumbar spine surgery in the United States, 1979–1990. Spine 1994;19:1117–1124.
3. Bono C, Lee CK. Critical analysis of trends in fusion for degenerative disc disease over the last twenty years. Spine (Feb 2004).
4. Fritzell P, Hagg O, Wessberg P, et al. Swedish lumbar spine study group: complications in lumbar fusion surgery for chronic low back pain: comparison of three surgical techniques used in a prospective randomized study. A report from the Swedish Lumbar Spine Study. Eur Spine J 2003;12(2):178–189.
5. Rhyne AL III, Smith SE, Wood KE, et al. Outcome of unoperated discogram positive low back pain. Spine 1995;20:1997–2000.
6. McCoy CE, Selby DK, Henderson R, et al. Patients avoiding surgery: pathology and one year life status follow-up. Spine 1991;16S:198–200.
7. Lee CK, Vessa P, Lee JK. Chronic disabling low back pain syndrome caused by internal disc derangements. The results of disc excision and posterior lumbar interbody fusion. Spine 1995;20:356–361.
8. Lee CK, Langrana NA. Lumbar spinal fusion: a biomechanical study. Spine 1984;9:574–581.
9. Rolander SD. Motion of the spine with special reference to stabilizing effect of posterior fusion. Acta Orthop Scand Suppl 1966;90:1–144.
10. Weatherby CR, Pricket CP, O'Brien JP. Discogenic pain persisting despite solid posterior fusion. J Bone Joint Surg 1986;68B:142–143.
11. Barrick WT, Schorfferman JA, Reynolds JB. et al. Anterior lumbar fusion improves discogenic pain at levels of prior posterolateral fusion. Spine 2000;25:853–857.
12. Lee CK, Kopacz K. Discogenic pain and instability. In: Fardon, DF, Garfin, SR, Abitbol, JJ, et al., eds. Orthopaedic knowledge update. Spine 2. Rosemont, IL: American Academy of Orthopaedic Surgeons, 2002:333–342.
13. Kumar MN, Baklanov A, Chopin D. Correlation between sagittal plane changes and adjacent segment degeneration following lumbar spine fusion. Eur Spine 2002;10:314–319.
14. Lee CK, Thacker I. Surgeons factor. Paper presented at: Annual Meeting of the American Academy of Orthopaedic Surgeons; February 1995; Orlando, FL.
15. Lin PM. A technical modification of Cloward's posterior lumbar interbody fusion. Neurosurgery 1977;1:118–124.
16. Lin PM, Cautilli RA, Joyce MF. Posterior lumbar interbody fusion. Clin Orthop 1983;180:154–168.
17. Cloward RB. The treatment of ruptured lumbar intervertebral disc by interbody fusion. Indications, operative technique, aftercare. J Neurosurg 1953;10:154–168.
18. Cloward RB. Lesions of intervertebral disc and their treatment by interbody fusion methods. The painful disc. Clin Orthop 1963;27:51–77.
19. Cloward RB. Posterior lumbar interbody fusion updated. Clin Orthop 1985;193:16.
20. Hollowell JP, Wellner DG, Wilson CR, et al. Biomechanical analysis of thoracolumbar interbody fusion constructs. How important is the endplates? Spine 1996;21:1032–1036.
21. Closky RF, Parsons JR, Lee CK, et al. Mechanics of interbody fusion: analysis of critical bone graft area. Spine 1993;18:1011–1105.
22. Barnes B, Rodts GE, McLaughlin MR, et al. Threaded cortical bone dowels of lumbar interbody fusion: over 1 year mean follow up in 28 patients. J Neurosurg 2001;95[1 Suppl]:1–4.
23. Brantigan JW, Steffee AD. A carbon fiber implant to aid interbody lumbar fusion. Two-year clinical results in the first 26 patients. Spine 1993;18:2106–2107.
24. Brantigan JW, Steffee AD, Lewis ML, et al. Lumbar interbody fusion using the Brantigan I/F cage for posterior lumbar interbody fusion and the variable pedicle screw placement system: two-year results from a Food and Drug Administration investigational device exemption clinical trial. Spine 2000;25:1437–1446.
25. Csecsei GI, Klekner AP, Dobai J, et al. Posterior interbody fusion using laminectomy bone and transpedicular screw fixation in the treatment of lumbar spondylolisthesis. Surg Neurol 2000;53:2–6.
26. Hashimoto T, Shigenobu K, Kanayama M, et al. Clinical results of single level posterior lumbar interbody fusion using the Brantigan I/F carbon cage filled with a mixture of local morselized bone and bioactive ceramic granules. Spine 2002;27:258–262.
27. Kuslich SD, Ulstrom CL, Griffith SL, et al. The Bagby and Kuslich method of lumbar interbody fusion. History, techniques, and 2-year follow-up results of a United States prospective, multicenter trial. Spine 1998;23:1267–1278.
28. Ido K, Asada Y, Sakamoto T, et al. Use of an autologous cortical bone graft sandwiched between two intervertebral spacers in posterior lumbar interbody fusion. Neurosurg Rev 2001;24:119–122.
29. Ray CD. Threaded titanium cages for lumbar interbody fusions. Spine 1997;22:667–679.
30. Simmons JW. Posterior lumbar interbody fusion with posterior elements as chip grafts. Clin Orthop 1985;193:85–89.
31. Steffee AD, Sitkowski DJ. Posterior lumbar interbody fusion and plates. Clin Orthop 1988;227:99–102.
32. Hai Y, Kopacz K, Lee CK. Posterior lumbar interbody fusion with and without pedicle screw fixation. A comparison study for bone graft subsidence. Paper presented at: 12th Annual Meeting of the North American Spine Society; October 1997; New York.
33. Wong HK, Goh JC, Goh PS. Paired cylindrical interbody cage fit and facetectomy in posterior lumbar interbody fusion in an Asian population. Spine 2001;26:567–571.
34. Ma GWC. Posterior lumbar interbody fusion with specialized instruments. In: Lin PM, Gill K, eds. Lumbar interbody fusion. Rockville, MD: Aspen, 1989:243–249.
35. Lin PM. Techniques and complications of posterior lumbar interbody fusion. In: Lin PM, Gill K, eds. Lumbar interbody fusion. Rockville, MD: Aspen, 1989:171–199.
36. Lin PM. Posterior lumbar interbody fusion technique: complications and pitfalls. Clin Orthop 1985;193:90–102.
37. Uzi EA, Dabby D, Tolessa E, et al. Early retropulsion of titanium-threaded cages after posterior lumbar interbody fusion: report of two cases. Spine 2001;26:1073–1075.
38. Janssen ME, Lam C, Beckham R. Outcomes of allogenic cages in anterior and posterior lumbar interbody fusion. Eur Spine J 2001;10[Suppl 2]:S158–S168.
39. Elias WJ, Simmons NE, Kaptain GJ, et al. Complications of posterior lumbar interbody fusion when using a titanium threaded cage device. J Neurosurg 2000;93:45–52.
40. Okuyama K, Abe E, Suzuki T, et al. Posterior lumbar interbody fusion: a retrospective study of complications after facet joint excision and pedicle screw fixation in 148 cases. Acta Orthop Scand 1999;70:329–334.
41. Collis JS. The technique of total disc replacement: a modified posterior lumbar interbody fusion. In: Lin PM, Gill K, eds. Lumbar interbody fusion. Rockville, MD: Aspen, 1989:221–226.

CHAPTER 33

Operative Treatment of Anterior Procedures

Kambiz Hannani and Rick Delamarter

Low back pain has been a significant cause of disability. Disc pathology, such as degenerative disc disease and instability, is believed to contribute to chronic low back pain. Anterior lumbar interbody fusion (ALIF) addresses this issue by removal of the disc and stabilization of the vertebrae via bone graft or substitutes, including autograft or allograft bone or bone morphogenic protein. In the past 5 years, cages have been introduced in addition to bone grafting to improve anatomic alignment and provide stability. More recently, artificial disc replacement has been investigated for the anterior treatment of degenerative disc disease.

Axial pain caused by degenerative disc disease continues to be the main indication for stand alone ALIF. Multiple studies have demonstrated the presence of nociceptors in the anulus of the disc. The innervation of the disc is found to increase in discogenic disease (1). Therefore, the removal of the pain generator (disc) is a logical approach to improve patients' symptoms.

Determining which patients with low back discomfort have discogenic pain is challenging. Multiple factors, including the patient's signs and symptoms, radiographic findings, and provocative tests need to be combined to make an accurate diagnosis and treatment plan. Patients with discogenic disease tend to complain mainly of low back pain with minimal leg radicular symptoms. The pain usually worsens with flexion and on the return to the erect posture.

Radiographic findings may be subtle on X-ray films. Degenerative disc disease (DDD) can be identified radiographically by a decrease in disc space height and the presence of osteophytes. Magnetic resonance imaging (MRI) is helpful in identifying DDD. Magnetic resonance imaging findings of DDD include decreased signal of the disc on the T2-weighted images. A high-intensity zone (HIZ) may be identified, which is thought by some to be associated with positive discography and annular tears. Discography, although controversial, is helpful in identifying symptomatic DDD. Concordant pain during discography may respond to surgical fusion (2).

Multiple surgical options are available for the surgical treatment of symptomatic DDD. Anterior lumbar interbody fusion alone, combined ALIF and posterior fusion with instrumentation, posterior fusion alone or combined with posterior lumbar interbody fusion (PLIF) are all potential options available to the surgeon. Although many patients having fusion do well, the removal of the disc appears to improve the surgical outcome for DDD (3–6). The two approaches that allow for removal of the disc are ALIF and PLIF.

Cloward first reported on posterior interbody fusion in 1943 (7). In 1956, he described an anterior cervical interbody fusion (8). However, anterior lumbar interbody fusion was first reported by Paul Harmon in 1963, and Crock described a bilateral Dowel technique in 1982 (9,10). Although multiple options are available for the surgical treatment of DDD, ALIF has many advantages compared to other procedures. In contrast to posterolateral intertransverse fusions (PLIF), ALIF restores the disk height thereby allowing decompression of neuroforaminal stenosis. Anterior column support favors load transmission and places the bone graft volume under compression. Finally, ALIF removes the disc, which may be the painful structure (11). Compared to PLIF, ALIF affords a more complete discectomy and avoids dissection of the posterior paraspinal muscles. The operative time is significantly less with ALIF compared to PLIF, and it can be performed using minimally invasive procedures (11).

Allograft or autograft can be used for ALIF procedures. Historically, autograft has been the gold standard with excellent incorporation and high fusion rates. Good clinical outcomes with ALIF autograft have been reported. Penta reviewed 125 patients who underwent ALIF with iliac crest bone graft (ICBG) over a 10-year period (12). Sixty-eight percent of the patients were satisfied. The overall fusion rate was 72.4%, and varied from 91% for single level fusions to 51% for multilevel fusions. However, one drawback of ICBG is the risk of graft subsidence and collapse, which is less common with allograft struts (13,14). Furthermore, the iliac crest donor site is a significant source of morbidity.

Allograft bone has also been used as a stand-alone device with ALIF. Kozak reported excellent results with a combination of cortical and cancellous allograft with 97% fusion rate at 1-year follow-up. Recently, however, unfavorable results with this procedure were reported by Dawson et al. (15). Seven of 16 patients in that study

developed a pseudarthrosis that required posterior fusion. Additionally, all patients showed subsidence of their grafts within the first year, with the pseudarthrosis group having a threefold increase in subsidence compared to the fused group (Fig. 33-1).

The fusion rate increases when ALIF using autograft is combined with posterior instrumentation (16,17). Sarwat reviewed 43 patients undergoing combined antero-posterior fusions using femoral allograft rings packed with

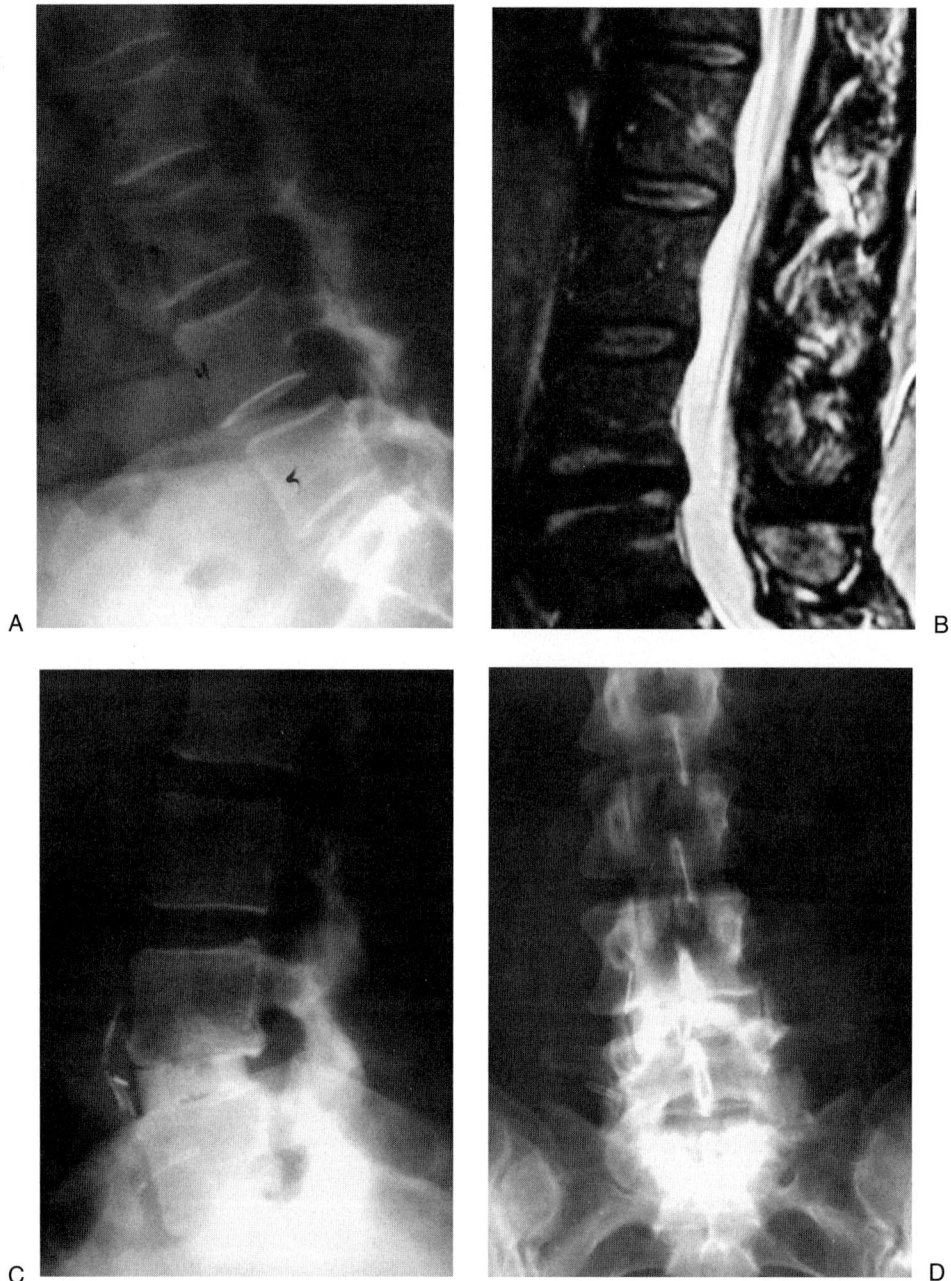

FIG. 33-1. A: Lateral X-ray of a lumbar spine illustrating instability and grade I spondylolisthesis at L4-5 with moderate disc space loss and degenerative disc disease at L5-S1 interspace. B: T2 sagittal magnetic resonance image confirming the degenerative disc disease at the lower two levels with decrease T2 signal and end plate changes at L4-5. C: Lateral X-ray of the lumbar spine following anterior lumbar interbody fusion using femoral ring allografts at the L4-5 and L5-S1 interspaces; the disc spaces have been restored with anatomic reduction of the spondylolisthesis at L4-5. D: Antero-posterior X-ray following anterior lumbar interbody fusion.

cancellous allograft with supplemental posterior stabilization (17). One hundred percent of the one level and 93% of the two level fusion were solid radiographically on follow-up. Allograft bone provided improved compressive strength but required more time for incorporation compared to autograft bone (18). At our institution, stand alone allograft ALIFs are not performed without supplemental posterior instrumentation.

Within the past decade, cages have been popularized for performing ALIF. Cages were initially introduced by Bagby for the treatment of wobbler's disease in horses in 1977. Multiple modifications of the original cage design have been made since 1988. The BAK cage, Ray Cage, and Interfix Device are all cylindrical cages that are packed with bone graft. Two cylindrical cages are inserted in the interspace and give excellent overall stability (Fig. 33-2).

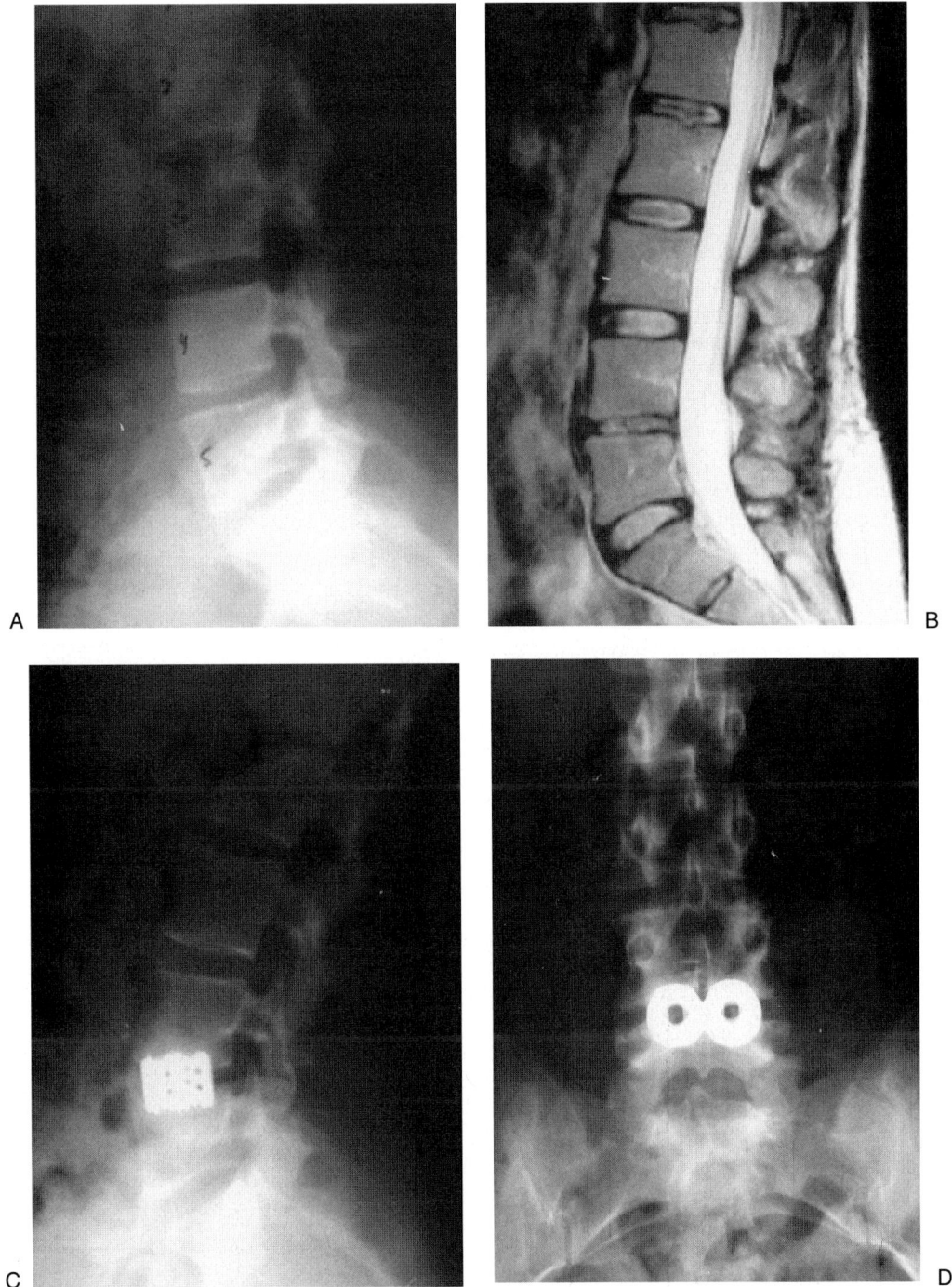

FIG. 33-2. A: Lateral X-ray of the lumbar spine illustrating a disc space narrowing at L4-5. **B:** Sagittal T2-weighted magnetic resonance image of the same patient showing decreased height and disc hydration consistent with degenerative disc disease. **C:** Lateral X-ray findings after a anterior interbody fusion using two cylindrical cages. **D:** Antero-posterior view of the cage construct seen in **C.**

Tapered threaded devices are also available and have the theoretical advantage of improved lordosis and anatomic alignment.

Cages have been shown to increase the stability of ALIF. In reviewing five types of cages, Tsantrizos concluded that cages decreased the range of motion at the interspace by an average of 63% in flexion and extension, 69% in lateral bending, and 23% in axial rotation (11). Cages have other advantages compared to other fusion methods. In a sheep study by Sandhu et al., a lower subsidence rate was shown with cages compared to autograft alone (19). Compared to PLF, ALIF using cages increases the axial stiffness of the interspace by 80% (compared to 40% seen in PLF). Moreover, higher nonunion rates have been reported with the PLF compared with ALIF (11). The increased stability is likely a function of increased disc space distraction seen with cage placement versus bone grafting alone.

The design of the cage also contributes to its stability. Cages with sharp teeth were found to exhibit higher pullout forces (20,21). Flexible cages constructed with carbon fiber reduce stress shielding of the bone graft. Stiffer cage constructs transmit less stress to the bone graft and the stress shielding effect of stiff cages may have a deleterious effect on bone graft incorporation (Fig. 33-3) (22).

The results of interbody fusion with cages have been reported in two Food and Drug Administration studies. Anterior lumbar interbody fusion was evaluated by Kuslich using the bar cage in 1998. Nine hundred forty-seven patients underwent ALIF using the BAK cage in that multicenter study. Bony fusion was noted in 86% of patients at 12 months, 91% at 24 months, and 98% at 3 years after surgery. More than 85% of the patients reported pain reduction and 91% had improved function by 24 months postsurgery. Seventy-eight percent of the employable patients were working at 24 months and 91% at 3 years after surgery (5). In 1997, Ray reported on 236 undergoing PLIF using the Ray cage. In this prospective study, functional improvement was excellent in 40%, good in 21%, fair in 21%, and poor in 14% of the subjects. The complication rate was less than 1%.

Kleeman reported on the use of bone morphogenetic protein (BMP) in laparoscopic ALIF. Using computed tomography and X-ray evaluation at 6 and 12 months postoperatively, he found that 100% of 22 patients were fused (23). Furthermore, all of the subjects were satisfied with the treatment at 12 months with relief of back pain and improved leg symptoms.

Currently, artificial disc replacement (ADR) is being evaluated for the treatment of lumbar DDD. Preliminary results in the United States and long-term results from Europe are encouraging. The advantage of ADR is that it allows motion at the involved level compared to fusion surgery and decreases stress on adjacent level with a hypothetical decrease in future adjacent level disease. One artificial disc is composed of cobalt-chrome alloy end plate elements, and an ultra–high molecular weight polyethylene inlay element. The disc functions based on the ball-and-socket joint principle (Fig. 33-4).

Multiple variations of the anterior approach are available for ALIF, including mini-open, endoscopic assisted,

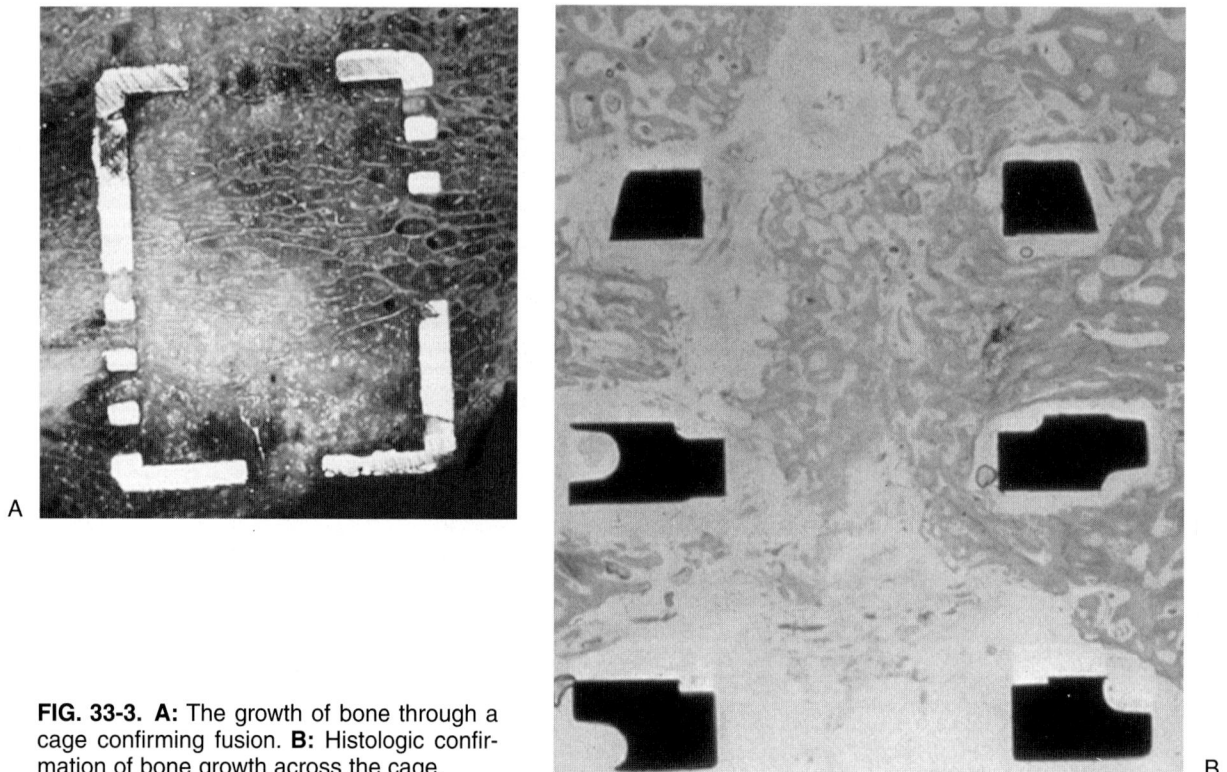

FIG. 33-3. A: The growth of bone through a cage confirming fusion. B: Histologic confirmation of bone growth across the cage.

A,B

C,D   E

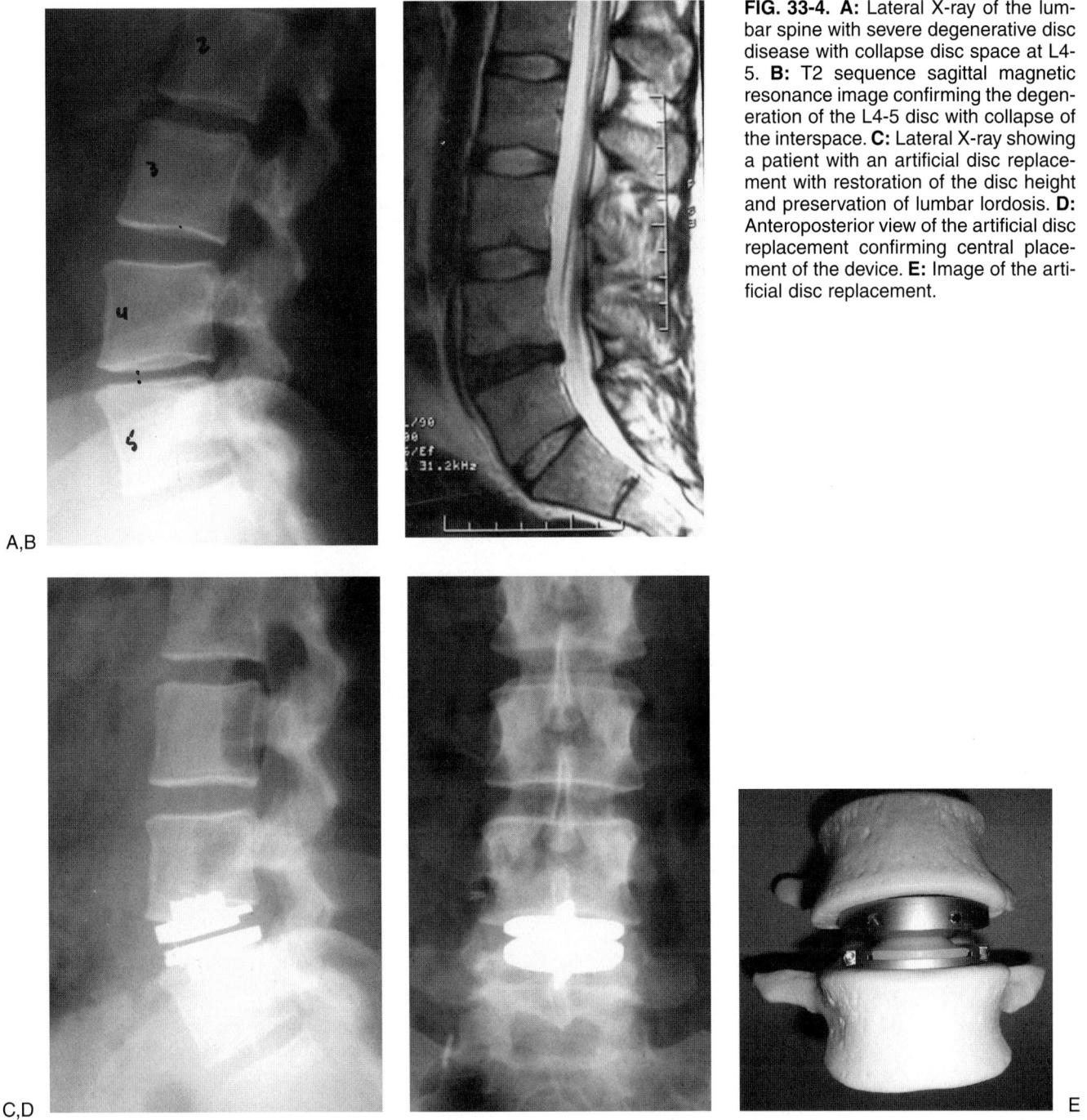

FIG. 33-4. A: Lateral X-ray of the lumbar spine with severe degenerative disc disease with collapse disc space at L4-5. **B:** T2 sequence sagittal magnetic resonance image confirming the degeneration of the L4-5 disc with collapse of the interspace. **C:** Lateral X-ray showing a patient with an artificial disc replacement with restoration of the disc height and preservation of lumbar lordosis. **D:** Anteroposterior view of the artificial disc replacement confirming central placement of the device. **E:** Image of the artificial disc replacement.

or microsurgically assisted (24–26). The most common surgical method is the retroperitoneal lumbar approach for anterior discectomy with interbody fusion. The retroperitoneal or transperitoneal approach can be used with minimal morbidity from extensive dissection of muscle, as seen with posterior procedures.

Multiple investigators have reported good results with laparoscopic ALIF (23,27). Regan compared laparoscopic with open ALIF with the BAK cage in a multicenter study (28). The laparoscopy group had a shorter hospital stay and reduced blood loss but increase operative time. Ten percent of the cases needed

to be converted to an open procedure. However, complication rates were comparable between open and laparoscopic procedure.

The laparoscopic approach at L4-5 interval is more challenging than at the L5-S1 level. Zdeblick compared the mini-open and laparoscopic approach in 50 consecutive patients undergoing ALIF at L4-5. He found that the rate of complications was significantly higher with the laparoscopic procedure (20% versus 4%). The operative time was 25 minutes longer for the laparoscopic group; furthermore, 16% of the laparoscopic group had inadequate exposure for the placement of two cages.

The anterior retroperitoneal approach can be complicated by venous injury requiring repair as well as development of subsequent thrombosis. Arterial occlusion of the internal iliac artery has also been reported (29). Patients that present with ongoing leg pain and weakness in a nondermatomal distribution following ALIF should be evaluated for iliac vessel thrombosis (30).

Complications are associated with the ALIF procedures. Bone graft collapse or extrusion and cage malposition or migration can result in poor alignment and pseudoarthrosis. Iliac crest bone graft donor site morbidity has been reported in up to 30% of patients that may last for years (11,16). Moreover, allograft bone has the potential for disease transmission and immunologic reaction. The risk of HIV infection, for example, has been estimated at less than 1/1,000,000 in properly screened donors (31).

Retrograde ejaculation results form injury to the superior hypogastric plexus. This plexus is responsible for bladder neck closure during ejaculation. Retrograde ejaculation has been reported in as many as 8% of patients with ALIF (32). In a review of 4,500 patients, 0.42% of patients experienced retrograde ejaculation (33). Regan found an incidence of retrograde ejaculation in 2.3% of his open versus 5.1% of his laparoscopic ALIF cases. Fifty percent of the patients had resolution of their symptoms at follow-up. Other rare complications reported in ALIF include pituitary apoplexy, urethral injury, and pancreatitis (29,34,35).

In summary, the disc may be a significant cause of chronic low back pain in degenerative disc disease. One surgical option for DDD is anterior lumbar interbody fusion using bone graft or substitutes with or without cage instrumentation. The anterior approach has multiple advantages over posterior procedures, including the avoidance of muscle dissection, excellent restoration of the disc space height and neuroforaminal decompression, and improved biomechanics. New technologies, such as BMP and ADR, have decreased the risk of iliac crest graft site morbidity and adjacent level disease.

REFERENCES

1. Freemont AJ, Peacock TE, Goupille P, et al. Nerve ingrowth into diseased intervertebral disc in chronic back pain. Lancet 1997;350(9072): 178–181.
2. Colhoun E, McCall IW, Williams L, et al. Provocation discography as a guide to planning operations on the spine. J Bone Joint Surg (Britain) 1988;70(2):267–271.
3. Turner JA, Ersek M, Herron L, et al. Patient outcomes after lumbar spinal fusions. JAMA 1992;268(7):907–911.
4. Barrick WT, Schofferman JA, Reynolds JB, et al. Anterior lumbar fusion improves discogenic pain at levels of prior posterolateral fusion. Spine 2000;25(7):853–857.
5. Kuslich SD, Ulstrom CL, Griffith SL, et al. The Bagby and Kuslich method of lumbar interbody fusion. History, techniques, and 2-year follow-up results of a United States prospective, multicenter trial. Spine 1998;23(11):1267–1278; discussion 1279.
6. Vamvanij V, Fredrickson BE, Thorpe JM, et al. Surgical treatment of internal disc disruption: an outcome study of four fusion techniques. J Spinal Disord 1998;11(5):375–382.
7. Cloward RB. Spondylolisthesis: treatment by laminectomy and posterior interbody fusion. Clin Orthop 1981;(154):74–82.
8. Cloward RB. Lesions of the intervertebral discs and their treatment by interbody fusion methods. The painful disc. Clin Orthop 1963;27(51).
9. Harmon PH. Anterior excision and vertebral body fusion operation for intervertebral disc syndromes of the lower lumbar spine. Clin Orthop Rel Res 1963;107–127.
10. Crock HV. Anterior lumbar interbody fusion: indications for its use and notes on surgical technique. Clin Orthop 1982;(165):157–163.
11. Tsantrizos A, Andreou A, Aebi M, et al. Biomechanical stability of five stand-alone anterior lumbar interbody fusion constructs. Eur Spine J 2000;9(1):14–22.
12. Penta M, Fraser RD. Anterior lumbar interbody fusion. A minimum 10-year follow-up. Spine 1997;22(20):2429–2434.
13. Soini J. Lumbar disc space heights after external fixation and anterior interbody fusion: a prospective 2-year follow-up of clinical and radiographic results. J Spinal Disord 1994;7(6):487–494.
14. Kumar A, Kozak JA, Doherty BJ, et al. Interspace distraction and graft subsidence after anterior lumbar fusion with femoral strut allograft. Spine 1993;18(16):2393–2400.
15. Patel S, Timon S, Dawson EG, et al. Anterior lumbar discectomy and fusion using femoral ring allografts. Presented at the American Academy of Orthopaedic Surgeons annual meeting. February 13–17, 2002. Dallas, TX, 2002.
16. Wimmer C, Krismer M, Gluch H, et al. Autogenic versus allogenic bone grafts in anterior lumbar interbody fusion. Clin Orthop 1999; (360):122–126.
17. Sarwat AM, O'Brien JP, Renton P, et al. The use of allograft (and avoidance of autograft) in anterior lumbar interbody fusion: a critical analysis. Eur Spine J 2001;10(3):237–2341.
18. Aaron AD, Wiedel JD. Allograft use in orthopedic surgery. Orthopedics 1994;17(1):41–48.
19. Sandhu HS, Turner S, Kabo JM, et al. Distractive properties of a threaded interbody fusion device. An in vivo model. Spine 1996;21 (10):1201–1210.
20. Lund T, Oxland TR, Jost B, et al. Interbody cage stabilisation in the lumbar spine: biomechanical evaluation of cage design, posterior instrumentation and bone density. J Bone Joint Surg Br 1998;80 (2):351–359.
21. Pilliar RM, Lee JM, Maniatopoulos C. Observations on the effect of movement on bone ingrowth into porous-surfaced implants. Clin Orthop 1986;(208):108–113.
22. Martz EO, Goel VK, Pope MH, et al. Materials and design of spinal implants—a review. J Biomed Mater Res 1997;38(3):267–288.
23. Kleeman TJ, Ahn UM, Talbot-Kleeman A. Laparoscopic anterior lumbar interbody fusion with rhBMP-2: a prospective study of clinical and radiographic outcomes. Spine 2001;26(24):2751–2756.
24. Boos N, Kalberer F, Schoeb O. Retroperitoneal endoscopically assisted minilaparotomy for anterior lumbar interbody fusion: technical feasibility and complications. Spine 2001;26(2):E1–E6.
25. Mayer HM. A new microsurgical technique for minimally invasive anterior lumbar interbody fusion. Spine 1997;22(6):691–699; discussion 700.
26. Zdeblick TA, David SM. A prospective comparison of surgical approach for anterior L4-L5 fusion: laparoscopic versus mini anterior lumbar interbody fusion. Spine 2000;25(20):2682–2687.
27. Lieberman IH, Willsher PC, Litwin DE, et al. Transperitoneal laparoscopic exposure for lumbar interbody fusion. Spine 2000;25(4): 509–514; discussion 515.
28. Regan JJ, Yuan H, McAfee PC. Laparoscopic fusion of the lumbar spine: minimally invasive spine surgery. A prospective multicenter study evaluating open and laparoscopic lumbar fusion. Spine 1999;24 (4):402–411.
29. Rajaraman V, Vingan R, Roth P, et al. Visceral and vascular complications resulting from anterior lumbar interbody fusion. J Neurosurg 1999;91(1 suppl):60–64.
30. Hackenberg L, Liljenqvist U, Halm H, et al. Occlusion of the left common iliac artery and consecutive thromboembolism of the left popliteal artery following anterior lumbar interbody fusion. J Spinal Disord 2001;14(4):365–368.
31. Buck BE, Malinin TI, Brown MD. Bone transplantation and human

immunodeficiency virus. An estimate of risk of acquired immunodeficiency syndrome (AIDS). Clin Orthop 1989;(240):129–136.

32. Christensen FB, Bunger CE. Retrograde ejaculation after retroperitoneal lower lumbar interbody fusion. Int Orthop 1997;21(3):176–180.

33. Flynn JC, Price CT. Sexual complications of anterior fusion of the lumbar spine. Spine 1984;9(5):489–492.

34. Liu JK, Nwagwu C, Pikus HJ, et al. Laparoscopic anterior lumbar interbody fusion precipitating pituitary apoplexy. Acta Neurochir (Wien) 2001;143(3):303–306; discussion 306–307.

35. Isiklar ZU, Lindsey RW, Coburn M. Ureteral injury after anterior lumbar interbody fusion. A case report. Spine 1996;21(20):2379–2382.

CHAPTER 34

Operative Treatment of Anterior and Posterior Fusion

Björn Strömqvist

PROS AND CONS

Although everybody dealing with lumbar spine fusion is aware that selection of the right patient is more important than selection of the surgical technique, this should not keep us from optimizing the technical aspects of the procedures and identifying the most appropriate procedure in each case. In spite of the fact that many patients with degenerative disc disease (DDD) experience the so-called "instability catch" (1), the lumbar spine with disc degenerative changes is inherently stable. Hypermobility has not been demonstrated except in isthmic spondylolisthesis (2) and radiostereometric analysis (RSA) has recently shown that patients with DDD have decreased segmental mobility (Axelsson et al., personal communication). Thus, the basic attitude toward fusion of DDD should be to select the least possible invasive procedure with the least morbidity that will address the underlying pathology. Recent randomized controlled trials have not been able to demonstrate instrumentation to improve the outcome of lumbar spine fusion (3,4). In the Swedish National Lumbar Spine Study, posterolateral uninstrumented fusion seemed to fare equivalently to posterior instrumented or 360° (anterior and posterior) fusion (5). The fact that his and other prospective randomized studies show posterolateral uninstrumented fusion to give results equal to combined techniques, however, does not mean that posterolateral fusion is the preferred operation in every case. Patients undergoing lumbar spine fusion are very heterogeneous in regard to indications, demographics, personality traits, and anatomic aspects (6); individual considerations may have to be made.

INDICATIONS

Combined anterior and posterior fusion may be considered under the following circumstances:

1. Facetectomy. If concomitant facetectomy is performed bilaterally or unilaterally, an unstable situation is present and the ability to obtain a facet fusion is lost (7,8).
2. Inability to cope with postoperative regimen. In patients who cannot tolerate postoperative orthotic treatment and spine immobilization, a combined procedure may be indicated to resist the loading forces on the stabilized segment and therefore reduce the risk for nonunion or implant failure. This also may apply to patients with high performance demands.
3. Revision surgery. Patients with unsuccessful prior surgery for degenerative lumbar spine disorders are given the diagnostic label failed back surgery syndrome. Some studies report good results with combined anterior and posterior fusion in such cases (9,10), although no randomized studies exist.
4. Other metabolic or anatomic variants (e.g., osteopenia, insufficient bone surfaces for bony fusion, and deficiency disorders) may indicate the need for a combined antero-posterior fusion.

SPINAL STABILIZATION

Comparing anterior, posterolateral, and posterior fusion, Lee and Langrana (11) in a biomechanical study concluded that the posterolateral fusion technique was the best method of providing stabilization to the fused segment and having the least effect on the adjacent unfused segment. The combined anterior and posterior fusion provides better stabilization from a biomechanical point of view, but whether or not this has any relationship to future adjacent segment problems is not known (12,13). Using the RSA technique to study *in vivo* kinematics (14), it has been possible to demonstrate a slow healing rate of uninstrumented posterolateral fusion,

338

which becomes stable between 6 and 12 months after surgery. With the addition of posterior transpedicular instrumentation, immediate stability is obtained (15). Stand-alone interbody cages demonstrate an intermediate time required for segmental stabilization (16). This fact may be interpreted as obviating the need for routine use of combined procedures in the inherently stable degenerative lumbar spine. Although increased surgery time and more blood loss occur (5,17), many nonrandomized studies, however, report very good outcomes with combined fusions. When combined fusions are considered, one prerequisite is that they should be performed by spine surgeons very familiar with the technique in order to minimize the complication rate. The risk of retrograde ejaculation and for sympathetic trunk disturbance, for example, is solely associated with anterior surgery and may be minimized by limiting the procedure to surgeons experienced with anterior procedures.

A major issue in surgery for axial pain is determining the location of the pain generator. The spine, being a three-joint complex, can have pain from the disc as well as facet joint–related pain. This has been one argument for including vertebral body fusion because some micromotion may remain over the disc even in the presence of a solid posterolateral fusion (18,19). In some instances, this micromotion produces pain.

SURGICAL OPTIONS

Posterior Fusion plus Anterior Lumbar Interbody Fusion

This procedure requires posterior fusion and instrumentation, either from the midline approach or via the Wiltse approach between the longissimus and multifidus muscles (Fig. 34-1). Anterior disc replacement is performed via the transperitoneal or retroperitoneal approach (20). These approaches have been described previously. If

compression of the interbody implant is desired, anterior disc resection and implant insertion must be done before posterior compression is applied to the anterior implant. This is a complex procedure, but provides the most pronounced stability to the segment immobilized. Posterior transpedicular fixation techniques with rods or plates are used, and are usually combined with bone harvesting from the iliac crest. Anterior cortical bone grafts in the form of either autografts or allografts may be used or metal cages or other types of metal implants (usually titanium) (Fig. 34-2). These implants are presented elsewhere in this and other chapters. Immediate mobilization and early rehabilitation without orthosis usually is permitted.

Posterior Lumbar Interbody Fusion

This procedure is described elsewhere in this text (Chapter 32), and is essentially a combined anterior and posterior procedure performed via a posterior approach (21). Typically, transpedicular instrumentation is used, and the cages are inserted in the axilla between the common dural sac and the exiting nerve root. This may necessitate some traction on the nerve root and also may be associated with troublesome venous plexus bleeding; therefore, this procedure requires experience with the technique. Compression of the interbody graft is achieved by the posterior construct.

Transforaminal Lumbar Interbody Fusion

Transforaminal lumbar interbody fusion (TLIF), or monoportal posterolateral intertransverse fusions (PLIF), has been described by Harms and Tabasso (22). This is an operation performed posteriorly. One of the facet joints is resected, the disc is removed, and intercorporeal implants are filled with cancellous bone and are inserted. Posteriorly transpedicular instrumentation is used and compres-

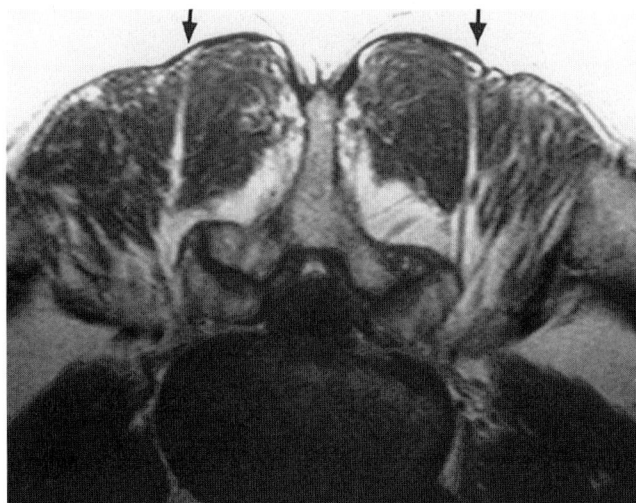

FIG. 34-1. Axial image of the lumbar spine showing (arrows) the Wiltse approach giving good access to pedicles and transverse processes when performing posterolateral fusion with and without instrumentation. The cleavage plane is between the longissimus and multifidus muscles.

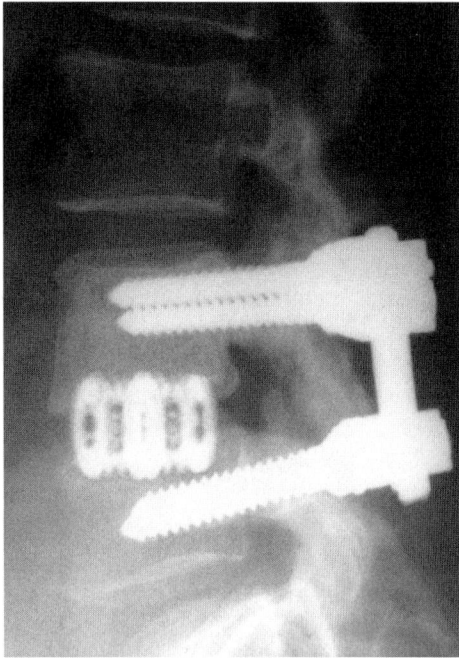

FIG. 34-2. Lateral radiograph after combined fusion using rods, pedicle screws, and autograft posteriorly and cages anteriorly.

sion is applied as with a PLIF. This approach provides access to the disc lateral to the nerve root, gives a wider access to the disc, and can reduce traction to the nerve root at the disc level.

A possible disadvantage of TLIF compared with PLIF is that one entire facet joint must be resected, although significant parts of both facet joints usually are resected

with PLIF. Threaded cages are less suitable for the TLIF procedure and smaller cages are used instead, for example, two Harms cages, which are inserted from the facet joint resection side; the first cage is moved to the contralateral side and the second is retained on the ipsilateral side (Fig. 34-3). Posterior compression is performed by the transpedicular system as in the other two procedures. To date this technique is not so well documented in the literature but seems like an attractive alternative when combined procedures are considered.

CONCLUSION

This chapter briefly described techniques for performing combined anterior and posterior (360°) fusions of the lumbar spine and discussed the advantages and disadvantages of combined fusion procedures in DDD. Combined procedures require surgical skill in the technical aspects of the procedure in order to minimize complications. Their indication is limited in the inherently stable degenerative spine; for example, in patients where concomitant facetectomy must be performed or in patients unable to tolerate the postoperative immobilization. Some studies have shown very good results from combined anterior and posterior procedures, especially in the failed back surgery syndrome, but in randomized controlled trials superiority of the technique has not been proved. Although an increased complication rate has been reported, this technique may be indicated in selected cases when performed by spine surgeons familiar with the technique. Future prospective studies may help to determine the optimal fusion procedure, taking into account biomechanical, biological, and psychosocial

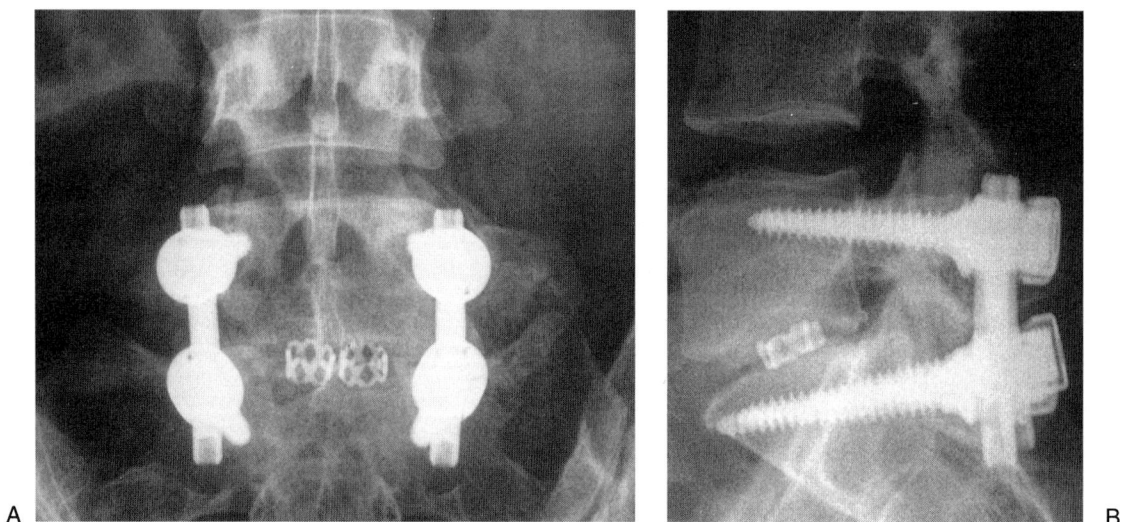

FIG. 34-3. Postoperative radiograph in patient operated on with a transforaminal lumbar interbody fusion technique. Posterior fixation is demonstrated with Diapason rod, screws, and autografting, interbody fusion with Harms cages, and autograft, both harvested from the posterior iliac crest. **A:** Anterior and posterior image. **B:** Lateral image.

clinical studies investigating the possible role of bone growth stimulators to enhance fusion with cages. However, in a study involving sheep implanted with titanium threaded fusion cages packed with autograft, bone growth stimulation was associated with a greater fusion rate (30). Other possible methods to enhance the fusion rate achieved with cages is the use of recombinant human bone morphogenetic protein-2 (rhBMP-2) (31–33), local gene therapy (34), and recombinant human osteogenic protein-1 (rhOP-1) (35). These materials have yielded high fusion rates in studies using animal models (31,35). In a small patient series, a 100% fusion rate was seen in a group of patients receiving BMP packed in tapered cylindrical cages (36). This material appear to be capable of achieving a high fusion rate and has the additional benefit of eliminating risk of complications and pain associated with harvesting iliac crest autograft. Larger series of patients are needed to determine if these promising early results can be maintained.

CLINICAL RESULTS

The clinical outcome achieved with fusion cages are difficult to evaluate due to inconsistency of the outcome measures used, use of nonstandardized and nonvalidated measurement tools, mix of diagnoses in the various studies, and different techniques and devices used within individual studies.

It should be noted that several of the large studies discussed in the following were performed as part of the approval process for sale of the devices in the United States. These studies have the benefits of enrolling a large number of patients, being closely monitored, and having a minimum of 2-year follow-up. However, such studies also tend to have some shortcomings that make it difficult to extrapolate the results to broader future applications. These include rigorous inclusion-exclusion criteria and their use by highly specialized and experienced surgeons recruited to participate in such studies.

Threaded Cylindrical Titanium Cages

In a large study of patients undergoing BAK cage fusion, Kuslich et al. reported a significant decrease in postoperative pain scores (22). However, only 32% of the group from which the preoperative scores were derived was included in the 24-month follow-up data. Four-year follow-up data on a subgroup of 185 patients has been reported (37). Pain and function were significantly improved at the 3-month follow-up compared to the preoperative values and did not deteriorate at 4-year follow-up. Work status improved from 44.1% preoperatively to 71.2% postoperatively. The results of this study have been criticized because some of the 17 patients who required additional surgery after the cage procedure were counted as having a good clinical outcome, and only 185 of the

original 947 patients enrolled in the original study were included in the analysis.

Results also have been reported on the 2-year follow-up of 226 of 236 patients who received the Ray threaded fusion cages (TFC) (26). Sixty-five percent of patients had good to excellent results and 65% had good to excellent function. Unfortunately, this study provided no data comparing the preoperative to postoperative function, so that conclusions concerning clinical improvement were not possible. Poor results were reported with the use of this cage in a series of only 13 patients, all operated at the L5-S1 level (38). Seven of the 13 patients went on to reoperation for symptomatic pseudarthrosis. The authors felt that the use of oversized cages, destruction of the anterior longitudinal ligament, and removal of part of the annulus contributed to the poor outcome.

Threaded Bone Dowels

Threaded bone dowels are similar in design to metal threaded fusion cages. Their potential benefit is that radiographic assessment is easier because of the lack of artifact created by cages. However, there are concerns about the consistency of the strength of these cages, which are made from allograft bone. Barnes et al reported 1-year follow-up on a series of 28 patients undergoing interbody fusion using threaded cortical bone dowels packed with autogenous iliac crest bone graft (39). Patients with disc-related pain alone underwent anterior interbody fusion, using the cages as stand-alone devices. In patients with concomitant spinal stenosis, decompression and posterior interbody fusion with supplemental posterior pedicle screws without bone graft was used. There was a relatively low rate of follow-up in the anterior interbody fusion group (67%). The rate of fusion was less in the anterior group than in the posterior group (13% versus 95%). Similarly, patient satisfaction was greater in the posterior group than in the anterior group (38% versus 70%). Based on their results, the authors strongly advocated the use of posterior fixation in addition with the threaded bone dowels.

There have been a few studies comparing the use of bone dowels to other fusion procedures. In one such study, laparoscopic anterior interbody fusion using threaded cortical bone dowels was compared to posterior fusion using pedicle screws (40). The laparoscopic group had shorter hospital stay, less blood loss, and less operative time than the posterior fusion group. However, it should be noted that the study was not randomized; therefore, there may have been differences in the patients treated with the two procedures. In a prospective randomized study, Schofferman et al. compared threaded titanium cylindrical cages packed with autograft to threaded bone dowel cages packed with demineralized bone matrix (41). At the 12-month follow-up, both groups improved significantly based on Oswestry and pain scores, and there were no significant differences in outcome between the two groups.

Carbon Fiber Cages

Carbon fiber cages are designed to be used in pairs and with posterior fixation. The carbon fiber allows for easier assessment of fusion status because this material is not visible on radiographic images and does not create artifact on CT scans. One disadvantage of carbon fiber cages is that they may fracture or collapse, which may result in release of some of the carbon fibers. Brantigan reported 2-year follow-up data for 221 patients receiving carbon fiber cages and pedicle screw fixation as part of a multicenter study (28). In the subgroup of 92 patients with a diagnosis of DDD, the fusion rate was 100% and 86% had a good clinical outcome; however, there were numerous complications in the series.

There have been other reports on the use of carbon fiber cages. One series included 71 patients with carbon fiber cages and posterior fixation (27). It reported a 90% fusion rate, but at the median follow-up of 28 months, only 66% of patients were satisfied with the results of the surgery and would have the procedure again for the same result. Two studies on the use of carbon fiber cages have reported fusion rates of 82% and 86%, but provided no clinical outcome data (29,42).

Mesh Cages

Mesh cages, also sometimes referred to as a type of vertical cage, can be cut to the height desired to fit into the disc space. The cages are packed with bone graft and inserted into the disc space. Reinforcement rings may be placed around the superior and inferior ends of the cage to provide axial support. There have been only a few reports on the clinical results of mesh cages, none of which deal specifically with disc-related pain. The patient population in these studies was typically a mixed group of patients with pseudoarthrosis, deformity, postlaminectomy syndrome, or disc-related pain. One study described the results of 50 patients undergoing combined antero-posterior lumbar fusion using mesh cages packed with coralline hydroxyapatite mixed with demineralized bone matrix (23). A buttress plate was placed anteriorly over the operated segment to prevent potential displacement of the cages. Pedicle screws or facet screws were used with the posterior fusion. The mean follow-up was 50 months, ranging from 36 to 64 months. The authors reported good results with the procedure, although there were several cases requiring posterior fixation removal.

One study evaluated the outcome following non-threaded cages (either Brantigan or Harms) for the treatment of single-level, disc-related pain was performed in a group of 15 active-duty servicemen (43). The cages were inserted posteriorly and packed with autogenous iliac

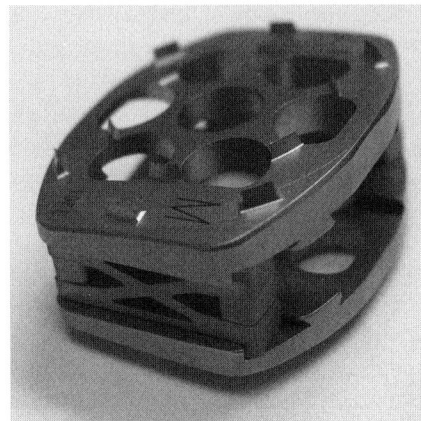

FIG. 35-2. Modular rectangular fusion cage.

crest graft and were supplemented with pedicle screw fusion. The authors reported that 12 of the 15 servicemen, 80%, returned to full duty. This compared favorably to the 36% who returned to active duty in a selected group who elected not to have surgery for their single-level symptomatic disc degeneration.

Modular Rectangular Cages

There is a rectangular, modular cage (InFix; Spinal Concepts, Austin, TX) (Fig. 35-2) designed to be used as a stand-alone device and to be implanted using an anterior approach to the spine. It consists of two plates with struts that are placed on the periphery of the plates to control the height and angulation between the plates, thereby allowing anatomic restoration of the disc height and lordosis. The plates have holes to allow bony ingrowth from the vertebral bodies to unite with the bone packed inside the cage. This device is being evaluated in a large, multicenter study, but currently no results from this study have been reported.

LAPAROSCOPIC LUMBAR INTERBODY FUSION

The introduction of fusion cages came at a time when laparoscopic spinal fusion was being developed. The cages complemented this evolving surgical technique. They were small enough to be passed through the cannulas used in the laparoscopic procedures. The role of laparoscopic spinal fusion has gained some acceptance but some still question if it reduces morbidity, reduces hospital stay, and reduces recovery time. The endoscopic technique has been criticized as having an increased complication rate, being too expensive, being too difficult to perform at the L4-5 level, and offering no benefit over open surgery.

Laparoscopic spine surgery requires developing new skills not typically learned by spine surgeons. They must manipulate the instruments based on what is viewed on a video monitor. Several authors have reported on the learning curve associated with laparoscopic spine surgery (44–46). In several reports, laparoscopic fusion is reported to have longer operating time but less blood loss than open anterior fusion (47,48). In both of these studies, laparoscopic surgery was also associated with reduced hospitalization time. There is debate concerning the effectiveness and safety of using endoscopic techniques to fuse the L4-5 level. Vraney reviewed radiographic vascular examinations performed for vascular conditions, and recorded the feasibility of accessing the L4-5 disc using laparoscopic techniques (49). He suggested that in only one-third of patients could the disc space be accessed safely because of the vascular anatomy. Zdeblick also expressed concern about the safety of accessing the L4-5 disc due to a greater incidence of complications (50). He advocated that laparoscopic fusion was feasible at L4-5 if the bifurcation of the vessels was above the L4-5 space and that an open approach should be used if the bifurcation was at or below the disc. Kathkouda et al. reported the feasibility of laparoscopic surgery at the L5-1 level (51), but discouraged its use for multilevel procedures because of difficulty accessing the L4-5 disc. However, it should be noted that they performed only 24 cases in the 3 years of their study. This small a number of cases may suggest that they had not overcome the learning curve associated with the technique. The laparoscopic approach to the L4-5 space was analyzed by Regan et al. (52), who found that by varying the approach to the L4-5 disc space, based on the location of the bifurcation of the great vessels, the disc space could be accessed safely laparoscopically. They noted that no patients were denied laparoscopic fusion because of vascular anatomy at the L4-5 level. The ability to safely assess the L4-5 disc laparoscopically has been reported by other authors as well (47,53).

Results from an animal study using mesh cages showed that laparoscopic fusion resulted in a less stiff spinal segment than that achieved by an open procedure (54). They attributed this difference primarily to the fact that less of a discectomy and less decortication of the end plates were performed laparoscopically than with an open procedure. The authors felt that these factors contributed to less bone growth into the cages, thereby reducing the stiffness of the fused segment. These laboratory findings were supported in a clinical study by McAfee et al. comparing the fusion rate achieved with partial versus complete discectomy (55). They found that the fusion rate was significantly greater in the group in whom a complete discectomy was performed than in patients having a partial discectomy. These results suggest that it is desirable to perform a complete discectomy when using fusion cages. This has been confirmed in another study (47).

There has been one published report of a large number of laparoscopic spine fusion cases performed using cages (48). The authors of this study reported on a multicenter series of 240 consecutive patients. The series was compared to a historical cohort of 591 consecutive patients undergoing open anterior lumbar interbody fusion using the same design of fusion cages. They found that the laparoscopic technique was associated with reduced hospital stay, less blood loss, but had greater operative time. Complications in the two groups were comparable.

There has been one prospective, randomized study directly comparing the results of laparoscopic to open anterior lumbar interbody fusion using the same design of interbody fusion cages (47). The authors reported that the laparoscopic procedure was associated with a longer operating time but reduced hospital stay. The hospital costs for the two techniques were similar. The laparoscopic group had a greater percentage of patients who returned to work and they did so more quickly than patients undergoing open fusion.

Surgeons considering performing laparoscopic fusions must have appropriate training in the technique and should do enough of the procedures to overcome the learning curve in order to attain and maintain a high skill level with this procedure.

ANTERIOR VERSUS POSTERIOR APPROACH FOR DEVICE IMPLANTATION

Several interbody fusion cages can be implanted from either an anterior or posterior approach to the disc space. There appears to be no recommended preference of approach based on clinical results from the procedure. Therefore, the decision regarding the approach generally is based on several other factors. One important factor is the training and experience of the surgeon. If there is neural compression, a posterior approach is preferable in order to address these problems. A posterior approach reduces the risk of injury to the major anterior vascular structures and also avoids damage to neural structures that can result in retrograde ejaculation. If the patient has significant calcification of the vessels or prior abdominal surgery in the vicinity of the disc level to be operated, anterior surgery may be risky. However, there are several advantages to the anterior approach. It provides a wider access to the disc space allowing more room to work. Posterior interbody fusion has a potential risk of injury to the nerve roots owing to overretraction and requires removal of some of the facet joints, which may contribute to instability if too much bone is removed. Finally, the posterior approach damages the posterior musculature, which may be a source of pain and disability.

DISTRACTION AND SUBSIDENCE

Interbody fusion should restore normal disc space height and prevent future collapse. Most fusion cages are strong enough to prevent failure and collapse. Disc space height may be lost if the cages subside into the adjacent vertebral bodies. In a study using a sheep model, it was found that fusion cages significantly distracted the disc space (56). Although there was subsidence for 2 months after surgery, by 4 months the operated levels were solidly fused and the disc space height was greater than it was preoperatively. Distraction and maintenance of the disc space height have been investigated in two recent clinical studies (57,58). Both studies reported reduction of initial disc space height following surgery, but the height remained greater than the preoperative height. Distraction of the disc space height also results in indirect decompression of the neural foramen. Results of a laboratory study showed that the implantation of interbody cages resulted in opening of the foramen (59). This finding was supported in a clinical study investigating changes in foraminal height when cages were inserted into collapsed disc spaces (60). These findings paralleled those of the studies on distraction of the disc space. That is, although the foraminal height decreased over the 2-year study period, it remained greater than the preoperative value.

LUMBAR LORDOSIS

It is desirable to create or maintain normal lumbar lordosis when fusing the spine. However, the impact of minor variation in alignment on clinical results has not been established. Klemme et al. compared the amount of lordosis produced by threaded devices alone to vertical cages with posterior fixation (61). They found that cylindrical fusion cages placed parallel to the end plates did not maintain lumbar lordosis as well as vertical mesh cages combined with pedicle screws. Another study investigated sagittal alignment with threaded fusion cages (62). The authors found that there was a significant decreased in lumbar lordosis at 2-year follow-up in patients with a posterior interbody fusion, although the values were within a normal range. They also found that lumbar lordosis was not related to ultimate clinical outcome. Another study compared the degree of lordosis achieved with wedged-shaped cages compared to rectangular cages (63). All cages were made of polyetheretherketone. The authors found that both cage designs improved the sagittal alignment and that there was no particular benefit with the wedge-shaped cages.

CAGES AS STAND-ALONE DEVICES

There is great debate concerning the use of fusion cages without supplemental posterior fixation. Biomechanical studies show that greater stability is achieved when posterior fixation is included. However, the question of how much immediate stability is needed to achieve good long-term outcome remains unanswered. The potential disadvantages of supplemental posterior

fixation include increased operating time, increased blood loss, increased cost, damage to the posterior musculature, and risk of mechanical failure and reoperations associated with the posterior instrumentation. In addition, the additional stiffness provided by supplemental posterior fixation may be associated with long-term accelerated breakdown of the adjacent segment. Several methods have been proposed to address some of these potential problems. There include use of pedicle screw fixation without bone graft, facet screw fusion, and use of translaminar screws without bone graft.

Although there is concern about the use of cages as stand-alone devices, there is little clinical evidence that there is a significant problem when using them in this manner. The clinical outcome reported from the large series of patients enrolled in the Food and Drug Administration Investigational Device Exemption (IDE) studies for the BAK and Ray TFC cages indicate that the devices perform well without supplemental posterior fixation. Hacker et al. compared the results of stand-alone posterior interbody fusion with titanium threaded fusion cages with combined antero-posterior fusion using allograft dowels (64). There was no significant difference in the percentages of patients reporting excellent or good results in the two groups. The total costs in the stand-alone cage group were less than in the combined group, although the follow-up time for the former was less than that of the combined antero-posterior fusion group.

O'Dowd et al. reported a revision rate of 31% at a mean of 17.8 months (range, 2 to 25 months) when using cages alone in anterior interbody procedures (65). In a review with 3- to 7-year follow-up of patients in whom cages were used as stand-alone devices, Tran et al. reported that 8.1% of patients underwent reoperation at the same level (66). However, 2.1% of this group underwent reoperation soon after the initial surgery to address problems with cage placement. Therefore, only 5.2% of the group underwent reoperation at the same level as the index surgery for unresolved or new onset pain. Their results support the concept that cages can be used effectively as stand-alone devices. In the large-scale studies reported by Kuslich et al. and Ray, in which cages were used as stand-alone devices, there was not a high reoperation rate to add supplemental posterior fixation (26,37).

In one small study of interbody fusion using cages only, cages supplemented with *in situ* posterolateral bone graft were compared to cages supplemented with posterolateral pedicle screw fixation (67). Cage subsidence was more common in the group without pedicle screw fixation, and device loosening was more common at the L3-4 and L4-5 levels. They suggested that pedicle screw fixation should be used when operating at levels above L5-1. However, this study did not compare clinical results to determine if there were any differences in outcome.

Carbon fiber cages were designed to be used with pedicle screw fixation (28). In Brantigan's study, the fusion rate was reported to be 100% in a subgroup of their patients, although their incidence of reoperation and complications was much greater than in the other studies using cylindrical titanium cages as stand-alone devices (26,37,66). There is a trend now among many clinicians to do combined antero-posterior fusions. Fusion cages in the proper clinical setting have proven useful as stand-alone devices. The best candidates are those who have relatively narrow disc height compared to those with normal heights.

COMPLETE VERSUS PARTIAL DISCECTOMY

There has been some discussion concerning the optimal preparation of a disc space prior to the implantation of threaded fusion cages. Some of these devices have been implanted after the removal of cylindrical plugs of disc tissue to make a space for the cages to be inserted. The primary theoretical benefit of this method is less damage to the anterior longitudinal ligament. The practicality of the situation is that once the surgeon finishes putting both cages of a dual cage construct, there is negligible anterior longitudinal ligament left. The potential benefits of complete removal of the disc are elimination of the pain generator and removal of disc tissue that might promote growth of fibrous tissue into the cage. The influence of complete versus partial discectomy in achieving solid fusion when using threaded titanium cages has been investigated in a randomized study (55). At the 2-year follow-up, all patients in whom a total discectomy was performed had a solid fusion compared to 86% fusion rate in group in whom a reamed channel discectomy was done. The importance of total discectomy was also discussed by Sachs et al., who reported a high fusion rate using the cages as stand alone devices (47). In general it makes intuitive sense to carry out a complete discectomy if a fusion is a desired end point.

COMPLICATIONS

Complications encountered in the treatment of symptomatic disc degeneration are discussed in detail in another chapter of this book (Blumenthal and Ohnmeiss). In general, the complications associated with the use of fusion cages are similar to those reported for other interbody fusion methods. We could not find any reports of frank device failure related to the use of threaded metal cylindrical cages. As expected, the anterior approach to the disc space is associated with problems related to injury of vascular and sympathetic structures as are encountered with fusion not involving cages. Posteriorly, complications have been related to retraction of the nerve roots to allow access to the disc space. There have been reports of a few cases of device migration or malpositioned cages requiring reoperation for revision. In a review of 20 patients with cage-related complications,

McAfee concluded that the problems were owing to technical error in all cases (68).

DISCUSSION

In recent years, a variety of fusion cages have been used as devices for interbody fusion procedures. They can provide initial stability to the operated segment and can increase the fusion rate. As with other spine surgery procedures, many questions remain concerning the use of the cages. There has been much discussion concerning optimal cage design. Items that have been discussed include the shape and modulus of elasticity of the cages, the optimal bone–implant interface area, the degree of penetration of the cage into the end plates of the vertebral bodies, and the use of posterior fixation. There have been attempts to address some of the issues in laboratory testing, but they have not been adequately addressed in clinical studies. The use of cages as stand-alone devices remains controversial. There are reports of good results with this method. However, although there has been much discussion concerning the potential problems with this procedure, there have been little or no data published on a large series of patients in whom the use of cages as stand-alone devices was related to poor results. Although routine use of posterior fixation may possibly minimize problems related to using cages as stand-alone devices, this increases costs, operative morbidity, and the potential for complications related to the additional instrumentation. As with other spine surgery procedures, there is a need for well-defined clinical outcome studies on cages investigating the impact of multiple factors such as approach and technique, posterior fixation, discectomy technique, graft material, device shape, size, and placement.

Although fusion cages have been reported to yield good results in many patients, surgeons must pay careful attention to patient selection and surgical technique. There needs to be a thorough diagnostic evaluation with correlative imaging studies. Patients should have failed an adequate course of nonoperative management prior to being considered a candidate for surgery. Patients with a poor psychological profile will likely do poorly with fusion using cages or any other operative intervention.

There is little doubt that the number of future interbody fusions will decrease as the use of disc prostheses increases. The indications for some of these devices will be similar to the indications for fusion cages in the treatment of disc-related pain. However, spinal fusion will continue to be performed for specific conditions and in patients who are not good disc replacement candidates. As discussed, the details of spinal fusion cage procedures needs further investigation, although based on the data currently available, these devices appear to have a significant role in the treatment of patients with back pain and remain an important part of the spine surgeon's armamentarium. We believe that in the properly selected patient, cages offer the surgeon a satisfactory option as a stand-alone device.

REFERENCES

1. Blumenthal SL, Baker J, Dossett A, et al. The role of anterior lumbar fusion for internal disc disruption. 1988;13:566–569.
2. Derby R, Howard MW, Grant JM, et al. The ability of pressure-controlled discography to predict surgical and nonsurgical outcomes. 1999;24:364–371.
3. Gill K, Blumenthal SL. Functional results after anterior lumbar fusion at L5-S1 in patients with normal fusion at L5-S1 in patients with normal and abnormal MRI scans. 1992;17:940–942.
4. Lee CK, Vessa P, Lee JK. Chronic disabling low back pain syndrome caused by internal disc derangements. The results of disc excision and posterior lumbar interbody fusion. 1995;20:356–361.
5. Linson MA, Williams H. Anterior and combined anteroposterior fusion for lumbar disc pain. A preliminary study. 1991;16:143–145.
6. Newman MH, Grinstead GL. Anterior lumbar interbody fusion for internal disc disruption. 1992;17:831–833.
7. Schechter NA, France MP, Lee CK. Painful internal disc derangements of the lumbosacral spine: discographic diagnosis and treatment by posterior lumbar interbody fusion. Orthopedics 1991;14:447–451.
8. Parker LM, Murrell SE, Boden SD, et al. The outcome of posterolateral fusion in highly selected patients with discogenic low back pain. 1996;21:1909–1916.
9. Wetzel FT, LaRocca SH, Lowery GL, et al. The treatment of lumbar spinal pain syndromes diagnosed by discography. Lumbar arthrodesis. 1994;19:792–800.
10. Abe E, Nickel T, Buttermann GR, et al. Lumbar intradiscal pressure after posterolateral fusion and pedicle screw fixation. Tohoku J Exp Med 1998;186:243–253.
11. Weatherley CR, Prickett CF, O'Brein JP. Discogenic pain persisting despite solid posterior fusion. J Bone Joint Surg (Britain) 1986;68:142–143.
12. Barrick WT, Schofferman JA, Reynolds JB, et al. Anterior lumbar fusion improves discogenic pain at levels of prior posterolateral fusion. 2000;25:853–857.
13. Block AR, Ohnmeiss DD, Guyer RD, et al. The use of presurgical psychological screening to predict the outcome of spine surgery. Spine 2001;1:274–282.
14. Jost B, Cripton PA, Lund T, et al. Compressive strength of interbody cages in the lumbar spine: the effect of cage shape, posterior instrumentation on bone density. Eur Spine J 1998;7:132–141.
15. Oxland TR, Lund T. Biomechanics of stand-alone cages and cages in combination with posterior fixation: a literature review. Eur Spine J 2000;9(suppl 1):S95–S101.
16. Hochschuler SH, Guyer RD, Ohnmeiss DD, et al. Anterior lumbar interbody fusion using donor femur bone grafts. Presented at the annual meeting of the North American Spine Society. August, 1990; Monterey, CA.
17. Holte DC, O'Brein JP, Renton P. Anterior lumbar fusion using a hybrid interbody graft. A preliminary radiographic report. Eur Spine J 1994;3:32–38.
18. Kozak JA, Heilman AE, O'Brein JP. Anterior lumbar interbody fusion options. Techniques and graft materials. Clin Orthop 1994;300:45–51.
19. Bagby GW. Arthrodesis by the distraction-compression method using a stainless steel implant. Orthopaedics 1988;11:931–934.
20. Cizek GR, Boyd LM. Imaging pitfalls of interbody spinal implants. 2000;25:2633–2636.
21. Heithoff KB, Mullin WJ, Holte D, et al. The failure of radiographic detection of pseudoarthrosis in patients with titanium lumbar interbody fusion cages. Presented at the International Society for the Study of the Lumbar Spine. June, 1999; Kona, HI.
22. Kuslich SD, Ulstrom CL, Griffith SL, et al. The Bagby and Kuslich method of lumbar interbody fusion. History, techniques, and 2-year follow-up results of a United States prospective, multicenter trial. 1998;23:1267–1278.
23. Thalgott JS, Giuffre JM, Klezl Z, et al. Anterior lumbar interbody fusion with titanium mesh cages, coralline hydroxyapatite, and demineralized bone matrix. Spine J 2002;2:63–69.
24. McAfee PC. Interbody fusion cages in reconstructive operations on the spine. J Bone Joint Surg (America) 1999;81:859–880.
25. Togawa D, Bauer TW, Brantigan JW, et al. Bone graft incorporation in radiographically successful human intervertebral body fusion cages. 2001;26:2744–2750.
26. Ray CD. Threaded titanium cages for lumbar interbody fusions. 1997;22:667–680.
27. Agazzi S, Reverdin A, May D. Posterior lumbar interbody fusion with cages: an independent review of 71 cases. J Neurosurg 1999;91(2 suppl):186–192.
28. Brantigan JW, Steffee AD, Lewis ML, et al. Lumbar interbody fusion using the Brantigan I/F cage for posterior lumbar interbody fusion and the variable pedicle screw placement system. 2000;25:1437–1446.
29. Tullberg T, Brandt B, Rydberg J, et al. Fusion rate after posterior lumbar interbody fusion with carbon fiber implant: 1-year follow-up of 51 patients. Eur Spine J 1996;5:178–182.
30. Toth JM, Seim HB III, Schwardt JD, et al. Direct current electrical stimulation increases fusion rate of spinal fusion cages. 2000;25:2580–2587.
31. Boden SD, Martin GJ Jr, Horton WC, et al. Laparoscopic anterior spinal arthrodesis with rhBMP-2 in a titanium interbody threaded cage. J Spinal Disord 1998;11:95–101.
32. Schimandle JH, Boden SD, Hutton WC. Experimental spinal fusion with recombinant human bone morphogenetic protein-2. 1995;20:1326–1337.
33. Sandhu HS, Toth JM, Diwan AD, et al. Histological evaluation of the efficacy of rhBMP-2 compared with autograft bone in sheep spinal anterior interbody fusion. 2002;27:567–575.
34. Boden SD, Titus L, Hair G, et al. Lumbar spine fusion by local gene therapy with a cDNA encoding a novel osteoinductive protein (LMP-1). 1998;23:2486–2492.
35. Cunningham BW, Kanayama M, Parker LM, et al. Osteogenic protein versus autologous interbody arthrodesis in the sheep thoracic spine. A comparative endoscopic study using the Bagby and Kuslich interbody fusion device. 1999;24:509–518.
36. Boden SD, Zdeblick TA, Sandhu HS, et al. The use of rhBMP-2 in interbody fusion cages. Definitive evidence of osteoinduction in humans: a preliminary report. 2000;25:376—381.
37. Kuslich SD, Danielson G, Dowdle JD, et al. Four-year follow-up results of lumbar spine arthrodesis using the Bagby and Kuslich lumbar fusion cage. 2000;25:2656–2662.
38. Pavlov PW, Spruit M, Havinga M, et al. Anterior lumbar interbody fusion with threaded fusion cages and autologous bone grafts. Eur Spine J 2000;9:224–229.
39. Barnes B, Rodts GE, McLaughlin MR, et al. Threaded cortical bone dowels for lumbar interbody fusion: over 1-year mean follow up in 28 patients. J Neurosurg 2001;95(1 suppl):1–4.
40. Kleeman TJ, Hiscoe AC. Critical analysis of laparoscopic ALIF vs. posterolateral fusion with instrumentation. Laparoscopic versus mini-ALIF. Presented at the annual meeting of the North American Spine Society. October, 1999; Chicago, IL.
41. Schofferman J, Slosar P, Reynolds J, et al. Anterior lumbar interbody fusion: Comparison of titanium threaded cages with threaded bone dowels. Presented at the annual meeting of the North American Spine Society. October, 1999; Chicago, IL.
42. Jun B-Y. Posterior lumbar interbody fusion with restoration of lamina and facet joint. 2000;25:917–922.
43. Molinari RW, Gerlinger T. Functional outcome of instrumented posterior lumbar interbody fusion in active-duty US servicemen: a comparison with nonoperative management. Spine J 2001;1:215–224.
44. Regan JJ, Ohnmeiss DD. Laparoscopic lumbar fusion: Single surgeon experience in 127 consecutive cases. Unpublished data. Poster presented at the annual meeting of the American Academy of Orthopaedic Surgeons. March, 2001; San Francisco.
45. Regan JJ, Ohnmeiss DD, Risk D. Laparoscopic anterior lumbar interbody fusion: analysis of learning curve and comparison to open cage procedures. Presented at the annual meeting of the International Society for the Study of the Lumbar Spine; June, 1999. Kona, HI.
46. Zucherman JF, Zdeblick TA, Bailey SA, et al. Instrumented laparoscopic spinal fusion. Preliminary results. 1995;20:2029–2034.
47. Sachs BL, McVoy J, Miller B, et al. A prospective, randomized comparison of laparoscopic to open anterior lumbar interbody fusion with cages. Presented at the Meeting of the Americas. April, 2002; New York.

48. Regan JJ, Yuan H, McAfee PC. Laparoscopic fusion of the lumbar spine: minimally invasive spine surgery. A prospective multicenter study evaluating open and laparoscopic lumbar fusion. 1999;24: 402–411.

49. Vraney RT, Phillips FM, Wetzel FT, et al. Peridiscal vascular anatomy of the lower lumbar spine. An endoscopic perspective. 1999;24: 2183–2187.

50. Zdeblick TA, David SM. A prospective comparison of surgical approach for anterior L4-5 fusion: Laparoscopic versus mini anterior lumbar interbody fusion. 2000;25:2682–2687.

51. Katkhouda N, Campos GM, Mavor E, et al. Is laparoscopic approach to lumbar spine fusion worthwhile? Am J Surg 1999;178:458–461.

52. Regan JJ, Aronoff RJ, Ohnmeiss DD, et al. Laparoscopic approach to L4-L5 for interbody fusion using BAK cages: experience in the first 58 cases. 1999;24:2171–2174.

53. Lieberman IH, Willsher PC, Litwin DEM, et al. Transperitoneal laparoscopic exposure for lumbar interbody fusion. 2000;25:509–514.

54. Riley LH 3rd, Eck JC, Yoshida H, et al. Laparoscopic assisted fusion of the lumbosacral spine. A biomechanical and histologic analysis of the open versus laparoscopic technique in an animal model. 1997;22: 1407–1412.

55. McAfee PC, Lee GA, Fedder IL, et al. Anterior BAK instrumentation and fusion: complete versus partial discectomy. Clin Orthop 2002;394: 55–63.

56. Sandhu HS, Turner S, Kabo JM, et al. Distractive properties of a threaded interbody fusion device: an in vivo model. 1996;21:1201–1210.

57. Brown A, Slosar P, Reynolds J, et al. Paired BAK Proximity cages versus standard BAKTM: subsidence and clinical failures. Presented at: North American Spine Society. October, 1999; Chicago, IL.

58. Ohnmeiss DD, Blumenthal SL, Guyer RD, et al. Analysis of threaded fusion cage subsidence. Presented at the annual meeting of the Inter-national Society for the Study of the Lumbar Spine. April, 2000; Adelaide, Australia.

59. Chen D, Fay LA, Lok J, et al. Increasing neuroforaminal volume by anterior interbody distraction in degenerative lumbar spine. 1995;20: 74–79.

60. Ohnmeiss DD, Blumenthal SL, Guyer RD, et al. Can foraminal height be increased and maintained with anterior lumbar interbody fusion using cages? Presented at the annual meeting of the International Society for the Study of the Lumbar Spine. April, 2000; Adelaide, Australia.

61. Klemme WR, Owens BD, Dhawan A, et al. Lumbar sagittal contour after posterior interbody fusion: threaded devices alone versus cages plus posterior instrumentation. 2001;26:534–537.

62. Goldstein JA, Macenski MJ, Griffith SL, et al. Lumbar sagittal alignment after fusion with a threaded interbody cage. 2001;26:1137–1142.

63. Diedrich O, Perlick L, Schmitt O, et al. Radiographic spinal profile changes induced by cage design after posterior lumbar interbody fusion. Preliminary report of a study with wedged implants. 2001; 26:E274–E280.

64. Hacker RJ. Comparison of interbody fusion approaches for disabling low back pain. 1977;22:660–666.

65. O'Dowd JK, Mullholland RC, Harris M. BAK cage: Nottingham results. Presented at the annual meeting of the North American Spine Society. October, 1998; San Francisco, CA.

66. Tran V, Ohnmeiss DD, Blumenthal SL, et al. Analysis of re-operations when using cages as stand-alone devices: Minimum three year follow-up study. Presented at the Meeting of the Americas. April, 2002; New York.

67. Shetty AP, Osti OL, Abraham G, et al. Cylindrical threaded cages for lumbar degenerative disc disease. A prospective long term radiological study. Presented at the annual meeting of the International Society for the Study of the Lumbar Spine. April, 2000; Adelaide, Australia.

68. McAfee PC, Cunningham BW, Lee GA, et al. Revision strategies for salvaging or improving failed cylindrical cages. 1999;24:2147–2153.

CHAPTER 36

Minimally Invasive Procedures for Anterior Column Fusion and Reconstruction

H. Michael Mayer

The term "minimally invasive" has been used in the surgical scientific literature since the introduction of microsurgical and endoscopic surgical approaches. It has been applied in various fields, mainly abdominal, gynecologic, and thoracic surgery (1–3). Although arthroscopic techniques in the peripheral joints or microsurgical techniques for discectomy or decompression have been used for many years in orthopedic surgery, the term "minimally invasive" was very rarely used or associated with these procedures. In fact, it has only come to our perception in recent years, when it was increasingly used to describe or characterize procedures or surgical approaches for the treatment of degenerative lumbar disc disorders.

It is important to distinguish between "true" minimally invasive procedures for diagnostic and therapeutic purposes and minimally invasive approaches for curative surgical procedures. Typical examples for minimally invasive diagnostic and therapeutic procedures include different kinds of infiltrations including epidural catheters, root blocks, facet joint block, discography, intradiscal electrothermal therapy, and others. These procedures, however, are either "diagnostic instruments" that are used to supplement information from noninvasive imaging techniques such as magnetic resonance imaging (MRI), or represent noncurative modalities with temporary therapeutic effects. They should thus be classified as semi-invasive conservative measures.

For the definitive surgical treatment of degenerative disorders of the lumbar spine, a variety of minimally invasive techniques have been developed over the last 15 years. All these techniques represent surgical *approaches* that are less invasive than the usual standard approaches (Table 36-1).

This leads to a very fundamental but important concept which should be appreciated to avoid misunderstandings and misinterpretations: minimally invasive surgery for the definitive curative treatment of segmental lumbar disc degeneration is a minimally invasive approach to perform "target surgery" such as disc excision, fusion, or disc replacement—procedures that are (maximally) invasive.

Wrong indications for surgery, undesired side effects, complications, and poor results are strongly influenced by the surgical approach to the target area (4,5). Less invasive techniques, in general, decrease the degree of "iatrogenic" surgical trauma. They ameliorate early postoperative morbidity and enable early and aggressive rehabilitation of the patient without an increase in complications. This chapter describes the rationale for surgery for degenerative lumbar spine disorders, the goals of surgical procedures, and the implementation of minimally invasive techniques into the surgical standard strategies.

RATIONALES FOR SURGERY

There is a long-standing controversy about the surgical treatment of degenerative lumbar disc "disease." Although there are no evidence-based data to support spinal fusion or reconstruction of the "functional spinal unit," surgery is performed worldwide with varying frequency depending on national or continental philosophies. The "gold standard" procedure has always been segmental spinal fusion. This can be performed by different techniques and has become one of the classic "experience-based" procedures with poorly predictable success rates due to the lack of an international consensus for patient selection, surgical approach, fusion technique, and postoperative management (6–9).

In the last 2 years, there has been a tremendous acceleration in the development and application of a new philosophy that is termed "spine arthroplasty." This term encompasses all surgical techniques that aim for a dynamic reconstruction and preservation of motion without performing a fusion (Table 36-2). Principles of some of these procedures are described in Chapters 38–40.

TABLE 36-1. *Minimally invasive access surgery for lumbar fusion and disc reconstruction*

Laparoscopic anterior lumbar interbody fusion (22,23)
Percutaneous posterolateral interbody fusion (12)
Mini-open microsurgical posterolateral fusion (13)
Mini-anterior lumbar interbody fusion (24)
Mini-open total disc replacement (26)

GENERAL PRINCIPLES

Disc degeneration may lead to clinical symptoms of pain ("discogenic" low back pain). However, low back pain due to disc degeneration is usually "multifactorial". Whereas young patients may present with pure discogenic back pain, the majority of patients present with a mixture of discogenic, arthrogenic, and musculoligamentous symptoms. Surgical procedures to deal with these symptoms have common goals: the excision or elimination of pain source(s), the elimination of biomechanical pain generating mechanisms, the restoration and retention of the physiologic segmental curvature, as well as the restoration of disc and foraminal height, especially in cases with lateral recess or foraminal stenosis. There is no doubt that these goals can be most reliably achieved by 360° or 270° fusion of one or several lumbar segments. Using this technique, all potential pain sources (disc, end plates, facet joints, facet joint capsules) are excised. Pathologic load patterns due to loss in disc height ("vertical instability") as well as macroinstabilities (e.g., degenerative spondylolisthesis) are eliminated by the fusion (Fig. 36-1). Disturbances of lumbar curvature in the sagittal (kyphosis, hyperlordosis) as well as frontal (degenerative lumbar scoliosis, segmental tilt) plane can be reduced and maintained by posterior instrumentation. Disc height and foraminal height can be restored in cases with root symptoms associated with low back pain. Thus spinal fusion is the only "curative" salvage procedure to treat degenerative low back pain.

TABLE 36-2. *Lumbar spine arthroplasty procedures*

Total disc replacement
  SB Charite disc (30)
  Prodisc (26,31)
  Acroflex (32)
Nucleus replacement
  Mechanical
    Prosthetic disc nucleus (33)
    Spiral nucleoplasty (34)
  Biological
    Autologeous disc chondrocyte transplantation (ADCT) (35)
Posterior Augmentation
  Graf ligaments (36)
  Dynesys (37)
  Wallis (38)

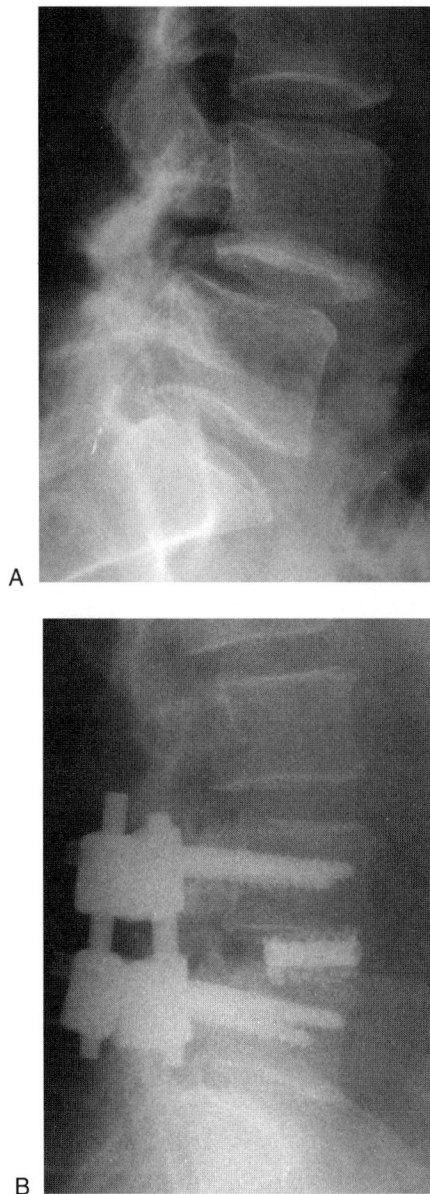

FIG. 36-1. Lateral X-ray of the lumbar spine. **A:** Preoperative–degenerative spondylolisthesis grade I. **B:** Postoperative–restoration of physiologic curvature with reduction and 270° lumbar fusion.

LUMBAR FUSION

The controversial discussion on the role of lumbar fusion is the result of an obvious discrepancy between the technical achievement of the surgical goals (discussed previously) and the clinical outcome. The majority of undesired side effects, complications, and poor outcome is determined or influenced by the surgical approach to the target area (4,5).

The main prognostic factors for outcome of lumbar fusion surgery are patient selection and surgical technique (7,10,11).

Patient Selection

The reader is referred elsewhere in the text (Chapters 28–35, 39, 45) to information on the current "state-of-the-art" treatment of degenerative low back pain. There is consensus that spinal fusion in degenerative conditions of the lumbar spine should be the last therapeutic step when noninvasive or semi-invasive conservative measures have failed. However, there is neither consensus on the identification of lumbar levels to be fused nor on the type of fusion (7,8,11,12). The most frequently used techniques are listed in Table 36-3.

Less Invasive Techniques for Lumbar Fusion

Microsurgical Posterolateral Fusion (13)

Posterolateral fusion has been the most widespread fusion technique for the past 25 years. It has been performed without instrumentation (11,14) or with instrumention (15), with varying clinical success and fusion rates. Decortication of laminae, facet joints, and transverse processes is followed by the application of autograft or allograft bone "posterolaterally" in order to achieve a solid bone bridge between adjacent segments. It is the easiest technique in fusion surgery, however, it also is the most traumatizing technique because of damage to the paravertebral muscles during the approach (16–18) (Fig. 36-2).

Unacceptably high pseudoarthrosis rates have limited the popularity of this fusion among spine surgeons in Europe (6,11,19).

In 1998 McCulloch described a microsurgical modification of the "classic" posterolateral/intertransverse lumbar fusion (13). Based on his experience with microsurgical discectomy, McCulloch described a minimally invasive paramedian approach to the intertransverse area. Soft-tissue dissection is reduced to a minimum. Preservation of a "soft tissue envelope" (paraspinal muscles, intertransverse ligament and muscle) is presumed to provide a vascularized bed for autologous bone graft. Decortication of the facet joints and the transverse processes is performed with high-speed drills. The use of autologous bone graft is recommended.

The clinical results described by McCulloch revealed the advantages of this minimal invasive technique: In a series of 22 patients with single-level degenerative disc disease, microsurgical posterolateral fusion was per-

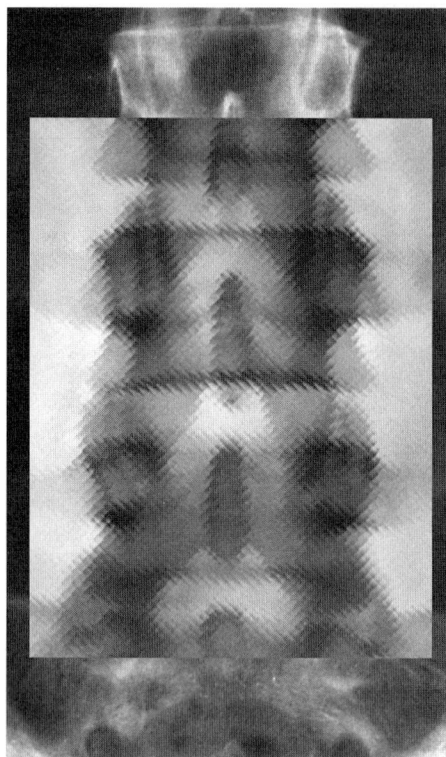

FIG. 36-2. X-ray lumbar spine, frontal view. Shaded area is necessary for muscle retraction for posterolateral L4-5 fusion.

formed. Follow-up after 2 years showed good and excellent results in 86.4% of the patients. The average hospital stay was less than 3 days, the average intraoperative blood loss less than 300 cc. There was only one pseudoarthrosis (13). In a similar series of 22 patients with degenerative spondylolisthesis and acquired spinal stenosis, the rate of satisfactory results was 91%. The pseudoarthrosis rate however was 14% (13).

Although this technique has not become very popular, it seems to be a reasonable alternative to the "classic" posterolateral type of fusion performed through the Wiltse approach.

Minimal Invasive Anterior Approaches for Interbody Fusion

In 1990 Obenchain first described a laparoscopic approach to the L5/S1 disc (20). This "key" publication triggered the development of a variety of less invasive anterior accesses to the lumbar spine that dominated the last decade. Laparoscopic surgery was associated with a variety of technical pitfalls and hazards and has never reached the status of a "routine-procedure" (21–23). However, the need for less invasive anterior approaches was obvious, since 360° or 270° fusion achieves the highest fusion rates of all techniques (5,10,24). In 1997, I described two "mini-open" access techniques to the lum-

TABLE 36-3. *Spinal fusion techniques*

Posterolateral (intertransverse)	180° posterior
TLIF/PLIF	270° posterior
Percutaneous PLIF	180° anterior
ALIF	180° anterior
Posterior/ALIF	270° posterior/anterior

ALIF, anterior lumbar interbody fusion; PLIF, posterior lumbar interbody fusion; TLIF, transforaminal lumbar interbody fusion.

bar levels for anterior interbody fusion (24). They were based on the application of microsurgical philosophy to the well-known standard anterior approaches.

Lateral Retroperitoneal Access to L2-L5

Monosegmental as well as multisegmental anterior fusion can be performed through a standard anterior approach to the lumbar levels L2-L5. With this technique, the abdominal muscle layers are cut, irrespective of their orientation, and the lumbar segment(s) are approached anterior to the psoas muscle (25).

Microsurgical (Mini-Open) Access

The mini-open anterior lumbar interbody fusion (ALIF) technique (mini-ALIF) has been described extensively (9,24), so only the basic principles are repeated here:

The patient is placed in a right lateral position (Fig. 36-3). The approach is from the left side. The operating table is tilted slightly posteriorly (20° to 40°) which facilitates the access to the lumbar spine through a small skin incision, even in very obese patients, since all abdominal contents and fat tissue "fall-away" anterior from the surgical field. The retroperitoneal cavity is entered through a 4 cm skin incision that is directed obliquely parallel to the direction of the external oblique abdominal muscle. The use of a bright head lamp (Xenon light source) and optical aids (surgical microscope, loupes) is recommended in special situations (e.g., obese patients, reoperation). The muscle layers (external oblique, internal oblique, transversus abdominus) are exposed by a blunt, muscle-splitting technique. The peritoneal sac is bluntly dissected from the psoas muscle and the disc space is exposed anterior and medial to the psoas muscle. The anterior circumference of the disc space is exposed from

the midline to approximately 2 cm lateral to the insertion of the anterior longitudinal ligament. This requires a small splitting (1 to 1.5 cm) of the medial insertions of the psoas. The anterolateral circumference of the disc space is exposed bluntly and kept free from surrounding tissue by insertion of frame-type retractors that are anchored in the adjacent vertebral bodies or by an external frame holder.

Fusion Technique

The type of anterior fusion performed is optional once the target area is exposed. All types of fusion techniques are possible (autologous bone graft, vertical cages with bank bone or autologous bone, femoral ring grafts, stand-alone ALIF cages, etc.) (Fig. 36-4A, B).

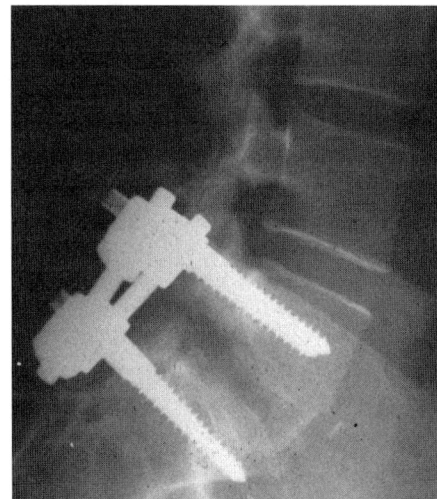

A

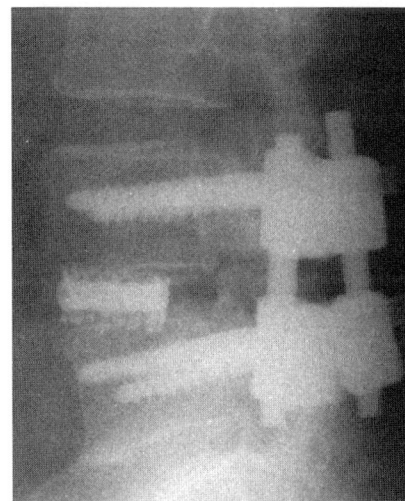

B

FIG. 36-4. A: A 360° instrumental fusion at L5-S1 with autologous bone graft. **B:** Both anterior approaches were done through a 6 cm skin incision at L4-5 with vertical titanium cage.

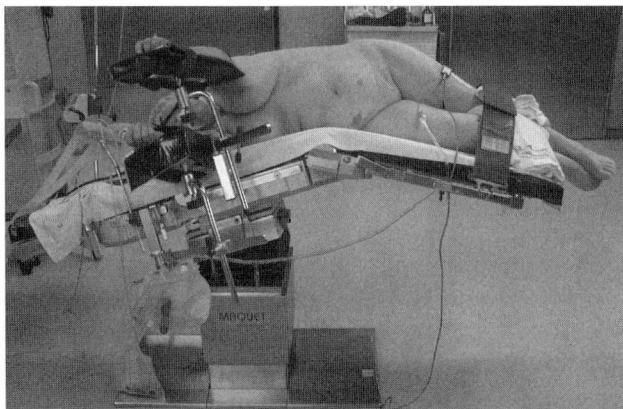

FIG. 36-3. Positioning of an obese patient for mini-open retroperitoneal approach to L2-L5.

Midline Retroperitoneal or Transperitoneal Access to the Lumbosacral Junction

The conventional approach to the lumbosacral junction is either through a midline longitudinal or transverse skin incision using a transperitoneal route or through a pararectal retroperitoneal approach. The patient is placed in a supine neutral position with the surgeon standing either on the left or right side of the patient

Mini-Open Access to L5-S1

Mini-open access to L5-S1 is performed through a 4 cm transverse or longitudinal skin incision in the midline and a mini-laparotomy. Patient positioning has been modified with the patient in a supine position with the legs abducted so that the surgeon can stand between the patient's legs.

Thus, the visual axis of the surgeon is parallel to the L5-S1 intervertebral space. The level of the skin incision can be marked in two different ways: in slim patients, the abdominal wall is slightly indented with a blunt metal marker and a lateral fluoroscopy is used to show the position of the marker over the L5-S1 disc space. In obese patients, the orientation and anterior border of the lumbosacral junction is identified by lateral fluoroscopy and a "corridor line" is drawn from there onto the abdomen. The transverse skin incision is placed 2 cm caudad to the corridor line (8).

The rectus sheath is exposed and split in the midline. L5-S1 can be approached through a retroperitoneal route either from the left or from the right side. To mobilize and shift the peritoneal sac, it is necessary to incise the posterior rectus sheath. In obese patients and in patients with previous abdominal surgery, a transperitoneal route is recommended. Dissection of the prevertebral part of the peritoneum should generally be from the right to the left. Electrocautery should be avoided to minimize the risk of injury to the superior hypogastric plexus and retrograde ejaculation in men. The anterior circumference of L5-S1 is exposed between the common iliac veins. The median sacral vessels need to be either ligated or coagulated with bipolar electrocautery and dissected. L5-S1 is exposed with the help of special retractors. The options for fusion are the same as in the levels L2-L5.

Results

Results of mini-open anterior fusion have already been described (5,8,9). The combination of mini-open anterior fusion with pedicle instrumentation produces excellent and good results in 75% to 85% of the patients (5,8). The pseudoarthrosis rate is 3% and the rate of complications due to the anterior approach is 5.2%. Perioperative morbidity is extremely low with clinical results that seem to be comparable to conventional fusion techniques.

Minimal Invasive Midline Accesses for Total Disc Replacement

Total disc replacement for the treatment of painful degenerated lumbar disc is an alternative to lumbar fusion (26,27). The principles of minimal invasive access surgery can be applied to this new technology (26,28). However, total disc replacement requires a midline approach to all lumbar segments. This mandates a modification of the approach to the L4-5 and more proximal levels. The surgical approach technique for L4-5, L3-4, and L2-3 is described subsequently.

Positioning of the patient and localization of the level are performed as previously described. Care must be taken to place the patient in a neutral supine position without hyperextension to prevent hyperlordosis that complicates implantation of the artificial disc.

L4-5 Level

A small transverse skin incision is centered over L4-5 or placed slightly left of the midline (28). The rectus sheath is exposed and can be split either longitudinally in the midline or transversely on the left side. In slim patients, midline splitting of the sheath can provide sufficient exposure to begin the retroperitoneal dissection from left to right (discussed previously). In obese patients, it is advisable to mobilize the rectus muscle circumferentially and begin the retroperitoneal dissection lateral to the muscle belly after incision of the posterior rectus sheath. It is important to first mobilize the common iliac artery and to identify the iliolumbar vein beneath the psoas muscle. Mobilization of the common iliac artery is performed with finger dissection and small peanut swabs. The iliolumbar vein must be identified, ligated, and cut before the common iliac vein is mobilized toward the midline (9,28). Once the vessels are mobilized toward the midline, the disc space can be palpated with the tip of the index finger. The segmental vessels of L4 on the left side then need to be identified and ligated if necessary (Fig. 36-5).

Thus, the anterior portion of L4-5 can be exposed and the retractor system can be inserted. Sharp retractor blades or pins should not be used since they could cause vascular injury (28,29).

L3-4 Level

The approach to L3-4 is performed the same way as for L4-5 except that a curved longitudinal incision is recommended if the L3-4 disc is at the level of the umbilicus. Usually the iliolumbar vein does not need to be identified, but the segmental vessels at L3 and L4 on the left must be ligated before the aorta and the vena cava are mobilized from left to right. Rarely, the L3-4 disc can be approached between the aorta and the vena cava. In this

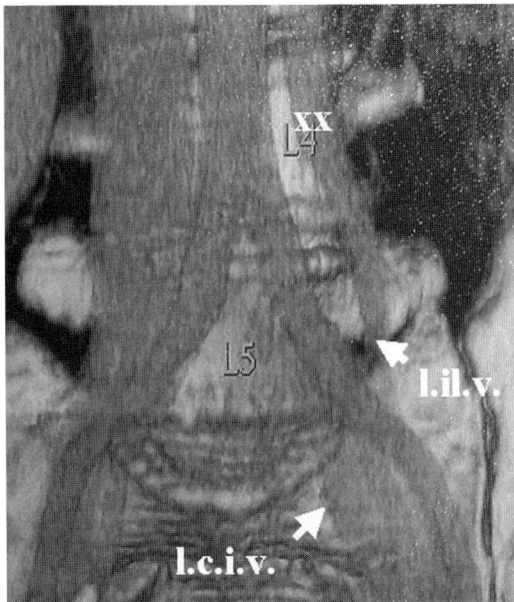

FIG. 36-5. Vessels to be identified for the midline approach at L4-5 as seen on three-dimensional computed tomography–angiography (*l.il.v.,* left iliolumbar vein; *l.c.i.v.,* left common iliac vein; *xx,* left segmental vessels L4).

case, the segmental vein(s) on the left and the segmental artery(s) on the right side must be ligated (26).

L2-3 Level

The approach to L2-3 for total disc replacement is rarely necessary since symptomatic disc degeneration at this segment is unusual. The skin incision is located at the level of or cranial to the umbilicus. A transperitoneal approach is recommended since retroperitoneal dissection is difficult. Care must be taken to avoid dissection through the mesenterium. The mesentery and small intestine are pushed cranially to the right and the prevertebral peritoneum is split in the midline. Care must be taken to avoid the renal artery.

Minimal Invasive Implantation of the Prodisc Implant

The Prodisc Total Disc (Spine Solutions, Inc., New York, NY) is the only implant that can be inserted through the minimal invasive approaches described in this chapter (Fig. 36-6). Once the anterior circumference of the disc space is exposed, the midline is marked and verified through anteroposterior fluoroscopy. A rectangular window is made in the disc space and the anterior annulus fibrosus is removed. The nucleus and the cartilaginous end plates are carefully removed with curettes. Preservation of the subchondral bone is of paramount importance. The trial implant can then be inserted (Fig.

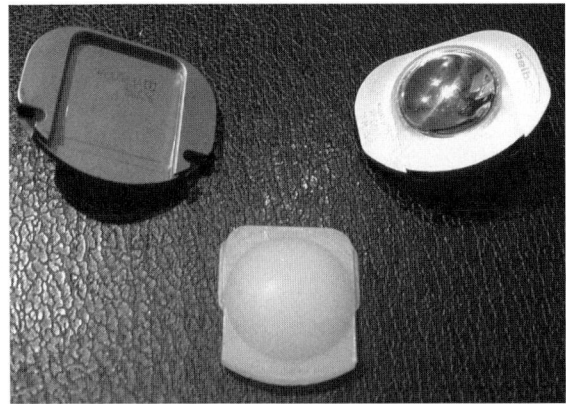

FIG. 36-6. The Prodisc implant (Spine Solutions, Inc., New York, NY), modular design: two metal end plates, ultra–high-molecular-weight polyethylene inlay.

36-7A, B). This trial implant determines the size, height, and degree of lordosis of the final implant. Once it is placed in the correct position, a groove is chiseled in the adjacent vertebral bodies for the two keels of the implant. After removal of the trial implant, the end plates of the modular total disc are implanted, the disc space is distracted, and a polyethylene insert is implanted (Fig. 36-8A,B).

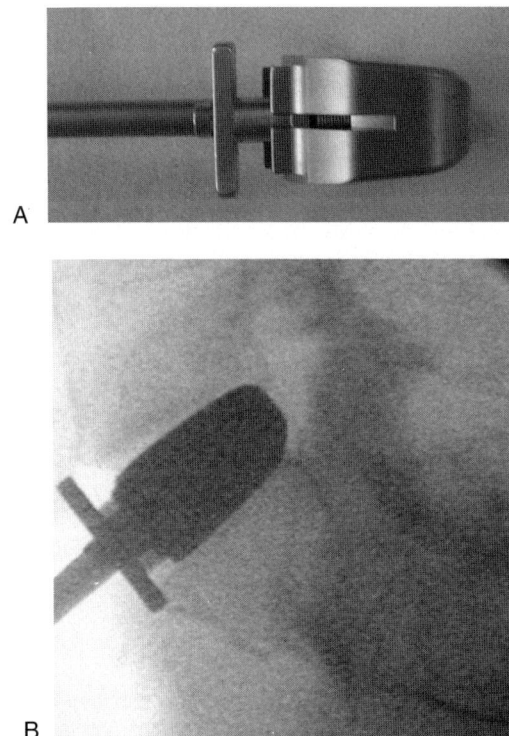

FIG. 36-7. A: Trial implant to determine size, height, and lordosis angle. B: Lateral X-ray, trial implant in place at L5-S1.

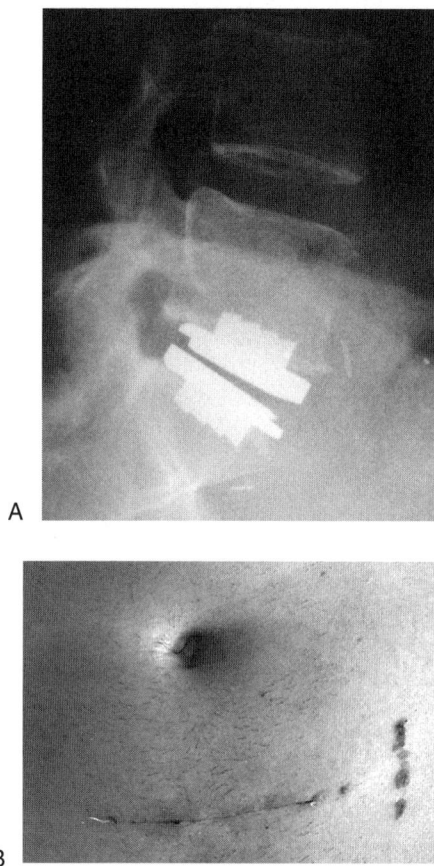

FIG. 36-8. X-ray postoperative lumbar spine. **A:** Implant in place (lateral view). **B:** Skin incision.

CONCLUSION

Minimally invasive surgical approaches for spinal fusion or reconstruction in degenerative diseases have been popularized within the last 10 years. Preoperative planning and modification of surgical strategies with innovative instruments and implants are key factors for performing safe and successful surgery. A vascular or general surgeon is extremely helpful in providing access to the surgical target area. The main advantages of minimal access surgery are the reduction in perioperative morbidity and the possibility of early and aggressive mobilization and rehabilitation of the patient. Although experience is still limited, disc replacement is a new and exciting application of less invasive surgical approaches.

REFERENCES

1. Mack MJ, Aronoff RJ, Acuff TE, et al. Present role of thoracoscopy in the diagnosis and treatment of diseases of the chest. Ann Thorac Surg 1992;54:403–409.
2. Reddick EJ, Olson DO. Laparoscopic laser cholecystectomy: a comparison with mini-lap cholecystectomy. Surg Endosc 1989;3:131–133.
3. Steptoe PC, ed. Laparoscopy in gynecology. Edinburgh: E&S Livingston, 1967.
4. Faciszewski T, Winter RB, Lonstein JE, et al. The surgical and medical perioperative complications of anterior spinal fusion surgery in the thoracic and lumbar spine of adults. Spine 1995;20:1592–1599.
5. Mayer HM, Korge A. Non-fusion technology in degenerative lumbar spinal disorders: facts, questions, challenges. Eur Spine J 2002;11 [Suppl 2]:85–91.
6. Axelsson P, Johnsson R, Strömqvist B, et al. Posterolateral lumbar fusion: outcome of 71 consecutive operations after 4 (2–7) years. Acta Orthop Scand 1994;65:309–314.
7. Greenough CG, Taylor LJ, Fraser RD. Anterior lumbar fusion: results, assessment techniques and prognostic factors. Eur Spine J 1994;3: 225–230.
8. Mayer HM. Microsurgical approaches for anterior interbody fusion of the lumbar spine. In: JA McCulloch, PA Young, eds. Essentials of spinal microsurgery. Philadelphia: Lippincott-Raven, 1998:633–649.
9. Mayer HM, ed. Minimally invasive spine surgery. Berlin-Heidelberg-New York: Springer-Verlag, 2000.
10. Grob D, Scheier HJG, Dvorak J, et al. Circumferential fusion of the lumbar and lumbosacral spine. Arch Orthop Trauma Surg 1991;111: 20–25.
11. Herkovitz HN, Kurz LT. Degenerative lumbar spondylolisthesis with spinal stenosis: a prospective study comparing decompression with decompression and intertransverse process arthrodesis. J Bone Joint Surg 1991;73A:802–808.
12. Kambin P. Arthroscopic lumbar interbody fusion. In: White AH, ed. Spine care. St. Louis: Mosby, 1996:1055–1066.
13. McCulloch JA. Posterolateral uninstrumented lumbar fusion. In: McCulloch JA, Young PA, eds. Essentials of spinal microsurgery. Philadelphia: Lippincott-Raven, 1998:531–552.
14. Turner JA, Herron, L, Deyo RA. Meta-analysis of the results of lumbar spine fusion. Acta Orthop Scand 1993;64 [Suppl 251]:120–122.
15. Bernhardt M, Swartz D, Clothiaux P. Posterolateral lumbar and lumbosacral fusion with and without pedicle screw internal fixation. Clin Orthop 1992;284:109–116.
16. Watkins MB. Posterior lateral fusion of the lumbar and lumbosacral spine. J Bone Joint Surg 1953;35A:1014–1019.
17. Wiltse LL, Spencer CW. New uses and refinements of the paraspinal approach to the lumbar spine. Spine 1988;13:696–706.
18. Zdeblick TA. A prospective randomized study of lumbar fusion. Preliminary results. Spine 1993;18:983–991.
19. Rompe JD, Eysel P, Hopf C. Clinical efficacy of pedicle instrumentation and posterolateral fusion in the symptomatic degenerative lumbar spine. Eur Spine J 1995;4:231–237.
20. Obenchain TG. Laparoscopic lumbar discectomy. J Laparoendosc Surg 1991;3:145–149.
21. Pellissé F, Puig O, Rivas A, et al. Low fusion rate after L5-S1—laparoscopic anterior lumbar interbody fusion using twin stand-alone carbon fiber cages. Spine 2002;27:1665–1669.
22. Regan JJ. Endoscopic applications of the BAK system. In: JJ Regan, McAfee PC, Mack MJ, eds. Atlas of endoscopic spine surgery. St. Louis: Quality Medical Publishing, 1995:321–331.
23. Sachs B, Schweitzberg SD. Lumbosacral discectomy and interbody fusion technique. In: JJ Regan, McAfee PC, Mack MJ, eds. Atlas of endoscopic spine surgery. St. Louis: Quality Medical Publishing, 1995: 275–291.
24. Mayer HM. A new microsurgical technique for minimally invasive anterior lumbar interbody fusion. Spine 1997;22:691–700.
25. Hodgson AR, Wong AK. A description of a technique and evaluation of results in anterior fusion for deranged intervertebral disk and spondylolisthesis. Clin Orthop 1968;56:133–161.
26. Mayer HM, Wiechert K, Korge A, et al. Minimally invasive total disc replacement: surgical technique and preliminary clinical results. Eur Spine J 2002;11[Suppl 2]:124–130.
27. Szplaski M, Gunzburg R, Mayer HM. Spine arthroplasty: a historical review. Eur Spine J 2002;11[Suppl 2]:65 – 84.
28. Brau SA. Mini-open approach to the spine for anterior lumbar interbody fusion: description of the procedure, results and complications. Spine 2002;2:216–223.
29. Baker JK, Reardon PR, Reardon MJ. Vascular injury in anterior lumbar surgery. Spine 1993;18:2227–2230.
30. Büttner-Janz K. The development of the artificial disc: SB Chariité. Dallas: Hundley & Associates, 1992.

31. Bertganoli R, Kumar S. Indications for full prosthetic disc arthroplasty: a correlation of clinical outcome against a variety of indications. Eur Spine J 2002;11[Suppl 2]:131–136.

32. Cunningham BW, Lowery GL, Serhan HA, et al. Total disc replacement arthroplasty using the AcroFlex lumbar disc: a non-human primate model. Eur Spine J 2002;11[Suppl 2]:115–123.

33. Ray CD. The PDN prosthetic disc nucleus device. Eur Spine J 2002;11[Suppl 2]:137–142.

34. Korge A, Nydegger T, Polard JL, et al. A spiral implant as nucleus prosthesis in the lumbar spine. Eur Spine J 2002;11[Suppl 2]: 149–153.

35. Ganey TG, Meisel J. A potential role for cell-based therapeutics in the treatment of intervertebral disc herniation. Eur Spine J 2002;11[Suppl 2]:206 – 214.

36. Gardner A, Pande KC. Graf ligamentoplasty: a 7-year follow-up. Eur Spine J 2002;11[Suppl 2]:157–163.

37. Stoll TM, Dubois G, Schwarzenbach O. The dynamic neutralization system for the spine: a multicenter study of a novel non-fusion system. Eur Spine J 2002;11[Suppl 2]:170–178.

38. Sénégas J. Mechanical supplementation by non-rigid fixation in degenerative intervertebral lumbar segments: the Wallis system. Eur Spine J 2002;11[Suppl 2]:164–169.

CHAPTER 37

Degenerative Disc Disease: Complications of Surgery

Scott L. Blumenthal and Donna D. Ohnmeiss

Many strategies for the surgical management of symptomatic disc degeneration have been developed. Potential advantages and disadvantages are associated with each of them. The development of fusion cages and artificial discs has brought renewed interest in surgery for symptomatic degenerative disc disease. The effectiveness of some of these techniques and devices is still in question. Another important issue is the safety of these devices and of the operative techniques required for them. In this chapter we will focus on the complications associated with lumbar fusion, particularly interbody fusion, artificial disc replacement, and intradiscal electrothermal therapy (IDET) used in the treatment of symptomatic disc degeneration. In order to focus this review on current techniques and instrumentation, the majority of the literature reviewed will cover the period from approximately 1990 to 2002. We tried to include information dealing specifically with the treatment of symptomatic degenerative disc disease; however, many articles involved a mixed group of diagnoses.

OVERVIEW OF POTENTIAL COMPLICATIONS

With most of the procedures discussed in this chapter, complications directly related to the surgery may arise from several sources. The greatest potential for complications is related to technical problems executing the surgery, poor implant selection, device failure, and poor patient selection. Technical problems can be grouped based on the operative approach used. With anterior lumbar interbody fusion, the most readily recognized risk is injury to the great vessels. This may occur by tearing or puncturing one of the structures with an instrument or during retraction. Other complications associated with anterior spine surgery include damage to the sympathetic chain resulting in temporary or permanent sexual dysfunction, urologic problems, or altered sensation in the lower extremities. When placing devices from the anterior approach, one must be

aware of the depth of the implant to avoid impingement of neural elements either directly by the device or by pushing disc tissue into the canal.

Posterior interbody fusion is also associated with potential significant complications. Injury to neural structures can result from making direct contact with an instrument or from retraction. Typically, bone must be removed from the posterior elements in order to gain access to the disc space, which has the potential to create or contribute to instability of the operated spinal segment. As with the anterior approach, the surgeon must be acutely aware of the depth of implants or bone graft since aggressive insertion of implants or graft can result in significant vascular injury. Other complications associated with posterior spine surgery include damage to the posterior musculature from dissection and retraction of these tissues. Also, screws placed posteriorly can penetrate the cortical bone of the pedicle injuring neural structures.

In surgeries using autogenous iliac crest bone graft, there are complications related to the donor site. These include injury to neural or vascular structures, fracture, infections, and persistent pain.

ANTERIOR APPROACHES TO THE LUMBAR SPINE

Interest in the anterior approach to the lumbar spine has increased dramatically in recent years due to the introduction of fusion cages, laparoscopic fusion techniques, and disc replacement. In this section we will review general complications as well as complications associated with specific devices implanted using an anterior approach.

Vascular Injuries

The risk of significant vascular complications during anterior lumbar interbody fusion is related to the proximity of the vena cava and aorta to the disc spaces. These structures are at greatest risk during the exposure of the disc space, but can also be injured by blunt contact or retraction during the placement of devices or bone graft. There is a great deal of individual variation with regard to the level of the vessel bifurcation that determines the approach. Surgery can either be above the bifurcation, below it, or in some cases between the vessels. Weiner at al. investigated variation in vascular anatomy with respect to anterior lumbar interbody fusion (1). They reported that in about 60% of cases, the vascular anatomy was predictable and the lumbosacral disc could be accessed below the bifurcation. In 30% of cases, there were minor variations in vascular anatomy, which did not significantly alter the approach to the spine. In the remaining 10% of cases, a significantly different approach to the disc was required due to variation in vascular anatomy. The altered surgical approach involved working above the bifurcation. In all of these cases, the operated level was a functional lumbosacral level above a fixed transitional vertebra.

One study reported the results of a retrospective review of 105 consecutive cases in which the retroperitoneal approach was used to gain access to the lumbar spine (2). These authors reported that the overall incidence of vascular complications was 15.6% (16/105). This included tears of the common iliac vein (10.5%), the inferior vena cava (3.8%), and the iliolumbar vein (0.9%). The authors found that the complication rate was almost twice as great with the hypogastric paramedian approach as with the anterolateral approach. The majority of complications occurred during the surgical exposure. Fortunately, these complications resulted in only one case of deep vein thrombosis, and there were no cases of pulmonary embolism or catastrophic blood loss.

In a detailed review of general surgery complication in anterior spinal fusion, the rate of vascular injury was found to be 6.6% (3). In two cases, venous injury occurred during the exposure of the disc space, and in one case, the injury occurred during graft placement. In all three cases, the problem was addressed intraoperatively with no serious sequelae. The other vascular injury occurred during the exposure in a case to revise or remove a malpositioned cage. That injury was attributed to dense adhesions that had formed after the initial surgery. There was significant blood loss and the surgery was abandoned.

The risk of vascular injury was of particular concern as laparoscopic fusion was being developed. With this procedure, injury to a major vessel has the potential for more severe consequence since it cannot be repaired directly. There was concern about whether or not the endoscopic procedure could be rapidly converted to an open procedure to repair a damaged vessel before the situation became critical. Tears of vessels have been reported during laparoscopic fusion (4). In the cases requiring con-

version to an open surgery, the vascular injury was addressed without serious sequelae. It was reported that among six cases converted to an open procedure due to iliac vein laceration or excessive bleeding, only one patient received a blood transfusion. When performing laparoscopic fusion, one must be acutely aware of the risk of vascular injury and have a plan to convert to an open procedure if needed. The equipment necessary for quick and safe conversion to an open procedure must be readily available.

Based on a review of abdominal vascular studies, Vraney et al. suggested that the L4-5 disc could be accessed laparoscopically in only approximately one-third of patients (5). The limiting factor was the location of the bifurcation of the great vessels with respect to the L4-5 disc space. The risk of vascular complications was thought to be too great in the remaining cases. However, Regan et al. reported that by varying the approach to the disc, to either above the bifurcation, below the bifurcation, or between the vessels, the disc space could be assessed in all cases and no patient had been denied a laparoscopic fusion based on the location of the vessel bifurcation (6).

A rare vascular complication of anterior lumbar interbody fusion is occlusion of the common iliac artery. This has been discussed in a few case reports (7–10). One case of aortic thrombosis following anterior-posterior fusion has been reported (11). The patient's condition continued to deteriorate after intensive treatment and she died 8 days after the spine surgery. In such cases, the vascular occlusion is usually caused by direct pressure of the vascular structures by the retractors. Vascular complications may be more likely or more severe in patients with risk factors such as smoking and vascular calcification.

Sexual Dysfunction

Retrograde ejaculation can occur with anterior spine surgery as a result of injury to the superior hypogastric plexus which is responsible for closing the bladder neck during ejaculation. This complication can be permanent; however, it typically resolves in 3 to 6 months after surgery, although it has been reported to take longer in some cases. The incidence and outcome of sexual dysfunction were studied in detail in a series of 41 men who underwent anterior lumbar interbody fusion using a retroperitoneal approach (12). The authors reported that 8% of the patients experienced retrograde ejaculation, but none had any alteration in attaining erection or achieving orgasm. Among the four patients in that study with retrograde ejaculation, two were permanent, one could not ejaculate for six months and had reduced ability to ejaculate thereafter, and the status of the other patient was unknown. In another study of complications related to anterior spine surgery, 9.6% of 31 male patients reported sexual dysfunction (two with retrograde ejaculation and one with reported impotence) following anterior spine surgery (3). Although impotence has been reported as a direct complication of anterior spine surgery, it is not very likely (3) since the parasympathetic plexus, which is responsible for erection, is located deep within the pelvis and should not be at risk during anterior spine surgery.

Ureteral Injury

Ureteral injury from blunt trauma can occur during anterior approaches to the lumbar spine. If not identified and addressed intraoperatively, the patient can experience severe abdominal pain from a large collection of urine in the abdomen. A few cases of ureteral injury related to anterior spine surgery have been reported (13–15). Bladder dysfunction from injury to the parasympathetic presacral nerve during the anterior portion of a combined anterior-posterior fusion has been reported (16). The patient was treated with self-catheterization and she ultimately regained bladder control in 3 months.

Neural Injury

Injury to the cauda equina or nerve roots may occur during anterior spinal surgery. This can be the result of passing instruments too deeply into the disc space, placing devices or bone graft too far posteriorly, by pushing disc tissue into the canal space, or by stretching the roots by over-distraction of the disc space.

In a cadaveric study, Taylor et al. investigated the occurrence of foraminal violation and nerve root impingement related to the use of anteriorly placed interbody fusion cages (17). Although the number of samples was small, the authors concluded that the occurrence of foraminal violation or neural impingement was reduced if a device was placed directly in the midline. The incidence of impingement was increased when the devices were placed 10% off midline, and increased further when the devices were placed 20% off midline.

Several studies have reported that the lateral placement of cages can cause disc tissue to be displaced posteriorly, resulting in nerve root compression (18,19). Patients with this complication generally complain of severe radicular pain immediately following surgery. Imaging can sometimes be difficult to interpret due to artifact from the metal cages. In a nonrandomized study comparing open to laparoscopic fusion using BAK cages, disc herniation was the only complication that was more common in the laparoscopic fusion group, occurring in 2.8% of cases (4).

Sympathetic sensory changes can occur and may result in a "warm leg", temperature variation, dysesthesia, discoloration, or swelling of the leg or foot (3,20). These patients should be evaluated carefully to rule out possible arterial complications. If the problem is not vascular, the altered sensations generally resolve over the course of several months.

Papastefanou et al. reported two cases of femoral nerve palsy due to patient positioning during anterior lumbar interbody fusion (21). The patients' symptoms resolved in 3 to 6 months. The authors attributed the injury to the patients being positioned intraoperatively with the spine and hip immobilized in a position of maximum stretch of the psoas muscle, compressing the femoral nerve.

COMPLICATIONS REPORTED IN VARIOUS ANTERIOR FUSION STUDIES

The reported incidence and types of complications related to anterior spine surgery vary greatly. This may be due to the different types of procedure performed, the type of graft or device used, the skill and experience level of the spine and access surgeons, the associated patient comorbidities present, and other factors. Presented herein is a review of complications reported in some studies of anterior lumbar spine surgery. The review deals primarily with publications since 1990 and those involving patients with symptomatic disc degeneration.

Newman and Grinstead reported a series of 36 patients undergoing anterior interbody fusion with autogenous graft specifically for discogenic pain (22). Complications in their series included one each of pulmonary embolism, retrograde ejaculation, donor-site wound hematoma, and graft extrusion. There were no vascular complications, although 16.7% of patients received a blood transfusion. Reoperation occurred in 8.3% of patients from extruded graft, symptomatic pseudoarthrosis, or for disc herniation above the fusion.

In one of the largest series of anterior lumbar interbody fusions, Kuslich et al. reported on 591 patients in whom BAK cages packed with autogenous iliac crest graft were used as a stand-alone device (23). The data were collected from the multicenter United States Food and Drug Administration Investigational Device Exemption (FDA IDE) trial. The incidence of complications reported in that series included neurologic injury (2.0%), superficial infection (3.1%), ileus (3.1%), new radicular pain (1.3%), retrograde ejaculation (4% of males), hematoma/seroma (1.5%), vessel damage/bleeding (1.7%), atelectasis/pneumonia (1.9%), urologic complications (1.4%), wound problems (1.2%), phlebitis/pulmonary embolism (0.7%), fatigue fracture of the S1 vertebral body (1.3%), and other complications (0.3%). In 0.8% of the study group, implant migration required reoperation. In an additional 1.5% there was implant migration not requiring reoperation. The authors did not provide data for the total reoperation rate in the patients undergoing anterior fusion with the cages. There were no cases of device failure, death, major paralysis, or deep infections. The low complication rate in this series was very impressive, since it represented the initial experience using this implant.

experienced the sudden onset of radiating leg pain, one at 2 months postoperatively and the other at 10 days postoperatively. X-rays showed that in both cases, both of the cages had migrated posteriorly. Reoperation was undertaken using pedicle screws to distract the disc space open. The retropulsed cages were then visualized and pushed anteriorly, and compression was then applied to the pedicle screws to lock the cages in place. The authors did not report the total number of cases in which the devices had been used and therefore the overall incidence of cage retropulsion could not be calculated.

Whitecloud et al. described their experience in a retrospective, nonrandomized study comparing a transforaminal posterior interbody fusion with combined anterior-posterior fusion (34). All procedures were performed using Harms cages packed with autogenous graft and pedicle screw fixation. Among the patients in the combined anterior interbody group, there was one iliac vein tear and six cases of ileus, only one of which prolonged the hospital stay. Twenty-three of the 40 patients received a blood transfusion, averaging 2.2 units. In the transforaminal group, there was one dural laceration, and six of the 40 patients received packed red blood cells, averaging 1.2 units. The transfusion rates in this study were much greater than reported in other studies and no reason for the high rate of transfusion could be determined.

Cages as Stand-Alone Devices

The use of titanium-threaded cylindrical cages as stand-alone devices without supplemental posterior fixation has been very controversial. However, there is little information suggesting significant problems using cages as stand-alone devices. One study reported a 31% reoperation rate among patients in whom the cages were used as stand-alone devices (35). The revision surgery was to add posterior fixation. This experience did not mirror that reported in some of the large series in which less than 8% of patients underwent reoperation at the same level to add supplemental posterior fixation (4,23,27). The reason for the discrepancies cannot be determined.

POSTERIOR FUSION

There is little literature available on the treatment of symptomatic disc degeneration using posterior fusion alone. Most surgeons think this is a suboptimal method for treating disc-related pain because the disc is not addressed directly. However, there have been a few reports on using this treatment method. Wood et al. reported on a series of 28 patients undergoing posterior fusion with pedicle screw and plate fixation and autogenous iliac crest bone graft (36). Reoperation for the removal of the internal fixation was performed in 14% of patients. There was a 32% complication rate including 6 wound infections (9.7%) (3 of which required reopera-

tion), phlebitis (3.2%), ileus (1.6%), pulmonary embolism (1.6%), urinary retention (1.6%), and wound necrosis (1.6%). Screw loosening occurred in 3 patients, but there were no cases of neurologic complications, pedicle breeches, or broken screws. However, it should be noted that this was a small series of patients, which makes it difficult to determine the true incidence of complications.

COMBINED ANTERIOR-POSTERIOR SPINE SURGERY

The term *combined anterior-posterior fusion* is synonymous with a 360° (circumferential) fusion, that is, an anterior interbody fusion combined with posterior fusion, with or without pedicle screw fixation. One benefit of 360° fusion is that it directly addresses the interbody space anteriorly, thereby avoiding the potential difficulties of posterior interbody fusion. The posterior fusion allows direct access to any posterior pathology, such as nerve root compression, and permits stabilization of the posterior column of the spine. The disadvantages of the combined procedure include the prolonged operative time, increased blood loss, greater risk of complications, and higher cost. The 360° fusions have typically been associated with a high fusion rate, but it has a greater risk of complications since two approaches to the spine are involved. There is also a risk of accelerated deterioration of the adjacent segment(s) due to the rigidity of the construct. The role of combined anterior interbody fusion with a posterior fusion is controversial. In recent years, however, it has gained popularity partially because of newer technologies, such as carbon fiber and other forms of cages, because of renewed interest in femoral ring allografts, and because of the use of minimally invasive posterior instrumented fusion, translaminar facet screw fusion, and other modifications.

Traditional 360° Fusion

Complications of traditional 360° fusions were reported by Gertzbein et al. in a series of 82 patients who underwent fusion with anterior allograft and posterior pedicle screw fusion (37). Complications included one death due to pulmonary embolism, two cases of deep vein thrombosis, two cases of paralytic ileus, and one case each of the following: iliac vein injury requiring repair, deep infection, superficial infection, dural tear, pneumonia, pulmonary edema, reflex sympathetic dystrophy, graft fracture, retroperitoneal hematoma, S1 nerve root injury, and wound dehiscence. Instrument-related complications included three broken screws and one broken rod. The posterior fixation was removed in two patients due to presumed symptoms.

Liljenqvist et al. reported their experience with 360° fusion using anterior femoral ring allograft and posterior translaminar screws in 41 patients (38). Complications included one of each of the following: peritoneal tear, common iliac vein tear, intraoperative fracture of the femoral graft, postoperative fracture of the femoral graft, deep vein thrombosis, dural tear, and retrograde ejaculation. One case of nerve root irritation required reoperation, as did one case of incisional abdominal hernia. Chronic graft donor-site pain was reported by 23.5% of patients.

Thalgott et al. reported on what was termed a "minimally invasive 360°" fusion (39). The technique combined endoscopic anterior interbody fusion with minimally invasive posterior screw fixation and fusion. Of the original 64 patients, 18 (28%) were converted to an open anterior fusion. Complications in the remaining 46 patients included one vessel laceration and six dural tears, all of which were repaired without event. There were four cases of interbody cage migration, none of which were of consequence. The authors noted that this series represented their initial experience with this new technique. The high rate of conversions to open surgery likely represents the authors' learning curve and a cautious approach to avoid significant complications.

Schofferman et al. reported on combined anterior-posterior fusion with pedicle screws, randomizing patients to receive either bone graft or no bone graft with the posterior instrumentation (40). Among the 26 patients in the group receiving bone graft, the complications included 1 case of deep vein thrombosis (3.8%) and 3 dural tears (11.5%). In the group of 22 patients who received instrumentation but no bone graft, the complications included 2 dural tears (9.1%). The reoperation rate to remove instrumentation was high in both groups at 62% and 64%, respectively, for residual low back pain associated with tenderness over the instrumentation.

POSTERIOR INTERBODY WITH POSTERIOR FUSION OR FIXATION

Some surgeons advocate combining PLIF with posterior fusion or fixation. This approach has the potential benefit of avoiding additional anterior spine surgery. There are several methods for accessing the disc space posteriorly as well as various types of posterior fixation, used either with or without bone graft.

Freeman et al. reported a 5-year follow-up of 60 patients undergoing combined posterior interbody and instrumented posterolateral fusion (41). In the majority of the interbody fusions, autogenous iliac crest graft was used. Complications in the series included four neurologic complications (6.7%), two of which resolved spontaneously, one of which required reoperation to reposition a pedicle screw, and one of which had bilateral foot drop, which resolved unilaterally. Three patients developed deep vein thrombosis, and there was one superficial wound infection.

There have been several studies reporting the use of carbon fiber cages and posterior fixation. Carbon fiber cages are typically rectangular and are used in pairs at each operated level with bone graft packed into the cages. They are designed to be used with posterior fixation, rather than as stand-alone devices. The potential benefit of carbon fiber cages compared to metal cages is that radiographic assessment is facilitated. The largest series of patients undergoing fusion with carbon fiber cages was published by Brantigan et al. (42) and involved 221 patients undergoing PLIF with supplemented pedicle screw fixation. There was a 13.5% rate of cage-related complications, including two cages that were cracked during implantation and 16 broken pedicle screws in 13 patients. Other complications in the series included two intraoperative deaths (one due to intraoperative bleeding and the other due to myocardial infarction), deep infections requiring reoperation (8 patients), deep vein thrombosis (2 patients), reflex sympathetic dystrophy (3 patients), increased motor deficit (3 patients), and myocardial infarction (1 patient). Two other patients in the study died of unrelated medical problems and two committed suicide. Additionally, the authors reported a 13.2% rate of what they described as "minor nondevice-related" complications and a 26.2% rate of what was termed "insignificant events" including 41 dural tears. The reoperation rate was 46.1%, including removal of the posterior instrumentation in 78 patients (35.2%). Other reoperations included repair of dural tears (6 patients), removal of retained drains (3 patients), the need to address pain coming from a different disc level (6 patients), and revision of pedicle screws or cages (5 patients). The complication rate in this series is greater than that reported in other studies. It cannot be determined if this is attributable to the devices themselves, the technique use to implant them, patient selection, or the skill level and training of the physicians involved. However, the data were from the FDA IDE study, which typically involves surgeons with a high level of expertise.

In a smaller series of 51 patients undergoing posterior interbody fusion using paired carbon fiber cages augmented with pedicle screw fixation, Tullberg et al. reported no cases of device failure (43). They reported three dural tears, one infection, and one case of screw loosening. Several years later, Tullberg published a case report involving a failed carbon fiber cage (44). During reoperation to remove the posterior fixation, a black discoloration of the dura and nerves was noted. The broken cages were later removed, and histologic analysis showed many carbon fiber particles but little inflammation around them. This case exemplifies one of the concerns of using carbon fiber implants, that is, fracture of the device with pieces of the cage infiltrating the area near neural structures.

In a series of 71 patients undergoing fusion using Ostaped carbon cages supplemented with posterior pedicle screw fixation (45) complications included seven neurologic complications (9.8%), two of which required reoperation for removal of the pedicle screw and plate fixation. Four additional patients underwent removal of the posterior fixation due to continued pain. The authors also reported two dural tears that were repaired intraoperatively.

In a study dealing primarily with psychological factors and surgical outcome, Tandon et al. reported on 58 patients who underwent interbody fusion using carbon fiber cages supplemented with posterior pedicle screw and plate fixation (46). Complications in this series included transient altered sensation in the foot (4), foot drop (1), malpositioned cages resulting in reoperation requiring piecemeal removal of the devices and fusion anteriorly (1), and one asymptomatic broken pedicle screw.

Some authors have advocated a transforaminal approach for posterior interbody fusion. Purported advantages of this technique include excellent access to the disc space and reduced risk of neurologic injury. Humphreys et al. compared the posterior and transforaminal approach for lumbar interbody fusion (47). Pedicle screw fixation was used in all cases. In the transforaminal cases, bone graft was packed anteriorly and a single Harms cage was placed in the middle and posterior portion of the interspace. In the posterior interbody group, a single cage was also used. The authors reported no complications in the group of 40 patients with transforaminal interbody fusion. Complications in the 34 patients with posterior interbody fusion included radiculitis (four cases), broken hardware (one case), screw loosening (one case), screw removal (two cases), superficial infection (one case), and pseudoarthrosis requiring reoperation (one case).

Jun et al. reported a small study of 36 patients undergoing posterior interbody fusion using a facetolaminotomy approach to the disc space (48). After placing carbon fiber cages and a block of autogenous iliac crest bone in the disc space, a facet fusion was performed using translaminar facet screws. The authors reported no neurologic complications or any screw breakage or loosening with this technique.

ADDRESSING FUSION CAGE PLACEMENT DIFFICULTIES

The large number of threaded cages has created the need to understand the genesis of complications and how to treat them. McAfee et al. reviewed a group of 20 patients who underwent reoperation for cage-related problems (19) and concluded that in all cases, the problems were due to technical error. In anterior procedures, the main problem was that the cage placement was too lateral, which pushed disc tissue from the space and resulted in compression of the nerve roots. When we encounter malpositioned cages placed too far anteriorly

and pushing disc tissue onto the nerve roots, we perform a posterior decompression and remove the compressing tissue (49). If the cage is positioned too far posteriorly, an anterior procedure can be performed to remove the cage and to replace it with bone graft, or to rotate the cage and move it more anteriorly. Typically, malpositioning problems are recognized early in the postoperative period, and anterior revision surgery is performed soon after the initial surgery. This allows the problem to be addressed as soon as possible before significant scar had formed. Repeat anterior surgery can be difficult as well as hazardous due to scarring and adhesions to vascular structures. In a review of complications related to anterior spine surgery, Rajaraman et al. reported significant difficulties when trying to retrieve a malpositioned cage (3). This resulted in a major vascular injury due to dense adhesions between the posterior vessel wall and the instrumentation. There was significant blood loss and the surgery had to be abandoned.

Reoperation to remove a migrated cage more than 14 months after posterior interbody fusion and pedicle screw and plate fixation has been reported (50). To avoid potential complications related to revising the cage through a posterior approach, an anterior approach was used. An osteotomy of the superior vertebral body was required because of bony ingrowth into one cage. The migrated cage was noted to have a fibrous union and was removed. During subsequent revision of the posterior fixation, it was noted that two of the four pedicle screws had breached the canal or foramen. The patient had a good result after the revision.

In some cases, two cages cannot be placed safely due to the degree of vessel retraction required to gain adequate access to the disc space (49). In such instances, a femoral ring allograft can instead be used without injury to the vessels. In some patients, the disc width cannot safely accept two cages of the diameter required to produce adequate purchase. Under such circumstances, one cage can be placed in the center of the disc space and bone graft placed on each side.

In a series of 35 patients, Hodges et al. reported intraoperative cage loosening in three patients (51). In these cases, the initially placed cage appeared to be well positioned and firmly seated. However, after the implantation of the second cage, the first cage was noted to be loose. In all three cases, the loose cage was replaced with a larger cage without subsequent problems. The loosening was only identified during a final check before closing. We have also noted cases where a loose cage fit was noted intraoperatively (49). Under such circumstances, the cage can be removed and replaced with bone graft.

In a review by McAfee et al. of malpositioned cages, posterior interbody procedures were associated with cage migration into the epidural space (19). This was attributed to the selection of too small of a cage to achieve adequate purchase into the vertebral bodies or the cages not being seated deeply enough into the disc space. The selection of small cages may have been related to the difficulty of trying to adequately access the disc space for fear of over-distracting the neural structures.

DONOR SITE COMPLICATIONS

One of the potential complications of lumbar spinal fusion is related to harvest of autogenous iliac crest graft. The reported incidence of donor-site pain varies in the literature that is likely related to variation in surgical technique, and the methodology for recording and defining pain. There are also other potential complications from the harvesting of autogenous iliac crest graft. Vascular injury, particularly to the superior gluteal artery, can occur. Neurologic injury can also occur at the donor site. The anterior nerve primarily at risk is the lateral femoral cutaneous nerve, although the ilioinguinal nerve may also be injured. The superior cluneal nerves are at risk with posterior iliac crest harvesting. Painful neuromas may occur with nerve injury. Fracture of the ilium may also occur, although this is not common. Fractures are typically seen in patients with osteoporosis, or in patients with previous injury to the ilium. There is a risk of deep or superficial infection, or hematoma formation.

One study compared the donor-site pain associated with two different harvest methods in two groups of 30 patients each (52). In one group of patients, harvesting included the outer cortex and cancellous bone beneath it. In the other group, a small opening was made in the cortex and only cancellous bone from between the cortices was taken. The authors found no statistically significant difference in donor-site pain with either method used. Two years after surgery, donor-site pain was reported in 17% in the first group and 20% in the second group.

In a prospective study of donor-site pain, Robertson and Wray reported relatively minor levels of donor-site pain (53). On a scale of 0 to 10, at 3 months after surgery, the mean score was 1.6, and at 12 months postoperatively it was only 1.2. A score of greater than 3 was reported by 12% of patients, while 55% of patients reported a score of 0. Although the mean pain values were low, the authors reported that 13% of patients had numbness at the scar, 10% had local sensory loss in the distribution of the cluneal nerves, and 35% had a palpable soft-tissue defect, many with related tenderness.

In another study involving 290 patients, 25% of patients had significant donor-site pain, 24% had an acceptable level of pain, and 51% had no pain (54). In a subgroup of 81 patients who returned for an assessment, significant numbness at the donor site was noted by 31% of patients, and an additional 17% had lesser degrees of numbness. Radiographs taken in another subgroup of 58 patients showed that none of the donor sites filled in with new bone to any significant degree, and in some patients, bony spikes had formed in the harvest area.

In a review of 414 patients, major donor-site complications occurred in 5.8% of patients (55). These included two donor-site hernias, three vascular injuries, six nerve injuries, seven deep infections, four deep hematomas, and two iliac fractures. Minor donor-site complications were reported in 10% of patients and consisted of superficial infections, seromas, and hematomas. The authors did not report on donor-site pain.

In a series of 147 patients, Fernyhough et al. found that 29% of patients had chronic donor-site pain at 1-year follow-up (56). They found no difference in the incidence of pain related to harvest technique when comparing a midline incision (harvesting through the same incision as the posterior fusion) versus a separate lateral incision to access the posterior iliac crest. Although an aching sensation was common in the entire study group, it was more common in the midline group, possibly because of the close proximity of the lateral incision to the cluneal nerves. The authors also reported that patients who underwent reconstructive surgery were twice as likely to have donor-site pain as patients who underwent surgery for traumatic injuries. This finding suggests that patients with chronic pain may be predisposed to more postoperative pain complaints that may be related to psychological or other factors.

In another study, two approaches to the posterior iliac crest for graft harvest were compared (57). In one group, an oblique incision was made parallel to the iliac crest (standard incision). In the other group, a more vertical incision was made parallel to the superior cluneal nerves and perpendicular to the posterior iliac crest (modified incision). At 1 month after surgery, 44% of the modified incision group and 74% of the standard incision group reported numbness at the donor site. At 6-month follow-up, these figures improved slightly in both groups to 42% and 68%, respectively. The percentages of patients reporting deep pain at 6 months was similar in the 2 groups (60% and 54%), although the modified incision group had less activity-related tenderness.

Another review of 225 patients reported no injuries to the superior gluteal artery or sciatic nerve. There were also no deep wound infections, herniation, meralgia paresthetica, instability, or fracture (58). Ten percent of patients had major complications, including two patients with wound drainage, one with a scar requiring revision surgery, twelve with unsightly scars, and three with chronic pain, limiting activities. Most of these patients also had local dysesthesia at the donor site. Minor complications were noted in 39% of patients. These included dysesthesia that resolved in 6 months, prolonged wound drainage, one superficial infection, and one retained drain. Of note is that many of the minor complications were identified by patient questionnaire but were not recorded during follow-up visits. This may suggest an under-reporting of problems unless the physician specifically addresses donor-site pain or scar problems during all follow-up visits. Several authors noted that scar problems emerged more than 6 months after surgery.

One potential method to avoid donor-site complications is the use of allograft. However, there may be concerns about the quality of allograft and risk of disease transmission. The use of allograft with fusion cages has not been investigated. For posterior fusion, the use of local autogenous graft has been reported to yield fusion rates similar to that using iliac crest graft (59). If enough local bone graft is not available, a graft extender or supplement can be used. Bone morphogenetic protein (BMP) and local gene therapy hold great promise for enhancing fusion rates and avoiding donor-site complications (60,61). BMP has yielded promising results in a small clinical series (62).

ARTIFICIAL DISCS

In recent years there has been a great deal of interest in artificial discs. The approach used to implant disc replacements is the same as is used for anterior interbody fusion using other devices. Disc replacement is most commonly used to treat symptoms related to internal disc disruption or disc degeneration that has failed to respond to nonoperative care. Currently, there are two total disc replacements and one disc nucleus replacement that have been used in large numbers of patients. One of the artificial discs, the Charité, has been used in Europe for more than 15 years. The third modification design of this device has been used for more than 10 years. This device is a polyethylene core placed between two metal plates. With the initial two designs of this disc, there were problems with subsidence. The third design addressed problems encountered with the earlier models. The other total disc replacement, the ProDisc, has been used in Europe for more than 10 years. There are several reports in the literature on complications related to these devices. In addition to complications related to any anterior spine surgery, the primary potential complications related to disc replacement devices are displacement, device failure, and wear debris.

With the early designs of the Charité disc, failure of the metallic endplates in occurred 31% of cases (63). In addition, anterior displacement of the device occurred in 22% of patients. In 31% of patients, the device subsided into the vertebral bodies. Redesign of the device (the Charité III) and subsequent experience have resulted in a much lower rate of complications. There have been no reported cases of device failure associated with the SB Charité III.

Evaluating the rate of complications from the Charité artificial disc is difficult due to overlap between authors of some of the series, which may have resulted in some

patients and complications being recorded more than once. In a series of 105 patients, Lemaire et al. noted a 10% complication rate (64). This included five vascular problems, two cases of neurologic deficits (one resolved spontaneously, the other required to revision surgery and fixation), and four cases of bone-related complications (one posttraumatic vertebral body endplate fracture, one case of subsidence into osteoporotic bone, and two cases of periprosthetic ossification). Cinotti et al. reported on a separate group of 46 patients (65). Implant subsidence occurred in four patients in whom too small of an implant was used, although this did not affect clinical outcome. Periprosthetic ossification was related to immobilization from a corset for 3 months postoperatively, and to malposition of the implant. David reported a 5-year follow-up of 96 patients, in which complications included one device removal and fusion for severe sciatica, one case of bone migration requiring reoperation and fusion, and eight cases requiring subsequent instrumented posterior fusion for device malpositioning and facet pain (66).

A multicenter review of the Charité III involving 93 patients and 139 disc levels revealed only one device-related problem, that being one case of deformation of the metal ring around the polyethylene core (67). This remained in place and posed no clinical risk to the patient. There was a 6.5% incidence of implant migration or subsidence due to using the wrong size implant. Other complications identified included phlebitis/leg thrombosis (2 cases), vein injury (6 cases), wound bleeding or dehiscence (2 cases), superficial infection (1 case), muscle atrophy (1 case), urinary tract infection (4 cases), incontinence (3 cases), constipation (4 cases), nausea (1 case), skin paresthesia (1 case), hematoma (11 cases), hypotension due to blood loss (1 case), retrograde ejaculation (1 case), reflex sympathetic dystrophy (1 case), paresthesia (1 case), unspecified neurologic problems (2 case), and pain (10 case). There were three reoperations in the group of 93 patients that included one case of percutaneous nucleotomy, one foraminotomy, and one combined anterior-posterior fusion. The authors did not describe if the fusion was at the same level as the prosthesis or at another segment.

Zeegers et al. reported a series of 50 patients in which there were 52 problems in 30 patients (68). Unresolved complications included dysesthesia into the legs (3 cases), sympathetic effect (4 cases), and malpositioned prosthesis (1 cases). Complications that did resolve included neurologic problems (7 cases), hematoma (12 cases), painful or numb scars (5 cases), abdominal problems (3 cases), new or progressive pain (5 cases), vascular problem (1 case), urinary tract infection (4 cases), retrograde ejaculation (1 case), and deep vein thrombosis (1 case). In one patient, repositioning of a malpositioned prosthesis was attempted and abandoned with subsequent fusion performed. There were instances of significant vascular injury during the procedure. In total, there was a 24% reoperation rate, primarily for pain control. The authors noted that this series consisted of their first 50 consecutive patients, and many of the problems encountered were likely attributable to a learning curve.

Sott and Harrison reported a series of 14 patients undergoing the Charité disc replacement (69). They found five patients (36%) with a "warm" left foot related to injury of the paravertebral sympathetic nerves, and one case of implant subsidence.

The other artificial disc that has been used for more than 10 years in Europe is the ProDisc. This design includes two metal plates with a polyethylene core between them. The core is flat on the inferior surface and slides into the inferior metal plate. There have been no reports of device failure related to this artificial disc, but there are only a few articles reporting on this device. In one study reporting 8- to 10-year follow-up, complications included one iliac vein tear that was uneventfully repaired intraoperatively, one case of appendicitis with peritonitis, and one disc herniation at the level above an ankylosed prosthetic disc (70).

One disc nucleus replacement, the Ray PDN (Prosthetic Disc Nucleus), has been used in large series of patients, although no reports on clinical experience with it have been published at this time. The device consists of a hydrogel material placed inside a woven restraining jacket. The hydrogel absorbs water and expands after being placed into the evacuated disc space. Two devices are placed at each operated level. The primary complication related to this device is migration, which has been reported in 10% of patients (71).

INFECTION

There has been little published on infection associated with surgery for the treatment of symptomatic disc degeneration. Several series report on the occurrence of superficial wound infections at the surgical site or the donor site. Of greater concern are deep infections. Fortunately these are rare. Glassman et al. investigated the treatment and outcome of 19 patients with deep infection related to spine surgery (72). The patients were treated with multiple irrigation and débridement procedures as well as antibiotic treatment. Outcome was assessed 12 to 42 months after the fusion surgery. Compared to their preoperative condition, 57.9% of patients were significantly improved, 21.0% were improved, and the remaining 21.1% were unchanged or worse than their preoperative condition (one of whom had a permanent neurologic injury during the surgery). Solid fusion was achieved in 73.6% of patients and in 21.0% fusion was probable. These results indicate that although deep infection related to spinal fusion is a significant problem, acceptable long-term results can be achieved with aggressive treatment.

INTRADISCAL ELECTROTHERMAL THERAPY

One relatively new method available for the treatment of disc-related pain is intradiscal electrothermal therapy (IDET). During this procedure, a catheter with a thermal coil is percutaneously placed into the disc. As the device heats up, it is thought to cause thermocoagulation of nociceptors in the disc annulus. It is also thought to modify the collagen in the disc as it heals. This is a new treatment with few reports on its outcome and complications. The most likely potential complication is injury to the nerve root during placement of the guide needle for the catheter. Other possible complications include thermal damage to the cord or nerve roots, and infection. Two reports on IDET published by the originators of the procedure noted no complications (73,74). A third paper by other authors did not comment on complications (75). One case of cauda equina injury during IDET has been reported (76). The presence or absence of complications associated with IDET has been addressed in less than 100 reported patients. This number is too small to adequately address the risk of occurrence of complications, particularly since these are the earliest reports using this device, many of which were performed and reported by the physicians who devised the procedure and were best acquainted with the device.

DISCUSSION

Many treatment options are available for symptomatic disc degeneration unresponsive to nonoperative treatment. The surgical treatment armamentarium for this condition continues to grow. In addition to traditional fusion, there are now a variety of different surgical approaches and devices to use. Avoiding complications is a primary goal in any operative procedure. In order to do so, one must consider the options available, the advantages and disadvantages of each—with particular application to the individual patient, and the surgeon's own level of training, experience, and comfort level associated with each option. As seen in this review, the type of complications and their incidence vary greatly. The reasons for this are not clear. It probably has to do with patient selection, patient comorbidities, skill and experience of the surgical team, the type of surgery used, and other factors. As discussed by Kain et al. in a review of complications of anterior lumbar interbody fusion, the complication rates appeared to be lower among surgeons with the largest group of patients (77). It may be that not only must one be properly trained in performing a technique, one must practice frequently enough to build and maintain an optimal skill level.

As described earlier, some potential complications can be avoided by altering the operative plan when difficulty is encountered. This is seen in laparoscopic cases where conversion to open surgery is done when there is difficulty with exposure, visualization, or other problems. When using cages, for example, difficulty placing a pair of cages or one of the devices may mandate altering the procedure to use allograft rather than a cage. One must plan to have proper equipment and graft materials readily available for unexpected changes in preoperative plans.

There are now many options available for the treatment of disc-related pain. There are various forms of fusion cages, some of which can be used as stand-alone devices, and others that are designed for use with posterior fixation. Other surgical options include disc replacement and IDET. It is likely that in the future, even more treatment options will be available. There are no definitive answers concerning which option is the best for any individual patient. IDET, for example, has the benefit of being a minimally invasive procedure. However, it is applicable to a relatively narrow spectrum of conditions and still needs further investigation. Artificial discs have been used with great success in Europe. The complications associated with these devices seem similar to those traditionally encountered with anterior interbody fusion. Artificial disc replacement is currently available in the United States only on a limited basis as investigational devices. Therefore, interbody fusion is currently the primary treatment option for symptomatic disc degeneration unresponsive to nonoperative care. The decisions concerning which fusion cage or allograft to use, which surgical approach to use, and whether or not to combine it with supplemental posterior fixation, are left to the discretion of the surgeon. The choice of treatment will vary based on the surgeon's training and experience, the patient's anatomy and history, and the details of the problem being treated. Surgeons must take every reasonable measure to reduce the risk including being aware of patient comorbidities and previous surgical history. One of the most important factors in reducing complications and the severity of their course is the surgeon's training and experience. New procedures should be undertaken only after the surgeon has undergone appropriate training. Important considerations include appropriate patient selection, the presence of anatomic variations and contraindications to the procedure, and hands-on training in the use of the instruments and surgical techniques. Despite enthusiasm over new techniques and devices, caution and appropriate training is mandatory to avoid complications.

REFERENCES

1. Weiner B, Walker M, Fraser RD. Vascular anatomy anterior to lumbosacral transitional vertebrae and implications for anterior lumbar interbody fusion. Spine J 2001;1:442–444.
2. Baker JK, Reardon PR, Reardon MJ, et al. Vascular injury in anterior lumbar surgery. Spine 1993;18:2227–2230.
3. Rajaraman V, Vingan R, Roth P, et al. Visceral and vascular complications resulting from anterior lumbar interbody fusion. J Neurosurg 1999;91:60–64.
4. Regan JJ, Yuan H, McAfee PC. Laparoscopic fusion of the lumbar spine: minimally invasive spine surgery. A prospective multicenter study evaluating open and laparoscopic lumbar fusion. Spine 1999;24:402–411.
5. Vraney RT, Phillips FM, Wetzel FT, et al. Peridiscal vascular anatomy of the lower lumbar spine. An endoscopic perspective. Spine 1999;24:2183–2187.
6. Regan JJ, Aronoff RJ, Ohnmeiss DD, et al. Laparoscopic approach to L4-L5 for interbody fusion using BAK cages: experience in the first 58 cases. Spine 1999;24:2171–2174.
7. Hackenberg L, Liljenqvist U, Halm H, et al. Occlusion of the left common iliac artery and consecutive thromboembolism of the left popliteal artery following anterior lumbar interbody fusion. J Spinal Disord 2001;14:365–368.
8. Khazim R, Boos N, Webb JK. Progressive thrombotic occlusion of the left common iliac artery after anterior lumbar interbody fusion. Eur Spine J 1998;7:239–241.
9. Marsicano J, Mirovsky Y, Remer S, et al. Thrombotic occlusion of the left common iliac artery after anterior retroperitoneal approach to the lumbar spine. Spine 1994;19:357–359.
10. Raskas DS, Delamarter RB. Occlusion of the left iliac artery after retroperitoneal exposure of the spine. Clin Orthop 1997;338:86–89.
11. Castro FP Jr, Hartz RS, Frigon V, et al. Aortic thrombosis after lumbar spine surgery. J Spinal Disord 2000;13:538–540.
12. Christensen FB, Bünger CE. Retrograde ejaculation after retroperitoneal lower lumbar interbody fusion. Int Orthop 1997;21:176–180.
13. Guingrich JA, McDermott JC. Ureteral injury during laparoscopy-assisted anterior lumbar fusion. Spine 2000;25:1586–1588.
14. Zekeriya ZU, Isiklar ZU, Lindsey RW, et al. Ureteral injury after anterior lumbar interbody fusion. A case report. Spine 1996;21:2379–2382.
15. Zdeblick TA, David SM. A prospective comparison of surgical approach for anterior L4-L5 fusion. Spine 2000;25:2682–2687.
16. Faraj AA, Webb JK, Lemberger RJ. Urinary bladder dysfunction following anterior lumbosacral spine fusion: case report and review of the literature. Eur Spine J 1996;5:121–124.
17. Taylor BA, Vaccaro AR, Hilibrand AS, et al. The risk of foraminal violation and nerve root impingement after anterior placement of lumbar interbody fusion cages. Spine 2001;26:100–104.
18. Regan JJ, Ohnmeiss DD. Laparoscopic lumbar fusion: single surgeon experience in 127 consecutive cases. Poster presented at the Annual Meeting of the American Academy of Orthopaedic Surgeons; March 2001; San Francisco, California.
19. McAfee PC, Cunningham BW, Lee GA, et al. Revision strategies for salvaging or improving failed cylindrical cages. Spine 1999;24:2147–2153.
20. Lieberman IH, Willsher PC, Litwin DEM, et al. Transperitoneal laparoscopic exposure for lumbar interbody fusion. Spine 2000;25:509–514.
21. Papastefanou SL, Stevens K, Mulholland RC. Femoral nerve palsy. An unusual complication of anterior lumbar interbody fusion. Spine 1994;19:2842–2844.
22. Newman MH, Grinstead GL. Anterior lumbar interbody fusion for internal disc disruption. Spine 1992;17:831–833.
23. Kuslich SD, Ulstrom CL, Griffith SL, et al. The Bagby and Kuslich method of lumbar interbody fusion. History, techniques, and 2-year follow-up results of a United States prospective, multicenter trial. Spine 1998;23:1267–1278.
24. Brown A, Slosar P, Reynolds J, et al. Paired BAK ProximityTM cages versus standard BAKTM: Subsidence and clinical failures. Presented at the Annual Meeting of the North American Spine Society; October 1999; Chicago, Illinois.
25. Davies MR, Geck MJ, Delamarter RB. Prospective comparison of fusion rates and subsidence between the BAK and BAK proximity cages. Presented at the Annual Meeting of the International Society for the Study of the Lumbar Spine; April 2000; Adelaide, Australia.
26. Pavlov PW, Spruit M, Havinga M, et al. Anterior lumbar interbody fusion with threaded fusion cages and autologous bone grafts. Eur Spine J 2000;9:224–229.
27. Tran V, Ohnmeiss DD, Blumenthal SL, et al. Analysis of re-operations when using cages as stand-alone devices: minimum three year follow-up study. Presented at the Meeting of the Americas; April 2002; New York, New York.
28. Sachs BL, McVoy J, Miller B, et al. A prospective, randomized com-

parison of laparoscopic to open anterior lumbar interbody fusion with cages. Presented at the Meeting of the Americas; April 2002; New York, New York.

29. Katkhouda N, Campos GM, Mavor E, et al. Is laparoscopic approach to lumbar spine fusion worthwhile? Am J Surg 1999;178:458–461.

30. Lee CK, Vessa P, Lee JK. Chronic disabling low back pain syndrome caused by internal disc derangements. The results of disc excision and posterior lumbar interbody fusion. Spine 1995;20:356–361.

31. Ray CD. Threaded titanium cages for lumbar interbody fusions. Spine 1997;22:667–680.

32. Elias WJ, Simmons NE, Kaptain GJ, et al. Complications of posterior lumbar interbody fusion with using a titanium threaded cage device. J Neurosurg 2000;93(Spine 1):45–52.

33. Uzi EA, Dabby D, Tolessa E, et al. Early retropulsion of titanium-threaded cages after posterior lumbar interbody fusion. A report of two cases. Spine 2000;26:1073–1075.

34. Whitecloud TS III, Roesch WW, Ricciardi JE. Transforaminal interbody fusion versus anterior-posterior interbody fusion of the lumbar spine: a financial analysis. J Spinal Disord 2001;14:100–103.

35. O'Dowd JK, Mulholland RC, Harris M. BAK cage: Nottingham results. Presented at the Annual Meeting of the North American Spine Society; October 1998; San Francisco, California.

36. Wood GW II, Boyd RJ, Carothers TA, et al. The effect of pedicle screw/plate fixation on lumbar/lumbosacral autogenous bone graft fusion in patients with degenerative disc disease. Spine 1995;20: 819–830.

37. Gertzbein SD, Betz R, Clements D, et al. Semirigid instrumentation in the management of lumbar spinal conditions combined with circumferential fusion. A multicenter study. Spine 1996;21:1981–1926.

38. Liljenqvist U, O'Brien JP, Renton P. Simultaneous combined anterior and posterior lumbar fusion with femoral cortical allograft. Eur Spine J 1998;7:125–131.

39. Thalgott JS, Chin AK, Ameriks JA, et al. Minimally invasive 360° instrumented lumbar fusion. Eur Spine J 2000;9[Suppl 1]:S51–S56.

40. Schofferman J, Slosar P, Reynolds J, et al. A prospective randomized comparison of 270° fusion to 360° fusions (circumferential fusions). Spine 2001;26:E207–E212.

41. Freeman BJC, Licina P, Mehdian SH. Posterior lumbar interbody fusion combined with instrumented postero-lateral fusion: 5-year results in 60 patients. Eur Spine J 2000;9:42–46.

42. Brantigan JW, Steffee AD, Lewis ML, et al. Lumbar interbody fusion using the Brantigan I/F cage for posterior lumbar interbody fusion and the variable pedicle screw placement system. Spine 2000;25: 1437–1446.

43. Tullberg T, Brandt B, Rydberg J, et al. Fusion rate after posterior lumbar interbody fusion with carbon fiber implant: 1-year follow-up of 51 patients. Eur Spine J 1996;5:178–182.

44. Tullberg T. Failure of a carbon fiber implant. A case report. Spine 1998;23:1804–1806.

45. Agazzi S, Reverdin A, May D. Posterior lumbar interbody fusion with cages: an independent review of 71 cases. J Neurosurg 1999;91[2 Suppl]:186–192.

46. Tandon VT, Campbell F, Ross ERS. Posterior lumbar interbody fusion. Association between disability and psychological disturbance in non-compensation patients. Spine 1999;24:1833–1838.

47. Humphreys SC, Hodges SD, Patwardhan AG, et al. Comparison of posterior and transforaminal approaches to lumbar interbody fusion. Spine 2001;26:567–71

48. Jun B-Y. Posterior lumbar interbody fusion with restoration of lamina and facet fusion. Spine 2000;25:917–922.

49. Blumenthal SL, Ohnmeiss DD, Regan JJ, et al. Addressing threaded fusion cage placement difficulties. Unpublished data; Texas Back Institute, Plano, Texas.

50. Glassman SD, Johnson JR, Raque G, et al. Management of iatrogenic spinal stenosis complicating placement of a fusion cage. Spine 1996; 21:2383–2386.

51. Hodges SD, Humphreys SC, Eck JC, Murphy RB. Intraoperative loosening of Bagby and Kuslich cages during anterior lumbar interbody fusion. J Spinal Disord 2000;13:535–537.

52. Mirovsky Y, Neuwirth MG. Comparison between the outer table and intracortical methods of obtaining autogenous bone graft from the iliac crest. Spine 2000;25:1722–1725.

53. Robertson PA, Wray AC. Natural history of posterior iliac crest bone graft donation for spinal surgery. A prospective analysis of morbidity. Spine 2001;1473–1476.

54. Summers BN, Eisenstein SM. Donor site from the ilium. A complication of lumbar spine fusion. J Bone Joint Surg [Br] 1989;677–680.

55. Arrington ED, Smith WJ, Chambers HG, et al. Complications of iliac crest bone graft harvesting. Clin Orthop 1996;329:300–309.

56. Fernyhough JC, Schimandle JJ, Weigel MC, et al. Chronic donor site pain complicating bone graft harvest from the posterior iliac crest for spinal fusion. Spine 1992;17:1474–1480.

57. Colterjohn NR, Bednar DA. Procurement of bone graft from the iliac crest. An operative approach with decreased morbidity. J Bone Joint Surg [Am] 1997;79:756–759.

58. Banwart JC, Asher MA, Hassanein RS. Iliac crest bone graft harvest donor site morbidity. A statistical evaluation. Spine 1995;20:1055–1060.

59. Hochschuler SH, Ohnmeiss DD, Hyde JA. Posterior lumbar fusion using local bone graft and pedicle screw fixation. Presented at the Annual Meeting of the International Society for the Study of the Lumbar Spine; June 2001; Edinburgh, Scotland.

60. Boden SD, Martin GJ Jr, Horton WC, Truss TL, Sandhu HS. Laparoscopic anterior spinal arthrodesis with rhBMP-2 in a titanium interbody threaded cage. J Spinal Disord 1998;11:95–101.

61. Boden SD, Titus L, Hair G, et al. Lumbar spine fusion by local gene therapy with a cDNA encoding a novel osteoinductive protein (LMP-1). Spine 1998;23:2486–2492.

62. Boden SD, Zdeblick TA, Sandhu HS, et al. The use of rhBMP-2 in interbody fusion cages. Definitive evidence of osteoinduction in humans: a preliminary report. Spine 2000;25:376–381.

63. Büttner-Janz K. The development of the artificial disc: SB Charité. Dallas: Hundley & Associates, 1992.

64. Lemaire JP, Skalli W, Lavaste F, et al. Intervertebral disc prosthesis. Results and prospects for the year 2000. Clin Orthop 1997;337:64–76.

65. Cinotti G, David T, Postacchini F. Results of disc prosthesis after a minimum follow-up period of 2 years. Spine 1996;21:995–1000.

66. David T. Lumbar disc prosthesis: five years follow-up study in 96 patients. Presented at the Annual Meeting of the North American Spine Society; October 2000; New Orleans, Louisiana.

67. Griffith SL, Shelokov AP, Buttner-Janz K, et al. A multicenter retrospective study of the clinical results of the Link SB Charité intervertebral prosthesis. The initial European experience. Spine 1994;19:1842–1849.

68. Zeegers WS, Bohnen LMLJ, Laaper M, et al. Artificial disc replacement with the modular type SB Charité III: 2-year results in 50 prospectively studied patients. Eur Spine J 1999;8:210–217.

69. Sott AH, Harrison DJ. Increasing age does not affect good outcome after lumbar disc replacement. Int Orthop 2000;24:50–53.

70. Marnay T. Lumbar disc arthroplasty: 8–10 years results using titanium plates with a polyethylene inlay component. Presented at the Annual Meeting of the American Academy of Orthopaedic Surgeons; March 2001; San Francisco, California.

71. Ray CD. Prosthetic disc nucleus 300 case update. Presented at the Annual Meeting of the Spinal Arthroplasty Society; May 2001; Munich, Germany.

72. Glassman SD, Dimar JR, Puno RM, et al. Salvage of instrumental lumbar fusions complicated by surgical wound infection. Spine 1996;21: 2163–2169.

73. Saal JS, Saal JA. Management of chronic discogenic low back pain with a thermal intradiscal catheter. A preliminary report. Spine 2000; 25:382–388.

74. Saal JA, Saal JS. Intradiscal electrothermal treatment for discogenic low back pain. Spine 2000;25:2622–2627.

75. Karasek M, Bogduk N. Twelve-month follow-up of a controlled trial of intradiscal thermal anuloplasty for back pain due to internal disc disruption. Spine 2000;25:2601–2607.

76. Hsia AW, Isaac K, Katz JS. Cauda equine syndrome from intradiscal electrothermal therapy. Neurology 2000; 55:320.

77. Kain C, Giesler B, Hochschuler SH. Anterior lumbar interbody fusion: lumbar approach, complications, and their prevention. Operative Tech Orthop 1993;3:225–231.

CHAPTER 38

Dynamic Stabilization in the Treatment of Low Back Pain Due to Degenerative Disorders

Dilip K. Sengupta

Several reports in the literature indicate that successful fusion may fail to improve chronic low back pain in a significant number of patients (1,2). This has renewed the interest in dynamic stabilization in the lumbosacral spine. Essentially, dynamic stabilization means instrumentation to control movement and load transmission through the motion segment. The terms *semirigid fixation*, *flexible stabilization*, and *soft stabilization* are apparently synonymous with dynamic stabilization. However, there is an essential difference between these terms. When the goal of stabilization is to improve the rate and quality of fusion without stress-shielding, the technique is called semirigid fixation. In contrast, when the goal is to preserve a controlled motion it is usually described as soft stabilization or flexible stabilization.

The following discussion elaborates the rationale, techniques, and evolution of the various dynamic stabilization systems in the treatment of chronic low back pain.

ROLE OF FUSION

The role of fusion in the treatment of degenerative low back pain is a matter of debate. In a review of the Cochrane databases for randomized controlled trials, Gibson et al. (1) concluded that for degenerative lumbar spondylosis there is no scientific evidence in favor of the effectiveness of any form of surgical decompression or fusion when compared with natural history, placebo, or conservative treatment. In contrast, in a multicenter randomized controlled trial, the Swedish Lumbar Spine Study Group reported that the outcome of fusion is significantly better than that of nonsurgical treatment. However, most authors agree that in a significant number of patients successful fusion may not produce adequate pain relief.

ETIOLOGY OF PERSISTENT BACK PAIN AFTER SUCCESSFUL FUSION

Chronic low back pain due to disc degeneration is believed to be generated by abnormal movement, abnormal load transmission, or both in the motion segment. When conservative treatment fails, the traditional surgical treatment is fusion. Theoretically, fusion should address both these mechanisms; load transmission is direct from bone to bone and there should be no movement after fusion. Instrumentation may be added to increase the fusion rate. Evolution of instrumentation techniques during the last decade has improved fusion rates to close to 95%. Unfortunately, this has not resulted in an equivalent success in the functional outcome (2).

It is unclear why pain persists in some patients following a successful fusion. The possible explanations that have been suggested by various authors may be summarized as follows:

1. Misinterpretation of pseudarthrosis as solid fusion
2. Adjacent segment disease
3. Abnormal load transmission despite fusion
4. Abnormal sagittal balance.

It has been well recognized that radiologic assessment of fusion is often unreliable (3–5). McAfee (6) reported that many cases of failed back syndrome following successful fusion were in fact a misinterpretation of pseudarthrosis. He emphasized that presence of the "sentinel sign", bridging bone in front of the cages, is the only definitive evidence of fusion. In a study involving 100 cases of failed back syndrome following apparent fusion, three-dimensional computed tomography (CT) uncovered incomplete fusion in 17%, transitional syndrome in 13%, and pseudarthrosis in 6% of cases (3). A solid fusion alters the biomechanics at the adjacent level, resulting in increased mechanical demands (7). There have been reports of increased rates of adjacent-level pathologic lesions after fusion, but these have not been taken into account for the natural history of degenerative changes (8,9). After solid fusion using metallic interbody cages, the mechanical stress at the contact surface of the end plate to the cages may be much higher than normal and may generate pain (10). Studies of finite element models have demonstrated that vertebral loads corresponding to certain activities may generate end-plate stresses at the control surface with cages that approach and exceed the failure stress for cortical bone (10,11). Loss of sagittal balance and "flat-back syndrome" following lumbar fusion may increase the stress at the adjacent segment leading to persistent back pain (12). In a review of 83 consecutive cases of spinal fusion, patients with abnormal C7 plumb line or abnormal sacral inclination in the immediate postoperative radiographs were found to have a much higher incidence of adjacent level degeneration compared with patients with normal sagittal balance (13). This has also been established in an *in vivo* study in a sheep fusion model (14).

ALTERNATIVE TO THE CONVENTIONAL FUSION PROCEDURES

Because of failure of fusion to relieve back pain, alternative surgical approaches have been developed. These may be broadly divided into three categories:

1. Semirigid stabilization—to achieve fusion without stress shielding
2. Artificial disc or nuclear prosthesis—to preserve motion and to stabilize the segment, while replacing a component of the motion segment
3. Dynamic stabilization—to preserve motion while stabilizing the segment, without replacement of any anatomic structure.

Semirigid Stabilization

As opposed to rigid stabilization, semirigid stabilization uses a somewhat flexible construct for fixation. The goal is to achieve fusion of the motion segment. The objective of semirigid implants is to avoid "stress shielding" which may discourage formation of the fusion mass, lead to osteoporosis, and cause loosening of implants. *In vitro* biomechanical studies showed semirigid devices share load with the anterior bone graft or cage to promote fusion (15,16).

Most authors describe semirigid rods between the pedicle screws. Musha et al. (17) reported over 97% successful fusion rate using a semirigid system consisting of rod and pedicle screws. Gertzbein et al. (18) reported 97% fusion rate using 4 mm threaded rod and polyaxial pedicle screw. They suggested that the system should only be used in conjunction with an anterior structural

support. Without this anterior support, the construct is expected to fail. Mochida et al. (19,20) described an ingenious method of using a Dacron ligament (Leeds Kieo Ligament, Neoligaments, Ltd., Leeds, UK) for spinal fusion, which was originally introduced for reconstruction of the anterior cruciate ligament. They described the technique as syndesmoplasty in which each end of the ligament is fed into a hole in the pedicle, crossed in a tunnel in the vertebral body, pulled out of the contralateral pedicle, and tied around the spinous process of the inferior segment. Their results were comparable to that with rigid fixation when the instability was small.

Artificial Disc or Nucleus Prosthesis

The goal of prosthetic replacement of the disc or the nucleus is to preserve motion. The pain is controlled by removing the pain generator, the diseased disc, and also by uniform load transmission through the end plate and the facet joints. The stabilization provided is indirect and is dependent on tensioning the remaining annulus and the ligamentous structure after insertion of the prosthesis. The artificial disc or nucleus differ from dynamic stabilization by prosthetic replacement of a section from the motion segment.

Artificial disc and nucleus have been discussed in Chapters 39 and 40.

Dynamic Stabilization

Due to the unpredictable outcomes of fusion procedures, spinal surgeons are showing an increasing interest in dynamic stabilization procedures. The goal of dynamic stabilization is to preserve motion while stabilizing the motion segment. It may be used alone or in conjunction with rigid stabilization, to "top off" the proximal segment adjacent to fusion to prevent its accelerated degeneration.

The ideal mechanism of dynamic stabilization has not been clearly defined in the literature. The issues of the degrees of restriction of motion and how much disc unloading is necessary have not been resolved. A clear understanding of the cause of low back pain in disc degeneration is needed before we may consider the ideal mechanism of dynamic stabilization.

ETIOLOGY OF CHRONIC LOW BACK PAIN DUE TO DISC DEGENERATION

Segmental Spinal Instability

The role of instability as a cause of chronic low back pain is not well understood. Panjabi (21) suggested that instability is a mechanical entity and is defined as a loss of stiffness to a given load. Frymore and Krag (22) echoed the same definition, as a loss of motion segment stiffness, such that application of force would produce greater than normal displacement. This may result in pain, progressive deformity, and neurologic deficit. However, biomechanical and radiological studies using open magnetic resonance imaging (MRI) in flexion and extension has shown that segmental motion either does not change significantly with the disc degeneration (23–25), or may in fact decrease, except during early stages of disc degeneration (26). Mulholland and Sengupta suggested that the era of back pain due to a disorder called "instability" was based on interpretation of spinal instability in a purely biomechanical sense, validated to some extent in other joints like the knee and shoulder, and fusion was seen as the appropriate solution (27).

In the clinical scenario of mechanical back pain, the instability concept fails to explain two commonly observed facts. First, patients with disc degeneration often experience episodes of acute exacerbations superimposed on a mild to moderate degree of baseline symptoms. If there were any abnormal translation or instability in the diseased segment, symptoms would be continuous. It is difficult to understand that if instability or abnormal movement is the cause of pain, why then is the acute pain only periodic rather than continuous. Secondly, manipulation by chiropractors, at least in some patients, results in dramatic relief of symptoms in an acute episode of low back pain. If instability is the etiology of the pain, it would not be reduced by manipulation. This also contradicts the notion that instability is the causative factor in low back pain secondary to disc degeneration.

Back Pain: Movement or Load-Related?

The intervertebral disc has two important biomechanical functions; it must transmit load and it must allow a controlled range of motion. This movement must not compromise the adjacent neural elements. Following disc degeneration, either the load transmission or the movement or both may become abnormal. The contribution of each of these to back pain in disc degeneration is unclear.

Load Transmission through Normal and Degenerated Discs

In the normal disc, the hygroscopic nature of the proteoglycan in the nucleus with intact annulus acts like an inflated car tire and helps in uniform distribution of load across the end plate. In a degenerated disc, the structure of the nucleus changes to a nonhomogeneous mixture of fragmented and condensed collagen, areas of fluid, and on occasion, areas of gas. Isolated fragments of annulus or end plate may add to the loose fragments inside the disc (28). The nucleus becomes depressurized and an increasingly larger load is transmitted through the annulus, which leads to splitting and inward folding of the annulus (29). The central area of the end plate overlying the depressurized nucleus now transmits lesser load, and corresponding end-plate changes, such as destruction and thinning of the trabeculae and thinning of the cartilaginous end plate (30,31), are noted in this area.

Mechanical Back Pain Related to Posture and Activity

The abnormal distribution of load across the disc space following disc degeneration as explained previously may causes baseline mild to moderate pain or discomfort. In the degenerated disc the principal area of load transmission becomes dependent on posture. In flexion, the anterior annulus bears major component of the load, while in extension the posterior annulus bears the major component. The abnormal high load transmission through the various areas of the annulus with changes in posture may explain the activity- and posture-related mechanical back pain.

Acute Episodes of Pain and "Stone in the Shoe" Hypothesis

It seems most likely that the acute episodes of back pain must be related to a movement of tissues within the disc. In a degenerated disc, the fragments of nucleus, end-plate cartilage, or annulus may move under the end plate, and become areas of high spot loading depending on their position within the disc. The best analogy for this theory is the "stone in the shoe," a concept proposed by Mulholland (27). When a stone moves under the heel, it causes high spot loading and pain, similar to an acute exacerbation of back pain. When the fragment shifts, the pain may subside. Manipulation of the lumbar spine by a chiropractor may, on occasion, dislodge the fragment from its weight-bearing position, bringing an immediate relief of acute pain (27).

McNally and Adams (32) demonstrated the nature of load distribution across the normal and degenerated disc. Disc pressure profilometry studies in cadaver spine shows that in the normal disc the load is evenly distributed, but in degenerated disc the nucleus is depressurized, higher load is transmitted near the peripheral annulus, and there are irregular areas of high spot loading. A subsequent in vivo study established that abnormal pressure profiles correlate with abnormal discograms with positive pain provocation (33).

THE RATIONALE AND PRINCIPLES OF DYNAMIC STABILIZATION

If the primary cause of back pain is abnormal load transmission, the aim for treatment should be unloading the disc. In particular, the abnormal high spot loading and abnormal high load transmission through the annulus should be prevented. Movement should be preserved since the transport of nutrients and metabolites in the disc is dependent on movement (34). However, any abnormal

GM Graph - Actuator 1

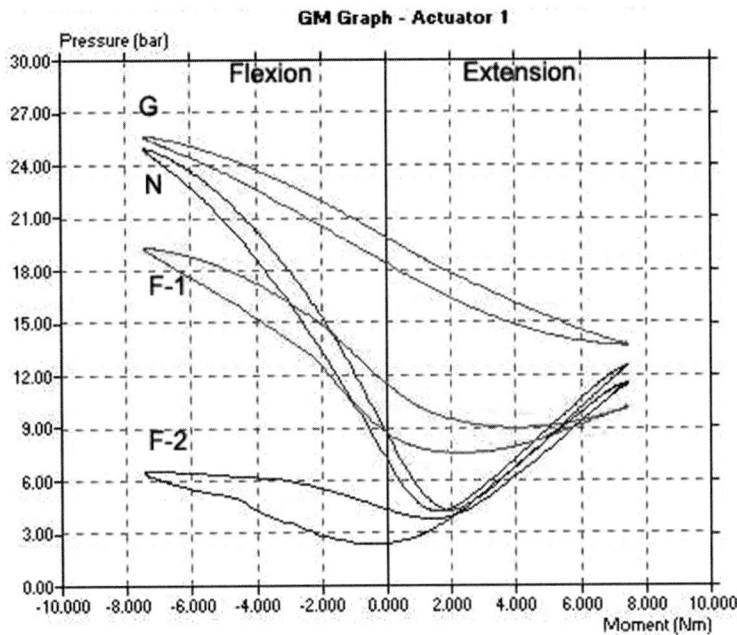

FIG. 38-1. The pressure tracing from the center of the disc in cadaver lumbar spine during flexion and extension movement. Normally *(N)* the pressure is lowest during the early phase of extension and rises both during flexion and extension. Following Graf ligament application *(G)*, the pressure was raised at neutral position. Following application of FASS system (described later) with moderate degree of compression by the ligament *(F-1)*, the disc was unloaded during flexion but not during extension. When the FASS system was applied with larger compression force by the ligament *(F-2)*, the system became rigid in flexion and unloaded the disc further, indicating a possibility that such a system would eventually fail. It should also be noted that with the FASS system there was very little effect on disc unloading in extension.

range or direction of motion may secondarily cause areas of spot loading, and therefore should be prevented.

The pertinent questions in the dynamic stabilization therefore are (a) how much disc unloading; (b) how much control of motion would be desirable; and (c) in the long-term, how can fatigue failure be prevented, in view of constant movement of the stabilized segment. Pseudarthrosis may lead to failure of rigid implant, but a flexible implant should be able to accommodate the movement without failure.

The fatigue life of a dynamic stabilization system will depend on two factors: (a) load-sharing property, and (b) instant axis of rotation (IAR). The system should share the load with the disc and facet joints uniformly throughout the range of movement. Let us consider arbitrarily that the system should bear around 30% of the load and allow the

remaining 70% of the load to be transmitted through the disc and facet joints. If at any time during the range of motion the implant system has to bear near 100% of the load, and unload the disc fully, the system would eventually fail (Fig. 38-1). Secondly, each spinal motion segment has an optimum IAR, depending on the anatomy of the disc and the facet joints. Similarly, every dynamic stabilization device has an optimum IAR, which can be determined in laboratory, when the system is implanted in two polyethylene blocks representing vertebral bodies, not connected by the disc or facet joints. If there is a mismatch in the location of the IAR of the motion segment and the device after implantation, they will tend to fight against each other during motion. This will lead to abnormal high stress to the device and the implant-bone junction, leading to the failure of the instrumentation in the long run. The ideal dynamic stabilization device should be a load-sharing device throughout the range of motion, and have an IAR close to that of the motion segment.

The various dynamic stabilization systems described in the literature are all posterior implants (35–43). Most of these devices aim at restriction of some motion but do not describe the mechanism of action or extent of disc unloading. Table 38-1 provides a classification of the currently described dynamic stabilization devices.

TABLE 38-1. *Classification of the dynamic stabilization devices in the treatment of low back pain, currently described in the literature*

I. Interspinous distraction devices
   a. Minns silicone distraction device
   b. Wallis system
   c. X-stop
II. Interspinous ligament devices
   a. Elastic ligament (Bronsard ligament across the spinous processes)
   b. Loop system
III. Ligaments across the pedicle screws
   a. Graf ligament
   b. Dynesis system
   c. Fulcrum-assisted soft stabilization system (FASS)
IV. Semirigid metallic devices across the pedicle screws
   a. Dynamic stabilization systems (DSS-I and DSS-II)

Modified from Sengupta DK. Dynamic stabilization devices in the treatment of low back pain. Orthop Clin North Am 2003; 35(1):43–56, with permission.

The Interspinous Distraction Devices

These are floating devices (i.e., not rigidly connected to the vertebrae). This avoids the possibility of loosening, a major concern for any implant that would have to survive against motion. The primary indication for interspinous distraction devices is degenerative spinal stenosis with neurogenic claudication in an older adult patient. By causing distraction between the spinous processes at the stenotic

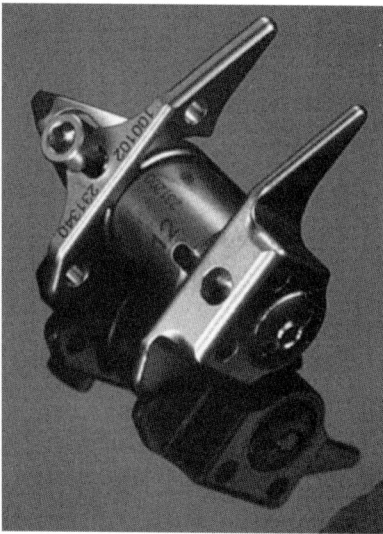

FIG. 38-2. The X-Stop titanium interspinous distraction system (St. Francis Medical Technologies, Inc., Concord, CA). (From Sengupta DK. Dynamic stabilization devices in the treatment of low back pain. Orthop Clin North Am 2003; 35(1):43–56, with permission.)

segment, an interspinous distraction device unfolds the buckled ligamentum flavum and posterior annulus, thereby relieving the stenosis. The device holds the segment in relative flexion, a posture adopted by these patients to relieve their symptoms. The posterior distraction may unload the facet joint joints and the posterior part of the disc. However, kyphosis of the segment may increase the load in the anterior part of the disc and these devices may not be suitable for primarily discogenic back pain.

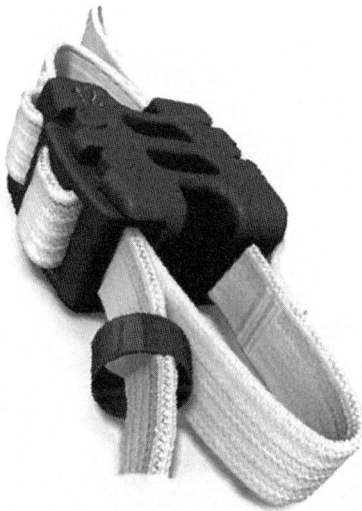

FIG. 38-3. The Wallis implant consists of polyetheretherketone interspinous spacer, anchored in its place by wrapping two woven Dacron ligaments around the spinous processes of the adjacent vertebrae under tension. (From Sengupta DK. Dynamic stabilization devices in the treatment of low back pain. Orthop Clin North Am 2003; 35(1):43–56, with permission.)

Minns and Walsh (35) described silicone interspinous spacers, which on biomechanical testing in the cadaver spine showed unloading the disc and correcting sagittal plane imbalance of the spine. No clinical application of this system has since been described by the authors. A titanium interspinous distraction device, X-Stop (Fig. 38-2) has been described by Lindsey et al. (SFMT, Concord, CA) (37). These are typically indicated for older adult patients with spinal stenosis presenting with neurogenic claudication. Senegas et al. (36) described an interspinous spacer made of polyetheretherketone (PEEK), "the Wallis implant" (Fig. 38-3), which is held between the spinous processes with Dacron tape. The addition of the Dacron tape provides further restriction of motion. The authors have advocated this system for treatment of early disc degeneration.

The Interspinous Ligaments

These devices are applied directly to the vertebrae, without using any metal anchorage. There is no rigid component to share the load. These devices do not unload the disc or the facet joint. Their primary mechanism of action is by limitation of the range of motion.

Caserta et al. (38) reported their experience of using elastic ligament using alone or to supplement the segment adjacent to fusion (Fig. 38-4). The authors have used the

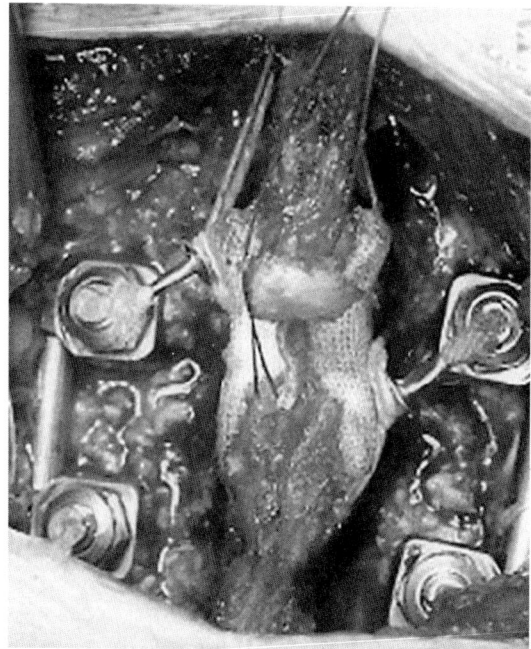

FIG. 38-4. The elastic interspinous ligament as described by Caserta et al. Peroperative picture of L4-5 elastic stabilization following rigid fixation of the L5-S1 segment. (From Caserta S, La Maida GA, Misaggi B, et al. Elastic stabilization alone or combined with rigid fusion in spinal surgery: a biomechanical study and clinical experience based on 82 cases. Eur Spine J 2002;11 Suppl 2:S192–197, with permission.)

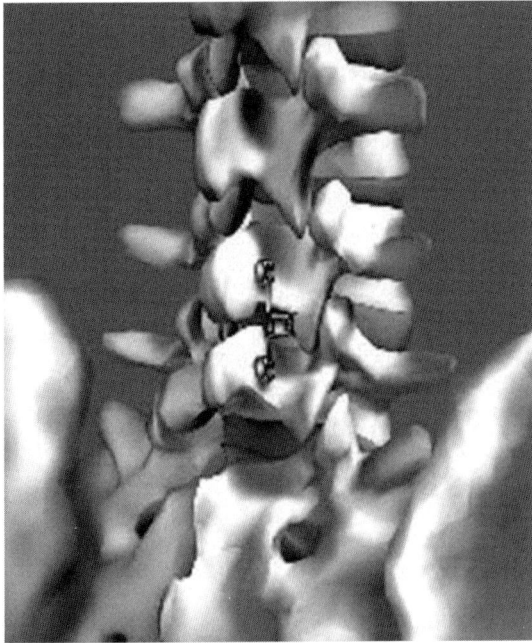

FIG. 38-5. The Loop system (Spinology, Inc., Stillwater, MN). (From Garner MD, Wolfe SJ, Kuslich SD. Development and preclinical testing of a new tension-band device for the spine: the Loop system. Eur Spine J 2002;11 Suppl 2:S186–191, with permission.)

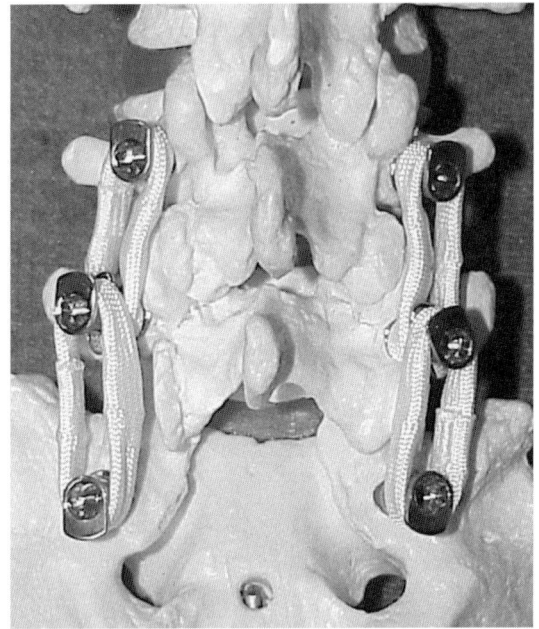

FIG. 38-6. The Graf ligament system (Neoligaments, Leeds, UK), applied between pedicle screws at L4-5 and L5-S1 segment in saw-bone. (From Mulholland RC, Sengupta DK. Rationale, principles and experimental evaluation of the concept of soft stabilization. Eur Spine J 2002;11[Suppl 2]:S198–205, with permission.)

system in 82 cases since 1994 and described encouraging results. Unfortunately, their report does not describe any detail of the implant material or the clinical results. Garner et al. (39) described a tension-band device, the Loop System (Spinology, Inc., Stillwater, MN), which consists of a braided polyethylene cable for stabilization of the spine across the spinous processes. The polymer cable provides high fatigue strength, in addition to tensile strength similar to that of metallic cables (Fig. 38-5).

Ligaments across Pedicle Screws

These devices are designed to be anchored to the vertebral bodies through the interface of pedicle screws. A fabric ligament connects the screw heads to restrict the motion of the spinal segment. In addition to the ligament, some of these devices may have a semirigid component.

The Graf ligament (Neoligaments, Leeds, UK), described by Henry Graf in 1989 (40), is the most commonly used device in this group (Fig. 38-6). This system consists of a pair of Dacron ligaments applied to the pedicle screws with a predetermined compression force. It immobilizes the spine in lordosis and locks the facet joints into full extension. No biomechanical study on the effect of this system has been published by the inventor. The system restricts motion but does not unload the disc. An independent biomechanical study shows that, in fact, it increases the load in the posterior part of the disc and

the annulus (45). The Graf ligament has been used by several independent surgeons in Europe and Asia, who reported with clinical success comparable to that of fusion (45–51). The proposed clinical indications include back pain due to segmental instability, to supplement a direct repair of low-grade spondylolisthesis, and in combination with fusion to stabilize an adjacent segment. In the author's experience the Graf ligament was found to be most useful for stabilizing multisegment disc disease in younger patients, where fusion has obvious disadvantages. One common complication with the Graf ligament is postoperative leg pain due to narrowing of the foramen or buckling of the posterior annulus secondary to hyperlordosis; a prophylactic decompression of the nerve roots has been recommended in these situations. The initial encouraging clinical results tend to deteriorate during next 2 years of follow-up (45) and the long-term results have been reported to be disappointing compared to fusion (52). This is probably because the Graf ligament increases the load in the posterior part of the disc and the facet joints causing accelerated degeneration and also that the ligament stretches over time and becomes ineffective (52).

The Dynesys (the dynamic neutralization system [Centerpulse Spine-Tech, Minneapolis, MN]) was described by Gilles Dubois (41) in 1994. The system consists of titanium alloy (Protasul 100) pedicle screws, polyester (Sulene-PET) cords, and polycarbonaturethane (Sulene-

five cases in the same segment and in seven cases for adjacent segment disease.

The distraction between the pedicle screw heads by the Dynesys system may force the segment into kyphosis and increase the load in the anterior part of the disc. The spinal extensor muscles may be able to restore the lordosis of the segment by distracting the disc space and unloading the disc. This will force the spacers to act as a load-bearing fulcrum. Therefore, the lordosis and load sharing by the plastic cylinder depends very critically on distraction produced by the implant, and on the ability of the patient to achieve lordosis with the extensor muscles (27).

The Fulcrum-Assisted Soft Stabilization (FASS) system (Fig. 38-8A, B) was introduced (42) to address what was perceived as disadvantage by the author of the Graf system. These include posterior compression leading to narrowing of the foramen and increased load over the posterior annulus.

In the FASS system a flexible fulcrum is placed between the pedicle screws, in front of the ligament to distract the posterior annulus. A fabric ligament, preferably of elastic material, placed posterior to the fulcrum, applies a compressive force across the pedicle screws and maintains lordosis. The fulcrum transforms this posterior compression force into an anterior distraction force, which distracts and unloads the disc, independent of muscle action. The degree of disc unloading depends on the relative tension and compression produced by the fulcrum and the ligament. For a given distraction by the fulcrum, the higher the compressive force applied by the ligament the greater would be the disc unloading. Laboratory experiments on spine models and cadaver spines demonstrated that, as greater unloading of the disc was achieved by adjustment of the tension in the ligament and the fulcrum, the system shared higher load, and the motion segment lost flexibility (42). An undue stiffness of the system may be unphysiologic and may cause early loosening of the screws or implant failure. The other disadvantage of the FASS system was that the polytetrafluoroethylene (PTFE) fulcrum was solid and although flexible from side to side, was not compressible along its long axis. The fabric ligament was also not elastic. The combination of such a fulcrum and ligament leads to a gross limitation of flexion, but almost no limitation in extension. Consequently, disc unloading was greater in flexion but very little in extension (Fig. 38-1). A second generation of the FASS system was tested, where the fulcrum was made up of a compressible titanium spring, but the ligament was the same. This spring-based FASS system unloaded the disc and resisted flexion and extension more uniformly throughout the range of motion (54). An ideal FASS system should consist of a flexible as well as compressible fulcrum, and an elastic ligament that would not creep significantly. Currently such a system is under development.

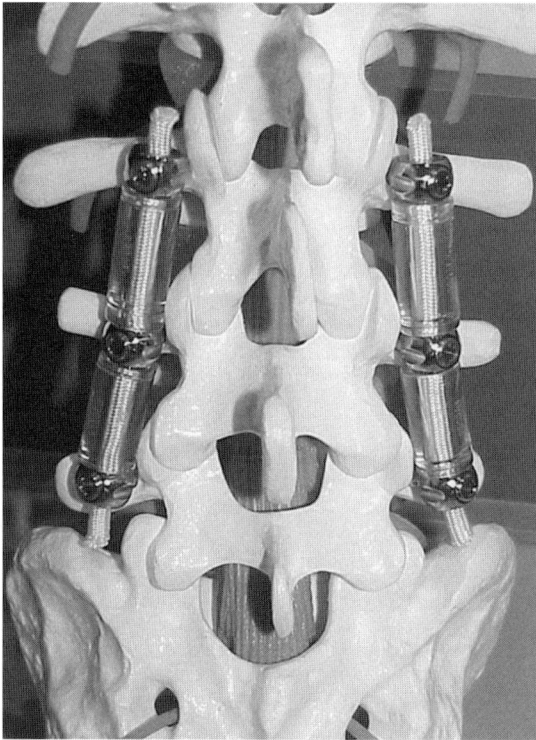

FIG. 38-7. The Dynesys system consists of pedicle screws, connected with a fabric cord, passed through the cylindrical spacers between the heads of the pedicle screws. (From Mulholland RC, Sengupta DK. Rationale, principles and experimental evaluation of the concept of soft stabilization. Eur Spine J 2002;11[Suppl 2]:S198–205, with permission.)

PCU) cylindric spacers (Fig. 38-7). The pedicle screw heads are connected by a cord under a given tension similar to the Graf ligament. The cord is threaded through the hollow cylindric spacers between the pedicle screws, which prevents excessive compression between the screw heads by the cord. The stabilizing cord carries tensile forces and the spacers resist compressive forces. The purpose of the system is to establish a mobile load transfer and control motion of the segment in all planes.

The biomechanical testing of the Dynesys system is mostly limited to fatigue testing of the whole construct and determining biocompatibility of the nonmetallic components. In a recent biomechanical study on cadaver spine, the Dynesys system was found to provide greater flexibility in extension and rotation but similar stiffness in flexion and lateral bending as compared to rigid fixation (53). There is no data available for the load-sharing characteristics of the spinal motion segments with the Dynesys system.

The initial clinical results in a multicenter trial have been encouraging and the device was found to be safe (41). However, unlike the Graf ligament, screw loosening was observed in seven cases. Early surgical intervention was needed in four cases, and late surgery was needed in

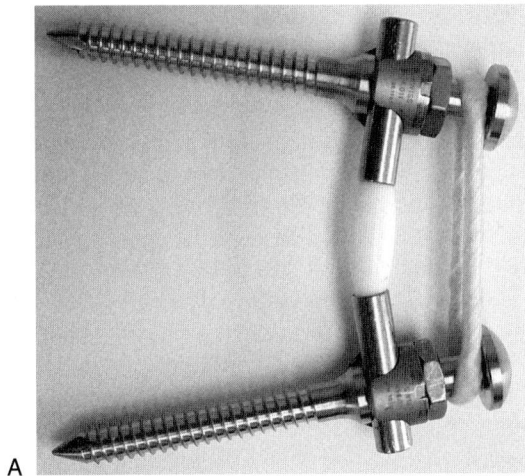

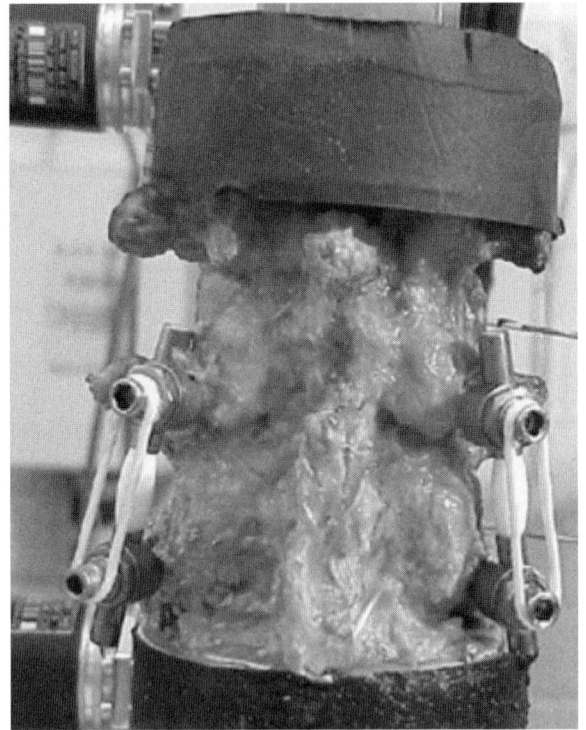

FIG. 38-8. A: The Fulcrum-Assisted Soft Stabilization (FASS) system. In this prototype, the fulcrum is made of flexible polytetrafluoroethylene and the ligament is made of an elastic fabric band containing polyurethane. **B:** The FASS system applied to a cadaver spine for biomechanical testing. (From Sengupta DK. Dynamic stabilization devices in the treatment of low back pain. Orthop Clin North Am 2003;35(1):43–56, with permission.)

Semirigid Metallic Devices across the Pedicle Screws

Currently there is no semirigid metallic device for soft stabilization without fusion available for clinical use. There are a few such devices under development.

The Dynamic Stabilization System (DSS) system (43) (Spinal Concepts, Inc., Austin, TX) is presently being tested in the laboratory. This system consists of a titanium spring connected to the vertebra with the pedicle screws. Two designs of the springs have been tested. The DSS-I system (Fig. 38-9A) consists of a "C"-shaped spring, 3 mm in cross-sectional diameter. The DSS-II system (Fig. 38-9B) consists of an elliptical coil spring of 3 to 4 mm in cross-sectional diameter. These

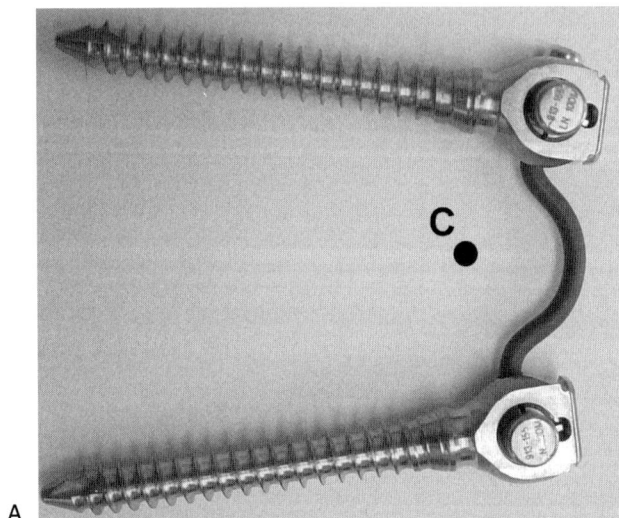

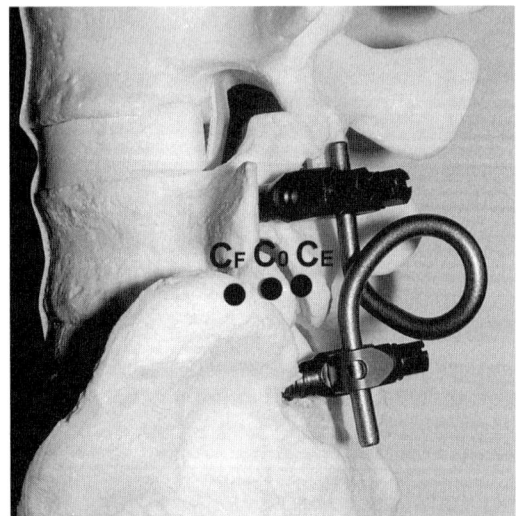

FIG. 38-9. The Dynamic Stabilization System (DSS) (Spinal Concepts, Inc., Austin, TX). **A:** DSS-I system consists of titanium spring in the shape of a "C", the straight ends of which are attached to the vertebral body with the pedicle screws. The axis of rotation of this spring is located at the center of the curvature of the spring at C both during flexion and extension. **B:** DSS-II system consists of a titanium coil spring. The axis of rotation of this spring lies in front of the coil spring, at C0 location in resting position, moves forward in flexion to CF, and backward in extension to CE locations.

systems may be applied to the motion segment, with an appropriate degree of distraction and lordosis, to produce a mild disc unloading at resting position. The stiffness of the spring limits the range of motion and unloads the disc further during motion.

As explained earlier, the uniform disc unloading throughout the range of motion will require the IAR of the spring to lie close to that of the motion segment. The axis of rotation of the DSS-I system is located close to the center of the "C" (Fig. 38-9A). In the DSS-II system, the axis of rotation is located in front of the coil, and moves forward and backward during flexion and extension, respectively, resembling the translation of IAR of a spinal motion segment (Fig. 38-9B). Therefore, the DSS-II system unloads the disc more uniformly during flexion-extension motion. This has been established in a continuous record of disc pressure from the center of the disc in cadaver lumbar spine, following application of the two spring systems (Fig. 38-10). Normally, the disc pressure at the center of the disc is lowest at the early phase of extension, and rises both in flexion and in extension because the anterior part of the disc is compressed in flexion and the posterior part in extension. Biomechanical testing on cadaver spine shows that the DSS-I system unloads the disc and restricts motion favorably during flexion. However, in extension the system forces the entire disc into distraction, resulting in greater restriction of motion and also lowest disc pressure at full extension. This is because the IAR of the DSS-I lies far behind that of the motion segment, and it becomes a full load-bearing structure toward the end of extension. This indicates that DSS-I is more likely to experience fatigue failure or loosening. The IAR of the DSS-II system translates like that of a normal spinal motion segment. Therefore, application of DSS-II system causes a more uniform disc unloading and restriction of motion in flexion and extension (43) (Fig. 38-10).

Semirigid metallic devices across the pedicle screws have a unique advantage over the other dynamic stabilization devices. They may be applied with the initial pretension, to distract the disc, when disc unloading is intended. Conversely, it may be applied with an elastic compression force on the disc, when a fusion is intended. Therefore DSS-I may be used in conjunction with an interbody graft to keep the graft under compression, and to resist the instability in extension caused by excision of the annulus in anterior lumbar interbody fusion.

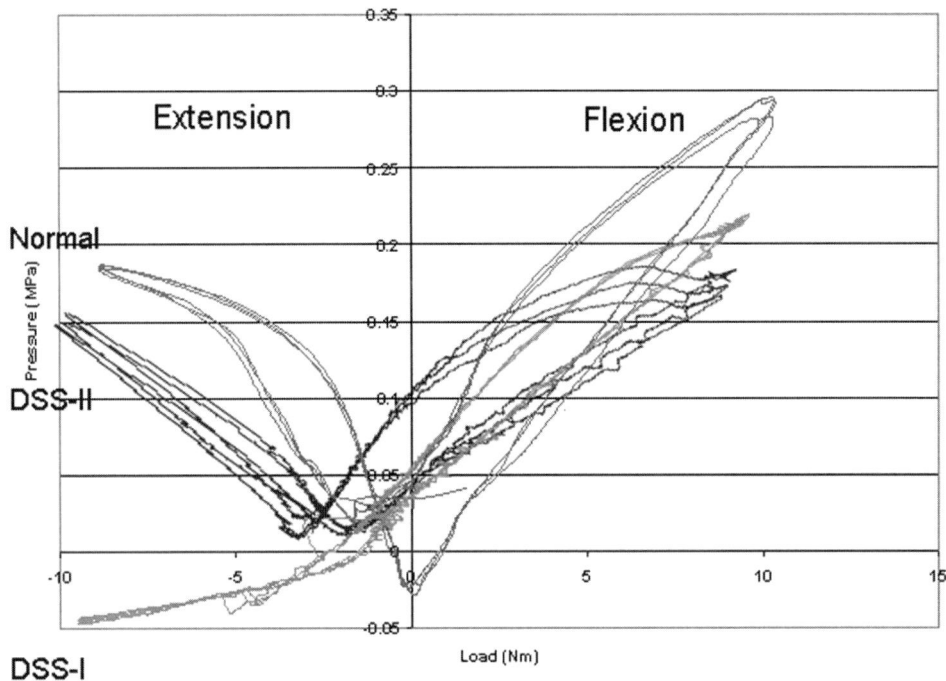

FIG. 38-10. The disc pressure tracing at the center of the disc in cadaver lumbar spine during flexion-extension movement, with 10 Nm pure moment, in a 6° freedom spine tester. Normally the pressure rises both in flexion and extension and is lowest during the early phase of extension. Following stabilization with DSS-II system the disc was partly unloaded both in flexion and extension, because of uniform load sharing with the disc. Following DSS-I stabilization the disc was partly unloaded in flexion, but fully unloaded in extension, which indicates that the implant becomes a fully load-bearing structure in extension, and therefore is more likely to experience fatigue failure or loosening.

SOFT STABILIZATION AS AN ADJUNCT TO DISC PROSTHESIS

Prosthetic disc replacement is an equivalent of a partial joint replacement. In the presence of significant facet joint arthritis, disc replacement may not relieve pain. When radicular pain warrants decompression involving partial facetectomy, prosthetic disc replacement may destabilize the motion segment. A posterior dynamic stabilization system may add the necessary stability for disc prosthesis to work in this situation. In effect, addition of a posterior dynamic stabilization system may convert disc replacement into a total joint replacement.

SOFT STABILIZATION AND DISC REPAIR

If a favorable environment may be created in the motion segment by unloading the disc and permitting near normal motion, the disc may be able to repair itself. Gene therapy in degenerative disc diseases, either by promoting enzymes to produce proteoglycans, or by preventing enzymes like proteases that damage the disc, is an emerging technology with much promise. Soft stabilization may further enhance the reparative process activated by the gene therapy.

SUMMARY

In summary, dynamic stabilization appears to have an important role in the treatment of the degenerative lumbar spine. Fusion of one or two motion segments does not make a significant difference in the total range of motion of the lumbar spine. However, preserving flexibility of a motion segment may prevent adjacent segment disease. Dynamic stabilization is more physiologic and may deliver a better clinical outcome in chronic low back pain than fusion. Additionally, it may permit disc replacement, even when facet joints need to be excised. If a favorable environment is created in the motion segment by unloading the disc and permitting motion by dynamic stabilization, the disc may be able to repair itself or may supplement reparative potential of gene therapy.

Despite all these bright prospects, a cautious approach is recommended before accepting any new implant system. The implant for fusion only has to serve a temporary stabilization until fusion takes place. Implant loosening is not uncommon in the presence of pseudarthrosis. After soft stabilization, the implant has to provide stability for an indefinite period, and also stay anchored to the bone despite allowing movement. This sounds like a daunting task. This may only be possible if the dynamic stabilization device functions only as a load-sharing device throughout the range of motion and does not become a load-bearing structure at a certain range. To achieve uniform load sharing and disc unloading, the instant axis of rotation of the implant has to lie close to that of the motion segment. Any mismatch between the kinematics of the implant system and the motion segment would result in an early implant failure or loosening. Therefore, the need for a strict bench test in the laboratory cannot be overemphasized. The few dynamic stabilization systems that have been used clinically have been reported to produce clinical outcomes comparable to that of fusion. No prospective randomized controlled trial has been reported yet, which is essential for the practice of evidence-based medicine.

REFERENCES

1. Gibson JN, Grant IC, Waddell G. The Cochrane review of surgery for lumbar disc prolapse and degenerative lumbar spondylosis. Spine 1999;24(17):1820–1832.
2. Boos N, Webb JK. Pedicle screw fixation in spinal disorders: a European view. Eur Spine J 1997;6(1):2–18.
3. Zinreich SJ, Long DM, Davis R, et al. Three-dimensional CT imaging in postsurgical "failed back" syndrome. J Comput Assist Tomogr 1990;14(4):574–580.
4. Shah RR, Mohammed S, Saifuddin A, et al. Comparison of plain radiographs with CT scan to evaluate interbody fusion following the use of titanium interbody cages and transpedicular instrumentation. Eur Spine J 2003;12(4):378–385.
5. Etminan M, Girardi FP, Khan SN, et al. Revision strategies for lumbar pseudarthrosis. Orthop Clin North Am 2002;33(2):381–392.
6. McAfee PC. Interbody fusion cages in reconstructive operations on the spine. J Bone Joint Surg Am 1999;81(6):859–880.
7. Weinhoffer SL, Guyer RD, Herbert M, et al. Intradiscal pressure measurements above an instrumented fusion. A cadaveric study. Spine 1995;20(5):526–531.
8. Eck JC, Humphreys SC, Hodges SD. Adjacent-segment degeneration after lumbar fusion: a review of clinical, biomechanical, and radiologic studies. Am J Orthop 1999;28(6):336–340.
9. Nakai S, Yoshizawa H, Kobayashi S. Long-term follow-up study of posterior lumbar interbody fusion. J Spinal Disord 1999;12(4):293–299.
10. Polikeit A, Ferguson SJ, Nolte LP, et al. The importance of the endplate for interbody cages in the lumbar spine. Eur Spine J 2003;12(6):556–561.
11. Adam C, Pearcy M, McCombe P. Stress analysis of interbody fusion—finite element modelling of intervertebral implant and vertebral body. Clin Biomech (Bristol, Avon) 2003;18(4):265–272.
12. Lazennec JY, Ramare S, Arafati N, et al. Sagittal alignment in lumbosacral fusion: relations between radiological parameters and pain. Eur Spine J 2000;9(1):47–55.
13. Kumar MN, Baklanov A, Chopin D. Correlation between sagittal plane changes and adjacent segment degeneration following lumbar spine fusion. Eur Spine J 2001;10(4):314–319.
14. Oda I, Cunningham BW, Buckley RA, et al. Does spinal kyphotic deformity influence the biomechanical characteristics of the adjacent motion segments? An in vivo animal model. Spine 1999;24(20):2139–2146.
15. Pfeiffer M, Hoffman H, Goel VK, et al. In vitro testing of a new transpedicular stabilization technique. Eur Spine J 1997;6(4):249–255.
16. Goel VK, Pope MH. Biomechanics of fusion and stabilization. Spine 1995;20[24 Suppl]:85S–99S.
17. Musha Y, Okajima Y, Motegi M. Lumbar spinal fusion using the Diapason system. J Spinal Disord 1995;8[Suppl 1]:S7–S14.
18. Gertzbein SD, Betz R, Clements D, et al. Semirigid instrumentation in the management of lumbar spinal conditions combined with circumferential fusion. A multicenter study. Spine 1996;21(16):1918–1925; discussion 25–26.
19. Mochida J, Toh E, Suzuki K, et al. An innovative method using the Leeds-Keio artificial ligament in the unstable spine. Orthopedics 1997;20(1):17–23.
20. Mochida J, Suzuki K, Chiba M. How to stabilize a single level lesion of degenerative lumbar spondylolisthesis. Clin Orthop 1999;(368):126–134.

21. Panjabi MM. Clinical spinal instability and low back pain. J Electromyogr Kinesiol 2003;13(4):371–379.
22. Frymoyer JW, Krag MH. Spinal stability and instability: definitions, classification, and general principles of management. In: Kahn A, ed. The unstable spine. New York: Grune & Stratton; 1986.
23. Okawa A, Shinomiya K, Komori H, et al. Dynamic motion study of the whole lumbar spine by videofluoroscopy. Spine 1998;23(16): 1743–1749.
24. Murata M, Morio Y, Kuranobu K. Lumbar disc degeneration and segmental instability: a comparison of magnetic resonance images and plain radiographs of patients with low back pain. Arch Orthop Trauma Surg 1994;113(6):297–301.
25. Paajanen H, Tertti M. Association of incipient disc degeneration and instability in spondylolisthesis. A magnetic resonance and flexion-extension radiographic study of 20-year-old low back pain patients. Arch Orthop Trauma Surg 1991;111(1):16–19.
26. Fujiwara A, Tamai K, An HS, et al. The relationship between disc degeneration, facet joint osteoarthritis, and stability of the degenerative lumbar spine. J Spinal Disord 2000;13(5):444–450.
27. Mulholland RC, Sengupta DK. Rationale, principles and experimental evaluation of the concept of soft stabilization. Eur Spine J 2002;11 [Suppl 2]:S198–S205.
28. Moore RJ, Vernon-Roberts B, Fraser RD, et al. The origin and fate of herniated lumbar intervertebral disc tissue. Spine 1996;21(18): 2149–2155.
29. McNally DS. The objectives for the mechanical evaluation of spinal instrumentation have changed. Eur Spine J 2002;11[Suppl 2]:S179–S185.
30. Keller TS, Hansson TH, Abram AC, et al. Regional variations in the compressive properties of lumbar vertebral trabeculae. Effects of disc degeneration. Spine 1989;14(9):1012–1019.
31. Simpson EK, Parkinson IH, Manthey B, et al. Intervertebral disc disorganization is related to trabecular bone architecture in the lumbar spine. J Bone Miner Res 2001;16(4):681–687.
32. McNally DS, Adams MA. Internal intervertebral disc mechanics as revealed by stress profilometry. Spine 1992;17(1):66–73.
33. McNally DS, Shackleford IM, Goodship AE, et al. In vivo stress measurement can predict pain on discography. Spine 1996;21(22): 2580–2587.
34. Katz MM, Hargens AR, Garfin SR. Intervertebral disc nutrition. Diffusion versus convection. Clin Orthop 1986(210):243–245.
35. Minns RJ, Walsh WK. Preliminary design and experimental studies of a novel soft implant for correcting sagittal plane instability in the lumbar spine. Spine 1997;22(16):1819–1825; discussion 26–27.
36. Senegas J. Mechanical supplementation by non-rigid fixation in degenerative intervertebral lumbar segments: the Wallis system. Eur Spine J 2002;11[Suppl 2]:S164–S169.
37. Lindsey DP, Swanson KE, Fuchs P, et al. The effects of an interspinous implant on the kinematics of the instrumented and adjacent levels in the lumbar spine. Spine 2003;28(19)2192–2197.
38. Caserta S, La Maida GA, Misaggi B, et al. Elastic stabilization alone or combined with rigid fusion in spinal surgery: a biomechanical study and clinical experience based on 82 cases. Eur Spine J 2002;11[Suppl 2]:S192–S197.
39. Garner MD, Wolfe SJ, Kuslich SD. Development and preclinical testing of a new tension-band device for the spine: the Loop system. Eur Spine J 2002;11[Suppl 2]:S186–S191.
40. Graf H. Lumbar instability. Surgical treatment without Fusion. Rachis 1992;412:123–37.
41. Stoll TM, Dubois G, Schwarzenbach O. The dynamic neutralization system for the spine: a multi-center study of a novel non-fusion system. Eur Spine J 2002;11[Suppl 2]:S170–S178.
42. Sengupta DK, Ohnmeiss D, Guyer RD, et al. Fulcrum assisted soft stabilisation in the treatment of low back pain—a new concept. Paper presented at: ISSLS Annual Meeting; 1999 June; Kona, Hawaii.
43. Sengupta DK, Demetropoulos CK, Herkowitz HN, et al. Loads sharing characteristics of two novel soft stabilization devices in the lumbar motion segments—a biomechanical study in cadaver spine. Paper presented at: Spine Arthroplasty Society Annual Conference, 2003; Scottsdale, AZ.
44. Sengupta DK, Mehdian S, Mulholland RC, et al. Biomechanical evaluation of immediate stability with rectangular versus cylindrical interbody cages in stabilization of the lumbar spine. BMC Musculoskelet Disord 2002;3(1):23.
45. Grevitt MP, Gardner AD, Spilsbury J, et al. The Graf stabilisation system: early results in 50 patients. Eur Spine J 1995;4(3):169–175.
46. Gardner A, Pande KC. Graf ligamentoplasty: a 7-year follow-up. Eur Spine J 2002;11[Suppl 2]:S157–S163.
47. Kanayama M, Hashimoto T, Shigenobu K, et al. Adjacent-segment morbidity after Graf ligamentoplasty compared with posterolateral lumbar fusion. J Neurosurg 2001;95[1 Suppl]:5–10.
48. Brechbuhler D, Markwalder TM, Braun M. Surgical results after soft system stabilization of the lumbar spine in degenerative disc disease—long-term results. Acta Neurochir (Wien) 1998;140(6):521–525.
49. Hadlow SV, Fagan AB, Hillier TM, et al. The Graf ligamentoplasty procedure. Comparison with posterolateral fusion in the management of low back pain. Spine 1998;23(10):1172–1179.
50. Legaye J, De Cloedt P, Emery R. [Supple intervertebral stabilization according to Graf. Evaluation of its use and technical approach]. Acta Orthop Belg 1994;60(4):393–401.
51. Guigui P, Chopin D. [Assessment of the use of the Graf ligamentoplasty in the surgical treatment of lumbar spinal stenosis. Apropos of a series of 26 patients]. Rev Chir Orthop Reparatrice Appar Mot 1994; 80(8):681–688.
52. Rigby MC, Selmon GP, Foy MA, et al. Graf ligament stabilisation: mid- to long-term follow-up. Eur Spine J 2001;10(3):234–236.
53. Schmoelz W, Huber JF, Nydegger T, et al. Dynamic stabilization of the lumbar spine and its effects on adjacent segments: an in vitro experiment. Spine 2003;28[Suppl]:418–423.
54. Sengupta DK, Ohnmeiss D, Webb JK, et al. Can soft stabilization in the lumbar spine unload the disc and retain mobility?—a biomechanical study with fulcrum assisted soft stabilization on cadaver spine. Paper presented at: ISSLS Annual Meeting; June 2001; Edinburgh, UK.

CHAPTER 39

Lumbar Artificial Disc Replacement: Rationale and Biomechanics

Geoffrey M. McCullen and Hansen A. Yuan

Stability of the vertebral motion segment is dependent upon the structural integrity of the disc, facet joints, and the musculoligamentous complex. Intervertebral discs transmit 85% of the axial load and provide rotational/translational support and shock absorption (1,2). In a standing position, the intradiscal pressure at L3-4 is 1,000 N, increasing to 3,000 N when sitting, leaning forward, or carrying 20 kg (3,4). The estimated number of walking cycles a person performs is approximately 2 million per year (5). Each walking cycle loads the disc 150 to 1,250 N in compression and −40 N to +450 N in shear (5). The estimated number of lifting cycles is 125,000 per year, each producing an estimated compressive load between 200 and 2,250 N (5).

The magnitude and frequency of such imposed loads on the spinal motion segment will inevitably lead to wear and degenerative changes over time. Three sequential clinical and biomechanical stages of spinal degeneration have been proposed: dysfunction, instability, and stabilization (6,7). Segmental motion increases with the severity of disc degeneration (8) and facet degeneration most typically follows (9,10). Segmental axial rotation motion increases with the degree of cartilage degeneration within the facet joints (8). Stabilization occurs with advanced disc collapse associated with marked end-plate sclerosis and osteophytosis.

RATIONALE FOR THE ARTIFICIAL DISC

Spinal arthrodesis significantly alters the biomechanics of the spine and results in an increased compensatory motion and mechanical loading in the adjacent free segments, particularly within the facet joints (11–15). Changes in the adjacent segments become more pronounced as the fixation range extends and as the rigidity of the construct increases (13,16,17). A 45% increase in intradiscal pressure occurs adjacent to a fusion (17,18).

Elevated intradiscal pressure acts to alter the diffusion characteristics of nutrients into the disc (19,20) and leads to biochemical changes including an elevation of type 1 collagen and a decrease in proteoglycan chondroitin sulfate, type 2 collagen content, and water content (2,21). Single photon emission computed tomography imaging 4 years after lumbar fusion demonstrates 62% with increased uptake within the vertebral bodies and facet joints in the free motion segment adjacent to the fused segment (22). Symptomatic juxtafusion degeneration is estimated to occur in 35% of postfusion patients (23).

Discectomy adversely affects the mechanical properties of the segment and alters coupled motions within adjacent segments (24,25). The level above a discectomy experiences an increased anterior-posterior translation in flexion and increased lateral translation with lateral bending irrespective of the amount of disc removed (24). Removal of the nucleus from the disc causes the inner margins of the annulus to bulge inward rather than outward during loading causing delamination of the fibers and further degeneration (26–28). Subtotal discectomy induces significantly less abnormal motion than total discectomy in all loading modes (24,25).

The aim of an artificial disc is to decrease pain, provide stability while maintaining near-physiologic motion, and diminish the likelihood of adjacent-level degenerative cascade. Two artificial disc interventions have evolved: (a) a total disc replacement (nucleus and annulus) and (b) a nucleus substitute. Many designs have been suggested. Few devices have been analyzed in biomechanical or clinical studies.

TOTAL DISC REPLACEMENTS

Total disc replacements are used to treat degenerative disc disease when removal of all possible sources of discogenic pain, including the annulus, is desired. The elective indications for a total disc replacement are single- or double-level degenerative disc disease, juxtafusion degeneration, and postdiscectomy axial pain that have failed a significant trial of nonoperative care. Absolute contraindications include: local or systemic presence of tumor or infection; osteoporosis (dual energy X-ray absorptiometry T-score less than −2.5); obesity (body mass index: weight (kg)/height (m) greater than 40); overlying thoracolumbar kyphosis; spondylolisthesis (greater than grade 1); disabled posterior elements unable to contribute in load-sharing with the prosthesis; and facet osteoarthritis and facet-mediated pain patterns (Table 39-1).

The natural spine triple joint complex provides six degrees of freedom: (a) compression, (b) distraction, (c) flexion, (d) extension, (e) lateral bending, and (f) rotation. For the total disc replacement, the degree of "constraint" refers to the relative range of motion of the prosthetic joint compared with the healthy intact joint within each of these degrees of freedom (5,29). An "unconstrained" device provides no mechanical restraint or limit. An "under-constrained" device imposes limits to motion outside of the naturally occurring constraint of motion. With a "critically" constrained implant, motion is allowed within the physiologic range but blocked beyond. The "over-constrained" prosthesis prohibits natural motion by imposing limits within the normal range of motion.

Many current total disc devices are rotationally unconstrained and require intact posterior elements (facets and musculoligamentous complex) for load sharing and biomechanical stability. Over time, such a device risks overloading, injury and degeneration of the posterior elements, particularly the facets. Alternatively, designs with rotational over-constraint would off-load the facets at the expense of increasing stress at the implant-host interface. In addition, the majority of current devices have high compressive stiffness (over-constraint in axial compression) resulting in decreased shock-absorbing capacity and increased risk of vertebral body fracture with significant loading.

All total disc replacements are implanted through anterior open approach (transperitoneal or retroperitoneal). During implantation, the anterior longitudinal ligament

TABLE 39-1. *Biomechanical contraindications for the artificial disc*

Osteoporosis
Obesity
Significant deformity
Spondylolisthesis (> grade 1)
Disc height <5 mm
Facet incompetence, facet mediated pain
Posterior ligament compromise
Additional contraindications for nucleus replacement:
    Incompetent anulus
    End-plate sclerosis, Schmorl nodes

and the anterior annulus are excised. These two anterior ligamentous structures provide a balanced tensile resistance to rotation on the opposite side of the center of rotation from the facets (30). Methods of retaining or reconstructing the anterior longitudinal ligament may lead to restoration of normal load sharing and segmental stiffness (30). Ligament tensioning is the key to restoring segmental sagittal balance. Restoring the "normal" disc height can cause over-stretching of the spinal ligaments that would limit ultimate segmental motion. To avoid over-distraction, it is advisable not to increase the height of a degenerated disc by more than 3 mm (31).

The total disc implant requires support from the peripheral cortical shell of the vertebral body. The end-plate periphery is stronger while the center is weaker (32,33). The device end-plate "foot print" should cover the largest possible area of the vertebral end plate for optimal load distribution and to decrease the formation of heterotopic ossification occurring at the end-plate margins.

Improvements in material and design specifications are leading slowly toward the ideal artificial disc (Table 39-2). Material properties to be considered are cytotoxicity, fatigue strength, and the modulus of elasticity. The design must attempt to approximate the natural disc dynamics, plan for compatibility between materials, use safe insertion technique, and have a reliable fixation between host and implant.

Metal Devices

The primary advantage for using an all-metal total disc replacement is the optimal fatigue strength. Biocompatibility has been shown in other orthopedic applications including joint arthroplasty. Designs include the springs with hinge and the ball-in-socket.

Kostuik has developed a device that uses two springs coiled between plates with a posterior hinge allowing flexion and extension (34) (Fig. 39-1). This device allows 15° to 20° of axial rotation in the sagittal plane, 3° of lateral bending, and less than 1° of axial rotation (5). The hinge pin has a decreasing diameter as the ends of the pin are approached. This feature, combined with elongated holes in which the pin rotates, is intended to allow a small amount or rolling lateral rotation (3° to 6°) (5). The springs sit in pockets that are designed to minimize off-axis loading and provide for a mechanical stop to prevent the springs from being loaded to the point that the coils touch (5). The springs are made of titanium alloy and are designed to provide adequate stiffness in both flexion and extension with a combined resistive torque in sagittal plane rotations of 2.24 N per degree (5). The springs have been successfully tested to more than 100 million full deflection cycles without failure (5). Hot isostatically pressed cobalt chrome alloy, with high carbon content to improve wear characteristics, is employed in the remain-

TABLE 39-2. *Total disc device comparison*

	Kostuik metal spring-hinge	Salib metal ball-socket	Lee nonmetal elastomer composite	Marnay metal, polyethylene cup-cap	Buettner-Janz metal, polytheylene two moving articulations
Shock absorption	Yes	No	Yes	No	No
Axial rotation	Over constrained	Unconstrained	Critically constrained	Unconstrained	Unconstrained
Translation	Over constrained	Over constrained	Unknown	Over constrained	Critically constrained
Flexion-extension	Under constrained	Under constrained	Critically constrained	Critically constrained	Under constrained
Center of rotation	Fixed	Fixed	Moves	Fixed	Moves, replicates instantaneous axis of rotation
Potential problems	Galvanic corrosion, bulky, difficult, insertion	Metal-on-metal, wear	Material delamination, Device-host fixation	Polyethylene, wear	Polyethylene, wear

der of the device. Vertically projecting tabs are placed at the front and side of the plate members through which screws are placed for fixation. Using different metals, galvanic corrosion is a concern but minimal corrosive issues have been seen in short duration animal models (5). In a sheep model, with histologic analysis at 6 months, fibrous tissue does not grow between hinges or around coils (35). If such an in-growth were to occur, it would be expected to significantly interfere with the disc mechanics.

Reminiscent of hip arthroplasty, a prosthetic device shaped as a ball and socket has been proposed (36) (Fig. 39-2) and has subsequently been redesigned. The Maverick (Medronic, Sofamor Danek, Memphis, TN) is made entirely of cobalt chrome and is axially rigid. There is no inherent rotational stiffness (unconstrained). Finite element analysis (FEA) has predicted that surgical variables will modulate the loads transmitted through the posterior elements after implantation (30). When the Maverick is placed anteriorly, the FEA predicts that facet loads will increase 2.5 times. A Maverick implanted posteriorly within the intervertebral space will successfully unload the facets in axial compression.

Nonmetal Devices

Whereas the principal advantage of metals is fatigue strength, the primary benefit of using nonmetals such as rubber and the elastomers (silicone, polyurethane, polyethylene) is the biomechanical similarity to the natural disc (37). By using a material with a lower modulus of elasticity, it is easier to replicate disc dynamics, attenuate shocks, and distribute loads evenly across the end plates. Difficulties, however, arise when attempting to develop a long-lasting nonmetal component that has a stable host-device interface. In addition, a polymer disc prosthesis that has optimal rigidity in axial compression may possess insufficient torsional rigidity. Alternatively, a polymer disc that is suitably rigid in torsion frequently becomes too rigid axially (38). Polymers do not allow the defining of a stable center of rotation for a disc implant. Lastly, delamination commonly occurs between polymer materials.

In 1975, Stubstab and Urbaniak introduced a total disc constructed entirely of synthetic nonmetal materials (39). Silicone or other elastomers such as polyurethane were formed into the general kidney shape with a fluid-filled

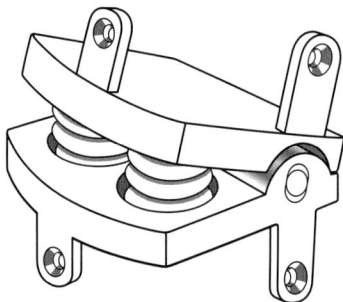
FIG. 39-1. Kostuik's all-metal device with two springs coiled between plates with a posterior hinge allowing flexion and extension (34).

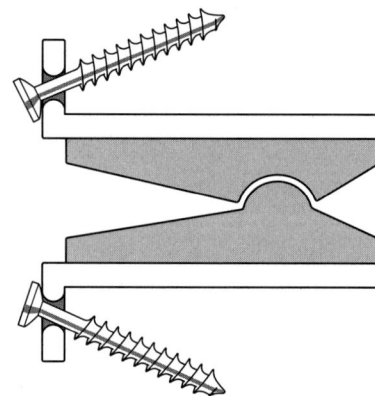
FIG. 39-2. All-metal ball-and-socket design by Salib (36).

core between flat superior and inferior elastomeric plates. Simulating the annulus, the device was covered by a weave of Dacron fibers creating pores for tissue ingrowth. This device has been implanted into eight chimpanzees followed for one year (40). Erosion and reactive end-plate bone formation have been attributed to an unstable host-implant interface.

Lee and Parsons (41,42) have designed what has been referred to as the "New Jersey disc" (Fig. 39-3). Two material designs have been described. In the first, a soft elastomer central core is surrounded by a fiber-reinforced polyurethane (12 layers of Dacron with alternating multi-directional pattern: −45, 0, −45). In the second, the core is surrounded by a nonfiber reinforced polymer, C-flex (polysiloxane-styrene-ethylene-styrene-butylene) (Concept Polymer Technologies, Clearwater, FL) (38,43). Two stiff end plates using elastomer or hydroxyapatite frame the disc. This disc has been studied both *in vitro* and in finite element models (43,44). Questions remaining for the New Jersey disc include: material biocompatibility, fatigue, and wear resistance; and the adequacy of short- and long-term implant fixation.

The "3-DF" disc is a three-dimensional fabric woven with an ultra–high-molecular-weight polyethylene (UHMWPE) fiber and a surface spray-coated with bioactive ceramics (45,46). Made of one material, the device avoids a composite interface. No changes in biomechanical parameters have occurred after 2 million loading cycles with compressive loading of 200 N (45). Creep-relaxation testing has demonstrated a viscoelastic strain-time curve almost identical to the normal intervertebral disc (45). The "3-DF" device has been studied using an *in vivo* sheep model (46). Highlighting the problems inher-

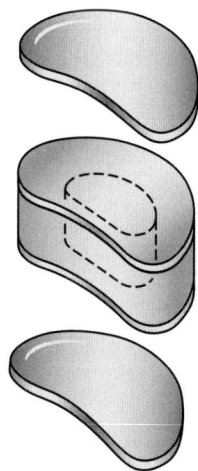

FIG. 39-3. The New Jersey disc designed by Lee et al (41). A soft, central elastomer core is surrounded by either a fiber-reinforced polyurethane or a nonfiber- reinforced polymer. Two stiff end plates using elastomer or hydroxyapatite frame the disc.

ent in animal models, complete removal of the end plates was required in order to fit the 10 mm artificial disc. This created a different implant-host interface than is clinically intended. The segmental biomechanics and interface histology were evaluated at 4 and 6 months. Implant displacement without complete dislodgement was noted. Those devices implanted with temporary internal fixation (Kanada one-rod Smooth Rod system) were firmly in place and demonstrated a successful bony bonding to the host. Work is now being directed toward the creation of a supplemental bioabsorbable spinal fixation device.

Combination Metal and Nonmetal Devices

To overcome the shortcomings found when using metals or nonmetals alone, designs have combined the materials. Most commonly, this has taken the form of a metal-polymer-metal sandwich disc. The metal tray is employed to improve fixation with spikes, tabs with screws, or porous coating for bony ingrowth. With the component thus stable and fixed, the central polymer provides the needed flexibility.

In 1991, Steffee developed the Acroflex disc (DePuy, Acromed Corporation, Cleveland, OH) (47). This disc replacement consists of a hexane-based, carbon black–filled, polyolefin rubber core vulcanized to the two titanium plates. Fixation is accomplished with a porous coating promoting ingrowth and four 7-mm cone-shaped posts that extend into the vertebral body. A significant subsurface shear is experienced at the rubber-metal junction producing failures with fracture of the rubber core (48).

The ProDisc (Spine Solutions, Inc., New York, NY) is a cap-cup matching articulation designed by Marnay (49) (Fig. 39-4). The end plates are made of a cobalt chrome molybdenum alloy with a central fixation keel projecting through the vertebral end plates. The convex bearing surface is made of UHMWPE that snaps into the inferior end plate. The device has a fixed center of rotation and is critically constrained in flexion-extension, unconstrained in rotation, and over-constrained in translation.

Buettner-Janz and Schellnack developed the Link SB Charité disc (Waldemar LINK GmbH and Co., Hamburg, Germany) (Fig. 39-5) (50). Since the first design in 1984, three revisions have been made. The current device (Link SB Charité III) includes two symmetric end plates made of cobalt chromium alloy. Immediate fixation is by anchoring teeth projecting from the outer end plate. For bony ingrowth, the end plates are porous coated with two layers of thin sintered titanium beads (pore size ranging from 75 to 300 microns) covered by electrochemically bonded hydroxyapatite. A primate model has demonstrated ingrowth over 48% of the end-plate surface (51).

The inner end-plate surface contour is an oval-shaped concave surface that articulates with a central high-density polyethylene core [modulus of elasticity 420 to 1,200

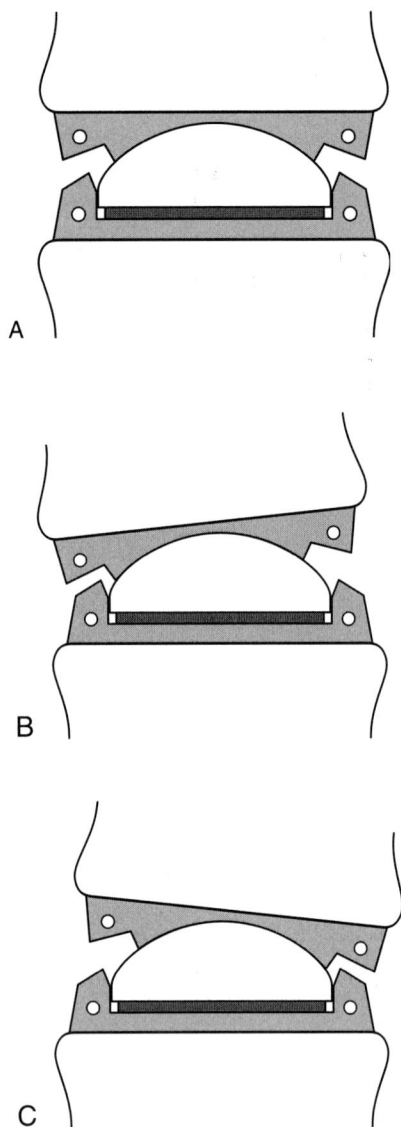

FIG. 39-4. The Marnay device (49). **A:** The polyethylene cups snaps into the inferior end plate. The device is unconstrained in axial rotation. **B, C:** The device in flexion and extension with movement occurring around a fixed center of rotation.

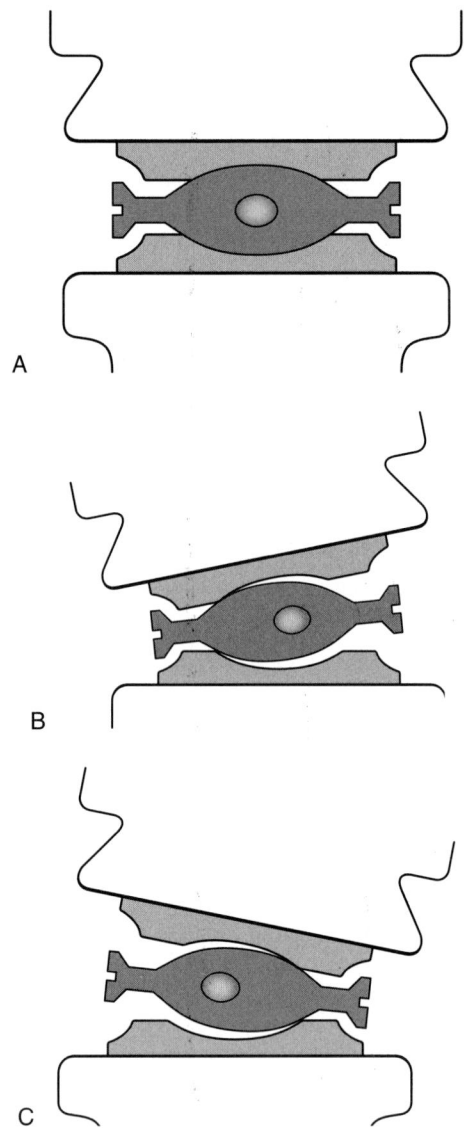

FIG. 39-5. The SB Charité disc (50). **A:** Both top and bottom inner end-plate surfaces articulate with the central polyethylene. With flexion, the polyethylene moves posteriorly. **B:** In extension, the polyethylene moves anteriorly, changing the instantaneous axis of rotation. **C:** The device allows 20° of motion in flexion-extension and lateral rotation and is unconstrained in axial rotation.

mega Pascals (MPa)] (52). The device allows 20° of motion in flexion-extension and lateral bending (underconstrained). There is no limit to motion in axial rotation (unconstrained) (53). Hysteresis (the conversion of strain energy into heat formation during cyclic loading) of the polyethylene occurs at loads less than 4.2 kN with incipient irreversible polyethylene deformation occurring with loads between 6 and 8 kN (53).

With movement in flexion and extension, the polyethylene core moves: in flexion the polyethylene moves posteriorly and in extension it moves anteriorly. This changing of the instant axis of rotation (IAR) is meant to replicate the natural disc (52). Because of the changing IAR, the Link SB Charité disc needs to be placed poste-

riorly within the intervertebral disc space. Anterior positioning of the device will significantly decrease the available motion (52,54).

In a human cadaveric biomechanical study, the Link SB Charité prosthesis showed an average percentage increase in segmental axial rotational range of motion of 44% when compared to the intact control (55). The increase in axial rotation reflects the excision of the anterior longitudinal ligament required during insertion and the unconstrained nature of the disc in axial rotation. Flexion and extension range-of-motion between the in-

TABLE 39-3. *Factors affecting* in situ *total disc device motion*

Preoperative segmental stiffness
Facet and ligament degeneration, end-plate osteophytes
Device positioning
Anterior positioning decreases motion
Device sizing
Over-stretching ligaments decreases motion
Under-sized "foot print"
Device subsidence
Heterotopic ossification formation
Bracing
Best to avoid

tact specimen and a segment implanted with the Link SB Charité disc were not significantly different. The disc preserved the normal mapping of segmental motion at the operative level and at the adjacent levels.

Clinically, postoperative segmental motion is equal to preoperative motion (54,56). The motion permitted by the implanted prosthesis appears to be determined by the extent of the degenerative changes in the adjacent structures such as the facet joints and neighboring spinal ligaments. The average postoperative range-of-motion for the SB Charité III is 9° of flexion and extension (52,54,56). At the L4-5 level 9.6° flexion, 3.4° extension, and 4° lateral bending motion has been reported (52). At L5-S1 these values are decreased with 6° flexion, 3.5° extension, and 3.2° of lateral bending (52). Clinical studies confirm that anterior device positioning decreases postoperative motion (54). Over-distraction causes excessive tightening of the posterior ligaments and decreases segmental motion. To obtain and maintain available motion, early postoperative motion is encouraged (54) (Table 39-3).

In published series, further surgery has been required in up to 24%, the majority for "pain control" as a result of ongoing or developing facet-mediated pain (56). Device dislocation/migration occurs in 2% to 6.5%, usually secondary to poor size selection (54,57). Eight percent of the devices have subsided most commonly because of an undersized device "footprint" (54).

NUCLEUS REPLACEMENTS

There are two potential indications for nucleus replacement: (a) as a adjunct to discectomy (open and percutaneous nucleotomy), addressing the biomechanical alterations of discectomy; and (b) to relieve back pain resulting from early stage degenerative disc disease that has failed to improve with nonoperative means.

Nucleus substitutes should be made of biocompatible materials; restore intervertebral height and tension the annulus with normal end-plate load distribution; recreate the intradiscal hydraulic pumping mechanism for pressure modulation and nutrient delivery to the remaining nucleus and the inner annulus; and demonstrate safe, possibly minimally invasive implantation with a revision strategy in cases of failure.

Nucleus replacement requires the satisfactory condition of the annulus and the vertebral end plates. Sufficient annular containment is essential to stabilize the device in the disc space and to avoid excessive motion that could lead to migration and an elevated rate of wear on end-plate or implant surface. When end plates are weakened by osteoporosis or Schmorl nodes or challenged by obesity (weight greater than 90 kg or body mass index greater than 30) subsidence of the implant into the vertebral body can occur.

Successful tensioning of the annulus will depend upon the implant modulus of elasticity and the implant/cavity conformity. The inward bulging of the annulus after nucleotomy is reversed by a nuclear implant with Young's modulus of elasticity of 3 MPa (range 0.2 to 40 MPa) (27). Restoration of intervertebral disc height with a nucleus replacement can best be accomplished if the starting disc height is greater than or equal to 5 mm. In late stage disc disruption, with failure of the annulus, end plate and facets, a nucleus replacement would certainly be ineffective. Annulus repair and methods to achieve annulotomy healing remain elusive.

Fernstrom developed the first nucleus replacement in 1966 (58). These devices were spheric, solid, stainless steel balls, up to 16 mm in diameter that were meant to serve as intervertebral spacers while allowing movement. Contact area with the vertebral bodies was small. No pressure modulation was possible with position change. The device did not restore the normal load distribution across the end plate and was ultimately abandoned because of implant migration or subsidence.

In the 1960s, work began with the injection of self-curing silicone and polyurethane into the disc space (3). The potential advantages of this technique were the minimally invasive, percutaneous route of insertion resulting in reduced annular injury and the *in situ* polymer curing that offered the possibility of obtaining good end plate–implant conformity. The problems encountered included: long polymerization reaction times; incomplete polymerization; exothermic reaction temperatures; high injection pressures; polymer containment; and the production of particulate wear debris (59). Subsequent efforts in nucleus replacement have been directed toward developing contained systems that allow a more reproducible fabrication and accurate prosthetic placement.

In 1988, Ray introduced the Prosthetic Disc Nucleus, or "PDN", (Raymedica, Minneapolis, MN) with dual disc cylinders resting side-by-side (60). In the original procedure, a trephine was used, from the posterior approach, to bore a passage into the center of the disc. After nucleotomy, the cylinders were slid into position and filled with a water-absorbing gel held within a semipermeable membrane. Prefilled devices have subsequently replaced *in situ* fill of the cylinders. The outer device layer of the PDN is constructed with a flexible but inelastic polyethylene fiber jacket that constrains the ultimate swelling of the hydrogel.

The PDN implants have passed U.S. Food and Drug Administration guidelines for biologic safety, cytotoxicity, carcinogenicity and long-term animal implantation. Fatigue studies to greater than 50 million cycles under simulated physiologic loads (200 to 800 N) have been successful (61). After nucleotomy *in vitro* insertion of the PDN has restored the segmental mobility in all movement/directions (62).

The first PDN clinical trials began in 1996. Initially, the PDN used a hydrogel polymer, HYPAN 68 (polyacrylonitrile-polyacrylamide), which absorbs 68% of its weight in water. Early analysis indicated that this device was too rigid, promoting pressure concentrations on the cartilaginous end plate (61). In 1998, a change was made to HYPAN 80, which absorbs more water and thus is softer. A higher rate of implant migration with a 38% revision rate was recognized (61). Further changes in design and surgical protocol followed. PDN devices are now two differently shaped units: a tapered anterior unit and a rectangular posterior unit placed transversely and connected by tethering sutures (Fig. 39-6). To accommodate the two units the end-plate anteroposterior diameter must be 37 mm or greater (61).

For device containment, the annulotomy must be kept as small as possible with a sequential annular dilating technique rather than a cut entry. Using lateral decubitus positioning and a lateral retroperitoneal exposure,

Bertagnoli has developed the anterolateral transpsoas approach (ALPA). The annulus is cut to create a hinged flap. The overlying psoas muscle covers the lateral annulotomy site, diminishing the risk of implant extrusion (63). A restricted postoperative protocol with the use of a brace for 6 weeks is recommended (63).

Moderate to severe end-plate remodeling, likely due to changes in load distribution, has been noted in some patients implanted with the PDN (63). Sixty patients with PDN have been followed with postoperative MRI (64). Six weeks postoperatively there is an increase in degenerative end-plate changes in 27% of the implanted levels (64,65). At one year, the incidence of such changes increases further to 70%. Advanced degenerative changes within the end plate at 1 year are seen in 7%. The clinical implications of these radiographic changes have yet to be determined.

Other nucleus replacements are emerging in various stages of early development. Bao has designed a polyvinyl alcohol (PVA) hydrogel nucleus replacement in the form of beads held within a retaining membrane (66) (Aquarelle Hydrogel Nucleus, Stryker/Howmedica, Mahwah, NJ). It is inserted in the dehydrated form, through a 5 mm cannula. Water, drawn from the surrounding tissues, fills the membrane to a 70% water content and the prosthesis nearly doubles in size. This *in situ* expansion creates an interference fit. Like the natural nucleus, the hydrogel replacement is able to absorb and relinquish water with changes in applied load. Biomechanical studies have confirmed restoration of disc function after hydrogel implantation (67,68). Preventing implant migration and extrusion remains a problem. The Newcleus (Sulzer SpineTech, Edina, MN) is an elongated, elastic memory-coiling, spiral-shaped polycarbonate urethane (69,70). It is inserted into the disc through a cannula device to create a spiral coil of the material. The Prosthetic Intervertebral Nucleus, or "PIN" (Disc Dynamics, Minnetonka, MN) is a polyurethane balloon inserted in deflated form into the disc and then inflated with an incompressible liquid (71). The size and shape of the nucleus prosthesis can be significantly altered during implantation and regained or restored after implantation.

DEVICE LONGEVITY

The generation of particulate debris can occur as a result of wear and corrosion and should be expected any time an artificial disc implant is used. The accumulated magnitude of the debris over time and the resultant clinical sequelae after disc replacement has yet to be determined. In long-term patient outcomes for total knee and hip replacements, microscopic wear fragments have disseminated to the liver, spleen, and paraaortic lymph nodes (72). Local wear debris can incite a local cytokine-mediated [tumor necrosis factor-α, prostaglandin-E2, interleukin (IL)-1, IL-2 or IL-6] immunologic reaction

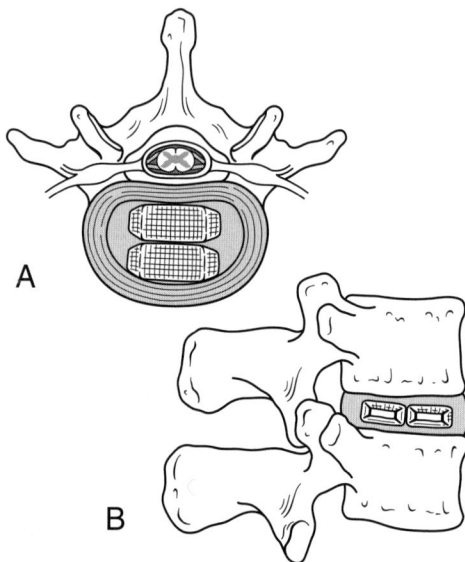

FIG. 39-6. The PDN devices (62). **A:** Sagittal view. **B:** Axial view demonstrating a tapered anterior unit and a rectangular posterior unit placed transversely and connected by tethering sutures. The annulus and end plates must be in satisfactory condition.

that causes destruction of bone at the prosthetic-bone interface (73). The optimal particle size to disseminate and to incite macrophages to release cytokines is 1 to 5 microns (72,73).

Among the metals implanted in the spine, titanium debris fragments appear to be the most reactive in eliciting a cytokine-mediated response (73,74). Polyolefin rubber compound particles have been generated *in vitro* and placed in subcutaneous pouches in rats and adjacent to the lumbosacral dura in sheep (75). A local foreign body reaction was created but no particle migration from the site of implantation was identified and no apparent local or systemic toxic effects resulted.

In a nonhuman primate study with the Link SB Charité III, histochemical assays showed no accumulation of particulate debris (no titanium, UHMWPE, or cobalt chrome) and no cytokines 6 months after implantation (51). The lack of long-term evaluation or anatomic differences including the absence of synovial fluid in the disc may be the reason why particulates have not been generated.

The SB Charité disc has more than 10 years of clinical use but no long-term clinical outcome studies. Neither osteolysis nor late loosening has been reported in clinical studies. It is a possibility that some cases will be identified with longer duration follow-up. Repeat anterior retroperitoneal approaches are fraught with potential hazard because of the development of a thick scar enveloping the spine and vascular structures. Therefore, when total disc devices fail, the safest revision strategy is a posterior spinal instrumented fusion.

CONCLUSIONS

With innovations in materials and design, the artificial disc is becoming a reality. Optimal short-term clinical results will depend upon patient selection.

Poor clinical results are expected when disc replacement is applied to advanced degeneration (76). Long-term outcome will depend upon the ability of the device to replicate natural kinematics and to withstand the repetitive loads over time. Long-term clinical evaluations after disc replacement will be essential to identify the rate and extent of progressive degenerative change within the facet joints and the adjacent segments.

For accurate comparability between developing devices, biomechanical terminology and methodology for the artificial disc must become standardized. The optimal device constraint for particular clinical situations must be determined.

REFERENCES

1. Adams MA, Green TP, Dolan P. The strength in anterior bending of the lumbar intervertebral discs. Spine 1994;19(19):2197–2203.
2. Hutton WC, Toribatake Y, Elmer WA, et al. The effect of compressive force applied to the intervertebral disc in vivo. Spine 23 1998;(23):2524–2537.
3. Nachemson A, Morris JM. In vivo measurements of intradiscal pressure. J Bone Joint Surg 1964;46A:1077.
4. Wilke HJ, Neef P, Caimi M, et al. New in vivo measurements of pressures in the intervertebral disc in daily life. Spine 1999;24(8):755–762.
5. Kostuik JP. Intervertebral disc replacement. Clin Orthop Rel Res 1997;33:727–741.
6. Farfan HF, Gracovetrsky S. The nature of instability. Spine 1984;9(7):714–719.
7. Kirkaldy-Willis WH, Wedge JH, Yong-Hing K, et al. Pathology and pathogenesis of spondylosis and stenosis. Spine 1978;3:319–328.
8. Fujiwara A, Lim TH, An HS, et al. The effect of disc degeneration and facet joint osteoarthritis on the segmental flexibility of the lumbar spine. Spine 2000;25(23):3036–3044.
9. Butler D, Trafimow JH, Andersson GB, et al. Discs degenerate before facets. Spine 1990;15:111–113.
10. Dunlop RB, Adams MA, Hutton WC. Disc space narrowing and the lumbar facet joints. J Bone Joint Surg 1984;66B:706–710.
11. Dekutoski MB, Schendel MJ, Ogilvie JW, et al. Comparison of in vivo and in vitro adjacent segment motion after lumbar fusion. Spine 1994;191:745–751.
12. Lee CK. Accelerated degeneration of the segment adjacent to a lumbar fusion. Spine 1988;13(3):375–377.
13. Nagata H, Schendel MJ, Transfeldt EE, et al. The effects of immobilization of long segments of the spine on the adjacent and distal facet force and lumbosacral motion. Spine 1993;182:471–479.
14. Quinnel RC, Stockdale HR. Some experimental observations of the influence of a simple lumbar floating fusion on the remaining lumbar spine. Spine 1981;6:263.
15. Hambly MF, Wiltse LL, Raghavan N, et al. The transition zone above a lumbosacral fusion. Spine 1998;23:1785–1792.
16. Shono Y, Kaneda K, Abumi K, et al. Stability of posterior spinal instrumentation and its effects on adjacent motion segments in the lumbosacral spine. Spine 1998;23:1550–1558.
17. Weinhoffer SL, Guyer RD, Hebert M, et al. Intradiscal pressure measurements above an instrumented fusion: a cadaveric study. Spine 1995;20:526–531.
18. Chow DHK, Luk KD, Evans JH, et al. Effects of short anterior lumbar interbody fusion on biomechanics of neighboring unfused segments. Spine 1996;21:549–555.
19. Eck JC, Humphreys C, Lim TH, et al. Biomechanical study on the effect of cervical spine fusion on adjacent-level intradiscal pressure and segmental motion. Spine 2002;27(22):2431–2434.
20. Buckwalter JA. Aging and degeneration of the human intervertebral disc. Spine 1995;20:1307–1314.
21. Urban JPG, McMullin JF. Swelling pressure of the lumbar intervertebral discs: influence of age, spinal level, composition and degeneration. Spine 1988;13(2):179–187.
22. Even-Sapir E, Martin RH, Mitchell MJ, et al. Assessment of painful late effects of lumbar spinal fusion with SPECT. J Nucl Med 1994;35(3):416–422.
23. Rahm MD, Hall BB. Adjacent-segment degeneration after lumbar fusion with instrumentation: a retrospective study. J Spinal Disord 1996;9(5):392–400.
24. Goel VK, Goyal S, Clark C, et al. Kinematics of the whole lumbar spine: effect of discectomy. Spine 1985;10:543–554.
25. Goel VK, Nishiyama K, Weinstein JN, et al. Mechanical properties of lumbar spinal motion segments as affected by partial disc removal. Spine 1986;11:1008–1012.
26. Brinckmann P, Grootenboer H. Change of disc height, radial disc bulge and intradiscal pressure from discectomy. Spine 1991;16(6):641–646.
27. Meakin JR, Reid JE, Hukins DW. Replacing the nucleus pulposus of the intervertebral disc. Clin Biomech 2001;16(7):560–565.
28. Hanley EN, Shapiro DE. The development of low-back pain after excision of a lumbar disc. J Bone Joint Surg 1989;71A:719–721.
29. Hedman TP, Kostuik JP, Fernie GR, et al. Design of an intervertebral disc prosthesis. Spine 1991;16:S256–S260.
30. Dooris AP, Goel VK, Grosland NM, et al. Load-sharing between anterior and posterior elements in a lumbar motion segment implanted with an artificial disc. Spine 2001;26(6):E122–E129.
31. Eijkelkamp MF, van Donkelaar CC, Veldhuizen AG, et al. Requirements for an artificial disc. Int J Artificial Organs 2001;24(5):311–321.

32. Aharinejad S, Bertagnoli R, Wicke K, et al. Morphometric analysis of vertebrae and intervertebral discs as a basis of disc replacement. Am J Anat 1990;189 (1):69–76.

33. Silva MJ, Keaveny TM, Hayes WC. Load sharing between the shell and centrum in the lumbar vertebral body. Spine 1997;22 (2):140–150.

34. Hedman TP, Kostuik JP, Fernie GR, et al. Artificial spinal disc. United States Patent: 4,759,769 (July 26, 1988).

35. Hellier W G, Hedman TP, Kostuik JP. Wear studies for the development of an intervertebral disc prosthesis. Spine 1992;17(6);S86–S96.

36. Salib RM, Pettine KA. Intervertebral disk arthroplasty. United States Patent: 5,258,031 (November 2, 1993).

37. Bao QB, McCullen GM, Hingham PA, et al. The artificial disc: theory, design and materials. Biomaterials 1996;17:1157–1167.

38. Lee CK, Langrana NA, Parsons JR, et al. Development of a prosthetic intervertebral disc. Spine 1991;16:S253–S255.

39. Stubstad JA, Urbaniak JR, Kahn P. Prosthesis for spinal repair. United States Patent: 3,867, 728 (February 25, 1975).

40. Urbaniak JR, Bright DS, Hopkins JE. Replacement of intervertebral discs in chimpanzees. J Biomed Mater Res 1973;7(3):165–186.

41. Lee CK, Langrana NA, Alexander H, et al. Functional and biocompatible intervertebral disc spacer. United States Patent: 4,911,718 (March 27, 1990).

42. Parsons JR, Lee CK, Langrana NA, et al. Functional and biocompatible intervertebral disc spacer containing elastomeric material of varying hardness. United States Patent: 5,171,281 (December 15, 1992).

43. Langrana NA, Lee CK, Yang SW. Finite-element modeling of the synthetic intervertebral disc. Spine 1991;16(6):S245–S252.

44. Langrana NA, Parson JR, Lee CK, et al. Materials and design concepts for the intervertebral disc spacer: I fiber-reinforced composite design. J Appl Biomaterials 1994;5:125–132.

45. Kadoya K, Kotani Y, Abumi K, et al. Biomechanical and morphologic evaluation of the three-dimensional fabric sheep artificial intervertebral disc: in vitro and in vivo analysis. Spine 2001;26(14):1562–1569.

46. Kotani Y, Abumi K, Shikinami Y, et al. Artificial intervertebral disc replacement using bioactive three-dimensional fabric: design, development and preliminary animal study. Spine 2002;27 (9):929–935.

47. Steffee AD. Artificial disc. United States Patent: 5,071,437 (December 10, 1991).

48. Enker P, Steffee A, McMillan C, et al. Artificial disc replacement: preliminary report with a three year minimum followup. Spine 1993;18: 1061–1070.

49. Marnay T. Prosthesis for intervertebral discs and instruments for implanting it. United States Patent: 5,314,477 (May 24, 1994).

50. Buettner-Janz K, Helisch HJ, Schellnack K, et al. Intervertebral disc endoprosthesis. United States Patent: 4,759,766 (July 26, 1988).

51. McAfee PC, Cunningham BW, Shimamoto N, et al. General principles of porous ingrowth total disc replacement arthroplasty compared with diarthrodial total: joint arthroplasty, a nonhuman primate model. Spine J 2002;2(2S):22,

52. Lemaire JP, Skalli W, Lavaste F, et al. Intervertebral disc prosthesis. Clin Orthop Rel Res 1997;337:64–76.

53. Buettner-Janz K, Schellnack K, Zippel H. Biomechanics of the SB Charite lumbar intervertebral disc endoprosthesis. Int Orthop 1989;13: 173–176.

54. Cinotti G, David T, Postacchini F. Results of disc prosthesis after a minimum follow-up period of two years. Spine 1996;21(8):995–1000.

55. Cunningham B, Gordon J, Dmitriev A, et al. Biomechanical evaluation of total disc arthroplasty: an in-vitro human cadaveric model. Spine J 2002;2 (5S):104.

56. Zeegers WS, Bohnen LM, Laaper M, et al. Artificial disc replacement with the modular type SB Charite III: 2-year results in 50 prospectively studies patients. Eur Spine J 1999;8 (3):210–217.

57. Griffith SL, Shelokov AP, Buettner-Janz K, et al. A multicenter retrospective study of the clinical results of the LINK-SB Charite intervertebral prosthesis. Spine 1994;19:1842–1849,

58. Fernstrom U. Arthroplasty with intercorporal endoprosthesis in herniated disc and painful disc. Acta Chir Scand 1966;355:154–159.

59. Garcia A, Lavignolle B, Morlier P, et al. Intravertebral polymerization: preliminary results of chemical and biomechanical studies. In: Brock M, Mayer HM, Weigel K, eds. The artificial disc. Berlin: Springer-Verlag, 1991:39–43.

60. Ray CD, Corbin TP. Prosthetic disc and method of implanting. United States Patent: 4,772,287 (September 20, 1988) and 4,904,260 (February 27, 1990).

61. Klara PM, Ray CD. Artificial nucleus replacement: clinical experience. Spine 2002;27(12):1374–1377.

62. Eysel P, Rompe J, Schoenmayr R, et al. Biomechanical behavior of a prosthetic lumbar nucleus. Acta Neurochir 1999;141(10):1083–1087.

63. Bertagnoli R, Schonmayr R. Surgical and clinical results with the PDN prosthetic disc-nucleus device. Eur Spine J 2002;11[Suppl 2]:S143–S148.

64. Meyers M, Weinandt B. Understanding end plate changes associated with disc surgery. Spine J 2002;2(5S):112S–113S.

65. Modic MT, Steinberg PM, Ross JS, et al. Degenerative disc disease: assessment of changes in vertebral body marrow with MR imaging. Radiology 1988;166:193–199.

66. Bao, QP. Hydrogel intervertebral disc nucleus. United States Patent: 5,047,055 (September 10, 1991) and 5,192,326 (March 9, 1993).

67. Ordway NR, Han ZH, Bao QP, et al. Biomechanical evaluation of the intervertebral hydrogel nucleus. Paper presented at: Ninth Annual Meeting of the North American Spine Society; October 19–22, 1994; Minneapolis, Minnesota.

68. Ordway NR, Han ZH, Bao QP, et al. Restoration of biomechanical function with the hydrogel intervertebral disc implant. Paper presented at: Twenty-first Annual Meeting of the International Society of the Study of the Lumbar Spine; June 21–25, 1995; Seattle, Washington.

69. Baumgartner W. Intervertebral prosthesis. United States Patent: 5,171, 280 (December 15, 1992).

70. Korge A, Nydegger T, Polard JL, et al. A spiral implant as nucleus prosthesis in the lumbar spine. Eur Spine J 2002;11[Suppl 2]:S149–S153.

71. Bao QB, Yuan HA. Nucleus replacement. Spine 2002;27:1245–1247.

72. Urban RM, Jacobs JJ, Tomlinson MJ, et al. Dissemination of wear particles to the liver, spleen, and abdominal lymph nodes of patients with hip or knee replacement. J Bone Joint Surg 2000;82-A:457–477.

73. Archibeck MJ, Jacobs JJ, Roebuck KA, et al. The basic science of periprosthetic osteolysis. Instr Course Lect 2001;50:185–195.

74. Cunningham BW, Orbegoso CM, Dimitriev AE, et al. The effect of spinal instrumentation particulate wear debris: an in vivo rabbit model and applied clinical study of retrieved instrumentation cases. Spine J 2002;2(5S):69–70.

75. Moore RJ, Fraser RD, Vernon-Roberts B, et al. The biologic response to particles from a lumbar disc prosthesis. Spine 2002;27(19):2088–2094.

76. Bertagnoli R, Kumar S. Indications for full prosthetic disc arthroplasty: a correlation of clinical outcome against a variety or indications. Eur Spine J 2002;11[Suppl 2]:S131–S136.

CHAPTER 40

Lumbar Disc Replacement: Current Model, Results, and the Future

Robert D. Fraser

More than 100 different designs for a disc prosthesis have been patented or described in publications (1) since Fernstrom first replaced the nucleus with a metal bearing ball in the late 1950s (2). Very few of these devices have been used clinically, however, reflecting the difficulty of translating the success of hip and knee arthroplasty to the spine. The prostheses that have been implanted in humans can be classified as (a) nucleus devices or spacers, (b) mechanical devices with moving parts, and (c) elastomeric implants that aim to reconstruct the normal elastic properties of the disc.

NUCLEUS PROSTHESES

The nucleus replacement device used most extensively in humans is the Prosthetic Disc Nucleus, or PDN (Raymedica, Minneapolis, MN). This consists of a hydrogel pellet contained within a woven polyethylene jacket. The hydrophilic properties of hydrogel provide this device with the capacity to absorb fluid and expand. Hydrogel is a copolymer of polyacrylonitrile (nonhydrophilic) and polyacrylamide (hydrophilic); the ability to absorb and bind water is determined by the ratio of these polymers. The current design permits the pellets to absorb 80% of their weight in water, giving the PDN device the potential to restore or maintain disc height. The aim of the woven polyethylene jacket is to limit swelling and to minimize horizontal spreading (3).

The recommended technique involves the coronal placement of two parallel devices within the enucleated disc space, either by the posterior (hemilaminotomy) or lateral (transpsoas) routes. The developers state that this device is not intended for use in cases of severe disc degeneration or where end plate defects are present (3).

Initial trials during the mid-1990s, with two implants placed side by side in a sagittal plane, demonstrated a high expulsion rate with 38% of subjects requiring revi-

sion (4). The PDN shape and surgical protocol were subsequently modified to minimize the extrusion rate, and further clinical trials are in progress. Encouraging results are claimed with the use of PDN (3–5), although in each paper details of the methodology are insufficient to permit critical review.

Other nuclear replacements implanted clinically include the Aquarelle (Stryker Howmedica, Mahwah, NJ), a polyvinyl alcohol material and the Newcleus (Sulzer Spine-Tech, Edina, MN), a polycarbonate urethane elastomer, but to date there are no published results of these devices.

Nucleus prostheses may be inserted through a relatively minimally invasive or potentially percutaneous approach. While this increases the appeal of the procedure, nucleus replacement does not address pathology related to the annulus or end plate, both of which may be important components of a painful degenerative process. Furthermore, nucleus devices are intended to work in conjunction with the annulus to restore the biomechanical function of the disc. To insert such a device, an annulus lesion must either be made or already exist. Although special dilators to minimize annulus damage have been used for the phase IV trials of the PDN, it is unclear whether the benefits of nucleus replacement will outweigh the effects of damage caused to the annulus.

MECHANICAL DISC PROSTHESES

The prime aim of mechanical disc replacement is to restore the normal kinematics of the motion segment. The designs of two mechanical disc prostheses tested in clinical trials are based on the principle of low-friction polyethylene on metal articulations developed for total hip and knee arthroplasty. A third device, similarly designed on the basis of the success of prostheses developed for large synovial joints but with a metal/metal (chrome cobalt) interface and a posterior rotation axis, is being

393

tested in a multicenter clinical trial (6). In general these prostheses are intended to replace almost the entire disc, are inserted using an approach similar to an anterior lumbar interbody fusion, and rely on large spikes or fins plus bony ingrowth for stability against the vertebral end plates. Mechanical artificial discs lack elasticity and cannot replicate the normal compressive stiffness of the natural disc. Instead they depend on the restoration of a mobile lordosis to absorb compressive loads across the lumbar spine (7). Moreover their articulating surfaces provide little resistance to torsion, a function of the motion segment that is impaired by the necessary removal of most of the annulus.

Schellnack and Buttner-Janz were responsible for the development of the first version of the Link SB Charité (Waldemar Link GmbH & Co., Hamburg) artificial disc in 1982 (8). Over the next five years there were two revisions of the design. Consisting of a biconvex polyethylene spacer articulating with two concave cobalt-chromium alloy end plates, the prosthesis allows rotation in all three planes. Changing centers of rotation are allowed by the sliding of the polyethylene core, similar to that which is achieved in mobile-bearing total knee replacements. First implanted in 1987, the latest model of the Link SB Charité has been used more extensively than any other disc prosthesis. Approximately 4,000 prostheses have been implanted (7); the report from the largest case series of 105 patients describes a satisfactory outcome with the procedure (8).

The ProDisc (Spine Solutions, New York, NY) was first described by Marnay in 1991 (9). It consists of a polyethylene cap articulating with two titanium alloy end plates. The cap over cup design of the metal-polyethylene-metal articulation permits motion in all three planes. Bertagnoli and Kumar reported on a series of 108 patients with follow-up ranging between 3 months to 2 years (10). In this, the only published paper on the outcome with the ProDisc, an overall success rate of 90.8% was claimed, increasing to 98% in patients considered to have "prime" indications.

ELASTOMERIC DISC PROSTHESES

The attraction of elastomeric discs is their potential to replicate the elasticity of the normal human disc. Not only would it be feasible to restore the normal compressive stiffness of the natural disc, but also if firm attachments to the bony end plates could be achieved, it would provide resistance to torsion and shear.

With these goals in mind, Steffee designed the Acro-Flex (DePuy, Acromed Corporation, Cleveland, OH) artificial disc using a polyolefin-based rubber core vulcanized between two titanium end plates. Not only did the rubber core provide range of motion, but it also enabled replication of normal disc elasticity. In theory, this design

should allow for better absorption of loads. However, this advantage of elastomers is offset by their potentially inferior wear characteristics as demonstrated by the relatively high rates of failure. In the original series of six patients, two were reported as failures due to debonding of the rubber core (11). A second-generation device, using a silicone core instead of rubber, was implanted in eight patients with one mechanical failure. All failures occurred at levels with increased stress, either due to adjacent fusion levels or scoliosis. The AcroFlex is now in its third generation of design, reverting back to the rubber core optimized with improved processing and bonding techniques, and refined indications for surgery. Although functional outcomes following implantation have been generally satisfactory, further trials with the third generation prosthesis were abandoned with the detection of early failure of the rubber core on thin-section computed tomography (CT) scans (12).

The thin-section CT scans used in the AcroFlex study also identified a significant number of patients with periprosthetic heterotopic ossification. Limiting range of motion may be another potential source of failure for any disc replacement. It is therefore recommended that future studies include the use of thin-section CT and relate this to range of motion on standing flexion and extension radiographs.

BASIS FOR CURRENT INDICATIONS

For any spinal operation, including total disc arthroplasty, patient selection should be based on a careful consideration of many factors. A successful outcome is more likely to be achieved with the precise correlation of the patient's history, physical examination, and radiographic investigations, in conjunction with psychosocial and medical backgrounds. Bearing this in mind, indications were developed for a trial of the AcroFlex lumbar disc prosthesis (12). Only patients with one- or two-level symptomatic disc degeneration at either L4-5 or L5-S1 were included. Patients had to complain of disabling low back pain, with or without referral type leg symptoms that had been present for a minimum of 12 months and had failed to respond to nonoperative treatment. Furthermore, the symptomatic degenerative level had to be convincingly localized by provocative discography. For inclusion in the study discography had to demonstrate (a) internal disc disruption at the target level, (b) reproduction of the patient's typical pain at the target level, and (c) failure to reproduce typical pain at the control levels adjacent to the target level. Because of uncertainty about the long-term results only patients between the ages of 30 and 55 were considered (12).

The contraindications to disc replacement surgery are made up of technical and patient selection considerations. Patients should be excluded if there is a history of previous lumbar infection or an active infection elsewhere. Because disc replacement surgery does not address posterior element pathology, patients with spondylitic spondylolisthesis, significant facet arthritis, lateral recess stenosis, or central stenosis should be considered unsuitable. Technical considerations that impede or prevent disc arthroplasty include patients with a steep lumbosacral angle at the target level, osteopenia, previous abdominal radiation or vascular graft, and morbid abdominal obesity. Lastly, patient factors such as significant medical comorbidity, ongoing litigation or compensation issues, substance abuse, presence of three or more Waddell behavioral signs (13), or psychiatric illness may be the major factors influencing eventual outcomes. The presence of any of these factors should be regarded a contraindication to disc replacement surgery.

Despite the suggestion that in time disc replacement will be a solution for multilevel degeneration or degeneration adjacent to a fused segment, this has not been considered an ideal indication. Additionally, given the increased stresses placed on the prosthesis in a patient with structural scoliosis or adjacent-level fusion, such conditions are considered relative contraindications.

Bertagnoli and Kumar tried to correlate preoperative clinical findings to outcome with a view to formulating appropriate indications for disc replacement (10). They conducted a retrospective review of 108 patients who underwent total disc arthroplasty with the ProDisc prosthesis. The patients were separated into accordingly into four groups, those who were considered to have "prime", "good", "borderline", or "poor" indications for surgery. Patients with a "prime" indication had a disc height greater than 4 mm, absence of facet joint arthritis, no adjacent-level degeneration, and intact posterior elements. Patients with adjacent-level fusions were considered to have "borderline" indications. While there appears to be a gradient of improved successful outcomes in patients with better indications, no statistical analyses were performed. However, it also seems that patients with "better indications" were those with minimal degeneration and they may well have achieved better outcomes no matter what form of treatment was employed.

REPORTED CLINICAL RESULTS

In a critical assessment of the evidence related to lumbar disc replacement, Wai et al. (14) carried out a thorough search of both the Pubmed and Ovid Medline databases up to October 2002, and identified papers concerned with the current clinical use of disc prostheses. Their assessment, summarized in Table 40-1, recorded factors important to the outcome of disc replacement, namely: (a) restoration of disc function, (b) preservation of adjacent levels, (c) overall clinical function, and (d) complications. The follow-up for all papers reviewed

averaged just less than 2 years with the conclusions often based on patients followed up for a much shorter period.

Although a follow-up of 2 years is generally considered acceptable for publishing surgical results, it is quite inadequate when assessing the outcome of disc replacement surgery. This is particularly the case when assessing the safety of implants used for total disc replacement. Their large dimensions and location close to major vessels makes anterior low-lumbar revision surgery hazardous, particularly when this is performed for complications related to mechanical failure.

In their critical review, Wai et al. (14) found a wide discrepancy in the definitions of clinical outcome, many of which were poorly defined, with reported success rates ranging from 63% to 95% after disc replacement. Overall, these results are similar to those from case series reports for spinal fusion (15–21), and for common forms of nonoperative care (22–26). Certainly, randomized controlled trials, using validated and independent assessments of outcome and safety are necessary to establish the efficacy of disc replacement compared with the current standard of care. Clearly, because of the large influence on function of factors other than disc pathology, a major effect from disc replacement would be needed to reach statistically significant differences. The Swedish Lumbar Spine Study Group published a report of a randomized controlled trial on fusion for back pain (15). From the published data, Wai et al. (14) estimated that more than 500 subjects would be needed to determine a 10% improvement in outcome for a 2:1 study design with a power of 0.8.

Even though there may be no significant difference in clinical outcomes between fusion and disc replacement in the short term, the latter has the theoretical advantage of restoring the function of the motion segment, hence protecting the adjacent levels. Almost all of the published studies have described restoration of disc height and return of motion for both nuclear and total disc replacement surgeries (14). Although protection of adjacent disc levels is considered of prime importance to the rationale for disc replacement, only three studies have assessed this potential benefit. Cinotti et al. performed magnetic resonance imaging (MRI) on 10 patients from their original cohort of Link SB Charité III prostheses and found no adjacent level degeneration (27). As more than 75% of their study population has not been assessed, it is not valid to draw any conclusions from their report. In the report of their experience with the ProDisc, Bertagnoli and Kumar mention that 4.6% of patients developed radiographic evidence of adjacent-level degeneration within 3 to 24 months of implantation (10). With such a short follow-up and without a control group, it is unclear if this represents the natural history of disc degeneration or is significantly less than would have occurred had the patients undergone a lumbar fusion. Many investigations of

TABLE 40-1. *Summary of published peer-reviewed clinical papers on disc replacement arthroplasty*

Author/year	Disc	Sample size (no. of discs)	Months of follow-up (range if stated)	Study quality	Restoration of normal mechanics	Preservation of adjacent levels	Clinical success	Complications
Enker, 1993	Acroflex	6	40	—	8° avg. ROM	N/A	66% success	33% implant failure
Griffith, 1994	Charité SB III	93 (139)	12 (1–37)	—	N/A	N/A	65% improvement in back pain	4.3% migration/dislocation; 1% core failure
Cinotti, 1996	Charité SB III	46 (56)	38 (48–60)	IR, NC	12° avg. ROM	No degeneration on MRI for 10 patients	63% good or excellent, 17% required eventual fusion	26% placed too anterior; ROM affected if malpositioned
Lemaire, 1997	Charité SB III	105	51	NC	7° avg. ROM, >50% restoration of disc height and lordosis	N/A	79% excellent	2.9% related to implant (1 subsidence, 2 ossification)
Zeegers, 1999	Charité SB III	46 (75)	48	NC	74% good technical radiographic result	24% required adjacent level OR	70% improved	1 required conversion to fusion
Sott, 2000	Charité SB III	15	48 (18–68)	NC	N/A	N/A	80% good or fair results	None related to implant
Bertagnoli, 2002	ProDisc	108 (134)	(3–48)	VQ, NC	10° avg. ROM	4.6% adjacent level degeneration	90.8% excellent	None related to implant
Hopf, 2002	Charité SB III	35	15	NC	Correction of avg. lordosis by 7°	N/A	80% reduction in pain medication	None related to implant
Bertagnoli, 2002	PDN—phase III trials	168	6 (3–24)	VQ	Preservation of disc height	N/A	88% success	26% required revision for migration
Hochshuler, 2002	Charité SB III	22	12	VQ	N/A	N/A	40% improvement in Oswestry	None related to implant
Klara, 2002	PDN—all phases	423	Up to 48[a]	VQ	Increase in disc height by an avg. of 1.8 mm reported in 7 patients[b]	N/A	43.7% improvement of Oswestry scores reported in 7 patients	10% overall explant rate
Buttner-Janz, 2002	Charité SB III	20	46 (6–156)	VQ	7° avg. ROM	N/A	95% reduction in pain	None related to implant

IR, reported that outcomes assessed independently; MRI, magnetic resonance imaging; NC, no conflict of interest stated; OR, operation; ROM, range of motion; VQ, validated questionnaire (e.q., SF36, Oswestry) used in clinical assessment.

Reproduced from Wai E, Selmon G, Fraser RD. Disc replacement arthroplasties: can the success of hip and knee replacements be repeated in the spine? Semin Spine Surg 2003;(15)4:473–482.

[a]Clinical results of patients with shorter follow-up not reported.

[b]Not clearly stated for radiographic details but implied since 7 patients reported for Oswestry.

adjacent-level degeneration after fusion have used MRI or have longer follow-up times (28–31).

The work of Kumar et al. is the most similar in methodology to the study by Bertagnoli et al. but with a much longer follow-up period (32). They found an 8% incidence of radiographically determined adjacent-level disease in patients 5 years following lumbar fusion with a normal sagittal alignment. Furthermore, in an MRI study we carried out 10 years after anterior lumbar interbody fusion (28), the adjacent disc was found to be free of degeneration in 68% of cases. We examined the pattern of degeneration in the remainder of the lumbar spine, including the presence of skip lesions, comparing this with the reports of MRI findings in normal asymptomatic populations. Based on this comparison, we concluded that adjacent-level degeneration was determined more by constitutional factors than by the presence of a solid fusion.

Further challenging the ability of disc replacement to preserve the adjacent levels, a study by Zeegers found that 24% of patients required adjacent-level surgery within 2 years of having an SB Charité III prosthesis inserted (33). While this high incidence may represent a failure to adequately rule out adjacent-level pathology before performing the index procedure, it is much higher than any reported for lumbar fusion. In any event, there is clearly no evidence to date that disc replacement protects against adjacent level degeneration.

FOOD AND DRUG ADMINISTRATION STATUS

At the present time, the U.S. Food and Drug Administration (FDA) has not approved disc replacement devices for routine marketing, and currently the use of these devices is for investigational purposes only. To obtain approval for general use the manufacturer is required to demonstrate to the FDA's satisfaction that their prosthesis is as substantially equivalent (as safe and effective) to an already approved device. Specific guidelines concerning the indications, *in vivo* biomechanical testing, and clinical results of devices have been published for spinal implants (34).

Two separate multicenter, randomized controlled clinical trials are in progress in the United States under the FDA's Investigational Device Exemption. The SB Charité III is being compared with anterior interbody fusion using the Bagby and Kuslich (BAK) device, while the ProDisc is being tested against combined anterior and posterior fusion using pedicle screws and an interbody fusion construct (35). Both trials intend to recruit between 300 and 500 patients and the manufacturers hope to achieve FDA approval within the next few years. The initiation of a FDA-approved trial in the United States is pending. The PDN has been given approval by the Canadian Therapeutic Directorate to begin a clinical trial and three Canadian centers are recruiting patients for a prospective evaluation of the PDN (4).

It is expected that these trials will address short-term safety issues related to the prostheses and whether the clinical efficacy is similar to fusion at 2 years. As mentioned previously, these studies are unlikely to have sufficient power to detect a difference with fusion unless there is a large clinical effect. It is therefore essential that long-term follow-up of the studies be carried out to determine efficacy, the overall safety of the implants, and their ability to protect adjacent levels.

THE FUTURE OF DISC REPLACEMENT

It is the spectacular success of arthroplasty of the hip and knee that has continued to drive the development of artificial disc technology. Further enthusiasm has been generated by the demonstration that a number of prostheses have restored range of motion to the disc and by the clinical use of the Link SB Charité device for over 10 years. However, this measure of technical success and implant longevity does not necessarily mean that the future of disc replacement is certain. It is only if it can be shown in the long term to perform at least as well as fusion, without compromise from implant failure, heterotopic bone formation or excessive facet degeneration leading to stenosis, that the place of disc replacement will be finally assured.

From the reported results of case series described herein, it seems likely that current FDA trials will demonstrate short-term efficacy and safety, leading to approval of these devices for routine marketing. Because of anticipated demand, the expected FDA approval is likely to be followed by extensive and widespread clinical usage of these devices. Based on the experience associated with the release of other spinal implants as well as the knowledge gained from hip and knee arthroplasty, it will be only a matter of time before surgeons are confronted with problems created by implant failure. There is, however, one major advantage for the spinal surgeon compared with the hip or knee surgeon undertaking revision procedures for a failed prosthesis. Unlike surgery for the hip and knee, there is unlikely to be a great functional disadvantage in converting spinal arthroplasty to arthrodesis; moreover, it may be possible to circumvent the surgical site by retrieving the situation with a posterolateral fusion. However, when it is necessary to remove a large lumbar interbody device anteriorly, the proximity of the major vessels and other vital organs, the scarring from the original surgery, and the pathology associated with implant failure all combine to make the revision procedure extremely difficult and potentially disastrous (12).

Clearly the introduction of these devices into the community should be with caution. The current "gold standard" investigations for diagnosis of discogenic back pain, MRI, and discography have significant high false-positive rates. A large potential for misdiagnosis resulting in surgery for pain not arising from the disc exists; hence the unsatisfactory outcomes often reported for treatment of discogenic back pain.

Combined anterior and posterior fusion has been promoted by many spinal surgeons for the management of back pain since it deals with many different potential pain sources, including not only the disc but also the ligaments and facet joints. In contrast, disc arthroplasty targets only the disc. It is, therefore, more vulnerable to the effects of misdiagnosis leading to the replacement of a nonpainful disc rather than dealing with the actual pain source. This is countered by the restoration of the functional spinal unit's range of motion. However, it is unclear whether the extra few degrees of range of motion offered by a disc replacement over fusion is functionally significant, especially given the motion available at adjacent levels and hip joints.

Future models of spinal arthroplasty will no doubt aim to replicate the elastic properties of the disc without incurring the problem of wear particles, and also will attempt to address facet joint pathology. It will take a great deal of time and carefully controlled long-term trials to determine whether or not these devices offer the best alternative for patients undergoing surgery for discogenic low back pain.

REFERENCES

1. Szpalski M, Gunzburg R, Mayer M. Spine arthroplasty: a historical review. Eur Spine J 2002;11:S65–S84.
2. Fernstrom U. Arthroplasty with intercorporal endoprosthesis in herniated disc and in painful disc. Acta Orthop Scand 1966;10:S287–S289.
3. Ray CD. The PDN prosthetic disc-nucleus device. Eur Spine J 2002; 11:S137–S142.
4. Klara PM, Ray CD. Artificial nucleus replacement—clinical experience. Spine 2002;27:1374–1377.
5. Bertagnoli R, Schonmayr R. Surgical and clinical results with the PDN prosthetic disc-nucleus device. Eur Spine J 2002;11:S143–S148.
6. Matthews H, Le Huec JC, Bertagnoli R, et al. Design, rationale and early multicenter evaluation of Maverick total disk arthroplasty. Paper presented at: International Meeting on Advanced Spine Technologies; May 2002; Montreux, France.
7. Lemaire JP, Skalli W, Lavaste F, et al. Intervertebral disc prosthesis. Results and prospects for the year 2000. Clin Orthop 1997;337:64–76.
8. Link HD. History, design and biomechanics of the Link SB Charite artificial disc. Eur Spine J 2002;11:S98–S105.
9. Marnay T. L'arthroplastie intervertebrale lombaire. Med Orthop 1991; 25:48–55.
10. Bertagnoli R, Kumar S. Indications for full prosthetic disc arthroplasty: a correlation of clinical outcome against a variety of indications. Eur Spine J 2002;11:S131–S136.
11. Enker P, Steffee A, McMillin C, et al. Artificial disc replacement. Preliminary report with a 3-year minimum follow-up. Spine 1993;18:1061–1070.
12. Fraser RD, Ross ER, Lowery G. AcroFlex: design and results. Spine J 2004 (in press).
13. Waddell G, McCulloch JA, Kummel E, et al. Nonorganic physical signs in low-back pain. Spine 1980;5:117–125.
14. Wai E, Selmon G, Fraser RD. Disc replacement arthroplasties: can the success of hip and knee replacements be repeated in the spine? Semin Spine Surg 2003;15(4):473–482.
15. Fritzell P, Hagg O, Wessberg P, et al. 2001 Volvo award winner in clinical studies: lumbar fusion versus nonsurgical treatment for chronic low back pain. A multicenter randomized controlled trial from the Swedish Lumbar Spine Study Group. Spine 2001;26:2521–2534.
16. Bjarke-Christensen F, Stender-Hansen E, Laursen M, et al. Long-term functional outcome of pedicle screw instrumentation as a support for posterolateral spinal fusion: randomized clinical study with a 5-year follow-up. Spine 2002;27:1269–1277.
17. Kuslich SD, Ulstrom CL, Griffith SL, et al. The Bagby and Kuslich method of lumbar interbody fusion. History, techniques, and 2-year follow-up results of a United States prospective, multicenter trial. Spine 1998;23:1267–1278.
18. Kuroki H, Tajima N, Kubo S. Clinical results of posterolateral fusion for degenerative lumbar spinal diseases: a follow-up study of more than 10 years. J Orthop Sci 2002;7:317–324.
19. Liljenqvist U, O'Brien JP, Renton P. Simultaneous combined anterior and posterior lumbar fusion with femoral cortical allograft. Eur Spine J 1998;7:125–131.
20. O'Beirne J, O'Neill D, Gallagher J, et al. Spinal fusion for back pain: a clinical and radiological review. J Spinal Disord 1992;5:32–38.
21. Kleeman TJ, Ahn UM, Talbot-Kleeman A. Laparoscopic anterior lumbar interbody fusion with rhBMP-2: a prospective study of clinical and radiographic outcomes. Spine 2001;26:2751–2756.
22. Cherkin DC, Deyo RA, Battie M, et al. A comparison of physical therapy, chiropractic manipulation, and provision of an educational booklet for the treatment of patients with low back pain. N Engl J Med 1998;339:1021–1029.
23. Nelemans PJ, Bie RA, deVet HCW, et al. Injection therapy for subacute and chronic benign low back pain. Cochrane Database of Systematic Reviews. 2002;4.
24. Saal JA, Saal JS. Intradiscal electrothermal treatment for chronic discogenic low back pain: prospective outcome study with a minimum 2-year follow-up. Spine 2002;27:966–973.
25. Tulder MW, Cherkin DC, Berman B, et al. Acupuncture for low back pain. Cochrane Database of Systematic Reviews. 2002;4.
26. Tulder MW, Malmivaara A, Esmail R, et al. Exercise therapy for low back pain. Cochrane Database of Systematic Reviews. 2002;4.
27. Cinotti G, David T, Postacchini F. Results of disc prosthesis after a minimum follow-up period of 2 years. Spine 1996;21:995–1000.
28. Penta M, Sandhu A, Fraser RD. Magnetic resonance imaging assessment of disc degeneration 10 years after anterior lumbar interbody fusion. Spine 1995;20:743–747.
29. Hanley EN, Shapiro DE. The development of low-back pain after excision of a lumbar disc. J Bone Joint Surg 1989;71-A:719–721.
30. Kumar MN, Jacquot F, Hall H. Long-term follow-up of functional outcomes and radiographic changes at adjacent levels following lumbar spine fusion for degenerative disc disease. Eur Spine J 2001;10: 309–313.
31. Nakai S, Yoshizawa H, Kobayashi S. Long-term follow-up study of posterior lumbar interbody fusion. J Spinal Disord 1999;12:293–299.
32. Kumar MN, Baklanov A, Chopin D. Correlation between sagittal plane changes and adjacent segment degeneration following lumbar spine fusion. Eur Spine J 2001;10:314–319.
33. Zeegers WS, Bohnen LM, Laaper M, et al. Artificial disc replacement with the modular type SB Charité III: 2-year results in 50 prospectively studied patients. Eur Spine J 1999;8:210–217.
34. Food and Drug Administration. FDA Guidance for Spinal System 510(k)s: U.S. Department of Health and Human Services, 2000.
35. Hochshuler SH, Ohnmeiss DD, Guyer, et al. Artificial disc: preliminary results of a prospective study in the United States. Eur Spine J 2002:11:S106–S110.

CHAPTER 41

Disc Herniation: Definition and Types

Tom Bendix

Disc herniation used to be considered as a local bulge on a disc surface, causing pressure on a nerve root. This was based largely on the fact that myelogram was the only way to establish the diagnosis. As myelogram is a highly invasive procedure, which also exposes the patient to significant radiation levels, it is considered ethically unacceptable in the examination of asymptomatic individuals. Today, computed tomography (CT) and magnetic resonance imaging (MRI) studies in asymptomatic individuals have shown that the presence of a local bulge on the disc surface certainly does not correlate convincingly with the classic symptoms of disc herniation (Fig. 41-1) (1–6).

Such studies have sparked a totally new era for this diagnosis. It is likely that disc herniation symptoms are predominantly initiated by nuclear tissue coming into physical contact with the nerve root, whereas a (local) bulge does not normally cause nerve damage (Fig. 41-1). Moreover, after a passed clinical cause the bulge consists of scar tissue, forming the morphologic "herniation" (7).

Several terms have been used to describe this condition: disc herniation, herniated nucleus pulposus (HNP), prolapse, and slipped disc are those most often used. Time has come, however, to redefine the condition as a syndrome characterized by nerve damage, primarily caused by irritation from nuclear tissue, giving rise to a production of a variety of cytokines and other inflammatory or autoimmune components (8–21), leading to secondary pressure hypersensitivity (22,23).

While lifetime prevalence of sciatica of any etiology is about 40% (24), no authors have been able to give a serious frequency of lifetime prevalence of lumbar disc herniation (LDH). This may be in agreement with the vague definitions described later in the chapter that the most frequent rough estimate is about 3% to 4%. The 1-year incidence has been estimated at 0.1% to 0.5% (25). Of patients with acute low back pain, only 1% have nerve-root symptoms (26). Age distribution has its peak close to 40, and male: female ratio is probably close to 1:1 for all

LDH, whereas for those operated upon it is 1.5:1 to 2:1 (5,27,28).

In this chapter only lumbar annular (not end plate) disc herniation is addressed.

The onset of annular rupture is usually the end point of gradual disc degeneration, which in turn seems more related to genetic issues than to physical loads (29). Of physical factors, flexion plays the greatest role, but even this factor is not impressive (30).

DEFINITIONS

Considering the aforementioned poor correlation between clinical and imaging findings, different aspects of definitions have to be considered.

Patho-Anatomic Types

In accordance with today's knowledge (as discussed later in the chapter), the aspect of the nucleus being contained or not seems most relevant as the primary nerve damage is most likely associated with the inflammatory influence of free nucleus pulposus tissue on the nerve root. If nerve damage resulted primarily from pressure, it is not likely that so many silent disc herniations are seen in MRI studies. Pressure is, however, obviously important secondarily, as pressure on any inflamed structure causes pain. But as the primary lesion, pressure alone only rarely seems to be relevant (Fig. 41-2).

Contained

The disc bulges locally, but the outermost layer is still intact. In most cases it is questionable whether this condition causes root damage, rather than referred discogenic pain. If the bulge compresses the dorsal ganglion of the intervertebral nerve root, however, it is likely that the presence of nuclear material directly touching the root

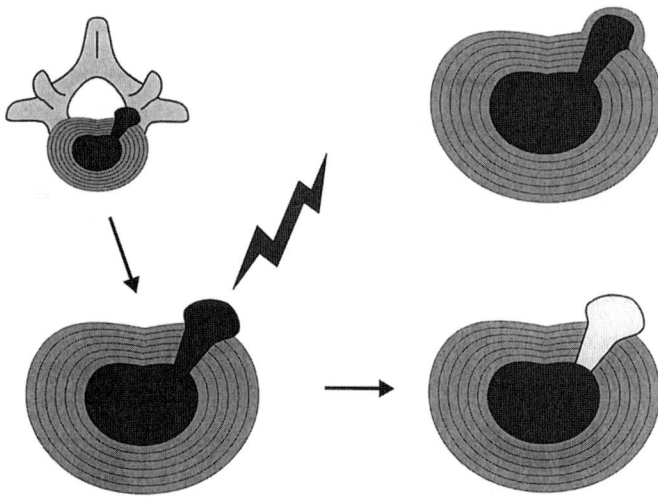

FIG. 41-1. The three disc herniations shown here are identical on computed tomography or magnetic resonance imaging. Clinically only the one with chemical irritation of the nerve root **(bottom, left)** produces symptoms. **Bottom right:** A healed, but now clinically silent herniation.

may not be necessary (31,32). This is substantiated by research demonstrating that the threshold for compression-induced neuronal firing is about half that for other parts of the nerve root (33). Likewise, if a chemically inactive bulge causes compression over such a wide area of the nerve root that the root suffers ischemia (33), this may also sensitize the nerve root without any chemically induced lesion (34–36) (Fig. 41-3).

It seems as if contained disc herniations or more diffuse disc herniation displacements (5,37,38) represent a poorer prognosis as opposed to a more well-defined herniation, probably because the first condition is only a small part of a more substantial degeneration (Fig. 41-6). Some authors also divide "contained disc herniations" into "soft" and "hard" categories. Thus, pain from a primary contained disc herniation is most likely rather a "simple" discogenic pain, which causes back pain that dominates over optional leg pain. Such leg pain can be "radicular"/dermatomal in its perceived location (39), but will most often be diffuse in its distribution.

Contained

Complete

or

Sequestered

"No-bulge herniation" (?)

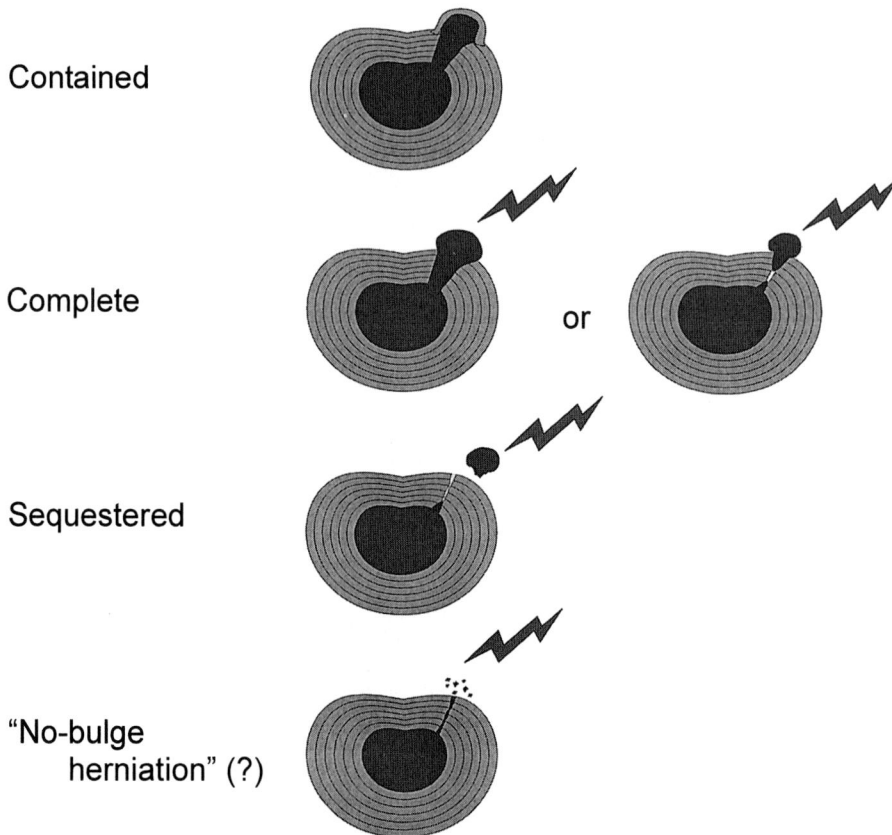

FIG. 41-2. The different types of disc herniations.

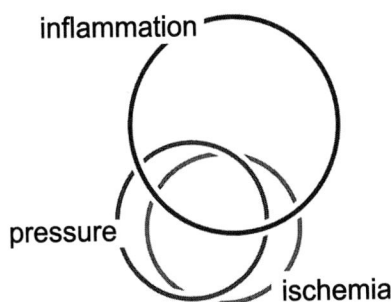

FIG. 41-3. The main basic pathology in disc herniation is inflammation. Pressure on the ganglion and ischemia (widespread compression) may also cause a primary lesion, but plays a greater role as secondary irritation when existing inflammation has caused nerve damage.

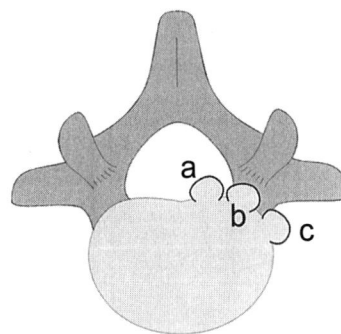

FIG. 41-4. The location in the segment can be intraspinal (a), foraminal (b), or extraforaminal (c).

Complete = Protruded = Free

The nuclear material has broken through the outermost layer of annulus fibrosus, and can be seen in the canal, and is therefore no longer contained. It is extruded from the fissure of the disc, whether or not it is in continuum with the central nuclear tissue. It is not quite clear from literature if a herniation that has passed the outermost annulus layer, but still remains subligamentous (40), is considered "free". Those protruding through the ligament are called "transligamentous" (40).

Sequestered

A free nucleus fragment, no longer in contact with the annular canal it originated from, is clinically meaningful in the interpretation of fluctuating symptoms, and during surgery.

"No-Bulge Herniation"

It seems likely that some nucleus-tissue–induced nerve damage is caused by leakage of nuclear chemicals that do not physically form a bulge on the disc (Olmarker, personal communication). As with other nerve-root lesions, a mechanical component is needed to cause the leakage.

Radiologic Types

Radiologically, LDH is defined as a localized bulge on a disc. Several researchers have tried to make a strict distinction between prolapse and disc protrusion by means of deciding how much of the entire intervertebral-disc circumference is taken up by the bulging "dome". The reason why no consensus has ever been made is most likely that it has become clearer that the correlation between a certain "dome" and the clinical symptoms is small (1).

Another radiologic categorization refers to the location of the LDH on the circumference (Fig. 41-4).

The intraspinal herniation is most often paramedian as shown on Fig. 41-4, but can be median as well. "Extraforaminal" herniation is also known as "extreme lateral", and seems to cause a higher degree of pain than the other types (41).

Clinical Types

The classic disc herniation starts after a period with only back pain, or back pain that dominates over leg pain/sciatica. When leg pain takes over and dominates, the course of a disc herniation begins (Fig. 41-5).

It may be argued that the clinical disc herniation begins with the initial back pain. However, when a period of (dominating) back pain of discogenic origin starts, it is only seldom that it is followed by a disc herniation. Moreover, dominating leg pain may follow shortly after the onset of back pain, or after months or years with back pain. Probably the short course corresponds to a single, and "clean" annular rupture, whereas a long-lasting "prodrome" may correspond to a herniation in a disc that is highly degenerated (Fig. 41-6).

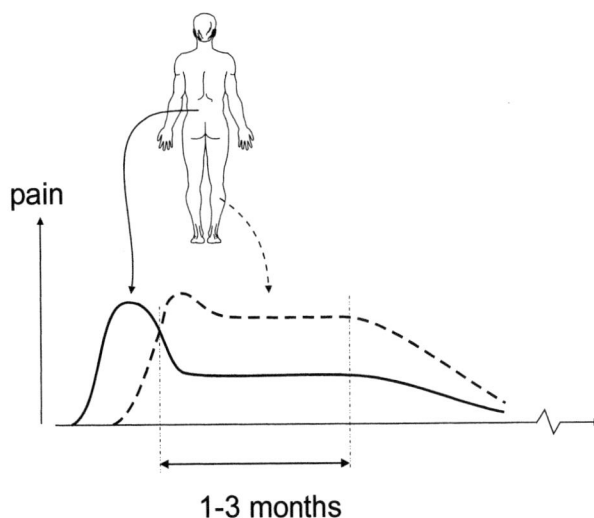

FIG. 41-5. A typical course of a disc herniation. See text.

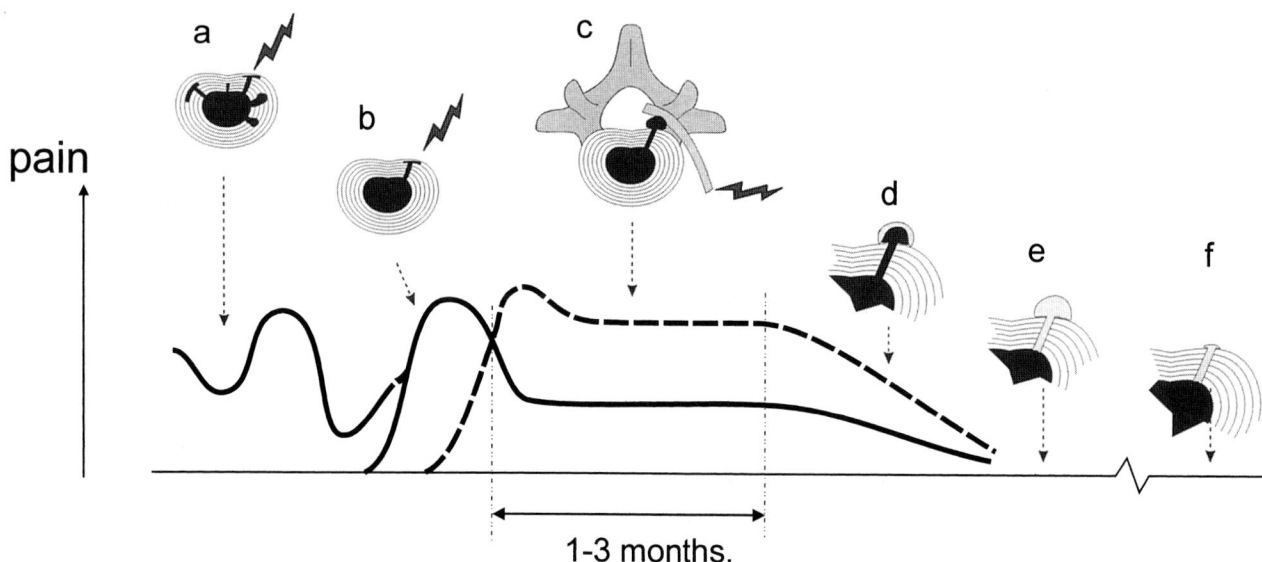

FIG. 41-6. The clinical course of a disc herniation in relation to the different stages of what happens in the disc. See text.

The distribution of leg pain usually follows the root leaving the spinal canal one level caudal to the herniation (Fig. 41-7). If the herniation is more centrally located, the root leaving two levels below will occasionally be affected. A central herniation may even damage the roots that exit several levels below, as seen in the "cauda equina syndrome" (see below). Or it may simply cause—or take part in—spinal stenosis, most often when the canal is already narrow at that level (see Chapters 1 and 48).

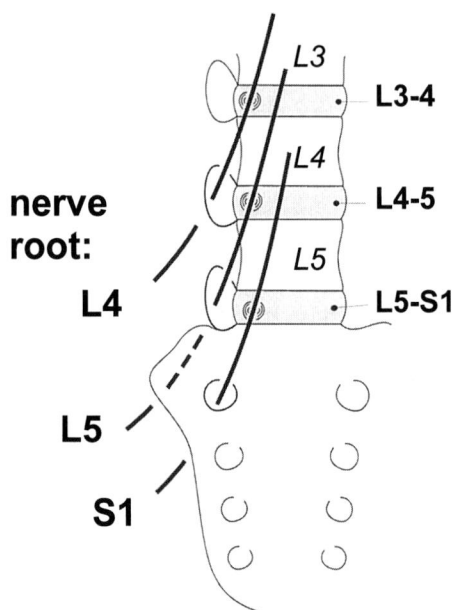

FIG. 41-7. The typical root irritations with paramedian lumbar disc herniation at various levels.

If the herniation is foraminal or extraforaminal, the nerve root taking off at the same level may be affected.

About 95% of lumbar herniations are located in the two lower discs, 5% at L3-4, and only very few above that level.

The symptoms of "cauda equina syndrome", where several sacral roots are involved, include flatus incontinence, urinary incontinence, and groin hypoanesthesia. The influence on the vesica urticaria sphincter is most often retention. Urinary incontinence may either be seen because of retention in terms of overflow, or as a primary neurologic disturbance. Groin hypoanesthesia can be unilateral or bilateral.

NATURAL HISTORY

The natural course of LDH has certainly not been accurately stated (42). It varies with:

- different intensity of clinical symptoms including the degree of paresis
- coexisting pathology, particularly whether the actual disc is highly degenerated or not, but also recess or spinal stenosis, spondylolisthesis, and so forth (43)
- psychosocial factors (e.g., employment and higher social group correlates to a faster recovery) (44).

The course does not seem influenced by sex or age (44), the latter at least not with complete herniation (5).

It is problematic that the clinical courses described in various studies represent a variety of definitions of LDH, most likely including many without actual nuclear herniation. The literature makes no conclusions on an average course of the different phases.

Thus, the "about-average" natural history (described subsequently) is largely based on clinical experience, and a mixture of literature information (28,37,43,45,46). The onset of dominating leg pain is usually the period with the most intense pain. Commonly, the pain fades out to some extent after a few weeks and then tends to remain at about the same level for a total of approximately 1 to 3 months. Thereafter, the symptoms generally abate over another few months, and (almost) disappear in 50% to 70% of nonsurgical cases (28,37,46), and in about the same number of surgical cases in most reports (5,47,48), with as many as 80% to 90% in a few reports (28,49) (Fig 41-5). The remaining patients experience:

- long-lasting discogenic pain, which also tends to fade off, but over a period of some years (50,51)
- peripheral neurogenic leg pain due to root damage (52)
- domination of a central nervous system component of the pain (53).

Among these, psychosocial factors are associated with the majority of the pain (37).

Formation of a fibrous layer (54,55) is followed by a gradual reduction of the scar bulge (56) (Fig. 41-6). The rate of recurrent LDH is about 3% to 14% (54,57).

History and Physical

Several relevant issues of the clinical examination will be presented, but not all. For further details on clinical usefulness of history and physical signs, test repeatability, and so forth see Andersson and Deyo (58), Hunt et al. (59), or Vroomen et al. (60).

From the history taking, one of the most important questions is probably whether leg pain or paraesthesia dominates over back pain or vice versa. The distribution of the leg pain—radicular or diffuse—does not allow a clear distinction between disc herniation or other causes of sciatica to be made, as diffuse sciatica has often been reported where herniation has subsequently been verified at surgery.

As paresis in gradual progress is an indication for acute surgery, this should be explored during history taking, as should possible cauda equina symptoms, where the sequence of symptoms most often is flatus incontinence, urinary retention, and groin hypoesthesia.

"Bowel strain" is also described to be reasonably indicative for herniation.

Whereas painful forward bending is highly correlated to herniation, there does not seem to be a consistent correlation with lying or sitting. Especially in the acute stage night pain is common, probably due to increased temperature and inflammation. Sitting has been thought to aggravate a herniation due to the increased intradiscal pressure (IDP), but is not often the most pain-free posture. A possible explanation could be that the advantage of more space around the herniation due to reduced lor-

dosis—or even kyphosis—caused by sitting (61) exceeds the disadvantage from a small increase in herniation size (62) (Fig. 41-8). Moreover, the increase in IDP is probably smaller than previously believed (63), and when sitting backwardly inclined with a backrest, the IDP is at least not higher than when standing (64).

Conversely, lumbar extension is generally omitted due to the reduction in the foramen size (65).

Of the physical signs, the sagittal lumbar curve in standing is also influenced by the same principle: the lumbar curvature is flattened or even kyphotic, automatically arranged by a posterior rotation of the pelvis. This is done to enable the described mechanism of optimizing the space for the nerve root. Such a kyphotic curve might also be obtained by forward bending of the trunk. However, in that case the addition of static back-muscle activity compresses the herniated disc to an uncomfortable level. Thus, erect posture with flattened or kyphotic loin, or a supported (e.g., hands on the thighs) forward bended posture is characteristic.

A scoliotic list seems only moderately correlated to operative findings (66–68). In particular, the Finneson hypothesis that a certain side location of the herniation and the nerve root should cause a specific list direction does not seem valid (67).

A painful forward bending may distinguish disc herniation from recess stenosis, where leg pain also may dominate over back pain, but where forward bending usually relieves the sciatica (69). A lateral shift—usually away from the side of the LDH—during forward bending is often seen in LDH, but does not provide much help in distinguishing between herniation or recess stenosis.

Side bending toward the opposite side of the pain usually relieves the pain (Fig. 41-8).

The straight leg-raising (SLR) test with radiating pain below knee level seems reasonably associated to disc herniation (38), although the test reliability—like that for the ranges of motion mentioned earlier—seems lower than commonly believed (59). With the surgical finding as the

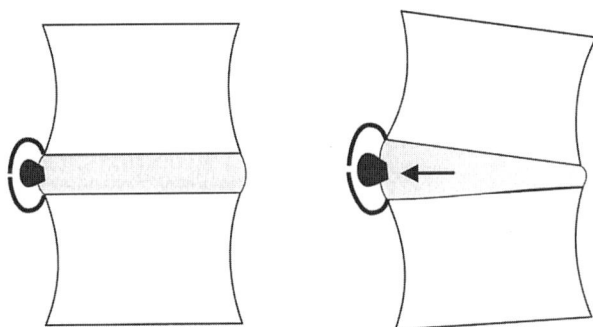

FIG. 41-8. With reduction of the lordotic curvature, and with lateral bending, the size of the herniation increases, but the enlargement of the intervertebral foramen is even more pronounced.

"gold standard," and without letting SLR influence the indication for surgery, the following was registered by Kosteljanetz et al. (48) (Fig. 41-9): Root compression, if present, was estimated to be caused by disc herniation in two-thirds of the patients in this study. This is the case for those patients with dominating leg pain of more than 6 weeks' duration. It may be differently distributed in another group of patients, characterized otherwise.

The literature on SLR is confusing regarding the degree of leg angle and clinical symptoms. Some authors report that the smaller the SLR angle, the more intense the symptoms (70), whereas others do not find such correlation (71).

SLR is not very sensitizing to an extraforaminal herniation (41). The crossed SLR sign (lifting the symptom-free leg, increasing contralateral pain) seems highly correlated to LDH, especially to complete and large herniations (5,67,72).

For a herniation affecting nerve root L4—or L2-L3, which are rare—the "femoral-nerve stretch test" may be valid if carried out correctly: the patient is in a prone position and the 90° flexed knee is lifted causing hip extension. To avoid co-movements of the lumbar spine, the pelvis is fixated by pressing on the lower third of the sacral bone.

The springing test is a "segmental lordosing" pressure placed successively on all lumbar segments with the patient lying prone. If it is painful, it may indicate which segment of the leg pain originates from, and may also help to differentiate pain arising in areas such as the sacroiliac joint.

Obviously neurologic signs—altered sensibility, reflexes, muscle strength, and muscle atrophy—should be tested (refer to neurologic textbooks for more information).

Consideration of the piriformis muscle may be worthwhile. In many patients with disc herniation piriformis myosis may contribute to some of the buttock

and leg pain, especially for herniation at L5-S1, because the S1 root innervates this muscle. There has been some discussion whether leg pain is caused by "self-strangulation" in the major ischiadicus foramen where swelling of the muscle causes compression of the sciatic nerve, or whether it is simply referred pain. Piriformis involvement can be tested with (a) palpating the muscle for tenderness or (b) placing the ipsilateral foot on the other knee, fixating the pelvis with the "heel of the hand" on the anterior superior iliac spine (ASIS), and then pushing the knee toward the contralateral side, and asking for stretch pain.

Dynamic testing *ad modem* McKenzie should be performed. With extension, an increase in radicular pain indicates an active herniation (73). As the herniation increases, and the foramen decreases (65), possible centralization of the pain with repeated extension indicates either that the healing has begun, or at least that the prognosis is good (74).

It seems likely that future tests may include blood samples elucidating whether or not an inflammatory process of the disc is present. Serum tested for glycosphingolipid is already optional, but its applicability in practice is still unclear (75).

REFERENCES

1. Boos N, Rieder R, Schade V, et al. The diagnostic accuracy of magnetic resonance imaging, work perception and psychosocial factors in identifying symptomatic disc herniations. Spine 1995;20(24):2613–2625.
2. Fraser RD, Sandhu A, Gogan WJ. Magnetic resonance imaging findings 10 years after treatment for lumbar disc herniation. Spine 1995; 20:710–714.
3. Jensen R, Bliddal H, Hansen SE, et al. Severe low-back pain. II: Changes in CT scans in the acute phase and after long-term observation. Scand J Rheumatol 1993;22:30–34.
4. Karppinen J, Malmivaara A, Kurunlahti M, et al. Periradicular infiltration for sciatica: a randomized controlled trial. Spine 2001;26: 1059–1067.
5. Spangfort E. The lumbar disc herniation—a computer-aided analysis of 2,504 operations. Acta Orthop Scand Suppl 1972;142:1–95.
6. Wiesel SW, Tsourmas N, Feffer HL, et al. A study of computer-assisted tomography. I. The incidence of positive CAT scans in an asymptomatic group of patients. Spine 1984;9:549–551.
7. Jensen TT, Overgaard S, Thomsen NO, et al. Postoperative computed tomography three months after lumbar disc surgery. A prospective single-blind study. Spine 1991;16:620–622.
8. Brisby H, Olmarker K, Larsson K, et al. Proinflammatory cytokines in cerebrospinal fluid and serum in patients with disc herniation and sciatica. Eur Spine J 2002;11:62–66.
9. Nishimura K, Mochida J. Percutaneous reinsertion of the nucleus pulposus. An experimental study. Spine 1998;23:1531–1538.
10. Olmarker K, Blomquist J, Strömberg J, et al. Nucleus pulposus cells and indomethazin in nucleus pulposus-induced microvascular inflammatory reactions in the hamster cheek-pouch. International Society of the Study of the Lumbar Spine, Burlington Vermont, June 25–29, 1996.
11. Olmarker K, Brisby H, Yabuki S, et al. The effects of normal, frozen, and hyaluronidase-digested nucleus pulposus on nerve root structure and function. Spine 1997;22:471–475.
12. Olmarker K, Nordborg C, Larsson K, et al. Ultrastructural changes in spinal nerve roots induced by autologous nucleus pulposus. Spine 1996;21:411–414.
13. Olmarker K, Rydevik B. Selective inhibition of tumor necrosis factor-alpha prevents nucleus pulposus-induced thrombus formation, intra-

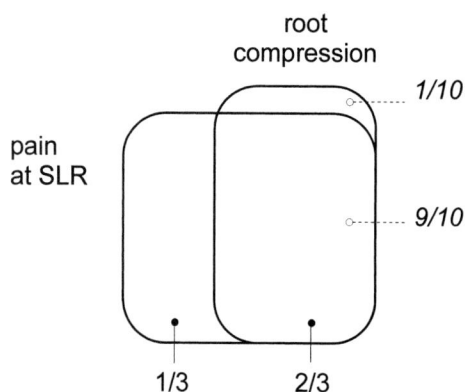

FIG. 41-9. One indication of sensitivity and specificity for straight leg raising.

neural edema, and reduction of nerve conduction velocity: possible implications for future pharmacologic treatment strategies of sciatica. Spine 2001;26:863–869.

14. Olmarker K, Rydevik B, Nordborg C. Autologous nucleus pulposus induces neurophysiologic and histologic changes in porcine cauda equina nerve roots [see Comments]. Spine 1993;18:1425–1432.
15. Olmarker K, Storkson R, Berge OG. Pathogenesis of sciatic pain: a study of spontaneous behavior in rats exposed to experimental disc herniation. Spine 2002;27:1312–1317.
16. Otani K, Arai I, Mao GP, et al. Experimental disc herniation: evaluation of the natural course. Spine 1997;22:2894–2899.
17. Park JB, Chang H, Kim KW. Expression of Fas ligand and apoptosis of disc cells in herniated lumbar disc tissue. Spine 2001;26:618–621.
18. Rannou F, Corvol MT, Hudry C, et al. Sensitivity of anulus fibrosus cells to interleukin 1 beta. Comparison with articular chondrocytes. Spine 2000;25:17–23.
19. Satoh K, Konno S, Nishiyama K, et al. Presence and distribution of antigen-antibody complexes in the herniated nucleus pulposus. Spine 1999;24:1980–1984.
20. Specchia N, Pagnotta A, Toesca A, et al. Cytokines and growth factors in the protruded intervertebral disc of the lumbar spine. Eur Spine J 2002;11:145–151.
21. Yabuki S, Kikuchi S, Olmarker K, et al. Acute effects of nucleus pulposus on blood flow and endoneurial fluid pressure in rat dorsal root ganglia. Spine 1998;23:2517–2523.
22. Ozawa K, Atsuta Y, Kato T. Chronic effects of the nucleus pulposus applied to nerve roots on ectopic firing and conduction velocity. Spine 2001;26:2661–2665.
23. Takebayashi T, Cavanaugh JM, Cuneyt OA, et al. Effect of nucleus pulposus on the neural activity of dorsal root ganglion. Spine 2001;26:940–945.
24. Frymoyer JW, Pope MH, Clements JH, et al. Risk factors in low-back pain. An epidemiological survey. J Bone Joint Surg Am 1983;65:213–218.
25. Kelsey JL, White AA III. Epidemiology and impact of low-back pain. Spine 1980;5:133–142.
26. Frymoyer JW. Back pain and sciatica. New Engl J Med 1988;318:291–300.
27. Kelsey JL, Githens PB, O'Conner T, et al. Acute prolapsed lumbar intervertebral disc. An epidemiologic study with special reference to driving automobiles and cigarette smoking. Spine 1984;9:608–613.
28. Weber H, Holme I, Amlie E. The natural course of acute sciatica with nerve root symptoms in a double-blind placebo-controlled trial evaluating the effect of piroxicam. Spine 1993;18:1433–1438.
29. Battié MC, Videman T, Gibbons L, et al. Determinants of lumbar disc degeneration—a study of lifetime exposures and magnetic resonance imaging findings in identical twins. Spine 1995;20:2601–2612.
30. Simunic DI, Broom ND, Robertson PA. Biomechanical factors influencing nuclear disruption of the intervertebral disc. Spine 2001;26:1223–1230.
31. Aota Y, Onari K, An HS, et al. Dorsal root ganglia morphologic features in patients with herniation of the nucleus pulposus: assessment using magnetic resonance myelography and clinical correlation. Spine 2001;26:2125–2132.
32. Pedrini-Mille A, Weinstein JN, Found EM, et al. Stimulation of dorsal root ganglia and degradation of rabbit annulus fibrosus. Spine 1990;15:1252–1256.
33. Sugawara O, Atsuta Y, Iwahara T, et al. The effect of mechanical compression and hypoxia on nerve root and dorsal root ganglia. Spine 1996;21(18):2089–2094.
34. Cornefjord M, Olmarker K, Rydevik R, et al. Mechanical and biochemical injury of spinal nerve roots: a morphological and neurophysiological study. Eur Spine J 1996;5:187–192.
35. Olmarker K, Rydevik B, Holm S. Edema formation in spinal nerve roots induced by experimental, graded compression. An experimental study on the pig cauda equina with special reference to differences in effects between rapid and slow onset of compression. Spine 1989;14:569–573.
36. Rydevik BL, Myers RR, Powell HC. Pressure increase in the dorsal root ganglion following mechanical compression. Closed compartment syndrome in nerve roots. Spine 1989;14:574–576.
37. Hasenbring M, Marienfeld G, Kuhlendahl D, et al. Risk factors of chronicity in lumbar disc patients. A prospective investigation of biologic, psychologic, and social predictors of therapy outcome. Spine 1994;19:2759–2765.

38. Thelander U, Fagerlund M, Friberg S, et al. Straight leg raising test versus radiologic size, shape, and position of lumbar disc hernias. Spine 1992;17:395–399.
39. Ohnmeiss D, Vanharanta H, Ekholm J. Degree of disc disruption and lower extremity pain. Spine 1997;22:1600–1605.
40. Ahn SH, Ahn MW, Byun WM. Effect of the transligamentous extension of lumbar disc herniations on their regression and the clinical outcome of sciatica. Spine 2000;25:475–480.
41. Ohmori K, Kanamori M, Kawaguchi Y, et al. Clinical features of extraforaminal lumbar disc herniation based on the radiographic location of the dorsal root ganglion. Spine 2001;26:662–666.
42. Andersson GB, Brown MD, Dvorak J, et al. Consensus summary of the diagnosis and treatment of lumbar disc herniation. Spine 1996;21:75S–78S.
43. Saal JA, Saal JS, Herzog R. The natural history of lumbar intervertebral disc extrusions treated nonoperatively. Spine 1990;15:683–686.
44. Rasmussen C. Lumbar disc herniation: social and demographic factors determining duration of disease. Eur Spine J 1996;5:225–228.
45. Bush K, Cowan N, Katz DE, et al. The natural history of sciatica associated with disc pathology. A prospective study with clinical and independent radiologic follow-up. Spine 1992;17:1205–1212.
46. Weber H. The natural course of disc herniation. Acta Orthop Scand Suppl 1993;251:19–20.
47. Espersen JO, Kosteljanetz M, Halaburt H, et al. Predictive value of radiculography in patients with lumbago-sciatica. A prospective study (Part II). Acta Neurochir (Wien) 1984;73:213–221.
48. Kosteljanetz M, Espersen JO, Halaburt H, et al. Predictive value of clinical and surgical findings in patients with lumbago-sciatica. A prospective study (Part I). Acta Neurochir (Wien) 1984;73:67–76.
49. Pappas CT, Harrington T, Sonntag VK. Outcome analysis in 654 surgically treated lumbar disc herniations. Neurosurgery 1992;30:862–866.
50. Krämer J. Presidential address: natural course and prognosis of intervertebral disc diseases. Spine 1995;20:635–639.
51. Weber H. Lumbar disc herniation. A controlled, prospective study with ten years of observation. Spine 1983;8:131–140.
52. Nakamura SI, Myers RR. Injury to dorsal root ganglia alters innervation of spinal cord dorsal horn lamina involved in nociception. Spine 2000;25:537–542.
53. Hunt JL, Winkelstein BA, Rutkowski MD, et al. Repeated injury to the lumbar nerve roots produces enhanced mechanical allodynia and persistent spinal neuroinflammation. Spine 2001;26:2073–2079.
54. Ahlgren BD, Lui W, Herkowitz HN, et al. Effect of anular repair on the healing strength of the intervertebral disc: a sheep model. Spine 2000;25:2165–2170.
55. Carragee EJ. Point of view. Spine 2001;26:651–651.
56. Doita M, Kanatani T, Ozaki T, et al. Influence of macrophage infiltration of herniated disc tissue on the production of matrix metalloproteinases leading to disc resorption. Spine 2001;26:1522–1527.
57. Nykvist F, Hurme M, Alaranta H, et al. A prospective 5-year follow-up study of 276 patients hospitalized because of suspected lumbar disc herniation. Int Disabil Stud 1989;11:61–67.
58. Andersson GBJ, Deyo RA. History and physical examination in patients with herniated lumbar discs. Spine 1996;21:10S–18S.
59. Hunt DG, Zuberbier OA, Kozlowski AJ, et al. Reliability of the lumbar flexion, lumbar extension, and passive straight leg raise test in normal populations embedded within a complete physical examination. Spine 2001;26:2714–2718.
60. Vroomen PC, de Krom MC, Knottnerus JA. Consistency of history taking and physical examination in patients with suspected lumbar nerve root involvement. Spine 2000;25:91–96.
61. Bendix T. Adjustment of the seated workplace—with special reference to heights and inclinations of seat and table. Dan Med Bull 1987;34:125–139.
62. Fujiwara A, An HS, Lim TH, et al. Morphologic changes in the lumbar intervertebral foramen due to flexion-extension, lateral bending, and axial rotation: an in vitro anatomic and biomechanical study. Spine 2001;26:876–882.
63. Wilke H, Neef P, Hinz B, et al. Intradiscal pressure together with anthropometric data—a data set for the validation of models. Clin Biomech (Bristol, Avon) 2001;16[Suppl 1]:S111–S126.
64. Andersson GBJ, Örtengren R, Nachemson A, et al. Lumbar disc pressure and myoelectric activity during sitting. I: Studies on an experimental chair. Scand J Rehabil Med 1974;6:104–114.
65. Adams MA, May S, Freeman BJ, et al. Effects of backward bending on

lumbar intervertebral discs. Relevance to physical therapy treatments for low back pain. Spine 2000;25:431–437.

66. Matsui H, Ohmori K, Kanamori M, et al. Significance of sciatic scoliotic list in operated patients with lumbar disc herniation. Spine 1998;23:338–342.

67. Suk KS, Lee HM, Moon SH, et al. Lumbosacral scoliotic list by lumbar disc herniation. Spine 2001;26:667–671.

68. Takahashi K, Shima I, Porter RW. Nerve root pressure in lumbar disc herniation. Spine 1999;24:2003–2006.

69. Jenis LG, An HS. Spine update. Lumbar foraminal stenosis. Spine 2000;25:389–394.

70. Jonsson B, Stromqvist B. The straight leg raising test and the severity of symptoms in lumbar disc herniation. A preoperative evaluation. Spine 1995;20:27–30.

71. Jensen R, Bliddahl H, Hansen SE, et al. Severe Low-back pain. II: Changes in CT-scans in the acute phase and after long-term observation. Scand J Rheumatol 1993;22:30–34.

72. Kosteljanetz M, Bang F, Schmidt-Olsen S. The clinical significance of straight-leg raising (Lasegue's sign) in the diagnosis of prolapsed lumbar disc. Interobserver variation and correlation with surgical finding. Spine 1988;13:393–395.

73. Donelson R, Aprill CN, Medcalf R, et al. A prospective study of centralization of lumbar and referred pain: a predictor of symptomatic discs and anular competency? Spine 1997;22:1115–1122.

74. Werneke M, Hart DL. Centralization phenomenon as a prognostic factor for chronic low back pain and disability. Spine 2001;26:758–764.

75. Brisby H, Balague F, Schafer D, et al. Glycosphingolipid antibodies in serum in patients with sciatica. Spine 2002;27:380–386.

CHAPTER 42

Disc Herniation: Imaging

Josef Assheuer and Klaus-Peter Schulitz

PLAIN RADIOGRAPH

Following the Quebec Task Force on Spinal Disorders (1), a radiograph of the lumbar spine is of limited value in the first 7 weeks after onset of low back pain. Even with the pain radiating to the extremities with neurologic signs, radiography can delineate loss of disc height, vacuum phenomena, and calcification, as well as sclerosis of the end plates, osteophytes, and focal end plate defects. Those signs are not specific for herniation; they are hardly found in acute disc herniation.

A radiographic examination is not recommended when disc herniation is suspected. It is the main purpose of radiographic evaluation to exclude low back pain (LBP), which was specifically caused by tumors, infections, inflammatory spondylarthropathies, and fractures (2).

Functional radiographs can delineate instability. Some biomechanical studies (3) showed increased hypermobility after open discectomy at the level of operation. How-

ever, hypermobility can be found preoperatively at the same rate at the level of herniation as in adjacent levels (4–7). Postoperatively, no significant changes in hypermobility were found. Therefore, hypermobility does not seem to be a consequence of discectomy. Instability in the levels above or beneath the level of herniation is caused by increased stress in the moving segment caused by changes in motion pattern at these levels (4,5).

MYELOGRAPHY

Myelogram delineates the cerebrospinal fluid (CSF) space of the thecal sac including the subarachnoidal space of the nerve roots. An indentation or occlusion of this space can be regarded as an indirect sign of disc herniation and must be differentiated from other space-occupying lesions (Fig. 42-1). Therefore, it is of minor importance for the diagnosis of herniation.

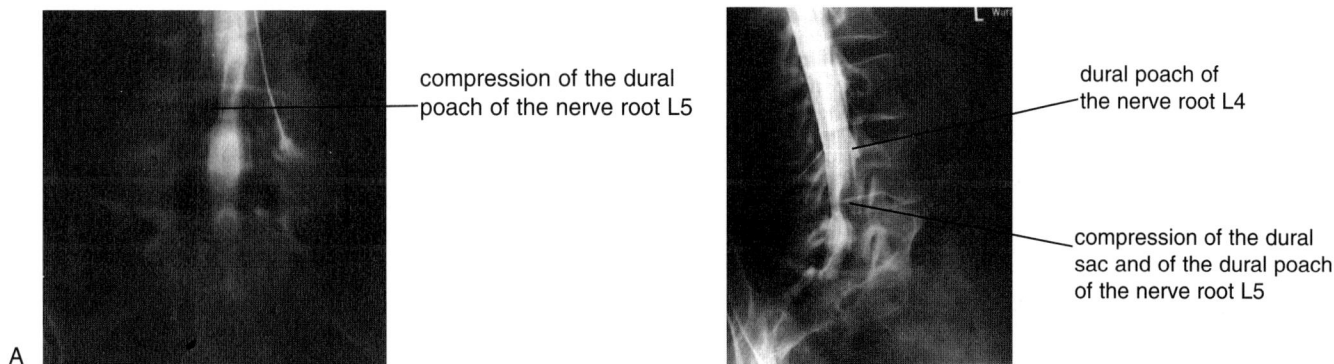

A

compression of the dural poach of the nerve root L5

dural poach of the nerve root L4

compression of the dural sac and of the dural poach of the nerve root L5

B

FIG. 42-1. A: The right dural poach of the nerve root L5 is not filled because of compression by a herniation (myelography antero-posterior view). B: The mass compressing the dural sac and poach of the L5 nerve root can not be identified. It is probably a herniation according to the position of the mass (myelography, right oblique view).

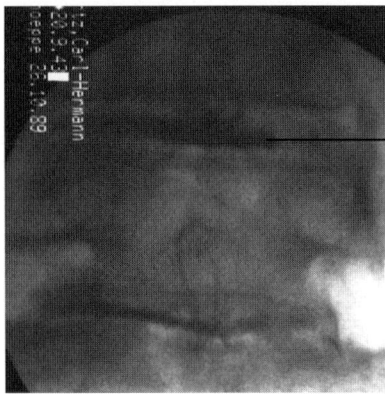

radial fissure extending right side into the outer annulus

FIG. 42-2. Discography L4-5 antero-posterior view. The intradiscal injected contrast media extends in both levels into the outer annulus according to grade 4.

Nerve root entrapment beyond the termination of the nerve root sheath caused by lateral or foraminal disc herniation cannot be detected. High radiation exposure and invasive procedure as well as possible complications also have to be taken into account.

Myelography may be the only method to evaluate disc herniation and other stenosing diseases in patients having metal implants.

Functional myelography may be indicated to evaluate so-called dynamic entrapment in disc herniation in patients showing motion-dependent pain patterns. In future, functional myelography may be replaced by positional magnetic resonance imaging (MRI) (8,9).

DISCOGRAPHY

Discography mainly demonstrates the internal state of the disc and it is very useful to classify types of internal derangement. The contrast medium injected into the center of the disc pushes the disc matrix aside and forms pools. The locations and patterns of these pools are the criteria for the staging of disc degeneration (10–12). Five different types of discograms are distinguished based on consistently identifiable features in the shape and extension of the radiopaque shadow (13,14). There are different classifications. According to the pathoanatomic classification of Adams et al. (13), type 1 does not show any signs of degeneration (cotton ball), type 2 is a mature disc with the nucleus starting to coalesce into fibrous lumps (lobular or sandwich), type 3 demonstrates a degenerated disc with fissures and clefts in the nucleus and inner annulus (irregular), type 4 is a degenerated disc with radial fissures extending into the outer edge of the annulus (fissured) (Fig. 42-2), and type 5 has complete radial fissures that allow injected fluids to escape (ruptured) (Fig. 42-3). Injection is done into at least two segments depending on the pain pattern. Herniation cannot be visualized directly but if type 4 and 5 are found, herniation is likely, especially if the contrast medium forms a pool beyond the intervertebral interspace (Figs. 42-3, 42-4). The leakage of the contrast medium beneath the posterior longitudinal ligament (PLL) is not a relevant sign for herniation. Therefore,

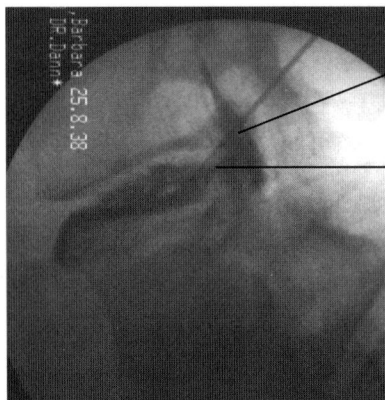

Leakage of contrast media into the extradural space

Complete fissure of the annulus

FIG. 42-3. Discography L4-5 reveals total degeneration of the disc with rupture of the annulus, allowing the intradiscal injected contrast media to escape into the epidural space according to grade 5.

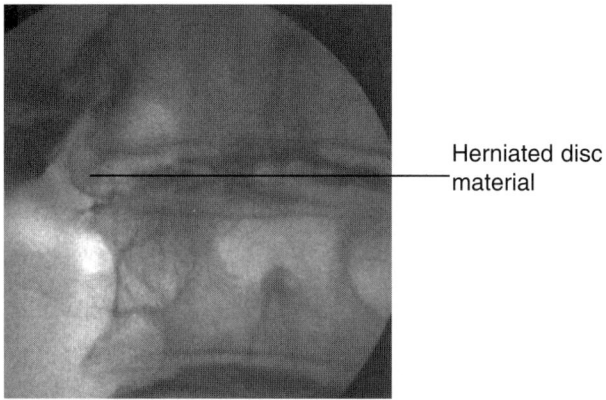

FIG. 42-4. Discography L4-5. The rim of the herniated disc is marked by contrast media.

discography is not a relevant imaging modality to demonstrate herniation. Discography is widely used as a pain reproduction test to identify the segment causing the low back pain and sciatica. The reliability of this test is controversial because the referred pain depends to a high degree on the psychological profile of the patient (15–21).

COMPUTED TOMOGRAPHY

Computed tomography discriminates with high contrast between bone structures and soft tissue. High resolution computed tomography (HRCT) visualizes the subarachnoidal sac, nerve root sleeves, and ligamentum flavum (Fig. 42-5) (22). Disc material can well be detected inside and outside the spinal canal. However, CT does not differentiate between nuclear and annular tissue (Fig. 42-6). There is a high contrast between herniated disc material and epidural fat tissue (23,24). Contrast media after intravenous (i.v.) administration enhance vascular structures and delineate tissue with disturbances of the blood-tissue barrier. This is helpful in the diagnosis of vascular malformations and certain tumors such as meningiomas (25,26). Sometimes, after i.v. administration of contrast medium, a rim of enhancement is observed at the margins of the herniated disc material. This may be related to epidural veins or edema of the neighboring tissue (27,28). Swelling and displacement of ganglia and nerve roots can be visualized as well as the indentation of the dural sac (Fig. 42-7). However, swollen nerve roots and ganglia with high content of water may have the same Hounsfield Units (HU) as disc material and it may be difficult to distinguish one from the other.

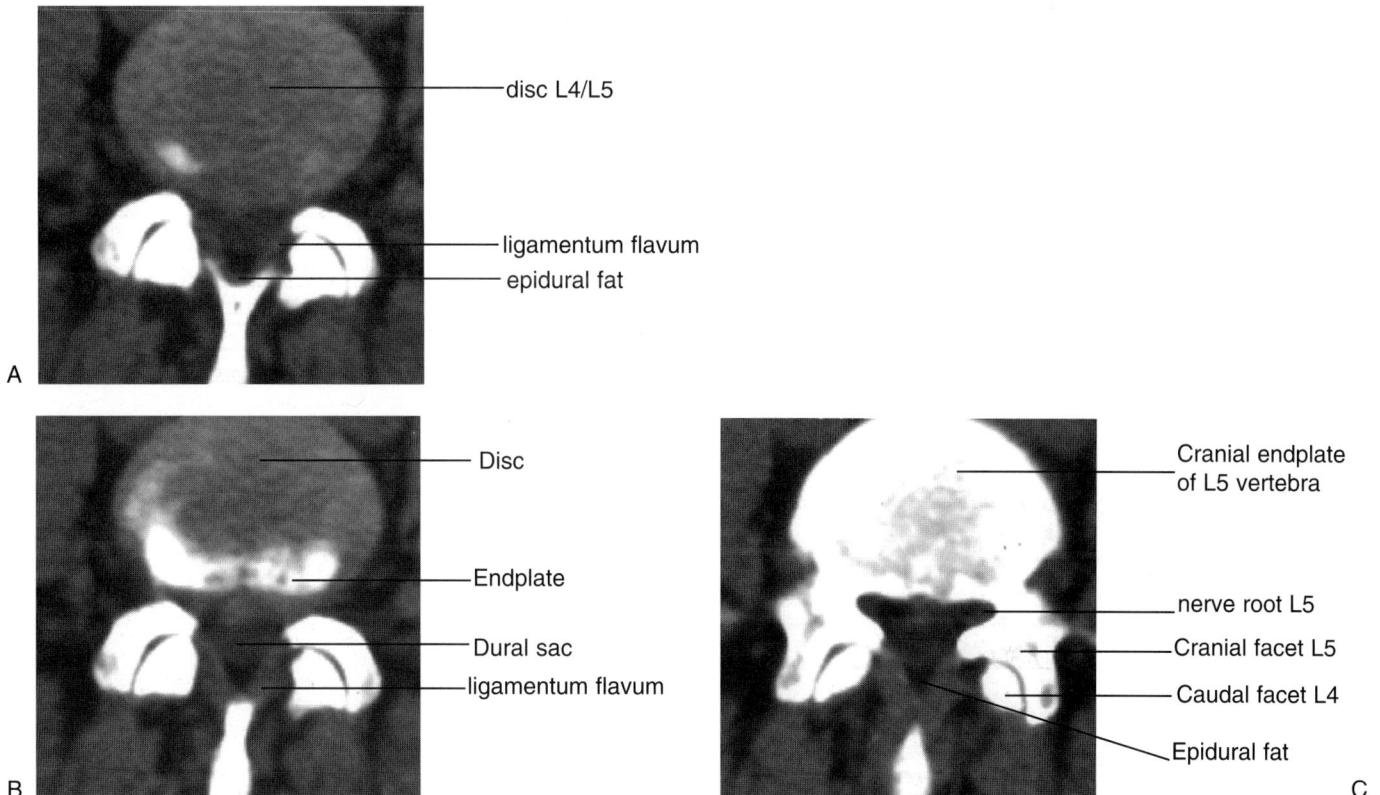

FIG. 42-5. A: Computed tomography of the disc level L4-5. **B:** Computed tomography of the level L4-5 4 mm below Figure 42-5A. **C:** Computed tomography of the level L4-5 8 mm below Figure 42-5A.

focal extension of disc material

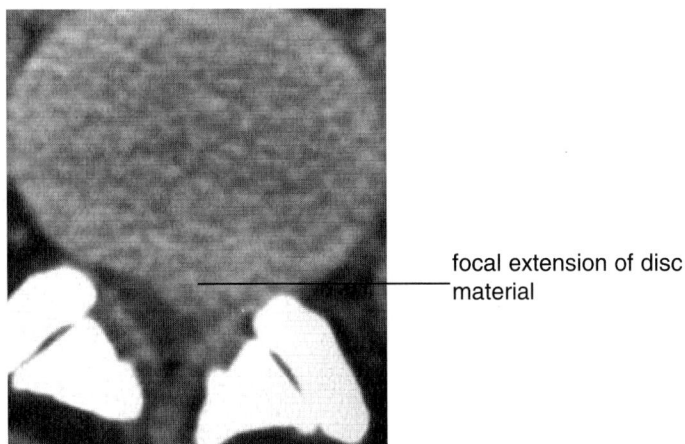

FIG. 42-6. By computed tomography herniation is delineated as focal extension of the disc. Differentiation between nucleus and annular tissue as well as between protrusion and extrusion is not possible.

Multiplanar reconstruction is helpful in these cases, especially with foraminal disc herniations (23,29).

Conjoined nerve roots occurring on the L5-S1 level are likely to have the same attenuation as disc material and may be misinterpreted as a disc herniation (30,31). An accurate analysis of successive CT slices demonstrates this anatomic variant. It can be seen how two nerve roots outside the dura join the same dural sheath cranially. Both nerve roots occasionally leave the spinal canal by the same neuroforamina (32). The process is unilateral. A rounded lateral recess is always found with it. Intrathecal administration of contrast media verifies the diagnosis, showing the common dural recess (33). This anomaly was found in 2% of the cases within a CT study, and in 14% within an autopsy series (32).

Most hematomas of the lumbar spine are located epidurally or subdurally. They may be confounded with disc herniations. The epidural mass has indistinct margins and extends over the surface of a vertebral body, being largest at the mid-vertebral level. The hematomas are isodense with the thecal sac and are indistinguishable from the nerve root and ganglia. They may arise from a tear of the fragile epidural veins because of disc disruption. Computed tomography follow-ups show a regression of

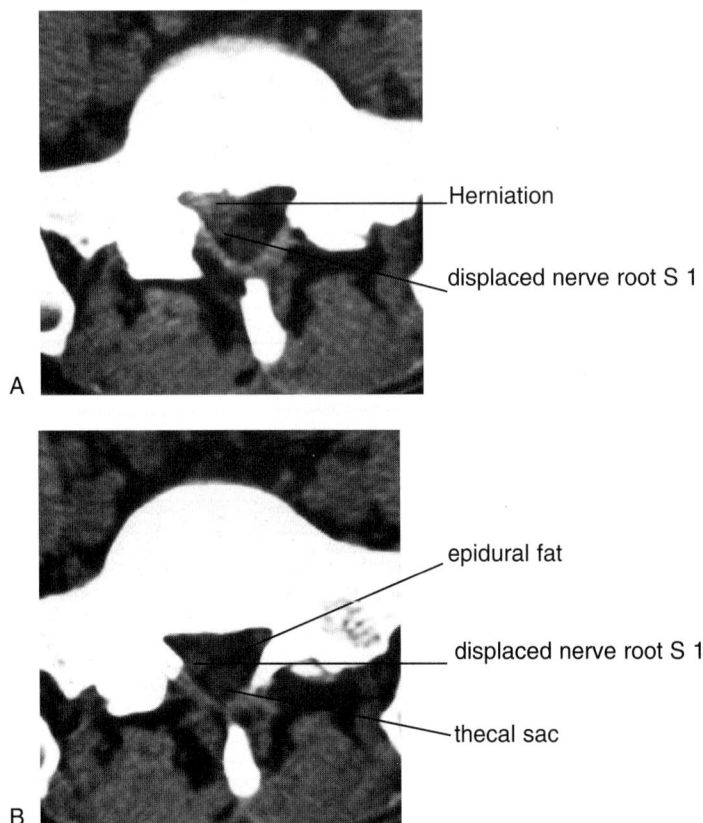

Herniation

displaced nerve root S 1

A

epidural fat

displaced nerve root S 1

thecal sac

B

FIG. 42-7. A: Computed tomography of the level L5-S1. A right side disc herniation displacing the right nerve root S1 dorsally. The nerve root is nearly indistinguishable from the herniated disc material. **B:** Computed tomography of the level L5-S1 3 mm beneath the level of Figure 42-11A. The displaced nerve root is delineated by the surrounding epidural fat of low density.

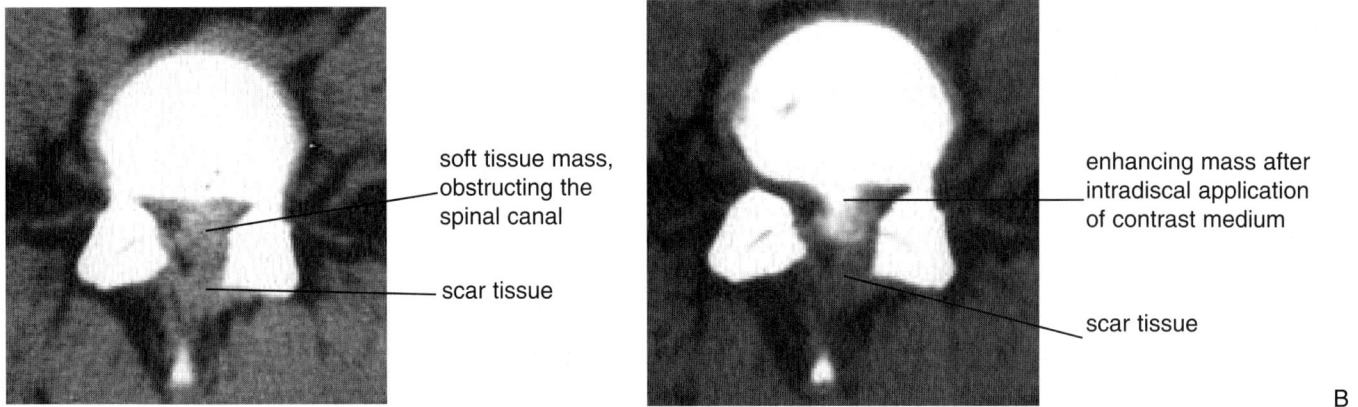

FIG. 42-8. A: Differentiation between scar tissue and possible reherniation is not possible (computed tomography native at the level L4-5). **B:** The enhancement of the intraspinal mass after intradiscal administration of contrast medium reveals reherniation and differentiation from scar tissue (computed tomography discography at the level of L4-5).

hematomas with the underlying disc herniation remaining (34–36). Epidural and subdural hematomas also may originate from hematologic disorders, hypertension, and atherosclerotic vascular diseases (36–38).

Because of their location, synovial cysts and synovial ganglia of degenerated facet joints may mimic disc fragments. They are broad-based to the zygapophyseal joint, mostly rounded, emerging into the central canal or subarticular recess. The mass may exhibit internal gas or a calcified rim (39–42). The thickened and protruding ligamentum flavum and capsule are isodense with the disc and may cause diagnostic problems. Injection of contrast media into the relevant facet joint shows the communication of the cyst with the joint space (43). Occasionally cysts can also emerge out of a degenerated disc and are difficult to differentiate from herniation. They may result from resorption or mucoid degeneration of an already existing herniation (44).

Perineural cysts (45), occurring beneath the perineurium at the level or beyond the dorsal root ganglion, and subarachnoidal cysts (cystic nerve root sleeve dilatation or meningeal diverticulum) (46) located proximally to the nerve root ganglion, should not be misinterpreted as herniation. They can be distinguished from herniation when the pressure erosion of the surrounding bone is regarded and contrast medium is filled in after intrathecal administration (47,48).

Nerve sheath tumors may be confounded with lateral herniations and because of their locations are only Schwannomas (49).

The main question with postoperative backaches (failed back surgery syndrome) is to find out whether the nerve root compression results from reherniation or scar tissue, especially epidural fibrosis. Native CT is not suitable to answer this question (Fig. 42-8) (50). It shows

both scar tissue and reherniated disc material with identical density. The location of both processes does not permit discrimination either, because scar tissue normally extends epidurally and laterally to the posterior aspect of the operated disc (51,52). Therefore, CT discography is necessary to clarify this condition (Fig. 42-8). If postoperative spine hemorrhage and noninfectious inflammatory processes arise, they can be well visualized. Contrast enhancement of scar tissue depends on the time that passed between operation and CT examination with older scar enhancing less. Nevertheless, the diagnosis improves by 20% up to 3 years after operation (53,54).

PATHOMORPHOLOGIC DEFINITIONS AND NOMENCLATURE OF DISC HERNIATION

The grading of disc herniation mainly depends on the internal disarrangement of nucleus and annulus; the displacement of nuclear material is the most important feature.

Resnick and Niwayama (55) and other authors (56) propose the following schema for disc herniation:

Annular bulge: Annular fibers are intact and the disc protrudes beyond the intervertebral interspace around the end plate (Fig. 42-9).
Protrusion: Nuclear material protrudes through torn fibers of the annulus, with the outermost fibers remaining intact (Fig. 42-6).
Extrusion: The nuclear material penetrates all of the fibers of the annulus fibrosus and lies under the PLL (Fig. 42-10).
Discal sequestration: The nucleus material penetrates the posterior longitudinal ligament (PLL) and lies within the epidural space or the nucleus material does not

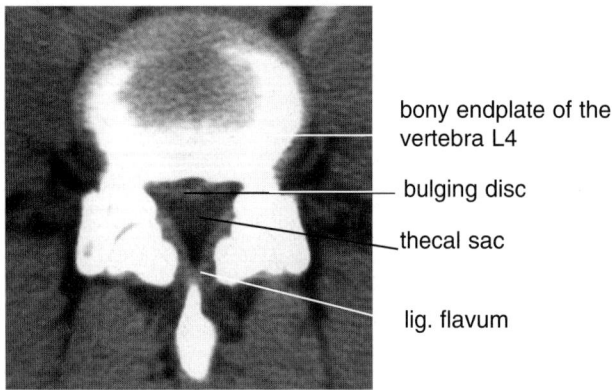

bony endplate of the vertebra L4

bulging disc

thecal sac

lig. flavum

FIG. 42-9. Computed tomography at the border of the disc L3-4 to the vertebra L4. The disc exceeds symmetrically and uniformly the contour of the margin of the vertebra.

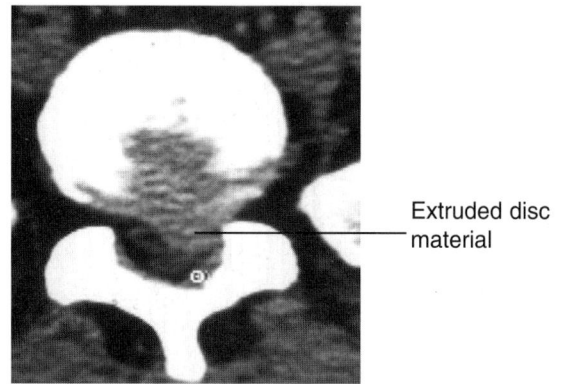

Extruded disc material

FIG. 42-10. Computed tomography of the level L5-S1. The extruded disc material is clearly depicted. Possible rupture of the posterior longitudinal ligament cannot be visualized.

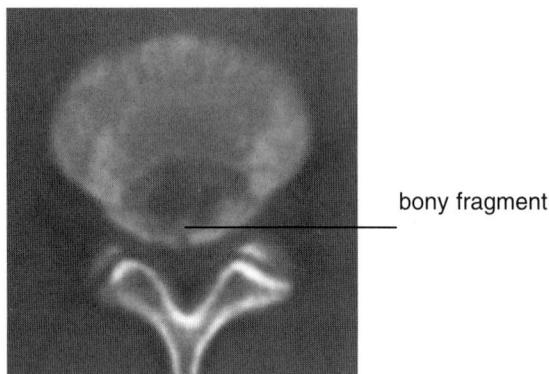

bony fragment

FIG. 42-11. Computed tomography of the level L4-5 (bony window). A bony fragment has extruded together with disc material into the subligamentous space of a 15-year-old trampoline jumper.

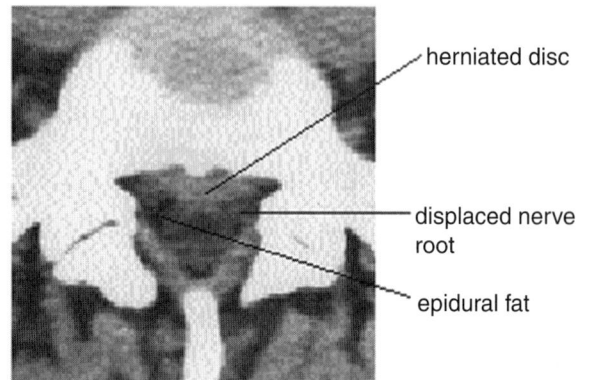

herniated disc

displaced nerve root

epidural fat

FIG. 42-12. Computed tomography of the level L5-S1. The herniation has displaced the left nerve root S1 dorsally. The epidural fat on the left side has nearly disappeared.

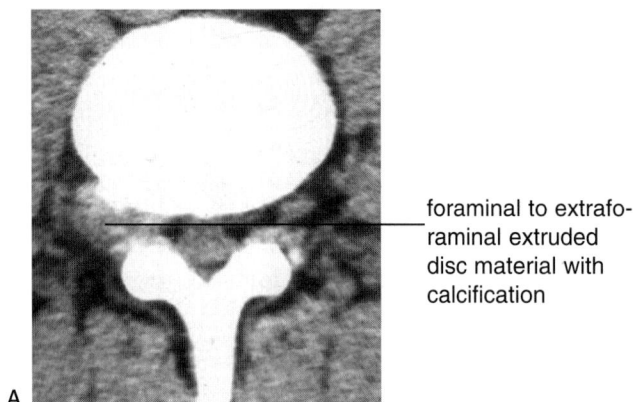

foraminal to extrafo-raminal extruded disc material with calcification

A

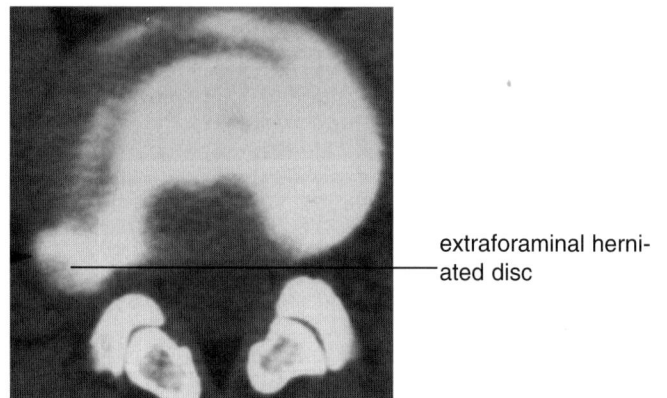

extraforaminal herni-ated disc

B

FIG. 42-13. A: Computed tomography of the level L3-4. An extruded mass of disc material extends from foraminal to extraforaminal with calcification. **B:** CT-discography ascertains extraforaminal herniation suspected by discography.

penetrate the PLL and migrates beneath the PLL cranially or caudally as a fragment and is separated from the remaining portion intervertebral disc.

The schema proposed by Herzog (57) is more related to practical experience concerning protrusion and extrusion.

Protrusion is a herniation of disc material and not only nuclear material. It results in a focal contour abnormality of the disc margin (Fig. 42-6).

Extrusion means penetration of the outer annulus of any disc material, including possible bony fragments (Figs. 42-10, 42-11). This material may remain beneath the PLL and is called subligamentous extrusion. If it penetrates through the PLL it is called transligamentous extrusion. Once the extruded material looses contact with the parent disc, it is called a sequestered disc fragment, which can be transligamentous or subligamentous.

Because CT examination cannot discriminate between nuclear and disc material or outer annular fibers and PLL (Fig. 42-10), the pathomorphologic schema should be used only with restrictions.

Bulging occurs when the disc symmetrically and uniformly exceeds the contour of the margin of the vertebra (Fig. 42-9) (22,58,59). The differentiation between protrusion and extrusion as well as subligamentous and transligamentous extrusion is uncertain (Fig. 42-10). A distinct focal extension of disc material of remarkable volume and clear lateral position is probably an extrusion. A protrusion normally has a broader base with regard to its extension (Fig. 42-12) (60). A sequester has to be assumed when there is clear loss of continuity of extruded disc material in successive slices. Reformatting of the axial slices into sagittal orientated views are helpful in demonstrating a sequestered extrusion. Therefore, a CT description of herniation is mainly restricted to the localization of the herniated material. This may be central, lateral, intraforaminal, and extraforaminal and can extend into cranial and caudal direction. The extent of herniated disc material is better visualized by CT discography (Fig. 42-13). The relation of disc herniation contact and displacement to the nerve root can be depicted.

COMPUTED TOMOGRAPHY DISCOGRAPHY

To get more information about the pathoanatomy of the degenerative disc, discography may be followed by CT examination (12,61–64). When performing a CT immediately after discal injection, the annular fissures are mainly filled with contrast media. When a CT 4 to 6 hours after the injection is performed, mainly the nuclear material is stained. On the base of the discography grading (13,14), it may be useful for CT discography-staging to subdivide type 4 into a, b, and c, where in (a) the derangement extends to less than half of the cross-section

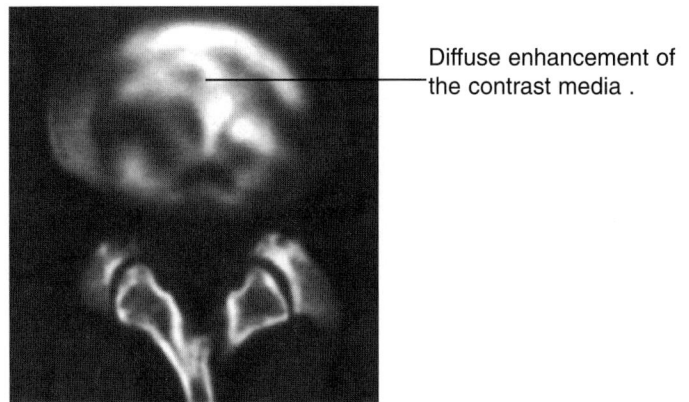

FIG. 42-14. CT-discography of L4-5. Patches of enhancement of contrast media in internal disc disruption. No herniation.

of the disc; (b) the unstained annulus amount is still one third of the disc radius; and (c) the contrast medium extends to the outer fibers of the annulus (Fig. 42-14). Leakage is possible in this case (Fig. 42-15). Type 5 is also subdivided into a, b, and c groups, where (a) means protrusion (Fig. 42-16); (b) subligamentous extrusion (Fig. 42-17); and (c) transligamentous extrusion (Fig. 42-18). Types 5 b and c include sequestration (63,65). Small and broad-based disc herniation can be defined (66). The amount of contrast-medium uptake in the herniated portion can be evaluated (67). Because of the high information value, CT discography is regarded as golden standard in evaluating disc degeneration and herniation for other imaging procedures.

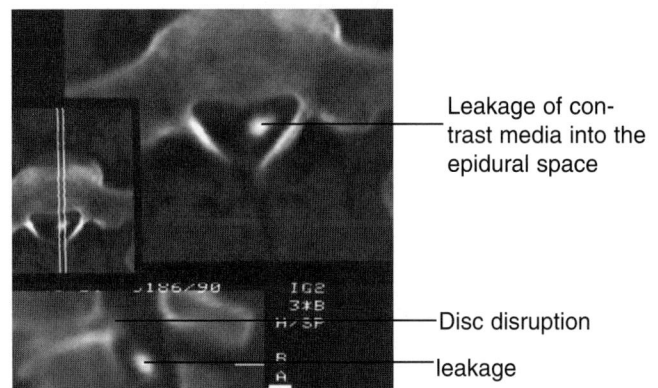

FIG. 42-15. CT-discography of the level L5-S1. Axial view in the upper part of the image and sagittal reconstruction in the lower part. The leakage may mimicry straining of sequestrated disc herniation.

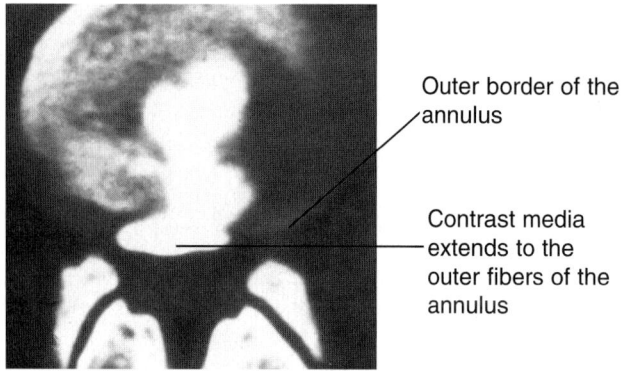

Outer border of the annulus

Contrast media extends to the outer fibers of the annulus

FIG. 42-16. CT-discography of the level L4-5. The intradiscal applied contrast media extends with a broad base to the dorsal border of the disc according to type Va.

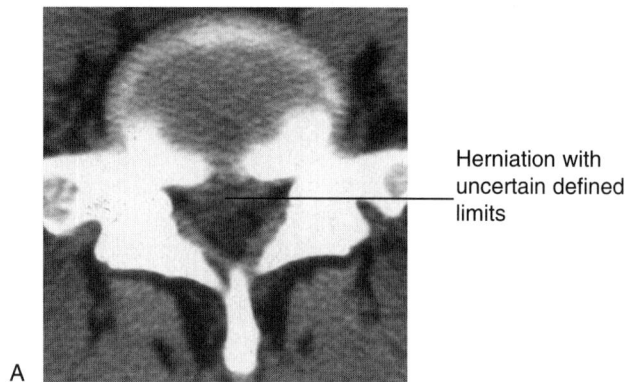

A

Herniation with uncertain defined limits

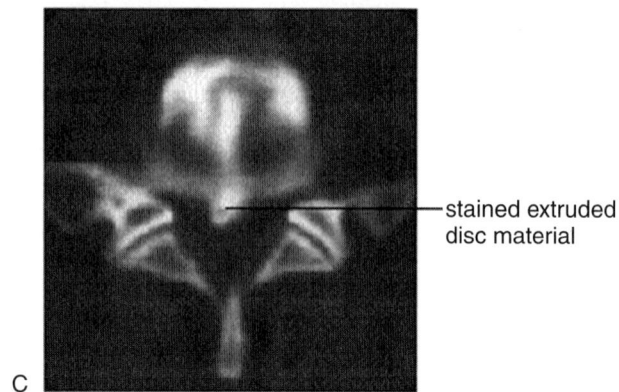

nerve root

small based extrusion of disc material stained with contrast media

B

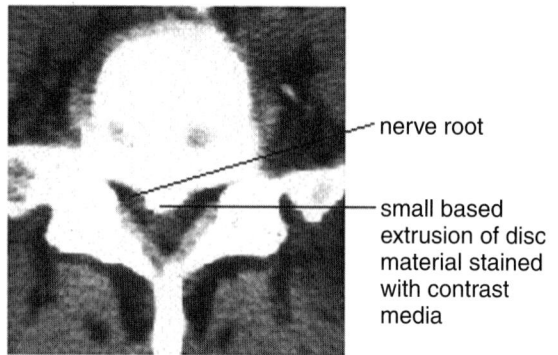

C

stained extruded disc material

FIG. 42-17. A: Computed tomography of the level L5-S1. The herniation has uncertain defined limits. Distinction from nerve root is not possible. **B:** CT-discography of the level L5-S1 displayed in the soft-tissue window defines clearly the border of the extruded disc material. **C:** CT-discography of the level L5-S1 displayed in the bony window. The bony structures are better defined CT-discography.

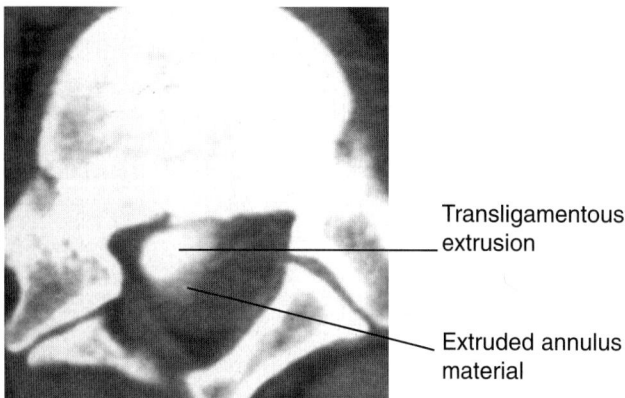

Transligamentous extrusion

Extruded annulus material

FIG. 42-18. CT-discography L4-5 displayed with soft-tissue window shows a transligamentous extrusion with staining of the disc material. The extruded annulus material has less uptake of contrast media.

MAGNETIC RESONANCE IMAGING

Up to now, MRI has become the most frequently used method to depict disc herniation. In contrast to CT, MRI can directly produce slices in every chosen plane. In CT as in all X-ray modalities, the electron density is the contrast-determining parameter. In MRI there are at least three intrinsic parameters (proton density, spin-spin, and spin-lattice relaxation) with a multitude of extrinsic parameters (echo-time (TE), repetition-time (TR), inversion-time (TI), flip angle, field-strength, receiver-coils, etc.).

This allows to show the different spinal tissues with remarkable different signal intensities and results in high contrasts (Fig. 42-19). The nucleus, which is indistinguishable from the annulus in T1-weighted images, becomes very bright in strongly T2-weighted images. The

annulus, ligaments, and nerve roots with fiberlike structures are bright in gradient-echo sequences, out of phase, and T1-weighted and dark in T1- and T2-weighted SE-images. Epidural and intraforaminal fat appears very bright in T1-weighted images and less bright in T2-weighted images. It is dark with fat-suppression techniques. Cerebrospinal fluid has very low signal intensity on T1-weighted images and gets higher signal intensity with more T2 weighting. Because of identical values for T1 and T2 relaxation as for proton density, it is impossible to differentiate the outer annulus PLL complex. The resolution is equal to high-resolution CT. Inherent artifacts, mainly chemical shift (68) and pulsation, have to be considered because they can affect morphometric and signal intensity analysis. For signal intensities are no absolute values, ratios of the signal intensity of interest-

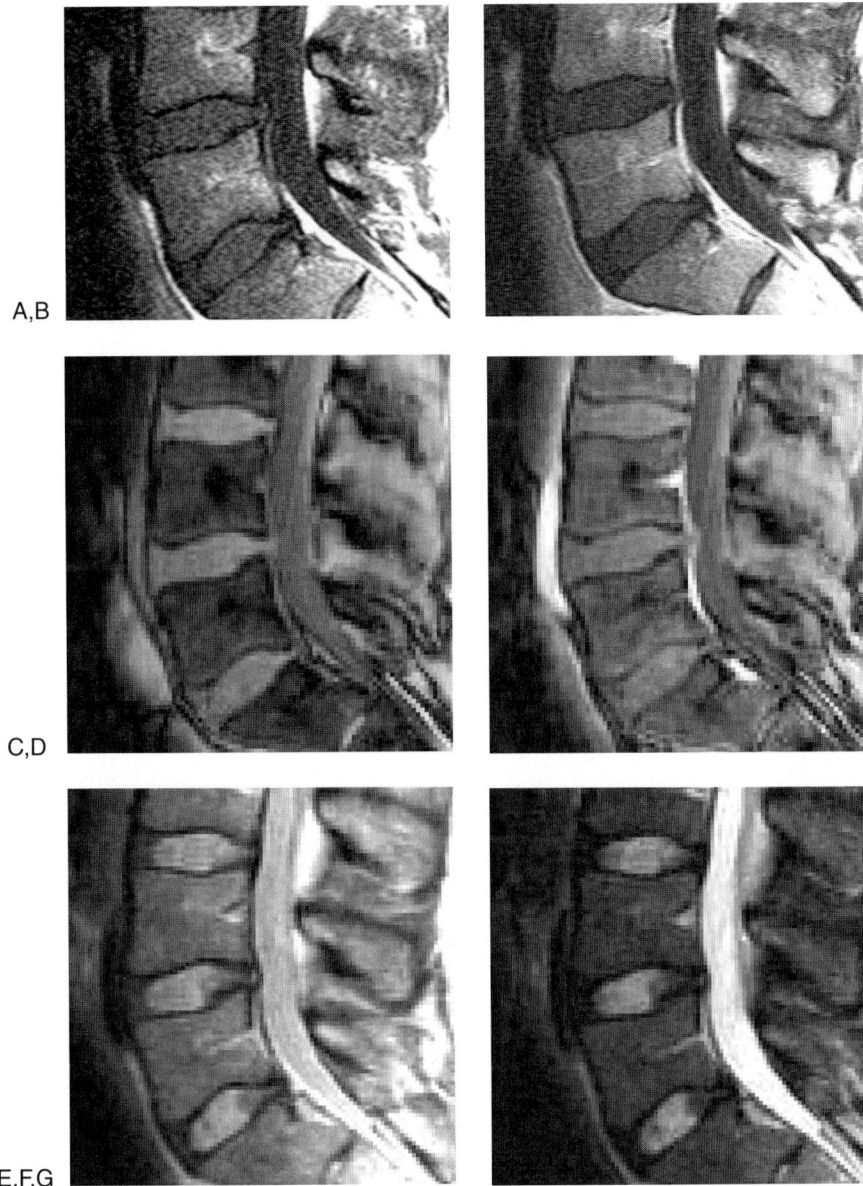

A,B
C,D
E,F,G

FIG. 42-19. Appearance of disc, vertebrae, and neuronal structures in differently weighted sequences. A slight protrusion exists in L4-5 and L5-S1. A: T1-weighted image. B: Enhanced vascular structures after intravenous (i.v.) application of gadolinium (Gd) contrast medium. C: T1-weighted opposed phased image. D: Better delineation of the vascular structures after i.v. application of Gd contrast medium. E: Proton density weighted image. F: T2-weighted image. G: Fat suppression with appearance of heavily T2 weighting.

ing tissue to the signal intensity of a reference tissue, are used to describe physiologic or pathologic changes; for example, the change of signal intensity of the aging or degenerated disc. Cerebrospinal fluid, adjacent vertebral marrow, or intensity of the nucleus of obviously normal disc segments mostly are taken as reference tissues (69–73). Because of the multitude of parameters that influence tissue contrast, there is no commonly accepted protocol for image-based investigation of the lumbar spine. T1- and T2-weighted images are included in most studies. The guidelines for quality control of the German Board of Medicine (Bundesärztekammer) list the spinal structures that have to be delineated and require in-plane resolution of 1 × 1.5 mm with a slice thickness less than 4 mm (74).

Different classification systems are used to describe the degeneration process of the disc. The used parameters are the signal intensity of the nucleus, which decreases with growing age and degeneration, and the height of the intervertebral interspace. There is no commonly accepted procedure to determine stages of the intervertebral disc degeneration. Classification schemata, as proposed by Battié (69) and Pfirrmann (72), include the signal intensity of the nucleus, disc height, and morphologic description of the nucleus, and seem to be most appropriate to evaluate the degree of degeneration.

Herniated material may contain nuclear, annular, and end plate tissues. The classification schema of Brant-Zawadzki (60) for herniation, which is purely based on morphologic criteria, is widely accepted. These authors give the following definitions:

Normal: No disc extension beyond the interspace
Bulge: Circumferential extension beyond the interspace (Fig. 42-20). If a spondylolisthesis occurs, the axial images can lead to misinterpretation of the disc fixed on the upper end plate, and the adjacent non-dislocated vertebra as protrusion (pseudoprotrusion) (Fig. 42-21).
Herniation: Any focal extension beyond the interspace. Subdivisions:
(a) *Protrusion:* Focal or asymmetric extension beyond interspace into the canal, base is broader than any other diameter of the protrusion (Fig. 42-22);
(b) *Extrusion:* Focal, obvious extension beyond interspace; the base against the parent disc is narrower than the diameter of the extruding material itself, or there is no connection to parent disc at all (Fig. 42-23).

To eliminate a false-positive diagnosis it seems important not to use the global term "herniation," but rather its subgroups.

The subdivisions of extrusion in transligamentous and subligamentous herniation as described by Herzog (57) are not included in the preceding schema, probably because of the difficulty of depicting the outer annulus PLL complex. An exact differentiation between these two subgroups can only be done when the rupture of this complex is clearly demonstrated (75,76). For the same reason, differentiation between protrusion and

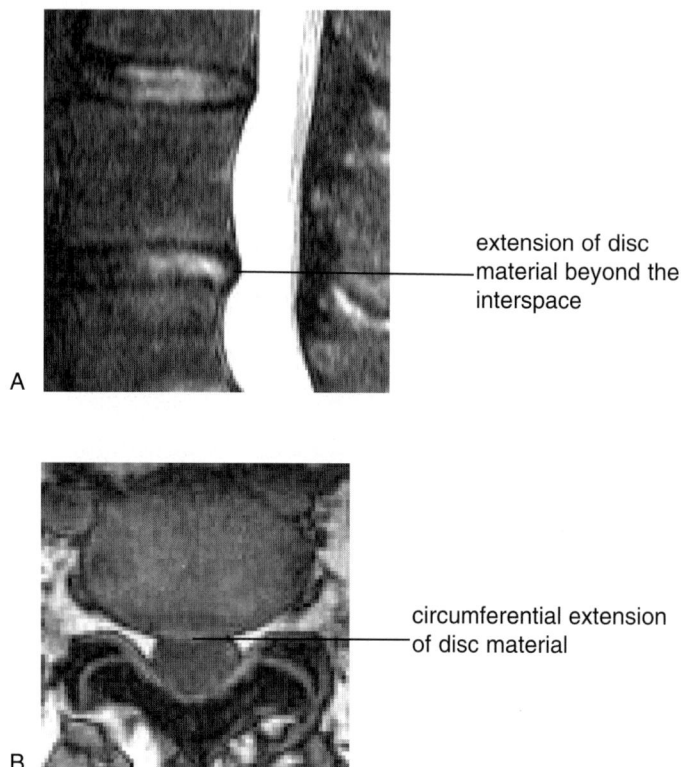

A

extension of disc material beyond the interspace

FIG. 42-20. **A:** The bulging disc slightly dents the dural sac (sagittal image, STIR 2000/150/20). **B:** The convex shape of the disc is characteristic for bulging disc (transverse image, GRE 500/7 out of phase). **C:** We report the enhancement of the outer annulus fibers to the elevated tension of the annulus (transverse image, GRE 500/7 out of phase after intravenous administration of gadolinium contrast medium).

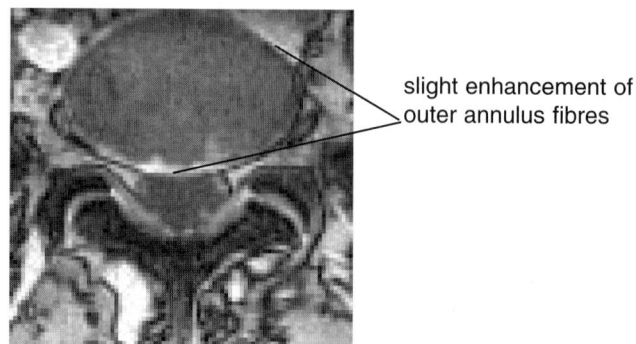

B

circumferential extension of disc material

slight enhancement of outer annulus fibres

C

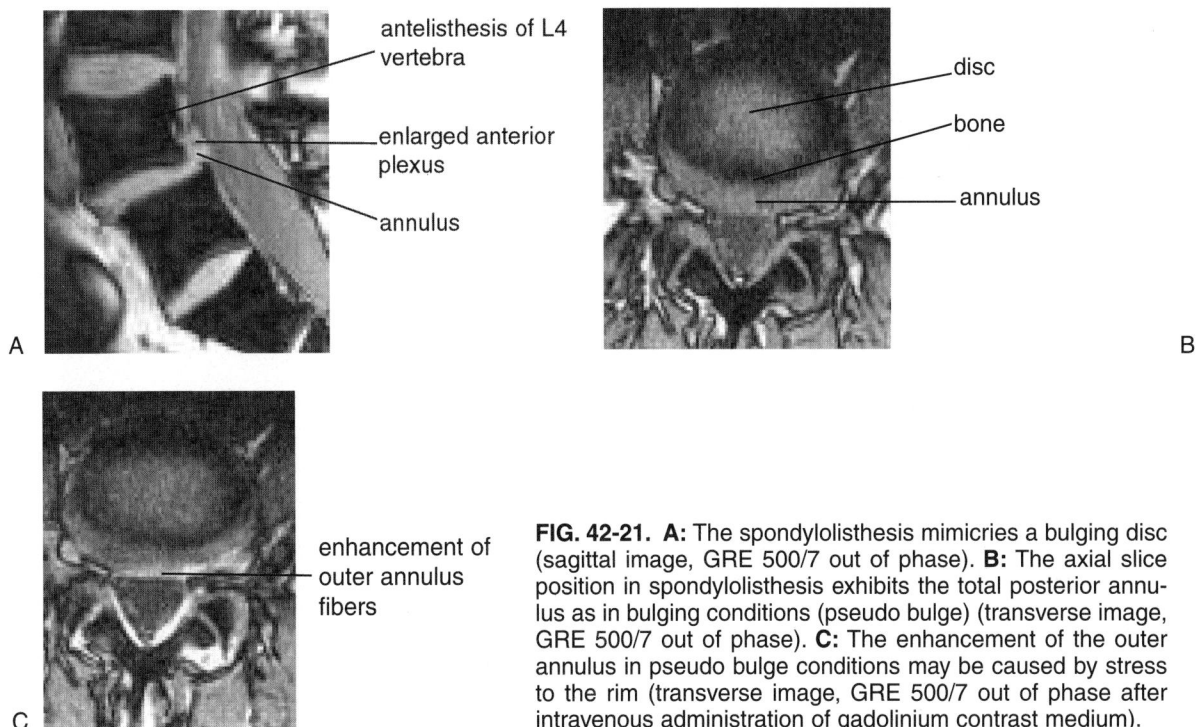

antelisthesis of L4 vertebra

enlarged anterior plexus

annulus

disc

bone

annulus

enhancement of outer annulus fibers

FIG. 42-21. **A:** The spondylolisthesis mimicries a bulging disc (sagittal image, GRE 500/7 out of phase). **B:** The axial slice position in spondylolisthesis exhibits the total posterior annulus as in bulging conditions (pseudo bulge) (transverse image, GRE 500/7 out of phase). **C:** The enhancement of the outer annulus in pseudo bulge conditions may be caused by stress to the rim (transverse image, GRE 500/7 out of phase after intravenous administration of gadolinium contrast medium).

extrusion may be difficult (60). Extrusion is more likely if the herniated material contains nuclear fragments with high signal intensity on T2-weighted images (Fig. 42-23). With older extrusions, the nuclear fragment tends to become dark by resorption and desiccation (76,77). There may be different opinions when defining a bulge or protruded disc (77). The divergence from the concentric contour cannot be clearly identified in every case. Foraminal and extraforaminal herniations are difficult to classify into protrusion and extru-

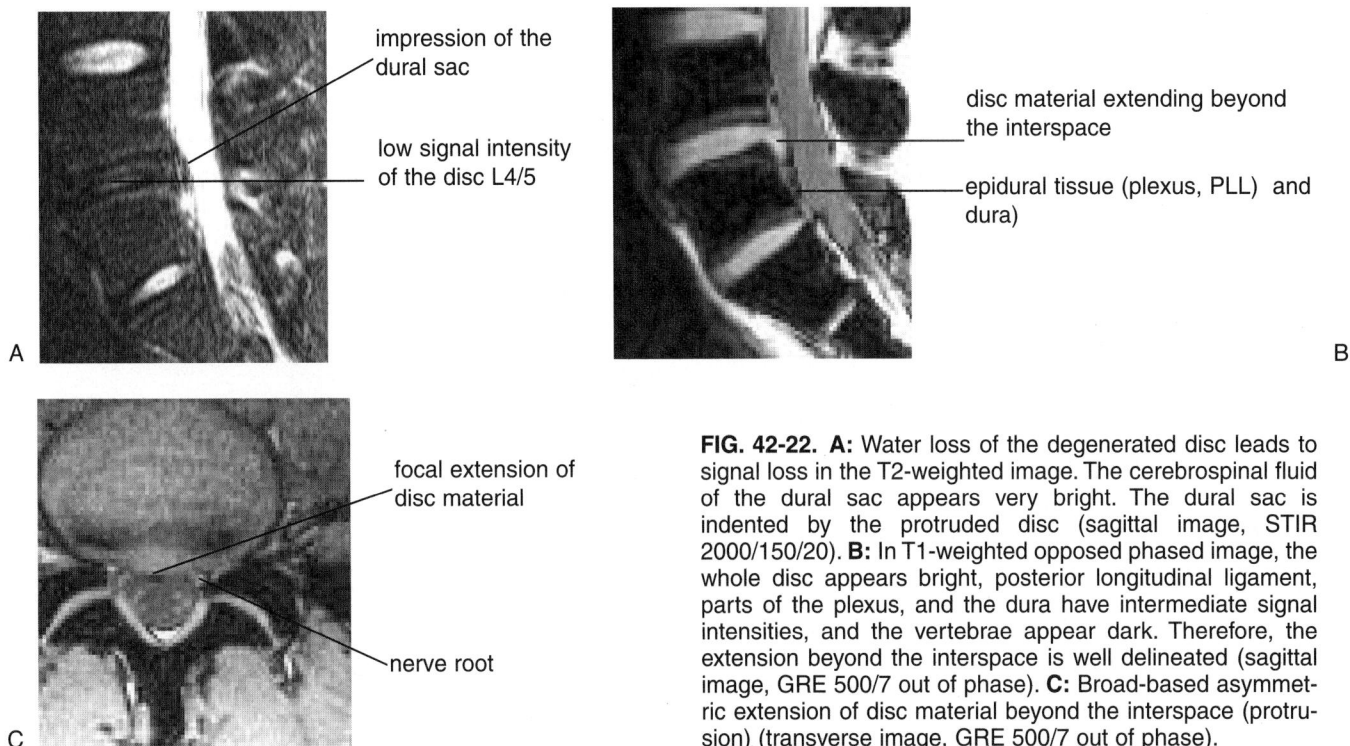

impression of the dural sac

low signal intensity of the disc L4/5

disc material extending beyond the interspace

epidural tissue (plexus, PLL) and dura)

focal extension of disc material

nerve root

FIG. 42-22. **A:** Water loss of the degenerated disc leads to signal loss in the T2-weighted image. The cerebrospinal fluid of the dural sac appears very bright. The dural sac is indented by the protruded disc (sagittal image, STIR 2000/150/20). **B:** In T1-weighted opposed phased image, the whole disc appears bright, posterior longitudinal ligament, parts of the plexus, and the dura have intermediate signal intensities, and the vertebrae appear dark. Therefore, the extension beyond the interspace is well delineated (sagittal image, GRE 500/7 out of phase). **C:** Broad-based asymmetric extension of disc material beyond the interspace (protrusion) (transverse image, GRE 500/7 out of phase).

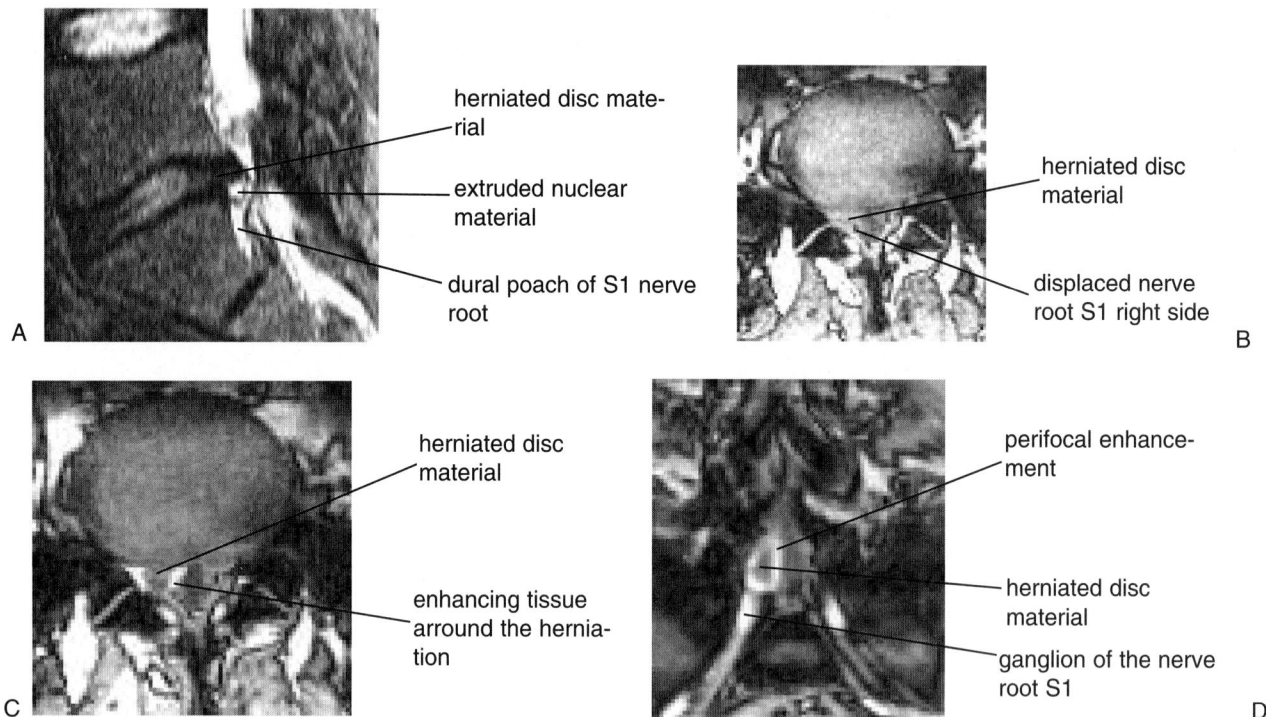

FIG. 42-23. A: Obvious compression of the dural poach of the nerve root S1 by herniated disc material. The herniated nuclear material has penetrated the outer fibers of the annulus (sagittal image, STIR 2000/150/20). **B:** The herniated disc obstructs the recessus S1 on the right side and displaces the nerve root (transverse image, GRE 500/7 out of phase). **C:** The uptake of contrast medium in the tissue adjacent to the herniation is caused by edema or hypervascularization (transverse image, GRE 500/7 out of phase after intravenous administration of gadolinium contrast medium). **D:** Coronal image may be helpful in delineating extension and position of the herniation with regard to the neuronal and bony structures (coronal image, GRE 500/7 out of phase after intravenous administration of gadolinium contrast medium).

sion, especially when nuclear material inside the herniation cannot be depicted (Figs. 42-24, 42-25). Sequestered intervertebral discs are well delineated by sagittal images (Fig. 42-26)(78).

The relationship of herniation and the neurovascular structures is of major clinical importance. The contact of the herniation with the nerve root and its possible deviation, mostly posteriorly, is well visualized in T1- and T2-weighted axial images. The term "nerve root compression" (79–81) does not seem to be adequate for these two conditions and is not convincingly presented in published images.

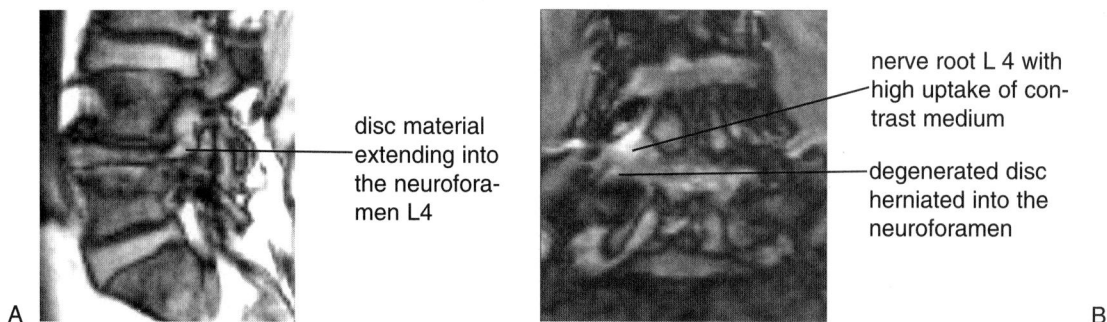

FIG. 42-24. A: The degenerated disc L4-5 extends laterally into the neuroforamina. Nerve root, intervertebral vessels, and intraforaminal fat cannot be differentiated by this sequence (sagittal image, GRE 500/7 out of phase). **B:** The coronal image after intravenous application of gadolinium (Gd)-contrast medium differentiates better between the affected nerve root and the intraforaminal herniation (coronal image, GRE 500/7 out of phase after intravenous administration of Gd contrast medium).

extraforaminal herniated disc material

extraforaminal herniated disc material with a rim of high contrast medium uptake

A

B

intravertebral vessel

displaced nerve root

herniated disc material

C

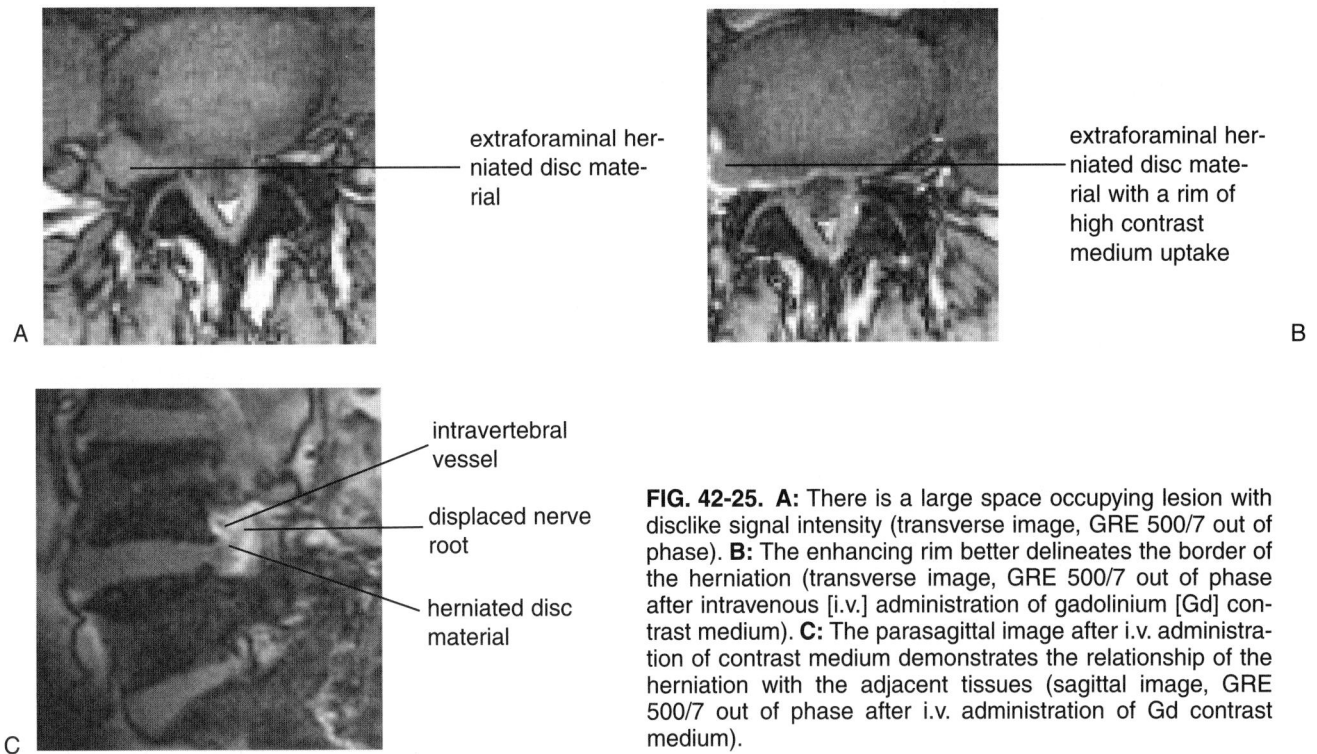

FIG. 42-25. A: There is a large space occupying lesion with disclike signal intensity (transverse image, GRE 500/7 out of phase). **B:** The enhancing rim better delineates the border of the herniation (transverse image, GRE 500/7 out of phase after intravenous [i.v.] administration of gadolinium [Gd] contrast medium). **C:** The parasagittal image after i.v. administration of contrast medium demonstrates the relationship of the herniation with the adjacent tissues (sagittal image, GRE 500/7 out of phase after i.v. administration of Gd contrast medium).

The effect of disc herniation on neurovascular structures may be visualized as swelling of the nerve root, possibly caused by edema. This effect is better demonstrated by enhancement after i.v. administration of gadolinium (Gd) contrast media (82–89). Enhancement is nearly always seen at the rim of the herniation (90,91). This is caused by neurovascularization. Together with dynamic examination, MR angiography allows the separation of vascularization from edema (Fig. 42-27) (92–94). Also, the venous stasis of the anterior venous plexus caused by the herniation that obstructs the spinal canal can be visualized (83,95).

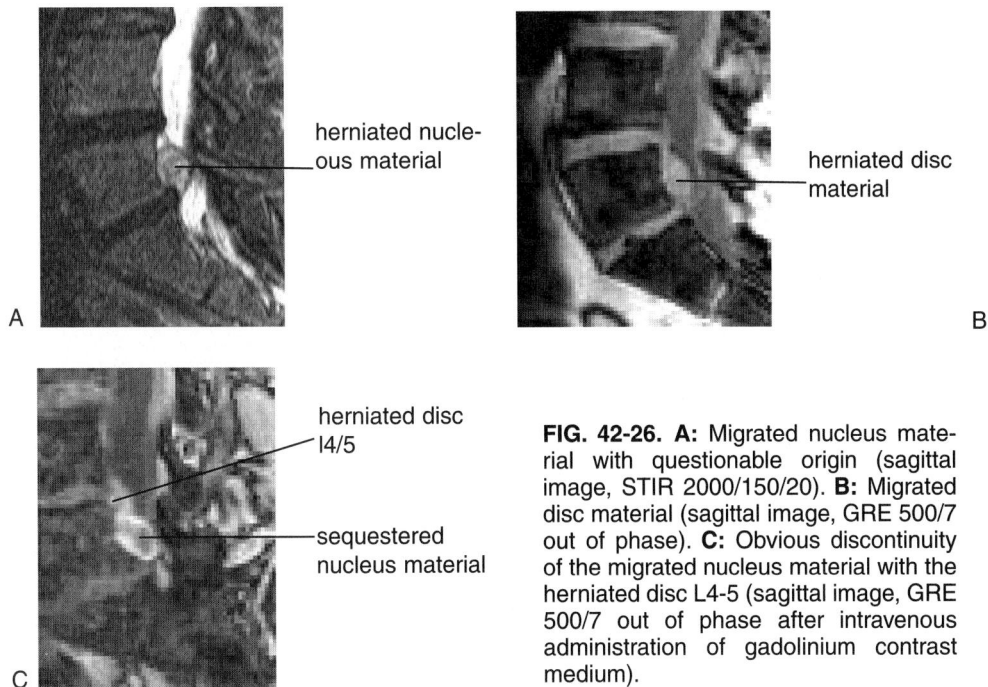

herniated nucleous material

A

herniated disc material

B

herniated disc l4/5

sequestered nucleus material

C

FIG. 42-26. A: Migrated nucleus material with questionable origin (sagittal image, STIR 2000/150/20). **B:** Migrated disc material (sagittal image, GRE 500/7 out of phase). **C:** Obvious discontinuity of the migrated nucleus material with the herniated disc L4-5 (sagittal image, GRE 500/7 out of phase after intravenous administration of gadolinium contrast medium).

A

B

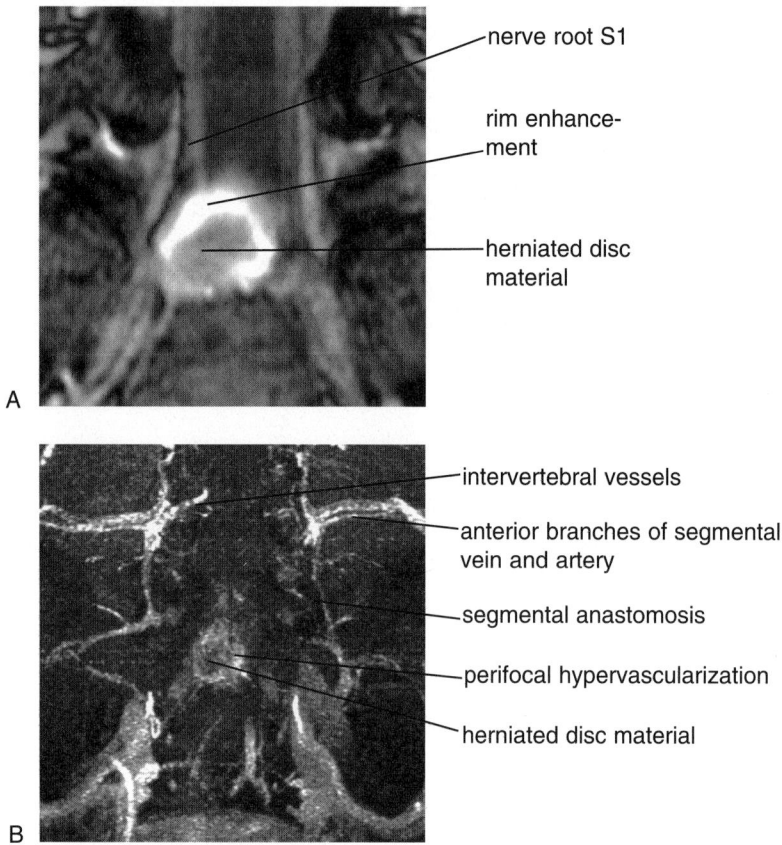

FIG. 42-27. **A:** The enhanced rim represents perifocal edema or vascularization (coronal image, GRE 500/7 out of phase after intravenous administration of gadolinium contrast medium). **B:** The arterial phase of angiography demonstrates the hypercapillarization of the perifocal tissue.

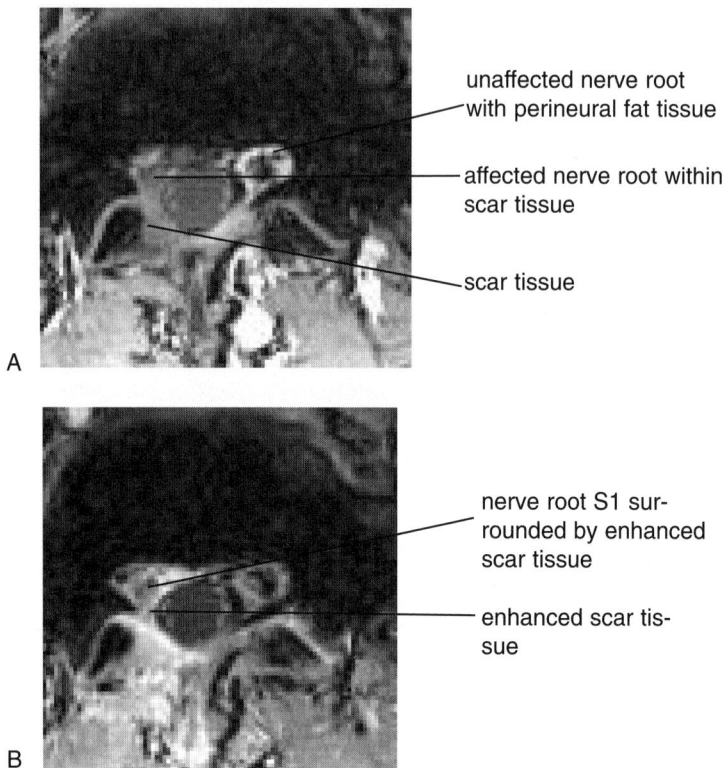

A

B

FIG. 42-28. **A:** Scar tissue appears with lower signal intensity than the normal ligamentum flavum at the opposite side (transverse image, GRE 500/7 out of phase). **B:** Scar tissue has high uptake of contrast medium and better delineation of the affected nerve root.

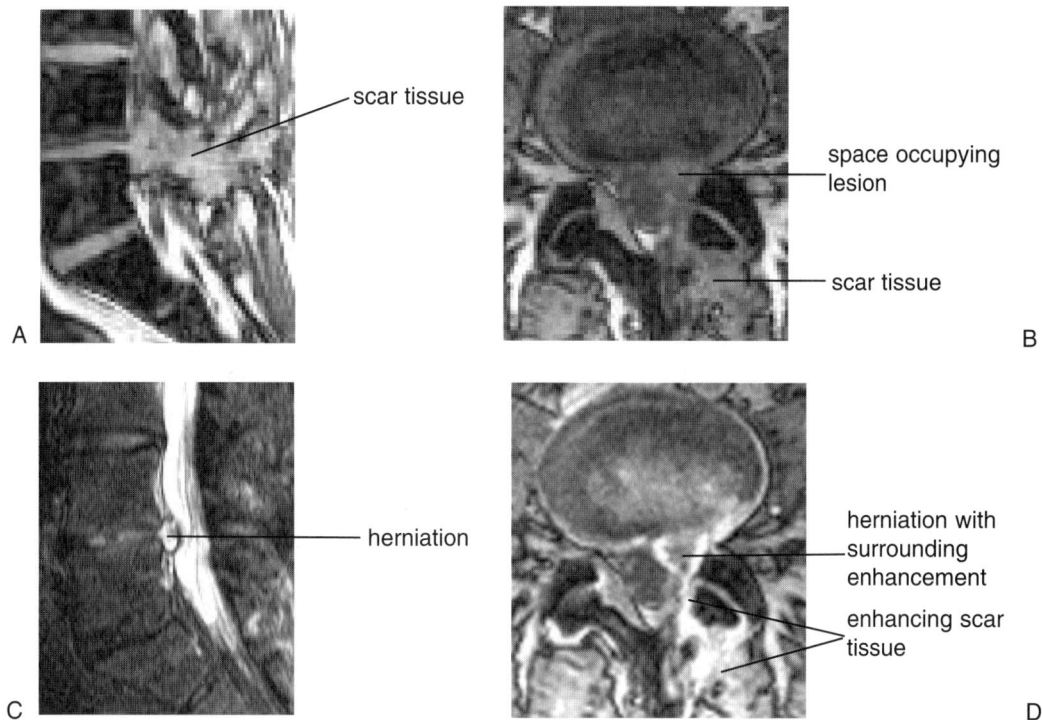

FIG. 42-29. A: Recurrent low back pain 9 months after discectomy. Epidural scar tissue with suspicion of reherniation (sagittal image, GRE 500/7 out of phase). **B:** The reherniated nucleus appears very bright in T2-weighted images, indicating recent herniation (sagittal image, STIR 2000/150/20). **C:** Foreign mass on the left side compressing dural sac (transverse image, GRE 500/7 out of phase). **D:** After intravenous (i.v.) administration of gadolinium (Gd) contrast medium, the reherniation is demarked by a rim of high enhancement (transverse image, GRE 500/7 out of phase after i.v. administration of Gd contrast medium).

Shortly after discectomy, scar tissue appears dark in T1- and bright in T2-weighted images because of its high water content. It appears enhanced after i.v. administration of Gd-contrast media (Fig. 42-28) (96,97). Gradually, scar tissue becomes brighter in T1- and darker in T2-weighted images. The enhancement of contrast does not change much. Differentiation of recurrent herniation and scar tissue can be difficult when the herniated disc material also enhances by ingrowth of vascular structures. Normally, the herniated material does not enhance (Fig. 42-29). The usefulness of Gd-contrast media is doubtful when the high resolution fast spin-echo sequences are used along with proton density–weighted images (98).

T1-weighted images before and after Gd-contrast application are not sufficient to investigate the origin of reappearing pain in the early postoperative period. In such cases, retrodiscal infection has to be taken into account. T1-weighted out-of-phase sequences before and after Gd administration show the inflammatory tissue with high enhancement (Fig. 42-30). Possibly re-herni-

ated disc material appears brighter than any possible abscess (Fig. 42-31) (99).

Perineural or neurogenic tumors, which might be confounded with lateral herniation in native MR images, are identified by their high uptake of contrast medium, which may be homogeneous, heterogeneous, or annular (Fig. 42-32) (100–102).

Synovial cysts and ganglia can be recognized easily by their high homogeneous signal intensity in T2-weighted images and various signal intensities on T1-weighted images. The signal intensity depends on the fluid composition ranging from serous to proteinaceous to hemorrhagic (Fig. 42-33). In most cases, the synovial tissue is enhanced after i.v. application of Gd-contrast media (42,103,104).

Hematomas may be confounded with herniation in T1- and T2-weighted images (34,76,105). Better differentiation is possible with T1-weighted GE out-of-phase sequences where hematomas appear very bright because of susceptibility effects.

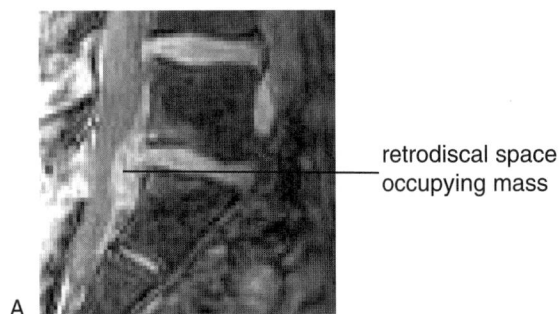

retrodiscal space occupying mass

A

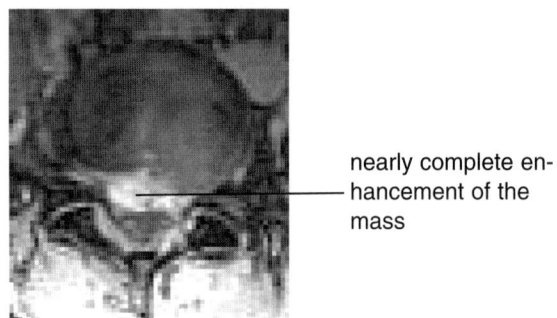

nearly complete enhancement of the mass

B

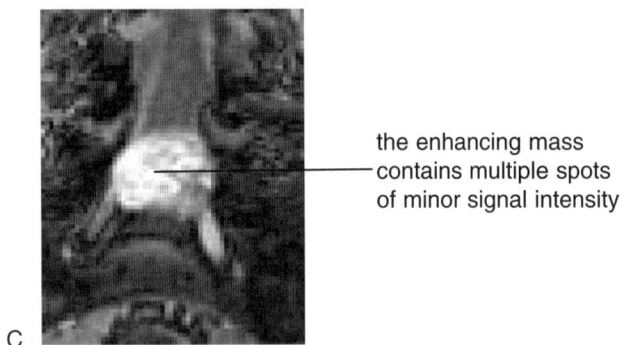

the enhancing mass contains multiple spots of minor signal intensity

C

FIG. 42-30. A: Five days after surgical intervention, the patient presented with acute low back pain. A bend-shaped retrodiscal structure can be seen with nearly disclike signal intensity (sagittal image, GRE 500/7 out of phase). **B:** The throughout enhanced mass after i.v. application of Gd-contrast media exclude a disc herniation (transverse image, GRE 500/7 out of phase after intravenous [i.v.] administration of gadolinium [Gd] contrast medium). **C:** At reoperation, the mass reveals to be infectious tissue with pus accumulation (coronal image, GRE 500/7 out of phase after intravenous administration of Gd contrast medium).

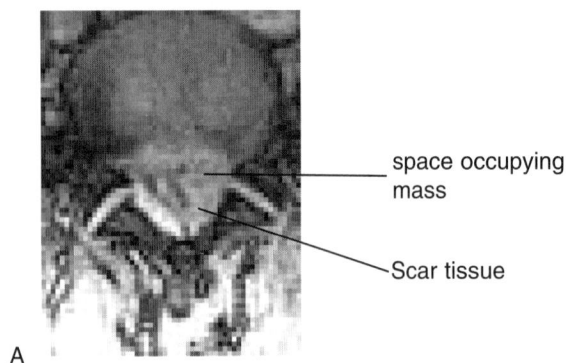

space occupying mass

Scar tissue

A

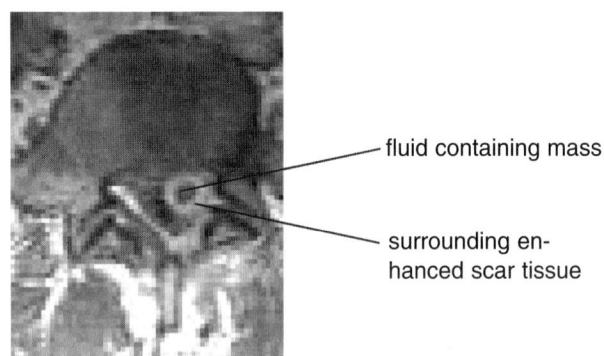

fluid containing mass

surrounding enhanced scar tissue

B

FIG. 42-31. A: The unenhanced T1-weighted opposed phased image shows a mass of uncertain origin (transverse image, GRE 500/7 out of phase). **B:** After intravenous (i.v.) application of gadolinium (Gd) contrast medium, an enhancing rim appears. The center has slightly lower signal intensity than disc material. At operation, the mass is revealed to be an abscess (transverse image, GRE 500/7 out of phase after i.v. administration of Gd contrast medium).

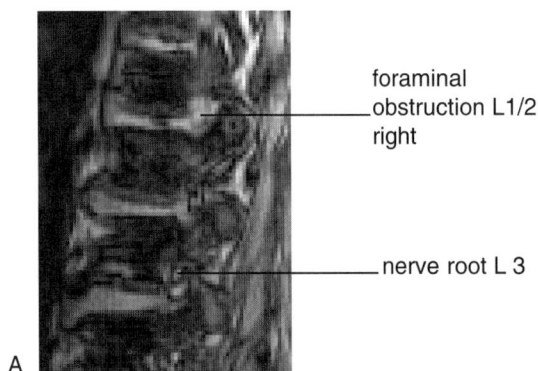

foraminal obstruction L1/2 right

nerve root L 3

A

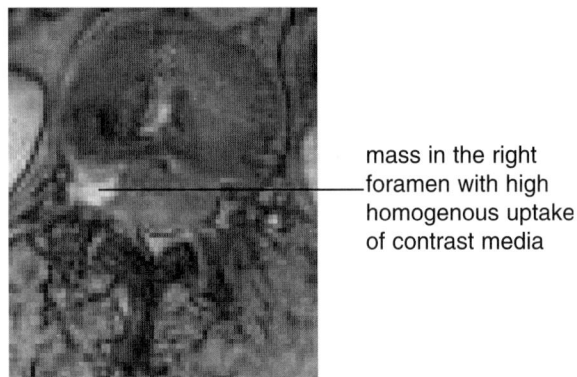

mass in the right foramen with high homogenous uptake of contrast media

B

FIG. 42-32. A: The foramen is obstructed by a mass of high-signal intensity equal to the intensity of the disc (sagittal image, GRE 500/7 out of phase). **B:** The homogenous high uptake of contrast media is characteristic for neurinomas (transverse image, GRE 500/7 out of phase after intravenous administration of gadolinium contrast medium).

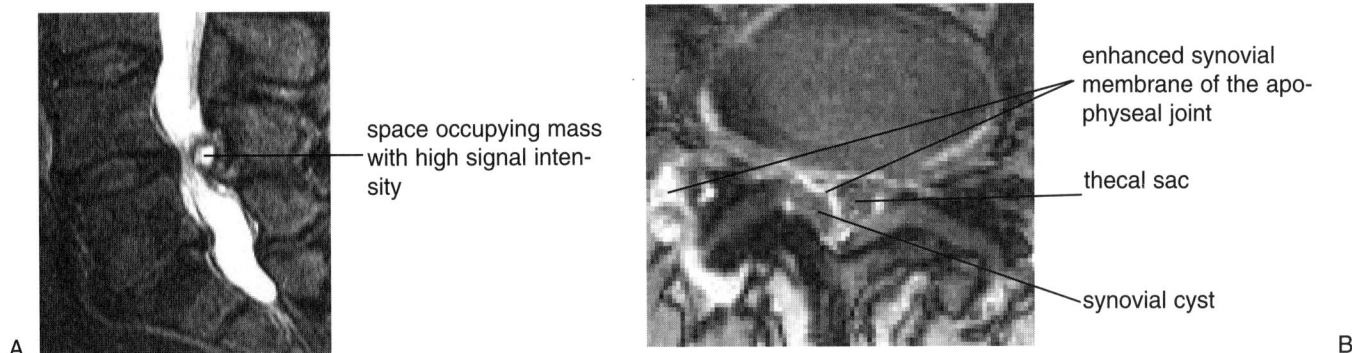

space occupying mass with high signal intensity

enhanced synovial membrane of the apophyseal joint

thecal sac

synovial cyst

A

B

FIG. 42-33. A: Well delineated space occupying lesion with high signal intensity (saggital image, STIR 2000/150/20). B: After intravenous (i.v.) application of gadolinium (Gd) contrast medium, there is a strong enhancement of the hypertrophic synovial membrane of the apophyseal joint. The synovial cyst compresses the thecal sac (transverse image, GRE 500/7 out of phase after i.v. administration of Gd contrast medium).

CLINICAL RELEVANCE

As shown, there are different imaging techniques to elucidate the pathomorphologic origin of low back pain and sciatica. The evaluation of methods regarding accuracy and predictive value highly depends on the technical performance (106) and the expertise of the persons interpreting the data.

A plain radiograph may show a narrowing of the disc space, osteophytes, and calcification. Therefore, it is not the method of choice when there are strong clinical hints for discal herniation, and no suspicion of consuming diseases is given.

Myelography demonstrates filling defects of the thecal sac and dural recess that may be caused by any stenosing process (discal, spondylotic, osteoarthritic, or tumorous). Therefore, this imaging procedure is only indicated today when patients have metal implants.

Discography describes the internal derangement of the discs, and rupture and herniation of the outer annulus. Major disadvantages of discography are: invasiveness, selectivity of examination, and no differentiation between subligamentous and transligamentous extrusion. It can be combined with the pain reproduction test to locate the painful segment. The reliability is controversial (19,21, 101,107–114). When discography is followed by CT examination, it is possible to precisely locate the herniation and determine the form and volume of herniated material (62,112). Because of invasiveness and inherent risks, discography and CT discography are image procedures that are secondary to CT and MRI.

Computed tomography delineates the outer contour of the disc as well as gas and calcification. It does not supply any information about the disc matrix. Sagittal and coronal views are only available by reconstruction. This demands thin contiguous axial section. Exposure to radiographs should not be neglected. Apart from MRI, this technique is the imaging modality of choice to demonstrate discus herniation and osseous stenosing processes, even when subligamentous and transligamentous extensions cannot be evaluated.

Magnetic resonance images correlate well with macroscopic anatomic sections (112). However, in 13% of the cases, discs that appear normal on MRI may show tears on discography (71). The high-intensity zone (HIZ) (115) does not seem to be a relevant feature for an aching disc (116). Annulus and nucleus can be distinguished. The location of herniation inside and outside the canal as well as its correlation with the neurovascular structures can be exactly identified. Subligamentous and transligamentous extrusions are hardly ever indistinguishable. Views of the whole lumbar spine can be taken from all angles without any risk for the patient. To sum up, it can be said that MRI has some advantages in comparison with CT regarding the diagnosis of disc herniation.

One has to review the ways that image information can explain patients' symptoms and therefore form the basis for treatment.

There is a high incidence of disc abnormalities, as described by CT and MR examinations in asymptomatic individuals (21,117–122).

Studies have shown that spontaneous regression of the hernia can occur with regression of radicular pain (76,77, 90,123–129). It seems that sequestered disc material has a greater potential for regression than extruded and protruded disc material (50). The contact of herniated material with the vascular system in the epidural space is probably responsible for this natural course of herniation (130–133). Therefore, conservative treatment should be considered for at least 2 months after onset of radicular pain (125,134–137).

The morphometric measurements and their ratios (volume or size of the herniation, diameters of the dural sac and spinal canal), and different types of herniation are considered for their predictive value for the outcome of conservative or surgical treatment (137–145).

A connection can be assumed of nerve root compression and swelling of the root and ganglia with location and severity of leg pain (78,117,120,146–148).

For the welfare of the patient, the collaboration between radiologists and clinicians is a sine qua non. For this purpose, the following demands have to be accomplished:

1. The technical performance has to be optimal.
2. Disc herniation has to be exactly characterized for morphology, location, and its relation to the neurovascular system.
3. A generally accepted nomenclature is necessary.
4. In the absence of disc abnormalities the imaging should be able to detect other reasons to explain the pain of the patient.
5. The results of imaging have to correlate with the patient's symptoms.

REFERENCES

1. Scientific approach to the assessment and management of activity-related spinal disorders: a monograph for clinicians. Report of the Quebec Task Force on Spinal Disorders. Spine 1987;12:S1–S59.
2. Tulder MW van, Assendelft WJJ, Koes BW, et al. Spinal radiographic findings and nonspecific low back pain. Spine 1997;22:427–434.
3. Goel VK, Goyal S, Clark C, Nishiyama K, et al. Kinematics of the whole lumbar spine. Effect of discectomy. Spine 1985;10:543–554.
4. Fink B, Kothe R, Browa A, et al. Die segmentale Hypermobilität der LWS vor und nach Disektomie. Z Orthop 1996;134:483–487.
5. Schultz KP, Fink B, Kothe R, et al. Segmental hypermobility in the lumbar spine following discectomy. International Society for the Study of the lumbar Spine, Abstract, Burlington VT. June 1996.
6. Stokes IAF, Wilder DG, Frymoyer JW, et al. Assessment of patients with low-back pain by biplanar radiographic measurement of intervertebral motion. Spine 1981;6:233–240.
7. Tibrewal SB, Pearcy MJ, Portek I, et al. A prospective study of lumbar spinal movements before and after discectomy using biplanar radiography. Correlation of clinical and radiographic findings. Spine 1985;10:455–460.
8. Weishaupt D, Zanetti M, Hodler J, et al. MR imaging of the lumbar spine: prevalence of intervertebral disk extrusion and sequestration, nerve root compression, end plate abnormalities, and osteoarthritis of the facet joints in asymptomatic volunteers. Radiology 1998;209:661–666.
9. Wildermuth S, Zanetti M, Duewell S, et al. Lumbar spine: quantitative and qualitative assessment of positional (upright flexion and extension) MR imaging and myelography. Radiology 1998;207:391–398.
10. Brodsky AE, Binder WF. Lumbar discography. Its value in diagnosis and treatment of lumbar disc lesions. Spine 1979;4:110–120.
11. Collis JS. Lumbar discography. Springfield, IL: Charles C Thomas, 1963.
12. Videman T, Malmivaara A, Mooney V. The value of the axial view in assessing discograms. An experimental study with cadavers. Spine 1987;12:299–304.
13. Adams MA, Dolan P, Hutton WC. The stages of disc degeneration as revealed by discograms. J Bone Joint Surg 1986;68B:36–41.
14. Erlacher PR. Nucleography. J Bone Joint Surg 1952;34B:204–210.
15. Carragee EJ, Tanner CM, Yank B, et al. False-positive findings on lumbar discography. Reliability of subjective concordance assessment during provocative disc injection. Spine 1999;24:2542–2547.
16. Carragee EJ, Chen Y, Tanner CM, et al. Provocative discography in patients after limited lumbar discectomy. A controlled, randomized study of pain response in symptomatic and asymptomatic subjects. Spine 2000;25:3065–3071.
17. Guyer RD, Ohnmeiss DD. Contemporary concepts in spine care lumbar discography. Position statement from the North American Spine Society Diagnostics and Therapeutic Committee. Spine 1995;20:2048–2059.
18. Heggeness MH, Watters WC, Gray PM. Discography of lumbar discs after surgical treatment for disc herniation. Spine 1997;22:1606–1609.
19. Holt EP. The question of lumbar discography. J Bone Joint Surg 1967;50A:720–726.
20. Schultz KP. Die neuroradiographische Diagnostik degenerativer Bandscheibenerkrankungen- Das Düsseldorfer diagnostische Diskusprogramm (DdD) II. Die Schmerzreproduktion durch Discographie. Z Orthop 1994;132:1–7.
21. Walsh TR, Weinstein JN, Spratt KF, et al. Lumbar discography in normal subjects. A controlled, prospective study. J Bone Joint Surg (Am) 1990;72:1081–1088.
22. Haughton VM, Syvertsen A, Williams AL. Soft-tissue anatomy within the spinal canal as seen on computed tomography. Radiology 1980;134:649–655.
23. Rosenthal DI, Stauffer AE, Davis KR, et al. Evaluation of multiplanar reconstruction in CT recognition of lumbar disc disease. AJR 1984;143:169–176.
24. Rovira M, Romero F, Ibarra B, et al. Prolapsed lumbar discs: value of CT in diagnosis. AJNR 1983;4:593–594.
25. Di Chiro G, Doppman JL, Wener L. Computed tomography of spinal cord arteriovenous malformations. Radiology 1977;123:351–354.
26. Nakagawa H, Huang YP, Malis LI, et al. Computed tomography of intraspinal and paraspinal neoplasms. J Comput Assist Tomogr 1977;1:377–390.
27. DeSantis M, Crisi G, Folchi Vici F. Late contrast enhancement in the CT diagnosis of herniated lumbar disk. Neuroradiology 1984;26:303–307.
28. Raininko R, Torma T. Contrast enhancement around a prolapsed disk. Neuroradiology 1982;24:49–51.
29. Glenn WV Jr, Rhodes ML, Altschuler EM, et al. Multiplanar display computerized body tomography applications in the lumbar spine. Spine 1979;4:282–352.
30. Helms CA, Dorwart RH, Gray M. The CT appearance of conjoined nerve roots and differentiation from a herniated nucleus pulposus. Radiology 1982;144:803–807.
31. Peyster RG, Teplick JG, Haskin ME. Computed tomography of lumbosacral conjoined nerve root anomalis: potential cause of false-positive reading for herniated nucleus pulposus. Spine 1985;10:331–337.
32. Kadish LJ, Simmons EH. Anomalies of the lumbosacral nerve roots: an anatomical investigation and myelographic study. J Bone Joint Surg 1984;66B:411–416.
33. Williams AL, Haughton VM, Daniels DL, et al. Differential CT diagnosis of extruded nucleus pulposus. Radiology 1983;148:141–148.
34. Gundry CR, Heithoff KB. Epidural hematoma of the lumbar spine: 18 surgically confirmed cases. Radiology 1993;187:427–431.
35. Heithoff KB. Myelography and computed tomography of the lumbar spine. In: Wiesel SW, Weinstein JN, Herkowitz HN, et al, eds. The lumbar spine. Philadelphia: WB Saunders, 1996:376-428.
36. Post MJ, Seminer DS, Quencer RM. CT diagnosis of spinal epidural hematoma. AJNR 1982;3:190–192.
37. Mattle H, Sieb JP, Rohner M, et al. Nontraumatic spinal epidural and subdural hematomas. Neurology 1987;37:1351–1356.
38. Wisoff HS. Spontaneous intraspinal hemorrhage. In: Wilkins RH, Rengachary SS, eds. Neurosurgery. New York: McGraw-Hill, 1985:1500–1503.
39. Fardon DF, Simmons JD. Gas-filled synovial cyst. A case report. Spine 1989;14:127–129.
40. Maupin WB, Naul LG, Kanter SL, et al. Synovial cyst presenting as a neural foraminal lesion: MR and CT appearance. AJR 1989;153:1231–1232.
41. Reust P, Wendling D, Lagier R, et al. Degenerative spondylolisthesis synovial cyst of the zygapophyseal joints, sciatic syndrome: report of two cases and review of the literature. Arthritis Rheum 1988;31:288–294.
42. Silbergleit R, Gebarski SS, Brungerg JA, et al. Lumbar synovial cysts: correlation of myelographic, CT, MR and pathologic findings. AJNR 1990;11:777–779.
43. Mariette X, Glon Y, Clerc D, et al. Medical treatment of synovial cysts of the zygophyzeal joints: Four cases with long-term followup. Arthritis Rheum 1989;32:660–661.
44. Chiba K, Toyama Y, Matsumoto M, et al. Intraspinal cyst communicating with the intervertebral disc in the lumbar spine. Discal Cyst Spine 2001;26:2112–2118.
45. Tarlov IM. Spinal perineurial and meningeal cysts. J Neurol Neurosurg Psychiatry 1970;33:833–843.

46. Neave VCD, Wycoff RR. Computed tomography of cystic nerve root sleeve dilatation: case report. J Comput Assist Tomogr 1983;7: 881–885.
47. Eisenberg D, Gomori JM, Findler G, et al. Symptomatic diverticulum of the sacral nerve root sheath: case note. Neuroradiology 1985;27: 183.
48. Naidich TP, McLone DG, Harwood-Nash DC. Arachnoid cysts, paravertebral meningoceles, and perineurial cysts. In: Newton TH, Potts DG, eds. Computed tomography of the spine and spinal cord. San Anselmo, CA: Clavadel Press, 1983:383–396.
49. Nikolic B, Abbara S, Heindel W, et al. Sakrale Perineuralzysten: gibt es radiologische Kriterien für eine Operationsindikation? Fortschr Röntghenstr 2000;172:1035–1042.
50. Ahn SH, Ahn MW, Byun WM. Effect of the transligamentous extension of lumbar disc herniations on their regression and the clinical outcome of sciatica. Spine 2000;25:475–480.
51. Haughton VM, Eldevik OP, Magnaes B, et al. A prospective comparison of computed tomraphy and myelography in the diagnosis of herniated lumbar disks. Radiology 1982;142:103–110.
52. Pfadenhauer K, Ebeling U, Bergleiter R, et al. Zuverlässigkeit der Computertomographie bei der Diagnostik von Rezidivbeschwerden nach lumbalen Bandscheibenoperationen. Fortschr Röntgenstr 1983; 139,2:127–131.
53. Claussen C, Grumme Th, Treisch J, et al. Die Diagnostik des lumbalen Bandscheibenvorfalls. Fortschr Röntgenstr 1982;136,1:1–8.
54. Weiss Th, Treisch J, Kazner E, et al. Intravenöse Kontrastmittelgabe bei der Computertomographie (CT) der operierten Lendenwirbelsäule. Fortschr Röntgenstr 1984;141:30–34.
55. Resnick D, Niwayama G. Degenerative disease of the spine. In: Resnick D, ed. Diagnosis of bone and joint disorders. Philadelphia: W.B.Saunders 1995:1424.
56. Chafetz N. Computed tomography of lumbar disk disease. In: HK Genant, N Chafetz, CA Helms, eds. Computed tomography of the lumbar spine. San Francisco: University of California Press, 1982: 125.
57. Herzog RJ. The radiologic assessment for a lumbar disc herniation. Spine 1996;21:19S–38S.
58. Williams AL, Haughton VW, Meyer GA, et al. Computed tomographic appearance of the bulging annulus. Radiology 1982;142: 403–408.
59. Williams JP, Joslyn JN, Butler TW. Differentiation of herniated lumbar disc from bulging annulus fibrosis. Use of reformatted images. J Comput Tomogr 1982;6:89–93.
60. Brant-Zawadzki MN, Jensen MC, Obuchowski N, et al. Interobserver an intraobserver variability in interpretation of lumbar disc abnormalities. Spine 1995;20:1257–1264.
61. McCutcheon ME, Thompson WC. CT scanning of lumbar discography. A useful diagnostic adjunct. Spine 1986;11:257–259.
62. Sachs BL, Vanharanta H, Spivey MA, et al. Dallas discogram description. A new classification of CT-discography in low back disorders. Spine 1987;12:287–294.
63. Schultz KP, Schöppe K, Wehling P. The correlation between CT-discography, MRI and surgical findings in sequestrated and non-sequestrated herniation. Presented at the International Society for the Study of the lumbar Spine, Miami, FL, May 1988.
64. Vanharanta H, Guyer RD, Ohnmeiss D, et al. Disc deterioration in low back syndromes. A prospective, multi-center CT-discography study. Spine 1988;13:1349–1351.
65. Schultz KP, Schöppe K. Die neurographische Diagnostik degenerativer Bandscheibenerkrankungen. Das Düsseldorfer diagnostische Discusprogramm. I. Das Computer-Discogramm. Z Orthop 1994;132:25–32.
66. Castro WHM, Jerosch J, Hepp R, et al. Restriction of indication for automated percutaneous lumbar discectomy based on computed tomographic discography. Spine 1992;17:1239–1243.
67. Edwards WC, Orme TJ, Orr-Edwards G. CT discography: prognostic value in the selection of patients for chemonucleolysis. Spine 1987; 12:792–795.
68. Whitehouse RW, Hutchinson CE, Laitt R, et al. The influence of chemical shift artifact on magnetic resonance imaging of the ligamentum flavum at 0.5 tesla. Spine 1997;22:200–202.
69. Battié MC, Videman T, Gibbons LE, et al. 1995 Volvo Award in Clinical Sciences. Determinants of lumbar disc degeneration. A study relating lifetime exposures and magnetic resonance imaging findings in identical twins. Spine 1995;20:2601–2612.
70. Luoma K, Vehmas T, Riihimäki H, et al. Disc height and signal intensity of the nucleus pulposus on magnetic resonance imaging as indicators of lumbar disc degeneration. Spine 2001;26:680–686.
71. Milette PC, Fontaine S, Lepanto L, et al. Differentiating lumbar disc protrusions, disc bulges, and discs with normal contour but abnormal signal intensity. Spine 1999;24:44–53.
72. Pfirrmann CWA, Metzdorf A, Zanetti M, et al. Magnetic resonance classification of lumbar intervertebral disc degeneration. Spine 2001; 26:1873–1878.
73. Raininko R, Manninen H, Battié MC, et al. Observer variability in the assessment of disc degeneration on magnetic resonance imaging of the lumbar and thoracic spine. Spine 1995;20:1029–1035.
74. Bundesärztekammer. Leitlinien der Bundesärztekammer zur Qualitätssicherung der Magnet-Resonanz-Tomographie. Deutsches Ärzteblatt 2000;97:A2557–A2568.
75. Grenier N, Greselle JF, Vital JM, et al. Normal and disrupted lumbar longitudinal ligaments: correlative MR and anatomic study. Radiology 1989;171:197–205.
76. Komori H, Shinomiya K, Nakai O, et al. The natural history of herniated nucleus pulposus with radiculopathy. Spine 1996;21:225–229.
77. Bozzao A, Gallucci M, Masciocchi C, et al. Lumbar disk herniation: MR imaging assessment of natural history in patients treated without surgery. Radiology 1992;185:135–141.
78. Masaryk TJ, Ross JS, Modic MT, et al. High-resolution MR imaging of sequestered lumbar intervertebral disks. AJR 1988;150: 1155–1162.
79. Beattie PF, Meyers SP, Stratford P, et al. Associations between patient report of symptoms and anatomic impairment visible on lumbar magnetic resonance imaging. Spine 2000;25:819–828.
80. Rankine JJ, Fortune DG, Hutchinson CE, et al. Pain drawings in the assessment of nerve root compression: a comparative study with lumbar spine magnetic resonance imaging. Spine 1998;23:1668–1676.
81. Weishaupt D, Schmid MR, Zanetti M, et al. Positional MR imaging of the lumbar spine: does it demonstrate nerve root compromise not visible at conventional MR imaging? Radiology 2000;215:247–253.
82. Aota Y, Onari K, An HS, et al. Dorsal root ganglia morphologic features in patients with herniation of the nucleus pulposus. Spine 2001;26:2125–2132.
83. Assheuer J, Sissopoulos A, Schulitz KP. Visualisation of venous stasis, edema and granulation tissue in narrowing conditions of the lumbar spine by MRI. Chicago: International Society for the Study of the Lumbar Spine, 1992.
84. Crisi G, Carpeggiani P, Trevisan C. Gadolinium-enhanced nerve roots in lumbar disk herniation. AJNR Am J Neuroradiol 1993;14:1379–1392.
85. Jinkins JR. MR of enhancing nerve roots in the unoperated lumbosacral spine. AJNR Am J Neuroradiol 1993;14:193–202.
86. Kobayashi S, Yoshizawa H, Hachiya Y, et al. Vasogenic edema induced by compression injury to the spinal nerve root. Distribution of intravenously injected protein tracers and gadolinium-enhanced magnetic resonance imaging. Spine 1993;18:1410–1424.
87. Lane JI, Koeller KK, Atkinson JL. Enhanced lumbar nerve roots in the spine without prior surgery: radiculitis or radicular veins? AJNR Am J Neuroradiol 1994;15:1317–1325.
88. Taneishi H, Abumi K, Kaneda K, et al. Significance of Gd-DTPA-enhanced magnetic resonance imaging for lumbar disc herniation: the relationship between nerve root enhancement and clinical manifestations. J Spinal Disord 1994;7:153–160.
89. Toyone T, Takahashi K, Kitahara H, et al. Visualisation of symptomatic nerve roots. Prospective study of contrast-enhanced MRI in patients with lumbar disc herniation. J Bone Joint Surg (Br) 1993;75-B:529–533.
90. Komori H, Okawa A, Haro H, et al. Contrast-enhanced magnetic resonance imaging in conservative management of lumbar disc herniation. Spine 1998;23:67–73.
91. Ross JS, Modic MT, Masaryk TJ. Tears of the anulus fibrosus: assessment with Gd-DTPA-enhanced MR imaging. AJNR Am J Neuroradiol 1989;10:1251–1254.
92. Assheuer J, Crock H, Forutan F, et al. Lumbar spinal MR angiography in the normal and pathological spine. International Society for the Study of the Lumbar Spine, Adelaide, Australia, April 2000.
93. Assheuer J. Magnetic resonance imaging examination for degenerative disease of the lumbar spine in lumbar disk herniation. In: Szpalski M, Gunzburg R, eds. Baltimore: Lippincott Williams & Wilkins, 2002:111–124.
94. Castro WHM, Assheuer J, Schulitz KP. Haemodynamic changes in lumbar nerve root entrapment due to stenosis and/or herniated disc of

the lumbar spine canal: a magnetic resonance imaging study. Eur Spine J 1995;4:220–225.

95. Sager M, Assheuer J. Imaging of pathophysiological aspects after disc herniation in dogs. Second Annual Congress of the European Association Veterinary Diagnostics Imaging (EAVDI), Alghero, Sept.1993.

96. Cavanagh S, Stevens J, Johnson J. High-resolution MRI in the investigation of recurrent pain after lumbar discectomy. J Bone Joint Surg (Br) 1993;75:524–528.

97. Hueftle MG, Modic MT, Ross JS, et al. Lumbar spine: postoperative MR imaging with Gd-DTPA. Radiology 1988;167:817–824.

98. Mullin WJ, Heithoff KB, Gilbert TJ, et al. Magnetic resonance evaluation of recurrent disc herniation. Spine 2000;25:1493–1499.

99. Schulitz KP, Assheuer J. Discitis after procedures on the intervertebral disc. Spine 1994;10:1172–1177.

100. Demachi H, Takashima T, Kadoya M, et al. MR imaging of spinal neurinomas with pathologic correlation. J Comput Assist Tomogr 1990;14:250–254.

101. Ohnmeiss DD, Vanharanta H, Guyer RD. The association between pain drawings and computed tomographic/discographic pain responses. Spine 1995;20:729–733.

102. Schroth G, Thron A, Guhl L, et al. Magnetic resonance imaging of spinal meningiomas and neurinomas. Improvement of imaging by paramagnetic contrast enhancement. J Neurosurg 1987;66:695–700.

103. Jackson DE, Atlas SW, Mani JR, et al. Intraspinal synovial cysts: MR imaging. Radiology 1989;170:527–530.

104. Yuh WTC, Drew JM, Weinstein JN, et al. Intraspinal synovial cysts. Magnetic resonance evaluation. Spine 1991;16:740–745.

105. Watanabe N, Ogura T, Komori K, et al. Epidural hematoma of the lumbar spine, simulating extruded lumbar disk herniation: clinical, discographic, and enhanced magnetic resonance imaging features. Spine 1997;22:105–109.

106. Jarvik GJ, Robertson WD, Wessbecher F, et al. Variation in the quality of lumbar spine MR images in Washington state. Radiology 2000; 215:483–490.

107. Schwarzer AC, Aprill CN, Derby R, et al. The prevalence and clinical features of internal disc disruption in patients with chronic low back pain. Spine 1995;20:1878–1893.

108. Block AR, Vanharanta H, Ohnmeiss DD, et al. Discographic pain report. Influence of psychological factors. Spine 1996;21:334–338.

109. Carragee EJ, Tanner CM, Khurana S, et al. The rates of false-positive lumbar discography in select patients without low back symptoms. Spine 2000;25:1373–1381.

110. Klenerman L, Slade PD, Stanley IM, et al. The prediction of chronicity in patients with an acute attack of low back pain in a general practice setting. Spine 1995;20:478–484.

111. Massie W, Stevens D. A critical evaluation of discography. J Bone Joint Surg (Am) 1967;49:1243–1244.

112. Vanharanta H, Sachs BL, Spivey M. A comparison of CT/discography, pain response and radiographic disc height. Spine 1988;13: 321–324.

113. Vanharanta H, Sachs BL, Spivey MA, et al. The relationship of pain provocation to lumbar disc deterioration as seen by CT-discography. Spine 1987;12:295.

114. Zindrick MR, Lorenz MA, Noonan C, et al. The Correlation MRI, Discogram and Pain Reproduction. Presented at the International Society for the Study of the Lumbar Spine Meeting, Rome, Italy, May 1987.

115. Aprill C, Bogduk N. High-intensity zone: a diagnostic sign of painful lumbar disc on magnetic resonance imaging. Br J Radiol 1992;65: 361–369.

116. Carragee EJ, Paragioudakis SJ, Khurana S. 2000 Volvo Award winner in clinical studies. Lumbar high-intensity zone and discography in subjects without low back problems. Spine 2000;25:2987–2992.

117. Boden SD, Davis DO, Dina TS, et al. Abnormal magnetic resonance scans of the lumbar spine in asymptomatic subjects. J Bone Joint Surg (Am) 1990;72:403–408.

118. Boos N, Rieder R, Schade V, et al. 1995 Volvo Award in Clinical Sciences. The diagnostic accuracy of magnetic resonance imaging, work perception, and psychosocial factors in identifying symptomatic disc herniations. Spine 1995;20:2613–2625.

119. Buirski G, Silberstein M. The symptomatic lumbar disc in patients with low back pain: magnetic resonance imaging appearances in both symptomatic and control population. Spine 1993;18:2153–2162.

120. Jensen MC, Brant ZM, Obuchowski N, et al. Magnetic resonance imaging of the lumbar spine in people without back pain. N Engl J Med 1994;331:69–73.

121. Modic MT, Masaryk TJ, Ross JS. Magnetic resonance imaging of the spine, 1st ed. St. Louis: Mosby, 1989.

122. Wiesel SW, Tsourmas N, Feffer HL, et al. A study of computer-assisted tomography. I. The incidence of positive CAT scans in an asymptomatic group of patients. Spine 1984;9:549–551.

123. Bush K, Cowan N, Katz DE, et al. The natural history of sciatica associated with disc pathology: A prospective study with clinical and independent radiologic follow-up. Spine 1992;17:1205–1212.

124. Delauche-Cavallier MC, Budet C, Laredo JD, et al. Lumbar disc herniation. Computed tomography scan changes after conservative treatment of nerve root compression. Spine 1992;17:927–933.

125. Dullerud R, Nakstad PH. CT changes after conservative treatment for lumbar disk herniation. Acta Radiol 1994;35:415–419.

126. Matsubara Y, Kato F, Mimatsu K, et al. Serial changes on MRI in lumbar disc herniations treated conservatively. Neuroradiology 1995;37: 378–383.

127. Saal JA, Saal JS, Herzog RJ. The natural history of lumbar intervertebral disc extrusions treated nonoperatively. Spine 1990;15:683–686.

128. Teplick JG, Haskin ME. Spontaneous regression of herniated nucleus pulposus. Am J Roentgenol 1985;145:371–375.

129. Yukawa Y, Kato F, Matsubara Y, et al. Serial magnetic resonnance imaging follow-up study of lumbar disc herniation conservatively treated for average 30 months: relation between reduction of herniation and degeneration of disc. J Spinal Disord 1996;9:251–256.

130. Doita M, Kanatani T, Harada T, et al. Immunohistologic study of the ruptured intervertebral disc of the lumbar spine. Spine 1996;2: 235–241.

131. Hirabayashi S, Kumano K, Tsuiki T, et al. A dorsally displaced free fragment of lumbar disc herniation and its interesting histologic findings. Spine 1990;15:1231–1233.

132. Ikeda T, Nakamura T, Kikuchi T, et al. Pathomechanism of spontaneous regression of the herniated lumbar disc. Histologic and immunohistochemical study. J Spinal Disord 1996;9:136–140.

133. Ito T, Yamada M, Ikuta F, et al. Histologic evidence of absorption of sequestration-type herniated disc. Spine 1996;2:230–234.

134. Ellenberg MR, Ross ML, Honet JC, et al. Prospective evaluation of the course of disc herniations in patients with proven radiculopathy. Arch Phys Med Rehabil 1993;74:3–8.

135. Ito T, Takano Y, Yuasa N. Types of lumbar herniated disc and clinical course. Spine 2001;26:648–651.

136. Maigne JY, Rime B, Deligne B. Computed tomographic follow-up study of forty-eight cases of nonoperatively treated lumbar intervertebral disc herniation. Spine 1992;17:1071–1074.

137. Saal J, Saal J. Nonoperative treatment of herniated lumbar intervertebral disc with radiculopathy: an outcome study. Spine 1989;14: 431–437.

138. Carragee EJ, Kim DH. A prospective analysis of magnetic resonance imaging findings in patients with sciatica and lumbar disc herniation correlation of outcomes with disc fragment and canal morphology. Spine 1997;22:1650–1660.

139. Dvorak J, Gaucha M, Valach L. The outcome of surgery for lumbar disc herniation: I. A 4–17 year followup with emphasis on somatic aspects. Spine 1988;13:1418–1422.

140. Eismont F, Currier B. Surgical management of lumbar intervertebral-disc disease. J Bone Joint Surg (Am) 1989;71:1266–1271.

141. Enzman D. On low back pain. Am J Neuroradiol 1994;15:109–113.

142. Fagerlund M, Thelander U, Friberg S. Size of lumbar disc hernias measured at computer tomography in relation to sciatica symptoms. Acta Radiol 1990;31:555–558.

143. Junge A, Dvorak J, Ahrens S. Predictors of bad and good outcomes of lumbar disc surgery. Spine 1995;20:460–486.

144. Nachemson A. Lumbar disc herniation: conclusions. Acta Orthop Scand Suppl 1993;251:49–50.

145. Pople I, Griffith H. Prediction of an extruded fragment in lumbar disc patients from clinical presentations. Spine 1994;19:156–158.

146. Jarvik JJ, Hollingworth W, Heagerty P, et al. The longitudinal assessment of imaging and disability of the back (LAIDBack) study. Spine 2001;26:1158–1166.

147. Takata K, Inoue S, Takahashi K, et al. Swelling of the cauda equina in patients who have herniation of a lumbar disc. J Bone Joint Surg (Am) 1988;A70:361–368.

148. Weishaupt D, Zanetti M, Hodler J, et al. MR imaging of the lumbar spine: prevalence of intervertebral disk extrusion and sequestration, nerve root compression, end plate abnormalities, and osteoarthritis of the facet joints in asymptomatic volunteers. Radiology 1998;209: 661–666.

CHAPTER 43

Disc Herniation: Nonoperative Treatment

Kevin P. Singer and Peter J. Fazey

"... surgical treatment of spinal disorders produces the best results when clinical symptoms and signs are congruous and confirmed by carefully selected imaging studies, and when they have resulted in an unequivocal diagnosis amenable to surgical management. An additional and important caveat is that the surgical result ought to be better than the 'natural history' of the disease being treated."

—J.W. Frymoyer, 1997

Herniations of the intervertebral disc (IVD) have probably afflicted man since earliest times, with the associated backache entrenched within folklore. The depiction by Luschka in 1885 of a central nuclear herniation of a lumbar IVD (1) (Fig. 43-1) is perhaps the first illustration of a specific spinal pathology that continues to command the attention of modern societies. The fact that, for tens of thousands of years, humans have been reliant upon nature underscores the challenge from John Frymoyer (2) to not disadvantage the individual if the natural history of spinal disease may be better in the long term than surgical interventions. The early clinical reports by Lindblom and Hultquist (3), and Hakelius (4), which identified progressive recovery following sciatica, have been quantified by others using cross-sectional computed tomography (CT) and magnetic resonance imaging (MRI) (5,6). These observations of the spontaneous regression of disc herniations have since prompted investigation into the physiology of this process.

The natural history of disc herniation describes a process of resolution both of symptoms and often a diminution of the herniation itself; which may be aided pharmacologically through epidural steroids and nerve root sleeve blocks or through rest and other conservative interventions. The purpose of this chapter is to review the natural history of lumbar disc herniation and principles of nonoperative management of this clinical problem. A case study report of the sequence to spontaneous regression of a large central disc herniation at L4-5 in a 32-year-old woman is provided to illustrate the natural course of this condition.

In the case of established herniated nucleus pulposus (HNP) there is an abundance of literature that confers advantage to conservative management (7). The efficacy of nonoperative management, observed through spontaneous regression of disc herniation, has been reported not only for the lumbar (8–10), but also thoracic (11–13) and cervical disc herniations (14,15). Further reinforcement for the principle of management by "watching and waiting" stems from the numerous reports of disc herniation and related disease in a large proportion of asymptomatic individuals.

In the 10-year controlled follow-up study reported by Weber (16), similar patterns of neurologic recovery in groups treated surgically and conservatively were demonstrated. In contrast, the 5-year follow-up study by Atlas et al. (17) determined that patients with moderate or severe sciatica, who had lower functional status at baseline, reported better outcomes following surgery compared with nonoperated patients. Irrespective of the extent of the initial neurologic deficit, a trend favoring nonoperative treatment was reported by Saal and Saal (18) who confirmed the capacity of HNP to resolve clinically without surgery or chemonucleolysis. The trend for larger herniations and sequestrated fragments to show an enhanced capacity for regression was supported by subsequent reports (9,19–21). Importantly, a 10-year review by Fraser et al. (22) clearly indicated that long-term improvement of a patient's symptoms of HNP could occur with or without regression of the herniation.

EVALUATION OF DISC HERNIATION

Early postmortem studies of the thoracic and lumbar spine by Andrae (23) and Schmorl (24) indicated that HNP was a frequent occurrence (Fig. 43-2). Since the advent of plain radiography, a high prevalence of spinal disease has been identified within asymptomatic individuals (25). Similarly, CT and MRI have highlighted the extent to which advanced pathology of the IVD, includ-

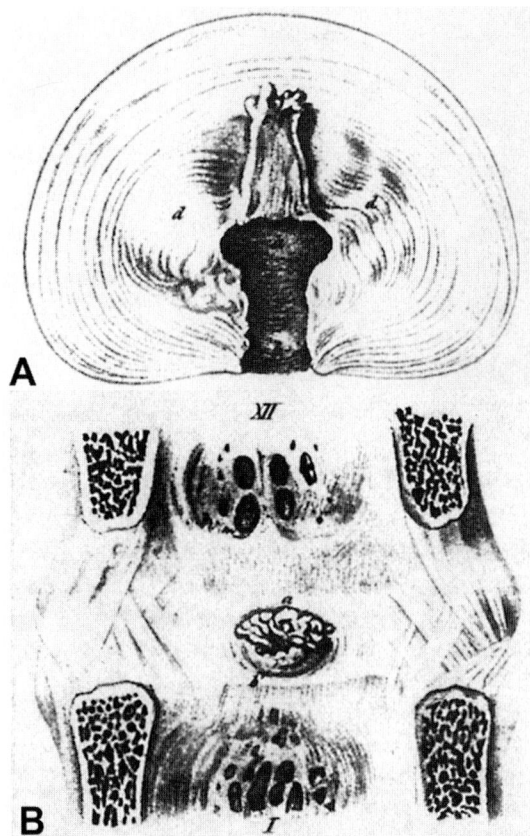

FIG. 43-1. Depiction of posterior disc herniation, as represented by Luschka (1) showing a nuclear fissure (reflected) passing through the posterior anulus (A) and protruding into the vertebral canal (B).

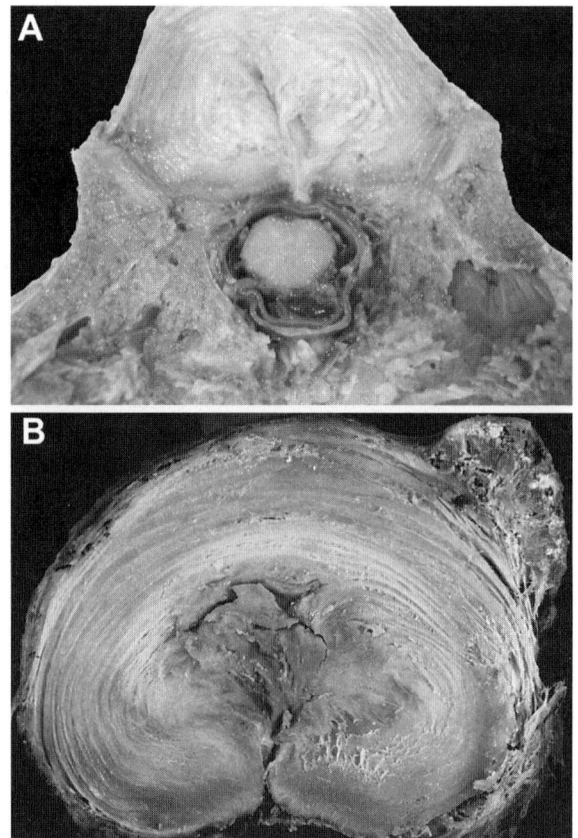

FIG. 43-2. Axial views of the thoracic (A) and lumbar (B) cadaveric discs, depicting a midline radial fissure through the posterior anulus with degeneration and dissication in the nuclear region of the disc. Apart from a localized osteophyte to the right side of the vertebral body in B, and the radial anular defect, the anulus appears relatively normal.

ing disc herniations, are present in asymptomatic study cohorts (26–30). These observations make more difficult the interpretation of results from diagnostic procedures used to investigate individual patients presenting with low back pain. According to Beauvais et al. (31), CT imaging did not predict the outcome of lumbar IVD herniation. Although a larger herniation or free fragment was found in the group with the best clinical outcome, the differences at 3 months were not significant in conferring any prognostic value. In contrast, a review by Henmi et al. (32), which followed the conservative management of 10 individuals with HNP, found signal intensity ratios derived from T2-weighted MRI sequences in the acute and late follow-up phases that predicted the pattern of HNP reduction. These authors reported that those HNPs with lower signals did not show size reductions.

MODEL OF DISC RESORPTION

Although the mechanisms of disc resorption remain unclear, it has been proposed that, following HNP and its immediate postinflammatory sequence, intrinsic hydrophilic capacity is impaired which leads to progressive

desiccation. End stages of the inflammatory cascade are phagocytosis and eventual resorption (33). Larger isolated disc fragments may regress more readily given their tendency to migrate and regress due to the inflammatory mediated response (34,35). Fibroblast growth factor, inducing neovascularization, appears to be one potent source for this functional change in morphology of the fragment (36). In a study by Bozzao et al. (37), reductions of more than 70% were recorded for large and medium herniations, averaged across an 11-month follow-up period. Similar observations have been noted by Ito (7). In an interesting study by Boos et al. (38), 22 symptomatic and asymptomatic disc herniations, matched according to age, gender, disc level, and the extent of disc herniation, were compared using MRI (T1 and T2 relaxation times). In the symptomatic disc herniations, significantly reduced T1 and T2 relaxation times were recorded compared with the matched asymptomatic herniations. In addition, the symptomatic disc herniations were associated with more advanced levels of disc degeneration. These results suggest that symptomatic and morphologically matched asymptomatic disc herniations differ with regard to the matrix composition of the whole disc.

An early consideration during the acute phase of HNP is the role of epidural steroid injection, either local to the site of the HNP, or nerve root sleeve injections (39). Epidural steroids introduced specifically into the epidural space adjacent to the HNP can aid the inhibition of inflammatory mediators, moderate pain, and facilitate the resorption process (40). Although there has been considerable debate over the years, recent reviews provide support for spinal epidurals and nerve root sleeve blocs, respectively, as adjuncts to the conservative management of disc herniation and radiculopathies (40,41).

DISC HERNIATION AND SURGERY

The lifetime prevalence for lumbar radicular syndrome has been estimated at approximately 5% (42). However, there are marked regional and international differences in rates for surgery and conservative management of this problem that reflect a wide range of issues (2). Candidates for surgery following lumbar disc herniation account for a relatively small proportion of all spinal cases. Classic indications include: cauda equina syndrome, functional weakness of the lower extremity, and severe pain (2). In selecting surgical cases, many factors have been found to be predictive of outcome including unequivocal radicular symptoms and associated sensory changes, motor weakness, and straight-leg raising (SLR) test reduced to less than 30°, with positive tension signs from contralateral SLR, all of which must be confirmed by concordant positive imaging studies (43). An increasingly important consideration of presurgical screening is the determination of psychosocial factors that can moderate the outcome (44).

While the study by Weber (16) provided evidence that discectomy produced better clinical outcomes at 1 year, delaying surgery in cases where indications were uncertain to monitor the natural recovery did not produce long-

term harm. The reviews by Hoffman et al. (45) and Stevens et al. (46) reiterate the importance of careful patient selection and confirm clinical empiricism that the principal benefit of surgery for HNP is the rapid relief of sciatica in those individuals who have failed to improve under conservative care. Consideration of the state of the involved disc as a whole may be important given the observations by Boos et al. that symptomatic HNP cases tended to be associated with more advanced disc degeneration (38). It is valuable to determine, during the physical examination, whether peripheral (radicular) symptoms can change to a more central location following repeated movements (47). If symptoms can be changed with mechanical maneuvers, such a finding should encourage a "wait and watch" approach.

The astute clinician is able to identify salient indications for surgery based principally upon symptomology, while recognizing that patient preference and psychosocial indicators also play a role in determining outcomes (48,49).

PRINCIPLES OF CONSERVATIVE MANAGEMENT

As a consequence of the burden of back pain on health care systems, a diverse range of nonoperative management options exist. At present, not all interventions have an established scientific basis, however this deficiency is progressively changing through the impetus of systematic reviews of published literature and randomized controlled studies into specific therapies (50). The Cochrane Back Review Group maintains a comprehensive resource of contemporary systematic reviews of many of these therapeutic strategies (51), which is updated and expanded according to the cyclic review process (46, 52–57) (Table 43-1). In addition, other published nonsystematic reviews are available from this resource (58).

The goals associated with many conservative interventions are: reduction of disability, symptomatic management of pain and gradual restoration of premorbid levels

TABLE 43-1. *Selected Cochrane reviews and protocols related to spine surgery and rehabilitation (51,58)*

Author (yr)	Title of review
Hagen KB et al., 1999	Bed rest for acute low back pain and sciatica
Gibson JNA et al., 2000	Surgery for lumbar disc prolapse
Ostelo RWJG et al., 2000	Rehabilitation after lumbar disc surgery
van Tulder MV et al., 2000	Traction for low back pain with or without radiating symptoms
Hilde G et al., 2001	Advice to stay active as a single treatment for low back pain and sciatica
Karjalainen K et al., 2001	Multidisciplinary biopsychosocial rehabilitation for subacute low back pain among working age adults
Rozenberg et al., 1999[a]	Efficacy of epidural steroids in low back pain and sciatica; a critical appraisal by a French Task Force of randomized trials
Faas et al., 1996[a]	Exercises: Which ones are worth trying, for which patients, and when?

[a]Nonsystematic reviews.
From Cochrane Back Review Group. Available at: http://www.cochrane.iwh.on.ca/review.htm. Accessed October 30, 2003, with permission.

of spinal motion, cardiovascular fitness, muscle strength, motor coordination, and function. Conservative therapeutic options for the management of disc herniation are many and mirror, in part, the strategies that are employed for mechanical back pain, namely (a) limited bed rest, physical therapy including exercise prescription, manual therapy, and forms of electric stimulation for pain management; (b) local and systemic analgesic and antiinflammatory medications; and (c) holistic groupings of rehabilitation strategies which include cognitive behavioral approaches (53).

The need to guide patients to an informed decision, based upon careful monitoring of the severity of the clinical presentation and their tolerance of symptoms over the first 2 months, is crucial to successful conservative outcome (Table 43-2). Understanding the physiologic sequelae of the natural history (7), and imparting this information objectively and positively to the patient is essential to optimize outcomes. The issue of psychological support to this patient group is particularly important (50,53,56,59). This process has been likened to that of a coach motivating a patient throughout the rehabilitation program (60). In addition to describing the expected natural history of recovery as it relates specifically to the individual, there is the need to provide accurate information regarding the various progressions that the rehabilitation program will involve (60). Such programs need to be modified according to the extent and location of the HNP. If the chosen approach is one of a conservative rehabilitation strategy, the patient can be encouraged to progressively avoid prolonged bed rest and to increase activity levels within pain limits. The role of pain and antiinflammatory medications should be explained, along with promoting an expectation that recovery will occur, and that surgery may not be required. Careful selection of a combination of interventions such as manual therapy, including mobilization, manipulation and traction of spinal segments in the involved area; active exercises for range of motion and trunk stabilization; in addition to education concerning back care and short-term rest during exacerbations will be necessary, along with ongoing reassurance. According to some investigations, specific supervised retraining of trunk stabilizing muscles appears superior to general exercise programs in restoring spinal function and preventing recurrence of symptoms (61,62). However, general exercise in the form of supervised gym cir-

cuits may combine elements of many of these interventions and contribute positively in terms of social interactions with others who are well.

As disc herniation is a relative contraindication to manipulation, such forms of manual treatment are not usually recommended, particularly at the affected intervertebral level or in the presence of protective muscle spasm (63). However, in carefully selected individuals screened for contraindications to manipulation, symptomatic relief can be achieved and sustained over the medium term from such therapy (64). For example, manual traction or specific mobilization may be effective in relieving symptoms by decreasing mechanical stress on sensitized structures and encouraging local physiologic responses to assist in reduction of edema and inflammatory reaction (65). Some forms of lateral flexion mobilization of the lumbar spine, popularized by McKenzie (66), may be helpful in correcting a scoliotic list, producing improvement which may be short-lived but beneficial. Of interest are the reports that find certain types of spinal manipulation can achieve marked symptomatic relief in patients with HNP (64,67,68). Even short-term reduction in symptoms may reassure patients that their pain is able to be managed and, importantly, increase their expectation of a favorable prognosis. Symptom control will also expedite return to functional activity.

Although focusing on back pain of mechanical origin, *The Back Book* (69) conveys essential conservative back care information (48,70), which can benefit individuals with disc herniation, particularly if additional cautions are emphasized during the acute period according to the severity of symptoms. The principles of such advice for patients regarding conservative management of herniated disc are summarized in Table 43-3.

The effect of HNP on the spinal musculature is an important consideration of rehabilitation following injury. In parallel with pain arising from HNP marked muscle atrophy can occur, particularly in multifidus and adjoining paraspinal muscles. This atrophy can be unilateral, associated with a specific segmental level (71), and persist well beyond the time of injury and symptom resolution (72,73) (Fig. 43-2). Although this observation was confirmed by Kader et al. (74) in a retrospective analysis of 78 patients with mixed spinal symptoms, the associations between muscle atrophy, radicular symptoms, root compression, HNP, and degenerated discs were not

TABLE 43-2. *Assessment criteria for conservative versus surgical management for herniated lumbar disc, according to SINS*

Severity:	Self-reported severity of symptoms, using a visual analog scale; confirmed by responses during examination of active and passive spinal motion, and nerve tension testing.
Irritiability:	The ease with which symptoms are aggravated and their duration, which determines physical capacity and treatment options. Key indicators: intractable pain, limited range of pain-free motion and functional activity, poor quality sleep.
Nature:	Characteristics of symptoms in relation to local and referred pain, and symptomatic response to compression or traction, or positioning which may caution against activity.
Stage	Is the presentation improving, stable, or progressively worsening?

TABLE 43-3. *Principles of patient advice regarding conservative management of disc herniation*

Be aware of the "red flags" and report them if they arise. These include: bladder and bowel problems, progressive increase in pain, loss of sensation, progressive peripheral muscle weakness.

Take it easy initially. When pain is acute, rest is necessary but avoid prolonged bed rest.

Believe that you will get better, but be aware that it may take several months.

Pain management is important: epidural and nerve root sleeve injections may help.

Maintain general spinal movements, avoiding positions or directions that increase symptoms. This will assist recovery and not worsen the problem.

Traction or gentle passive treatment may help during exacerbations but may offer only short-term relief. Active movement and general exercise are important for the long term.

Keep mobile without aggravating pain levels. Initial light activity can be gradually extended to include exercises to restore spinal muscle strength and endurance, and cardiovascular fitness. Hydrotherapy may be helpful in the early stages of recovery.

Minimize prolonged static weight-bearing postures.

Avoid unnecessary lifting.

Surgery may not produce better outcomes than conservative care in the longer term. Unless "red flags" are evident, watchful waiting may be better than early surgery.

After 2 months of conservative management, surgery is much less likely to be required.

Adapted from Buchbinder R, Jolley D, Wyatt M. Population based intervention to change back pain beliefs and disability: three part evaluation. BMJ 2001;322:1516–1520; Nachemson A. Back pain: delimiting the problem in the next millennium. Int J Law Psychiatry 1999;22:473–490; and Weinstein SM, Herring SA. Lumbar epidural sterioid injections. Spine J 2003;3:37S–44S, with permission.

strong. The morphologic effects of spinal muscle damage and atrophy following surgery and arising from other forms of back pain have been examined in a series of investigations (75–77). Similarly, profound effects of deconditioning on paraspinal muscles have been docu-

mented after disc injury (78). Minimization of muscle atrophy must be balanced with the need for adequate initial bed rest. Following the acute phase, a graduated active exercise program, which may include hydrotherapy, should be encouraged and reinforced with education. Restoration of muscle strength and endurance through specific back exercises appears to be achieved initially through neuromuscular adaptations rather than overt changes in muscle morphology (77), which have a longer time course for recovery. Abdominal stabilizing exercises have been demonstrated to play a key role in recruitment of muscles that sustain lumbar mechanical function (61,79,80). Aerobic exercise is a recommended component of the rehabilitation in most cases as an aide to restoration of trunk, spinal, and lower extremity musculature (60).

Effective management of pain is a very important consideration during the acute phase (Fig. 43-3), given its profound inhibitory effect upon function and muscle morphology (81,82). The model of structural pathology imposing pain inhibition on joint movement, and contributing to local muscle atrophy, subsequently creating a vicious cycle of ongoing mechanical pain and dysfunction is a well-recognized sequence for many musculoskeletal systems (83) (Fig. 43-4). Some gentle forms of passive movement during the acute stage may also be helpful but must be guided by the symptomatic response of the individual with consideration of the key elements of the severity of the clinical presentation, presented in Table 43-2. Graduated mobilization and some forms of manipulation for pain-induced limitation of spinal movement may be indicated in the postacute stage of rehabilitation (64,65).

The natural history of HNP is presented in the following clinical case which highlights the process of symptom reduction and functional improvement and concomitant changes in MR images. The rehabilitation approach in this case included initial rest and analgesia followed by a graduated exercise program, including hydrotherapy, which was moderated according to symptom changes.

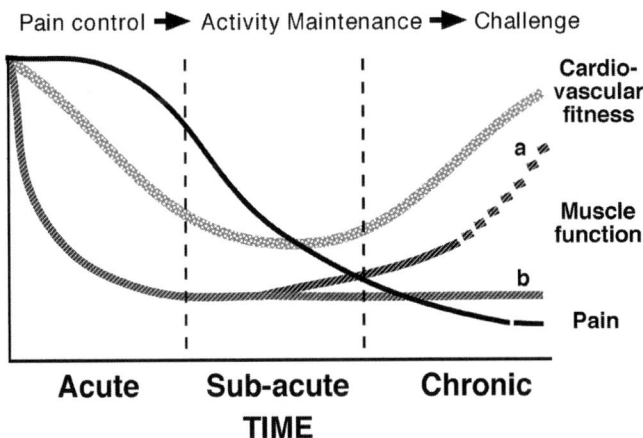

FIG. 43-3. Schematic representation of the interrelationship between pain, muscle function, and cardiovascular fitness following disc herniation. Initial chemical pain and related inhibition can result in early and profound spinal muscle disuse (atrophy), which may contribute to decreased stability of the involved segment(s). General deconditioning resulting from reduced functional activity must be addressed if the rehabilitation program is to be successful. An early focus on pain management is important in the acute phase followed by progressive cardiovascular maintenance exercise and muscle endurance/strength. Unless specific muscle stabilization and strengthening protocols are implemented *(A)* there is the potential for chronically inhibited and atrophic spinal musculature *(B)* following herniated nucleus pulposus. Exercise can also contribute to pain control through improved functional capacity and endurance.

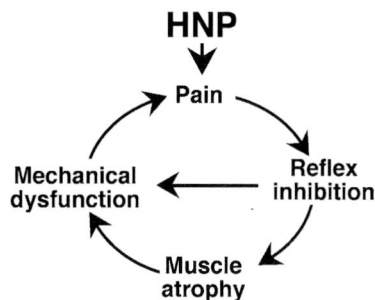

FIG. 43-4. A "vicious cycle" of pain-mediated inhibition on the musculoskeletal system is depicted. Initial chemical pain from the herniated nucleus pulposus produces profound suppression of motor function that may directly contribute to dramatic muscle atrophy and disturbed mechanics of the motor segment. This compromise can induce further mechanical disruption and pain that perpetuates the cycle. (Adapted from Young A, Stokes M, Iles JF. Effects of joint pathology on muscle. Clin Orthop 1987;18:21–27.)

Case Study

A 32-year-old woman presented with severe back pain, radiating to her left buttock, posterior thigh, and lateral leg as far as the left ankle. This followed an incident involving shifting of frozen food products from a low refrigerated container into storage with a time imperative to avoid deterioration of the frozen goods. This work required repetitive lifting in a sustained stooped posture. Over the next 24 hours, progressive worsening of back pain and leg symptoms forced her to stop work and seek urgent medical attention. At no time were bladder or bowel symptoms reported.

On physical examination, at 3 weeks following the onset of sciatic symptoms, sitting was not tolerated and the patient preferred to stand and move around during interview. She reported that sleep was frequently disturbed. Static standing posture showed a list to the right.

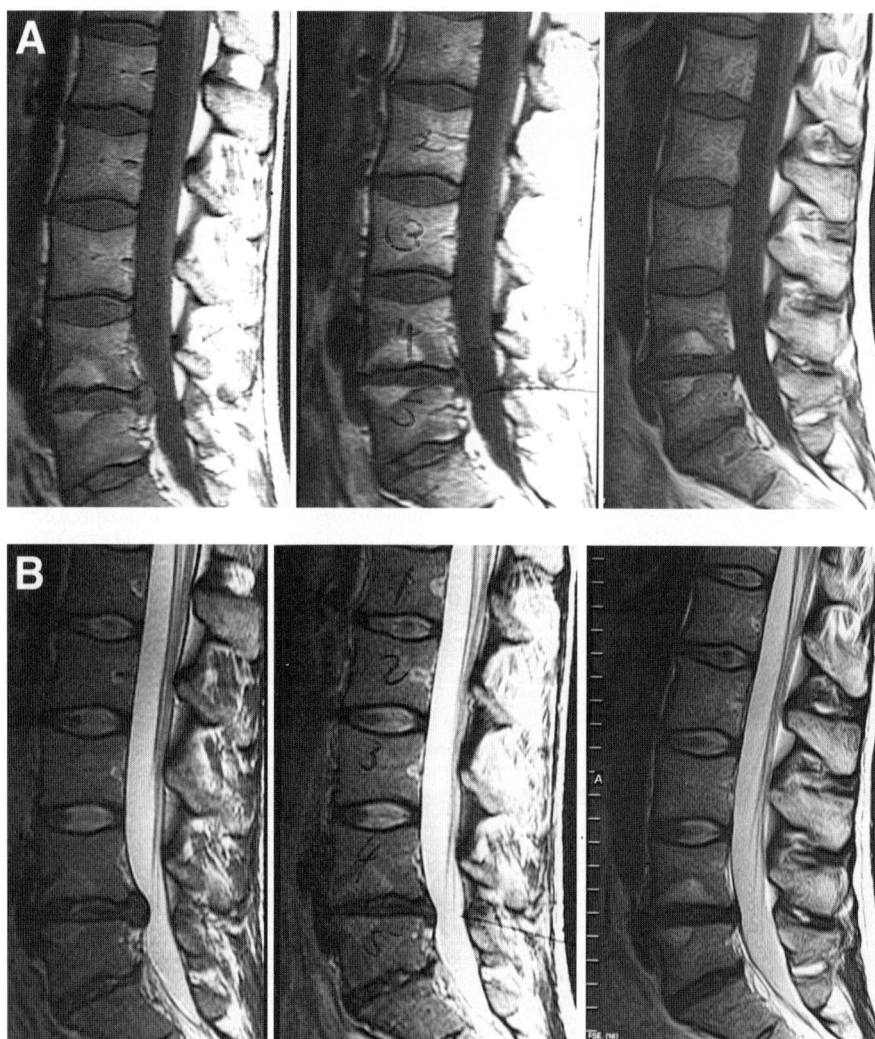

FIG. 43-5. Sagittal T1- **(A)** and T2- **(B)** weighted magnetic resonance images depicting the extent of the central disc protrusion at L4-5 in a 32-year- old woman. The initial imaging was performed 4 weeks after the incident **(left)**, with subsequent investigations at 6 months **(middle)** and 4 years **(right)**, respectively. Degenerative changes of the L5-S1 disc are also noted.

All spinal movements were markedly restricted. Forward flexion was arrested by pain with fingertips reaching above the knees. Extension was limited to less than 50%. Sensation was impaired over the L5 distribution into the region of the posterolateral leg. In supine lying, there was marked restriction of SLR (45°) bilaterally, with crossover sign from the right causing left buttock pain. Reflexes were diminished at the knees and could not be elicited at either ankle. Lower limb perfusion was normal.

Plain films demonstrated long-standing degenerative changes at L4-5 with some anterior osteophytes and loss of disc height. A large posterior central disc protrusion at L4-5 was demonstrated on initial CT. The bony canal dimensions were good and adjacent disc levels were satisfactory. At 4 weeks post-onset, lumbar MRI sequences confirmed the extent of the central disc herniation with migration of disc material inferior to the L5 superior end plate, causing compression of the ventral aspect of the thecal sac (Figs. 43-5, 43-6). At this time the patient had epidural steroid injection under radiologic guidance at the left L4-5 level which resulted in marked improvement in local and referred pain.

On review at 8 weeks post-onset, SLR was still reduced to 45° on the left and 60° on the right. Standing posture was normal and only a mild limp was noticeable.

Although surgery was discussed with the patient she refused this option preferring to continue with conservative physical therapy, including hydrotherapy and antiinflammatory medications as required. Due to persisting radicular symptoms and sleep disturbance, a second L4-5 epidural was given at 9 weeks achieving further good effect. At this time forward flexion was still limited by pain to fingertips reaching the knees. While spinal extension was reduced to approximately 75% of the expected range for her age, SLR had increased to 60° on the left.

A repeat MRI examination at 6 months demonstrated more than 70% reduction in the size of the central disc prolapse (Figs. 43-5, 43-6). On review at 12 months following the injury near normal lumbar extension was achieved and on forward flexion, fingertips reached to mid-shins. SLR was now approximately 75° bilaterally with negative nerve root tension signs. Subtle reduction in sensation persisted over the lateral aspect of the left leg.

Repeated MRI at 4.5 years demonstrated further reduction in the extent of the L4-5 disc prolapse since the 6-month assessment (Figs. 43-5, 43-6). Mild reduced sensation persisted along the L5 distribution. Spinal mobility was slightly limited although movements were pain-free. Symptoms had reduced to a significant extent, apart from

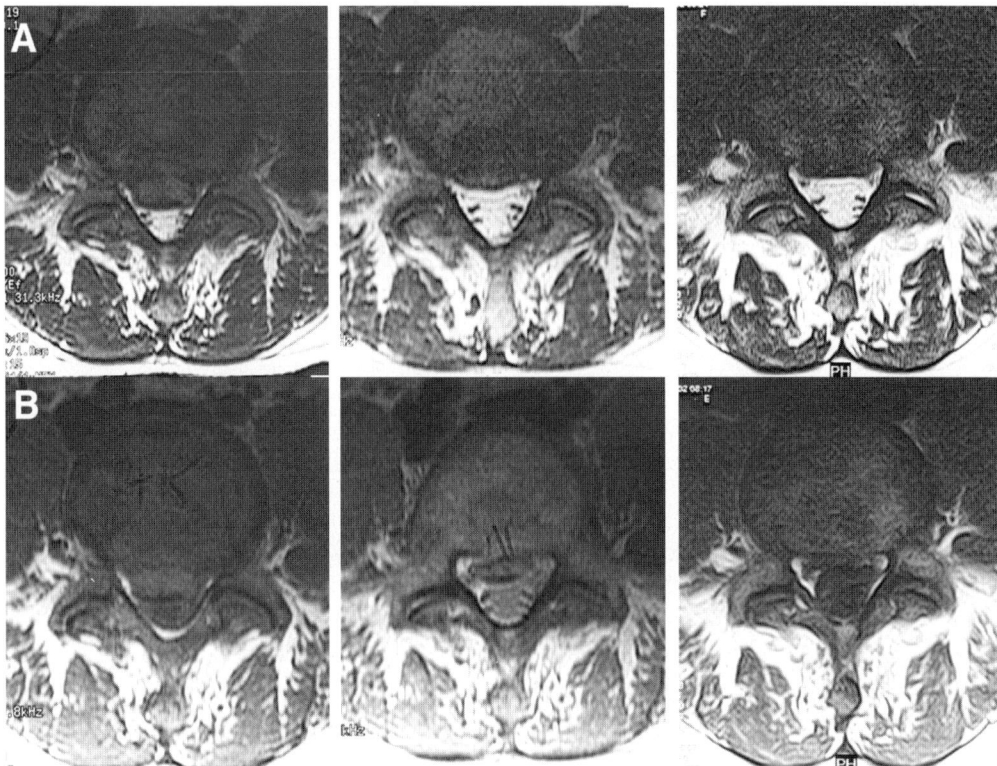

FIG. 43-6. Axial T1- **(A)** and T2- **(B)** weighted magnetic resonance (MR) images depicting the extent of the large paracentral disc protrusion at L4-5 resulting in marked displacement of the thecal sac. Comparison with the initial MR images clearly shows the substantial reduction in size of the disc extrusion, particularly in the anteroposterior dimension. Note the serial changes in muscle cross-sectional area with marked increase in the relative fatty infiltration and coincident bilateral muscle atrophy.

occasional activity related low back pain, in parallel with restoration of normal activity levels.

It is interesting to note that profound muscle atrophy persists almost 5 years after this acute disc herniation at L4-5 (Figs. 43-5, 43-6). This may in part result from modification of the patient's occupation and functional activities to accommodate the requirement for more conservative spinal loading during the postinjury period.

SUMMARY

Epidemiologic and clinical studies show the potential for the majority of IVD prolapses to regress naturally over time with conservative management alone. In carefully selected patients with sciatica due to lumbar HNP that fail to resolve with conservative care, there is good evidence that surgical discectomy achieves effective clinical relief of symptoms; although the scientific evidence on the optimal timing for surgery is limited. Even less clear is the balance of risks associated with delayed intervention, of relative complication rates over the intermediate years following disc injury, and of the longer term clinical outcomes due to the natural history of nonoperated disc herniation.

The immediate challenge is to improve the planning and execution of controlled trials of nonoperative management, with particular attention to areas such as blinded assessment, randomization, follow-up period, and the use of discriminating clinical outcome measures. Perhaps the single major need is to support longer-term reviews into the lifetime natural history of disc disease, including HNP, which can then be referenced to specific diagnostic groups. In this regard, the work of Boos et al. (38) in differentiating the characteristics of symptomatic HNP appears helpful.

Nonoperative management of disc herniation can result in successful resolution of symptoms in a large proportion of individuals although the time course to initial recovery may be variable and longer than that achieved with early surgery. While the late results appear similar, the operated cohort may be more disposed to subsequent mechanical back pain (43). The initial evaluation for serious pathology and monitoring for the onset of significant complications, such as neurologic defects, progressive cauda equina syndrome, or refractory pain, are critical in the optimal management of disc herniation. The recommendation for a conservative strategy should persist because a large number of operations performed currently are unnecessary when the late outcomes and morbidity following surgical intervention are considered (43,50).

In the absence of clear indications for surgery, conservative management, at least for the first 2 months, is recommended to determine the initial progression of the problem.

In this regard, careful education of each patient is mandatory as is the patient's involvement in the decision-making process (84–86). Further, clinical education models employing decision leaders can positively influence surgical intervention patterns (87).Throughout the often prolonged rehabilitation following HNP, biopsychosocial issues need to be considered. Acknowledgment that perseverance is necessary is important when counseling patients to consider a conservative rather than an operative strategy.

ACKNOWLEDGMENTS

We gratefully acknowledge the input of Dr. Swithin Song, MD, head of the MRI Unit, Department of Radiology and Mr. Peter Woodland, FRACS, spinal surgeon, Sir George Bedbrook Spinal Unit and the Department of Orthopaedics at Royal Perth Hospital.

REFERENCES

1. Luschka H. Die Halbgelenke des menschlichen Körpers. Berlin: Reimer, 1858.
2. Frymoyer JW, Radiculopathies: lumbar disc herniation: patient selection, predictors of success and failure, and non-surgical treatment options. In: Frymoyer J, ed. The adult spine. Philadelphia: Raven-Lippincott, 1997:1937–1946.
3. Lindblom K, Hultquist G. Absorption of protruded disc tissue. JBJS 1950;32A:557–560.
4. Hakelius A. Prognosis in sciatica. A clinical follow-up of surgical and non-surgical treatment. Acta Orthop Scand Suppl 1970;129:1–76.
5. Guinto FC, Jr., Hashim H, Stumer M. CT demonstration of disk regression after conservative therapy. Am J Neuroradiol 1984;5:632–633.
6. Teplick JG, Haskin ME. Spontaneous regression of herniated nucleus pulposus. Am J Roentgenol 1985;145:371–375.
7. Ito T, Takano Y, Yuasa N. Types of lumbar herniated disc and clinical course. Spine 2001;26:648–651.
8. Dullerud R, Nakstad PH. CT changes after conservative treatment for lumbar disk herniation. Acta Radiol 1994;35:415–419.
9. Matsubara Y, Kato F, Mimatsu K, et al. Serial changes on MRI in lumbar disc herniations treated conservatively. Neuroradiology 1995;37: 378–383.
10. Slavin KV, Raja A, Thornton J, et al. Spontaneous regression of a large lumbar disc herniation: report of an illustrative case. Surg Neurol 2001;56:333–336; discussion 337.
11. Coevoet V, Benoudiba F, Lignieres C, et al. Spontaneous and complete regression in MRI of thoracic disk herniation. J Radiol 1997;78: 149–151.
12. Wood KB, Blair JM, Aepple DM, et al. The natural history of asymptomatic thoracic disc herniations. Spine 1997;22:252–530.
13. Morandi X, Crovetto N, Carsin-Nicol B, et al. Spontaneous disappearance of a thoracic disc hernia. Neurochirurgie 1999;45:155–159.
14. Kobayashi N, Asamoto S, Doi H, et al. Spontaneous regression of herniated cervical disc. Spine J 2003;3:171–173.
15. Mochida K, Komori H, Okawa A, et al. Regression of cervical disc herniation observed on magnetic resonance images. Spine 1998;23: 990–995; discussion 996–997.
16. Weber H. The natural history of disc herniation and the influence of intervention. Spine 1994;19:2234–2238; discussion 2233.
17. Atlas SJ, Keller RB, Chang Y, et al. Surgical and nonsurgical management of sciatica secondary to a lumbar disc herniation: five-year outcomes from the Maine Lumbar Spine Study. Spine 2001;26: 1179–1187.
18. Saal JA, Saal JS. Nonoperative treatment of herniated lumbar intervertebral disc with radiculopathy. An outcome study. Spine 1989;14: 431–437.
19. Maigne JY, Rime B, Royer P, et al. X-ray computed tomographic study

of the outcome of lumbar disk hernia after conservative medical treatment (34 cases). Rev Rhum Mal Osteoartic 1991;58:355–359.

20. Maigne JY, Rime B, Deligne B. Computed tomographic follow-up study of forty-eight cases of nonoperatively treated lumbar intervertebral disc herniation. Spine 1992;17:1071–1074.
21. Ellenberg MR, Ross ML, Honet JC, et al. Prospective evaluation of the course of disc herniations in patients with proven radiculopathy. Arch Phys Med Rehabil 1993;74:3–8.
22. Fraser RD, Sandhu A, Gogan WJ. Magnetic resonance imaging findings 10 years after treatment for lumbar disc herniation. Spine 1995; 20:710–714.
23. Andrae R. Über Knorpelknötchen am hinteren Ende der Wirbelbandscheiben im Bereich des Spinalkanals. Beitrage zur Pathologischen Anatomie und zur Allemeinen Pathologischen 1929;82:464–474.
24. Schmorl G. Zür pathologische Anatomie der Wirbelsäule. Klinik Wochenscrift 1929;8:1243–1249.
25. Hitselberger WF, Witten RM. Abnormal myelograms in asymptomatic patients. J Neurosurg 1968;28:204–206.
26. Wiesel SW, Tsourmas N, Feffer HL, et al. A study of computer-assisted tomography. I. The incidence of positive CAT scans in an asymptomatic group of patients. Spine 1984;9:549–551.
27. Boden SD, Davis DO, Dina TS, et al. Abnormal magnetic-resonance scans of the lumbar spine in asymptomatic subjects. A prospective investigation. J Bone Joint Surg Am 1990;72:403–408.
28. Greenberg JO, Schnell RG. Magnetic resonance imaging of the lumbar spine in asymptomatic adults. J Neuroimaging 1991;1:2–7.
29. Jensen MC, Brant-Zawadzki MN, Obuchowski N, et al. Magnetic resonance imaging of the lumbar spine in people without back pain. N Engl J Med 1994;331:69–73.
30. Boos N, Rieder R, Schade V, et al. 1995 Volvo Award in clinical sciences. The diagnostic accuracy of magnetic resonance imaging, work perception, and psychosocial factors in identifying symptomatic disc herniations. Spine 1995;20:2613–2625.
31. Beauvais C, Wybier M, Chazerain P, et al. Prognostic value of early computed tomography in radiculopathy due to lumbar intervertebral disc herniation. A prospective study. Joint Bone Spine 2003;70: 134–139.
32. Henmi T, Sairyo K, Nakano S, et al. Natural history of extruded lumbar intervertebral disc herniation. J Med Invest 2002;49:40–43.
33. Arai Y, Yasuma T, Shitoto K, et al. Immunohistological study of intervertebral disc herniation of lumbar spine. J Orthop Sci 2000;5: 229–231.
34. Matsui Y, Maeda M, Nakagami W, et al. The involvement of matrix metalloproteinases and inflammation in lumbar disc herniation. Spine 1998;23:863–868; discussion 868–869.
35. Minamide A, Hashizume H, Yoshida M, et al. Effects of basic fibroblast growth factor on spontaneous resorption of herniated intervertebral discs. An experimental study in the rabbit. Spine 1999;24: 940–945.
36. Haro H, Kato T, Komori H, et al. Vascular endothelial growth factor (VEGF)-induced angiogenesis in herniated disc resorption. J Orthop Res 2002;20:409–415.
37. Bozzao A, Gallucci M, Masciocchi C, et al. Lumbar disk herniation: MR imaging assessment of natural history in patients treated without surgery. Radiology 1992;185:135–141.
38. Boos N, Dreier D, Hilfiker E, et al. Tissue characterization of symptomatic and asymptomatic disc herniations by quantitative magnetic resonance imaging. J Orthop Res 1997;15:141–149.
39. Cowan NC, Bush K, Katz DE, et al. The natural history of sciatica: a prospective radiological study. Clin Radiol 1992;46:7–12.
40. Barnsley L. Steroid injections: effect on pain of spinal origin. Best Pract & Res Clin Anaesthesiol 2002;16:579–596.
41. Weinstein SM, Herring SA. Lumbar epidural steroid injections. Spine J 2003;3:37S–44S.
42. Group Standards Advisory Group. Epidemiology review: the epidemiology and cost of back pain. London: HMSO, 1994.
43. Postacchini F. Lumbar disc herniation: a new equilibrium is needed between nonoperative and operative treatment. Spine 2001;26:601.
44. Junge A, Frohlich M, Ahrens S, et al. Predictors of bad and good outcome of lumbar spine surgery. A prospective clinical study with 2 years' follow up. Spine 1996;21:1056–1064.
45. Hoffman RM, Wheeler KJ, Deyo RA. Surgery for herniated lumbar discs: a literature synthesis. J Gen Intern Med 1993;8:487–496.
46. Stevens CD, Dubois RW, Larequi-Lauber T, et al. Efficacy of lumbar

discectomy and percutaneous treatments for lumbar disc herniation. Soz Praventivmed 1997;42:367–379.
47. Wetzel FT, Donelson R. The role of repeated end-range/pain response assessment in the management of symptomatic lumbar discs. Spine J 2003;3:146–154.
48. Burton AK, Waddell G, Tillotson KM, et al. Information and advice to patients with back pain can have a positive effect. A randomized controlled trial of a novel educational booklet in primary care. Spine 1999;24:2484–2491.
49. Kendall NA. Psychosocial approaches to the prevention of chronic pain: the low back paradigm. Baillieres Best Pract Res Clin Rheumatol 1999;13:545–554.
50. Nachemson A. Back pain: delimiting the problem in the next millennium. Int J Law Psychiatry 1999;22:473–490.
51. Cochrane Back Review Group reviews. Available at: http://www.cochrane.iwh.on.ca/review.htm. Accessed November 3, 2003.
52. Gibson JN, Grant IC, Waddell G. Surgery for lumbar disc prolapse. Cochrane Database Syst Rev 2000: CD001350.
53. Guzman J, Esmail R, Karjalainen K, et al. Multidisciplinary bio-psycho-social rehabilitation for chronic low back pain. Cochrane Database Syst Rev 2002: CD000963.
54. Hagen KB, Hilde G, Jamtvedt G, et al. Bed rest for acute low back pain and sciatica. Cochrane Database Syst Rev 2000: CD001254.
55. Hilde G, Hagen KB, Jamtvedt G, et al. Advice to stay active as a single treatment for low back pain and sciatica. Cochrane Database Syst Rev 2002: CD003632.
56. Ostelo RW, de Vet HC, Waddell G, et al. Rehabilitation after lumbar disc surgery. Cochrane Database Syst Rev 2002: CD003007.
57. van Tulder MW, Malmivaara A, Esmail R, et al. Exercise therapy for low back pain. Cochrane Database Syst Rev 2000: CD000335.
58. Cochrane Back Review Group. Non-Cochrane systematic reviews for chronic low back pain. Available at: http://www.cochrane.iwh.on.ca/systematic.htm. Accessed November 3, 2003.
59. Burton AK, Waddell G. Clinical guidelines in the management of low back pain. Baillieres Clin Rheumatol 1998;12:17–35.
60. Saal JA, Saal JS. Physical rehabilitation of low back pain. In: Frymoyer J, ed. The adult spine. Philadelphia: Raven-Lippincott: 1997:1805–1819.
61. O'Sullivan PB, Twomey LT, Allison GT. Evaluation of specific stabilizing exercise in the treatment of chronic low back pain with radiologic diagnosis of spondylolysis or spondylolisthesis. Spine 1997; 22:2959–2967.
62. Danneels LA, Vanderstraeten GG, Cambier DC, et al. Effects of three different training modalities on the cross sectional area of the lumbar multifidus muscle in patients with chronic low back pain. Br J Sports Med 2001;35:186–191.
63. Singer KP, Contraindications to spinal manipulation. In: Giles L, Singer KP, eds. Clinical anatomy and management of low back pain. Oxford: Butterworth-Heinemann, 1997:387–391.
64. Burton AK, Tillotson KM, Cleary J. Single-blind randomised controlled trial of chemonucleolysis and manipulation in the treatment of symptomatic lumbar disc herniation. Eur Spine J 2000;9:202–207.
65. Edmondston S, Elvey R. Physiotherapy management of low back pain. In: Giles L, Singer KP, eds. Clinical anatomy and management of low back pain. Oxford: Butterworth-Heinemann, 1997:387–391.
66. McKenzie RA. The lumbar spine—mechanical diagnosis and therapy. Waikanae, New Zealand: Spinal Publications, 1981.
67. Mathews JA, Yates DA. Reduction of lumbar disc prolapse by manipulation. BMJ 1969;3:696–697.
68. Cassidy JD, Thiel HW, Kirkaldy-Willis WH. Side posture manipulation for lumbar intervertebral disk herniation. J Manipulative Physiol Ther 1993;16:69–103.
69. Roland M, Waddell G, Moffat J, et al. The back book. London: Stationery Office, 1996.
70. Buchbinder R, Jolley D, Wyatt M. Population based intervention to change back pain beliefs and disability: three part evaluation. BMJ 2001;322:1516–1520.
71. Hides JA, Stokes MJ, Saide M, et al. Evidence of lumbar multifidus muscle wasting ipsilateral to symptoms in patients with acute/subacute low back pain. Spine 1994;19:165–172.
72. Cooper RG, St Clair Forbes W, Jayson MI. Radiographic demonstration of paraspinal muscle wasting in patients with chronic low back pain. Br J Rheumatol 1992;31:389–394.
73. Hides JA, Richardson CA, Jull GA. Multifidus muscle recovery is not

automatic after resolution of acute, first-episode low back pain. Spine 1996;21:2763–2769.

74. Kader DF, Wardlaw D, Smith FW. Correlation between the MRI changes in the lumbar multifidus muscles and leg pain. Clin Radiol 2000;55:145–149.

75. Lehto M, Hurme M, Alaranta H, et al. Connective tissue changes of the multifidus muscle in patients with lumbar disc herniation. An immuno-histologic study of collagen types I and III and fibronectin. Spine 1989; 14:302–309.

76. Danneels LA, Vanderstraeten GG, Cambier DC, et al. CT imaging of trunk muscles in chronic low back pain patients and healthy control subjects. Eur Spine J 2000;9:266–272.

77. Kaser L, Mannion AF, Rhyner A, et al. Active therapy for chronic low back pain: part 2. Effects on paraspinal muscle cross-sectional area, fiber type size, and distribution. Spine 2001;26:909–919.

78. Rantanen J, Hurme M, Falck B, et al. The lumbar multifidus muscle five years after surgery for a lumbar intervertebral disc herniation. Spine 1993;18:568–574.

79. O'Sullivan PB. Lumbar segmental 'instability': clinical presentation and specific stabilizing exercise management. Man Ther 2000;5:2–12.

80. Hodges PW. Changes in motor planning of feedforward postural responses of the trunk muscles in low back pain. Exp Brain Res 2001;114:261–266.

81. Cousins M, ed. Acute pain management: scientific evidence. Canberra: National Health & Medical Research Council of Australia, 1999.

82. Lipetz JS. Pathophysiology of inflammatory, degenerative, and compressive radiculopathies. Phys Med Rehabil Clin N Am 2002;13: 439–449.

83. Young A, Stokes M, Iles JF. Effects of joint pathology on muscle. Clin Orthop 1987;18:21–27.

84. Deyo RA. Nonsurgical care of low back pain. Neurosurg Clin N Am 1991;2:851–862.

85. Deyo RA. Tell it like it is: patients as partners in medical decision making. J Gen Intern Med 2000;15:752–754.

86. Phelan EA, Deyo RA, Cherkin DC, et al. Helping patients decide about back surgery: a randomized trial of an interactive video program. Spine 2001;26:206–211; discussion 212.

87. Goldberg HI, Deyo RA, Taylor VM, et al. Can evidence change the rate of back surgery? A randomized trial of community-based education. Eff Clin Pract 2001;4:95–104.

CHAPTER 44

Operative Treatment of Disc Herniation: Natural History and Indications for Surgery

Charles G. Greenough

In 1985, Frymoyer and Donaghy (1) reported the 50-year follow-up of a case of surgical treatment of lumbar disc herniation. This was a 25-year-old man with a 2-year history of left leg pain, commencing after a skiing accident. On examination the straight leg raise was 25 degrees and the ankle jerk was absent. A myelogram (Lipiodol) was negative, the cerebrospinal fluid protein was 108 mg with a pressure of 145 mm HG and there was a slow rise with jugular compression. Operation was undertaken with osteotomy of the spinous processes and left hemilaminectomies from L2-S1. The dural sac was opened and no abnormalities were seen. Beneath the sheath of the L5 root, a 1-cm nodule was found arising from disc L5-1, which was excised. The patient required transfusion. He was discharged in a brace 19 days following surgery. Fourteen years later he presented with recurrent leg pain that responded to conservative treatment. A further episode of leg pain occurred 19 years later; at 50 years he was symptom free. The excised specimen was originally reported as a chondroma, but the pathologist then remarked on the lack of cellular material and was able to make the correct diagnosis after comparison with sections of normal disc material.

"K.N. is of particular interest as he is the first patient in whom a ruptured intervertebral disc was recognized as such and as a cause of sciatica. Therefore, he is the man who started all the damn trouble" (2).

Excision of lumbar disc herniation is the most common spinal operation undertaken and, with precisely defined indications, one of the most successful.

Prolapsed intervertebral disc is rare in adolescents and most common in the third, fourth, and fifth decade. Usually occurring at L5-S1 or L4-5, the prolapse most often consists of nuclear material and is frequently unilateral within the central canal. Commonly the root exiting immediately below the affected level is involved, the direct pressure leading to root dysfunction (loss of sensation or motor power), and the inflammation leading to radicular pain. Urgent referral is indicated for bowel or bladder disturbance

ASYMPTOMATIC DISC PROLAPSE

The correlation of radiologic findings to clinical symptoms and examination findings is vital. The incidence of asymptomatic disc prolapse in the lumbar spine is significant and without careful clinical correlation, the surgeon may make the mistake of operating on purely archeological findings.

Boden et al. (3) noted the presence of asymptomatic lumbar disc prolapse on magnetic resonance imaging (MRI) in 20% of subjects under 60 and in 36% of subjects over 60. These findings were confirmed by Jensen et al. (4), who noted protrusion in 27% of 98 volunteers and one patient with extruded disc. Boos et al. (5) examined a cohort of subjects matched by age, sex, and work intensity to a group of patients who presented with symptomatic disc prolapse. These asymptomatic matched subjects were found to have abnormalities in 76% of the 46 volunteers, 27 volunteers had a protrusion and three an extrusion. Therefore, it is clear that radiologic disc prolapse is common, particularly in subjects whose work environment is associated with an increased incidence of prolapsed intervertebral disc.

Follow-up of patients with asymptomatic disc prolapse has been undertaken. Boos et al. (6) followed 41 of their original 46 matched volunteers for a period of 5 years. At follow-up the subjects underwent MRI scanning and completed a questionnaire. There was almost no change in the radiologic classification of the disc prolapse (Table 44-1). Magnetic resonance images also were assessed for severity and at follow-up 31 out of 41 subjects were rated

TABLE 44-1. *Asymptomatic disc prolapse, progression over 5 years*

	Baseline	Follow-up
No prolapse	11	11
Protrusion	27	26
Extrusion	3	4
Neural compromise	29	29

Source: Adapted from Boos N, Semmer N, Elfering A, et al. Natural history of individuals with asymptomatic disc abnormalities in magnetic resonance imaging: predictors of low back pain-related medical consultation and work incapacity. Spine 2002;21:1484–1492, with permission.

TABLE 44-2. *Immunological assay*

Culture→ Serology ↓	Positive	Negative	Total
Positive	13	6	19
Negative	34	55	89
TOTAL	47	61	108

Source: Adapted from Stirling A, Worthington T, Mathur K, et al. Association between sciatica and skin commensals. Presented at the Annual Meeting of the Society of Back Pain Research, Manchester, UK, 2001, with permission.

the same and 10 rated radiologically worse. However, multiple regression analysis of these subjects indicated that presence or absence of asymptomatic disc prolapse or its type and extent had no predictive value for duration of low back episodes during the follow-up period, for consultations with health care professionals for low back pain or time off work. These findings were corroborated by Borenstein (7), who performed a 7-year follow-up of 50 subjects with a symptomatic disc prolapse. During the follow-up period, 20 reported low back pain; in seven patients this was a duration of more than 7 weeks. However, no correlation was found with the MRI appearances.

Thus, it appears that asymptomatic disc prolapse is not only relatively common, but when present does not appear to progress significantly over time in the majority of subjects. Therefore, it is not clear why some disc prolapses are symptomatic and others are not. Recently an intriguing hypothesis has been suggested by a research group in Birmingham, England. Stirling et al. (8) made use of an enzyme-linked immunosorbent assay (ELISA) incorporated with lipid S antigen, an antigen that is present in the cell wall or membrane of gram-positive cocci. This assay has already been established in gram-positive bacterial endocarditis and other deep-seated staphylococcal infections. The assay was being investigated for suitability in diagnosing and monitoring spinal infection. However, an unexpectedly high incidence of positive results was found in a group of disc prolapse patients who had been used as controls. In a formal trial, 108 patients undergoing surgery for prolapsed intervertebral disc were studied. Forty-seven positive cultures were obtained from excised disc material taken under the strictest of aseptic precautions. Nineteen patients were found to have a positive immunologic assay (Table 44-2). There was a significant association between positive culture and positive assay ($p < 0.01$). The bacteriologic species cultured are given in Table 44-3. Although these findings need to be replicated in other centers, it remains possible that at least some cases of symptomatic disc prolapse are related to subclinical bacteriologic infection.

Turning to the natural history of symptomatic disc prolapse some information is available. In 1992, Gogan and

Fraser (9) perform a randomized control of Chymopapain against placebo (saline injection) for prolapsed intervertebral disc. Thirty subjects were injected with saline. Twenty-six of these subjects were reviewed at 10 years; approximately half subsequently underwent surgery (10). Of the remaining 12, six were symptom free at review, four were significantly improved, and two were not improved.

In his seminal paper, Weber (11) found that in patients with radiologically proved disc prolapse, 70% reported decreased pain and 60% returned to work within 4 weeks during initial conservative management. Further, on long-term (10-year) follow-up, they were able to show that patients with good long-term results with conservative therapy had demonstrated significant improvement within 3 months of onset. This study remains the only controlled trial of surgical intervention against conservative therapy. A group of 126 patients with proved disc prolapse and "uncertain indications" for surgery was defined. Of these 66 were allocated to conservative treatment and 60 were treated surgically. Of the randomized subjects at 1 year, those allocated to surgical treatment were significantly better. At 4 years, improvement was still noted but less marked and statistically nonsignificant. At 10 years, the results were identical. This trial may be criticized on a number of grounds, particularly because there was no blinding and a crossover of some 26% of the conservative group to surgery in the first year. However, it did provide evidence that surgery may improve the outcome in the short term. Subsequently it

TABLE 44-3. *Positive cultures (47 cases)*

Propionibacterium acnes	29 (62%)
Coagulase negative staphylococcus	8 (17%)
Propionibacterium + CNS	6 (13%)
Mixed CNS	1 (2%)
Coryne Prop.	1 (2%)
Coryne sp./micrococcus	1 (2%)

CNS, central nervous system.
Source: Adapted from Stirling A, Worthington T, Mathur K, et al. Association between sciatica and skin commensals. Presented at the Annual Meeting of the Society of Back Pain Research, Manchester, UK, 2001, with permission.

was estimated by Malter et al. (10) that operative treatment for lumbar disc prolapse provided 5 months of healthy life as compared with conservative treatment.

Hakelius (12) retrospectively examined 583 patients with sciatica. He noted that surgically treated patients had a better result initially but this advantage over conservatively treated cases was not demonstrable at 6 months. However, at 7 years the conservatively treated group had more back pain, recurrences, and time lost from work.

Radiologic appearances also can change with time, but not consistently (13,14). Delauche-Cavallier et al. (13) performed repeat scans at 12 months and found that in 21 patients with disc prolapse, five had completely disappeared, five had undergone major reduction, four minor reduction, and no significant change was observed in seven. At 1 year, Matsubara found the size of the herniation decreased by more than 20% in 11 patients (34%), by 10% to 20% in eight (28%), and was unchanged in 12 (38%). Even after treatment, in some cases the radiologic appearance remains unchanged. Fraser et al. (15) rescanned 39 patients 10 years after therapy. Twelve had been treated by saline injection alone, 14 by chemonucleolysis alone, and 13 had subsequently required laminectomy for a failed intradiscal injection. The signal of the treated disc was absent in all cases in each group. Thirty-seven percent of patients were found to have a persistent herniated disc and the incidence was similar in all three treatment groups. The presence or absence of radiologic herniation at 10 years had no significant bearing on a successful outcome.

Not all patients who recover spontaneously go onto have permanent improvement. Following the first attack of sciatica, some 5% of subjects experience a recurrent attack. Following the second attack, the incidence of recurrence rises to 20% or 30%, and following the third or subsequent attack, recurrence occurs in 70% of patients (G. Findlay, personal communication).

DIFFERENTIAL DIAGNOSIS

Differential diagnosis in the spine includes conus and cauda equina lesions, infection at the vertebral body or disc, arachnoiditis, and intracanal neoplasia. Extraspinal differential diagnosis includes peripheral vascular disease, gynecologic conditions, orthopedic conditions (e.g., osteoarthritis of the hip or sacroiliac disease), neoplasia involving the lumbosacral plexus, mononeuropathy, conditions involving the sciatic nerve itself, and shingles.

INVESTIGATION

Magnetic resonance imaging is the tool of choice today. Computed tomography scanning may be used but lesions outside the area actually scanned cannot be visualized (e.g., cauda equina lesions). With exact concordance of CT findings with clinical findings, CT remains

a satisfactory method of investigation. It is important that scanning is undertaken from pedicle to pedicle rather than simply at disc space level to ensure sequestrated fragments are visualized. There is no place for myelography, radiculography, or discography in the diagnosis of prolapsed lumbar intervertebral disc.

CLINICAL INDICATIONS FOR SURGERY

Increasing Neurologic Deficit

If neurologic deficit is progressive, then intervention is indicated.

General indications for surgical intervention in herniated lumbar discs are well understood. Disc excision surgery is far most successful in relieving leg pain than back pain. It has been outlined in the preceding that the natural history in this condition is favorable; 70% report decreased pain and 60% have returned to work within 4 weeks of the onset of symptoms. This is not dependent on the size or location of the prolapse radiologically. Long-term success with conservative management is indicated by substantial improvement within 3 months. Except in the case of profound motor deficit, there is little indication for operative intervention within 6 weeks of the onset of symptoms. Further, little improvement may be expected in patients with neurologic deficit that is pain free, because neurologic recovery is unusual.

The criteria of Macnab or "the Rule of Five" (16) have withstood the test of time and still remain the gold standard for indications for disc excision surgery (Table 44-4).

Careful examination is required to confirm the presence of neurologic deficit and sciatic tension signs according to Macnab's criteria. Muscle spasm and spinal tilt do not add independent prognostic significance.

TECHNICAL INDICATIONS

Technical factors had been thought to influence the results of surgical procedure for prolapsed lumbar intervertebral disc, and thus had been relative indications for surgery. The size of the prolapse and presence of spinal

TABLE 44-4. *The "rule of five"*

2 Symptoms	1 Leg pain, greater than back pain
	2 Specific neurologic symptoms (paraesthesia)
2 Signs	3 Straight leg raising <50% of normal or positive crossover test or positive bowstring test
	4 Two of four neurologic signs (altered reflex, wasting, weakness, sensory loss)
1 Investigation	5 Positive concordant imaging

Source: Adapted from McCulloch J, Macnab I. Sciatica and chymopapain. Baltimore: Williams & Wilkins, 1983.

TABLE 44-5. *Results of surgical discectomy*

	Facet Joint Degeneration	No Facet Joint Degeneration
Excellent	3	23
Improved	5	15
Poor	5	3

$p < 0.01$.

Source: Adapted from Jensen TT, Overgaard S, Thomsen NO, et al. Postoperative computer tomography three months after lumbar disc surgery, a prospective single applicance study. Spine 1991;16:620–622, with permission.

TABLE 44-6. *Results of surgical management of discectomy*

	Compensation	Non-compensation
Excellent	3	31
Good	7	68
Fair	20	43
Poor	35	29

$p < 0.001$.

Source: Adapted from Tregonning GD, Transfeldt EE, McCulloch JA, et al. Chymopapain versus conventional surgery for lumbar disc herniation. 10-year results of treatment. J Bone Joint Surg (Br) 1991;73-B:481–486, with permission.

stenosis were felt to have an important influence; the larger the prolapse or the smaller canal, the worse the results (17,18). More recent studies in large patient groups, however, have failed to confirm these findings. Van Leeuwen et al. (19) could not find any predictive value in the size of the herniation or dimensions of the spinal canal in patients treated by chemonucleolysis. In a large study of 148 patients, Garreau (20) made a careful analysis of type and size of herniation and the shape and size of the spinal canal. The overall dimensions of the canal were examined together with the shape and size of the lateral recess. They were unable to demonstrate any relationship of canal size or hernia size with the results of chemonucleolysis. Thus, the radiologic size of the prolapse does not appear to constitute an indication for surgery.

Jensen et al. (21) reported no association of postoperative results with epidural fibrosis or appearance of residual or recurrent disc prolapse. However, they were able to demonstrate an association of overall result with facet joint degenerative disease (Table 44-5).

PATIENT-RELATED INDICATIONS

Patient-related factors also provide important modifiers to the indications for surgery, because they appear to have significant influence on the outcome of surgery. In a well-conducted study, Spengler et al. (22) examined the influence of neurologic signs, sciatica tension signs, personality factors, and imaging studies on the outcome of surgical discectomy. Careful evaluation of the history, examination, and investigation findings was performed and points were awarded in each category according to a strictly defined protocol. Personality factors were evaluated using the Minnesota Multiphasic Personality Inventory. Overall, the preoperative assessment scores were highly predictive of the surgical outcome. Forty-seven patients with good results had a mean preoperative score of 86, whereas four patients with fair results had a preoperative score of 73 and 10 patients with poor results scored only 62. However, more detailed analysis revealed different contributions of the four factors to the overall outcome. The best predictor of the operative findings was the imaging studies. Thirty-nine

percent of the variance was explained of which imaging studies contributed to 26%. Neurologic signs and sciatic tension signs were much less predictive at 8% and 5% respectively. However, the clinical result was overwhelmingly predicted by the personality factors. Total variance explained all four factors were 40%, of which personality factors contributed 26%. Imaging studies contributed 10%, but neurologic signs and sciatic tension signs contributed only 3% and 1%, respectively.

Another large study by Junge et al. (23) examined a large number of possible predictive factors. The factors that in his analysis were of prognostic significance, however, did not include specific examination findings or investigations. Eighty percent of good and poor results in this study were predicted by physical mobility, pain intensity, other pain locations, compensation, and socioeconomic group. They found no prognostic significance in age or sex, sciatic tension signs or imaging appearances.

In 1991 Tregonning et al. (24) found the presence of a compensation claim had a significant impact on the overall results (Table 44-6).

ADMISSION AND POST OPERATIVE CARE

The management of patients during the operative treatment has also been studied. A number of reports have examined the performance of micro-discectomy under day case conditions (25-28). One case series has also been reported examining fenestration and discectomy without a microscope undertaken as a day case (29). Recently a prospective randomized controlled trial has further examined the use of day case management in conventional fenestration and discectomy surgery (30). Patients were randomized to day case surgery or to overnight admission. All patients were admitted on the day of surgery. Significant advantages in mobility on the day of surgery, daytime hours spent in bed on the first post-operative day and walking distance at two weeks were demonstrated. Patient's opinion of the length of stay was good. No increase in complications was noted. Thus, there is evidence that conventional fenestration and discectomy surgery for prolapsed lumbar intervertebral disc may be safely and with benefit undertaken as a day case.

Postoperative management of patients undergoing surgical treatment for prolapsed intervertebral disc is also controversial. Fear of recurrence, re-injury, or instability has lead to the suggestion of several post operative protocols to restrict activity. However, a study by Carragee et al, (31) has indicated that these may not be necessary. In this study, patients were allowed to determine their own levels of activity post operatively and no postoperative restrictions were imposed. All were urged to return to full activity as soon as possible. The mean time from surgery to return to work was 1.7 weeks and 25 percent of patients returned to work the following day. 97 percent of those working at the time of surgery returned to full duty by eight weeks. At two years, no patient had changed employment because of back or leg pain. Recurrent disc prolapse occurred in six percent (three patients) of whom one required surgical intervention. Thus when freed from restrictions imposed by health care professionals, patients returned to activities and work much more rapidly and in apparent safety. Magnusson et al (32) have found no rational basis for lifting restrictions after lumbar spine surgery.

In a recent review of rehabilitation after lumbar disc surgery (33) the authors found strong evidence that intensive exercise programs commencing 4 to 6 weeks following surgery were more effective in improving functional status and produced a faster return to work as compared to mild exercise programs (34, 35). However, there was also strong evidence that this influence was not maintained into the long-term. No evidence was found of the effectiveness of supervised training as compared with home exercises. There was also no strong evidence of the effectiveness of multi-disciplinary rehabilitation over the usual care. Limited evidence indicated that exercises were more effective in improving low back function status than physical agents, joint manipulations, or no treatment.

CONCLUSIONS

Surgery for prolapsed intervertebral disc is principally indicated on clinical grounds. The radiologic appearances do not appear to add significant independent predictive value but patient-related factors are important.

REFERENCES

1. Frymoyer JW. Donaghy RM. The ruptured intervertebral disc. Follow-up report on the first case fifty years after recognition of the syndrome and its surgical significance. J Bone Joint Surg 1985;67:1113–1116.
2. Mixter J, 1946. quoted in Frymoyer JW, Donaghy RM. The ruptured intervertebral disc. Follow-up report on the first case fifty years after recognition of the syndrome and its surgical significance. J Bone Joint Surg 1985;67:1113–1116.
3. Boden SD, McCowin PR, Davis DO, et al. Abnormal magnetic-resonance scans of the cervical spine in asymptomatic subjects. A prospective investigation. J Bone Joint Surg 1990;72:1178–1184.
4. Jensen MC, Brant-Zawadzki MN, Obuchowski N, et al. Magnetic resonance imaging of the lumbar spine in people without back pain. N Engl J Med 1994;331:69–73.
5. Boos N, Rieder R, Schade V, et al. 1995 Volvo Award in clinical sciences. The diagnostic accuracy of magnetic resonance imaging, work perception, and psychosocial factors in identifying symptomatic disc herniations. Spine 1995;20:2613–2625.
6. Boos N, Semmer N, Elfering A, et al. Natural history of individuals with asymptomatic disc abnormalities in magnetic resonance imaging: predictors of low back pain-related medical consultation and work incapacity. Spine 2000;21:1484–1492.
7. Borenstein G, O'Mara JW, Boden SD, et al. A 7-year follow up study of the value of lumbar spine MR to predict the development of low back pain in asymptomatic individuals. Presented at the 25th Annual meeting of the International Society for the Study of the Lumbar Spine, Brussels, Belgium, June 9–13, 1998
8. Stirling A, Worthington T, Mathur K, et al. Association between Sciatica and skin commensals. Presented at the Annual meeting of the Society of Back Pain Research, Manchester, UK, 2001
9. Gogan WJ, Fraser RD. Chymopapain. A 10-year, double-blind study. Spine 1992;17:388–394.
10. Malter AD, Larson EB, Urban N, et al. Cost-effectiveness of lumbar discectomy for the treatment of herniated inter-vertebral disc. Spine 1996;21:1048–1055.
11. Weber H. Lumbar disc herniation. A controlled, prospective study with ten years of observation. Spine 1983;8:131–140.
12. Hakelius A. Prognosis in sciatica. A clinical follow-up of surgical and non-surgical treatment. Acta Orthop Scand 1970;129(Suppl):1–76.
13. Delauche-Cavallier MC, Budet C, Laredo JD, et al. Lumbar disc herniation. Computed tomography scan changes after conservative treatment of nerve root compression. Spine 1992;17:927–933.
14. Matsubara Y, Kato F, Mimatsu K, et al. Serial changes on MRI in lumbar disc herniations treated conservatively. Neuroradiology 1995;37:378–383.
15. Fraser RD, Sandhu A, Gogan WJ. Magnetic resonance imaging findings 10 years after treatment for lumbar disc herniation. Spine 1995;20:710–714.
16. McCulloch J, Macnab I. Sciatica and Chymopapain. Baltimore: Williams & Wilkins, 1983.
17. Mulawka S, Weslowski DP, Herkowitz HN. Chemonucleolysis, the relationship of the physical findings, discography and myelography to the clinical result. Spine 1996;4:391–396.
18. Postecchini F, Lami R, Massoberio N. Chemonucleolysis versus surgery in lumbar disc herniations: correlation of the results to pre-operative clinical pattern and size of the herniation. Spine 1987;12:87–96.
19. van Leeuwen RB, Hoogland PH, de Weerd AW. Chemonucleolysis. Predictive factors. Spine 1992;17:838–841.
20. Garreau C, Dessarts I, Lassale B, et al. Chemonucleolysis: correlation of results with the size of the herniation and the dimensions of the spinal canal. Eur Spine J 1995;4:77–83.
21. Jensen TT, Overgaard, Thomsen NOB, et al. Post operative computer tomography three months after lumbar disc surgery, a prospective single appliance study. Spine 1991;16:620–622.
22. Spengler DM, Ouellette EA, Battie M, et al. Elective discectomy for herniation of a lumbar disc. Additional experience with an objective method. J Bone Joint Surg (Am) 1990;72-A:230–237.
23. Junge A, Dvorak J, Ahrens S. Predictors of bad and good outcomes of lumbar disc surgery. A prospective clinical study with recommendations for screening to avoid bad outcomes. Spine 1995;20:460–468.
24. Tregonning GD, Transfeldt EE, McCulloch JA, et al. Chymopapain versus conventional surgery for lumbar disc herniation. 10-year results of treatment. J Bone Joint Surg (Br) 1991;73-B:481–486.
25. Bookwalter JW, Bush H, Nicely D. Ambulatory surgery is safe and effective in radicular disease. Spine 1994;19:526–530.
26. Griffiths HB. The 100th Day case Disc. West of England Medical Journal 1992;7:43–44.
27. Griffith HB. Results of day case surgery for lumbar disc prolapse. British Journal of Neurosurgery 1994;8:47–49.
28. Zahrawi F. Microlumbar discectomy. Is it safe as an out-patient procedure? Spine 1994;19:1070–1074.
29. Newman NM. Out patient conventional laminotomy and disc excision. Spine 1995;20:353–355.
30. Gonzalez-Castro A, Shetty A, Nagendar K, et al.. Day Case Conventional Discectomy—a Randomised Controlled Trial. European Spine Journal 2002;11:67–70.

31. Carragee EJ, Han MY, Yang B, et al. Activity restrictions after posterior lumbar discectomy. A prospective study of outcomes in 152 cases with no postoperative restrictions. Spine, 1999; 24:2346–51.

32. Magnusson ML, Pope MH, Wilder DG, et al. Is there a rational basis for post-surgical lifting restrictions? 1. Current understanding. Eur. Spine J 1999;8:170–178.

33. Ostelo RWJG, de Vet HCW, Waddell G, et al. Rehabilitation after lumbar disc surgery (Cochrane Review). In: The Cochrane Library, Issue 2, 2002. Oxford: Update Software.

34. Davis RA. A long-term outcome analysis of 984 surgically treated herniated lumbar discs. Journal of Neurosurgery 1994; 80:415–421.

35. Manniche C, Skall HF, Braendholt L, et al. Clinical trial of postoperative dynamic back exercises after first lumbar discectomy. Spine 1993; 18:92–97.

CHAPTER 45

Operative Treatment of Disc Herniation: Laminotomy

Charles G. Greenough

The first operation undertaken to remove a lumbar disc herniation involved osteotomy of the spinous processes and hemilaminectomies from L2 to S1. A transdural approach was employed (1). Significant refinements of surgical technique took place in the following 70 years. Open discectomy now requires only excision of or raising of a flap of ligamentum flavum and minimal resection of the adjacent borders of the laminae. In contrast to the 19-day hospitalization of the first surgery, patients now may be subjected to open discectomy on an outpatient basis (2).

TECHNIQUE

Open discectomy is undertaken under endotracheal general or spinal anesthesia. The patient is generally positioned prone, although a small number of surgeons prefer to perform the surgery in the lateral position. However, in the latter case, it can prove awkward if intraoperative extension or exploration on the opposite side is required. Relevant scans and other investigations must be available, and the surgeons should use them to confirm level and side of the prolapse. Careful assessment should be made for the presence of segmentation abnormality. Note should be taken of the relative position of the iliac crests and involved disc space. The direction and extent of the prolapse must be identified, together with any possible sequestrated fragments.

Controversy has existed over whether or not the use of the microscope improves outcome. Proponents of the microscope point to the improved illumination, provision of binocular vision, and magnification. Others express concerns about the difficulty of seeing pathology outside the field of view and the possible increased risk of infection. Three randomized controlled trials have failed to show any significant differences between the two techniques (3–5).

The positioning of the patient should allow some reduction of the normal lumbar lordosis to increase the interlaminar space and should also allow decompression of the abdomen to reduce epidural bleeding. A number of positioning techniques are available, each of which has advantages and disadvantages. The surgeon employs the one with which he or she is most familiar and is most convenient in the operative working environment. The knee/chest position provides excellent abdominal decompression but can place the thoraco-lumbar fascia under tension. In addition, considerable manual handling of the patient is required; with heavy patients this can present a risk both to the patient and staff. A modification of this technique is to use a Salford seat where the patient's weight is taken on the buttocks and the table is tilted foot down to produce a more sitting posture. Both of these positions require increased positioning time. A Wilson frame is convenient, but in obese patients it does not provide abdominal decompression as satisfactorily as other devices. A four-post support system with supports under the antero-superior iliac spines and shoulders provides good abdominal decompression but less reduction in lumbar lordosis. In addition, pressure complications have been reported with this frame. The Montreal mattress is convenient and easy to employ and elimination of lordosis can be achieved by breaking the operating table. However, in obese patients insufficient room may be available for the abdomen to hang freely to produce good decompression. Shorter patients on a thick mattress can develop pressure-related complications across the upper anterior thigh.

Once the patient is properly positioned, the skin is prepared and consideration given to identification of level. Some surgeons rely on identification of the sacrum at the time of surgery when undertaking L5-S1 or L4-5 surgery. This is not possible to do with confidence at L3-4 unless one makes a large excision and employs radiologic iden-

443

tification of level. X-rays may be taken with a percutaneous needle, leaving the needle *in situ* or injecting methylene blue to mark the tissues. Even this method is not foolproof; exploration of the wrong level can occur despite placing a needle in the right interspace and using it as a dissection guide.

It should be borne in mind that two of the most common errors in disc surgery are operating on the wrong side and operating at the wrong level. Experience has shown that when the wrong level is operated on it is usually above the intended level. The surgeon must remain alert to this possibility throughout the approach; if the intraoperative findings do not agree with the preoperative imaging, then a careful review of the level is mandatory. This may include further radiologic confirmation or exposure to the sacrum to count and confirm the level.

If no radiologic confirmation is being used, then the position for the incision may be estimated relative to the position of the iliac crests. The incision is carried down to the thoraco-lumbar fascia once hemostasis is obtained. A self-retaining retractor is placed in the fat layer.

Using cutting diathermy, an incision made vertically in the thoraco-lumbar fascia, immediately adjacent to the supraspinous ligament and the side of the spinous process. To allow tension-free retraction of the musculature, the length of this excision should be adequate, usually 4 or 5 cm. This fascial incision may be longer than the skin incision. Muscle then is carefully dissected from the spinous processes and interspinous ligament using cutting diathermy under direct vision. Dissection is carried out on the superior and inferior laminae, taking care to divide the muscular attachments as close to the bone as possible. Stripping of the muscle using a Cobb or flat periosteal elevator results in avulsion of tendonous attachments from the muscle because the instrument cannot conform to the complex shape of the laminae. Avulsion of these tendonous slips may cause bleeding, which may result in postoperative stiffness and discomfort.

If radiographic confirmation has not been done, the level is then confirmed by identification of the sacrum. The sacrum produces a different sound under percussion than L5, and usually presents a continuous bony surface. The inferior margin of the L5 lamina often is sharp, whereas those laminae above are blunt. Identification may be made of the lowest mobile segment by use of a large Cob or other instrument. None of these indicators is pathognomic; confirmatory radiographs should be obtained if the operating surgeon has any doubt. Having identified the correct level, the ligamentum flavum and adjacent laminae are cleared of all soft tissue with a large pituitary rongeur or curette.

The attachment of the ligamentum flavum to the adjacent laminae is significantly different at each end of the lamina. Caudally it is attached to the superior edge of the lamina; cranially it is attached to the superior edge and the deep surface of the lamina. Therefore, access to the canal can be obtained by careful use of a small Cobb or similar instrument to detach the fibers of the ligamentum flavum from the superior border of the caudal lamina. A smooth instrument (e.g., a McDonald dissector) can be introduced immediately beneath the lamina to ensure that no adhesions are present. The ligamentum flavum then can be excised with a Kerrison rongeur, taking care to ensure that no adhesions are present as removal proceeds. Some surgeons prefer to raise the ligamentum flavum as a medially based flap.

The most important landmark is then the medial border of the caudal pedicle. The superior border of the lamina and, if necessary, part of the medial portion of the base of the superior facet may be carefully excised with a Kerrison rongeur until the pedicle can be positively identified. To preserve stability, it is important not to allow bony dissection to stray lateral to the medial border of the pedicle at any point. The nerve root is identifiable adjacent to the medial border of the pedicle. Care should be taken to ensure that there is no conjoined root, because the superior portion of this often exits in contact with the superior border of the pedicle. The nerve root then can be traced proximally and carefully mobilized medially off the disc prolapse. It is safer to identify the root at the point where it approaches the pedicle because, with a large prolapse, the root can be thinned and stretched to such an extent that the edge can become difficult to identify at the level of the disc.

Once the root is safely mobilized medially, the disc space may be opened and all loose disc material removed. Careful examination is then made anterior to the root and for any sequestrated fragments identified on the scan. Curettage of the end plates is not necessary.

It must always be borne in mind that the great vessel is immediately in front of the anterior annulus. Particular care should be taken that a rongeur is not introduced deeper than the anterior annulus. On occasion a preexisting defect may be present in the anterior annulus; this represents a significant hazard.

At the end of the procedure the surgeon should examine the excised material and compare with this with the amount and location of the disc prolapse visible on the preoperative scan as a final assessment of completeness of disc removal. An assessment also should be made of the dimensions of the lateral recess. It may be necessary to perform an undercutting facetectomy to decompress the lateral recess. This facetectomy should not be carried lateral to the medial border of the pedicle. Before closure, careful review of the operative field is necessary to ensure that the nerve root is freely mobile and free from compression. A probe is passed down the intervertebral canal and superiorly and inferiorly in the spinal canal. Gentle elevation of the root is performed to allow examination anterior to the root itself. Careful and gentle palpation through the dura is undertaken to detect any subligamentous residual fragment or the rare intradural fragment.

Hemostasis of epidural bleeding is obtained with bipolar diathermy. Recently, interest has been expressed in the use of materials to reduce the fibrosis following disc surgery. However, although there is good evidence that such substances do reduce postoperative fibrosis, the evidence that this results in any clinical improvement is conflicting. BenDebba et al. (6) studied 298 patients who underwent surgery for lumbar disc herniation in a randomized, controlled, double-blind multicenter clinical trial using the scar-inhibiting substance ADCON-L. Those patients receiving ADCON-L at surgery developed significantly less scar ($p = 0.01$) and experienced less activity-related pain than the control group ($p = 0.05$). Logistic regression analysis demonstrated a significant association ($p = 0.02$, odds ratio = .7) showing that the odds of extensive scar decreased by 30% for every 31% decrease in activity-related pain score. Similar results were noted by Geisler (7), but no such effects were found by Richter (8). Hieb (9) noted an increased risk of cerebrospinal fluid (CSF) leakage with ADCON-L.

The thoraco-lumbar fascia is repaired and the superficial fascia within the fat layer is sutured. The skin wound is closed and the wound may be infiltrated with local anesthetic.

Postoperatively, patients are mobilized on the day of surgery and can be discharged the same day (2). Carragee (10) has demonstrated that when encouraged to return early to normal activities, patients return to work very early. Twenty-five percent of his cases returned to work the day following surgery, and the average time to return to work was 1.7 weeks. No increase in complications or recurrent disc herniation was observed. Magnusson et al. (11) have found no rational basis for lifting restrictions after lumbar spine surgery.

In a recent Cochrane review (12) intensive exercise programs commencing 4 and 6 weeks postoperatively also were found to be more effective for improved functional status and more rapid return to work than mild exercise programs.

RESULTS OF SURGERY AND FUNCTIONAL OUTCOME

The results of modern minimally invasive open discectomy are the gold standard against which other treatments are measured. Sciatica from disc herniation is more amenable to discectomy than is low back pain and results are maintained over 24 months. Weber (13) performed the only randomized study of discectomy against conservative care. At 1 year, surgically treated patients were statistically significantly better than patients randomized to conservative treatment, but at 4 years the difference was not statistically significant.

The results of surgery are influenced by many factors. Howe and Frymoyer (14) used 14 different outcome measures to assess the 10-year follow-up results of 244 patients who had undergone lumbar disc surgery. They found that the percentage of "satisfactory outcomes" ranged from 60% to 97%, depending on the outcome measure employed. In general, measures examining patient satisfaction provided a higher success rate than measures using more objective criteria, such as return to previous occupation. This range of satisfactory results is substantially greater than the difference among many techniques used in the surgical management of lumbar disc herniation. Therefore, it is essential that only direct comparisons using validated instruments be used to compare outcomes.

Loupasis et al. (15) analyzed 109 patients with surgically documented herniated lumbar disc over 12 years. The late results were satisfactory in 64% of patients, but 28% still complained of significant back or leg pain. Ninety-four percent of patients were very satisfied or satisfied with their results. The reoperation rate was 7.3%, about one third of which resulted from recurrent disc herniation. Sociodemographic factors predisposing to unsatisfactory outcome included female gender, low vocational education, and jobs requiring significant physical strength.

Atlas et al. (16) retrospectively examined 507 patients with sciatica, 275 surgically treated and 232 non–surgically treated. On average, surgically treated patients had more severe symptoms, signs, and imaging findings than non–surgically treated patients. At 1 year, surgically treated patients reported significantly greater improvement in symptoms, functional status, and disability. Seventy-one percent of surgically treated and 43% of non–surgically treated patients reported definite improvement ($p < .001$), an effect increased after adjustment for differences between treatment groups at entry (relative odds of definite improvement, 4.3; $p < .001$). However, little difference in the employment or workers' compensation status of patients treated surgically versus non–surgically was observed at 1 year (5% versus 7% unemployed, 46% versus 55% receiving workers' compensation, respectively).

Davis (17) was able to examine 98% of 984 patients operated on for a herniated lumbar disc with a mean follow-up period of 10.8 years. L4-5 and L5-S1 discs were involved with equal frequency (47%). The recurrence rate was 6%, one third of which developed during the first year after operation. The complication rate was 4%, with no intraoperative vascular or intestinal injuries. The outcome was good in 89% of patients, defined as a Prolo score of 8 in 10%, 9 in 19%, and 10 in 60% of patients. Patients who did sedentary work and homemakers had a statistically higher total and economic Prolo scores ($p < .01$) than those who did strenuous work. Risk factors for a poor result were pending legal or workers' compensation claims and psychological distress.

Two large reviews (18,19) have indicated consistent surgical success rates of 65% to 90% in clinical series, but have emphasized that careful selection of patients is of great importance.

TABLE 45-1. *Incidence of complications in open discectomy*

Complication	Incidence (percentage)
Cauda equina syndrome	0.2
Thrombophlebitis	1
Pulmonary embolism	0.4
Wound infection	2.2
Pyogenic spondylitis	0.07
Postoperative discitis	2
Dural tears	1.6
Nerve root injury	0.5

Modified from Spangfort.
Adapted from Spangfort EV. The lumbar disc herniation: a computer aided analysis of 2,504 operations. Acta Orthop Scand 1972;142(suppl):1, with permission.

COMPLICATIONS

In 1972, Spangfort (20) analyzed 2,504 operations and recorded the incidence of complications (Table 45-1).

Cauda equina syndrome may result from excessive compression of the dural contents during surgery. In the presence of a very large disc fragment, the exposure should be widened to allow the fragment to be removed without excessive traction on the dura. It should be remembered that diabetic patients are more vulnerable to this complication, and extra care is required for such patients.

Wound infection and postoperative discitis may be reduced by use of prophylactic antibiotics. Rohde (21) studied 1,642 patients in whom 1,712 discectomies were performed. In 508 patients, no prophylactic antibiotics were given; in 1,134 patients, a collagenous sponge containing gentamicin was placed in the cleared disc space. A postoperative spondylodiscitis developed in 19 of the 508 patients who were not treated with antibiotic prophylaxis (3.7%), whereas none of the 1,134 patients who received antibiotic prophylaxis developed infection ($p < .00001$). A single dose of intravenous antibiotics at induction of anesthesia may be as effective as other regimens.

Dural tear occurs in a small percentage of surgeries. Pseudomeningocele and fistula formation following dural tears should be repaired. It is essential that the exposure be widened to provide a good view of, and access to, the whole length of the tear. With loss of CSF the cauda equina is much more sensitive to pressure, and extreme caution should be exercised. Suction should be avoided inside the dural cavity and over the area of any prolapsed nerve roots. Suction through a patty is permissible. Dural tears should be repaired with continuous monofilament, nonabsorbable suture, taking care not to narrow the dural sac. Large defects can be repaired with dural replacement material and fibrin glue. Postoperative patients with dural repairs should be maintained on bed rest for 48 to 72 hours.

Penetration of the anterior annulus is a rare complication that can be associated with vascular or visceral damage (22). Constant monitoring of the depth of the rongeur is mandatory. If penetration of the anterior annulus is suspected, careful postoperative monitoring of blood pressure, pulse, and abdominal signs is indicated. Laparotomy should be undertaken without hesitation in the presence of adverse physical signs.

REFERENCES

1. Frymoyer JW, Donaghy RM. The ruptured intervertebral disc. Follow-up report on the first case fifty years after recognition of the syndrome and its surgical significance. J Bone Joint Surg 1985;67:1113–1116.
2. Gonzalez-Castro A, Shetty A, Nagendar K, et al. Day case conventional discectomy: a randomised controlled trial. Eur Spine J 2002;11:67–70.
3. Henrikson L, Schmidt V, Eskesen V, et al. A controlled study of microsurgical versus standard lumbar discectomy. Br J Neurosurg 1996;10:289–293.
4. Kahanovich N, Viola K, McCulloch JA. Limited surgical discectomy and microdiscectomy: a clinical comparison. Spine 1989;14:79–81.
5. Lagarrigue J, Chaynes P. A comparative study of disk surgery with or without microscopy. A prospective study of 80 cases. Neurochirurgie 1994;40(2):116–120.
6. BenDebba M, Augustus van Alphen H, Long DM. Association between peridural scar and activity-related pain after lumbar discectomy. Neurol Res 1999;21(suppl 1):S37–S42.
7. Geisler FH. Prevention of peridural fibrosis: current methodologies. Neurol Res 1999;21(suppl 1):S9–S22.
8. Richter HP, Kast E, Tomczak R, et al. Results of applying ADCON-L gel after lumbar discectomy: the German ADCON-L study. J Neurosurg 2001;95(2 suppl):179–189.
9. Hieb LD, Stevens DL. Spontaneous postoperative cerebrospinal fluid leaks following application of anti-adhesion barrier gel: case report and review of the literature. Spine 2001;26:748–751.
10. Carragee EJ, Han MY, Yang B, et al. Activity restrictions after posterior lumbar discectomy. A prospective study of outcomes in 152 cases with no postoperative restrictions. Spine 1999;24:2346–2351.
11. Magnusson ML, Pope MH, Wilder DG, et al. Is there a rational basis for post-surgical lifting restrictions? 1. Current understanding. Eur Spine J 1999;8:170–178.
12. Ostelo RWJG, de Vet HCW, Waddell G, et al. Rehabilitation after lumbar disc surgery (Cochrane review). Oxford, UK: The Cochrane Library, 2002.
13. Weber H. Lumbar disc herniation. A controlled, prospective study with ten years of observation. Spine 1983;8:131–140.
14. Howe J, Frymoyer JW. The effects of questionnaire design on the determination of end results in lumbar spine surgery. Spine 1985;10:804–805.
15. Loupasis GA, Stamos K, Katonis PG, et al. Seven- to 20-year outcome of lumbar discectomy. Spine 1999;24:2313–2317.
16. Atlas SJ, Deyo RA, Keller RB, et al. The Main Lumbar Spine Study, Part II. One-year outcomes of surgical and no surgical management of sciatica. Spine 1996;21:1777–1786.
17. Davis RA. A long-term outcome analysis of 984 surgically treated herniated lumbar discs. J Neurosurg 1994;80:415–421.
18. Hoffman RM, Wheeler KJ, Deyo RA. Surgery for herniated lumbar discs: a literature synthesis. J Gen Int Med 1993;8:487–496.
19. Stevens CD, Dubois RW, Larequi-Lauber T, et al. Efficacy of lumbar discectomy and percutaneous treatments for lumbar disc herniation. Soz-Pravedtivmed 1997;42:367–379.
20. Spangfort EV. The Lumbar disc herniation: a computer aided analysis of 2,504 operations. Acta Orthop (Scand) 1972;142(suppl):1.
21. Rohde V, Meyer B, Schaller C, et al. Spondylodiscitis after lumbar discectomy. Incidence and a proposal for prophylaxis. Spine 1998;23:615–620.
22. Goodkin R, Laska LL. Vascular and visceral injuries associated with lumbar disc surgery: medicolegal implications. Surg Neurol 1998;49:358–370.

CHAPTER 46

Chymopapain and Chemonucleolysis

Jeremy Fairbank

Chemonucleolysis is one of the best investigated interventions for the treatment of spinal disorders. There is good evidence of efficacy, and yet its use has declined sharply in North America in recent years. It is still used in Europe. Recently, manufacture was discontinued although it is likely to resume shortly.

Chemonucleolysis dates back to the early 1960s when Lyman Smith first injected a purified extract of the papaya fruit into the intervertebral disc to treat intervertebral disc prolapse (1,2). Chymopapain was first extracted in 1941. In 1959 Hirsch was the first to propose the use of a proteolytic enzyme to dissolve the intervertebral disc. Chemonucleolysis has been the subject of a series of randomized controlled trials. Its use has been fashionable in various countries at various times. It reputation was damaged because of complications that generally turned out to be either due to poor technique of needle placement or to unrecognized comorbidity. Intradural injection of the enzyme with serious neurologic sequelae has occurred, but experienced radiologic technique should make this complication extremely unlikely. There was also anxiety in the United States because of anaphylaxis. This is unusual in Europe, perhaps because meat tenderizer (based on the same enzyme) is not widely used (3,4). A lower dosage was also used in Europe. In the United States some surgeons have been reluctant to use chemonucleolysis because of reimbursement issues.

The most serious complication of chemonucleolysis is transverse myelitis. This occurs in 1:18,000 to 1:25,000 cases (note that this is less than the risk of cauda equina damage in surgically treated cases. Litigation in California is four times more common following discectomy than following chemonucleolysis.

Figure 46-1 shows needle placement and pre-injection discography in a 23- year-old woman with a 1-year history of back and leg pain. The symptoms and signs in this patient were consistent with a disc prolapse at L5-S1. She was frightened of surgery and eventually chose chemonucleolysis. This gave her good relief of leg pain, but her back pain persisted. A 3-month postintervention magnetic resonance (MR) scan showed that the disc prolapse had largely dissolved. A 9-month scan showed complete resolution. The back pain was managed conservatively.

BIOCHEMISTRY

Chymopapain is a sulfhydryl protease found in papaya latex. It closely resembles papain in its ability to hydrolyze a wide variety of substrates but at slower rates. Chymopapain was so named because it was thought to have a higher ratio of milk clotting to proteolytic activity when compared to papain. The clotting capacities of the two enzymes are in fact equal. It is supplied as a partially purified, lyophilized powder. Its activity is measured in units, where 1 unit hydrolyzes 1 μmol of benzoyl-L-arginine ethyl ester per minute at 25°C and pH 6.2 after activation in a solution containing 1.1 μm EDTA, 0.067 μm mercaptoethanol, and 5.5 μM cysteine-HCl for 30 minutes (5).

In humans there are measurable rises in keratin sulfate levels for 5 days following chymopapain injection (6).

INDICATIONS

The indications for chemonucleolysis parallel those for the surgical treatment of disc prolapse. The McCulloch criteria are widely used (7). McCulloch's series of 480 patients showed 70% success in those patients fulfilling his criteria. He suggested that candidates for chemonucleolysis should meet three or more of the following:

1. Unilateral leg pain in a typical sciatic root-type distribution, including discomfort below the knee. The leg pain has to be more severe than, or at least equal to, the severity of the associated back pain. If the roots of the femoral nerve are involved, pain in the front of the thigh is produced.

447

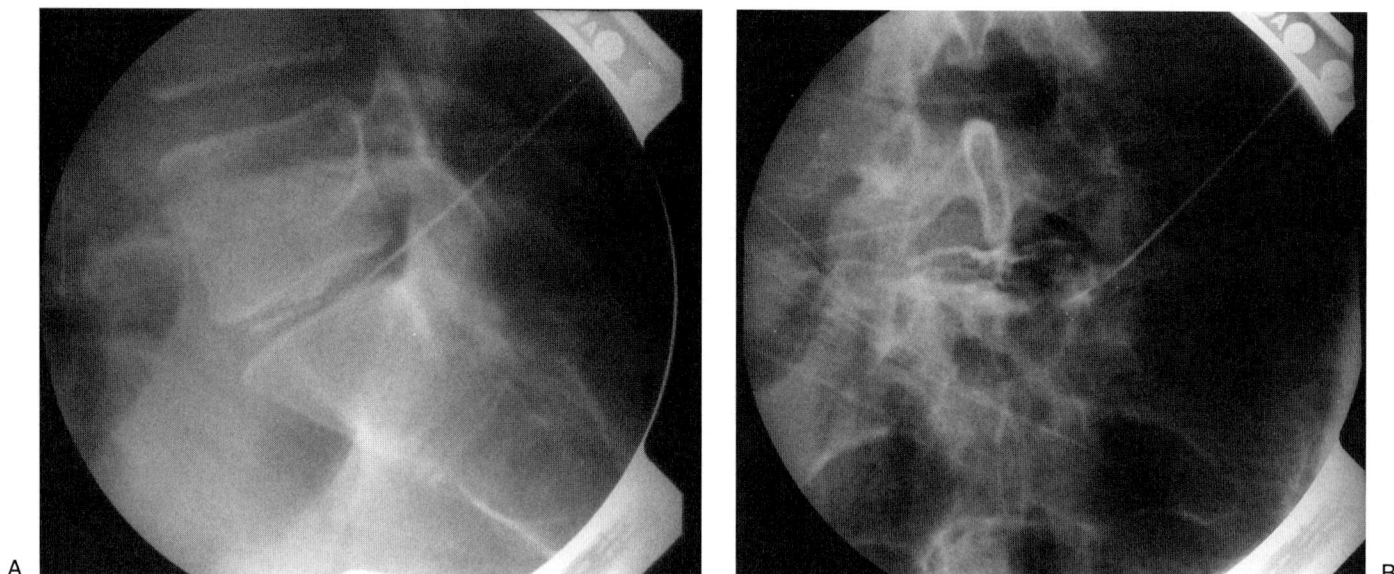

FIG. 46-1. A: A lateral radiograph of the L5-S1 disc to show needle placement and a pre-chymopapain injection of contrast (discogram) in a 23-year-old woman with a 1-year history of back and right leg pain. **B:** An anteroposterior radiograph of the same patient.

2. Specific neurologic symptoms incriminating a single nerve (e.g., numbness over the dorsum of the foot or over the great toe region or flopping of the foot on walking, signifying the involvement of the fifth lumbar nerve).

3. Limitation of straight-leg raising, due to pain in the leg, by at least 50% of normal; crossover pain from the unaffected leg to the symptomatic leg; or radiating thigh or back discomfort or calf and foot numbness on bowstring pressure over the medial or lateral popliteal nerve.

4. At least two of four possible neurologic changes: muscle wasting, muscle weakness, sensory alteration, and reflex changes.

5. A positive myelogram showing a disc herniation at the level suspected clinically.

These criteria continue to hold up today. Number 5 can be reasonably substituted by findings on an MR scan confirming disc herniation. Lateral recess compression and exit foraminal stenosis have become contraindications. Even though these were not detected on the myelogram of the 1970s, McCulloch's report emphasized the clinical importance of spinal stenosis and lateral recess stenosis as a cause of failure. Other contraindications were nonorganic back pain and disc degeneration. Chymopapain should only be injected at an additional level in the unusual situation where the same criteria apply.

CONTRAINDICATIONS

This intervention depends on the chymopapain reaching the proteoglycan element of the herniated nucleus pulposus. This cannot occur if there is a sequestrated fragment surrounded by fibrosis or a posterior ligament defect closed by fibrosis. If the offending herniation consists of annulus, its predominantly collagenous content will not be reduced by chymopapain. Spinal stenosis, whether central or lateral, may be exacerbated by chemonucleolysis rather than helped. This is because the disc space always narrows following chemonucleolysis and may produce neural compression from foraminal narrowing. It tends to regain some of its height after a year (8,9). The disc may be dose-dependent (10).

Allergy to chymopapain occurs. In the past chymopapain has been used as a meat tenderizer, and this may have led to undetected exposure to the antigen. Skin testing using subcutaneous chymopapain has been described by Grammer et al. (1988) (11). They used 10 mg per mL chymopapain on 540 chemonucleolysis candidates, of whom 6

TABLE 46-1. *Absolute or relative contraindications to chemonucleolysis*

Sequestrated discs
"Hard" discs
Lateral recess stenosis
Foramenal stenosis
Fibrosis due to prior surgery
Arachnoiditis
Neurologic disease
Polyneuritis of diabetic origin
Tumors
Cauda equina syndrome
Severe spondylolisthesis
Known chymopapain or papaya allergy

were positive. These individuals were excluded. None of the negative patients developed unequivocal anaphylaxis to chymopapain. If anaphylaxis occurs it should respond to normal treatment including the use of adrenalin.

The full list of contraindications is listed in Table 46-1.

COMPLICATIONS

In the United States, between 1982 and 1991, 121 adverse events were reported in approximately 135,000 patients having chemonucleolysis (12). This included seven cases of fatal anaphylaxis, 24 patients with infection, 32 patients with hemorrhage, 32 neurologic events, and 15 miscellaneous occurrences with an overall mortality rate of 0.019%. Of the 121 events, 105 reported to the U.S. Food and Drug Administration (FDA) occurred before the end of 1984. Among these, were six cases reported as acute transverse myelitis. It is likely that two of these were due to previously unrecognized multiple scleroses. There were one each of cauda equina syndrome, diabetic neuropathy, intrathecal injection, and postviral myelitis. Three of the six patients recovered.

Overall it was found that 47 instances of the complications (out of the 135,000 patients exposed) were probably related to chymopapain, 38 were probably not related, and in the remaining instances, there was insufficient information to decide.

In all of the categories investigated, there was a lesser incidence of complications with chemonucleolysis than that seen following laminectomy. This report was important and was an accurate record of complications because of the supervision of the FDA. This meant that the data for chemonucleolysis were far more accurate than the available data on laminectomy and discectomy. The early neurologic complications and anaphylaxis cases dealt the reputation of the procedure a serious blow. This was only overcome by showing that the neurologic problems were associated with poor technique and that anaphylaxis could be avoided by careful history taking and sensitivity testing. In fact, anaphylaxis has been reduced from an early 0.5% to 0.25%, and there have been no reported deaths or major neurologic complications between 1987 and 1996 (13).

In a series from Austria, Deutman reported one case in 2,000 of anaphylaxis and seven "sensitivity" reactions. All survived with appropriate treatment (14).

DISCITIS

When discitis was first described, it was thought to be a "chemical" discitis. Fraser demonstrated conclusively that this discitis was due to bacterial contamination (15,16). The use of a double-needle technique and prophylactic antibiotics has virtually eliminated this complication. It is not always easy to grow bacteria from disc space biopsies, so some surgeons still believe in chemical discitis when there is a negative culture (17). Poynton et al. reported discitis in 6 of 105 patients (5.7%) (18). Only two had a positive culture (*Escherichia coli*). None had long-term sequelae. Endplate changes can be detected on MR after chemonucleolysis (19).

TECHNIQUE

McCulloch advocated a posterolateral approach under local anesthesia (7). Anaphylaxis should be treated if it arises. Other authors have preferred a general anesthetic and watchful waiting for complications. In our institution, we use local anesthesia and sedation with an anesthesiologist in attendance. A transdural approach to the disc is strongly contraindicated. Some authors use discography to check needle position. Others believe that this has an adverse effect on the enzyme, although this has not been substantiated.

In the past back spasm was common after chemonucleolysis. The incidence of inflammatory changes can be reduced with smaller dosages (20). Dosage has been reduced from 3,000 to 4,000 U per disc down to 2,000 U per disc, or even to 500 U per disc by some (21). Pain and spasm may be reduced by injecting bupivacaine (8 to 10 mL, 0.25%) during needle withdrawal or by using intravenous corticosteroids just before the chymopapain injection. Antibiotic prophylaxis is essential (15).

The disc height decreases following injection by chymopapain by about one-fourth of the pre-injection height (22). It may recover some or all of the lost height over the course of a year.

Walking remains the best exercise post-chemonucleolysis. Swimming is encouraged. Most can return to a light or sedentary type of work within 2 to 4 weeks, and heavier work in 6 to 12 weeks.

LONG-TERM RESULTS: CLINICAL TRIALS/REVIEWS

The most compelling evidence that chemonucleolysis is a safe and effective treatment for herniation of the nucleus pulposus is found in well-designed and conducted prospective, randomized, double-blind studies in the United States and Australia. One of these double-blind studies has been carried out for 10 years without code break or loss of follow-up (23,24).

In Australia, Fraser (24) randomized 60 patients to chemonucleolysis or intradisc saline. In the chemonucleolysis group 80% regarded treatment as successful compared with 34% in the saline group. In the chemonucleolysis group, 20% were operated on compared with 47% in the saline group. These patients were also assessed by an independent observer who concluded that 77% of the chemonucleolysis group and 38% of the saline group had "moderate" improvement. One patient in each group developed discitis.

Success prevailed in 77% of patients receiving chemonucleolysis compared with only 38% for the placebo group ($p < .004$). Only 6 of the patients receiving chemonucleolysis had required laminectomy compared with 14 in the placebo group ($p < .028$) (24).

A European study (25) reported the success rate at 1 year for chemonucleolysis at 88% and for laminectomy at 76%. Chemonucleolysis continued to be superior to surgery after an additional year. In a 9- to 11-year prospective, randomized study comparing patients with these two methods, surgically treated patients who had done well initially deteriorated with time, whereas those who did well following chemonucleolysis maintained a successful outcome in the long term ($p < .041$).

The long-term results of surgery after failed chemonucleolysis are similar to those obtained after primary disc excision, indicating that failure to respond to chemonucleolysis does not compromise surgical discectomy, should it be necessary. In comparing long-term follow-up of patients who have undergone postchymopapain laminectomy versus patients who have undergone repeat laminectomy, better results were obtained in post-chemonucleolysis laminectomy which were statistically significant (26).

In trials versus placebo, there is a clear advantage for chymopapain (27,28). Trials against surgery (observational and randomized controlled trials) show slightly less efficacy of chemotherapy over surgery in the short term, fewer complications, and fewer long-term recurrences. In the longer term the results are comparable (23,29–33).

Nordby and Wright reviewed 45 studies (observational and randomized controlled trials) made between 1985 and 1993 (27). There were 7,335 patients. On average 76% reported a benefit with chymopapain compared with 88% in patients having open surgery.

Javid reported a prospective cohort design of 200 selected patients, 100 having chemonucleolysis and 100 undergoing surgery (26). Of chemonucleolysis patients 82% saw immediate benefit; 92% surgical patients saw immediate benefit. By 1 year 88% chemonucleolysis patients and 85% of surgical patients had benefited from the respective procedures. In this study chemonucleolysis was more cost-effective than surgery.

Observational studies are helpful for investigating efficacy and complications. Bouillet reviewed 43,662 cases from 316 centers. The overall complication rate was 3.7%, with 0.45% serious complications (34). Other observational data are reported by various authors (35–37).

JUVENILE DISC PROLAPSE

Bradbury et al. reported a long-term observational study of 60 adolescents (13 to 19 years) with disc pro-

lapses (38). All were treated with chemonucleolysis initially. There were 18 failures (30%) treated by open discectomy. Follow-up in all cases was more than 5 years (mean follow-up: chemonucleolysis 8.5 years, surgery 7.2 years). Pain relief was successful in all the chemonucleolysis patients and 16 of 18 of the surgical patients. Failures are due to large prolapse, sequestrated disc, lateral recess stenosis, facet arthropathy, and osteophytes (7,31,39,40).

The authors concluded that chymopapain injection was an effective first-line treatment for this group of patients. Surgery can then be confined to failures of this treatment with, in most cases, a good clinical outcome. Both this study and that of Javid (26) suggest that more chemonucleolysis patients are employed than those who have surgery. This may represent some selection bias.

DISC PROLAPSE IN OLDER ADULTS

Evidence shows that chymopapain is effective in older adults with disc prolapse (14,41). Associated pathology, such as lateral stenosis or root canal stenosis, is more likely than in younger patients. This can preclude a good outcome.

HEALTH ECONOMICS

It is likely that chemonucleolysis is less expensive than surgery, especially when done as outpatient procedure; it also may be more cost-effective (42). Short-term efficacy is slightly less than surgery, but in the long-term, it is as effective. It is likely that there are fewer recurrences with chemonucleolysis. The health economics of this issue have been investigated in various studies. None have been designed to investigate the current practice of low dose outpatient day care chemonucleolysis or have looked at the question of long-term recurrence. Malter et al. concluded that surgical treatment was cost-effective and that there was a cost-utility benefit (43). The cost-utility of surgery was just under $30,000 per quality adjusted life year gained compared with nonoperative treatment. This compares favorably with coronary artery bypass grafting. These authors had insufficient data to make a conclusion on chemonucleolysis, but they thought that it would have comparable findings.

This view is contested by a study by Muralikuttan et al. (29). This study involved 92 patients randomized to surgery or chemonucleolysis. Nine of 46 chemonucleolysis patients came to surgery (19%) and only 1 surgery of the 46 was a failure. By 1 year there was no detectable difference between the groups. In this study the chemonucleolysis patients were kept in the hospital for a mean of 7 days and the surgical patients for a mean of 8 days. There was a demonstrated cost-benefit and cost-utility benefit for surgery and no advantage for chemonucleolysis. The prolonged inpatient stays make this study of little relevance today. This matter is also reviewed by Javid (26) and Norton (44).

In a European study, Launois et al. (45). reported the success rate at 1 year for chemonucleolysis at 88% and for laminectomy at 76%. Chemonucleolysis continued to be superior to surgery after an additional year.

ALTERNATIVES

Alternatives to chymopapain have been sought. There is some evidence to support the use of collagenase: in a 5-year randomized study of 100 patients comparing collagenase to chymopapain, collagenase was effective in relieving pain in 52% patients compared with 72% of patients treated with chymopapain. Surgery rates were 24% and 18%, respectively (46). Other agents, such as chondroitinase ABC have not shown efficacy. Chemonucleolysis is superior to automated percutaneous discectomy (47,48).

CONCLUSIONS

I have used both chemonucleolysis and surgery in managing patients with disc prolapses when other interventions have failed. This requires waiting a minimum of 6 weeks from the onset of symptoms. Chemonucleolysis is safer than surgery, but its success rate is less. I prefer to use chemonucleolysis in my younger patients (under 25 years of age), but there is evidence of efficacy in older patients as well (41). Sequestrated discs will not respond to chemonucleolysis. Chemonucleolysis does generate significant back pain in the first 6 weeks (so does surgery, but patients find postsurgical back pain easier to accept, and it is expected that strong opiate analgesia will be used). This means there is not much to choose between the interventions in recovery time. This risk of recurrence is probably less with chemonucleolysis compared with surgery (which is about 10% in 10 years). The size of the disc prolapse is irrelevant to outcome.

The complete rejection of chymopapain in the United States is difficult to comprehend when the results of treatment are carefully reviewed. Low-dose day treatment for a symptomatic disc prolapse should be offered as a treatment option to all eligible patients with sciatica from a contained disc prolapse that has not responded to nonoperative treatment.

REFERENCES

1. Smith L, Garvin P, Gesler R, et al. Enzyme dissolution of the nucleus pulposus. Nature 1963;198:1311.
2. Smith L. Enzyme dissolution of the nucleus pulposus in humans. JAMA 1964;197:137–140.
3. Dando P, Sharp S, Buttle D, et al. Immunoglobulin-E antibodies to papaya proteinases and their relevance to chemonucleolysis. 1995;20:981–985.
4. Renoux M, Carter H, Menkes C. Incidence of chymopapain (CP) allergy in a series of 629 chemonucleolyses. XVIII Congress Rheumatol 1993:412(abst); Barcelona, Spain.
5. Gesler R. Pharmacologic properties of chymopapain. Clin Orthop 1969;67:47–51.
6. Muralikuttan K, Adair I, Roberts G. Serum keratin sulfate level following chemonucleolysis. Spine 1991;16:1078–1080.
7. McCulloch J. Chemonucleolysis. J Bone Joint Surg 1977;59-B:45–52.
8. Patt S, Brock M, Mayer H-M, et al. Nucleus pulposus regeneration after chemonucleolysis with chymopapain. Spine 1993;18:227–231.
9. Jerosch J, Castro W, Halm H, et al. Long-term changes after chemonucleolysis in the MRI. Z Orthop 1994;132:1–8.
10. Melrose J, Taylor T, Ghosh P, et al. Intervertebral disc reconstitution after chemonucleolysis with chymopapain is dependent on dosage. An experimental study in beagle dogs. Spine 1996;21:9–17.
11. Grammer L, Schafer M, Bernstein D, et al. Skin testing using sub-cutaneous chymopapain. Clin Orthop 1988;234:12–15.
12. Nordby E, Wright P, Schofield S. Safety of chemonucleolysis. Adverse affects reported in the United States 1982–1991. Clin Orthop 1993;293:122–134.
13. Nordby E, Fraser R, Javid M. Spine update. Chemonucleolysis. Spine 1996;21:1102–1105.
14. Deutman R. Chemonucleolysis. In: Gunsberg R, Szpalski M, eds. Lumbar disc herniation. Philadelphia: Lippincott, Williams & Wilkins, 2002:151–163.
15. Fraser R. Discitis following chemonucleolysis: an experimental study. Spine 1986;11:679–87.
16. Fraser R, Osti O, Vernon-Roberts B. Discitis following chemonucleolysis. Spine 1986;11:679–87.
17. Eggen P, Bruggen J, Wein B, et al. Aseptic spondylodiscitis: a complication of chemonucleolysis. Spine 1993;18:2358–2361.
18. Poynton A, O'Farrell D, Mulcahy D, et al. Chymopapain chemonucleolysis: a review of 105 cases. J R Coll Surg Edinburgh 1998;43:407–409.
19. Kato F, Ando T, Kawakami M, et al. The increased signal intensity at the vertebral body end-plates after chemonucleolysis demonstrated by magnetic resonance imaging. Spine 1993;18:2276–2281.
20. Kiester D, Williams J, Andersson G, et al. The dose-related effect of intradiscal chymopapain on rabbit intervertebral discs. Spine 1994;19:747–751.
21. Benoist M, Bonneville J-F, Lassalle B, et al. A randomized double-blind study to compare low dose with standard dose chymopapain in the treatment of herniated lumbar intervertebral discs. Spine 1993;18:28–34.
22. Konings J, Williams F, Deutman R. Computed tomography (CT) analysis of the effects of chemonucleolysis. Clin Orthop 1986;206:32–36.
23. Fraser R. Chymopapain for treatment of intervertebral disc herniation. Spine 1982;7:608–612.
24. Gogan W, Fraser R. Chymopapain. A 10 year double-blind study. Spine 1992;17:388–394.
25. Launois R, Henry B, Marty J, et al. Chemonucleolysis versus surgical discectomy for sciatica secondary to lumbar disc herniation. A cost and quality-of-life evaluation. Pharmacol Econ 1994;6:453–463.
26. Javid M. Chemonucleolysis versus laminectomy. A cohort comparison of effectiveness and charges. Spine 1995;20:2016–2022.
27. Nordby E, Wright P. Efficacy of chymopapain in chemonucleolysis. A review. Spine 1994;19:2578–2583.
28. Javid M, Nordby E, Ford L, et al. Safety and efficacy of chymopapain (Chymodiactin) in herniated nucleus pulposus with sciatica: results of a randomized, double blind study. JAMA 1983;249:2489–2494.
29. Muralikuttan K, Hamilton A, Kernohan W, et al. A prospective randomised trial of chemonucleolysis and conventional disc surgery in single level lumbar disc herniation. Spine 1992;17:381–387.
30. VanAlphen H, Braakman R, Bexemer D, et al. Chemonucleolysis versus discectomy: a randomised multi-centre trial. J Neurosurg 1989;70:869–875.
31. Weinstein J, Lehmann T, Henjna W, et al. Chemonucleolysis versus open discectomy: a 10-year follow-up study. Clin Orthop 1986;206:50–55.
32. Tregonning G, Transfeldt E, McCulloch I, et al. Chymopapain versus conventional surgery for lumbar disc herniation: 10-year results of treatment. J Bone Joint Surg[Br] 1991;73-B:1–6.
33. Weinstein J, Spratt K, Lehmann T, et al. Lumbar disc herniation: a comparison of the results of chemonucleolysis and open discectomy after 10 years. J Bone Joint Surg [Am] 1986;68-A:43–54.
34. Bouillet R. Treatment of sciatica: a comparative survey of complications of surgical treatment and nucleolysis with chymopapain. Clin Orthop 1990;251:145–152.

35. Javid M. Efficacy of chymopapain chemonucleolysis. A long-term review of 105 patients. J Neurosurg 1985;62:662–666.

36. Dabexies E, Beck C, Shoji H. Chymopapain in perspective. Clin Orthop 1986;206:10–14.

37. Nordby E. An 8–13 year follow-up evaluation of chemonucleolysis patients. Clin Orthop 1986;206:18–23.

38. Bradbury N, Wilson L, Mulholland R. Adolescent disc protrusions. A long-term follow-up of surgery compared to chymopapain. Spine 1996;31:372–377.

39. McManus F. Chemonucleolysis of prolapsed intervertebral discs. Ir Med J 1982;75:234–235.

40. Smith L. Failures with chemonucleolysis. Orthop Clin North Am 1975; 6:255–258.

41. Benoist M, Parent H, Nizard M, et al. Lumbar disc herniation in the elderly: long-term results of chymopapain chemonucleolysis. Eur Spine J 1993;2:149–152.

42. Ramirez L, Javid M. Cost-effectiveness of chemonucleolysis versus laminectomy in the treatment of herniated nucleus pulposus. Spine 1985;10:363–367.

43. Malter A, Larson E, Urban N, et al. Cost-effectiveness of lumbar discectomy for the treatment of herniated intervertebral disc. Spine 1996;1996:1048–1054.

44. Norton N. Chemonucleolysis versus surgical discectomy: comparison of costs and results in workers compensation claimant. Spine 1986;11: 440–443.

45. Launois R, Rebous-Marty J, Henrey B, et al. Cost-utility analysis after seven years of treatment of lumbar discal hernia. J Econ Med 1992; 10:307–325.

46. Wittenberg R, Oppel S, Rubenthaler F, et al. Five-year results from chemonucleolysis with chymopapain or collagenase: a prospective randomized study. Spine 2001;26:1835–1841.

47. Chatterjee S, Fox P, Findlay G. Report of a controlled clinical trial comparing automated percutaneous discectomy and micro-discectomy in the treatment of lumbar disc herniation. Spine 1995;20: 734–738.

48. Revel M, Payan C, Vallee C, et al. Automated percutaneous lumbar discectomy versus chemonucleolysis in the treatment of sciatica. A randomized multi-center trial. Spine 1993;18:1–7.

CHAPTER **47**

Microscopic Lumbar Discectomy

Robert Kraemer, Alexander Wild, Holger Haak, Joerg Herdmann, and Juergen Kraemer

MICRODISCECTOMY OR MACRODISCECTOMY

Open lumbar discectomy is still the most frequent and most important intervention in spine. The question is how to perform open disc surgery—with a small or wide exposure: microdiscectomy or macrodiscectomy? The choice of procedure depends on the expected pathology:

- Is it multisegmental?
- Is there a concomitant spinal stenosis?
- Is there a tumor or postoperative fibrosis?

A monosegmental disc prolapse is the most frequent cause for lumbar disc surgery. The surgical approach should be as small as possible and wide as necessary. Besides less trauma, less postoperative pain, and more rapid mobilization, a small approach reduces the amount of scaring which is important to prevent perineural fibrosis which is a cause of the failed back surgery syndrome. The interlaminar approach is similar for both microdiscectomy and macrodiscectomy, but the wound and scar formation might be more extensive in a wide approach. Using a microscope provides better illumination and better three-dimensional visualization, and is a better teaching tool. Several studies report good outcome with shorter hospital stay and earlier return to work rates compared to conventional disc surgery (1–3). On the other hand, there are reports of comparable outcome with both procedures, as well as concerns about specific complications (4,5).

There are potential pitfalls and errors with microdiscectomy. The limited exposure makes it easier to operate at the wrong level, to overlook free fragments, and to decompress inadequately. Technical difficulties and inexperience with the microscope can result in inadvertent injury to neural structures and vessels in the spinal canal. Because of these issues, many surgeons prefer a wide exposure for open disc surgery that permits better intra-operative orientation and visualization. It is a challenge for a spine surgeon to abandon a wide exposure for microdiscectomy without a loss of quality. Optimal intra-operative orientation with a small exposure can be achieved by precise preoperative planning of the incision and X-ray localization with a needle. A small incision provides a better illumination of the operative field than can be achieved by a headlamp. Surgery through a small approach can be facilitated by special bayonet-shaped instruments.

Microscopic lumbar discectomy is a four-step procedure starting from the skin to the anterior epidural space that provides clear visualization of each layer and segment. The overlapping of the lamina over the disc space varies by level and must be recognized. The disc space at L5-S1 is interlaminar in location; at L4-5 the disc is partially covered by the lamina of L4; and at L3-4 and higher the disc space is completely covered by the superior lamina. The skin must therefore be appropriate: for an infradiscal L4-5 herniation the disc prolapse is below the spinal process, for supradiscal L5-S1 herniation the disc prolapse is at the level of the spinal process. For microdiscectomy, it is extremely important to visualize the pathology in the center of the wound. In microdiscectomy the surgeon must be oriented as to the precise location of the foramen, nerve roots, and pedicles.

For foraminal and lateral disc herniation the skin incision is placed 3 cm lateral to the midline and the approach is between the transverse process.

In conclusion, the surgical incision and approach should be as small as possible and as wide as necessary. One way to progress to microdiscectomy is to start with a headlamp and to use microinstruments. The surgeon should use the procedure with which he or she is most comfortable. It is better for a patient to be operated upon by an experienced macrosurgeon than by an inexperienced microsurgeon.

CLASSIFICATION OF LUMBAR MOTION SEGMENTS FOR MICRODISCECTOMY

For a better correlation between preoperative and intraoperative findings in microscopic discectomy it is helpful to have anatomic landmarks that can be easily identified both on radiographic images as well as intraoperatively. In most classifications, posterior elements such as facet joints, laminae, and pedicles are key structures for the surgical approach to the lumbar spine (7–11). McCulloch (9) related his classification to the pedicles and compared the lumbar segments to the stories of a house. The disc level was the first story, the infrapedicle level the second story, and the pedicle level the third story of the house. Wiltse (11) added a suprapedicle level, which could be considered the upper part of McCulloch's third story, and laterally (horizontally), a subarticular zone. For orientation during interlaminar lumbar disc microsurgery, the surgeon has only a few anatomic landmarks. Exposure of the facet joint should be avoided in order to maintain the vascularization and innervation of its capsule and to avoid damage to the joint itself.

For the routine interlaminar approach to the lower lumbar spine, disc-related orientation is more useful, especially for less experienced surgeons. After identifying the inferior border of the lamina and the disc space by its relation to an intraoperative localizing needle on an X-ray film, it is easy to find the pedicles, foramen, and nerve roots.

The main difference from the classifications of McCulloch (9) and Wiltse (11) is that the intraoperative orientation is related only to the disc, not the foramen, pedicles and facet joints, which cannot be seen in most microsurgical approaches.

DISC-RELATED CLASSIFICATION

A disc and the adjacent vertebrae form a segment (the Junghans motion segment) that is divided vertically into levels and horizontally into zones (Fig. 47-1).

At the center of a segment is the disc level, with the supradiscal level above and the infradiscal level below. Supradiscal and infradiscal levels border on the middle of the vertebra, which is identical with a line between the inferior borders of the pedicles. Protruded disc material can stay at the disc level or dislocate in a supradiscal or infradiscal direction.

From the midline of the segment in a lateral direction, there are three zones: medial, paramedial, and lateral. The medial zone has a right and a left part. The middle of the paramedial zone is identical with the center of the interlaminar approach at L5-S1 and, after removing parts of the upper lamina, also at L4-5 and higher segments. Most contained or noncontained disc herniations are in this area. They lie under or close to the traversing nerve root at the disc level or the supradiscal or infradiscal level. If pathology medial to the traversing root is closer to the segment midline, it lies in the medial zone.

The lateral zone begins at the medial border of the pedicle and includes the foraminal area and the extraforaminal (far out) area. Disc herniations that lie lateral to the traversing root usually have contact with the exiting root in the foramen, causing a double-root syndrome. All levels have the same zones except the infradiscal level, which does not really have a lateral zone due to presence of the pedicles.

Myelogram and anteroposterior reconstructions on magnetic resonance imaging (MRI) show the dural sac and nerve roots with bony structures.

In the lower lumbar segments, the nerve roots traverse the disc and infradiscal area before they exit the spinal canal through the intervertebral foramen of the segment below. The vertical part of the nerve root that passes the paramedial zone is called the traversing root until it enters the lateral zone at the medial border of the pedicle. From there on it is the exiting root.

The interlaminar approach to the lumbar spine always exposes the traversing root centrally and the exiting root cranially and laterally within the intervertebral foramen. The pedicle is caudally and laterally located. The travers-

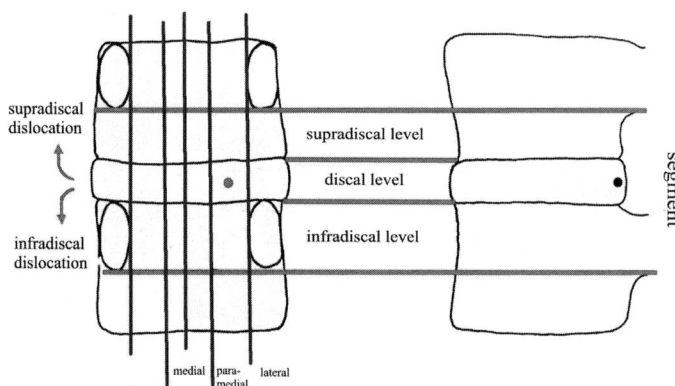

FIG. 47-1. Disc-related classification of the segment. Above the disc level is the supradiscal level, and below it is the infradiscal level; these border on the middle portion of the vertebra. In the lateral direction are the medial, paramedial, and lateral zones.

ing roots are intrathecal until they leave the dural sac and enter the nerve root sheath at the axilla of the root. The main part of the lumbar traversing root lies intrathecally. The lumbar traversing roots course past the disc and supradiscal levels intrathecally. The sheath-surrounded part of the L3-4 and L5 traversing roots is very short. The entrance point into the nerve root sheath (axilla point) for the L5 root is infradiscal medial to the L5 pedicle, and for the L3 and L4 roots it is caudal to the pedicle. For the S1 root, it is just below the L5-S1 disc. This means that in microscopic lumbar discectomy an approach to the discal and supradiscal level in L3-4 and L4-5 segments and to the supradiscal level at L5-S1 exposes only the lateral part of the dural sac with the traversing root inside, not surrounded by a nerve root sheath. A medial part of traversing root does not exist at these levels of the spinal canal and separation should therefore not be attempted. Only an interlaminar approach to the disc and infradiscal levels of L5-S1 and sometimes the intradiscal levels of L4-5 show sheath-surrounded traversing nerve roots. Traversing nerve roots are most sensitive to mechanical strain in their sheath-surrounded part, especially at the entrance point, because they can be manipulated as easily as in their intrathecal part.

Exiting roots have a nerve root sheath that naturally adheres to the posterior surface of the vertebra and the pedicle. They are also sensitive to any kind of mechanical strain because they cannot move. Exiting roots are located craniolaterally to the interlaminar approach and the disc. They pass around the pedicle into the superior (upper) part of the intervertebral foramen. The exiting nerve root and the pedicle adjacent to it have the same name: the L5 root passes beneath the L5 pedicle, the L4 root around the L4 pedicle, and so forth.

Fragment dislocation in the supradiscal direction often causes double-root involvement, with simultaneous compression of the traversing and the exiting root. This involves the intrathecal traversing root and the exiting root from the segment above.

APPROACH TO THE LAMINA

After incision of the skin and fascia, contact with the spinous process with a bone rasp leads to the upper corner of the interlaminar window. The bone rasp passes along the inferior part of the spinous process to the inferior part of the lamina and then to the upper interlaminar corner. With the 30° oblique view the surgeon looks at the lower part of the spinous process and the medial part of the inferior lamina which form the upper interlaminar corner (Fig. 47-2). The highest point of this corner has specific relation to the disc space of the segment. At L5-S1 this point lies above the disc, at L4-5 it lies at the disc level, and at L3-4 and higher it lies below the disc space.

The inferior part of the lamina in the upper interlaminar corner is not covered by the ligamentum flavum. The

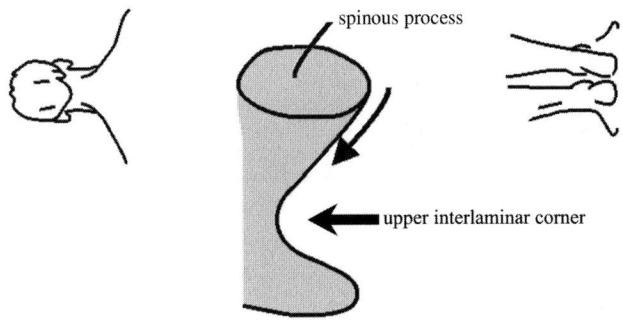

FIG. 47-2. A surgeon's 30° oblique view of the upper areas of a left-sided interlaminar window. Bony contact with the inferior part of the spinous process leads directly to the upper interlaminar corner.

superior part of the lamina in the lower interlaminar corner is much thinner and is partially covered by the ligamentum flavum. Before entering the spinal canal by flavectomy it is useful to take another X-ray with a dissector in the upper interlaminar corner, which is much closer to the disc than the needle used to radiographically localize the proper level for skin incision.

SURGICAL VIEW THROUGH INTERLAMINAR WINDOW AND DISTRIBUTION OF FRAGMENT LOCATION

After removal of the ligamentum flavum from the lateral interlaminar area, epidural fat and the lateral portion of the dura and the traversing root appear. It is not necessary to remove the ligamentum flavum in the medial interlaminar area in order to expose nerve roots. The L5-S1 disc lies in the middle of the interlaminar approach to L5-S1, directly under the traversing S1 root. In the middle of the interlaminar approach to L4-5, directly under the traversing L5 root, lies the infradiscal area of the L5 vertebral bone surface.

Exiting roots cannot be seen from this approach, they can only be estimated. On a left-sided approach, the foramen and exiting root are on the surgeon's left, and on a right-sided approach they are on the surgeon's right. The segmental pedicle is on the opposite side (Fig. 47-3A,B).

In addition to the four main directions—cranial, caudal, medial, and lateral—there are intermediary planes (craniomedial, craniolateral (foraminal), and caudomedial) for describing fragment migration. Caudolateral position of a fragment is not possible because of the presence of the pedicles. Even if a fragment lies lateral to the traversing root in the infradiscal area, it is still in the paramedial zone because the lateral border to this zone is the pedicle. Infradiscal caudal herniations are the most frequent indication for open surgery (59%). The disc fragment lies between bone and the traversing root, which is immobile because of the presence of the pedicle laterally. Hernia-

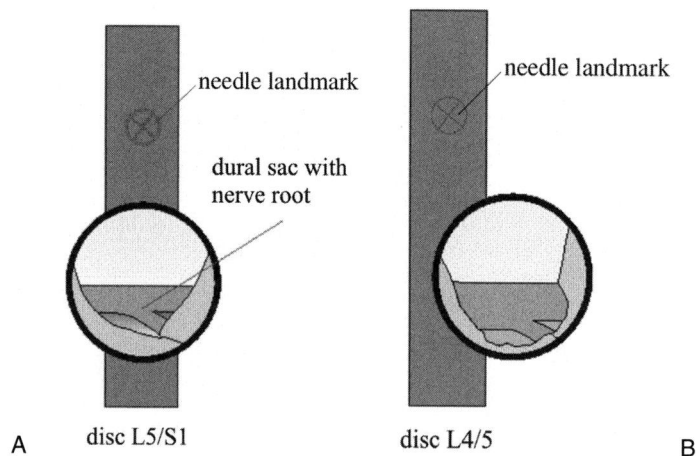

FIG. 47-3. A, B: Left-sided microscopic interlaminar approach to the lumbar spine. In front of the approach is the dural sac with the traversing root inside. Only at the disc and infradiscal levels of L5-S1, and sometimes at the infradiscal level of L4-5, is there a traversing nerve root surrounded by a nerve root sheath.

tions in other directions less frequently come to surgery. The distribution of fragment migration in patients who have been treated conservatively is completely different from that in surgically treated patients (12).

FOUR STEPS TO THE DISC

First Step: Skin

Needle localization with X-ray is generally more accurate than localization by palpation. The needle should be placed at a 90°-angle to the skin, approximately 2 to 3 cm paramedically on the contralateral side (Fig. 47-4).

Palpation of iliac crest and spinous processes is often misleading because of anatomic variations and difficulty in palpating bony landmarks in obese patients. The 3 cm skin incision is placed centrally at the appropriate level. For supradiscal and discal herniations of L3-4, L4-5, or L5-S1 the incision is placed at the level of the spinous process. For infradiscal herniations, the incision should be slightly below the spinous process.

Second Step: Ligamentum Flavum

After incision of the fascia and stripping aside the back muscles, palpation along the inferior part of the spinous process leads to the upper interlaminar corner (Fig. 47-2). The highest point in this upper interlaminar corner is the best place to enter the spinal canal. When the skin incision is correctly centered over the L5-S1 disc, the upper interlaminar corner is the cranial part of the approach; for the L4-5 disc it is in the middle of the approach. For L3-4 discs and higher the upper interlaminar corner is in the caudal part of the approach (Fig. 47-5). A modified Casper retractor is inserted to maintain exposure.

Before opening the spinal canal the upper interlaminar corner of the inferior part of the lamina has to be identi-

fied in relationship to the needle landmark in order to know where to find roots pedicle and discs in microscopic discectomy without further exposure.

Third Step: Posterior Epidural Space

The spinal canal should be opened to reach the parent disc even if fragments have migrated. After removal of ligamentum flavum and parts of the lamina the posterior epidural space can be visualized. In the lateral part of the interlaminar window at L5-S1 the surgeon has a direct view on the transversing S1 root that is sometimes covered or surrounded by epidural fat. At L4-5, and in higher segments, the interlaminar window is more medial and the dural sac wider so that the transversing root is covered by the lateral dural sac.

Fourth Step: Anterior Epidural Space

Medialization of the transversing root with a lone nerve root retractor allows a direct view of the disc level at L5-S1 after flavectomy and of the L4-5 and more proximal levels after additional bone removal of the lamina in the upper interlaminar corner. At L4-5 and higher levels a flavectomy without laminotomy exposes the anterior epidural space on the vertebral bony surface of the infradiscal zone. This area has many epidural veins and should not be exposed if the pathology is at the disc or supradiscal level. Medialization of the dura and nerve root, extraction of the disc prolapse, and wound closure are the same as with conventional discectomy. A specialized disc extractor with a depth block is recommended in order to avoid anterior perforation of the annulus fibrosus with possible injury to the abdominal vessels (Fig. 47-6).

A

B

C

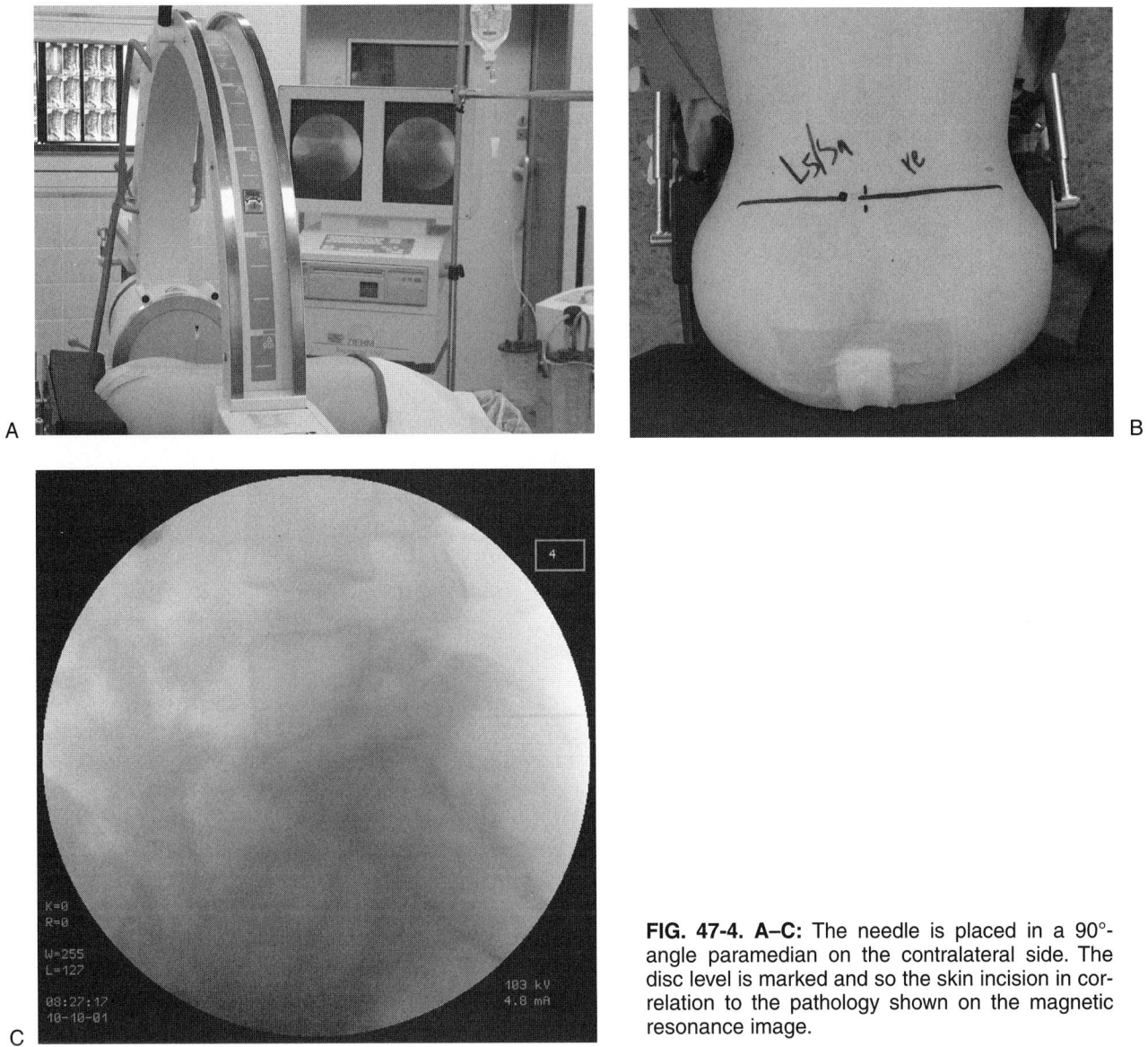

FIG. 47-4. A–C: The needle is placed in a 90°-angle paramedian on the contralateral side. The disc level is marked and so the skin incision in correlation to the pathology shown on the magnetic resonance image.

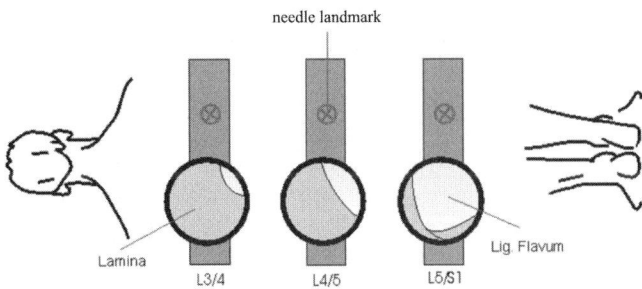

FIG. 47-5. Second step: lamina flavum at the disc level. When the skin incision is centered over the disc at L5-S1 the approach exposes the ligamentum flavum with the upper interlaminar corner cranially located. At L4-5 the upper interlaminar corner is in the middle and at L3-4 it is caudal and medial.

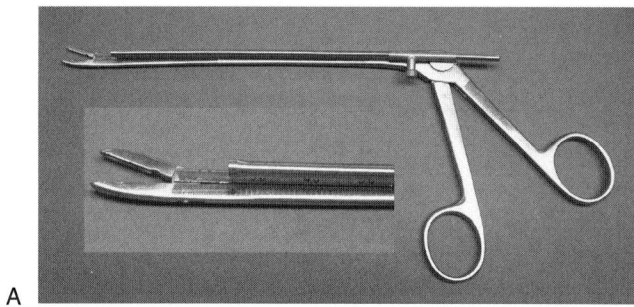

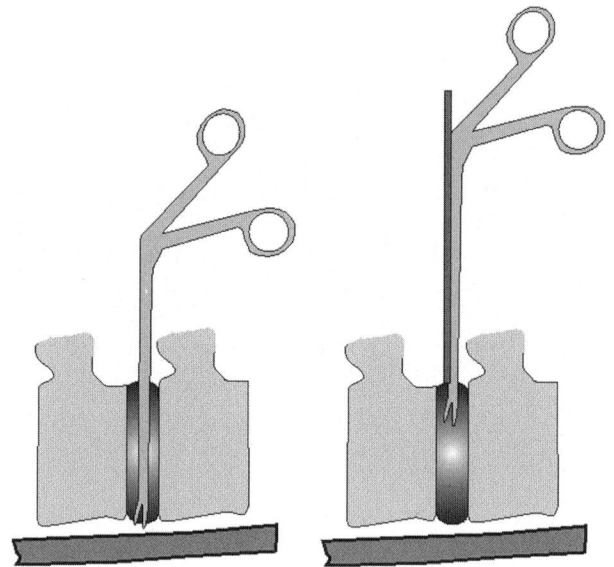

FIG. 47-6. A, B: Rongeur with a depth guard for intradiscal maneuvers to avoid anterior vessel injury (Aesculap).

LIGHT SOURCES

Good lighting is mandatory for a microsurgical approach. If there is no microscope available, a headlamp can be useful, although only the surgeon will have an adequate view. The use of a microscope is excellent for teaching conditions—the assistant has the same view as the surgeon —and it also provides optimal illumination and magnification of the operating field. Performing surgery with an operating microscope (Fig. 47-7) demands a certain level of training and the learning curve may vary between surgeons. The adapting time can be individually different. Nevertheless, a surgeon who uses a microscope should be able to switch over to the head lamp if technical problems with the microscope occur.

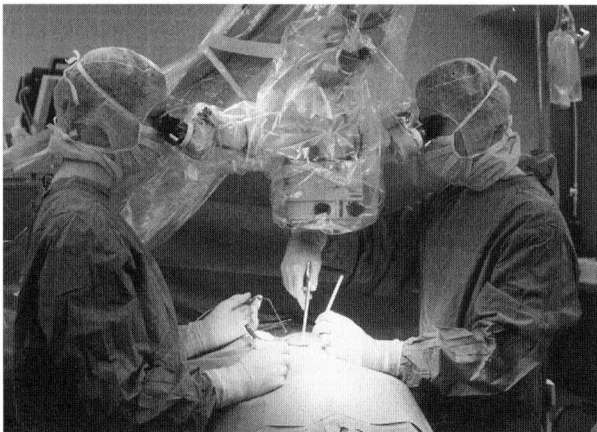

FIG. 47-7. Operating microscope. Surgeon and assistant have the same view.

INSTRUMENTS

The standard instruments used for the microsurgical approach to the lumbar disc are designed for manipulation in the spinal canal and are thin with a special angular shape.

RESULTS

The reported results of microscopic lumbar discectomy vary. These variations are the result of different indications for surgery and different outcome measures. Results after microsurgical procedures are reported by Caspar (13), Kahanovitz (14), Krämer (15,16), McCulloch (6), Silvers (2), Williams (17), Wilson (18), and Zahrawi (19).

Two trials were conducted comparing microdiscectomy with standard discectomy, both included clinical outcomes that were similar (20,21). Because of different outcome measures, metaanalysis is generally not possible (22).

EARLY COMPLICATIONS IN MICROSCOPIC LUMBAR DISCECTOMY

The complications of open disc surgery and microscopic discectomy are discussed mainly in books of experienced spine surgeons (6,23).

In the European Spine Society questionnaire (24) to evaluate a risk and value score for different diagnostic and therapeutic procedures in the spine, open discectomy had the highest effectiveness for pain relief, but a negative overall risk value score because of complications and poor results. Our recent studies evaluated different factors that influenced the outcome of open lumbar disc surgery (24,25).

Classification

Complications of open lumbar disc surgery may be classified as intraoperative, immediate postoperative, and late postoperative according to when they are apparent rather than when they occur. Complications of lumbar spine surgery can either be general, and therefore common to any type of surgery, such as thrombosis, embolism, and anesthetic problems, or they may be specific for spine surgery.

Intraoperative complications are recognized immediately by the surgeon and should be recorded. Operative reports are not always complete so their true frequency remains uncertain. Many of these problems can be avoided by meticulous preoperative planning. Some intraoperative complications are common, such as epidural bleeding and durotomy, and can be managed quite easily. Other complications, such as anterior vessel and visceral injury, are severe, but fortunately extremely rare.

Immediate postoperative general complications such as vomiting, thrombosis, and circulatory problems can occur after any kind of surgery. Some of the specific spine complications occurring during the operation may be initially unrecognized by the surgeon and become symptomatic and obvious in the days following surgery. These include complications secondary to patient positioning, abdominal symptoms, and bladder disturbances.

Late postoperative complications after lumbar disc surgery may become obvious after the patient leaves the hospital. These include general complications like thromboembolism as well as specific complications such as recurrent disc herniation, spondylodiscitis, and the failed back surgery syndrome due to peridural fibrosis and instability. Late complications can only be evaluated by questionnaires or follow-up studies with patient examination since not all patients consult their surgeon when these complications arise.

Intraoperative Complications

Missed Preoperative Checklist

The surgeon performing a lumbar disc operation should examine the patient just prior to the surgical procedure to verify any recent change in symptoms or new findings. Symptoms can change in a short time because of fragment migration or resorption. A difference in visualization between MRI and intraoperative X-ray findings must be recognized. Sometimes a lumbosacral segment can be seen on MRI but not on X-ray. General anesthesia should commence only when all preoperative imaging is complete including an X-ray with the needle localization.

Wrong Level Exploration

Precise preoperative planning is one of the main prerequisites for successful microsurgery and avoiding

wrong level exploration. For McCulloch (6) it is the most important prerequisite. In our comparative study (25), wrong level exploration occurred 1.2% of the time in a group of very experienced surgeons and 3.3% of the time in a group of less experienced surgeons.

Wrong level exploration is more likely to occur at L4-5 and higher segments than at L5-S1. In all cases the correct segment was ultimately identified intraoperatively by X-ray. As described previously it is useful to take a second X-ray with a dissector in the upper interlaminar corner before flavectomy.

Missed Pathology

Missed pathology means that the compressive pathology causing the clinical symptoms was not adequately addressed. This can happen when wrong level exploration is not recognized and other nonsignificant pathology is removed. Under such circumstances the patient awakes with the same pain or worse than before surgery.

If the suspected intraoperative pathology is not found, an intraoperative myelogram can be considered.

Other Pathology

Other pathology means the surgeon finds a different pathologic entity than what was expected but which could have caused the clinical symptoms. This could be an undiagnosed neurinoma or a synovial cyst from the facet joint. In these cases a closer look at the imaging pictures should be undertaken. In some cases it might be necessary to perform an intraoperative X-ray or myelogram to identify missed pathology.

Bleeding or Epidural Hematoma

Epidural hematoma causing symptomatic neurologic compression or cauda equina syndrome is one of the most feared complications of spine surgery. During a posterior approach, lumbar spinal canal arterial bleeding from the back muscles and epidural venous bleeding are the most important causes for such bleeding. Intraoperative bleeding can be minimized by positioning the patient prone with the abdomen hanging freely.

Arterial bleedings from the back muscles should be identified and coagulated carefully.

At the end of the surgical procedure, after the muscle retractor is removed, the muscle walls should be checked for bleeders because prolonged muscle retraction may temporarily occlude potentially significant muscle bleeders, which could begin bleeding after muscle layer closure. When an epidural hematoma is identified, surgical intervention must be performed as soon as possible to evacuate the hematoma.

Epidural vein bleedings do not cause compression of the dural sac, but do cause cauda equina syndrome. Some experienced spine surgeons (26–28) believe that epidural vein bleeding often stops when the disc fragment is removed and after wound closure. We prefer to tamponade as long as possible before using bipolar cautery. Excessive cautery of epidural veins may inhibit the nutrition of the nerve roots and may be the cause of epidural fibrosis and postdiscectomy syndrome (failed back syndrome).

An epidural hematoma, even if it does not compress the dural sac, can also cause epidural fibrosis. The main reason to prevent and stop bleeding from epidural veins is that they obscure the visual field. Because of the limited approach in microdiscectomy, even a small amount of bleeding may appear as a major hemorrhage under the microscope and make it difficult to perform a safe and adequate discectomy. Therefore the following precautions should be followed to prevent intraoperative bleeding:

- positioning of the patient with abdomen hanging freely
- avoid exploring the posterior surface of the vertebra if it is not necessary
- retract epidural veins with the retractor before entering the disc space
- cauterize veins if they are in the way.

If epidural vein bleeding occurs it may be better to remove as much of the protruded disc material as possible before taking care of the bleeding. The bleeding during this maneuver could be managed by continuous suction and the use of cotton tamponades. After removal of the disc prolapse, it is easier to expose the bleeding vein and cauterize it if necessary.

For continuous bleeding from cancellous bone we use a small amount of bone wax.

In our series excessive bleeding occurred in 7.1% of patients treated by the group of experienced surgeons and in 3.5% of the patients treated by the group of very experienced surgeons. In all cases, excessive epidural vein bleeding did not cause intraoperative or immediate postoperative complications (25).

Durotomy

Injuries to the dura with loss of cerebrospinal fluid (CSF) occur in many types of spine surgery. Clear fluid in the wound should not automatically mean dural tear. It could also arise from a puncture hole from previous myelography, from a spinal anesthetic, or from inadvertent dural puncture from an epidural injection days before surgery. Other causes of intraoperative fluid include synovial fluid from facet joints (6) or from a wet cotton patty.

Unfortunately presence of clear fluid usually means CSF from inadvertent durotomy by surgical instruments. Most commonly this occurs during opening of the dura by incision of the ligamentum flavum. This can happen when the ligamentum flavum is very thin, which

occurs with lumbosacral anomalies (6), or when a big disc herniation displaces the dural sac posteriorly under the ligamentum flavum. This is why we prefer a two-step flavotomy with a special semi-sharp dissector. Under special conditions, intentional durotomy is necessary to deal with intradural pathology, which is rare in lumbar disc surgery (6).

When a CSF leak is recognized, localization and assessment of the injury must be determined: Is it medial or lateral, caused by incision or punch, are nerve roots involved? When the durotomy is localized, it is better to avoid it in order not to inadvertently enlarge the hole. After the disc herniation is removed, there is more space and less tension on the dura and suture repair is easier. A head down/back up position reduces dural tension and empties the dural sac. Tears of more than 3 mm in length should be closed with 6-0 sutures. Usually, the microsurgical exposure must be extended. Small punctures can be left alone. We prefer to put a small free fat graft from the subcutaneous fat to the dural repair. The patient should have intravenous antibiotics and be kept in bed for 3 days.

Complications of dural tears include headache due to CSF loss, CSF fistula, and postoperative pseudomeningocele, which can be seen by MRI. Our own experience with a follow-up study comparing patients who had intraoperative dural tears with a control group showed better results in the control group (25). With a two-step blunt perforation of the ligamentum flavum, appropriate instrumentation, and good visualization of the lateral dura and nerve root border it should be possible to reduce the number and extent of dural tears in lumbar microdiscectomy to a minimum. In conclusion, durotomies are a matter of experience. They occurred in the group of less experienced surgeons 7.2% of the time and among the very experienced surgeons 0.8% ($p < .001$) of the time (25).

Nerve Root Lesion

The incidence of nerve root lesions after lumbar spine surgery has been estimated at 0.2% (29). Such injury may be suspected postoperatively by the presence of a new or increased neurologic deficit. Iatrogenic intraoperative nerve root injuries are classified by the site where they occur, proximal to the foramen or extraforaminal, and by the way in which the injury occurs: open by sharp instrumentation or closed by excessive traction, compression, or heat from electrocautery. Poor visibility, perineural adhesions, and congenital neural anomalies such as conjoined nerve roots are the most common causes of damage to the nerve roots. Therefore, it is absolutely necessary to define the lateral border of the root and dural sac before removing any material from the spinal canal. Even when the neural elements are safely retracted by a nerve root retractor, the tissue in the anterior epidural space should be identified by the 2 mm dissector. The bright white of disc material should not be mistaken for epidural fat and vessels.

Rootlets may herniate through a durotomy. After reduction of the rootlets the dura must be repaired. Small defects may be covered by a free fat graft especially if a suture could strangle the nerve root. The most vulnerable area for an open nerve root legion is the axilla of the exiting nerve root. Thus effects to remove intradiscal fragments should not take place medial to the nerve root in the axilla. One of the principles of microdiscectomy is to stay lateral to the nerve root in order to avoid axillary injury.

Anterior Vessel Injury, Visceral Injuries

When a rongeur penetrates the anterior annulus fibrosus, it may contact a major vessel that lies immediately in front of the lower lumbar discs. Grasping maneuvers in order to clean out the disc material may rupture the vessels. The most frequent lesion is an isolated injury to the left common iliac artery (30) caused by surgery of the L4-5 disc. The overall complication rate for anterior vessel injury is 0.045% (31). Only 50% of such injuries are immediately apparent with a dramatic unexplained fall in blood pressure and excessive hemorrhage from the disc. In these cases disc surgery has to be stopped immediately, the wound closed, and the patient turned over for a laparotomy and repair of the injured vessel.

In 50% of the patients the symptoms of anterior vessel injury and other abdominal injuries are recognized later in the recovery room with extreme hypotension and painful abdominal swelling. In these cases, laparotomy must be performed immediately. Even with prompt action, the mortality of this complication is approximately 50% (6). Prevention of this major complication is possible if intradiscal maneuvers are performed only with rongeurs that cannot be inserted deeper than 25 mm. This leaves an adequate safety margin since the anteroposterior disc diameter is 35 to 40 mm on average (Fig. 47-6).

Immediate Postoperative Complications

Postoperative Leg Pain and Neurologic Deficits (Table 47-1)

Although not usually considered a complication in most series, persistent or residual leg pain after nerve root decompression surgery of the lumbar spine can be considered a complication. If the correct level was operated upon, and if neurologic symptoms are not severe or progressive, one can wait.

It is important, however, to consider the possibility of a residual disc fragment or a recurrent herniation. Indications for a careful postoperative neurologic examination and a repeat computed tomography (CT) or MRI study are:

- severe leg pain lasting more than 2 to 3 days

- progressing neurologic deficit
- cauda equina syndrome.

When a nerve root has been compressed for a long time by a disc herniation or an osteophyte it may not become asymptomatic immediately after decompression. The reasons for residual symptoms are not completely understood, but include the duration of compression, the presence of comorbidities such as diabetes, intraoperative nerve injury, compression from a hematoma, inadequate postoperative pain medication, and individual pain sensitivity.

In addition to wrong level exposure, missed additional pathology at the current level is another cause of failed lumbar disc surgery. Additional disc fragments can be missed or concomitant bony stenosis may not be appreciated and thus decompressed. The patient may awake from surgery with the same pain or it might even be worse because of additional operative trauma and postoperative hematoma. Repeat CT or MRI should be performed to detect the missed fragment or other pathology.

Continued postoperative leg pain and neurologic symptoms of the same or increased intensity as before surgery can be caused by either missed pathology or by an early recurrent disc herniation. This could be caused by abdominal pressure such as by coughing during the immediate postoperative period.

Usually symptoms from a recurrent disc prolapse occur after a pain-free interval. It may occur when the patient begins to stand and axially load the spine with more frequency. In our series we had 0.2% rate of recurrent disc herniation in the first week after surgery. Once a new herniation is verified by repeat CT or MRI conservative management or revision surgery at the same level may be considered. The risk of recurrent disc herniation cannot be eliminated by extensive disc curettage (6,29,30). It is generally recommended that all disc material under the annulus perforation that could lead into a recurrent herniation be removed at the time of the initial surgery.

All variations of the kneeling position that are used in lumbar disc surgery can produce compression on the skin and neurologic structures. Brachial plexus stretch injuries and compression of the radial and ulnar nerve can develop by the hyperabduction of the arm. Bernsmann (32) observed two cases of slight brachial plexus dysfunction in our series, all of which disappeared in the first few days following surgery. Severe lesions from position-

---

TABLE 47-1. *Causes for postoperative leg pain*

Residual symptoms from original condition
Intraoperative nerve root injury
Residual fragment disc, foreign body retention
Early recurrent disc herniation
Nerve irritation secondary to intraoperative positioning

ing, such as cervical myelopathy from hyperextension of the neck, or visual disturbances (6,33,34) from failure to protect the eyes during surgery and in the prone position are very rare and should be avoided by proper head positioning.

There is a wide range of possible cauda equina symptoms, from slight bladder disturbances to the fully developed cauda equina syndrome with perineal anesthesia, urinary incontinence and decreased rectal tone, and bilateral progressive leg weakness.

The absence of any of these clinical features does not rule out a developing cauda equina syndrome.

Injury to the cauda equina can occur at surgery from direct damage to the nerves or postoperatively from hematoma. We have not seen a cauda equina syndrome from fat graft compression in our large prospective randomized study of free fat graft versus no fat graft for epidural scarring (9), although this condition has been reported by others.

Concern about a possible cauda equina syndrome mandates a thorough neurologic examination and immediate CT or MRI. If a compression lesion is found, immediate surgery to decompress the cauda equina is necessary, although a study showed that there is no statistically significant difference in outcome between patients who had decompressive surgery within the first 20 hours after the onset of cauda equina syndrome and those who had surgery 24 to 48 hours after onset (35).

The reported incidence of disc space infection ranges from 0.13% to 0.9% (6,30,36–38). Most studies recommend infection prophylaxis with antibiotics.

It has been claimed that microdiscectomy has a higher infection rate than standard disc surgery because of contamination by the microscope. However, publications on microdiscectomy surgery (30) and our own experience show that the deep wound infection rate in microdiscectomy surgery is not significantly higher than with traditional discectomy.

CONCLUSIONS

It is impossible to avoid all complications in any surgery, including lumbar microdiscectomy. According to McCulloch (6), the two major criticisms of microdiscectomy are wrong level exploration and missed pathology. If wrong level exposure is not recognized, pathology will be missed. The risk of complications with lumbar microdisc surgery can be minimized if meticulous attention is given to preoperative, intraoperative, and postoperative details (24). It is helpful for spine surgeons to master the microsurgery learning curve by working with other experienced spine microsurgeons and to read the literature about how to avoid intraoperative complications and how to manage them if they occur.

The outcome of lumbar disc surgery depends heavily upon proper patient selection (Table 47-2). The right

TABLE 47-2. *Ways to avoid complications in lumbar microdisc surgery*

Proper patient selection
Surgeon training
Preoperative planning
Systematic 4-step surgical approach
Infection prophylaxis
Postoperative care

patient with the right indication for microscopic disc surgery will have a good result if a well-trained surgeon removes the disc fragment using a standard approach. The learning curve in micro-decompression surgery can be improved upon in special training courses that provide instruction for working with the microscope on cadaver spines. Infection can be decreased by careful draping of the microscope and by the use of prophylactic antibiotics. Recurrent disc herniation is an uncommon but important complication in lumbar disc surgery that may result in another operation with a greater risk for complications and scar formation. In many cases it is the beginning of a failed back surgery syndrome.

REFERENCES

1. Findlay G. 10 year follow study after lumbar microdiscectomy: a comparative study. Paper presented at ISSLS Meeting; 1997; Singapore.
2. Silvers R. Microsurgical versus standard lumbar discectomy. Neurosurg 1988;22: 837–841
3. Wilson D, Harbaugh R. Microsurgical and standard removal of protruded lumbar disc: a comparative study. Neurosurgery 1981;8: 422–427
4. Caspi I. Percutaneous discectomy of lumbar spine. Int Orthop 1987;2: 331.
5. Fager C. Comments on microsurgical and standard removal of the protrudes lumbar disc. A comparative study. Neurosurgery 1987;8: 426–427.
6. McCulloch J, Young PH. Essentials of spinal microsurgery. Philadelphia: Lippincott-Raven, 1998.
7. Akkerveeken PF. A taxonomy of lumbar stenosis with emphasis on clinical applicability. Eur Spine J 1994;3:130.
8. Finneson B. Low back pain. Philadelphia: JB Lippincott, 1980.
9. McCulloch J. Principles of microsurgery for lumbar disc disease. New York: Raven, 1990.
10. White A, Watkins R, Ray C. Surgical anatomy and nomenclature. In: White A, Rothmann R, Ray C, eds. Lumbar spine surgery. St. Louis: Mosby, 1987.
11. Wiltse 1992
12. Krämer J. A new classification of lumbar motion segments for microdiscotomy. Eur Spine J 1995;4:327–334.
13. Caspar W. A new surgical procedure for lumbar disc herniation causing less tissue damage though a microsurgical approach. Adv Neurosurg 1977;4:74–80.
14. Kahanovich N, Viola K, McCulloch JA. Limited surgical discectomy and microdiscectomy: a clinical comparison. Spine 1989;14:79– 81.
15. Krämer J, Ludwig J. Die operative Behandlung des lumbalen bandscheibenvorfalls. Der Orthopädie 1999;28:579–584.
16. Krämer J (1990) Intervertebral disc disease. Causes, diagnosis, treatment and prophylaxis, 2nd ed. Stuttgart/New York: Georg Thieme/Verlag.
17. Williams R. Microlumbar discectomy: a conservative surgical approach to the virgin herniated lumbar disc. Spine 1978;3:175–182.
18. Wilson DH 1979.
19. Zahrawi F. Microlumbar discectomy. Is it safe as an outpatient procedure? Spine 1994;9:1070–1074.
20. Henrikson L, Schmidt V, Eskesen V et al. A controlled study of micro-

surgical versus standard lumbar discectomy. Br J Neurosurg 1996;10: 289–293.

21. Lagarrigue J, Chaynes P (1994). Comparative study of disk surgery with or without microscopy: a prospective study of 80 cases [in French]. Neurochirurgie 1994;40:116–120.

22. Nachemson A, Jonsson E. Neck and back pain. Philadelphia: Lippincott Williams & Wilkins, 2000.

23. Postacchini F 1999.

24. Krämer J. The LIRCE principle: a risk value score for the spine. Eur Spine J 1998;7:353–357.

25. Bernsmann 1997.

26. Dyke 1998.

27. Findlay G, Neurosurgeon in Liverpool UK. Personal communication, 1998.

28. Yoshizawa 1998.

29. Bell G. Complications of lumbar spine surgery. In: Wiesel S, Weinstein J, eds. The lumbar spine, 2nd ed. Philadelphia: WB Saunders, 1996.

30. Postacchini F. Lumbar disc herniation. Wien/New York: Springer-Verlag, 1998.

31. Wildförster 1991.

32. Bernsmann K, Krämer J, Ziozious I, et al. Lumbar microdisc surgery with and without autologous fat graft. Arch Orthop Trauma Surg 2001; 121:476–480.

33. Lee A. Ischemic optic neuropathy following lumbar spine surgery. J Neurosurg 1995;83:348–349.

34. Wolfe 1992.

35. Ahn V, et al. Meta-analysis of studies on cauda equina syndrome. AAOS Abstracts 1999;Back letter 14.6.61.

36. Haaker R, Senkal M, Kielich T, et al. Percutaneous lumbar discectomy in the treatment of lumbar discitis. Eur Spine J 1997;6:98–101.

37. Rompe JD, Eysel P, Zoellner J, et al. Intra- und postoperative risikoanalyse nach lumbaler bandscheibenoperation. Ztsch Orthop 1999;137:201–205.

38. Roberts MP. Complications of lumbar disc surgery. Spinal Surg 1988; 2:13–19.

CHAPTER 48

Classification, Natural History, and Clinical Evaluation

Yong Hai

Lumbar spinal stenosis is defined as the reduction in the diameter of the spinal canal, lateral nerve canals, or neural foramina. The stenosis may occur as a part of a generalized disease process and involve multiple areas of the canal and multiple levels or, conversely, may be localized or segmental. The reduction in the diameter of the spinal canal or neural outlets may be attributable to bone hypertrophy, ligamentous hypertrophy, disc protrusion, spondylolisthesis, or any combination of these elements. This clinical entity is used to describe a complex set of symptoms, physical findings, and radiographic abnormalities caused by a narrowed spinal canal. Pain in the back and leg(s) and, in particular, claudication caused by compression and ischemia of nerve roots are the main symptoms. Although it is one of the most common spinal disorders in people older than 65 years, and frequently causes significant functional impairment (1), there is still some uncertainty in diagnosing and treating lumbar canal stenosis, including:

1. Though nearly all people in this age group have radiographic evidence of degenerative disc and joint disease, the incidence of clinically symptomatic lumbar canal stenosis is unknown.
2. The diagnosis is largely clinical. Although imaging studies can confirm the diagnosis, they often show abnormalities in people with no symptoms.
3. Treatment is mostly empiric. Although lumbar canal stenosis is the most common reason for spinal surgery in this older population group (2) and accounts for inpatient expenses approaching $1 billion per year (3), no comparison of surgical versus nonsurgical treatment has ever been done.

Lumbar spinal stenosis has been known for more than 100 years, but for a long time it was simply not addressed. This occurred because the association between herniated vertebral discs and sciatica received most of the attention after it was discovered by Mixter (4) in 1934. However, since the early 1950s, starting with the studies of Verbiest (5), this has changed, and lumbar spinal stenosis now is an accepted clinical entity and a well-recognized spinal disorder.

Stenosis is most frequently a sequela of the aging process, usually readily identifiable on imaging studies as evidenced by the high incidence of positive radiographic findings in asymptomatic patients (6–8). The presence of a narrow canal on radiographic imaging studies does not by itself define the syndrome. Rather, the syndrome is defined by a complex set of symptoms and clinical findings that must be supported by radiographic evidence. Patients with spinal stenosis patients often present with few objective physical findings. Up to 95% of patients treated surgically have only subjective symptoms, mainly pain (9,10). Accurate diagnosis and treatment decisions must be based on a thorough knowledge of the clinical syndrome and natural history (11–15). Vascular claudication in particular (16) must be considered in the differential diagnosis, in addition to lumbar spondylosis, peripheral vascular disease, and peripheral neuropathy.

CLASSIFICATION

The classification of lumbar stenosis is important because of the implications of the underlying etiology of the condition and when forming a therapeutic strategy, specifically directing surgical approaches (17).

Spinal stenosis may be classified by either its etiology or location. The classification of spinal stenosis proposed by Arnoldi (18) in 1976 remains useful and is still the most widely used classification. He divided lumbar stenosis into two major groups: congenital or developmental stenosis, and acquired stenosis. Congenital stenosis (primary stenosis) is present at birth as part of a malformation and is divided into idiopathic and achondroplastic etiologies. In contrary, acquired stenosis (secondary stenosis) is present in patients with symptoms and signs of stenosis but with normal dimensions of the original vertebral canal and is further classified into degenerative, combined congenital and degenerative, spondylotic and spondylolisthetic, iatrogenic posttraumatic, and metabolic. Degenerative stenosis of the lumbar region is the most common type of spinal stenosis. Symptomatic lumbar stenosis typically occurs in patients in the fifth to seventh decades of life with a reported incidence from 1.7% to 10%, and as the population ages, a greater number of patients will need to be treated for this condition (19–23). Although there may be a structural predisposition to spinal stenosis (congenitally short pedicles), symptomatic narrowing of the spinal canal usually is seen in association with osteoarthritic changes of the lumbar spine. Men and women seem to be affected equally with spinal stenosis; however, women are afflicted with associated degenerative spondylolisthesis four times more often than men (24).

Anatomic classification refers to central canal stenosis, lateral recess stenosis, or neural foraminal stenosis.

Central stenosis refers to a narrowing of the spinal canal across the anteroposterior diameter, the transverse diameter, or both (17,25,26). The central canal is enclosed anteriorly by the posterior portion of the vertebral body and the vertebral disc and posteriorly by the lamina and the base of the spinous process. Central canal stenosis, commonly occurring at an intervertebral disc level, defines midline sagittal spinal canal diameter narrowing that may elicit neurogenic claudication or pain in the buttock, thigh, or leg. Such stenosis results from ligamentum flavum hypertrophy, inferior articulating process, facet hypertrophy of the cephalad vertebra, vertebral body osteophytosis, and herniated nucleus pulposus (27,28). Stenosis at multiple levels is more common than strictly segmental stenosis. In approximately 40% of cases, central stenosis is caused by soft tissue hypertrophy. On computed tomography (CT) scans, midsagittal lumbar canal diameters less than 10 mm represent absolute stenosis and midsagittal lumbar canal diameters less than 13 mm represent relative stenosis (29).

Entrapment and compression of the nerve root in its pathway through the spine, referred to as the nerve root canal, is termed *lateral stenosis* (17,25,26,30,31). The nerve root canal begins where the nerve root exits the dura and ends where the nerve root leaves the intervertebral foramen. The nerve root canal is bordered by the pedicle of the vertebra above and the pedicle of the vertebra below. The anterior side of the canal is formed by the vertebral body and vertebral disc. The posterior side of the canal is formed by the facet joint structures of the vertebrae above and below. Lateral stenosis occurs when the spinal nerve is compressed within the nerve root canal or the vertebral foramina (32). As the disc narrows, the pedicle may move in an inferior direction, narrowing the lateral recess and pinching the spinal nerve (33,34). MacNab (35) originally described this entrapment and compression of the nerve root between a diffuse lateral bulge of the disc and the pedicle above as pedicular kinking. Narrowing of the lateral recess can also be the result of facet hypertrophy or enlargement and ossification of the ligamentum flavum. Radiculopathy, or decreased function of a nerve root, is commonly observed with lateral stenosis.

Lateral recess stenosis (i.e., lateral gutter stenosis, subarticular stenosis, subpedicular stenosis, foraminal canal stenosis, intervertebral foramen stenosis) is defined as narrowing (less than 3 to 4 mm) between the facet superior articulating process and posterior vertebral margin. Such narrowing may impinge the nerve root and subsequently elicit radicular pain. This lateral region has been compartmentalized by several authors into entrance zone, mid-zone, exit zone, and far-out stenosis (30,31,36).

The *entrance zone* lies medial to the pedicle and superior articulating process, and, consequently, arises from facet joint superior articulating process hypertrophy. Other causes include developmentally short pedicle and facet joint morphology, as well as osteophytosis and herniated nucleus pulposus anterior to the nerve root. The lumbar nerve root compressed below superior articulating process retains the same segmental number as the involved vertebral level (e.g., L5 nerve root is impinged by L5 superior articulating process).

The *mid-zone* extends from the medial to the lateral pedicle edge. Mid-zone stenosis arises from osteophytosis under the pars interarticularis and bursal or fibrocartilaginous hypertrophy at a spondylolytic defect.

Exit zone stenosis involves an area surrounding the foramen and arises from facet joint hypertrophy and subluxation, as well as superior disc margin osteophytosis. Such stenosis may impinge the exiting spinal nerve.

Far-out (extraforaminal) stenosis entails compression lateral to the exit zone. Such compression occurs with far lateral vertebral body end-plate osteophytosis and when the sacral ala and L5 transverse process impinge on the L5 spinal nerve (8).

In order to correlate the classification of lumbar spinal stenosis with surgical planning, Hansraj et al. (37,38) introduced a classification of typical and complex lumbar spinal stenosis. Typical lumbar spinal stenosis was classified in those patients:

- who did not undergo previous lumbar spine operations
- who did not have radiographic evidence of instability
- who had degenerative spondylolisthesis at most grade 1, with no instability, if present
- who had degenerative scoliosis with a curve less than 20°, if present.

In their study, patients with typical lumbar spinal stenosis were treated with decompressive surgery. Complex lumbar spinal stenosis was classified in patients with

- lumbar spine operations with evidence of radiographic instability, if present
- radiographic evidence of postoperative junctional stenosis, if present
- degenerative spondylolisthesis greater than grade 1 with instability, if present
- degenerative scoliosis with a curve greater than 20°, if present.

These patients were treated with decompressive surgery and also underwent surgical stabilization.

NATURAL HISTORY

The natural history of lumbar spinal stenosis is not well understood. A slow progression appears to occur in all affected individuals. Even with significant narrowing, such persons are very unlikely to develop an acute cauda equina syndrome in the absence of significant disc herniation. Anecdotally, the clinical course varies considerably. In most patients, the course is chronic and benign (32,39,40).

Only one study has been concentrated on the natural course of lumbar spinal stenosis. In 1992, Johnsson et al. (40) reported on 32 patients followed up for an average of 49 months (range, 10–103 months). Fifteen percent of the patients were improved, 70% were the same, and 15% were worse. The patients received no specific nonoperative therapy. Two of the patients were not operated on because of advanced cardiovascular disease, and the remainder of the patients refused surgical treatment. No proof of deterioration was found after 4 years, and the authors concluded that the condition of the majority of patients with lumbar stenosis who were treated conservatively remained unchanged over a period of 4 years. However, the patients did not improve either, so surgical decompression may be an option as decompression of the symptomatic level yields a high rate of improvement.

Numerous other nonoperative outcome studies for lumbar spinal stenosis have been published. In 1996, Atlas et al. (41) assessed the outcomes of 81 patients who were treated surgically and 67 patients who were treated conservatively after 12 months. Although the conditions of patients who underwent surgery were worse clinically and radiographically at the start of the study, their results were better after treatment than the results of the patients who were treated conservatively. For 28% of patients who were treated conservatively, pain was better to completely gone, and for 15%, the pain was much worse. In 2000, the same authors (42) reported their results of 4 years' follow-up in their perspective study of surgical or conservative treatment of lumbar spinal stenosis. Among 119 patients, 67 were treated surgically and 52 were treated conservatively. After 4 years, 70% of the surgically treated and 52% of the conservatively treated patients reported that their predominant symptom, either leg or

back pain, was better. Satisfaction of patients with their current state at 4 years was reported by 63% of the surgically treated and 42% of the conservatively treated patients. Surgical treatment remained a significant determinant of 4-year satisfaction. For the conservatively treated patients, there was no significant change in outcomes over 4 years, whereas the initial improvement seen in the surgically treated patients modestly decreased over the subsequent 4 years.

Swezey (43) reported on the outcomes of 47 patients who had been evaluated 5 years earlier for lumbar spinal stenosis. Patients had symptoms of neurogenic claudication, and CT or MRI findings of moderate to severe stenosis (43 patients) or severe spondylosis by plain radiographs (4 patients). Treatments included instruction of ergonomics and flexion exercise, analgesic medications, intermittent pelvic traction (11 patients), and epidural steroids (13 patients). Eleven patients required laminectomy. Of the patients who were treated conservatively, 43% were improved. Symptoms of neurogenic claudication were unchanged in 30%.

Simotas et al. (44) reported 49 patients with lumbar stenosis treated conservatively with an average follow-up of 3 years. At 3 years following treatment, 9 of the 49 patients had undergone surgical intervention. Of the remaining 40 unoperated patients, it is reported that two suffered significant motor deterioration, one of whom still reported overall symptoms as mild improvement, and the other as definite worsening. Five of the 40 unoperated patients reported feeling overall symptoms as probably or definitely worse, 12 reported no change, 11 reported only mild improvement, and 12 reported sustained improvement. Twelve of the 40 unoperated patients also had no pain or only mild pain. The authors concluded that aggressive nonoperative treatment for spinal stenosis remains a reasonable option.

In a randomized study by Amundsen et al. (39), 100 patients with symptomatic lumbar spinal stenosis were given surgical or conservative treatment and followed for 10 years. Nineteen patients with severe symptoms were selected for surgical treatment and 50 patients with moderate symptoms for were chosen for conservative treatment, whereas 31 patients were randomized between the conservative (18 patients) and surgical (13 patients) treatment groups. After a period of 3 months, relief of pain had occurred in most patients. Some had relief earlier, whereas for others it took 1 year. After a period of 4 years, excellent or fair results were found in half of the patients selected for conservative treatment, and in four-fifths of the patients selected for surgery. Patients with an unsatisfactory result from conservative treatment were offered delayed surgery after 3 to 27 months (median, 3.5 months). The treatment result of delayed surgery was essentially similar to that of the initial group. The treatment result for the patients randomized for surgical treatment was considerably better than for the patients randomized for conservative treatment. Clinically significant deterioration of symptoms during the final 6 years of the follow-up period was not observed. Patients with multilevel afflictions that were either surgically treated or not did not have a poorer outcome than those with single-level afflictions. Clinical or radiologic predictors for the outcome were not found. The authors concluded that the outcome was most favorable for surgical treatment, but an initial conservative approach seems advisable for many patients because those with an unsatisfactory result can be treated surgically later, with a good outcome.

As the population becomes older, this condition is encountered more frequently. The diagnosis accuracy has improved and the number of cases detected is increasing. Because of the relative unpredictability of surgical treatment, good knowledge of natural evolution and of the predictive factors influencing the course of the disease is crucial. Unfortunately, and in contrast with numerous surgical series, few studies have dealt with natural evolution. Only one randomized study (39) has compared short- and long-term results of medical versus surgical treatment. Most of these studies are retrospective, with methodologic flaws and are difficult to compare. At the present time no scientifically based recommendations can be made to lumbar spinal stenosis patients at diagnosis. Similarly, predictors of success of medical and surgical treatment still need to be identified. However, results of the studies published suggest that a substantial proportion of patients do not automatically deteriorate and will remain unchanged or even improved by medical means. Randomized studies with the necessary ethical precautions are needed to obtain clear-cut conclusions.

HISTORY AND CLINICAL EVALUATION

Recognition of spinal stenosis depends primarily on the description of the leg symptoms. The history and physical examination are an essential component in the assessment of patients with lumbar spinal stenosis. Physical examination occasionally demonstrates neurologic deficits or exacerbation of symptoms with spinal positioning. However, many patients with spinal stenosis have no abnormal findings on examination. Spinal imaging confirms the clinical impression. Because many people who have no symptoms are found to have radiographic abnormalities, clinical correlation is critical.

Patients with lumbar spinal stenosis usually undergo a "staged" diagnosis (Fig. 48-1). The first diagnostic stage is the physician visit, during which the patient receives a physical examination. Results of the physical are combined with information from the patient history in a preliminary diagnosis. Lumbar spinal stenosis is not definitively diagnosed at this stage, so the diagnostic results are described as "consistent with" spinal stenosis or not consistent with spinal stenosis.

History

Spinal stenosis typically affects persons over 50 years of age (45). It is uncommon in younger people unless they are anatomically predisposed by a congenitally narrowed canal, previous spine trauma or surgery, spondylolisthesis, or even scoliosis. The classic symptom of central canal stenosis is pseudoclaudication, also known as neurogenic claudication (1–3,45–47). Patients typically complain of pain, paresthesia, weakness, or heaviness in the buttocks radiating into the lower extremities with walking or prolonged standing, relieved with flexion or sitting. Though many patients have significant lumbar pain due to degenerative joint and disc changes, most have more lower extremity discomfort rather than spinal pain. The most important aspect of neurogenic claudication is the relationship of symptoms to posture. Symptoms occur with spinal extension and are relieved in flexion. Patients usually have no symptoms or have minimal discomfort when seated or supine. They can walk longer distances with less pain in a forward flexed position, such as when using a grocery cart while shopping (the "grocery cart sign"). They may be able to exercise using a stationary bicycle in the seated flexed position for a much longer time than when walking in the erect position on a treadmill. In a review of 68 patients with myelographically proven, surgically confirmed spinal stenosis (47), the most common symptoms were pseudoclaudication and standing discomfort (94%), followed by numbness (63%) and weakness (43%). Symptoms were bilateral in 68%. Discomfort was felt both above and below the knee in 78%, in the buttocks or thigh in 15%, and below the knee in 7%. Historic features correlating most strongly with a confirmed diagnosis of spinal stenosis (likelihood ratio 3:2) include age greater than 65 years, severe lower extremity pain, and absence of pain when seated (13).

Physical Examination

The most important features of the physical examination are the motor, reflex, and the palpatory examinations. The physical examination in patients with lumbar canal stenosis is frequently normal or demonstrates only nonspecific findings. Many older people have reduced spinal mobility, with or without spinal canal stenosis. Extension is usually more limited than flexion (12,15). Patients with stenosis often have lumbar, paraspinal, or gluteal tenderness, probably related to underlying degenerative changes, muscle spasms, and poor posture. Some assume a characteristic "simian stance", with their hips and knees slightly flexed and the trunk stooped forward (45). This semiflexed posture allows patients to stand or walk for longer distances. Hamstring tightness is often present and may produce a false-positive straight leg-raise test. The neurologic examination typically is normal or reveals only subtle abnormalities such as mild weakness, sensory changes, and reflex abnormalities. This is

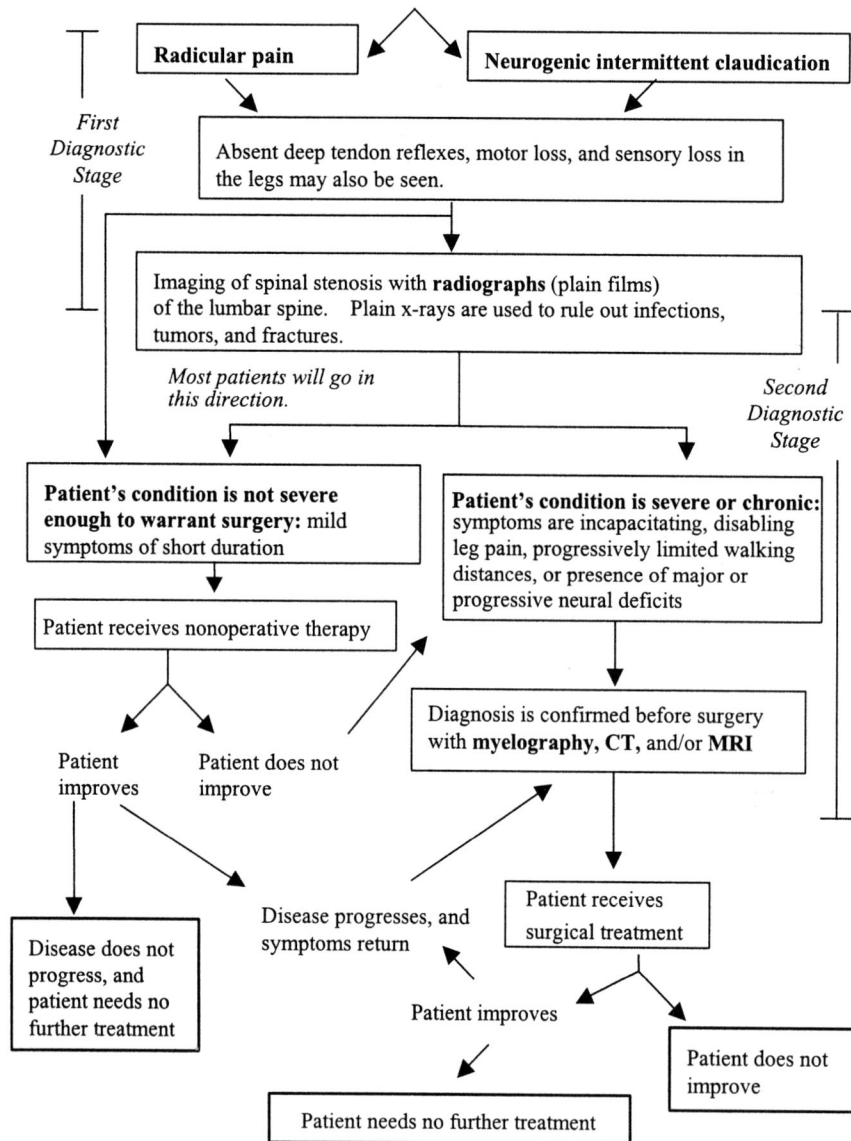

FIG. 48-1. Diagnosis and treatment of lumbar spinal stenosis. Clinical symptoms at the time of presentation to the physician. Patient may have one or all of the symptoms.

particularly true if the patient has rested in the seated position before the physical examination begins. These subtle findings may be unmasked if the patient is examined after walking until developing leg and buttock symptoms similar to the presenting complaint (46).

Ankle reflexes are diminished in 43% to 65% of patients, while knee reflexes are abnormal in 18% to 42% (13,15). The straight leg-raising test and other nerve root tension signs are usually negative unless there is concomitant disc herniation. A careful motor examination should be done. Leg weakness is generally mild and overwhelmingly in the distribution of the L4, L5, or S1 nerve roots. Objective evidence of subtle weakness can usually be demonstrated in about 50% of persons with spinal stenosis (2). Weakness of the muscles innervated by the

L5 nerve root is the most common finding (46), and weakness of great toe extensors (extensor hallucis longus) and hip abductors should be sought, the latter by the Trendelenburg test (46).

The Trendelenburg test is performed by having the patient stand on one leg; if the gluteus medius is not functional or is denervated, the pelvis drops on the side opposite the damaged muscle. This is shown clinically by an abnormal, waddling gait called the "Trendelenburg gait", caused by trying to compensate for a drooping pelvis. The gait should be carefully observed. Difficulty in walking on the toes suggests S1 root involvement. Difficulty with heel walking suggests L4 or L5 nerve dysfunction. Sensory abnormalities may be present in 46% to 51% of preoperative spinal stenosis patients (2,12).

Katz et al. (13) found a positive lumbar extension test to be strongly predictive of imaging confirmed spinal stenosis. This test is performed by asking the standing patient to hyperextend the lumbar spine for 30 to 60 seconds. A positive test is defined by reproduction of the buttock or leg pain. Katz et al. (13) examined the value of the history and physical examination in the diagnosis of degenerative lumbar spinal stenosis. In this study, 93 patients over 40 years of age with symptoms of low back pain were examined by attending physicians who were then asked the extent to which they were certain the patient had lumbar spinal stenosis. The diagnostic impressions of expert clinicians and imaging, when available, were used as a reference standard to evaluate the attending physician's diagnosis. Severe lower extremity pain, absence of pain when seated, a wide-based gait, thigh pain following 30 seconds of lumbar extension, and neuromuscular deficits were all strongly associated with patients with lumbar spinal stenosis. No pain when seated and wide-based gait had the highest specificity, 93% and 97%, respectively. The highest sensitivity came from age greater than 65 (77%), pain below buttocks (88%), and no pain with flexion (79%).

Fritz (48) has developed a treadmill test as a clinical diagnostic tool for the differentiation of neurogenic claudication due to lumbar spinal stenosis from other pathologies that may produce similar symptoms. Spinal extension and weight bearing that occur during walking narrow the spinal canal and exacerbate the symptoms of lumbar spinal stenosis. Spinal flexion or nonweight-bearing postures that occur while sitting increase the dimensions of the spinal canal and reduce symptoms. The treadmill test involves having the patient walk on a level surface and an inclined surface. The time until onset of symptoms, total walking time, and time until symptoms return to baseline are recorded for each surface. Walking on an inclined plane produces spinal flexion and may be better tolerated by patients with lumbar spinal stenosis. The treadmill test was evaluated using 45 subjects with low back pain of varying etiologies and self-reported limitations in walking. Diagnostic images with MRI or CT were used as the gold standard for diagnosis. Twenty-six of the subjects were diagnosed by imaging as being stenotic. Self-reported sitting to relieve symptoms was significantly related to diagnosis. The sensitivity of this self-reported measure was 88.5% [95% confidence interval (CI) of 76.2 to 100], but specificity was 38.9% (95% CI of 16.4 to 61.4). For the treadmill test, earlier onset of symptoms with level walking, greater total walking time during inclined walking, and prolonged recovery after level walking were significantly related to a diagnosis of lumbar spinal stenosis. The sensitivity and specificity for earlier onset of symptoms with level walking were 68.0% (95% CI of 49.7 to 86.3) and 83.3% (95% CI of 66.1 to 100), respectively; for larger total walking time during

inclined walking they were 50.0% (95% CI of 37.5 to 62.5) and 92.3% (95% CI of 77.8 to 100), respectively; and for prolonged recovery after level walking they were 81.8% (95% CI of 5.7 to 97.9) and 68.4% (95% CI of 47.5 to 89.3), respectively. The authors concluded that a two-stage treadmill test might be more useful in the differential diagnosis of lumbar spinal stenosis compared to patients' self-reports of posture.

Use of the treadmill-bicycle test for the differential diagnosis of neurogenic claudication was also examined by Tenhula et al. (49). In their study, 32 patients with documented lumbar spinal stenosis were evaluated before and after surgery. Patients were found to have a significant increase in their symptoms from the start to the end of the treadmill test but fewer patients were found to have significant symptoms on bicycle testing. Two years after surgery, patients had an improvement in their walking ability on treadmill testing, but showed no improvement in their ability to bicycle. The authors believe the treadmill-bicycle test may be a useful tool for the differential diagnosis of neurogenic claudication.

CENTRAL CANAL STENOSIS VERSUS LATERAL STENOSIS

Symptoms of pseudoclaudication are associated primarily with central lumbar stenosis. In contrast, patients with purely lateral recess stenosis:

- usually do not develop symptoms of neurogenic claudication (15)
- typically have radicular symptoms in a specific dermatomal pattern (30)
- often have pain at rest, at night, and with the Valsalva maneuver (30)
- tend to be younger (mean age 41 years) than patients with central canal stenosis (mean age 65 years) (15).

DIFFERENTIAL DIAGNOSIS

The differential diagnosis is broad, and many conditions may be ruled out with a thorough evaluation (Fig. 48-2). Peripheral neuropathy, arteriovascular disease, and hip arthritis are common entities with similar symptoms. In older patients with back or leg pain, diagnostic possibilities differ from those in younger patients; nonmechanical causes of back pain such as malignancy, infection, or abdominal aortic aneurysm are more common in older patients than in younger patients (11,14).

Malignancy

Red flags that should raise the suspicion of underlying malignancy include significant weight loss, intractable night pain unrelieved by change in posture or pain medicine, or history of malignancy (50).

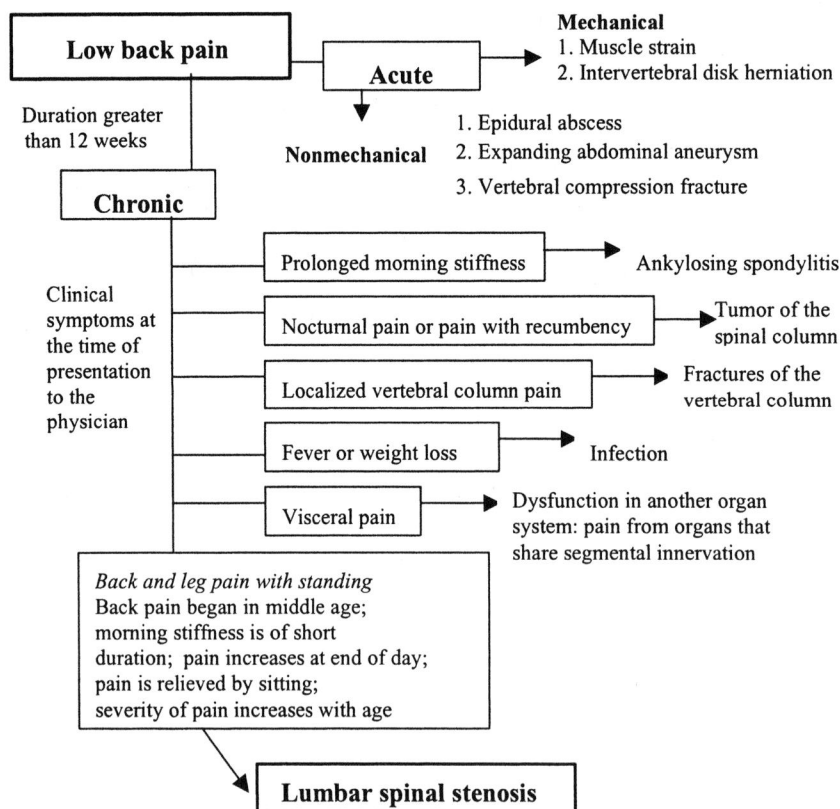

FIG. 48-2. Differential diagnosis of lumbar spinal stenosis. *Arrows* indicate the possible or most likely condition associated with the described symptoms. Many of these symptoms overlap, and an individual may need additional testing to determine the exact cause of low back pain.

Infection

Fever with localized back tenderness, recent systemic infection, or history of an invasive spinal procedure should raise the possibility of a spinal infection (11).

Vascular Claudication

When evaluating leg pain in older adults, neurogenic claudication must be distinguished from vascular claudication (Table 48-1).

Peripheral Neuropathy

Peripheral neuropathy may also superficially mimic features of spinal stenosis. However, patients with periph-

eral neuropathy usually have a stocking-glove distribution of pain or paresthesia. There may be a bilateral symmetric reflex loss. Vibratory sensation is frequently diminished (46). Numbness is typically constant with peripheral neuropathy.

Hip Disease

Hip disease may produce gait difficulty and leg symptoms. A careful examination of the hips and surrounding soft tissue should be done to exclude significant hip arthritis and gluteal or trochanteric bursitis.

Although clinicians consider a combination of results of the history and physical examination and imaging findings to be the most effective means of diagnosing lumbar spinal

TABLE 48-1. *Findings in neurogenic claudication and vascular claudication*

Finding	Neurogenic claudication	Vascular claudication
Symptoms with walking	Yes	Yes
Symptoms with standing	Yes	No
Variable walking distance before symptoms	Yes	No
Relief with flexion	Yes	No
Relief with sitting	Yes	Yes
Peripheral pulses diminished	No	Yes

stenosis, no objective criteria for using the history and physical examination have been reported. In addition, there are no reported clinical trials of the effectiveness of such a composite diagnosis. The only quantitative evidence correlating diagnostic information with outcomes is for the imaging findings. Clinical decision making should be based on a collection of data, including the history and physical findings, functional status, imaging and electrodiagnostic studies, and other adjunctive studies.

REFERENCES

1. Spivak J. Degenerative spinal stenosis. J Bone Joint Surg 1998:80: 1053–1066.
2. Katz J, Dalgas M, Stucki G, et al. Diagnosis of lumbar canal stenosis. Rheum Dis Clin North Am 1994:20:471–483.
3. Garfin S, Herkowitz H, Mirkovic S. Spinal stenosis. AAOS Instr Course Lect 2000;49:361–374.
4. Mixter WJ, Barr JS. Rupture of the intervertebral disc with involvement of the spinal canal. N Engl J Med 1934;211:210–215.
5. Verbiest H. A radicular syndrome from developmental narrowing of the lumbar vertebral canal. J. Bone Joint Surg Br 1954;36:230–237.
6. Boden S, Davis D, Dina T, et al. Abnormal magnetic resonance scans of the lumbar spine in asymptomatic subjects. J Bone Joint Surg Am 1990;72:403–408.
7. Ullrich CG, Binet EF, Sanecki MG, et al. Quantitative assessment of the lumbar spinal canal by computed tomography. Radiology 1980; 134:137–143.
8. Wiesel SW, Tsourmas N, Feffer HL. A study of computer-assisted tomography. I. The incidence of positive CAT scans in an asymptomatic group of patients. Spine 1984;9(6):549–551.
9. Pheasant HC, Dyck P. Failed lumbar disc surgery: Cause, assessment, treatment. Clin Orthop 1982;164:93.
10. Ray CD. Extensive lumbar decompression: Patient selection and results. In: White AH, Rothman RH, Ray CD, eds. Lumbar Spine Surgery. St. Louis; C.V. Mosby Co., 1987.
11. Deyo RA, Cherkin DC, Loeser JD. Morbidity and mortality in association with operations on the lumbar spine. The influence of age, diagnosis, and procedure. J Bone Joint Surg Am 1992;74(4): 536–543.
12. Johnsson B, Stromqvist B. Symptoms and signs in degeneration of the lumbar spine. A prospective, consecutive study of 300 operated patients. J Bone Joint Surg Br 1993;75:381–385.
13. Katz JN, Dalgas M, Stucki G. Degenerative lumbar spinal stenosis. Diagnostic value of the history and physical examination. Arthritis Rheum 1995;38(9): 1236–1241.
14. Mazanec D. Diagnosis and management of low back pain in older adults. Clin Geriatr 2000:8:63–71.
15. Turner J, Ersek M, Herron L, et al. Surgery for lumbar spinal stenosis. Attempted meta-analysis of the literature. Spine 1992;17:1–8.
16. Hawkes CH, Roberts GM. Neurologic and vascular claudication. J Neurol Sci 1978;38:337–345.
17. Postacchini F. Surgical management of lumbar spinal stenosis. Spine 1999;24:1043–1047.
18. Arnoldi CC, Brodsky AE, Cauchoix J, et al. Lumbar spinal stenosis and nerve root entrapment syndromes: definition and classification. Clin Orthop 1976;115:4–5.
19. De Villiers PD, Booysen EL. Fibrous spinal stenosis: a report on 850 myelograms with a water-soluble contrast medium. Clin Orthop 1976; 115:140–144.
20. Fanuele JC, Birkmeyer NJ, Abdu WA, et al. The impact of spinal problems on the health status of patients: have we underestimated the effect? Spine 2000;25(12):1509–1514.
21. Hart LG, Deyo RA, Cherkin DC. Physician office visits for low back pain. Frequency, clinical evaluation, and treatment patterns from a U.S. national survey. Spine 1995;20(1):11–19.
22. Long DM, BenDebba M, Torgerson WS, et al. Persistent back pain and

sciatica in the United States: patient characteristics. J Spinal Disord 1996;9(1):40–58.
23. Roberson GH, Llewellyn HJ, Taveras JM. The narrow lumbar spinal canal syndrome. Radiology 1973;107:89–97.
24. Rosenberg NJ. Degenerative spondylolisthesis: predisposing factors. J Bone Joint Surg 1975;57A:467–474.
25. Gunzburg R, Szpalski M, eds. Lumbar spinal stenosis. Hagerstown, MD: Lippincott Williams & Wilkins, 1999.
26. Woolsey RM. Lumbar spinal stenosis. Semin Neurol 1986;6(4): 385–389.
27. Bolander NF, Schonstrom NSR, Spengler DM. Role of computed tomography and myelography in the diagnosis of central spinal stenosis. J Bone Joint Surg 1985;67A:240–246.
28. Carrera CF, Williams AL. Current concepts in evaluation of lumbar facet joints. CRC Crit Rev Diagn Imaging 1985;21:85–104.
29. Verbiest H. The significance and principles of computerized axial tomography in idiopathic developmental stenosis of the bony lumbar vertebral canal. Spine 1979;4(4):369–378.
30. Jenis LG, An HS. Spine update: lumbar foraminal stenosis. Spine 2000;25(3):389–394.
31. Lee CK, Rauschning W, Glenn W. Lateral lumbar spinal canal stenosis: classification, pathologic anatomy and surgical decompression. Spine 1988;13(3):313–320.
32. Fritz JM, Delitto A, Welch WC. Lumbar spinal stenosis: a review of current concepts in evaluation, management, and outcome measurements. Arch Phys Med Rehabil 1998;79(6):700–708.
33. Jane JA Sr, Jane JA Jr, Helm GA, et al. Acquired lumbar spinal stenosis. Clin Neurosurg 1996;43:275–299.
34. Mirkovic S, Garfin SR. Spinal stenosis: history and physical examination. Instr Course Lect 1994;43:435–440.
35. MacNab I. Backache. Baltimore: Williams & Wilkins, 1977.
36. Crock H. Normal, pathologic anatomy of the lumbar spinal nerve root canals. J Bone Joint Surg [Br] 1981;63:487–490.
37. Hansraj KK, Cammisa FP, O'Leary PF, et al. Decompressive surgery for typical lumbar spinal stenosis. Clin Orthop 2001;384:10–17.
38. Hansraj KK, O'Leary PF, Cammisa FP, et al. Decompressive surgery for typical lumbar spinal stenosis. Clin Orthop 2001;384:18–25.
39. Amundsen T, Weber H, Nordal H, et al. Lumbar spinal stenosis: conservative or surgical management? A prospective 10-year study. Spine 2000;25:1424–1436.
40. Johnsson KE, Rosen I, Uden A. The natural course of lumbar spinal stenosis. Clin Orthop 1992;279:82–86.
41. Atlas SJ, Deyo RA, Keller RB, et al. The Maine Lumbar Spine Study: Part III. 1-year outcomes of surgical and nonsurgical management of lumbar spinal stenosis. Spine 1996;21:1787–1795.
42. Atlas SJ, Keller RB, Robson D. Surgical and nonsurgical management of lumbar spinal stenosis: four-year outcomes from the Maine Lumbar Spine Study. Spine 2000;25(5):556–562.
43. Swezey RL. Outcomes for lumbar stenosis: a 5-year followup study. J Clin Rheumatol 1996;2(3):129–134.
44. Simotas AC, Dorey FJ, Hansraj KK. Nonoperative treatment for lumbar spinal stenosis. Clinical and outcome results and a 3-year survivorship analysis. Spine 2000;15:25(2):197–203.
45. Bridwell K. Lumbar spinal stenosis. Diagnosis, management, and treatment. Clin Geriatr Med 1994;10:677–701.
46. Arbit E, Pannullo S. Lumbar stenosis—a clinical review. Clin Orthop 2001;384:137–143.
47. Hall S, Bartleson J, Onofrio B, et al. Lumbar spinal stenosis—clinical features, diagnostic procedures, and result of surgical treatment in 68 patients. Ann Intern Med 1985;103:271–275.
48. Fritz JM, Erhard RE, Delitto A, et al. Preliminary results of the use of a two-stage treadmill test as a clinical diagnostic tool in the differential diagnosis of lumbar spinal stenosis. J Spinal Disord 1997;10(5): 410–416.
49. Tenhula J, Lenke LG, Bridwell KH, et al. Prospective functional evaluation of the surgical treatment of neurogenic claudication in patients with lumbar spinal stenosis. J Spinal Disord 2000;13(4):276–282.
50. Deyo R, Diehl A. Cancer as a cause of back pain—frequency, clinical presentation, and diagnostic strategies. J Gen Intern Med 1988;3: 230–238.

CHAPTER 49

Imaging of Spinal Stenosis and Degenerative Lumbar Spondylolisthesis with Stenosis

Donald L. Renfrew and Kenneth B. Heithoff

There is no universally accepted definition of the term spinal stenosis. Gunzburg et al. (1), in an article correlating computed tomography (CT) findings with decompression surgery, state, "Lumbar spinal stenosis is . . . a clinical condition and not a radiologic finding or diagnosis." Nonetheless, the same authors also affirm, "CT or MRI [magnetic resonance imaging] combined with myelography has become the standard tool for iconographic evaluation of (spinal stenosis)." In an article on conservative treatment of spinal stenosis published in 2000, Simotas et al. (2) state, "No validated system for radiographic rating of stenosis exists." Although we recognize that this controversy exists, we offer this chapter to explain and illustrate our approach to the imaging of spinal stenosis.

Many authors (3–5) use the term stenosis to signify *any* reduction of size of the spinal canal or neural foramina, whether from chronic bone, cartilage, or degenerative changes or from acute disc herniation, tumor, or epidural abscess. Others (6,7) reserve use of the term stenosis for bony reductions in canal size. Most clinical cases of spinal stenosis follow from degenerative changes of the intervertebral discs and facet joints. Although osteophytes along the disc and facet joints contribute to narrowing, degenerative soft-tissue abnormalities usually account for more of the narrowing than do bony abnormalities (5). Degenerative soft-tissue abnormalities include thickening of the ligamentum flavum (8), bulging of the disc, and capsular swelling of the facet joints. Therefore, we use the term stenosis for fixed bony or relatively fixed soft-tissue reductions in canal size. Used in this manner, the term is descriptive and does not name a disease process. Most cases of stenosis defined in this way result from degenerative disc bulging, osteophytic spurring, and facet arthropathy (Fig. 49-1), but stenosis may be caused by any of several other processes. Examples include foraminal stenosis from scoliosis (Fig. 49-2) or lytic spondylolisthesis (Fig. 49-3), and spinal canal stenosis from closed arch spondylolisthesis (Fig. 49-4) or after surgery (Fig. 49-5).

CLASSIFICATION AND NOMENCLATURE

Classification systems of stenosis may use cause (e.g., congenital, degenerative, or combined) or location (e.g., spinal canal, subarticular recess, and foramen) (Fig. 49-6). Another method of classification is by severity (mild, moderate, or severe). When reporting an imaging study, we grade spinal canal, subarticular, and foraminal stenosis not only relative to other levels in the same patient (and, when necessary because of an inherently small canal, an idealized norm from other patients), but also taking into account the degree of neural compression (Table 49-1; Figs. 49-1 to 49-5, 49-7) (9). Reliance solely on percentages of narrowing overrates the severity of stenosis in patients with inherently large spaces (canals, subarticular recesses, and foramina) while underrating the severity of stenosis in patients with small spaces (Tables 49-2 to 49-4). In addition to grading the degree of stenosis, note may be made in appropriate cases that the spinal canal has a trefoil configuration, a characteristic of congenital or developmental (short pedicle) spinal stenosis (Fig. 49-8).

Grading spinal canal stenosis and lumbar foraminal stenosis and neural compression may be done relatively easily on most scans. Grading lumbar subarticular recess stenosis is more difficult because of either scan quality (for technical or patient related reasons) or crowding of neural structures. As an alternative to grading subarticular stenosis using a mild–moderate–severe scale, it may be preferable to note simply that narrowing is present, and estimate whether compression of the associated neural structure is likely or not.

(Text continued on page 479)

472

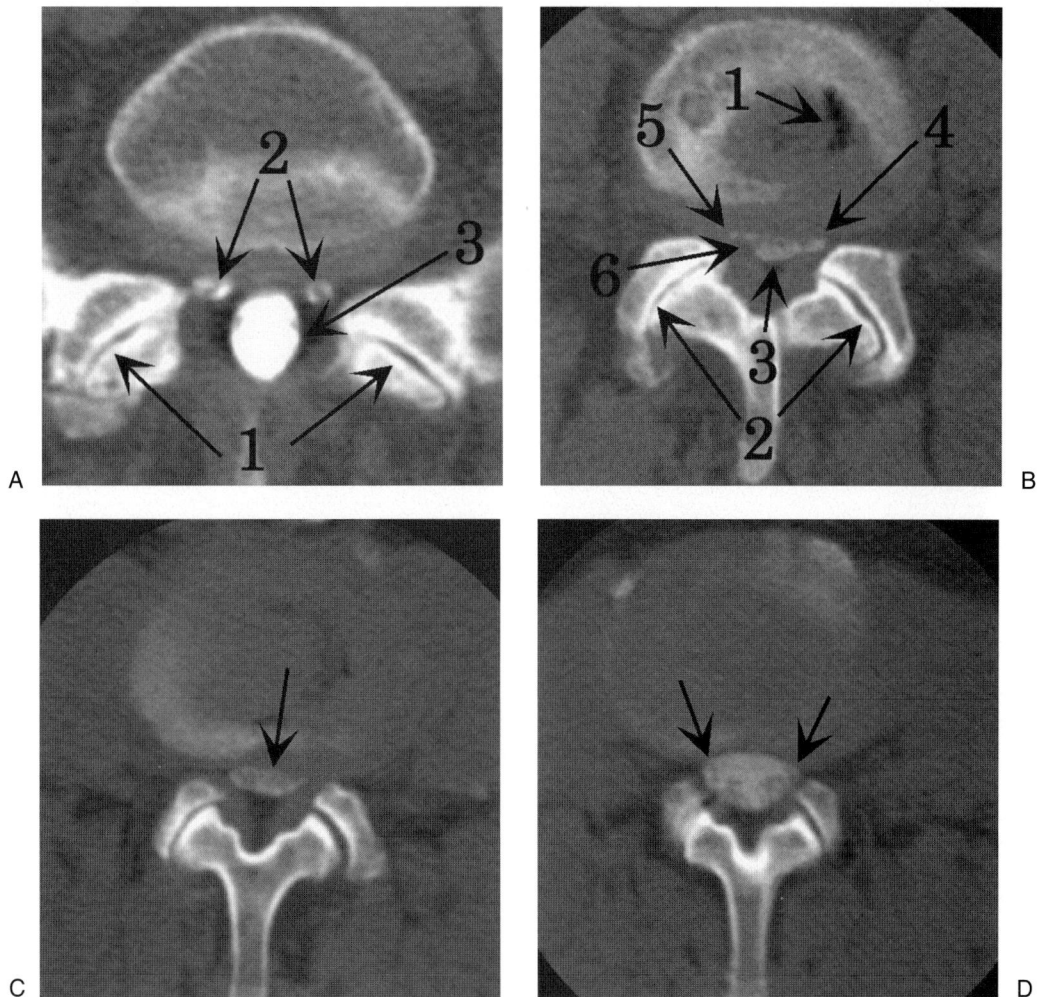

FIG. 49-1. Degenerative spinal canal and subarticular recess stenosis demonstrated on a myelogram-computed tomography (myelo-CT). This 45-year-old man had low back and bilateral leg pain. **A:** Axial 3-mm CT at the L5-S1 level following injection of intrathecal contrast demonstrates moderate facet arthropathy *(arrow 1)* but no spinal canal or subarticular recess stenosis. The degenerative abnormalities do not distort the S1 nerve root sleeves *(arrow 2)* or thecal sac *(arrow 3)*. **B:** Axial 3-mm CT at the L4-5 level following intrathecal contrast demonstrates degenerative disc bulging with a vacuum phenomenon *(arrow 1)* and bilateral severe facet arthropathy *(arrow 2)*. There is resultant severe (>50% antero-posterior diameter reduction) spinal canal stenosis *(arrow 3)* and severe left *(arrow 4)* and moderate right *(arrow 5)* subarticular recess stenosis. A focal abnormality of the facet joint capsule on the right *(arrow 6)* further narrows the subarticular recess; this may represent a small synovial cyst. **C:** Axial 3-mm CT at the L3-4 level following intrathecal contrast demonstrates findings similar (but less severe) to those seen at the L4-5 level, with degenerative disc bulging and facet arthropathy combining to cause severe spinal canal and subarticular recess stenosis *(arrow)*. **D:** Axial 3-mm CT at the L2-3 level following intrathecal contrast demonstrates that the spinal canal and subarticular recesses *(arrows)* have normal caliber at this level. (From Renfrew DL. Atlas of spine imaging. Philadelphia: Elsevier, 2003, with permission.)

A

B

C

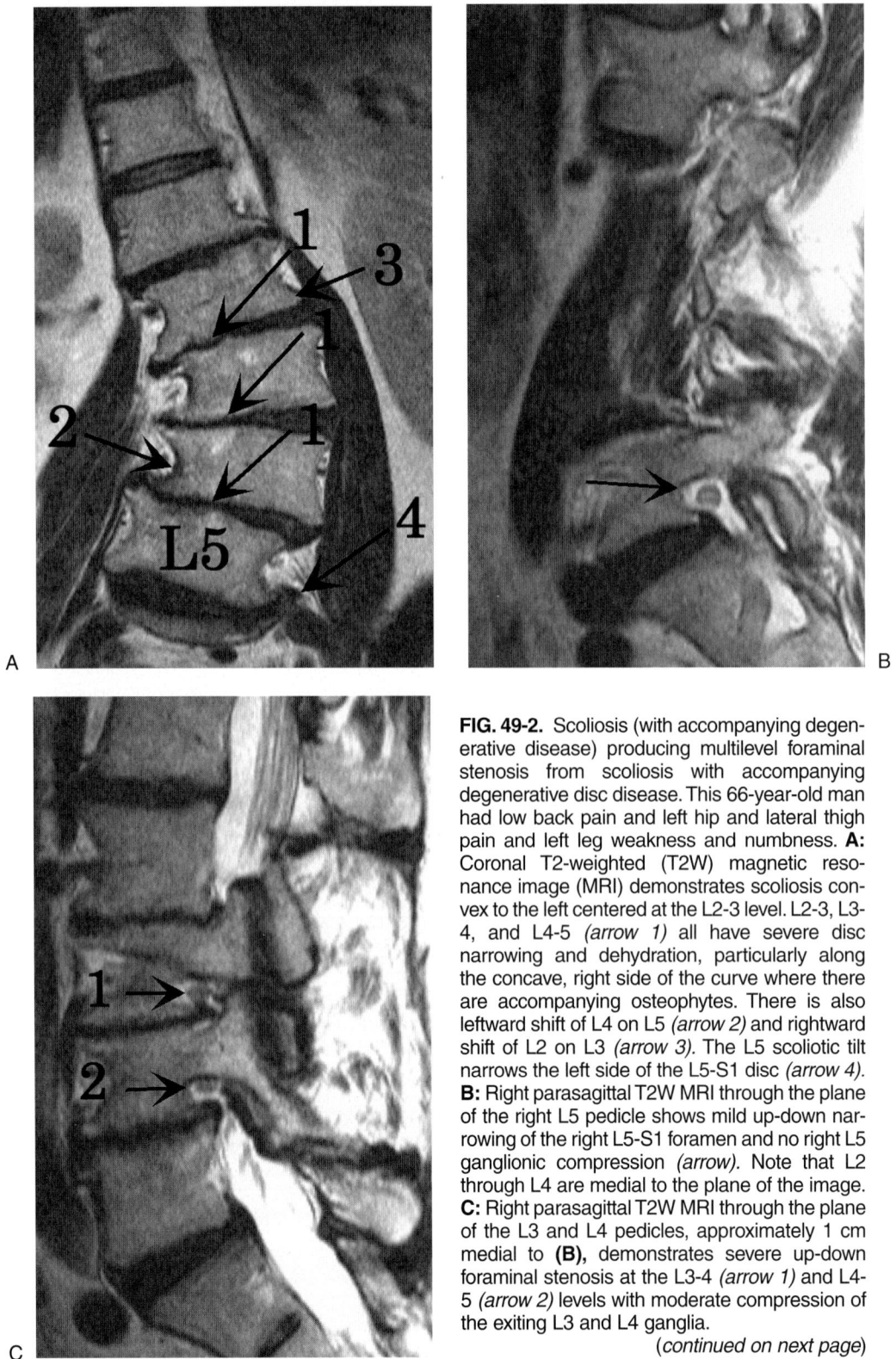

FIG. 49-2. Scoliosis (with accompanying degenerative disease) producing multilevel foraminal stenosis from scoliosis with accompanying degenerative disc disease. This 66-year-old man had low back pain and left hip and lateral thigh pain and left leg weakness and numbness. **A:** Coronal T2-weighted (T2W) magnetic resonance image (MRI) demonstrates scoliosis convex to the left centered at the L2-3 level. L2-3, L3-4, and L4-5 *(arrow 1)* all have severe disc narrowing and dehydration, particularly along the concave, right side of the curve where there are accompanying osteophytes. There is also leftward shift of L4 on L5 *(arrow 2)* and rightward shift of L2 on L3 *(arrow 3)*. The L5 scoliotic tilt narrows the left side of the L5-S1 disc *(arrow 4)*. **B:** Right parasagittal T2W MRI through the plane of the right L5 pedicle shows mild up-down narrowing of the right L5-S1 foramen and no right L5 ganglionic compression *(arrow)*. Note that L2 through L4 are medial to the plane of the image. **C:** Right parasagittal T2W MRI through the plane of the L3 and L4 pedicles, approximately 1 cm medial to **(B),** demonstrates severe up-down foraminal stenosis at the L3-4 *(arrow 1)* and L4-5 *(arrow 2)* levels with moderate compression of the exiting L3 and L4 ganglia.

(*continued on next page*)

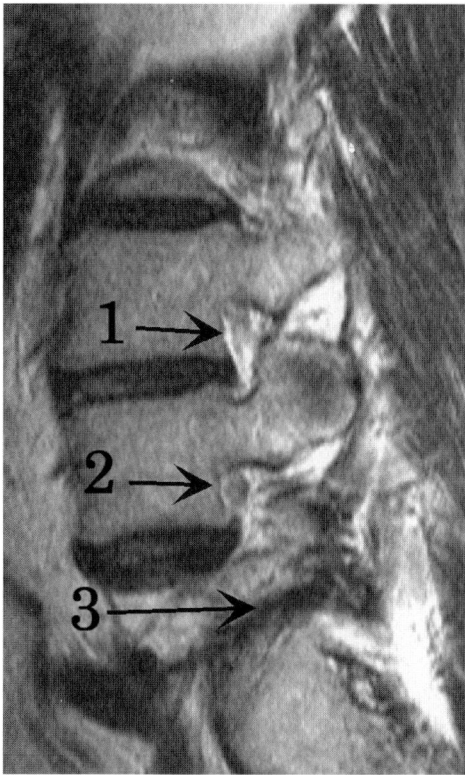

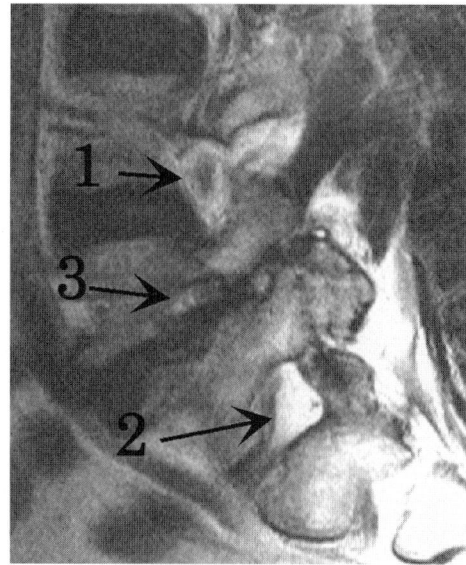

FIG. 49-3. Lytic spondylolisthesis with severe up-down foraminal stenosis. This 71-year-old man had right back pain and right leg tingling. This patient had 20% lytic spondylolisthesis and severe loss of disc height and hydration at L4-5. Right parasagittal T2-weighted (T2W) magnetic resonance image (MRI) at the level of the neural foramina shows normal up-down dimension of the L3-4 *(arrow 1)* and L5-S1 *(arrow 2)* foramina with severe up-down narrowing of L4-5 *(arrow 3)* foramen with associated moderate compression of the exiting L4 ganglion. (From Renfrew DL. Atlas of spine imaging. Philadelphia: Elsevier, 2003, with permission.)

FIG. 49-2. *(continued).* **D:** Left parasagittal T2W MRI through the plane of the left L4 and L5 pedicles, on the convex side of the curve, demonstrates little narrowing of the L3-4 *(arrow 1)* and L4-5 *(arrow 2)* neural foramina. However, the L5-S1 neural foramen is severely stenotic *(arrow 3),* with abutment of the L5 pedicle and sacral ala and resulting severe compression of the L5 ganglion. (From Renfrew DL. Atlas of spine imaging. Philadelphia: Elsevier, 2003, with permission.)

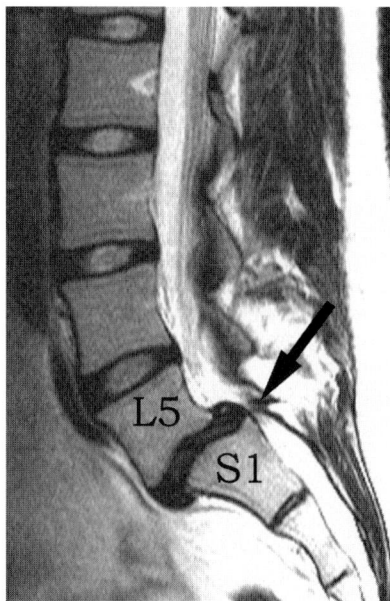

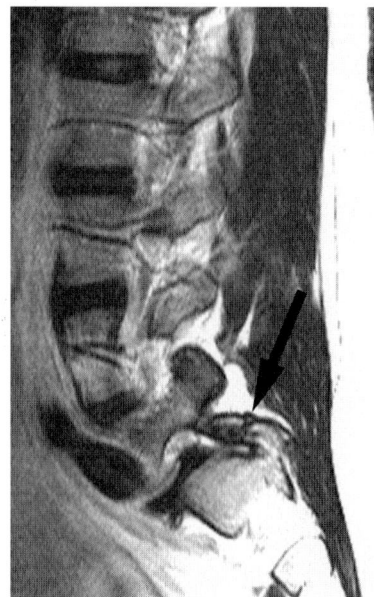

FIG. 49-4. Spinal canal stenosis from closed arch spondylolisthesis. This 25-year-old man had low back and bilateral leg pain. **A:** Sagittal T2-weighted (T2W) magnetic resonance image (MRI) demonstrates 40% spondylolisthesis of L5 on S1. The posterior elements of L5 are directly adjacent to the dorsal L5-S1 disc margin and dorsal superior aspect of the S1 vertebra, causing severe spinal canal stenosis *(arrow).* **B:** Parasagittal T2W MRI demonstrates a dysplastic (but otherwise intact) L5 pars *(arrow).* Usually, spondylolisthesis in young people is associated with pars defects that allow the posterior elements to remain in place while the remainder of the vertebra subluxes anteriorly, resulting in no spinal canal stenosis. In this case, the intact pars resulted in forward movement of the posterior elements as well, causing severe spinal canal stenosis.

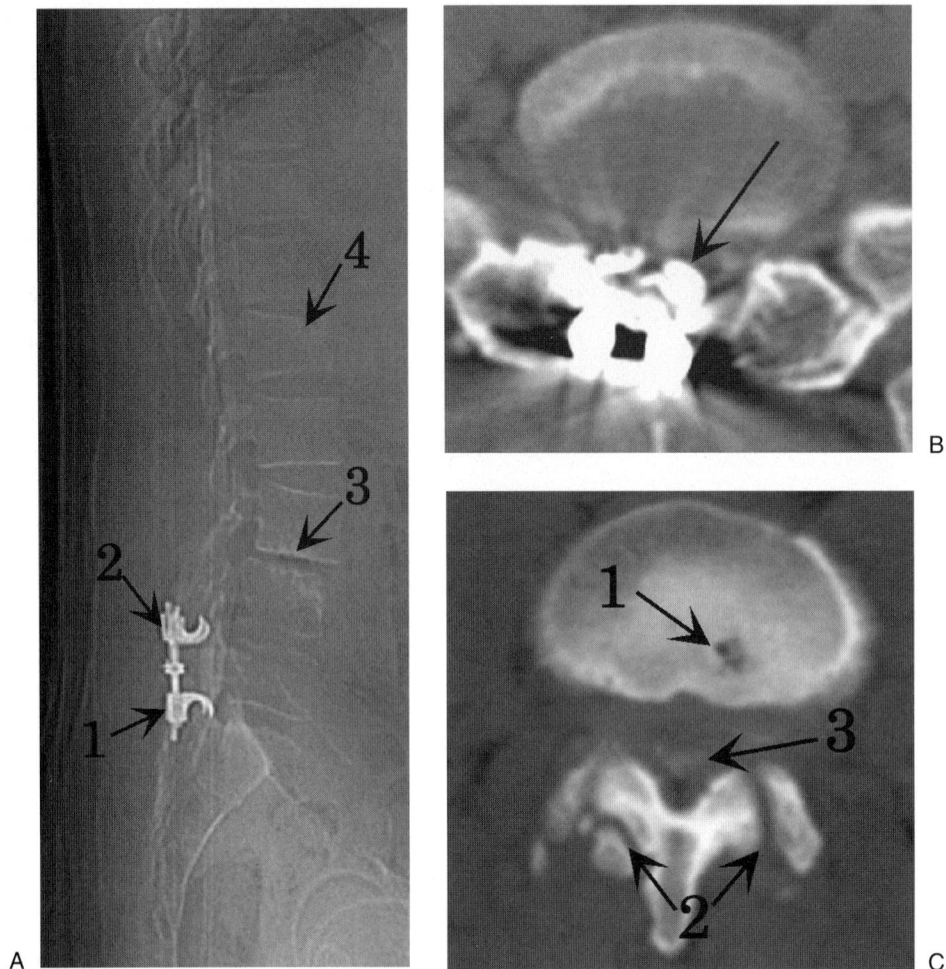

FIG. 49-5. Spinal canal stenosis following surgery, with additional adjacent segment degenerative stenosis. This 43-year-old man had undergone remote posterior fusion with instrumentation at the L5-S1 level. The patient returned with low back pain with lower extremity pain on ambulation. **A:** A lateral scout digital radiograph from myelo-CT (myelography-computed tomography) study demonstrates posterior hardware with two sets of paired laminar hooks. The lower set is over the S1 laminae *(arrow 1)* and the upper set beneath the L4 laminae *(arrow 2)*. Also noted is L3-4 degenerative disc narrowing with a vacuum phenomenon *(arrow 3)* and 15% degenerative spondylolisthesis, and wedging of L1 *(arrow 4)*. **B:** Axial 3-mm myelo-CT image at the L5-S1 intervertebral disc level demonstrates solid dorsal fusion, posterior instrumentation, and severe spinal canal stenosis at the level of the laminar hooks *(arrow)*. **C:** Axial 3-mm myelo-CT image through the L3-4 (superior adjacent segment) demonstrates degenerative disc disease with a vacuum phenomenon *(arrow 1)* and disc bulging combining with severe facet arthropathy *(arrow 2)* and degenerative spondylolisthesis to produce severe spinal canal and subarticular recess stenosis *(arrow 3)*. The patient tolerated the spinal canal stenosis at L5-S1 relatively well until development of adjacent segment degenerative stenosis at L3-4. (From Renfrew DL. Atlas of spine imaging. Philadelphia: Elsevier, 2003, with permission.)

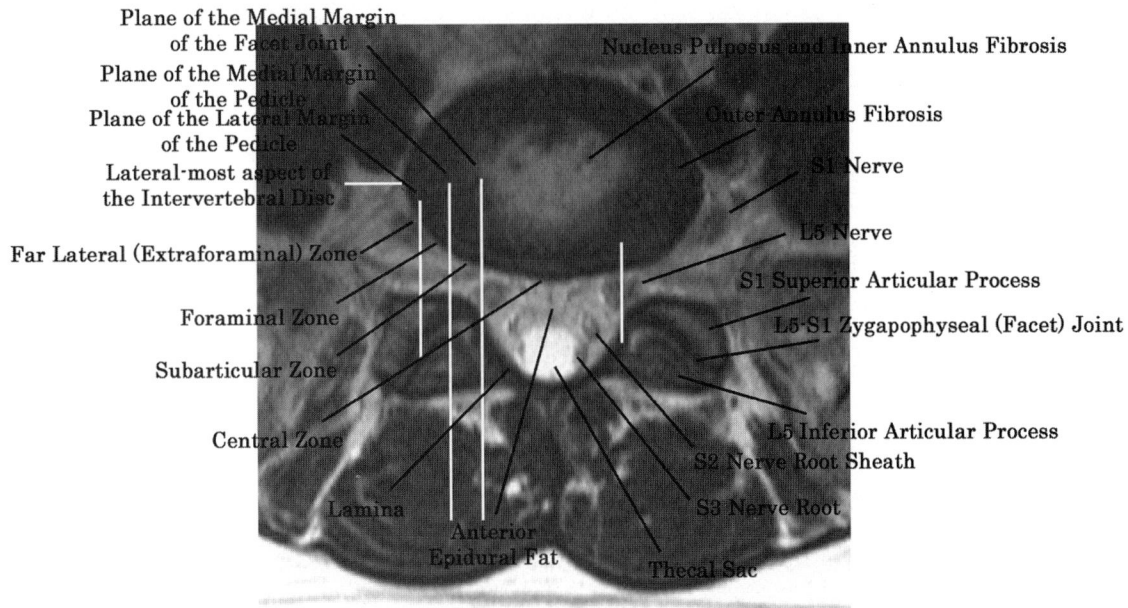

FIG. 49-6. Illustration demonstrating anatomic nomenclature. Axial magnetic resonance imaging at the L5-S1 level illustrating anatomic terms. The spinal canal (also called the central zone) is bounded anteriorly by the posterior disc margin, posteriorly by the laminae, and laterally by a plane drawn through the medial margin of the facet (zygapophyseal) joint. The subarticular recess (also called the subarticular zone) is bounded anteriorly by the disc margin, posteriorly by the superior articular facet of the S1 level, medially by a plane drawn through the medial margin of the facet joint, and laterally by another plane drawn through the medial margin of the pedicle. The foramen (also called the foraminal zone) is bounded anteriorly by the disc margin, posteriorly by the S1 superior articular process, medially by a plane drawn through the medial margin of the pedicle, and laterally through another plane drawn through the lateral margin of the pedicle. Note that the foramen also has a superior margin (the inferior aspect of the L5 pedicle) and an inferior margin (the superior aspect of the S1 pedicle), but that the subarticular space and spinal canal have no superior and inferior margins, although discussion of these spaces is generally about their configuration at the level of the disc. Also note that the lateral recess is defined as the space medial to the pedicle, and thus does not exist at the level of the disc, spinal canal, subarticular recess, or foramen (where most stenosis occurs). (From Renfrew DL. Atlas of spine imaging. Philadelphia: Elsevier, 2003, with permission.)

TABLE 49-1. *Neural compression definitions*

Term	Definition
Mild	75%–99% of normal diameter of the structure is maintained
Moderate	50%–74% of the normal diameter of the structure is maintained
Severe	<50% of the normal diameter of the structure is maintained

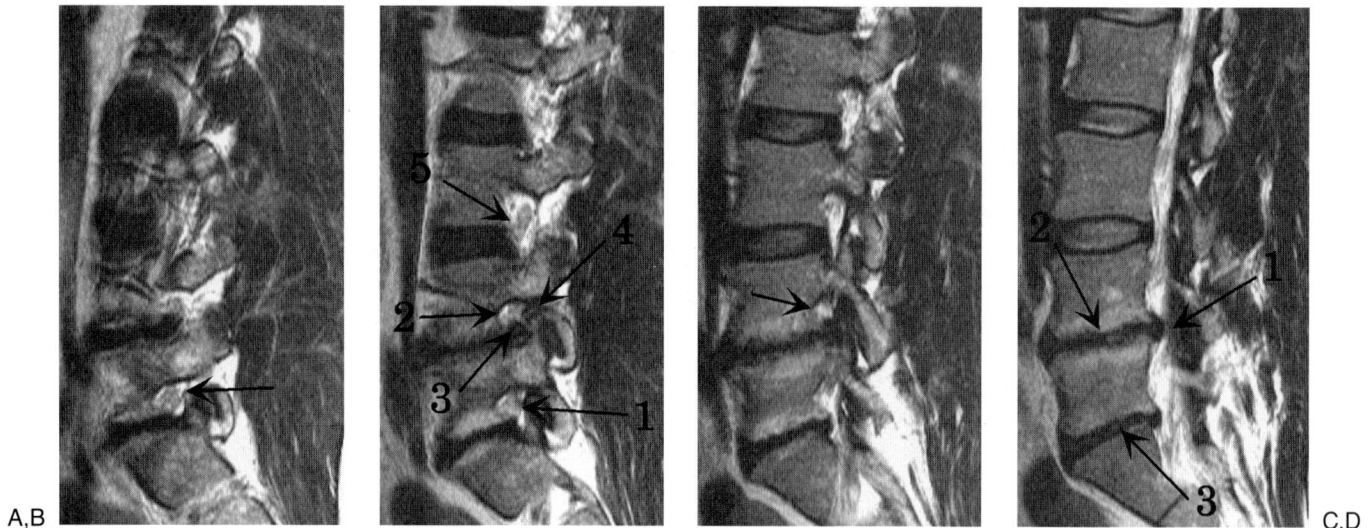

FIG. 49-7. Foraminal stenosis. This 42-year-old man had low back and right hip pain numbness in left foot. Sequential right parasagittal T2 weighted images (T2WI) from the lateral aspect of the L5 pedicle past the medial aspect of the pedicle to the right side of the spinal canal. **A:** Right parasagittal T2-weighted (T2W) magnetic resonance image (MRI) shows greater than 50% reduction in the up-down dimension of the L5-S1 foramen *(arrow);* however, no associated ganglionic deformity is present, so the stenosis is graded as moderate (see text). **B:** Right parasagittal T2W MRI medial to **(A)** demonstrates moderate stenosis is again seen at L5-S1 *(arrow 1).* At L4-5, there is severe combined up-down and front-back foraminal stenosis *(arrow 2)* from a combination of degenerative disc narrowing, degenerative disc bulging *(arrow 3),* and facet arthropathy *(arrow 4).* These degenerative processes result in mild compression of the L4 ganglion. No L3-4 narrowing is identified *(arrow 5).* **C:** Sagittal T2W MRI at the level of the medial aspect of the neural foramina shows no L5-S1 narrowing but there continues to be severe L4-5 narrowing *(arrow).* **D:** Sagittal T2W MRI at the lateral aspect of the spinal canal shows subarticular recess stenosis at the L4-5 level *(arrow 1).* There is severe loss of disc height and disc dehydration at L4-5 *(arrow 2)* and L5-S1 *(arrow 3),* and subchondral Modic type II degenerative changes at L4-5. (From Renfrew DL. Atlas of spine imaging. Philadelphia: Elsevier, 2003, with permission.)

TABLE 49-2. *Spinal canal stenosis grading scheme*

Term	Description
Mild	The spinal canal has >75% of the antero-posterior dimension of a normal level. The nerve roots are evenly distributed without crowding.
Moderate	The spinal canal has 50%–74% of the antero-posterior dimension of a normal level.[a] The nerve roots "crowded" or closer together than at a normal level.
Severe	The spinal canal has less than 50% of the antero-posterior dimension of a normal level. Typically, there is no visible cerebrospinal fluid (CSF) around the nerve roots at the level of severe stenosis.[b]

[a]If the patient has an inherently small spinal canal and this degree of narrowing produces a crowded appearance of the nerve roots with scant CSF around the nerve roots, the degree of stenosis should be upgrade to "severe." If the patient has an inherently large spinal canal and there is abundant CSF around the nerve roots, the stenosis should be graded as "mild."

[b]If the patient has an inherently large spinal canal so that there is still abundant CSF around the nerve roots with little crowding of these structures, the stenosis should be graded as "moderate."

TABLE 49-3. *Subarticular recess stenosis grading scheme*

Term	Description
Mild	The subarticular recess has 75%–99% of the antero-posterior dimension of a normal level, and the traversing nerve root has ample surrounding cerebrospinal fluid (CSF), without displacement or compression of the nerve root.
Moderate	The subarticular recess has 50%–74% of the antero-posterior dimension of a normal level.[a]
Severe	The subarticular recess has less than 50% of the antero-posterior dimension of a normal level. There is no visible CSF around the nerve root at the level of severe stenosis.[b]

[a]If the patient has an inherently narrow subarticular recess and this degree of narrowing produces compression of the traversing of the nerve root, the degree of stenosis should be upgraded to "severe." If the patient has an inherently generous subarticular recess and there is abundant CSF around the nerve root, the stenosis should be graded as "mild."

[b]If the patient has an inherently generous subarticular recess so that there is still abundant CSF around the nerve root, the stenosis should be graded as "moderate."

TABLE 49-4. *Foraminal stenosis grading scheme*

Term	Description
Mild	The neural foramen has 75%–99% of the antero-posterior *and* cephalocaudad dimension of a normal level, and the traversing nerve root has ample surrounding cerebrospinal fluid (CSF) or perineural fat, without displacement or compression of the nerve root.
Moderate	The neural foramen has 50%–74% of the antero-posterior *and* cephalocaudad dimension of a normal level. There may be up to mild (<25%) compression of the ganglion or nerve root.[a]
Severe	The neural foramen has less than 50% of the antero-posterior dimension of a normal level. There is no visible perineural fat around the nerve root at the level of maximal stenosis.[b]

[a]If the patient has an inherently small neural foramen and this degree of narrowing produces at least moderate (>25%) compression of the exiting nerve root or ganglion, the degree of stenosis should be upgraded to "severe." If the patient has an inherently generous neural foramen and there is abundant perineural fat or CSF around the nerve root and ganglion, the stenosis should be graded as "mild."

[b]If the patient has an inherently large neural foramen so that there is still abundant fat or CSF around the nerve root and ganglion and there is no neural compression, the stenosis should be graded as "moderate."

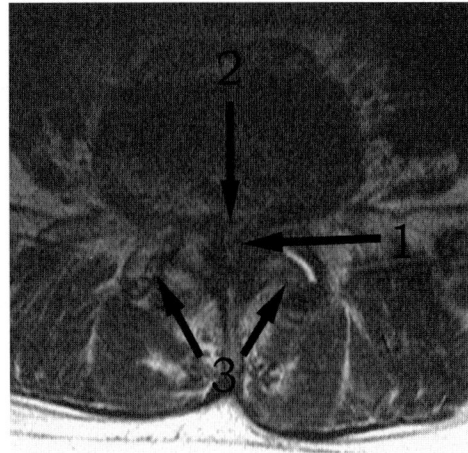

FIG. 49-8. Trefoil spinal canal with severe stenosis. This 76-year-old man with long-standing low back and bilateral leg pain and weakness. Axial T2-weighted magnetic resonance image at the L4-5 disc level demonstrates severe spinal canal and subarticular recess stenosis. Complete effacement of cerebrospinal fluid makes it difficult to identify the small, trefoil spinal canal *(arrow 1)*. Note degenerative disc bulging *(arrow 2)* and bilateral facet arthropathy *(arrow 3)*.

The direction as well as the degree of lumbar foraminal stenosis may be noted. Loss of disc height or disc margin osteophytic spurring and degenerative disc bulging causes the overwhelming majority (>90%) of cases of lumbar foraminal stenosis (10). Disc disease produces loss of the cephalocaudal dimension (craniocaudal or up-down) stenosis (Figs. 49-3, 49-7). On the other hand, facet arthropathy causes antero-posterior (AP) narrowing, and the stenosis may be termed either AP or front-back. A combination of both is called, logically enough, combined stenosis.

Although almost all causes of bony neural compression occur within the confines of the spinal canal or within the subarticular recesses or foramina, occasionally such compressions occur lateral to the foramen. Causes of this phenomenon include: (a) bony stenosis between the transverse process of L5 and the sacral ala (11); (b) a pseudoarthrosis between a transitional transverse process or sacral ala and the vertebral body of the next higher segment (Fig. 49-9); or (c) a lateral osteophyte formation off of the L5-S1 disc with narrowing of the space between the disc margin and ipsilateral sacral ala (Fig. 49-10).

In addition to the imaging findings of reduction of size of the normal spinal canal, subarticular recess, foramen; or extraspinal space and narrowing of neural structures,

Hacker et al. (12) have described an additional sign in spinal stenosis consisting of redundant nerve roots in the thecal sac (Fig. 49-11). They posited that such redundancy follows repeated stretching of the nerve roots above a level of stenosis, with failure of passage of the nerve roots back past the level of stenosis once pulled through.

DEGENERATIVE SPONDYLOLISTHESIS

Degenerative spondylolisthesis is a common cause of spinal stenosis. In this condition, degeneration of the facet joints and intervertebral disc may cause spondylolisthesis, or forward displacement of one vertebra relative to the next lower level. Degenerative spondylolisthesis occurs most frequently at the L4-5 level in middle-aged to elderly women (13–19). Overly sagittal (20) or axial (13,18) alignment of the facet joints may produce degenerative spondylolisthesis. Whether abnormally aligned or not, the facets almost invariably demonstrate moderate or severe degenerative changes in degenerative spondylolisthesis. A combination of spondylolisthesis, facet arthropathy, and associated degenerative disc disease produces associated stenosis, particularly of the subarticular recesses and spinal canal and usually somewhat less dramatically of the neural foramina (Figs. 49-12 to 49-14). Sequential images may

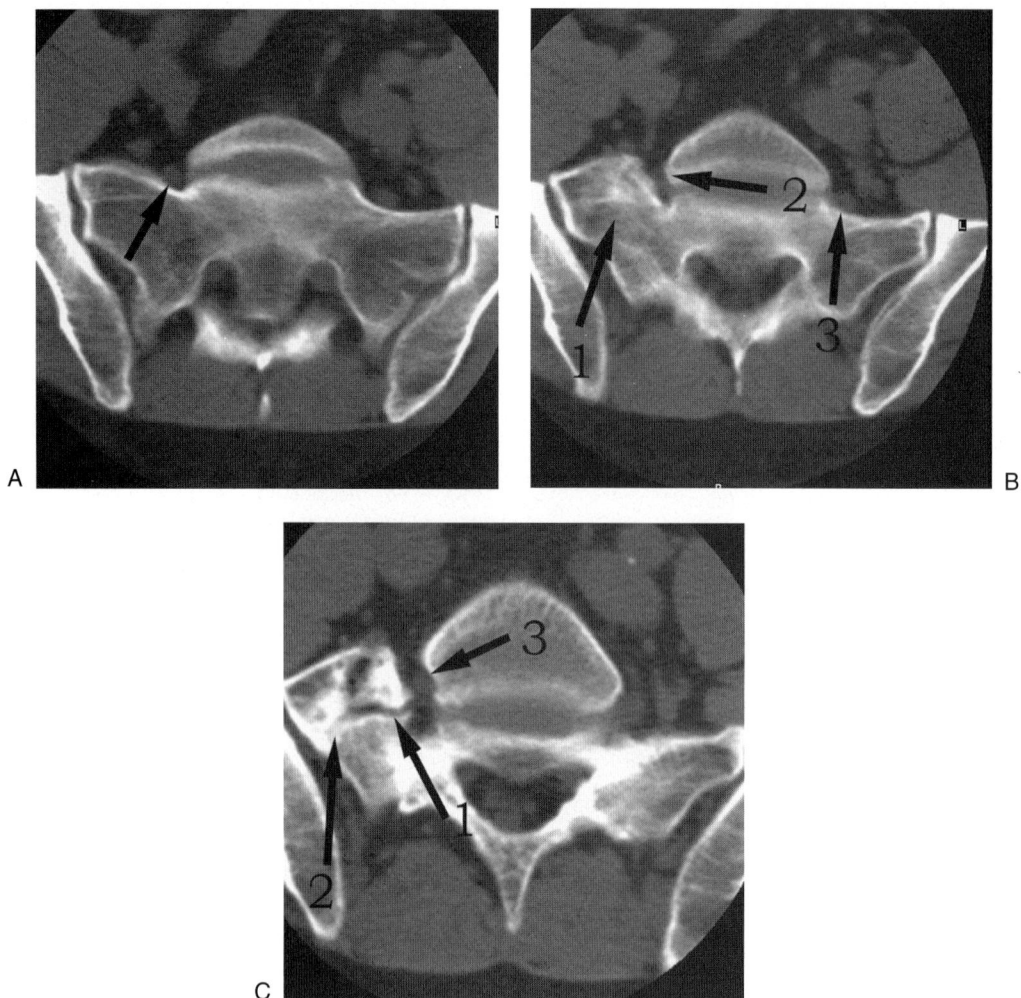

FIG. 49-9. Stenosis between a pseudoarthrosis and the next higher vertebral body. This 50-year-old man had low back and right leg pain. Plain films (not shown) demonstrated transitional anatomy with sacralization of the right side of the L5 segment. **A:** Axial 3-mm computed tomography (CT) examination at the level of the upper sacrum demonstrates asymmetry of the sacral ala. The right L5 ventral ramus *(arrow)* is located in a notch along the medial aspect of the right sacral ala. **B:** Axial 3-mm CT examination superior to **(A)**, demonstrating the sacralized right side of the L5 vertebra *(arrow 1)* and a narrow channel for passage of the right L5 ventral ramus *(arrow 2)*. Note that the contralateral left L5 ventral ramus *(arrow 3)* sits along the anterior aspect of the sacrum. The right L5 ventral ramus is in a position where it could be compressed between the L5 vertebral body and disc and the anomalous lateral mass. **C:** Axial 3-mm CT examination superior to **(B)**. Note the anomalous articulation between the right L5 lateral mass and S1 sacral ala *(arrow 1)*. There are reactive or degenerative changes along the lateral margin at this level *(arrow 2)*. At this level, the space between the lateral mass and L5 vertebra *(arrow 3)* is much larger than in **(B)**.

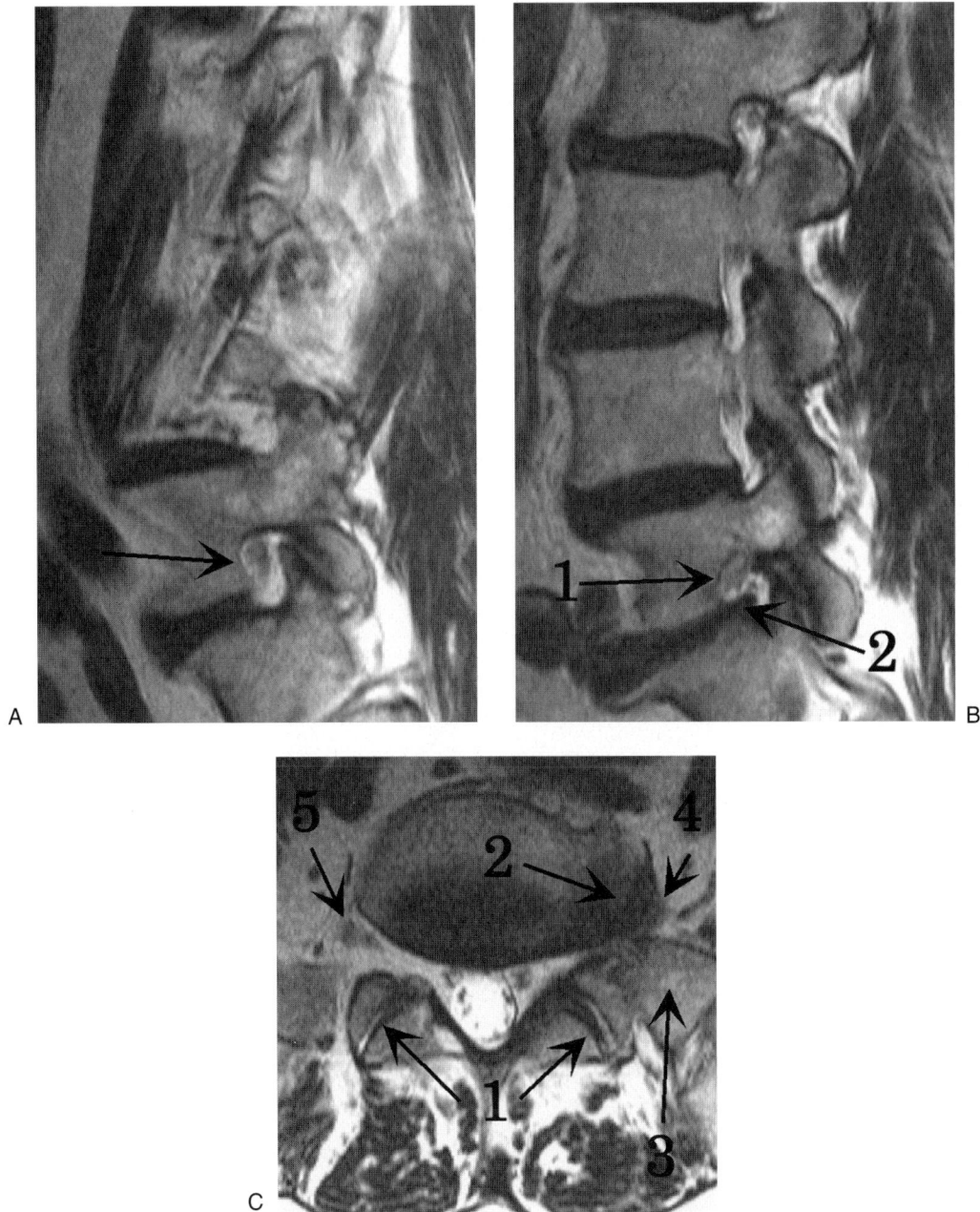

FIG. 49-10. Stenosis between lateral osteophyte formation and the sacral ala with radicular pain. This 67-year-old man had low back and left leg pain in the hip, lateral thigh, and lateral calf. **A:** Right parasagittal T2-weighted (T2W) magnetic resonance image (MRI) demonstrates a widely patent neural foramen *(arrow)* without L5 ganglionic compression. **B:** Left T2W MRI shows severe up-down foraminal stenosis *(arrow 1)* secondary to loss of disc height and osteophyte formation *(arrow 2),* with associated mild flattening of the exiting right L5 ganglion. **C:** Axial T2WI through the L5-S1 intervertebral disc demonstrates moderate facet arthropathy *(arrow 1)* and degenerative disc bulging. Furthermore, there is extensive left-sided osteophyte formation *(arrow 2),* which projects along the left lateral aspect of the L5 vertebral body and narrows the space between the vertebral body and the left sacral ala *(arrow 3),* with displacement and compression of the L5 ventral ramus *(arrow 4).* (Compare to the position of the left L5 ventral ramus *[arrow 5].*) The stenosis is lateral to the plane in **(B),** and lateral to the parasagittal images obtained in routine lumbar MRI. (From Renfrew DL. Atlas of spine imaging. Philadelphia: Elsevier, 2003, with permission.)

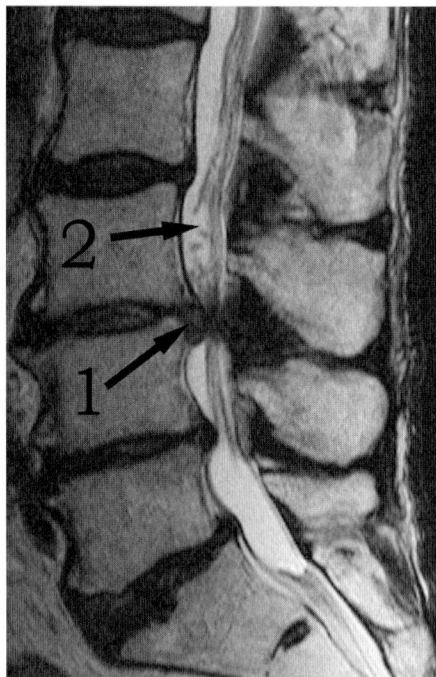

FIG. 49-11. Redundant nerve roots above a level of stenosis in the lumbar spine. This 68-year-old man had low back and bilateral leg pain. Sagittal T2-weighted (T2W) magnetic resonance image (MRI) demonstrates severe L3-4 spinal canal narrow/stenosis *(arrow 1)* secondary to a combination of degenerative disc disease and facet arthropathy with a superimposed caudally dissecting disc extrusion. Superior to the level of the stenosis, there is redundancy of the nerve roots within the thecal sac *(arrow 2)*. This redundancy is thought to be secondary to a lack of free movement through the level of stenosis (see text).

demonstrate progression of degenerative spondylolisthesis through time (Fig. 49-15). Table 49-5 lists imaging features differentiating degenerative and lytic spondylolisthesis, but note that the two processes may coexist at different levels in the same patient (Fig. 49-16).

The development of synovial cysts sprouting off of degenerated facet joints in patients with degenerative spondylolisthesis frequently contributes to symptoms (10); this complication should be suspected when a patient develops superimposed radicular pain on long-standing

(Text continued on page 487)

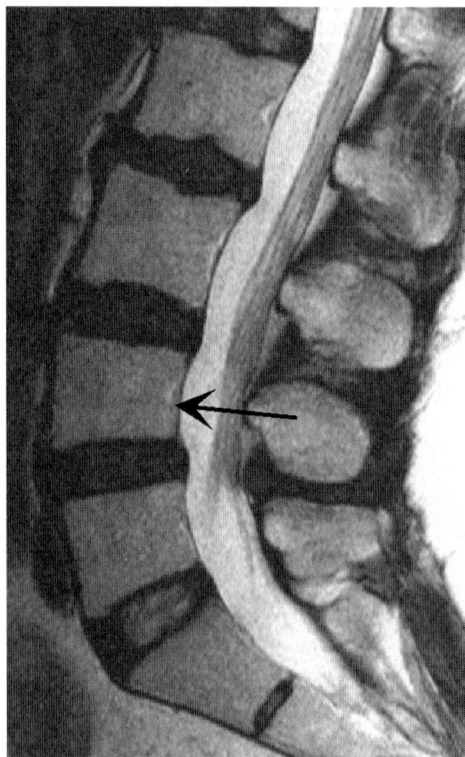

FIG. 49-12. Magnetic resonance image (MRI) of mild degenerative spondylolisthesis. This 59-year-old woman had central low back pain radiating into both legs. **A:** Sagittal T2-weighted (T2W) MRI minimal (<5%) degenerative spondylolisthesis: Note the forward shift of L4 on L5 *(arrow)*. The examination also demonstrates multilevel degenerative disc disease with disc dehydration and Schmorl node formation.

(continued on next page)

A

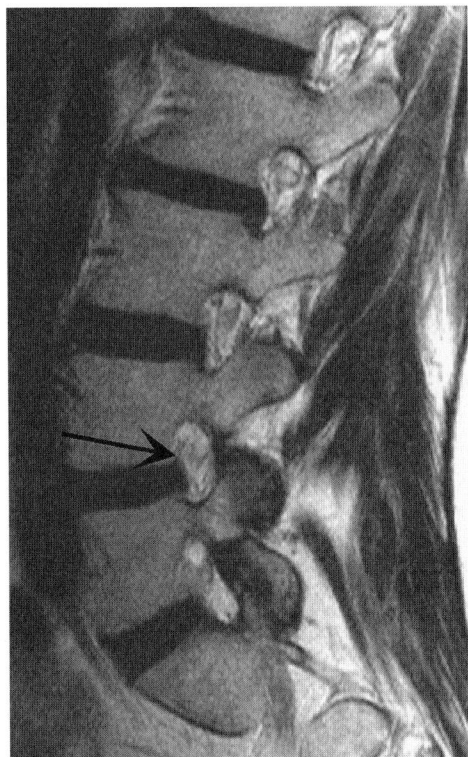

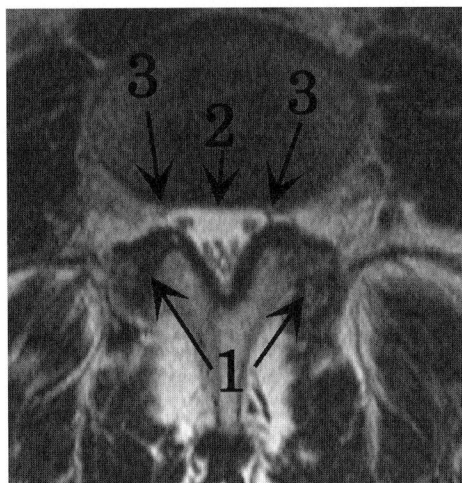

FIG. 49-12. (*continued*) **B:** Right parasagittal T2W MRI through the level of the foramina show no foraminal stenosis *(arrow).* **C:** Axial T2W MRI at the level of the L4-5 disc shows moderate facet arthropathy *(arrow 1),* mild spinal canal *(arrow 2),* and mild subarticular recess *(arrow 3)* stenosis. No neural compression is present. (From Renfrew DL. Atlas of spine imaging. Philadelphia: Elsevier, 2003, with permission.)

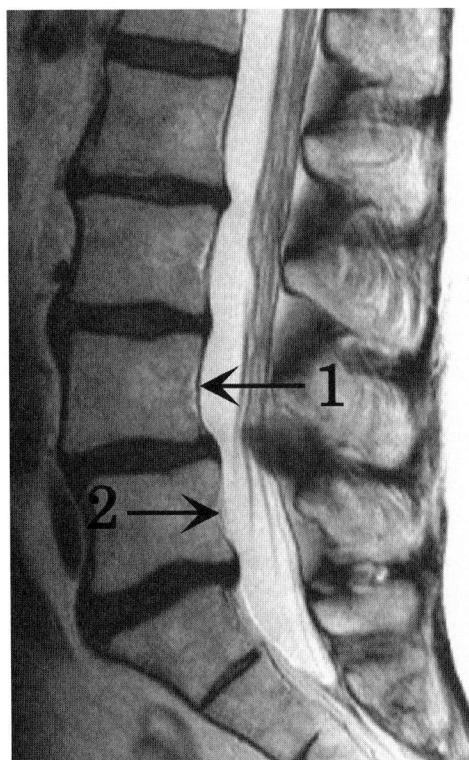

FIG. 49-13. Magnetic resonance image (MRI) of moderate degenerative spondylolisthesis. This 74-year-old woman had a constant backache with radiation of pain into both hips and legs, and superimposed sharp pain with walking. **A:** Sagittal T2WI shows multilevel degenerative disc disease, 15% degenerative spondylolisthesis at L4-5 *(arrow 1),* and 3 mm of retrolisthesis at L5-S1 *(arrow 2).*

(continued on next page)

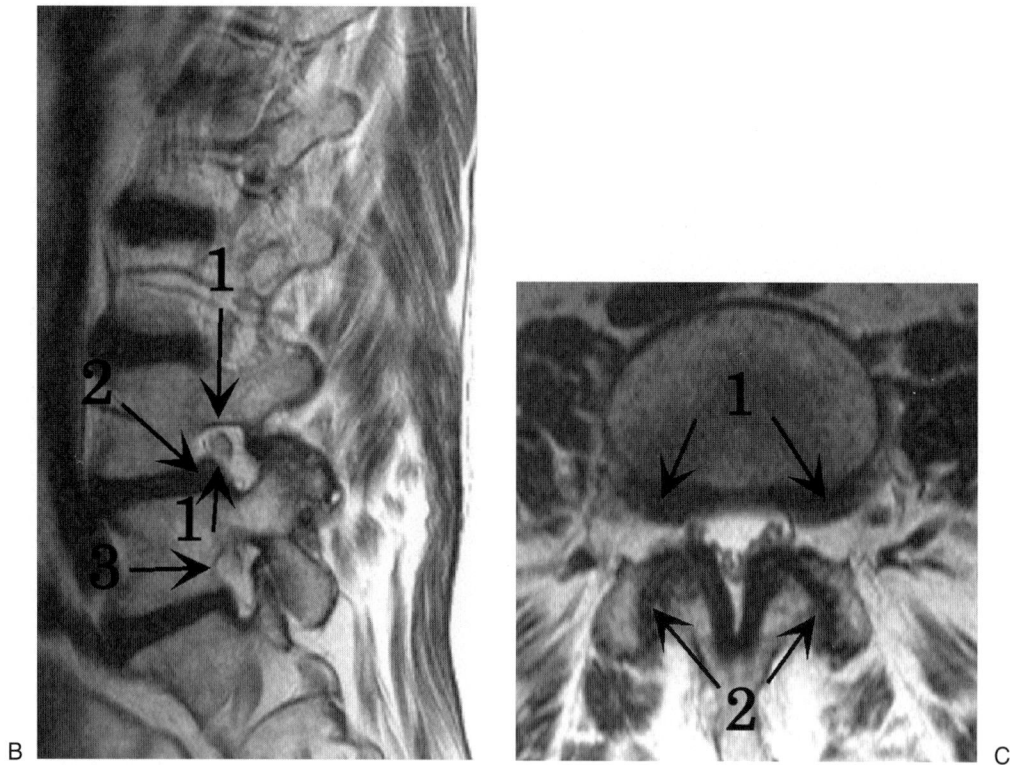

FIG. 49-13. (*continued*) **B:** Parasagittal right T2-weighted (T2W) MRI shows mild L4-5 up-down narrowing *(arrow 1)* from a foraminal disc protrusion *(arrow 2)* and a patent L5-S1 foramen *(arrow 3)*. **C:** Axial T2W MRI at the superior margin of the L4-5 disc shows a pseudodisc appearance because of spondylolisthesis *(arrow 1),* moderate facet arthropathy *(arrows 2),* and mild spinal canal and subarticular recess stenosis. The pseudodisc appearance is secondary to volume averaging through two adjacent segments on axial images. (From Renfrew DL. Atlas of spine imaging. Philadelphia: Elsevier, 2003, with permission.)

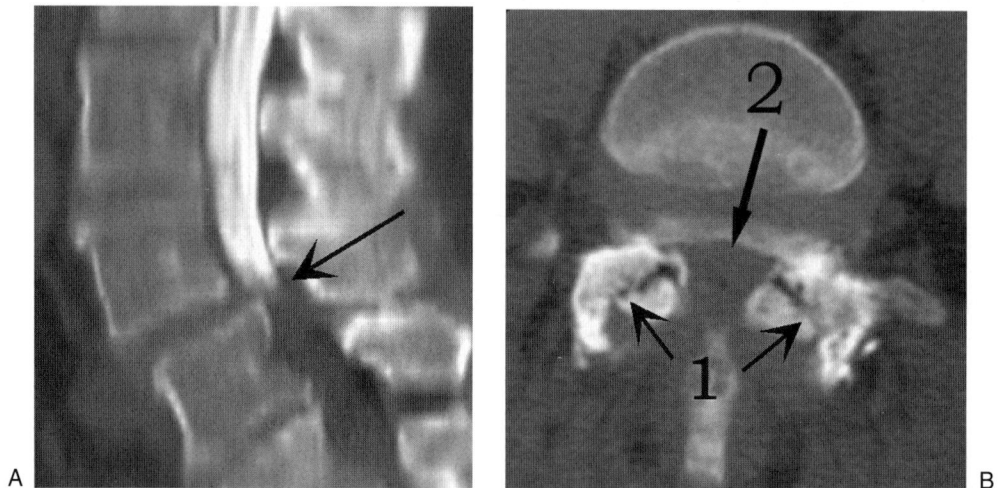

FIG. 49-14. Computed tomography-myelogram (Myelo-CT) of severe degenerative spondylolisthesis. This 62-year-old woman with low back pain had bilateral leg pain and right leg weakness. **A:** Sagittal reconstruction CT examination shows moderate L4-5 and severe L5-S1 disc narrowing. There is 20% degenerative spondylolisthesis of L4 on L5 and complete block to flow of myelographic contrast material at the L4-5 level *(arrow)*. **B:** Axial 3-mm CT cut at the level of the L4-5 intervertebral disc shows severe facet arthropathy *(arrow 1)*. Note the volume averaging through the L4 and L5 levels and severe spinal canal stenosis, with no myelographic contrast within the spinal canal *(arrow 2)*. (From Renfrew DL. Atlas of spine imaging. Philadelphia: Elsevier, 2003, with permission.)

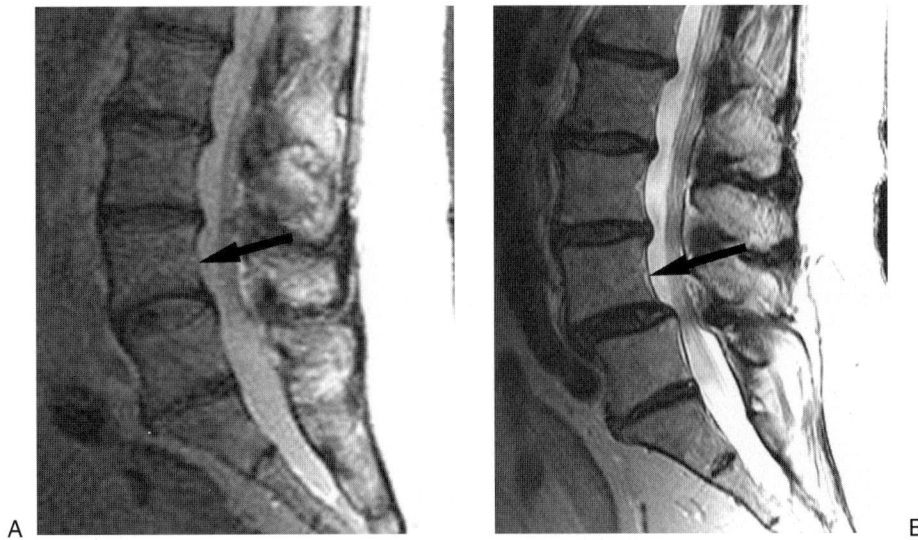

FIG. 49-15. Progression of degenerative spondylolisthesis through time. **A:** Sagittal T2-weighted (T2W) magnetic resonance image (MRI) demonstrates multilevel degenerative disc disease. Minimal degenerative spondylolisthesis of L4 on L5 is seen *(arrow)*. **B:** Sagittal T2W MRI done 5 years later demonstrates 15% degenerative spondylolisthesis *(arrow)*. Note ongoing degenerative disc disease and improved image quality with technologic advancements in the interval since the prior study. The patient originally had exclusively back pain, but developed leg symptoms by the time of the second scan.

TABLE 49-5. *Differentiation of degenerative and lytic spondylolisthesis*

	Degenerative spondylolisthesis	Lytic spondylolisthesis
Usual location	L4-5	L5-S1
Facet arthropathy	Moderate or severe	Usually none; the joints beneath the level of lysis tend to be atrophic
Spinal canal diameter	Decreased	Increased
Pars interarticularis	Intact	Interrupted

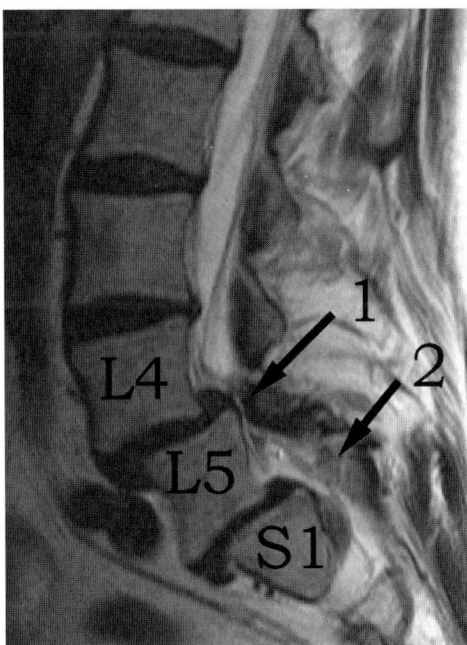

FIG. 49-16. Coexistent lytic and degenerative spondylolisthesis. This 73-year-old woman had low back pain with right leg pain and tingling. **A:** Sagittal T2-weighted (T2W) magnetic resonance image (MRI) shows multilevel degenerative changes with lumbar disc dehydration and L4-5 and L5-S1 disc narrowing. There is 20% spondylolisthesis of L4 on L5 and L5 on S1. Note spinal canal stenosis at L4-5 *(arrow 1)* at a level of degenerative spondylolisthesis and lack of spinal canal stenosis at L5-S1 *(arrow 2)* at a level of lytic spondylolisthesis.

(continued on next page)

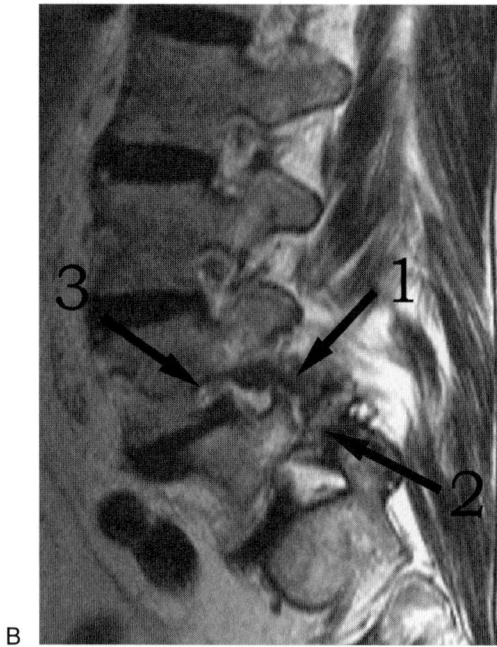

FIG. 49-16. *(continued)* **B:** Right parasagittal T2W MRI demonstrates L4-5 facet arthropathy *(arrow 1)* and a pars defect at L5 *(arrow 2)*. Note that the L4-5 foramen demonstrates severe stenosis *(arrow 3)*, whereas there is less stenosis at L5-S1. **C:** Axial T2W MRI through the level of the L5 pars demonstrates fibroproliferative changes along the pars margins *(arrow 1)* and asymmetric and dysplastic posterior elements *(arrow 2)*. **D:** Axial T2W MRI through the level of the L4-5 intervertebral disc demonstrates severe facet arthropathy *(arrow 1)* with a pseudodisc anteriorly and moderate spinal canal and subarticular recess stenosis *(arrow 2)*.

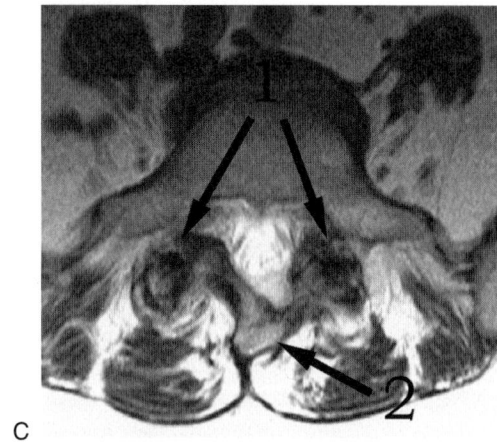

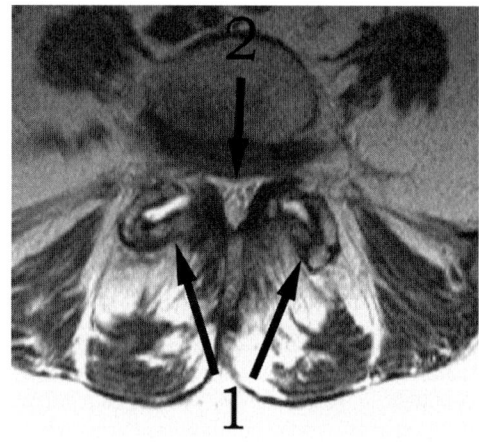

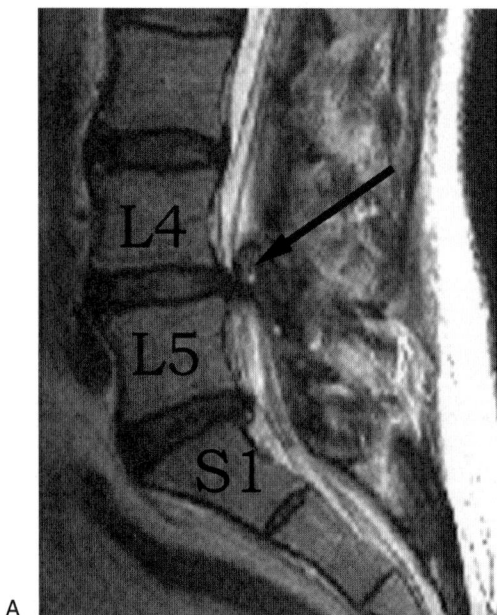

FIG. 49-17. Degenerative spondylolisthesis with radicular pain secondary to synovial cyst formation. This 52-year-old woman had new onset of low back and right leg pain. **A:** Sagittal T2-weighted (T2W) magnetic resonance image (MRI) shows 5% degenerative spondylolisthesis of L4 on L5 and L5-S1 mild disc degeneration and bulging. In addition, there is a dorsal soft-tissue mass within the spinal canal at the L4-5 level *(arrow)*.

(continued on next page)

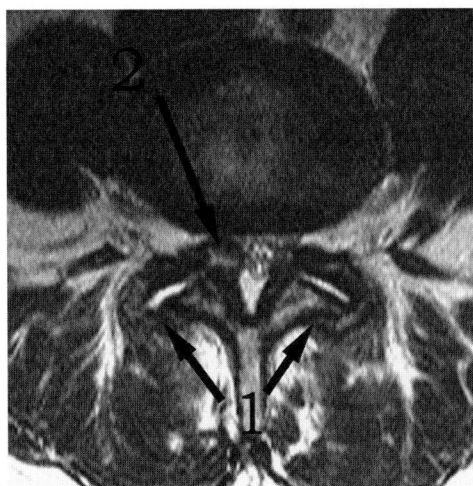

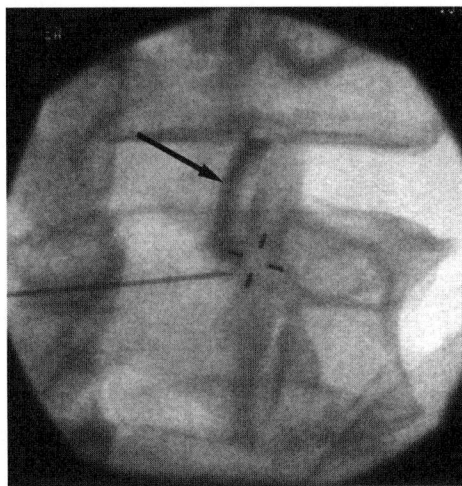

FIG. 49-17. *(continued)* **B:** Axial T2W MRI demonstrates bilateral L4-5 facet joint arthropathy *(arrow 1)*. In addition, a synovial cyst *(arrow 2)* projects off the anteromedial aspect of the right joint. **C:** Oblique fluoroscopic image from an L4-5 facet joint injection. A 22-gauge needle is at the inferior aspect of the L4-5 facet joint and contrast flows through the joint *(arrow)*. With injection of a small volume of local anesthetic and steroid, the patient had a brief recurrence of her typical pain followed by long-standing, complete pain relief, consistent with synovial cyst rupture.

low back pain (Fig. 49-17). Of course, an acute disc herniation may be seen in the same clinical scenario, and imaging is required to make the differentiation (Fig. 49-18).

IMAGING MODALITIES AND CONTROVERSIES

The classification system proposed here applies regardless of the imaging modality used. Myelography, CT, MRI, and myelography with CT (myelo-CT) have all been used for evaluation of spinal stenosis. We typically use MRI to evaluate stenosis, supplemented by myelo-CT in some cases. Bartynski et al. (21) recently published a study suggesting that both MR imaging and myelo-CT significantly underestimated spinal stenosis 28% to 38% of the time, and that standard myelography performed much better, underestimating spinal stenosis in only about 6% of cases. This finding runs counter to the trend of using MR imaging for diagnosis of stenosis. In addition, the outperformance of myelo-CT by plain film myelography suggests that myelography may always or nearly always have an appearance of spinal stenosis. We could determine whether myelography was in fact often a false-positive test if we had a reliable reference standard; however, we do not. Measurements typically are not obtained at the time of surgery as to the AP diameter of the spinal canal, subarticular recess, or foramen, and it is questionable whether such measurements would be considered reliable. We can use surgical outcome as the reference standard of whether someone has spinal stenosis, and assume that those who fare well following surgery are "disease-positive" for stenosis and those who do not are "disease-negative." In Bartynski et al.'s study, all patients were relieved of symptoms following surgery. Differentiating which of the three imaging methods evaluated in Bartynski's study (MRI,

myelo-CT, and myelography) probably would be best evaluated using receiver operating characteristic curve analysis, but this topic is beyond the scope of this chapter. Note that at least three problems arise if we use such surgical outcome as the reference standard: (a) Patients achieving symptom relief might be getting it through a placebo mechanism. (b) Patients who fail to achieve symptom relief may still have stenosis but also have or develop other conditions producing similar symptoms (including failed back surgery). (c) Other studies have shown no relationship between relief of symptoms and improvement of stenosis as depicted by imaging. Attempts to find a specific fixed numerical value for a given measurement (either AP diameter or cross-sectional area) predictive of symptom production or surgical outcome have not been successful (5,7,22–24). Use of only bony measurements makes little sense in light of the contributions of soft tissue to spinal canal narrowing (5,22). Use of dural sac dimensions makes more sense, but is still not predictive of surgical results (1,25). In fact, some studies have shown poorer outcomes when operating on more severe degrees of narrowing, perhaps because of the permanent damage of the nerve roots before operation. Thus, although absolute measurements of a linear dimension or (with markedly greater difficulty) cross-sectional area of the spinal canal, subarticular recess, or neural foramen may be reported, their significance in a given case is questionable. Factors contributing to the lack of correlation between measurements of narrowing and symptoms or surgical outcomes include the necessity of a second location of stenosis for symptom production (26,27), the rapidity of onset of stenosis (slowly progressive stenosis is better tolerated than rapidly progressive stenosis), superimposed minor trauma (10), positional narrowing of the structure in question (28,29), and

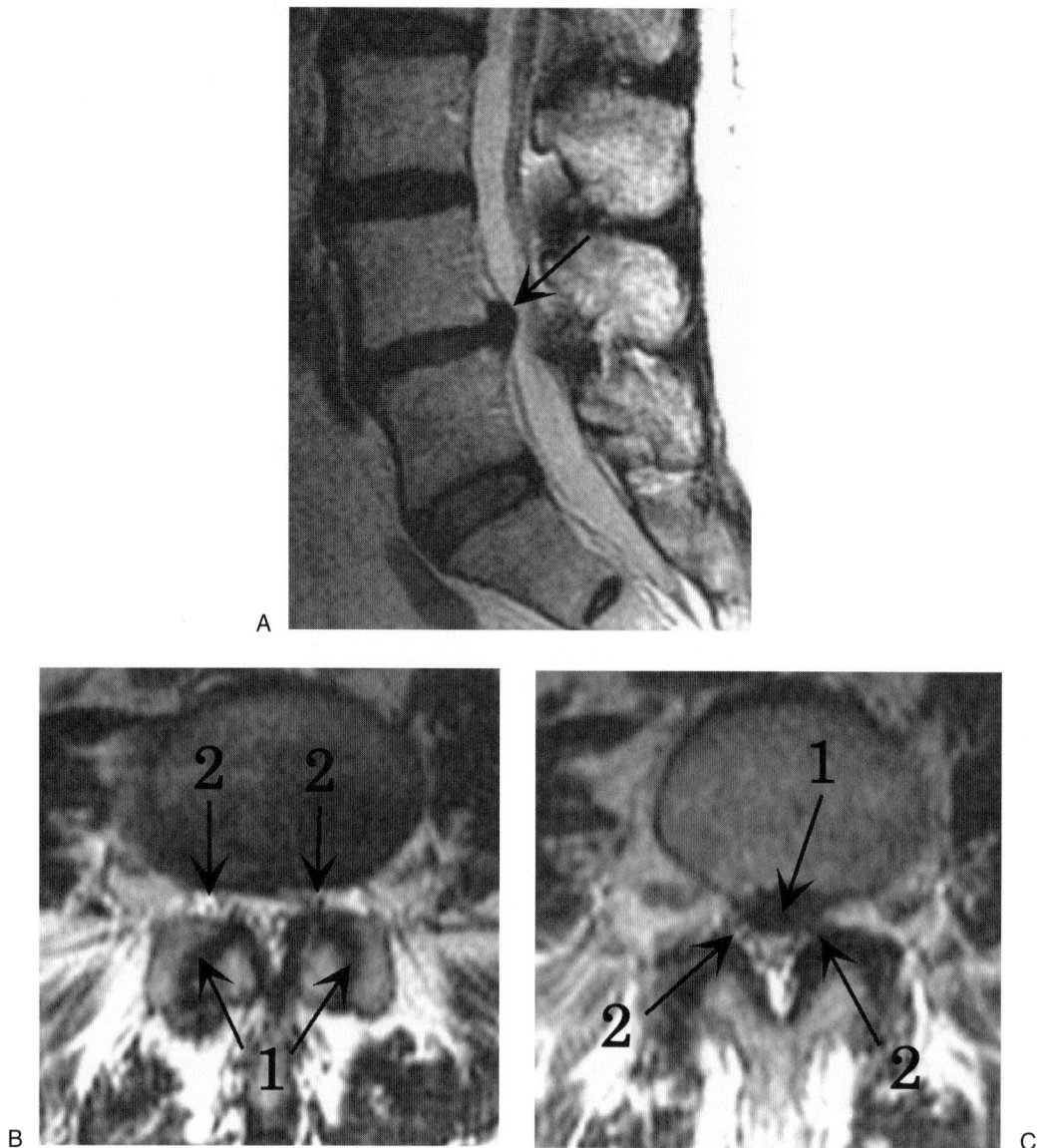

FIG. 49-18. Degenerative spondylolisthesis with superimposed disc herniation. This 66-year-old woman with chronic low back pain had new onset left leg pain. **A:** Sagittal T2-weighted (T2W) magnetic resonance image (MRI) demonstrates multilevel degenerative disc disease with 5% degenerative spondylolisthesis at L4-5. There is a superimposed cranially dissecting 6-mm disc extrusion *(arrow)*. **B:** Axial T2W MRI at the level of the L4-5 disc demonstrates severe facet arthropathy *(arrow 1)* and moderate spinal canal and subarticular recess stenosis *(arrow 2)* with a trefoil appearance of the spinal canal. **C:** Axial T2W MRI just above the level of the L4-5 disc demonstrates the cranially dissecting disc extrusion *(arrow 1)* with severe spinal canal and bilateral subarticular recess narrowing *(arrow 2)* with compression of the traversing L5 nerve roots, left greater than right. (From Renfrew DL. Atlas of spine imaging. Philadelphia: Elsevier, 2003, with permission.)

poor interobserver and intraobserver agreement among interpreters of imaging studies (30–32). Our terminology and the illustrations offered in this chapter are our attempt to address the last concern.

TREATMENT

Treatment of spinal stenosis varies greatly. Many publications have supported conservative treatment (2,33) with a combination of exercise, nonsteroidal antiinflammatory drugs, or epidural steroid injection (2,4,34–35). Because symptom production follows from not only single level narrowing, but also from any additional areas of narrowing (26,36), the rapidity of onset of the narrowing of such superimposed soft-tissue abnormalities as disc herniations, synovial cysts, minimal trauma (10), and additional as yet unidentified factors, addressing only the stenosis at a single level does not invariably lead to a favorable outcome. However, in a meta-analysis of 74 articles on spinal stenosis, Turner et al. (37) found favorable outcomes reported in an average of 64% of cases. In a more recent publication, Atlas et al. (38) compared 4-year outcomes in a matched prospective observational study and found that surgical treatment was associated with a greater improvement in patient-reported outcomes than nonsurgical treatment. The decision to perform surgery usually hinges more on clinical symptoms (particularly on neurogenic claudication interfering with activities of daily living or progressive neurologic dysfunction) (39), than it does on imaging appearance. Controversy continues regarding whether fusion should accompany decompression (40,41).

In the special case of degenerative spondylolisthesis, Vogt et al. (17) in a population study found no relationship between anterolisthesis and back pain. Kauppila et al. (42) found it problematic to ascribe back pain to degenerative spondylolisthesis, and Matsunaga et al. (16) felt autostabilization prevented progression of disease and that the natural history of the disease was thus benign. Iguchi et al. (43) found most patients did well even without surgery. On the other hand, Moller et al. (19) found that surgery provided better pain relief and functional outcome than an exercise program.

REFERENCES

1. Gunzburg R, Keller TS, Szpalski M, et al. A prospective study on CT scan outcomes after conservative decompression surgery for lumbar spinal stenosis. J Spinal Disord Techniques 2003;3:261–267.
2. Simotas AC, Dorey FJ, Hansraj KK, et al. Nonoperative treatment for lumber spinal stenosis: clinical and outcome results and a 3-year survivorship analysis. Spine 2000;25:197–204.
3. Arnoldi CC, Brodsky AE, Cauchoix J et al. Lumbar spinal stenosis and nerve root entrapment syndromes. Clin Orthop Rel Res 1976;115:2–3.
4. St Amour TE, Hodges SC, Laakman RW, et al. Osteomyelitis of the spine. In: St Amour TE, Hodges SC, Laakman RW, et al., eds. MRI of the spine. New York: Raven Press, 1994;593–607.
5. Schonstrom NSR, Bolender NF, Spengler DM. The pathomorphology of spinal stenosis as seen on CT scans of the lumbar spine. Spine 1985;10:806–811.
6. Verbiest H. Neurogenic intermittent claudication in cases with absolute and relative stenosis of the lumbar vertebral canal (ASLC and RSLC), in cases with narrow lumbar intervertebral foramina, and in cases with both entities. Clin Neurosurg 1973;20:204–214.
7. Verbiest H. Stenosis of the lumbar vertebral canal and sciatica. Neurosurg Rev 1980;3:75–89.
8. Yoshida M, Shima K, Taniguchi Y, et al. Hypertrophied ligamentum flavum in lumbar spinal canal stenosis: pathogenesis and morphologic and immunohistochemical observation. Spine 1992;11:1353–1360.
9. Renfrew DL. Atlas of spine imaging. Philadelphia: Elsevier, 2003.
10. Heithoff KB, Ray C, Schellhas KP, et al. CT and MRI of lateral entrapment syndromes. In: Genant HK, ed. Spine Update 1987, Radiology Research and Education Foundation. San Francisco, CA: The University of California Press, 1987;203–236.
11. Wiltse LL, Guyer RD, Spencer CW, et al. Alar transverse process compression of the L5 spinal nerve: the far-out syndrome. Spine 1984;9:31–41.
12. Hacker DA, Latchaw RE, Yock DH Jr, et al. Redundant lumbar nerve root syndrome: myelographic features. Radiology 1982;143:457–461.
13. Macnab I. Spondylolisthesis with an intact neural arch-the so-called pseudo-spondylolisthesis. J Bone Joint Surg 1950;32-B:325–333.
14. Newman PH. The etiology of spondylolisthesis. J Bone Joint Surg 1955;45B:39–59.
15. Rosenberg NJ. Degenerative spondylolisthesis: predisposing factors. J Bone Joint Surg 1975;57-A:467–474.
16. Matsunaga S, Sakou T, Morizono Y, et al. Natural history of degenerative spondylolisthesis: pathogenesis and natural course of the slippage. Spine 1990;15:1204–1210.
17. Vogt MT, Rubin D, Valentin SR, et al. Lumbar olisthesis and lower back pain symptoms in elderly white women: the study of osteoporotic fractures. Spine 1998;23:2640–2647.
18. Nagaosa Y, Kikuchi S, Hasue M, et al. Pathoanatomic mechanisms of degenerative spondylolisthesis: a radiographic study. Spine 1998;23:1447–1451.
19. Moller H, Hedlund R. Surgery versus conservative management in adult isthmic spondylolisthesis. A prospective randomized study: Part 1. Spine 2000;25:1711–1715.
20. Grobler LJ, Robertson PA, Novotny JE, et al. Etiology of spondylolisthesis: assessment of the role played by lumbar facet joint morphology. Spine 1993;18:80–91.
21. Bartynski WS, Lin L. Lumbar root compression in the lateral recess: MR imaging, conventional myelography, and CT myelography comparison with surgical confirmation. AJNR 2003;24:348–360.
22. Bolender NF, Schonstrom NSR, Spengler DM. Role of computed tomography and myelography in the diagnosis of central spinal stenosis. J Bone Joint Surg 1985;67-A:240–246.
23. Weisz GM, Lee P. Spinal canal stenosis: concept of spinal reserve capacity: radiologic measurements and clinical applications. Clin Orthop Rel Res 1983;179:134–140.
24. Amundsen T, Weber H, Lilleas F, et al. Lumbar spinal stenosis: clinical and radiographic features. Spine 1995;10:1178–1186.
25. Herno A, Saari T, Suomalainen O, et al. The degree of decompressive relief and its relation to clinical outcome in patients undergoing surgery for lumbar spinal stenosis. Spine 1999;24:1010–1014.
26. Olmarker K, Rydevik B. Single- versus double-level nerve root compression. Clin Orthop Rel Res 1992;279:35–39.
27. Porter RW, Ward D. Cauda equina dysfunction: the significance of two-level pathology. Spine 1992;17:9–15.
28. Fujiwara A, An HS, Lim T-H, et al. Morphologic changes in the lumbar intervertebral foramen due to flexion-extension, lateral bending, and axial rotation: an in vitro anatomic and biomechanical study. Spine 2001;26:876–882.
29. Weishaupt D, Schmid MR, Zanetti M, et al. Positional MR imaging of the lumbar spine: does it demonstrate nerve root compromise not visible at conventional MR imaging? Radiology 2000;215:247–253.
30. Drew B, Bhandari M, Kulkarni AV, et al. Reliability in grading severity of lumbar spinal stenosis. J Spinal Disord 2000;13:253–258.
31. Yousem DM, Atlas SW, Goldberg HI, et al. Degenerative narrowing of the cervical spine neural foramina: evaluation with high-resolution 3DFT gradient-echo MR imaging. AJNR 1991;156:229–236.
32. Stafira JS, Sonnad JR, Yuh WTC, et al. Qualitative assessment of cervical spinal stenosis: observer variability on CT and MR images. Am J Neuroradiol 2003;24:760–769.
33. Johnsson KE, Rosen I, Uden A. The natural course of lumbar spinal stenosis. Acta Orthop Scand 1993;64(suppl 251):67–68.
34. Ferrante FM. Epidural steroids in the management of spinal stenosis. Semin Spine Surg 1989;1:177–181.
35. Jenis LG, An HS. Lumbar foraminal stenosis. Spine 2000;25:389–394.
36. Porter RW. Spinal stenosis and neurogenic claudication. Spine 1996;17:2046–2052.
37. Turner JA, Ersek M, Herron L, et al. Surgery for lumbar spinal stenosis: attempted meta-analysis of the literature. Spine 1992;17:1–8.
38. Atlas SJ, Keller RB, Robson D, et al. Surgical and nonsurgical management of lumbar spinal stenosis. Spine 2000;25:556–562.
39. Herkowitz HN, Garfin SR. Decompressive surgery for spinal stenosis. Semin Spine Surg 1989;1:163–167.
40. Grob D, Humke T, Dvorak J. Degenerative lumbar spinal stenosis: decompression with and without arthrodesis. J Bone Joint Surg 1995;77-A:1036–1041.
41. McCullouch JA. Microdecompression and uninstrumented single-level fusion for spinal canal stenosis with degenerative spondylolysthesis. Spine 1998;23:2243–2252.
42. Kauppila LI, Eustace S, Kiel DP, et al. Degenerative displacement of lumbar vertebrae: a 25 year follow-up study in Framingham. Spine 1998;17:1868–1874.
43. Iguchi T, Kurihara A, Nakayama J, et al. Minimum 10-year outcome of decompressive laminectomy for degenerative lumbar spinal stenosis. Spine 2000;25:1754–1759.

CHAPTER 50

Spinal Stenosis Without Deformity: Nonoperative Treatment

Arto Herno

The nonoperative treatment of lumbar spinal stenosis (LSS) is a very current and practical topic because the aging of the general population is increasing the number of patients with this degenerative spinal disorder. Even now degenerative LSS is a major cause of low back and lower extremity pain as well as functional limitation in elderly persons (1–3). Research on the nonoperative treatment of LSS patients has been very modest compared with the large number of studies on the operative treatment of LSS (2,4,5). In fact, surgery has been the treatment of choice since the 1950s, when Verbiest (6) published his first report; however, at present it seems unreasonable that this increasing number of LSS patients could be left to surgical management alone. The basic problem with the nonoperative treatment of LSS is that little is known about the efficacy of nonoperative therapy modalities and the factors that are associated with a better outcome (2). Until now, LSS patients with mild to moderate symptoms have been treated conservatively, and patients with severe symptoms have been treated surgically (7). Recently, more reports concerning nonoperatively treated LSS patients have been published. In these comparative cohort studies between nonoperative and operative treatment, the results were more favorable to operative than to conservative treatment. However, regardless of treatment, unsatisfactory outcomes were common: 20% to 40% of patients treated operatively, and 50% to 70% of patients treated nonoperatively had unsatisfactory outcomes after 4 years (4,5,8,9).

THE PATHOANATOMY AND PATHOPHYSIOLOGY OF LUMBAR SPINAL STENOSIS

Lumbar spinal stenosis is a posture-dependent functional and structural disorder caused by the progressive degenerative and reparative stenotic process of the lum-

bar spine resulting in continuous reduction of the central and lateral canal spaces. This process is slow and gradual, taking many years to occur and deteriorate. These degenerative changes dominate at the level of the mobile portion of the lumbar segment (i.e., at the level of the three-joint complex) (10), and mostly at the three lower lumbar levels (11). In patients with initially diminished size of the spinal canal (i.e., preexisting developmental relative stenosis) (12), symptomatic LSS generally occurs before the age of 50 because these patients have limited reserve space to accommodate the degenerative encroachment. Although various radiologic measurements of the lumbar spinal canal and the dural sac are useful as guidelines, the degree of impingement on the neural elements by the bone and soft tissues is more important. The cross-sectional area of the caudal fibers varies from 62 mm^2 at L1 to 30 mm^2 at L5 in men, and 50 mm^2 and 32 mm^2 in women, respectively (13).

The physiology of the lumbar spine is characterized by space changes in the spinal canal during various lumbar positions. The available space within the spinal canal decreases in extension and axial loading (minimum size of the canal), and increases in flexion and axial distraction of spine (maximum size of the canal) (14). In healthy subjects, the relative narrowing of the antero-posterior diameter of the dural sac from lumbar flexion to extension decreases about 10% but in patients with mild, moderate, or severe LSS this diameter decreases 32%, 45%, and 67%, respectively. Thereby, the more the canal is structurally narrowed by the stenosing process, the more it will be functionally narrowed by additional lumbar extension. Penning (13) called this phenomenon "the rule of progressive narrowing."

The decisive turning point for symptomatic LSS is when the available reserve space of the spinal canals for the nerve roots has been used up. Schönström (14) called this point to the critical size of the spinal canal. In practice, this means that the ability of the nerve roots to receive their needed nutrition and blood supply is reducing when the spinal canal dimensions are decreasing to this point. For instance, if the patient has moderate stenosis, the spinal canal enters this critical size only in extension of the lumbar spine (i.e., walking and standing), but when the spinal canals are reduced, the patient has to bend her or his back in order avoid the canal to enter the critical point and escape symptoms (15). It is obvious that in most LSS patients this stenosing process is not continuously progressive but stabilizes at a certain individual level of stenosis.

The functional pathophysiology of LSS explains the posture-dependency of the LSS patient's symptoms: Pain is exacerbated in lumbar extension (i.e., on prolonged standing and walking), and pain is relieved in lumbar flexion (i.e., on standing or sitting with the trunk in flexion, or lying down with knees flexed) (7–18). These posture-dependent changes can be proved by various functional radiographies (i.e., functional myelography, dynamic computed tomography [CT], axially loaded CT-myelography, MRI, and positional MRI) (13,19–21). Takahashi et al. (17,18) demonstrated that this functional phenomenon is more sophisticated by measuring the changes of the local epidural pressure at the stenotic level in various body postures and during walking.

CLINICAL EVALUATION OF PATIENTS WITH LUMBAR SPINAL STENOSIS

Symptomatic LSS is a dynamic and structural syndrome in which the symptoms are dependent on the patient's posture. Although the symptoms of LSS may be variable, bizarre, and vague, their typical feature is the relationship between symptoms and body posture. This "symptom-posture" analysis is a keystone when diagnosing LSS because radiographic findings are meaningful diagnostically only if they are accompanied by the clinical syndrome of neurogenic claudication or chronic nerve root compression (16). However, the basic clinical problem is that symptoms, signs, and radiologic findings of patients with LSS are not associated with each other (11). Further, if pain and other symptoms of LSS are solely related to compression of the cauda equina, nearly all elderly people would suffer from symptoms of stenosis because the pathoanatomic changes related to LSS are a function of the aging process (7). Hence, it is important that the physician listens closely to the patient's symptoms and pays attention to the relationship between symptoms and body postures. Furthermore, the extension test of the lumbar spine (16) and the treadmill test (22) with pain analysis may help to verify the clinical diagnosis of LSS.

Before the clinician is able to reliably diagnose LSS, she or he has to reconcile the patient's symptoms, signs, clinical tests, and imaging findings, to exclude other condition mimicking LSS symptoms and identify the etiol-

ogy and coexisting pain syndromes of LSS (16,23). Consequently, the most demanding task of the clinician is to estimate how much the aging patient's symptoms and lowered functional capacity is related to her or his radiologically confirmed stenotic findings, and how much is related to coexisting spinal, other musculoskeletal, and medical comorbidities (16,24). The conclusion of this thinking process is critical to appropriate selection of therapy for the patient. Optimal treatment begins with accurate identification of the condition.

NONOPERATIVE TREATMENT OF LUMBAR SPINAL STENOSIS

The nonoperative treatment of LSS is not supported by controlled studies, but has to apply a practical and rational understanding of the pathoanatomic and pathophysiologic changes that are taking place in LSS patients during aging.

When a patient comes to the physician with pain in the back and lower extremities related to LSS, she or he is most likely requesting some form of treatment (7). At present, the primary treatment of LSS is mostly nonoperative because many patients respond well to this treatment (4,25,26). Although nonoperative treatment is less successful in patients who have more severe pain, functional limitation, and neurologic dysfunction, the nonoperative approach is recommended because a delay of surgery for some months does not worsen the prognosis of these patients (3,4). Also the rapid symptomatic or functional decline is unexpected in patients with LSS but a traumatic distortion of the lumbar spine or a lumbar disc herniation may temporarily exacerbate the LSS patient's symptoms. Further, although an attack of cauda equina syndrome is very rare in LSS patients, the physician has to keep this possibility in mind because these patients have to be operated on as soon as possible.

The nonoperative option is the only chance for an LSS patient who refuses surgical treatment or in whom surgical treatment is contraindicated because of the patient's medical condition. Currently, we have more and more elderly LSS patients who have many other diseases (i.e., heart disease, asthma, other lung diseases, aortoiliac occlusive disease, osteoarthritis of hip and knee joints, diabetes, severe obesity, peripheral neuropathy, rheumatoid arthritis, osteoporosis, etc.). Thus, the physician has to have a good overall picture of the LSS patient and her or his other diseases when considering appropriate therapy for alleviation of LSS symptoms.

NONOPERATIVE TREATMENT OPTIONS OF LUMBAR SPINAL STENOSIS

Nonoperative treatment is based on the rational application of the pathoanatomic and pathophysiologic findings for the nonoperative therapy plan. The treatment is aimed at acting on these biomechanical and musculoskeletal alterations and on inflammatory processes to alleviate the patient's pain and discomfort and improve functional capacity. Simotas (27) proposed that nonoperative treatment is divided into three independent but overlapping phases: pain control, stabilization, and a conditioning phase. Thus, it is often necessary to combine many treatment options and time them properly so that therapy can be effective on various etiologic factors.

Little is known about the efficacy of nonoperative therapy of LSS and which factors are associated with better outcome (2). Nonetheless, there is a rational reason to suppose that the current nonoperative treatment can have an effect on those pathoanatomic and pathophysiologic mechanisms that cause symptoms in patients with LSS. It is reasonable to suppose that we attain better results by using concurrent or overlapping treatment options.

Medical Treatment

Nonsteroidal Antiinflammatory Drugs

The use of nonsteroidal antiinflammatory drugs (NSAIDs) is based on the presumption that mechanical and structural alteration combined with local inflammatory changes lead to pain in LSS patients (28). Thus, NSAIDs are aimed at relieving the LSS patient's pain and inflammation to relax the muscle tension, and in this way to improve the functional cooperation of the lumbar spine, pelvis, and lower extremities. These drugs are effective for acute low back pain, but sufficient evidence on chronic low back pain and on LSS is still lacking (29,30).

We have several NSAIDs, as well as cox-2 specific drugs, in clinical use at the present time. However, the efficacy of various NSAIDs is roughly equivalent (28,30). The most common side effects of NSAIDs are gastrointestinal irritation and bleeding, which one has to pay to attention in older patients. These drugs can also deteriorate renal function because of the inhibition of renal prostaglandin synthesis.

Analgesic Drugs

Most LSS patients have chronic low back pain caused by degenerative changes of the lumbar spine (11). There are various pathogenetic mechanisms for this chronic pain (e.g., vascular damage, neuromodulation, and the extensive nerves innervating degenerative discs). Degenerative discs have more extensive innervation than normal discs; these additional nerves may have nociceptive properties (31). It is rational to suppose that the same pain mechanisms play a role in LSS. Centrally acting analgesics should be effective for chronic low back pain and sciatica. Schnitzer et al. (31) showed that tramadol was very effective for the treatment of chronic low back patients. Tramadol also can be used in combination with NSAIDs for a double-active antiinflammatory and analgesic effect.

These centrally acting analgesics are valuable additions to our drug arsenal; however, because of the potential for addiction, sedation, constipation, and other adverse effects (e.g., nausea, dizziness, somnolence, and headache), their use among older patients is limited.

Muscle Relaxants

Muscle relaxant drugs are a logical approach for muscle tension, which may be one of the important etiologic roles in the pathogenesis of chronic low back pain (28,31). However, there is limited evidence for the effectiveness of these drugs in the treatment of chronic low back pain. Further, it is debated whether muscle relaxants offer additive relief when combined with analgesics or NSAIDs (28).

Antidepressant Drugs

Originally, the efficacy of antidepressant drugs was demonstrated in patients with painful diabetic neuropathy. Thus, their use in patients with LSS, including radiculopathy and neuropathic pain, seems to be reasonable, although there is no evidence for the use of antidepressants in LSS. Also, the evidence of their effect is conflicting in chronic low back pain patients. But two other reasons support the use of these drugs for chronic pain of LSS patients: antidepressive effect for subclinical depression and sedating effect for improving sleep. Newer antidepressant drugs (i.e., serotonin reuptake inhibitors) have not been well evaluated in the treatment of chronic pain syndromes (28).

Calcitonin

The effect of salmon calcitonin on LSS pain is probably based on central analgesic effect, improvement of cauda equina blood flow, or antiinflammatory effect (32). Calcitonin has some beneficial analgesic effect on LSS patients with spinal claudication (33,34), but its use has not become standard for LSS nonoperative treatment. However, the use of calcitonin is reasonable in LSS patients with osteoporosis or Paget disease.

Physical Therapy

All treatment options of physical therapy are based on a rational understanding of the degenerative process of the lumbar spine resulting in LSS. Thus, the goal of physical therapy is to counteract the mechanisms of the degenerative process causing symptomatic LSS.

In practice, the physiotherapist has to apply this knowledge to various treatment modalities because currently little is known about the efficacy of physical therapy options. Because LSS patients are often elderly people, the physiotherapist also should have an understanding of age-related changes in the musculoskeletal tissues and their relationship to musculoskeletal impairment (35).

Manual Traction

The therapeutic goal of the manual lumbar traction is aimed at increasing space of the lumbar spinal canal in order to reduce the pressure on the cauda equina (15). It is obvious that traction causes axial movement on discs and facet joints to mobilize and stretch the stiff three-joint complex. If this traction therapy relieves pain, the patient can continue this therapy at home by hanging from the horizontal bar.

Therapeutic Exercise

Therapeutic exercise includes stretching, strengthening, and conditioning, as well as postural education (36). The biomechanical goal of therapeutic exercises is aimed at decreasing the anterior pelvic tilt to decrease the extension the lumbar spine in order to increase space of the lumbar spinal canals (25). The prescription of proper therapeutic exercise should be based on the specific limitations detected during the physical examination and on the understanding of the age-related changes in the musculoskeletal tissues and their relationship to musculoskeletal impairment (35,37). Lindgren et al. (38) showed that therapeutic exercise does not influence segmental instability seen on functional radiography, whereas functional electromyographic (EMG) findings were significantly improved. Further, Arokoski et al. (39) showed by using the surface EMG measurement that simple therapeutic exercises were effective in activating both abdominal and paraspinal muscles.

Transcutaneous Electrical Nerve Stimulation

Transcutaneous electrical nerve stimulation (TENS) is a noninvasive therapeutic option used for pain relief by electrically stimulating peripheral nerves via skin surface electrodes. The goal of TENS in LSS patients is to relieve pain, reduce muscle spasms, improve range of motion, and advance functional ability (40).

The evidence from randomized controlled trials does not support the use or nonuse of TENS alone in the treatment of the chronic pain. Transcutaneous electrical nerve stimulation is likely useful to employ concurrently with other physical therapy modalities because patients in the TENS groups consistently report less pain, better functional status, and greater satisfaction (40). Thus, it is reasonable to suppose that LSS patients benefit from these concurrent treatments.

Epidural Steroid Injection Therapy

Favorable outcomes from some controlled and many uncontrolled studies suggest that epidural steroid injections reduce lumbar radicular pain caused by lumbar disc herniation and LSS. The therapeutic benefit of this therapy may be best attained with concurrent use of other nonoperative treatment (e.g., physical therapy) (41).

The mechanical compression of the nerve root may cause microvascular injury, resulting in formation of nerve root edema, which is likely to cause various neural changes and may be involved in the production of pain in nerve roots (42). The alleged rationale for using epidural steroids is that they reduce the edema and inflammation around nerve roots. However, there is weak evidence in the scientific literature supporting the use of epidural steroids in the management of LSS.

Lumbar spinal stenosis usually occurs in the elderly population in which the surgical risk may be considerable. Because of such risk factors the treating physician may consider alternative treatment options (42). In a descriptive, prospective study of 30 patients with a mean age of 76 years and 10-month follow-up, the caudal epidural injection offered significant pain relief for up to 10 months (43).

Epidural injections should be performed by experienced physicians, and fluoroscopically monitored injections are recommended. Further, no absolute orders can be made regarding the most effective type and dosage of steroid, timing or number of injections, or route of administration (41).

Other Nonoperative Treatment Options

Lumbar Belts

The use of lumbar belts in LSS patients has two goals: to maintain the lumbar spine in slight flexion in order to decrease the compression of the cauda equina and to mitigate irritation or inflammation of the nerve roots, and to improve the motion control in order to result in more stable motion patterns of the functional spinal unit.

Current definitions of spinal instability are based on a loss of stiffness (44). The degeneration of the three-joint complex considerably alters spinal dynamics (44), resulting in abnormal kinematics of the motion segment that may produce irritation or inflammation of the spinal nerves and cauda equina (3,7). Further, a gradual increase in lordosis of the lumbar spine is one sequela of degenerative disc disease. Thus, lumbar supports that decrease lumbar lordosis could be helpful (1).

Ultrasound Therapy and Trigger Point Injections

Myofascial pain syndrome is very likely one of pain expression that arises from the irritated and inflamed source of the degenerative lumbar spine. Both ultrasound therapy and trigger point injections (1% lidocaine) with stretching were found to be effective in reducing pain intensity, increasing pain threshold of myofascial trigger points, and improving range of motion (45).

SUMMARY

Lumbar spinal stenosis is a common and increasing clinical entity because of the growing number of elderly people. The pathoanatomic verification of LSS is practical and easy by means of CT or MRI equipment, but the accurate reconciling the patient's complaints with radiologic changes is not verifiable by clinical means. Further, these elderly patients may have much concurrent pathology. However, the functional nature of LSS, the extension test, and the treadmill test help the physician to unite compatible symptoms and signs with radiologic findings for the clinical diagnosis of LSS.

The management of LSS is not established. The treatment is aimed at alleviating the severity of pain to guarantee the patient's functional capacity in everyday life. In practice, conservative treatment is often adequate in patients with mild or moderate pain, whereas in patients with severe pain surgical decompression is a noteworthy option after 3 months of conservative treatment. The increasing number of LSS patients should motivate us to carry out all-round functional studies on the conservative treatment of LSS.

REFERENCES

1. Berthelot J-M, Bertrand-Vasseur A, Rodet D, et al. Lumbar spinal stenosis: a review. Rev Rhum (English edition) 1997;64:315–325.
2. Simotas AC, Dorey FJ, Hansraj KK, et al. Nonoperative treatment for lumbar spinal stenosis. Clinical and outcome results and a 3-year survivorship analysis. Spine 2000;25:197–204.
3. Spivak JM. Degenerative lumbar spinal stenosis. J Bone Joint Surg 1998;80-A:1053–1066.
4. Amundsen T, Weber H, Nordal H, et al. Lumbar spinal stenosis: conservative or surgical management? A prospective 10-year study. Spine 2000;25:1424–1436.
5. Atlas SJ, Keller RB, Robson D, et al. Surgical and nonsurgical management of lumbar spinal stenosis. Four years outcomes from the Maine Lumbar Spine Study. Spine 2000;25:556–562.
6. Verbiest H. A radicular syndrome from developmental narrowing of the lumbar vertebral canal. J Bone Joint Surg 1954;36-B:230–237.
7. Garfin SR, Herkowitz HN, Mirkovic S. Spinal stenosis. J Bone Joint Surg 1999;81-A:572–586.
8. Mariconda M, Fava R, Gatto R, et al. Unilateral laminectomy for bilateral decompression of lumbar spinal stenosis: a prospective comparative study with conservatively treated patients. J Spinal Dis Tech 2002;15:39–46.
9. Mariconda M, Zanforlino G, Celestino GA, et al. Factors influencing the outcome of degenerative lumbar spinal stenosis. J Spinal Dis 2000;13:131–137.
10. Rauschning W. Pathoanatomy of lumbar disc degeneration and stenosis. Acta Orthop Scand 1993;(Suppl 251)64:3–12.
11. Amundsen T, Weber H, Lilleås F, et al. Lumbar spinal stenosis. Clinical and radiologic feature. Spine 1995;20:1178–1186.
12. Verbiest H. Stenosis of the lumbar vertebral canal and sciatica. Neurosurg Rev 1980;3:75–89.
13. Penning L. Functional pathology of lumbar spinal stenosis. Clin Biomech 1992;7:3–17.
14. Schönström N, Lindahl S, Willen J, et al. Dynamic changes in the dimensions of the lumbar spinal canal: an experimental study in vitro. J Orthop Res 1989;7:115–121.
15. Schönström N. The narrow lumbar spinal canal and the size of the cauda equina in man. A clinical and experimental study. Thesis, University of Gothenburg, 1988.
16. Katz JN, Dalgas M, Stucki G, et al. Diagnosis of lumbar spinal stenosis. Rheum Dis Clin North Am 1994;20:471–483.
17. Takahashi K, Kagechika K, Takino T, et al. Changes in epidural pressure during walking in patients with lumbar spinal stenosis. Spine 1995;20:2746–2749.
18. Takahashi K, Miyazaki T, Takino T, et al. Epidural pressure measurements. Relationship between epidural pressure and posture in patients with lumbar spinal stenosis. Spine 1995;20:650–653.
19. Sortland O, Magnaes B, Hauge T. Functional myelography with metrizamide in the diagnosis of lumbar spinal stenosis. Acta Radiol 1977;355(suppl):42–54.
20. Wildermuth S, Zanotti M, Duewell S, et al. Lumbar spine: quantitative and qualitative assessment of positional (upright flexion and extension) MR imaging and myelography. Radiology 1998;207:391–398.
21. Willen J, Danielson B, Gaulitz A, et al. Dynamic effects on the lumbar spinal canal. Axially loaded CT-myelography and MRI in patients with sciatica and/or neurogenic claudication. Spine 1997;22:2968–2976.
22. Fritz JM, Erhard RE, Delitto A, et al. Preliminary results of the use of a two-stage treadmill test as a clinical diagnostic tool in the differential diagnosis of the lumbar spinal stenosis. J Spinal Dis 1997;10:410–416.
23. Moreland LW, Lopez-Mendez A, Alarcon GS. Spinal stenosis: a comprehensive review of the literature. Semin Arthritis Rheum 1989;19:127–149.
24. Haegerstam GAT. Pathophysiology of bone pain. A review. Acta Orthop Scand 2001;72:308–317.
25. Nagler W, Hausen HS. Conservative management of lumbar spinal stenosis. Identifying patients likely to do well without surgery. Postgrad Med 1998;103:69–88.
26. Truumees E, Herkowitz HN. Lumbar spinal stenosis: treatment options. AAOS Instr Course Lect 2001;50:153–161.
27. Simotas AC. Nonoperative treatment for lumbar spinal stenosis. Clin Orthop Rel Res 2001;384:153–161.
28. Deyo RA. Drug therapy for back pain. Which drugs help which patients? Spine 1996;21:2840–2850.
29. Koes BW, Scholten RJ, Mens JM, et al. Efficacy of non-steroidal anti-inflammatory drugs for low back pain: a systematic review of randomised clinical trials. Ann Rheum Dis 1997;56:214–223.
30. van Tulder MW, Scholten RJP, Koes BW, et al. Nonsteroidal anti-inflammatory drugs for low back pain. Spine 2000;25:2501–2513.
31. Schnitzer TJ, Gray WL, Paster RZ, et al. Efficacy of tramadol in treatment of chronic low back pain. J Rheumatol 2000;27:772–778.
32. Marcotte PJ, Virella A. Lumbar spinal stenosis: treatment options and results. Semin Neurosurg 2000;11:231–244.
33. Eskola A, Pohjolainen T, Alaranta H, et al. Calcitonin treatment in lumbar spinal stenosis: a randomized, placebo-controlled, double-blind, cross-over study with one-year follow up. Calcif Tissue Int 1992;50:400–403.
34. Porter RW, Hibbert C. Calcitonin treatment for neurogenic claudication. Spine 1983;8:585–592.
35. Buckwalter JA, Woo SL-Y, Goldberg VM, et al. Soft-tissue aging and musculoskeletal function. J Bone Joint Surg 1993;75-A:1533–1548.
36. Bodack MP, Monteiro M-E. Therapeutic exercise in hte treatment of patients with lumbar spinal stenosis. Clin Orthop Rel Res 2001;384:144–152.
37. Rosomoff HL, Rosomoff RS. Nonsurgical aggressive treatment of lumbar spinal stenosis. State Art Rev 1987;1:383–399.
38. Lindgren K-A, Sihvonen T, Leino E, et al. Exercise therapy effects on functional radiographic findings and segmental electromyographic activity in lumbar spine instability. Arch Phys Med Rehabil 1993;74:933–939.
39. Arokoski JP, Valta T, Airaksinen O, et al. Back and abdominal muscle function during stabilization exercises. Arch Phys Med Rehab 2001;82:1089–1098.
40. Brosseau L, Milne S, Robinson V, et al. Efficacy of the transcutaneous electrical nerve stimulation for the treatment of chronic low back pain. A meta-analysis. Spine 2002;27:596–603.
41. Weinstein SM, Herring SA, Derby R. Contemporary concepts in spine care. Epidural steroid injections. Spine 1995;20:1842–1846.
42. Rydevik BL, Cohen DB, Kostuik JP. Spine epidural steroids for patients with lumbar spinal stenosis. Spine 1997;22:2313–2317.
43. Ciocon JO, Galindo-Ciocon D, Amaranath L, et al. Caudal epidural blocks for elderly patients with lumbar spinal stenosis. J Am Geriatr Soc 1994;42:593–596.
44. Ogon M, Bender BR, Hooper DM, et al. A dynamic approach to spinal instability. Part I: Sensitization of intersegmental motion profiles to motion direction and load condition by instability. Spine 1997;22:2841–2858.
45. Esenyel M, Caglar N, Aldemir T. Treatment of myofascial pain. Am J Phys Med Rehab 2000;79:48–52.

CHAPTER 51

Indications for Surgery and Laminotomy Procedures

Franco Postacchini

Lumbar spinal stenosis has been defined as a "narrowing of the osteoligamentous vertebral canal and/or the intervertebral foramen causing compression of the thecal sac and/or the caudal nerve roots; at a single level, narrowing may affect the whole canal or part of it" (1–3). This definition implies a clear-cut distinction between a narrow spinal canal in which the neural structures are not compressed and a stenotic canal causing compression of the caudal nerve roots (Fig. 51-1A, B).

Spinal stenosis includes developmental, degenerative, and combined (developmental and degenerative) stenosis.

Developmental stenosis can be achondroplastic or constitutional. The former is the pathologic narrowing that can be found in achondroplastic dwarfs. The latter, which has also been called idiopathic developmental stenosis (4), is characterized by an abnormal narrowing of the bony vertebral canal that cannot be ascribed to any known etiologic factor. A narrow spinal canal may transform into stenosis in the presence of minor degenerative changes of the intervertebral disc or the articular processes and is unable to cause compression of the neural structures in a spinal canal that primarily is of normal size.

Degenerative stenosis is most often associated with deformities such as degenerative spondylolisthesis or scoliosis. The form not associated with deformities may be called simple degenerative stenosis. The latter is due to degenerative changes of the articular processes or osteophytosis of the vertebral end plates in the presence of a spinal canal originally of normal size.

Each condition includes spinal canal stenosis and isolated nerve root canal stenosis, which correspond, respectively, to the so-called central stenosis and lateral stenosis (Fig. 51-1B, Fig. 51-2). Stenosis of the intervertebral foramen, which should not be identified with lateral stenosis, is usually associated with one of the two other types of stenosis (5).

INDICATIONS FOR SURGERY

Natural History

Johnsson et al. (6) compared 19 untreated patients with 30 patients who underwent surgery. They were followed for a mean of 31 and 53 months, respectively; all patients in both groups had lumbar stenosis of moderate severity. One-third of the untreated patients were improved and two-thirds were unchanged or had worsened. Porter et al. (7) reviewed 169 patients with lateral stenosis, most of whom had no treatment. After a mean of 2 years, radicular symptoms persisted in 78% of cases, but had improved in 90%. In the vast majority of preoperative patients, however, there was no evidence of neurologic deficits, and in no instances was clinical diagnosis confirmed by imaging or neurophysiologic studies.

Conservative Management

In a retrospective study (8) of 49 patients followed for a mean of 33 months, it was found at the latest follow-up that 9 patients had undergone surgery, 7 had worsened, 12 were unchanged, and 21 were slightly or significantly improved.

In a prospective study (9), 19 patients with severe symptoms were selected for surgery and 50 patients with moderate symptoms for conservative treatment, whereas 31 were randomized between the conservative and surgical treatment groups. At 3-month follow-up, relief of pain had occurred in most patients. After 4 years, satisfactory results were observed in half of the patients in the conservative group and in four-fifths of those treated surgically. After 10 years, the results showed no significant deterioration in both groups. The results in the patients randomized for surgery were considerably better than in those randomized for conservative management. In another prospective study (10), 67 patients treated surgi-

495

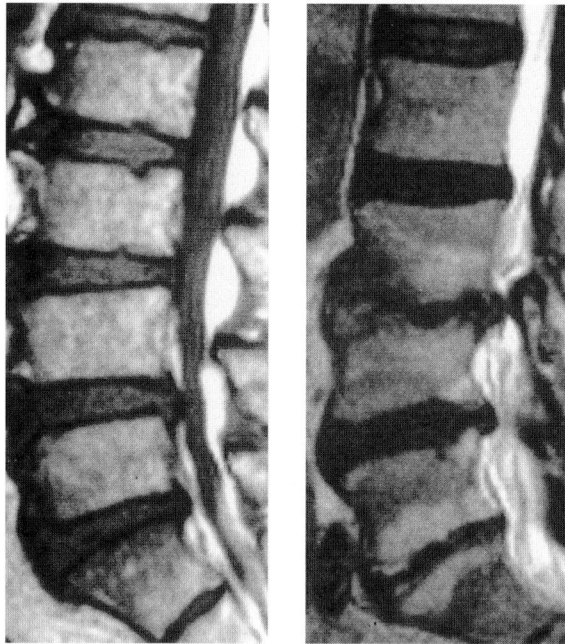

FIG. 51-1. A: T1-weighted magnetic resonance imaging (MRI) sagittal scan showing a narrow spinal canal. The thecal sac has small anteroposterior diameters, particularly at the lower three lumbar levels, but the neural structures show no osteoligamentous compression. **B:** T2-weighted sagittal MRI scan showing severe stenosis at L2-L3 level and less marked stenosis at L4-L5.

cally and 52 nonsurgically were followed for 4 years. At the latest follow-up, satisfactory results were reported by 63% of the patients in the surgery group and 42% of those treated conservatively.

In my experience, most patients with severe central stenosis do not improve or show temporary relief after

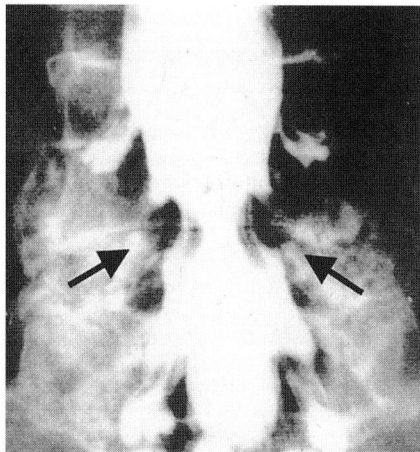

FIG. 51-2. Anteroposterior myelogram showing lateral stenosis at L4-L5 level. The L5 root is not filled with contrast medium bilaterally *(arrows)* and the thecal sac shows a mild indentation on both sides.

conservative management. Conversely, patients with central stenosis causing posterior or posterolateral compression of the thecal sac, but no significant nerve root compression in the radicular canal, often show a significant improvement, which is probably due to the natural course of the disease. The same is true for lateral stenosis: if narrowing of the radicular canal is severe and responsible for significant neurologic changes, conservative management does not usually lead to significant improvement, particularly in the long term.

Candidates for Surgery

There is no indication for surgery in patients with only a narrow spinal canal. Similarly, surgery is usually not indicated in stenotic patients who complain only of back pain, in the absence of deformities, such as degenerative spondylolisthesis or scoliosis, or vertebral instability. In patients with an unstable motion segment who have only back pain it is usually sufficient to carry out a fusion alone if stenosis is mild, because it is very unlikely that neural compression will significantly increase and become symptomatic over time once the motion segment has been stabilized. Conversely, neural decompression should be performed if stenosis is severe, because the modifications of reciprocal position of the articular processes, as a result of fusion, can be responsible for postoperative onset of radicular symptoms.

In patients with radicular symptoms, surgery is indicated when conservative management protracted for at least 3 months has led to no significant improvement.

In the presence of motor deficits only, it can be difficult to decide whether there is an indication for decompression. Surgery is usually indicated when stenosis is severe and the deficits are severe and of less than a few months' duration. In the presence of paresis lasting more than 6 to 8 months, there can be no indication for decompression because there are few or no chances of improvement of muscle function.

The best candidates for surgery are those patients under the age of 70 years with no comorbid diseases, who have a severe or very severe stenosis, long-standing radicular symptoms associated with severe intermittent claudication, moderate, or no motor deficits, and mild or no back pain. On the opposite side of the spectrum are patients who have mild stenosis, mild or inconstant leg symptoms with no precise radicular distribution, a history of claudication after several hundred meters or longer, no motor deficit, and back pain of similar severity to, or more severe than, leg symptoms. In these cases, surgery usually involves high risk of a poor result and should be thus avoided or delayed as long as possible. Between the two extremes there are numerous situations in which the surgical indication should be evaluated individually, based on several factors, which may or may not influence the decision.

Advanced Age

Several studies have shown that surgical decompression also may offer significant relief of symptoms to patients older than 70 years (6,11–13). In my experience, there is no significant difference in the results of surgery between patients in early older adulthood (60 to 70 years) and those who are older (over 80 to 90 years), provided the stenosis is severe and the patient is in satisfactory general health.

Comorbidity

In one study (12), a high rate of comorbid illnesses was found to be inversely related to the rate of satisfactory results after surgery. Another study (14) compared the long-term results of surgery in 24 diabetic and 22 nondiabetic patients. In the diabetic group there was a 41% rate of satisfactory results, compared with 90% in the nondiabetic group. Different results, however, were observed in a similar study (15), in which the outcome was satisfactory in 72% of the diabetic and 80% of the nondiabetic patients. Neither the duration of the diabetes before surgery nor its type correlated with the outcome. A mistaken preoperative diagnosis was the main cause of failure in diabetic patients, in whom diabetic neuropathy or angiopathy may mimic the symptoms of stenosis.

Previous Surgery

Surgery for spinal stenosis tends to give less favorable results in patients who previously underwent decompressive procedures in the lumbar spine (11,16–18). This is particularly true when stenosis is at the same level or levels at which the previous surgery for disc herniation or stenosis had been performed (3). In these cases, decompressive surgery should usually be undertaken in the presence of severe compression of the neural structures and severe symptoms well correlated with the vertebral level or levels that appear stenotic on the imaging studies.

Disc Herniation

A concomitant disc herniation in the stenotic area does not influence the indications for surgery. However, the presence of multiple, markedly bulging discs associated with only mild posterolateral compression of the neural structures exposes the patient to the risk of persistent anterior compression of the nerve roots after a posterior decompression.

Type of Stenosis

There is no significant difference in terms of indications for surgery between the various types of central stenosis. However, patients with degenerative or combined stenosis at a single level appear to be the best candidates to surgery because they tend to have a better outcome compared to those with stenosis at multiple levels. In patients with constitutional stenosis, the intervertebral disc may play a significant role in the compression of the neural structures. When the disc bulges considerably in the spinal canal, but is not truly herniated, it may be impossible to eliminate the anterior compression of the neural structures and this may lead to less satisfactory results compared with the cases in which the neural compression is caused exclusively by the articular processes. Patients with lateral stenosis tend to have better results than those with central stenosis in terms of relief of both radicular symptoms and back pain, particularly when stenosis, as usually occurs, is at a single level.

Certainty of the Diagnosis

It is sometimes difficult, in patients with leg symptoms, to determine whether the symptoms are related to compression of a nerve root and which root is involved. This often occurs in patients with mild or moderate narrowing of the central or lateral spinal canal and no motor deficits or reflex changes. In these cases, in which magnetic resonance imaging (MRI) and computed tomography (CT) may be unhelpful, there is an indication for myelography. When myelography is inconclusive, nerve root injection with local anesthetic may be indicated. Even the latter, however, may leave the diagnosis uncertain. These patients are the worse candidates for surgery. Surgical management can be taken into consideration only when other diseases, particularly hip conditions and peripheral neuropathies, are excluded and the clinical symptoms and preoperative investigations indicate that there are enough possibilities that a given spinal root is the cause of symptoms.

Spinal Fusion

Fusion of motion segments decompressed bilaterally is unnecessary, unless (a) the motion segment, albeit in the absence of degenerative spondylolisthesis, is preoperatively unstable, as shown by flexion-extension X-rays; (b) at surgery, the articular processes have completely been removed, accidentally or purposely, on both sides; or (c) the articular processes have been excised on one side and discectomy has been performed bilaterally in a patient complaining of chronic back pain, particularly when the latter probably originated from the decompressed motion segment. These guidelines, previously indicated based of the clinical experience (3), were confirmed by a prospective randomized study (19).

SURGICAL TREATMENT

Definition of Terms

Decompression of the lumbar spinal canal can be carried out by central laminectomy—also defined as bilateral or complete laminectomy—or by laminotomy. The latter—also called keyhole laminotomy or hemilaminectomy or partial hemilaminectomy—consists in the removal of the caudal portion of the proximal lamina, the cranial portion of the distal lamina and a varying portion of the articular processes, together with a part of, or the entire, ligamentum flavum on the side of surgery.

The term *foraminotomy* indicates removal of a part of the posterior wall of the intervertebral foramen, while the term *foraminectomy* refers to complete excision of the wall of the foramen.

Unilateral Laminotomy at a Single Level

Indications

The main indication is lateral stenosis at a single level on one side.

The preoperative planning may be difficult when lateral stenosis is severe and symptomatic on one side and mild and asymptomatic on the opposite side. In these cases, the advantage of performing a unilateral decompression is more to preserve the stability of the motion segment and to avoid the risk of onset of radicular symptoms on the asymptomatic side after surgery. There are patients who complain of radicular pain for several weeks or months after decompression on the asymptomatic side. A possible explanation is that the surgical trauma and the scarring tissue may irritate a nerve root which is not significantly compressed before surgery, while these factors have no detrimental effect on a compressed root.

Unilateral decompression may also be indicated in the presence of severe lateral stenosis on both sides in older patients with unilateral symptoms who are in poor general health or when there are high chances that bilateral decompression may lead to vertebral instability and spinal fusion is, for any reason, not indicated.

In patients with central stenosis at a single level or multiple levels, unilateral laminotomy may be indicated in the presence of monoradicular symptoms, particularly when nerve root injection with a local anesthetic has shown that a single root is symptomatic or when a more extensive decompression appears unnecessary or contraindicated.

Technique

The surgical technique is similar to that used to remove a herniated disc. When using the operating microscope, the skin incision is some 4 cm in length. I usually begin by removing the caudal half of the cranial lamina and the medial half of the inferior articular process of the vertebra above using an osteotome. There is no risk in using the osteotome for removal of the inferior articular process because the underlying superior articular process of the vertebra below protects the emerging nerve root. The lig-

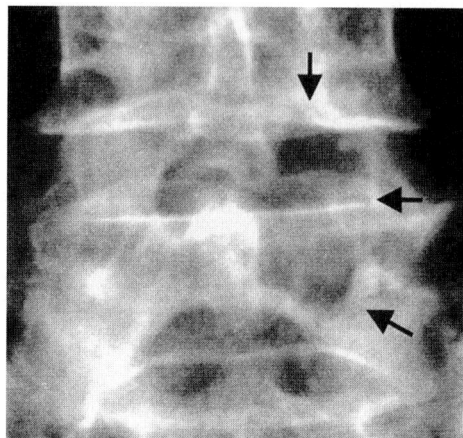

FIG. 51-3. Postoperative radiograph of a patient with lateral stenosis at L4-L5 level on the left side who underwent laminotomy on that side *(arrows)*. Note the wide decompression performed on the transverse plane.

amentum flavum can now be seen and detached from the border of the caudal lamina and the superior articular process with a curette. The osteotome can also be used to remove the proximal half of the caudal lamina and the superior articular process. When removing the latter, attention must be paid to place the blade of the osteotome in the most lateral part of the process and to orient the osteotome 15° to 20° obliquely in a medial-lateral direction to avoid damage to the underlying root (17). Alternatively, a Kerrison rongeur is used for piecemeal removal of the caudal lamina and the superior facet. Once the emerging root and the thecal sac are exposed, bone removal from the lateral part of the canal is continued using the osteotome obliquely until the neural structures are completely free of compression. Complete excision of the articular processes must be avoided. However, when laminotomy is performed on one side only, decompression can be generous because there is no risk to destabilize the motion segment, if this is stable preoperatively (Fig. 51-3). The disc is inspected and excised if it is soft and protrudes markedly. The final step is to use a probe to determine whether the emerging nerve root is compressed in the intervertebral foramen and to remove bone until it is completely free of compression, paying attention to not perform an unnecessary foraminectomy.

Bilateral Laminotomy at a Single Level

Indications

The advantage of bilateral laminotomy at a single level, compared with central laminectomy, is that laminotomy preserves vertebral stability to a greater extent than laminectomy by preserving the supraspinous and interspinous ligaments and the central portion of the vertebral arch.

This procedure is the treatment of choice in patients with lateral stenosis at a single level in the presence of bilateral leg symptoms. In central stenosis, bilateral laminotomy is indicated when narrowing of the spinal canal is mild or moderate, particularly when discectomy on one side or both sides is performed due to concomitant disc herniation or marked disc bulging. This often occurs in constitutional stenosis, in which bilateral laminotomy should usually be preferred to central laminectomy. In degenerative central stenosis, there is an indication for laminotomy when narrowing of the spinal canal is not exceedingly severe. When stenosis is marked, bilateral laminotomy may lead to persistence of radicular symptoms due to inadequate decompression of the thecal sac in the central portion of the spinal canal.

Technique

The technique is similar to that described for unilateral laminotomy. More attention must be taken to preserve the outer third of the articular processes because total or subtotal arterectomy, particularly when bilateral, entails a high risk of postoperative instability.

Laminotomies at Multiple Levels

Indications

Patients with constitutional central stenosis often have stenosis at multiple levels. Usually they are middle-aged or in early older adulthood and in many cases stenosis is of moderate severity and the intervertebral discs are normal in height. Furthermore, the discs often play an important role in the compression of the neural structures by protruding in the spinal canal. In these patients, central laminectomy exposes the patient to the risk of postoperative vertebral instability, particularly when discectomy is carried out or stenosis involves the high lumbar levels, where it is more difficult, with central laminectomy, to preserve the articular processes. In these cases, laminotomies at multiple levels allow vertebral stability to be preserved, thus avoiding fusion procedures at two or more levels.

The same considerations are valid for degenerative central stenosis. In this type of stenosis, however, it is less often necessary to make any effort to preserve vertebral stability and avoid spinal fusion because the presence of intervertebral osteophytes or a marked decrease in height of the discs exposes the patient less to the risk of postoperative instability. Furthermore, narrowing of the spinal canal may be much more severe than in constitutional stenosis and laminectomy thus ensures a more complete neural decompression. However, in patients with degenerative stenosis there is also often an indication for multiple laminotomies. This occurs when central laminectomy is a risk to destabilize the motion segments, or

stenosis, although involving the whole canal, is particularly severe in the nerve root canal. An advantage of laminotomy is that decompression is focused on the nerve root emerging from the thecal sac and it can therefore be more effective in terms of clinical results, because in stenotic patients the radiated symptoms are often caused by compression of the emerging root, rather than the thecal sac.

Occasionally, the two procedures can be combined, when stenosis is very severe at one or two levels and moderate and essentially lateral at one or two additional levels.

Technique

The spine is exposed using the same technique employed for central laminectomy. The interlaminar spaces are cleaned of residual muscle tissue using a curette. Beginning on one side, laminotomy is performed, as described earlier, at the most stenotic level and then at the cranial or caudal levels needing decompression. The same procedure is successively carried out on the opposite side (Fig. 51-4). When performing laminotomy at two adjacent levels, care should be taken not to remove the entire lamina on one side and particularly on both sides at the same level, since in the latter case the spinous process becomes unstable and should be removed. If complete arthrectomy is inadvertently carried out on one side, at least the outer third of the articular processes on the opposite side should be preserved and discectomy should be avoided, particularly on both sides.

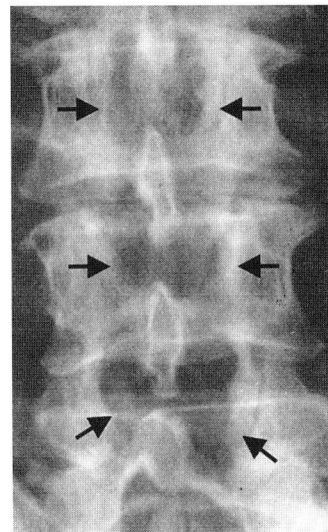

FIG. 51-4. Radiograph taken 2 years postoperatively in a patient with constitutional stenosis at L2-L3 to L4-L5. The *arrows* indicate the laminotomies performed at the stenotic levels.

Results of Laminotomies

In a prospective randomized study comparing central laminectomy with multilevel laminotomy in central lumbar stenosis, Postacchini et al. (20) found laminotomy to give similar overall results to total laminectomy. Patients submitted to laminotomy had less back pain and none had vertebral instability postoperatively, but they also had less subjective improvement for radicular symptoms, although the difference was not significant. It was concluded that multiple laminotomy is the treatment of choice when narrowing of the spinal canal is mild or moderate.

In a prospective study of patients with central or lateral stenosis, 96% were satisfied with tier treatment at a mean of 4 years after surgery (21). Aryanpur and Ducker (22) obtained satisfactory results in the vast majority of their 32 patients with lateral stenosis. None of these individuals experienced surgical complications. However, Young et al. (23), using multiple laminotomy with an operating microscope in 32 patients with lateral or central stenosis reported a 9% incidence of dural tears. In the series of patients mentioned above, we found a higher incidence of postoperative neural deficits with laminotomy than with central laminectomy and in most cases neural complications occurred in patients with severe stenosis.

REFERENCES

1. Postacchini F. Lumbar spinal stenosis and pseudostenosis. Definition and classification of pathology. Ital J Orthop Traumat 1983;9:339–351.
2. Postacchini F. Management of lumbar spinal stenosis. J Bone Joint Surg 1996;78B:154–164.
3. Postacchini F. Lumbar spinal stenosis. Vienna: Springer-Verlag, 1989.
4. Verbiest H. Results of surgical treatment of idiopathic developmental stenosis of the lumbar vertebral canal. A review of twenty-seven years experience. J Bone Joint Surg 1977;59B:181–188.
5. Cinotti G, De Santis P, Nofroni I, et al. Stenosis of the intervertebral foramen. Anatomic study on predisposing factors. Spine 2002;27: 223–229.
6. Johnsson KE, Udén A, Rosén I. The effect of decompression on the natural course of spinal stenosis. A comparison of surgically treated and untreated patients. Spine 1991;16:615–619.
7. Porter RW, Hibbert C, Evans C. The natural history of root entrapment syndrome. Spine 1984;9:418–421.
8. Simotas Ac, Dorey FJ, Hansraj KK, et al. Nonoperative treatment for lumbar spinal stenosis. Clinical and outcome results and a 3-year survivorship analysis. Spine 2000;25:197–204.
9. Amundsen T, Weber H, Nordal HJ, et al. Lumbar spinal stenosis: conservative or surgical management? A prospective 10-year study. Spine 2000;25:1424–1436.
10. Atlas SJ, Keller RB, Robson D, et al. Surgical and nonsurgical management of lumbar spinal stenosis. Four-year outcome from the Maine Lumbar Spine Study. Spine 2000;25:556–562.
11. Herron LD, Mangelsdorf C. Lumbar spinal stenosis: results of surgical treatment. J Spinal Disord 1991;4:26–33.
12. Katz IN, Lipson SJ, Larson MG, et al. The outcome of decompressive laminectomy for degenerative lumbar stenosis. J Bone Joint Surg 1991; 73A:809–811.
13. Sanderson PL, Wood PLR. Surgery for lumbar spinal stenosis in old people. J Bone Joint Surg 1993;75B:393–397.
14. Simpson JM, Silveri CP, Balderstone RA, et al. The results of operations on the lumbar spine in patients who have diabetes mellitus. J Bone Joint Surg 1993;75A:1823–1829.
15. Cinotti G, Postacchini F, Weinstein JN. Lumbar spinal stenosis and diabetes. Outcome of surgical decompression. J Bone Joint Surg 1994; 76B:215–219.
16. Boccanera L, Pelliccioni S, Laus M. Stenosis of the lumbar vertebral canal (a study of 25 cases operated on). Ital J Orthop Traumat 1984; 10:227–236.
17. Getty CJM. Lumbar spinal stenosis. The clinical spectrum and the results of operation. J Bone Joint Surg 1980;62B:481–485.
18. Nasca RJ. Rationale for spinal fusion in lumbar spinal stenosis. Spine 1989;14:451–454.
19. Grob D, Humke T, Dvorak J. Degenerative lumbar spinal stenosis. Decompression with and without arthrodesis. J Bone Joint Surg 1995; 77A:1036–1041.
20. Postacchini F, Cinotti G, Perugia D, et al. The surgical treatment of central lumbar stenosis. Multiple laminotomy compared with total laminectomy. J Bone Joint Surg 1993;75B:386–392.
21. Kleeman TJ, Hiscoe AC, Berg EE. Patient outcomes after minimally destabilizing lumbar stenosis decompression. The "port-hole" technique. Spine 2000;25:865–870.
22. Aryanpur J, Ducker T. multilevel lumbar laminotomies: an alternative to laminectomy in the treatment of lumbar stenosis. Neurosurgery 1990;26:429–433.
23. Young S, Veerapen R, O'laoire SA. Relief of lumbar canal stenosis using multilevel subarticular fenestration as an alternative to wide laminectomy: preliminary report. Neurosurgery 1988;23:628–633.

CHAPTER 52

Laminectomy for Spinal Stenosis

Brian J. C. Freeman

Spinal stenosis maybe defined as a narrowing of the central spinal canal, the lateral recess, or the neural foramina. Normal canal size has been reported as a midsagittal diameter of greater than 11.5 mm and a cross-sectional area of greater than 1.45 cm^2 (1,2). *Absolute stenosis* is said to occur when the midsagittal diameter of the canal is less than 10 mm and *relative stenosis* is said to occur when the midsagittal diameter of the canal is between 10 and 13 mm (3).

Spinal stenosis may be primary or secondary. Primary spinal stenosis may be congenital or developmental (e.g., achondroplastic stenosis or constitutional spinal stenosis). Secondary stenosis occurs in a canal of normal dimension and is acquired as a result of conditions such as spondylosis. Degeneration in the three joint complexes typically starts this process. Synovitis commencing in the facet joints leads to the thinning of articular cartilage and loosening of the joint capsule (4). This leads to greater spinal motion accelerating degeneration in the disc. Disc height is lost leading to a reduction in the size of the neural foramina (so called up-down stenosis). The ligamentum flavum becomes redundant with infolding further contributing to a reduction in canal dimensions (5). Osteophytes on the superior articular facet narrow the lateral recess; osteophytes on the inferior articular facet narrow the central canal. Reduction in canal volume can compromise vascular supply to the neural elements leading to an ischemic neuritis (6), and direct compression of nerve roots may lead to demyelination causing unremitting pain. Spinal stenosis may be present in isolation or in combination with other conditions such as degenerative spondylolisthesis or degenerative scoliosis. The natural history of spinal stenosis remains unclear. There are few longitudinal prospective studies documenting the course in untreated patients (7). Existing literature suggests that symptoms progress in approximately 20% (8) to 33% (7) of nonoperated patients.

INDICATIONS FOR SURGERY

Patients present with an insidious onset of back, buttock, thigh, and calf pain. Typically in neurogenic claudication, back, and leg pain are increased when standing and walking. Patients may sit or bend forward to relieve this pain. These postural changes result in an increase in the size of the canal. Walking is increasingly restricted and ultimately rest pain or a neurogenic bladder may develop. Vascular claudication may be confused with neurogenic claudication. The patient with vascular insufficiency has pain that is increased by walking and lying down but is often decreased by standing. The patient with spinal stenosis may be able to cycle a considerable distance because the lumbar spine is flexed during this activity. The patient with vascular insufficiency however is likely to provoke symptoms during such activity. A search for risk factors such as cigarette smoking and diabetes, plus a careful examination of peripheral pulses will usually help to distinguish the two conditions.

Physical examination in a patient with spinal stenosis typically reveals a loss of lumbar lordosis, increased pain on extension, and reduced pain on flexion. Specific neurologic signs are rare, but may be provoked by exercise. Passive straight leg raise is often negative. The shuttle walking test (9) and the exercise treadmill (10) have been used to measure baseline functional status and surgical outcome objectively. Patients with hip, groin, or knee pain may have osteoarthritis of the hip or knee. If doubt exists, plain radiographs of the lumbar spine, pelvis, and knee will help to confirm the pain source. Patients with diabetes commonly have symptoms of peripheral neuropathy. Electromyograms (EMGs) and nerve conduction studies may help with the diagnosis. Finally it should be remembered that there is an associated cervical stenosis in approximately 5% of patients with lumbar stenosis (11).

Conservative management should always be considered before surgery. Nonsteroidal antiinflammatory medication can reduce both back and leg pain. Physiotherapy working on trunk stabilization and flexion exercises may be beneficial. General fitness work including cycling, swimming, and walking in water may improve a patient's symptoms. The use of epidural steroids remains controversial. They may relieve acute pain, but long-term results have been disappointing. Others suggest epidural steroids should be considered as a nonsurgical alternative, especially in the older adult patient where surgery carries greater risk (12). There is circumstantial evidence that calcitonin is beneficial for approximately 40% of patients with neurogenic claudication, particularly in those with spinal Paget disease (13). Simotas et al. studied 49 patients with lumbar spinal stenosis who were treated with aggressive nonoperative treatment including exercise, analgesics, and epidural steroids (14). They reported 25% of patients were significantly better after a 3-year period, and that neurologic deterioration was rare.

Patients who fail conservative treatment and persist with moderate or severe intractable leg pain should be considered for surgery. Patients who are unable to stand upright, and have a significant reduction in walking distance, and who find this degree of disability unacceptable should also be considered for elective surgery. The patient should be medically fit and able to tolerate a general anesthetic, the prone position, and the estimated blood loss. Occasionally, among older adults multiple comorbidities may preclude surgery. A delay in surgery of months or even years does not appear to adversely affect the result of surgery (15). Patients with rest pain or acute onset of urinary retention or fecal incontinence should be considered for *urgent* surgery.

Imaging studies are of prime importance in defining the level and degree of stenosis. Plain radiographs may show a narrow interpedicular distance on the anteroposterior view and short pedicles on the lateral view in congenital stenosis. They may also reveal a degenerative spondylolisthesis or a degenerative scoliosis. Water-soluble myelography combined with computed tomography (CT) has until recently been regarded as the gold standard. However, this invasive technique has largely been replaced by fine-cut CT scan (Figs. 52-1, 52-2) and magnetic resonance imaging (MRI) (Figs. 52-3 through 52-7). The latest generation two-dimensional CT scanners allow soft tissue and bony windows of both axial and sagittal orientation. However, there is still the difficulty of surveying the whole spine with CT. MRI is noninvasive and allows surveillance of the whole spine. Its use is contraindicated in the presence of ferromagnetic implants. Bony detail and extent of foraminal stenosis is still best observed on a good CT scan. CT and MRI remain complementary investigations, with the majority of surgeons opting for MRI as the initial investigation.

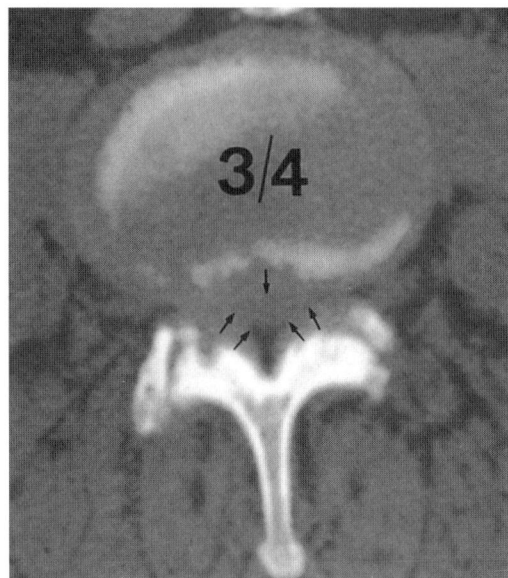

FIG. 52-1. Case 1. An 81-year-old man with bilateral leg pain, maximum walking distance 100 yards. Computed tomography of the spine, axial section at L3-L4, showing moderate central and lateral recess stenosis. Circumferential disc bulge *(arrow)* and hypertrophic degenerative changes in the facet joints with associated flaval ligament thickening *(arrow)*.

Before proceeding with surgery all imaging should demonstrate clear evidence of neural compression that is *congruent* with the patient signs and symptoms. If doubt exists regarding the extent of decompression, electrodiagnostic testing can help. EMGs show changes in approximately 80% of patients with spinal stenosis and may help

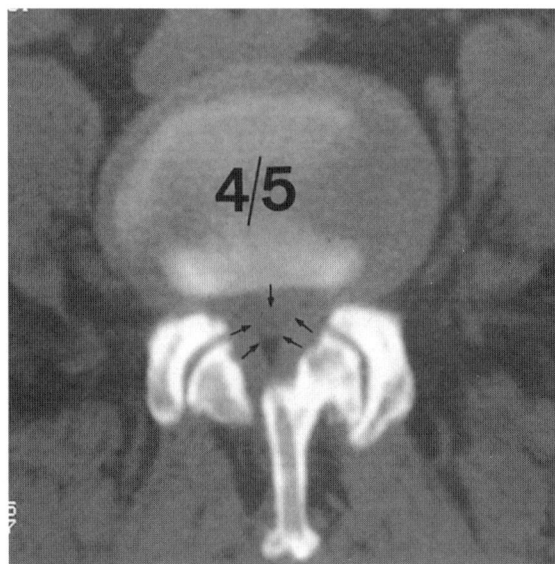

FIG. 52-2. Case 1. Computed tomography of the spine, axial section at L4-L5, showing further central canal and lateral recess stenosis.

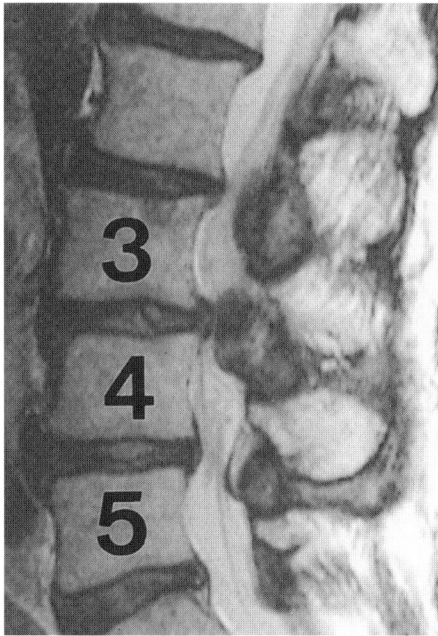

FIG. 52-3. Case 2. An 80-year-old man with weakness in both legs when walking more than 3 yards. Midline sagittal T2-weighted magnetic resonance image scan showing critical central canal stenosis L3-L4, relative stenosis L2-L3, and L4-L5.

to localize surgery (16). Somatosensory evoked potentials have been used, but have a high false-positive rate. Motor evoked potentials may also play a role in the assessment of the complex patient. The response to lumbar epidural steroids can predict the outcome of decompressive surgery.

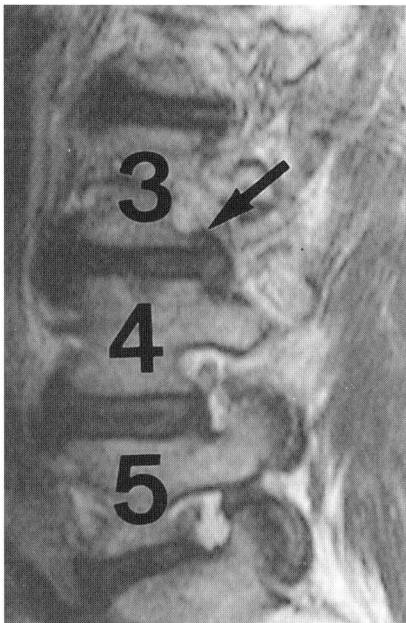

FIG. 52-5. Case 2. Axial T2-weighted magnetic resonance image through L3-L4. Central and lateral canal stenosis. Note facet joint hypertrophy and thickening of ligamentum flavum.

In one series, patients who had pain for less than 12 months and in whom epidural steroids reduced leg pain by 50% for more than 1 week, a good result was observed in 95% 12 months after surgery (17). On the other hand if symptoms were present for more than 1 year, and the

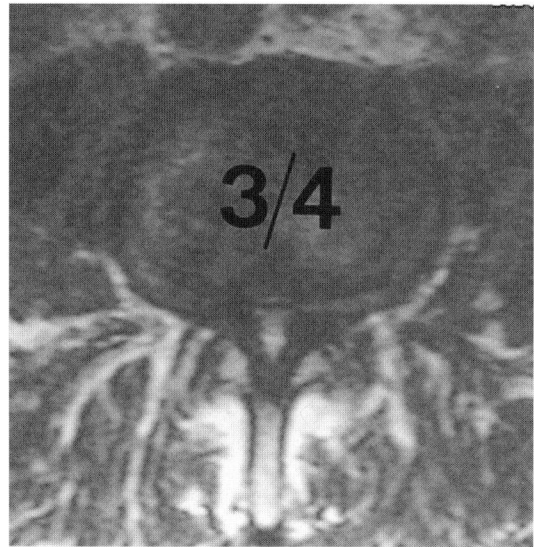

FIG. 52-4. Case 2. Right parasagittal T2-weighted magnetic resonance image showing foraminal stenosis, right L3-L4 (arrow).

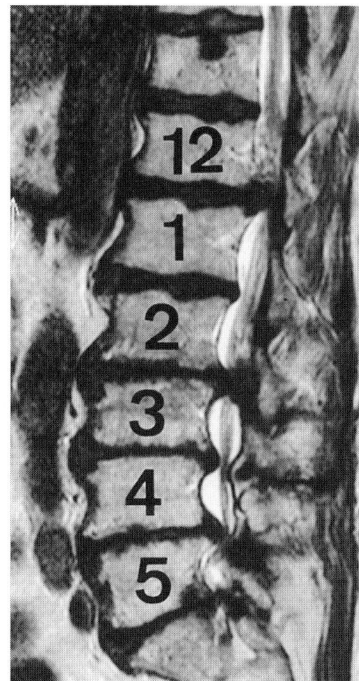

FIG. 52-6. Case 3. A 76-year-old man unable to stand straight, intense bilateral leg pain. Walking distance 3 yards. Midline T2-weighted magnetic resonance image scan showing multilevel severe central stenosis due to degenerative discs and narrow central canal.

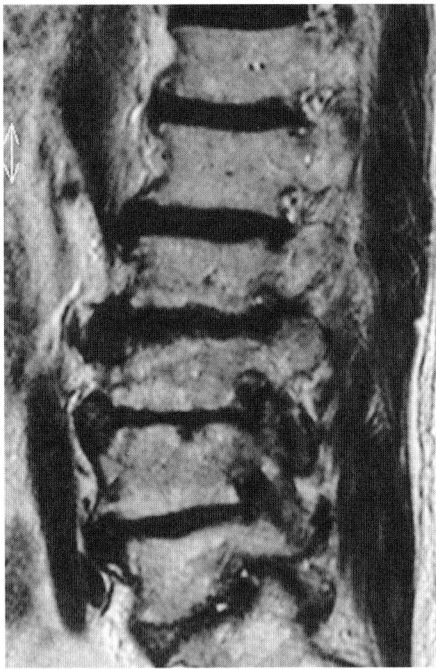

FIG. 52-7. Case 3. Right parasagittal T2-weighted magnetic resonance image scan showing multilevel foraminal stenosis, right L2-L3, L3-L4, L4-L5, L5-S1. Contrast with the foramina at L1-L2 and above. This patient underwent a five-level spinal decompression facilitated by a spinous process osteotomy. Estimated blood loss 800 to 900 mL. Patient was discharged from hospital on postoperative day 6.

improvement after epidural was less than 50% and only 5% were improved by surgery. Diagnostic nerve root blocks can be helpful in predicting the outcome of localized decompression. Preoperatively, if the patient can find relief by postural changes such as sitting or bending forward, a good outcome can be predicted (18). If postural changes do not produce relief, only 50% of patients can be expected to improve with surgical decompression.

SURGICAL TECHNIQUE

Patients are fitted with thromboembolic deterrent (TED) stockings. A general anesthetic is administered and a urinary catheter is inserted. The patient is positioned in mild lordosis on well-padded rolls. The abdomen must be free to reduce venous distension and potential epidural venous bleeding. We routinely use hypotensive anesthesia and intraoperative cell salvage to minimize the need for homologous blood transfusion. I prefer to use Loupe magnification (2.5×) with a fiberoptic light source.

The Approach

I commonly use a spinous process osteotomy (19) to facilitate lumbar decompressive surgery. The multifidus is taken down unilaterally approaching on the most clinically symptomatic side. Care is taken not to extend the subperiosteal dissection beyond the medial aspect of the facet joint, thereby preserving the medial branch of the dorsal ramus. Using a broad curved osteotome, an osteotomy is made through the involved segments just superficial to their junction with the lamina. The spinous processes with the attached interspinous and supraspinous ligament are then retracted to reveal the lamina. The technique affords excellent visualization with a wide area available for Kerrison use while minimizing destruction to the tissues. Weiner et al. discuss the advantages of this approach including reduction in paraspinal denervation, preservation of the supraspinous/interspinous ligament complex, reduction of dead space, and preservation of the median furrow, which may be of cosmetic concern to the patient (20). I believe the procedure saves time when compared to a bilateral take down of multifidus and results in significantly lower blood loss. An average blood loss is 250 mL (range 125 mL to 1,100 mL) for two, three, four and five level decompressions, a figure similar to that reported by Weiner et al. (20).

Laminectomy

Laminectomy addresses the global degenerative process by allowing decompression of the central canal, lateral canal, and neural foramina across multiple levels. The extent of the decompression will depend on the preoperative imaging. The most frequent error is to decompress too little (21). Most decompressions are carried out for degenerative changes. These changes will continue after surgery and it is easier to fully and adequately decompress on the first occasion. The laminectomy is most easily performed with a Leksell rongeur. This double-action rongeur is particularly good for hard bone. When the majority of the bony work has been done, checks should be made for any adhesions between the remaining lamina and the dural sac with a Watson-Cheyne dissector. The laminectomy is then completed with a Kerrison rongeur. The decompression should always begin away from the area of maximal stenosis. The lamina can safely be removed out to the most medial portion of the articular facets. Care is taken to preserve the pars interarticularis. When the central canal has been decompressed for the planned distance it is advisable to place a Kocher tissue forceps at the most cranial and at the most caudal extent of the decompression and take an X-ray (Fig. 52-8). This provides clear documentation of the limits of decompression and allows for any intraoperative adjustment to the length of decompression (Fig. 52-9). The decompression is now moved out laterally. A partial facetectomy is best achieved with a 1 to 2 cm osteotome angled away from the dura commencing cranially and moving to the most caudal limit of the decompression. The loose bone is then removed with a pituitary

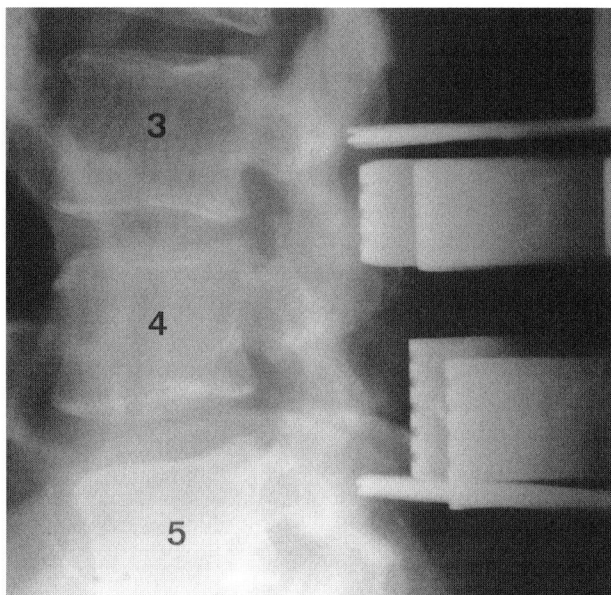

FIG. 52-8. Case 1. Operative marker film showing Kocher tissue forceps on the cranial and caudal extent of the planned decompression.

rongeur. Up to 50% of the facet joint can be removed without significantly compromising stability. Finally, the nerve root canals are checked and further decompressed with a Kerrison rongeur. At this point it is helpful if the assistant retracts the dura protected by a pattie, with a fine-tipped sucker in one hand and a nontoothed forceps in the other. Epidural bleeding may be controlled by judicious use of bipolar diathermy. After decompression of the nerve root a 3 to 4 mm probe should easily pass out the nerve root foramen and it should be possible to

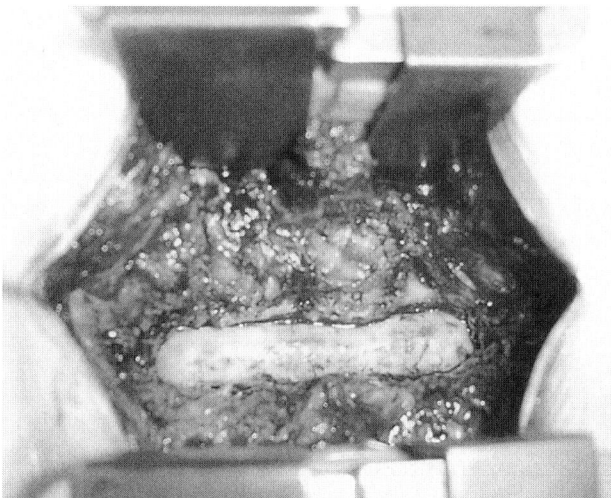

FIG. 52-9. Case 1. Operative picture showing the extent of decompression. Partial laminectomy L3, and total laminectomy L4 and L5 have been performed.

demonstrate a 1 cm medial displacement with a root retractor. One should check for concomitant disc herniation that may be contributing to the neural compression. Rarely is it necessary to perform a discectomy in addition to a laminectomy. However, if laminectomy and discectomy are performed simultaneously, then a spinal fusion should be considered to prevent the risk of postoperative instability. I prefer to avoid the placement of Gelfoam, Surgicel, Floseal, or other hemostatic sealant on the dura. There are reports of cauda equina and spinal cord compression caused by such agents (22,23).

Hemilaminectomy

Hemilaminectomy involves the unilateral removal of bone and ligamentum flavum. It is appropriate for patients with unilateral symptoms from a unilateral stenosis. Hemilaminectomy allows the ipsilateral exiting and the traversing nerve root to be decompressed, while preserving the spinous process and the interspinous and the supraspinous ligaments. To improve visualization, the table can be tilted away from the surgeon. Foraminal stenosis may be decompressed with an upbiting Kerrison. Total facetectomy can decompress this region, but concern regarding postoperative stability will mean that stabilization and fusion will usually be necessary.

Extraforaminal stenosis is best dealt with by the paraspinal approach described by Wiltse (24). Decompression may require total facetectomy, removal of the transverse process, and partial removal of the pedicle.

The Closure

When closing a spinous process osteotomy, the retractors are removed and the spinous process remnant checked for any sharp bone spikes. If present, these are removed with a rongeur. A deep drain is placed and the dorsolumbar fascia is resutured to the supraspinous ligament/fascial complex with the osteotomized spinous process resuming its native position, maintaining the posterior midline furrow.

Postoperative Care

Patients are mobilized the next morning. The drains are removed at 24 to 48 hours. If concern exists about stability, a lumbosacral orthosis may be worn for the first 6 weeks. Patients are usually discharged within 3 to 5 days. Physiotherapy to increase range of motion and restore trunk stability is offered at 6 weeks. Patients may return to light work at 6 weeks and heavy manual work at 3 months.

RESULTS

Johnsson et al. compared 44 patients with lumbar spinal stenosis treated surgically to 19 patients with lumbar spinal stenosis treated without surgery (7). The study was not prospective, nor randomized. They found 59% of operated patients to be clinically improved, compared to 32% of nonoperated patients. However, a greater percentage of the surgical group compared to the nonsurgical group (25% versus 10%) was worse at follow-up. Katz et al. reported retrospectively on 88 consecutive patients who underwent laminectomy for degenerative lumbar stenosis and were followed for 2.8 to 6.8 years (25). Repeat operations for instability or stenosis were required for 17% of patients and 30% had severe pain at the latest follow-up. Risk factors for poor outcome included preoperative comorbidity and limited single-level decompression. They concluded the long-term outcome of decompressive laminectomy was less favorable than had been previously reported.

Turner et al. reviewed 74 articles reporting on the outcome of surgery for spinal stenosis. Overall they found 64% of patients had a good or excellent result (26). The results in those with degenerative spondylolisthesis were good or excellent in 83% to 85% of patients. Atlas et al. reported the 1-year outcome of surgical and nonsurgical management of lumbar spinal stenosis in a prospective, nonrandomized cohort study (27). They concluded that patients with severe lumbar spinal stenosis treated surgically had greater improvement than patients treated nonsurgically. They subsequently reported the 4-year outcome (28). Of 119 patients with 4-year follow-up, 67 were treated surgically (the vast majority with laminectomy) and 52 were treated nonsurgically. The surgical group had more severe symptoms and worse function at baseline. Even after control for baseline differences, surgically treated patients reported better outcome at 4 years compared to nonsurgically treated patients: 70% of the surgical group compared to 52% of the nonsurgical group reported that their predominant symptom (either leg or back pain) was better. Satisfaction was greater in the surgical group: 63% compared to 42% in the nonsurgical group. The relative benefit of surgery declined over time with differences in outcome narrowing between the two groups over the four years. Nevertheless, the relative benefit of surgery remained superior to nonsurgical treatment.

In comparing the technique of multiple laminotomies versus total laminectomy, Postacchini et al. reported a longer operating time for bilateral laminotomy at two or three levels compared to total laminectomy at an equal number of levels (29). They reported a higher incidence of neural complications in the laminotomy group and a higher incidence of instability in the laminectomy group. At present Postacchini reports that 70% to 80% of patients have a satisfactory result from surgery, but the outcome tends to deteriorate in the long term (30). Iguchi et al. reported a minimum 10-year outcome following decompressive laminectomy for degenerative lumbar spinal stenosis (31). Over 50% of patients in this series were evaluated as good or excellent.

Comorbidities including osteoarthritis, cardiac disease, rheumatoid disease, and chronic pulmonary disease have a detrimental effect on outcome following surgery according to Katz et al. (25). Ragab et al. reported on 118 patients over the age of 70 years who had surgery on the lumbar spine for spinal stenosis (32). In this study advanced age and the presence of comorbidity did *not* affect the overall outcome of pain relief and resumption of daily activities, with 91% of patients experiencing good or excellent results. Similarly, Sanderson and Wood reported good or excellent results in 81% of patients 65 years of age or older undergoing decompression for degenerative lumbar stenosis (33). Diabetes mellitus was associated with poor results in one series (34), however Cinotti et al. showed similarly successful outcomes following spinal decompression in diabetic and nondiabetic patients (35). There is a strong association between self-rated health and surgical outcome reported by Katz et al. (36).

Gibson et al., in the Cochrane Review, concluded there was no acceptable evidence of the efficacy of any form of decompression for degenerative lumbar spondylosis or spinal stenosis (37). There is an urgent need for properly conducted prospective randomized controlled trials with subjective and objective outcome measures to assess the efficacy of decompressive surgery for spinal stenosis.

COMPLICATIONS

Dural Tears

Dural tears occur in approximately 5% of primary decompressions for spinal stenosis. This rate may increase in revision decompression procedures to 13.2% (38). Tears should be repaired with a 4-0 to 6-0 running suture (I prefer 5-0 Vicryl) and the repair should be tested with a Valsalva maneuver (positive pressure inspiration for several seconds). Fibrin glue may be used to supplement the repair, or indeed if the tear is small, fibrin glue alone may be sufficient. A deep drain is placed and allowed to drain under the effects of gravity. A careful watertight closure of the dorsolumbar fascia, subcuticular tissues, and skin is strongly recommended. Patients are kept lying flat for 48 hours, at which point the drain is usually removed. Dural tears that are recognized and treated appropriately do not lead to long-term sequelae (39).

Neural Injury

Primary neural injury is extremely rare with primary lumbar decompressions but less so with revision procedures. The surgeon must suspect a nerve injury when a cerebrospinal fluid leak is observed and a close inspection should be made. Patients on aspirin may develop a postoperative hematoma that can compress the thecal sac leading to a delayed cauda equina syndrome. Particularly, if the case was associated with a dural tear, the cauda equina seem less resilient to compression by an expanding hematoma. The operating surgeon should, as a matter of routine, perform a complete neurologic assessment of postoperative patients in the recovery area and document this in the medical records. Repeated neurologic assessment should be performed over the following 24 to 48 hours. Any significant deterioration in lower extremity power, loss of sensation in the perineal area, inability to void, or fecal incontinence must be investigated *urgently* with MRI and the appropriate action taken immediately.

Infection

The risk of infection in primary lumbar decompressions is about 1% to 2%, however this figure may rise to 5% in revision procedures. Suspected cases should be taken to the operating theatre and have both the superficial and deep tissues explored and cultured. A thorough débridement should be performed and deep drains left *in situ*. A low threshold for repeated débridement should be operated. For deep infections, it is common to require 3 weeks of the intravenous antibiotics, dependent on the organism and the measured response of the patient's inflammatory markers.

Iatrogenic Instability

Instability following laminectomy is uncommon. White and Wiltse reported a 2% incidence of postoperative iatrogenic spondylolisthesis (40). Johnsson et al. however reported 10 out of 31 patients (32%) in their series developing a slip following radical decompression (41). Postoperative slips greater than 2 mm were associated with poorer results and slips appeared to be more common in females. Robertson et al. stressed the importance of facet joint orientation and dimensions rather than the absolute amount of the joint removed (42). More sagittally aligned facets were more likely to result in slippage when compared to the more coronally aligned facets. Extensive decompressions over multiple levels with subtotal or near total facetectomies and discectomies are much more likely to slip. These cases should be considered for preoperative fusion. However, it is generally accepted that fusion is not required following decompressive surgery provided there is no evidence of segmental instability. This is confirmed by Grob et al. who prospectively evaluated 45 patients undergoing decompression of the spine with and without arthrodesis for the treatment of lumbar spinal stenosis without instability (43). They concluded that in the absence of segmental instability, arthrodesis was not necessary after decompression of the lumbar spine, provided the stabilizing posterior elements of the spine are preserved during the operation. This is possible with a spinous process osteotomy as previously described. Those patients with

preoperative spondylolisthesis and degenerative scoliosis are special cases and ones in which spinal fusion should more readily be contemplated.

Epidural Fibrosis

This may be associated with heavy epidural bleeding and the excessive use of the bipolar diathermy. It is diagnosed as a worsening of leg pain and may be diagnosed by MRI with the administration of a contrast agent such as gadolinium. Treatment options include drugs such as amitriptyline, carbamazepine, or gabapentin, X-ray–targeted foraminal epidural steroid injections, or occasionally revision surgery and neurolysis.

Arachnoiditis

This is characterized by intrathecal fibrosis and responds poorly to treatment. It may be minimized by careful handling of neural tissue and frequent release of retracted nerve roots during surgery. The risk of arachnoiditis is thought to increase with epidural bleeding. Larger epidural vessels should be controlled with bipolar diathermy, smaller vessels with temporary placement of patties, or absorbable hemostats (e.g., Surgicel).

Failure to Relieve Pain

This may occur with long-standing ischemic neuritis, inadequate decompression, bony regrowth (44), postoperative instability, pseudarthrosis, flat back syndrome, and neural injury. Some of these problems are correctable. Many, however, are not and these patients should be referred appropriately to pain management programs.

SUMMARY

Decompression without arthrodesis is the preferred treatment for spinal stenosis without instability. The spinous process osteotomy does much to facilitate decompressive surgery, while preserving the stabilizing posterior elements. Laminectomy allows a global decompression of the central canal, lateral canal, and neural foramen. Laminotomy is not suitable for congenital stenosis or constitutionally narrow canals. If more than one facet joint is sacrificed or the disc is removed then prophylactic fusion should be considered. Advances in anesthetic and surgical techniques mean the procedure may safely be offered to patients well over 80 years of age, provided multiple comorbidities have been taken into account. There is an urgent need for properly conducted randomized controlled trials to assess the efficacy of decompressive surgery versus conservative treatment of spinal stenosis.

REFERENCES

1. Aryanpur J, Ducker T. Multilevel lumbar laminotomies: an alternative to laminectomy in the treatment of lumbar stenosis. Neurosurgery 1990;26:429–433.
2. Ullrich CG, Binet EF, Sanecki MG, et al. Quantitative assessment of the lumbar spinal canal by computed tomography. Radiology 1980; 134:137.
3. Eisenstein S. The morphometry and pathological anatomy of the lumbar spine in South African Negroes and Caucasians with specific reference to spinal stenosis. J Bone Joint Surg [Br] 1977;59:173.
4. Yong-Hing K, Kirkaldy-Willis WH. The pathophysiology of degenerative disc disease of the lumbar spine. Orthop Clin North Am 1983;14: 491–504.
5. Yoshida M, Shima K, Taniguchi Y, et al. Hypertrophied ligamentum flavum in lumbar canal stenosis. Spine 1992;17:1353.
6. Rauschning W. Normal and pathological anatomy of the lumbar root canals. Spine 1987;12;1008.
7. Johnsson KE, Uden A, Rosen I. The effect of decompression on the natural course of lumbar spinal stenosis: a comparison of surgically treated and untreated patients. Spine 1991;16:615–619.
8. Bell GR. Surgical management of lumbar spinal stenosis and degenerative spondylolisthesis. In: Fardon DF, Garfin SR, eds. Orthopaedic knowledge update: spine, 2nd ed. Illinois: American Academy of Orthopaedic Surgeons, 2002:343–352.
9. Pratt RK, Fairbank JCT, Virr A. The reliability of the Shuttle Walking Test, the Swiss Spinal Stenosis Questionnaire, the Oxford Spinal Stenosis Score, and the Oswestry Disability Index in the assessment of patients with lumbar spinal stenosis. Spine 2002;27:1:84–91.
10. Deen HG, Zimmerman RS, Lyons MK, et al. Use of the exercise treadmill to measure baseline functional status and surgical outcome in patients with severe lumbar spinal stenosis. Spine 1998;23:244–248.
11. Epstein N, Epstein JA. Individual and coexistent lumbar and cervical spinal stenosis. In: Hopp E., ed. Spine: state of the art reviews. Vol 1. Philadelphia: Hanley and Belfus, 1987:401.
12. Rydevik BL, Cohen DB, Kostuik JP. Spine epidural steroids for patients with lumbar spinal stenosis. Spine 1997;22(19):2313–2314.
13. Porter RW. Spinal stenosis and neurogenic claudication. Spine 1996; 21:17:2046–2052.
14. Simotas AC, Dorey FD, Hansraj KK, et al. Nonoperative treatment for lumbar spinal stenosis. Spine 2000;25(2):197–204.
15. Amundsen T, Weber H, Nordal HJ, et al. Lumbar spinal stenosis: conservative or surgical management? A prospective 10-year study. Spine 2000;25(11):1424–1436.
16. Eisen A, Hoirch M. The electrodiagnostic evaluation of spinal root lesions. Spine 1983;8:98.
17. Derby R, Kine G, Saal J, et al. Response to steroid and duration of radicular pain as predictors of surgical outcome. Spine 1992;17:176.
18. Ganz J. Lumbar spinal stenosis: postoperative results in terms of preoperative posture related pain. J Neurosurg 1990;72:71.
19. Yong-Hing K, Kirkaldy-Willis WH. Osteotomy of the lumbar spinous process to increase surgical exposure. Clin Orthop 1978;134:218–220.
20. Weiner BK, Fraser RD, Peterson M. Spinous process osteotomies to facilitate lumbar decompressive surgery. Spine 1999;24(1):62–66.
21. Whiffen JR, Neuwirth MG. Spinal Stenosis. In: Bridwell KH, DeWald RL, eds. The textbook of spinal surgery, 2nd ed. Vol 2. Philadelphia: Lippincott-Raven, 1997:1561–1580.
22. Friedman J, Whitecloud TS 3rd. Lumbar cauda equina syndrome associated with the use of Gelfoam: case report. Spine 2001;26(20): E485–E487.
23. Alander DH, Stauffer ES. Gelfoam-induced acute quadriparesis after cervical decompression and fusion. Spine 1995;20(8):970–971.
24. Wiltse LL, Spencer CW. New uses and refinements of the paraspinal approach to the lumbar spine. Spine 1988;13:696–706.
25. Katz JN, Lipson SJ, Larson MG, et al. The outcome of decompressive laminectomy for degenerative lumbar stenosis. J Bone Joint [Am] 1991;73A(6):809–816.
26. Turner JA, Ersek M, Herron L, et al. Surgery for lumbar spinal stenosis: attempted meta-analysis of the literature. Spine 1992;17:1.
27. Atlas SJ, Deyo R, Keller RB, et al. The Maine Lumbar Spine Study, Part III. 1-Year outcomes of surgical and non-surgical management of lumbar spinal stenosis. Spine 1996;21:1787–1794.
28. Atlas SJ, Keller RB, Robson D, et al. Surgical and non-surgical management of lumbar spinal stenosis: four-year outcomes from the Maine Lumbar Spine Study. Spine 2000;25(5):556–562.
29. Postacchini F, Cinotti G, Perugia D, et al. The surgical treatment of central lumbar stenosis. Multiple laminotomy compared to total laminectomy. J Bone Joint Surg [Br] 1993;75B(3):386–392.
30. Postacchini F. Spine update: surgical management of lumbar spinal stenosis. Spine 1999;24(10):1043–1047.
31. Iguchi T, Kurihara A, Nakayama J, et al. Minimum 10-year outcome of decompressive laminectomy for degenerative lumbar spinal stenosis. Spine 2000;25(14):1754–1759.
32. Ragab AA, Fye MA, Bohlman HH. Surgery of the lumbar spine for spinal stenosis in 118 patients 70 years of age or older. Spine 2003; 28(4):348–353.
33. Sanderson PL, Wood PLR. Surgery for lumbar spinal stenosis in old people. J Bone Joint Surg [Br] 1993;75B(3):393–397.
34. Simpson JM, Silveri CP, Balderston RA, et al. The results of operations on the lumbar spine in patients who have diabetes mellitus. J Bone Joint Surg [Am] 1993;75A:1823–1829.
35. Cinotti G, Postacchini F, Weinstein JN. Lumbar spinal stenosis and diabetes. Outcome of surgical decompression. J Bone Joint Surg [Br] 1994;76B(2):215–219.
36. Katz JN, Stucki G, Lipson SJ, et al. Predictors of surgical outcome in degenerative lumbar spinal stenosis. Spine 1999;24(21):2229–2233.
37. Gibson JNA, Grant IC, Waddell G. The Cochrane review of surgery for lumbar disc prolapse and degenerative lumbar spondylosis. Spine 1999;24(17):1820–1832.
38. Sell P. National audit of dural tears. Paper presented at: Annual Meeting of the British Association of Spinal Surgeons; 2003; London.
39. Cammisa FP, Gerardi FP, Sangani PK, et al. Incidental durotomy in spine surgery. Spine 2000;25(20):2663–2667.
40. White A, Wiltse LL. Postoperative spondylolisthesis. In: Weinstein P, ed. Lumbar spondylolysis. Chicago: Year Book, 1977:184.
41. Johnsson KE, Redlund-Johnell I, Uden A, et al. Preoperative and postoperative instability in lumbar spinal stenosis. Spine 1989;14:591.
42. Robertson PA, Grobler LJ, Novotny JE, et al. Post-operative spondylolisthesis at L4-5: the role of facet joint morphology. Spine 1993;18: 1483.
43. Grob D, Humke T, Dvorak J. Degenerative lumbar spinal stenosis: decompression with and without arthrodesis. J Bone Joint Surg [Am] 1995;77A(7):1036–1041.
44. Postacchini F, Cinotti G. Bone regrowth after surgical decompression for lumbar spinal stenosis. J Bone Joint Surg [Br] 1992;74B(6): 862–869.

CHAPTER 53

Laminoplasty

Yoshiharu Kawaguchi and Masahiko Kanamori

Extensive laminectomy has been used widely for the treatment of lumbar spinal stenosis. However, results of laminectomy were not consistent because of postoperative instability of the lumbar spine and laminectomy membrane into the spinal canal. To resolve these problems, the technique of lumbar expansive laminoplasty was developed in 1981 (1). This operation enlarges the spinal canal and preserves the posterior spinal structure for the adequate decompression of spinal nerve and reinforcement of spinal stability (2). This procedure has been used in patients who are active physically with combined lumbar stenosis, including developmental or degenerative stenosis, spinal stenosis with multiple ossification of intraspinal ligaments or herniated nucleus pulposus, and degenerative stenosis accompanied by segmental instability (3–5). In this chapter, we describe the indication, operative procedure, postoperative management, results, and complications of lumbar laminoplasty.

INDICATIONS

Laminoplasty is usually carried out on active patients who have multilevel spinal stenosis. Recently, we have also used laminoplasty on older patients (over 70 years) who had spinal stenosis with segmental instability.

Other indications for laminoplasty include:

1. Multilevel degenerative spinal stenosis accompanied by developmental spinal stenosis in patients in whom heavy physical activity is required in daily living.
2. Multilevel combined spinal stenosis accompanied by herniated nucleus pulposus or intraspinal ossified masses (bony spur formation at the posterior vertebral edge, peridiscal ossification, ossification of the posterior longitudinal ligament, or ligamentum flavum) in active patients.
3. Cauda equina tumor in young or middle-aged patients (less than 60 years).

4. Multilevel degenerative spinal stenosis with instability of the segment in patients who require reinforcement of stability of the lumbar spinal segment.
5. Migrated lumbar disc herniation.

OPERATIVE PROCEDURE

Groove Making in the Laminae

The spinous process is carefully removed at its base and used as a bone graft. The target laminae are cut by high-speed air drill. The outer edge of the bilateral grooves is made to reach the lateral one-third of the articular facet. The groove on the hinged side should be wider and more conical than the groove on the open side.

Tunnel Making for Wiring (Fig. 53-1A)

Just prior to mobilization of the laminae, small holes are made in each lamina on the open side, using a special awl, a pusher, and a perforator.

Rotating the Laminae

The laminae are completely cut off along the groove on the open side using a diamond burr and the ligamentum flavum is also dissected on the same side with a knife. Then, the laminae are turned up to an angle of at least 45°. In the hinged side, an incomplete separation of the laminae is recommended by means of an interrupted perforation of the internal cortex using a diamond burr.

Intraspinal Intervention

If there is a symptomatic herniated nucleus pulposus or cauda equina tumor, discectomy or tumor extirpation is performed through the open gap.

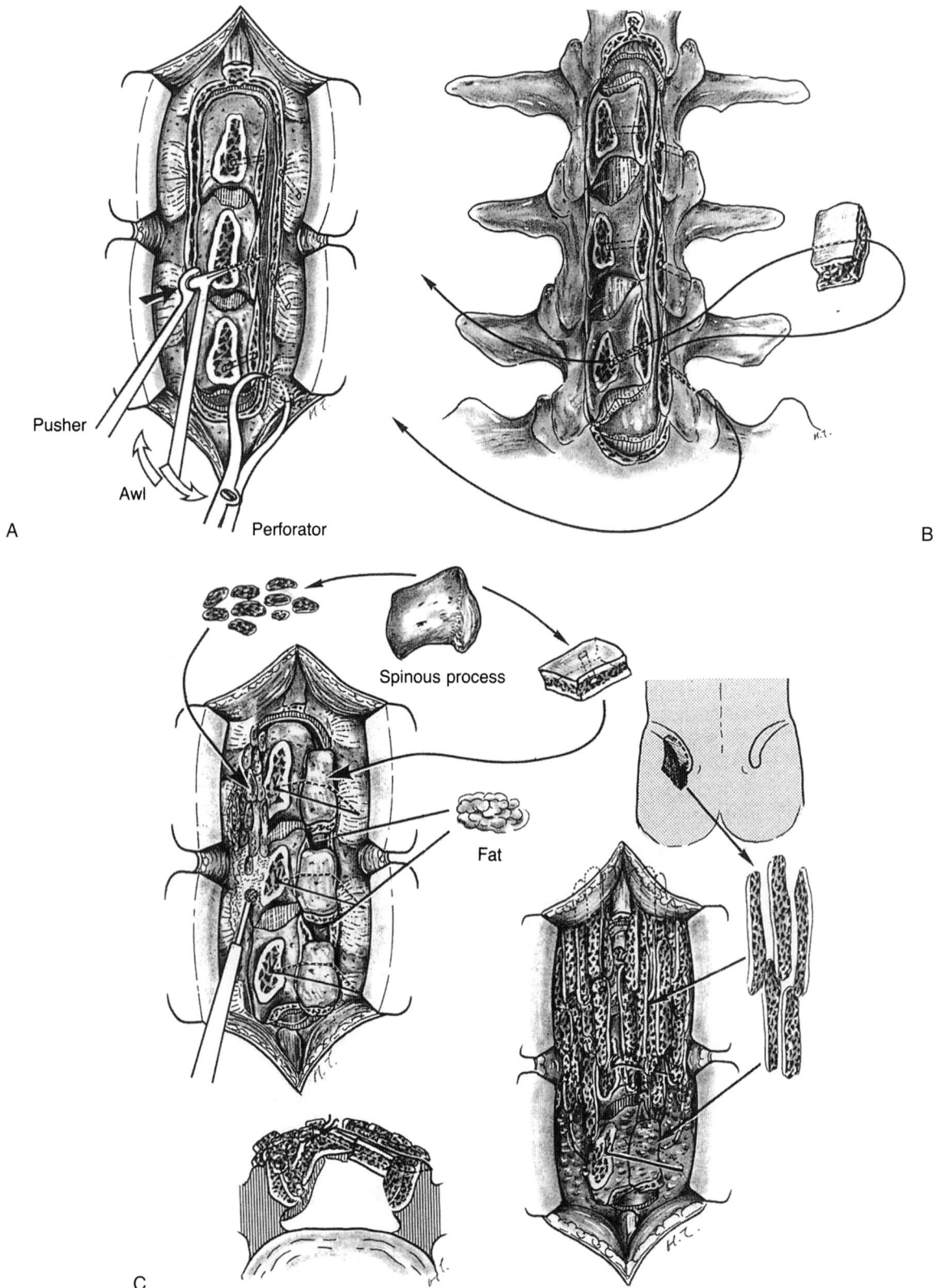

Pusher

Awl

Perforator

A

B

Spinous process

Fat

C

FIG. 53-1. A–C: Schematic representation of the procedure of expansive laminoplasty. [From Tsuji H. Expansive laminoplasty. In: Tsuji H, Dawson E, eds. Comprehensive atlas of lumbar spine surgery. St. Louis: Mosby-Year Book, 1991:116–119, with permission. (This edition published by arrangement with Nankodo Co, Ltd, Tokyo.)]

Trimming of the Cut Surface

The edge of the groove facing the lateral recess of the spinal canal is trimmed with a rongeur and curette, and the remaining ligamentum flavum is removed as completely as possible.

Wiring (Fig. 53-1B)

A 0.3-mm braided steel wire or 1.0 braided nylon is passed through each hole. Using a small-diameter steel burr, the orifice of each hole is sufficiently widened to facilitate each passage of the wire or the nylon. A curved blunt needle is used to pass the wire or nylon through the hole in the bone.

Bone Grafting and Fat Tissue Grafting (Fig. 53-1C)

The spinous processes are reformed into cubes measuring 15 to 20 mm × 10 to 15 mm for bone grafts, and a transverse hole is made in each graft. One end of the steel wire or the nylon, first passed through the lamina, is also passed though the bone graft and the articular process. The wire or the nylon is tied after the bone graft is interposed into the gap on the open side. The laminae, including the articular processes are thoroughly decorticated with an air drill. The bone chips for the spinous process or posterior iliac bone are translated on both sides. Free fat tissue is also grafted onto the epidural areas of the open gap. After a suction drain is placed, the wound is closed.

POSTOPERATIVE MANAGEMENT

The suction drain is removed 48 hours after surgery. Assisted turning of the patient and active exercise of the lower extremities are begun on the second postoperative day. The patient is permitted to walk 1 to 2 weeks after surgery wearing a body cast or hard corset. The cast or hard corset is worn for 4 weeks, followed by a soft corset for 8 weeks.

RESULTS

Neurologic Results

54 patients with lumbar spinal stenosis were operated on from 1981 to 1999. The average length of follow-up was 5.5 years with a range from 2 to 13 years. The local pathologic findings included 25 patients with degenerative stenosis, 12 with combined stenosis, and 6 with hyperostotic stenosis. Thirteen patients revealed spondylolisthesis and 12 had scoliosis (Cobb angle greater than 10°). The operation time and blood loss per one lamina were 60 minutes and 214 mL, respectively. Twenty-four patients (44%) received blood transfusion.

The Japanese Orthopaedic Association (JOA) proposed a scoring system for low back pain (Table 53-1).

Neurologic results were assessed by the system and evaluated based on the postoperative score and the recovery rate was calculated using the following formula:

The recovery rate (%) =

$$\frac{(\text{postoperative score} - \text{preoperative score}) \times 100}{29 \ (\text{full score} - \text{preoperative score}}$$

The preoperative and postoperative JOA scores and recovery rate are shown in Table 53-2. The average recovery rate at the last follow-up was 69.2%±21.1% in degenerative stenosis, 66.5%±44.5% in combined stenosis, and 65.2%±26.1% in hyperostotic stenosis. That was 54.7%±37.4% in the patients with spondylolisthesis and 63.7%±29.5% with scoliosis. The recovery tended to be poor in the patients with spondylolisthesis, but there was no statistical difference. As yet, long-term result has not been clarified, because this procedure developed in the early 1980s. In our follow-up series of more than 5 years, 6 patients showed spinal instability at the adjacent level of expansive laminoplasty.

Roentgenographic Results

Using computed tomography, the shape of the spinal canal was enlarged with a rectangular shape (Fig. 53-2). The average cross-sectional area was expanded from 1.8 cm²±0.9 cm² to 3.0 cm²±0.9 cm² after surgery. None of the patients showed kyphotic change of the lumbar spine, but five patients revealed progression of degenerative spondylolisthesis. Laminar fusion was achieved in 21 patients (43%). In the patients without laminar fusion, the range of flexion-extension motion of the operated spinal area was reduced to 58% of preoperative range.

Complications: How to Avoid/Treat

Surgical trauma in lumbar laminoplasty is not as limited as with laminectomy, however, there were no major general or neurologic complications experienced intraoperatively or postoperatively. Blood transfusion was required in 44% of the patients, but in the more recent cases, autologous blood transfusion was introduced and allogenic transfusion was avoided.

Expansive lumbar laminoplasty is most suitable for central canal stenosis. Decompression of the nerve root is usually difficult in patients with lateral stenosis in the ordinary procedure. Lateral recess decompression can be performed at the open side in the same manner as laminectomy. When decompression of the lateral recess at the hinge side is required, decompressive fenestration should be performed before lifting up the laminae. For decompression of the nerve root tunnel, unroofing of the tunnel can be performed.

In long-term follow-up of more than 5 years, spinal instability at the adjacent level of the laminoplasty was observed in 6 patients. This may be a disadvantage of

TABLE 53-1. *The evaluation system for the treatment of low back disorders devised by the Japanese Orthopaedic Association (JOA score)*

	Score
Subjective symptoms	
Low back pain	
None	3
Occasional mild pain	2
Frequent mild or occasional severe pain	1
Frequent severe pain	0
Leg pain or numbness	
None	3
Occasional mild leg pain or numbness	2
Frequent mild or occasional severe leg pain or numbness	1
Frequent severe leg pain or numbness	0
Walking capacity	
Normal	3
Able to walk >500 m with leg pain or numbness	2
Able to walk for 100–500 m	1
Able to walk <100–500 m	0
Clinical signs	
Straight leg raising test	
Normal	2
30°–70°	1
<30°	0
Motor function	
Normal	2
Slight weakness (MMT: good)	1
Severe weakness (MMT: less than good)	0
Sensory function	
Normal	2
Slight disturbance	1
Severe disturbance	0
Bladder function	
Normal	0
Mild dysuria	−3
Severe dysuria	−6

	Impossible	Difficult	Easy
Restriction of activities of daily living			
Tossing about in bed	0	1	2
Standing up	0	1	2
Washing face	0	1	2
Half-sitting posture	0	1	2
Sitting	0	1	2
Lifting	0	1	2
Running	0	1	2
Total for normal			29

MMT, Manual Muscle Testing.

TABLE 53-2. *Results of expansive laminoplasty*

	JOA score (point)	Recovery rate (%)
Preoperative	11.2 ± 4.1	NA
Postoperative 6 months	21.3 ± 3.9	55.4 ± 22.6
Postoperative 1 year	23.3 ± 4.3	69.0 ± 21.7
Last follow-up	23.0 ± 5.6	65.6 ± 31.3

JOA, Japanese Orthopaedic Association; NA, not applicable.

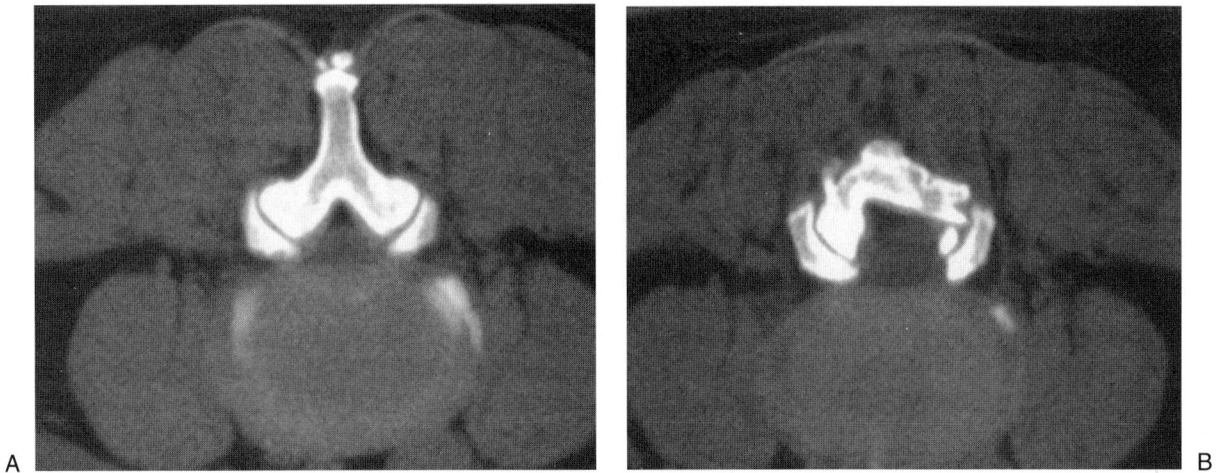

FIG 53-2. A: Preoperative computed tomography (CT). **B:** Postoperative CT.

spinal fusion by laminoplasty. Thus, it is necessary to evaluate disc degeneration in the whole lumbar spine and the operative area should be determined according to the level of stenosis and the condition of the disc degeneration.

REFERENCES

1. Tsuji H. Laminoplasty for patients with compression myelopathy due to so-called spinal canal stenosis in cervical and thoracic region. Spine 1982;7:28–34.

2. Tsuji H. Expansive laminoplasty. In: Tsuji H, Dawson E, eds. Comprehensive atlas of lumbar spine surgery. St. Louis: Mosby-Year Book, 1991:116–119. [This edition published by arrangement with Nankodo Co, Ltd, Tokyo.]

3. Tsuji H, Itoh T, Sekido H, et al. Expansive laminoplasty for lumbar spinal stenosis. Int Orthop 1990;14:309–314.

4. Matsui H, Tsuji H, Sekido H, et al. Results of expansive laminoplasty for lumbar spinal stenosis in active manual workers. Spine 1992;17: S37–S40.

5. Matsui H, Kanamori M, Ishihara H, et al. Expansive lumbar laminoplasty for degenerative spinal stenosis in patients below 70 years of age. Eur Spine J 1997;6:191–196.

CHAPTER 54

Degenerative Lumbar Spondylolisthesis with Spinal Stenosis: Natural History, Diagnosis, Clinical Presentation, and Nonoperative Treatment

Mohamed Mostafa Mossaad

Forward displacement of a proximal vertebra in relation to its adjacent vertebra in association with an intact neural arch, and in the presence of degenerative changes is known as degenerative spondylolisthesis (1). The term is derived from the Greek word *spondylous,* meaning vertebra and *olisthesis,* meaning to slip or slide down a slippery incline.

Degenerative spondylolisthesis is usually a result of long-standing instability; it is most common at the junction of the fourth and fifth lumbar vertebrae. The instability is a result of a combination of disc degeneration and facet joint degeneration. The displacement results from a failure of the apophyseal joints to restrain shear (2,3). In 1950 MacNab showed that the displacement occurs in the sixth decade, and patients generally attend with symptoms around 60 years of age. He also postulated that the displacement is limited, and a slip ratio of more than 15% is unusual (4). The degenerative changes at the facet joints and disc degeneration add to subluxation of the facet joints, which allow forward or posterior movement of one vertebra over the other.

Degenerative spondylolisthesis narrows the spinal canal, and symptoms of spinal stenosis are most common. Hypertrophic facet arthrosis is a frequent cause of foraminal stenosis (1). The symptoms of lumbar spinal canal stenosis, particularly a complaint of neural claudication, serve as the most common operative indication (5).

Because the appearance of a significant deformity or neural claudication is often antedated by significant and recurring episodes of low back pain, sometimes the condition is considered a prototype for spinal segmental

instability. However, the radiographic abnormality may occur without current or prior symptoms (Fig. 54-1) (5).

NATURAL HISTORY

Degenerative spondylolisthesis occurs when a vertebra is displaced in relation to that immediately below it, with no disruption of the neural arch, no congenital anomaly, and in the presence of degenerative changes in a spine not previously subjected to surgical or traumatic insult (6).

In 1997 Marchetti and Bartolozzi showed that there are two main types of degenerative spondylolisthesis: primary, in a spine without congenital or acquired pathologic conditions; and secondary, as a result of congenital or acquired pathologic conditions, both with degenerative changes at the facet joints and disc spaces (6).

They showed that primary degenerative spondylolisthesis occurs mainly in patients over or around the age of 60 years, most involving L4. The initial pathologic condition is usually degeneration of the posterior articular process, which is the cause of segmental instability and involves the disc space as well.

Most of these patients present a translational olisthesis that resembles lumbar spinal stenosis in clinical and radiographic assessment.

The disc may protrude posteriorly into the spinal canal. Symptoms start to appear gradually and develop slowly with severe back pain and radicular pain. Nonoperative treatment generally provides a satisfactory result, with indication for surgery when this fails.

Secondary degenerative spondylolisthesis occurs because of a congenital or acquired pathologic condition

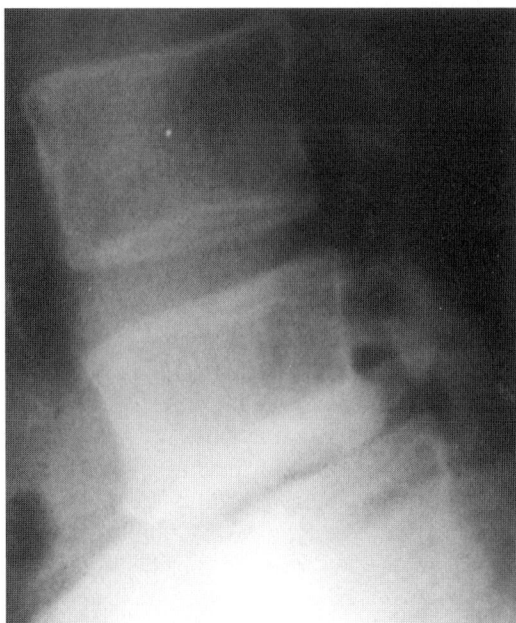

FIG. 54-1. Lateral radiograph of a patient with degenerative spondylolisthesis at L4-5. The disc space is shown to be reduced with bony sclerosis and forward displacement of body of L4, with an intact neural arch. There is deformity of the superior articular facet of L5 and deformation of the central canal, root canal, and intervertebral foramen.

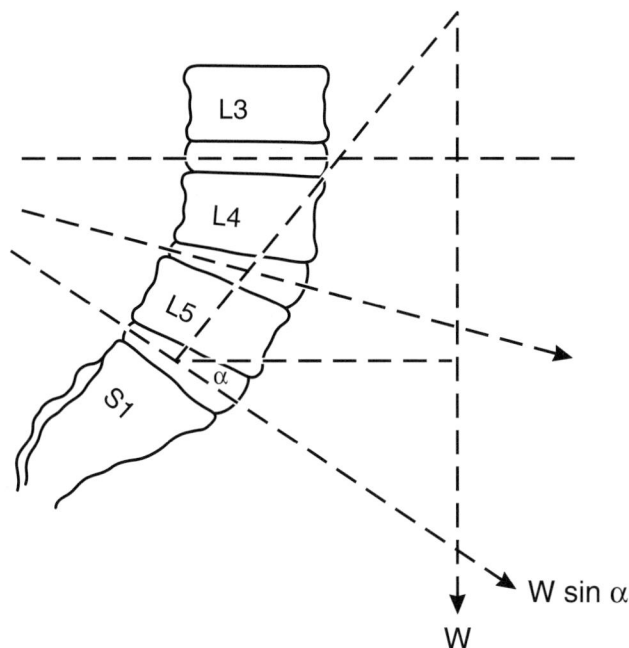

FIG. 54-2. Diagram to show sheer through the lumbosacral disc, where W is the body weight above and disc, and α is the lumbo-sacral angle. (From Porter RW. Management of back pain, 1st ed. Edinburgh: Churchill Livingstone, 1986:40, with permission.)

localized above or below the olisthetic vertebra, which is not clinically important. Marchetti and Bartolozzi reported that this condition is mild, presented with mild symptoms, and has little tendency to deteriorate. Nonoperative treatment is usually the treatment of choice and is appropriate. Surgery has never proved to be necessary in their or our experience (6).

In 1997 Bridwell reported that degenerative spondylolisthesis is variable as it is for all degenerative disc disease, but in 1990 Sakou et al. reported a gradual tendency toward loss of disc height and narrowing of spinal canal. They also mentioned that it is uncommon for an unoperated degenerative spondylolisthesis to slip more than 50% (7,8).

Forward displacement results from a failure of the apophyseal joints to restrain shear. They are orientated in the sagittal plane in the upper lumbar spine, and become progressively more coronally orientated toward the lower lumbar spine (Table 54-1; Fig. 54-2) (3).

TABLE 54-1. Forward displacement

	Mean facet angle (degrees)	
L1	66.5	±13.3
L2	61.3	6.8
L3	54.4	10.0
L4	41.5	10.8
L5	38.8	7.4

The most frequent site for degenerative spondylolisthesis is at L4-5, where the shearing forces are not adequately restrained by the apophyseal joints. Microfractures and remodeling occur in the subchondral bone of the joints. The vertebra slowly displaces forward, with gradual bony deformity, loss of disc integrity, and stretching of the ligaments. The causative factors and their related importance are uncertain. Osteoporosis has been implicated in the sagittal orientation of the joints and disruption of the disc. There is no evidence that joint laxity is significant (9,10).

An intact neural arch is essential for the apophyseal joints to effectively restrain shear. The fact that spondylolysis can be present with no vertebral displacement suggests that spinal structures other than neural arch play a significant point in resisting shear forces (9,10).

The increasing shear forces in the lower lumbar lordotic spine are balanced by the progressively efficient restraint of the coronally orientated lumbar facet. L4-5 appears to be the level where the joints may fail to restrain shear. Several possible factors cause this failure:

1. Constitutional variation in the orientation of the apophyseal joints. Those individuals whose L4-5 facets are more sagittally orientated than the rest of the population are more prone to displacement (11).
2. Osteoporosis of the subchondral bone of the facet joints is vulnerable to microfractures, with deformity of the facet joints. It was suggested by Junghanns and

MacNab that an increased angle between the pedicle and inferior articular facet allows forward subluxation of the upper vertebra (2,4); however, Newman found no increase of this angle in the slipping vertebra. He suspected that progressive widening of the angle may accompany the progressive slip from remodeling in response to microfractures (3).

3. A degenerative disc less effectively restrains shear (12).
4. Increased lumbar lordosis increases the force of shear, but there is no evidence that these patients have an increased lumbosacral angle. Posture may be significant, especially in pregnant women, in whom the ligamentous restraint is less effective (11).
5. Newman believed that poor spinal and abdominal muscles place proportionally greater strain on the apophyseal joints, and the facets give way from an acquired instability of the soft tissues, especially the interspinous and supraspinous ligaments. He also thought the high incidence of spina bifida occulta is significant (3).
6. Obesity disproportionate to muscle strength increases the shear.
7. Diabetic patients (especially women) who have undergone oophorectomy are also at significantly higher risk (5).

Several of the mentioned causative factors in combination may explain the higher incidence of degenerative spondylolisthesis in women, especially obese women.

The proximal vertebra steadily displaces forward, deforming the vertebral canal, root canal, and intervertebral foramina (Fig. 54-3). If the central canal is already constitutionally narrow, then vertebral displacement with an intact neural arch will deform the dura and its contents. The root canal can become critically narrow, especially at the exit of the foramina. If a dynamic element is superimposed on the reduction of the space for the neural contents, pathologic changes develop in the dura and nerve roots, producing symptoms (11).

Degenerative changes develop in the apophyseal joints and at the margins of the vertebral bodies until a degree of stability occurs. These osteophytic changes can encroach on the root canal. It is interesting that the vertebral body does not become wedge shaped as in the displaced body of an isthmic spondylolisthesis; the former displacing in adult life, the latter during growth (11).

The major instability is not flexion-extension instability (in other words, tilt), but axial rotational and anteroposterior (AP) transitional instability (13).

In 1994 Frymoyer mentioned that radiographic surveys showed that degenerative spondylolisthesis is more common in patients with hemisacralization. This finding is thought to be of etiologic significance because the immobility of the L5-S1 level shifts mechanical stress to the adjacent level of L4-5 (5).

An important requisite for degenerative spondylolisthesis is relative immobility of the lumbar segment below the lesion. The immobility is most commonly caused by hemisacralization, but can result from advanced disc degeneration at the level of L5-S1 (Fig. 54-4). Spinal fusion is an iatrogenic cause for immobility. The forward slip occurs many years after the original fusion. Surprisingly, many patients are asymptomatic despite the deformity (Fig. 54-5) (14).

Degenerative spondylolisthesis with a canal stenosis has been shown by Frymoyer to be more common in diabetic women who have undergone oophorectomy. These observations are clinically relevant because the orthopedist faced with a patient with degenerative spondylolisthesis, diabetes, and leg pain often has to determine whether diabetic neuropathy or spinal stenosis is the cause of the leg pain. The relationship to oophorectomy suggests that estrogen replacement might prevent or slow the onset of the deformity and symptoms. The higher prevalence in diabetic patients is thought to result from weakened collagen cross-linking. Other mechanical theories suggest that congenital or acquired abnormalities in the orientation of the facets predispose to forward displacement. Unfortunately, the various pathoanatomic theories have no utility for designing specific prevention strategies (5).

Degenerative spondylolisthesis is the result of long-standing intersegmental instability (15,16). As the slip progresses, the articular processes change direction and become more horizontal (17). Degenerative spondylolisthesis occurs six times more commonly in women than in men, six to nine times more frequently at the L4 interspace than at adjoining levels, and four times more frequently when the L5 is sacralized than when it is not.

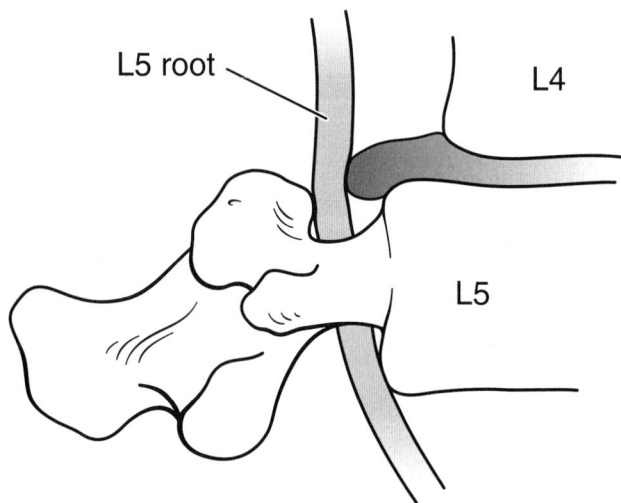

FIG. 54-3. Diagram to show that the L5 nerve root can be affected in the central canal from a rim of L4-5 disc in degenerative spondylolisthesis. (From Porter RW. Management of back pain, 1st ed. Edinburgh: Churchill Livingstone, 1986: 147, with permission.)

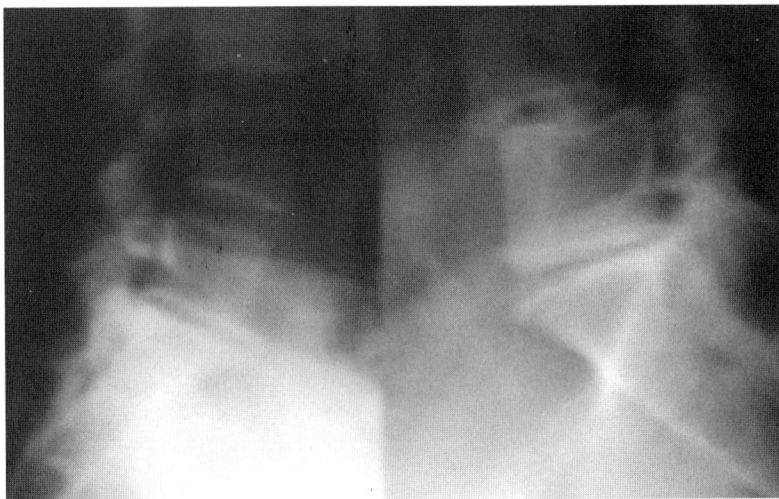

FIG. 54-4. Lateral radiograph of a patient with degenerative spondylolisthesis at L4-5 with the L5-S1 space extremely narrowed. (From Frymoyer JW. Degenerative spondylolisthesis: diagnosis and treatment. J Am Acad Orthop Surg 1994:2;10, with permission.)

When the lesion is at L4, the L5 vertebra is more stable and exhibits less lordosis than is average (17,18).

Knutsson believed that flexion and extension views also reveal dynamic instability, a frequent precursor of degenerative spondylolisthesis, at even earlier ages (19).

Degenerative spondylolisthesis with an intact neural arch, which is a secondary form of lumbar stenosis, is more common at the L4-5 level, and followed in descending order of occurrence at the L3-4, the L2-3, and the L5-S1 interspaces (20–22).

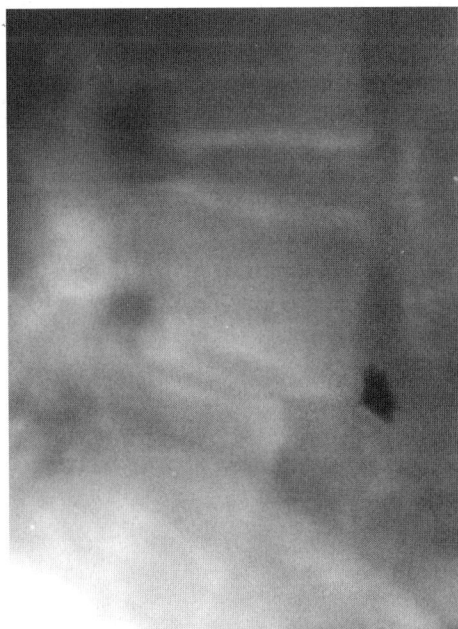

FIG. 54-5. Lateral radiograph of a patient who had fusion from L5 to the sacrum, sometime previously. Displacement of L3 over L4 above the solid fusion is demonstrated *(arrow)*. (From Frymoyer JW. Degenerative spondylolisthesis: diagnosis and treatment. J Am Acad Orthop Surg 1994:2;10, with permission.)

Interestingly, the slip in degenerative spondylolisthesis seldom exceeds 30% unless there has been surgical intervention (19).

Sakou et al. found that progression of slipping was observed in 30% of 40 patients followed for longer than 5 years, but the progression was not necessarily associated with deterioration of the patient's condition (8).

DIAGNOSIS

As always, a careful history and physical examination are the first steps in the diagnosis of degenerative spondylolisthesis with lumbar canal stenosis. The description of the pain is helpful and important in the diagnosis. There may be sensory loss or leg weakness. Hamstring tightness is always a common finding. Patients with spondylolisthesis may exhibit a type of waddling gait.

As in most patients with lumbar spinal stenosis, the clinical examination findings often are nonspecific. The loss of lumbar lordosis can be detected by inspection if the patient is experiencing significant spine or neurologic symptoms (5). When stenotic symptoms are severe, a fixed forward-flexed posture, sometimes accompanied by hip-flexion contractures, can be observed. Except in very thin patients, the step deformity usually is not palpable (23).

Surprisingly, some patients with degenerative spondylolisthesis retain a normal spinal mobility or in some instances, hypermobility. It has been suggested that patients with this condition have generalized ligamentous laxity, which might be of etiologic significance (23).

The neurologic examination may be useful when the patient has an isolated unilateral radiculopathy. The knee jerk reflex may be reduced or absent when the L4 nerve root is involved. Unilateral dorsiflexion or quadriceps weakness and the pattern of sensory loss are important findings. However, a positive nerve root tension sign is uncommon, particularly in the older population. More commonly, the neurologic findings are nonspecific and

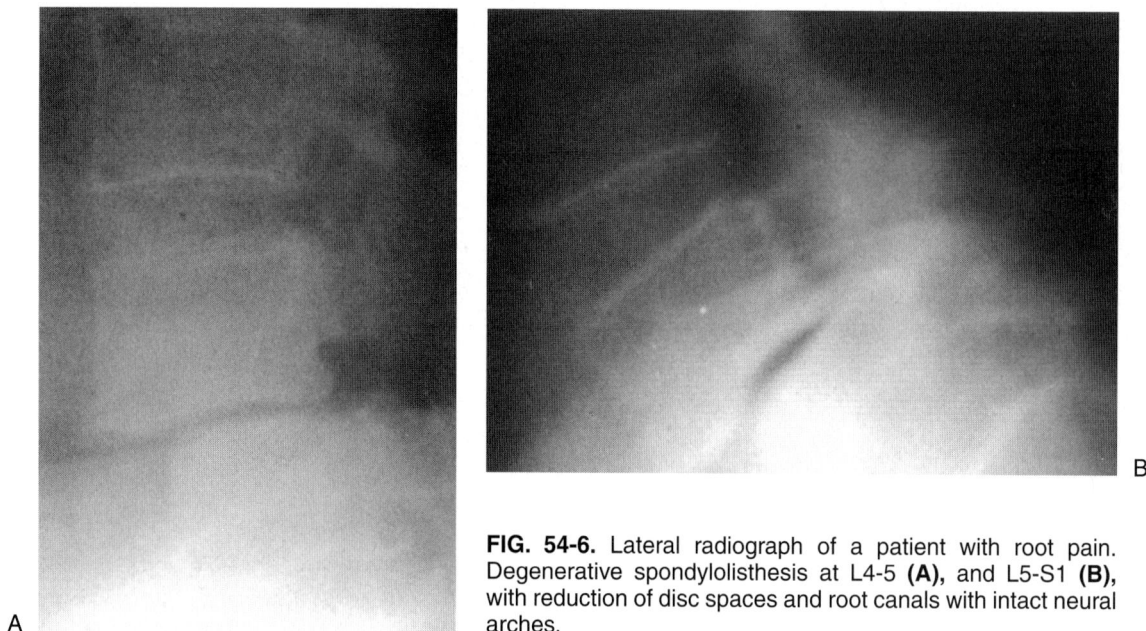

FIG. 54-6. Lateral radiograph of a patient with root pain. Degenerative spondylolisthesis at L4-5 **(A)**, and L5-S1 **(B)**, with reduction of disc spaces and root canals with intact neural arches.

may include bilaterally absent reflexes, spotty sensory losses, as well as muscle atrophy or weakness.

Plain roentgenogram (Fig. 54-6) include the essential finding of demonstrating the forward displacement of L4 on L5, the most common level at which this disorder occurs, or more rarely, L5 on S1 or L3 on L4 in the presence of an intact neural arch. Isthmic spondylolisthesis also may occur at this level, and plain X-ray should help to rule out this entity. Concomitant degenerative changes include disc space narrowing, end plate irregularities, sclerosis, osteophytes, and traction spurs (Fig. 54-7). Facet sclerosis and hypertrophy should all be noted on the plain X-ray film. Patients with isthmic spondylolisthesis are quite likely to be young and have neurologic symptoms. The AP radiograph often, but not always, demonstrates the accompanying hemisacralization of L5.

Dynamic flexion-extension views may be obtained but rarely demonstrate significant additional translational instability. Several authors have suggested recumbent supine or prone lateral flexion-extension radiographs for patients who are too uncomfortable to endure standing dynamic X-ray studies (24).

The alternative approach to demonstrate instability is the traction-compression radiographs, which has been described by Friberg (25). In this technique, a lateral lumbar radiograph is taken first after the application of a standard axial load and then after traction. The difference in displacement between these two views is correlated with back pain and instability, and is considered by Friberg to be of prognostic significance (25).

Further roentgenographic evaluation is not warranted for patients with predominantly mechanical back pain that responds to the usual conservative modalities. However, additional imaging studies may be warranted if sig-

nificant back pain persists that is unresponsive to nonoperative means or if significant radicular pain intervenes, with progressive neurologic claudication or radiculopathies and clinical suspicion that another condition (e.g., metastatic disease) may be causative. The presence of bladder or bowel complaints is an absolute indication.

The imaging alternatives include computed tomography (CT), myelography, contrast material–enhanced CT,

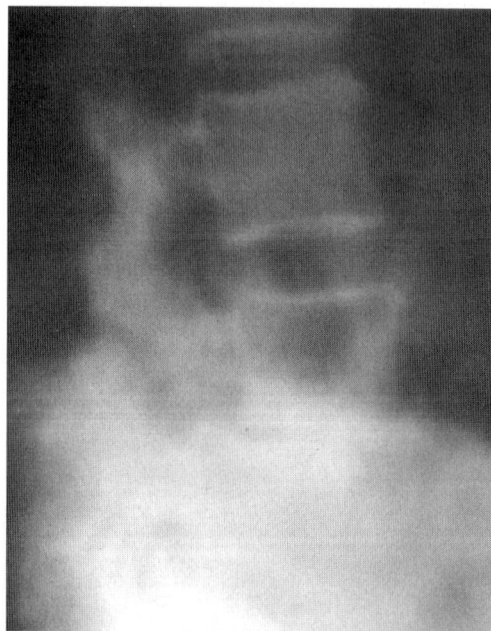

FIG. 54-7. Lateral radiograph of a patient with L4-5 ischemic spondylolisthesis with an advanced slip. Note the defect in the pars. (From Frymoyer JW. Degenerative spondylolisthesis: diagnosis and treatment. J Am Acad Orthop Surg 1994: 2;10, with permission.)

and magnetic resonance imaging (MRI). Typically, there is a diminished cross-sectional area at the level of the spondylolisthesis. There also may be hypertrophy of the superior facet with subarticular entrapment of the L5 nerve root. Soft-tissue abnormalities include thickening of the ligamentum flavum and posterior translation of a disc fragment.

Sagittal plane MRI is best for displaying the abnormal anatomy of spondylolisthesis, T2-weighted images for the canal and T1-weighted images for the pars interarticularis and neural foramina. The MRI sagittal view clearly shows the degree of subluxation and the relationship of the intervertebral disc to the adjacent vertebral bodies and spinal canal. Parasagittal images are excellent for showing encroachment of the nerve root in the foramina by disc or hypertrophic bone. Loss of the normal fat signal cushioning the nerve root is a sign for significant foraminal stenosis.

Ulmer et al. proposed the "wide canal sign" to distinguish between isthmic and degenerative spondylolisthesis (26). Using a midline sagittal section, they noted that the sagittal canal ratio (maximum anteroposterior diameter at any level divided by the diameter of the canal at L1) did not exceed 1:25 in normal controls and in subjects with degenerative spondylolisthesis. The measurement always exceeded 1:25 in patients with spondylolysis.

Technetium bone scanning was more commonly ordered before the advent of MRI scanning to rule out possible metastatic diseases. However, currently bone scanning is less commonly used in the initial evaluation of patients with degenerative spondylolisthesis.

Local anesthetic injections may be useful in specific cases. The best indication is concomitant degenerative spondylolisthesis and hip osteoarthritis. Relief of symptoms following an intra-articular hip injection suggests that the hip is the most probable origin for the symptoms.

DIFFERENTIAL DIAGNOSIS

Epidemiologic studies have suggested that degenerative spondylolisthesis is often an asymptomatic roentgenographic finding. This fact is of enormous importance because there is a natural tendency for clinicians to ascribe symptoms to an obvious structural lesion. Numerous spinal entities can give rise to similar symptoms, including spinal stenosis, central disc herniation, and degenerative scoliosis. One study demonstrated that a high percentage of patients with degenerative scoliosis also had degenerative spondylolisthesis (27). In patients with coronal plane abnormalities, who are frequently elderly, neurologic symptoms may suggest multilevel involvement.

Disease of cervical spine commonly produces symptoms that radiate to the lower extremities in elderly people. In all patients who are being evaluated (especially for surgery) cervical abnormalities should be ruled out with flexion-extension plain radiographs and possibly an MRI

scan of the cervical spine if the physical examination raises any question of cervical problems.

Osteoarthritis of the hip joint occurs in 11% to 17% of patients with degenerative spondylolisthesis, and can mimic the anterior thigh pain of an L4 nerve root entrapment (16). Therefore, the hip needs to be carefully examined for an alternative cause for symptoms of leg pain. Also, medial knee pain from degenerative disease or a torn meniscus may stimulate an L4 radiculopathy and produce considerable confusion for the clinician.

Peripheral vascular disease is common in elderly persons, who are also candidates of degenerative spondylolisthesis. Pain with ambulation is a typical finding, but it is much more closely related to decreased oxygen-carrying capacity of circulation to the lower extremities than to activity. Patients with vascular disease typically have more problems walking uphill than do patients with degenerative spondylolisthesis or spinal stenosis. In addition, patients with peripheral vascular disease typically have increased pain when riding a stationary bicycle, whereas patients with spinal stenosis typically are able to ride a stationary bicycle for a prolonged period because they can flex the lumbar spine. Patients with peripheral vascular disease need only to stop walking to alleviate their symptoms; patients with degenerative spondylolisthesis often must sit down and flex the lumbar spine to relieve their symptoms.

Unfortunately, elderly patients often have both diseases. They should have Doppler studies if there is any question of diminished blood flow to the lower limbs. With equal degrees of vascular and neural involvement from spinal stenosis, the vascular problem is usually addressed first.

Diabetic neuropathy rarely produces a painful radiculopathy. Electromyelographic and neural conduction studies should be performed in patients with diabetes mellitus. The surgical outcome for radiculopathy may not be as good in diabetic as in nondiabetic patients.

A less common coexistent condition is diffuse idiopathic skeletal hyperostosis. This condition is characterized by multilevel bridging osteophytes and commonly affects middle-aged and older men, who frequently are diabetic and uricemic. If surgery is required, these patients can be far more challenging than those with standard degenerative spondylolisthesis.

Other disorders that may resemble the symptoms of degenerative spondylolisthesis include metastatic disease of the spine or the presence of retroperitoneal tumor. Because of the age group affected and the substantial differential diagnosis, it is important to perform a current and complete medical evaluation before proceeding with definitive treatment of the spinal disorder (5).

CLINICAL PRESENTATION

Back pain is the most common chief complaint in patients with degenerative spondylolisthesis. Often the pain has been episodic and recurrent for many years. The course of the back pain in the patient's history may be highly variable and usually is unrelated to trauma. Few patients can recall a specific traumatic event. The back pain usually is mechanical and may be relieved with rest. Back pain usually is noted early as the superior vertebral body translates anteriorly with forward displacement of its inferior articular process (28). Radiation into the posterolateral thighs also is common and is independent of neurologic signs and symptoms. The second most common presenting symptom is neurogenic claudication. The advent of leg symptoms is the most common reason why patients and referring physicians become concerned and seek specialized medical attention. This results from further thecal compression by the posterior articular facets, as well as posterior displacement of the intervertebral disc level at the level of olisthesis (29). The pain is usually diffuse in the lower limbs, involving dermatomes and muscles innervated by the L4-5 and S1 nerve roots. Another type of presentation is a monoradicular nerve pain pattern usually involving an L5 spinal nerve root. The leg pain is always accentuated by walking and relieved by rest. These symptoms of spinal stenosis are reported by 42% to 82% of patients who seek help from spine surgeons (23). Typically, the leg pain is also relieved by forward flexion of the spine. Additional complaints include cold feet, altered gait, and "drop episodes" wherein the patient unexpectedly falls while walking (23).

Genitourinary findings are uncommon, but patients with these complaints should undergo imaging studies.

Interference with bladder and bowel control can occur with extreme stenosis, as was reported by Kostuik et al. in 3% of their patients (30). Unlike the acute and often devastating bladder and bowel symptoms of cauda equina syndrome in lumbar disc herniation, spinal stenosis often has an insidious and subtle presentation. The unwary examiner is at risk of attributing these symptoms to age-related conditions, such as cystocele in women and prostatism in men.

Stenotic symptoms are the result of mechanical and vascular factors. As the slip progresses, facet hypertrophy, buckling of the ligamentum flavum, and diffuse disc bulging contribute with forward displacement to compression of the cauda equina (Fig. 54-8). As in any stenotic condition, the relief of symptoms that follows forward spinal flexion is thought to be related to the increase in the AP diameters of the spinal canal that occurs in that posture. In extreme cases, patients may report the need to sleep in the fetal position to relieve leg symptoms.

The significant vascular component in complaints of leg pain may lead to restless legs syndrome sometimes called "vesper's curse" (31). In this condition, patients are awakened by aching pain in the calves, restlessness, an irresistible urge to move the legs, and fasciculations. This syndrome is reported to be exacerbated by congestive heart failure, which in turn may increase pressure in the arteriovenous anastomoses that characterizes the lumbar nerve-root microcirculation. Accordingly, if the patient reports increasing night cramps, it is worthwhile to obtain a thorough cardiovascular examination. Other associated neurologic symptoms (e.g., numbness and weakness) are present variably. The patients also may note a sudden episode of weakness, altered gait, or numbness. The pain may be progressive and incapacitating and may occur much more frequently with positional changes of the lumbar spine unrelated to significant exertion. For example, a patient may inadvertently extend the lumbar spine during sleep and produce such severe pain that significant sleep disturbance results (32,33). Progressive motion weakness and symptoms and signs of cauda equina syndrome are indications for emergent decompression surgery.

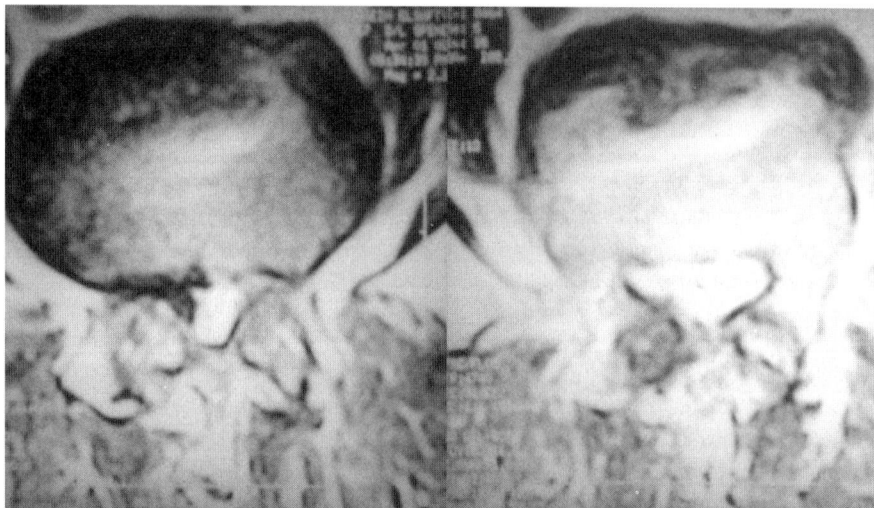

FIG. 54-8. Magnetic resonance imaging scan demonstrates the relationship of the caudal sac and nerve roots and facet degeneration. Note the marked narrowing of the lateral recesses.

The physical examinations findings in patients with degenerative spondylolisthesis (as in patients with spinal stenosis) may be nonspecific. In the standing position, the patient may decompensate anteriorly to allow a more flexed position of the lumbar spine. Inspection and palpation of the lumbar spine may reveal a palpable step off at the level of the olisthesis. The iliolumbar ligaments, sacral iliac joints, sciatic notches, other spinous processes, and trochanteric bursae should all be palpated and the presence of symptoms noted.

Range of motion of the lumbar spine usually is normal, and many patients can flex forward without difficulty. The examiner should attempt to extend the lumbar spine fully and, if possible, the patient should be asked whether the symptoms are being reproduced (33,34).

As noted, some patients present with degenerative spondylolisthesis above a spinal fusion (35). A long symptom-free interval is followed by the onset of nerve-root symptoms and stenosis emanating from the level above their previous fusion (35).

The neurologic examination may reveal a focal nerve deficit. The quadriceps tendon reflex may be reduced with an L4 radiculopathy. Less commonly, there is quadriceps weakness and possibly atrophy. Extensor hallucis longus weakness also may be encountered with an L5 spinal nerve root abnormality. However, most commonly, the results of neurologic examination are nonspecific, with symmetric motor findings and symmetrically depressed reflexes noted in the elderly population.

NONOPERATIVE TREATMENT

Nonoperative management is the primary treatment for patients with low-grade adult degenerative spondylolisthesis who present with acute or chronic low back pain (36).

Nonoperative treatment should include reducing environmental pain generators, various physical therapy modalities, non-narcotic medications, immobilization, and occasionally multidisciplinary pain clinics (37). This nonoperative management regimen is similar for all populations with other types of mechanical low back symptoms and should be pursued diligently both by the patient and surgeon (38).

The initial recommendations include practicing healthy back care, including proper lifting and bending techniques, and avoiding periods of prolonged sitting or driving (39). Decreasing or eliminating tobacco use and pursuing an ideal body weight benefit the patient.

Nonoperative treatment of degenerative spondylolisthesis is similar to the nonoperative management of other mechanical disorders of the lumbar spine. No prospective randomized studies confirm a preferred method of nonoperative treatment. However, there is recent evidence that the natural history of degenerative spinal stenosis and degenerative spondylolisthesis may be more favorable than previously thought.

Johnsson et al. followed 32 patients with clinical symptoms and myelographically confirmed stenosis for an average of 49 months. No patient had significant deterioration, and surprisingly many patients improved (40). In patients who have predominantly back pain, the usual conservative modalities of appropriate rest, the use of anti-inflammatory nonsteroidal medication may have a significant beneficial impact.

MEDICATION

Anti-inflammatories

This group of medications, which specifically aims to decrease inflammation in tissues, can be quite effective in mild and moderate pain. Side effects (aside from allergic reactions) may include stomach upset, gastritis, ulcer problems, and kidney and liver problems.

Analgesics

This group of medications aims to reducing the sensation of pain without any specific action at the source of the pain. In a sense, this covers or dampens the pain but does not treat the site of the problem.

Muscle Relaxants

These medications aim to loosen the tension and irritability of muscle tissue. By relaxing a very tense muscle, the pain caused by spasm and cramping can be reduced. Some patients become very drowsy with these medications.

Combination Drugs

These combine different types of medication to offer pain relief and anti-inflammatory effects.

Narcotics

These pain medications are quite strong and act on the brain and spinal cord to decrease the sensation of pain. Because of addiction potential and risks of overdose, these medications should be restricted in use.

Antidepressants

In some cases mild doses of antidepressant medication may offer added relief from chronic nerve related pain.

The second nonoperative measure that deals with pain in patients with degenerative spondylolisthesis is the encouragement of aerobic conditioning, on the premise that exercise may improve arterial circulation to the cauda equina because walking often aggravates symptoms. A stationary bicycle is a good alternative, particularly if the handle bars and seat are set up to allow the forward-flexed position.

AEROBIC CONDITIONING

Physical Therapy

Physical therapy for spinal conditions includes pain modality treatments such as transcutaneous electrical nerve stimulation (TENS), massage and ultrasound, acupuncture and traction, and structured guided strengthening programs for restoring good muscle function. There are many different types of exercise programs. Particular focus on isometric strengthening appears to be beneficial for many patients. Isometric exercises involve activities that stimulate contraction of a muscle (working the muscle) while maintaining the length of that muscle (i.e., no significant motion across the span of the muscle). Vigorous movements or extremes of motion are often avoided in physical therapy approaches to spinal care.

Exercise

Most patients are advised to maintain some form of regular exercise on a long-term basis. Even patients with mild or intermittent back pain and no severe underlying problem may benefit from regular exercise. A number of studies have shown that regular aerobic activity reduces the change of developing repeated back injuries. Clear advantages of one type of sport over another have not been shown. Therefore, it may be more important to find an activity that is enjoyable and easy to maintain on a regular schedule, such as swimming, fast walking, and running.

Weight Reduction

The third method of nonoperative therapy in managing back pain from degenerative spondylolisthesis is weight reduction. This strategy often minimally affects neurologic complaints. Careful management of osteoporosis may be helpful. Additional strategies include the judicious use of braces.

ADDITIONAL STRATEGIES

There are a wide variety of binders, belts braces, and other devices designed to offer relief from back pain. There effectiveness in most cases has not been clearly proven, and yet many patients do feel some relief from their pain with some of these applied devices. However, long-term wear of back braces may lead to gradual weakening of the supportive muscles owing to the effect of unloading the spine; therefore, this may not be desirable.

Epidural block and extended bed rest appear to be of little value and carry a significant risk of morbidity, especially in elderly patients. Likewise, there is no information to support the use of manipulative therapy, which may be contraindicated, particularly in osteoporotic patients.

Many studies suggest that radicular pain is much less amenable to the same nonoperative management strategies that are applicable when radiculopathy is related to a herniated disc. In general, patients with predominantly leg pain require a longer trial of nonoperative care to evaluate the efficacy of treatment. For patients with significant leg pain, administration of epidural steroids is an appropriate temporizing measure (36–39).

Patients with low-grade degenerative spondylolisthesis may present with a multitude of physical, emotional, and psychological symptoms, and these patients often are best handled by a multidisciplinary pain center approach. This includes input from different services, including anesthesia, physiatry, psychiatry, physical therapy, occupational and behavioral therapy, and social work. It was found that this multidisciplinary approach is useful in both previously operated and nonoperated patients (41).

REFERENCES

1. Wiltse LL, Newman PH, MacNab I. Classification of spondylolysis and spondylolisthesis. Clin Orthop Rel Res 1976;117:23–29.
2. Junghanns H. Spondylolisthesen ohne spalt imzwischengelenkstuck. Archiv fur Orthopadische und Unfall Chirurgie 1930;29:118.
3. Newman PH. The etiology of spondylolisthesis. J Bone Joint Surg 1963;45B:39—59.
4. MacNab I. Spondylolisthesis with an intact neural arch so called pseudospondylolisthesis. J Bone Joint Surg 1950;32–B:325.
5. Frymoyer JW. Degenerative spondylolisthesis: diagnosis and treatment. J Am Acad Orthop Surg 1994;2:9–15.
6. Marchetti PG, Bartolozzi P. Classification of spondylolisthesis as a guideline for treatment. In: Bridwell KH, Dewald RL, eds. The text book of spinal surgery, 2nd ed. Philadelphia: Lippincott-Raven, 1997:1250–1253.
7. Bridwell KH, Sedgewick TA, Obrien MF, et al. The role of fusion and instrumentation in the treatment of degenerative spondylolisthesis with spinal stenosis. J Spinal Disord 1993;6:461–472.
8. Matsunaga S, Sakou T, Morizono Y, et al. Natural history of degenerative spondylolisthesis pathogenesis natural course of the slippage. Spine 1990;15:1204.
9. Farfan HF. The biomechanical advantage of lordosis and hip extension for upright man as compared with other anthropoids. Spine 1978;3:336.
10. Farfan HF. The mechanical disorders of the lower back. Philadelphia: Lea and Febiger, 1973.
11. Porter RW. Management of back pain. Edinburgh: Churchill Livingstone, 1986.
12. Larson SJ. Degenerative spondylolisthesis. Neurosurgery 1983;13:561.
13. Mimura M, Moriya H, Takahashi K. Rotational instability in degenerative spondylolisthesis. A possible mechanical etiology of the disease. Presented at the International Society for the Study of the Lumbar Spine Meeting, Marseiles, France, June 1993.
14. Valkenburg HA, Haanen HCM. The epidemiology of low back pain. In: White AA III, Gorden SL, eds. American Academy of Orthopaedic Surgeons Symposium on Idiopathic Low Back Pain. St. Louis: CV Mosby, 1982:9–22.
15. Herkowitz HN, Kurz LT. Degenerative lumbar spondylolisthesis with spinal stenosis: a prospective study comparing decompression with decompression and intertransverse process arthrodesis. J Bone Joint Surgery Am 1991;73:802–808.
16. Rosenberg NJ. Degenerative spondylolisthesis: predisposing factors. J Bone Joint Surg Am 1975;57:467–474.
17. Rosenberg NJ. Degenerative spondylolisthesis. Surgical treatment. Clin Orthop 1976;117:112.
18. Cyron RM, Hutton WC. Articular trophism and stability of the lumbar spine. Spine 1980;5:168–172.
19. Knutsson F. Instability associated with disc degeneration. Acta Radiol 1944;15:593.
20. Fritzgerald JAW, Newman PH. Degenerative spondylolisthesis. J Bone Joint Surg 1976;58B:184–192.
21. Epstein BS, Epstein IA, Jones MD. Degenerative spondylolisthesis with an intact neural arch. Radio Clin North Am 1977;15:227–239.

22. Wiltse LL. Salvage of failed lumbar spinal stenosis surgery. In Hopp E, ed. Spine: state of the art reviews. Philadelphia: Hanly-Belfus, 1987: 421–450.
23. Frymoyer JW. Degenerative spondylolisthesis. In: Andersson GBT, McNell TW, eds. Lumbar spinal stenosis. St. Louis: Mosby Year Book, 1992.
24. Whiffen JR, Neurwith MG. Degenerative spondylolisthesis. In: Bridwell KH, Dewald RL, eds. The text book of spinal surgery, vol. 2. Philadelphia: JB Lippincott, 1991:657–674.
25. Friberg O. Lumbar instability: a dynamic approach by traction-compression radiography. Spine 1987;12:119–129.
26. Ulmer JL, Elster AD, Mathews VP, et al. Distinction between degenerative and isthmic Spondylolisthesis on sagittal MR images: importance of increased anteroposterior diameter of the spinal canal ("wide canal sign"). Am J Rontgenol 1994;163:411–416.
27. Pritchett JW, Bortel DT. Degenerative symptomatic lumbar scoliosis. Spine 1993;18:700–703.
28. Satomi K, Hirabayashi K, Toyamo Y, et al. A clinical study of degenerative spondylolisthesis radiographic analysis and choice of treatment. Spine 1992;17:1329–1336.
29. Herron LD, Trippi AC. Degenerative spondylolisthesis. The results of treatment by decompressive laminectomy without fusion. Spine 1989; 14:534–538.
30. Kostuik JP, Harrington I, Alexander D, et al. Cauda equina syndrome and lumbar disc herniation. J Bone Joint Surg Am 1986;68:386–391.
31. Laban MM, Viola SL, Femminineo AF, et al. Restless legs syndrome associated with diminished cardiopulmonary compliance and lumbar spinal stenosis: a motor concomitant of "Vespers curse." Arch Phys Med Rehabil 1990;71:384–388.
32. Lombardi JS, Wiltse LL, Reynolds J, et al. Treatment of degenerative spondylolisthesis. Spine 1985;10:821–827.
33. Grobler LJ, Robertson PA, Novotny JE, et al. Decompression for degenerative spondylolisthesis and spinal stenosis at L4-5. The effect on facet joint morphology. Spine 1993;18:1475.
34. Katz JN, Lipson SJ, Larson MG, et al. The outcome of decompressive laminectomy for degenerative lumbar stenosis. J Bone Joint Surg Am 1991;73:809–816.
35. Frymoyer JW, Hanley EN Jr, Howel J, et al. A comparison of radiographic findings in fusion and non—fusion patients ten or more years following lumbar disc surgery. Spine 1979;4:435–440.
36. Barr W. Spondylolisthesis. J Bone Joint Surg (Am) 1955;37:878.
37. Magora A. Conservative treatment of spondylolisthesis. Clin Orthop 1978;117:74.
38. Boachie-Adjei O. Conservative treatment of spondylolysis and spondylolisthesis. Semin Spine Surg 1989;1:106.
39. Gramse RR, Sinaki M, Ilstrup DM. Lumbar spondylolisthesis: a rational approach to conservative treatment. Mayo Clin Proc 1980;55(11):681.
40. Johnsson KE, Rosen I, Volen A: The natural course of lumbar spinal stenosis. Clin Orthop 1992;279:82–86.
41. Capner N. Spondylolisthesis. Br J Surg 1932;19:347.

CHAPTER 55

Decompression

Bo Jönsson

Degenerative spondylolisthesis mostly occurs at the L4-L5 level and has a gender-related difference in prevalence, being four to five times more frequent in women. Radiographic cross-sectional studies of older adult women have demonstrated an incidence of anterior slip of 29% in the lumbar spine, but without correlation between pain and olisthesis (1). There was an increasing prevalence of L4-L5 olisthesis with increasing patient age.

The proportion of patients with degenerative spondylolisthesis in articles dealing with spinal stenosis shows a rather wide variation. Turner et al. (2) noted that 28 out of 74 articles on spinal stenosis included data on degenerative spondylolisthesis, with a mean proportion of 50% (range 0 to 100). Their compilation included, however, four articles containing only patients with degenerative spondylolisthesis and therefore 50% probably does not reflect the true prevalence. In a prospective, consecutive long-term study on spinal stenosis including 105 patients with radiographic reassessment of all patients (3), 32 out of 105 patients (30%) had degenerative spondylolisthesis. Katz et al. (4) have retrospectively analyzed a group of 88 patients with spinal stenosis regarding long-term result; of these 88 patients, 22 had a degenerative spondylolisthesis (25%). In a study on postoperative instability after lumbar decompression by Johnsson et al. (5), 20 out of 45 patients (44%) had a preoperative olisthesis. Katz et al. (6) presented another prospective, multicenter study including 272 patients with spinal stenosis, where 93 patients (34%) had a spondylolisthesis of 5 mm or more.

ANATOMY

Patients with degenerative spondylolisthesis often have a specific laminar configuration predisposing for the vertebral slipping (7). The articular surface of the superior articular process is facing medially and the laminae are converging distally toward the inferior articular processes, which are medially located with their joint surfaces facing laterally. Due to this configuration of the

articular processes, the facet joints are more or less sagittally oriented. This configuration is more easily recognized in younger patients without degenerative changes (Fig. 55-1).

A number of radiographic studies have demonstrated a correlation between degenerative spondylolisthesis and sagittally angled facet joints (8–10). Grobler at al. (11) described the increased angles in patients with degenerative spondylolisthesis, but also the reduced coronal dimension after decompression, with increased risk for instability.

In a recent study (10) on orientation and osteoarthritis of the lumbar facet joints, the authors found a significant correlation between sagittally oriented joints and osteoarthritis, even in patients without olisthesis. The degenerative changes in patients with spondylolisthesis, however, were more severe.

Love et al. (12) confirmed the sagittal orientation of facet joints in patients with degenerative spondylolisthesis, but interpreted this joint configuration more as a consequence of arthritic remodeling.

RADIOGRAPHIC FINDINGS

In a study of 105 patients with spinal stenosis by Jönsson et al. (3) the radiographic findings were assessed for all patients. There were 32 patients with degenerative spondylolisthesis, 4 at level L3-L4, 25 at L4-L5 and 3 at L5-S1 (Fig. 55-2). Patients with degenerative spondylolisthesis had a more pronounced narrowing of the spinal canal with an anteroposterior-diameter of 5.6 mm compared with 6.7 mm in patients with no spondylolisthesis. The site of the spondylolisthesis was the narrowest site in most (24 of 32) patients.

DECOMPRESSION

The standard surgical procedure consists of a midline laminectomy extended laterally toward the edge of the

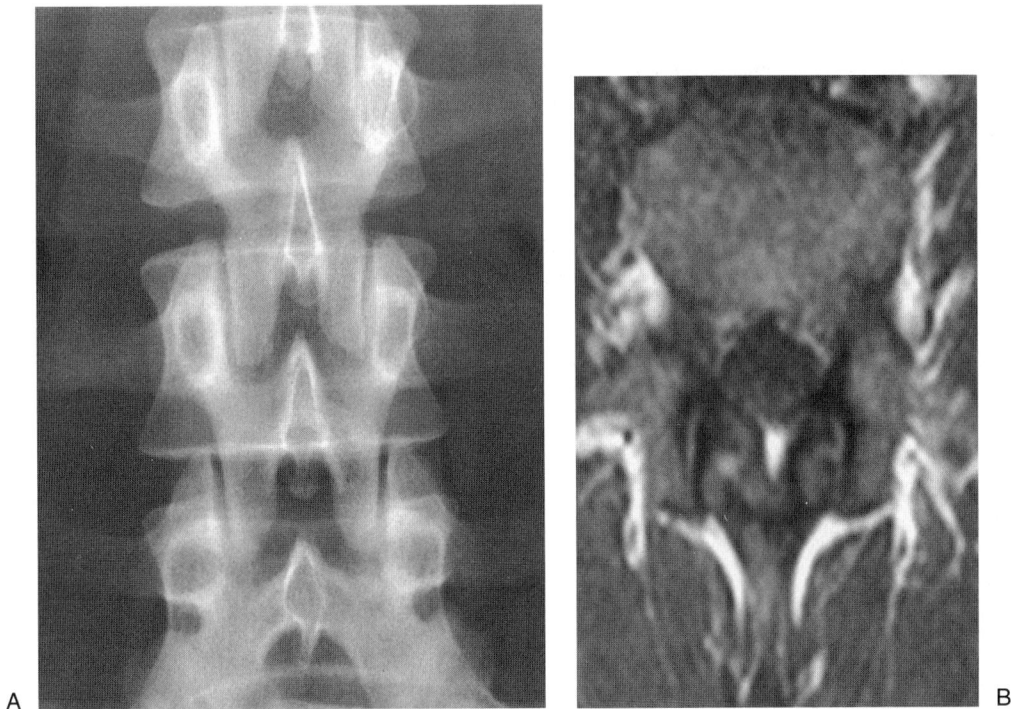

FIG. 55-1. A: Plain X-ray demonstrating laminar configuration in a patient with sagittally oriented facet joints. **B:** Magnetic resonance imaging, axial view demonstrating sagittal angles of facet joints.

dural sac. In order to decompress the single nerve roots, the decompression is extended laterally-distally including the medial part of the facet joints without violating the stability. In patients with facet joints orientated in the coronal plane (and no degenerative spondylolisthesis), nerve root impingement may occur in the lateral recess (i.e., below the superior articular process). Decompression is obtained by the undercutting technique. In patients with sagittally oriented facet joints and degenerative spondylolisthesis, root compression may be caused by the anteriorly displaced inferior articular process, necessitating resection of the medial/anterior part of this process (Fig. 55-3).

Results of Decompression

In 1992, Turner et al. presented a survey of 74 articles on results after decompression for spinal stenosis (2). Good to excellent results were on average reported by 64% of the patients; there was, however a wide variation in outcome. The authors noted better outcome in studies including more patients with degenerative spondylolisthesis. There were four reports including only patients with degenerative spondylolisthesis and good to excellent result was noted by 83% to 85% in these articles. Some of these articles however included patients who underwent spinal arthrodesis.

A corresponding meta-analysis including only studies dealing with spinal stenosis and degenerative spondy-

lolisthesis was presented by Mardjetko et al. (13). Their analysis included 25 papers published between 1970 and 1993. Superior results were found in patients who underwent a concomitant spinal arthrodesis; satisfactory results were noted in 69% of patients who were treated with decompression only, while 86% to 90% of those who underwent fusion reported satisfactory results.

Herron and Trippi (14) evaluated 24 patients, all with degenerative spondylolisthesis treated with laminectomy

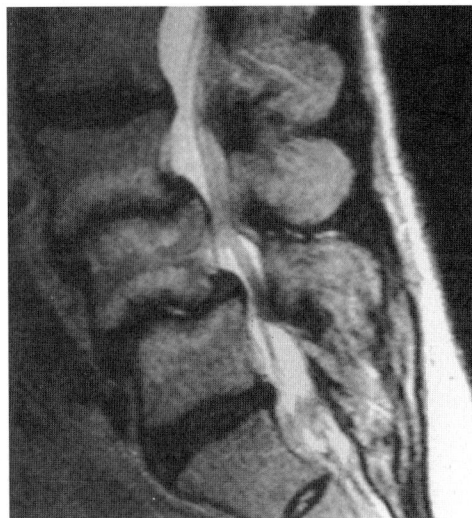

FIG. 55-2. Degenerative spondylolisthesis is most commonly seen at level L4-L5, but may occur at multiple levels.

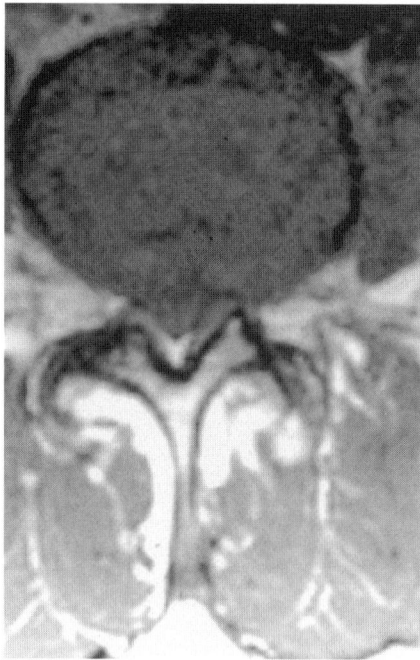

FIG. 55-3. Magnetic resonance imaging, axial view at L4-L5 in a 70-year-old woman with degenerative spondylolisthesis and spinal stenosis. Note anterior displacement of inferior articular process.

alone. At follow-up (18 to 71 months after surgery) 20 out of 24 patients (83%) reported good result.

Epstein (15) has reported the results of decompression alone in 290 patients treated over a 25-year period. Excellent result was obtained in 69% and good result in 13%. Secondary spinal arthrodesis was performed in 8 (2.7%) of the patients.

In a prospective and consecutive study of 105 patients operated on due to spinal stenosis (16), 32 patients had a degenerative spondylolisthesis. Follow-up examinations were performed 4 months and 1, 2, and 5 years postoperatively. All radiographs were reassessed by a neuroradiologist, who had no information regarding surgical results. Predictors of good outcome were sought using logistic regression analysis. In this study design, the most important factors were, in this order: a low anteroposterior (AP) diameter of the spinal canal, absence of comorbid disease affecting walking, and less than 4 years of leg symptoms. Most patients with degenerative spondylolisthesis had a more pronounced narrowing of the spinal canal and reported good results at follow-up.

POSTOPERATIVE PROGRESSIVE SLIP AFTER DECOMPRESSION ONLY

Johnsson et al. studied postoperative slipping after lumbar decompression (5). In the patient group with degenerative spondylolisthesis, progressive slip occurred in 65% of the patients without influencing the surgical

results. During this period, many authors recommended a wide, radical decompression and total facetectomies were performed in more than 50% of the patients in this study.

Another study of postoperative stability after surgery using a facet-preserving undercutting technique (17) demonstrated better results with progressive slip in only 32% of patients with spondylolisthesis preoperatively. Also in this study, no correlation between surgical result and progressive slip was seen.

Recently, two studies using alternative decompressive procedures have reported good results and low risk of increased instability postoperatively. Kinoshita et al. (18) evaluated 51 patients who underwent decompression through a unilateral approach and found no increased slip postoperatively. Kleeman et al. (19) described their results in 54 patients who underwent decompression through the "port-hole" technique. Good to excellent result was noted in 88% and there was no statistical difference regarding result in patients with or without degenerative spondylolisthesis. Progressive slip was noted in 13% of the patients.

Matsanuga et al. (20) studied the natural course of slippage and described 30% progressive slippage in a study of 40 patients.

DISCUSSION

During the last decade, randomized, controlled studies have demonstrated superior surgical outcome in patients operated on with concomitant spinal arthrodesis. The results of these procedures are described in Chapters 56 and 58. Spinal stenosis, with or without degenerative spondylolisthesis afflicts an older adult patient group, and is the main indication for spinal procedures in the elderly. With increasing age, the incidence of concomitant cardiovascular and other degenerative diseases increase, with associated potential risks for anesthesiologic/surgical complications. The complication rate is higher in patients who are treated with a concomitant spinal fusion (21). In the clinical situation, the spinal surgeon has to include these considerations in the surgical decision making. In a study on patient selection, costs and outcomes, Katz et al. (6) noted that patients who underwent spinal fusion were significantly younger.

A national registry of lumbar spine surgery due to degenerative diseases has been evolved in Sweden (21). According to data from surgical procedures performed in the year 2000, 15% of patients with spinal stenosis underwent a concomitant spinal fusion, indicating that in common clinical practice, half or less than half of the patients with spinal stenosis and degenerative spondylolisthesis are selected for spinal arthrodesis in conjunction with decompression. Interestingly, Katz et al. (6) noted similar figures, with 50% of patients with spondylolisthesis greater than 5 mm or scoliosis greater than 15° being treated with laminectomy alone.

Studies on patients with spinal stenosis and degenerative spondylolisthesis have evaluated this patient group as a homogenous entity. The number of patients included in randomized studies, as in the Herkowitz study (22), has been too few to allow analysis of subgroups. In the clinical situation, however, the spinal surgeon encounters situations with a wide variation of symptoms within the same group of diagnosis. There are, for example, patients with minor or no back pain at all despite a radiologically verified olisthesis. Is there a need for fusion in these patients? Or consider the patient in whom physiologic stabilization has reduced the vertebral mobility at the slipped level. Does this patient need a fusion?

There is still no consensus regarding treatment of this patient group and there are different opinions between spinal researchers, exemplified by two recently published surveys (23,24). There is a need for further research with the aim to create more precise scientific guidelines regarding treatment of the different subgroups.

REFERENCES

1. Vogt MT, Rubin D, Valentin RS, et al. Lumbar olisthesis and lower back symptoms in elderly white women. The study of osteoporotic fractures. Spine 1998;23:2640–2647.
2. Turner J, Ersek M, Herron L, et al. Surgery for lumbar spinal stenosis. Attempted meta-analysis of the literature. Spine 1992;17:1–8
3. Jönsson B, Annertz M, Sjöberg C, et al. A prospective and consecutive study of surgically treated lumbar spinal stenosis. Part I: Clinical features related to radiographic findings. Spine 1997;24:2932–2937.
4. Katz JN, Lipson SJ, Chang LC, et al. Seven to 10-year outcome of decompressive surgery for degenerative lumbar spinal stenosis. Spine 1996;1:92–98.
5. Johnsson KE, Uden A, Jonsson K. Postoperative instability after decompression for lumbar spinal stenosis. Spine 1986;11:107–110.
6. Katz JN, Lipson SJ, Lew RA, et al. Lumbar laminectomy alone or with instrumented or noninstrumented arthrodesis in degenerative lumbar spinal stenosis. Patient selection, costs and surgical outcomes. Spine 1997;10:2640–2647
7. Sato K, Wakamatsu E, Yoshizumi A, et al. The configuration of the laminas and facet joints in degenerative spondylolisthesis. A clinicoradiologic study. Spine 1989;11:1265–1271.
8. Boden SD, Riew KD, Yamaguchi K, et al. Orientation of the lumbar facet joints; association with degenerative disc disease. J Bone Joint Surg 1996;78A:403–411.
9. Dai LY. Orientation and tropism of lumbar facet joints in degenerative spondylolisthesis. Int Orthop 2001;25(1):40–42.
10. Fujiwara A, Kazuya T, An Howard S, et al. Orientation and osteoarthritis of the lumbar facet joint. Clin Orthop 2001;385:88–94.
11. Grobler L, Robertson P, Nolomy J, et al. Etiology of lumbar spondylolisthesis: assessment of the role played by lumbar facet joint morphology. Spine 1993;18:80–92.
12. Love TW, Fagan AB, Fraser RD. Degenerative spondylolisthesis. Developmental or acquired? J Bone Joint Surg Br 1999;81(4):670–674.
13. Mardjetko SM, Connoly PJ, Shott S. Degenerative lumbar spondylolisthesis. A meta-analysis of literature 1970–1993. Spine 1994;20S: 2256S–2265S
14. Herron LD, Trippi AC. L4-5 degenerative spondylolisthesis. The results of treatment by decompressive laminectomy without fusion. Spine 1989;14:534–538.
15. Epstein NE. Decompression in the surgical management of degenerative spondylolisthesis: advantages of a conservative approach in 2290 patients. J Spinal Disord 1998;11(2):116–122.
16. Jönsson B, Annertz M, Sjöberg C, et al. A prospective and consecutive study of surgically treated lumbar spinal stenosis. Part II: Five-year follow-up by an independent observer. Spine 1997;24:2938–2944.
17. Jönsson B, Åkesson M, Jonsson K, et al. Low risk for vertebral slipping after decompression with facet-joint preserving technique for lumbar spinal stenosis. Eur Spine J 1992;1:90–94.
18. Kinoshita T, Ohki I, Roth KR, et al. Results of degenerative spondylolisthesis treated with posterior decompression alone via a new surgical approach. J Neurosurg 2001;95:11–16.
19. Kleeman TJ, Hiscoe AC, Berg EE. Patient outcome after minimally destabilizing lumbar stenosis decompression: the "port-hole" technique. Spine 2000;25:865–870.
20. Matsanuga S, Sakou T, Morizomo Y, et al. Natural history of degenerative spondylolisthesis. Pathogenesis and natural course of slippage. Spine 1990;15:1204–1210.
21. Strömqvist B, Jönsson B, Fritzell P, et al. National Register for Lumbar Spine Surgery. Acta Orthop Scand 2001;72:99–106.
22. Herkowitz HN, Kurz LT. Degenerative lumbar spondylolisthesis. A prospective study comparing decompression and intertransverse arthrodesis. J Bone Joint Surg [Am] 1991;73-A:802–808.
23. Bassewitz H, Herkowitz H. Lumbar stenosis with spondylolisthesis. Current concepts of surgical treatment. Clin Orthop 2001;384:54–60.
24. Postacchini F. Spine update. Surgical management of lumbar spinal stenosis. Spine 1999;10:1043–1047.

CHAPTER 56

Decompression with Posterolateral Fusion

Gianluca Cinotti

INDICATIONS

As in any patients with spinal condition in whom the surgical option has been considered, a successful operation may be expected if a correct surgical indication has been made. A wrong surgical indication, in fact, is probably the most important factor responsible for poor surgical outcomes in patients with degenerative spinal conditions. This is particularly true in degenerative spondylolisthesis, since the condition may be asymptomatic, and thus not requiring any treatment, or cause a wide spectrum of symptoms including low back pain, radicular pain or both. As a result, in any patient with degenerative spondylolisthesis (DS) in whom surgery may be indicated, a careful clinical and radiologic evaluation should be carried out to confirm that patient's symptoms are due to the spondylolisthesis.

Preoperative Planning

Historically, a degenerative spondylolisthesis can be treated with decompression alone, decompression plus fusion with or without internal fixation and, in a few patients, with fusion alone. Decompression plus fusion is thought to be the treatment of choice by most surgeons since it allows reaching better results compared to decompression alone (1–6). This is certainly true when an unselected population of patients with DS is randomly treated with the two procedures. However, if a selection of patients who need fusion or decompression is carried out preoperatively, the surgical outcomes may further improve and unnecessary fusion be avoided. An accurate clinical and radiologic assessment before surgery may be helpful to this aim.

Clinical evaluation should assess whether predominant symptoms are due to nerve root compression (radicular pain is the predominant symptom), to spinal instability (back pain is the predominant symptom), or both. Radiologic evaluation should assess the degree of vertebral instability and the severity of stenosis at the spondylolis-

thetic level. In particular, standard and flexion-extension radiographs should determine the degree of vertebral slipping and whether a hypermobility of the olisthesic vertebra is present. Magnetic resonance (MR) scans should assess whether a narrowing of the spinal canal or a true stenosis, including a compression of the nervous structures, is present and, in the latter event, if this involves the lateral or central portion of the spinal canal. On axial MR scans, the orientation of facet joints in the horizontal plane and the amount of facet joint resection necessary to free the nerve root in the lateral canal should be also evaluated (7,8). Disc herniation below the spondylolisthetic vertebra is uncommon; however, since a false impression of disc herniation may be seen on both sagittal and axial scans, the presence of a posterolateral or lateral disc herniation associated to the spondylolisthesis should be ruled out. Finally, MR scans should evaluated whether degenerated discs are present at the levels adjacent to the spondylolisthesis since this may influence the choice of vertebral levels which have to be included in the fused area.

On the basis of preoperative investigations, a decompression with fusion is indicated in patients with one, or more, of the following requisites: low back pain is predominant or equal to radicular pain; a grade II spondylolisthesis is present; a hypermobility of the spondylolisthetic vertebra is seen on flexion-extension radiographs; severe central stenosis is present, whereby central laminectomy is needed; facet joints show a marked sagittal orientation in the horizontal plane, so that a tendency to vertebral slipping may be expected after decompression (although this event is often asymptomatic). Conversely, decompression alone may be indicated in the minority of patients with the following requisites: radicular pain is the only, or predominant, symptom; a grade I spondylolisthesis is present; flexion-extension radiographs show no evidence of hypermobility of the slipped vertebra; a lateral stenosis is present, whereby a unilateral or bilateral laminotomy may be adequate to decompress the nerve root; facet joints show a mild sagittal orientation in the horizontal plane, so that only a slight increase in vertebral slipping may be expected after decompression. Fusion alone is indicated in a few patients with DS in whom low back pain is the only symptom and no stenosis is present on MR scans.

Specific Indications to Decompression plus Posterolateral Fusion

In any patients with DS in whom fusion is indicated, a posterolateral arthrodesis may be performed successfully. Spinal instrumentation may be associated to fusion; however, since most of the patients with DS do not show a marked vertebral instability, the indication to perform an instrumented or a noninstrumented fusion rests entirely on discretion of the surgeon. Many surgeons are use to associate pedicle screws to posterolateral fusion to reduce postoperative pain, avoid a rigid orthosis, shorten the hospitalization time and accelerate the functional recovery. Internal fixation was also found to increase the fusion rate (1,9–11), possibly by reducing vertebral motion and subsequent unfavorable mechanical stresses (axial rotation and tension stresses) on the graft material. However, no significant difference was found in the clinical outcomes of patients submitted to instrumented or noninstrumented fusion (9,12).

Posterolateral non-instrumented fusion may be advantageous in any patient with DS showing degenerative processes at the levels adjacent to the spondylolisthesis, since in these cases a less rigid fusion mass reduces mechanical stresses at the adjacent levels compared to an instrumented fusion. A noninstrumented posterolateral fusion may also be advantageous in severely osteoporotic patients in whom a poor fixation of pedicle screws may be expected.

Interbody devices may be associated to posterolateral fusion and pedicle screws to increase the fusion rate, reduce vertebral slipping, and restore the height of the disc space. However, there is no evidence that these factors may influence the surgical results in patients with DS. In particular, no prospective randomized study demonstrated better clinical outcomes after 360° fusion, nor that the reduction of olisthesis may improve the results in patients with DS. The restoration of the foraminal height subsequent to the insertion of interbody devices has little clinical effects on the nerve root (13), particularly in DS patients in whom the olisthesis may cause lateral or central stenosis whereas the foraminal dimensions are not affected by the condition. Patients with DS may be treated with interbody devices, along with pedicle screws, as alternative to posterolateral fusion, to eliminate the need for harvesting autogenous bone graft from the iliac crest. However, since the type of fixation (biological or mechanical) achieved with interbody cages has not well established yet, further studies should assess whether this procedure can yield surgical outcome as good as those reported by patients submitted to posterolateral fusion at long- and very long-term follow-ups.

OPERATIVE TREATMENT

Whatever support is used the patient should be positioned on the operative table so that the abdomen is maintained free during the operation in order to avoid compression on large abdominal vessels and reduce intraoperative bleeding.

The posterolateral approach described by Wiltse (14) or the posterior approach can be used. The former allows a better exposure of the fusion area and reduces intraoperative bleeding; the second is more frequently used when a decompression of the nervous structures has to be associated to fusion, that is, in the majority of cases. With the posterior approach the skin incision should be extended one or two levels proximally and distally to the fusion area so that an adequate muscular retraction to expose the transverse processes is achieved. If a decompression of the nervous structures has to be performed this is usually carried out before fusion to limit the blood loss.

Decompression

In the most frequent situation (i.e., degenerative spondylolisthesis of L4), the vertebral slipping causes a compression of L5 nerve root in the lateral canal. If severe slipping is present, or if the sagittal dimension of the spinal canal is extremely narrow, the olisthesis may also cause central stenosis at the disc level due to the forward slipping of the posterior vertebral arch.

Nerve decompression can be performed with several techniques, but the most commonly used are central laminectomy and unilateral, or bilateral, laminotomy (15). Central laminectomy is indicated in patients with severe stenosis and in any patients in whom fusion has been planned. The procedure entails initially the excision of the spinous process of the slipped vertebra so that laminectomy can be started in the middle portion of the spinal canal and then extended laterally on both sides. This reduces the risk of damaging the nervous structures during decompression since the sagittal dimension of the spinal canal is larger, and stenosis less severe, in the central portion of the spinal canal than in the lateral portion. The ligamentum flavum, which can be normal or hypertrophic, is removed at this stage and the dural sac exposed. Partial facetectomy is then carried out to free the emerging nerve root that may be compressed by the superior or inferior facet joint. The extension of facetectomy varies depending on the severity of stenosis. Usually, in the presence of severe central stenosis both the inferior and superior facets should be extensively resected (approximately the medial two-thirds of the facet joints) whereas a less extensive facetectomy may be performed in patients with moderate isolated lateral stenosis. The orientation of facet joints in the horizontal plane also affects the extension of facetectomy. When facet joints show a coronal, or slight sagittal, orientation, lateral stenosis is mainly due to a hypertrophic superior facet joint (Fig. 56-1A). In this case partial facetectomy may be accomplished by removing initially the medial one-half or two-third of the inferior facet with a small osteotome, and then the medial one-half or two-third of the superior facet with a pituitary rongeur. When facet joints show a marked sagittal orientation, stenosis is often caused by the forward slipping of the inferior facet (Fig. 56-1B). In this case, only the anterior portion of the inferior facet needs to be excised. Total facetectomy should be avoided, even if fusion has been planned, because it is usually unnecessary and it may cause marked postoperative instability that may increase the risk of pseudarthrosis, particularly in non-instrumented fusion. Laminectomy should be extended cranially, approximately 1 cm beyond the inferior endplate of the slipped vertebra, and caudally, until the emerging nerve root is entirely free in the lateral canal. Foraminotomy is usually not necessary in these patients. Nerve decompression is performed in a similar fashion when a unilateral or bilateral laminotomy is carried out. However, in these cases, the spinous process with the supraspinous and intraspinous ligaments are preserved, whereby decompression consists in a unilateral or bilateral fenestration of the spinal canal including a small removal of the lamina along with partial facetectomy as described before. Laminotomy is the treatment of choice in patients with DS in whom decompression alone has been planned or in those in whom posterolateral fusion has been planned but radicular symptoms involve only one leg, so that a unilateral opening of the spinal canal can be performed.

Preparation of the Bed Graft

The bed graft for posterolateral fusion is prepared by dividing, with a diathermy blade, the insertions of the longissimus muscle from the lateral aspect of the articular apophyses. Two arteries may be found at this phase: one is located laterally to the pars interarticularis and one at the junction between the superior border of the transverse process and the pedicle. Both these arteries can be coagulated using bayonet forceps. The lateral portion of the articular apophysis is palpated with the index finger and the transverse process identified and exposed.

The bed graft should be carefully prepared and as large as possible to increase the amount of blood supply and osteoinductive factors available for the graft material. To achieve this goal the decortication should include, other than the transverse processes, the lateral portion of the superior facet joint and the pars interarticularis, so that a continuous bony bridge between the adjacent vertebrae will more likely occur (Fig. 56-2).

Decortication can be performed either manually or by using a high-speed burr. A manual decortication is preferred by some surgeons because the high-speed burr may cause thermal necrosis of the decorticated bone that could negatively affects the result of fusion. If a manual decortication is performed, a bone rongeur can be ini-

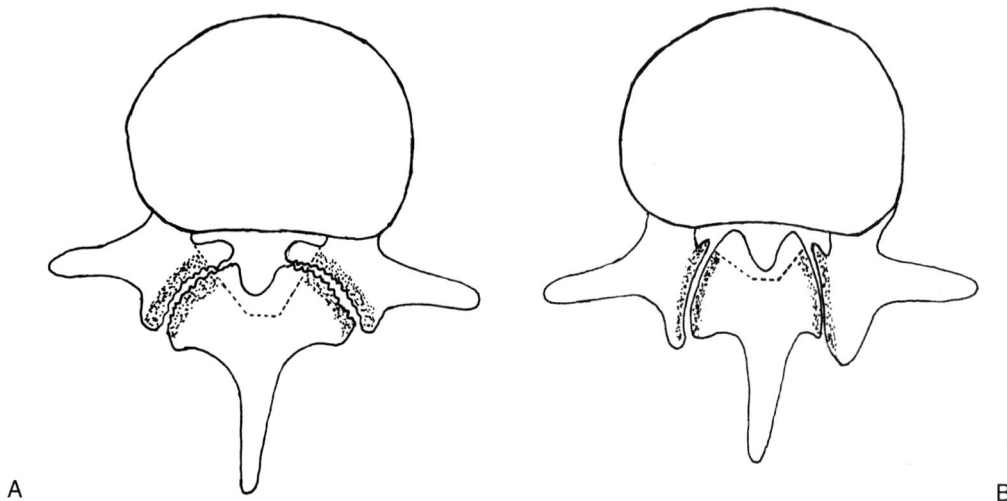

FIG. 56-1. A: In degenerative spondylolisthesis (DS) patients showing facet joints coronally oriented, hypertrophic changes of the superior facet are often responsible for lateral stenosis. In these cases, facetectomy includes the removal of the medial one-half of the inferior and superior facet joint. **B:** In DS patients showing facet joints sagittally oriented, the forward slipping of the inferior facet is often responsible for lateral or central stenosis. In these cases facetectomy may be limited to the removal of the ventral portion of the inferior facet providing no further compression is caused by the superior facet joint.

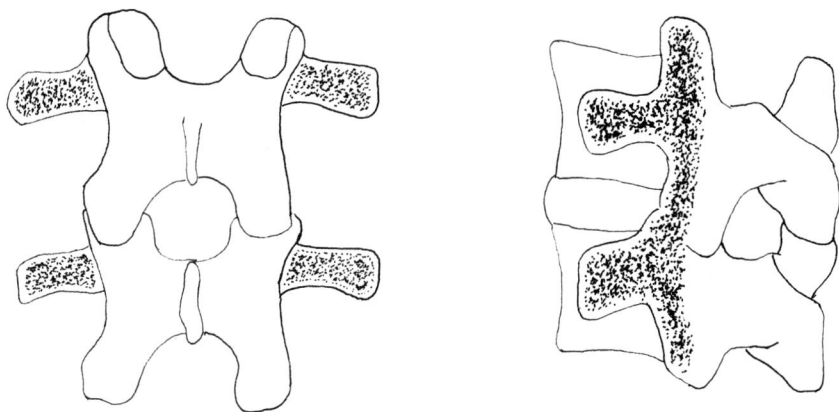

FIG. 56-2. Decortication of the bed graft in posterolateral fusion. The bed graft should include the transverse processes, the lateral portion of the superior facet joint and the pars interarticularis.

tially used to interrupt the thin cortical wall of the transverse processes, taking care to avoid its complete fracture. The decortication is then extended to the entire transverse process with a small curette. The pars interarticularis and the lateral aspect of the superior articular apophyses can be decorticated with a curved osteotome, a large curette or a bone rongeur. The preparation of the bed graft is completed when bleeding bone has been exposed throughout the fusion area and when soft tissues that might interpose between the bone graft and the decorticated bone have been carefully removed.

Harvesting and Positioning of Graft Material

Autograft and allograft are currently used for posterolateral fusion. This author currently use autogenous bone graft from the iliac crest since, at the present, this seems to be the best graft material for spinal fusion. This is particularly true in degenerative spondylolisthesis in which a one level fusion is usually performed and unilateral harvesting of bone graft from the iliac crest is sufficient for the entire bed graft. Alternative graft materials, including osteoinductive and osteoconductive substances, are under investigations; however, further studies are needed to evaluate their effectiveness compared to autograft.

Autogenous bone graft is usually harvested from the iliac crest. Some surgeons are used to expose the iliac crest from the same skin incision of laminectomy. However, this implies that a wide subcutaneous dissection has to be performed to expose the iliac crest, with possible occurrence of subcutaneous seromas and delay in the healing of the surgical wound. It is preferable to perform a second skin incision, 3 to 4 cm lateral from the posterior iliac spine, with an oblique direction from cranial to caudal and from medial to lateral. This skin incision is perpendicular to the iliac crest, and thus limits the amount of bone graft which may be harvested, but is in the same direction of the cluneal nerves which lie subcutaneously in this region (Fig. 56-3). On the other hand, a skin incision parallel to the iliac crest allows harvesting a larger amount of bone graft but entails higher risks of transect-ing the cluneal nerves, with possible occurrence of painful neuroma, compared to the previous skin incision.

Once the iliac crest is exposed, a subperiosteal dissection is carried out on the external portion of the iliac wing. Care must be taken to avoid a subperiosteal dissection, and elevator positioning, too close to the sciatic notch, since at this level the superior gluteal artery and vein may be damaged (Fig. 56-3). Although this complication is uncommon, the surgeon should be well aware of it because it can be difficult to control the bleeding, particularly if the transected vessel retracts within the pelvis. In this event treatments include: (a) a caudal enlargement of the surgical wound in order to elevate subperiosteally, and retract laterally, the gluteus maximus, to expose the piriformis muscle and, at its superior border, the superior gluteal artery which at this point can be ligated (16); (b) embolization of the superior gluteal artery (17); (c) direct ligation of the artery by turning the patient in supine position and reaching the arterial origin through an anterior retroperitoneal or transperitoneal approach.

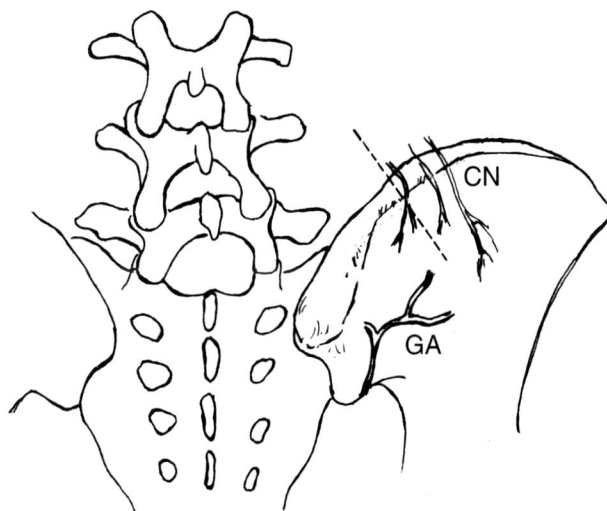

FIG. 56-3. Anatomic structures which can be injured during harvesting autogenous bone graft from the iliac crest. *CN,* cluneal nerves; *GA,* gluteal artery.

Harvesting of bone graft consists in taking cortical bone and cancellous bone separately. Cortical bone is removed by performing vertical and horizontal cuts with a straight osteotome on the cortical wall of the iliac wing. A curved osteotome is then used to remove cortical chips while cancellous bone is usually taken with a gouge. Small bone chips are then prepared and placed in the bed graft, first positioning a layer of cancellous bone directly in contact with the decorticated bone and then positioning a layer of cortical bone over the cancellous bone. Paraspinal muscles are then replaced over the bone graft taking care to avoid a displacement of bone chips into the spinal canal. To prevent this from occurring, the dural sac should always be protected with hemostatic sponges before the positioning of the bone graft. Before skin closure, bone wax should be placed over the decorticated area of the iliac wing until bone bleeding is arrested and a drain is positioned in both surgical wounds.

POSTOPERATIVE MANAGEMENT

Standing and walking is allowed from the first operative day as tolerated by the patient. We encourage six walks of 5 minutes from the second postoperative day and as long as possible from the fourth day after the operation. A plaster cast or corset is worn 24 hours before hospital discharge, that is, between the seventh and tenth day after surgery. This hospitalization time is substantially reduced (3 to 6 days) in patients submitted to instrumented fusion. The corset is usually removed 4 months after surgery but physical exercises are not allowed until 6 months from the operation.

RESULTS

Although degenerative spondylolisthesis is probably the most frequent condition requiring spinal fusion in the adult population, few studies analyzed in detail the results of this procedure in DS patients.

Feffer et al. (2) analyzed the surgical outcome in 19 patients with DS treated in two different Hospitals. Eight patients underwent decompression and fusion, and 11 decompression alone. All patients had leg pain equal to or greater than their back pain and radiologic investigations showing a compression of the nervous structures. Length of follow-up ranged from 12 to 72 months. In the fused group, the clinical result was rated as good in 5 patients and fair in 3. In the decompressed group, the clinical result was rated as good in 5, fair in 3 and poor in 3 patients. Lombardi et al. (5) analyzed the surgical outcome in 47 patients with DS treated with wide decompression (bilateral total facetectomy) in 6 patients, standard decompression (partial facetectomy) in 20 patients, and decompression with partial facetectomy plus posterolateral fusion in 21 patients. The follow-up ranged from 24 months to 7 years. The surgical outcome was rated as excellent or good in 30% of the patients who had wide decompression, 80% of those who had standard decompression, and in 90% of those who had decompression plus fusion. Postoperative increase in vertebral slipping did not correlate with the clinical result except when postoperative slip approached 50%.

We evaluated the clinical and radiologic results of 16 patients with DS (included in a larger group of patients with spinal stenosis) after a mean follow-up of 8.6 years (range 5 to 19 years) (18). The clinical outcome was rated as excellent or good in eight of the ten patients who had decompression and fusion and in two of the six who had decompression alone. A reconstitution of the posterior vertebral arch excised at surgery was found to occur more frequently in spondylolisthetic patients than in stenotic patients without spondylolisthesis and, in the spondylolisthetic group, in those who had decompression alone compared to those who had decompression and fusion.

Herkowitz and Kurz (4) analyzed prospectively the surgical outcome in patients with DS. Of the 50 patients included in the study, 25 were treated with decompression alone and 25 with decompression and fusion. The length of the follow-up ranged from 2.4 to 4 years. The clinical outcome was rated as excellent or good in 96% of the patients in the fused group and in 44% of those in the decompressed group. A pseudarthrosis was noted in 36% of the patients of the fused group; however, all these patients reported an excellent or good result.

A prospective randomized study analyzed the effectiveness of decompressive laminectomy and posterolateral fusion with or without spinal instrumentation in patients with degenerative spondylolisthesis (9). In the 67 patients available for a 2-year follow-up the clinical outcome was rated as excellent or good in 85% of patients who had a noninstrumented fusion and in 76% of those who had an instrumented fusion. However, a successful arthrodesis was found in 45% and 82% of the patients who had, respectively, a noninstrumented and an instrumented fusion. An excellent or good result was reported by 83% of patients with pseudarthrosis after noninstrumented fusion.

A meta-analysis of literature on DS patients treated with laminectomy alone or laminectomy and instrumented or noninstrumented fusion, revealed satisfactory results in 69% of those who had laminectomy alone, and 90% and 86% of those who had laminectomy with noninstrumented and instrumented fusion, respectively (6). The reported fusion rate was 86% in those who had a noninstrumented fusion and 93% in those who had an instrumented fusion.

McCulloch retrospectively reviewed 21 patients with degenerative spondylolisthesis who had a decompression and noninstrumented unilateral fusion (19). After an average follow-up of 38 months, the overall satisfactory outcome was 76%. Twenty of twenty-one patients had relief of their claudicant leg pain and the overall fusion rate was 86%.

Kuntz et al. analyzed the cost-effectiveness of fusion with and without instrumentation for patients with degenerative spondylolisthesis and spinal stenosis (20). The results showed that the cost-effectiveness of laminectomy with non-instrumented fusion compares favorably with decompressive alone and with decompressive plus instrumented fusion.

In conclusion, data on the surgical outcome in patients with DS are largely incomplete due to methodologic limitations of the studies. Most of the series are retrospective, did not analyze the functional outcome, did not address possible causes of failures, and are based on short-term follow-ups. Nevertheless, most of the studies show that DS is one of the spinal condition in which the result of the surgical treatment is more predictable and that posterolateral fusion is one of the most effective procedures in the treatment of DS. A correct surgical indication, including an evaluation of the psychological profile of the patient, is one of the most important factors in determining the success of the operation. Preoperative assessment should also include a radiologic investigation at the levels adjacent to the spondylolisthesis, to avoid missing a concomitant spinal condition at another vertebral level.

COMPLICATIONS

Decompression and posterolateral fusion is though to be a safe procedure with a low complication rate. In keeping with this, no surgically related complications were reported in a meta-analysis of literature on DS patients treated with decompression and non-instrumented fusion (6).

Complications may be related to decompression or fusion. The former are similar to those reported by stenotic patients, including dural tear, motor deficits and infections. These complications are uncommon and their incidence is usually lower than in stenotic patients without spondylolisthesis, since in the latter decompression is more likely to be performed at multiple levels compared with patients with DS in whom stenosis is often present at a single level.

Complications related to posterolateral fusion are also rare. They are usually associated to the harvesting of iliac crest bone graft rather than to posterolateral fusion in itself. Their reported incidence was found to range between 0.7% and 25% for major complications and between 9.4% and 24% for minor complications (21,22). In a large retrospective study, none of the patients had major perioperative complications such as superior gluteal artery injury, sciatic nerve injury or deep infection, nor did patients report major late complications such as herniation at the donor site, meralgia paresthetica, pelvic instability or fractures (23). However, 18 patients (10%) had other major complications, including prolonged sterile drainage, subcutaneous seroma, unsightly scar revision and chronic pain limiting physical activities. In the same series, 39% of the patients had minor complications, including temporary dysesthesia, wound drainage, and superficial infection (23). In a consecutive series of patients in whom autogenous bone graft was harvested through a skin incision perpendicular to the posterior iliac crest (study group) and, for comparison, through a skin incision parallel to the posterior iliac crest (controls), the patients in the study group reported significantly lower numbness, tenderness and pain at the donor site compared with the controls (24).

In conclusion, major complications, including superior gluteal artery injury, sciatic nerve injury, meralgia paresthetica etc. are uncommon and often published as case reports. Minor complications occur more frequently, particularly persistent donor site pain. This complication usually does not limit physical activities but may affect, in some way, the overall clinical outcome in approximately 10% to 30% of patients. The amount of bone graft harvested from the iliac crest with related soft tissue dissection, the accuracy in the surgical procedure and the type of skin incision used to expose the iliac crest seem to be the most important factors affecting donor site complications.

REFERENCES

1. Bridwell KH, Sedgewick TA, O'Brien MF, et al. The role of fusion and instrumentation in the treatment of degenerative spondylolisthesis with spinal stenosis. J Spinal Disord 1993;6:461–472.
2. Feffer HL, Wiesel SW, Cuckler JM, et al. Degenerative spondylolisthesis. To fuse or not to fuse. Spine 1985;10:287–289.
3. Fox MW, Onofrio BM, Hanssen AD. Clinical outcomes and radiological instability following decompressive lumbar laminectomy for degenerative spinal stenosis: a comparison of patients undergoing concomitant arthrodesis versus decompression alone. J Neurosurg 1996; 85:793–802.
4. Herkowitz HN, Kurz LT. Degenerative lumbar spondylolisthesis with spinal stenosis. A prospective study comparing decompression and intertransverse process arthrodesis. J Bone Joint Surg [Am] 1991;73: 802–808.
5. Lombardi JS, Wiltse LL, Reynolds J, et al. Treatment of degenerative spondylolisthesis. Spine 1985;10:821–827.
6. Mardjetko SM, Connolly PJ, Shott S. Degenerative lumbar spondylolisthesis: a meta-analysis of literature 1970–1993. Spine 1994;19: S2256–S2265.
7. Cinotti G, Postacchini F, Fassari F et al. Predisposing factors in degenerative spondylolisthesis. A radiographic and CT study. Intern Orthop 1997;21:337–342.
8. Grobler LJ, Robertson PA, Novotny JE, et al. Decompression for degenerative spondylolisthesis and spinal stenosis at L4-L5. The effects of facet joint morphology. Spine 1993;18:1475–1482.
9. Fischgrund JS, Mackay M, Herkowitz HN, et al. Degenerative lumbar spondylolisthesis with spinal stenosis: a prospective, randomized study comparing arthrodesis with and without instrumentation. Spine 1997; 22:2807–2812.
10. Yuan HA, Garfin SR, Dickman CA, Mardjetko SM. A historical cohort study of pedicle screw fixation in thoracic, lumbar and sacral spinal fusions. Spine 1994;20S:2279S–2296S.
11. Zdeblick TA. A prospective, randomized study of lumbar fusion. Preliminary results. Spine 1993;18:983–991.
12. Thomsen K, Christensen FB, Eiskjaer SP, et al. The effects of pedicle screw instrumentation on functional outcome and fusion rates in posterolateral lumbar spinal fusion. A prospective randomized clinical study. Spine 1997;22:2813–2822.

13. Cinotti G, De Santis PF, Nofroni I, et al. Stenosis of lumbar interverte-bral foramen. anatomic study on predisposing factors. Spine 2002;27: 223–229.
14. Wiltse LL, Spencer CW. New uses and refinements of the paraspinal approach to the lumbar spine. Spine 1988;13:696–706.
15. Postacchini F, Cinotti G, Perugia D, et al. The surgical treatment of cen-tral lumbar stenosis. Multiple laminotomy compared with total laminectomy. J Bone Joint Surg [Br] 1993;75:386–392.
16. Shin AY, Moran ME, Wenger DR. Superior gluteal artery injury sec-ondary to posterior iliac crest bone graft harvesting. A surgical tech-nique to control hemorrhage. Spine 1996;21:1371–1374.
17. Lim EVA, Lavadia WT, Roberts JM. Superior gluteal artery injury dur-ing iliac bone grafting for spinal fusion. A case report and literature review. Spine 1996, 21:2376–2378.
18. Postacchini F, Cinotti G. Bone regrowth after surgical decompression for lumbar spinal stenosis. J Bone Joint Surg 1992;74-B:862–869.
19. McCulloch J A. Microdecompression and uninstrumented single-level fusion for spinal canal stenosis with degenerative spondylolisthesis. Spine 1998;23:2243–2252.
20. Kuntz KM, Snider RK, Weinstein JN, et al. Cost-effectiveness of fusion with and without instrumentation for patients with degenerative spondylolisthesis and spinal stenosis. Spine 2000;25:1132–1139.
21. Keller EE, Triplett WW. Iliac crest bone graft: review of 160 consecu-tive cases. J Oral Maxillofac Surg 1987;45:11–14.
22. Summers BN, Eisenstein SM. Donor site pain from the ilium. A com-plication of lumbar spine fusion. J Bone Joint Surg [Br] 1989;71: 677–680.
23. Banwart JC, Asher MA, Hassanein RS. Iliac crest bone graft harvest donor site morbidity. A statistical evaluation. Spine 1995;20:1055–1060.
24. Colterjohn NR, Bednar DA. Procurement of bone graft from the iliac crest. An operative approach with decreased morbidity. J Bone Joint Surg [Am] 1997;79:756–759.

CHAPTER 57

Anterior Lumbar Interbody Fusion

Mamoru Kawakami and Tetsuya Tamaki

Degenerative spondylolisthesis is a clinical term characterized by the forward translation of a vertebra on the inferior vertebra in the presence of an intact neural arch. The pathoanatomic elements of degenerative facet arthropathy, anterolisthesis, narrowing of the disc space, and ligamentum flavum redundancy contribute to the development of spinal stenosis, including the central canal, lateral recess, and foraminal zones (1). It may be a source of low back pain with insidious onset of radicular or referred leg pain or intermittent claudication. Although there are many reports with regard to surgical results for patients with degenerative spondylolisthesis, evaluating the outcomes of surgical treatments requires knowledge of the natural history of the untreated condition. However, little is known of the natural history of, or the optimal surgical treatment for, degenerative lumbar spondylolisthesis.

When deciding on operative treatment for degenerative lumbar spondylolisthesis, it is essential to choose the appropriate surgical procedure based on the stage and pathogenesis (2). In the early stage of degenerative lumbar spondylolisthesis, the initial symptom is mainly low back pain, while pain of the lower extremities can also occur. These symptoms are thought to be related to either disc degeneration or degenerative arthritis of the facet joints. In the middle stage of degenerative lumbar spondylolisthesis, the dural sac is constricted, causing central canal stenosis because of the anterior shift of the inferior articular process of the slipping vertebra and posterior bulging of the intervertebral disc materials. During this stage, the patient suffers from low back pain associated with radicular pain of the lower extremities, and intermittent claudication. By late and end-stage degenerative lumbar spondylolisthesis, osteophytes have formed on the medial and ventral sides of the superior articular process of the lower spine, preventing the displacement from progressing further, and these osteophytes become one of the causes of lateral stenosis. Although low back pain occasionally abates because of the decrease in instability, this is accompanied by the simultaneous development of numbness or paresis of the lower extremities at rest (2–4).

There does not appear to be a clear consensus for the optimal surgical treatment of degenerative lumbar spondylolisthesis. Most studies show that the clinical outcome is better when decompression is accompanied by fusion using the posterior approach (5). However, sufficient decompression and fusion may be obtained by the anterior lumbar interbody fusion in some condition or stage of degenerative lumbar spondylolisthesis. The mechanism of neural decompression is indirect, with restoration of disc space height, reduction of listhesis, and foraminal enlargement, which are achieved by intervertebral distraction and maintained by a structural anterior interbody fusion (1). An experimental study using cadaveric lumbar spines also demonstrated that interbody distraction using anteriorly inserted plugs, immediately improved the narrowed canal area and increased the spinal canal and the foraminal volume, in lumbar degenerative spondylolisthesis (6). An intervertebral fusion takes advantage of the large surface area for graft contact of both contiguous vertebral end plates, assists in maintaining or improving disc space height, and allows placement of the graft under compression, which biomechanically is a more suitable environment for graft maturation.

Using a meta-analysis of the literature from 1970 to 1993, Mardjetko et al. evaluated the results of anterior interbody fusion for patients with degenerative lumbar spondylolisthesis (7). They found that only three articles met the inclusion criteria and that pooling the data from these three studies yielded a 94% fusion rate, with an 86% rate of patient satisfaction (7). Two of these three papers are Japanese in origin and there are many reports in Japanese with regard to the anterior lumbar interbody fusion for degenerative lumbar spondylolisthesis. In this chapter, we review the indications and the clinical outcomes, including radiologic assessments and complications of anterior lumbar interbody fusion, for degenerative lumbar spondylolisthesis.

INDICATIONS FOR ANTERIOR LUMBAR INTERBODY FUSION

Surgical treatment is indicated when appropriate conservative treatments fail to control clinical symptoms such as low back pain, leg pain, numbness, and intermittent claudication. Anterior interbody fusion involves an anterior retroperitoneal approach. Adhesion of the peritoneum is thus a factor of contraindication. It has been reported that patients can expect satisfactory results up to about 65 years of age (1,8,9). Anterior interbody fusion is indicated for younger patients (i.e., those under 50 years), but is not generally indicated for older patients (10–12). Patients with osteoporosis have a lower success rate for correction and are at risk of collapse of the bone grafts (12). Degeneration of the adjacent segment at the time of surgery may possibly cause enhanced degeneration after surgery (13). The indication is for patients without osteoporosis or degeneration of the adjacent segments (13,14). Anterior interbody fusion is not recommended for patients with an apparent multilevel involvement (1,9,10,14). A patient with a single-level lesion, symptoms and signs that usually appear or worsen after activities such as standing or walking, or who has neurologic symptoms and signs in the leg but no leg pain in the resting position, is a good candidate for this surgery (15). A patient whose clinical symptoms can be relieved by the application of a carefully molded body cast or corset in a flexed position is also a good candidate for this surgery (1,9). A poorer functional outcome may be found in patients who have responded poorly to a preoperative test brace.

An indication for this surgery, using data from dynamic X-rays, is lumbar instability of the affected segments but not severe stenosis, where posterior elements such as the facet joint are involved (10–12,15). A need for decompression can possibly occur in patients with stenosis of the lateral recess. The staging in degenerative spondylolisthesis proposed by Satomi et al., using computed tomography (CT) scanning after myelography, is very useful to evaluate the cause of dural sac compression (8,16,17). Stage 1 images exhibit posterior distension of the intervertebral disc with vertical inclination of the articular facets. In stage 2, the inferior articular process of the slipping vertebra shifts anterior to the superior articular process of the lower vertebra. In stage 3, osteophytes form anterior and posterior to the superior articular process of the lower vertebra. The anterior shift of the inferior articular process of the slipping vertebra can improve with reduction of slippage and restoration of the intervertebral disc height secondary to the anterior interbody fusion (stages 1 and 2). However, the anterior interbody fusion is not effective in those cases where the superior articular process of the lower vertebra is involved in the clinical symptoms (stage 3) (8).

POSTOPERATIVE MANAGEMENT

Postoperative bed rest is recommended for 3 weeks after surgery (2,14). Supplementation with Arbeitsgemeinschaft für Osteosynthasefragen (AO) screwing and wiring (18) can reduce the time of bed rest after surgery (13,16) to 2 weeks. A body cast is applied for 4 to 6 weeks after bed rest (2,14,19), followed by a corset for about 6 months until bony fusion is obtained (14). Postoperative management should be very strict and is important because there is no optimal anterior instrumentation. An interbody cage, including threaded cylinders and monobloc devices from the anterior may give stabilization of the lumbar spine immediately after surgery and reduce the time of bed rest. Biomechanical studies reveal that the cage decreases intervertebral motion in flexion, axial rotation, and lateral bending compared with uninhibited motion (20). However, the cage does not stabilize the spine in extension (20). Supplementary posterior fixation including pedicle screw fixation and translaminar fixation substantially improves the stabilization (21,22). Therefore, supplementary posterior fixation can reduce the time of bed rest, and eliminates the need for a body cast. Supplementation with pedicle screw fixation to the anterior interbody fusion can reduce the period of bed rest to only 2 to 3 days in patients with degenerative lumbar spondylolisthesis (15).

CLINICAL OUTCOMES

Functional Results

Takahashi et al. have reported that long-term results have been achieved with anterior interbody fusion for the treatment of degenerative spondylolisthesis (1,9). They used the score rating system of the Japanese Orthopaedic Association (JOA) for clinical evaluation (23), a full score being 29 points. They classified patients with a score of 25 points or more as "satisfactory", while those with a score of 24 points or less were classified as "unsatisfactory". Using a Kaplan-Meier survivorship analysis at an average follow-up of 12 years and 7 months, Takahashi et al. reported a 76% rate of satisfactory results at 10 years, a 60% rate of satisfactory results at 20 years, and a 52% rate of satisfactory results at 30 years (1,9). All patients in their 30s (average age at surgery, 36.5 years) maintained satisfactory results at least until their final examination, with an average follow-up of 24 years, 11 months after surgery (range, 20 years to 29 years, 10 months). Results were also satisfactory in 80% of patients in their 40s (average age at surgery, 44.7 years) for up to 16 years, and 73% of patients in their 50s (average age at surgery, 54.8 years) for up to 10 years. However, results were satisfactory in only 4 of the 7 patients 60 years of age or older (average age at surgery, 65.2 years) immediately after surgery. The authors concluded that these results indicate that regardless of patient age at surgery, patients can expect satisfactory results up to about 65 years of age, and that anterior interbody fusion is a treatment that can guarantee a good lifelong course for patients with degenerative spondylolisthesis.

Satomi et al. compared the results of anterior interbody fusion with or without AO screwing and wiring to patients who underwent posterior decompression with or without spinal fusion (8,16,17). They used the degree of recovery or recovery rates, which were calculated from preoperative and postoperative JOA scores. The mean follow-up period was 3 years, 2 months. Clinical improvement was seen in 77% of the group undergoing anterior interbody fusion compared with only 55.7% of patients in the group undergoing posterior decompression. Since their indications were different for patients with degenerative spondylolisthesis as described previously, it is questionable to compare these functional outcomes.

Nishizawa and Fujimura retrospectively reviewed 58 patients (13 men and 45 women) with degenerative spondylolisthesis treated with anterior lumbar interbody fusion. The follow-up period ranged from 28 to 128 months, averaging 63 months, and the mean recovery rate was 78%. They found that the recovery rate for low back pain and gait was better than for leg pain or tingling, clinical signs, and urinary bladder function (2).

Tanaka et al. reported surgical results for minimally invasive anterior lumbar interbody fusion (24) with a supplemental pedicle screw system for degenerative spondylolisthesis, compared with those of posterior lumbar interbody fusion (15). They found that the mean recovery rate was 76.8% in patients treated with minimally invasive anterior lumbar interbody fusion with a supplemental pedicle screw system, compared with 70.9%.

Nishizawa et al. reported on results following anterior interbody fusion for lumbar degenerative spondylolisthesis (19). The mean follow-up period was 11 years, 10 months. They found that the mean recovery rates were 76%, 80.9%, 81.6%, 73.1%, and 68.8%, in follow-ups at 1 year, 3 years, 5 years, and 10 years after treatment, and at the final follow-up, respectively. Long-term results showed some deterioration of functional outcomes in patients treated with anterior interbody fusion (1,9,19). The deterioration of the JOA score is thought to be attributable to age-related general weakness (1,9).

Kim et al. reported six patients with degenerative spondylolisthesis treated with anterior interbody fusion (25). Their evaluation was a pain rating only: excellent, good, fair, and poor, where there was little or no pain, mild pain, moderate pain, and severe pain, respectively. One, three, and two patients had excellent, good, and fair results, respectively. Four patients were satisfied with the surgical results. Functional results using the recovery rates are summarized in Table 57-1. These results were obtained from retrospective studies.

The indications for anterior interbody fusion are different from those for posterior decompression with or without posterolateral fusion or posterior interbody fusion. Although reports from Japan have used the JOA score and recovery rates, the instrument for functional measures is also different from that reported in other countries. It is questionable whether these functional results of anterior interbody fusion are superior to those of the posterior approach for patients with degenerative lumbar spondylolisthesis.

Radiologic Results

Inoue et al. performed anterior interbody fusion on 36 patients with degenerative lumbar spondylolisthesis to remove the diseased intervertebral disc (4). They reported a correction in sagittal malalignment with restoration of disc space height in the majority of patients. Fusion was successful in all single-level fusions and in 85% of double-level fusions (4). Takahashi et al. found 4 cases of nonunion in 10 patients treated with double-level fusions (1,9). Nishizawa et al. reported that bony union was achieved in 55 of 58 patients (95%), including fusion *in situ* for 39 patients (67%), collapsed fusion for 16 patients (28%) and nonunion for 3 patients (5%). They found that the recovery rate was 85% in patients with fusion *in situ*, 66% in those with collapsed union, and 46% in those with nonunion ($p < .05$) (2).

TABLE 57-1. *The periods of follow-up and recovery rates in anterior interbody fusion for degenerative lumbar spondylolisthesis*

	Total	Mean follow-up period (mos)	Mean recovery rates (%)
Takahashi et al. (1)	19	151	71
Satomi et al. (17)	27	38	77
Nishizawa & Fujimura (2)	58	63	78
Tanaka et al. (15)	18[a]	14	76.8
Nishizawa et al. (19)	27	142	68.8
Hirofuji et al. (11)	28	104	52.8
Total:	177	85	70.7

[a]Minimally invasive anterior lumbar interbody fusion with supplemental pedicle screw system.

Satomi et al. reported that the average percentage of vertebral slippage improved from 18.5% preoperatively to 7.4% postoperatively in the anterior interbody fusion group, and that the reduction rate of the slippage was 62.1% (16,17). Nishizawa et al. reported in their long-term follow-up study that the union rate was 92.6% (18). Nonunion was found in two patients treated with double-level fusion; both had poor outcomes. In their series, the average percentage of vertebral slippage improved from 19.1% preoperatively to 6.8% immediately after surgery, and to 9.2% at follow-up. The mean collapse rate was 22.4% and was not related to the recovery rate.

Rates of fusion reported in the literature are summarized in Table 57-2. According to the definition of fusion proposed by Fujimura (10), 16 patients (26%) were classified as collapsed fusion, where the collapse rate calculated from the disc heights immediately after surgery and at follow-up was more than 20%. Forty-two patients (69%) were classified as fusion *in situ*, where the collapse rate was less than 20%, and three patients (5%) had nonunion. The mean recovery rates were 86%, 67%, 47% in fusion *in situ*, collapsed union, and nonunion, respectively (10).

Collectively, these reports demonstrate that anterior interbody fusion for degenerative spondylolisthesis can improve and restore the percentage of anterior vertebral slippage and maintain the sagittal alignment at the fusion level. It has been reported that the facet angle and the spread ratio of the intervertebral disc space are factors influencing the collapse of bone grafts (26). In patients with osteoporosis, some countermeasures are required to prevent the collapse of bone grafts, due to a small facet angle and the need to spread the intervertebral disc space excessively. If there is a suspicion of incipient pseudoarthrosis, patients with spondylolisthesis should be treated by fusion with either intralaminal screw fixation or pedicle screw fixation, by posterior spondylodesis, or by posterolateral fusion. The combined use of bone graft substitutes, such as hydroxyapatite-based ceramic or an interbody cage, with autologous bone may prevent collapse of the grafting bone and improve fusion rates and functional outcomes after anterior interbody fusion.

COMPLICATIONS

Anterior interbody fusion involves an anterior retroperitoneal approach along with its attendant complications. The most serious complication has been death because of pulmonary embolism. Surgical injury to the presacral sympathetic nerves may result in either retrograde ejaculation or ejaculatory dysfunction. There is the possibility of vascular injury through the anterior approach, especially in older patients with fragile vessels. Usually, this is considered a temporary and very rare complication when the retroperitoneal approach is performed. No procedure-related complications were reported in two papers published by Takahashi et al. (9) and Satomi et al. (17). Nishizawa and Fujimura reported that 9 of 58 patients treated with anterior interbody fusion had complications including iliac donor-site pain (n = 3), wire breakage of AO screwing and wiring (n = 2), liver dysfunction (n = 2), deep vein thrombosis (n = 1), and pulmonary embolism (n = 1) (2). Anterior interbody fusion may be also complicated by injury to the lateral femoral nerve in connection with harvesting of the bone graft.

The iliac crest was used as the donor site. In 26 patients treated with anterior interbody fusion, Nakai and Abe found that 17 suffered complications: neurologic complication (n = 1); donor site complications (meralgia paresthetica (n = 7), fracture (n = 2); deep vein thrombosis (n = 2); and edema in left leg (n = 4) (12). Rates of complications are summarized in Table 57-2.

For anterior intervertebral fusion, bone graft substitutes such as allografts or hydroxyapatite instead of autologous bone or an interbody cage may be useful to prevent donor site complications. The rate of nonunion after anterior interbody fusion for patients with degenerative lumbar spondylolisthesis has been previously described. Anterior interbody fusion may result in enhanced degeneration in the adjacent segments of the fusion site. Long-term follow-up is needed to assess possible disc degener-

TABLE 57-2. *Fusion rate, complications, and reoperation in anterior interbody fusion for degenerative lumbar spondylolisthesis*

	Total	Fusion (%)	Complications (%)	Reoperation
Takahashi et al. (1)	39	35 (89.7)	ND	ND
Satomi et al. (17)	27	26 (96.3)	ND	ND
Nishizawa & Fujimura (2)	58	55 (94.8)	9 (15.5)	ND
Tanaka et al. (15)	18[a]	18 (100)	0 (0)	ND
Nishizawa et al. (19)	27	25 (92.6)	ND	3
Hirofuji et al. (11)	28	28 (100)	ND	3
Nakai & Abe (12)	26	25 (96.2)	16 (61.5)	2
Total:	223	212 (95.1)		

ND, not described.
[a]Minimally invasive anterior lumbar interbody fusion with supplemental pedicle screw system.

ation, including herniated disc and instability. Nishizawa et al. clearly demonstrated that the lesion of the adjacent segments did not result from anterior interbody fusion, because there were no significant differences in mobility of the intervertebral disc space and in disc height between the age-matched groups after the surgical and conservative treatments (19).

We have reported that lumbar sagittal alignment influences the clinical outcome after decompression and posterolateral spinal fusion for degenerative lumbar spondylolisthesis (27). Even in patients treated with anterior interbody fusion, imbalance of the sagittal alignment of the spine may result in enhanced disc degeneration in the adjacent segments. Further study is needed to evaluate whether the sagittal alignment of the spine influences the surgical result after anterior interbody fusion. Although there can be serious complications such as pulmonary embolism, the number of complication events is small. It is important to evaluate complication rates in large series and compare with the posterior approach to make clear the effectiveness and safety of anterior interbody fusion for patients with degenerative lumbar spondylolisthesis.

CONCLUSION

The consensus throughout the literature about surgical approaches is that anterior interbody fusion in the surgical management of degenerative lumbar spondylolisthesis improves clinical outcomes and achieves solid fusion. However, surgical indications for this procedure should be limited because of the differing stages of degenerative spondylolisthesis. Although several comparative studies of anterior interbody fusion and posterior approaches have been undertaken, the indication was different and the results varied. Functional outcomes, fusion rates, and complications should be compared for both the anterior and posterior approaches. Prospective randomized studies addressing this issue have yet to be performed. The role of new bone graft substitutes and interbody cages should be made clear in anterior interbody fusion for degenerative lumbar spondylolisthesis.

REFERENCES

1. Takahashi K, Kitahara H, Yamagata M, et al. Long-term results of anterior interbody fusion for treatment of degenerative spondylolisthesis. Spine 1990;15:1211–1215.
2. Nishizawa T, Fujimura Y. A clinical study of anterior lumbar interbody fusion for degenerative spondylolisthesis. J Orthop Surg 1997;5:21–27.
3. Farfan HF. The pathological anatomy of degenerative spondylolisthesis: a cadaver study. Spine 1980;5:412–418.
4. Inoue S, Watanabe T, Goto S, et al. Degenerative spondylolisthesis pathophysiology and results of anterior interbody fusion. Clin Orthop 1988;227:90–98.
5. Bell GR. Surgical management of lumbar spinal stenosis and degenerative spondylolisthesis. In Fardon DF, Garfin SR, Abitbol JJ, et al., eds. Orthopaedic knowledge update: spine 2. Rosemont, IL: The American Academy of Orthopaedic Surgeons, 2002:343–352.
6. Vamvanij V, Ferrara LA, Hai Y, et al. Quantitative changes in spinal canal dimensions using interbody distraction for spondylolisthesis. Spine 2001;26:E13–E18.
7. Mardjetko SM, Connolly PJ, Shott S. Degenerative lumbar spondylolisthesis: a meta-analysis of literature, 1970–1993. Spine 1994;19 [Suppl 20]:2256S–2265S.
8. Satomi K, Hirabayashi K, Fujimura Y, et al. Pathogenesis and choice of treatment on degenerative spondylolisthesis. Rinshoseikeigeka 1990;25:399–406 [in Japanese].
9. Takahashi K, Kitahara H, Yamagata M, et al. Clinical results of anterior interbody fusion for degenerative lumbar spondylolisthesis. Rinshoseikeigeka 1990;25:473–478 [in Japanese].
10. Fujimura Y. Anterior interbody fusion for degenerative lumbar spondylolisthesis. Kansetsugeka 1997;16:1520–1526 [in Japanese].
11. Hirofuji E, Miyazaki K, Onosaki A, et al. Evaluation of our surgical treatment for lumbar degenerative spondylolisthesis. Cent Jpn J Orthop Surg Traum 1996;39:87–88 [in Japanese].
12. Nakai O, Abe M. Posterior decompression and posterolateral fusion using pedicle screw instrumentation for lumbar degenerative spondylolisthesis. Kansetsugeka 1997;16:1527–1533 [in Japanese].
13. Tokioka T, Yasuda S, Imai K. Choice of surgical methods and their results for degenerative lumbar spondylolisthesis. Seikei Saigaigeka 1991;34:471–479 [in Japanese].
14. Abe E, Satoh K, Shimada Y, et al. Comparative study of anterior spinal fusion and posterolateral fusion for degenerative spondylolisthesis. East Jpn J Clin Orthop 1990;2:18–21 [in Japanese].
15. Tanaka M, Nakahara S, Koura H, et al. Minimally invasive anterior lumbar interbody fusion for degenerative spondylolisthesis. Seikeigeka 1999;50:1384–1388 [in Japanese].
16. Satomi K, Hirabayashi K, Nagayama N, et al. Pathogenesis and treatment of degenerative spondylolisthesis: significance of the anterior spinal body fusion. Seikeigeka 1988;39:1863–1876 [in Japanese].
17. Satomi K, Hirabayashi K, Toyama Y, et al. A clinical study of degenerative spondylolisthesis radiographic analysis and choice of treatment. Spine 1992;17:1329–1336.
18. Hirabayashi K, Wakano K, Suzuki N, et al. Anterior lumbar spinal body fusion with addition of A-O screwing and wiring. Neuro-Orthop 1986;2:15–20.
19. Nishizawa T, Chiba K, Watanabe M, et al. Long-term results following anterior interbody fusion for lumbar degenerative spondylolisthesis. Sekitsuisekizui 2000;13:709–714 [in Japanese].
20. Oxland TR, Lund T. Biomechanics of stand-alone cages and cages in combination with posterior fixation: a literature review. Eur Spine J 2000;9[Suppl 1]:S95–S101.
21. Lund T, Oxland TR, Jost B, et al. Interbody cage stabilization in the lumbar cage stabilization in the lumbar spine: biomechanical evaluation of cage design, posterior instrumentation and bone density. J Bone Joint Surg Br 1998;80:351–359.
22. Rathonyi GC, Oxland TR, Gerich U, et al. The role of supplemental translaminar screws in anterior lumbar interbody fixation: a biomechanical study. Eur Spine J 1998;7:400–407.
23. Izumida S, Inoue S. Assessment of treatment for low back pain. J Jpn Orthop Assoc 1986;60:391–394 [in Japanese].
24. Mayer HM. A new microsurgical technique for minimally invasive anterior interbody fusion. Spine 1997;22:691–700.
25. Kim NH, Kim HK, Suh JS. A computed tomographic analysis of changes in the spinal canal after anterior lumbar interbody fusion. Clin Orthop 1993;286:180–191.
26. Nishizawa T, Fujimura Y, Suzuki N, et al. Clinical results of spondylolisthesis treated with anterior interbody fusion: with special reference to the influencing on collapse of grafted bone. East Jpn I Clin Orthop 1995;7:234–236 [in Japanese].
27. Kawakami M, Tamaki T, Ando M, et al. Lumbar sagittal alignment influences the clinical outcome after decompression and posterolateral spinal fusion for degenerative lumbar spondylolisthesis Spine 2002;27:59–64.

CHAPTER 58

Decompression with Instrumented Fusion

Dilip K. Sengupta and Harry N. Herkowitz

A consensus has been formed that degenerative lumbar spondylolisthesis with stenosis benefits from decompression, with significant reduction of radicular pain and claudication, if nonsurgical treatment fails. But there is no general agreement about the indications for fusion. Indications for instrumentation are even more controversial. Generally speaking, the goals for decompression are to relieve radicular symptoms and neurogenic claudication. The goals for fusion are to relieve back pain from a degenerated disc and elimination of instability. The goals for instrumentation are to promote fusion and to correct listhesis or kyphotic deformity.

INDICATIONS FOR INSTRUMENTATION

The factors leading to the decision for fusion and instrumentation may be based on (a) preoperative condition and (b) intraoperative assessment of stability of the motion segment.

There are four preoperative factors to consider:

1. Disc height
2. Degree of kyphosis
3. Degree of instability
4. Degree of listhesis.

There are four intraoperative factors to consider:

1. Extent of decompression procedure
2. Previous laminectomy
3. Adjacent segment disease
4. Available bone stock

Disc Height

When the disc height is completely collapsed to only 1 or 2 mm, then progression of the spondylolisthesis after decompression is less likely (1). When the preoperative disc height is greater than 2 mm, an instrumented fusion is recommended to prevent progression of listhesis.

Degree of Kyphosis

Normal sagittal Cobb angle at the L4-5 level varies between −8° to −17° (2). Degenerative spondylolisthesis results in a relative segmental hypolordosis. Presence of frank kyphosis is considered an indication of restoration of lordosis. Instrumentation is always indicated whenever a correction of deformity is intended at surgery.

Degree of Instability

Presence of abnormal motion at the listhetic segment exceeding 5 mm is an indication for instrumentation to achieve fusion. The best way to demonstrate the pathologic motion is controversial. The instability may be assessed radiologically by flexion-extension films in either supine or sitting posture. An alternate method is to compare lateral radiographs in standing position versus in a supine hyperextended position on a pillow. However, even in absence of preoperative demonstrable motion, many observers noted as much as 20% to 40% reduction of listhesis, when the patient is positioned prone on table after general anesthesia (3,4).

Degree of Listhesis

Degenerative listhesis rarely exceeds grade I or grade II. In occasional cases, listhesis may progress beyond 50%, even in absence of previous surgery.

Degenerative listhesis following previous laminectomy, or when involving an adjacent segment to previous fusion may exceed grade II. An instrumented fusion is indicated when listhesis exceeds 50%, whether or not a correction of deformity is indicated.

Extent of Decompression

The stabilization structures in a motion segment include the disc anteriorly, the facet joints posteriorly, and the pars. The exact degree of instability engendered by a given decompression is difficult to predict. However, previous reports in the literature show that removal of one-third to one-half of the facet joints on both sides or all of one facet joint at a given level is often tolerated, without progression of the listhesis (5,6). Abumi et al. (7) demonstrated in a biomechanical study in cadaver spine that removal of greater than 50% of each facet joint led to an unacceptable movement of the motion segment. Therefore, when facet excision in excess of 50% in each side is required for adequate decompression, an instrumented fusion is recommended. When adequate decompression warrants violation of the pars, or bilateral discectomy in addition to partial removal of the facet joints, progress of listhesis may be anticipated. An instrumented fusion is indicated in such cases as well.

Recurrent Stenosis after Previous Laminectomy

Degenerative listhesis may progress beyond 50% in the presence of previous laminectomy. Even if the listhesis has not progressed, a revision decompression at the same level often requires significant removal of the remaining facet joints, indicating an instrumented fusion. On the other hand, previous decompression surgery may achieve a spontaneous facet joint fusion that may add stability and may not need further fusion.

Adjacent Segment Disease

Degenerative lumbar spondylolisthesis with stenosis at an adjacent level to a caudal fusion segment is subjected to additional stress and is more likely to progress unless instrumented.

Available Bone Stock

In order to achieve successful fusion without instrumentation, adequate bone graft needs to be applied on a sufficiently large bed. In patients with small transverse processes, meaningful transverse process fusion becomes unlikely. To accomplish facet fusion disruption of the facet joint capsule an articular cartilage is needed, which predisposes to further instability. Instrumentation is indicated in these situations to achieve fusion. Significant osteoporosis is a contraindication to instrumentation.

TYPE AND EXTENT OF INSTRUMENTATION

Posterior Pedicle Screw Fixation Alone

Only posterior pedicular instrumentation is adequate for most cases of degenerative lumbar spondylolisthesis with stenosis, where instrumentation is indicated. Although it is conventional to instrument both sides, there has been no difference in the fusion rate or clinical outcome after unilateral versus bilateral pedicle fixation (8). For multilevel fusion it is preferable to instrument both sides. End vertebrae should be instrumented, but it is not mandatory to insert pedicle screws in all the levels (Fig. 58-1). Many surgeons deliberately skip the middle vertebrae during pedicle fixation, if the bone quality is good and pedicle fixation appears firm at surgery. This

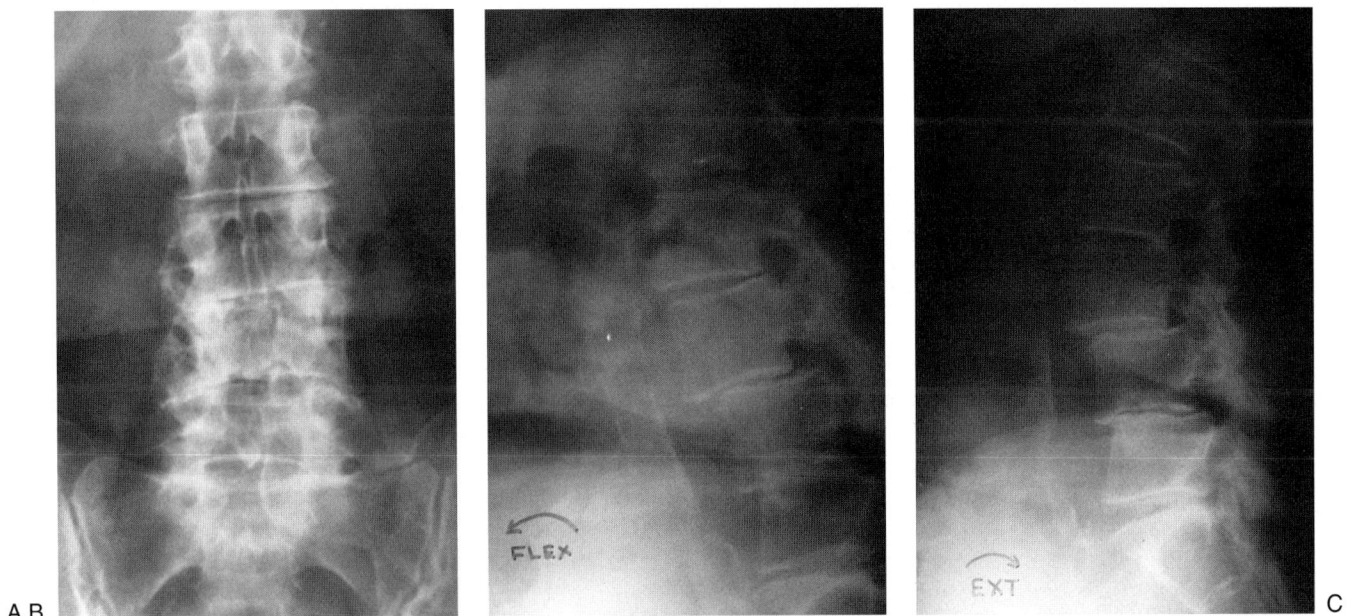

A,B

C

FIG 58-1. A: A 72-year-old female patient with degenerative spondylolisthesis at L3-4 and L4-5 segments presented with mechanical back pain and neurogenic claudication. B, C: Flexion-extension views show translation at both the levels. (*continued*)

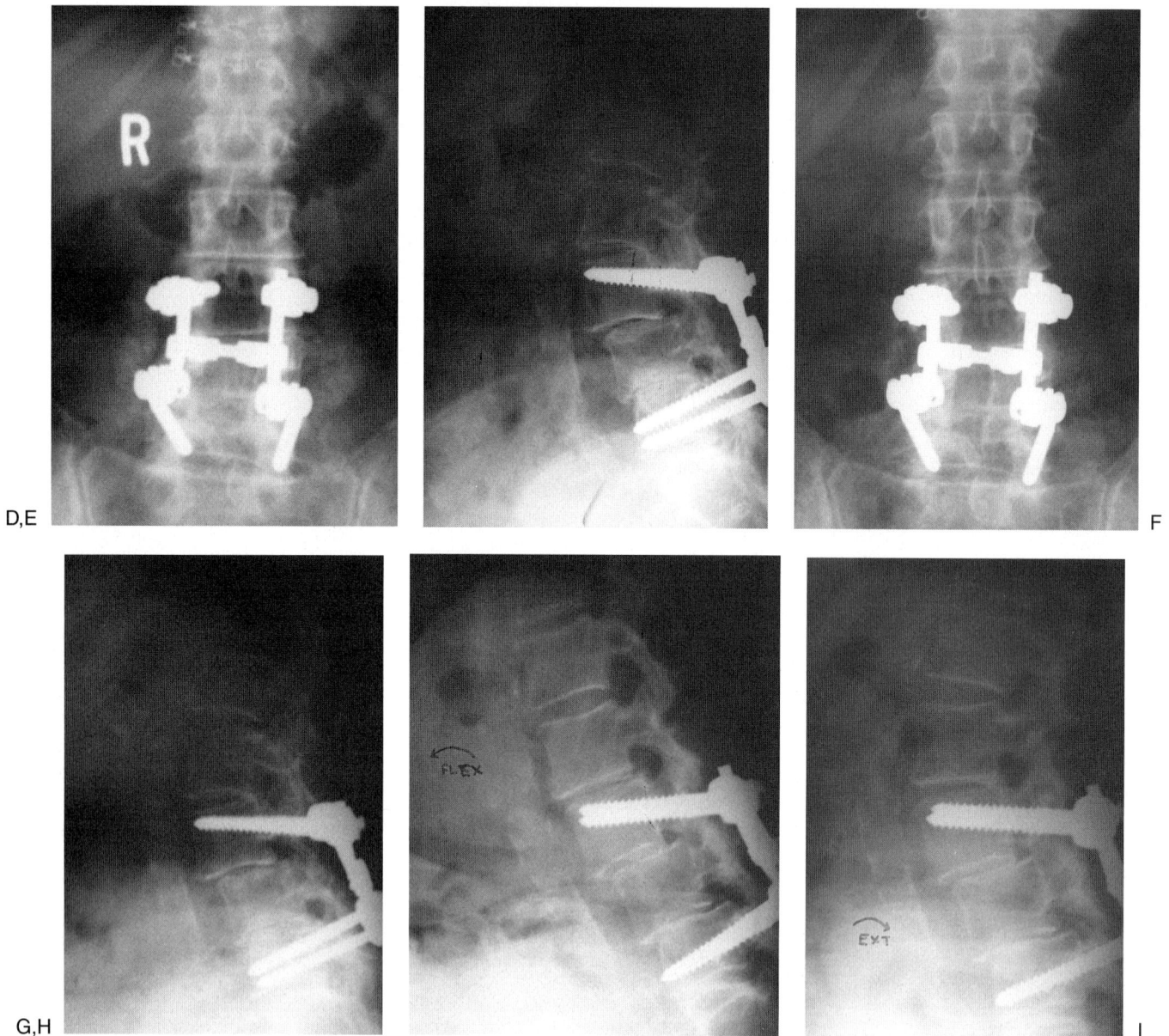

FIG 58-1. (*Continued*) **D, E:** The patient was treated with decompression and posterior instrumentation fusion from L3 to L5 segments. Since L4-5 disc space was completely collapsed, no screw was inserted at this level. **F, G:** At 2-year follow-up, the instrumented segments maintained stability. Consolidation of bone graft is difficult to interpret from these plain radiographs. **H, I:** Flexion-extension lateral radiographs show no movement at the instrumented segment, indicating a possible fusion.

reduces the cost of instrumentation as well as avoids unnecessary complication associated with pedicle screw insertion.

Selective Fusion

In the presence of multiple level spinal stenosis associated with degenerative spondylolisthesis it is not necessary to fuse all the segments. In a prospective randomized study in 45 patients with spinal stenosis without instability undergoing decompression alone, decompression with selective fusion or decompression with fusion of all the segments, Grob et al. (9) found no difference in outcome between the different groups. They concluded that arthrodesis was not justified in the absence of radiographically proven instability. Herkowitz et al. also suggest decompression of all the symptomatic stenotic levels, but instrumented fusion of only the listhetic segment with instability (10) (Fig. 58-2).

Interbody Fusion

When correction of listhetic segment is intended because of grade II slip or higher, or restoration of lordo-

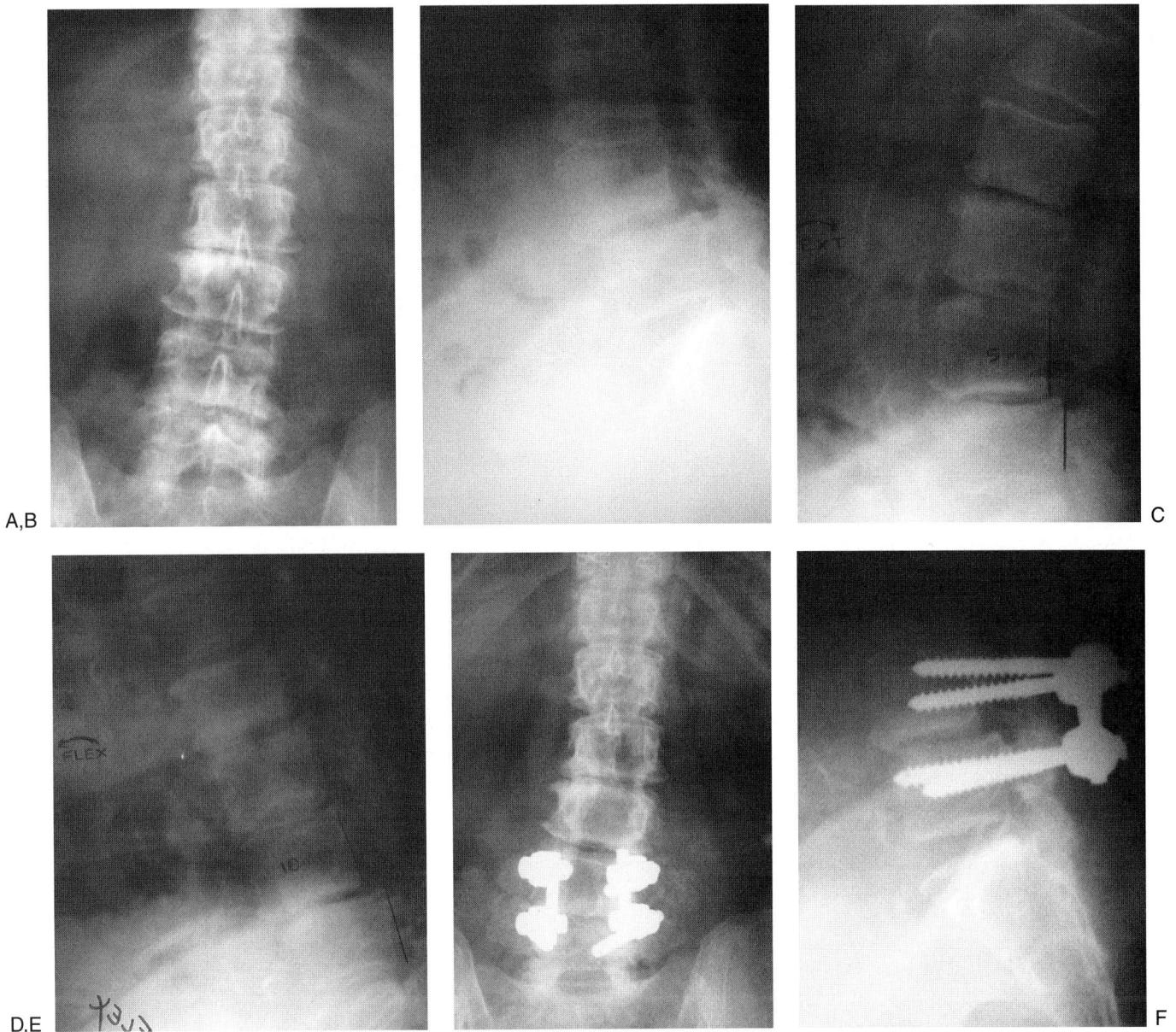

FIG. 58-2. A, B: A 68-year-old male patient with mechanical back pain and neurogenic claudication. Anteroposterior and lateral radiographs show degenerative spondylolisthesis at L4-5 segment and stenosis at L3 to S1 segment. **C, D:** Flexion-extension lateral radiographs clearly demonstrate 5 mm translation at L4-5 segment. **E, F:** The patient was treated by decompression from L2 to S1 segment, but stabilization of the unstable L4-5 segment only. *(continued on next page)*

sis is intended due to presence of frank kyphosis, only posterior pedicle fixation may not be adequate. The pedicle screws are subjected to excessive stress in these situations, unless supported by an interbody device. This may be accomplished by either posterior lumbar interbody fusion or by an additional anterior interbody fusion.

An alternative to interbody fusion is to extend the fusion to an additional segment caudally. For example, correction of spondylolisthesis or slip angle at L4-5 level may be achieved by additional interbody fusion of L4-5

level alone or by extending posterior pedicle fixation from L4 to S1 levels.

Posterior Instrumentation without Fusion

A small but increasing group of surgeons prefer to use soft stabilization procedures after decompression with posterior instrumentation but without fusion. Gardner et al. (11,12) described the Graf ligamentoplasty (13) procedure with long-term follow-up (11) in degenerated disc

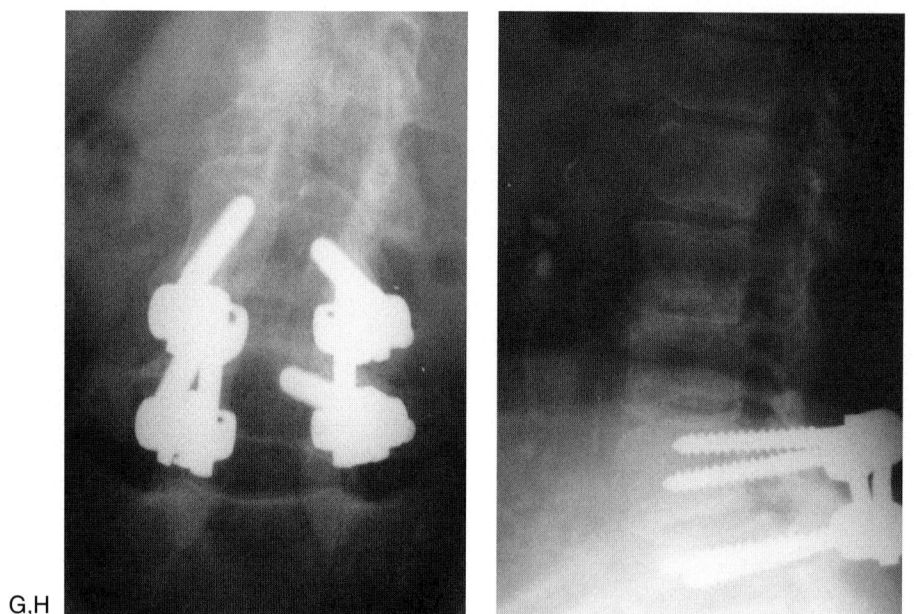

FIG. 58-2. (*Continued*) **G, H:** Anteroposterior and lateral radiographs at 3-year follow-up show the lumbar spine maintains stability, despite short segment fusion only.

diseases with or without spondylolisthesis. This procedure involves attachment of a Dacron ligament to the pedicle screws across the unstable segment. The disadvantage of this procedure is that it increases the lordosis by compressing the posterior segment of the disc, which may cause further narrowing of the foramen. The recently described Dynamic Neutralization System (Dynesys) implant (14), which involves insertion of a similar ligament, but with a plastic cylinder around it, may produce the distraction of the disc space. However, since the distraction is produced by an implant lying posterior to the axis of flexion-extension, this system may lead to loss of lordosis. Restoration of lordosis of the motion segment then depends on the muscle action by the spinal extensor muscles. Mochida et al. (15) reported an innovative method of posterior stabilization in which the Leeds-Keio artificial ligament was used as a nonrigid implant to stop movement in degenerative spondylolisthesis.

POSTOPERATIVE MANAGEMENT

The average duration of surgery for decompression and instrumented posterolateral fusion is approximately 2 to 3 hours. Single-level fusion may be performed under spinal anesthesia. The patients are mobilized to a chair on the evening of surgery and ambulation begins the next day with the help of physical therapy. Deep vein thrombosis prophylaxis is done by sequential pumps and compression stockings around the legs and by early mobilization. Braces are typically not used. Drains are removed in the first or second postoperative day. The average hospital stay is 2 to 4 days. Most patients may be discharged home. Some older adult patients may require inpatient rehabilitation. The patients are advised against bending, lifting, and twisting motion of the spine for 6 to 12 weeks. Return to work may vary between 6 to 12 weeks depending on the nature of job. Nonsteroidal antiinflammatory drugs should be avoided in all fusion patients.

RESULTS

Traditionally, the surgical management of degenerative lumbar spondylolisthesis involves decompressive laminectomy alone. Superiority of fusion over decompression alone was being reported in the literature. A prospective randomized study comparing the role of arthrodesis versus decompression alone was lacking until 1991, when Herkowitz and Kurz published a prospective study in 50 cases, comparing decompressive laminectomy alone with additional intertransverse fusion for single level spinal stenosis with degenerative spondylolisthesis. The results of this study showed a significantly better outcome and a lesser chance of progression of the slip in the fusion group.

Several studies compared the role of instrumentation. The critical issues in adding instrumentation to a fusion are whether the fusion rate will increase and whether the clinical outcome will improve. This must be balanced against increased cost of the implants and potential complications of instrumentation.

In a prospective randomized study in 124 patients (including 56 with degenerative or isthmic spondylolisthesis) in 1993, Zdeblick (16) reported significantly better fusion rate in the instrumented group. However, no breakdown of the number of patients with degenerative spondylolisthesis was made. Subsequently, Bridwell et al. (17) reported a study on 44 patients who underwent fusion after decompression for degenerative stenosis with spondylolisthesis. They compared a decompression group, decompression and uninstrumented fusion group, and fusion with instrumentation group. The instrumentation group showed a much higher fusion rate, better functional outcome, and improved restoration of sagittal alignment compared to the uninstrumented group, (87% and 30%, respectively).

In 1994 Mardjetko et al. (18), in a meta-analysis of literature between 1970 and 1993, reviewed 25 papers on degenerative spondylolisthesis, which met the inclusion criteria. This study compared fusion rate and clinical outcome between five groups, which were decompression alone, decompression and uninstrumented fusion, decompression, and fusion with control instrumentation (Harrington hook-rod construct, Luque segmental fixation with sublaminar wires), and decompression and fusion with pedicle screws. They found a 69% satisfactory outcome in the nonfusion group compared to a 90% satisfactory outcome in the fusion group, which was statistically significant. The fusion rate in the instrumented group varied from 93% to 96% and was significantly higher compared to uninstrumented group (86%). The clinical outcome (satisfaction rate) between instrumented groups (86% to 90%) and uninstrumented group (90%) was not significantly different. They concluded that spinal fusion rate is enhanced by adjunctive spinal instrumentation, with no significant difference between control devices and pedicle screws. Possibly, this reflected early results of pedicle fixation, and also a difference in the number of segments fused, with control devices versus pedicle screws.

Yuan et al. (19) published an historical cohort study of 2,684 patients with degenerative spondylolisthesis with 81% of patients being treated by pedicle screw fixation. They observed a significantly higher and faster fusion rate (89.1% versus 70.4%) in the instrumentation group, and in addition, a better maintenance of spinal alignment. The pedicle screw fixation group also demonstrated a higher rate of neurologic and functional improvement compared to the uninstrumented control group. Rechtine et al. (20) reported a prospective study with instrumented fusion for degenerative spondylolisthesis, and compared the results with a literature-based control group of degenerated spondylolisthesis with uninstrumented *in situ* fusion. They concluded that fusion was more than three times more likely to occur with instrumentation compared to the uninstrumented *in situ* fusion group.

Although these studies indicated a higher fusion and better clinical outcome rate with instrumentation over uninstrumented fusion, there was no conclusive evidence, in absence of a prospective randomized controlled study. Finally, Fischgrund et al. (21) presented a randomized controlled study, comparing decompressive laminectomy

and fusion with or without spinal instrumentation using pedicle screw in 67 patients with single-level degenerative spondylolisthesis with stenosis. Clinical outcome was excellent to good in 82% of the uninstrumented group, and 76% of the instrumented group. The difference was not significant ($p < .45$). Successful fusion was observed in 45% of the uninstrumented group, and 82% of the instrumented group, and the difference was significant ($p < .0015$). Overall, successful fusion did not influence patient outcome ($p < .435$). They concluded that instrumentation certainly improves fusion rate but not necessarily improves clinical outcome. The long-term implications of pseudarthrosis and adjacent segment disease in this patient population remain to be studied.

COMPLICATIONS

The potential complications of decompression and pedicle instrumentation include wound infection, dural tear, and complications related to malplacement of pedicle screws. Recurrent stenosis and junctional stenosis need further discussion.

Adjacent segment stenosis has been reported to be around 42% in a long-term follow-up study of lumbar fusion by Lehmann et al. (22). Whitecloud et al. (23) reported a study of 14 patients with adjacent-level stenosis, treated with decompression and fusion. They found an 80% pseudoarthrosis rate with uninstrumented fusion compared to only 17% with instrumentation.

Patel et al. (24) reviewed 42 cases in our institute that required surgery for adjacent-level stenosis and found that the symptom of adjacent-segment stenosis developed more frequently and at an earlier period when the initial surgery involved instrumentation compared to the uninstrumented fusion. Of the 42 cases reviewed, 12 had an uninstrumented fusion at the initial operation; they developed adjacent segment stenosis at an average of 143 months, compared to 30 cases with primary instrumented fusion that developed symptoms at an average of 62 months. Adjacent segment stenosis was found to be more frequent in the proximal segment. Some 24 cases had a floating fusion; 20 developed stenosis at the proximal level; 3 developed stenosis at the distal level; and one case developed stenosis at both the adjacent levels. While all these cases had decompression at the second operation, 33 of the 42 cases required extension of fusion to the adjacent level. The authors suggested, in absence of instability and when no significant facet excision is necessary, stenosis above a previous fusion may be treated with decompression alone; otherwise, instrumentation is recommended.

Recurrent stenosis may also be produced by laminar regrowth. Postacchini and Cinotti (25) reported some degree of bone regrowth in 88% of cases treated with laminectomy or laminotomy with or without fusion in 40 patients. They reported symptomatic restenosis in as much as 40% of cases with moderate or severe degree of bony regrowth.

CONCLUSION

Although there is some consensus for indications for fusion in the surgical treatment of degenerative spondylolisthesis with stenosis, indications for additional instrumentation remain controversial. Generally, presence of significant movement in the listhetic segment indicates instrumentation. Any intention for correction of listhesis or kyphosis of the listhetic segment warrants either interbody fusion or extension of fusion down to the sacrum, with instrumentation. Recurrent stenosis of a previous laminectomy level or adjacent segment disease often indicates instrumented fusion. Instrumentation certainly improves the successful fusion rate but there is no conclusive evidence that it improves clinical outcome.

REFERENCES

1. Matsunaga S, Sakou T, Morizono Y, et al. Natural history of degenerative spondylolisthesis. Pathogenesis and natural course of the slippage. Spine 1990;15(11):1204–1210.
2. Bernhardt M, Bridwell KH. Segmental analysis of the sagittal plane alignment of the normal thoracic and lumbar spines and thoracolumbar junction. Spine 1989;14(7):717–721.
3. Montgomery DM, Fischgrund JS. Passive reduction of spondylolisthesis on the operating room table: a prospective study. J Spinal Disord 1994;7(2):167–172.
4. Bridwell KH. Acquired degenerative spondylolisthesis without lysis. In: DeWald RL, ed. The text book of spinal surgery, 2nd ed. Vol 2. Philadelphia: Lippincott-Raven Publishers, 1996:1299–1315.
5. White AA, Wiltse LL. Spondylolisthesis after extensive lumbar laminectomy. Paper presented at: Annual Meeting of the American Academy of Orthopaedic Surgeons; 1976; New Orleans.
6. Boden SD, Martin C, Rudolph R, et al. Increase of motion between lumbar vertebrae after excision of the capsule and cartilage of the facets. A cadaver study. J Bone Joint Surg Am 1994;76(12):1847–1853.
7. Abumi K, Panjabi MM, Kramer KM, et al. Biomechanical evaluation of lumbar spinal stability after graded facetectomies. Spine 1990;15(11):1142–1147.
8. Suk KS, Lee HM, Kim NH, et al. Unilateral versus bilateral pedicle screw fixation in lumbar spinal fusion. Spine 2000;25(14):1843–1847.
9. Grob D, Humke T, Dvorak J. [Significance of simultaneous fusion and surgical decompression in lumbar spinal stenosis]. Orthopade 1993;22(4):243–249.
10. Herkowitz HN, Abraham DJ, Albert TJ. Management of degenerative disc disease above an L5-S1 segment requiring arthrodesis. Spine 1999;24(12):1268–1270.
11. Gardner A, Pande KC. Graf ligamentoplasty: a 7-year follow-up. Eur Spine J 2002;11[Suppl 2]:S157–S163.
12. Grevitt MP, Gardner AD, Spilsbury J, et al. The Graf stabilisation system: early results in 50 patients. Eur Spine J 1995;4(3):169–175; discussion 35.
13. Graf H. Lumbar instability. Surgical treatment without fusion. Rachis 1992;412:123–137.
14. Stoll TM, Dubois G, Schwarzenbach O. The dynamic neutralization system for the spine: a multi-center study of a novel non-fusion system. Eur Spine J 2002;11[Suppl 2]:S170–S178.
15. Mochida J, Suzuki K, Chiba M. How to stabilize a single level lesion of degenerative lumbar spondylolisthesis. Clin Orthop 1999(368):126–134.
16. Zdeblick TA. A prospective, randomized study of lumbar fusion. Preliminary results. Spine 1993;18(8):983–991.
17. Bridwell KH, Sedgewick TA, O'Brien MF, et al. The role of fusion and instrumentation in the treatment of degenerative spondylolisthesis with spinal stenosis. J Spinal Disord 1993;6(6):461–472.
18. Mardjetko SM, Connolly PJ, Shott S. Degenerative lumbar spondylolisthesis. A meta-analysis of literature 1970–1993. Spine 1994;19[20 Suppl]:2256S–2265S.
19. Yuan HA, Garfin SR, Dickman CA, et al. A historical cohort study of pedicle screw fixation in thoracic, lumbar, and sacral spinal fusions. Spine 1994;19[20 Suppl]:2279S–2296S.
20. Rechtine GR, Sutterlin CE, Wood GW, et al. The efficacy of pedicle screw/plate fixation on lumbar/lumbosacral autogenous bone graft fusion in adult patients with degenerative spondylolisthesis. J Spinal Disord 1996;9(5):382–391.
21. Fischgrund JS, Mackay M, Herkowitz HN, et al. 1997 Volvo Award winner in clinical studies. Degenerative lumbar spondylolisthesis with spinal stenosis: a prospective, randomized study comparing decompressive laminectomy and arthrodesis with and without spinal instrumentation. Spine 1997;22(24):2807–2812.
22. Lehmann TR, Spratt KF, Tozzi JE, et al. Long-term follow-up of lower lumbar fusion patients. Spine 1987;12(2):97–104.
23. Whitecloud TS 3rd, Davis JM, Olive PM. Operative treatment of the degenerated segment adjacent to a lumbar fusion. Spine 1994;19(5):531–536.
24. Patel C, Truumees E, Gitlin J, et al. Symptomatic spinal stenosis adjacent to a previous lumbar fusion. Spine J 2002;2(5S):54S.
25. Postacchini F, Cinotti G. Bone regrowth after surgical decompression for lumbar spinal stenosis. J Bone Joint Surg Br 1992;74(6):862–869.

Degenerative Lumbar Spinal Stenosis with Scoliosis-Kyphosis: Surgical Techniques, Results, and Complications

Hirokazu Ishihara and Hisao Matsui

Degenerative lumbar spinal stenosis with scoliosis is a relatively new concept of the disease. In 1976, Arnoldi et al. (1) defined the international classification of lumbar spinal stenosis and nerve root entrapment syndromes. In their classification, lumbar spinal stenosis was defined as the following: congenital stenosis (idiopathic, achondroplastic) and acquired stenosis (degenerative, combined, spondylolisthetic/spondylolytic, iatrogenic, posttraumatic, Paget disease, fluorosis). The concept of degenerative lumbar spinal stenosis with scoliosis had not yet been described. Due to the longer life span and greater expectations during this life span, the number of patients being treated for this condition is increasing. It is important to differentiate degenerative scoliosis from other degenerative spinal stenosis syndromes because the pathogenesis of nerve root or cauda equina compression and treatment considerations are quite different. Despite the number of studies that have focused on degenerative lumbar spinal stenosis with scoliosis, considerable confusion continues to persist as to the optimal method of the treatment. This study defines the pathogenesis as well as the appropriate surgical techniques for degenerative scoliosis based on the current literature and our surgical experience.

PATHOGENESIS OF CAUDA EQUINA AND NERVE ROOT COMPRESSION

Lumbar spinal stenosis refers to any narrowing of the spinal canal, resulting in highly variable signs and symptoms. In addition to the central canal containing cauda equina, there are three potential zones that may affect the nerve roots: the lateral recess zone, the foraminal zone, and the extraforaminal zone (2). Central canal and lateral recess stenosis may occur with any one or a combination of disc prolapse, facet degeneration and hypertrophy, ligamentum flavum hypertrophy or degenerative spondylolisthesis, and may cause cauda equina and nerve root compression. In addition to these changes, loss of lumbar lordosis, an increase of apical rotation, lateral vertebral slip, as well as foraminal stenosis as a result of disc collapse, pedicle approximation and facet joint subluxation (the superior articular process of the inferior vertebra subluxates anteriorly and superiorly, diminishing the area of the foramen) can occur with the progression of degenerative scoliosis (2). Hasegawa et al. (3), in a cadaveric study, showed that significant foraminal stenosis is commonly associated with a foraminal height of 15 mm or less and a posterior disc height of 4 mm or less. Nerve root entrapments can also be caused by pedicular kinking (the root is kinked and over stretched by downward pedicle migration on the concave side concomitant with disc collapse) (Fig. 59-1). Foraminal or extraforaminal disc herniation can occur at the compression site (concave site) of the curve (4) (Fig. 59-2). Thus, it is very common for the nerve roots in the foraminal or extraforaminal zone to be compressed in patients with degenerative scoliosis. Many authors have stated that nerve root compression is almost always seen on the concave side of the scoliosis (5–7), and L4 and L5 nerve roots are the most often involved (8). We have analyzed the relationship between nerve root compression and the pattern of the scoliotic curve in 22 consecutive degenerative scoliosis patients. L3 root was affected in 23% of patients; L4 root in 68%, L5 root in 55%, and S1 root in 18%. Of these, both L3 and L4 roots and both L5 and S1 roots were affected in 23% and 18% of patients, respectively. L3 and L4 roots were more compressed by foraminal or extraforaminal

A,B

C

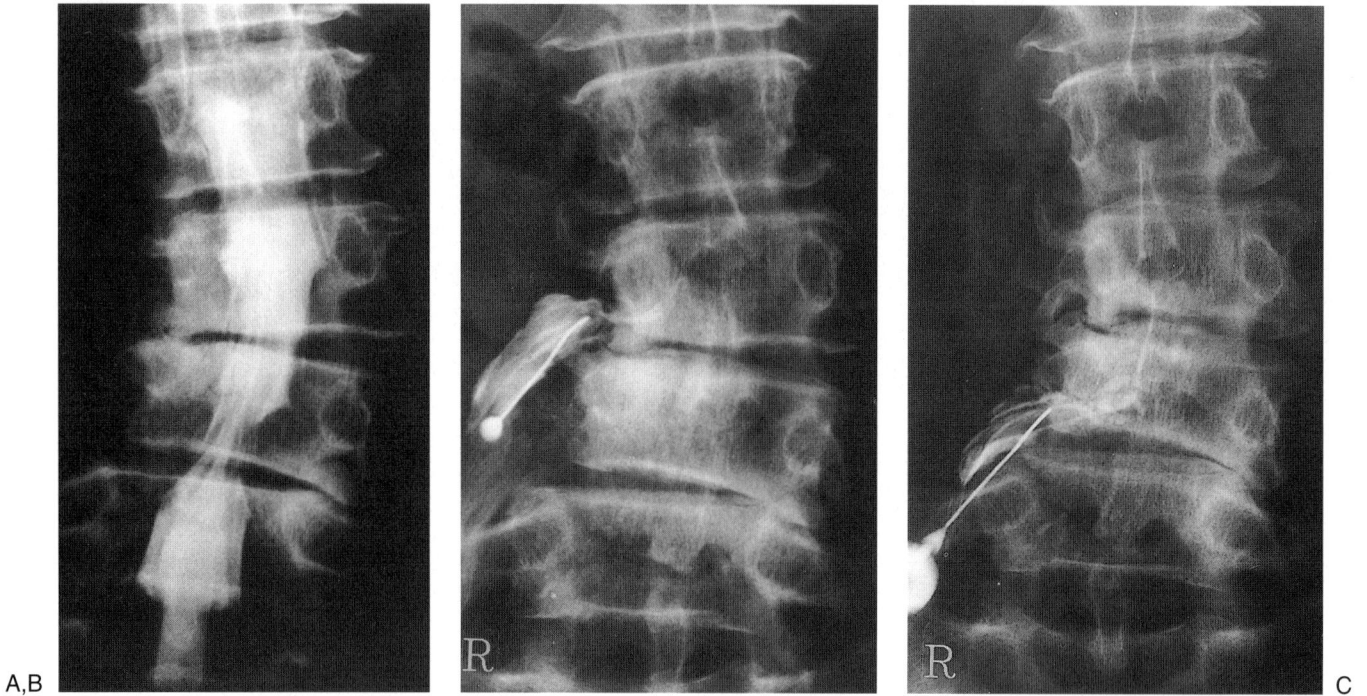

FIG. 59-1. A 54-year-old man complained of right leg pain. Neurologic examination indicated that the symptomatic nerve roots were L3 and L4. Lumbar spine radiographs show a left lumbar scoliosis from L1 to L4 of 23° with the apex at L3. **A:** On myelography, there is no remarkable compressive factor for L3 and L4 roots. **B, C:** Right L3 and L4 radiculographies reveal the compression and elongation of the nerve roots due to pedicular kinking.

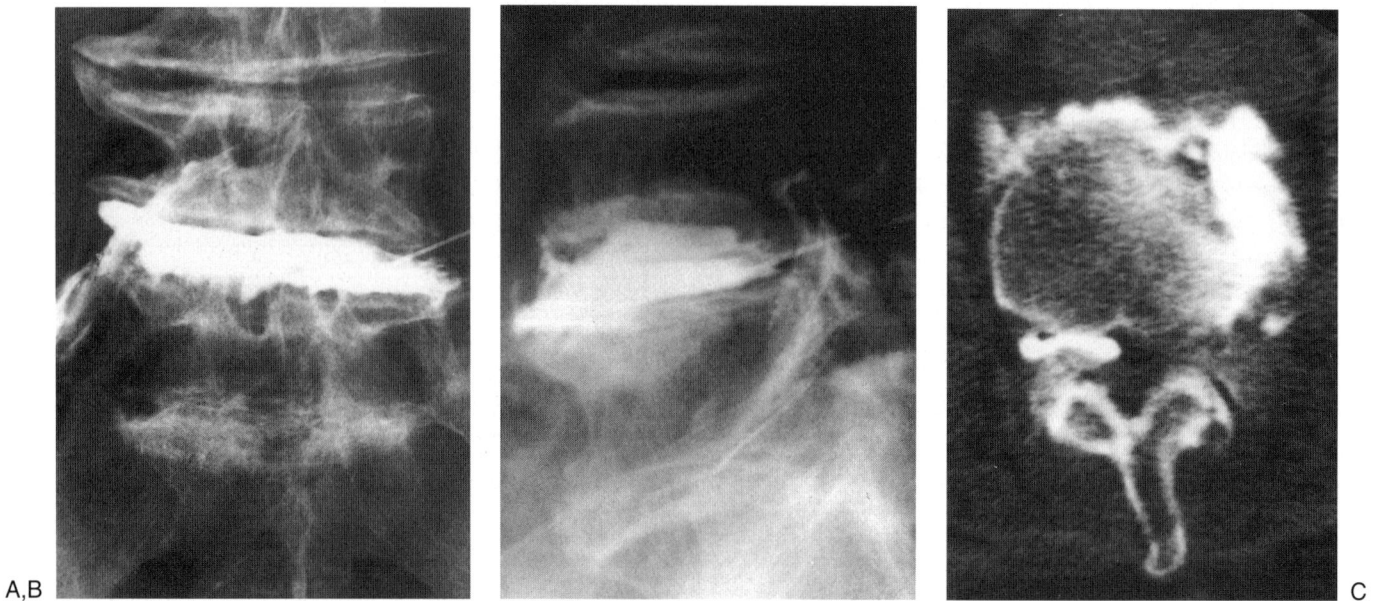

A,B

C

FIG. 59-2. A 76-year-old woman presented with right L4 radiculopathy. L4-L5 discography **(A, B)** and computed tomography after discography **(C)** disclose L4-L5 foraminal intervertebral disc herniation with leakage of the contrast medium to the right L4 root sheath.

stenosis on the concave side of the curve, while L5 and S1 roots were commonly affected by lateral recess stenosis on the convex side. The Cobb angle of the curve and the lateral slip of the apex or next to the apex vertebra of the cases in which L3 or L4 root was affected by foraminal or extraforaminal stenosis were significantly larger than those of the cases in which L5 or S1 root was compressed by lateral recess stenosis (8a).

DIAGNOSTIC STRATEGY

It is necessary to determine the symptomatic nerve roots and their compressive factors. The symptomatic nerve roots can be determined by the pain distribution, neurologic findings, and nerve root infiltration using lidocaine. In plain radiographs, the pattern of scoliosis, such as the upper and lower end vertebrae, the apex vertebrae, Cobb angle of the curve, and the rotation and lateral slip of vertebrae are determined. Intervertebral disc space narrowing, osteophyte formation, shortening of the pedicles with pedicular thickening, and facet joint arthrosis are also important findings (6). Segmental instability is assessed by lateral flexion-extension and anteroposterior lateral bending radiographs (dynamic radiographs). The generally accepted standard criteria for instability are more than 4 mm of translation and more than 10° of angularity when compared with the adjacent proximal or distal levels (9).

The central canal and lateral recess stenosis are relatively easy to diagnose by magnetic resonance imaging (MRI) or myelograms, however, in foraminal or extraforaminal herniation, discography, computed tomography after discography (CTD), and nerve root infiltration are necessary in addition to MRI and myelography (Fig. 59-2). The use of CT allows detection of bony encroachment on the foramen. Although the shape of the foramen is not well seen on axial images, parasagittally reconstructed images, including bony and soft tissue windows, allow better definition of the presence of bony spurs arising from the posterolateral vertebral body or facet joint and extending into the foramen (2). The parasagittal and coronal images of MRI may allow visualization of the foramina along the length of the lumbar spine. The most suggestive finding is a paucity of perineural fat surrounding the nerve root on T1-weighted images (10) (Fig. 59-3). However, scoliosis sometimes makes it difficult to read these images correctly. Radiculography may show a filling defect or deformity of the nerve root sleeves (Fig. 59-1). However, sometimes it may be difficult to demonstrate the foraminal stenosis from the neuroradiologic point of view. Foraminal stenosis is sometimes concluded based on the negative findings (e.g., radiculography demonstrated pain recurrence and disappearance after nerve root infiltration by lidocaine), but no obvious root compression was found in the lateral recess zone or extraforaminal zone. It is also necessary to consider the double crush syndrome (e.g., the same nerve root is compressed at both the lateral recess zone and the foraminal zone).

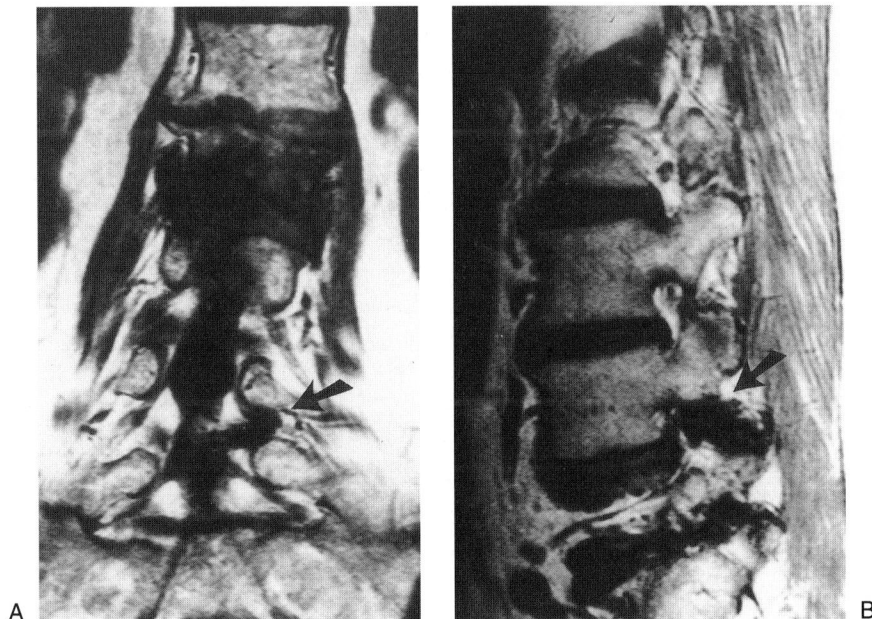

FIG. 59-3. Coronal and parasagittal T1-weighted magnetic resonance images of a 70-year-old patient with left L4 radiculopathy due to L4-5 foraminal stenosis. Note the presence of fat signal around the right L4 root in a coronal image **(A)** or L2 and L3 nerve roots in a parasagittal image **(B)**, but the absence of fat signal around the left L4 root *(arrow)*.

INDICATIONS FOR SURGERY

Conservative treatment must be tried. Pitchett et al. (8) stated that nonsteroidal antiinflammatory drugs reduced symptoms in 54% of patients. Bracing, bed rest, exercise, traction, and application of heat were effective in relieving pain in 46% of patients. Indications for surgery include progressive neurologic deficit or severe pain that is refractory to conservative treatments.

DECOMPRESSION ALONE

In 1974, Epstein et al. (11) first reported the surgical treatment of nerve root compression caused by degenerative lumbar scoliosis. Four patients between the ages of 58 to 80 years were followed for 6 to 18 months. Laminectomy or hemilaminectomy was performed with unroofing of the lateral recesses and foramina by medial facetectomy or total facetectomy, and lasting relief of pain was achieved. The authors concluded that because of associated spondyloarthrosis, advanced disc degeneration, and spontaneous interbody fusion in this age group, the spinal column is stable and can tolerate facet removal.

San Martino et al. (12) also performed hemilaminectomy, with foraminotomy and medial facetectomy in 12 patients and laminectomy with bilateral decompression of multiple nerve roots including facetectomy in 8 patients. The patients were followed up for 4 years and in 16 patients the results were considered excellent with return of function and no restriction regarding occupational activities. No patient suffered a recurrence of major symptoms and no one required additional surgery.

On the contrary, Benner and Ehni (5) also performed laminectomy, hemilaminectomy, and foraminotomy in 14 patients between the ages of 50 to 85 years. The results were generally quite good and relief of radiculopathy was obtained. However, occasionally low back pain and sacroiliac pain persisted and four patients in this group developed progression of scoliosis. These patients underwent additional Harrington instrumentation and fusion. Katoh et al. (13) compared the results of decompression alone (fenestration, laminectomy, or hemilaminectomy) and decompression with posterior fusion using Harrington instrumentation in degenerative lumbar scoliosis. Three patients were treated with laminectomy alone and seven were treated with laminectomy and posterior fusion. The mean age at surgery was 65 years (range, 54 to 75), and the curve measured between 15° and 50°. At follow-up (mean of 4.2 years), overall satisfactory clinical results with pain relief and improved walking distance were noted in the patients treated with laminectomy and posterior fusion. However, all patients treated with decompression alone needed reoperation because of recurrence of leg symptoms due to the progression of scoliosis.

Recently, many papers have stated that with decompression alone, without any form of stabilization as the treatment of degenerative scoliosis, additional problems usually occur as does the progression of deformity. Such treatment does not yield a long-term satisfactory result (14).

INDICATIONS FOR SPINAL FUSION

The selection criteria for which patients with degenerative scoliosis should be fused are not clear and are somewhat controversial. The average age of the patients is relatively high and a number of patients have some complications such as hypertension, diabetes mellitus, or heart problems. Thus, most surgeons prefer to avoid an operative procedure that causes prolonged and excessive bleeding.

Postacchini (15) stated that in a few older adult patients who present little or no back pain with mild scoliosis, there can be an indication for decompression alone; however, in patients who present with severe scoliosis and low back pain, there is an indication for wide decompression and spinal fusion using pedicle screw instrumentation. Because back pain is related to a loss of lumbar lordosis and trunk unbalance in severe degenerative scoliosis, a primary aim of the surgery is the correction of the curve and restoration of body balance. Hansraj et al. (16) stated that the spinal fusion and instrumentation is needed for degenerative scoliosis with a curve of greater than 20°. Gelalis and Kang (9) stated that each patient must be treated on an individual basis depending on the age of the patient, whether there has been documentation of progression of the scoliosis curve, the amount of low back pain versus the amount of radicular symptoms, and finally the experience of the spine surgeon. If the patient predominantly has stenosis symptoms with a minimal degree of scoliosis (less than 25° to 30°), in most instances a simple laminectomy along with foraminotomy without fusion is all that is necessary and a good outcome is achieved. If a patient has a more pronounced deformity (greater than 30°), with any degree of lateral translational listhesis, a fusion should be performed at the time of decompression. This becomes especially true if the main reason for the surgical treatment was to treat the spinal stenosis symptoms (17). The surgeons nevertheless must keep in mind the potential for destabilization of the spine during the decompression procedure, particularly if excessive amounts of facet joints are resected. However, it is difficult to predict which patients with subtle degenerative scoliosis will develop progression of the deformity after decompression surgery (9).

EXPANSIVE LAMINOPLASTY WITH POSTERIOR SPINAL FUSION

Tsuji et al. (18,19) have developed lumbar expansive laminoplasty. This technique provides reinforcement of the stability of the lumbar spine as well as decompression of the nerve roots by expanding the cross-sectional area of the spinal canal. The merits of this method are that it is minimally invasive, applicable for older patients who have other comorbid medical problems, and the use of instrumentation can be avoided. However, the method is limited to some extent in the decompression of the hinged side; thus, indications are limited. It is impossible to correct the deformity by this method. We have applied this procedure to treat lumbar spinal stenosis with scoliosis.

The spinous process is removed from its origin and used as a bone graft. The lamina is cut wider as the outer edge of the groove reaches the lateral one-third or one-half of the facets. The groove at the hinged side is outlined as a cone in the horizontal plane. Small holes are made in each lamina and in the articular processes on the open side using an awl, pusher, and perforator. The laminae are then detached completely at the open side in order to obtain sufficient rotation of the laminae. The lateral recess of the spinal canal is trimmed, and the remaining ligamentum flavum is removed completely. The medial facetectomy or partial pediculectomy are added in case of necessity. The bone grafts from the spinous processes are fitted into the gap of the open side and held in place by No.1 nylon threads. At least a 45° rotation angle of the lamina is necessary. The cross-sectional shape of the canal is altered from triangular to square. All of the open epidural space between the laminae is shielded by free fat grafting. The

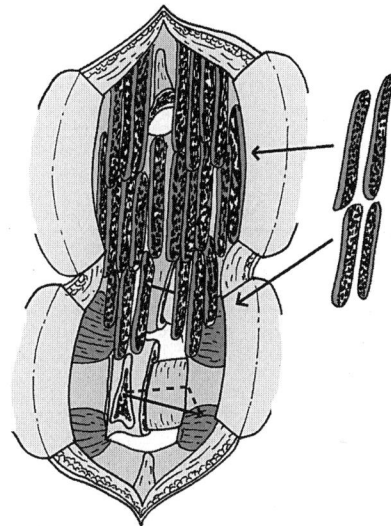

FIG. 59-5. In performing a posterior spinal fusion, the joint capsules are completely removed, and the laminae and the articular processes are decorticated bilaterally, including adjacent intact laminae, using a high-speed air drill. Corticocancellous bone sticks from the posterior ilium are carefully grafted.

joint capsules are completely removed, and the lamina and the articular processes are decorticated bilaterally, including adjacent intact laminae, using a high-speed air drill. Corticocancellous bone sticks from the posterior ilium are carefully grafted (Figs. 59-4, 59-5).

Matsui et al. (20) reviewed the clinical and radiologic results of 27 patients who underwent expansive laminoplasty with a mean follow-up of 5.6 years. There was marked recovery of clinical symptoms, and nearly 80% of patients obtained good or excellent results. Only one patient (4%) required additional surgery, which involved discectomy at the caudal level of the laminoplasty. Radiographic evaluation revealed that postoperative changes of scoliosis were slight both in the expanded area and at the L1-L5 levels (Fig. 59-6).

DECOMPRESSION AND POSTEROLATERAL FUSION (PLF) OR POSTERIOR LUMBAR INTERBODY FUSION (PLIF) WITH PEDICLE SCREW INSTRUMENTATION

Pedicle screw instrumentation is the best method to fuse and correct the deformity, because it has the best biomechanical advantage, acting through the three columns of the spine and also providing the best fixation in the bony substrate (14). Aebi (21) described the techniques of degenerative scoliosis correction using the Arbeitsgemeinschaft für Osteosynthasefragen (AO) internal spinal fixator system. The pedicle screws are inserted into the pedicles of both neutral vertebrae and the apex vertebra. The pedicles of the intermediate vertebrae are then supplemented by additional screws. Next, complete

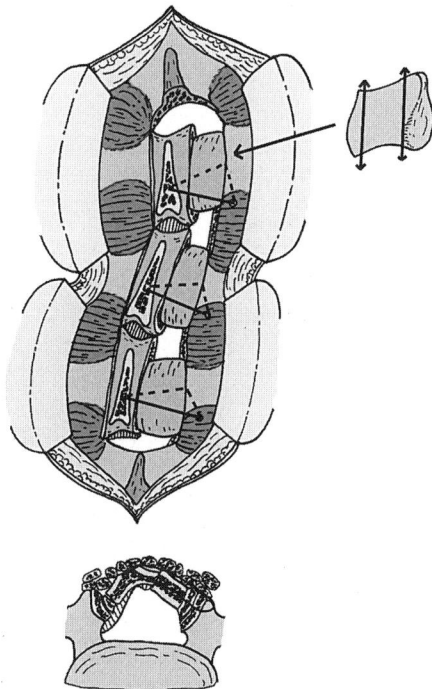

FIG. 59-4. Lumbar expansive laminoplasty. Small holes are made in each lamina and the articular processes on the open side using an awl, pusher, and perforator. The bone grafts from the spinous processes are fitted into the gaps of the open side and held in place by nylon threads.

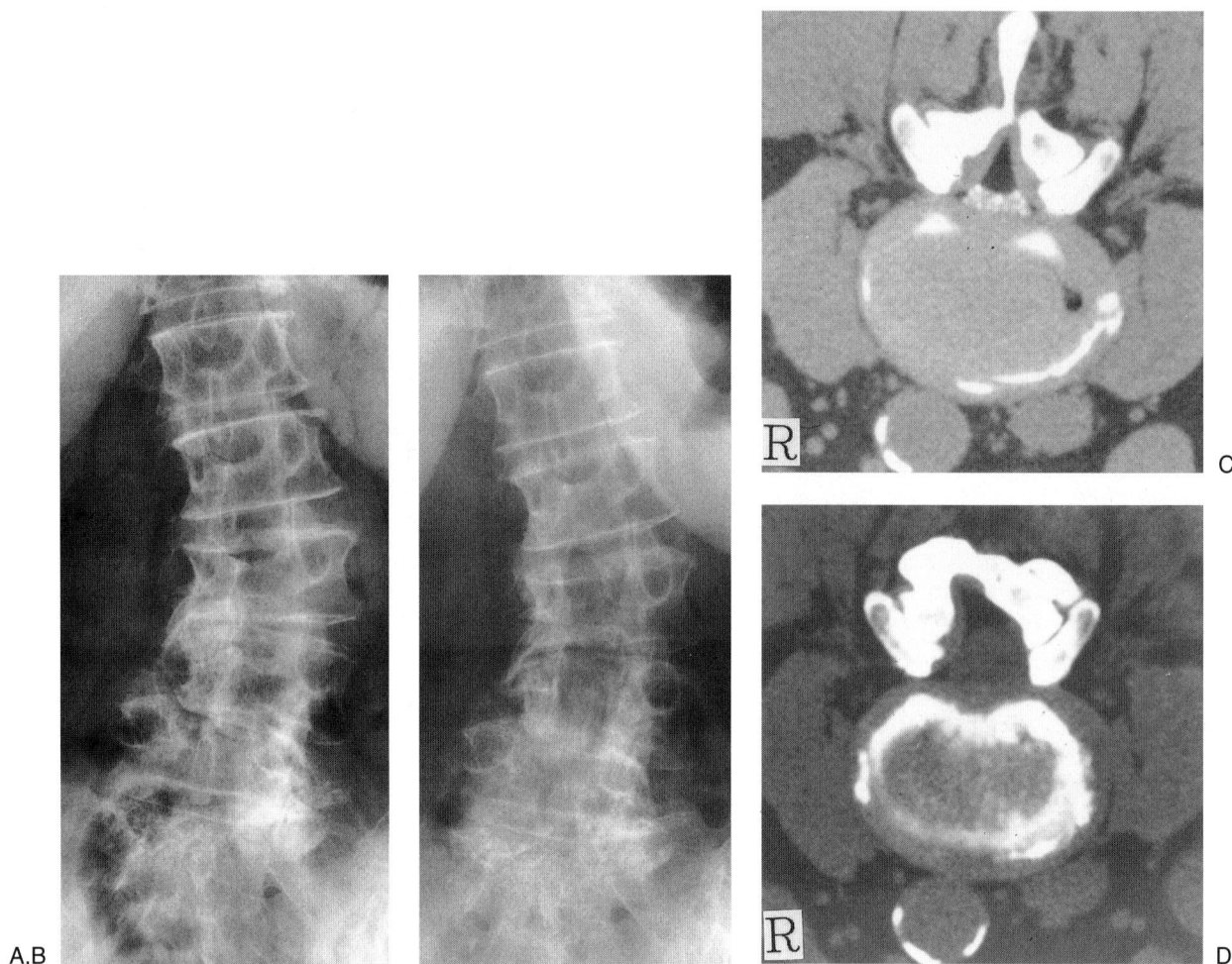

FIG. 59-6. A 76-year-old woman complained of left leg pain and low back pain. Neurologic examination and root block revealed that her symptomatic nerve root was right L4. **A:** Lumbar spine radiographs show a right lumbar scoliosis from L2 to L4 of 24° with the apex at L3. There is a 10 mm lateral slip of L3 on L4 vertebra on the preoperative anteroposterior view. **B:** L3-5 laminoplasty with L4-5 medial facetectomy, L4 partial pediculectomy and posterior spinal fusion was performed. A 2-year follow-up anteroposterior radiograph indicates that the posterior fusion is accomplished. Postoperative computed tomography (CT) **(D)** shows that the spinal canal is enlarged into a rectangular shape, comparing with preoperative CT **(C)**.

posterior soft tissue release over the involved spine is achieved to mobilize the curve. The distracter is then mounted on the concave side of the curve with attachment being made to the end vertebrae screws. Gentle distraction is performed with this device as the pedicle screws in the apex vertebra and the screws in the remaining intermediate vertebrae are used to mobilize the deformity manually, segment by segment, through repeated rotatory movements toward the midline. A long threaded rod is inserted on the pedicle screws on the convex side of the curve and fixed by a clamp. The apex vertebra is derotated as far as possible by this mechanism. The sagittal plane deformity, irrespective of the coronal plane curve, can then be corrected by pushing forward or pulling back on the pedicle screw.

The author pointed out sagittal curve correction and restoration of body balance are the most important factors influencing the incidence of low-back pain. The persistence of a flat back after surgery clearly correlates with continuous lumbar pain. Furthermore, the convexity of the curve can be reduced by compressing the pedicle screws of the neutral end vertebrae along the threaded rod toward the apex vertebrae. The screws in the intermediate vertebrae are tightened against the rod. The femoral distracter is removed and a second threaded rod with hinged clamps is inserted into the screws on the concave side. The screws in the remaining vertebrae are tightened in the same manner as on the convex side. A bilateral PLF using iliac crest autograft bone is then performed in a routine fashion. Nerve root exploration and decompression is performed after the spine is completely instrumented.

Aebi (21) has performed this operation for 8 patients who ranged in age from 44 to 74 years. The postoperative follow-up time was 1 to 3 years. The curves ranged from 22° to 48°. Seven of these eight patients subjectively rated the overall outcomes of their surgery as good or excellent and believed that surgery significantly improved the quality of their daily life. One patient was dissatisfied with the results and had expected greater relief from pain. The overall correction of curves was greater than 50%. There was no infection, no evidence of pseudoarthrosis, and no instrumentation-related complications.

Marchesi (22) reviewed the result of segmental pedicle screw instrumentation in degenerative lumbar scoliosis. The AO internal fixator was used for 9 patients and the Cotrel-Dubousset (CD) instrumentation was used for 18 cases. Mean age at surgery was 60 years (range, 40 to 88), and the curve measured between 22° and 82°. At follow-up (mean of 56 months for the AO Internal Fixator and 42 months for CD instrumentation), the average curve correction was better than 50%. Overall, satisfactory clinical results with pain relief and improved walking distance were noted in 86% of the patients. Using this technique, no postoperative deaths or neurologic deficits occurred. Only a few complications and a 4% pseudoarthrosis rate could be observed.

Liew and Simmons (7,14) described the two general techniques for correction of degenerative scoliosis. One is a technique used for patients with short degenerative collapsing curves with reasonably well-maintained lumbar lordosis or minimal loss of lordosis. This involves some distraction on the concave side with the rod carefully contoured to maintain lordosis and a neutralization rod on the convex side (Fig. 59-7). The other technique is a rod derotation maneuver as used for patients with idiopathic curves. This technique is useful for patients with longer degenerative curves and for patients with more significant loss of lumbar lordosis. In these patients, the derotation maneuver will convert the scoliotic curve in the coronal plane into a lordotic curve in the sagittal plane. The overriding principle for both of these techniques is to end up with a spine that is balanced above the sacrum with the areas that have been decompressed well stabilized within the instrumented segments. Another important principle is to avoid ending the instrumentation at an area of junctional kyphosis or at a level of a spondylolisthesis.

Simmons and Simmons have performed this operation for 40 patients with degenerative scoliosis. The average follow-up was 44 months. Satisfactory outcome was noted in 93%. The mean correction of the curve was 19°. No instrument-related failure or pseudoarthrosis occurred (23).

Zurbriggen et al. (24) also reported a surgically treated series of 40 patients with degenerative scoliosis. The surgical techniques applied consisted of decompression of neural elements by laminectomy and partial scoliosis correction with CD instrumentation and PLF with autologous bone graft. The series included 18 males and 22 females with a mean age of 62.8 years. Final evaluation was possible in 30 patients at a mean period of observation of 59.5 months. Following a very precise diagnostic and therapeutic protocol, excellent, good, and satisfactory results were obtained in 13 (43.3%), 16 (53.3%), and 1 (3.3%) patients, respectively. While scoliosis was converted from a mean preoperative Cobb angle of 18.7° to 7.6°, mean preoperative lumbar lordosis was slightly augmented from 37° to 41.5°. The results suggested that maintenance or correction of lumbar lordosis is more important than the correction of the scoliosis.

Oguma et al. (25) stated that PLIF using threaded titanium interbody fusion cage with pedicle screw instrumentation was better to correct and maintain lumbar lordosis. They compared the results of PLF with pedicle screw instrumentation (15 cases) and PLIF using threaded titanium fusion cage with pedicle screw instrumentation (35 cases) in degenerative scoliosis. The average follow-up period was 44 months, and successful fusion was observed in all cases. There was no significant difference about the correction and correction loss of scoliosis between PLF and PLIF cases. However, the mean correction loss of lumbar lordosis was 13.2° in PLF cases and 1.9° in PLIF cases.

The complications of these instrumentation surgeries include blood loss, infection, nerve root or cauda equina injury, and the pseudoarthrosis with or without instrumentation failure. The risk of adjacent segment degeneration is also higher when lengthy fusion with rigid instrumentation is performed. In a review of 125 patients, Etebar and Cahill (26) noted a 14% incidence of symptomatic adjacent-segment degeneration after lumbar fusion with pedicle screw instrumentation. A 78% incidence of adjacent segment degeneration occurred after fusion encompassing three or more segments.

CONCLUSION

The appropriate surgical techniques for degenerative scoliosis remain one of the most controversial topics in spine surgery. It is important to determine the symptomatic nerve roots and their compressive factors. The nerve roots in the foraminal or extraforaminal zone are compressed frequently by pedicular kinking, foraminal stenosis because of disc collapse, pedicle approximation and facet joint subluxation, or foraminal and extraforaminal disc herniation. The decompression alone without some form of stabilization usually will have additional problems and progression of the deformity and will not yield a long-term satisfactory

A,B

C

D

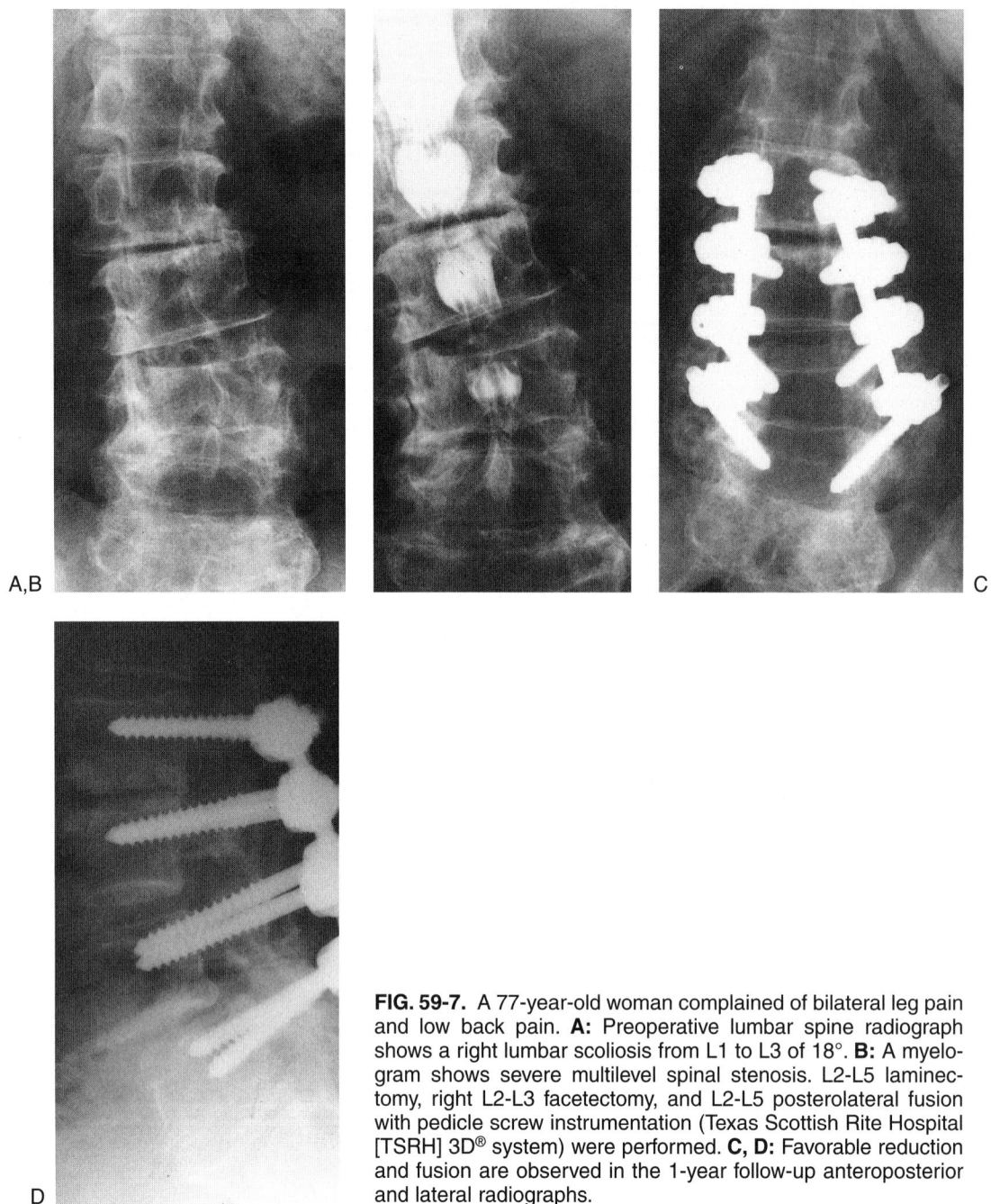

FIG. 59-7. A 77-year-old woman complained of bilateral leg pain and low back pain. **A:** Preoperative lumbar spine radiograph shows a right lumbar scoliosis from L1 to L3 of 18°. **B:** A myelogram shows severe multilevel spinal stenosis. L2-L5 laminectomy, right L2-L3 facetectomy, and L2-L5 posterolateral fusion with pedicle screw instrumentation (Texas Scottish Rite Hospital [TSRH] 3D® system) were performed. **C, D:** Favorable reduction and fusion are observed in the 1-year follow-up anteroposterior and lateral radiographs.

result. Expansive laminoplasty with posterior spinal fusion or decompression and PLF or PLIF with pedicle screw instrumentation will result in a successful outcome.

REFERENCES

1. Arnoldi CC, Brodsky AE, Cauchoix J, et al. Lumbar spinal stenosis and nerve root entrapment syndromes. Clin Orthop 1976;115:4–5.
2. Jenis LG, An HS. Spine update. Lumbar foraminal stenosis. Spine 2000;25:389–394.
3. Hasegawa T, An HS, Haughton V, et al. Lumbar foraminal stenosis: critical heights of the intervertebral discs and foramina. J Bone Joint Surg [Am] 1995;77:32–38.
4. Simmons EH, Jackson RP. The management of nerve root entrapment syndromes associated with the collapsing scoliosis of idiopathic lumbar and thoracolumbar curves. Spine 1979;4:533–541.
5. Benner B, Ehni G. Degenerative lumbar scoliosis. Spine 1979;4:548–552.
6. Epstein JA, Epstein BS, Jones MD. Symptomatic lumbar scoliosis with degenerative changes in the elderly. Spine 1979;4:542–547.
7. Liew SM, Simmons ED, Jr. Thoracic and lumbar deformity. Rationale for selecting the appropriate fusion technique (anterior, posterior, and 360 degree). Orthop Clin North Am 1998;29:843–858.
8. Pitchett JW, Bortel DT. Degenerative symptomatic lumbar scoliosis. Spine 1993;18:700–703.
8a. Liu H, Ishihara H, Kanamori M, et al. Characteristics of nerve root compression caused by degenerative lumbar spinal stenosis with scoliosis. Spine J 2003;3:524–529.
9. Gelalis ID, Kang JD. Thoracic and lumbar fusions for degenerative disorders. Orthop Clin North Am 1998;29:829–842.

10. Maher CO, Henderson FC. Lateral exit-zone stenosis and lumbar radiculopathy. J Neurosurg (Spine 1) 1999;90:52–58.
11. Epstein JA, Epstein BS, Lavine LS. Surgical treatment of nerve root compression caused by scoliosis of the lumbar spine. J Neurosurg 1974;41:449–454.
12. San Martino A, D'andria FM, San Martino C. The surgical treatment of nerve root compression caused by scoliosis of the lumbar spine. Spine 1983;8:261–265.
13. Katoh Y, Morita Y, Kanamori M, et al. Lumbar spinal stenosis associated with degenerative scoliosis. Rinsho Seikei Geka 1992;27:421–427 [in Japanese].
14. Simmons ED. Surgical treatment of patients with lumbar spinal stenosis with associated scoliosis. Clin Orthop 2001;384:45–53.
15. Postacchini F. Spine update. Surgical management of lumbar spinal stenosis. Spine 1999;24:1043–1047.
16. Hansraj KK, O'Leary PF, Cammisa FP, et al. Decompression, fusion, and instrumentation surgery for complex lumbar spinal stenosis. Clin Orthop 2001;384:18–25.
17. Grubb SA, Jipscomb HJ, Suh PB. Results of surgical treatment of painful adult scoliosis. Spine 1994;19:1619–1627.
18. Matsui H, Tsuji H, Sekido H, et al. Results of expansive laminoplasty for lumbar spinal stenosis in active manual workers. Spine 1992;17:S37–40.
19. Tsuji H. Posterior lumbar surgery. In: Tsuji H, Dawson E, eds. Comprehensive atlas of lumbar spine surgery. St. Louis: Mosby-Year Book, 1991:64–175.
20. Matsui H, Kanamori M, Ishihara H, et al. Expansive lumbar laminoplasty for degenerative spinal stenosis in patients below 70 years of age. Eur Spine J 1997;6:191–196.
21. Aebi M. Correction of degenerative scoliosis of the lumbar spine. A preliminary report. Clin Orthop 1988;232:80–86.
22. Marchesi DG, Aebi M. Pedicle fixation devices in the treatment of adult lumbar scoliosis. Spine 1992;17:S304–309.
23. Simmons ED Jr., Simmons EH. Spinal stenosis with scoliosis. Spine 1992;17:S117–120.
24. Zurbriggen C, Markwalder TM, Wyss S. Long-term results in patients treated with posterior instrumentation and fusion for degenerative scoliosis of the lumbar spine. Acta Neurochir 1999;141:21–26.
25. Oguma T, Hatayama A, Kanayama M, et al. Clinical results of posterior lumbar interbody fusion with threaded interbody fusion cage for degenerative lumbar kyphoscoliosis—a preliminary report. Spine Spinal Cord 1999;12:255–262 [in Japanese].
26. Etebar S, Cahill DW. Risk factors for adjacent-segment failure following lumbar fixation with rigid instrumentation for degenerative instability. J Neurosurg (Spine 2) 1999;90:163–169.

CHAPTER 60

Nondegenerative Spondylolisthesis: Epidemiology and Natural History, Classification, History and Physical Examination, and Nonoperative Treatment of Adults

James Rainville

Spondylolisthesis is defined as a displacement of a vertebral body on the one below it. The term is derived from the Greek *spondylos* (vertebra) and *olisthesis* (a slippage or falling). The term was first used by Kilian in 1854 (1), though this spinal deformity was first described by Herbinaux in 1782 (2). Both descriptions were in obstetric literature as cases of severe anterior displacement of the fifth lumbar vertebra on the sacrum that were noted to compromise the pelvic inlet during labor and delivery.

The most common direction of spondylolisthesis, and the alignment abnormality that will be implied when the term is used in this chapter, is a forward or anterior displacement of the superior vertebral body, sometimes referred to as anterolisthesis. Posterior vertebral displacement termed *retrolisthesis,* and lateral displacement termed *laterolisthesis* are also commonly observed abnormalities of vertebral alignment.

The intact neural arches of the lumbar vertebrae add stability to the spinal motion segments, in part through the function of the inferior and superior articular processes of the facet joints. In the lumbar region, anterior displacement of the superior vertebra of each motion segment is resisted through overlapping of its inferior articular processes with the superior articular processes of the vertebra below (3). In 1855, Robert zu Koblenz first recognized that the presence of spondylolisthesis indicated failure of this essential function (4). When spondylolisthesis is noted, a systemic evaluation of the posterior aspect of the vertebra is required to determine the cause of that failure.

CLASSIFICATION OF SPONDYLOLISTHESIS

The causes of spondylolisthesis can be categorized into distinct categories. Classification of spondylolisthesis into five categories was derived from the collaborative work of Wiltse, Newman, and MacNab (5), and expanded into six by Wiltse and Rothman (6). The classification is based on anatomic characteristics of the neural arch for the first two types, and on acquired pathologic conditions for the last four types. Following presentation of this classification, this chapter will focus mainly on issues relevant to congenital and isthmic spondylolisthesis.

Type I: Congenital or Dysplastic Spondylolisthesis

Congenital abnormalities of the lumbosacral junction can permit slippage of L5 on the sacrum. These are divided into three subtypes.

Subtype IA

Here the articular processes of the facet joints are poorly developed and have a horizontal (axial) orientation, making them ineffective at preventing forward displacement of the lumbar vertebra above (Fig. 60-1) (5). It is often accompanied by spina bifida of L5 and S1. Although the pars may remain unchanged in this type, critical narrowing of the spinal canal could potentially occur if slip exceeds 25% as the posterior neural arch moves forward. However,

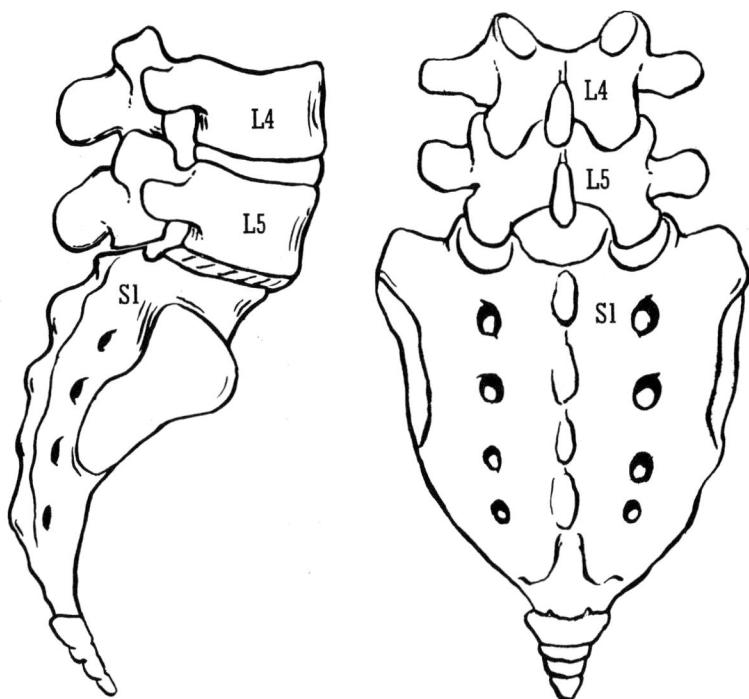

FIG. 60-1. Type IA congenital spondylolisthesis where the facet joints have a horizontal (axial) orientation, making them ineffective at preventing forward displacement of the lumbar vertebra above.

A,B

usually the pars articularis is also hypoplastic and often it either elongates or comes apart, thus preventing critical canal narrowing (6). When abnormalities of the pars interarticularis are combined with this congenital subtype, it is difficult to distinguish this type from the isthmic spondylolisthesis listed below (5).

Subtype IB

In this type the articular processes have a sagittal malorientation but the neural arch is usually intact (Fig. 60-2). The intact neural arch usually prevents high degrees of forward slippage in this type (6).

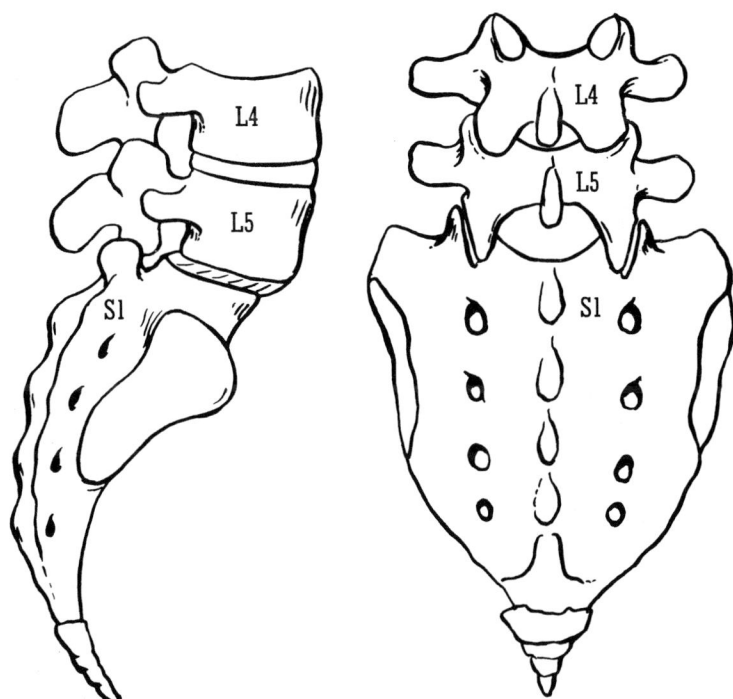

FIG. 60-2. Type IB congenital spondylolisthesis caused by the articular processes having a sagittal malorientation.

A,B

Subtype IC

This group includes all other congenital malformation of the lumbosacral junction, including congenital kyphosis due to congenital failure of vertebral body formation (6).

Type II: Isthmic Spondylolisthesis

In this type of spondylolisthesis, the location of structural failure is the pars interarticularis—the isthmus or bridge of bone between the superior and inferior articular processes of the neural arch. Two subtypes are recognized.

Subtype IIA

By far, the most common abnormality of the pars interarticularis is a bony defect that completely disrupts its integrity, termed *spondylolysis* [Greek: *spondylos* (vertebra) and *lysis* (loosening)] (Fig. 60-3). Spondylolysis can occur bilaterally or unilaterally. When bilateral spondylolysis is present, the inferior articular processes and the lamina are structurally dissociated from the remainder of the vertebra. This compromises the ability of the facet joints to control vertebral movement and alignment at that segment, thus allowing spondylolisthesis to occur (5).

Subtype IIB

Spondylolisthesis can also result from elongation of the pars interarticularis without separation (Fig. 60-4).

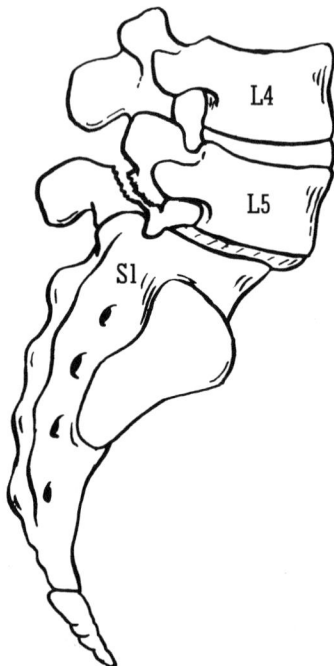

FIG. 60-3. Type IIA isthmic spondylolisthesis caused by bony defects of the pars interarticularis.

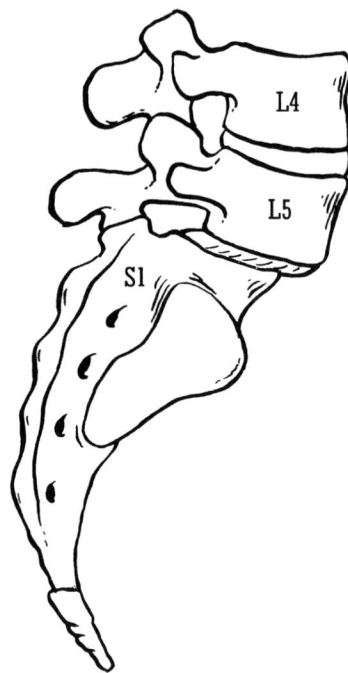

FIG. 60-4. Type IIB isthmic spondylolisthesis caused by elongation of the pars interarticularis.

The elongation is thought to develop from repeated fracturing and healing of the pars that occurs as the vertebral body slides forward (6).

Type III: Degenerative Spondylolisthesis

Long-standing degeneration of the lumbar motion segment can lead to failure of the ability of the facet joints to maintain normal sagittal vertebral alignment. This is discussed in Chapters 54 through 58.

Type IV: Traumatic Spondylolisthesis

This condition results from severe trauma, with acute fractures often involving multiple parts of the pedicles and neural arch. The resulting structural incompetence allows forward slippage to develop over a period of weeks or longer (6).

Type V: Pathologic Spondylolisthesis

In the presence of local or generalized bony disease, abnormalities can develop in the pedicles and neural arch leading to their failure to resist the forward thrust of the upright spine, resulting in spondylolisthesis (6). Basu et al. presented two cases of spondylolisthesis in patients with osteogenesis imperfecta caused by pathologic elongation of the pedicles (7).

Type VI: Postsurgical Spondylolisthesis

During spinal surgery performed to decompress compromised neural elements, large amounts of the posterior supporting structures including the facet joints can be removed in order to obtain adequate decompression. In approximately 4% of cases, this can lead to incompetence of the neural arch and facet joints (and in some cases stress fractures of the weakened inferior articular process) and resulting spondylolisthesis (6,8).

EPIDEMIOLOGY AND NATURAL HISTORY OF SPONDYLOLYSIS

Spondylolysis is an acquired condition, as it has never been documented in fetal dissections or at birth (9–12). Spondylolysis can occur soon after birth however and has been reported in infants less than 1 year of age (13,14). The majority of cases of spondylolysis are thought to occur in young children. Radiographic screenings of children entering first grade (ages 5 to 7) have identified defects in 4.4 % of that population (13,15). By 18 years of age, 6% of that same population was observed to have spondylolysis, suggesting that an additional 1% to 2% of people developed spondylolysis during later childhood and adolescents (13). Few additional cases are thought to occur throughout adult life, and the prevalence of 6% has been documented in radiographic screening of large numbers of adult spines (16). Spondylolysis is almost twice as common in males than females (7.7% versus 4.6%), (13,17), and is more frequently seen in white than black populations (12).

Higher prevalence of spondylolysis has been reported in some populations. Clinical studies of Alaskan Eskimo and archeologic studies of some Eskimo and Native American skeletons have noted a rate of spondylolysis of ranging from 17% to 53% (18–20). Children and adolescents aggressively participating in certain activities such as gymnastics (21–23), throwing sports (23), football (24), wrestling (25), dance (21), and swimming breast and butterfly strokes (26) are suspected to have a higher incidence of acute spondylolysis caused by the mechanical stresses of those sports on the pars interarticularis.

Spondylolysis occurs most frequently at the L5 vertebra, where about 90% of the cases are found, and then with decreasing frequency at higher lumbar levels (13,17,27).

Numerous factors have been implicated in the etiology of spondylolysis. Wiltse suggested that the basic lesion was a stress fracture of the pars interarticularis (28). His theory postulates that significant forces were transmitted through the pars interarticularis during vigorous activities and that either from repeated minor trauma, or occasionally after a single traumatic incident, a stress fracture develops. When this stress fracture fails to unite, spondylolysis results. Wiltse's theory implies that the pars inter-

articularis of some individuals is structurally susceptible to fracture under physiologic stresses that are common to active children and adolescents.

This theory has received some support by histologic studies of the lumbar vertebrae of human fetuses performed by Sagi et al. (29). They noted that after 12 to 13 weeks of gestation, ossific nuclei of the neural arch for the lower lumbar vertebrae were present in the region of the pars interarticularis and resulted in uneven distribution of trabeculation and cortication in these regions. This results in the development of a potential area of weakness, or a stress riser, that would be susceptible to failure under repeated stress or micro trauma. Of interest, in the upper lumbar spine, where spondylolysis is infrequently observed, the ossific nuclei were noted to be at the base of the pedicles and more uniform trabeculation of the pars was observed (29).

It seems likely that the upright posture and resulting lumbar lordosis are required to deliver sufficient stress to the pars interarticularis in order to induce spondylolysis. This is supported by the lack of spondylolysis in the lumbar spines of neurologically impaired individuals who have never walked (30), and the absence of neural arch defects in any species other than humans, the only species with lordosis in the lumbar spine (14).

A genetic predisposition to spondylolysis has long been suspected. Relatives of index cases of spondylolysis have been observed to have a greater incidence of this finding that ranges from 19% to 69% (5,13,31–33). Perhaps it is some morphologic feature of the pars interarticularis that is genetically transmitted which results in a predisposition to the formation of the pars defect (28,31,33).

EPIDEMIOLOGY AND PROGRESSION OF SPONDYLOLISTHESIS

Radiographic evidence of spondylolisthesis is present in many children and adolescents at the time of diagnosis of spondylolysis. Fredrickson et al. noted spondylolisthesis in 68% of children with spondylolysis detected by radiographic screening at entry to first grade (13). For those who developed spondylolysis after first grade, Fredrickson et al. only noted spondylolisthesis in 35%. Higher prevalence of spondylolisthesis may occur in patients with spondylolysis who present for medical care. Wiltse et al. suggested that spondylolisthesis developed in about 50% of older children and adolescents who presented with symptoms of back pain suggestive of acute spondylolysis (28). Studies headed by both Danielson and Frennered noted spondylolisthesis in over 80% of children who were evaluated in a hospital clinic for spondylolysis (34,35). In contrast to these studies, Ishida et al. observed a much lower rate of spondylolisthesis of 40% in a review of 325 radiographs of patients with spondylolysis (36).

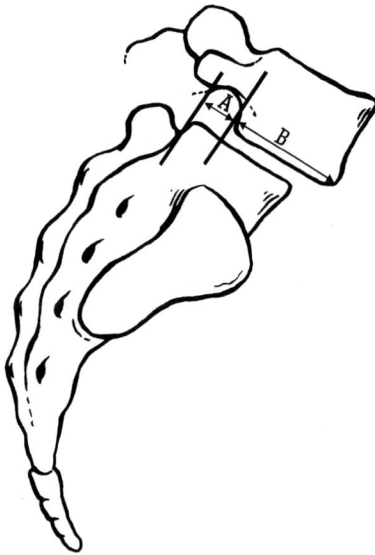

FIG. 60-5. The percent of slippage of spondylolisthesis is calculated by measuring the distance between the posterior borders of L5 and S1 at the level of the superior end plate of S1. This measurement is divided by the sagittal length of the inferior end plate of L5 and expressed as a percentage.

The degree of spondylolisthesis can be described in several ways. The slippage can be quantified by measuring the distance between the posterior borders of L5 and S1 at the level of the superior end plate of S1. This measurement is divided by the sagittal length of the inferior end plate of L5 and expressed as a percentage (Fig. 60-5) (34). At least 5% slippage must be present to confer a diagnosis of spondylolisthesis (36). In clinical practice, slippage is more commonly categorized into five grades:

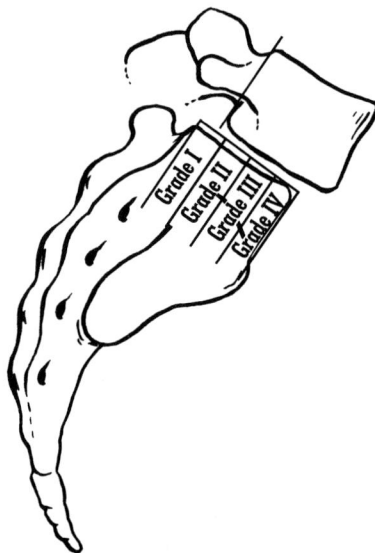

FIG. 60-6. Meyerding classification of spondylolisthesis into grades is based on the amount of slippage of the superior vertebral body on the vertebrae below.

grade I indicates slippage from 5% to 25%; grade II, 26% to 50%; grade III, 51% to 75%; and grade IV over 75% (Fig. 60-6) (37). Grade V, termed *spondyloptosis*, refers to complete dislocation of L5 on S1.

The vast majority of cases of spondylolisthesis (60% to 75%) are classified as grade I, with 20% to 38% classified as grade II, and less than 2% of all cases grade III, IV, or V (17,36,38,39).

Progression of Slippage

Following diagnosis, substantial concern about possible progression of spondylolisthesis is common. Fortunately, progression of slippage has received considerable study.

Evidence suggests that most progression of spondylolisthesis occurs in the immature skeleton. In a follow-up study of spondylolysis in children and adolescents that did not heal with conservative treatment, Sairyo et al. observed progression of slippage in 80% of children in the cartilaginous stage of skeletal development, and in 17% during the apophyseal stage of development. After skeletal maturity, no progression was noted (40). These findings that connect slip progression with skeletal maturity help explain the observation of others who have noted that most progression occurs during childhood and the early teenage years (13,41), and only minor progression occurs after skeletal maturity (42,43).

Prognostic factors are lacking to predict progression of spondylolisthesis (34,35). In a study of slip progression of 311 young patients (less than age 30) with mean observation time of 3.8 years, no radiographic or demographic predictor of progression could be found (34). When observed, only rarely was the slip progression greater than 20%. High initial slip correlated with a combination of high slip angle, convexity of the upper end plate of S1, low lumbar index and disc height reduction, but these factors did not predict further slippage. Instead these factors are suspected to be the consequences of high-degree spondylolisthesis (34). Participation in competitive sports does not influence progression of spondylolisthesis (44).

Several recent studies have noted an anatomic finding that may influence spondylolisthesis. It has been observed that spondylolisthesis was rare in cases of spondylolysis in which there was an increased vertical thickness of the L5 transverse process (45,46). They found that this increased thickness of the transverse process was associated with increased size of the posterior band of the iliolumbar ligament, and postulated that this increased stability of the L5 vertebra, thus preventing anterior displacement (45). The same findings were noted to predict adjacent disc degeneration in older subjects with spondylolysis. Those with slender L5 transverse processes were found to have advanced degeneration at L5-S1, and those with thicker transverse processes had little degeneration at L5-S1 but advanced degeneration at L4-5 (36).

Progression of spondylolisthesis in adults has been noted in several studies. Spondylolisthesis may develop or progress with advancing age, though the amount of slippage is generally small (36,46). Fredrickson et al. noted a slip progression of 2%, 5%, and 1% during the third, fourth, and fifth decades, respectively (42). Floman reported on a series of 18 spondylolytic patients presenting with back pain. He demonstrated progression of a mean of 15% in vertebral slippage over an average of 7 years (47). In adults, disc degeneration at the level of the defect occurs with greater frequency in individuals with spondylolysis and spondylolisthesis (48,49), and when it occurs is associated with slip progression (39,42,47). Neither the degree of disc degeneration nor the amount of spondylolisthesis is associated with the prevalence of back pain (39) and no study has linked progression of slip with pain symptoms.

Symptoms and Disability

It is apparent that the development of spondylolysis in toddlers and young children produces only minor symptoms, if any symptoms at all, for complaints of back pain are not acknowledged by the adults responsible for their care. Because of this, the development of spondylolysis is rarely detected in this age group (13,14,28).

For older children and adolescents, back pain occurring with the development of spondylolysis is a more common complaint, especially in those with acute stress reactions or acute stress fractures of the pars interarticularis. The intensity of pain can range from mild to severe (35), therefore, this diagnosis must be considered in all children and adolescents presenting with back pain, especially those participating in aggressive physical activities (28,35,50,51). Sciatica has been reported in a small percentage of adolescents with spondylolysis but neurologic deficits are rare (13,35,42).

In adults, an association between spondylolysis and spondylolisthesis with pain symptoms has been hard to establish (17). The soft tissue at the site of spondylolysis contains sensory nerve fibers and neuropeptides with potential to generate pain (52,53). Several epidemiologic studies (13,17,39,42), along with case series (38,47,49, 54–56) of subjects with spondylolysis and spondylolisthesis, confirm that some have back pain complaints. Saraste observed that low back pain symptoms were more frequently reported in the subpopulation of young adults with spondylolisthesis of greater than 25% (grade 2 or higher), with a high slip angle, with spondylolysis at the L4 level, or with early disc degeneration (48). In contrast, no relationship was noted between the grade of slippage and back pain in older adults (39). Abnormal motion or instability at the spondylolytic level has not been demonstrated to occur in adults with back pain (57,58). Clearly, most people with spondylolysis and spondylolisthesis are asymptomatic, and the incidence of back pain in adults

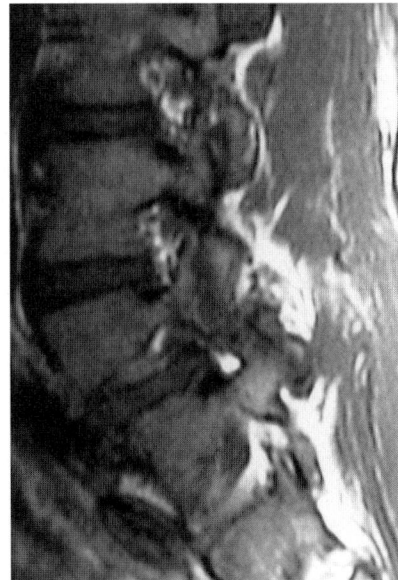

FIG. 60-7. Neuroforaminal stenosis caused by disc material entrapping the L3 nerve root under the pedicle above.

with these problems is similar to that in the population in general (13,17,31,33,39,56,59,60).

Some patients with spondylolisthesis develop progressive neuroforaminal encroachment, most commonly by disc material pushing upward toward the root from below and trapping it under the pedicle above, that can ultimately cause nerve root entrapment with resultant signs and symptoms (Fig. 60-7) (61–63). The most commonly involved roots are L5. The rate of occurrence of lumbar radiculopathies in spondylolisthesis is not reported, but is most likely quite low, but certainly not rare.

For women, spondylolysis and spondylolisthesis were not found to be risk factors for pregnancy complications, nor was pregnancy associated with slip progression or increased low back pain symptoms (64).

Disability because of back pain is not more prevalent in adults with spondylolysis and spondylolisthesis than in the general public (38,39,60). In studies of young athletes with spondylolysis and spondylolisthesis, frequent problems related to pain or disability were not observed, even in those participating in contact sports (44,65).

Regardless of the low frequency of symptoms with spondylolysis and spondylolisthesis, some patients do present with back pain or sciatica attributable to these structural problems. When patients do develop symptoms, spondylolysis and spondylolisthesis may be considered within the context of the patient's complex spinal situation, and viewed as concurrent factors but not necessarily the cause of symptoms.

PHYSICAL EXAMINATION

The physical examination in spondylolysis and spondylolisthesis has few specific or sensitive findings.

Detection of spondylolisthesis on physical examination is difficult except in the rare cases of grade III or greater slips. Here a "step off" of the spinous processes can be seen or palpated at the level of the spondylolisthesis. In grade I and II spondylolisthesis, the "step off" is much more difficult to detect, and not a reliable finding in our experiences. Painful trunk range of motion is often noted with children and adolescents with symptoms from acute spondylolysis. This is especially noted for trunk extension, as this motion shifts load to the facet joints and neural arch and thus through the region of the pars (66). Limitation of range of motion for trunk extension has been observed (38,67), and palpation of the back may reveal local tenderness at the lumbosacral junction (38). Unfortunately, these findings are common to other spinal disorders, and are not specific for spondylolysis.

Neurologic deficits and positive straight leg-raising tests are rarely found in cases of spondylolisthesis, including cases with sciatica (38). When neurologic deficits are noted, they usually involve the L5 roots that can become irritated within their neuroforamina (38,61,62).

CONSERVATIVE TREATMENT OF ADULTS WITH SPONDYLOLYSIS AND SPONDYLOLISTHESIS

Spondylolysis and spondylolisthesis are often first detected in adults when they present for evaluation and treatment of back or leg pain complaints. When discovered, these findings must be considered within the context of the complete clinical picture, and only with caution should the patient's symptoms be attributed to these bony abnormalities.

In general, evaluation and treatment of acute back pain in adults with spondylolysis and spondylolisthesis should follow recommendation for nonspecific low back pain, including avoidance of bed rest and rapid return to activities (68–71). No studies have addressed the use of commonly prescribed medication, modalities, and manual therapies for treatment of symptoms in this population. Some researchers have advocated extension bracing for adults with back pain including those with spondylolisthesis (72), but convincing evidence of efficacy is lacking.

Exercise

Exercise is commonly prescribed for the treatment of back pain. Several studies have evaluated exercise as a treatment for back pain with associated spondylolysis and spondylolisthesis.

Möller and Hedlund randomized a population of 111 adults with isthmic spondylolisthesis to one of three groups: an exercise program, posterolateral fusion, or posterolateral fusion with transpedicular fixation (38).

The exercise group underwent a program consisting of eight simple exercises that did not require equipment and four exercises that required a pulley and leg press machine. Exercises focusing on strengthening both the back and abdominal muscles and postural training were performed 3 times per week for 6 months, and then twice a week for the next 6 months under the guidance of a physical therapist. At 1- and 2-year follow-up, the exercise group demonstrated a small reduction in pain, and no change in disability. Both function and pain were significantly better in the two surgical groups. Return to work rates were similar for both groups at 2 years (54% versus 55%).

Another study compared flexion versus extension exercises in 48 adults with spondylolisthesis (73). The study reports randomly assigning patients to different physicians who prescribed (or perhaps preferred) either flexion or extension exercises. Flexion exercises consisted of pelvic tilts and the seated chest to thigh maneuvers, and extension exercises consisted of upper trunk extension and hip extension performed in the prone position. The study does not report on the type of instruction, the frequency and duration of the exercises, exercise compliance, or the methods used for conducting follow-up. Short- and long-term results strongly favored the flexion exercise group. Unfortunately, methodologic shortcomings make the findings interesting but in need of further study before full endorsement of flexion exercises can be given.

O'Sullivan et al. studied stabilization exercises in a group of patients with chronic back pain and spondylolysis or spondylolisthesis (74). They randomized 44 patients to a specific stabilization exercise treatment or uncontrolled care directed by their treating practitioner. The stabilization exercise group underwent 10 weekly sessions of physical therapy aimed at training the specific contraction of the deep abdominal muscles, namely the internal oblique and the transverse abdominus with coactivation of the lumbar multifidus muscles, presumably selectively proximal to the pars defect. After accurate patterns of co-contractions were achieved, these were incorporated into daily activities. The control group received variable exercises and passive treatment. Their results showed that the stabilization exercise group experienced significant reduction in pain intensity and disability scores compared to the control group. These results were maintained at 30-month follow-up.

Rainville and Mazzaferro reported on a group of 48 patients with spondylolysis and spondylolisthesis with chronic low back pain who were treated with exercise (75). This exercise program was based on the functional restoration model, where physiologically intensive exercises are prescribed to eliminate impairments in trunk flexibility, strength, and endurance. The exercise program was not altered because of the presence of spondylolysis and spondylolisthesis Exercises were supervised by a physical therapist, consisting of resistive training, stretching and endurance activities, and were done in both flexion and extension directions. Patients were encouraged to continue exercising in the presence of tolerable pain (76). Treatment time averaged 6 weeks. Outcomes included measurements of flexibility, strength, pain, and disability. Significant improvements in flexibility and strength were noted, and were similar to those observed in patients without these abnormalities. During treatment, pain score decreased by an average of 36%, and disability scores by 46%. Long-term outcomes were not reported.

Injections

The use of spinal injection for the treatment of spondylolysis or spondylolisthesis has not been studied. Some clinicians do use injection with corticosteroid or local anesthetic agents into the facet joints adjacent to the pars defects, and others directly into the pars defects as potentially therapeutic interventions for back pain symptoms in these patients, but efficacy has not been validated. Some clinicians use selective injections as tools to diagnose the specific pain generator in spondylolysis. The lack of joint capsules at the pars defects, and the potential for uncontrolled spread of injected material may limit the conclusions that can be drawn regarding specific pain generators from these injection procedures (77,78).

In cases of radicular pain and foraminal stenosis, selective nerve root blocks with local anesthetic agents or corticosteroids may be used to try to confirm the source of pain generation or to treat the radicular symptoms. We are unaware of any studies that address this procedure in spondylolysis and spondylolisthesis.

CONCLUSION

Conservative treatment options for adults with pain symptoms and spondylolysis and spondylolisthesis have received sparse study. In general, following the common treatment guidelines for back pain seems merited. Some evidence suggest that exercise may be useful, with programs using flexion exercises, spine stabilization, and aggressive stretching and strengthening all having some advocates. Diagnostic and therapeutic selective spinal injections may be of some use, but have not been studied in this population.

REFERENCES

1. Kilian HF. De spondylolisthesi gravissimae pelvagustiae caussa nuper detecta. Commentario anatomico-obstetrica. Bonn: C Georgii Co, 1854.
2. Herbrinaux G. Traité sur divers accouchements laborieux, et sur les polypes de al matrice. Brussels: J.L. DeBoubers, 1782.
3. Hollinshead WH. Anatomy for surgeons: volume 3—the back and limbs. New York: Harper & Row, 1982.
4. Robert zu Koblenz. Eine eigentümliche angeborene Lordose wahrscheinlich bedingt eine Verschiebung des Korpers des letzten Linden-
worbels auf die vorderee Flache des ersten Kreuheinwirbels (Spondylolisthesis, Kilian) nebst Bemerkungen über die Mechanik dieser Beckenformation. Monatsschr Geburtskd Frauenkrank 1885;5:891–894.
5. Wiltse LL, Newman PH, MacNab I. Classification of spondylolysis and spondylolisthesis. Clin Orthop 1976;117:23–29.
6. Wiltse LL, Rothman LG. Spondylolisthesis: classification diagnosis and natural history. Semin Spine Surg 1993;5:264–280.
7. Basu PS, Hilali Noordeen MH, et al. Spondylolisthesis in osteogenesis imperfecta due to pedicle elongation: report of two cases. Spine 2001;26:E506–509.
8. Lee CK. Lumbar spinal instability (olisthesis) after extensive posterior spinal decompression. Spine 1983;8:429–433.
9. Batts M. The etiology of spondylolisthesis. J Bone Joint Surg 1939;21:879–884.
10. Chandler FA. Lesions of the "isthmus" (pars interarticularis) of the laminae of the lower lumbar vertebrae and their relation to spondylolisthesis. Surg Gynecol Obstet 1931;53:273–306.
11. Hitchcock HH. Spondylolisthesis. Observations on its development, progression and genesis. J Bone Joint Surg 1940;22:1–16.
12. Rowe GG, Roche MB. The etiology of separate neural arch. J Bone Joint Surg 1953;35A:102–111.
13. Fredrickson BE, Baker D, McHolick WJ, et al. The natural history of spondylolysis and spondylolisthesis. J Bone Joint Surg 1984;66A:699–707.
14. Wertzberger KL, Peterson HA. Acquired spondylolysis and spondylolisthesis in the young child. Spine 1980;5:437–442.
15. Baker DR, McHolick WJ. Spondyloschisis and spondylolisthesis in children. J Bone Joint Surg 1956;38A:933–934.
16. Virta L, Rönnemaa T, Österman K, et al. Prevalence of isthmic lumbar spondylolisthesis in middle aged subjects form eastern and western Finland. J. Clin Epidemiol 1992;45:917–922.
17. Österman K, Schlenzka D, Poussa M, et al. Isthmic spondylolisthesis symptomatic and asymptomatic subjects, epidemiology, and natural history with special reference to disc abnormalities and mode of treatment. Clin Orthop Rel Res 1993;297:65–70.
18. Bridges PS. Spondylolysis and its relationship to degenerative joint disease in the prehistoric southeastern United States. Am J Phys Anthropol 1989;79:321–329.
19. Simpler LB. Spondylolysis in Eskimo skeletons. Acta Orthop Scand 1986;57:78–80.
20. Stewart T. The age incidence of neural arch defects in Alaskan natives, considered from the standpoint of etiology. J Bone Joint Surg 1953;35A:937–950.
21. Hutchinson MR. Low back pain in elite rhythmic gymnasts. Med Sci Sports Exerc 1999;31:1686–688.
22. Jackson DW, Wiltse LL, Ciricincione RJ. Spondylolysis in female gymnast. Clin Orthop 1976;117:68–73.
23. Soler T, Calderon C. The prevalence of spondylolysis in the Spanish elite athletes. Am J Sports Med 2000;28:57–61.
24. McCarroll JR, Miller JM, Ritter MA. Lumbar spondylolysis and spondylolisthesis in college football players. A prospective study. Am J Sports Med 1986;14:404–406.
25. Granhed H, Morelli B. Low back pain among retired wrestlers and heavyweight lifters. Am J Sports Med 1988;16:530–533.
26. Nyska M, Constantini N, Cale-Benzoor M. Spondylolysis as a cause of low back pain in swimmers. Int J Sports Med 2000;21:3775–3779.
27. Rothman SL, Glenn WV. CT multiplanar reconstruction in 253 cases of lumbar spondylolysis. Am J Neuroradiol 1984;5:81–90.
28. Wiltse LL, Widell EH, Jackson DW. Fatigue fracture: the basic lesion in isthmic spondylolisthesis. J Bone Joint Surg 1975;57A;17–22.
29. Sagi HC, Jarvis JG, Uhthoff HK. Histomorphic analysis of the development of the pars interarticularis and its association with isthmic spondylolysis. Spine 1999;23:1635–1640.
30. Rosenberg NJ, Bargar WL, Friedman B. The incidence of spondylolysis and spondylolisthesis in nonambulatory patients. Spine 1981;6:35–38.
31. Albanese M, Pizzutillo PD. Family study of spondylolysis and spondylolisthesis. J Pediatr Orthop 1982;4:495–499.
32. Shahriaree H, Sajadi KM, Rooholamini SA. A family with spondylolisthesis. J Bone Joint Surg 1979;61A:1256–1258.
33. Wynne-Davies R, Scott JHS. Inheritance and spondylolysis. J Bone Joint Surg 1979;61B:301–305.
34. Danielson BI, Frennered AK, Irstam LKH. Radiologic progression of

isthmus lumbar spondylolisthesis in young patients. Spine 1991:16: 422–425.

35. Frennered AK, Danielson BI, Nachemson AL. Natural history of symptomatic isthmic low-grade spondylolisthesis in children and adolescents: a seven-year follow-up study. J Pediatr Orthop 1991;11: 209–213.

36. Ishida Y, Ohmori K, Inoue H, et al. Delayer Vertebral slip and adjacent disc degeneration in isthmic defect of the fifth lumbar vertebra. J Bone Joint Surg 1999;81B:240–244.

37. Meyerding HW. Spondylolisthesis. Surg Gynecol Obstet 1932;54: 371–377.

38. Möller H, Hedlund R. Surgery versus conservative management in adult "isthmic spondylolisthesis" a prospective randomized study: part I. Spine 2000;25:1711–1715.

39. Virta L, Rönnemaa T. The association of mild-moderate isthmic lumbar spondylolisthesis and low back pain in middle-age patients is weak and it only occurs in women. Spine 1993;18:1496–1503.

40. Sairyo K, Katoh S, Ikata T, et al. Development of spondylolytic olisthesis in adolescents. Spine J 2001;1:171–175.

41. Seitsalo S, Österman K, Hyvarinen H et al. Progression of spondylolisthesis in children and adolescents—a long-term follow-up of 272 patients. Spine 1991;16:417–421.

42. Fredrickson BE, Baker D, Murtland AM, et al. The natural history of spondylolysis and spondylolisthesis: 45-year follow-up. Paper presented at: North American Spine Society 15th Annual Meeting; October 26, 2000; New Orleans.

43. Ikata T, Miyake R, Katoh S, Morita T, Musase M. Pathogenesis of sports-related spondylolisthesis in adolescents—radiographic and magnetic resonance imaging study. Am J Sports Med 1996;24:94–98.

44. Muschik M, Hahnel H, Robinson PN. Competitive sports and the progression of spondylolysis. J Pediatr Orthop 1996;16:364–369.

45. Moriya H, Shimada Y. Does the iliolumbar ligament prevent anterior displacement of the fifth lumbar vertebra with defects of the pars? J Bone Joint Surg 2000;82B:846–850.

46. Ohmori K, Ishida Y. Takatsu T, et al. Vertebral slip in lumbar spondylolysis and spondylolisthesis. Long-term follow-up of 22 adult patients. J Bone Joint Surg 1995;77B:771–773.

47. Floman Y. Progression of lumbosacral isthmic spondylolisthesis in adults. Spine 2000;25:342–347.

48. Saraste H. Long-term clinical and radiological follow-up of spondylolysis and spondylolisthesis. J Pediatr Orthop 1987;7:631–638.

49. Szypryt EP, Twining P, Mulholland RC, et al. The prevalence of disc degeneration associated with neural arch defects of the lumbar spine assessed by magnetic resonance imaging. Spine 1989;14:977–981.

50. Micheli LJ. Back injuries in dancers. Clin Sports Med 1983;2: 473–484.

51. Morita T, Ikata T, Katoh S, et al. Lumbar spondylolysis in children and adolescents. J Bone Joint Surg 1995;81B:620–625.

52. Eisenstein SM, Ashton IK, Roberts S, et al. Innervation of the spondylolysis "ligament". Spine 1994;19:912–916.

53. Nordström D, Santavirta S, Seitsalo S, et al. Symptomatic lumbar spondylolysis. Neuroimmunologic studies. Spine 1994;19:2752–2758.

54. Apel DM, Lorenz MA, Zindrick MR. Symptomatic spondylolisthesis in adults: four decades later. Spine 1989;14:345–348.

55. Harris IE, Weinstein SL. Long-term follow-up of patients with grade-III and grade-IV spondylolisthesis—treatment with or without posterior fusion. J Bone Joint Surg 1987;69A:960–969.

56. Porter RW, Hibbert CS. Symptoms associated with lysis of the pars interarticularis. Spine 1984;9:755–758.

57. Axelsson P, Johnsson R, Strömqvist B. Is there increased intervertebral mobility in isthmic adult spondylolisthesis? A matched comparative study using roentgen stereophotogrammetry. Spine 2000;25: 1701–1703.

58. Pearcy M, Shepherd J. Is there instability in spondylolisthesis? Spine 1985;10:175–177.

59. Congeni J, McCulloch J, Swanson K. Lumbar spondylolysis: a study of natural progression in athletes. Am J Sports Med 1997;25:248–253.

60. Frennered K. Isthmic spondylolisthesis among patients receiving disability pension under the diagnosis of chronic low back pain syndromes. Spine 1994;19:2766–2769.

61. Jinkins JR, Matthews JC, Sener RN, et al. Spondylolysis, Spondylolisthesis, and associated nerve entrapment in the lumbosacral spine: MR evaluation. Am J Roentgenol 1992;159:799–803.

62. Jinkins JR, Rauch A. Magnetic resonance imaging of entrapment of lumbar nerve roots in spondylolytic spondylolisthesis. J Bone Joint Surg 1994;76A:1643–1648.

63. Rijk PC, Deutman R, De Jong TE. Spondylolisthesis with sciatica. Magnetic resonance findings and chemonucleolysis. Clin Orthop 1996;326:146–152.

64. Saraste H. Spondylolysis and pregnancy—a risk analysis. Acta Obstet Gynecol Scand 1986;65:727–729.

65. Semon RL, Spengler D. Significance of lumbar spondylolysis in college football players. Spine 1981;6:172–174.

66. Yamane T, Yosida T, Mimatsu K. Early diagnosis of lumbar spondylolysis by MRI. J Bone Joint Surg 1993;75B:764–768.

67. McGregor AH, Cattermole HR, Hughes SPF. Global spinal motion in subjects with lumbar spondylolysis and listhesis. Does the grade or type of slip affect global spinal motion? Spine 2001;26:282–286.

68. Bigos SJ (chair). Acute low back problems in adults: clinical practice guideline. Rockville: US Department of Health and Human Services, Agency for Health Care Policy and Research, 1994.

69. Deyo RA, Diehl AK, Rosenthal M. How many days of bed rest for acute low back pain? A randomized clinical trial. N Engl J Med 1986; 315:1064–1070.

70. Gilbert JR, Taylor DW, Hildebrand A, et al. Clinical trial of common treatments for low back pain in family practice. Br Med J 1995;291: 789–794.

71. Malmivaara A, Hakkinen U, Aro T, et al. The treatment of acute low back pain-bed rest, exercises or ordinary activity? N Engl J Med 1995; 332:351–355.

72. Spratt KF, Weinstein JN, Lehmann TR, et al. Efficacy of flexion and extension treatments incorporating braces for low-back pain patients with retrodisplacement, spondylolisthesis, or normal sagittal translation. Spine 1993;18:1839–1849.

73. Sinaki M, Lutness MP, Ijjlstrup DM, et al. Lumbar spondylolisthesis: retrospective comparison and three-year follow-up of two conservative treatment programs. Arch Phys Med Rehabil 1989;70:594–598.

74. O'Sullivan PB, Twomey LT, Allison GT. Evaluation of specific stabilizing exercise in the treatment of chronic low back pain with radiologic diagnosis of spondylolysis or spondylolisthesis. Spine 1997;22:2959–2967.

75. Rainville J, Mazzaferro R. Evaluation of outcomes of aggressive spine rehabilitation in patients with back pain and sciatica from previously diagnosed spondylolysis and spondylolisthesis. Arch Phys Med Rehabil 2001;82:1309.

76. Rainville J, Sobel J, Hartigan C, et al. Decreasing disability in chronic low back pain through aggressive spine rehabilitation. J Rehabil Res Develop 1997;34:383–393.

77. Park WM, McCall IW, Benson D, et al. Spondylarthrography: the demonstration of spondylolysis by apophyseal joint arthrography. Clin Radiol 1985;36:427–430.

78. Maldague B, Mathurin P, Malghan J. Facet joint arthrography in lumbar spondylolisthesis. Radiology 1981;40:29–36.

CHAPTER 61

Imaging in the Evaluation of Lumbar and Lumbosacral Spondylolysis and Spondylolisthesis

Stephen L. Gabriel Rothman and Leon L. Wiltse

Spondylolysis and spondylolisthesis continue to fascinate the medical community, with an ever-increasing mass of information being published each year (1). As imaging techniques become more sophisticated, more detailed information is available to the clinician. Thin section computed tomography (CT) with reformations (2,3) and magnetic resonance imaging (MRI) allow detailed analysis of the abnormal motion segment as never before. This chapter reviews the classification of spondylolisthesis and spondylolysis and illustrates how modern imaging studies have expanded our understanding of the group of disorders.

ANATOMIC CLASSIFICATION

The classification adopted here is based primarily on the previous work of Wiltse et al., slightly modified from previous editions of the compendium. The classification is anatomic without regard to underlying etiology.

1. Congenital
    A. Juvenile dysplastic spondylolisthesis—This is type of spondylolisthesis occurs in young children. The articular processes of the affected motion segment are axially oriented. The anomalous articular processes are often associated with spina bifida of the upper sacral segment. This unstable anatomic situation may lead to forward slippage (4,5).
    B. Adult facet misalignment—Congenital or developmental asymmetry of the articular processes occurs in two general forms. The articular processes may be sagittally oriented and therefore parallel to one another or they may be anomalous

in their orientation and asymmetric (Fig. 61-1). In both of these instances, the articular processes are free to glide forward one upon the other causing slippage in adult life as the joints begin to degenerate.
    C. Other congenital anomalies of the lumbar spine allow spondylolisthesis to occur. Congenital kyphosis is the most common anomaly (6).
2. Isthmic spondylolisthesis—The lesion is within the pars interarticularis. There are three variants.
    A. Lytic spondylolisthesis—The most common type of spondylolisthesis is a stress fracture of the pars interarticularis that has not healed (7).
    B. Healed lytic spondylolisthesis—Slippage is due to elongated pars interarticularis caused by healing of a previous stress fracture of the pars.
    C. Acute fractures of the pars. These are very rare and are associated with other fractures of the neural arch or articular processes.
3. Degenerative spondylolisthesis—This type is due to articular subluxation caused by 4. Postsurgical spondylolisthesis.
    A. Slippage due to surgical removal of most or all of the articular processes.
    B. Postoperative stress fractures of the base of the articular processes at the junction with the lamina. This occurs in patients with extensive partial facetectomy.
5. Posttraumatic spondylolisthesis—This condition is always due to very severe trauma of the neural arch other than the pars.
6. Pathologic spondylolisthesis—Slippage is due to deformity of the pars caused by a bone softening disease.

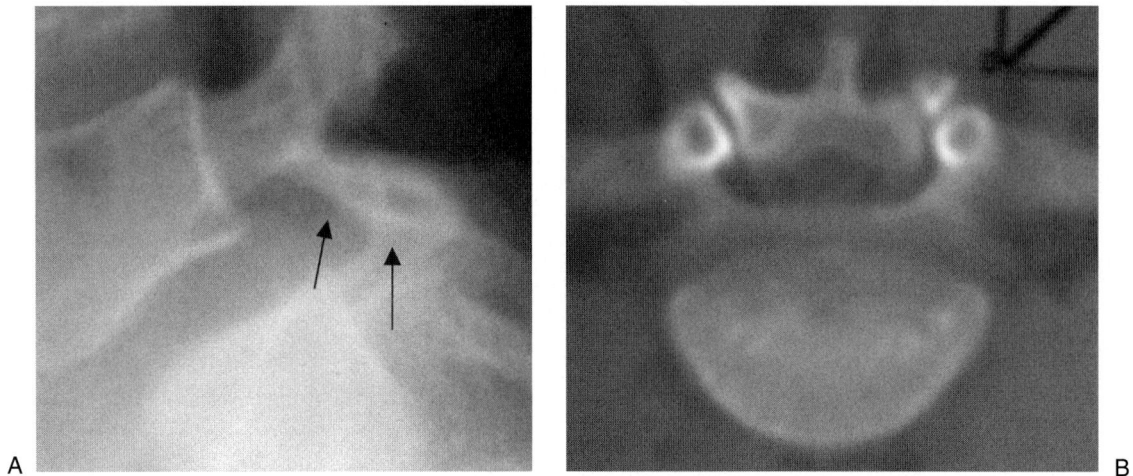

FIG. 61-1. Elongated but intact pars: **A:** Lateral radiograph showing elongation of the pars. There is no localized callus formation and no clear signs of pseudarthrosis. There is no open pars defect. **B:** Axial computed tomography scan shows dysplasia of the articular processes.

TYPES OF SPONDYLOLISTHESIS

Congenital Spondylolisthesis

Type A

Congenital spondylolisthesis of the lumbosacral area in young children is due to hypoplasia or dysplasia of the superior sacral segment. This most commonly manifests itself as a combination of spina bifida occulta of S1 and deformity of the sacral articular processes. The superior articular processes of the sacrum are axially oriented and very short. There is concomitant deformity of the inferior articular processes of L5 (Fig. 61-2). The inferior articular processes of L5 parallel the horizontally oriented sacral facets. This axial orientation produces a pair of joints, which allow forward slippage, because the articular processes cannot check the forward gliding of L5 on the sacrum. With flexion, the weight of the body bearing down upon the axial-oriented facets causes forward deformity and spondylolisthesis. The pars interarticularis remains intact in this disorder. Consequently, if the slippage significantly exceeds 35%, cauda equina compression is likely to occur. This manifests itself as tightness of the hamstrings.

On occasion there may be more pronounced anomalies of the first sacral segment and L5. The more the sacrum is hypoplastic the more likely there is to be slippage. Zembo et al. (8) reported a series in infants, two of who had the condition at birth. These lesions are different from congenital kyphosis, which usually occurs in the thoracolumbar area.

Type B

Adult congenital spondylolisthesis is a disorder of the articular processes. Slippage probably occurs because of an unstable orientation of the articular processes (Fig. 61-3). Typically, the articular processes are sagittally oriented. In most normal people, a line drawn along the plane of the joint surfaces of the lumbosacral facets will intersect within the spinal canal or vertebral body. Because of this orientation, the inferior articular processes prevent excessive forward gliding of the superior articular processes upon flexion. There is bone against bone contact throughout the range of motion. When the articular processes are sagittally oriented, there is no bone on bone contact in flexion. The soft tissues of the joint capsules bear the force of flexion and allow forward subluxation. In some patients, the articular processes are parallel to each other. This may also allow spondylolisthesis.

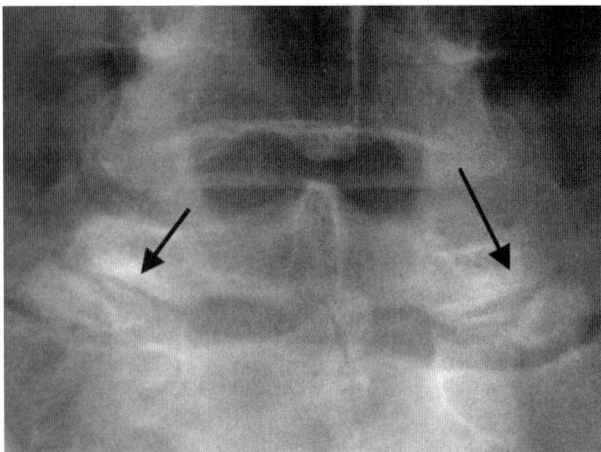

FIG. 61-2. Congenital spondylolisthesis. Frontal radiographs on a patient with flat, axially oriented articular processes. Note the hypoplasia of the superior surface of the sacrum with spina bifida occulta.

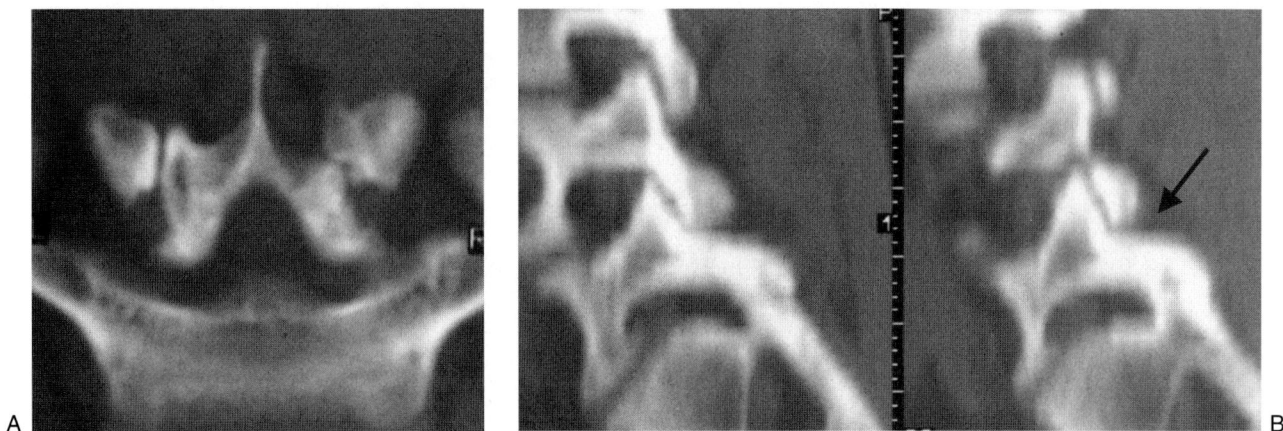

FIG. 61-3. Adult congenital spondylolisthesis. Axial computed tomography scan **(A)** and sagittal reformation **(B)** reveal abnormal orientation of the articular processes. The right articular processes is sagittally angulated and the left is hypoplastic.

Type C

Other severe congenital anomalies may be associated with spondylolisthesis. Congenital kyphosis is the most common member of this group. Congenital failure of formation of a vertebral body, congenital failure of segmentation, and combinations of complex anomalies may all lead to spondylolisthesis (9).

ISTHMIC SPONDYLOLYSIS AND SPONDYLOLISTHESIS

Spondylolysis is one of the most common disorders of the lumbar spine. It is firmly established that lytic defects of the pars interarticularis are stress fractures of childhood. There are fewer than five reported cases of spondylolysis in very young children. There is a report on a child of 8 months with a defect in the pars interarticularis whose father had a similar lesion (10). Boukow and Kleiger (11) reported on a child whose defect was diagnosed at 4 months of age.

The fractures typically begin to make their appearance around the age of 5. There is an occurrence peak between the beginning of kindergarten and the end of the second grade. Baker and McHolick (12) and Frederickson et al. (13) reviewed radiographs on a large number of children at approximately 5 years of age and again 2 years later. Approximately 4.4% of children developed pars defects in this age group. The same authors reviewed films on the same group of patients and proved that approximately 2% more will develop spondylolysis by age 19, with a peak in the teenage years.

Spondylolysis is not caused by a single traumatic event. It is due to the repeated stresses of life. In teenagers, there is usually a history of sports-related back pain. The disorder is extraordinarily common in gymnasts, divers, and other participants in bending and twist-

ing activities. The etiology is unknown. There is a definite genetic propensity for developing pars fractures. Approximately 30% of Northern Slope Alaskan Eskimos have defects in the pars. There are numerous publications documenting the incidence in other populations.

IMAGING ANALYSIS

In children, the diagnosis of spondylolysis can be made with regular X-rays or nuclear bone scan. The evolving fracture is obvious, especially on single photon emission computed tomography (SPECT) scans. It is not often that CT or MRI is necessary. It is possible to differentiate recent, evolving pars fractures from subacute and chronic lesions by CT. In the acute phase, the fracture line is sharp and jagged. As the lesion progresses the edges of the fracture become indistinct. Although pars fractures can be identified on almost any imaging study, CT is the procedure of choice for defining the subtleties of the bony abnormalities. It is usually possible to define nearly all the bony abnormalities on MRI but it requires more interpretive skill and high-quality images. Subtle signal changes can be seen in the pars on MRI during the acute phase similar to other fractures but they are hard to define. Bright signal is noted on the T2-weighted sequences in the pars and adjacent lamina and pedicle. Low signal is noted on the T1 scans. Abnormal signal within the pars and adjacent pedicle may be the earliest signs on MRI even before the fracture is obvious. There is occasionally abnormal signal noted within the adjacent pedicle in adults with spondylolysis. This is thought to represent increased fat in the marrow space (Fig. 61-4).

L5 Spondylolysis

Having reviewed MR images and CT scans on more than 3,000 patients with spondylolysis and spondylolis-

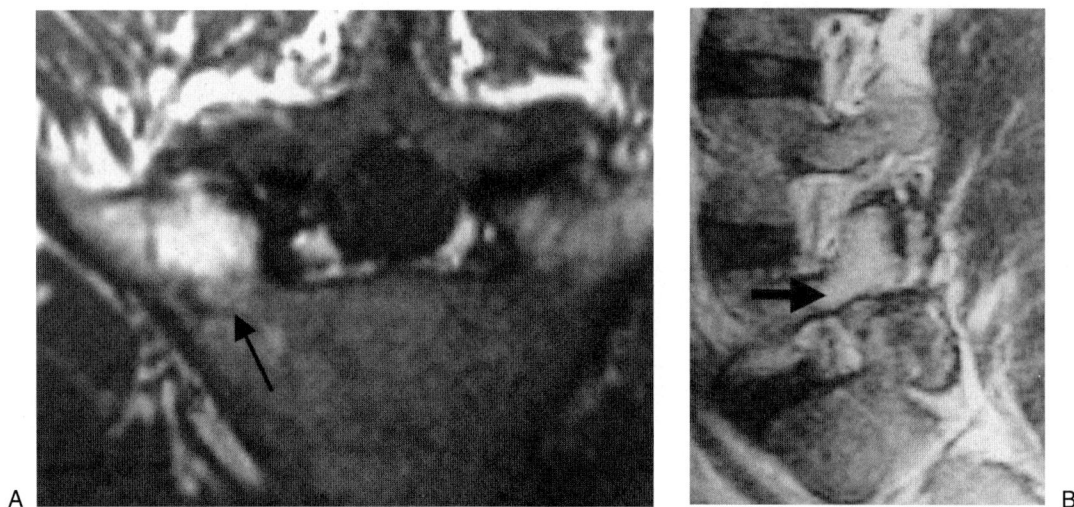

FIG. 61-4. **A:** Axial T1-weighted magnetic resonance (MR) scan with abnormal bright signal with the pedicles adjacent to pars defects. **B:** Sagittal T2 MR scans show similar bright signal within the pedicle and adjacent bone.

thesis, a theory has evolved regarding the etiology of stress fractures of the neural arch. It has long been realized from routine radiographs, that anomalies of the superior sacral segment were very common in spondylolysis. Spina bifida occulta, for example, is extremely common. What was not obvious from regular X-rays is that another manifestation of superior sacral dysplasia is hypoplasia of the superior articular processes of the sacrum.

Children who develop pars fractures between the ages of 5 and 7 rarely have any clinical signs. The diagnosis was made based on imaging studies. Teenagers who develop pars fractures will usually have back pain. Nuclear bone scans in this painful period will be positive because of the body's attempt to heal the fractures. It is therefore reasonable to presume that there must be some difference in the cause or mechanism of fracture development.

A review of 250 consecutive reformatted CT scans of the lumbar spines in patients with L5 spondylolysis revealed two distinct anatomic patterns that suggest a unifying theory of the etiology of pars fractures and appears to explain the difference in clinical presentation.

Axial CT scans on patients with L5 spondylolysis reveal that approximately two-thirds will have hypoplastic superior articular processes of the first sacral segment (Fig. 61-5). Other minor and occasional major anomalies are also noted in this group of patients. Spina bifida occulta is the most common. One-third of patients with L5 spondylolysis have normal articular processes and neural arch (Fig. 61-6). This ratio of two-thirds with hypoplastic facets and one-third with normal facets is the same ratio Frederickson et al. (13) showed between the occurrence rate peaks in young children between the ages of 5 and 7 and the second teenage peak. We believe that this is not mere happenstance.

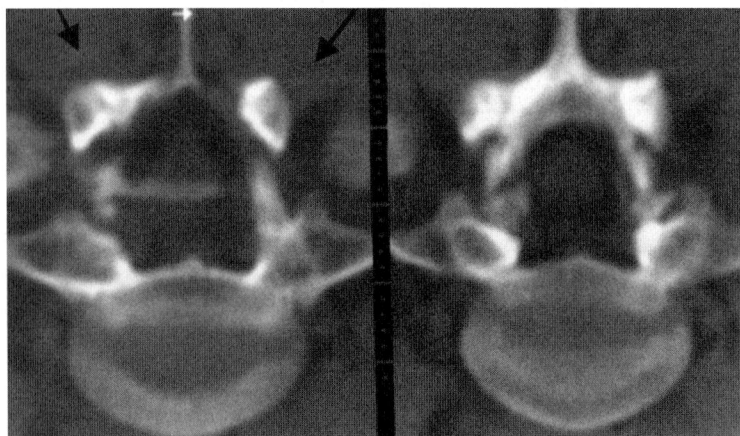

FIG. 61-5. Axial computed tomography scans showing marked symmetric hypoplasia of the sacral articular processes with forward slippage of L5 on the sacrum.

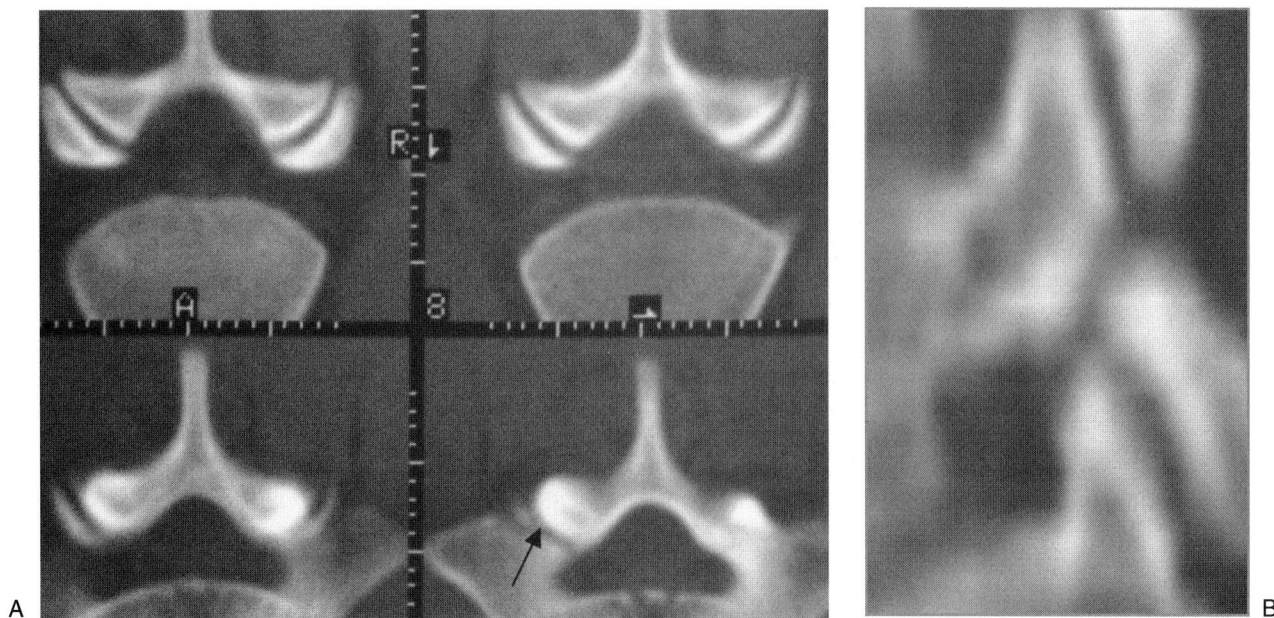

FIG. 61-6. A: Axial computed tomography scan demonstrates normal sacral articular processes and spondylolysis. **B:** Sagittal reformation shows the normal position of the superior articular process of the sacrum with respect to the pars.

In our series, the teenage patients with a known history of vigorous sports activity always had normal neural arches and normal sacral articular processes. None of the patients with an obvious sports-related clinical syndrome had hypoplastic articular processes. We were able to scan a number of children early in the course of a bout of severe back pain. In some of these children, recent fractures with sharp edges were visualized on the sagittal reformations. In several instances, fracture lines were visualized that had not gone completely through the pars. They always occurred in the same location. The fracture was always open on the inferior surface on the pars. The superior surface of the pars was intact. Several of these children had follow up CT scans. In some cases the partial fracture was seen to progress to complete fracture. In some cases, the fracture was noted to heal. Figure 61-7 depicts a CT scan on a child who presented with recent back pain. The nuclear scan was positive unilaterally. Note the unilateral partial fracture of the pars on the axial images and the sagittal reformations. Approximately one month later, the scan was repeated because of increasing back pain. The repeat scan demonstrated bilateral open pars fractures. Contrast this with the pair of scans in Figure 61-8. This child was also scanned because of recent onset of severe back pain and a unilaterally positive bone scan. On the initial scan, a fracture is noted extending superiorly from the undersurface of the pars extending upward toward the pedicle but completely through the bone. A follow-up scan approximately 6 weeks later showed that the fracture had healed. The pars was scle-

rotic and slightly deformed. A small residual deformity was noted at the most inferior edge of the pars where the fracture began. This pattern of healing is quite common.

None of the patients with pars fractures, which were in a phase of active healing, had hypoplastic articular processes. According to Frederickson et al. (13), none of the children in their series who developed spondylolysis between the ages of 5 and 7 had any low back symptoms. We believe that the finding of hypoplastic articular processes on the CT or MRI scan indicates that the spondylolysis developed silently between the ages of 5 and 7. This would account for all the CT observations.

Unilateral Spondylolysis

A series of CT scans was reviewed on adult patients with unilateral spondylolysis. There are two possible causes for unilateral spondylolysis in adults. Either the patients had a single stress fracture that failed to heal or had bilateral stress fractures that healed on only one side. It is certainly probable that both scenarios occur (as we have shown previously two patients, one of whom healed the fracture and one who went on to develop bilateral fractures). We suspect that most adult patients who are diagnosed with unilateral spondylolysis originally had bilateral fractures with healing on one side. The evidence for this is twofold. The most telling fact is that there is frequently sclerosis and deformity of the contralateral neural arch in patients with unilateral spondylolisthesis (Fig. 61-9). This may be so striking as to be confused

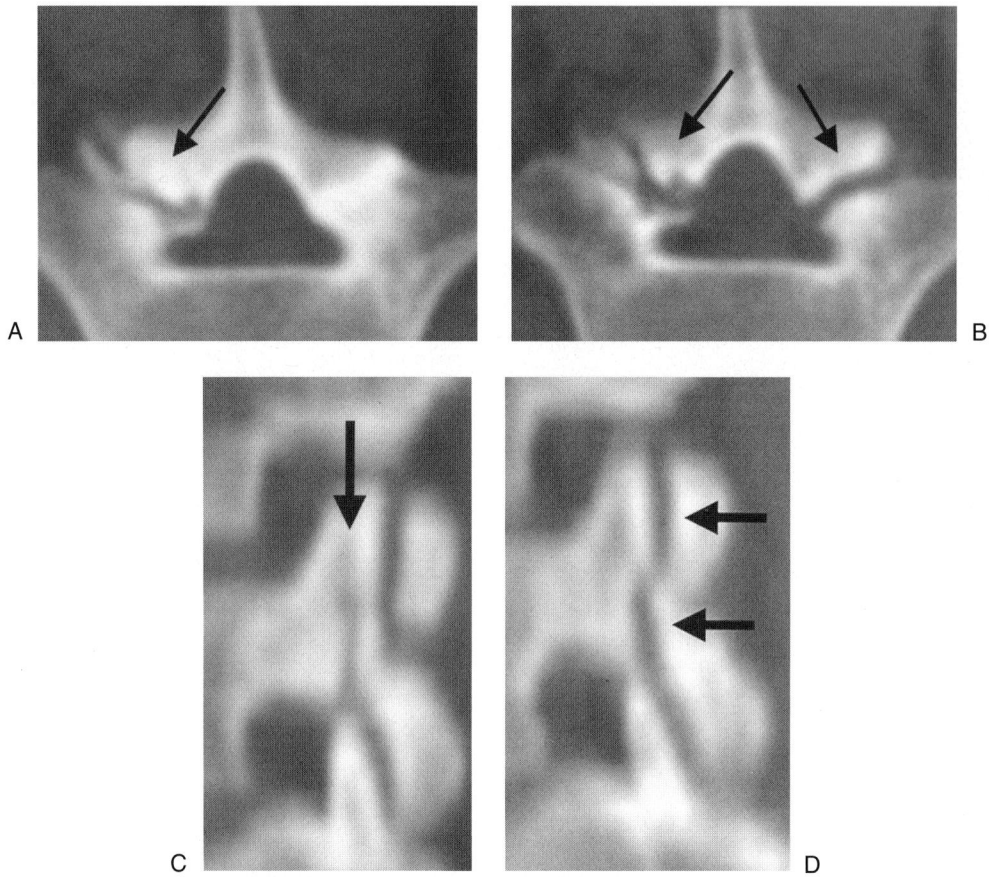

FIG. 61-7. Pars fracture in evolution **A:** Axial computed tomography (CT) taken near the onset of back pain. There is a unilateral right-sided pars fracture. The left pars is intact. **B:** Axial CT scan approximately 6 weeks later now shows bilateral pars fractures. **C:** Sagittal reformation of the first scan. The fracture line extends superiorly from the tip of the sacral articular process but does not extend completely through the pars. **D:** Sagittal reformation of the second scan. The fracture now extends completely through the pars and the defect has completely widened. The opposite pars looked identical.

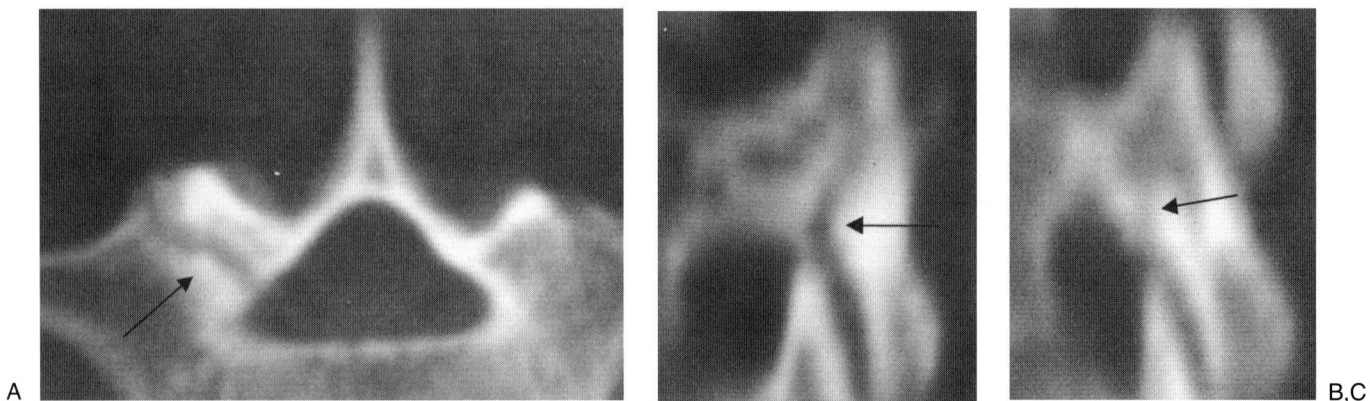

FIG. 61-8. Pars fracture in evolution. **A:** Axial computed tomography (CT) scan shows a very subtle lucency within the right pars *(arrow).* This is the evolving pars fracture. **B:** Sagittal reformation. The fracture extends partially through the pars pointing superiorly from the tip of the normal size sacral articular process. **C:** Sagittal reformation performed on a second CT scan done several months later shows that the fracture line has shortened and the bone is more sclerotic indicating healing.

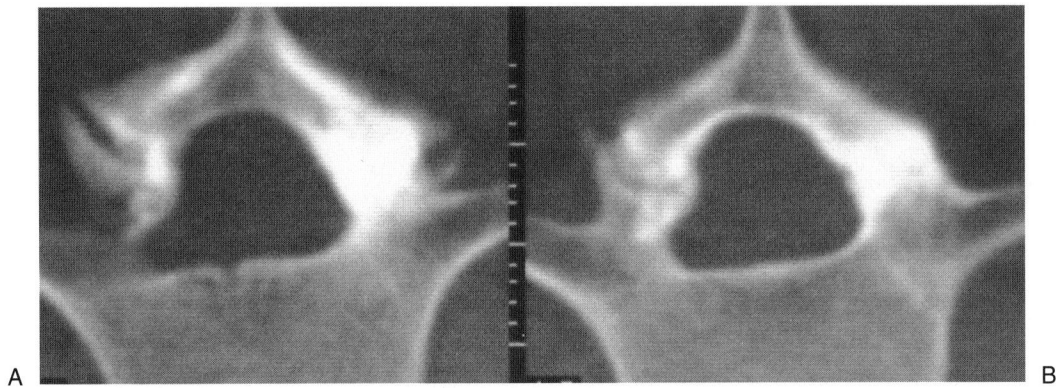

FIG. 61-9. Unilateral spondylolysis. Axial computed tomography scans demonstrate open pars defect on the right side and a dense, sclerotic lamina on the left. The lamina is diffusely thickened.

with osteoblastoma, the most common hyperostotic benign lesion of the neural arch. The explanation in the older literature was that the thickening of the neural arch and prominence of the trabeculae was due to the "stress effect" on the contralateral lamina. Based on CT observations on the many other neural arch stress fractures that will be discussed subsequently and on the numerous cases of proven healed spondylolysis, it seems obvious that this is not correct. Rather the sclerosis is due to a healed pars or laminar fracture.

The second interesting observation is that the majority of patients with unilateral spondylolysis have unilateral hypoplastic sacral articular processes. Occasionally the entire hemilamina is hypoplastic (Fig. 61-10). When we tabulated our data on this group of patients, we found the same two-thirds to one-third ratio of hypoplastic facets that was noted in the bilateral pars group. Remarkably, in the group with hypoplastic articular processes, the hypoplastic facet was always on the side of the open pars defect.

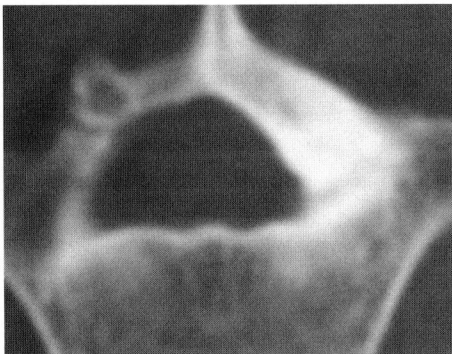

FIG. 61-10. Hypoplasia of the lamina and articular process on the side of an open pars defect. Axial computed tomography scans reveal a normal left articular process and lamina. The right lamina is hypoplastic and there is no recognizable joint.

Healed Spondylolysis

We easily diagnose patients with open pars defects and spondylolisthesis, as their abnormality is obvious. Patients with healed spondylolysis may be very difficult to diagnose. These patients have sustained injury to the lumbosacral motion segment. This may very well lead to early disc degeneration. The deformity of healed pars defects is less well known and may only be seen on high-quality reformatted CT scans. There is usually residual deformity with bone sclerosis. There are numerous adult patients whose CT scans reveal sclerosis and subtle deformity of the pars. This has been termed "hockey stick" deformity and usually represents healing of the fracture with slight lengthening of the pars. The older literature describes many patients with a diagnosis of congenital spondylolysis with intact neural arch. While this probably occurs due to microfractures that do not actually separate, we believe that the great majority of these patients have healed bilateral spondylolysis. The subtle changes of healing are obvious on high-quality reformatted CT. The previous generations of researchers could not possibly see these minor abnormalities commonly on regular radiographs.

There are two common patterns of healing definable by CT. The healing fracture may unite *in situ* with little or no slippage. The bone will appear sclerotic as previously demonstrated in Figure 61-8. That scan showed a fracture in the process of healing. A hint of the residual fracture line was seen in that patient and may remain for a long time. In adults with old healed spondylolysis, the pars will be sclerotic and usually deformed in the shape of an inverted hockey stick. In those instances, the fracture heals across the entire width of the fracture line. The CT scan in Figure 61-11 demonstrates the characteristic changes of this type of fracture healing. In some patients, the entire length of the fracture may not heal. Ossification of the ligamentum flavum (which is also the joint capsule

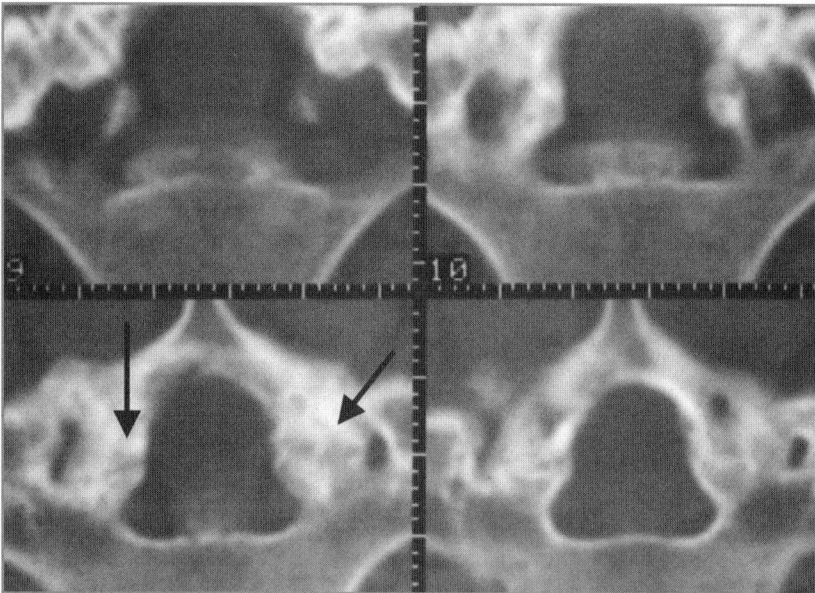

FIG. 61-11. Healed pars fracture in adults. Axial computed tomography demonstrates thickening and deformity of the pars. A faint residual line is noted in the area of the previous fracture.

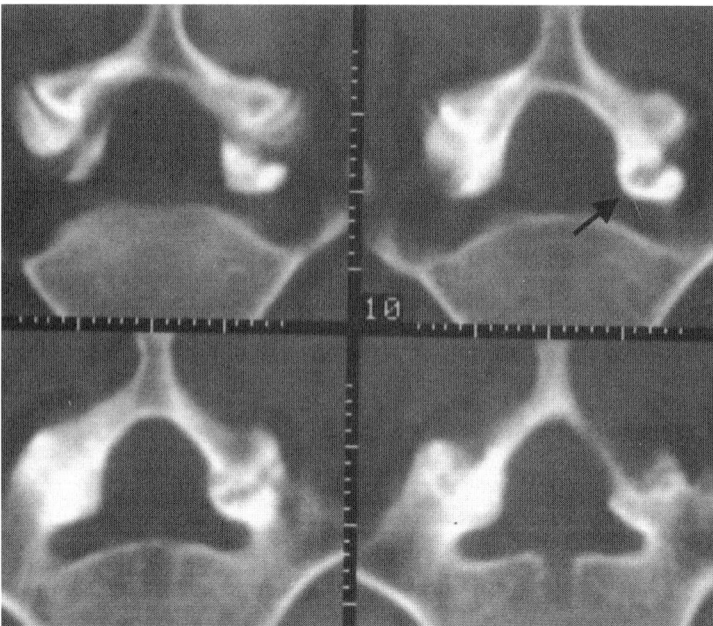

A

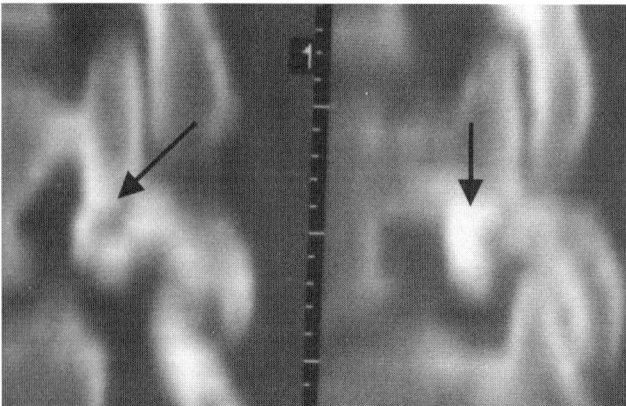

B

FIG. 61-12. A: Axial computed tomography scan on a patient with bilaterally healed pars fractures. The left pars and lamina are diffusely sclerotic, enlarged, and deformed. The entire length of the fracture has closed as in the previous figure. The right pars defect is still visible laterally but fused medially by a bridge of bone. **B:** Sagittal reformatted scan showing a portion of the residual open defect and the dense, downward projection of the bridge of bone which has formed in the ligamentum flavum.

of the zygapophyseal joint) may ossify and produce a medial projecting bridge of bone bridging the pars defect. This bar of bone may extend inferiorly into the neural foramen and compress the exiting L5 nerve (Fig. 61-12).

ADULT SPONDYLOLYSIS AND SPONDYLOLISTHESIS

It is virtually unheard of to find a patient over the age of 20 with recent pars fractures without other major trauma to the motion segment. One must consider the adult pars defect a pseudarthrosis. CT will therefore demonstrate the findings typical of a pseudarthrosis. Adult pars defects have smooth edges, much as we would expect from any pseudarthrosis. Disorganized callus is commonly seen projecting into the spinal canal.

The overwhelming majority of patients with spondylolysis are diagnosed as adults. They present with back pain, leg pain, or both. Frequently, the spondylolysis is unrelated to the cause of the back or radicular pain, which may be coming from an acute process at a higher level. In adults with a diagnosis of spondylolysis made in childhood, spinal imaging is usually performed for the elucidation of the causes of neural compression or for planning operative intervention.

Imaging studies *are useless* for the evaluation of back pain. It is a common logical flaw to presume that the cause of back pain can be diagnosed on CT or MRI. Back pain cannot be seen on scans. A painless spondylolysis and one that is hurting look identical. The amount of slippage says nothing about the existence of back pain because the patient's spine undoubtedly looked the same the day before the onset of back pain as it did the day the scan was performed. Furthermore, nearly all L5 discs will be degenerated in patients with spondylolisthesis. Painful and painless discs look the same. Since approximately 25% of patients with L5 spondylolysis will have disc protrusions at L4 greater than 5 mm, one cannot

even know if the back pain is coming from the next rostral or any other disc space. Furthermore, even seeing hypermobility of the motion segment on flexion and extension films does not allow one to diagnose that as the cause of back pain. Hypermobility and even instability develops over a very long time, and was undoubtedly present on days when there was no back pain. Therefore, seeing hypermobility does not allow one to conclude that it is the cause of back pain. A patient may be having back pain from any of the anatomic areas just mentioned, but one can never conclude from the imaging study that any of these abnormalities is the pain generator.

CAUSES OF RADICULOPATHY

The most common radicular syndrome is due to compression of the L5 nerve roots. This may occur anywhere from the nerve root origin near the L4/L5 disc, the lateral recess, along the course of the L5 neural foramen, and outward, beyond the foramen to the tip of the L5 transverse process. S1 radiculopathy is much less common. Forward slippage of the L5 body actually decompresses the S1 root because the neural arch remains behind with superior articular process of the sacrum. Consequently S1 radiculopathy is an unusual clinical finding. Disc herniation at the L5 level is also very rare.

The L5 root may be compressed at the L4/L5 disc space by a bulging or herniated disc. This is no different than the typical patient with L4/L5 disc herniation. The disc fragment compresses the origin of the L5 root as it exits from the thecal sac. At least one-fourth of patients with L5 spondylolisthesis will have up to 5 mm of disc protrusion at L4/L5. Compression of the L5 root also can occur in the subarticular gutter and the lateral recess due to buildup of fibrocartilaginous material at the pseudarthrosis. This bony callus can become very large. Figure 61-13 shows a patient in whom the callus is so large that the two masses nearly meet in the midline.

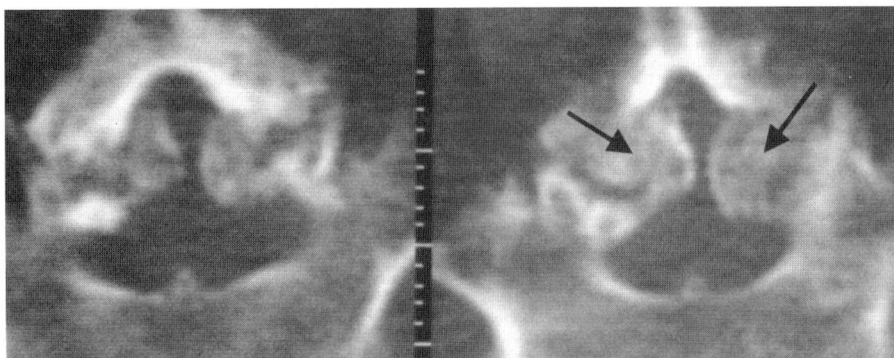

FIG. 61-13. Canal stenosis from fibrocartilaginous buildup at the pseudarthrosis. Axial computed tomography scans demonstrate amorphous lumps of bone projecting from the medial border of each of the pars defects. They nearly meet in the midline.

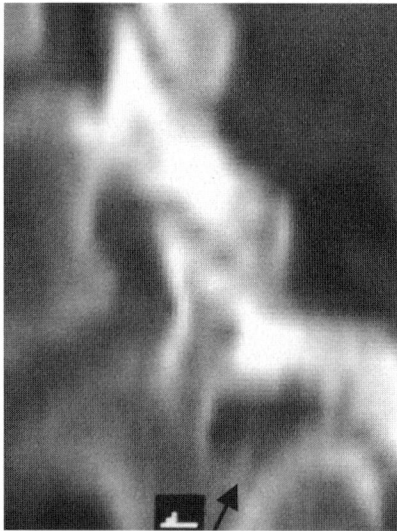

FIG. 61-14. The horizontal foramen of spondylolisthesis. Sagittal reformatted scan reveals normal orientation of the L4/L5 foramen. The L5/S1 foramen is flattened and horizontally oriented. Note the upward projecting spike of bone arising from the inferior end plate of L5.

The L5 root is most often compressed in the neural foramen. The foramen narrows and deforms in a characteristic way. As the L5 body slips forward, the pedicle descends relative to the sacrum and flattens the root against the bulging pseudo-disc and an osteophyte, which frequently projects upward from the superior edge of the sacrum. The shape of the neural foramen in spondylolisthesis is characteristic of vertebral slippage. This produces a horizontally oriented foramen rather than the typical keyhole-shaped foramen (Fig. 61-14). It is important to remember that the foramen is not simply a hole through which the nerve exits. It is a bony channel of at least 1 cm. The nerve root may be compressed throughout the length of the exit canal. Simply widening the entrance to the foramen does little to relieve compression of the L5 nerve. Furthermore, proper decompression of the foramen requires removal of the length of the S1 ridge projecting upward into the L5 nerve.

In patients with advanced slippage, the L5 root can be compressed beyond the exit zone of the neural foramen. This has been termed the "far-out syndrome". It is critical to recognize far-out root compression because routine foraminotomy will fail to cure the radiculopathy. The nerve root is compressed between the transverse process of L5, which has slid forward, and the ala of the sacrum. Proper surgical therapy requires decompression of the nerve root within the foramen as well as removal of the L5 transverse process.

AN ANATOMIC THEORY ON THE ETIOLOGY OF L5 SPONDYLOLYSIS

We believe that the anatomic analysis of the CT scans in our series leads to unifying theory on the etiology of spondylolysis. Since it is uniformly accepted that the basic lesion is a stress fracture, this theory must define a congenital anatomic variation, which should be the precursor of the fracture. We believe that hypoplasia of the sacral articular processes is anatomic malformation. The first premise is that the pars interarticularis is the weakest portion of the neural arch. The pars can be thought of as an inclined plane balanced on the tip of the superior articular process of the sacrum. The fulcrum of rotation is a point within the pars adjacent to the tip of the articular process (Fig. 61-15A, B). In children with normal articular processes, the rostral and caudal portions of the pars are of equal length and therefore balanced. In this balanced state, forces on the pars due to everyday motion are insufficient to fracture the pars.

In children with hypoplastic articular processes of S1, that portion of the pars in apposition to the tip of the articular processes is significantly displaced caudally. The fulcrum of rotation is therefore displaced caudally creating an asymmetric inclined plane with increased stress on the upper portion of the pars (Fig. 61-15C, D). The mobility of everyday life produces excess stress on the rostral end of the pars and causes silent stress fracture. This theory accounts for all of the previously described observations. Two-thirds of patients will develop silent stress fractures between the ages of 5 and 7 years. Two-thirds of patients with both unilateral and bilateral adult pars defects have hypoplastic facets. Finally, since none of the sports-related fractures occurred in patients with hypoplastic facets we can therefore conclude that in children with normal articular processes, the pars fractures are due to increased stress from vigorous sport, even in the face of normal anatomy.

OTHER STRESS FRACTURES OF THE LUMBAR VERTEBRAE

Although stress fractures most commonly occur in the pars interarticularis, any portion of the vertebral ring can fracture. These unusual fractures nearly always occur contralateral to a typical pars fracture and must be considered variants of the spondylolysis complex. The most common non-pars contralateral fracture occurs in the lamina. There are two types. The better-known lesion has been termed a "retro-isthmic cleft". Originally, these lesions were thought to be congenital clefts in the neural arch posterior to a normal pars. They appear as fairly well circumscribed linear lucent defects, which run perpendicular to the long axis of the lamina. They generally have slightly shaggy edges consistent with a pseudoarthrosis and inconsistent with the smooth, corticated edges expected in congenital clefts (Fig. 61-16). These lesions are visible on MRI scans although they are much more difficult to diagnose on MRI than on CT. The signal in the bone adjacent to the cleft is generally low on T1 because of the sclerosis present in the area.

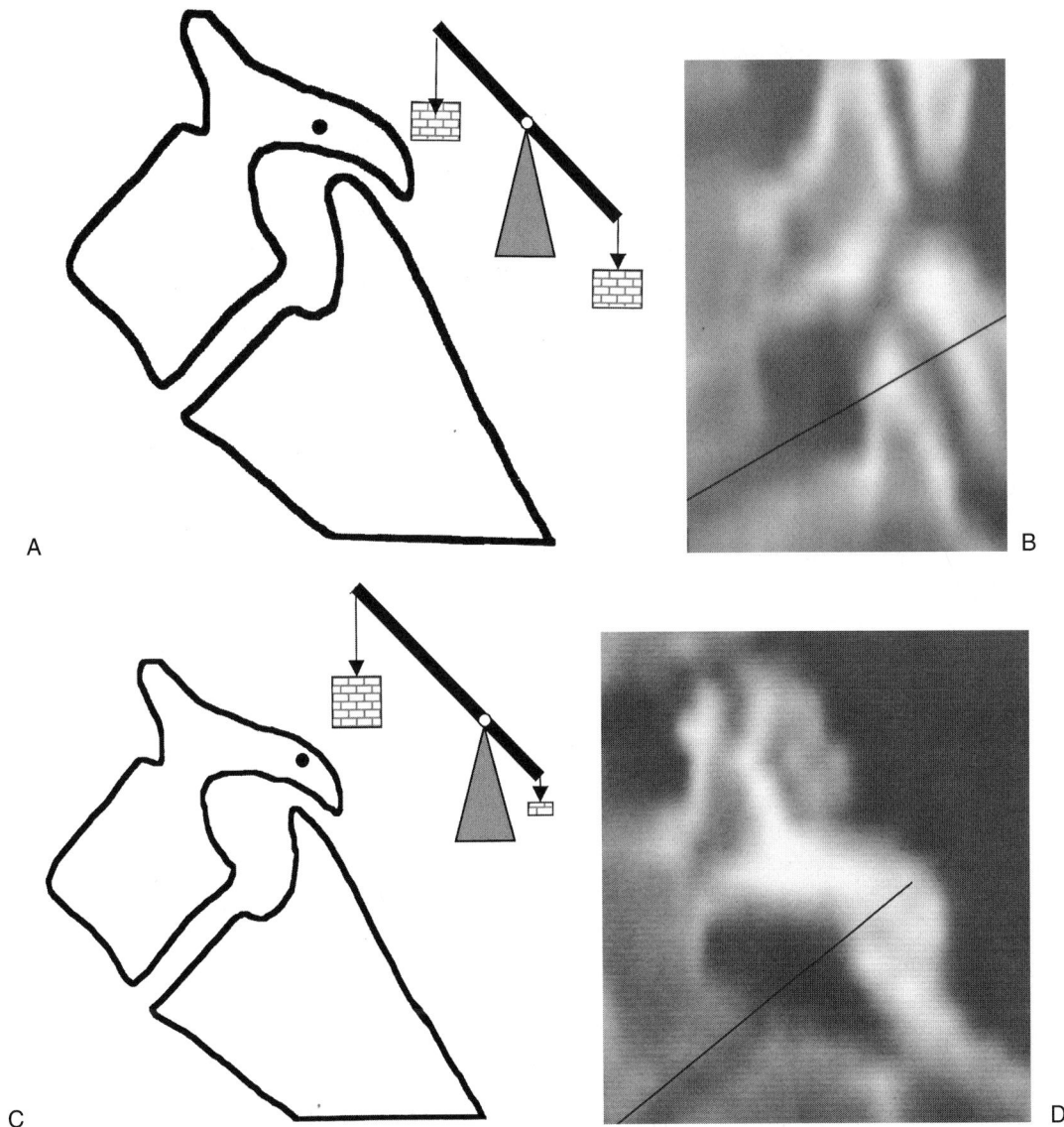

FIG. 61-15. Theory of the etiology of L5 spondylolysis. **A:** Diagrammatic representation of the forces on the pars in a patient with teenage spondylolysis with normal articular processes. Note that the forces on either end of the inclined plane will be balanced. The fulcrum is in apposition to the tip of the superior articular process. **B:** Sagittal computed tomography reformation on a patient with conforming anatomy. A line drawn through the L5/S1 disc passes well below the tip of the sacral articular process. **C, D:** Diagrammatic representation of the forces on the pars in a patient with hypoplastic sacral articular processes. The fulcrum descends along the length of the pars to a point just rostral to the tip of the articular process.

The second type of fracture is perhaps even more common but less well known. It is a spiral fracture through the lamina opposite a typical pars fracture. CT reveals the residual deformity of the fracture. The changes in the lamina are no different from those seen in healing fractures of other long bones (Fig. 61-17). It is probable that the thickened, sclerotic lamina in many patients with unilateral open pars defects are due to healed laminar fractures.

Much less commonly, defects occur within the pedicle on the contralateral side from a regular pars fracture. This is the least common neural arch fracture in our series, being seen in only two patients, one of who was a professional soccer player. Stress fractures of the pedicle can also occur following laminectomy and facetectomy due to weakening of the neural arch by the decompression (Fig. 61-18).

The literature defines a lucent cleft in the vertebral body just anterior to the pedicle as a "retrosomatic cleft". This was originally thought to be a congenital failure of fusion of the vertebral body ossification center to that of the pedicle. High-resolution CT has proven that incorrect. These are vertebral stress fractures. The typical retrosomatic cleft tends to be a well-defined lucent line between the pedicle and the posterior edge of the vertebral body (Fig. 61-19). The fusion plane of the

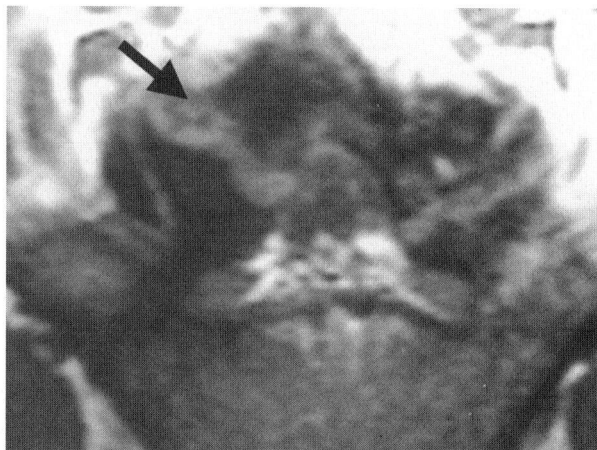

FIG. 61-16. Retro-isthmic cleft. Axial magnetic resonance imaging scan. There is a typical pars defect on the right and a retro-isthmic defect on the left. The edges of both fractures are irregular as seen in any pseudoarthrosis.

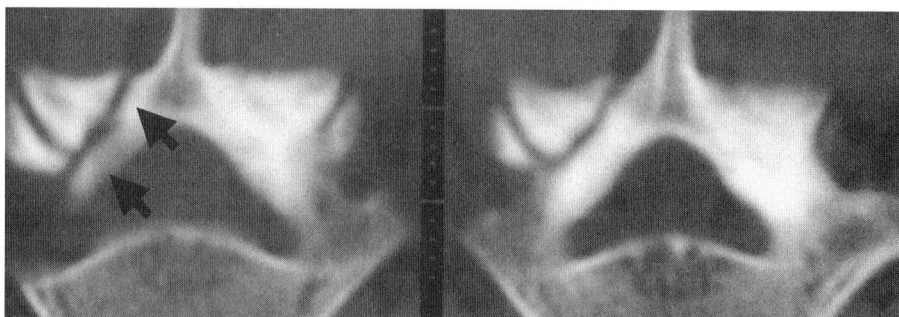

FIG. 61-17. Spiral fracture of the lamina. Axial computed tomography scans reveal an oblique fracture through the left lamina.

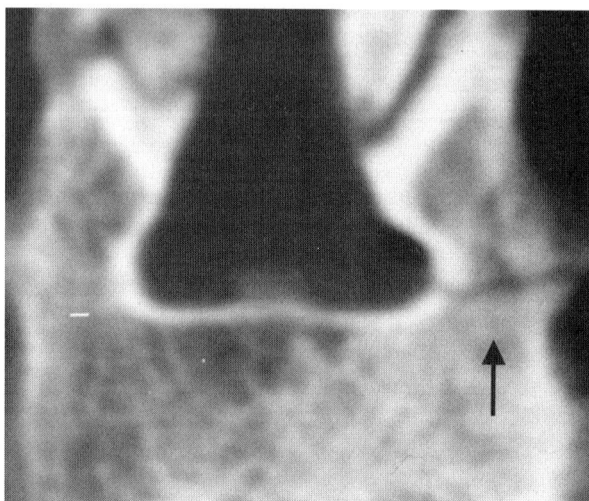

FIG. 61-18. Stress fracture of the pedicle. Axial computed tomography scan reveals sclerosis of the vertebra from degenerative disease. A stress fracture is seen in the right pedicle.

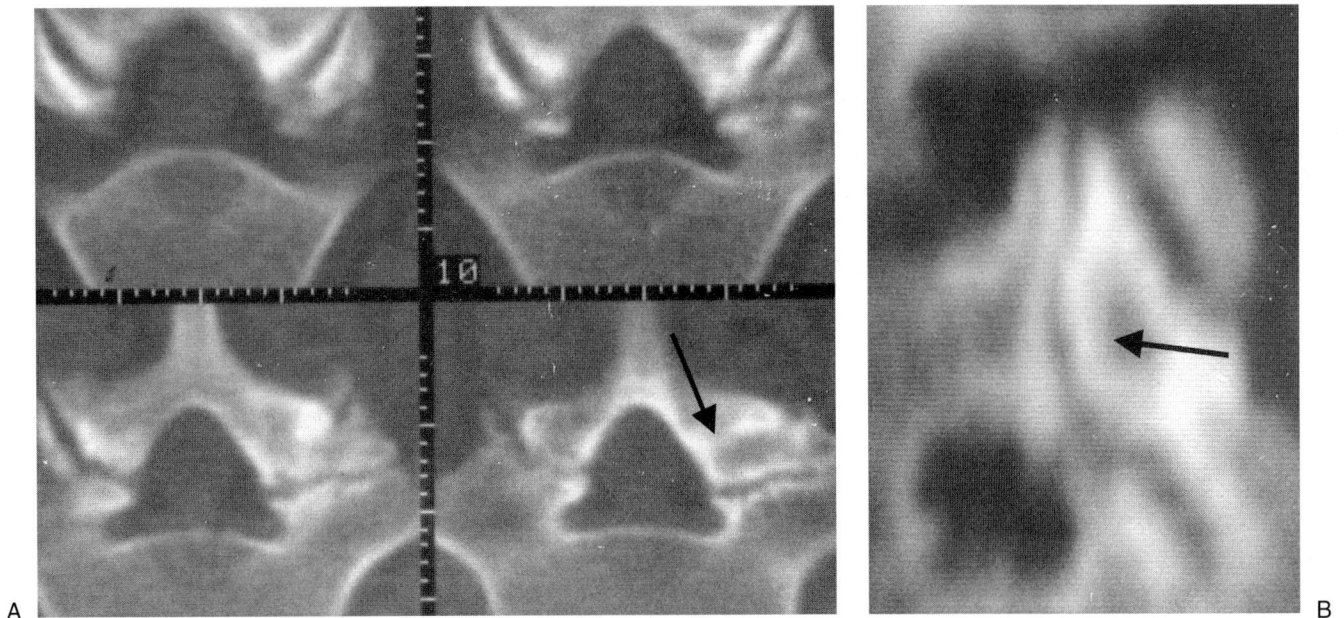

FIG. 61-19. Retrosomatic cleft. Axial **(A)** and **(B)** sagittal reformatted computed tomography scan. There is a typical pars defect on the left side and an irregular cleft on the right.

vertebral ossification center and the pedicular ossification center lies much farther anterior within the vertebral body. In many instances one can identify a faint, curvilinear, sclerotic line within the vertebral body representing the fusion plane of these ossification centers (Fig. 61-20). The retrosomatic fracture occurs posterior to this fusion plane.

Although not generally considered when one thinks of the neural ring, the posterior edge of the apophyseal ring of the vertebral body is the anterior margin of the neural canal. Separation of the posterior apophyseal ring is termed a *posterior limbus vertebra.*

Posterior limbus vertebra occurs when a fragment of disc material herniates through the ununited posterior apophyseal ring, fracturing a segment of the ring and displacing it into the spinal canal. While technically this may not be a stress fracture, it is useful to include it as the last of the neural ring fractures to be associated with spondylolysis. The combination of spondylolysis and posterior limbus vertebra may be associated with heavy sports activity such as weight lifting (Fig. 61-21).

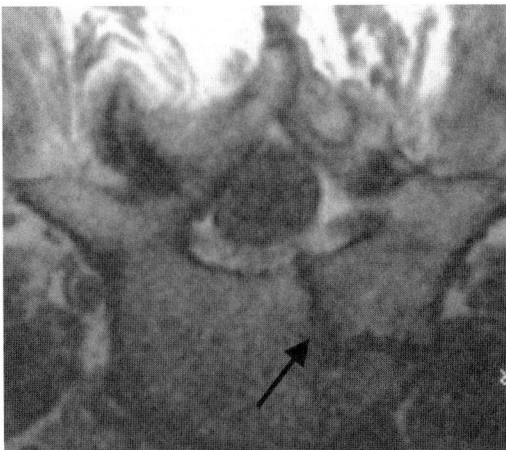

FIG. 61-20. Failure of complete fusion of the ossification centers of the vertebral body with that of the right pedicle. Axial T1-weighted magnetic resonance scan reveals a lucent crescentic line well within the vertebra.

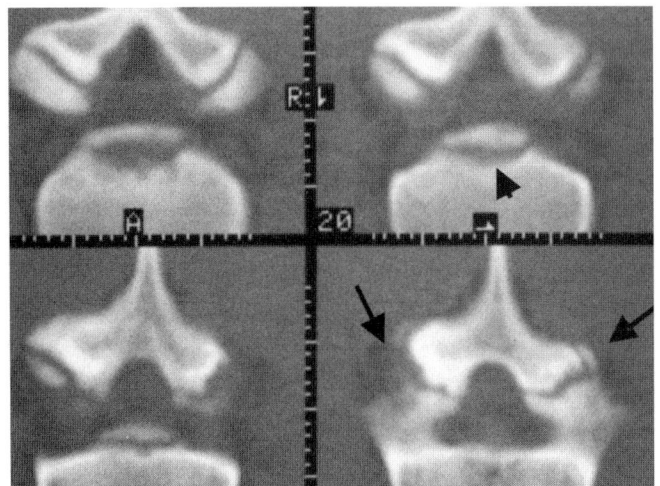

FIG. 61-21. Pars fractures and posterior limbus vertebra. Axial CT beside the typical bilateral pars defects, a crescentic bar of bone has displaced posteriorly from the vertebral body. This is a large segment of the apophyseal ring. This is due to herniation of disc material through the developing vertebral end plate prior to fusion of the apophyseal ossification center to the remainder of the vertebra.

CONCLUSION

Children between the ages of 5 and 7 years account for two-thirds of patients with spondylolysis. They likely fracture their pars because of increased forces on the pars due to the long lever caused by hypoplastic facets. There is usually no history of sports activity or unusual back activities. Teenagers account for one-third of patients. They fracture their pars through repeated vigorous activity and are often serious athletes. Although the pars is the most likely portion of the neural arch to fracture, any portion of the ring may be involved. Multiplanar CT is the procedure of choice for the evaluation of the bony anatomy in patients with spondylolysis, spondylolisthesis, and the stress fracture variants.

REFERENCES

1. Wiltse LL, Rothman SLG. Lumbar and lumbosacral spondylolisthesis, classification, diagnosis and natural history. In: The lumbar spine, 2nd ed. Philadelphia: WB Saunders, 1996.
2. Rothman SLG, Glenn WV. Multiplanar CT of the spine. Baltimore: University Park Press, 1984.
3. Rothman SLG, Glenn WV. CT multiplanar reconstructions in 253 cases of lumbar spondylolysis. AJNR 1984;5:81–90.
4. Newman PH. The clinical syndrome associated with severe lumbosacral subluxation. J Bone Joint Surg 1965;47B;472–481.
5. Pfeil J, Neithard F, Cotta N. Pathogenesis of pediatric spondylolisthesis. Z Orthop 1987;125:526–533.
6. Albinase M, Pizzutillo PD. Family study of spondylolisthesis. J Pediatr Orthop 1982;2;496–499.
7. Wiltse LL. Fatigue fracture: the basic lesion in isthmic spondylolisthesis. J Bone Joint Surg 1975;57A:17–22.
8. Zembo MM, Roberts JM, Burke SW, et al. Congenital spondylolisthesis. Paper presented at: 21st Annual Meeting of the Scoliosis Research Society; September 1986; Bermuda.
9. Winter RB. Congenital kyphosis. J Bone Joint Surg 1973;55A: 223–256.
10. Oakley RH, Carty H. Review of spondylolysis and spondylolisthesis in pediatric practice. Bone Joint Radiol 1984;57:877–885.
11. Borokw SE, Kleiger B. Spondylolisthesis in the newborn, a case report. Clin Orthop 1971;81:73–76.
12. Baker DR, McHolick W. Spondylolisthesis and spondylolysis in children. J Bone Joint Surg 1956;38A:933.
13. Frederickson BE, Baker D, McHolick WJ, et al. The natural history of spondylolysis and spondylolisthesis. J Bone Joint Surg 1984;66A: 699–707.

CHAPTER 62

Evaluation and Management of the Athlete with "Pars Fracture"

Robert Watkins III and Robert G. Watkins IV

A complaint of low back pain in a competitive athlete requires an in-depth investigation, specific diagnosis, and appropriate treatment. Lumbar pain in an athlete is a stress fracture until proven otherwise. While the incidence of stress fractures is higher in certain types of athletics compared to others, any athlete is potentially subjected to the repetitive twisting and extension motion that is identified with the etiology of spondylolysis. The typical spondylolytic lesion occurs in the par interarticularis, but may be present in the pedicle or articular process.

While there have been references made to a congenital predisposition to spondylolysis, environmental factors have clearly been shown to be a significant source of pathology in the young athlete. The sports frequently associated with a significantly increased incidence are diving, gymnastics, wrestling, and weightlifting (1). The incidence of pars interarticularis defects in female gymnasts is four times that of the general female Caucasian population. The incidence of pars defects is approximately 4.5% during the first year of school and is more common in boys than girls (2). There are certain familial predispositions to pars defects in young children and there is an increased incidence of spina bifida occulta in young athletes who have spondylolysis (3). Spondylolysis rarely leads to progressive high-grade spondylolisthesis. Progressive slip has a higher incidence between the ages of 9 and 12 in girls and 10 and 14 in boys (4). Cahill's evaluation of the young athlete documented an incidence of 0.8% of children without evidence of fatigue fractures developing such a fracture between the ages of 10 and 20 (15). McCarroll documented an incidence of 2.4% of acquired spondylolysis during a 4-year college football career (6). In answer to the question, "Is spondylolysis a fatigue fracture?" Hutton, Stott, and Cryon demonstrated that cyclic loading can produce a fatigue fracture of the pars interarticularis (19). Because of the increasing use of weightlifting as a training technique in all varieties of sports, many athletes suffer a fatigue fracture in the weight room as opposed to directly on the athletic field. There are still certain maneuvers in specific sports such as hyperextension in gymnasts, extension in anterior alignment in weightlifters, and extension with rotation in baseball pitchers that can lead to the repetitive loading that produces the fracture.

The pain source of acute spondylolysis is predominantly the fracture. Just as fractures hurt in other locations, the fracture of the pars interarticularis can produce pain. The location can be at any level of the spine. It is certainly more common at L5, because L5 is a transitional area between the fixed sacrum and the mobile lumbar spine. There is an abnormal distribution of forces at this level, and rotational forces may be inappropriately directed to the pars interarticularis at L5 (8). Shear forces at the lumbosacral junction have been shown to predispose the pars to fracture (7,9).

Athletes are often seen with asymptomatic spondylolysis. There is a high incidence of professional athletes with asymptomatic lesions not related to a specific complaint of low back pain. Bilateral defects with or without grade I spondylolisthesis can produce pain from the relative instability of the anterior column produced by the loss of inherent tensile and shear strength of the pars interarticularis. Symptomatic discogenic pain is a reality and certainly can be coupled with spondylolysis at the same level. The injured disc, innervated by the sinuvertebral nerve, undergoes annular tears and inflammation, which result in pain.

Often the patient arrives at the spinal specialist with a diagnosis, and is already improving after having stopped the sport activity. This patient needs the full history and physical examination afforded to every patient with back pain with testing for signs of nerve root impingement and a complete neurologic examination.

HISTORY AND PHYSICAL EXAMINATION

The key to a proper history and physical examination is to have a standardized form that accomplishes the needed specific objectives:

1. Quantitate the morbidity. Use a value scale of pain, function, and occupation. Converse with the patient and listen to the inflections and manner of pain description. Detail the time of disability and the time of origin of the pain. We use the Oswestry Scale and Disability Rating. The severity of the morbidity often determines the aggressiveness of the diagnostic and therapeutic plan.

2. Delineate the psychosocial factors. Know what psychologic effect the pain has had on the patient. Know the social, economic, and legal results of the patient's disability. We use the pain drawing on the initial visit and a detailed psychologic report in certain instances. Understand what can be gained by the patient's being sick or well. Derive an understanding of what role these factors are playing in the patient's complaints.

3. Eliminate the possibility of tumors, infections, and neurologic crisis. These conditions have a certain urgency that requires immediate attention and a diagnostic therapeutic regimen that is very different from that required for disc disease. Constant, unrelenting pain that becomes worse at night is an indication of tumor or infection. Ask about bowel, bladder, and sexual dysfunction and do a thorough examination.

4. Diagnose the clinical syndrome:

   a. *Nonmechanical back or leg pain*—Inflammatory, constant pain; minimally affected by activity; usually worse at night or in early morning.
   b. *Mechanical back or leg pain*—Made worse by activity; relieved by rest.
   c. *Sciatica*—Predominantly radicular pain; positive stretch signs, with or without neurologic deficit.
   d. *Neurogenic claudication*—Radiating leg or calf pain; negative stretch signs; made worse with ambulation and spinal extension; relieved by flexion.

Pinpoint the pathophysiology causing the syndrome. Three important determinations are:

1. What nerve (especially in radiculopathy)?
2. What level? Which neuromotion segment?
3. What pathology? What is the exact structure or disease process in that neuromotion segment that is causing the pain?

Some key factors in the history and physical examination are:

1. What caused the injury?
2. The time of day when the pain is worse?
3. A comparison of pain levels during walking, sitting, and standing.
4. The effects of Valsalva maneuver, coughing, and sneezing on pain.

5. The type of injury and duration of the problem.
6. The percentage of back versus leg pain. (We insist on getting an accurate estimate of the relative amount of discomfort in the back versus that in the legs. These two numbers must add up to 100%.)

The physical examination should address:

1. Maneuvers during the examination that reproduce the pain.
2. The presence of sciatic stretch signs.
3. The neurologic deficit.
4. Back and lower extremity stiffness and loss of range of motion.
5. The exact location of tenderness and radiation of pain or paresthesias.

The presentation of an athlete or adolescent with mechanical low back pain requires a thorough examination. Most athletes can identify the mechanical activity in their sport that produces the pain. At times, players will only have pain while throwing or only have pain while batting. Of course, if the inflammation is significant enough the athlete may have constant unrelenting pain, even interfering with sleep. Some athletes present with a long history of pain with activity—a chronic lumbar pain that intermittently flares up. At other times, athletes can specifically remember the types of activities they were performing when the pain started. Many athletes with spondylolysis will have pain both in flexion and extension. Coughing, sneezing, and straining may also cause pain for patients with severe inflammation.

The examination begins with finding the location of pain and tenderness. The patient frequently points to a unilateral lumbosacral location in the area of the posterosuperior iliac spine.

Typically, patients with acute spondylolysis do not have leg pain, although it can be present. They often have paraspinous spasm and hamstring tightness. Patients typically have more pain with extension and with extension and rotation toward the painful side. The one-legged lumbar extension maneuver in which the patient stands on one leg and bends backward is a commonly used test to accentuate the pain from an acute spondylolysis.

RADIOGRAPHS

X-ray evaluation is limited in the ability to pinpoint an area of acute spondylolysis. Areas of sclerosis may be an impending fracture or a more ominous osteoid osteoma or osteoblastoma (10). Oblique X-rays may demonstrate the presence of a spondylolysis. Because some defects are seen better at 30° and others at 60°, and because the presence or absence of an established spondylolysis has little correlation with the exact etiology of pain, we stopped the use of oblique X-rays on patients with lumbar pain (11).

The key to diagnosis in the athlete and adolescent with back pain is a lumbar single photon emission computed tomography (SPECT) scan (12). The tomography of the bone scan is a very accurate test for identifying an impending or established acute spondylolysis. The radionucleotide is picked up by bone-forming cells. These cells may be in response to a fracture or impending fracture. It can also be associated with arthritis in a lumbar facet joint (13). A chronic spondylolysis that is negative on the SPECT scan should not be the etiology of that patient's pain.

Our typical workup for the young athlete with back pain of more than 3 weeks' duration includes a lumbar SPECT scan. If it is positive for reaction, we order a lumbar CT scan to identify what area is positive. Is this an osteoid osteoma, osteoblastoma, injured facet joint, arthritic facet joint, or a stress fracture in the pedicle, pars, or articular facet? If the SPECT scan is negative, we order a magnetic resonance imaging (MRI) to rule out disc degeneration, infection, or tumor.

Use of the MRI to diagnose acute spondylolysis has been presented in a number of different forums. Proper technique with the MRI can identify acute bone edema. This certainly can be a method of identifying an acute spondylolysis. There is certainly less radiation exposure using the MRI. However, the combination of the bone scan and CT scan is a visual demonstration to parents and the patient of their exact back problem. The CT scan allows a clear-cut definition of what is positive on the bone scan and it allows one to determine how long the defect has been present. A very early defect is most likely to heal regardless of treatment. A well-established defect is less likely to heal. A CT scan offers a way of following this in the future that is much more specific than the MRI.

TREATMENT

When the young athlete comes to you for care, it is the obligation of the clinician to properly demonstrate the lesion to the patient and the parents and devise an appropriate treatment program for the patient's complaints. Treatment begins with identification of the etiology of the problem. If the etiology of the problem is one specific maneuver in a sport, stop that maneuver. If it is participation in the sport, stop the participation in the sport. Stopping the motion that causes the problem is the first step in treatment.

For many years, conservative treatment has consisted of avoidance of physical activity and the use of orthoses to immobilize and support the back. Such treatment has been only minimally effective. For example, in looking at pars defects in 185 spondylolytic adolescent athletes, Morita et al. classified the defects into early, progressive, and terminal stages, depending on degree of severity, as revealed by CT (10). Patients wore a lumbosacral support

corset for periods as long as 6 months. The defect healed in 73% of the early cases, but only 38.5% of the progressive cases and none of the terminal cases. The subject of pain relief was not addressed in their report.

However, as early as 1976 physicians such as Magora in Israel advised that orthoses be used only to train the patient in building good postural habits, not for support in treating spondylolysis or asymptomatic spondylolisthesis (9). An orthosis may produce some relief from pain because of the limitation of movements and general feeling of support it provides. However, as Magora observed, as soon as the orthosis is removed the tenderness tends to increase, the back and abdominal muscles are weakened and atrophied, and some movements of the lumbosacral spine are limited, all of which result in a more prolonged and painful therapy. Only in the case of severe low back pain did Magora prescribe bed rest. When pain was mild to moderate, he recommended an immediate return to normal daily activities, albeit with some modifications to those activities, combined with an exercise program to strengthen back and abdominal musculature (15).

Others agree with this stance and, like Hensinger (18) and Johnson (26), maintain that when symptoms are related to activity, stabilization of the spine alone will achieve excellent long-term remission of symptoms and minor neurologic findings.

The trunk stabilization program offers an early return to sports without the use of a lumbosacral brace. It comprises a combination of activities that work to bring the spine back to a position of balance and power in injured athletes. By training muscles of the trunk to work in coordination, the program produces biomechanically sound spinal function. It uses special isometric strengthening exercises to develop specific trunk muscles that are molded in response to proprioceptive feedback. Muscle function based on balance and coordination, not strength alone, is the result. Initially, the athlete is taught to attain a very safe, neutral, pain-free, and controlled position. He or she then moves through a series of exercises that combine balance and coordination. Gradually, the athlete, while maintaining good trunk control, is moved in incremental steps through increasingly advanced exercises. In each succeeding exercise, the patient assumes a somewhat more precarious position than he or she had experienced in the one that preceded it. There are eight categories of exercises:

1. Dead bug
2. Partial sit-ups
3. Bridging
4. Prone
5. Quadripedal
6. Wall slides
7. Ball exercises
8. Aerobics.

Each of these categories consists of five levels, with each level of difficulty amplifying the intensity of perfor-

TABLE 62-1. *Watkins-Randall scale*

	Dead bug A	Partial situps B	Bridging C	Prone D	Quadriped E	Wallslide F	Ball G	Aerobic H
1	Supported arms over head Two minutes Marching	Forward—Hands on Chest 1 × 10	Slow Reps Double Leg 2 × 10	Gluteal Squeeze Alternating arm or leg lifts 1 × 10 reps	Upper Ext. or Lower Ext Hold 1 × 10	Less than 90 degree Reps × 10	Balance on Ball Leg Press	Walk Land and Water
2	Unsupported Arms over Head/ one leg Extended × 3 min	3 × 10 Fwd Hands on Chest	Slow Reps Double Leg Weight on Hips 2 × 20	Alternating Arm/ Leg Lift 2 × 10 Hold	Arm & Leg 2 × 10 Hold	90 degree Hold 20 sec × 10	Leg press w/ arms over head Sit-ups forward No hold Run	10 Min. Cycle Water
3	Unsupported Arms 7 Min. Over alternate Leg Extended with Weights	3 × 10 Fwd 3 × 10 Rt. 3 × 10 Lt.	Single Leg 3 × 20 Hold Double w/ wts. Double on ball	Ball Flys Swims Superman 2 × 10	Arm & Leg 3 × 20 Hold 5 Sec. W/Weights	90 degree Hold 30 sec × 10 Lunges/no wts.	Ball sit ups × 20 Fwd, Rt.Lt.	20–30 Min. Swim & Nordic Track
4	Unsupported UES #/LE 10 min Alt. leg ext	3 × 20 Fwd. 3 × 20 Rt. 3 × 20 Lt. Weights on Chest	On Ball Single Leg 4 × 20 Hold dbl on ball w/wts feet on ball double bridge	Ball 10 × 20 Hold Superman w/wts Prayer Pushups Walkouts	Arm & Leg 2 × 20 Hold 10 Sec. W/Weights Body blade	90 degree Hold 15 sec W/Weights × 10 Lunges w/ wts	Ball, Situps Fwd, Rt, Lt w/wts 3 × 20 Wand Manual Resistance, Pulleys	45 Min. Versaclimeber also Step Skip rope
5	Unsupported Bil. LE ext 15 min total Increased wts Bil.UE w/ bil LE extension	3 × 30 Fwd. 3 × 30 Rt. 3 × 30 Lt. Unsupported Weights Over head & behind	On Ball Single Leg 5 × 20 w/ wts holding dbl w/ feet on ball and bil knees flex	Ball, All Exercises W/Weights 4 × 20 Body blade Body blade	Arm & Leg 3 × 20 Hold 15 Sec. W/Weights	90 degree Hold Arms Extended w/ wts × 10 Lunges w/ wts Hold 1 min	Ball Overhead & Lateral Pull through Sports Stick Pulleys Body blade	60 Min. also Run

mance, increasing the number of repetitions of the exercise performed, varying the body positions, adding resistance when exercising, and so forth (Table 62-1).

TREATMENT

Certain spondylolytic defects will heal. Acute lesions have a higher chance of healing than chronic defects (18). Use of a Boston brace has never statistically been demonstrated to enhance healing of the spondylolytic defect (19,20). At our institution, follow up X-rays and CT scans are of no practical value in spondylolytic patients who are responding favorably to a back strengthening rehabilitation program and whose symptoms have subsided. Radiographically following spondylolisthesis is only important in young athletes. From the ages of 9 to 13, in the presence of occulta spinal bifida and with a doming of the sacrum, spinal optosis can occur. After the age of 16, this would be a rare occurrence. This can be followed with a simple lateral radiograph. General guidelines are that, with a slip of less than 50%, there are no restrictions necessary. With a slip of 50% or more, high-risk sports are not recommended until the growth stops. As a practical matter, those with high-grade slips are seldom able to participate in high-velocity sports.

Our experience in the use of bracing versus stabilization in adolescent athletes consists of an unpublished series of 31 athletes evaluated for return to full activity. The athletes were divided into two groups: group A, 19 patients treated only with the trunk stabilization and group B, 12 patients treated with a rigid lumbosacral orthosis, followed by a trunk stabilization program. The patients were selected randomly. Group A was treated purely with stabilization training. Group B wore the brace without physical therapy for 2 months before beginning physical therapy. Group A patients returned to full activity at 3 months, and group B patients at 4 months. The two groups reached the same excellent functional recovery rate. As a result, we have not used a lumbosacral orthosis in the last 15 years.

Return to sport after acute spondylolysis is based on the Watkins-Randle 1 through 5 rating scale of trunk stabilization exercises. An adolescent athlete should be able to do a full level 3 workout and college and professional athletes should be able to do level 4 or 5 workouts before practice. Steps in returning an athlete to play are as follows:

1. Complete the appropriate level of the stabilization program
2. Be in excellent aerobic condition compatible with the sport through aerobic conditioning while doing the stabilization program
3. Work with the coaching staff and training staff in a series of sport-specific exercises for the individual sport

4. Return slowly to the sport with playing time or position changes as needed and specific to the sport
5. Maintain the same level of stabilization training after return to the sport for a period of 6 months to a year.

SURGICAL TREATMENT

There are very limited indications for the surgical treatment of spondylolysis. In 20 years of treating spondylolysis in adolescent, college, and professional athletes, we have resorted to surgery two times. One was in a minor league baseball pitcher with a unilateral defect who had already missed one season and was in danger of missing another. The other was for bilateral spondylolysis in a minor league pitcher. The incidence of symptomatic acute spondylolysis not responding to stabilization training and allowing a return to the sport is rare. Experiences with extremely demanding activities such as cricket bowlers may be different.

Direct repair of the spondylolytic defect has been shown to be effective (21–26). Many different techniques have been described such as hook screws (21,22,26), translaminar screws (21,26), wiring (26), and pedicle screws with a V-shaped rod (27). Our operation of choice is a lag screw across the spondylolytic defect and grafting of the defect with minimal exposure. A prerequisite for a spondylolysis repair is that the disc is normal (23). This can be determined with MRI or discography. Other operations such as the Hamby modification of the Cole and Scott technique for tension bind wiring and bone grafting for bilateral defects (28) is certainly acceptable in treating the problem.

Patients with significant disc degeneration may need a one-level fusion. We have performed two fusions in professional athletes for spondylolisthesis with a 50% effectiveness rate. Lumbar spinal fusion in professional athletes is not a very successful operation because of the high demands placed on adjacent levels, the amount of time out from the sport for the fusion to heal, and the aggressive demands put on the spine in the early-healed phase. Artificial disc replacement for spondylolisthesis is an unknown factor at this time.

REFERENCES

1. Elliot S, Hutson MA, Wastie ML. Bone scintigraphy in the assessment of spondylolysis in the patients attending a sports injury clinic. Clin Radiol 1988;39:269.
2. Sales de Gauzt J, Vadier F, Cahuzac JP. Repair of lumbar spondylolysis using Morscher material: 14 children followed for 1–5 years. Acta Orthop Scand 2000;71(3):292–296.
3. Dandy DJ, Shannon MJ. Lumbo-sacral subluxation (group 1 spondylolysthesis). J Bone Joint Surg 1971;53B:578.
4. Lament LE, Einola S. Spondylolysthesis in children and adolescents. Acta Orthop Scand 1961;28:45.
5. Sys J, Michielsen J, Bracke P, et al. Nonoperative treatment of active spondylolysis in elite athletes with normal x-ray findings: literature review and results on conservative treatment. Eur Spine J 2001;10(6):498–504.

6. McCarroll JR, Miller JM, Ritter MA. Lumbar spondylolysis and spondylolisthesis in college football players. AM J Sports Med 1986:14:404.

7. Rossi F. Spondylolysis, spondylolisthesis, and sports. J Sports Med Phys Fitness 1978;18:317.

8. Hambly MF et al. Tension band wiring-bone grafting for spondylolysis and spondylolisthesis: a clinical biomechanical study. Spine 1989;14:455.

9. Magora A. Conservative treatment in spondylolisthesis. Clin Orthop Rel Res 1976;117:74–79.

10. Morita T, Ikata T, Katoh S, et al. Lumbar spondylolysis in children and adolescents. J Bone Surg 1995;77B:620–625.

11. Micheli LJ. Back injuries in gymnastics. Clin Sports Med 1985;4:85.

12. Chen JF, Lee ST. A physiologic method for the repair of young adult simple isthmic lumbar spondylolysis. Changgeng Yi Xue Za Zhi 2000; 23(2):92–98.

13. De Maeseneer N, Lenchik L, Everaert H, et al. Evaluation of lower back pain with bone scintigraphy and SPECT. Radiographics 1999;19 (4):901–912.

14. Swaid L, et al. Spondylolysis and the sacrohorizontal angle in athletes. Acta Radiol 1989;30:359.

15. Cahill BR. Chronic orthopedic problems in the young athlete. J Sports Med 1973;3:36.

16. Saifuddin A, White J, Tucker S, et al. Orientation of lumbar pars defects: implications for radiological detection and surgical management. J Bone Joint Surg 1998;80B(2):208–211.

17. Jackson DW, Wiltse LL, Cirincione RJ. Spondylolysthesis in the female gymnast. Clin Orthop 1976;117:68.

18. Hensinger RN, Lang JR, MacEwen GD. Surgical management of spondylolisthesis in children and adolescents. Spine 1976;1:207–216.

19. Hutton WC, Stott JRR, Cryon BM. Is spondylolysis a fatigue fracture? Spine 1977;2:202.

20. Schulitz KP, Niethard FU. Strain on the interarticular stress distribution. Arch Orthop Trauma Surg 1980;96:197.

21. Prasartritha T. Surgical repair of pars defects in spondylolisthesis. J Med Assoc Thai 2001:84(9):1235–1240.

22. Chang JH, Lee CH, Wu SS, et al. Management of multiple level spondylolysis of the lumbar spine in young males: a report of six cases. J Formos Med Assoc 2001;100(7):497–502.

23. Dai LY, Jia LS, Yuan W, et al. Direct repair of defect in lumbar spondylolysis and mild isthmic spondylolysthesis by bone grafting, with or without facet joint fusion. Eur Spine J 2001;10(1):78–83.

24. Sherman FC, Wilkinson RH, Hall JE. Reactive sclerosis of a pedicle and spondylolysis in the lumbar spine. J Bone Joint Surg 1977;59A:49.

25. Micheli LJ, Hare JE. Miller ME. Use of a modified Boston brace for back injuries in athletes. Am J Sports Med 1980;8:351.

26. Johnson JR, Kirwan EO. The long-term results of fusion in situ for severe spondylolisthesis. J Bone Joint Surg 1983;65B:43–46.

27. Gillet P, Petit M. Direct repair of spondylolysis without spondylolysthesis, using a rod-screw construct and bone grafting of the pars defect. Spine 1999;24(12):1252–1256.

28. Wu SS, Lee CH, Chen PQ. Operative repair of symptomatic spondylolysis following a positive response to diagnostic pars injection. J Spinal Disord 1999;12:10–16.

CHAPTER 63

Indications for Surgery in Spondylolysis and Spondylolisthesis in Adults and Surgery for Low-Grade Spondylolisthesis

Dahari D. Brooks and Bruce E. Fredrickson

The goal of this chapter is twofold: (a) present and discuss the indications for operative management of low-grade nondegenerative slips; and (b) present and discuss surgical options for the treatment of low-grade nondegenerative slips. For the purposes of this chapter, we will discuss the indications and procedures as they relate to low-grade, nondegenerative causes of spondylolisthesis only. Nonoperative treatment modalities, and the evaluation and management of high-grade (III through V) slips will not be addressed in this chapter.

The term *spondylolysis* is defined as the breaking down of a vertebral structure; and is derived from the Greek "spondylos" (vertebra) and "lysis" (dissolution). *Spondylolisthesis*, derived from the Greek "spondylos" (vertebra) and "oblishtesis" (a slipping), refers to any forward slipping of one vertebra onto the one below it. The underlying pathology that predisposes to this forward slippage includes spondylolysis, disc degeneration, elongated pars intra-articularis, or pedicles, and congenital arch defects. In 1963, Newman reviewed 319 cases of lumbar spondylolisthesis and described three categories (1):

1. Congenital (dysplastic)
2. Isthmic (spondylolytic)
3. Degenerative spondylolisthesis.

Since the publication of this classification scheme, Wiltse devised a classification scheme based on etiologic and anatomic factors (Fig. 63-1) (2):

1. Traumatic spondylolisthesis
2. Congenital or dysplastic
3. Isthmic
4. Pathologic spondylolisthesis
5. Iatrogenic (postsurgical) spondylolisthesis.

In congenital or dysplastic spondylolisthesis displacement occurs early in life and is often severe. Overall, congenital slips account for approximately 15% of cases, and affects females to a greater extent (1). The pars may remain intact, but is usually underdeveloped.

Isthmic spondylolisthesis is the most common form of spondylolisthesis. Isthmic spondylolisthesis is defined as an anterior slip of the upper lumbar vertebrae, as well as separation of the anterior aspect of the vertebrae from the posterior neural arch (3,4). The fibrous defect in the pars allows for the future displacement (2,3,5–10).

Degenerative slips typically occur at the L4-5 level, and result from long-standing instability secondary to disc and facet degeneration (1).

Traumatic spondylolisthesis refers to slips secondary to an acute injury pars/facet complex. Posterior element destruction secondary to a lytic process such as malignancy or infection, results in a pathologic spondylolisthesis. And finally, excessive surgical removal of the supporting bony and ligamentous structures results in an iatrogenic spondylolisthesis.

The severity of the slip, despite the various etiologies, has been historically based upon the slip percentage. The slip percentage is determined in a number of ways. The classically described method involves the division of the inferior end plate of the superior vertebra into four equal segments (each representing 25%). The numbers of segments anteriorly displaced determine the slip grade. Slips are classified as either low- or high-grade based upon this percentage. A low-grade slip indicates that the amount of anterior translation is less than or equal to 50%; whereas a high grade slip indicates that the amount of anterior translation exceeds 50%.

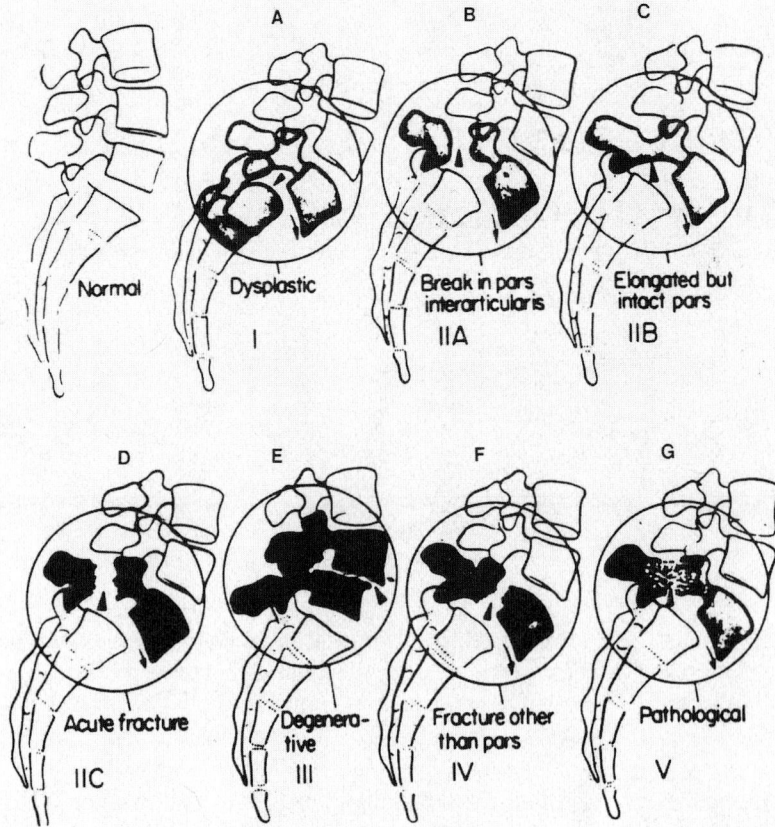

FIG. 63-1. Classification scheme for spondylolisthesis based on etiology and radiographic appearance. (From Frymoyer JW, ed. The adult spine: principles and practice. New York: Raven Press, 1991, with permission.)

INDICATIONS

Natural history studies have demonstrated that the majority of individuals with a pars defect remain asymptomatic. While radiographic evidence of slip progression in the adult is possible, the likelihood of this translating into clinical symptoms is low. Although patients may experience back pain with or without extremity pain, the overall incidence of low back symptoms is not significantly higher than that of the general population (4,11,12).

The treatment options are quite variable for those individuals with significant complaints despite an adequate course of supervised conservative management. Clinically, patients can present with a variety of symptoms.

1. Mechanical low back pain with normal neurologic examination
2. Mechanical low back pain with extremity pain and normal neurologic examination
3. Mechanical low back pain and either unilateral or bilateral radicular leg pain (13).

In addition to back or leg pain, patients may also complain of postural changes, or hamstring tightness. Radiographs are helpful in this situation to determine whether the slip has progressed. Slip progression can cause or intensify radicular or back pain (6,14).

It is commonly accepted that patients who present with intractable low back pain with or without lower extremity symptoms despite adequate conservative therapy, or radicular symptoms are appropriate surgical candidates (15). Conservative management in general consists of an exercise protocol, with emphasis on trunk stability and strength training. In addition, activity/lifestyle modifications, weight loss, epidural or selective nerve root injections, and aerobic conditioning have also been shown to improve long-term function (16). Modalities such as ultrasound, massage, or traction have not been shown to make a statistical difference with respect to outcome.

TABLE 63-1. *Surgical options*

Posterior	Anterior
Gill decompression	Anterior lumbar interbody fusion (ALIF)
In situ fusion	Combined ALIF and posterior fixation
Decompression and *in situ* fusion	
In situ fusion with instrumentation	
Decompression and instrumented fusion	
Direct repair of pars defect	

Once the decision for operative management has been made, the treating surgeon has several available options (Table 63-1). Surgical intervention can provide superior long-term results for appropriately selected patients (13,17–21).

POSTERIOR DECOMPRESSION

In 1965, Gill published a study of 20 adult patients with symptomatic isthmic spondylolisthesis treated with posterior decompression consisting of wide excision of the loose lamina and inferior facets and foraminal decompression (Gill decompression) (22). It was noted that the most common root involved in this condition was L5. It appeared that compression of the fifth lumbar root resulted from the buildup of fibrocartilaginous tissue at the site of the pars defect, and that the presence of a slip, either preoperatively or postoperatively, did not reliably correlate with symptoms. At an average follow-up of 36 months, Gill noted no slip progression, and only 3 fair/unsatisfactory outcomes (22a). In 1984, Gill reevaluated 52 patients (including those of the original study) ranging in age from 14 to 57 years. Twenty-one individuals demonstrated slip progression, with an average increase of 5.9% in males and 16% in females. Despite the progression, only 10% of these patients were symptomatic. Furthermore, good/excellent results were noted in 82% of those individuals without radiographic evidence of progression.

DECOMPRESSION AND *IN SITU* FUSION

Despite such encouraging reports of posterior decompression, the increased risk of slip progression has prevented this technique from gaining greater support. The addition of a posterolateral *in situ* fusion allows one to address this added risk of progression (Fig. 63-2). Long-term results demonstrate low rates of slip progression, excellent patient pain relief and satisfaction, and relatively low complications. Various authors have evaluated this procedure and report an approximate 80% to 85% success rate, with few (if any) reports of slip progression (13). Furthermore, those individuals with poor surgical outcomes had a significantly higher pseudoarthrosis rate (15,17). Thus, successful clinical outcomes relied heavily on the presence of a solid fusion mass (15,17,20).

Fusion *in situ*

Realizing that the success of surgical management of low-grade nondegenerative spondylolisthesis is dependent largely upon obtaining a solid arthrodesis; *in situ* posterolateral fusion without decompression has been performed as a reliable, rapid, and easy means of treatment (23,24). Various reports demonstrate similar success rates as those seen with decompression and fusion. The only identifiable factor that has been shown to impact outcome is the presence of a pseudoarthrosis. Individuals with a nonunion were more likely to have a poor outcome as has been shown in the past.

The addition of a Gill decompression to arthrodesis for the treatment of low-grade isthmic spondylolisthesis in patients who do not demonstrate significant radicular symptoms does not appear to improve clinical outcomes.

POSTERIOR INSTRUMENTATION AND FUSION

Given the strong correlation between radiographic fusion and clinical outcome, pedicle screw fixation is often used to increase fusion rates in this subset of patients (25–28). The use of tobacco products and nonsteroidal antiinflammatory drugs (NSAIDs) postoperatively has been demonstrated to adversely affect fusion rates. The use

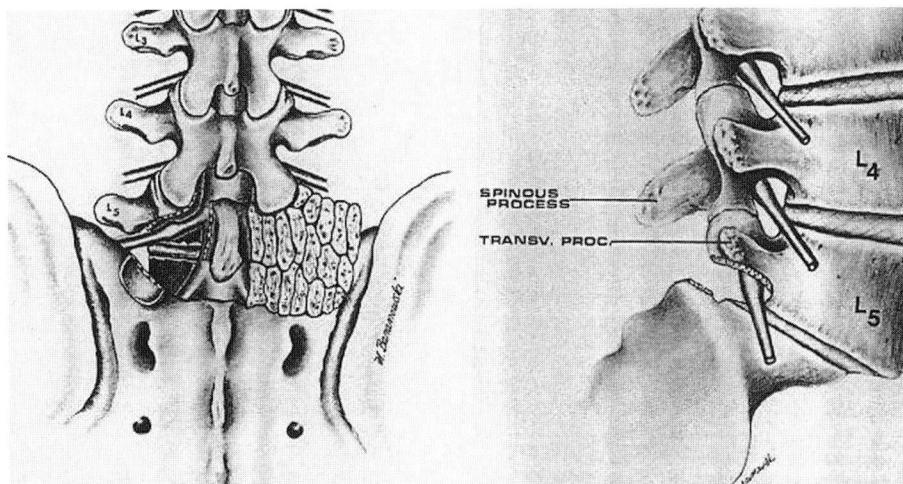

FIG. 63-2. Illustration of a posterolateral decompression and *in situ* fusion. (From Frymoyer JW, ed. The adult spine: principles and practice. New York: Raven Press, 1991, with permission.)

of supplementary instrumentation in addition to decompression, and autologous posterolateral arthrodesis has been shown to improve the clinical outcome and fusion rate for those patients who are smokers, have an iatrogenic slip, or require revision secondary to an established pseudoarthrosis (29). It should be noted that for those individuals without such predisposing risk factors, there is no significant advantage of transpedicular screw fixation in improving fusion rates or clinical outcome (29).

DIRECT REPAIR OF THE PARS INTRA-ARTICULARIS

Direct pars defect repair allows for the preservation of lumbar motion segments, and restoration of the normal anatomy (30–36). In addition to the previously stated indications for operative treatment, when considering direct repair, particular attention should be paid to the quality of the disc and facets (5,37). In the setting of degenerative disc disease (DDD) there is inherit instability and abnormal motion which can lead to early facet degeneration, spur formation, and nerve root compression. Therefore, preservation of the degenerated lumbar motion segment increases the likelihood of a poor outcome (30,34,36). Direct repair is best suited for younger, symptomatic patients without concomitant DDD (36).

In addition to DDD, the incidence of spina bifida occulta among those individuals with low- grade isthmic spondylolisthesis at L5/S1 is increased. These congenital defects or absence of the posterior elements can present technical difficulties that prevent direct pars repair. Special attention should be paid to those patients in whom repair is considered at the L5/S1 level.

Overall, the reported results for direct repair in appropriate patients are quite encouraging (30–35,38). Individuals with back pain secondary to either spondylolysis or grade I spondylolisthesis treated with direct repair typically have excellent results. Reports indicate the presence of a solid bony union at approximately 6 months as well as no significant limitation in lumbar motion (30,34). Direct repair of the pars defect has been shown to provide satisfactory results with few complications, as well as the added benefit of maintaining normal lumbar motion (30,34).

ANTERIOR LUMBAR INTERBODY FUSION (ALIF)

Interbody fusion involves complete anterior discectomy and interbody fusion of the affected level. Advocates of this technique indicate that the associated degenerative disc disease and instability is best addressed anteriorly (39–42). The ability to excise the disc, fuse, and possibly reduce the slipped level allows for encouraging results with relatively few postoperative complications. Not only do patients appear to improve initially, long-term results demonstrate improvement for up to 10

years after surgery (41,42). Despite such positive reports, the potential for significant complications does exist, and is increased when reduction maneuvers are attempted. Complications include vascular as well as neurologic injury. Reports range from a 0 to 30% incidence of L5, S1 nerve root injury, or cauda equina syndrome. The incidence of pseudoarthrosis secondary to shear forces is greater than that reported from posterolateral *in situ* fusion. Despite the potential risks of ALIF, no statistically significant difference in fusion rates or clinical outcome has been demonstrated when compared with posterior decompression and fusion with pedicle screw fixation (41).

COMBINED ALIF AND POSTERIOR INSTRUMENTATION

The trend for higher pseudoarthrosis rates secondary to shear forces with ALIF alone lead to the use of supplemental posterior pedicle screw fixation and fusion (43). Fusion rates did appear to improve; however, the overall success rate was similar to that of either ALIF or posterior fusion. In addition, increased operative times and blood loss makes this surgical option less appealing.

DISCUSSION

To date there have been many studies evaluating surgical management of low-grade nondegenerative spondylolisthesis. Regardless of the method employed, the indications for surgical intervention are quite uniform. These are low back pain with or without lower extremity pain despite an adequate trial of conservative treatment, or symptomatic slip progression.

The authors recommend the following approach to the evaluation and treatment of those individuals with symptomatic low-grade nondegenerative slips. Clinical symptoms/signs of low back pain and nerve root irritation consistent with spondylolisthesis should be documented. Anteroposterior (AP), lateral, and oblique lumbosacral plain radiographs are obtained for the purposes of classifying the type and grade of slip. The first line of treatment should be conservative; it is important to stress to the patient that nonoperative treatment does not equate to no treatment. Conservative management consists of supervised physical therapy, weight reduction, activity modification, pain blocks, and if applicable, job retraining.

For that subset of patients who complete the 6-month course of conservative care and continue to be symptomatic, surgical intervention is pursued. A magnetic resonance (MR) image and dynamic LS spine films are obtained preoperatively. Flexion/extension films provide a rough estimate of the degree of instability present and the potential need for instrumentation. The presence and extent of disc and facet degeneration can be evaluated on

MRI. In addition, discography, selective nerve root, facet, or pars blocks can better delineate the source of the patient's pain.

For young individuals (between the age of 16 and 30) with no evidence of DDD, with complaints primarily of low back pain, we recommend direct pars repair for those lesions of L4 and above. The presence of other congenital posterior defects at L5 often prohibits repair. Only in rare circumstances in which the posterior and anterior elements are normal do we recommend repair of the L5 defect. Preoperative MRI evaluation is an excellent means of evaluating the integrity of the posterior and anterior elements. In addition to plain radiographs and MRI, we also recommend diagnostic pars blocks to help differentiate the source of the patient's symptoms and signs. Although more technically demanding, the maintained motion and restoration of normal alignment provide excellent long-term patient satisfaction.

For those patients who are not candidates for direct repair, we further subclassify them based on presenting signs and symptoms. Patients can typically be separated into one of three categories:

1. Category A—mechanical low back pain with normal neurologic examination
2. Category B—mechanical low back pain with extremity pain and normal neurologic examination
3. Category C—mechanical low back pain and either unilateral or bilateral radicular leg pain.

For those patients who fall into either category A or B we recommend posterolateral *in situ* fusion with autologous bone graft as the primary surgical treatment. This can be accomplished either through a midline posterior approach or a Wiltse posterior muscle splitting approach (which is our preferred method). We do not, however, recommend dual skin incisions. Removal of the facet capsule and articular cartilage and insertion of bone graft is an important part of the procedure. We do recommend the addition of pedicle screw fixation in those individuals who have identifiable risk factors for pseudoarthrosis or demonstrate excessive motion on dynamic radiographs. Risk factors for nonunion include tobacco use, revision procedures secondary to an established nonunion, iatrogenic slip, or long-term NSAID use for other medical problems.

For patients who present with symptoms and signs consistent with a radiculopathy (category C), we elect to perform a single-level decompression and *in situ* fusion with autologous bone graft. Once again, instrumentation is used for individuals who are at greater risk of nonunion or demonstrate excessive motion.

CONCLUSION

Each intervention presents a unique set of technical demands, potential risks, and complications. Whether one chooses to address the condition anteriorly, posteriorly, or some combination thereof, success is directly related to achieving a solid fusion. For those individuals without degenerative disc disease or evidence of advanced facet arthritis, direct pars repair provides satisfactory results with limited loss of lumbar motion. The success rate in the presence of preexisting degenerative disc disease or abnormal facets has been clearly demonstrated to significantly diminish over time.

We recommend posterior *in situ* fusion for those symptomatic patients with evidence of disc or facet abnormality. The addition of a posterior decompression in the setting of leg pain without radicular findings does not significantly improve the results and should be avoided. The results in the presence of a true radiculopathy do improve with combined posterior decompression and fusion. Supplemental instrumentation should be considered for those patients at higher risk of developing a pseudoarthrosis, or who demonstrate motion on dynamic radiographs.

In conclusion, the key points when treating patients with symptomatic low-grade slips are to determine whether they are suitable surgical candidates, and to determine what is the most efficacious, reliable, and safest means of addressing the pathology. Regardless of the surgical procedure performed, the ability to obtain a solid fusion and thereby reduce pathologic motion and the risk of progression provides the patient with the best chance for a positive outcome.

REFERENCES

1. Newman PH. The etiology of spondylolisthesis. J Bone Joint Surg (Am) 1963;45B:39–59.
2. Wiltse LL, Jackson DW. Treatment of spondylolisthesis and spondylolysis in children. Clin Orthop 1976;117:92–100.
3. Fredrickson BE. The natural history of spondylolysis and spondylolisthesis. J Bone Joint Surg 1984;66A:699.
4. Osterman K, Schlenzka D, Poussa M, et al. Isthmic spondylolisthesis in symptomatic and asymptomatic subjects, epidemiology, and natural history with special reference to disk abnormality and mode of treatment. Clin Orthop 1993;297:65–70.
5. Deutman R, Diercks RL, de Jong TE, et al. Isthmic lumbar spondylolisthesis with sciatica: the role of the disc. Eur Spine J 1995;4:136–138.
6. Floman Y. Progression of lumbosacral isthmic spondylolisthesis in adults. Spine 2000;25:342–347.
7. Moon MS. The pathomechanism of isthmic lumbar spondylolisthesis: a biomechanical study in immature calf spines. Spine 1999;24:731–732.
8. Wiltse LL, Hutchinson RH. Surgical treatment of spondylolisthesis. Clin Orthop 1964;35:116–135.
9. Wiltse LL, Newman PH, Macnab I. Classification of spondylolisis and spondylolisthesis. Clin Orthop 1976;117:23–29.
10. Wiltse LL, Widell EH Jr, Jackson DW. Fatigue fracture: the basic lesion is isthmic spondylolisthesis. J Bone Joint Surg Am 1975;57:17–22.
11. Vaccaro AR, Martyak GG, Madigan L. Adult isthmic spondylolisthesis. Orthopedics 2001;24:1172–1177; quiz 1178–1179.
12. Vaccaro AR, Ring D, Scuderi G, et al. Predictors of outcome in patients with chronic back pain and low-grade spondylolisthesis. Spine 1997;22:2030–2034; discussion 2035.
13. Johnson LP, Nasca RJ, Dunham WK. Surgical management of isthmic spondylolisthesis. Spine 1988;13:93–97.
14. Ohmori K, Ishida Y, Takatsu T, et al. Vertebral slip in lumbar spondy-

lolysis and spondylolisthesis. Long-term follow-up of 22 adult patients. J Bone Joint Surg Br 1995;77:771–773.

15. Hanley EN Jr. Indications for fusion in the lumbar spine. Bull Hosp Joint Dis 1996;55:154–157.

16. Frennered K. Isthmic spondylolisthesis among patients receiving disability pension under the diagnosis of chronic low back pain syndromes. Spine 1994;19:2766–2769.

17. Hanley EN Jr, Levy JA. Surgical treatment of isthmic lumbosacral spondylolisthesis. Analysis of variables influencing results. Spine 1989;14:48–50.

18. Lauerman WC, Cain JE. Isthmic spondylolisthesis in the adult. J Am Acad Orthop Surg 1996;4:201–208.

19. Lenke LG, Bridwell KH, Bullis D, et al. Results of in situ fusion for isthmic spondylolisthesis. J Spinal Disord 1992;5:433–442.

20. Moller H, Hedlund R. Surgery versus conservative management in adult isthmic spondylolisthesis—a prospective randomized study: part 1. Spine 2000;25:1711–1715.

21. Mooney V. Re: Surgery versus conservative medical and adult isthmic spondylolisthesis (Spine 2000;25:1711–1715). Spine 2001;26:594–595.

22. Gill GG, White HL. Surgical treatment of spondylolisthesis without spine fusion. A long term follow-up of operated cases. Acta Orthop Scand 1965;85[Suppl]:5–99.

22a. Gill GG. Long-term follow-up evaluation of a few patients with spondylolisthesis treated by excision of the loose lamina with decompression of the nerve roots without spinal fusion. Clin Orthop 1984;182:215–219.

23. de Loubresse CG, Bon T, Deburge A, et al. Posterolateral fusion for radicular pain in isthmic spondylolisthesis. Clin Orthop 1996;323:194–201.

24. Deguchi M, Rapoff AJ, Zdeblick TA. Posterolateral fusion for isthmic spondylolisthesis in adults: analysis of fusion rate and clinical results. J Spinal Disord 1998;11:459–464.

25. Harrington PR, Dickson JH. Spinal instrumentation in the treatment of severe progressive spondylolisthesis. Clin Orthop 1976;117:157–163.

26. Nooraie H, Ensafdaran A, Arasteh MM. Surgical management of low-grade lytic spondylolisthesis with C-D instrumentation in adult patients. Arch Orthop Trauma Surg 1999;119:337–339.

27. Ohmori K, Suzuki K, Ishida Y. Translamino-pedicular screw fixation with bone grafting for symptomatic isthmic lumbar spondylolysis. Neurosurgery 1992;30:379–384.

28. Ricciardi JE, Pflueger PC, Isaza JE, et al. Transpedicular fixation for the treatment of isthmic spondylolisthesis in adults. Spine 1995;20:1917–1922.

29. Schnee CL, Freese A, Ansell LV. Outcome analysis for adults with spondylolisthesis treated with posterolateral fusion and transpedicular screw fixation. J Neurosurg 1997;86:56–63.

30. Bonnici AV, Koka SR, Richards DJ. Results of Buck screw fusion in grade I spondylolisthesis. J R Soc Med 1991;84:270–273.

31. Buck JE. Direct repair of the defect in spondylolisthesis. Preliminary report. J Bone Joint Surg Br 1970;52:432–437.

32. Dai LY, Jia LS, Yuan W, et al. Direct repair of defect in lumbar spondylolysis and mild isthmic spondylolisthesis by bone grafting, with or without facet joint fusion. Eur Spine J 2001;10:78–83.

33. Jeanneret B, Miclau T, Kuster M, et al. Posterior stabilization in L5-S1 isthmic spondylolisthesis with paralaminar screw fixation: anatomical and clinical results. J Spinal Disord 1996;9:223–233.

34. Johnson GV, Thompson AG. The Scott wiring technique for direct repair of lumbar spondylolysis. J Bone Joint Surg Br 1992;74:426–430.

35. Nicol RO, Scott JH. Lytic spondylolysis. Repair by wiring. Spine 1986;11:1027–1030.

36. Winter M, Jani L. Results of screw osteosynthesis in spondylolysis and low-grade spondylolisthesis. Arch Orthop Trauma Surg 1989;108:96–99.

37. Seitsalo S, Schlenzka D, Poussa M, et al. Disc degeneration in young patients with isthmic spondylolisthesis treated operatively or conservatively: a long-term follow-up. Eur Spine J 1997;6:393–397.

38. Salib RM, Pettine KA. Modified repair of a defect in spondylolysis or minimal spondylolisthesis by pedicle screw, segmental wire fixation, and bone grafting. Spine 1993;18:440–443.

39. Cheng CL, Fang D, Lee PC, et al. Anterior spinal fusion for spondylolysis and isthmic spondylolisthesis. Long term results in adults. J Bone Joint Surg Br 1989;71:264–267.

40. Ishihara H, Osada R, Kanamori M, et al. Minimum 10-year follow-up study of anterior lumbar interbody fusion for isthmic spondylolisthesis. J Spinal Disord 2001;14:91–99.

41. Kim NH, Lee JW. Anterior interbody fusion versus posterolateral fusion with transpedicular fixation for isthmic spondylolisthesis in adults. A comparison of clinical results. Spine 1999;24:812–6; discussion 817.

42. Tsuji H, Ishihara H, Matsui H, et al. Anterior interbody fusion with and without interspinous block implementation for lumbar isthmic spondylolisthesis. J Spinal Disord 1994;7:326–330.

43. Kim SS, Denis F, Lonstein JE, et al. Factors affecting fusion rate in adult spondylolisthesis. Spine 1990;15:979–984.

CHAPTER 64

Surgery for High-Grade Spondylolisthesis

Marek Szpalski and Robert Gunzburg

Spondylolisthesis is a common condition reported in 5% to 6% of Caucasian males and 2% to 3% of Caucasian females (1). It can be encountered in up to 50% in Alaskan Inuits (2). In the latter case, Stewart suggested that this high frequency could be due to repeated falls on the ice may be associated with a predisposing weakness of the pars (3).

This chapter discusses high slippage isthmic spondylolisthesis classified by Wiltse as IIA (4). In the Meyerding classification, those high-grade slippages are classified as III and IV, meaning a displacement of more than 50% (5). A further degree consisting of the fall of the vertebra in front of the sacrum is referred to as spondyloptosis. Progression of slip is usually reported at 6% in adult life, so a relatively small number of subjects will fall into this category.

The existence of type I or congenital spondylolysis is controversial. Dysplastic articular process may predispose to pars elongation and separation, but we did not find any published report of spondylolysis found at birth. Spondylolysis does not therefore appear to be a congenital lesion and developmental errors are not considered relevant to its etiology (6). It does not appear that spondylolysis was ever described in newborns or very young infants. Repetitive stress seems to be the main etiologic factor although hereditary factors may predispose to the injury (7,8). Once separation of the pars occurs, however, so-called type I is indistinguishable from type IIA.

Contrary to other stress fracture locations, spondylolysis only rarely heals spontaneously.

In the vast majority of subjects, the condition is present at the L5S1 level. The frequency is higher in subjects presenting frequent lumbar hyperlordosis—dancers, gymnasts, weight lifters, javelin throwers, football linemen, and so forth.

Higher grade lesions will provoke different mechanical or neurologic problems. On the neurologic point, root impingement and stenosis (foraminal, lateral, or central) can be encountered. This can be made worse by the frequent degenerative changes and disc bulge accompanying spondylolisthesis. The tension of the dural sac over the upper edge of the S1 vertebra can even induce a cauda equina syndrome.

Higher slippage degree will influence the sagittal spinopelvic alignment and balance that may be very disabling, as it will eventually involve knee flexion and spine hyperextension.

Although even high-grade lesions can be silent, symptomatic high-grade spondylolisthesis will often require adequate surgical treatment.

The surgical options will include simple decompression, fusion *in situ* with possible decompression, reduction, and fusion. Fusion can be anterior or posterior and reduction can be accompanied by partial or total resection of the slipped vertebra.

INDICATIONS FOR SURGERY

In children and adolescents, all subjects with a slip over 50% or with documented progression of a slip from 25% to 50%, regardless of symptoms, will be candidates for surgery (9). Patients with L1 to L4 spondylolisthesis often have a poorer prognosis than those with a lower lesion. However some authors have described a very long-term follow-up of high-grade spondylolisthesis patients treated conservatively with good results, although surgical treatment resulted in a higher and faster symptomatic improvement (10).

In adults the main indication for surgery will be based on the importance of the symptoms, persistent leg pain, neurologic deficits, or cauda equina syndrome are definitive indications. The same applies in cases in which major sagittal imbalance induces severe standing, walking, or visual difficulties (11). Although back pain is more frequent in patients with higher slip (12), surgery for isolated back pain is still discussed as the exact source of nociception is unclear. Highly disabling back pain is a relative indication; however, the patient must be aware

591

that a full resolution of pain is not certain. Caution should be exercised before deciding to operate for isolated back pain in even high-grade spondylolisthesis patients. Only realistic surgeon and patient expectation will avoid major and some times medicolegal disappointments.

Goals of surgery in symptomatic high-grade spondylolisthesis comprise the resolution of back and leg pain as well as the restoration of anatomic balance and function by the fusion of the affected levels. This surgery, however, is extremely challenging and accompanied with a high rate of complications. The aim of achieving an anatomic reduction may lead to an increase in back or leg pain. Surgical therapy should therefore always be considered with the utmost caution.

High-grade spondylolisthesis is relatively rare and large series, especially randomized comparative studies, difficult to perform. Possible techniques include decompression, posterior fusion *in situ*, posterior decompression and posterolateral fusion without reduction, 360° *in situ* fusion, 360° fusion after reduction, L5 resection, and L4 to S1 fusion.

Decompression

Some authors have advocated isolated decompressive laminectomy and presented satisfactory results (13) when they performed an associated partial facetectomy. However, this study treated degenerative lesions of moderate grade. Other studies present a success rate around 70% (14,15).

Laminectomy alone (even total) does not seem sufficient to decompress all the neural structures and more specifically the foramen. It is often necessary to remove the remaining pars interarticularis and all callus fragments (Gill nodules) (14). At the L5-S1 level it will sometimes be necessary to resect the sacral dome anterior to the cauda equina.

Moreover further slippage, with worsening of symptoms, often occurs after isolated decompressive surgery (16–18).

For all these reasons it appears that decompression alone does not seem an adequate treatment of high-grade spondylolisthesis (19), and significant decompression should be followed by fusion (12).

Fusion *in situ*

Fusion *in situ* is a widely accepted treatment for lumbosacral spondylolisthesis (20). It is a safe and reliable procedure and excellent results have been reported in the cases of high-grade displacements. It is the most common type of surgery performed in the treatment of spondylolisthesis. Posterior, anterior, and combined procedures have been described. The number of levels involved in the fusion has been subject to discussion. It is generally

believed that in case of severe displacement at L5-S1 (Meyerding grade III and IV) the fusion should include L4 and down to the sacrum. Some authors even advocate L4-S1 fusion in lower-grade lesions (21).

Posterolateral Fusion

Posterolateral *in situ* fusion has been routinely recommended (18,22,23), in spite of relatively high pseudoarthrosis rates (24–26).

This procedure can be performed by midline or bilateral lateral approach. In the presence of neurologic signs or symptoms, decompression will be realized. Ricciardi et al. reported good results after transpedicular fixation combined with systematic L5 root decompression (27). However, adjuvant extensive decompression may favor pseudoarthrosis and Carragee found no advantages in performing decompression in patients without serious neurologic deficits (19).

As in all posterolateral fusions obesity or a history of smoking induces of higher risk of pseudoarthrosis. In presence of nonfusion, slippage can gradually increase. Among the complications described, acute cauda equina syndrome in the early postoperative period is a rare but dramatic event. Neurologic complications and even cauda equina syndrome can also occur after *in situ* fusion (28). In a series of 189 patients, Schoenecker et al. reported a 6% cauda equina incidence in patients who had no neurologic dysfunction before surgery (28).

Some authors have attributed cauda equina lesions to mechanical damage endured during decortication before bone grafting (29). Nevertheless, good functional results have been reported at long-term follow-up. Johnson and Kirwan report an average follow-up of 14 years with favorable outcome (23). It appears that even though there is no correction of the sagittal pelvic balance, kinematic and temporal parameters of gait can be normalized after *in situ* fusion (30).

Instrumentation is widely used and transpedicular fixation appears to be the material of choice. However, the use of instrumentation remains a controversial subject. Many studies present good results with instrumentation (31), however, few are prospective and controlled. Some prospective controlled studies have reported better fusion rates but no change in outcome with instrumentation than with noninstrumented fusion (19,32). In a mixed cohort of diverse indications including spondylolisthesis, Zdeblick reported better fusion rates and outcomes (33). However, in another study Thomsen did not show any differences in fusion rate or outcome (34). The same results where reported by France in a mixed cohort (35). McGuire showed no difference in fusion rate between instrumented and noninstrumented fusion (36).

A metaanalysis of the available controlled trials showed a slightly significant advantage of instrumentation to produce bone fusion and a nonsignificant trend toward better outcomes (37). A Cochrane Review of surgery for degenerative spondylolisthesis shows no advantage of surgical treatment over conservative alternatives (38).

However, those controlled studies usually refer to low-grade or degenerative spondylolisthesis and there does not appear to be similar controlled work in the area of higher grade lesions. In slips, over 50% adjunction of instrumentation seems a reasonable and safe alternative. (17). Nevertheless, the reported pseudoarthrosis rates are high, ranging from 17% to 40%. Bending of the fusion mass and instrumentation failure have also been described and increased slippage can occur in the absence of fusion even with the use of adequate instrumentation.

Posterior Interbody Fusion (PLIF)

The use of PLIF has been described in grade I and II spondylolisthesis (39,40) and in grade III and IV after reduction (41) but does not appear to have been described in grade III and IV *in situ* fusion.

Bohlman and Cook described a fibular strut placed posteriorly from the sacrum into the body of L5. This technique appears interesting in the stabilization of higher grade lesions (42). A similar technique has been used by Esses et al. (43).

Anterior Interbody Fusion (ALIF)

Isolated ALIF has been suggested (44) and described for the treatment of lower-grade spondylolisthesis since the 1930s (45), and ALIF cages have been used routinely (26,46).

Some authors report a high rate of progressive slippage after ALIF when slippage is over 50% (11). In high displacement cases, the size of the contact surfaces available for fusion is very limited. It does not appear that cages have been used in the *in situ* fusion of high-grade lesions.

Verbiest has described a technique using a fibular graft placed between L4 and the sacrum in the stabilization of high-grade spondylolisthesis (47). This technique provides a good anterior column support and the anterior fibular graft has been used with success by other authors (48).

The addition of an anterior fibular strut has also been described as a salvage procedure in the treatment of failed isolated posterior fusion with good reported results (49,50).

Isolated anterior intervertebral cages or dowels are not appropriate in the treatment of spondylolisthesis as they are unable to stand the constant high shear loads encountered in lumbosacral spondylolisthesis combined with an immobile sacral segment and highly mobile lower lumbar area (51,52).

Circumferential Fusion (360°)

Several authors propose a combined anterior and posterior stabilization, especially in the adult patient and if a wide decompression has been performed (48). Smith and Bohlamn described good results with a combined *in situ* fusion through a single posterior approach, partial resection of the first sacral segment and an anterior interbody fibular graft combined with a posterolateral fusion (53). Roca et al. (54) have also reported favorable results with the same technique in a group of patients presenting with an average slip of 77% and a slip angle of 36°.

It appears that circumferential fusion has been mostly described in combination with a reduction of the slippage.

Reduction of Spondylolisthesis

The first trials of reducing spondylolisthesis were reported in the 1930s (55); however, poor results and major neurologic complications led to the abandonment of those procedures in favor of *in situ* fusions. In the 1970s, reduction through a two-step posterior and anterior approach with the use of Harrington rods is described (56). Other techniques describe the preoperative reduction by plaster casts followed by posterior instrumentation and fusion with good results (57). The more recent evolution of surgical techniques and efficient instrumentations brought a new interest in reduction of severe spondylolisthesis.

Several reasons can be put forward to advocate reduction of spondylolisthesis. The cosmetic appearance is a first factor to consider as *in situ* fusion does not restore the sagittal balance. Therefore, reduction will improve this cosmetic aspect (58). However, many studies have shown that cosmetic deformity was not considered a major problem by the majority of patients (10,23,31). Some authors even reported that patients who had undergone reduction were less satisfied with their appearance than those who had simple *in situ* fusion (59).

The high pseudarthrosis rate and progression of slippage associated with *in situ* fusion can be improved by performing a reduction (60,61) and avoiding high tensile shear forces across the fusion mass. Yet, this maneuver increases risk of neurologic injury, particularly to nerve root L5 (17). According to Kozak (62), routine release of the lumbosacral ligament in order to avoid injury to the L5 nerve root seems prudent. Molinari et al. (63) found *in situ* fusion to give poor results when severe dysplasia of the posterior elements of L5 are present, in particular small transverse process surfaces.

In a recent retrospective analysis of six cases in which partial lumbosacral kyphosis reduction, posterior decompression, and pedicle screw fixation were performed, Boachie-Adje et al. found that it is the partial reduction of the slip angle and not the percentage of slip that is important in obtaining optimal results (64). With a similar technique using fibular allograft for the posterior interbody fusion, Smith et al. (65) had good clinical and radiologic results in nine cases.

According to Molinari et al. (63) the addition of long iliac screws reduces the risk of instrumentation failure. Experimental biomechanics studies have shown the advantages of screws purchasing the iliac bone down to the acetabular column (66). Other authors have advocated the use of a second set of sacral fixation points (67). Klöckner stresses the fact that the dome-shaped surface of the sacrum needs to be resected, thus allowing a monosegmental reduction (68).

Grade III and IV spondylolisthesis cases, in which the kyphosis has led to an impairment of the full upright standing position with extended hips and knees, are a primary indication for reduction. Such a reduction can be achieved by either a posterior instrumented approach, a combined anterior and posterior approach (360°), or a vertebral body resection. Slow gradual reduction by means of an external fixator followed by internal fusion and fixation has also been described (69,70). Using this method, Wild et al. report good results, an 84.5% correction of the slip and no neurologic complications (70). Only experienced surgeons should perform these operations and neurologic monitoring is certainly not a luxury. Based on a retrospective analysis of 93 cases of grade III or IV spondylolisthesis, Seitsalo et al. (18) suggested that an attempt to reduce an increased slip angle was warranted in some cases.

Some authors however believe that in adults the risks of reduction outweigh the benefits (53,71,72). These risks consist primarily of neurologic compromise of the cauda equina or the L5 nerve root by lengthening and traction or by impingement against the iliolumbar ligament. The frequency of neurologic complications reported in the literature varies from 6% to over 50% (17,24,63,67,73–76).

An experimental study Petraco et al. suggests that partial reduction be advocated since the risk of stretch injury to the L5 root is not linear and sharply increases during the second half of reduction. Reductions greater than 50% of the width of the L5 body demonstrated the higher root tension and potential for neurologic injury (77).

It appears that reduction of the slip angle is more important than reduction of the percentage slip and that partial reduction of the slip angle is often sufficient to reduce kyphosis and enable stable fixation while decreasing the neurologic problems associated with more complex reduction maneuvers (64). Furthermore, reduction of slip angle allows easier decompressive maneuvers and places the fusion mass in a more compressive position, thus decreasing the risk of fusion mass elongation and pseudoarthrosis. Furthermore, for some authors, such a partial reduction allows the use of isolated posterior fusion without the need for additional anterior exposure. Smith and Bohlman report good results with partial reduction and fixation with a posterior interbody fibula interposition supplemented by a pedicular fixation (63). Those techniques using an isolated posterior approach decrease the burden and risk of neurologic and vascular complications associated with anterior approaches.

The advantage of the posterior reduction techniques is that they can be completed in one stage. A thorough decompression has to be performed before the reduction is attempted and a fixation by transpedicular screw is mandatory to maintain the position. It is more important to correct the kyphosis than to correct the translation (64). In a report on prospective cases Steffee and Brantigan (78) noted clinical success in 86% of patients with spondylolisthesis.

With posterolateral surgery the fusion mass is under tension. This has led to many cases of nonunion when severe slippage was present. Hu et al. (67) reported on 16 patients and found hardware failure in 5 cases. Boos et al. (79) reported 83% implant failure and pseudarthrosis rate in patients where postreduction stabilization was performed by an isolated posterolateral fusion. They recommend a combined interbody and posterior fusion since they believe that pedicular fixation systems alone do not allow permanent stabilization.

Due to the problems reported with isolated posterior fixation, many authors have advocated the use of anterior column support (67). Molinari et al. found largely superior results after reduction in those patients with added anterior support compared with those treated by posterior fusion alone. The rate of nonfusion in the latter group was 39% compared to none in the 360° group (25). DeWald et al. also reported a very high rate of solid fusion after 2 years' follow-up after reduction and 360° fusion (24).

Indeed, the combination with anterior surgery where the graft is under compression answers a biomechanical rationale adopted by many (11,24,80,81). These two operative stages can either be performed in one or two separate stages with a one-week interval. Anterior fusion can be obtained by the use of an array of devices ranging from autologous bone (fibula, iliac crest) and allografts to cages of varying shapes and composition. Louis and Maresca have described a technique with a specific instrumentation allowing L5 to be tilted back on to S1 and progressively pushed back in place (61).

Laursen et al. reported good results following partial reduction and fixation by anterior interbody fusion and posterior pedicular screws. There were no complications and good functional outcome (82).

Circumferential fusion also decreases the occurrence of hardware failure.

Reduction of severe spondylolisthesis is a demanding and very long surgery; surgical duration is often around 8 hours (67) and blood loss may be critical. The results of reduction in severe spondylolisthesis are satisfactory but must be balanced by the risk of permanent neurologic complications. Although for some authors this risk is acceptably low it is, nevertheless, present and much higher than in cases of *in situ* fusion. Therefore care must be taken, in postoperative planning, to compare this risk with the importance of the expected benefits.

Vertebral Body Resection

Total resection of the fifth vertebral body and fusion of L4 to S1 has been proposed by Gaines and Nichols (83). The rationale was that the shortening would facilitate the sagittal balance realignment and reduce the risk of neurologic impairment. A high rate of complications precluding the wide application of the technique was later reported (84). Out of 16 patients, 12 had early postoperative neurologic troubles and 5 had permanent neurologic motor deficit. Four patients had a revision surgery for pseudarthrosis or fixation failure. This procedure has also been advocated by other authors (85).

The indications for this type of surgery are exceptional. Wild et al. present such a procedure for the treatment of spondyloptosis in an 18-month-old patient with good results after 10 years of follow-up (86).

CONCLUSIONS

The goal of surgery in high-grade spondylolisthesis is to improve pain, neurologic deficits, and avoid further displacement. Restoration of sagittal balance will be a major goal if kyphosis disallows the patient to stand, walk, or look forward. Patients presenting with such severe sagittal imbalance are at risk of further slippage and subsequent neurologic damage. Cosmetic criteria do not appear to be major surgical indications in most subjects (31).

However, surgery for high-grade spondylolisthesis, and more specifically reduction techniques, carries a high incidence of major complications, mainly neurologic, which are sometimes permanent. Likewise, the incidence of revision procedures for fixation failure is high. In those conditions the risk/benefit ratio for this surgery has to be assessed carefully.

The exceptional nature of this surgery and the small sample sizes encountered in most studies make true randomized controlled studies hardly feasible. The lack of an instrument to record specific outcome makes the problem even more complex. Some authors (65) have applied the Scoliosis Research Society (SRS) outcome questionnaire described by Haher et al. (87) and modified by Asher et al. (88). However, the SRS instrument was only validated for adolescent scoliosis and validation of the same or another instrument in the context of high-grade spondylolisthesis would be welcome.

Fusion *in situ* appears indicated for pain and minor walking disturbances in the absence of neurologic symptoms or deficits. Reduction (essentially partial) will be indicated in more severe cases. Complete reduction or vertebrectomy will only be indicated in a few extremely severe cases.

Surgery in high-grade spondylolisthesis and spondyloptosis is a high-risk surgery and should be restricted to those cases where conservative treatment could not significantly reduce invalidating complaints of low back pain and radiculopathy or walking or forward vision is not possible because of severe sagittal plane imbalance. It should be performed only by experienced surgeons in well-equipped centers.

REFERENCES

1. Rowe GG, Roche MB. The etiology of separate neural arch. J Bone Joint Surg 1953;35A:102–110.
2. Kettlekamp DB, Wright GD. Spondylolysis in the Alaskan Eskimos. J Bone Joint Surg 1971;53-A:563–566.
3. Stewart TD, Washington DC. The age incidence of neural-arch defects in Alaskans natives considered from the standpoint of etiology. J Bone Joint Surg 1953;35-A:937–950.
4. Wiltse LL, Winter RB. Terminology and measurement of spondylolisthesis. J Bone Joint Surg 1983;65-A:768–772.
5. Meyerding HW. Spondylolisthesis. Surg Gynecol Obstet 1932;54: 372–377.
6. Krenz J, Troup JDG. The structure of the pars interarticularis of the lower lumbar vertebrae and its relation to the etiology of spondylolisthesis. J Bone Joint Surg 1973;55-B:735–741.
7. Haukipuro K, Keranen N, Koivisto E, et al. Familial occurrence of lumbar spondylolysis and spondylolisthesis. Clin Genet 1978;13:471–476.
8. Wynne-Davis R, Scott JH. Inheritance and spondylolisthesis: a radiographic family survey. J Bone Joint Surg Br 1979;61-B:301–305.
9. Amundsen G, Edwards CC, Garfin SR. Spondylolisthesis. In: Herkowitz HN, Garfin SR, Balderston RA, et al., eds. Rothman-Simeone the spine. Philadelphia: WB Saunders, 1999;835–885.
10. Harris IE, Weinstein SL. Long-term follow-up of patients with grade-III and IV spondylolisthesis. Treatment with and without posterior fusion. J Bone Joint Surg Am 1987;69:960–969.
11. Boxall D, Bradford DS, Winter RB, et al. Management of severe spondylolisthesis. J Bone Joint Surg 1979;61A:479–495.
12. Lauerman WC, Cain JE. Isthmic spondylolisthesis in the adult. J Am Acad Orthop Surg 1996;4:201–208.
13. Herron LD, Trippi AC. L4-5 degenerative spondylolisthesis: the results of treatment by decompressive laminectomy without fusion. Spine 1989;14:534–538.
14. Gill GG. Spondylolisthesis and its treatment: excision of loose lamina and decompression. In Runge D, Wiltse LL, eds. Spinal disorders: diagnosis and treatment. Philadelphia: Lea & Febiger, 1977:218–222.
15. Lapras C, Pierluca P, Pernot P, et al. Treatment of spondylolisthesis (stage I-II) by neurosurgical decompression without either osteosynthesis or reduction. Neurochirurgie 1984;30:147–152.
16. Davis IS, Bailey RW. Spondylolisthesis. Long-term follow-up study of treatment with total laminectomy. Clin Orthop 1972;88:46–49.
17. Hensinger RN. Spondylolysis and spondylolysthesis in children and adolescents. J Bone Joint Surg 1989;71-A:1098–1107.
18. Seitsalo S, Osterman K, Hyvarinen H, et al. Severe spondylolisthesis in children and adolescents. A long-term review of fusion in situ. J Bone Joint Surg Br 1990;72:259–265.
19. Caragee E. Single level postero lateral arthrodesis, with or without posterior decompression for the treatment of isthmic spondylolisthesis in adults: a prospective randomized study. J Bone Joint Surg 1997;79-A: 1175–1180.
20. Smith JA, Hu SS. Management of spondylolysis and spondylolisthesis in the pediatric and adolescent population. Orthop Clin North Am 1999;30:487–499.
21. Hanley EN, Levy JA. Surgical treatment of isthmic lumbosacral spondylolisthesis. Analysis of variables influencing results. Spine 1989;14:48–50.

22. Frennered AK, Danielson BI, Nachemson AL, et al. Midterm follow-up of young patients fused in situ for spondylolisthesis. Spine 1999; 16:409–416.

23. Johnson JR, Kirwan EO. The long-term results of fusion in situ for severe spondylolisthesis. J Bone Joint Surg Br 1983;65:43–46.

24. DeWald RL, Faut MM, Taddonio RF, et al. Severe lumbosacral spondylolisthesis in adolescents and children. Reduction and staged circumferential fusion. J Bone Joint Surg Am 1981;63:619–626.

25. Molinari RW, Bridwell KH, Lenke LG, et al. Anterior column support in surgery for high-grade, isthmic spondylolisthesis. Clin Orthop 2002; 394:109–120.

26. Van Rens TJ, van Horn JR. Long-term results in lumbosacral interbody fusion for spondylolisthesis. Acta Orthop Scand 1982;53:383–392.

27. Ricciardi JE, Pflueger PC, Isaza JE, et al. Transpedicular fixation for the treatment of isthmic spondylolisthesis in adults. Spine 1995;20: 1917–1922.

28. Schoenecker PL, Cole HO, Herring JA, et al. Cauda equina syndrome after in-situ arthrodesis for severe spondylolysthesis at the lumbosacral junction J Bone Joint Surg 1990;72-A:369–377.

29. Maurice HD, Morley TR . Cauda equina lesions following fusion in situ and decompressive laminectomy for severe spondylolisthesis. Four case reports. Spine 1989;14:214–216.

30. Meyers LL, Dobson SR, Wiegand D, et al. Mechanical instability as a cause of gait disturbance in high-grade spondylolisthesis: a pre- and postoperative three-dimensional gait analysis. J Pediatr Orthop 1999; 19:672–676.

31. Freeman BL 3rd, Donati NL. Spinal arthrodesis for severe spondylolisthesis in children and adolescents. A long-term follow-up study. J Bone Joint Surg Am 1989;71:594–598.

32. Fischgrund JS, Mackay M, Herkowitz HN, et al. Degenerative lumbar spondylolisthesis with spinal stenosis: a prospective, randomized study comparing decompressive laminectomy and arthrodesis with and without spinal instrumentation. Spine 1997;22:2807–2812.

33. Zdeblick TA. A prospective, randomized study of lumbar fusion. Preliminary results. Spine 1993;18:9839–9891.

34. Thomsen K, Christensen FB, Eiskjaer SP, et al. The effect of pedicle screw instrumentation on functional outcome and fusion rates in posterolateral lumbar spinal fusion: a prospective, randomized clinical study. Spine 1997;22:2813–2822.

35. France JC, Yaszemski MJ, Lauerman WC, et al. A randomized prospective study of posterolateral lumbar fusion. Outcomes with and without pedicle screw instrumentation. Spine 1999;24:553–560.

36. McGuire RA, Amundson GM. The use of primary internal fixation in spondylolisthesis. Spine 1993;18:1662–1672.

37. Nachemson AL, Johnson EJ. Neck and back pain. Philadelphia: Lippincott Williams & Wilkins, 2000:318–321.

38. Gibson JNA, Waddell G, Grant IC. Surgery for degenerative lumbar spondylosis. Cochrane Database Syst Rev 2000;(3):CD001352.

39. Hashimoto T, Shigenobu K, Kanayama M, et al. Clinical results of single-level posterior lumbar interbody fusion using the Brantigan I/F carbon cage filled with a mixture of local morselized bone and bioactive ceramic granules. Spine 2002;27:258–262.

40. Lerat JL, Rubini J, Vincent P, et al. Results of posterior lumbar intersomatic fusion in the treatment of isthmic spondylolisthesis. Apropos of 27 cases followed over more than 10 years Rev Chir Orthop Reparatrice Appar Mot 1996;82:475–489.

41. Klockner C, Weber U. Correction of lumbosacral kyphosis in high grade spondylolisthesis and spondyloptosis. Orthopade 2001;30:983–987.

42. Bohlman HH, Cook SS. One-stage decompression and posterolateral and interbody fusion for lumbosacral spondyloptosis through a posterior approach. Report of two cases. J Bone Joint Surg Am 1982;64:415–418.

43. Esses SI, Natout N, Kip P. Posterior interbody arthrodesis with a fibular strut graft in spondylolisthesis. J Bone Joint Surg Am 1995;77: 172–176.

44. Capener N. Spondylolisthesis. Br J Surg 1932;19:374–386.

45. Burns BH. An operation for spondylolisthesis. Lancet 1933;1:1233.

46. Ishihara H, Osada R, Kanamori M, et al. Minimum 10-year follow-up study of anterior lumbar interbody fusion for isthmic spondylolisthesis. J Spinal Disord 2001;14:91–99.

47. Verbiest H. The treatment of lumbar spondyloptosis or impending lumbar spondyloptosis accompanied by neurologic deficit and/or neurogenic intermittent claudication. Spine 1979;4:68–77.

48. Whitecloud TS 3rd, Butler JC. Anterior lumbar fusion utilizing transvertebral fibular graft. Spine 1988;13:370–374.

49. Jones AM, McAfee PC, Robinson RA, et al. Failed arthrodesis of the spine for severe spondylolysthesis. J Bone Joint Surg 1988;70-A:25–30.

50. Majd ME, Holt RT. Anterior fibular strut grafting for the treatment of pseudoarthrosis in spondylolisthesis. Am J Orthop 2000;29:99–105.

51. Cunningham BW, Polly DW Jr. The use of interbody cage devices for spinal deformity: a biomechanical perspective. Clin Orthop 2002; 394:73–83.

52. Potvin JR, Norman RW, Mc Gill SM. Reduction in anterior shear forces on the L4-L5 disc by the lumbar musculature. Clin Biomech 1991;6:88–96.

53. Smith MD, Bohlamn HH Spondylolisthesis treated by a single-stage operation combining decompression with in situ posterolateral and anterior fusion. An analysis of eleven patients who had long-term follow-up. J Bone Joint Surg 1990;72:415–421.

54. Roca J, Ubierna MT, Caceres E, et al. One-stage decompression and posterolateral and interbody fusion for severe spondylolisthesis. An analysis of 14 patients. Spine 1999;24:709–714.

55. Jenkins JA. Spondylolisthesis. Br J Surg 1936;24:80–85.

56. Morsher E. Two-stage reposition and fixation of spondyloptosis with Harrington instrumentation and anterior intercorporal spondylodesis. Arch Orthop Unfallchir 1975;83:323–334.

57. Scaglietti O, Frontino G, Bartolozzi P. Technique of anatomical reduction of lumbar spondylolisthesis and its surgical stabilization. Clin Orthop 1976;117:1651–1675.

58. Bradford DS. Closed reduction of spondylolisthesis. An experience in 22 patients. Spine 1988;13:580–587.

59. Seitsalo S, Osterman K, Hyvarinen H, et al. Surgical treatment of severe isthmic spondylolisthesis in adolescents. Reduction or fusion in situ. Spine 1993;18:894–901.

60. Fabris DA, Constantini S, Nena U. Surgical treatment of severe L5-S1 spondylolisthesis in children and adolescents. Results of intraoperative reduction, posterior interbody fusion, and segmental pedicle screw fixation. Spine 1996;21:728–733.

61. Louis R and Maresca C. Les arthrodèses stables de la charnière lombosacrée. Rev Chir Orthop 1976;62[Suppl 2]:70–79.

62. Kozak JA. Isthmic spondylolisthesis: reduction vs. in-situ fusion. Backup 2002:2.

63. Smith MD, Bohlman HH. Spondylolisthesis treated by a single-stage operation combining decompression with in situ posterolateral and anterior fusion. An analysis of eleven patients who had long-term follow-up. J Bone Joint Surg 1990;72-A:415–421.

64. Boachie-Adje OI, Do O, Rawlings BA. Partial lumbosacral kyphosis reduction, decompression, and posterior lumbosacral transfixation in high-grade isthmic spondylolisthesis. Spine 2002;27:E161–E168.

65. Smith JA, Deviren V, Berven S, et al. Clinical outcome of trans-sacral interbody fusion after partial reduction for high-grade L5-S1 spondylolisthesis. Spine 2001;26:2227–2234.

66. McCord DH, Cunningham BW, Shono Y, et al. Biomechanical analysis of lumbosacral fixation. Spine 1992;17[8 Suppl]:S235–S243.

67. Hu SS, Bradford DS, Transfeldt EE, et al. Reduction of high-grade spondylolisthesis using Edwards instrumentation. Spine 1996;21: 367–371.

68. Klöckner C. Die Operation der hochgradigen spondylolisthesis und spondyloptoser. Operat Orthop Traumatol 2002;14:49–62.

69. Hohmann F, Sturz H. Differential indications for lumbosacral fusion and reposition operation in spondylolisthesis. Orthopade 1997;26:781–789.

70. Wild A, Jager M, Webb JK. Staged reposition and fusion with external fixator in spondyloptosis. Z Orthop Ihre Grenzgeb 2001;139:152–156.

71. Bradford DS, Gotfried Y. Staged salvage reconstruction of grade IV and V spondylolisthesis. J Bone Joint Surg 1987;69-A:191–202.

72. Dick WT, Schnebe BL. Severe spondylolisthesis. Reduction and internal fixation. Clin Orthop 1988;232:70–79.

73. Ani N, Keppler L, Biscup RS, et al. Reduction of high-grade slips (grades III–V) with VSP instrumentation. Report of a series of 41 cases. Spine 1991;16[6 Suppl]:S302–S310.

74. Bradford DS, Boachie-Adjei O. Treatment of severe spondylolisthesis by anterior and posterior reduction and stabilization. A long-term follow-up study. J Bone Joint Surg Am 1990;72:1060–1066.

75. Matthiass HH, Heine J. The surgical reduction of spondylolisthesis. Clin Orthop 1986;203:34–44.

76. Transfeldt EE, Dendrinos GK, Bradford DS. Paresis of proximal lumbar roots after reduction of L5-S1 spondylolisthesis. Spine 1989;14: 884–887.

77. Petraco DM, Spivak JM, Cappadona JG, et al. An anatomic evaluation of L5 nerve stretch in spondylolisthesis reduction. Spine 1996;21: 1133–1138.
78. Steffee AD, Brantigan JW. The variable screw placement spinal fixation system: report of a prospective study of 250 patients enrolled in Food and Drug Administration clinical trials. Spine 1993;18:1160–1172.
79. Boos N, Marchesi D, Zuber K, et al. Treatment of severe spondylolisthesis by reduction and pedicular fixation: a 4–6 year follow-up study. Spine 1993;18:1655–1661.
80. Balderston RA, Bradford DS. Technique for achievement and maintenance of reduction for severe spondylolisthesis using spinous process traction wiring and external fixation of pelvis. Spine 1985;10: 376–382.
81. Ohki I, Inoue S, Murata T, et al. Reduction and fusion of severe spondylolisthesis using halo-pelvic traction with wire reduction device. Int Orthop 1980;4:107–113.
82. Laursen M, Thomsen K, Eiskjaer SP, et al. Functional outcome after partial reduction and 360 degree fusion in grade III-V spondylolisthesis in adolescent and adult patients. J Spinal Disord 1999;12:300–306.
83. Gaines RW, Nichols WK. Treatment of spondyloptosis by two-stage L5 vertebrectomy and reduction of L4 onto S1. Spine 1985;10:680–686.
84. Lehmer S, Steffee AD, Gaines RW. Treatment of L5-S1 spondyloptosis by staged L5 resection with reduction and fusion of L4 onto S1. Spine 1994;19:1916–1925.
85. Dimar JR, Hoffman G. Grade 4 spondylolisthesis. Two-stage therapeutic approach of anterior vertebrectomy and anterior-posterior fusion. Orthop Rev 1986;15:504–509.
86. Wild A, Jager M, Werner A, et al. Treatment of congenital spondyloptosis in an 18-month-old patient with a 10-year follow-up. Spine 2001;26:E502–E505.
87. Haher TR, Gorup JM, Shin TM, et al. Results of the Scoliosis Research Society instrument for evaluation of surgical outcome in adolescent idiopathic scoliosis. A multicenter study of 244 patients. Spine 1999;24 (14):1435–1440.
88. Asher MA, Min Lai S, Burton DC. Further development and validation of the Scoliosis Research Society (SRS) outcomes instrument. Spine 2000;25:2381–2386.

CHAPTER 65

High-Grade Spondylolisthesis: Slip Reduction versus *in situ* Fusion

William C. Lauerman and Steven C. Scherping

Isthmic spondylolisthesis occurs because of a defect in the pars interarticularis that allows the forward slippage of one vertebra, most commonly L5, on the level below. This defect, called spondylolysis, is presumed to be a fatigue fracture, for the development of which there is a hereditary predisposition, and which is caused by repetitive hyperextension stresses (1).

Spondylolysis is common, with a prevalence of 5% to 6% of the population at skeletal maturity. Approximately 75% of individuals with spondylolysis are seen to have an associated slip, the large majority of which are in the Meyerding grade I (0 to 25%) or less commonly grade II (26% to 50%) categories. Only a small percentage of cases of spondylolisthesis involve slips that progress beyond 50%, into the realm of high-grade spondylolisthesis (2).

The occasional case of true high-grade spondylolisthesis differs from the more common lower-grade cases in several ways. While spondylolysis and isthmic spondylolisthesis, on the whole, are twice as common in males as in females, high-grade slips occur in women as much as four times as frequently as in men. Furthermore, the pathoanatomy of the high-grade slip involves more than just anterior translation of L5 on S1, a fact that has major significance in terms of presentation and, in some instances, treatment. As the L5 vertebral body translates anteriorly it also, once it passes about 50% translation, rolls anteriorly into kyphosis. This lumbosacral kyphosis, measured by the slip angle (Fig. 65-1), alters the biomechanics of the entire lumbar spine; in order to balance the trunk over the pelvis hyperlordosis, above L5, is necessary. The hyperlordosis can then lead to long-term problems including pain, facet joint arthrosis, and central and lateral recess stenosis above the lumbosacral level (3).

The well-described cosmetic alterations seen in high-grade spondylolisthesis are also a function, in large part, of this lumbosacral kyphosis. The kyphotic forward roll of the body of L5 usually induces a backward rotation of the sacrum, measured by the sacral inclination (Fig. 65-1), with concomitant backward rotation of the entire pelvis. This accounts for the flattening of the buttocks and transverse abdominal crease, which are often cosmetically objectionable in these patients (4).

Finally, in cases of high-grade spondylolisthesis, patterns of nerve root or cauda equina compression differing from those usually seen should be considered. While L5 nerve root entrapment in the L5-S1 foramen is common in the adult with isthmic spondylolisthesis of any grade, it appears to be more common in higher grade slips. Patients with high-grade spondylolisthesis, particularly when there is significant lumbosacral kyphosis, may also manifest cauda equina symptoms due to stretching of the sacral nerve roots over the L5-S1 disc and the posterior aspect of the dome of the sacrum (5). This picture is quite rare in slips below 50%. Finally, it is not uncommon to see stenosis develop above the L5-S1 level, particularly when there has been a previous fusion, in patients with high-grade slips and compensatory proximal hyperlordosis.

SURGICAL INDICATIONS

The adult patient with spondylolisthesis may present with back or leg pain; failing nonoperative treatment these are the most common indications for surgery in all grades of slip. Patients with higher-grade slips may also present with symptoms of cauda equina syndrome, which are usually mild and chronic and may be easy to overlook. Clear-cut evidence of urinary retention would represent an absolute indication for surgical treatment. Cosmetic considerations may also play a role in treatment decision making. While it is easy to assume that the adult has come to accept his or her deformity, this may not be the case and the patient's perception of the relative impor-

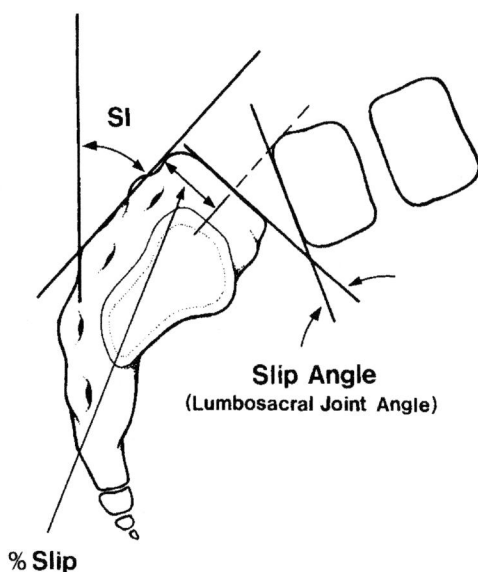

FIG. 65-1. Drawing illustrating the pertinent measurements to quantify the deformity in spondylolisthesis. *SI*, the sacral inclination, describes the orientation of the sacrum and pelvis. The slip angle, when positive, measures lumbosacral kyphosis. The percent slip measures the anterior translation of L5 on S1. (From Miller MD, Brinker MR. Review of orthopaedics, 3rd ed. Philadelphia: WB Saunders, 2000:367, with permission.)

tance of his or her appearance must factor into selection of the appropriate operation. In the adult slip progression can occur, although it is uncommon in the absence of prior surgery (6). The presence of progressive spondylolisthesis represents an indication for surgery, however, and current radiographs should be compared to old films, if available, always taken with the patients standing.

SURGICAL OPTIONS

The surgical treatment of the patient with high-grade spondylolisthesis falls into two categories: fusion *in situ* or reduction and fusion. Nerve root, and sometimes cauda equina, decompression are commonly performed as part of either of these two types of surgeries; radicular or cauda equina symptoms may constitute part of the patient's symptom complex or decompression may be undertaken as a prophylactic measure. Nerve root decompression is universally recommended when reduction is undertaken and is employed by some surgeons when performing *in situ* fusion.

Fusion *in situ* is most commonly performed through a posterior approach, although circumferential fusion may be employed. Anterior fusion for high-grade spondylolisthesis is rarely employed as a stand-alone primary operation. Nerve root decompression is usually necessary as an adjunct in case of fusion *in situ* as most adults presenting

with high-grade spondylolisthesis have signs or symptoms of radiculopathy.

Posterolateral *in situ* fusion for high-grade slips generally extends from L4-S1 and the use of pedicle screw instrumentation, in addition to autologous bone grafting, is now routine in such cases. The rationale for extending the fusion to L4 in children and adults stems from the mechanically disadvantaged position of the L5 transverse processes, which are also commonly quite small, relative to the sacral ala. Extension of the bone grafting up to L4 is considered necessary in order to create a fusion bed that is under compression (L4-S1) rather than under tension (L5-S1) (4).

A significant risk of nonunion exists with posterolateral fusion, with or without instrumentation, for high-grade spondylolisthesis (7). To offset this risk Smith and Bohlman have described fusion of both the anterior and posterior columns, through a single posterior approach. In addition to traditional posterolateral fusion a fibula dowel graft is introduced through a drill hole in the sacrum, across the L5-S1 disc, and into the body of L5 (8) (Fig. 65-2). A more commonly employed alternative to the posterolateral fusion is a combined anterior and posterior approach. Transperitoneal or retroperitoneal exposure of the L5-S1 level allows for discectomy and grafting. Alternatively, a fibular strut graft can be introduced into the body of L5, across the disc space, and into the sacrum. Either anterior technique is followed by posterolateral fusion and instrumentation.

The techniques used for slip reduction have evolved over the last quarter century, and much of the experience reported has been in adolescents. Many techniques, particularly those involving cast reduction, traction, or other indirect means, are rarely employed at this time and are unsuitable for the adult patient.

The major risks of reduction of high-grade spondylolisthesis include neurologic injury and instrumentation failure, with loss of reduction (3,7,9–11). Both of these may be minimized by, and most authors stress the importance of, accepting less than complete reduction. This clearly lessens the risk of nerve root injury, a finding that Petraco et al. have explained in a study on cadavers demonstrating the disproportionate strain in the L5 root occurring during the last 50% of reduction (12). Since it is the lumbosacral kyphosis, in a high-grade slip, which causes most of the mechanical problems, it is now well accepted that kyphosis reduction, rather than complete reversal of the anterior translation, should be the primary goal of surgery (12,13).

Currently the options commonly used for reduction include a posterior instrumented reduction using gradually applied distraction, posterior translation of L5, and lumbosacral extension (Fig. 65-3). This technique, originally pioneered by Edwards, takes advantage of viscoelastic stress-relaxation and is not suitable for some

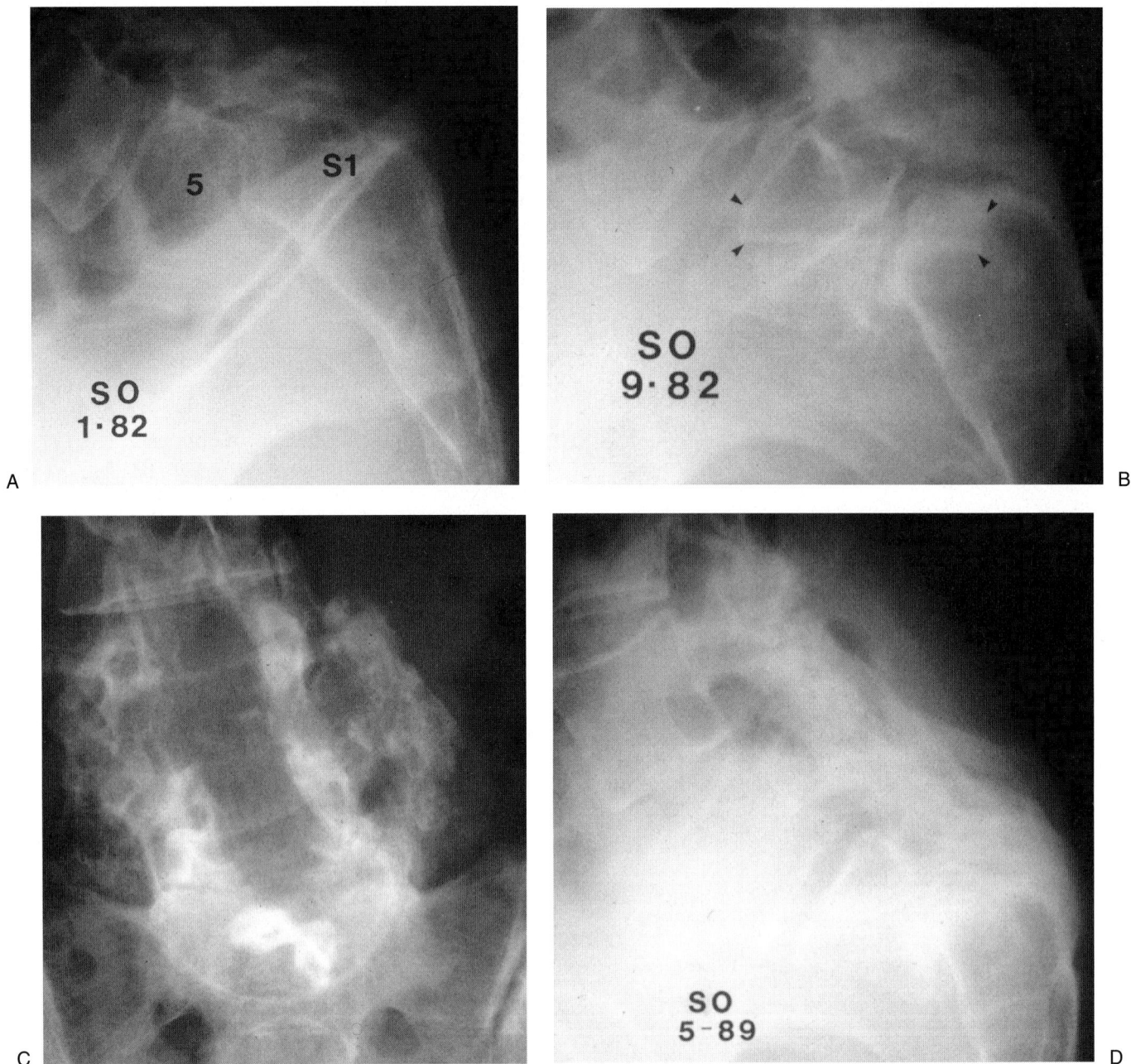

FIG. 65-2. A 46-year-old woman with progressive spondylolisthesis following a prior attempt at fusion. **A:** Marked lumbosacral kyphosis with an almost vertical sacrum. **B:** The patient's lateral radiograph shortly after the Bohlman procedure. The *arrowheads* mark the corners of the fibular strut graft. **C, D:** The anteroposterior and lateral views 7 years after the patient's second surgery. She had excellent relief of her pain. Note, however, the persistent lumbosacral kyphosis and compensatory hyperlordosis proximally.

adults with more rigid curves or who have had prior attempts at fusion (3).

Transforaminal interbody fusion techniques can facilitate reduction and enhance arthrodesis rates when used in conjunction with instrumented posterior reduction. Following foraminotomy and distraction, subtotal L5-S1 discectomy, working through both foramina, is performed.

This serves to increase flexibility of the deformity at the time of posterior translation and extension. The disc space can then be grafted, with a structural graft if desired, to provide fusion in both the anterior and posterior columns (14).

An alternative approach is to combine anterior L5-S1 and L4-L5 discectomy with instrumented posterior

A–B

C

D–E

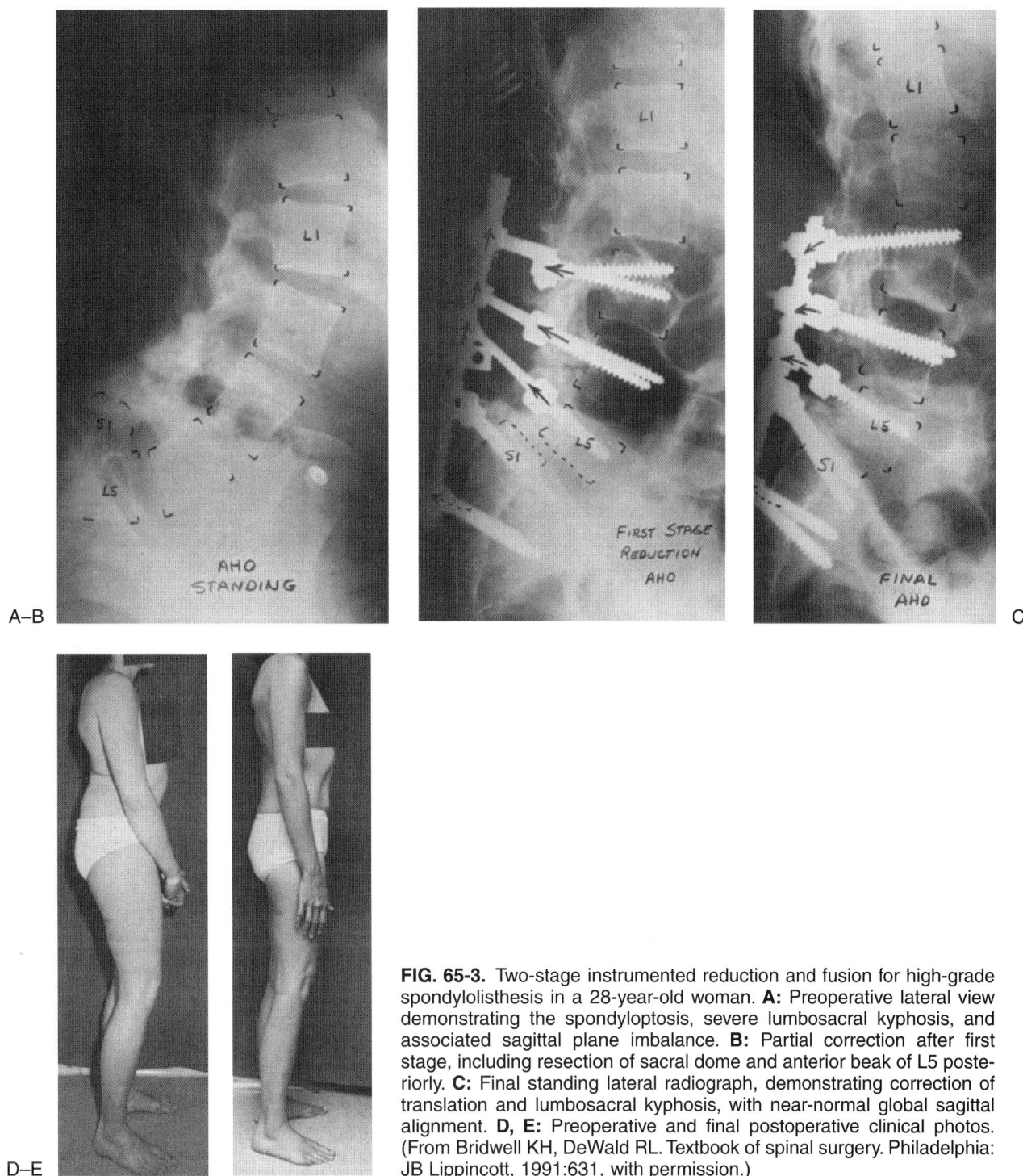

FIG. 65-3. Two-stage instrumented reduction and fusion for high-grade spondylolisthesis in a 28-year-old woman. **A:** Preoperative lateral view demonstrating the spondyloptosis, severe lumbosacral kyphosis, and associated sagittal plane imbalance. **B:** Partial correction after first stage, including resection of sacral dome and anterior beak of L5 posteriorly. **C:** Final standing lateral radiograph, demonstrating correction of translation and lumbosacral kyphosis, with near-normal global sagittal alignment. **D, E:** Preoperative and final postoperative clinical photos. (From Bridwell KH, DeWald RL. Textbook of spinal surgery. Philadelphia: JB Lippincott, 1991:631, with permission.)

reduction and fusion. Greater flexibility, lending to easier reduction, is achieved with this method. In higher grade slips or cases of spondyloptosis, however, it can be exceedingly difficult to visualize the L5-S1 disc that becomes trapped between the L5 vertebral body and the front of the sacrum.

A final alternative, popularized by Gaines, is resection of the entire L5 vertebrae through a combined anterior and posterior approach, followed by reduction of L4 onto the sacrum and instrumented L4-S1 fusion. The advantages ascribed to this technique include lesser risk of neurologic injury and ease of achieving reduction (15), although mechanical and neurologic complications have been reported (16). The Gaines procedure probably represents, however, the most reliable reduction procedure available for high-grade slips when there has been a previous attempt at fusion or when there is severe lumbosacral kyphosis resulting in the L5 vertebral body descending anterior to the sacrum (17).

Essentially all authors who describe modern techniques of slip reduction stress the importance of thorough neural decompression (3,4,12). Even in patients without overt radiculopathy, aggressive foraminotomy allows visualization of the L5 nerve roots that must be checked and rechecked many times throughout the course of the reduction of the slip. In some cases resection of the L5-S1 disc and even partial resection of the dome of the sacrum is employed to decompress the sacral roots and facilitate reduction.

Fusion *in situ* versus Reduction

No aphorism is more appropriate, when considering the right treatment for the adult with high-grade isthmic spondylolisthesis, than that admonishing the surgeon to "fit the operation to the patient, not the patient to the operation." Selecting the right operation requires considering individual factors in the patient's presenting complaints and past history as well as physical findings and radiographic criteria.

What does the patient want from surgery? Most adults are reluctant to identify cosmesis as a major part of their concern. The surgeon, therefore, needs to present the effect that one operation, or another, is likely to have on the patient's appearance. Where is the pain? While either approach is likely to relieve low back pain or leg pain, some patients have chronic fatigue pain in the upper lumbar and thoracolumbar region. This often is caused by sagittal plane imbalance induced by the lumbosacral kyphosis and relief may be less predictable with *in situ* techniques (Fig. 65-4) (3).

Has the patient had surgery before? The timing and type of such surgery may have an impact on the optimal procedure. A recent decompression without fusion with rapid slip progression often lends itself to attempted reduction. On the other hand an established nonunion at the lumbosacral junction, without motion, often requires extensive surgery to achieve reduction and may be better suited to *in situ* fusion techniques.

Physical findings typically supplement factors in the history. Marked sagittal plane imbalance, manifested by compensatory hyperlordosis and a "crouched posture", often results in fatigue-type pain in the mid-back and is only likely to be altered significantly with reduction. Other physical findings consistent with severe spondylolisthesis and sagittal plane decompensation include flattening of the buttocks, a transverse abdominal crease, and trunk shortening with the lower ribs sitting on the lateral iliac crests; these rarely improve with *in situ* fusion. Finally, certain radiographic findings favor one approach or the other, although the radiographs typically reflect what is seen on physical examination. Some patients have

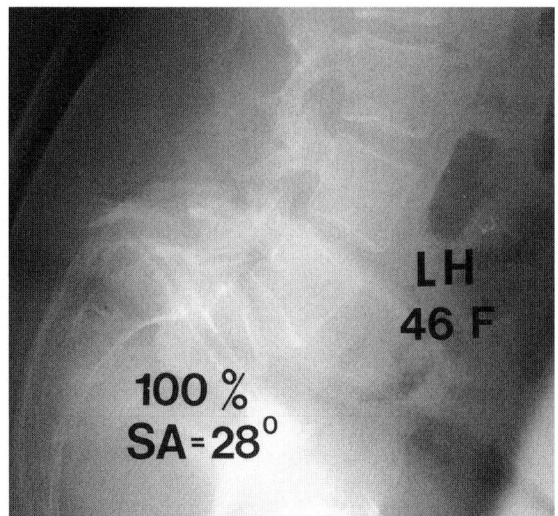

FIG. 65-4. A 46-year-old woman, approximately 30 years after *in situ* fusion for high-grade isthmic spondylolisthesis. Lateral radiograph demonstrates sagittal plane imbalance and hyperlordosis from L1 to L5. She has chronic thoracolumbar and lumbar fatigue-type pain.

relatively high-grade slips but do not develop a particularly severe lumbosacral kyphosis; in these individuals, who often have less dramatic physical findings, *in situ* fusion is advantageous. Other patients have such severe kyphosis, and sagittal plane decompensation, that even a fusion from the transverse processes of L4 to the sacral ala would lie outside the compressive "anatomic zone", described by Bradford as the imaginary proximal extension of the sacrum (17). These patients require either circumferential fusion *in situ* or reduction (at least partial) to establish a favorable fusion environment.

The major clear-cut advantage of *in situ* fusion is safety (3–5,9,10). While nerve root injury and even cauda equina syndrome have been reported following fusion *in situ*, major permanent deficits are uncommon. Virtually all reports of spondylolisthesis reduction, however, note the occurrence of neurologic complications. These deficits have been reported following all techniques as well, including noninstrumented reduction, L5 vertebrectomy, combined anterior and posterior approaches, and gradual instrumented reduction. The reported incidence of root deficits, usually at L5, ranges from 0 to 40% (3,4). Cauda equina syndrome following reduction is less common. The majority of neurologic deficits, including root and cauda equina, improve but most larger series contain patients with permanent disability. Amundson et al. have proposed several maneuvers that may be used at surgery to minimize the risk of neurologic injury. These include either staged reduction (with a 1- to 2-week interval) or spine shortening by virtue of a sacral dome osteotomy in cases where excessive axial lengthening, particularly of rigid deformities, is anticipated (Fig. 65-2). Neurologic monitoring, including one or more wake-up tests, can be used to alert the surgeon to root compromise (5). As a final safeguard, accepting partial reduction often lessens the neurologic risk (13).

Other advantages of *in situ* fusion are less clear-cut. It would appear that reduction is technically more complex, with increased operating room time and cost, increased blood loss, and monitoring expenses. Some *in situ* techniques, however, call for a combined anterior and posterior approach, require extending the fusion cephalad, and may have a higher long-term failure rate from nonunion or slip progression. These "costs" may offset the complexity of reduction.

Heller et al. have described a number of potential advantages of reduction, fixation, and fusion for spondylolisthesis. These include reduced risk of postoperative progression, more rapid pain relief, the ability to more aggressively decompress the nerve roots without fearing instability, increased fusion rates, limited fusion length, and the restoration of normal spine mechanics and body posture with improved appearance (7). Only the last of these advantages is universally accepted, while the others have not been fully documented. Fusion *in situ* for spondylolisthesis has a nonunion rate reported to be between 0 and 40%, with a risk of slip progression as high as 50%. The reported incidence of nonunion following reduction and fusion for high-grade spondylolisthesis varies from 0 to 38%, sometimes with slip progression. It should be noted, however, that some of these reports, such as Bradford and Gotfried's series in which 6 of 16 patients developed delayed union, do not involve the use of more modern instrumentation techniques (11). Other putative advantages of reduction, while potentially valid, depend somewhat on surgeon bias; advocates of *in situ* fusion do not compromise the extent of their nerve root decompression in most cases and would likely agree that the rare patient in whom partial sacrectomy, or extensive discectomy is needed to achieve adequate decompression requires instrumentation and fusion.

CONCLUSION

Many factors in a given patient's history, physical examination, and radiographic evaluation need to be considered when determining *if* surgery is necessary, and if so what procedure is best *for that patient*. Younger adults with high-grade isthmic spondylolisthesis frequently require surgical treatment and there is no one option that is right for all such patients. Advocates of *in situ* fusion cite numerous advantages, the most widely accepted of which would be a decreased risk of neurologic injury. Instrumented reduction and fusion, while offering a number of potential benefits, clearly is able to restore more normal mechanics to the lumbar spine, resulting in an improved appearance and posture. Careful analysis of the patient's pathologic anatomy, signs, and symptoms allows the surgeon to offer the patient the procedure with the most favorable risk/benefit ratio.

REFERENCES

1. Lauerman WC, Cain JE. Isthmic spondylolisthesis in the adult. J Am Acad Orthrop Surg 1996;4:201–208.
2. Fredrickson BE, Baker D, McHolick WJ, et al. The natural history of spondylolysis and spondylolisthesis. J Bone Joint Surg Am 1984;66: 699–707.
3. Edwards CC, Curcin A. Instrumented reduction of high-grade spondylolisthesis. Semin Spine Surg 1994;6:34–45.
4. Bradford DS. Spondylolysis and spondylolisthesis. In: Lonstein SE, Bradford DS, Winter RB, et al., eds. Moe's textbook of scoliosis and other spinal deformities, 3rd ed. Philadelphia: WB Saunders, 1995: 399–430.
5. Amundson G, Edwards CC, Garfin SR. Spondylolisthesis. In: Rothman RH, Simeone FA, eds. The spine, 13th ed. Philadelphia: WB Saunders, 1992:913–969.
6. Floman Y. Progression of lumbosacral isthmic spondylolisthesis in adults. Spine 2000;25:342–347.
7. Heller JG, Schimandle JH, Garfin SR. The operative reduction of spondylolisthesis: indications, results, complications. Semin Spine Surg 1994;6:22–33.
8. Smith MD, Bohlman HH. Spondylolisthesis treated by a single-stage operation combining decompression with in situ posterolateral and anterior fusion: an analysis of eleven patients who had long term follow-up. J Bone Joint Surg Am 1990;72:415–421.
9. Edwards CC, Bradford DS. Controversies—instrumental reduction of spondylolisthesis. Spine 1994;13:1535–1537.
10. Amundson G. The advantages of reduction in spondylolisthesis. Semin Spine Surg 1994;6:46–57.
11. Bradford DS, Gotfried Y. Staged salvage reconstruction of grade IV and V spondylolisthesis. J Bone Joint Surg 1987;69A:191–202.
12. Petraco DM, Spivak JM, Cappadona JG, et al. An anatomic evaluation of L5 nerve stretch in spondylolisthesis reduction. Spine 1996;21: 1133–1139.
13. Boachi-Adjei O, Twee D, Rawlins B. Partial lumbosacral kyphosis reduction, decompression, and posterior lumbosacral transfixation in high-grade isthmic spondylolisthesis. Clinical and radiological results in six patients. Spine 2002;27:161–168.
14. Molinari MW, Bridwell KH, Leuke LG, et al. Complications in the surgical treatment of high-grade, isthmic dysplastic spondylolisthesis. A comparison of three surgical approaches. Spine 1999 1701–1711.
15. Gaines RW, Nichols WK. Treatment of spondyloptosis by two stage L5 vertebrectomy and reduction of L4 onto S1. Spine 1985;10:680–686.
16. Lehmer SM, Steffee AD, Gaines RW. Treatment of spondyloptosis by staged L5 resection with reduction and fusion of L4 onto S1 (Gaines procedure). Spine 1994;19:1916–1925.
17. Bradford DS, Boachie-Adjei O. Reduction of spondylolisthesis. In: Evarts CM, ed. Surgery of the musculoskeletal system, 2nd ed. New York: Churchill Livingstone, 1990:2129–2142.

CHAPTER 66

Adult Scoliosis

Yizhar Floman

For many years scoliosis was considered a condition that starts exclusively during skeletal growth either in childhood or adolescence, not in adult life. Indeed, scoliosis is common in adolescence (4% of the population) and may carry forward into adult years as an untreated condition. However, more recently it has been recognized that scoliosis also can start *de novo* during adult life. For practical reasons, adult scoliosis is defined as a presentation of spinal deformity after skeletal maturity (usually after the age of 20 years). Adult scoliosis may start before skeletal maturity, but treatment may not be sought until later in adult life; alternatively, it may present as a *de novo* spinal deformity in adult life. The most frequent type, present before skeletal maturity, is idiopathic scoliosis. On the other hand, *de novo* scoliosis usually arises because of advanced degenerative disc disease, osteoporosis, or both. Adults also may present with a spinal deformity following a previous surgery for degenerative disc disease (DDD) or as a sequel to a previous fusion surgery (e.g., adjacent level disc degeneration with scoliosis or iatrogenic flat back).

The predominance of the literature dealing with scoliosis remains focused on adolescent spinal deformities. The natural history of adult spinal deformities is less known. Nevertheless, as more adults with scoliosis seek treatment, more interest and research focus on the natural history of these complex deformities in adult life and their management. Aside from the disfigurement caused by the spinal deformity, pain and disability may become a major problem. The recent awareness of the public toward quality of life issues and not just longevity may bring adult scoliosis into the focus of attention; the condition may soon become a significant health care problem.

PREVALENCE

The prevalence of adult scoliosis is probably on the rise because of increased longevity in the Western world.

Lonstein estimated that there are about half a million adults with spinal curves (including thoracic curves) 30° or greater in the United States (1). The two most common types of curves that are encountered in adult life are idiopathic and degenerative scoliosis. The former is a condition that starts in childhood or adolescence, and progresses over the years with superimposed DDD that becomes symptomatic in adult life. On the other hand, degenerative scoliosis is a *de novo* type scoliosis secondary to DDD that developed on a formerly straight spine. Scoliosis may be the result of the asymmetric involvement of disc degeneration, facet arthrosis, and disc collapse (2). Although it is obvious that the etiology of the two conditions is completely different, adult idiopathic scoliosis and degenerative scoliosis coexist and may share a common final pathway (i.e., increasing disc degeneration with increasing spinal deformity accompanied by pain and disability).

The prevalence of adult scoliosis in the general population has been estimated to be 2% to 15% (3–7). The wide variation in the reported prevalence of adult spinal deformities is because most published reports were based on different population surveys, different gender studies, different age groups, and various inclusion criteria. Strayer (8) reviewed routine chest X-rays of 928 postpartum women and obtained standing antero-posterior (AP) views of the spine of those appearing to have a spinal deformity in the coronal plane (scoliosis). Five percent of the entire study group had curves measuring 10° to 19° and 2% had curves exceeding 20°. The vast majority of women in the study population (77%) were thought to have idiopathic scoliosis (8). Kostuik and Bentivoglio (9) studied 5,000 intravenous pyelograms of patients older than 20 years. Thoracolumbar or lumbar scoliosis greater than 10° was found in 3.9% of the study population. The incidence of lumbar curves was 2.5%, whereas the incidence of thoracolumbar curves was 1.4 % (9). Vanderpool et al. (10) found an even higher incidence of scoliosis (6%) in people 50 years of age and older. Most identified curves in the study of Kostuik and Bentivoglio (86%) were idiopathic in nature; however, some curves were secondary to congenital or neuromuscular etiologies (9). Biot and Perdrix found 12% prevalence of lumbar curves in a retrospective study of abdominal X-rays (3). Robin (6), in a study of 3,600 persons aged 45 to 84 years who were chosen at random from electoral lists, found that 15% had a thoracolumbar or lumbar curve of more than 10°. Perennou et al. (5) described the frequency and characteristics of adult lumbar scoliosis in a prospective clinical and radiologic study. They studied 671 adults (49.8% M, 50.2% F) who were admitted to a spine rehabilitation unit for back pain during an 8-month period (5). The mean age of the patients was 50 years; 30% were older than 60 years. The prevalence of curves greater than 10° was 7.5% (55 out of the 671 patients in the study group). Seventy-two percent of the scoliotic patients were females (2:1 sex ratio). The prevalence of lumbar scoliosis increased with age: It was found to be 2% before age 45, 6% between 45 and 59 years, 15% in patients older than 60 years (5). The mean Cobb angle was 21°. Only 14% of the patients reported about a known deformity in their adolescent years. Korovesis (4) in a similar study on adult scoliosis found that right-sided lumbar curves were as common as left sided curves (as opposed to the predominance of left-sided lumbar curve in adolescent idiopathic scoliosis).

In summary, it may be noted that the prevalence of adult scoliosis rises with age. More recent studies show more equal numbers of degenerative and idiopathic type curves while early surveys reported that the majority of adult curves were idiopathic. There are a significant number of right lumber curves and the female to male ratio is smaller than in comparable series of patients with adolescent idiopathic scoliosis.

PATHOGENESIS AND CLASSIFICATION

Adult scoliosis can be divided into two main subgroups; individuals with previous history of scoliosis before the end of skeletal maturity and individuals whose scoliosis started in adult life (de novo) (Figs. 66-1,66-2). Contributing factors for adult onset scoliosis are degenerative disc disease, osteoporosis (10,11), and prior back surgery. Although the association between adult scoliosis and DDD is obvious, it is less so in relationship to osteoporosis. Velis et al. (12) found a significant reduction in bone mineral content in young women with idiopathic scoliosis. The incidence of adult scoliosis in women with osteoporosis also is higher (10,13). Vanderpool et al. (10), Healy and Lane (13), and Velis and Thorne (14) found a positive correlation between osteoporosis and increased prevalence of scoliosis in an older adult population. Robin et al. were some of the few investigators to find no correlation between degenerative scoliosis and osteoporosis (6). Nevertheless, it is well established that vertebral osteo-

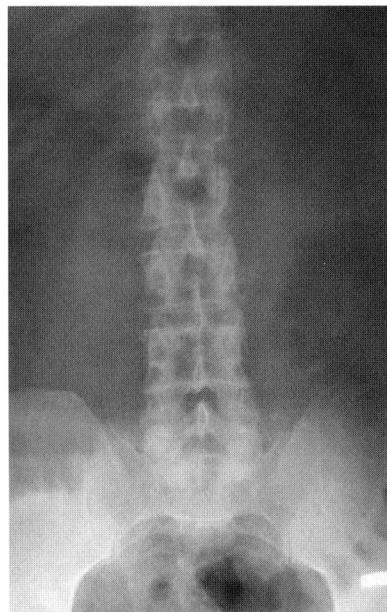

FIG. 66-1. Antero-posterior X-ray of the lumbar spine in a 55-year-old woman with low back pain. Note that the lumbar spine is straight with no apparent deformity.

porosis and disc degeneration with facet joint arthrosis coexist in the elderly population (15).

Regardless of the etiology, adult scoliosis is characterized by vertebral structural changes with translatory shifts (i.e., lateral olisthesis accompanied by degenerative

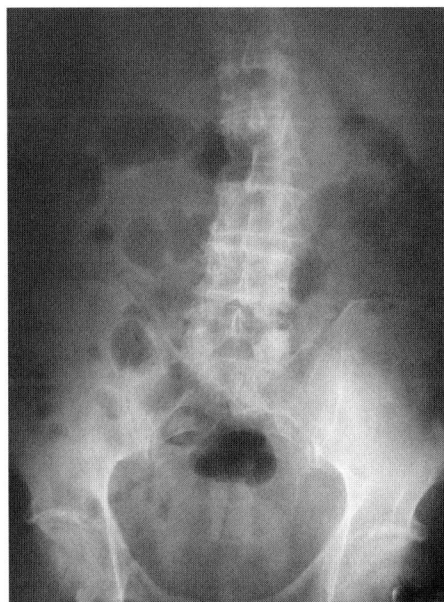

FIG. 66-2. Antero-posterior X-ray of the lumbar spine of the same patient as in Figure 66-1, 7 years later. Note that a scoliotic curve has evolved (de novo scoliosis) with marked rotation at L2.

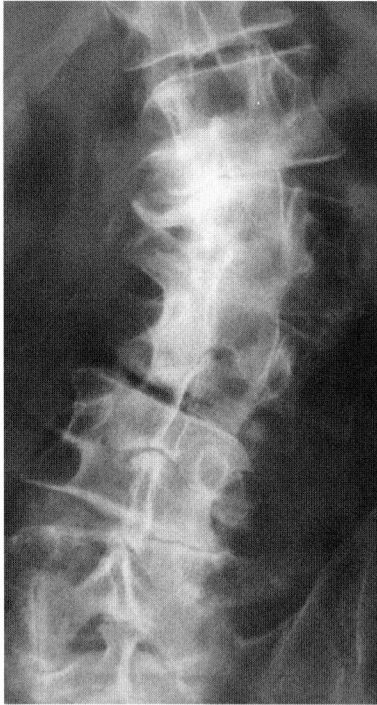

FIG. 66-3. Antero-posterior X-ray of the lumbar spine in a 64-year-old woman with low back pain. Note the marked degenerative lumbar scoliosis with lateral spondylolisthesis at L2-3.

disc and facet joint arthrosis). Although the magnitude of these curves usually is mild, only 10% develop curves that exceed 30°; lateral vertebral subluxation (lateral spondylolisthesis) is observed more frequently (Fig. 66-3) (13,14). The degenerative process is either the primary event leading to a spinal deformity or superimposed as a secondary event on a preexisting curve that started before skeletal maturity.

Therefore, adult thoracolumbar or lumbar scoliosis may be classified as follows:

1. Primary adult curves: true adult onset deformity (*de novo* scoliosis) resulting from degenerative disc disease, osteoporosis, or both. This type of deformity is often associated with loss of lumbar lordosis (16).

2. Secondary adult curves:
   a. On the top of a previous stable adolescent curve (at the end of skeletal growth, up to 30° to 40°). In these cases, a previously stable curve becomes unstable because of superimposed degenerative changes with or without osteoporosis.
   b. On top of a previous unstable progressive adolescent curve (at the end of skeletal growth). The curve continues to increase in magnitude in adult life because of its inherent biomechanical behavior and also as a result of superimposed degenerative process.

In both primary and secondary adult scoliosis, the degenerative process plays a central role in the loss of lumbar lordosis and may even result in thoracolumbar kyphosis (Fig. 66-4).

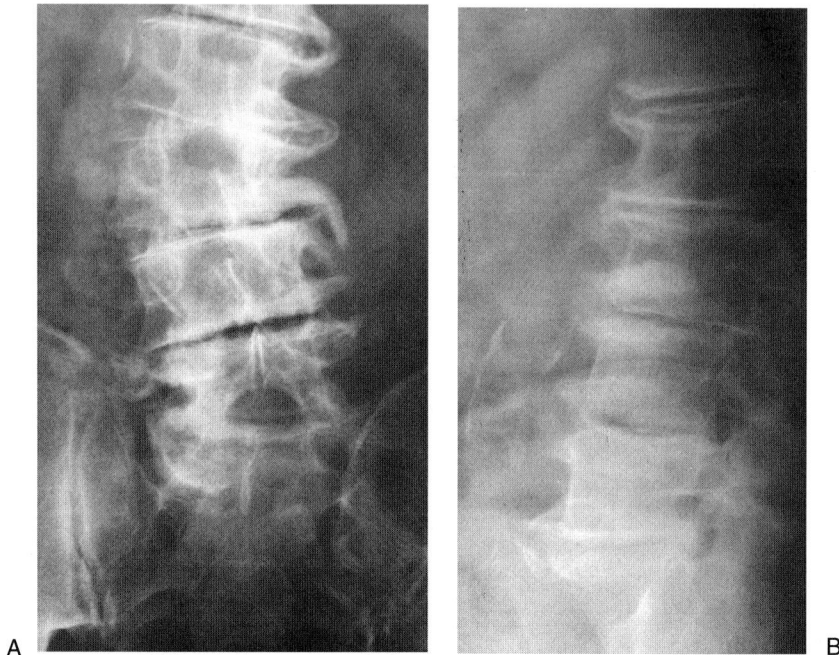

A   B

FIG. 66-4. A: Antero-posterior X-ray of the lumbar spine in a 72-year-old woman with low back pain. Note the lumbar scoliosis with advanced disc degeneration. **B:** Lateral lumbar spine X-ray of the same patient as in Figure 66-4A. Note the true lumbar kyphosis.

CLINICAL PRESENTATION

It is common for the spinal health care provider to be presented with an adult patient with a spinal deformity accompanied by loss of lumbar lordosis, trunk imbalance, and significant mechanical back pain. When obtaining the history it is important to establish whether curve progression has taken place. Previous radiographs are not available in many cases (or are inadequate to determine if curve progression took place). Important clues in the history taking are loss of height or altered waistline, increase in the size of the lumbar paraspinal hump, or the need to alter clothing. Although adult idiopathic scoliosis patients are predominantly women, the percentage of men with *de novo* degenerative scoliosis is greater.

It is well established that adult scoliosis can lead to a painful progressive spinal deformity. Pain may arise not only from DDD and facet arthritis leading to symptoms of spinal stenosis, but also from muscle fatigue caused by the altered biomechanics secondary to the deformity. The latter muscle problem arises from the coronal as well as the sagittal imbalance caused by the progressive spinal deformity. In general, the incidence of back pain in the adult scoliosis patient is about equal to that in age matched controls (9,17–19). Also, the vast majority (91%) of older patients with long-standing adolescent idiopathic scoliosis exhibited degenerative changes of the involved vertebrae (20). Kostuik and Bentivoglio (9) found that 60% of adults with scoliosis had back pain; the same figure was noted in adults without spinal deformity.

However, adult patients with lumbar curves have greater pain intensity (21). When the curve progressed above 45°, prevalence and severity of pain increased (22). Patients with thoracolumbar or lumbar curve patterns, especially with lateral olisthesis tend to have a greater incidence of back pain (23). In reports from more recent studies, chronic back pain was present in 61% of the scoliotic patients versus 35% in control subjects (24). Pain may arise at the apex of the deformity or be referred lower down. A radicular component may be present, especially with advanced degenerative changes (25). Root entrapment is common and occurs more often on the concavity of the curve (5,17).

Pritchett et al. (26) studied 200 patients with degenerative scoliosis. All 200 patients had back pain aggravated by standing and walking, and 142 (72%) had lower limb symptoms including complaints of spinal claudication. Forty-five percent of the patients had neurologic symptoms, mostly paresthesias (26).

Schwab et al. (27) studied 95 patients with adult scoliosis: 33 men and 62 women, whose average age was 59 years. Most had significant back pain (74%); the average visual analog scale (VAS) of pain was 58. Fifty-four percent of the curves were classified as degenerative and 46% as idiopathic. The average lumbar curve magnitude was 36°. The authors found a highly significant correlation between the VAS of pain and the presence on radiographs of lateral olisthesis and obliquity of the L3 or L4 end plates (Fig. 66-5).

Likewise, loss of lumbar lordosis and thoraco-lumbar kyphosis were positively correlated with the self-reported

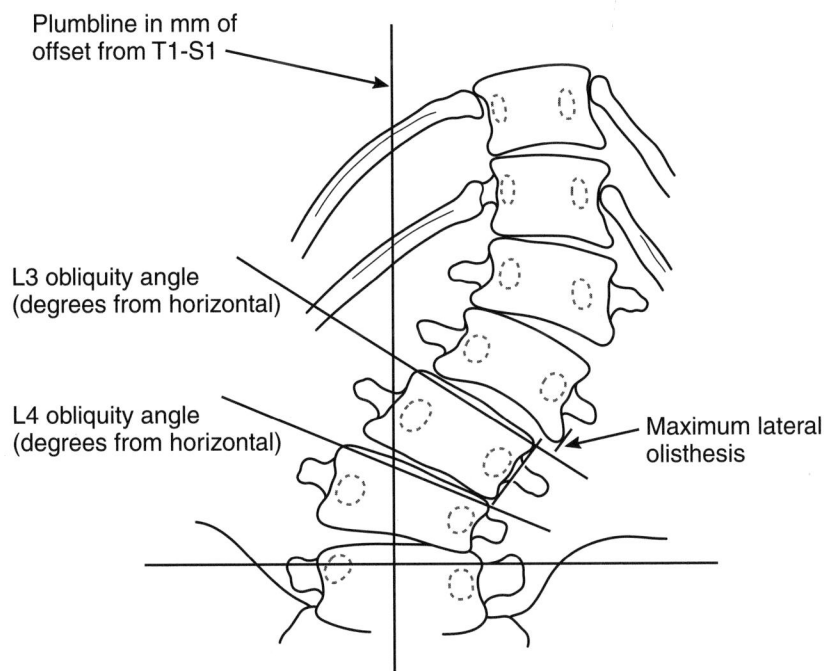

FIG. 66-5. Important radiographic measurements in the assessment of lumbar scoliosis taken from a standing antero-posterior X-ray of the lumbar spine. (From Schwab FJ, et al. Adult scoliosis: a quantitative radiographic and clinical analysis. Spine 2002;27:388, with permission.)

pain. On the other hand, the magnitude of the Cobb angle, the sagittal pelvic tilt index, and the plumbline offset showed no statistically significant correlation with the self-reported pain by the VAS. Symptomatic lumbar curves tended to be larger in the idiopathic group (40° versus 25° in the degenerative group).

Although the disfigurement caused by the lumbar deformity may have adverse psychological consequences, most middle-aged adults cope well with the deformity (23).

In summary, the incidence of back pain has been shown to be similar among adults with and without scoliosis although patients with lumbar curves with lateral olisthesis tend to have a greater incidence of back pain. Also, the severity and chronicity of back pain has been reported to be greater among adults with lumbar scoliosis as compared to age-matched controls without spinal deformity (17,28–31). Symptoms of neurogenic claudication are common in adults with lumbar scoliosis; however, history of pain relief by bending forward or sitting is less reliable than in patients with lumbar spinal stenosis without scoliosis (26).

NATURAL HISTORY

The natural history of adult scoliosis should be analyzed according to the classification of adult deformities i.e. idiopathic or degenerative. It is recognized however that the two conditions may co-exist.

IDIOPATHIC CURVES

In a review of 161 patients observed for an average of 40 years at the university of Iowa, 68% of the curves progressed after maturity (19,23,32,33). This trend continued 10 years later (total follow-up time of 50 years!) (24). Although thoracic curves progressed 1° per year, thoracolumbar curves progressed 0.5° per year and lumbar curves even less (.24° per year) (32). From this long-term study, Weinstein and Ponseti (32) identified multiple factors that were associated with curve progression (Table 66-1). For example, lumbar curves of more than 30° with apical vertebral rotation of more than 30% progressed the

TABLE 66-1. *Features associated with progression in curves >30 degrees at skeletal maturity*

Lumbar	Thoracolumbar
Cobb angle >30	Cobb angle >30
Apical vertebral rotation >30%	Apical vertebral rotation >30%
Curve direction	Translatory shifts
Relation of L5 to intercrestal line	
Translatory shifts	

Source: Adapted from Weinstein SL. Naural history. Spine 1999;24:2592–2600, with permission.

most. Right-sided lumbar curves tended to progress twice as much as left lumbar curves (32). Also, marked vertebral rotation combined with translatory shift (lateral olisthesis) was associated with significant curve progression. The thoracolumbar curve pattern manifested the most pronounced amount of apical vertebral rotation. The incidence of translatory shifts increased with time. At 50 years of follow-up, 71% of patients had at least one translatory shift (24). Combined curves tended to balance with age, although the lumbar part tended to progress more than the thoracic counterpart. Weinstein and Ponseti (32) noted greater progression in lumbar curves if L5 was not well seated over the sacrum and apical vertebral rotation was more than 33%.

DE NOVO DEGENERATIVE CURVES

Robin (6) studied AP X-rays of a randomly chosen population of 3,600 subjects aged 45 to 84 years. These individuals were part of a population survey for osteoporosis in the city of Jerusalem. The authors found that scoliosis was much more common in the elderly population than the reported incidence of scoliosis in school children. Indeed the incidence of scoliosis in various reported series shows a constant rise from childhood to old age. Although the prevalence of adolescent idiopathic scoliosis in the at-risk population (i.e., children 10 to 16 years old) is approximately 2% to 3% (19) and only 10% to 15% of these have lumbar curves, 15% of individuals over 60 years of age have lumbar curves (5).

Robin et al. (7) further analyzed 554 individuals longitudinally for 7 to 13 years (315 women, and 239 men, age range 50 to 84 years). Each individual had one supine AP X-ray of the lower thoracic and lumbar spine. One hundred seventy-nine individuals (113 F, 66 M) had curves exceeding 10°. Fifty-five individuals (10%) developed *de novo* scoliosis during this period (curve range, 1° to 20°). Left-sided curves were common in women; the sex ratio (F:M) increased with curve size. Rotatory olisthesis was found in 34% of the patients, most common at the L3-4 and L4-5 levels. In the supine position, most curves were reduced by about 30%. Korovessis et al. (4) identified 137 individuals with adult scoliosis among a group of 1,154 patients with low back pain during a 3-year period. They excluded from the study group patients with a positive history of spinal deformity, curves smaller than 10°, and osteoporotic vertebral fractures. Ninety-one patients out of the 137 (66%) were available for follow-up evaluation (18 men and 73 women, mean age 67 years). Right-sided lumbar curves were most common (55%). Average curve size was 16.5° (range, 10° to 36°). Lateral spondylolisthesis was present in most cases. Risk factors directly related to curve progression were lateral olisthesis at the apical vertebra, a high Harrington factor (Cobb angle divided by the number of vertebrae included in the curve), and the disc index (4).

TABLE 66-2. *Risk factors for curve progression in degenerative lumbar curves*

Factor	Curve progression	No curve progression
Patients 41 (100%)	30 (73%)	11 (27%)
Cobb angle	>30 Degrees	<30 Degrees
Rotation	Grade 2–3	Grade 1–2
Intercrestal line	Through L5	Through L4
Vertebral translation	≥6 mm	<6 mm

Source: Adapted from Pritchett JW, Bortel DT. Degenerative symptomatic lumbar scoliosis. Spine 1993;18:700–703, with permission

Various authors calculated the annual curve progression rate to range from .3° to 3° (4,5,26). Korovessis et al. (4) noted progression of 5° or more in 72% of the curves during an average follow-up period of 3.7 years. Perennou et al. (5) studied 41 patients with a follow-up period spanning 10 to 30 years (mean, 12 years) and found that 73% of the patients showed curve progression of 10° or more (2° to 6° per year, average 3°).

Pritchett and Bortel (26) examined 200 patients with degenerative lumbar scoliosis. Inclusion criteria were a curve greater than 10° with no previous history of spinal deformity. Of the entire patient population, 151 were women and the mean age of the study population was 69 years (range, 50 to 89) (Table 66-2). Curve range was 14° to 60° (mean, 24°). Curve size was greater than 35° in about 20% of the patients. The number of vertebrae involved in the curve was 3 to 6 (mean, 3). Sixty-eight percent of the curves were left-sided. The apex of the curve was most commonly located between L2 and L3. In 67% the Moe-Nash grade of vertebral rotation was 2. An interesting finding was that *degenerative spondylolisthesis* was noted as well in more than half of the patients. (Indeed, many patients with neurogenic claudication caused by spinal stenosis also have some degree of degenerative scoliosis.) An even more common finding was a lateral spondylolisthesis (78% of the patients). Average lateral translation was 8 mm (range, 3 to 8 mm). The lumbar scoliosis was associated with a reduction in the size of lumbar lordosis in 85% of patients. Mean lumbar lordosis was 18° (range, 7° to 45°). All curves with the intercristal line passing through L5 or L4-5 interspace with vertebral rotation of 2 or more (Moe-Nash) had curve progression. Curves greater than 30° with lateral translatory shift of 6 mm or more also had continued curve progression. Most progression occurred in curves with apices between L2-4 (26).

ASSESSMENT: IMAGING

Full-length standing radiographs (35 × 91 cm) (postero-anterior [PA] and lateral) allow a thorough assessment of the entire length of the spinal column in both the coronal and sagittal planes. If surgical curve correction is considered, PA and lateral supine-bending films should be taken to assess curve rigidity and flexibility. In rigid curves that do not significantly correct on side bending views, traction views have been suggested to provide better information regarding curve correctability during surgery (34,35). Others have advocated the "push-prone" view (manual lateral forced correction) for assessment of curve flexibility (36). Recently, Luk et al. (37) advocated the fulcrum bending view as a better predictor of curve correctability (the patient lies in a lateral decubitus position with the apex of the major curve placed over a large bolster) (37).

Patients with symptoms of radiculopathy, without or with neurologic deficit, are traditionally evaluated by myelography followed by post-myelography computed tomography (CT). An alternative to myelography is magnetic resonance imaging (MRI) scans. Magnetic resonance imaging may provide detailed information on central, lateral, and foraminal neural encroachment. Magnetic resonance imaging scans also may provide information regarding disc degeneration and may dictate the extent of spondylodesis. If surgery is contemplated, provocative discography may add further information as to the extent of arthrodesis needed (38). Although provocative discography remains a controversial diagnostic procedure, leading authorities such as Kostuik (39) and Bradford et al. (20,40) recommend its use in conjunction with MRI to determine the extent of distal spondylodesis. However, the lack of prospective clinical studies that prove that the use of provocative discography leads to better clinical results makes the use of discography disputable. Occasionally flexion-extension views as well as facet block injections may be considered as well to determine the extent of instrumentation and fusion (39).

EVALUATION OF CORONAL AND SAGITTAL BALANCE

Coronal Balance

The Cobb angle and number of vertebrae in the curve are recorded (Figs. 66-6,66-7). Next, the end plate obliquity (from the horizontal) of the apical and the end vertebra are measured. Also, the maximal lateral olisthesis (translatory shift) is recorded as well. The central sacral line (from the spinous process of S2) is erected. The plumb line (a parallel line to the center sacral line) is drawn bisecting the center of C7 or T1. The distance between the central sacral line and the plumb line is the coronal decompensation measurement. For certain thoracolumbar curves it is better to evaluate the lateral trunk shift (LTS) (Fig. 66-8). This is calculated by first drawing a horizontal line to the edges of the ribs of the apical vertebra. A perpendicular line bisects the horizontal line. The distance between the perpendicular line and the center sacral line represents LTS (41,42).

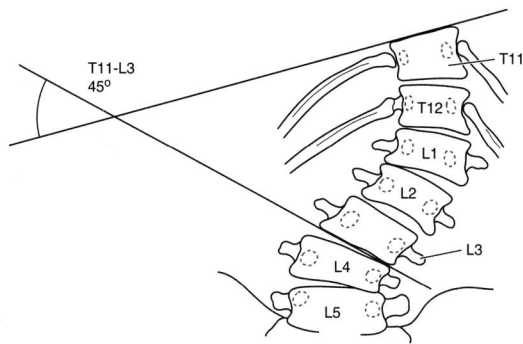

FIG. 66-6. Evaluation of the coronal balance. The Cobb angle and the number of vertebrae in the curve are recorded. (Modified from Spine 2002;27:388.)

Apical vertebral translation also can be evaluated by measuring the lateral distance of the apical vertebra from the plumb line.

Sagittal Balance

Before the 1980s, little attention was paid to the sagittal contour of the spine and assessment, and treatment of spinal deformities focused almost exclusively on the frontal or coronal plane of the spine. The sagittal contours

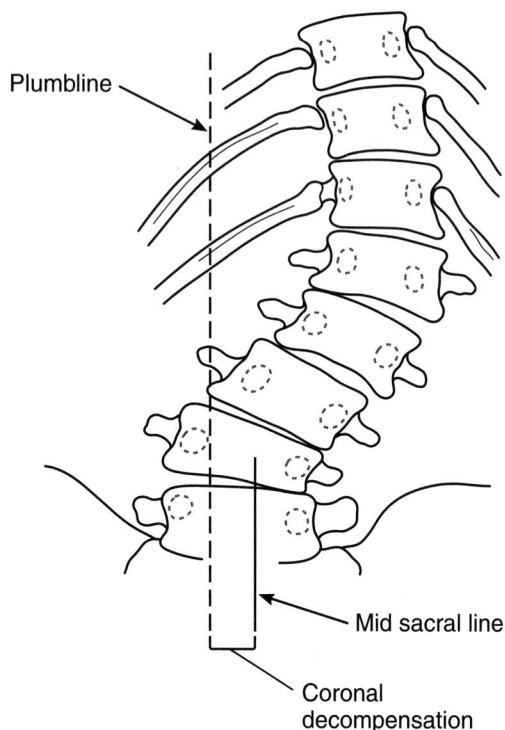

FIG. 66-7. The plumb line is drawn bisecting the center of C7 or T1. Also the central sacral line is erected. The distance between the central sacral line and the plumb line is the coronal decompensation. (Modified from Spine 2002;27:388.)

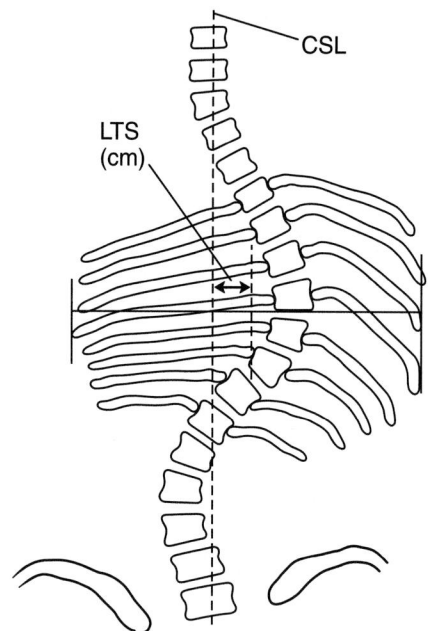

FIG. 66-8. Evaluation of the lateral trunk shift (LTS). This is calculated by first drawing a horizontal line to the edges of the ribs of the apical vertebra. A perpendicular line bisects the horizontal line. The distance between the perpendicular line and the center sacral line represents LTS. (From Katz DC, Durrani AA. Factors that influence outcome in bracing large curves in patients with adolescent idiopathic scoliosis. Spine 2001;26:2354–2361; Floman Y, Penny NJ, Micheli LJ, et al. Osteotomy of the fusion mass in scoliosis. J Bone Joint Surg 1982;64A:1307–1312; Spine 2001;26:2356.)

of the spine and global sagittal balance have emerged in recent years as crucial factors in assessing spinal deformities. This is especially true when one deals with thoraco-lumbar or lumbar deformities where changes in the lateral profile of spine have a central role in the severity of symptoms in patients with adult lumbar deformities. Indeed, there is a spectrum of involvement in the sagittal contour of the spine in adult scoliosis from hypolordosis to true segmental kyphosis. Therefore, the evaluation of the sagittal balance of the spine is extremely important.

Regional intervertebral relationships are important when assessing the sagittal plane balance, but the global alignment of the spine is even more important. There is a close relationship between the intervertebral angulations in the various regions of the spine (cervical, thoracic, and lumbar) and the global sagittal balance. For example, the lumbar spine compensates with lordosis if the thoracic kyphosis increases. In order to maintain a normal overall sagittal balance (a negative vertical sagittal alignment; see the following) the lumbar lordosis should exceed the thoracic kyphosis by 20° to 30° (Fig. 66-9). This is also true with cervical lordosis. The normal cervical lordosis is about 40°, to which the occipito-atlantal junction contributes about 30° (43). The mean thoracic kyphosis from

T1-12 (apex T6-7) is 27° to 39°, each disc contributing 1° to 3° of kyphosis (44). The thoracolumbar junction is a transition zone connecting the kyphotic thoracic spine to the lordotic lumbar counterpart. The L1-2 disc is the first lordotic segment. The global sagittal alignment at the thoracolumbar junction (T12-L2) is either neutral or slightly lordotic.

The simplest assessment of the sagittal contour is the lateral plumb line, which is dropped from C7 and normally falls posterior to the postero-superior corner of the lumbosacral disc (45). This is referred to as the sagittal vertical axis (SVA) and quantifies the global sagittal balance of the spine (Fig. 66-9). The SVA normally falls anterior to the thoracic spine and through or slightly posterior to the apical lumbar bodies. When the SVA falls anterior to the S1 body, it is considered positive and if it falls behind the S1 body it is considered negative. The normal SVA in adults usually is negative.

The lumbar spine is lordotic; the apex is located at the L3-4 interspace (44,45). The L4-5 and the L5-S1 segments provide for about 60% of the total lumbar lordosis. The lumbar discs provide for 47° of lordosis and the vertebral bodies only 12° (46). Adolescents have a greater negative sagittal spinal balance than asymptomatic adults (47).

Studies of normal subjects have demonstrated a clear relationship between standing sagittal sacropelvic angulation (sacral inclination) and lumbar lordosis (Fig. 60-10) (48). Jackson and McManus (48) found that sacral inclination correlated with total lumbar lordosis and standing hip extension (hip axis). The pelvic hip axis is located midway along a line drawn between the centers of the femoral heads on the lateral radiograph. These correlations appear to be valid not only in normal volunteers but also in patients with low back pain and DDD (45,48). As segmental lordosis and total lordosis decrease in patients with DDD of the lumbar spine, the vertical sacral inclination increases with increased hip extension. The sacral angulation is an indicator of standing hip extension through the acetabular or hip axis. In patients with DDD, the sacropelvis rotates posteriorly around the hip axis as both the segmental and total lordosis decrease. This results in more vertical sacral inclination with associated hip extension. The sacrum acts as a sixth lumbar vertebra and translates around the hip axis (Fig. 66-10).

The vertical plumb line measurements have no correlation with the sacral inclination. Therefore, it is important to assess both the vertical line balance and the sacropelvic and hip axis. These important biomechanical relationships in the standing position should be kept in mind when assessing patients for fusion surgery. Preservation of lumbar lordosis and normal alignment of the thoracolumbar junction are believed to be crucial factors for the well being of the spine and also affect the long-term results of spinal fusion (49). In a case of hip flexion contracture the compensatory mechanism of spinal balance through hip extension and sacral translation may be compromised (50).

More recently, Lagaye and Duval-Beaupere described the pelvic incidence as the most important radiographic parameter in maintaining an "economical" sagittal balance (51). The pelvic incidence is the angle between the perpendicular to the sacral plate at its midpoint and the line connecting this point to the middle axis of the femoral heads (Fig. 66-11). These authors (51) found that the pelvic incidence has a key importance in the regulation of sagittal balance not only in "normal" subjects but also in scoliotic patients. The greater the apical rotation and the Cobb angle in scoliotic subjects, the lower is the pelvic incidence; the ability to maintain an "economical" sagittal balance also is reduced.

In summary, the assessment of the sagittal contours of the spine and global sagittal balance are of utmost importance in the management of spinal deformities. The sagittal vertical axis and its relationship to the lumbar spine and sacrum, the vertical sacral inclination, and the pelvic incidence are important tools in evaluation of thora-

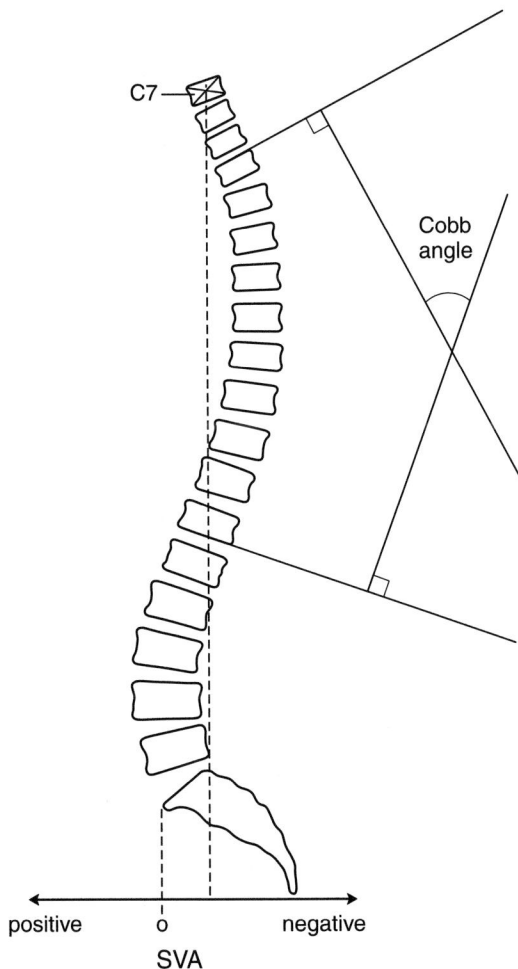

FIG. 66-9. The sagittal vertical axis. (From Gelb DE, et al. Spine 1995;20:1351–1358, with permission.)

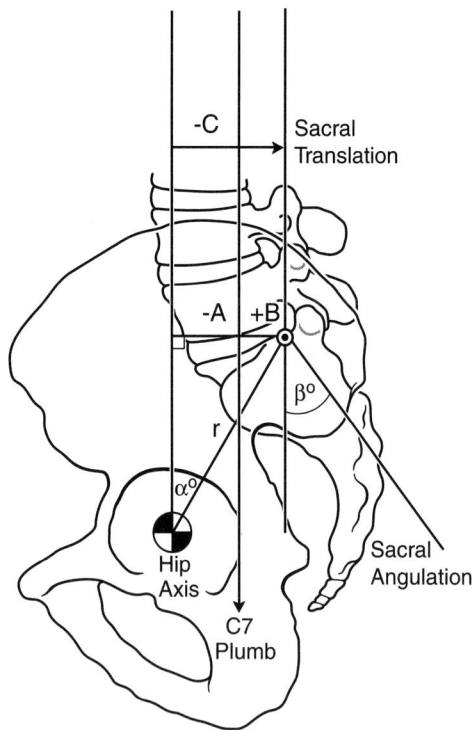

FIG. 66-10. Measurement of the sagittal lumbopelvic alignment. (From Jackson RP. Spine: state of the art review 1997;11:39, with permission.)

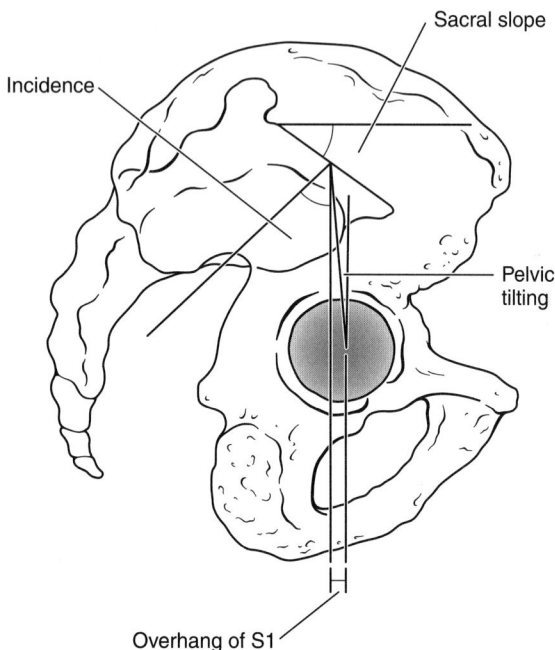

FIG. 66-11. The pelvic incidence. (From Lagaye J, et al. Pelvic incidence: A fundamental pelvic parameter for three-dimensional regulation of spinal sagittal curves. Eur Spine J 1998;7:99–103, with permission.)

columbar and lumbar deformities. Thus, pelvic morphology has been found to affect standing lumbosacral lordosis and pelvic balance in adult volunteers, individuals with low back pain, and scoliosis patients (51,52).

REFERENCES

1. Lonstein JE. Adult scoliosis. In: Lonstein JE, Bradford DS, Winter RB, et al., eds. Moe's textbook of scoliosis and other spinal deformities, 2nd ed. Philadelphia: WB Saunders, 1987.
2. Simmons ED, Simmons EH. Spinal stenosis with scoliosis. Spine 1992;17:S117–S120.
3. Biot B, Perdrix D. Frequence de la scoliose lombaire a l'age adulte. Ann Med Phys 1982;25:251–254.
4. Korovessis P, Piperos G, Sidiropuolos P, et al. Adult idiopathic lumbar scoliosis. A formula for prediction of progression and a review of the literature. Spine 1994;19:1926–1932.
5. Perennou D, Marcelli C, Herisson C, et al. Adult lumbar scoliosis. Spine 1994;19:123–128.
6. Robin GC, Span Y, Makin M, et al. Scoliosis in the elderly: idiopathic or osteoporotic. Proceedings of the 5th Zorab Scoliosis Symposium. London, 1976.
7. Robin GC, Span Y, Steinberg R, et al. Scoliosis in the elderly. A follow-up study. Spine 1982;7:355–359.
8. Strayer LM. The incidence of scoliosis in the postpartum female on Cape Cod. J Bone Joint Surg 1973;55A:436.
9. Kostuik JP, Bonteviglio J. The incidence of low back pain in adult scoliosis. Spine 1981;6:268–273.
10. Vanderpool DW, James JIP, Wynne-Davis R. Scoliosis in the elderly. J Bone Joint Surg 1969;51A:446–455.
11. O'Brien MF, Bridwell KH, Lenke LG, et al. Adult degenerative scoliosis: classification and treatment. Dublin: Scoliosis Research Society, 1993.
12. Velis KP, Healy JH, Schneider R. Peak skeletal mass assessment in young adults with idiopathic scoliosis. Spine 1989;14:706.
13. Healy JH, Lane J. Structural scoliosis in osteoporotic women. Clin Orthop 1985;195:216–223.
14. Velis KP, Thorne RP. Lateral spondylolisthesis in idiopathic scoliosis. J Bone Joint Surg Orthop Trans 1979;3:282.
15. Margulies JY, Payzer A, Nyska M, et al. The relationship between degenerative changes and osteoporosis in the lumbar spine. Clin Orthop 1996;324:145–152.
16. Grubb SA, Lipscomb HJ, Coonard RW. Degenerative adult onset scoliosis. Spine 1988;13:241–245.
17. Jackson RP, Simmons EW, Stripinis D. Coronal and sagittal plane spinal deformities correlating with back pain and pulmonary function in adult idiopathic scoliosis. Spine 1989;14:1391–1397.
18. Nachemson A. Adult scoliosis with back pain. Spine 1979;4:513–517.
19. Weinstein SL. Natural history. Spine 1999;24:2592–2600.
20. Bradford DS, Tay BK-B, Hu SS. Adult scoliosis: surgical indications, operative treatment, complications and outcomes. Spine 1999;24:2617–2629.
21. Briard JL, Jegon D, Cauchoix J. Adult lumbar scoliosis. Spine 1979;4:526–532.
22. Kostuik JP, Gleason TF, Errico TY, et al. The surgical correction of the flat back syndrome. J Bone Joint Surg Orthop Transac 1985;9:131.
23. Weinstein SL, Zavala DC, Ponseti IV. Idiopathic scoliosis: Long term follow up and prognosis in untreated patients. J Bone Joint Surg 1981;63A:702–712.
24. Weinstein SL, Dolan LA, Spratt KF, et al. Natural history of adolescent idiopathic scoliosis: back pain at 50 years. Annual Meeting of the Scoliosis Research Society. New York, 1998.
25. Simmons EH, Jackson RP. The management of nerve root entrapment syndrome associated with the collapsing scoliosis of idiopathic lumbar and thoracolumbar curves. Spine 1979;4:533–541.
26. Pritchett JW, Bortel DT. Degenerative symptomatic lumbar scoliosis. Spine 1993;18:700–703.
27. Schwab FJ, Smith VA, Biserni M, et al. Adult scoliosis: a quantitative radiographic and clinical analysis. Spine 2002;27:387–392.
28. Collis DK, Ponseti IV. Long term follow up of patients with idiopathic scoliosis not treated surgically. J Bone Joint Surg 1969;51A:425–445.

29. Jackson RP, Simmons EW, Stripinis D. Incidence and severity of back pain in adults with idiopathic scoliosis. Spine 1983;8:749–756.

30. Liebholt JD, Ballard A. The disability of lumbar curves in adulthood. J Bone Joint Surg 1974;56A:444.

31. Nachemson AL. A long term follow up study of non treated scoliosis. Acta Orthop Scand 1968;39:456–465.

32. Weinstein SL, Ponseti IV. Curve progression in idiopathic scoliosis. Long term follow up. J Bone Joint Surg 1983;65A:447–455.

33. Weinstein SL. Idiopathic scoliosis. Natural history. Spine 1986;11: 780–783.

34. Polly DW Jr, Sturm PF. Traction versus supine side bending. Which technique best determines curve flexibility? Spine 1998;23:804–808.

35. Bradford DS, Vaughan JJ, Winter RB, et al. Comparison of the use of supine bending and traction radiographs in the selection of the fusion area in adolescent idiopathic scoliosis. Spine 1996;21:2469–2473.

36. Bridwell KH, McAllister JW, Betz R, et al. Coronal decompensation produced by the Cotrel-Dubousset derotation maneuver for idiopathic thoracic scoliosis. Spine 1991;16:769–777.

37. Luk KD, Cheung KM, Lu DS, et al. Assessment of scoliosis correction in relation to flexibility using fulcrum bending correction index. Spine 1998;23:2303–23037.

38. Grubb SA, Lipscomb HJ, Coonard RW. Diagnostic findings in painful adult scoliosis. Spine 1992;17:518–527.

39. Kostuik JP. Adult scoliosis. In: Frymoyer JW, Ducker TB, Hadler NM, et al., eds. The adult spine, 2nd ed. New York: Lippincott-Raven, 1997:1579–1622.

40. Bradford DS. Adult scoliosis. Current concept of treatment. Clin Orthop 1988;229:70–87.

41. Floman Y, Penny NJ, Micheli LJ, et al. Osteotomy of the fusion mass in scoliosis. J Bone Joint Surg 1982;64A:1307–1312.

42. Katz DE, Durrani AA. Factors that influence outcome in bracing large curves in patients with adolescent idiopathic scoliosis. Spine 2001;26: 2354–2361.

43. Hardacker JW, Shuford RF, Capicotto PN, et al. Radiographic standing cervical segmental alignment in adult volunteers without neck symptoms. Spine 1997;22:1472–1479.

44. Bernhardt M, Bridwell KH. Segmental analysis of the sagittal plane alignment of the normal thoracic and lumbar spines and the thoracolumbar junction. Spine 1989;14:717–721.

45. Gelb DE, Lenke LG, Bridwell KH, et al. An analysis of sagittal spinal alignment in 100 asymptomatic middle and older aged volunteers. Spine 1995;20:1351–1358.

46. Wambolt A, Spencer DA. A segmental analysis of the distribution of lumbar lordosis in the normal spine. Orthop Trans 1987;11:92–93.

47. Vedantam R, Lenke LG, Keeney JA, et al. Comparison of standing sagittal alignment in asymptomatic adolescents versus adults. Spine 1998;23:211–215.

48. Jackson RP, McManus AC. Radiographic analysis of sagittal plane alignment and balance in standing volunteers and patients with low back pain matched for age, sex, and size: a prospective controlled clinical study. Spine 1994;19:1611–1618.

49. Herkowitz HN. Lumbar spinal stenosis: indications for arthrodesis and spinal instrumentation. Instr Course Lect 1994;43:425–433.

50. Rand N, Patlas M, Floman Y. Sagittal alignment of the spine in patients with advanced osteoarthrosis of the hips. ISSLS 1996;64(abstract).

51. Lagaye J, Duval-Beaupere D, Hecquet J, et al. Pelvic incidence: a fundamental pelvic parameter for three-dimensional regulation of spinal sagittal curves. Eur Spine J 1998;7:99–103.

52. Jackson RP, Kanemura T, Kawakami N, et al. Lumbopelvic lordosis and pelvic balance on repeated standing lateral radiographs of adult volunteers and untreated patients with constant low back pain. Spine 2000;25:575–586.

CHAPTER 67

Adult Scoliosis: Indications for Surgery

James A. Antinnes and Serena S. Hu

Adult scoliosis is defined as a curve that presents or undergoes treatment after the onset of skeletal maturity. Adult scoliosis can be classified into two groups. The first group is a curve that arose before skeletal maturity but is being treated as an adult curve. Most of these patients have idiopathic scoliosis; rarely congenital or paralytic curves may not require treatment until adulthood.

The second group includes curves that present *de novo*, after skeletal maturity. It may be difficult to differentiate between adult idiopathic scoliosis and *de novo* scoliosis, however the principles of treatment are the same and will be discussed in this chapter. The *de novo* type of curve is typically secondary to degeneration, but may also be due to osteoporosis, or is seen after prior spinal surgery. Patients can develop deformity after wide decompression for spinal stenosis, particularly if a pars fracture develops, but may also present as a complication of a prior fusion. Patients in the latter category may have adjacent segment degeneration or iatrogenic flatback deformities.

Conservative care is usually the initial treatment for management of pain in adult scoliosis. Advancements in spinal instrumentation, improvements in anesthetic techniques, spinal cord monitoring, and postoperative care have improved the ability to safely address complex deformities in patients with adult scoliosis.

INDICATIONS FOR SURGERY

The indications for surgery can be based on the following criteria:

- back pain failing conservative care
- progressive leg pain or neurologic deficit
- muscle fatigue secondary to spinal imbalance
- curve progression
- progressive pulmonary compromise secondary to deformity
- severe deformity.

As with any patient with mechanical back pain, initial treatment is conservative. A physical therapy program to improve aerobic capacity, strengthen muscles, and improve flexibility and joint motion is the mainstay of treatment (1–6). Local modalities, including heat and massage, as well as nonsteroidal antiinflammatory drugs (NSAIDs), and possibly bracing may provide some relief although none has been shown to prevent curve progression (7). Finally, injections such as corticosteroid injections in facet joints, epidural space, or nerve root blocks may be of value in helping relieve a patient's pain. If surgery is eventually needed despite conservative measures, patient outcomes may be enhanced by improving baseline activity and aerobic activity prior to undertaking surgery.

Obtaining successful surgical outcomes in adult spinal deformity requires an understanding of surgical principles and how these factors apply to each patient's needs and expectations. In general, the goals of surgery in adult scoliosis are to decrease pain, to stabilize the curve, and to halt progression or improve neurologic symptoms.

Pain is the most common presenting complaint, accounting for up to 85% of surgical cases (8–12). Back pain in the area of spinal curvature is thought to be related to the degree of disc degeneration, with subsequent facet arthropathy, rotatory subluxation, and lateral listhesis. Generalized back pain is often related to muscle fatigue from either coronal or sagittal imbalance (13).

Claudicatory leg pain can be due to central lateral recess or foraminal stenosis and often corresponds to the concavity of the curve. Magnetic resonance imaging (MRI) or computed tomography (CT)-myelogram are helpful for diagnosing central lateral recess or foraminal stenosis. Foraminal stenosis can also be suspected with disc space narrowing. Rotatory subluxation can also compromise nerve roots, especially in the concavity at the apex of the curve (14). All of these mechanisms can be dynamic and relieved to some extent by position.

Curve progression in the adult with an idiopathic curve pattern has been well documented (2,7,15–17). Weinstein and Ponsetti studied 40-year follow-up data on patients with idiopathic curve patterns. Thoracolumbar curves between 50° and 75° at maturity increased an average of 22.3°. Lumbar curves had the most progression, especially when the fifth lumbar vertebra was not well seated and when the apical rotation was greater than 33% (17,18). The findings of Kostuik et al. showed similar results (19–21). Furthermore, Kostuik and Bentivoglio found that when the curves were greater than 45°, the prevalence and severity of pain increased significantly (22). This is in contrast to the research of Nachemson and Nilsonne who reported that there was not a strong correlation between curve magnitude and pain intensity (4,13). Most studies do agree that the majority of pain emanates from the lumbar spine, increasing in severity if the curve is greater than 45° at skeletal maturity (22–24).

Pain may be improved by up to 70% after successful fusion, but the frequency of the pain does not necessarily improve (25,26). Complete recovery from an involved long segment decompression and fusion can take up to 2 years, especially in older or debilitated patients (27). Therefore an open dialog with the patient prior to undertaking any surgical intervention is crucial in providing the patient with reasonable expectations. As with any elective orthopedic procedure, the more certain the cause of the pain, the more likely one is of a successful outcome.

Finally, a discussion of cosmesis as an indication in the adult with scoliosis is warranted. Johnson and Holt followed 100 patients for over 10 years after a spinal fusion and retrospectively reported that body image and cosmesis played a larger role in the patient's decision to proceed with surgery than was thought at the time of the operation (10,28). While previously thought to be an uncommon indication for surgery, it may be considered after thorough discussions with patients and their families about the goals and expectations. Posterior segmental instrumentation with or without thoracoplasty (29) can often yield excellent correction of the deformity.

Adult patients appear to fall into two categories when considering surgical intervention. Patients under the age of 40 with curves greater than 50° to 60° with chronic pain not relieved by conservative management may opt for surgery. Patients with significant deformity that is unacceptable to them may also be considered for surgery.

In patients over the age of 50 with adult scoliosis it is more common to find complaints of curve progression, back and radicular pain, or pain that is claudicatory in nature. Some patients with curves greater than 90° may benefit from surgery if there is a progressive loss of pulmonary function that is not attributable to an underlying pulmonary disorder. This is not a problem with lumbar scoliosis.

SURGICAL PLANNING

As part of the surgical planning, many factors need to be considered and the overall health of the patient as well as their expectations must not be overlooked. While many of the basic principles are the same, there are many factors that make surgery for adult scoliosis different and often more challenging than the surgical correction of adolescent idiopathic scoliosis. The presence of disc degeneration, facet arthropathy, and osteopenia are just some of the challenges of surgery in the adult population.

There is also a greater tendency for adjacent segment problems in the adult population. Progressive kyphosis at the end of constriction most commonly occurs proximally. Attention to avoiding ending a fusion at a kyphotic segment can prevent this problem, but may still occur in osteoporotic patients.

Osteopenia is a major concern, especially in older adult females, but should not be overlooked in male patients or any patient with a paralytic curve. Multiple fixation levels and supplemental fixation with sublaminar wires can be helpful (30). For curvatures in which significant correction is obtained, care must be taken not to place too much force on the end vertebra as fixation failure and fracture are certainly possible in osteopenic bone. Segmental fixation can provide increased purchase and creates a larger area for force transmission in deformity correction. A combination of transpedicular screws in the lumbar spine with either segmental hooks and sublaminar wires in the thoracic are typically used. Lumbar pedicle screws have been shown to be superior to hooks with better curve correction and greater correction of compensatory curves below the instrumented levels (31,32). Recent studies suggest that the pullout strength of thoracic pedicle screws is superior to hooks and their use in experienced hands may be warranted when increased strength is needed (33,34).

The possibility for coronal and sagittal imbalance in adults is greater as curves are stiffer than those found in adolescents. Therefore any imbalance is less tolerated in the adult population and flexibility should be assessed preoperatively with bend films and balance assessed intraoperatively with full-length radiographs. It is important to remember that in the adult patient, achievement or maintenance of coronal and sagittal balance is more important than curve correction (15,23,33–38).

In general, adult patients are at an increased risk for developing perioperative complications when compared to adolescents. Major complications include residual pain (5% to 15%), neurologic injury (up to 5%), infection (1% to 5%), pseudoarthrosis (5% to 27%), and thromboembolic event (1% to 20%) (16,21,27,36,37,39–45).

The surgical instrumentation should provide maximum stability and allow early mobilization. For combined surgery, same day procedures are preferable to staged procedures if physiologically and technically feasible. There have been several studies, most notably by Dick et al., which showed that combined procedures had a lower infection rate than did staged procedures (46). This difference was attributed to patient malnourishment and subsequent inability to fight potential pathogens. Hu et al. further found that total parenteral nutrition improved nutritional status in patients undergoing staged anterior-posterior surgeries (47). Furthermore, Lenke et al. demonstrated that nutritional status did not return to baseline for up to 6 to 12 weeks after surgery (47a).

SURGICAL TECHNIQUES

Thoracolumbar and Lumbar Curves

Patients with thoracolumbar or lumbar curves with flexible secondary curves are ideal candidates for anterior correction and fusion with segmental instrumentation (Fig. 67-1). The anterior procedure has many advantages in this setting which include fusing fewer motion segments, obtaining superior correction, and obtaining higher fusion rates (49). It is important in the lumbar spine to maintain or produce lordosis by the use of structural interbody grafts or cages placed as far anteriorly as possible in the disc space (20,50).

When choosing this technique, it is crucial to make certain that the secondary curves are flexible. If there is a fixed secondary curve, especially a fixed oblique lumbosacral take-off, this procedure will result in a significant coronal imbalance.

In patients with either spinal stenosis or radiculopathy, decompression is required and in this case a posterior or combined approach is preferable. Generally, these patients are older and often have poor bone quality. Often their curves are quite stiff, and these patients are better served by a combined approach. In this set of patients, it is important to follow certain principles. Firstly, the fusion should not end at a kyphotic segment to decrease the risk of junctional kyphosis (23,51). It may be necessary to extend the fusion proximally to the upper thoracic level in some older patients.

Double Thoracic and Lumbar Curves

In this group of patients, it is important to remember the overall goals in adult deformity surgery: achieve spinal balance, provide pain relief, and obtain a solid fusion. With that in mind, for patients with balanced curves in the thoracic and lumbar regions, posterior instrumentation, and fusion usually leads to a successful result. These patients will often have curves of less than 60°.

In more severe curves, particularly if associated with imbalance, a combined anterior and posterior procedure is preferred. In the first stage, an anterior discectomy and fusion of the lower thoracic and lumbar levels is performed, using structural allografts or mesh cages to restore lordosis. The allografts are prevented from migrating with cancellous 6.5 mm AO (Arbeitsgemeinschaft für Osteosynthesefragen) with plastic washers as interference screws. They are supplemented with autogenous local graft. In the second stage, posterior instrumentation with generous iliac crest bone graft is performed.

Fusion to the Sacrum

There is some controversy regarding fusion to the sacrum in adult scoliosis, with most reports claiming a higher complication rate and lower patient satisfaction rate when patients are fused to the sacrum (27,42,43, 52–55). Some recent studies reported no increase in complications or decreases in patient satisfaction in long fusions to the sacrum (42,56).

There are certain special conditions for which fusion to the sacrum should be considered:

- an unbalanced lumbosacral curve that does not correct on side bending radiographs
- the presence of substantial degeneration of the L4-5 and L5-S1 motion segments
- the need to decompress the lumbosacral junction below a lumbar fusion.

Long fusion to the sacrum always requires a circumferential fusion, generally with an anterior procedure. The allograft femoral rings can be shaped to preserve lumbar lordosis, which is important as 66% of the lumbar lordosis arises from the lowest two levels, L4-L5 and L5-S1. Structural grafting at the L4-L5 and L5-S1 levels improves fusion rates and decreases stress on the sacral screws (Fig. 67-2). If needed, the fusion can be extended to the pelvis using the Galveston technique, iliac screws, or intrasacral rods (43,52,54,55,57). S2 screws have been shown to decrease the strain on the S1 screws (57). Extension to the pelvis can provide a crucial fixation point in osteoporotic patients (43), but the iliac fixation can be prominent in thin patients and may need to be removed after fusion is achieved. For patients with good bone stock, strong anterior structural graft and sagittal balance, bicortical sacral screws may be adequate. Transforaminal or posterior interbody graft can obviate the need for a separate anterior procedure, and can also restore foraminal height and interpedicular distance (50,52,55,58,59). These results are too preliminary to endorse this technique.

If a fusion to the sacrum is undertaken, it is of utmost importance to achieve both coronal and sagittal balance (60). Care must be taken not to over correct either the thoracic or lumbar curve to prevent ending up with a fixed pelvic obliquity and severe imbalance. We routinely

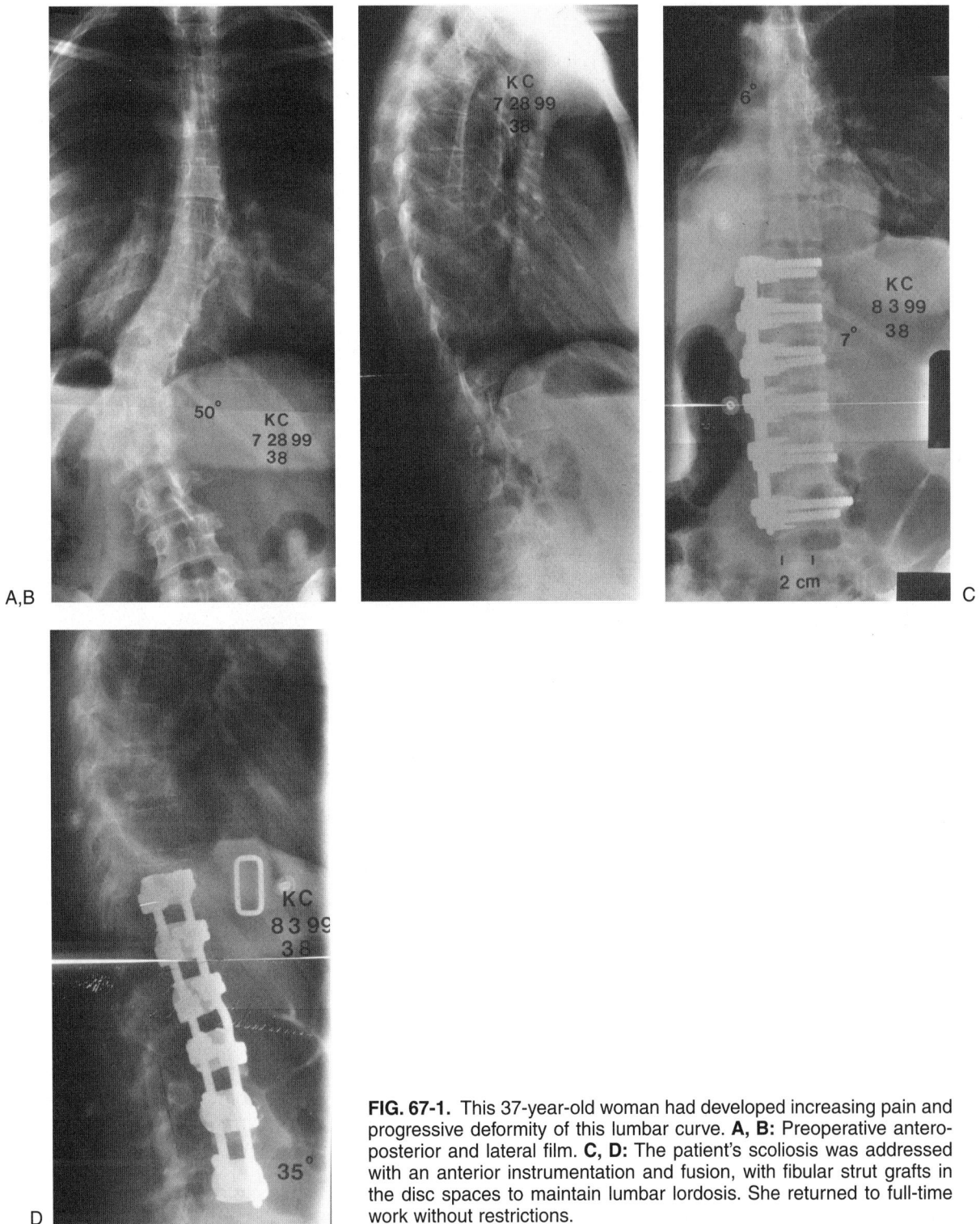

FIG. 67-1. This 37-year-old woman had developed increasing pain and progressive deformity of this lumbar curve. **A, B:** Preoperative antero-posterior and lateral film. **C, D:** The patient's scoliosis was addressed with an anterior instrumentation and fusion, with fibular strut grafts in the disc spaces to maintain lumbar lordosis. She returned to full-time work without restrictions.

take long cassette intraoperative anterior-posterior and lateral X-rays to assess balance.

Patients who undergo extensions of their fusions to the sacrum for pain or progression of scoliosis can also have a high rate of successful outcomes. Kostuik and others showed good and fair postoperative results in up to 93%

of patients, as long as a solid fusion was obtained and lumbar lordosis was restored (42,53,54). Our experience has also been similar, however, some maintain there is a higher complication rate when fusing to the sacrum, and the decision to fuse to the sacrum should not be taken lightly (42,43).

A,B

C

D

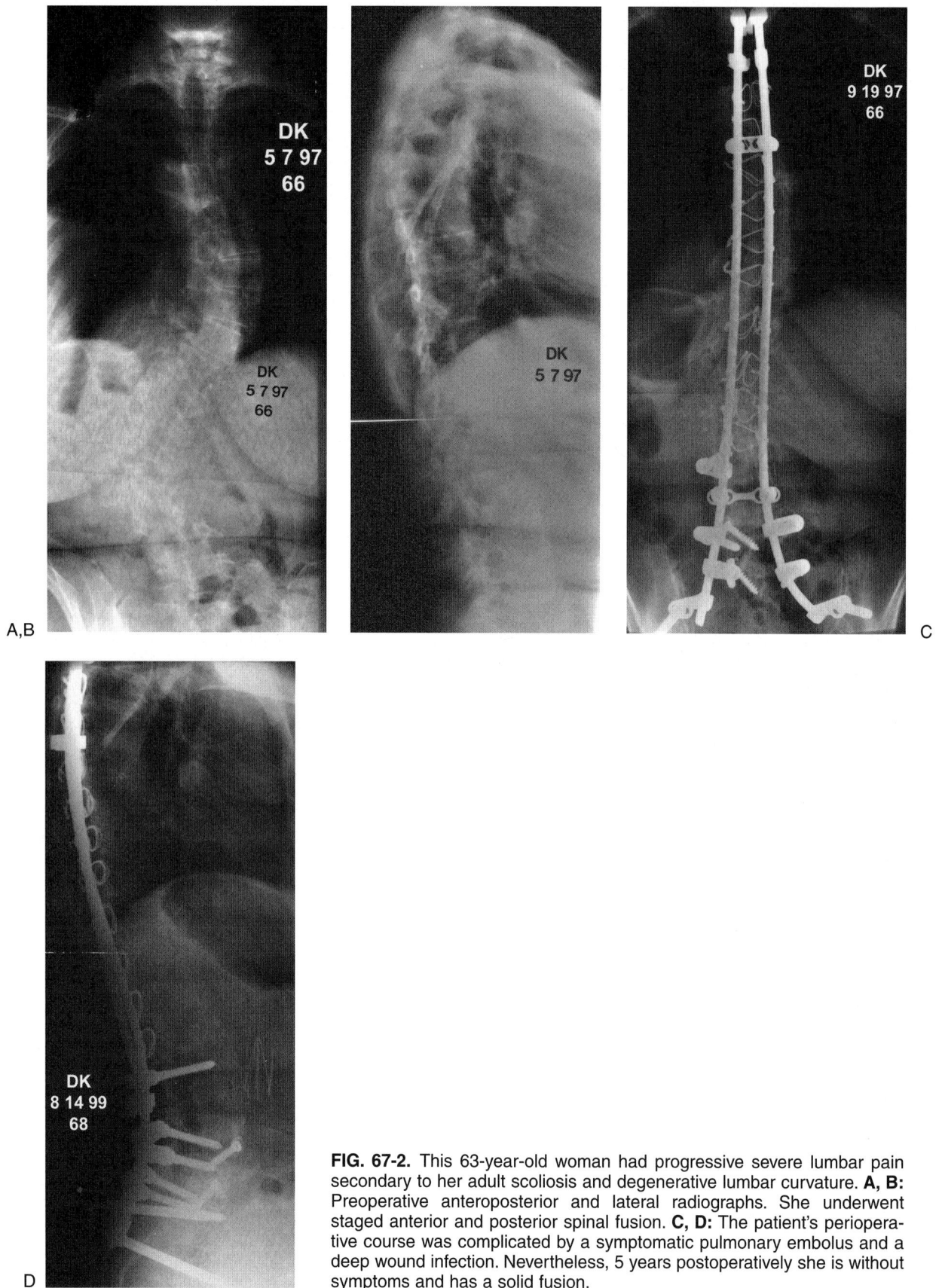

FIG. 67-2. This 63-year-old woman had progressive severe lumbar pain secondary to her adult scoliosis and degenerative lumbar curvature. **A, B:** Preoperative anteroposterior and lateral radiographs. She underwent staged anterior and posterior spinal fusion. **C, D:** The patient's perioperative course was complicated by a symptomatic pulmonary embolus and a deep wound infection. Nevertheless, 5 years postoperatively she is without symptoms and has a solid fusion.

As stated earlier in the chapter, determining the precise source of pain in adult scoliosis patients can be challenging. The use of lumbar discography continues to be controversial as a diagnostic tool (61,62). It is known that concordant pain in the lumbar spine may not be relieved by disc excision and interbody fusion at the concordant level. Discography, when correlated with the complete clinical picture, may provide additional information. In general we prefer to use coronal balance rather than discography to decide the distal extent of our fusion including whether to fuse to the sacrum.

DEGENERATIVE SCOLIOSIS

Surgical treatment of degenerative scoliosis has several goals, which include decompression of the neural elements, and achieving a balanced, stable spine. In patients with stenosis and minimal curvature, decompression alone can be performed. In these patients, great care must be taken to preserve the pars interarticularis and the facet joints as much as possible. In older patients a weakened pars can later fracture and result in progressive deformity (Fig. 67-3). The presence of any signs of instability, such

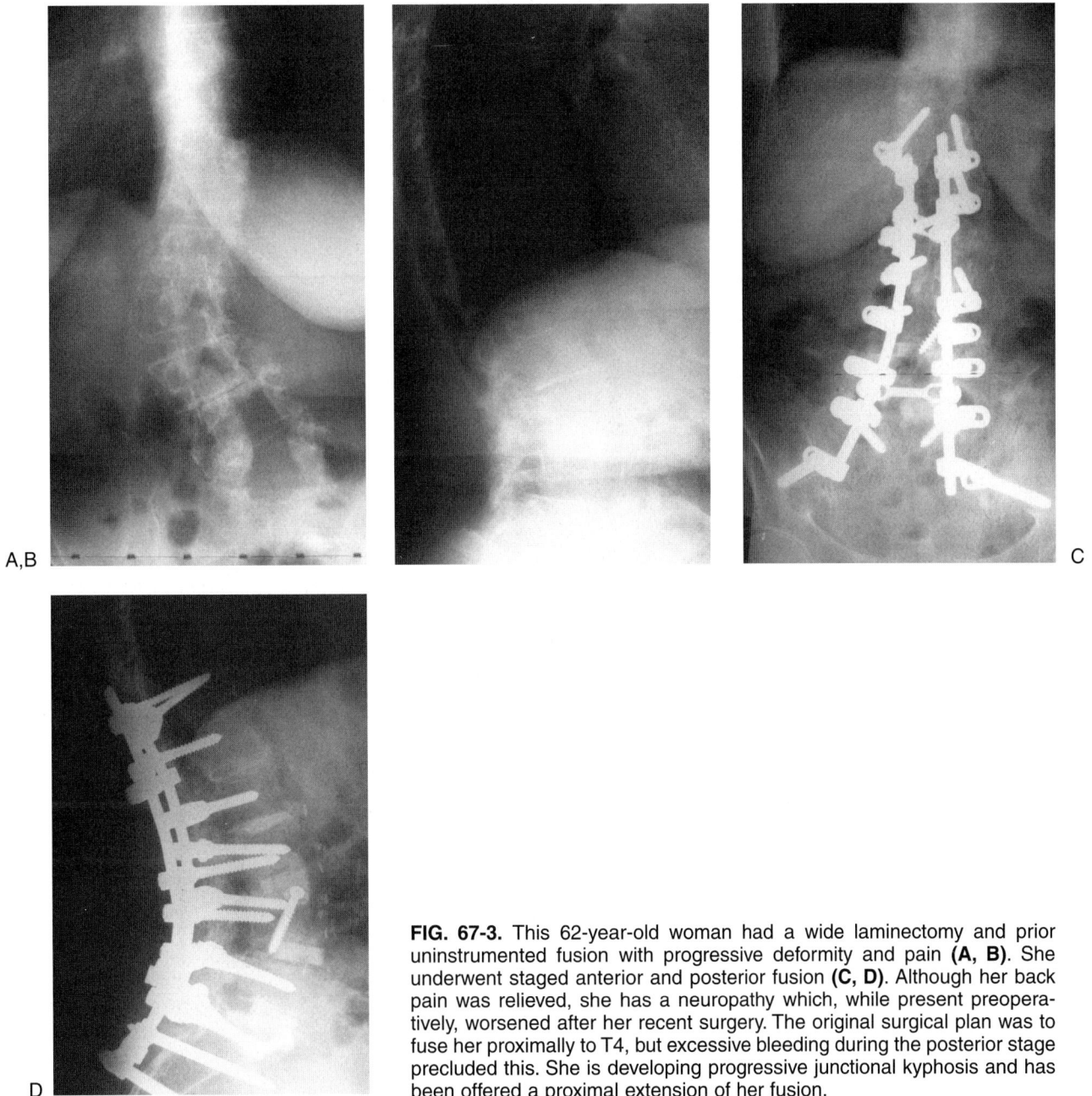

FIG. 67-3. This 62-year-old woman had a wide laminectomy and prior uninstrumented fusion with progressive deformity and pain **(A, B)**. She underwent staged anterior and posterior fusion **(C, D)**. Although her back pain was relieved, she has a neuropathy which, while present preoperatively, worsened after her recent surgery. The original surgical plan was to fuse her proximally to T4, but excessive bleeding during the posterior stage precluded this. She is developing progressive junctional kyphosis and has been offered a proximal extension of her fusion.

as rotatory subluxation, lateral listhesis or spondylolisthesis, usually requires the addition of a fusion to the decompression. Patients with curves greater than 30°, if the patients are of generally good health, should be considered for fusion for the entirety of the curve.

If the patient has significant loss of lumbar lordosis with clinically significant sagittal decompensation, anterior release with an anterior fusion may be necessary in conjunction with a posterior decompression and fusion. By using structural graft, the disc height can be restored allowing more room at the foraminal level for nerve roots, and lumbar lordosis can be maintained. The morbidity of combined procedures in older adults should not be understated and careful consideration should be placed on not only the pathology, but the patient's overall needs as well. The surgeon should always keep in mind that spinal stenosis in itself causes patients to have a forward lean and that most patients with spinal stenosis and loss of lumbar lordosis do not need combined procedures.

Salvage Procedures

Revision and salvage procedures for previous spinal deformities provide spine specialists with some of the most challenging and complex spine cases. Failed spinal deformity cases can result from several conditions and the indications for revision scoliosis surgery in the adult include:

- painful pseudoarthrosis with instrumentation failure
- pseudoarthrosis with progressive deformity
- flatback syndrome
- symptomatic adjacent segment degeneration
- unacceptable residual deformity or deformity secondary to adjacent segment degeneration
- painful hardware.

Each of the above situations requires careful consideration as each can present significant challenges. The goals of salvage surgery are the same as in primary surgery—to obtain a solid fusion, provide rigid internal fixation, and to achieve spinal balance in coronal and sagittal planes.

Pseudoarthrosis

Management of painful pseudoarthroses depends on several conditions, including the level of pseudoarthrosis, the status of present fixation, associated deformity, and the level of pain for the patient. Any hardware failure and indeed many cases of "painful hardware" should be assumed to have a pseudoarthrosis unless thorough exploration demonstrates otherwise. In general, a painful pseudoarthrosis associated with progressive deformity and loss of fixation is a clear indication for revision surgery through a combined approach. Single-level pseudoarthrosis, particularly in the thoracic spine, with-

out loss of correction or fixation can often be treated with single-stage anterior or posterior revision with significant autogenous bone graft. As newer bone morphogenetic proteins and osteoinductive materials are developed, different techniques for salvage of pseudoarthrosis without loss of balance may emerge. In the presence of multiple pseudoarthroses, a thorough exploration of the fusion mass should be performed. In these cases reinstrumentation is the method of choice with augmentation anteriorly if not already performed. In these cases, copious autogenous bone graft is necessary (51,63,64).

Progressive Deformity

Adult deformity may progress secondary to a pseudoarthrosis, a primary fusion that did not include the entire curve, or degeneration of levels above or below a prior fusion. For minor deformities, extension of the prior fusion with instrumentation can be performed.

Junctional kyphosis can occur above or below the level of prior fusions. Progressive deformity often ensues and patients can complain of pain or note difficulty walking secondary to the imbalance. Junctional kyphosis can be addressed with an appropriate extension of the fusion with or without osteotomies of segments in the previously fused spine.

For patients with fixed spinal deformities and spinal imbalance, a combined anterior and posterior approach is necessary. In many cases, anterior or posterior osteotomies may be required. A pedicle subtraction osteotomy can provide a significant amount of sagittal, and to lesser degrees, coronal balance (65). For severe, rigid deformities, a spinal shortening procedure may be necessary (66,67).

Flatback Syndrome

In general, lumbar lordosis is lost as a part of the natural aging process (68). Successful fusion with distraction instrumentation, as is typical with Harrington rod instrumentation, can create an iatrogenic flatback, especially when the fusion is created in the lumbar spine. The condition leads to a crouched position, with fatigue in the thigh musculature. Often there is associated degeneration of adjacent segments and sometimes spinal stenosis across these levels.

If there is a solid fusion posteriorly, there are several options. Multilevel Smith-Peterson osteotomies can provide correction if there is not evidence of an anterior fusion. These may need to be supplemented with anterior grafting. If osteotomies are performed across pseudoarthrosis levels, anterior fusion should also be performed. A Thomasen pedicle subtraction osteotomy can provide up to 30° to 40° of correction (Fig. 67-4) (69), and is especially useful when there is a solid anterior fusion (65).

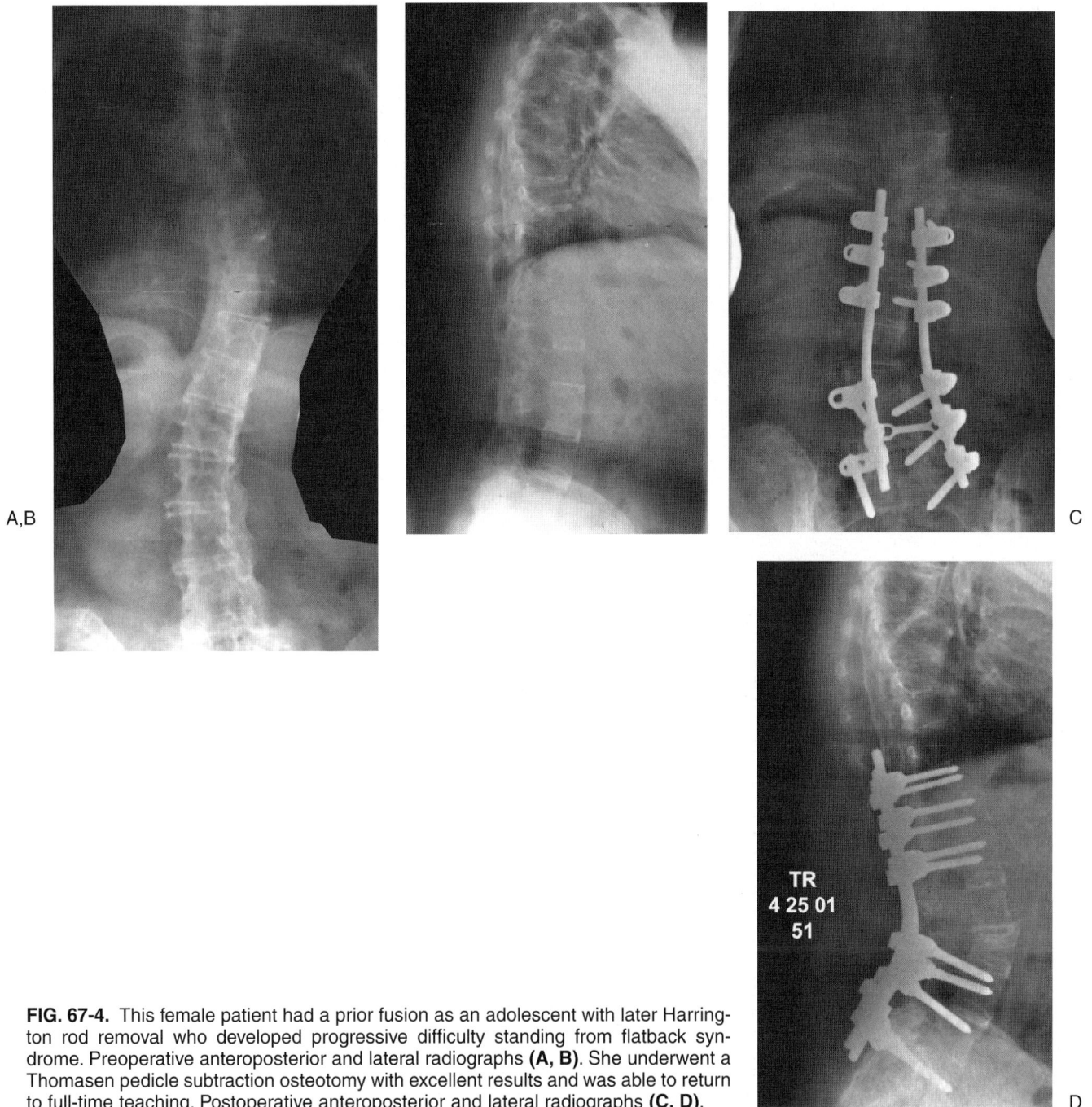

A,B

C

D

FIG. 67-4. This female patient had a prior fusion as an adolescent with later Harrington rod removal who developed progressive difficulty standing from flatback syndrome. Preoperative anteroposterior and lateral radiographs **(A, B)**. She underwent a Thomasen pedicle subtraction osteotomy with excellent results and was able to return to full-time teaching. Postoperative anteroposterior and lateral radiographs **(C, D)**.

Special Reconstruction Techniques

Anterior and Posterior Osteotomies

Reconstruction techniques include anterior osteotomies, posterior osteotomies, decancellation or pedicle subtraction osteotomies, and vertebral column resection. Anterior osteotomies are performed through the area of a fused disc space. Care must be taken to identify the foramen and the pedicles, especially in patients with a rotational component to the deformity. The posterior cortex is then removed with curettes or a Kerrison rongeur.

Posterior osteotomies can be performed by resecting bone in the area of the prior fusion at the fused facet joints, removing osteophytes until mobility is achieved. If the facets are completely fused and cannot be mobilized, Kerrison rongeurs are used to remove bone from the midline through the intertransverse foramen. It may be necessary to open the midline either with a laminectomy or at the edge of a prior laminectomy. Posterior osteotomies over multiple levels can achieve a significant amount of correction over a large area (70).

Spinal Shortening (Spinal Column Resection)

This procedure is only used for severe and rigid deformities with significant truncal decompensation. The first stage consists of an anterior approach on the convex side of the curve. Multiple osteotomies are performed proximally and distally to the intended resection level. An osteoperiosteal flap is raised over the apical first to third vertebrae after which the vertebral bodies are decancellated back to the posterior longitudinal ligament. The convex and concave pedicles are removed as far back as possible without risking damage to the dura or the exiting nerve roots. Gelfoam is placed over the dura and the decancellated bone is morselized and loosely laid down

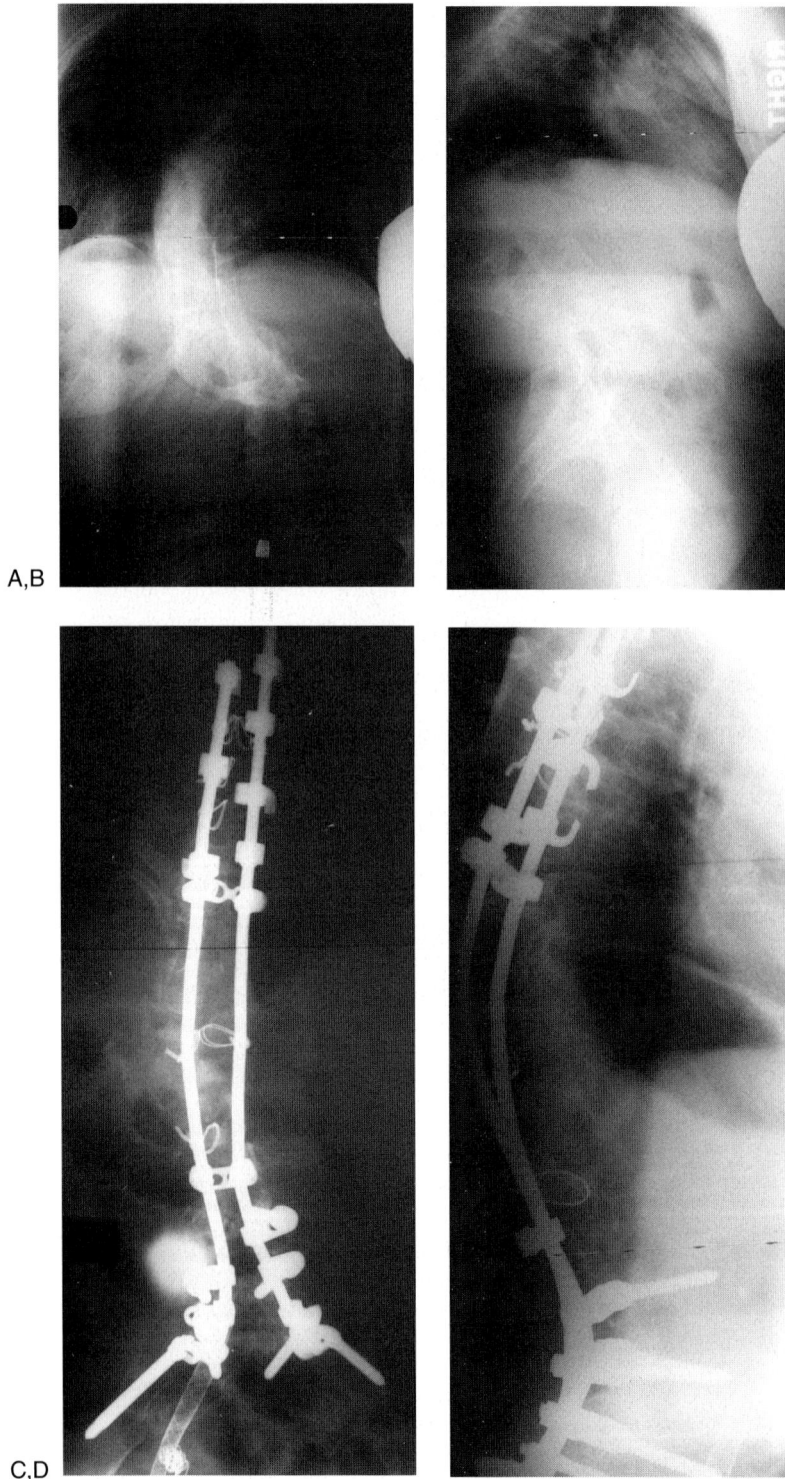

FIG. 67-5. This patient had several prior anterior and posterior fusions for her neurofibromatosis-related scoliosis and presented with severe back pain, truncal imbalance, and progression of her deformity **(A, B)**. She underwent a vertebral column resection with excellent correction of coronal and sagittal imbalance **(C, D)**.

into the defect. The osteoperiosteal flap is then sutured over the top (66,67). Either at the same setting or typically 5 to 7 days later, the posterior procedure is performed. After proximal and distal osteotomies are completed posteriorly, the remainder of the spinal elements over the anteriorly resected segments (lamina and remaining pedicles) are removed. Thoracoplasty is performed on the convex side and the apical ribs are resected on the concave side. The convex rod is fixed to the upper portion of the curve above the level of the resection using segmental fixation and is then carefully cantilevered to

the spine distally, correcting the curvature and effectively shortening the vertebral column. Dural pulsations should be monitored during the cantilevering process and a wake-up test is carried out after fixation of the rod distally. If electrophysiologic monitoring is available, this can provide continuous neurologic information. Following a satisfactory wake-up test, the concave rod is inserted to help secure the correction with additional points of fixation. Additional correction is not attempted. A second wake-up test is then performed. The implants are then secured and bone grafting completed (Fig. 68-5).

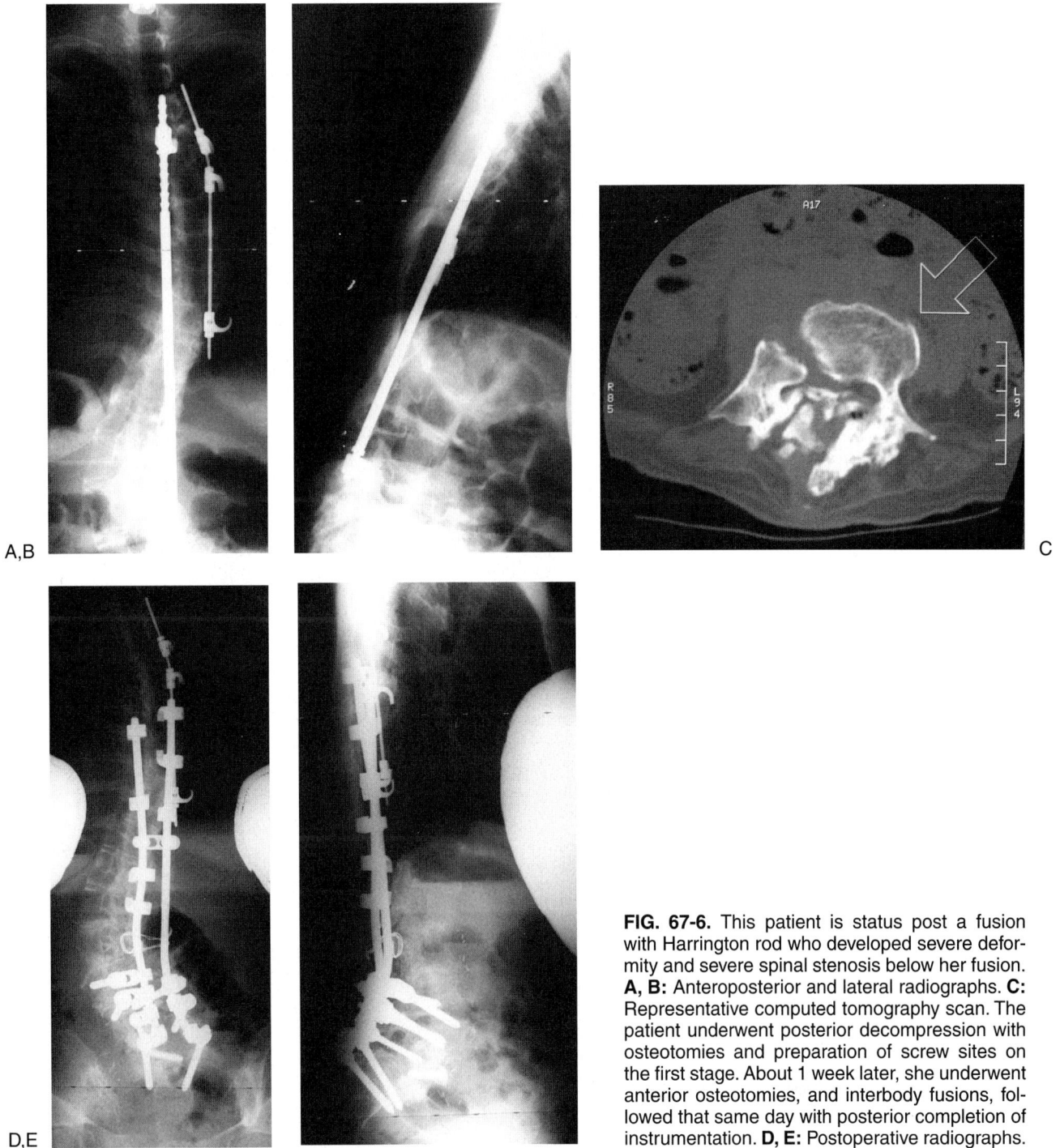

FIG. 67-6. This patient is status post a fusion with Harrington rod who developed severe deformity and severe spinal stenosis below her fusion. **A, B:** Anteroposterior and lateral radiographs. **C:** Representative computed tomography scan. The patient underwent posterior decompression with osteotomies and preparation of screw sites on the first stage. About 1 week later, she underwent anterior osteotomies, and interbody fusions, followed that same day with posterior completion of instrumentation. **D, E:** Postoperative radiographs.

The goal is to achieve coronal and sagittal plane balance by shortening the spine and avoiding spinal cord distraction. An alternative to this procedure is the posterior eggshell approach, decancelling multiple vertebrae through the pedicles. It is effective in obtaining correction, but anterior arthrodesis may be difficult to achieve.

Special Considerations and Controversies

Indications for Combined Surgery

A carefully designed operative plan includes deciding on performing combined anterior and posterior surgery versus posterior fusion alone. Most surgeons would favor combined surgeries for the following conditions:

- failed posterior fusion in lumbar spine
- rigid deformity requiring anterior release
- long fusion to sacrum
- lumbar or thoracolumbar kyphosis requiring anterior structural grafting.

While single-stage posterior fusion is attractive, combined surgery allows for both better correction and permits the reestablishment of lumbar lordosis with anterior structural grafts. This has the added benefit of increasing the probability of successful fusion. When a thoracolumbar fusion is extended across the lumbosacral junction, anterior interbody fusion becomes a requirement as the pseudoarthrosis rate can be as high as 40% to 60% with posterior fusion alone (27,53).

On some rare occasions, posterior osteotomies should be performed before anterior osteotomies, such as in cases of correction of severely decompensated, fused, rigid deformities. It is usually possible to complete the three stages under two anesthetics. The first stage includes posterior osteotomies and insertion of hardware without connecting the rods. If there is any question as to pedicle screw placement, 4.5 mm AO cortical screws can be placed as radiographic markers so that postoperative radiographs or CT can confirm screw placement. Most pedicle screws for implantation are too prominent to be placed at this time in patients with severe kyphosis. At the second stage, 5 to 7 days later, anterior release and osteotomies are accomplished and interbody fusion is performed. In the same setting, the patient is instrumented posteriorly and final correction is carried out (Fig. 68-6). It has been our experience that a two-stage procedure is better tolerated with only a slightly higher risk of infection and increased blood loss which is also advocated in the recent literature (36,46,52).

RESULTS AND COMPLICATIONS

Even when the major goals of adult deformity surgery are met, pain may not be completely relieved. Residual pain after complex spinal reconstructive surgery varies between 5% and 15%.

The challenges in this type of surgery are great, but improvements in anesthesia techniques, neuromonitoring, internal fixation, and intensive care medicine have improved perioperative care such that the majority of cases can be performed with acceptable risk. Mortality remains low, but not insignificant, at less than 1%.

Neurologic injury is relatively uncommon and occurs in less than 1% to 5% of cases. Significant risk factors for major intraoperative neurologic deficits include combined anterior and posterior surgery, severe rigid curves, and hyperkyphosis (40). Direct injury of neural elements can result from instrumentation or from indirect causes, such as ischemic insult or neuropraxia from distraction. Delayed postoperative paraplegia is another devastating complication following extensive spinal reconstructive surgery that can occur several hours after the completion of the procedure. This phenomenon has been attributed to ischemia of the spinal cord from postoperative hypovolemia, mechanical tension of spinal blood vessels on the concavity of the curve, and preexisting atherosclerosis, and can often be reversed if rapid improvement of perfusion pressure and correction of anemia is performed (72). Delayed paresis may also occur with postoperative hematoma. Thus, repeat neurologic exams after completion of the surgery are essential.

Myers has reported 37 cases of visual loss as a complication of spinal reconstructive surgery that occurred as the result of ischemic optic neuropathy, retinal artery occlusion, or cerebral ischemia (44). The visual losses that were reported often did not fully resolve.

The incidence of pulmonary embolism varies from 1% to 20%, depending upon the series and appears to be increased after anterior procedures in older patients (73–75).

Infection is a relatively rare event, occurring between 1% and 8% of patients. Infection after anterior surgery alone is about 1% (18). However, the sequelae of deep postoperative infection are substantial. The use of preoperative broad-spectrum antibiotics, meticulous wound handling, and providing nutritional supplementation and augmentation for patients undergoing staged procedures decreases infection and wound healing complications. Redosing intravenous antibiotics with significant blood loss has also been shown to be an effective adjunct to help decrease infection rates (76).

Failed fusion is the most common complication of adult deformity surgery, with the highest rates occurring after revision surgery. Other factors that have been found to increase pseudoarthrosis rates include the use of allograft bone and the use of nonsegmental instrumentation in a distraction mode. Weis reported a pseudoarthrosis rate of 38% at 37-month follow-up (18). Gertzbein reported poor clinical outcomes after circumferential fusion to treat lumbar pseudoarthrosis. Only 52% of his patients reduced their pain a full category and only 53% returned to work. These poor outcomes occurred despite a 100% fusion rate (77). We noted that patients who required reoperation at 6 months were more likely to be dissatisfied with their result (78). Persistent pain was the most commonly cited reason for dissatisfaction.

Spinal decompensation is most often the result of improper selection of fusion levels. Progressive decompensation below a fusion is possible if the fusion is stopped short of the stable vertebra or if there is significant residual obliquity of the last instrumented vertebra. As previously noted, ending a fusion at a kyphotic segment can result in junctional kyphosis and sagittal decompensation. Decompensation may result secondary to a failure to fuse all structural curves.

When dealing with the osteoporotic spine, multiple fixation points need to be used to reduce the chance of fixation failure at the bone/implant interface (30). Pedicles provide excellent fixation but may sometimes need to be supplemented with laminar hooks or sublaminar wires in severely osteoporotic spines (34,50,71,79,80).

POSTOPERATIVE MANAGEMENT

Postoperatively, patients are mobilized within 24 to 48 hours, depending on their pain level and medical condition. Many patients with long-term narcotic usage can present a challenge in terms of pain management in the immediate postoperative period. Patient-controlled analgesia is widely used in these patients. We have also found it helpful to arrange preoperative interviews between the patient and our pharmacology department, who then assist in managing postoperative pain. Postoperative pain in fusion patients is never managed with NSAIDs, as their use been shown to adversely affect fusion rates (81). All patients are treated with full-length antiembolic compression stockings and sequential compression devices to lower the rate of thromboembolic events. High-risk patients or those with known history of deep vein thrombosis may be considered for a vena cava filter prior to surgery as pharmacologic anticoagulation has potential for significant complications (72).

All staged patients are started on nutritional supplementation such as hyperalimentation or tube feeding until such a time after the second stage that they are able to consume enough calories to forego the supplementation. It has been shown that proper perioperative nutritional status correlates with a lower infection rate (47,48).

Patients are fitted for a custom thoracolumbosacral orthosis (TLSO) as soon as they are able to stand for a long enough period to make proper measurements, typically on the second or third postoperative day. Patients are instructed to wear the orthosis for at least 3 months whenever they are out of bed. Weaning off the brace depends upon surgeon preference, clinical improvement, and radiographic evidence of fusion mass. Thigh extensions for fusions to the sacrum are not well tolerated, but consideration for their use is given when distal fixation is subop-

timal. Patients average a 5- to 7-day hospital stay for single procedures, with staged procedures requiring a longer hospital stay. Follow-up clinic appointments are performed at 6 weeks, 3 months, 6 months, 1 year, and 2 years, with full-length radiographs obtained at each visit to ensure progression of fusion mass and to evaluate stability of the construct and overall alignment.

CONCLUSION

Surgery for patients with adult scoliosis requires careful preoperative evaluation and planning. The technical aspects of surgical correction and restoration of coronal and sagittal balance are challenging and complex. In addition, the number and types of complications that can occur during adult spinal reconstructive surgery are greater than those in the adolescent. Combined surgery is recommended for rigid deformities, those that involve the lumbar spine, or long fusions to the sacrum. Rigid, segmental instrumentation that will allow minimal postoperative support is advantageous and a careful preoperative workup and plan is needed.

The primary goal of surgery is the achievement of a balanced correction and a solid arthrodesis. Patients may take 6 to 12 months to fully recover from these procedures and improvement can occur for up to 2 years. Finally, proper patient selection with a frank discussion between surgeon and patient as to realistic expectations is vital to the achievement of a satisfactory outcome.

If coronal and sagittal balance is achieved and maintained with a solid fusion after the primary surgery, the outcomes are generally excellent. Correction of curvature varies from 30% to 60% and is very dependent on the nature of the preoperative curve, its flexibility, and the technique used for correction. Despite these relatively modest gains, patient satisfaction is generally high and can reach up to 90%. We retrospectively evaluated outcomes in patients over 40 years of age who underwent major spinal reconstructive surgery and found over 81% patient satisfaction with significant improvements in many areas of functional status (77). Dickson compared the outcomes of 81 adult patients undergoing operative treatment for idiopathic scoliosis with 30 patients who declined operative management (82). At an average of 5 years' follow-up, he found that treated patients reported a significantly greater decrease in pain and fatigue with improvement in self-image and functionality as compared to the nontreated group. Albert has also shown statistically significant improvements in functional outcome, pain, and body image in adults following spinal reconstructive surgery (1,83).

Outcomes tools are still being developed for evaluation of patients undergoing surgery for adult scoliosis. Most of the data available suggest that there is an improved quality of life for patients who have been carefully accepted into this type of treatment program.

REFERENCES

1. Albert TJ, Balderston RA. Treatment of adult scoliosis. J South Orthop Assoc 1996;5(3):229–237.
2. Ascani E, Bartolozzi P, Logroscino CA, et al. Natural history of untreated idiopathic scoliosis after skeletal maturity. Spine 1986;11(8):784–789.
3. Collins DK, Ponseti IV. Long-term follow-up of patients with idiopathic scoliosis not treated surgically. J Bone Joint Surg Am 1969;51(3):425–445.
4. Ogilvie JW. Adult scoliosis: evaluation and nonsurgical treatment. Instr Course Lect 1992; 41:251–255.
5. Pashman RS, Hu SS, Schendel MJ, et al. Sacral screw loads in lumbosacral fixation for spinal deformity. Spine 1993;18(16):2465–2470.
6. Vanderpool DW, James JI, Wynne-Davies R. Scoliosis in the elderly. J Bone Joint Surg Am 1969;51(3):446–455.
7. Chuah S, Kareem BA, Selvakumar K, et al. The natural history of scoliosis: curve progression of untreated curves of different aetiology, with early (mean 2 year) follow up in surgically treated curves. Med J Malaysia 2001;56[Suppl C]:37–40.
8. Jackson RP, Simmons EH, Stripinis D. Incidence and severity of back pain in adult idiopathic scoliosis. Spine 1987;8(7):749–756.
9. Korovessis P, Piperos G, Sidiropoulos P, et al. Adult idiopathic lumbar scoliosis. A formula for prediction of progression and review of the literature. Spine 1994;19(17):1926–1932.
10. Kostuik JP. Recent advances in the treatment of painful adult scoliosis. Clin Orthop 1980;(147):238–252.
11. Polly DW Jr, Meter JJ, Brueckner R, et al. The effect of intraoperative blood loss on serum cefazolin level in patients undergoing instrumented spinal fusion. A prospective, controlled study. Spine 1996;21(20):2363–2367.
12. Taylor BA, Webb PJ, Hetreed M, et al. Delayed postoperative paraplegia with hypotension in adult revision scoliosis surgery. Spine 1994;19(4):470–474.
13. Nachemson AL, Bjure JC, Grimby LG, et al. Physical fitness in young women with idiopathic scoliosis before and after an exercise program. Arch Phys Med Rehabil 1970;51(2):95–98 passim.
14. Bridwell KH. Degenerative scoliosis. In: Bridwell KH, DeWald RL, eds. The Textbook of Spinal Surgery, 2nd ed. Philadelphia: Lippincott-Raven Publishers, 1997.
15. Bradford DS. Adult scoliosis. Current concepts of treatment. Clin Orthop 1988;(229):70–87.
16. Robin GC, Span Y, Steinberg R, et al. Scoliosis in the elderly: a follow-up study. Spine 1982;7(4):355–359.
17. Weinstein SL, Ponseti IV. Curve progression in idiopathic scoliosis. J Bone Joint Surg Am 1983;65(4):447–455.
18. Weis JC, Betz RR, Clements DH 3rd, et al. Prevalence of perioperative complications after anterior spinal fusion for patients with idiopathic scoliosis. J Spinal Disord 1997;10(5):371–375.
19. Kostuik JP. Decision making in adult scoliosis. Spine 1979;4(6):521–525.
20. Kostuik JP, Errico TJ, Gleason TF. Techniques of internal fixation for degenerative conditions of the lumbar spine. Clin Orthop 1986;(203):219–231.
21. Kostuik JP, Israel J, Hall JE. Scoliosis surgery in adults. Clin Orthop 1973;93:225–234.
22. Kostuik JP, Bentivoglio J. The incidence of low back pain in adult scoliosis. Acta Orthop Belg 1981;47(4–5):548–559.
23. Jackson RP, Simmons EH, Stripinis D. Coronal and sagittal plane spinal deformities correlating with back pain and pulmonary function in adult idiopathic scoliosis. Spine 1989;14(12):1391–1397.
24. Voos K, Boachie-Adjei O, Rawlins BA. Multiple vertebral osteotomies in the treatment of rigid adult spine deformities. Spine 2001;26(5):526–533.
25. Simmons ED Jr, Kowalski JM, Simmons EH. The results of surgical treatment for adult scoliosis. Spine 1993;18(6):718–724.
26. Sponseller PD, Cohen MS, Nachemson AL, et al. Results of surgical treatment of adults with idiopathic scoliosis. J Bone Joint Surg Am 1987;69(5):667–675.
27. Grubb SA, Lipscomb HJ, Suh PB. Results of surgical treatment of painful adult scoliosis. Spine 1994;19(14):1619–1627.
28. Johnson JR, Holt RT. Combined use of anterior and posterior surgery for adult scoliosis. Orthop Clin North Am 1988;19(2):361–370.
29. Geissele AE, Ogilvie JW, Cohen M, et al. Thoracoplasty for the treatment of rib prominence in thoracic scoliosis. Spine 1994;19(14):1636–1642.
30. Hu SS. Internal fixation in the osteoporotic spine. Spine 1997;22[24 Suppl]:43S–48S.
31. Barr SJ, Schuette AM, Emans JB. Lumbar pedicle screws versus hooks. Results in double major curves in adolescent idiopathic scoliosis. Spine 1997;22(12):1369–1379.
32. Wood KB, Kos PB, Abnet JK, et al. Prevention of deep-vein thrombosis after major spinal surgery: a comparison study of external devices. J Spinal Disord 1997;10(3):209–214.
33. Gayet LE, Pries P, Hamcha H, et al. Biomechanical study and digital modeling of traction resistance in posterior thoracic implants. Spine 2002;27(7):707–714.
34. Luk KD, Cheung KM, Lu DS, et al. Assessment of scoliosis correction in relation to flexibility using the fulcrum bending correction index. Spine 1998;23(21):2303–2307.
35. Boachie-Adjei O, Lonner B. Spinal deformity. Pediatr Clin North Am 1996;43(4):883–897.
36. Bradford DS, Tay BK, Hu SS. Adult scoliosis: surgical indications, operative management, complications, and outcomes. Spine 1999;24(24):2617–2629.
37. Byrd JA 3rd, Scoles PV, Winter RB, et al. Adult idiopathic scoliosis treated by anterior and posterior spinal fusion. J Bone Joint Surg Am 1987;69(6):843–850.
38. Swank S, Lonstein JE, Moe JH, et al. Surgical treatment of adult scoliosis. A review of two hundred and twenty-two cases. J Bone Joint Surg Am 1981;63(2):268–287.
39. Boachie-Adjei O, Girardi FP, Bansal M, et al. Safety and efficacy of pedicle screw placement for adult spinal deformity with a pedicle-probing conventional anatomic technique. J Spinal Disord 2000;13(6):496–500.
40. Bridwell KH, Lenke LG, Baldus C, et al. Major intraoperative neurologic deficits in pediatric and adult spinal deformity patients. Incidence and etiology at one institution. Spine 1998;23(3):324–331.
41. Court-Brown CM, Stoll JE, Gertzbein SD. Thoracic facetectomy and bone grafting in the surgical treatment of adult idiopathic scoliosis. Spine 1987;12(10):992–995.
42. Eck KR, Bridwell KH, Ungacta FF, et al. Complications and results of long adult deformity fusions down to L4, L5, and the sacrum. Spine 2001;26(9):E182–E192.
43. Emami A, Deviren V, Berven S, et al. Outcome and complications of long fusions to the sacrum in adult spine deformity: Luque-Galveston, combined iliac and sacral screws, and sacral fixation. Spine 2002;27(7):776–786.
44. Myers MA, Hamilton SR, Bogosian AJ, et al. Visual loss as a complication of spine surgery. A review of 37 cases. Spine 1997;22(12):1325–1329.
45. Nachemson A. Adult scoliosis and back pain. Spine 1979;4(6):513–517.
46. Dick J, Boachie-Adjei O, Wilson M. One-stage versus two-stage anterior and posterior spinal reconstruction in adults. Comparison of outcomes including nutritional status, complications rates, hospital costs, and other factors. Spine 1992;17[8 Suppl]:S310–S316.
47. Hu SS, Fontaine F, Kelly B, et al. Nutritional depletion in staged spinal reconstructive surgery. The effect of total parenteral nutrition. Spine 1998;23(12):1401–1405.
47a. Lenke LG, Bridwell KH, Blanke K, et al. Prospective analysis of nutritional status normalization after spinal reconstructive surgery. Spine 1995;30(12):1359–1367.
48. Liljenqvist U, Hackenberg L, Link T, et al. Pullout strength of pedicle screws versus pedicle and laminar hooks in the thoracic spine. Acta Orthop Belg 2001;67(2):157–163.
49. Cotler JM, Cotler HB. Spinal fusion: science and technique. New York: Springer-Verlag, 1990.
50. Gertzbein SD, et al. Semirigid instrumentation in the management of lumbar spinal conditions combined with circumferential fusion. A multicenter study. Spine 1996;21(16):1918–1925; discussion 1925–1926.
51. Lapp MA, Bridwell KH, Lenke LG, et al. Long-term complications in adult spinal deformity patients having combined surgery a comparison of primary to revision patients. Spine 2001; 26(8):973–983.
52. Boachie-Adjei O, Dendrinos GK, Ogilvie JW, et al. Management of adult spinal deformity with combined anterior-posterior arthrodesis and Luque-Galveston instrumentation. J Spinal Disord 1991;4(2):131–141.

53. Horton WC, Holt RT, Muldowny DS. Controversy. Fusion of L5-S1 in adult scoliosis. Spine 1996;21(21):2520–2522.
54. Kostuik JP, Hall BB. Spinal fusions to the sacrum in adults with scoliosis. Spine 1983; 8(5):489–500.
55. Kostuik JP, Musha Y. Extension to the sacrum of previous adolescent scoliosis fusions in adult life. Clin Orthop 1999; (364):53–60.
56. Kuklo TR, Bridwell KH, Lewis SJ, et al. Minimum 2-year analysis of sacropelvic fixation and L5-S1 fusion using S1 and iliac screws. Spine 2001;26(18):1976–1983.
57. Perennou D, Marcelli C, Herisson C, et al. Adult lumbar scoliosis. Epidemiologic aspects in a low-back pain population. Spine 1994;19 (2):123–128.
58. Enker P, Steffee AD. Interbody fusion and instrumentation. Clin Orthop 1994;(300):90–101.
59. Glazer PA, Colliou O, Lotz JC, et al. Biomechanical analysis of lumbosacral fixation. Spine 1996;21(10):1211–1222.
60. Jackson RP, McManus AC. Radiographic analysis of sagittal plane alignment and balance in standing volunteers and patients with low back pain matched for age, sex, and size. A prospective controlled clinical study. Spine 1994;19(14):1611–1618.
61. Collins DK, Stack JP, O'Connell DJ. The role of discography in lumbar disc disease: a comparative study of MRI and discography. Clin Radiol 1969;42:252–257.
62. Ito M, Incorvaia KM, Yu SF, et al. Predictive signs of discogenic lumbar pain on magnetic resonance imaging with discography correlation. Spine 1998;23(11):1252–1258; discussion 1259–1260.
63. Buttermann GR, Glazer PA, Hu SS, et al. Revision of failed lumbar fusions. A comparison of anterior autograft and allograft. Spine 1997; 22(23):2748–2755.
64. Hansraj KK, O'Leary PF, Cammisa FP Jr, et al. Decompression, fusion, and instrumentation surgery for complex lumbar spinal stenosis. Clin Orthop 2001;(384):18–25.
65. Berven SH, Deviren V, Smith JA, et al. Management of fixed sagittal plane deformity: results of the transpedicular wedge resection osteotomy. Spine 2001;26(18):2036–2043.
66. Boachie-Adjei O, Bradford DS. Vertebral column resection and arthrodesis for complex spinal deformities. J Spinal Disord 1991;4 (2):193–202.
67. Bradford DS, Tribus CB. Vertebral column resection for the treatment of rigid coronal decompensation. Spine 1997;22(14):1590–1599.
68. Gelb DE, Lenke LG, Bridwell KH, et al. An analysis of sagittal spinal alignment in 100 asymptomatic middle and older aged volunteers. Spine 1995;20(12):1351–1358.
69. van Dam BE. Non operative treatment of adult scoliosis. Orthop Clin North Am 1988;19:347–351.
70. Weinstein SL. Bristol-Myers Squibb/Zimmer award for distinguished achievement in orthopaedic research. Long-term follow-up of pediatric orthopaedic conditions. Natural history and outcomes of treatment. J Bone Joint Surg Am 2000;82-A(7):980–990.
71. Simmons ED. Surgical treatment of patients with lumbar spinal stenosis with associated scoliosis. Clin Orthop 2001;(384):45–53.
72. Thomasen E. Vertebral osteotomy for correction of kyphosis in ankylosing spondylitis. Clin Orthop 1985;(194):142–152.
73. Cain JE Jr, Major MR, Lauerman WC, et al. The morbidity of heparin therapy after development of pulmonary embolus in patients undergoing thoracolumbar or lumbar spinal fusion. Spine 1995;20(14):1600–1603.
74. Dearborn JT, Hu SS, Tribus CB, et al. Thromboembolic complications after major thoracolumbar spine surgery. Spine 1999;24(14): 1471–1476.
75. Zheng F, Cammisa FP Jr, Sandhu HS, et al. Factors predicting hospital stay, operative time, blood loss, and transfusion in patients undergoing revision posterior lumbar spine decompression, fusion, and segmental instrumentation. Spine 2002;27(8):818–824.
76. Postacchini F. Surgical management of lumbar spinal stenosis. Spine 1999;24(10):1043–1047.
77. Gertzbein SD, Hollopeter MR, Hall S. Pseudarthrosis of the lumbar spine. Outcome after circumferential fusion. Spine 1998;23(21): 2352–2356; discussion 2356–2357.
78. Hu SS, Holly EA, Lele C, et al. Patient outcomes after spinal reconstructive surgery in patients > or < 40 years of age. J Spinal Disord 1996;9(6):460–469.
79. Butler TE Jr, Asher MA, Jayaraman G, et al. The strength and stiffness of thoracic implant anchors in osteoporotic spines. Spine 1994;19(17):1956–1962.
80. Halm H, Niemeyer T, Link T, et al. Segmental pedicle screw instrumentation in idiopathic thoracolumbar and lumbar scoliosis. Eur Spine J 2000;9(3):191–197.
81. Glassman SD, Rose SM, Dimar JR, et al. The effect of postoperative nonsteroidal anti-inflammatory drug administration on spinal fusion. Spine 1998;23(7):834–838.
82. Dickson JH, Mirkovic S, Noble PC, et al. Results of operative treatment of idiopathic scoliosis in adults. J Bone Joint Surg Am 1995;77 (4):513–523.
83. Albert TJ, Mesa JJ, Eng K, et al. Health outcome assessment before and after lumbar laminectomy for radiculopathy. Spine 1996;21(8): 960–962; discussion 963.

CHAPTER 68

The Surgical Treatment of Sagittal Plane Deformity

Thomas J. Errico, Orin Atlas, and Juan Carlos Rodriguez Olaverri

Spinal deformity can affect the coronal, sagittal, or multiple planes, causing symptomatic imbalance (1). These deformities present difficult management issues for spine surgeons. Sagittal plane deformities have many etiologies and can occur at multiple locations and levels. Etiologies include postural deformity; ankylosing spondylitis; diffuse idiopathic skeletal hyperostosis; Scheuermann disease; congenital kyphosis; postlaminectomy kyphosis; and postradiation and posttraumatic kyphosis; as well as osteoporosis and metabolic bone disease (through multiple compression fractures) (2).

Physiologic sagittal alignment implies that the sagittal plumb line dropped from the center of the odontoid or the center of the seventh cervical vertebral body falls anterior to the thoracic spine, crosses the thoracolumbar junction, and falls behind the lumbar spine, ending at the middle of the sacrum. A normal thoracic kyphosis measurement ranges from 25° to 55°, with the apex located at T6-7. The normal lumbar lordosis is 40° to 70°, with an apex located at the L3-4 interspace (3). Abnormalities of normal alignment may occur at specific regional anatomic locations such as the cervical, thoracic, or lumbar spine, as well as extraspinal locations. These alterations can affect regional or global alignment of the spine. Surgical correction of sagittal plane deformities shares many of the known challenges of the correction of coronal plane abnormalities, such as curve rigidity and spinal fixation. However, it also presents unique obstacles to the spine surgeon, especially in the rigidly fused spine of iatrogenic flat back syndrome.

Patients with fixed sagittal plane deformities are often quite disabled. They may have a primary spine deformity, or may present with a failed back after previous surgical procedures. A frequent cause is iatrogenic flat back syndrome, secondary to a previous spinal fusion, with the loss of normal lumbar lordosis. Prior surgeries using distraction instrumentation in the lower lumbar spine or malaligned lumbar fusions with a pseudoarthrosis are the main causes of disability and dysfunction in the iatrogenic group (4). Disability also may result from the use of modern segmental instrumentation, anterior release, and fusion without the use of structural graft for anterior column support, and moderate loosening of distal fixation. Patients seen at this institute, whose spinal disability condition is not related to scoliosis correction, are typically older patients, often with osteoporosis. Other less common causes are posttraumatic, neuromuscular, infectious, or degenerative conditions. Conditions not related to the spine, such as hip or knee flexion contractures, also can present with sagittal malalignment and must be ruled out.

Iatrogenic flat back syndrome is a postural disorder and a recognized complication following spine surgery, but most often occurs in the treatment of pediatric or adult scoliosis. For example, with distraction type instrumentation such as the Harrington rods, the posterior distraction force decreases the segmental and regional thoracolumbar and lumbar lordosis, resulting in sagittal imbalance (Fig. 68-1). It also may occur after surgery in adults for nonscoliotic degenerative processes or instability-related pathology. Loss of sagittal balance may be secondary to pseudoarthrosis within a fusion or degenerative changes below a previous fusion level. The degree of imbalance depends on several factors, including the alignment of the thoracic kyphosis and thoracolumbar junction, the flexibility of any mobile distal lumbar discs, and the flexibility of the hip joints. The resultant loss of lordosis results in forward inclination of the trunk, back pain, and the inability to stand erect without flexing the knees. This chapter reviews the diagnosis, pathogenesis, management, and prevention of lumbar sagittal plane deformity or flat back syndrome.

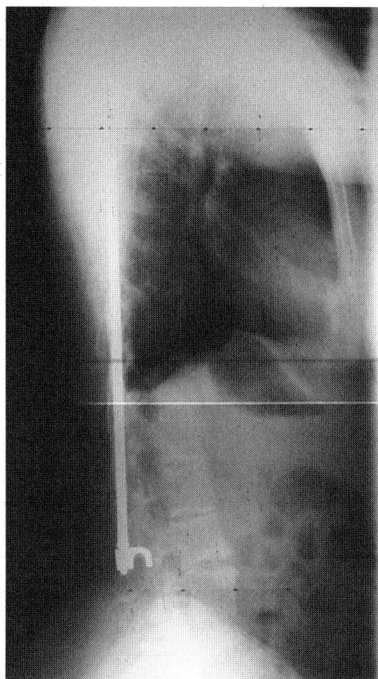

FIG. 68-1. A 35-year-old patient 20 years after insertion of a Harrington rod to L4. Note the loss of lumbar lordosis of the upper lumbar spine and the creation of actual kyphosis. The L4-5 disc has responded with hyperlordosis and disc degeneration.

CLINICAL PRESENTATION

Patients with flat back syndrome most commonly present in their late twenties to forties and have had surgery as a teenager for scoliosis. These patients present with a fixed forward inclination of the trunk and an inability to stand erect with their knees fully extended. To maintain an erect posture, the patient will flex the hips and knees and hyperextend the upper thoracic and cervical spine (Fig. 68-2). Presenting complaints usually are back pain, progressive fatigue, and, in severe cases, the classic signs of falling forward and difficulty maintaining a comfortable standing posture.

It is very important to distinguish fatigue- and alignment-related complaints from radicular complaints or pain related to instrumentation. In order to fully assess the patient, a detailed history that includes any prior diagnoses and surgical procedures should be performed. A detailed physical examination with a neurologic examination and balance assessment should be done.

PATHOGENESIS

The physical difficulty of maintaining an erect posture for patients with flat back places select muscle groups under a constant strain and results in pain and fatigue in the otherwise unaffected areas of the spine, thighs, and buttocks. The sagittal malalignment of the flat back places high demands on the muscles, ligaments, and discs of the vertebral column. Minimal disturbances in sagittal alignment are usually compensated for by muscle action to maintain a level gaze (horizontal visual field). However, increasing loss of normal lumbar lordosis leads to a decreased paraspinal muscles lever arm, and thus significant forces and energy expenditures are required to maintain an erect posture. The progressive decompensation in alignment can be theorized as a gradual process of failure of muscle mechanics (dynamic stabilizers) to maintain posture, followed by a gradual failure of the lig-

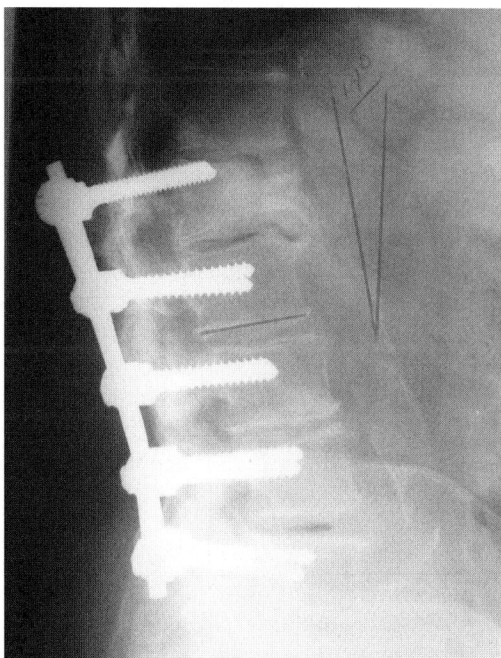

FIG. 68-2. A 72-year-old man with noted progressive difficulty standing erect after a four-level lumbar laminectomy and instrumented fusion of L1-5. The patient has subsequently developed a compression fracture of the upper-instrumented L1 vertebral body. **A:** Lateral X-ray of the lumbar spine with loss of normal lumbar lordosis.

(continued on next page)

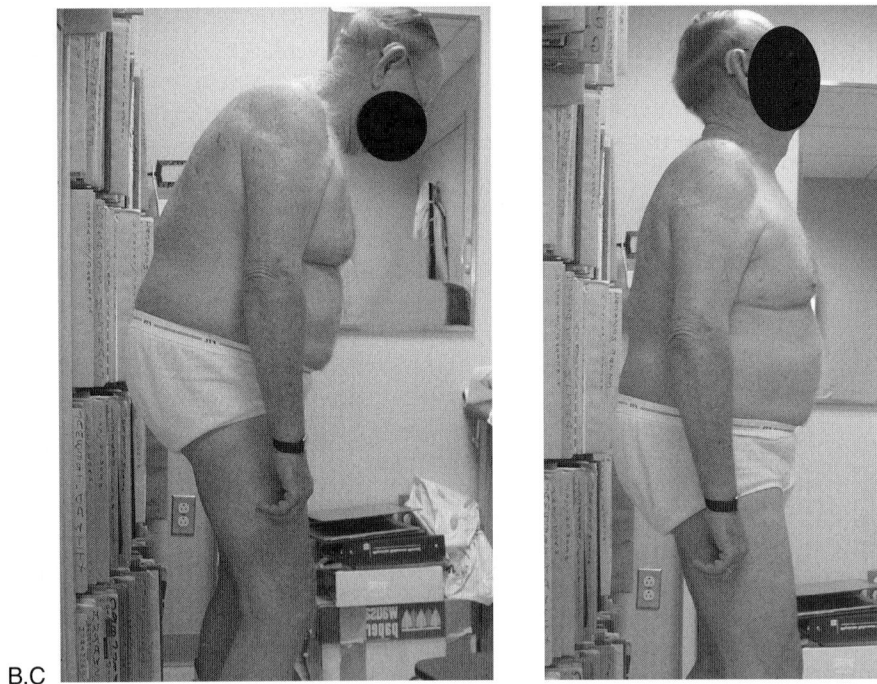

B,C

FIG. 68-2. (*Continued*) **B:** Relaxed clinical stance. **C:** Posture using maximal effort to stand erect requires bending of the knees and cervical hyperlordosis.

aments and capsular structures (rigid stabilizers). A progression of the deformity ensues, with persistent pain and limited function for the patient.

Scoliotic patients who otherwise have initially compensated well for their iatrogenic loss of correction often

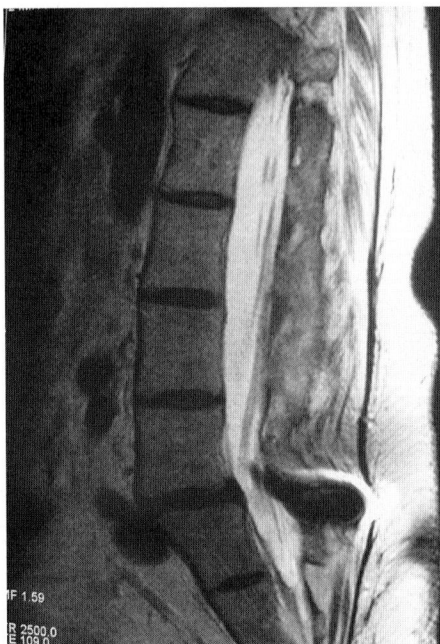

FIG. 68-3. Magnetic resonance image of a 41-year-old woman 26 years after fusion with a Harrington rod to L5. This patient has significant pain and flat back syndrome that has developed progressively over several years. Note the disc degeneration, translation, loss of disc height, and loss of the normal lordosis of the L5-S1 disc.

lose this ability in the third and fourth decades of life. The largest contributing factor is disc degeneration of the remaining disc or discs below the fusion. With loss of disc height the normal lordotic angulation of the important L4-5 and L5-S1 discs is lost. This angular disc space loss plus the inability of the lower extremity muscle groups to compensate create the clinically significant deformity in the previously compensated patient (Fig. 68-3) At this age, patients frequently begin to stoop forward. When they are evaluated with plain radiographs and magnetic resonance imaging (MRI), disc space narrowing, and degenerative changes are often found that can lead to spinal stenosis and degenerative spondylolisthesis at the first mobile level below the fusion.

Scoliosis patients are not the only patients to experience these problems. A similar syndrome of pain and a sensation of imbalance with sagittal malalignment can result from surgery in degenerative disease. Long lumbar fusions for instability associated with spinal stenosis may also create iatrogenic lumbar stenosis. These patients have poor compensatory mechanisms if their long fused lumbar segments are fused with loss of normal lordosis. They have generalized weak musculature for compensation and the adjacent disc levels are frequently flat with loss of normal disc angulation. In the osteoporotic patient, an adjacent segment compression fracture can push them over the edge into a pain kyphotic deformity.

RADIOGRAPHIC ASSESSMENT

Radiographic studies most useful in the evaluation of patients with sagittal plane imbalance include standing full-length (36-in.) antero-posterior (AP) and lateral radi-

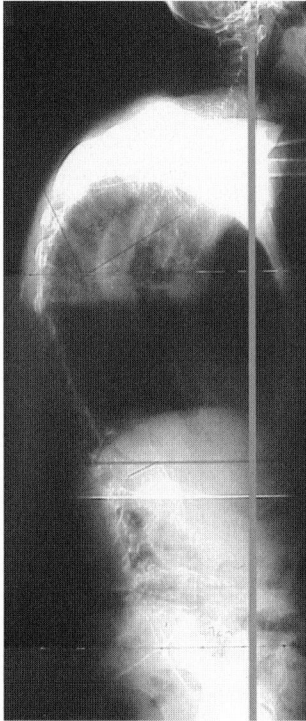

FIG. 68-4. Lateral 3-foot standing X-ray of a 78-year-old patient with kyphoscoliosis. Notice the loss of sagittal balance, with the plumb line dropped from C2 falling well anterior to the sacrum.

ographs of the entire spine. Lumbar radiographs alone are insufficient to evaluate for sagittal balance. A "reasonable" 35°- to 40°-lumbar lordosis may be totally adequate for a patient with a normal thoracic kyphosis but woefully inadequate for the patient with a 65°- to 70°-thoracic kyphosis. Full length radiographs permit calculation of the frontal and sagittal plane offset of the plumb line. Using the Cobb technique, thoracic kyphosis, lumbar lordosis, and thoracolumbar junctional measurements can be obtained. Most important is the overall sagittal balance. This is determined by dropping a plumb line from the center of the odontoid or seventh cervical vertebra and measuring the distance from the anterior aspect of the sacrum to this line. Normally, this plumb line should fall within 2 cm anterior or posterior to the anterior aspect of the sacrum (Fig. 68-4).

If other pathology, such as a nonunion, is suspected, additional radiographs may be needed, including dynamic studies, to assess junctional instability. Computed tomography, MRI, or myelograms may be needed if neurologic symptoms are present (5).

TREATMENT

Treatment options for flat back deformity evolve around obtaining global balance in the sagittal as well as the coronal plane. A complete physical and radiologic evaluation as well as the development of a preoperative plan is paramount to performing a successful correction for deformity. The goals of treatment are to: (a) enable the patient to resume a more erect posture that decreases the strain of adjacent cephalad and caudal muscle groups, (b) restore a horizontal visual field, (c) relieve compression of abdominal viscera, (d) improve diaphragmatic respiration, and (e) improve overall cosmesis (Fig. 68-5).

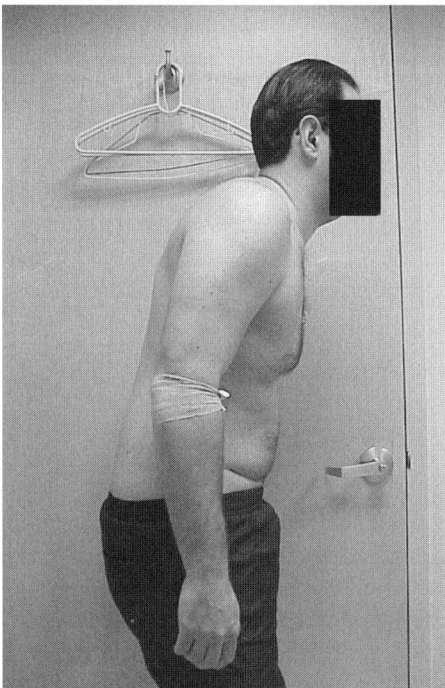

FIG. 68-5. A 42-year-old patient received posterior Harrington rods and fusion for an L1 burst fracture with significant neurologic deficit. The patient had near complete return of neurologic function but progressive incapacitating back pain. An extension of the fusion to the sacrum was attempted with posterior pedicle fixation supplemented by a single horizontal cage at L4-5 and L5-S1. The patient presented within 1 year of that procedure with worsening back pain and postural deformity. **A:** Lateral clinical view of the patient with classic flat back syndrome.

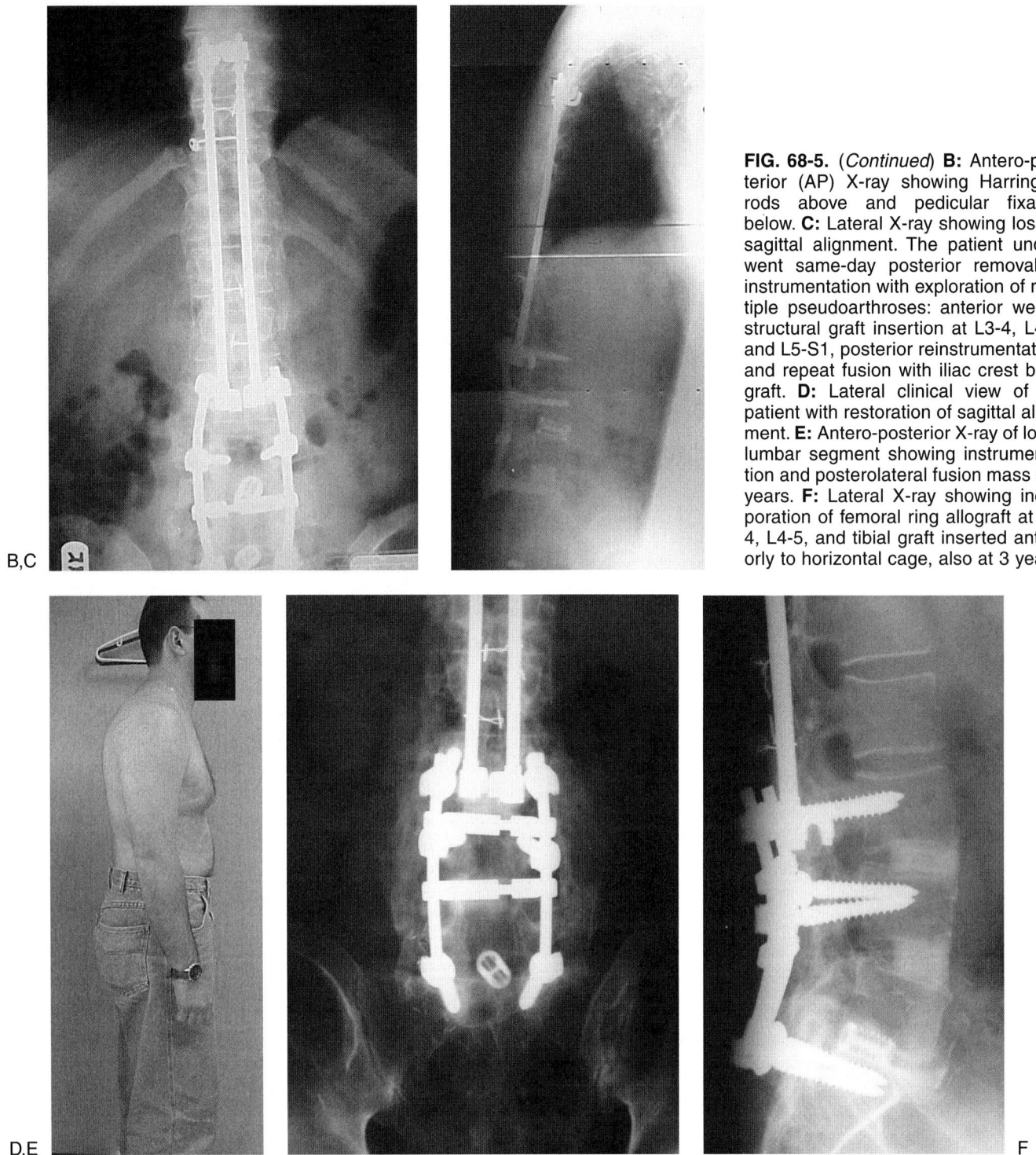

B,C

FIG. 68-5. (*Continued*) B: Antero-posterior (AP) X-ray showing Harrington rods above and pedicular fixation below. C: Lateral X-ray showing loss of sagittal alignment. The patient underwent same-day posterior removal of instrumentation with exploration of multiple pseudoarthroses: anterior wedge structural graft insertion at L3-4, L4-5, and L5-S1, posterior reinstrumentation, and repeat fusion with iliac crest bone graft. D: Lateral clinical view of the patient with restoration of sagittal alignment. E: Antero-posterior X-ray of lower lumbar segment showing instrumentation and posterolateral fusion mass at 3 years. F: Lateral X-ray showing incorporation of femoral ring allograft at L3-4, L4-5, and tibial graft inserted anteriorly to horizontal cage, also at 3 years.

D,E

F

NONOPERATIVE TREATMENT

Nonoperative treatment of flat back deformity is often first-line treatment for patients with minimal symptomatic complaints, nonprogressive deformity, or patients who are not operative candidates. There is no nonoperative treatment that corrects for lumbar lordosis abnormal-

ity, but treatment may provide some symptomatic relief of the symptoms. Patients with complicated medical problems may not be candidates for further surgery. A pharmacologic approach may include nonsteroidal antiinflammatory, non-narcotic pain medications, or even a long-term narcotic program, coordinated under the direct supervision of a pain management specialist. Rehabilitative measures, including abdominal strengthening, stretching, and range of motion exercises to the hips and trunk can often compensate for a decompensated trunk and improve paraspinal strength. It also optimizes the physical condition of preoperative patients. Farcy and Schwab documented a significant improvement in pain in 20 of 48 patients who underwent aggressive rehabilitation as an alternative to revision surgery (6). However, at 4-year follow-up, many of these patients' signs and symptoms had progressed, and surgical intervention was performed in seven out of the 20 patients who initially had been controlled with nonoperative care.

OPERATIVE TREATMENT

Surgical correction of flat back deformity involves general principles that are used in the correction of basic spinal deformities. The history of instrumentation for spinal deformity began with the correction of scoliotic curves. The original Harrington distraction rod was designed to lengthen the concavity of a scoliotic curve. Thus, the Harrington rod, which lengthened the "short side" (concavity) of a spinal curve with instrumentation was the first implant tool in the armamentarium of the modern spinal surgeon. Surgeons quickly grasped the concept that an additional tool to shorten the "long side" (convexity) of a spinal curve would be an additional benefit. The arrival of the Harrington compression rod system applied to the convexity of a scoliotic curve resulted in not only improved corrected force but also was historically closer to the more modern forms of segmental fixation. In scoliosis correction, because the "norm" is no curve, the surgeon aims for "lengthening" the short side and "shortening" the long side until ideally they are equivalent and the curve is eliminated.

Kyphotic deformities of the lumbar spine are similar but have an important difference. With a true kyphosis (not just loss of lordosis) of the lumbar spine, the surgeon aims to "lengthen" the short side (anterior column) and "shorten" the long side (posterior column) not just until they are equal but to push the correction further until the "long" side becomes the new "short" side and vice versa. In flat back syndrome this can be achieved in multiple ways. "Lengthening" of the anterior lumbar spine usually is achieved by discectomy, anterior wedging of the disc space, and maintaining correction with structural support (either structural allograft or vertical cages "shortening" of the posterior column (is achieved) through one (7) or multiple osteotomies (8). A combination procedure involving both anterior column lengthening and posterior column shortening allows for the greatest amount of overall correction of a kyphotic deformity. To maintain correction, all of these procedures must be performed with stabilizing instrumentation and fusion.

The surgical correction of the kyphotic deformity was first described, in 1945, by Smith-Peterson et al. with an osteotomy of the spine for ankylosing spondylitis (9). They described multiple wedge posterior osteotomies and posterior closure (shortening of the posterior column); resulting in rupture of the "brittle" anterior longitudinal ligament, thereby causing extension and opening through the disc spaces (elongation of the anterior column)—the final result producing lordosis in the lumbar spine. Significant complications have resulted from the relatively uncontrolled anterior column lengthening. These included paraplegia, catastrophic rupture of the anterior vascular structures, and gastrointestinal complications. Various surgeons have modified this technique (10,11).

La Chapelle, in 1946, described a two-stage osteotomy with combined anterior and posterior approaches (12). Briggs, in 1947, reported on a posterior wedge osteotomy with bilateral foraminotomies (13). Thomasen, in 1985, reported on a corrective osteotomy with removal of the neural arch of L2 and partial removal of the bone inside the vertebral body (14). This recreated lumbar lordosis by shortening the posterior column without excessive intra-abdominal distraction. This technique purportedly allowed for 30° to 50° of correction at a single level.

Heinig popularized the eggshell decancelation procedure (15). This procedure consists of removal of cancellous bone of the apical vertebral body through a bipedal approach in order to weaken the vertebral body and create a posterior column shortening with minimal force; an advantage is that it is performed under direct observation of the neural elements. The anterior part of the decancellized vertebra acts as a pivot point for closure of the gap, and because the pedicles have been removed, there is less of a chance of neurologic injury. As well, there is no stretching of the cauda equina and less stretching of the anterior vasculature. Bone grafting and rigid segmental instrumentation are applied in order to decrease the failure rate. Results published to date report a correction of 30° to 50° at a single level using this procedure, although most of these patients were among those with a diagnosis of ankylosing spondylitis. A key point to remember during the procedure is that segmental instrumentation, decompression, and bone graft harvesting should all be completed prior to the removal of cancellous bone because of the potential for rapid blood loss.

Pedicle subtraction osteotomy also has the goal of restoring sagittal balance and obtaining a fusion (16,17). This extension osteotomy shortens the posterior column without elongating the anterior column. The procedure is optimally performed at the L3-4 level because the L3-4 disc space is the physiologic apex of lumbar lordosis, and the osteotomy can be more safely performed at that level with retraction of the cauda equina rather than the conus medullaris. As well, the bifurcation of the vascular structures is below this level so there is a minimal risk of vascular injury. A single level osteotomy results in approximately 25° of sagittal plane correction and a high fusion rate, because it involves the vertebral body and adds bone grafting to the anterior column (18).

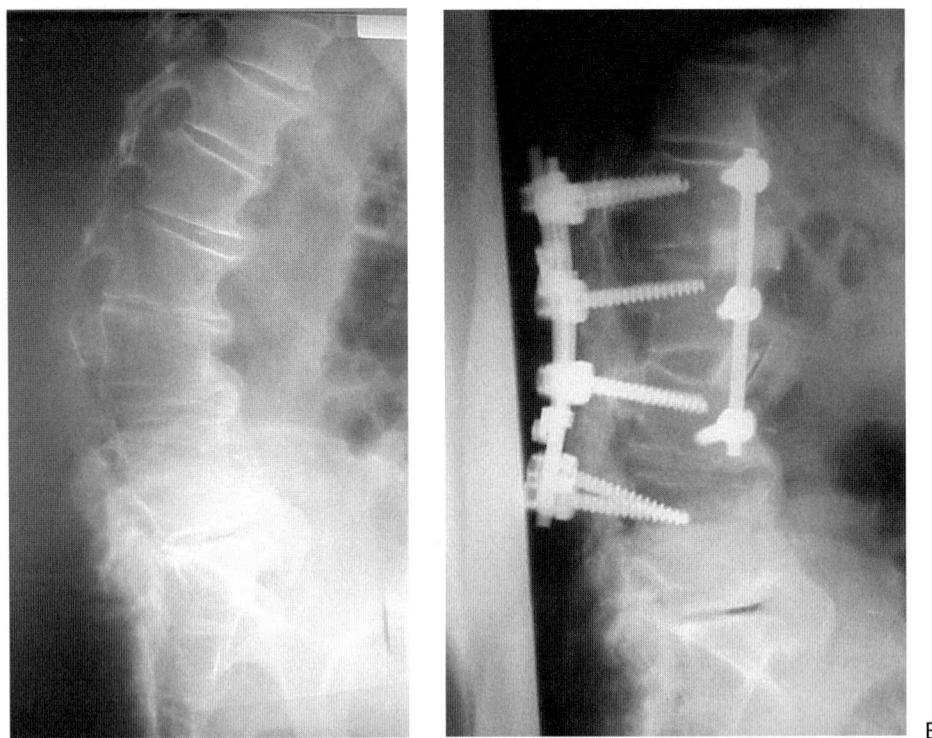

FIG. 68-6. A 75-year-old patient had a previous history of lumbar laminectomy and discectomy complicated by discitis or osteomyelitis, which resulted in a progressive kyphotic deformity. **A:** Lateral lumbar X-ray showing severe lumbar kyphosis. **B:** Postoperatively lateral lumbar film after multiple lumbar osteotomies, anterior structural wedge, grafts and instrumentation, and posterior compression pedicular fixation.

Combined anterior and posterior surgery in flat back treatment offers the advantage of a controlled lengthening of the anterior column in conjunction with posterior osteotomies and shortening of the posterior column (19). The anterior column can be lengthened and held either with wedge-shaped structural allograft such as femoral shafts or with wedge-shaped vertical cages. The posterior osteotomies can be closed down and thereby shortened with pedicular instrumentation. This technique usually demands a combined postero-anterior surgical procedure rather than a single posterior approach as with the pedicle subtraction osteotomy. In many cases, the anterior approach is necessary to provide anterior fusion and support to the areas adjacent to the posterior osteotomy. Furthermore, in cases of extreme kyphotic deformity, more correction is necessary than can predictably be obtained at one posteriorly based osteotomy (Fig. 68-6).

CONCLUSION

Flat back syndrome is an iatrogenic deformity in many cases that is usually easier to prevent than to correct. However, even in experienced hands, the deformity can develop because of loss of fixation, progressive degener-

ation, or compression fractures at the top or bottom of a surgical fusion. When surgical correction is warranted, the correction of the kyphotic deformity involves major spinal reconstructive surgery. There is no one procedure for all deformities. Certainly, vertebral wedge osteotomies are necessary either posteriorly based or in conjunction with anterior wedge strut grafting and instrumentation. The decisions are based on the surgeon's preference and experience, degree of correction needed, and location of the deformity. Single osteotomies may be used in relatively mild deformities when the principal deformity is in the mid to lower lumbar spine. Multiple osteotomies are preferred for more severe deformity to assure a better correction of the deformity, with less of a chance of neurologic injury. The decision for a combined anterior and posterior procedure often is necessitated in the patient with painful degenerated discs below long multisegment fusions with loss of lumbar lordosis, in order to not only restore sagittal balance but to relieve back pain and disability.

REFERENCES

1. Dewald RL. Revision surgery for spinal deformity. Adult spinal deformity. In: Eilert RE, ed. Instructional course lectures. San Francisco: American Academy of Orthopedic Surgeons, 1992:235–250.

2. LaGrone MO. Flat-back syndrome: avoidance and treatment. Semin Spine Surg 1998;10:328–338.
3. Kostuik JP. Adult scoliosis. In: Frymoyer JW, ed. The adult spine: principles and practice, 2nd ed. Philadelphia: Lippincott-Raven, 1997:1605–1613.
4. Denis F. The iatrogenic loss of lumbar lordosis. The flat back and the buttock syndromes. In: Farcy J-P, ed. Complex spinal deformities. Philadelphia: Hanley and Belfus, 1994:659–672.
5. Wu SS, Hwa SY, Lin LC, et al. Management of rigid post-traumatic kyphosis. Spine 1996;21:2260–2267.
6. Farcy JP, Schwab FJ. Management of flatback and related kyphotic decompensation syndromes. Spine 1997;22(20):2452–2457.
7. Noun Z, Lapresle L, Missenard G. Posterior lumbar osteotomy for flat back in adults. J Spinal Disord 2001;14:311–316.
8. Voos K, Boachie-Adjei OB, Rawling BA. Multiple vertebral osteotomies in the treatment of rigid adult spine deformities. Spine 2001;26:526–533.
9. Smith-Petersen MN, Larson CB, Aufranc OE. Osteotomy of the spine for correction of flexion deformity in rheumatoid arthritis. J Bone Joint Surg 1945;27:1–11.
10. Booth KC, Bridwell KH, Lenke LG, et al. Complications and predictive factors for the successful treatment of flatback deformity. Spine 1999;24:1712–1720.
11. Bradford DS, Tribus CB. Current concepts and management of patients with fixed decompensated spinal deformity. Clin Orthop Rel Res 1994;306:64–72.
12. LaChapelle EH. Osteotomy of the lumbar spine for correction of kyphosis in a case of ankylosing spondyloarthritis. J Bone Joint Surg 1946;28:851–858.
13. Briggs H, Keats S, Schlesinger PT. Wedge osteotomy of spine with bilateral intervertebral foraminotomy: correction of flexion deformity in five cases of ankylosing arthritis of the spine. J Bone Joint Surg (Br) 1947;29:1075–1082.
14. Thomasen E. Vertebral osteotomy for correction of kyphosis in ankylosing spondylitis. Clin Orthop 1985;194:142–152.
15. Heinig CA. Eggshell procedure. In: Luque ER, ed. Segmental spinal instrumentation. Thorofare, NJ: Slack, 1984:221–230.
16. Lowery GL, Bhat AL, Pennisi AE. Pedicle subtraction osteotomy and lumbar extension osteotomy for iatrogenic flat back. In: Margulies JY, Aebi M, Farcy J-PC, eds. Revision spine surgery. St. Louis: CV Mosby, 1999:576–588.
17. Boachie-Adjei OB, Girardi FP, Hall J. Posterior lumbar decancellation osteotomy. In: Margulies JY, Aebi M, Farcy J-PC, eds. Revision spine surgery. St. Louis: Mosby, 1999:568–588.
18. Murrey DB, Brigham CD, Kiebzak GM, et al. Transpedicular decompression and pedicle subtraction osteotomy (eggshell procedure): a retrospective review of 59 patients. Spine 2002;27(21):2338—2345.
19. Kostuik JP, Maurais GR, Richardson WJ, et al. Combined single stage anterior and posterior osteotomy for correction of iatrogenic lumbar kyphosis. Spine 1988;13(3):237–266.

CHAPTER 69

Spinopelvic Fixation

Joseph Y. Margulies and William O. Shaffer

Fixation to the pelvis has had limited usage, primarily in the treatment of spine deformity. Anchoring a rod to the pelvis has been very helpful in resisting coronal and sagittal plane imbalance. This has been especially helpful in neurologic-based spinal deformities such as cerebral palsy, myelomeningocele, and the muscular dystrophies. In these entities, the Galveston rod has become the standard and most useful technique to stabilize a neurogenic scoliosis to the pelvis.

Degenerative scoliosis is yet another difficult problem where an increasing use of fixation to the sacrum and the ilium has been realized. Here the Jackson intrasacral rod has proven useful in reinforcing the lower end of a long degenerative construct. The use of the sacral alar screw or the Chopin block have been attempts to further the anchorage to the sacrum to protect the lower S2 pedicle screw in such long constructs.

Trauma constructs have lagged behind the neuromuscular and degenerative constructs. Much of this has been because the trauma to the sacrum has come under orthopedic trauma surgeon purview for some fracture patterns and that of the orthopedic spine surgeon for other fracture patterns. Complicating this has been the lack of a comprehensive approach to these difficult fractures. Orthopedic trauma surgeons have approached sacral fractures and sacroiliac joint dislocations as a posterior pelvic ring disruption. In many cases, percutaneous iliosacral screws have been a good solution to this problem. Zone 1 and nondisplaced zone 2 sacral injuries (those lateral to the sacral foramina) are simply handled by this technique. However, when serious root and cauda equina injury occur there have been few durable solutions posed in the literature. Zone 2 fractures with radicular involvement and zone 3 fractures with either radicular or cauda equina injury demand a more comprehensive approach to neural decompression and skeletal stabilization.

In tumors of the sacrum and ilium, posterior pelvic ring instability is created by the necessary resection of the tumor and a margin of normal bone. Traditionally, allographic bone has been used to reconstruct these massive defects. Various anchors into the pelvis or remaining sacrum have been attempted and to a greater or lesser extent have been successful. However, in our experience pullout and hardware failure were all too often the result of the historical fixation such as iliac posts (rod or screw), iliac bars, iliac plates, or iliac threaded bars.

Dr. Marc Asher advanced the concept of spinal foundation for scoliosis and deformity correction in which two interconnected spinal anchors allow the forceful manipulation of the spine (1,2). The objective of this study was to develop a foundation to correct pelvic disassociation and rotation.

In 1996, we focused on the challenges of sacral tumor resections and complex sacral fractures resulting in pelvic dissociation, neurologic injuries, and severe lumbosacropelvic rotation. Reconstructive options were limited conceptually. A series of anchors were available to manipulate the pelvis or ilium but they did not allow the forceful manipulation of the pelvis in relation to the sacrum and the rest of the spine. Two possible exceptions are the Galveston rod technique (3) and the Jackson intrasacral rod (4,5). The Galveston technique, when placed in both ilia and interconnected, allows the coronal and sagittal planes in pelvic deformities to be manipulated. However, this technique suffers from a "windshield-wiper" effect because of cranial caudal pistoning of the anchor in the pelvis and the third plane was not controlled. Further, it meets the criteria for a foundation in scoliosis correction only. The Galveston rod technique cannot be applied in fracture or tumor work. The limits of all of the early pelvic anchors were related to the application of forces to the pelvis that overcame the bone implant interface in the ilium. The Jackson intrasacral rod technique places the anchors in the sacrum. The Jackson construct establishes a foundation only if the pelvis is intact, it is not an option for a disrupted pelvic ring.

636

This current system introduces a pelvic foundation that is applied to three distinct clinical situations. Two of these deal with pelvic dissociation. Tumor resections that sacrifice the sacrum and sacroiliac joint leave the ilium disconnected from the sacrum and the opposite ilium (6). Sacral fractures through or medial to the sacral foramina frequently result in devastating neurologic injury. The decompression of damaged neurologic structures requires reduction of these complex fractures and maintenance of the reduction requires a pelvic foundation. The third clinical situation deals with degenerative and neuromuscular scoliosis where pelvic rotations of obliquity and lumbosacropelvic kyphosis are difficult to control.

Technical guidelines have been established for constructing a foundation in the pelvis for spinopelvic fixation or for stabilizing the pelvis when loss due to tumors or fractures compromises pelvic stability.

Three distinct constructs are discussed:

1. The tumor construct consists of a two-screw iliac foundation connected either to a contralateral two-screw iliac foundation or to a spine foundation of pedicle screws.
2. The sacral fracture construct consists of a two-screw iliac foundation connected to a sacral, iliac, or lumbar anchor depending on the fracture pattern.
3. The scoliosis construct consists of a screw anchoring each ilium interconnected to form a pelvic foundation that is connected to a proximal lumbar foundation of pedicle screws.

Anatomy is the basis for modifications that have become the sacropelvic module of the spinal instrumentation system that allows the construction of the pelvic foundation (7).

VARIOUS OPTIONS

The preliminary study focused on the anatomic characteristics of the various sacropelvic anchors generally available at the time (8). They were examined to see if a pelvic foundation could be constructed. "Foundation" is defined as a solid combination with two interconnected construct elements (anchors) on each side that create a strong purchase in the bone to allow forceful manipulation of the anatomic structure. An "anchor" is a single implant element anchored in the bone. Possible anchors for constructing foundations in the spine are:

• Pedicle screws
• Hooks and claws
• Wires and cables.

Longitudinal members connect the installed anchors into the actual foundation. Usually they are rods but they can be plates as well. In the foundation scheme all the elements are interlocked to create a closed stable quadrilateral frame (Fig. 69-1). The interlocking mechanism consists of transverse connectors or any type of solid connection between the longitudinal elements on the right side and the left side. Any combination of connections spanned over one vertebra or more can be used to manipulate the spine.

Applying this approach to the pelvis poses the need for some adjustments. Anchors in the pelvis can be:

• S1 and S2 pedicle screws in all the possible angles suggested
• Jackson-type intrasacral rods
• Iliosacral transarticular screws
• Iliac screws
• Galveston posts
• S1-L5 transdiscal screws or dowels
• Sacral bars
• Hook claws
• Wires or cables
• Blocks (these are considered anchors because they enter the bone so close to each other that it can be considered one point).

In spite of the relatively large variety of anchors in the pelvis, application of any one of them is not always possible due to either poor bone condition or loss. Conceptually, the ideal technical solution is to create a device that uses all the available anchors to create a stable quadrilateral foundation. Integral to this concept is that the dissociated ilium in fractures and tumors can be manipulated independently of the proximal foundation. The technical solution is to design a family of rods with a variety of locking mechanisms at one of their ends. Custom rod connectors allow fixation of rod to rod. A new type of anchor with adequately sized iliac screws allows better purchase of the iliac wings. This system solidly connects all the available anchors into one true pelvic foundation (Fig. 69-2).

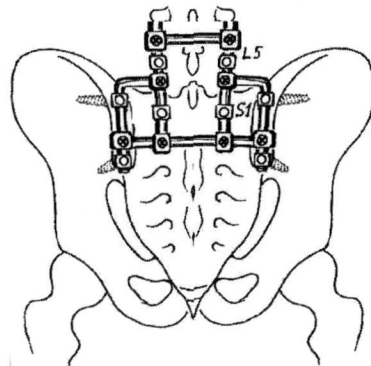

FIG. 69-1. The concept of the bilateral iliac foundation.

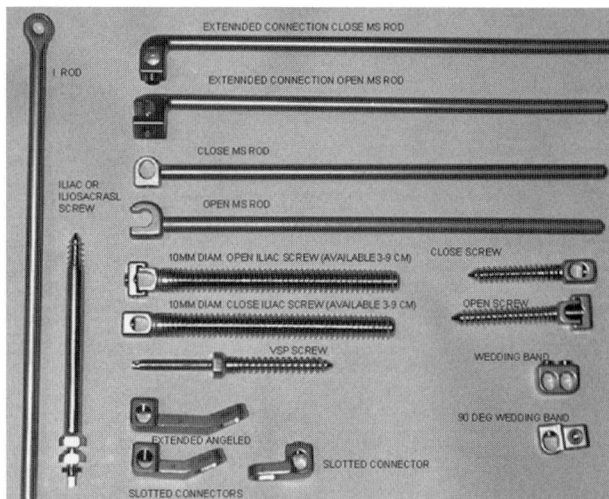

FIG. 69-2. Family of rods, anchors, and connectors.

CLINICAL INDICATION

The pelvis is instrumented in relatively rare clinical circumstances and this is as it should be. The major indications for instrumentation to the pelvis are:

- neuromuscular scoliosis
- degenerative scoliosis with deficient sacral bone stock
- sacral fracture with neurologic deficit
- sacral fracture where indirect reduction could lead to neurologic injury
- sacral tumors where posterior pelvic instability will result or pelvic dissociation is a risk.

MATERIALS AND METHODS

The basis of the module is a uniform locking mechanism of rods to anchors in open and closed versions. A sacropelvic module can be added to any existing spine/scoliosis system. Adapters can be introduced to combine elements from different systems. The newly developed kit contains a set of four rods with locking mechanisms on one end and a set of open and closed iliac screws 10 mm in

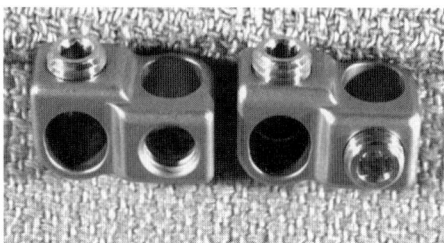

FIG. 69-3. 90°–90° wedding bands.

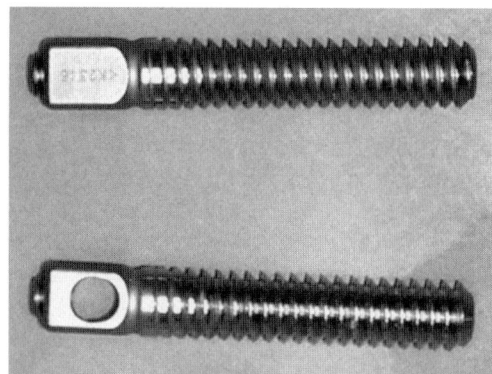

FIG. 69-4. Bolt (10 mm).

diameter. A large selection of adapters and 90°–90° wedding bands are included so that connectors can be rotated 90° to each other (Fig. 69-3). Specialized instruments to handle these specific implants are included.

Iliac Screws

Screws that are 10 mm in diameter (Fig. 69-4) were indicated after the preliminary anatomic study and later confirmed by the formal anatomic/computed tomography (CT) studies. The diameter size of the screw is intended to purchase the two iliac cortices. The screws are available in lengths ranging from 30 mm to 110 mm in 10 mm increments with closed and open locking mechanisms.

Rods

The rods are ¼-inch in diameter. The integral rod connectors are milled from ¾-inch bar stock (Fig. 69-5). This assures a strong transition from the rod to the connector. Rods with three types of locking mechanisms are available:

- Closed Isola-Groove Hollow Ground (VHG)
- Open Isola VHG type
- Side opening locking mechanism.

Each locking mechanism is attached to the rod in two ways:

- Directly at the axis of the rod
- Offset by about ½-inch to save the bending maneuver passing from the ilium medially to the sacrum

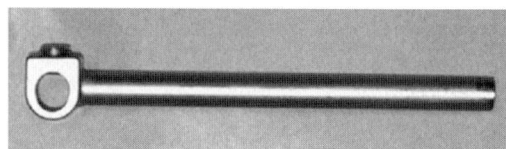

FIG. 69-5. Rod connector.

Instruments

Standard instruments are used with the addition of a tap for the 10 mm diameter screws.

Experimental Anatomic Study

Earlier spinopelvic instrumentation was a patchwork of anchors that attempted to fix the spine to the pelvis. Lebwohl et al. showed that iliac screws are the only ancillary fixation shown to protect S1 pedicle screws from cantilever stresses and pullout (9). To allow a better foundation and establish anchorage in the iliac bone, this study investigated alternative anchorage points and defined the dimensions of the upper and lower iliac columns (7) (Fig. 69-6). Seventeen iliac bones were sectioned in 10 mm increments to assess the cross-sectional dimensions (Fig. 69-7). The upper and lower iliac columns were measured directly on a General Electric CT workstation (Fig. 69-8).

The lower iliac column accommodates screws 10 mm in diameter to a depth of 100 mm in 100% of iliac bones. This includes even the smallest female pelvis of the series. The upper iliac column accommodates 10 mm screws up to 50 mm in length in 75% of the iliac bones. It accommodates 7.5 mm screws up to 50 mm in length in 95% of iliac bones. Preoperative CT can be used to determine the necessary screw sizes. Berry et al. have confirmed these dimensions in their study of the lower iliac column in the Hamann-Todd Osteological Collection at the Cleveland Museum of Natural History (10). Schwend et al. have recently published a confirmation of the use of the lower iliac column in neuromuscular scoliosis (11).

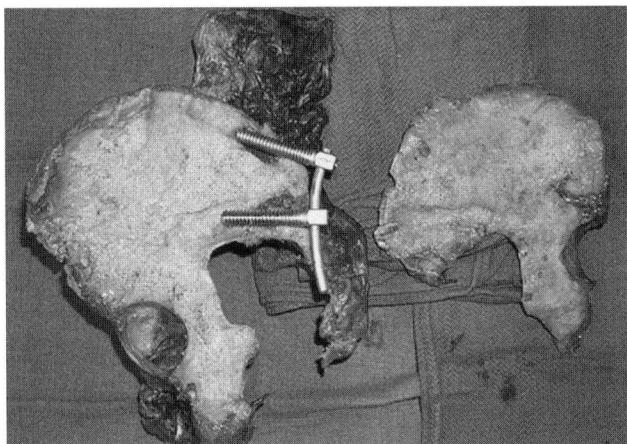

FIG. 69-7. Each hemipelvis was sectioned in 10 mm increments and the dimensions of the upper and lower iliac columns were directly measured.

The upper iliac column is as strong a structure for an anchor in the iliac crest as the lower column.

This module for reconstruction of the pelvic ring assures control over the iliac bone and builds a pelvic foundation that allows fusion of the spine to the pelvis.

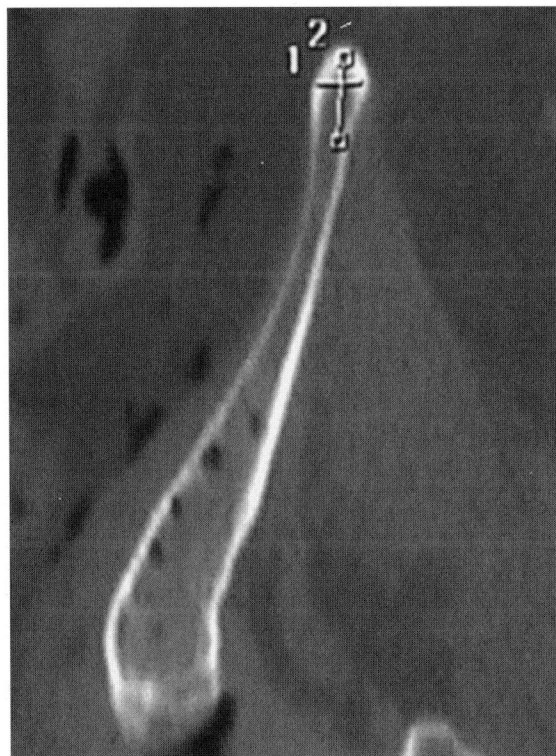

FIG. 69-6. The upper and lower iliac columns with an assembled two-bolt iliac foundation.

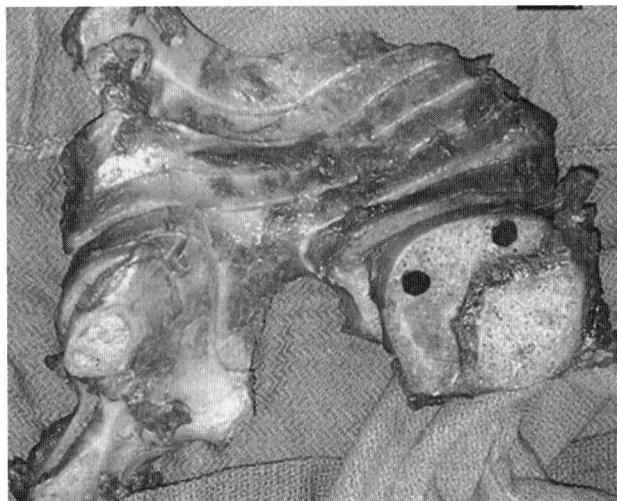

FIG. 69-8. The reconstructed ilium could be "electronically sliced" and the dimensions of the upper and lower iliac column were then measured on the workstation monitor.

Method of Application

Application is based on the available anchors and hence is subject to improvisation and creativity; however, the sequence is always to insert the anchors first and then to interconnect the anchors to construct a foundation.

Insertion of Anchors

Anchors are inserted according to the availability of insertion sites.

Iliac Approach

This is the fundamental technique for sacral fractures and tumor resections that leave the ilium dissociated from the sacrum on one or both sides. Insertion of superior and inferior iliac screws is possible (Fig. 69-1). The first screw placed is in the lower iliac column. The column will accept a 10 mm screw in almost all instances. Preparation of the starting point is important. The posterior superior iliac spine (PSIS) is essentially excised flush to the sacrum. This prepares the oval-shaped starting point for both the upper and lower iliac column approaches. This also provides an adequate graft for the fusion. The lower screw is placed in the traditional Galveston position, which is outward and slightly downward above the sciatic notch. The fingertip of the opposite hand is placed in the sciatic notch and an iliac probe is worked between the two cortical plates of the ilium just above the sciatic notch. The feel for this is akin to probing a pedicle in preparing for a pedicle screw. The average

distance accommodated is 70 mm, though the preliminary anatomic study suggested a 100 mm screw could be accommodated in most cases. The prepared channel is palpated with the ball feeler just as in the pedicle. The depth of the hole and any cortical broaches can thus be appreciated. The prepared channel is then tapped with a 10 mm tap.

The upper iliac column is approached at the superior end of the oval cancellous window created when the PSIS was excised. The iliac probe is directed outward between the iliac cortices at a slight inclination. The prepared channel is checked for depth and cortical break. The average depth is between 45 and 50 mm. The diameter of channel is assessed by direct comparison of a 7.5 versus 10 mm tap. The appropriate diameter tap is used to prepare the upper channel and a 7.5 or 10 mm screw is placed. The openings of the screws are rotated to face each other. An appropriate length of ¼-inch rod is cut and the rod is slightly contoured in order to place it through the connectors of each screw. Once unobstructed passage of the rod is confirmed the rod is withdrawn from one screw so the connector of the rod connector can be passed over the rod (Figs. 69-9A, B). Contouring of the rod connector will depend on the proposed construct. If it is to be connected across to the opposite ilium or sacrum slight bends will be needed. If the rod connector is to connect to the lumbar spine, an exaggerated lumbar lordotic curve will need to be placed in the rod. The geometry of the iliac fixation combined with the sacral pedicle screws shifts the fixation anterior, caudal, and cranial to the center of gravity of the spine, just in front of the sacrum. This placement of the instruments creates a powerful device

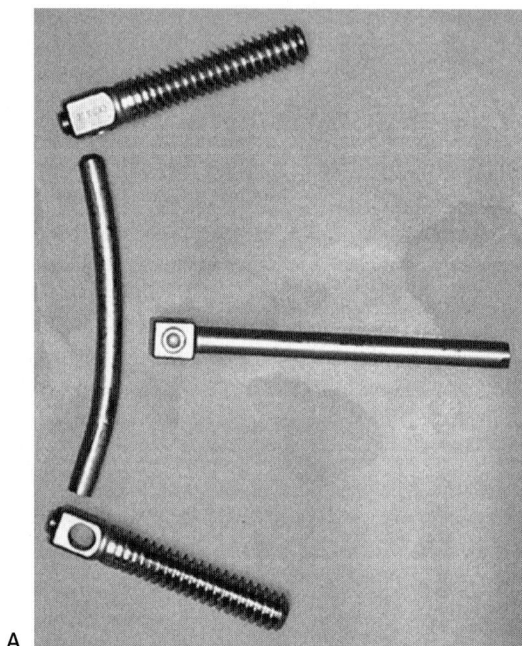

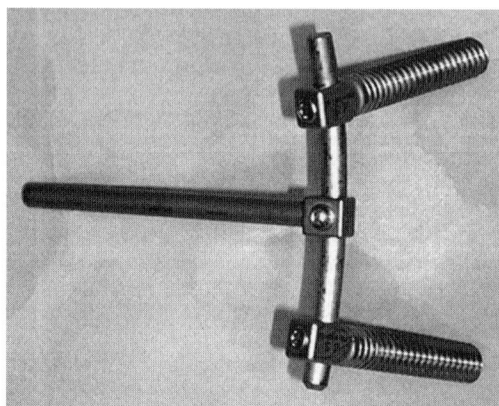

FIG. 69-9. **A:** Disassembled components of the two-bolt iliac foundation. **B:** The foundation assembled.

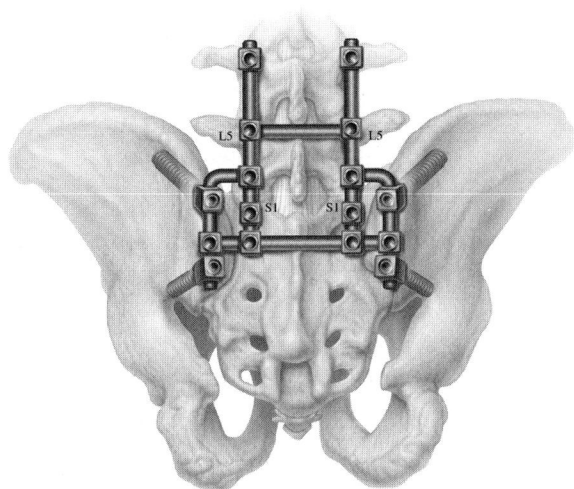

FIG. 69-10. Bilateral iliac foundation as may be used in a tumor or fracture construct.

controlling the pelvic rotations in all three planes of motion and all degrees of freedom of the pelvis in relationship to the spine.

Scoliosis Approach

The scoliosis approach is similar to the Galveston technique in that the anchors are placed into the iliac crests in the lower iliac column and S1 pedicles bilaterally. This distal placement allows the entire sacropelvis to be manipulated, rotated, and fixed to a lumbar foundation proximally.

Variable Approaches

Depending on the deformity and pathology with which one is dealing, two iliac screws may be fixed to both S1 or a contralateral S1 and S2 pedicle screw to complete a proximal anchorage. Once these two sites are connected, a transforaminal fracture is fixed. Effective fixation is accomplished by marrying the anchors with various connectors (Fig. 69-10).

Construction of Foundation

Rods, rod connectors, plates, or transverse connectors connect anchors. The desired assembly should use, as often as possible, straight segments of longitudinal members with the least possible bending maneuvers. Of the available sites to insert an anchor at least four are chosen. After all relevant considerations, the distance between the four should preferably be as long as possible for better stability. The anchors are interconnected in an attempt to close a quadrilateral shape. A spine construct may be fur-

ther connected to the pelvic "frame" by two rods at each side. Though the ideal construct consists of one or two pelvic quadrilateral frames and four rods to connect to the spinal construct, a less extensive one may suffice.

The constructs based on these foundations are characterized by three patterns discussed in the following sections.

Tumor Construct

In the treatment of sacroiliac tumor, tumor biology and specific tumor behavior must be clearly understood. Imaging studies reveal the anatomy of tumor involvement. Resection must be carefully planned with uninvolved normal spinal structures serving as resection margins. Nerve roots and stable joints often must be resected in order to achieve a curative margin.

The tumor construct consists of a two-screw iliac foundation connected either to the contralateral two-screw iliac foundation or to the spine by pedicle screw foundations (Fig. 69-10). This allows the dissociated ilium to be reduced against the remaining sacrum, or in the situation of a complete sacrectomy, the opposite ilium. The lumbar spine is connected to this substantial pelvic foundation.

Figure 69-11A shows a recurrent hemangiopericytoma of the sacrum. It was previously excised through a microscopic intralesional approach. Adequate revision required a hemisacrectomy and excision of the ilium resulting in a dissociation of the right hemipelvis from the sacrum. The S1-S5 roots on that side were excised as part of the resection. After dural repair, the pelvis was reconstructed. The distal foundation consisted of the iliac foundation described previously. The ilium was reduced to the remaining sacrum by a contralateral iliac foundation and rod connectors were attached through two wedding bands allowing the right ilium to be compressed against the remaining sacrum. This pelvic foundation was connected to a lumbar foundation consisting of the two L3 and L4 pedicle screws. Note the bend in the rod connector to connect the iliac foundation to the lumbar foundations (Figs. 69-11B, C).

Sacral Fracture Construct

Complex sacral fractures are approached surgically when neurologic deficit is present. Crushed roots require decompression of neural tissue. Stretch injuries to the neural structures require reduction of the fracture deformity.

The sacral fracture construct consists of a two-screw iliac anchor connected to a sacral, iliac, or lumbar anchor depending on the fracture pattern and whether the L5-S1 articulation is involved as often occurs with these shear fractures of the sacrum (Figs. 69-10, 69-12). The result is decompression of the damaged nerve roots and control of the fracture in all three planes of rotation. Anatomic

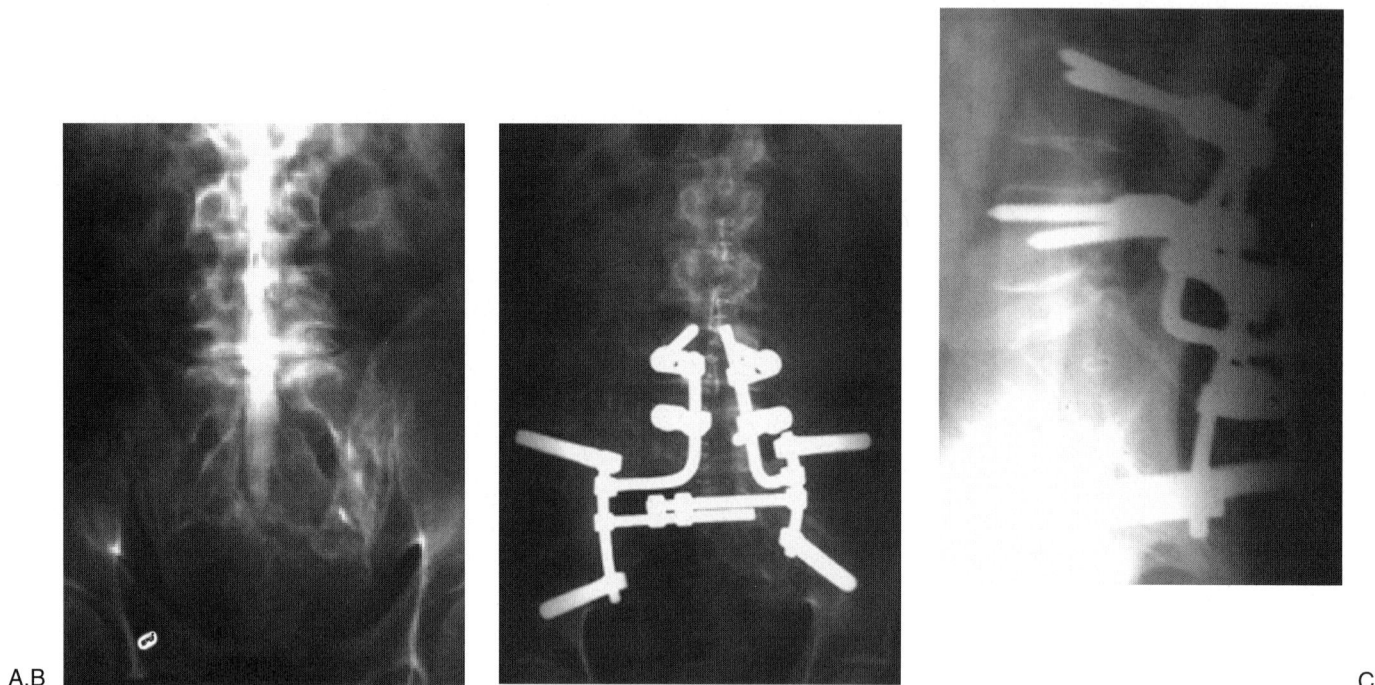

A,B

C

FIG. 69-11. A: Preoperative myelogram with involvement of the left sacral roots by the tumor. **B:** The antero-posterior radiograph of the reconstructed pelvis using the iliac foundation bilaterally. (WOS.) **C:** The lateral view of the construct. (WOS.)

reduction is achieved under direct vision while protecting the L5 nerve root anteriorly and the S1 root within the foramina.

Figures 69-13A–E demonstrate reduction of S1-S2 spondyloptosis. These constructs are based on four iliac

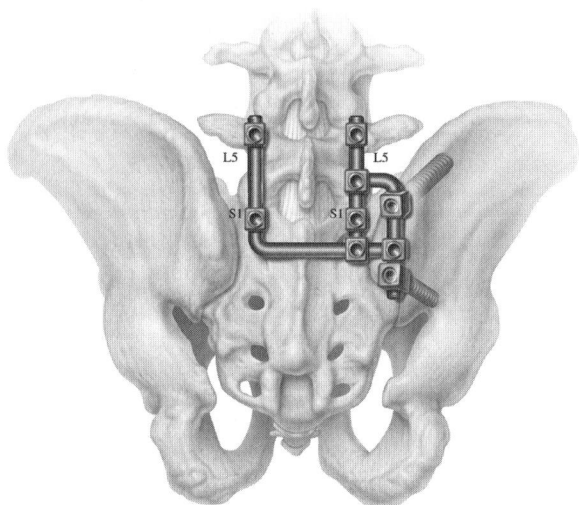

FIG. 69-12. Unilateral iliac foundation as may be used in a tumor or fracture construct.

screws as the distal foundations and L4-S1 screws as the proximal foundations in order to accomplish reduction. Reduction of S1 onto S2 can be predictably accomplished with a two-screw iliac post distal foundation. S1 and lumbar pedicle screws form the proximal foundation. A rod connector bridging these two foundations achieves reduction and controls the yaw, pitch, and vertical shear of these complex fractures (Figs. 69-14A–D).

The clinical example in Figures 69-15A and B show the difficulty with using standard components to treat transforaminal fractures with a severe S1 neurologic deficit and radicular pain. The S1 root was decompressed and a displaced butterfly fragment was retrieved from the S1 foramen. A modified Galveston rod and iliac screw foundation attached to proximal S1 screws stabilized the vertical shear component of the fracture. The rod required no fewer than three 90° bends to convert the distal Galveston post to engage both S1 pedicle screws and the upper iliac screw.

Figures 69-16A–D show the simplified approach to a similar transforaminal fracture with neurologic deficit using bilateral two-screw iliac anchors connected by a rod and wedding bands. This construct allows the rotation of the pelvis during reduction while controlling the neural structures within the foramen. Once the reduction is obtained the wedding band set screws are tightened and the rod connector is set to the two-bolt iliac post.

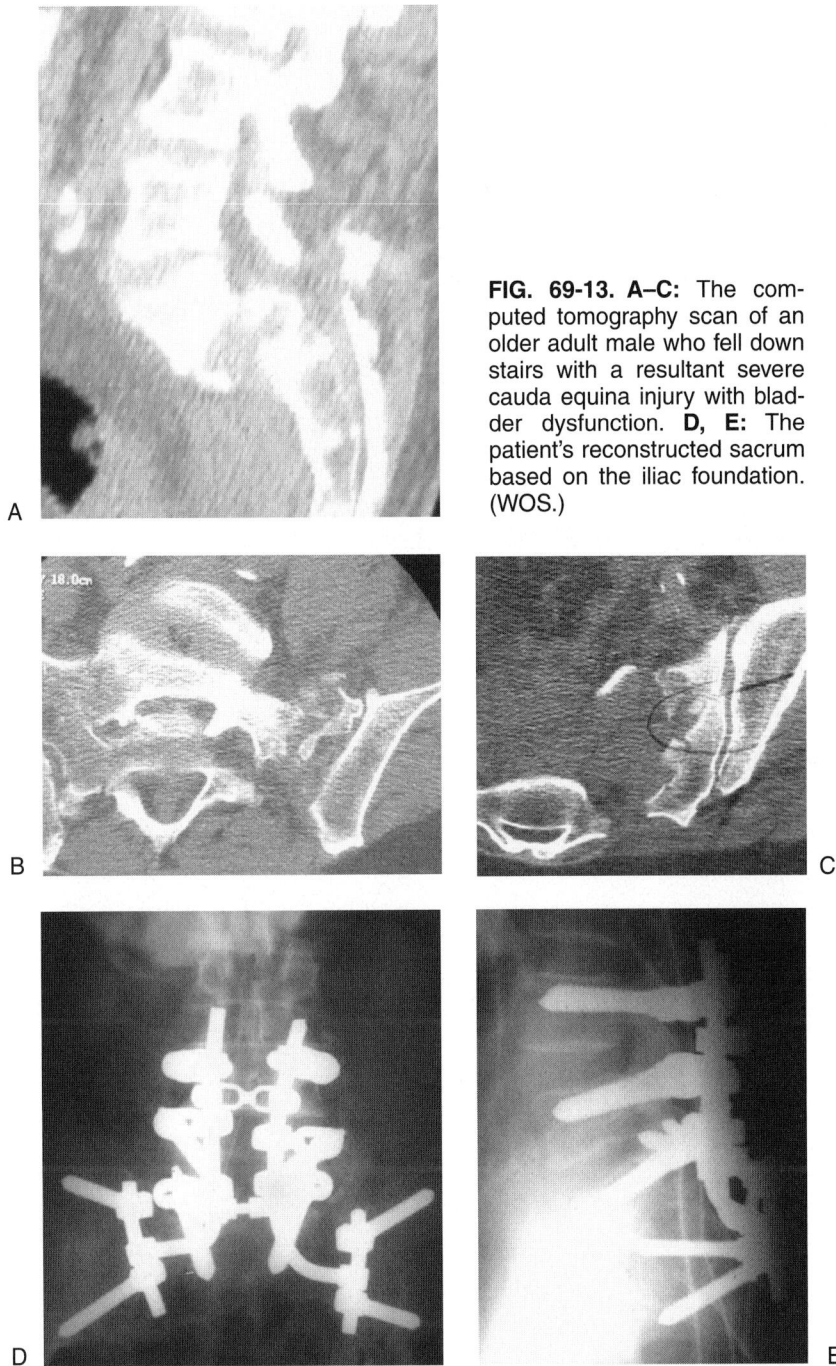

FIG. 69-13. A–C: The computed tomography scan of an older adult male who fell down stairs with a resultant severe cauda equina injury with bladder dysfunction. D, E: The patient's reconstructed sacrum based on the iliac foundation. (WOS.)

Scoliosis Construct

Reconstructive options have improved with modern spinal fixation. Lumbopelvic fixation must control the three planes of pelvic rotation: yaw, pitch, and vertical shear. The two-screw rod-connector foundation meets these goals.

The scoliosis construct consists of an iliac screw in each ilium interconnected with the S1 pedicle screw to form a pelvic foundation that is connected to a proximal lumbar pedicle screw–based foundation (Fig. 69-17A–C). This foundation allows coronal and sagittal plane sacropelvic rotations to be manipulated in relation to the proximal lumbar foundation. It is particularly helpful in controlling pelvic obliquities and lumbosacropelvic kyphosis and flat back.

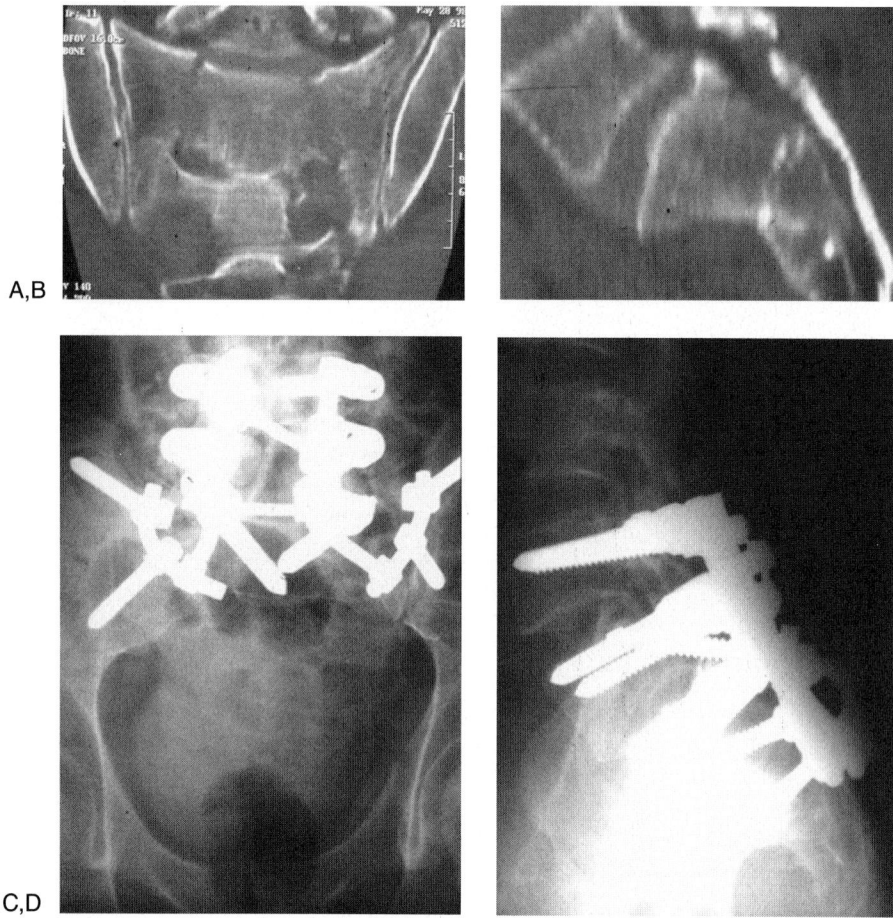

FIG. 69-14. **A, B:** The computed tomography scan views of a young man who fell from a silo while sitting in a boson's chair. Note the spondyloptosis of S1 on S2 and H fracture pattern. **C, D:** The reduced fracture using the iliac foundation distally and pedicle screws proximally. (WOS.)

RESULTS

Results of these techniques are preliminary. Kukio et al. (12) showed that "bilateral iliac screws coupled with bilateral S1 screws provide excellent distal fixation for lumbosacral fusions with a high fusion rate (95.1%) in high-grade spondylolisthesis and long fusions to the sacrum." Emami et al. have shown that there is an "unac-ceptable high rate of pseudarthrosis and this method [Galveston rod] is not recommended for adult deformities.... Emami recommend using iliac fixation, although there is a higher rate of painful hardware requiring removal" (13).

In our 24 patients with spinopelvic fixation most presented with neurologic deficits that were either radicular or cauda equina. There was a small group of injuries

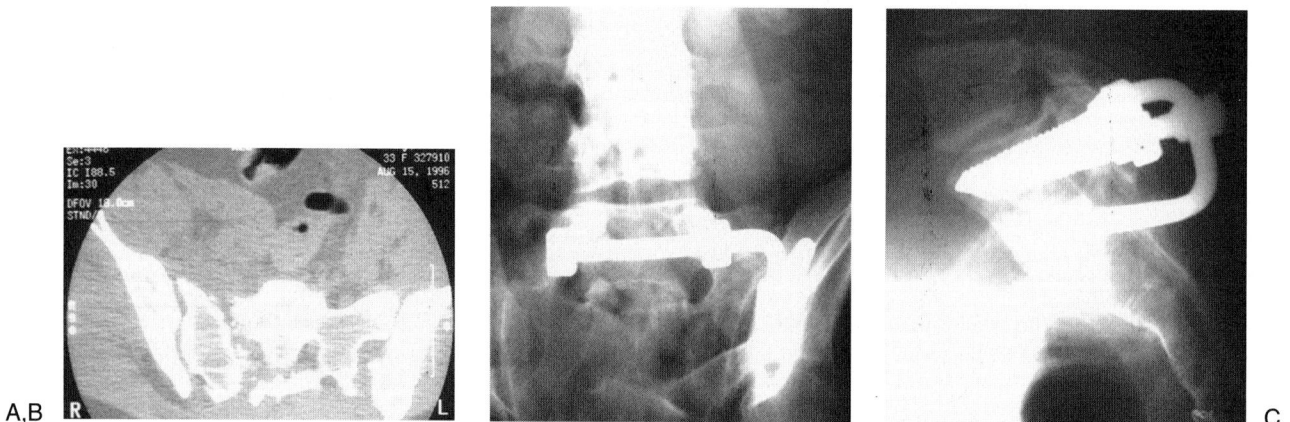

FIG. 69-15. **A:** The transforaminal fracture with the incarcerated fragment of bone in the neural foramen. **B, C:** The full decompression of the S1 foramen and the two S1 pedicle screws as the proximal foundation and the Galveston post and iliac bolt in the upper iliac column as the distal foundation. (WOS.)

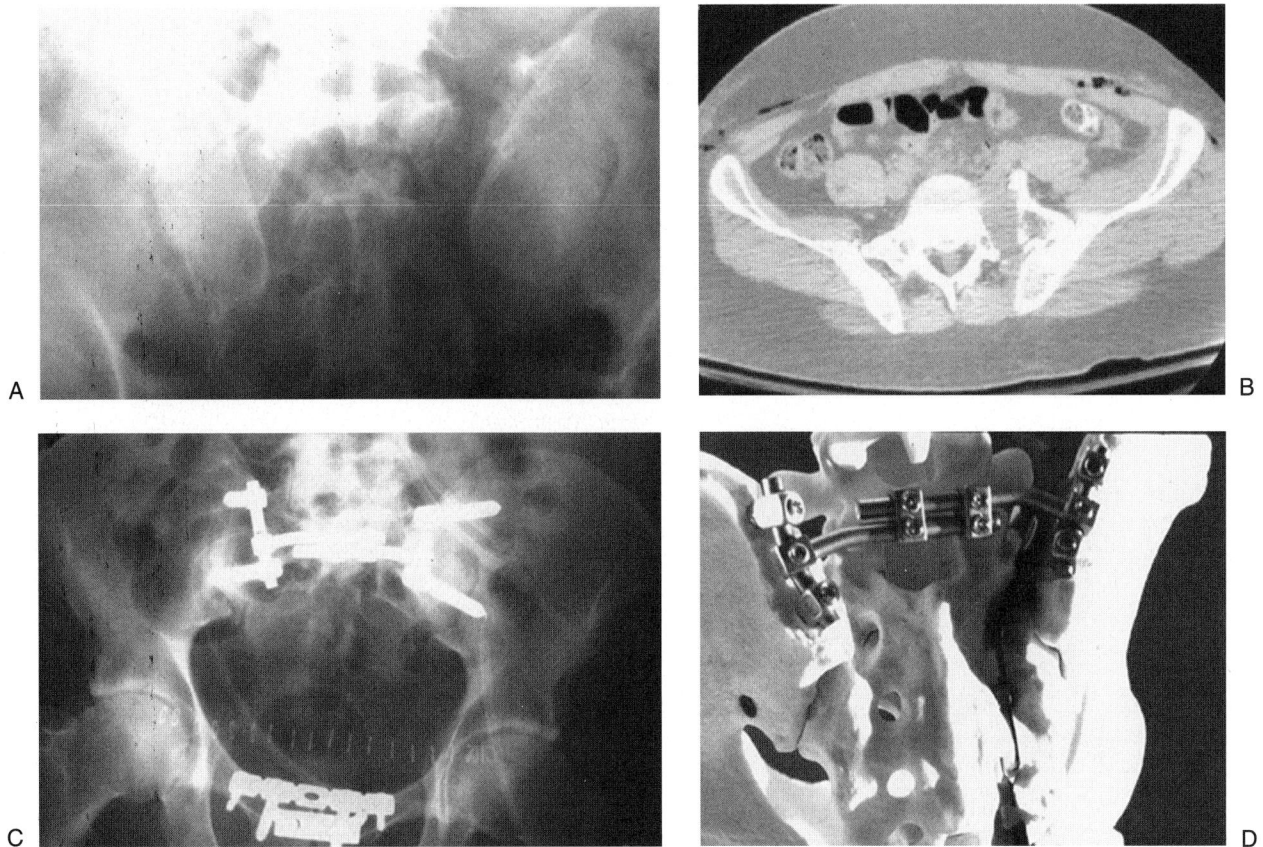

FIG. 69-16. A: The antero-posterior view of the sacrum showing the displaced transforaminal fracture with severe radiculopathy due to traction injury to the lumbar plexus. **B:** The computed tomography axial view of the injury. **C:** The reduction using the ipsilateral ilium for the distal foundation and the contralateral ilium for the proximal foundation. (WOS.) **D:** A model of this completed construct.

where zone 2 fractures presented with comminution at the S1 sacral foramina that increased the risk of neurologic injury with indirect and percutaneous techniques. A stable pelvis was achieved in all. This allowed the patient to be cared for without traction and mobilized 2 to 3 weeks after injury. If the injury was unilateral, the patient was allowed to weight bear on the uninjured hemipelvis immediately. If bilateral injury was fixed, the patient would be in bed then chair for 2 to 3 weeks prior to mobilization. Five patients suffered postoperative infections that were treatable with débridements, suction irrigation, and intravenous antibiotics. Six patients required explantation on an average of 2 years postoperatively. Neurologic improvement was seen in all patients except the two patients with cauda equina amputation. Bowel and bladder dysfunction improved or normalized in those patients without cauda equina amputation. Sexual function normalized in 70% of all patients, with better outcomes in women.

In the tumor cases we experienced one hardware failure in a patient in whom we used historical fixation anchors and two patients required explantation for infection.

COMPLICATIONS

Infection was high in our early experience. Our original incision was a midline incision where we detached the erector spinae from the sacral and iliac insertions. We now use a lambda incision where the major limb is formed on a midline incision over the back, which is gently curved to the PSIS of the most involved side of the pelvis. We then form a 90° arm to the other PSIS. The erector spinae is left attached distally and the hardware is tunneled underneath the erector spinae. This paralleled the experience of our pediatric orthopedist who found that tunneling the Galveston rod under the erector spinae resulted in less wound problems and infection.

Blood loss is expected. It is significant for fracture cases and can be catastrophic with tumor cases. In the tumor population we have experienced two deaths among nine patients. We have had one death from uncontrollable blood loss in a complete sacrectomy for a malignant tumor. Since that case we ligate the internal iliac during the anterior release and colostomy approach in all sacrectomies. This anterior procedure is staged 3 to 5 days before the posterior resection.

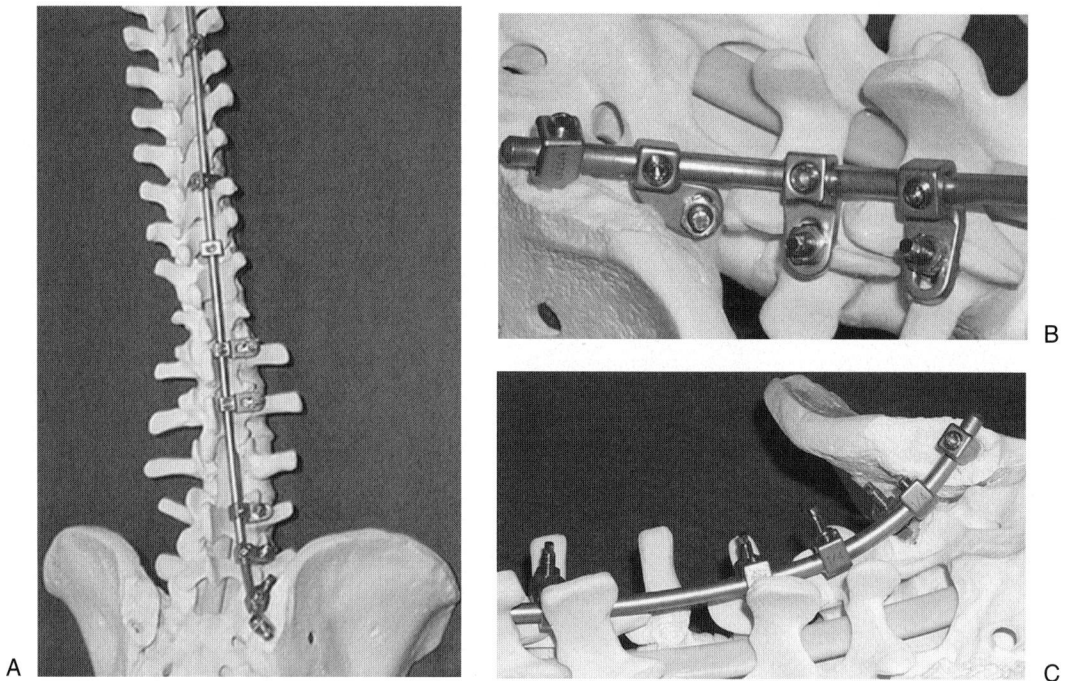

FIG. 69-17. A: The 10 mm bolt and S1 pedicle screw as the distal foundation connected to proximal claws and pedicle screws in this degenerative scoliosis model. **B:** Note the use of a thoracic slotted connector to allow the passage of the rod from the 10 mm bolt closely by the S1 pedicle screw. **C:** The rod bend is simply an exaggerated lordotic bend rolled out laterally.

Explantation is frequent as the hardware is prominent at the PSIS. Explantation was more frequent in our early experience because we were not removing the PSIS. Now that we take the entire PSIS down offering copious bone graft, the rate of explantation has lessened. However, in thin patients one can only plan to remove the iliac hardware once healing has occurred.

CONCLUSION

A pelvic foundation is indicated in cases where a solid foundation in the pelvis is needed for long spinal constructs and for tumors and fractures of the pelvis. It is fundamental to correcting the complexities of sacropelvic deficiencies. An assembly of available anchors and interlocking connectors achieves solid constructs. The sacropelvic module fixes pelvic dissociation, allows forceful manipulation and anatomic reduction of sacral fractures, and allows reduction of ilium to the resected sacrum. It is powerful enough to correct pelvic obliquities and lumbosacropelvic kyphosis and protects S1 pedicle screws from cantilever stresses and pullout.

REFERENCES

1. Asher MA. Lumbopelvic fixation with the Isola spinal implant system. In: Margulies JY, Floman Y, Farcy JPC, et al., eds. Lumbosacral and spinopelvic fixation. New York: Lippincott-Raven Press, 1996.
2. Asher MA, Strippgen WE. Anthropometric studies of the human sacrum relating to dorsal trans-sacral implant designs. Clin Orthop 1986;203:58–62.
3. Ferguson RL. Rod instrumentation. In: Weinstein SL, ed. The pediatric spine: principles and practice. New York: Raven Press, 1994.
4. Jackson RP. Jackson sacral fixation and contoured spinal correction techniques. In: Margulies JY, Floman Y, Farcy JPC, et al., eds. Lumbosacral and spinopelvic fixation. New York: Lippincott-Raven Press, 1996.
5. Jackson RP, McManus AC. The iliac buttress. A computed tomographic study of sacral anatomy. Spine 1993;18:1318–1328.
6. Shaffer WO. Revisions in spine tumor surgery. In: Margulies JY, Aebi M, Farcy JPC, eds. Revision spine surgery. St. Louis, Mosby, 1999:526–542.
7. Donovan J, Shaffer W, Marguiles J. Morphology of the ilium—the two bolt iliac foundation. In Brock M, Schwarz W, Wille C, eds. World Spine 1: First Interdisciplinary World Congress on Spinal Surgery and Related Disciplines. Berlin: Monduzzi Editore, 2000:153–156.
8. Margulies JY, Armour EF, Kohler-Ekstand C, et al. Revision of fusion from the spine to the sacropelvis: considerations. In: Margulies JY, Aebi M, Farcy JPC, eds. Revision spine surgery. St. Louis: Mosby, 1999:623–630.
9. Lebwohl NH, Cunningham BW, Dimitriev AE, et al. Biomechanical testing of sacro-pelvic fixation constructs in a calf spine model. Proceedings of the North American Spine Society, 16th Annual Mtg, Chicago, NASS, Oct. 31–Nov. 3, 2001;167–168. Isola Study Group; January 2001; Phoenix, Arizona.
10. Berry JL, Stahurski T, Asher MA. Morphometry of the supra sciatic notch intrailiac implant anchor passage. Spine 2001;26(7):E143–E148.
11. Schwend RM, Sluyters, R, Najdzionek J. The pylon concept of pelvic anchorage for spinal instrumentation in the human cadaver. Spine 2003;28(6):542–547.
12. Kukio, TR, Bridwell KH, Lewis SJ, et al. Minimum 2-year analysis of sacropelvic fixation and l5-s1 fusion using s1 and iliac screws. Spine 2001;26(18):1976–1983.
13. Emami A, Deviren V, Berven S, et al. Outcome and complications of long fusions to the sacrum in adult spine deformity "Luque-Galveston", combined iliac and sacral screws, and sacral fixation. Spine 2002;27:776–786.

CHAPTER 70

Paget Disease of the Spine and Its Management

Alexander G. Hadjipavlou, Ioannis N. Gaitanis, Pavlos G. Katonis, Michael N. Tzermiadianos, and George M. Tsoukas

The spine is the second most common site of involvement by Paget disease (PD) of the bone (1,2). This peculiar metabolic disorder of bone triggers abnormal bone remodeling and modeling processes that can predispose the spine to stenosis and facet joint arthritic changes.

ETIOLOGY (3,4)

PD of bone is a mono-ostotic or polyostotic nonhormonal osteometabolic disorder. Over a century after the original disease was described by Sir John Paget (5) in 1877, and despite recent intensive studies and widespread interest, its etiology still remains obscure.

The proclivity to sarcomatous transformation, the variability of osteoblasts (Fig. 70-1) (size, shape, and staining), the peculiarity of osteoclasts (Fig. 70-2) (size and number of nuclei, up to 100, seen also in giant cell tumors), and control of the disease by antimitotic agents such as plicamycin (also known as mithramycin) suggest that the disease may be a benign neoplasm of the mesenchymal osteoprogenitor cell, as was hypothesized by Ramussen and Bordier in 1973 (6).

It has been postulated that the disease may be caused by a viral infection (7–10). Electron microscopy of osteoclasts reveals viral intranuclear inclusion structures resembling those of an RNA-type virus related to measles or subacute sclerosing panencephalitis (Fig. 70-3). Immunologic studies show the presence of specific viral antigens in osteoclasts and cells grown from Pagetic bone (11). There is considerable evidence in support of a viral etiology for PD (9). A characteristic feature of paramyxoviruses is their ability to persist at

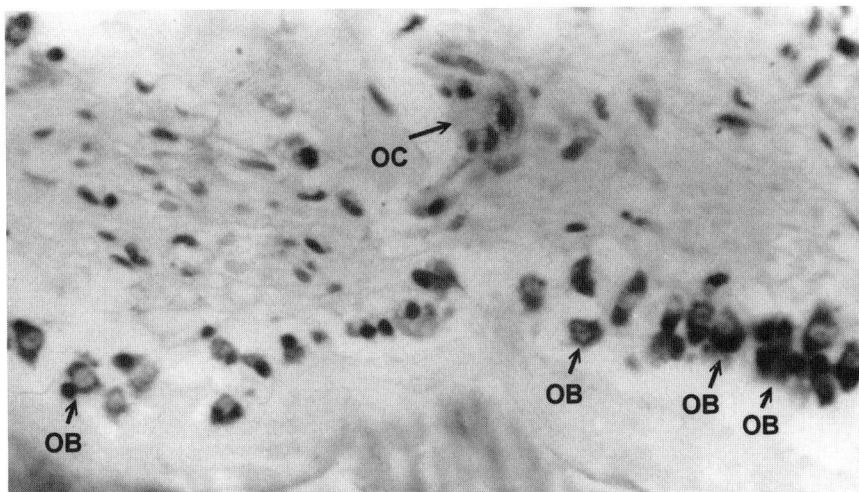

FIG. 70-1. Note the variable size of osteoblasts (OB) and osteoclasts (OC).

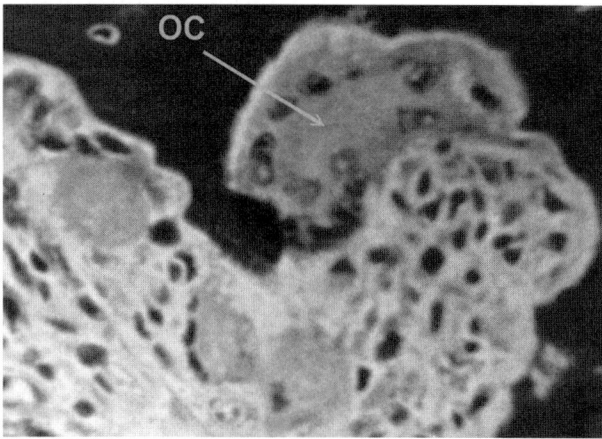

FIG. 70-2. Undecalcified bone demonstrating large osteoclasts (OC) with several nuclei. Black depicts old bone.

PREVALENCE, DISTRIBUTION, AND GENETIC FACTORS (3,4)

PD is found more commonly in populations of Anglo-Saxon origin. PD is rarely encountered in China, Japan, Iran, India, Scandinavia, Africa, or the Middle East (18); however, Singer (19) mentioned that 10% of PD patients in the Los Angeles area are of African decent. A survey of PD in Johannesburg, South Africa, revealed a prevalence of 1.3% among the black population and 2.4% among the white population (20). These findings suggest that PD may not be as uncommon in Africans as was previously believed. Autopsy reports indicated that the overall prevalence of PD is 3.0% to 3.7% (21,22), with a tendency to increase with age. At the age of 90, the expected prevalence is about 10% (22). Radiographic studies revealed a prevalence of 3.5% (23,24). A recent report on radiographic examination of the pelvis (25) revealed an estimated overall prevalence in the United States of 1% to 2%, with near equal distribution between whites and blacks and between sexes.

Genetic factors play a role in the pathogenesis of PD, which is inherited as an autosomal-dominant trait with high penetrance (26,27). PD often occurs in more than one member of a family (28). A positive family history in siblings of patients was reported in 12.3% of cases as compared to 2.1% of controls. The prevalence of PD was approximately seven times higher in relatives of cases than controls.

Studies in families with PD have shown linkage to a region of chromosome 18q near the polymorphic locus D 18S42, most likely due to gene mutation (26,29,30). Genetic heterogeneity is almost certainly present (26,31); data from some families with PD suggest the presence of at least one additional locus, which remains to be identified (26). Viral infection may also help explain the genetic predisposition, by gene mutation, of PD (9,32). Circumstantial evidence thus supports the plausible

very low levels and invade the host immune system. Factors that can be activated by virally induced Ross River virus (e.g., IL-6, C-fos, and Bcl-2) are all elevated in PD, strongly suggests viral infection.

Some reports have indicated that PD is a zoonosis, because it is associated with ownership of birds, dogs, cats, or cattle (12,13). These studies have suggested that canine distemper virus (a paramyxovirus closely related to measles), can contaminate human osteoclast cells, contributing to the development of PD (14,15). However, other studies (16,17) found no risk factors associated with animals. In addition, it should be noted that all of the claims mentioned here are only supported by circumstantial evidence garnered from electron microscopic, immunologic, and epidemiologic studies.

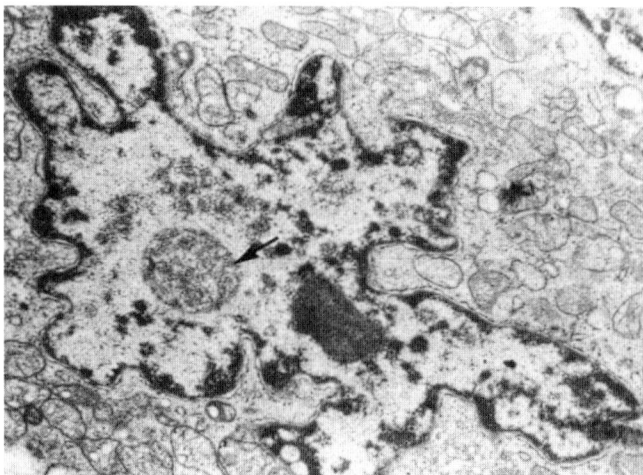

FIG. 70-3. Electron microscopic examination of portion of osteoclastic cell showing a nucleus. Osteoclastic inclusions, not containing membrane, arranged in paracrystalline array, 15 nm in diameter, are shown within the nucleus. (From Hadjipavlou A, Lander P. Paget's disease. In: White AH, Schofferman JA, eds. Spine care. St. Louis: Mosby, 1995:1720–1737, with permission.)

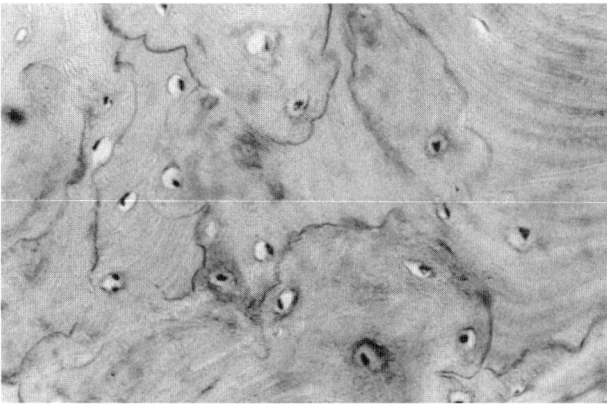

FIG. 70-4. Mosaic appearance of bone in Paget disease formed by cement lines of sequential reformation of new bone without formation of typical haversian systems. (From Hadjipavlou A, Lander P. Paget's disease. In: White AH, Schofferman JA, eds. Spinal care. St. Louis: Mosby, 1995: 1720–1737, with permission.)

hypothesis that viral infection may trigger the onset of PD as well as stimulating inheritable gene mutation. Future research hopefully will cast light on these issues.

HISTOPATHOLOGY (3,4)

The histopathology of PD is characterized by two entities: osseous lesions and bone marrow fibrosis. The former is characterized by its so-called mosaic appearance—the hallmark of pagetic lesion (Fig. 70-4). The pagetic cellularity consists of variable sizes of osteoblasts (Fig. 70-5) and large osteoclasts with multiple nuclei (up to 100) (6). Bone marrow fibrosis is not associated with anemia, because bone marrow hemopoietic activity can expand to the appendicular skeleton (Fig. 70-6) (2).

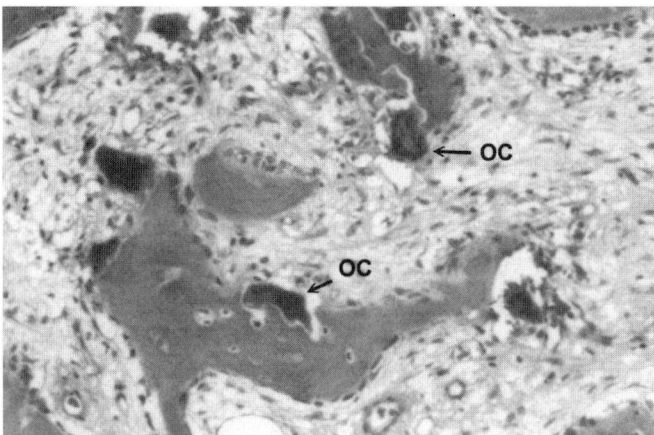

A

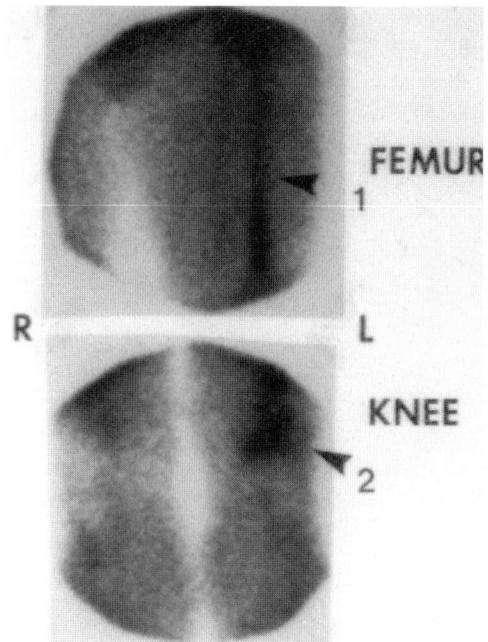

B

FIG. 70-6. A: Bone marrow scan reveals displacement of hemopoietic activity in the appendicular skeleton. **B:** Proven by biopsy.

Uncommonly, extramedullary hemopoiesis occurs in the thoracic cavity (31). These phenomena compensate for the extensive bone marrow fibrosis.

PREVALENCE OF BACK PAIN AND SPINAL STENOSIS (3)

The spine is the second most commonly affected site in PD (1,2,34,35), predisposing patients to low back pain

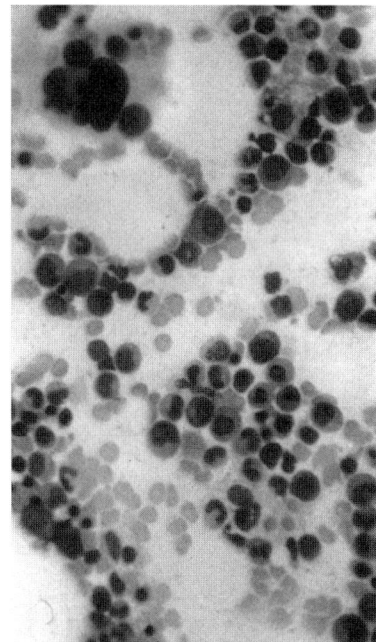

FIG. 70-5. Dense fibrous tissue with large osteoblast containing numerous nuclei eroding bone spicule. Note the variable size of osteoclasts (OC).

and spinal stenosis (36–39). Hartman and Dohn (40) have shown that 15.2% of patients with PD had involvement of the vertebrae, and 26% of these patients had symptoms of spinal stenosis. The reported incidence of back pain in PD ranges from 11% (41) to 34% (1), and 43% (42). The causal relationship between vertebral PD and back pain has been disputed by Altman et al. (25), who attribute the low back pain in PD to coexisting osteoarthritis of the spine in 88% of patients and to PD alone in only 12%. Others (43) consider PD to cause back pain even more rarely. However, in our population (44), 33% of patients with PD demonstrated pagetic involvement of the spine; 30% had clinical symptoms of spinal stenosis, and 54% of these patients suffered back pain (44) (24% attributed clearly to PD alone, 50% to degenerative changes, and 26% to a combination of PD and degenerative changes).

PATHOMECHANICS OF FACET JOINT ARTHROPATHY, SPINAL STENOSIS, AND PAIN (3)

PD can be defined as a disturbance of bone remodeling, which in turn leads to abnormal modeling. Frost (45) has defined remodeling as a constant bone renewal or turnover without changes in the size and shape of bone. Disturbance of the bone remodeling process, as seen in PD, changes the bone texture and gives rise to the four phases of the disease observed radiologically: the osteolytic, mixed, and osteoblastic phases, and the inactive osteosclerotic phase, characterized by normal or decreased bone scan activity (46). Bone modeling is a process that determines the shape and geometry of the bone (47) (Fig. 70-7). In PD, disturbed

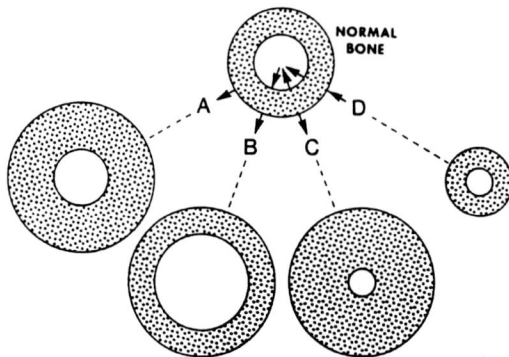

FIG. 70-8. Bone modeling of vertebra depicted diagrammatically to demonstrate tendency of bone expansion in all directions, leading to hypertrophic facet osteoarthropathy and spinal stenosis. (From Hadjipavlou A, Lander P. Paget's disease. In: White AH, Schofferman JA, eds. Spinal care. St. Louis: Mosby, 1995:1720–1737, with permission.)

modeling contributes to bone expansion that leads to spinal stenosis (46) (Fig. 70-8).

More specifically, pagetic spinal stenosis can be caused by posterior expansion of the vertebral body alone (least common) (Fig. 70-9), by the expansion of the neural arch and the overgrowth of the facet joints, or by a combination of these conditions (39,44,48) (Fig. 70-10).

Facet arthropathy can be produced by abnormal pagetic remodeling and modeling changes, causing the joint to become hypertrophic and incongruous, with destruction of articular cartilage, as may occur in other pagetic joints (36,49) (Fig. 70-11).

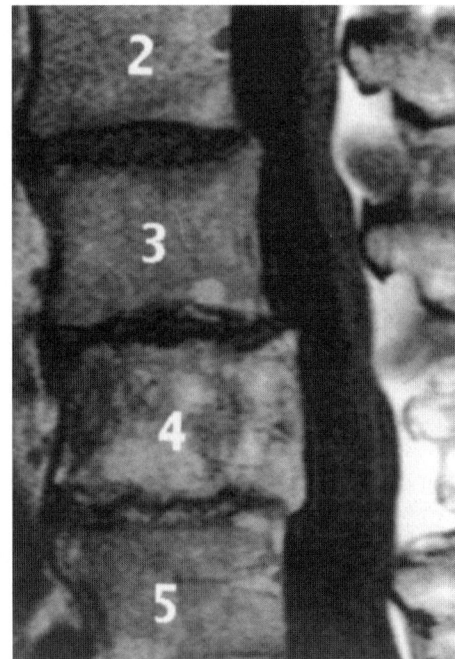

FIG. 70-7. Diagram of cross-sections of a long bone to demonstrate possible patterns of modeling in the periosteal and endosteal envelopes. The arrowheads show the direction of cortical drift due to bone apposition or absorption. Patterns *A*, *B*, and *C* all represent bone expansion. *A* shows apposition within the periosteal envelope, with the endosteum unchanged; *B* shows apposition within the periosteal envelope and absorption in the endosteal envelope resulting in a thin cortex; *C* shows apposition in both periosteal and endosteal envelopes, resulting in a thick cortex; *D* represents bone contraction; periosteal absorption with endosteal apposition causes a centripetal cortical drift. (From Lander P, Hadjipavlou A. A dynamic classification in Paget's disease. J Bone Joint Surg Br 1986;68:431–438, with permission.)

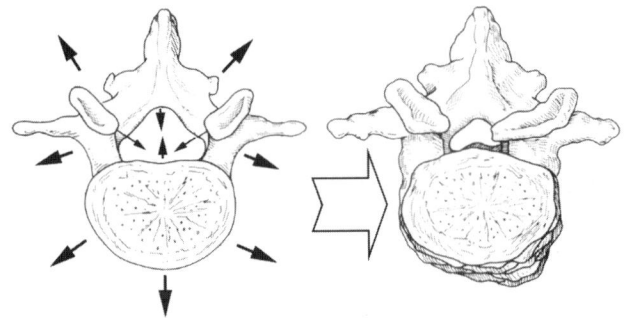

FIG. 70-9. T1-weighted magnetic resonance image showing posterior expansion of the vertebral body. (From Hadjipavlou A, Gaitanis I, Katonis P, et al. Paget's disease of the spine and its management. Eur Spine J 2001;10:370–384, with permission.)

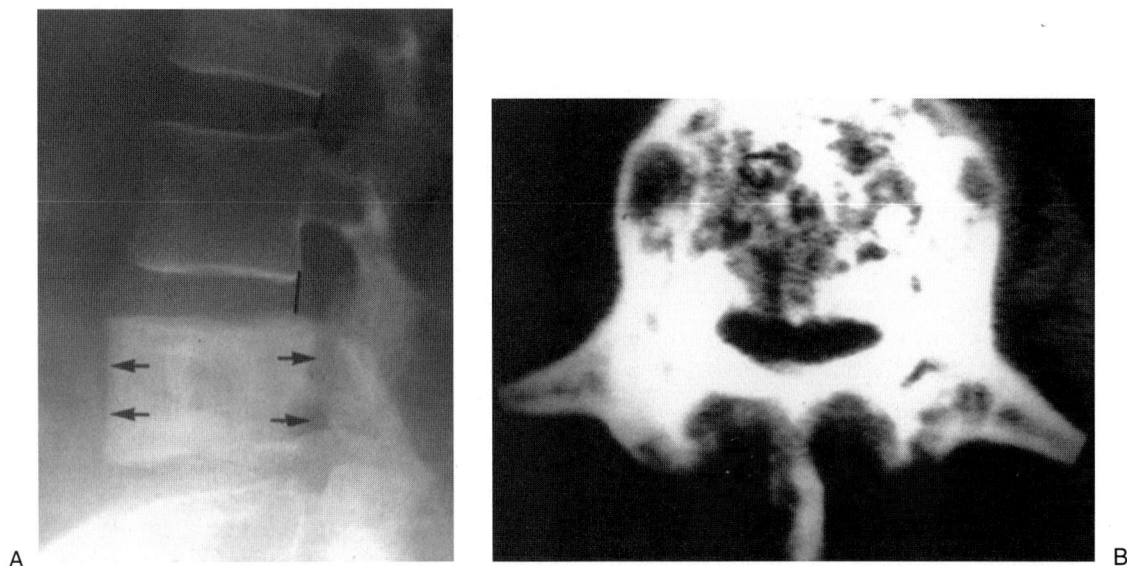

FIG. 70-10. A: Plain radiography demonstrating pagetic involvement of L4 vertebra with typical expansion in the mixed-blastic phase **B:** Axial computed tomography scan of the third lumbar vertebra, demonstrating circumferential expansion of a mixed-blastic-phase lesion of Paget disease causing severe spinal stenosis. (From Hadjipavlou A, Gaitanis I, Katonis P, et al. Paget's disease of the spine and its management. Eur Spine J 2001; 10:370–384, with permission.)

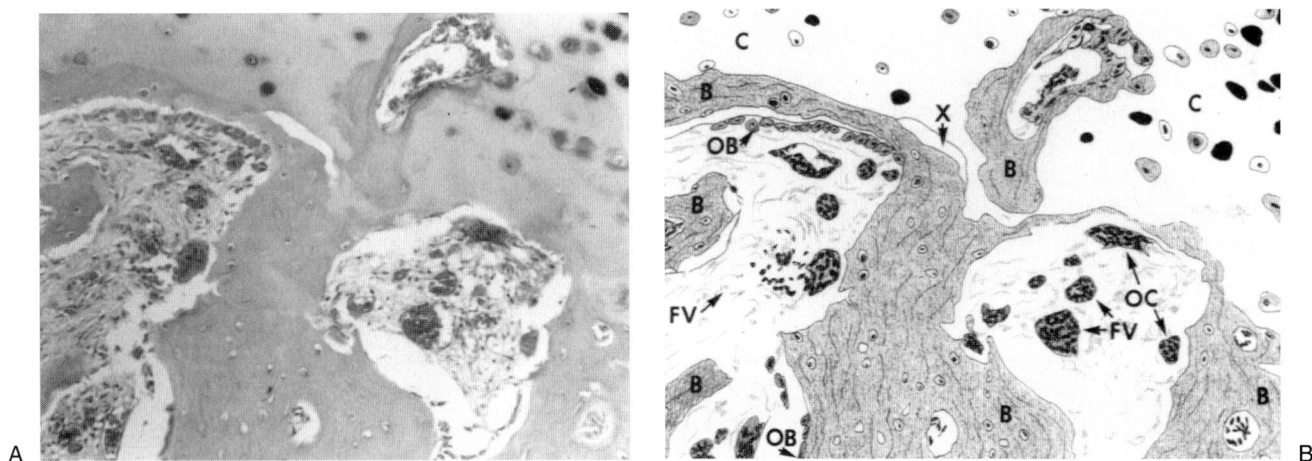

FIG. 70-11. A. Histologic section of articular cartilage showing invasion by the pagetic process. **B:** Schematic representation of **(A):** *C,* cartilage; *B,* subchondral bone; *OB,* osteoblasts; *FV,* fibrovascular tissue; *OC,* osteoclasts; *X,* artifact. (From Hadjipavlou AG, Lander PH, Enker P. Paget's disease of bone: orthopedic management. In: Uhthoff HK, ed. Current concepts of bone fragility. Arthritis pathology and management. Berlin/Heidelberg: Springer, 1986:237–262, with permission.)

SPINAL STENOSIS AND NEURAL DYSFUNCTION (3)

Several distinct mechanisms have been implicated as producing neural element dysfunction in the spines of patients affected by PD:

- Compression of the neural elements by pagetic process:
    - (a) pagetic bone overgrowth (25,44,50);
    - (b) pagetic intraspinal soft tissue (44,51) (Fig. 70-12);
    - (c) ossification of the epidural fat similar to ankylosing spondylitis (52).
- Neural ischemia produced by
    - (a) blood diversion, causing the so-called arterial steal phenomenon (38,40,53,54);
    - (b) interference with blood supply to the cord due to arterial compression by the expanding pagetic bone (55) or other factors not well defined (56).
- Vertebral fracture or atlantoaxial subluxation (55,57).
- Platybasia with impingement on the medulla (58).
- Formation of syringomyelia as a complication of PD of the spine, especially after cranial settling (basilar invagination) (59,60).
- Spinal cord compression by epidural hematoma from spontaneous bleeding (33,61,62).
- Rarely, neurocompression caused by pagetic sarcomatous degeneration (63,64).

About one-third of patients with spinal involvement exhibit symptoms of clinical spinal stenosis (44). Clinical spinal stenosis can be characterized as lateral or central stenosis. Lateral spinal stenosis manifests itself as constant or intermittent leg pain of variable intensity with specific radicular distribution associated with paraesthesias. This pain is exacerbated by walking, may improve with rest, and may be associated with motor weakness, reflex, and sensory changes. Central stenosis, on the other hand, is characterized by bizarre symptomatology, especially leg weakness and cramps with variable amounts of pain that is provoked by walking and improves with rest. Objective clinical signs are usually absent. A combination of central and lateral stenosis may also be present. Central stenosis with myelopathy is associated with upper motor neuron manifestations.

Several authors have mentioned that neural involvement is more commonly associated with PD of the thoracic spine (40,55,65) or the cervical spine (66), rather than the lumbar spine. This is attributed to the large size of the spinal cord in the thoracic and cervical regions relative to the capacity of the vertebral canal; therefore, the same proliferation of bone in all vertebrae would result in compression of the cervical and thoracic thecal sac sooner than it would in the lumbar spine (55). Involvement of the cervical and thoracic spine tends very often to predispose to clinical spinal stenosis with myelopathy (44).

Bone compression by the expanding pagetic vertebrae is by far the most common cause of neural dysfunction (44). It was first reported by Wyllie in 1923 (67). However, severe stenosis, as seen on computed tomographic (CT) scan, may remain asymptomatic, suggesting adaptability of the thecal sac and its neural elements to severe spinal stenosis without significant loss of function (44,55).

The mechanism of neural ischemia is, however, still theoretical and supported only by circumstantial evi-

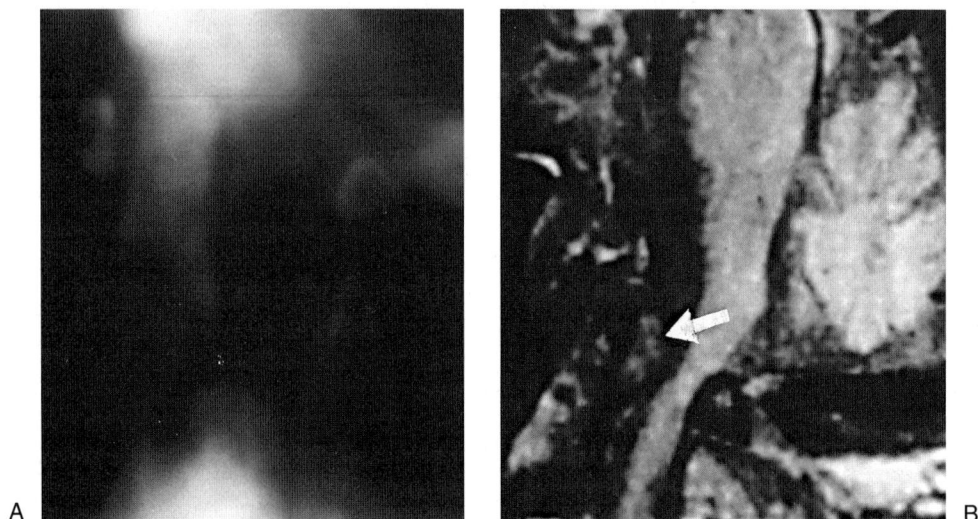

FIG. 70-12. A 63-year-old male patient with pagetic soft tissue expansion originating from the dens and compressing the medulla as seen on: **(A)** lateral computed tomogram of dens (bony element), and **(B)** soft tissue on magnetic resonance image *(arrow)*. The patient was treated successfully with surgical decompression.

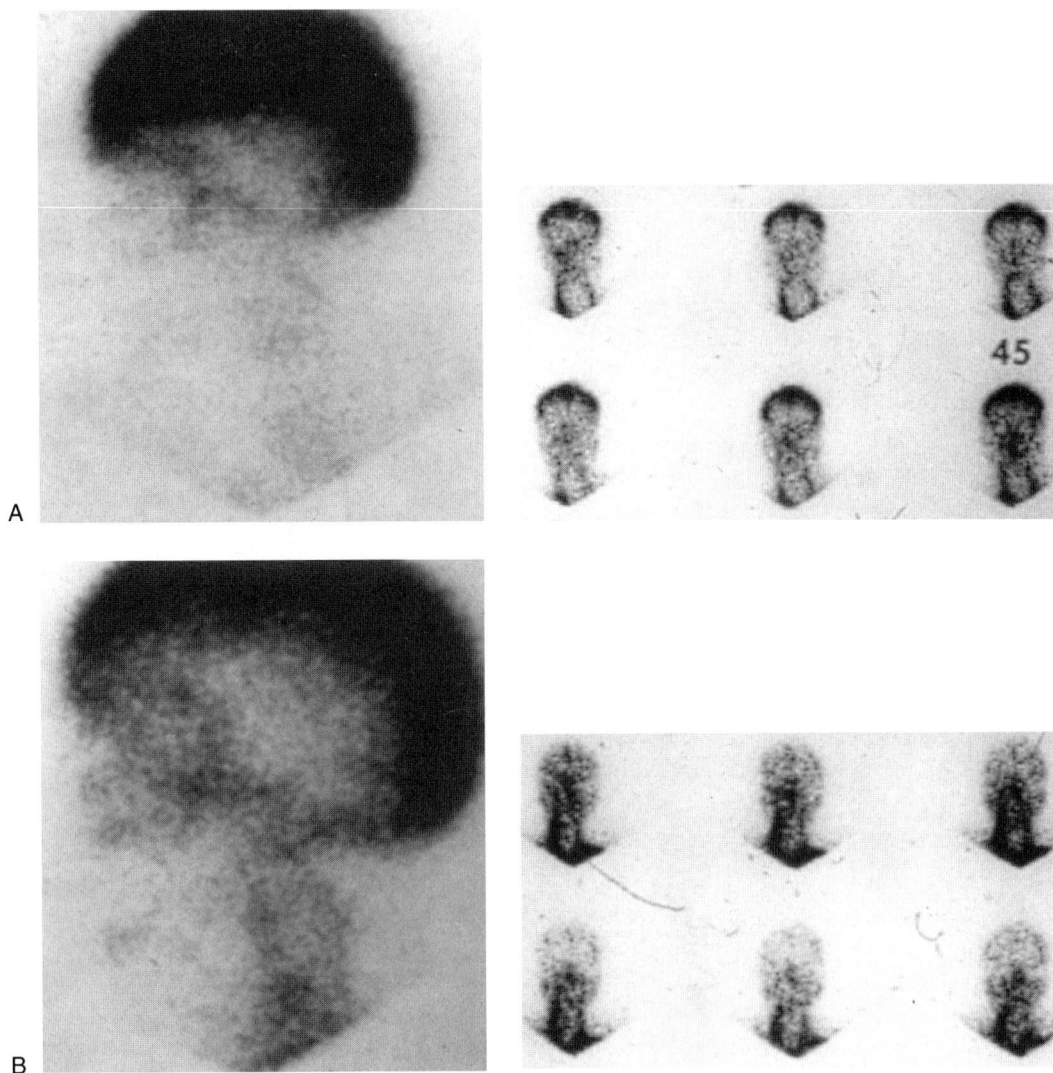

FIG. 70-13. A 78-year-old male patient presented himself with unsteady gait and confusion. **A:** Tc-99m-methylene diphosphonate bone scan revealed increased uptake in the skull, and bone-blood flow revealed increased engorgement of the skull. **B:** After treatment with i.v. mithramycin, bone scan activity somehow improved, however bone-blood flow was restored to normal. This coincided with improvement of the patient's gait and mental status, suggesting that most likely the brain was deprived of its blood supply (steal syndrome by the skull hypervascularity).

dence. For example, patients with spinal cord symptomatology respond to calcitonin treatment better than patients with spinal nerve root lesions (58); some patients experience progressive deterioration of neural function without evidence of myelographic block, which is not easily explained by mechanical effect alone (68); neurologic signs do not always correlate with the site of skeletal involvement; and rapid clinical improvement occurs in some patients with medical antipagetic treatment alone. These observations suggest that neural dysfunction in PD may also result from mechanisms other than simple bone encroachment on the neural element (38,48,50,54,67, 69–71), such as deprivation of blood supply to the neural elements by the rapidly remodeling hypervascular pagetic bone producing "arterial steal phenomenon" (Fig. 70-13).

SPINAL PAIN (BACK AND NECK PAIN) (3)

Pagetic facet arthropathy is a major contributing factor to both back pain and spinal stenosis, and the more advanced the facet joint arthropathy, the greater the likelihood that patients will suffer clinical spinal stenosis or back pain (44). However, this does not necessarily preclude the possibility that, though present, severe facet arthropathy may become asymptomatic (44). Back pain in PD may also be attributed to blood engorgement of the vertebral body caused by vascular and disorganized hyperactive remodeling processes (72). Other factors implicated in spinal pain may include invasion of the vertebral disc space by the pagetic process (72) and spinal stenosis (39). We hypothesize that microfractures of the pagetic vertebral bodies, especially in the osteolytic or mixed phase, can also lead to back pain (44).

OTHER ASSOCIATED CONDITIONS

Malignant Transformation (3)

Malignant transformation is relatively rare, occurring in about 0.7% (72) of cases. In our series of PD patients (73,64), we have not seen any cases with sarcomatous degeneration in the spine. In a series by Schajowicz et al. (64) of 62 patients with sarcomatous transformation, 5 malignancies occurred in the spine. These observations suggest that the incidence of malignant transformation in the spine is even more rare, and represents 7% of all sarcomatous degeneration in PD (64). The association between PD and osteosarcoma seems to be the result of a single gene or two tightly linked genes on chromosome 18q (29,30). A more recent study reported that both pagetic and sporadic osteosarcoma tumors showed loss of constitutional heterozygosity for all or part of the distal portion of chromosome 18q. Clinical presentation of Paget sarcoma-tous transformation is characterized by severe and persistent pain with rapid deterioration and eventual neurocompression and death (63). Surgical decompression offers little, if any, true relief of pain, with the longest survival reported at just over 5 months (63).

Less common is the appearance of "pseudosarcoma" or "pumice bone" in the spine, which is a localized extracortical periosteal bone expansion or a bulky juxtacortical soft tissue mass (usually seen in the long bones) giving the impression of sarcomatous transformation (26,75) (Fig. 70-14).

Rheumatic and Arthritic Conditions (4)

Forestier disease, or disseminated idiopathic hyperostosis (DISH), may affect patients with PD, and should not be confused with focal pagetic bone formation (46). The incidence of DISH in PD has been reported to range from 14% (44) to 30% (36). Pagetic tissue may invade the hyperostotic lesions produced by DISH and transform them into pagetic exostoses (44), which may then progress to vertebral ankylosis (76) (Fig. 70-15). Other rheumatic and arthritic conditions such as psoriatic or ankylosing spondylitis may coexist and be responsible for the clinical presentation (1,41). PD has also been noted to be associated with an increased incidence of gout (41) and pseudogout (77). Treatment with sodium etidronate may be responsible for the accumulation of pyrophosphate crystals in the synovial joint, producing pseudogout (78).

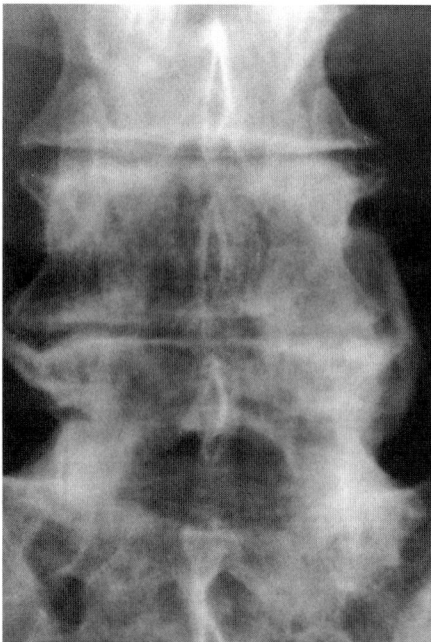

FIG. 70-14. Anteroposterior radiograph of the lumbar spine showing a localized bulky juxtacortical bone expansion of the lateral aspect of L4-L5 vertebrae and resulting in bone union. The appearance of the lesion can be misconstrued as sarcomatous degeneration (pseudosarcoma or pumice bone). The cortical margins are well defined in contrast to the usual appearance of sarcomatous transformation, which remains poorly delineated. (From Hadjipavlou A, Gaitanis I, Katonis P, et al. Paget's disease of the spine and its management. Eur Spine J 2001;10:370–384, with permission.)

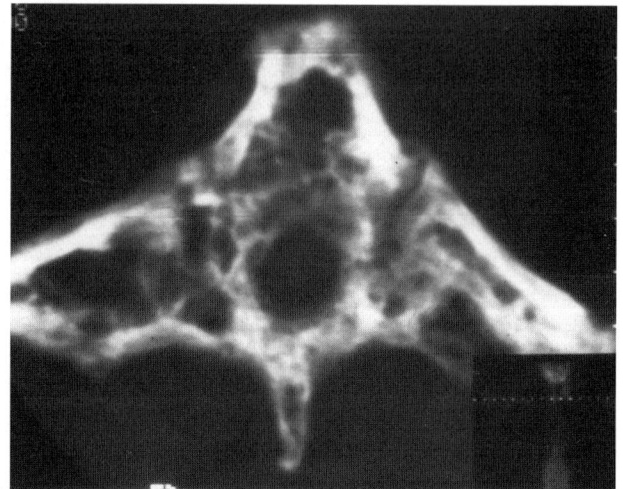

FIG. 70-15. Axial computed tomography scan of thoracic vertebra showing multidirectional expansion of Paget disease with transformation of flowing hyperostosis of Forestier (disseminated idiopathic hyperostosis) and contiguous with pagetic vertebral body. Note wide marrow spaces and thick cortices. (From Hadjipavlou A, Lander P. Paget's disease. In: White AH, Schofferman JA, eds. Spinal care. St. Louis: Mosby, 1995:1720–1737, with permission.)

Osteoarthritic changes in PD have been considered to be a nonspecific arthropathy, a coincidental finding (79), or a specific entity (80). Several distinct pathologic processes contribute to the degeneration and destruction of articular cartilage. Erosion of the subchondral bone may lead to collapse of the articular cartilage (80), which can also be eroded by accelerated endochondral ossification of the subchondral bone (81) or by invasion of aggressive pagetic change (82,83). Bone expansion and bone deformity may also produce incongruity of the articular cartilage, contributing to arthritic changes. Similarly aggressive pagetic tissue may invade and disinte-

grate the intervertebral disc (Fig. 70-16), a process that leads to fusion of the adjacent vertebrae and may be associated with pain. The incidence of intradiscal transgression in PD of the spine is reported to be 10.7% (72).

Pain originating in an arthritic Paget joint may be attributed to the occurrence of microfractures or to increased vascularity of the bone (80). Normalization of blood flow in the bone with antipagetic therapy may influence pain relief (70,84). Such treatment may also produce improvement in the appearance of bone scan and in the level of activity markers of bone remodeling, but if pain persists, conservative therapy has then failed.

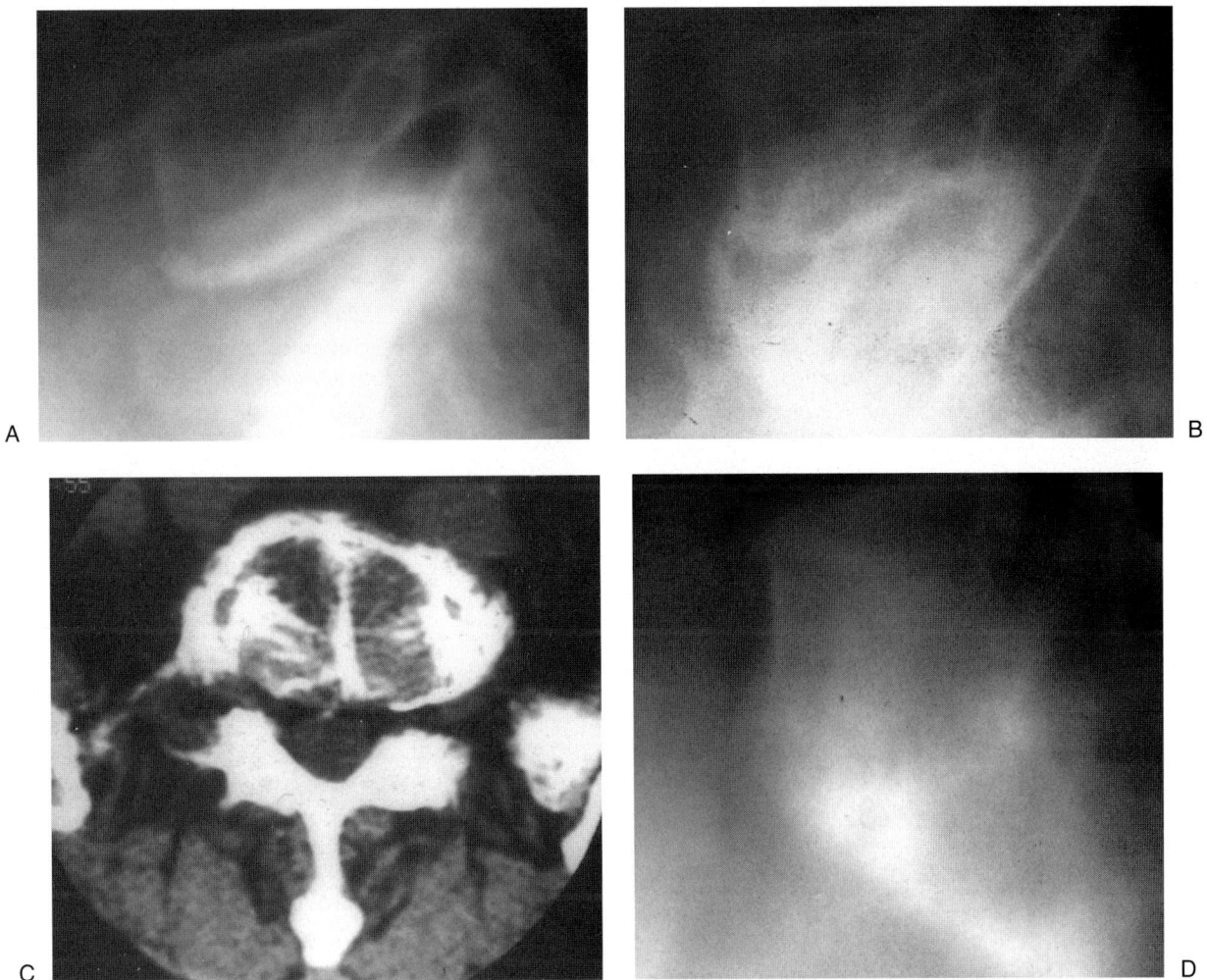

FIG. 70-16. A: Lateral radiograph of the lumbosacral junction demonstrating mixed phase Paget disease of the first sacral segment with moderate narrowing of the L5-S1 disc space. B: Pagetic bone extension across the disc space with adjacent anterior bridging with sclerotic bone noted 3 years after the initial radiograph. C: The corresponding axial computed tomography scan of the L5-S1 disc demonstrates pagetic bone within the disc D: Lateral computed tomogram demonstrating the intradiscal bone extension from the adjacent S1 vertebra resulting in complete bony ankylosis 4 years after the initial radiograph. (From Lander P, Hadjipavlou A. Intradiscal invasion of Paget's disease of the spine. Spine 1991;16:46–51, with permission.)

656 / SECTION V/SPECIFIC CLINICAL ENTITIES

TREATMENT

Treatment of Back Pain (4)

Care must be taken before attributing back pain to PD, otherwise the results of antipagetic treatment may be disappointing (85). Suppressive therapy with EHDP (disodium etidronate) is beneficial in about one-third of cases in patients with back pain and PD of the spine (76). This suggests that unless a well-defined focus of PD is related to low back pain, antipagetic therapy is not expected to be rewarding. If such therapy is ineffective within 3 months, a concomitant nonsteroidal antiinflammatory drug and other methods of treatment for back pain should be prescribed, especially when the pain is mechanical or arthritic in nature (86,87).

Treatment of Spinal Stenosis (3,4)

Treatment of the symptoms of spinal stenosis in PD should begin with medical therapy (3). Calcitonin, mithramycin, sodium etidronate, pamidronate disodium, and clodronate have been reported to either improve or completely reverse the clinical symptoms of spinal stenosis (3,57,74,88–90), but subsequent relapse is not uncommon (69,74,91). Patients should be closely monitored and cyclic therapy should be continued if necessary until biochemical bone indices are normal (37,92). If symptoms still persist, surgical intervention should be considered.

Decompression of spinal stenosis should be implemented promptly after failure of antipagetic therapy. Delay in decompression may result in irreversible myelopathy or radiculopathy (44,74). The results of surgery have shown variable improvement in 85% of patients (68), with frequent relapses, which may improve with subsequent medical treatment (53,74,88,90). Surgery may fail to reverse the neurologic deficit completely (3,74,93) and may be associated with serious complications such as dangerously profuse, if not massive, bleeding (94) and a mortality rate of 11% (68). Preoperative assessment of bone vascularity by means of radionuclide studies of bone- blood flow in the affected spinal region is a reliable, simple, and reproducible test (84). In order to decrease potential bleeding during surgery, when there is an increased vascularity in the affected region, a course of medical treatment should be administered until the blood flow in the bone is normal (70). This may take 2 to 3 months with calcitonin therapy or 2 to 3 weeks with mithramycin (70). The new generation of intravenous bisphosphonates can also be used effectively in this situation. In emergencies, embolization of the region may be considered. Because of the expected torrential bleeding during laminectomy, the use of a cell saver is also suggested (74).

Surgery for spinal stenosis, when indicated, should be tailored to the abnormality responsible for neural compression. If this is caused by the posterior vertebral elements, posterior decompression should be undertaken (70,86). If compression is caused by the posterior expansion of the vertebral body, especially when the cervical or thoracic spine is involved, an anterior approach with corpectomy and fusion should be carried out. An acute onset of spinal compression has a graver prognosis than the gradual development of symptoms (95). Surgery is also indicated as a primary treatment when neural compression is secondary to pathologic fracture, dislocation, epidural hematoma, syringomyelia, platybasia, or sarcomatous transformation (92).

PHARMACOLOGIC TREATMENT (4)

The progressive nature of PD, the severity of its associated complications, the potential negative impact on quality of life, and the availability of effective and relatively safe new drugs have led many experts to recommend treatment for asymptomatic patients who have active disease (86,96,97). However, there is no conclusive evidence to suggest that complications can be prevented by controlling bone remodeling by drug therapy (97). Patients who are clinically asymptomatic, but show increased activity of the disease as indicated by abnormal biochemical markers, bone-scan activity, or increased engorgement or radionuclide investigation, should be treated repeatedly until these indices return to normal values (92,96). Patients who are asymptomatic and inactive when assessed by biochemical and imaging investigations do not require treatment.

Five classes of drugs are available: bisphosphonates, calcitonin, mithramycin (plicamycin), gallium nitrate, and ipriflavone. Some of these are still under development and can be obtained only for use in clinical trials.

Several bisphosphonates have been investigated, but only those listed in Table 70-1 (39,98) have been approved for clinical use. Oral administration of alendronate has demonstrated efficacy, resulting in normalization of serum alkaline phosphatase in 63% of patients at a dose of 40 mg per day for 6 months (99). We assessed the effects of a higher dose (60 mg per day) of oral alendronate on PD over a shorter period (3 months) in 28 patients, 18 male and 10 female, with a mean age of 68 years. Ten patients had never been treated before, and 18 had previously received drug therapy. The mean period without treatment before alendronate was 14 months. Sites of PD were visually scored 1 to 4 for radiologic assessment. Quantitative uptake by region of interest (ratio of PD to normal bone) was also determined for scintigraphic examination.

Baseline alkaline phosphatase levels fell from 266.6 to 82.2 (mean difference 183.8, $p < .000$) Osteocalcin levels fell from a baseline of 5.1 to 8.7 (mean difference 3.6, p

TABLE 70-1. Bisphosphonates approved for clinical use

Drug	Dosage	Administration	Side effects	Comments
Disodium etidronate (EHDP)	5 mg/kg/d for 6 mos, or 10 mg/kg/d for 3 mos, or 20 mg/kg/d for 1 mo. Repeat every 6 mos until normalization of bone remodeling markers.	p.o i.v. also available	Osteomalacia, pathologic fractures	May become ineffective after 6 mos of treatment
Clodronate (Cl$_2$MBP)	800–1,600 mg/d for 6 mos, or 300 mg daily for 5 consecutive d	p.o. i.v.	Association with leukemia observed	Very potent bisphosphonate without mineralization defect
Pamidronate (ADP)	1,200 mg/d for 5 consecutive d, or 15–25 mg daily for 5–7 d, or 60 mg in 0.9 saline over 2 h, oral 180 mg/course over 3 d	p.o. i.v. i.v. i.v.	Transient febrile reactions with myalgias, transient hypocalcemia, neutropenia, and lymphopenia, mild thrombophlebitis, uveitis, scleritis. Appendicular bone loss (secondary hyperparathyroidism) close monitoring is required.	For severe forms of Paget disease, or refractory to other medications. Effective in healing lytic lesions. Further studies are needed to determine optimal dose, the length of treatment, and whether oral and i.v. therapies when combined, would allow for prolonged remission
Alendronate (amino-bisphosphonate)	40–60 mg/d for 3–6 mos, or 10 mg daily for 5 d	p.o. i.v.	Gastrointestinal (25%), esophagitis, esophageal ulcer or erosions	Potent amino-bisphosphonate. Effective in healing lytic lesions. Does not impair mineralization.
Risedronate (pyridinyl-bisphosphonate)	30 mg/d for 2–3 mos or less	p.o.	Gastrointestinal	Highly effective in osteolytic lesion after 6 mos of treatment
Neridronate (aminohexane biphosphonate, AHBP)	400 mg/d for 1–3 mos, or 15–20 mg daily for 5 d, or 200 mg in a single dose	p.o. i.v. i.v.	No significant	Long-lasting remission, successful when other bisphosphonates fail
Ibandronate	2 mg/d	i.v.	Fever, hypocalcemia, hypophosphatemia, gastrointestinal intolerance, flu-like symptoms	Long suppression, rapid action, no significant side effects
Tilludronate (chloro-4-phenylthiomethylene biphosphonate)	200–400 mg/d for 6 mos	p.o.	Hypophosphatemia, gastrointestinal intolerance, flu-like symptoms	Very potent 3rd generation bisphosphonate with rapid action
Aminohydroxybutylidene biphosphonate (ABDP)	5 mg/d for 4–5 d	i.v.	Fever, neutropenia, lymphopenia	New bisphosphonate with profound inhibition of bone resorption
Olpadronate (3-dimethylamino-1-dydroxypropylidene bisphosphonate	200 mg/d for 12 d	p.o.		One of the latest bisphosphonates. Potency is similar to aledronate, but more soluble in the digestive system
Zoledronate (dimethylamino-1-dydroxypropylidene bisphosphonate)	400 µg (single dose), or 200 mg/d for 10 d	i.v. p.o.		New, very potent, and promising bisphosphonate but merits further study to determine optimal dose and safety. Long-lasting effect.

From Hadjipavlou A, Gaitanis I, Kontakis G. Paget's disease of the bone and its management. *J Bone Joint Surg Br* 2002; 84-B:160–169, with permission.

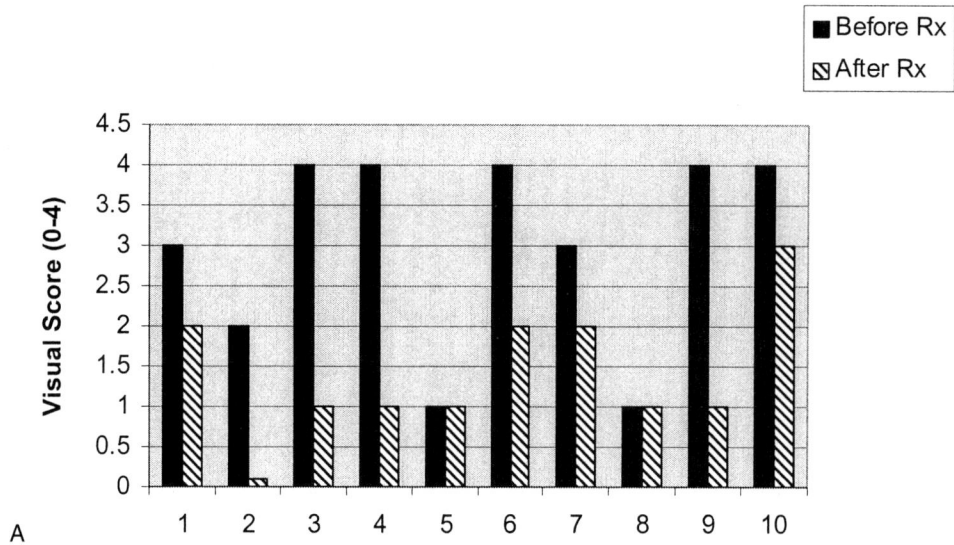

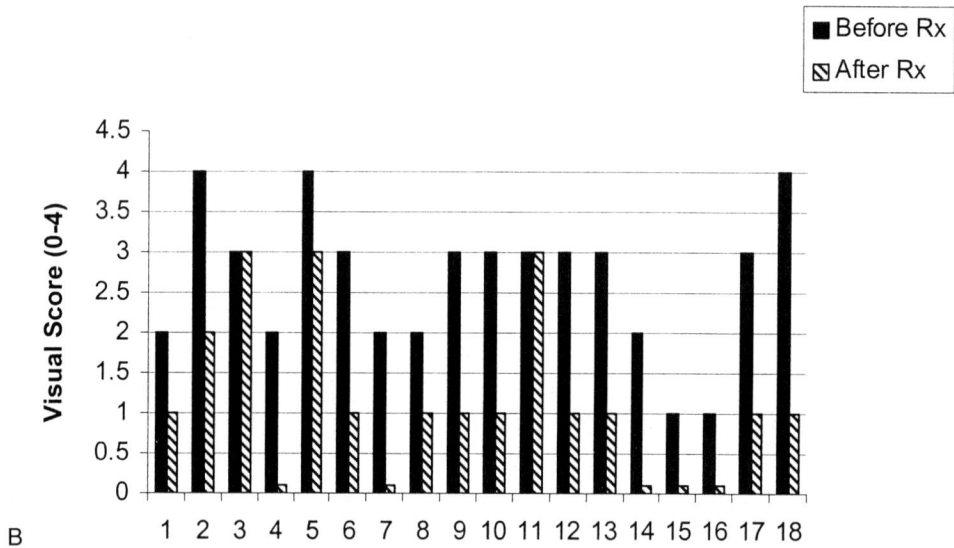

FIG. 70-17. Radiographic effects of alendronate treatment. Patients in group I **(A)** had never been treated before alendronate treatment. Group II patients **(B)** had previously received drug therapy. (From Hadjipavlou A, Katonis P, Tzermiadianos M, et al. Principles of management of osteometabolic disorders affecting the aging spine. Eur Spine J 2003;12(suppl);S113–S131, with permission.)

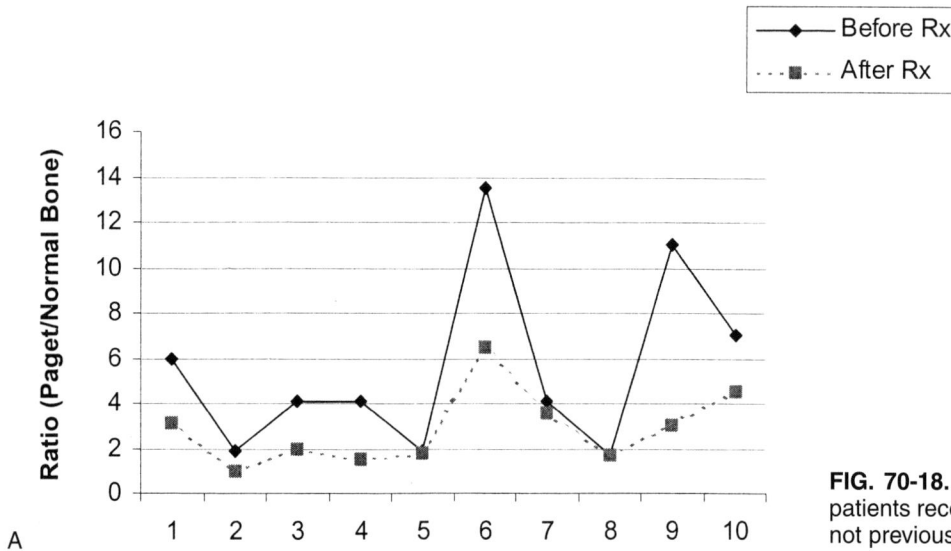

FIG. 70-18. Scintigraphic evaluation of group I patients receiving alendronate treatment **(A)** had not previously received drug therapy.

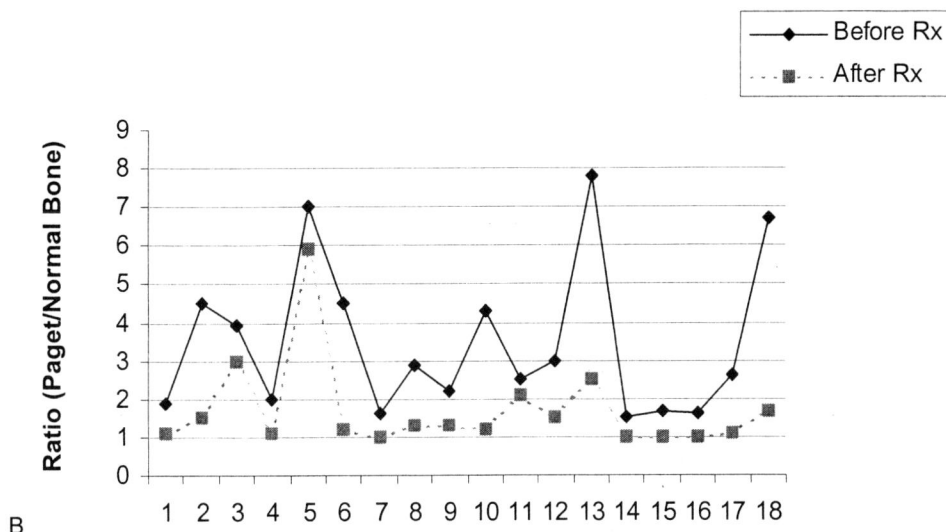

FIG. 70-18. (*Continued*) Group II patients **(B)** had previously received drug therapy. (From Hadjipavlou A, Katonis P, Tzermiadianos M, et al. Principles of management of osteometabolic disorders affecting the aging spine. Eur Spine J 2003;12(suppl);S113–S131, with permission.)

< .0002). All patients normalized their alkaline phosphatase levels. Follow-up was carried out on all 28 patients 2 years after the 3-month treatment. All but 3 were in remission, for a rate of 89.2%. No side effects were noted in any of the patients treated. The response to therapy was similar between patients who had previously received antipagetic therapy and those who had not. Similarly there was a marked radiologic (Fig. 70-17) and scintigraphic improvement (Fig. 70-18).

A major advantage of the bisphosphonates over calcitonin is that biochemical and histologic suppression of the disease activity may persist for many years after the cessation of treatment (100). Other antipagetic drugs are shown in Table 70-2 (39,98).

TABLE 70-2. *Other antipagetic drugs*

Drug	Dosage	Administration	Side effect	Comments
Calcitonin				
Human synthetic	0.25–0.5 mg/d for 6 mos	Subcutaneous		
Salmon calcitonin	100 MRC U/d	Subcutaneous	Mild allergic reaction	Clinical resistant
	200–400 MRC U/d for 6 mos	Nasal spray		
	300 U for 6 mos	Rectal		
Mithramycin (plicamycin)	15 µg/kg/d for 5 d (may be repeated after 7 d)	Intravenous	Toxic: liver, kidney, heart bone marrow, hypocalcemia	Very potent, with quick response, and sustained action. Indicated in severe cases especially complicated with myelopathy.
Ipriflavone (7-isoproxy-3-phenyl-4h-1-benzopyran-4-1)	600 mg/d for 30 d Oral intolerance	Gastrointestinal	Well-tolerated	
Gallium nitrate	2.5 µg/kg/d for 7 d	Intravenous	Transient hyperparathyroidism	Safe with lasting action
	0.25–0.5 µg/kg/d for 14 d (cyclic monthly repetition)	Subcutaneous		Safety and effectiveness have not yet been established

MRC, Medical Research Council.
From Hadjipavlou A, Gaitanis I, Kontakis G. Paget's disease of the bone and its management. J Bone Joint Surg Br 2002;84-B:160–169, with permission.

METHODS FOR CLINICAL ASSESSMENT AND MONITORING ANTIPAGETIC DRUG TREATMENT (4)

The effects of treatment are monitored by the patient's clinical response, imaging modalities, and bone remodeling markers (74,92).

A bone scan is recommended before and 6 months after treatment, and every 12 months thereafter depending on the behavior of the pagetic lesion. A 24-hour retention scan can be used as an adjunct to bone scan (84), allowing early and objective assessment of PD when evaluating the effects of therapy (101).

Biochemical markers of bone resorption are N-telopeptides, C-telopeptides, hydroxyproline, and collagen crosslinks pyridinoline and deoxypyridinoline. The serum tartrated-resistant acid phosphatase is a marker for osteoclastic activity. Markers of bone formation include bone-specific alkaline phosphatase, procollagen type I N-terminal polypeptide (PINP) and β-carboxyl-terminal telopeptide of type I collagen. Osteocalcin may indicate either formation when resorption and formation are coupled or turnover when they are uncoupled; therefore it is not a practical bone marker (102).

The serum markers of bone turnover show lower biologic variability than urinary markers, and are therefore more sensitive indices of the activity of the disease. Bone alkaline phosphatase and PINP seem to best reflect pagetic activity (103,104). The total alkaline phosphatase can also be considered as a sensitive and inexpensive marker for therapeutic monitoring of PD. However, more specific markers may improve the usefulness of the biochemical assessment in certain situations (105).

Bone markers should be checked every 3 to 6 months (1). Markers of bone resorption respond approximately at 1 to 3 months, whereas markers of bone formation usually respond at 6 to 9 months after treatment begins (106).

CONCLUSION

The natural history of PD affecting the spine is progressive. The altered remodeling unit in PD results in abnormal bone remodeling, producing structural changes precipitating or leading to facet joint osteoarthropathy and spinal stenosis (Fig. 70-4). Clinical entities are not always symptomatic. In the majority of cases, the clinical picture of pagetic spinal stenosis and facet osteoarthropathy is not expected to differ from that of degenerative spondylosis. A minority of patients (13%), however, exhibit constant spinal pain attributed to the pagetic pathologic remodeling process.

About one-third of patients with spinal involvement exhibit symptoms of clinical spinal stenosis. Ten distinct mechanisms have been implicated as producing neural element dysfunction. Bone compression by the expand-

ing pagetic vertebrae is by far the most common cause of neural dysfunction. However, severe stenosis, as seen on CT scan, may remain asymptomatic, suggesting adaptability of the thecal sac and its neural elements to severe spinal stenosis without significant loss of neural function. Pagetic facet arthropathy is a major contributing factor to both back pain and spinal stenosis, and the more advanced the facet joint arthropathy, the greater the likelihood that patients will suffer clinical spinal stenosis or back pain.

One must be careful before attributing back pain to PD, otherwise the results of antipagetic treatment may be disappointing. Treatment of pagetic spinal stenosis symptoms should start with medical antipagetic therapy. If the symptoms persist in spite of normalization of bone remodeling markers, surgery is the alternative treatment.

REFERENCES

1. Altman RD. Musculoskeletal manifestation of Paget's disease of bone. Arthritis Rheum 1980;23:1121–1127.
2. Danais S, Hadjipavlou A. Etude scintigraphique comparative des lesions osseuses et de la modelle osseuse dans la maladie de Paget. Union Med Can 1977;106:1100–1109.
3. Hadjipavlou A, Gaitanis I, Katonis P, et al. Paget's disease of the spine and its management. Eur Spine J 2001;10:370–384.
4. Hadjipavlou A, Gaitanis I, Kontakis G. Paget's disease of the bone and its management. J Bone Joint Surg (Br) 2002;84-B:160–169.
5. Paget J. On a form of chronic inflammation of bone (osteitis deformans). Trans R Med Chir Soc Lond 1877;60:36–43.
6. Ramussen H, Bordier P. The physiological cellular basis of metabolic bone disease. N Engl Med J 1973;184:25–29.
7. Basle MF, Rebel A, Fournier JG, et al. On the trail of paramyxoviruses in Paget's disease of bone. Clin Orthop 1987;217:9–15.
8. Hadjipavlou A, Begin LR, Abitbol JJ. Observations morfologiques, histochimiques et ultrastructulares de culture cellulaires in vitro d'os pagetique et normal. Union Med Can 1986;115:746–750.
9. Mee AP. Paramyxoviruses and Paget's disease: the affirmative view. Bone 1999;24[5 Suppl]:19–21.
10. Singer RF. Paget's disease of bone. New York: Plenum, 1977.
11. Mills BG, Singer FR. Critical evaluation of viral antigen data in Paget's disease of bone. Clin Orthop 1987;217:16–25.
12. Khan SA, Brennan P, Newman J, et al. Paget's disease of bone and unvaccinated dogs. Bone 1996;19:47–50.
13. Lopez-Abente G, Morales-Piga A, et al. Cattle, pets, and Paget's disease of bone. Epidemiology 1997;8:247–251.
14. Holdaway IM, Ibberston HK, Wattie D, et al. Previous pet ownership and Paget's disease. J Bone Miner Res 1990;8:53–58.
15. O'Driscoll JB, Buckler HM, Jeakurk J, et al. Dogs distemper, and osteitis deformans: a further epidemiological study. Bone Miner 1990;11:209–216.
16. Renier JC, Fanello S, Bos C, et al. An etiologic study of Paget's disease. Rev Rheum Engl Ed 1996;63:606–611.
17. Siris ES Kelsey JL, Flaster E, et al. Paget's disease of bone and previous pet ownership in the United States: dogs exonerated. Intern J Epidemiol 1990;19:455–458.
18. Barry HC. Paget's disease of bone. Edinburgh: Churchill Livingstone, 1969.
19. Singer RF, Millis BG. The etiology of Paget's disease of bone. Clin Orthop 1977;127:37–41.
20. Guyer PB, Chamberlain AT. Paget's disease of bone in South Africa. Clin Radiol 1988;39:51,52.
21. Collins DH. Paget's disease of bone: incidence and subclinical forms. Lancet 1956;2:51–56.
22. Schmorl G. Uber osteitis deformans Paget. Virchows Arch Anat Physiol 1932;183:694–701.
23. Maldaque B, Malghem J. Dynamic radiologic patterns of Paget's disease of bone. Clin Orthop 1987;217:126–151.

24. Pygott F. Paget's disease of bone: the radiological incidence. Lancet 1957;1:1170–1179.
25. Altman RD, Bloch DA, Hochberg MC, et al. Prevalence of pelvic Paget's disease of bone in the United States. J Bone Miner Res 2000; 15:461–465.
26. Haslam SI, Van Hul W, Morales-Piga A, et al. Paget's disease of bone: evidence for a susceptibility locus on chromosome 18q and for genetic heterogeneity. J Bone Miner Res 1998;13:911–917.
27. Hocking L, Slee F, Haslam SI, et al. Familial Paget's disease of bone: patterns of inheritance and frequency of linkage to chromosome 18q. Bone 2000;26:577–580.
28. Siris ES, Ottman R, Flasher E, et al. Familial aggregation of Paget's disease of bone. J Bone Miner Res 1991;6:495–500.
29. Cody JD, Singer FR, Roodman GD, et al. Genetic linkage of Paget disease of the bone to chromosome 18q. Am J Hum Genet 1997;61: 1117–1122.
30. Nellissery MJ, Padalecki SS, Brkanac Z, et al. Evidence for a novel osteosarcoma tumor-suppressor gene in the chromosome 18 region genetically linked with Paget disease of bone. Am J Hum Genet 1998;63:817–824.
31. Nance MA, Nuttall FQ, Econs M, et al. Heterogeneity in Paget disease of the bone. Am J Med Genet 2000;92:303–307.
32. Leach RJ, Singer FR, Cody JD, et al. Variable disease severity associated with a Paget's disease predisposition gene. J Bone Miner Res 1999;14[Suppl 2]:17–20.
33. Relea A, Garcia-Urbon MV, Arboleya L, et al. Extramedullary hematopoiesis related to Paget's disease. Eur Radiol 1999;9:205–207.
34. Kay HD, Levy-Simpson S, Riddoch G, et al. Osteitis deformans with roentgenologic section. Arch Intern Med 1934;53:208–212.
35. Meunier PJ, Salson C, Mathieu L, et al. Skeletal distribution and biochemical parameters of Paget's disease. Clin Orthop 1987;217:37–44.
36. Altman RD, Brown M, Gargano F. Low back pain in Paget's disease of bone. Clin Orthop 1987;217:152–161.
37. Hadjipavlou A. Paget's disease of bone: comments by eight specialist. Excerpta Medica, Princeton, 1988: 5.
38. Herzberg L, Bayllis E. Spinal cord syndrome due to compressive Paget's disease of bone: a spinal artery steal phenomena reversible with calcitonin. Lancet 1980;2:13–15.
39. Zlatkin MB, Lander PH, Hadjipavlou A, et al. Paget's disease of the spine: CT with clinical correlation. Radiology 1986;160:155–159.
40. Hartman JT, Dohn DF. Paget's disease of the spine with cord or nerve root compression. J Bone Joint Surg (Am) 1966;48-A:1079–1084.
41. Franck WA, Bress NM, Singer FR, et al. Rheumatic manifestations of Paget's disease of bone. Am J Med 1974;56:592–603.
42. Rosenkrantz JA, Wolf J, Kaicher JJ. Paget's disease (osteitis deformans). Arch Intern Med 1952;90:610–615.
43. Guyer PB, Shepherd DFC. Paget's disease of lumbar spine. Br J Radiol 1980;53:286–288.
44. Hadjipavlou A, Lander P. Paget's disease of the spine. J Bone Joint Surg (Am) 1991;73-A:1376–1381.
45. Frost H. Bone modeling and skeletal modeling errors. In: Orthopedic lectures, Vol 4. Springfield, IL: Charles C Thomas Publisher, 1973: 3–35.
46. Lander P, Hadjipavlou A. A dynamic classification in Paget's disease. J Bone Joint Surg (Br) 1986;68-B:431–438.
47. Gray RE. Paget's disease of bone: comments by eight specialists. Excerpta Medica, Princeton, 1988:5.
48. Turner JWA. Spinal complications of Paget's disease (osteitis deformans). Brain 1940;63:321–327.
49. Merkow RL, Lane JM. Paget's disease of bone. Orthop Clin North Am 1990;21:171–189.
50. Direkze M, Milnes JN. Spinal cord compression in Paget's disease. Br J Surg 1970;57:239,240.
51. Hadjipavlou A, Shaffer N, Lander P, et al. Pagetic spinal stenosis with extradural pagetoid ossification: a case report. Spine 1988;13: 128–130.
52. Clarke PR, Williams HI. Ossification in extradural fat in Paget's disease of the spine. Br J Surg 1975;62:571,572.
53. Chen JR, Richard SCR, Wallach S, et al. Neurologic disturbances in Paget's disease of bone: response to calcitonin. Neurology 1979;29: 448–457.
54. Porrini AA, Maldonado-Cocco JA, Morteo GO. Spinal artery steal syndrome in Paget's disease of bone. Clin Exp Rheumatol 1987;5: 377,378.
55. Schwarz GA, Reback S. Compression of the spinal cord in osteitis deformans (Paget's disease of the vertebrae). Am Roentgenol Radiat Ther 1939;42:345–347.
56. Mathe JF, Delobel R, Resche F, et al. Syndromes medullaire au cours de la maladie de Paget: role du facteur vasculaire. Nouv Presse Med 1976 ;5:2619–2621.
57. Whalley N. Paget's disease of the atlas and axis. J Neurol Neurosurg Psychiatry 1946;9:84–91.
58. Curran JE. Neurological sequel of Paget's disease of the vertebral column and skull bone. Australas Radiol 1975;19:15–19.
59. Elisevich K, Fontaine S, Bertrand C. Syringomyelia as a complication of Paget's disease. J Neurosurg 1987;67:611–613.
60. Goodman SJ. Syringomegalia in Paget's disease. J Neurosurg 1987; 67:790–793.
61. Lee KS, McWhorter JM, Angelo JN. Spinal epidural hematoma associated with Paget's disease. Surg Neurol 1988;30:131–134.
62. Richter RL, Semble EL, Turner RA, et al. An unusual manifestation of Paget's disease of bone: spinal epidural hematoma presenting as acute cauda equina syndrome. J Rheumatol 1990;17:975–978.
63. Huang TL, Cohen NJ, Sahgal SA, et al. Osteosarcoma complicating in Paget's disease of the spine with neurologic complication. Clin Orthop 1979;14:260–265.
64. Schajowicz F, Araujo SE, Berestein M. Sarcoma complicating Paget's disease of bone: a clinicopathology study of 62 cases. J Bone Joint Surg (Br) 1983;65:299–307.
65. Klenerman L. Cauda equina and spinal cord compression in Paget's disease. J Bone Joint Surg (Br) 1966;48-B:365–370.
66. Mawhinney R, Jones R, Worthington BJ. Spinal cord compression secondary to Paget's disease of the axis. Br J Radiol 1985;58: 1203–1206.
67. Wyllie WG. The occurrence in osteitis deformans of lesion of the central nervous system with a report of four cases. Brain 1923.46: 336–342.
68. Sadar SE, Walton RJ, Grossman HH. Neurological dysfunction in Paget's disease of the vertebral column. J Neurosurg 1972;37: 661–665.
69. Douglas DL, Duckworth T, Kanis JA, et al. Biochemical and clinical responses to dichloromethylene diphosphonate (Cl2MDP) in Paget's disease of bone. Arthritis Rheum 1980;23:1185–1192.
70. Hadjipavlou A, Tsoukas G, Siller T, et al. Combination drug therapy in treatment of Paget's disease of bone: clinical and metabolic response. J Bone Joint Surg (Am) 1977;59-A:1045–1051.
71. Kennedy BJ. Metabolic and toxic effects of mithromycin during tumor therapy. Am J Med 1970;48:494–503.
72. Lander P, Hadjipavlou A. Intradiscal invasion of Paget's disease of the spine. Spine 1991;16:46–51.
73. Hadjipavlou A, Lander P, Srulovitz H, et al. Malignant transformation in Paget's disease of bone. Cancer 1992;70:2802–2808.
74. Hadjipavlou AG, Lander PH. Paget's disease. In: White AH, Schofferman JA, eds. Spinal care. St. Louis: Mosby, 1995:1720–1737.
75. Lamovec J, Rener M, Spiler M, et al. Pseudosarcoma in Paget's disease of bone. Ann Diagn Pathol 1999;3:99–103.
76. Marcelli C, Yates AJ, Barjon MC, et al. Pagetic vertebral ankylosis and diffuse idiopathic skeletal hyperostosis. Spine 1995;20:454–459.
77. Radi I, Epiney J, Reiner M. Chondrocalcinose et maladie osseuse de Paget. Rev Rheum 1970;37:385–388.
78. Gallagher SJ, Boyle IT, Capell HA. Pseudogout associated with the use of cyclical etidronate therapy. Scott Med J 1991;36:49–54.
79. Guyer PB, Dewbury KC. The hip joint in Paget's disease (Paget coxopathy). Br J Radiol 1978;52:574–579.
80. Hadjipavlou A, Lander P, Srolovitz H. Pagetic arthritis: pathophysiology and management. Clin Orthop 1986;208:15–19.
81. Goldman AB, Bullough P, Kammeron S, et al. Osteitis deformans of the hip joint. Am J Radiol 1977;128:601–606.
82. MacGowan JR, Pringle J, Morris VH, et al. Gross vertebral collapse associated with long-term disodium etidronate treatment for pelvic Paget's disease. Skeletal Radiol 2000;29:279–282.
83. Resnick D, Niwayama G. Diagnostic of bone and joint disorders with emphasis on articular abnormalities. Philadelphia: WB Saunders, 1981:1738.
84. Boudreau RJ, Lisbona R, Hadjipavlou A. Observation on serial radionuclide blood flow studies in Paget's disease. J Nucl Med 1983;24:880–885.

85. Altman RD. Paget's disease of bone: rheumatologic complications. Bone 1999;24[5 Suppl]:47–48.
86. Hadjipavlou AG, Lander PH, Enker P. Paget's disease of bone: orthopedic management. In: Uhthoff HK, ed. Current concepts of bone fragility. Arthritis pathology and management. Berlin/Heidelberg: Springer/Verlag, 1986;237–262.
87. Stewart GO, Gutteridge DH, Price RI, et al. Prevention of appendicular bone loss in Paget's disease following treatment with intravenous pamidronate disodium. Bone 1999;24:139–144.
88. Alexandre C, Trillet M, Meunier P, et al. Traitement des paraplegics pagetiques par les disphosphonates. Ren Neurol (Paris) 1979; 135:625–632.
89. Eulry F, Poirier JM, Perard D, et al. Cauda equina syndrome with pagetic vertebral fusion. Clinical recovery under calcium-vitamin D supplementation plus clodronate after apparent failure of pamidronate and acquired resistance to etidronate. Rev Rheum (English ed.) 1997;64:495–499.
90. Ravichandran G. Neurologic recovery of paraplegia following use of salmon calcitonin in a patient with Paget's disease of the spine. Spine 1979;4:37–40.
91. Douglas DL, Duckworth T, Kanis JA, et al. Spinal cord dysfunction in Paget's disease of bone: has medical treatment a vascular basis? J Bone Joint Surg (Br) 1981;63-B:495–503.
92. Smidt WR, Hadjipavlou AG, Lander P, et al. An algorithmic approach to the treatment of Paget's disease of the spine. Orthop Rev 1994;23: 715–724.
93. Cantrill JA, Buckler HM, Anderson DC. Low dose intravenous 3-amino-hydroxy-prohylidene-1, bisphosphonate (APD) for the treatment of Paget's disease of bone. Ann Rheum Dis 1986;45:1012–1018.
94. Ryan MD, Taylor TKF. Spinal manifestations of Paget's disease. Aust N Z J Surg 1992;62:33–38.
95. Siegelman SS, Levine SA, Walpin L. Paget's disease with spinal cord compression. Clin Radiol 1968;19:421–425.
96. Meunier PJ, Vignot E. Therapeutic strategy in Paget's disease of bone. Bone 1995;17[5 Suppl]:489–491.
97. Tiegs RD. Paget's disease of bone: indications for treatment and goals of therapy. Clin Ther 1997;19:1309–1329.
98. Hadjipavlou A, Gaitanis I. Paget's disease of the bone and its management. In: Thorngren KU, Soukakos PN, Horan F, et al., eds. Eur Instr Course Lect 2001;5:110–123.
99. Siris E, Weinstein RS, Altman R, et al. Comparative study of alendronate versus etidronate for the treatment of Paget's disease of bone. J Clin Endocrinol Metab 1996;81:961–967.
100. Reginster JY, Lecart MP. Efficacy and safety of drugs for Paget's disease of bone. Bone 1995;17[5 Suppl]:485–488.
101. Pons F, Alvarez L, Peris P, et al. Quantitative evaluation of bone scintigraphy in the assessment of Paget's disease activity. Nucl Med Commun 1999;20:525–528.
102. Delmas PD. Biochemical markers of bone turnover in Paget's disease of bone. J Bone Miner Res 1999;14[Suppl 2]:66–69.
103. Alvarez L, Ricos C, Peris P, et al. Components of biological variation of biochemical markers of bone turnover in Paget's bone disease. Bone 2000;26:571–576.
104. Bonnin MR, Moragues C, Nolla JM, et al. Evaluation of circulating type I procollagen propeptides in patients with Paget's disease of bone. Clin Chem Lab Med 1998;36:53–55.
105. Wallace E, Wong J, Reid IR. Pamidronate treatment of the neurologic sequelae of pagetic spinal stenosis. Arch Intern Med 1995;155: 1813–1815.
106. Christenson RH. Biochemical markers of bone metabolism: an overview. Clin Biochem 1997;30:573–593.

CHAPTER 71

Osteopenia: Basic Science, Magnitude of Problem, Classification, Clinical Presentation, and Medical Therapy

Charles W. Cha and Scott D. Boden

The skeleton acts as the structural foundation for the body. Despite its demands for stability, the skeleton is not a static structure. Rather, it is a fluid and dynamic structure that is constantly changing and remodeling in response to mechanical stimulus. Apart from its mechanical duties, bone possesses a dual role, serving as a key endocrine organ involved in the regulation of calcium and phosphorus homeostasis. About 99% of the body's stores of calcium are harbored within the bone. The remaining 1% is in a soluble, ionized form. This free calcium has an important role in membrane function, especially in the cells that rely heavily on calcium metabolism for proper physiologic functioning. Calcium homeostasis must be strictly regulated in order to preserve and maintain proper muscle and cardiac function.

The regulation of calcium homeostasis depends on a complex interplay of hormones, which ultimately control the deposition and release of calcium from its stores within the bone. The large number of hormonal factors and the multiple organs involved reflect the level of complexity of this process. Parathyroid hormone (PTH), vitamin D_3, estrogens, corticosteroids, calcitonin, and thyroid hormone are all known to participate in the regulation of calcium homeostasis. They are produced by or act on organs such as the skin, liver, kidney, thyroid gland, parathyroid gland, gonads, adrenals, and the intestines.

The result of these endocrine interactions is the stimulation of either osteoblasts or osteoclasts within the bone, thereby stimulating bone deposition or resorption respectively. Bone mass is maintained when the level of bone deposition is equal to the level of resorption. Metabolic bone diseases occur when there is an imbalance between bone formation and destruction. Negative balance occurs when an excessive amount of bone is broken down or not enough bone is being formed. This leads to a loss of bone mass, which is simply described as osteopenia. When bone deposition surpasses bone removal, bone mass increases, which leads to increased density as seen in clinical syndromes such as osteopetrosis and Paget disease. This chapter will focus on the former scenario where bone mass is lost resulting in osteopenia. We will review the basics of mineral metabolism, define the magnitude of the problem that osteopenia poses, classify the different types of osteopenia, outline the clinical presentation, and summarize the current medical therapies.

BASICS OF MINERAL METABOLISM

Bone has both cortical and cancellous portions (1,2). Cortical bone accounts for about 80% of the skeleton (3). It is strong, stiff, and possesses a high resistance to bending and torsion. It is also marked by a very slow turnover rate. In contrast, cancellous bone is not nearly as dense as cortical bone. It has a spongy appearance with more elasticity than cortical bone and a smaller Young's modulus. Due to its higher turnover rate, cancellous bone is more susceptible to the factors that regulate bone remodeling. It is this portion of the bone that is primarily affected by the diseases of bone metabolism (Fig. 71-1).

There are three main cells that are present within bone: osteocytes, osteoblasts, and osteoclasts (4). The osteocytes reside within the mature matrix of the bone and represent former osteoblasts that become trapped within the matrix. They are interconnected with each other through canaliculi and interconnecting cytoplasmic processes (5). They are not as active as the osteoblasts and osteoclasts in matrix production, but do have a role in calcium and phosphorus metabolism through the action

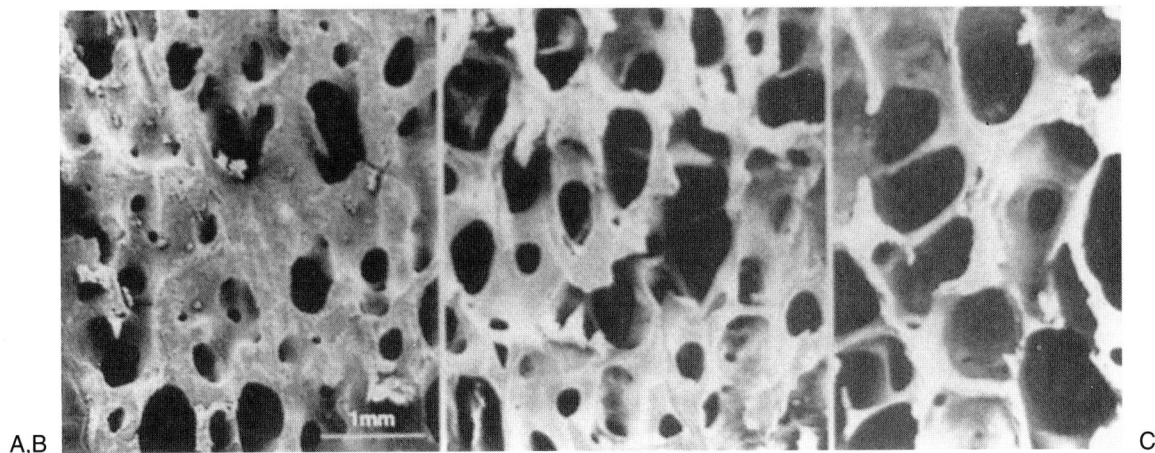

FIG 71-1. Changes in bone density and trabecular architecture related to aging in the lumbar spine. **A:** A 24-year-old female. **B:** A 63-year-old female. **C:** An 89-year-old female.

of calcitonin and PTH. The osteoblasts are primarily responsible for matrix production and are key cells in the maintenance of calcium and phosphorus homeostasis (3,6). Their action is directed through multiple hormonal receptors that are found on their surface. These cells respond directly to stimulation by PTH; 1,25 vitamin D$_3$; steroids; prostaglandins; and estrogen (7). While the osteoblasts are derived from mesenchymal stem cells, the osteoclasts have hematopoietic cell precursors (8–10). Osteoclasts are multinucleated giant cells and primarily act to resorb bone. The osteoclasts work within cavities known as Howship lacunae. They maintain a ruffled border underneath which an acidic environment essentially dissolves the hydroxyapatite crystals, thereby releasing the calcium and phosphate components. Osteoclasts possess receptors for calcitonin. In addition to the cells, the matrix is made up of additional organic components including collagen, proteoglycans, matrix proteins, growth factors, and cytokines. The remaining 60% of the dry weight of bone is the inorganic mineral component, which is the calcium hydroxyapatite (11,12).

For proper physiologic functioning, it is essential that the body maintain the calcium concentration within a strict window. The body depends on this maintained calcium concentration for muscular function (striated, smooth, and cardiac), blood coagulation, and intracellular signal transduction. Calcium homeostasis (13) is maintained at three main areas: dietary intake absorbed in the gut, renal reabsorption of excreted calcium, and release of calcium stored within the bone reservoir. The primary regulators of calcium metabolism—PTH; 1,25 vitamin D$_3$; and calcitonin—act by controlling the calcium traffic at these three areas.

Vitamin D is a naturally occurring steroid and, in general, acts to increase the plasma concentration of calcium through its actions on the kidney, gut, and bone. The metabolism of vitamin D is relatively complicated

(14–16). It begins at the skin where ultraviolet light from the sun converts 7-dehydrocholesterol into vitamin D$_3$, otherwise known as cholecalciferol. The vitamin D$_3$ that is produced at the skin and absorbed by the diet is then taken to the liver where it is converted into 25OH cholecalciferol. This is then metabolized in the kidney by 1-α-hydroxylase into 1,25 diOH cholecalciferol. This is the active metabolite of vitamin D that strongly stimulates the intestinal absorption of calcium. It also acts to release calcium from the stores within the bone by stimulating receptors that are located on the osteoblasts. Once stimulated the osteoblasts release a secondary signal that eventually culminates in calcium release from the bone. The production of 1,25 vitamin D is stimulated by elevated PTH levels, and decreased serum calcium and phosphorus. Conversely, low levels of PTH and elevated serum calcium and PO$_4$ inhibit 1,25 vitamin D$_3$ production.

PTH is produced within the parathyroid gland in the chief cells. In concert with vitamin D$_3$, PTH secretion acts to elevate the serum calcium. PTH stimulates the production of 1,25 OH vitamin D$_3$ at the kidney and also acts on the bone by signaling the osteoblasts to release a messenger to stimulate bone resorption. It also has direct effects on the kidney to promote calcium retention (7,17).

Calcitonin is produced by the parafollicular cells within the thyroid gland. It acts to decrease the serum calcium levels by directly inhibiting osteoclasts, thereby preventing the release of calcium from its body stores within the bone (18,19).

MAGNITUDE OF THE PROBLEM

The most common metabolic bone disease, osteoporosis, is a major health concern. This disease affects over 20 million people in the United States (20,21). The major medical morbidity associated with osteoporosis is the occurrence of fractures, most notably of the spine, hips, and wrists. In total, about 1.2 million fractures occur as a result of osteoporosis per annum. Five hundred thousand of these are vertebral compression fractures, another 200,000 are hip fractures, and 170,000 of these are wrist fractures (22,23). Each of these fractures takes a significant toll on the individual patient in terms of medical morbidity. There is a significant loss of function associated with these fractures and in the worst cases; these fractures can be a harbinger of death (24). In addition to the medical morbidities, there is a significant emotional cost associated with this disease due to pain, loss of function, and fear of future falls and fractures. Nearly half of all women over the age of 50 will sustain an osteoporosis-related fracture, and 13% of the men over age 50 face a similar fracture risk (25).

In 1984 the National Institutes of Health (NIH) produced a consensus statement and estimated the health care–related cost of osteoporosis in the U.S. to be around 3.8 billion dollars annually (26). Less than a decade later, this figure ballooned to an overall cost of 10 billion dollars annually. The current cost of fracture care is approaching 20 billion dollars (27). The overall medical costs will continue to increase given the current aging of our population, the number of people affected with this disease, and the number of fractures occurring because of this problem. It is projected that over the next 50 years, the number of people over the age of 65 is expected to double to 69 million. Some 15 million of these people will be over the age of 85. With these population figures, the estimated fracture associated costs could double or triple by 2050 (27–29).

CLASSIFICATION

Osteopenia is a generic term that describes a finding of decreased bone density on plain radiographs. This term relates only to the presence of the bone density loss itself and does not imply any specific cause for the bone loss. There are a variety of diseases that can lead to osteopenia, the two most notable of which are osteoporosis and osteomalacia.

The relative balance between the mineralized and unmineralized portions of bone distinguishes osteoporosis from osteomalacia. Osteomalacia occurs when the osteoid fails to mineralize during bone formation or remodeling. The excessive accumulation of unmineralized osteoid leads to a qualitative change in the bone rather than a quantitative change. The causes of osteomalacia are varied and result from a failure of the normal processes of bone metabolism such as vitamin D deficiency, impaired vitamin D production, metabolic acidosis, hypophosphatemia, kidney disfunction, and heavy metal intoxication.

In contrast to osteomalacia, which is a qualitative change in bone, osteoporosis is a quantitative loss of total bone mass. Both the mineralized and unmineralized por-

tions of the bone are lost in a proportionate fashion. This progressive loss of bone mass leads to bony fragility and ultimately to increased fracture risk. If an underlying causative factor for the osteoporosis can be identified, such as prolonged steroid use, then it is classified as secondary osteoporosis. Primary osteoporosis is a diagnosis of exclusion that is made when all of the causes of secondary osteoporosis have been ruled out.

Riggs and Melton (30) have further subclassified primary osteoporosis into two distinct categories. Type I, or postmenopausal osteoporosis, most commonly affects women between the ages of 51 to 65. The estrogen deficiency that accompanies the onset of menopause precipitates the bone loss. These patients lose about 2% to 3% of bone mass per year. Because mostly trabecular bone is affected, fractures occur in the skeletal regions with a high ratio of trabecular to cortical bone such as the vertebrae, distal radius, and femur. Type II, or senile osteoporosis, affects both men and women in a 2 to 1 ratio. It occurs in patients over the age of 75, and both aging and long- term calcium deficiency play a major etiologic role. In contrast to type I osteoporosis, type II osteoporosis affects cortical bone as well as trabecular bone. Therefore, fractures occur at sites with more cortical bone such as the hip, pelvis, proximal humerus, and proximal tibia.

The World Health Organization (WHO) has used bone mineral density as the main diagnostic criterion for osteoporosis (31). According to this criterion, a patient with a bone density that is below 2.5 standard deviations (SDs) from the mean density for a young adult reference population is diagnosed with osteoporosis. Osteoporotic patients who have insufficiency fractures are placed in the severe osteoporosis category. If the bone mineral density is between 1 and 2.5 SDs from the young adult mean, the patient is deemed to have low bone mass or osteopenia. These guidelines are useful for epidemiologic purposes, but they do not serve as an adequate guide for treatment.

CLINICAL EVALUATION

In most cases the presence of a metabolic bone disease, such as osteoporosis or osteomalacia, goes relatively unnoticed by the patient or the physician because of the generalized lack of associated symptoms. Suspicion for the presence of a metabolic bone disorder is aroused when a patient sustains a low-energy fracture of the ribs, wrists, hips, or spine (32,33). In the absence of an acute event, thoracic wedge compression fractures can be inadvertently detected on routine chest radiographs. Generalized osteopenia may be detected on routine radiographs when a mineralization loss of 30% to 50% has occurred (34,35). The presence of osteopenia should alert the clinician to the presence of a metabolic bone disorder and should prompt further clinical evaluation to identify the cause of the osteopenia.

Once the presence of metabolic bone disease is suspected, the clinical evaluation begins with a careful history and physical examination. A patient suffering from generalized osteoporosis is usually asymptomatic (36). Despite the lack of clinical symptomatology, the presence of associated risk factors can help support the diagnosis of osteoporosis. For example, a patient may relate a progressive loss of body height, or a change in body shape due to an increase in thoracic kyphosis (36). Caucasian females with light skin and hair, particularly of a northern European descent, are at an increased risk for the development of osteoporosis (37). Inquiries should also be made regarding the use of cigarettes, alcohol, and caffeine (38,39). These patients may be very thin, may have been very active at one point, and may have had exercise-induced amenorrhea or the early onset of menopause (40).

If the patient with osteoporosis is symptomatic at the time of presentation, the symptoms are usually directly attributable to an insufficiency fracture. During the evaluation, the clinician should localize the pain. With spinal insufficiency fractures, pain is usually localized to the lower thoracic or upper lumbar regions. However, the pain may be referred to the low lumbar, lumbosacral, or gluteal region. The onset of pain usually occurs with some low-energy activity although there may not be an inciting event. As the fracture heals, the pain will usually subside over the ensuing months. Unfortunately, despite successful fracture healing the patient rarely returns to the baseline status. These patients often develop generalized chronic low-grade back pain. Increased spinal kyphosis, prolonged inactivity, or altered muscular mechanics that occur after the fracture may contribute to the chronic symptoms (36). Chronic abdominal pain may also occur because the progressive spinal collapse diminishes space within the abdominal cavity (41). If the fracture fails to heal and a nonunion develops, the pain will remain severe, especially when in an upright position.

Clinically, patients with osteomalacia will have nonspecific complaints. They have generalized muscle weakness and generalized skeletal aches and pains. In contrast to osteoporosis, which predominantly affects the axial skeleton, osteomalacia predominates in the appendicular skeleton. Osteomalacia can be distinguished from osteoporosis radiographically by the presence of looser zones. These radiolucent areas are aligned perpendicular to the long axis of the bone. They represent complete cortical micro stress fractures that heal with unmineralized osteomalacic bone. The looser zones are usually bilateral and symmetric. Another distinguishing feature of osteomalacia is the presence of symmetric, pathologic fractures. The clinical evaluation should be targeted to finding the underlying cause of the osteomalacia. A variety of etiologies can lead to this disease process. The most common causes are chronic renal failure, disruption of the vitamin D pathway (either from deficient intake or impaired metabolism), hypophosphatemic syndromes, and heavy metal intoxications (42).

If a low-energy fracture or the presence of osteopenia on radiographs alerts the physician to the possibility of a metabolic bone disorder, the physician is obligated to determine the cause for the bone loss. With a low energy fracture, the first step is to rule out malignancy with magnetic resonance imaging (MRI), computed tomography (CT), or bone scan. After a malignant process has been eliminated, laboratory tests are obtained to delineate the diagnosis. Table 71-1 outlines the various laboratory values that are useful in establishing a cause for the osteopenia. A complete blood count with differential serum and urine protein electrophoresis, and an erythrocyte sedimentation rate will reveal any hematologic abnormalities. If any of these values are abnormal then a bone marrow aspirate is indicated. If these tests are negative, then the next step in the laboratory evaluation is to look for the presence of an endocrinopathy. Thyroid function tests, glucose level, cortisol level, and PTH levels help to identify the presence of Cushing disease, diabetes mellitus, hyperparathyroidism, or hyperthyroidism. If one of these diseases is discovered, they should be treated accordingly.

At this point in the evaluation, the clinician must distinguish between osteoporosis and osteomalacia as the cause of the bone loss. About 10% of these patients will have osteomalacia as the underlying diagnosis (22). Serum calcium, phosphorus, 24-hour urine calcium, parathyroid hormone, alkaline phosphatase, and 25OH vitamin D levels can help to identify about half of the cases of osteomalacia. Osteomalacia is suspected when the product of the serum calcium and serum phosphorus

---

TABLE 71-1. *Laboratory tests to evaluate osteopenia*

Hematologic
  Complete blood count with differential
  Erythrocyte sedimentation rate
  Serum protein electrophoresis
  Urine protein electrophoresis
Endocrine
  Thyroid function tests
  Glucose
  Parathyroid hormone level
  Cortisol level
Calcium metabolism
  Electrolytes
  Creatinine
  Blood urea nitrogen
  Calcium
  Phosphorus
  Alkaline phosphatase
  25(OH) vitamin D_3
  1,25(OH) vitamin D_3
Bone turnover
  Osteocalcin
  Procollagen-1 propeptides
  Urine pyridinoline
  Urine deoxypyridinoline

is less than 25 mL/dL², when bone-specific alkaline phosphatase is elevated, and when the 24-hour urine calcium is less than 50 mg (43). If all of the laboratory data are unable to establish a diagnosis, then a transiliac bone biopsy can make the final distinction between osteoporosis and osteomalacia (22). If the bone mineralization is found to be normal on biopsy, then the diagnosis of osteoporosis is established essentially by the exclusion of all other possibilities. Even in the setting of osteoporosis, the transiliac bone biopsy can distinguish between high turnover and low turnover osteoporosis. Additional laboratory assays are also helpful in assessing the metabolic activity of the bone with osteoporosis (44,45). Bone-specific alkaline phosphatase, osteocalcin, and procollagen-1 propeptides are indicative of bone formation. Urine pyridinoline, deoxypyridinoline, and the N-telopeptides are collagen breakdown products indicative of bone resorption or turnover.

RADIOGRAPHIC EVALUATION

The main goal guiding the treatment of the patient with osteopenia is to prevent the occurrence of fractures. However, the severity of the bone loss exists along a continuum, and the key to guiding treatment and preventing fractures is determining the threshold of bone loss below which fractures become imminent. A variety of noninvasive imaging tools are available which allow for an estimation of bone mineral density. These density measurements have been shown to correlate directly with fracture risk. For example, a 50-year-old woman whose bone density is 1 SD below the average for a woman has a 30% risk of fracture over her lifetime whereas that same 50-year-old woman with a 2 SD decrease in her bone mineral density has a 60% fracture risk over her lifetime (33). Before placing excessive emphasis on bone densitometry, it is important to realize that bone density is just one risk factor in a multitude of risk factors that can increase to fracture risk, such as cardiovascular status, geometry of the bone, force of the insult, risk of fall, and body habitus (46–48). There are many techniques to assess bone density and each has its relative merits and limitations. Factors to consider when assessing bone densitometry techniques include cost, radiation dose, and relative precision and accuracy as well as duration of the procedure.

Given the myriad options for assessing bone density, the question arises as to which technique to use. In a clinical setting where dual-energy X-ray absorptiometry (DEXA) or quantitative CT scan is unavailable, then radiogrametry or radioabsorptiometry are crude but effective methods for assessing bone density. DEXA is currently the method of choice to assess bone density in the osteopenic patient because it measures axial sites with high precision, high accuracy, low radiation dose, and low cost. However, in the older adult patient with osteoarthritis, adjacent calcifications, or a compression

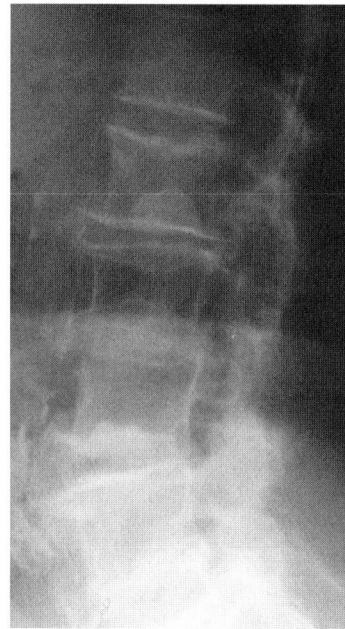

FIG. 71-2. Lateral lumbar radiograph of the lumbar spine in an 85-year-old patient with new onset of back pain reveals osteopenia and an insufficiency fracture of the second lumbar vertebra. Note the prevertebral calcifications, osteophytes, and end-plate sclerosis that can falsely elevate density measurements by dual-energy X-ray absorptiometry performed in the anteroposterior projection.

fracture, quantitative CT scan is still a viable option (Fig. 71-2).

TREATMENT

Simply put, the main goal of treatment for a patient with severe osteopenia is to prevent the occurrence of fractures by maintaining an adequate skeletal bone mass. Though declaring this goal is simple, achieving it is a more difficult matter. As outlined earlier in this chapter, the causes for significant osteopenia are varied. Currently, there are no existing means to completely replace lost bone mass, though certain medical therapies can effect some modest changes in bone mass. In addition, once the internal architecture is lost no clinical method to reestablish it exists. Since the metabolic bone diseases are clinically silent, the true denominator of the number of patients afflicted with this problem is unknown. This makes clinical investigations assessing therapeutic options difficult. Treatment of osteoporotic spine fractures, once they have occurred, will be discussed in Chapters 72 and 73.

Currently, the foundation for treatment of these disorders is to prevent skeletal bone loss. There are two ways to maximize bone mass during aging. The first is to maximize the peak bone mass obtained by an individual during growth and development. Most children do not currently receive adequate amounts of calcium in their diet (22), and this nutritional deficiency can lead to a lower peak bone mass at maturity. An ideal target for calcium supplementation during the stages of growth and development would be premenarchal adolescent girls (49). The second way to preserve bone mass later in life is to slow or stop the rate of decay of bone mass once skeletal maturity has been achieved.

A variety of factors are known to alter the rate of decline in bone mass. First, the patient needs to maximize their nutrition to make sure that they are getting adequate oral intake of minerals and hormones to maintain skeletal integrity. The diseases that are known to accelerate bone loss need to be identified and treated. Medications that stimulate bone loss should be avoided if possible, or used sparingly when necessary. These medications include steroids and the anticonvulsants (50,51). In the otherwise healthy individual without any underlying medical or pharmacologic cause for bone loss, cessation of smoking and alcohol intake are two factors that are easily addressed and can dramatically impact the rate of decay of bone mass. Impact loading exercise has been shown to positively effect bone mass (52,53). One hour of impact exercise two to three times per week can increase both the bone mineral content and the total body calcium (41). Conversely, it is well documented that sedentary people or people in antigravity settings such as astronauts can sustain a significant amount of bone loss secondary to the lack of skeletal loading (48,54). Since the ultimate goal is to prevent the occurrence of fractures, fall prevention is important in the older adult patient. Outfitting the patient's environment with appropriate assist devices for ambulation, avoiding medications that can negatively affect the mental status, and maximizing cardiovascular status can all help to lower the fall risk. Finally, there are a variety of pharmacologic interventions that can be instituted to slow down the rate of bone loss. These medical therapies are discussed subsequently in further detail.

Calcium is an essential nutrient to the body. A certain level of intake is required to maintain calcium homeostasis. The average woman requires 1 to 1.2 g per day in a premenopausal state and 1.5 g in the postmenopausal state (55). Unfortunately, the average woman does not meet these requirements. When the nutritional intake of calcium is deficient, the body will begin to deplete its store of calcium from the bone. Therefore, calcium supplementation can be beneficial by preventing this process from occurring. It has been shown to be helpful in the premenopausal patient (41). Also in the older adult patient with type II osteoporosis, calcium supplementation therapy, especially in combination with vitamin D, has been shown to lower the rate of hip fractures (56). It is interesting to note that the bone mass in these patients was unchanged and the effect may be related to crude bone quality or maintaining lower levels of PTH. Calcium supplementation therapy in the early post-

menopausal patient does not protect against bone loss (57,58). Here it seems that the effects of estrogen deficiency significantly overshadow any effect of nutritional deficiency. The current recommendations are for 1,200 mg of calcium supplementation in the premenopausal patient and 1,500 mg in the postmenopausal patient with an additional 400 to 800 units of vitamin D concurrently.

Estrogen plays a pivotal role in the development of type I osteoporosis. In the early postmenopausal period (i.e., the first 10 years) the absence of estrogen leads to a significant, accelerated bone loss. Bone responds to estrogen through receptors that are directly located in the bone (59). It also has a secondary antiresorptive effect by modulating certain cytokines, which ultimately promotes a positive calcium balance (60,61). Studies have shown that bone mass can be increased with estrogen therapy by 2% to 3% in the spine and that the fracture rate can be decreased by 50% (57,62,63). Unfortunately, this protective effect on the bone is not maintained when estrogen therapy is withdrawn. Additional benefits of estrogen therapy include treatment of the symptoms of menopause. It also imparts a cardioprotective effect by improving the cardiolipid profile (64). It also may improve cognition and decrease the risk of Alzheimer disease (65). However, estrogen therapy is not without its risk. The therapy is often poorly tolerated secondary to uterine bleeding. One of the more worrisome risks associated with estrogen therapy is the up to 30% increased risk of breast cancer that can occur with prolonged therapy (66,67). There is also an increased risk of developing uterine cancer. However, this risk can be negated by the use of combination therapy where the estrogen is given in conjunction with progestin (65). Finally, estrogen may have untoward effects on the liver, precipitating cholelithiasis.

A strong family history of osteoporosis, bone density less than 2.5 SDs below the norm, greater than 5% of bone loss per year, symptoms of menopause, and high cardiovascular risk are all indications for estrogen therapy. Contraindications to the use of estrogen therapy include a history of breast cancer regardless of receptor status, history of deep venous thrombosis (DVT) or pulmonary embolus (PE), and history of underlying liver disease or hypertension.

The selective estrogen receptor modulators (SERMs) can act either as an estrogen agonist or antagonist depending on the type of tissue that is being targeted. Their appeal rests in the ability to selectively stimulate estrogen receptors in bone, while simultaneously having an antiestrogenic effect on the breast. They therefore have the potential to retard bone loss and reduce breast cancer risk. Tamoxifen has primarily been used as a chemotherapeutic agent in women with receptor-positive breast cancer. A placebo-controlled trial in postmenopausal women revealed that tamoxifen therapy can precipitate mild increases in spinal bone mineral density (68). A second trial concluded that the overall occurrence of fractures could be reduced by 19% with tamoxifen therapy (69). Though the estrogenic effect of tamoxifen on bone is not as potent as regular estrogen therapy, other more potent SERMs are becoming available. Raloxifene increases bone density by 2.4% in the spine and hip when compared to placebo, and the reduction of new vertebral fractures was 30% at the low dose and 50% at the higher dose (70). These drugs maintain a positive effect on the cardiolipid profile, thereby having a beneficial effect on the heart. However, though raloxifene therapy has been shown to decrease spine fractures, the nonvertebral fracture rate remains unchanged. Further study is warranted with this class of drugs to better understand their physiologic effects and to guide development of future SERMs.

An exciting new class of drugs used in the battle against osteoporosis are the bisphosphonates. The bisphosphonates block the ability of the osteoclasts to resorb bone. A first generation bisphosphonate, etidronate, showed some promise in the early stage of treatment. However, it was becoming clear that with long-term treatment, etidronate may actually have inhibited bone mineralization (71). A second line of bisphosphonates is now available which does not inhibit mineralization long term as with the first generation bisphosphonates. Alendronate is taken orally in 5 to 10 mg doses. The main side effect is the development of upper gastrointestinal symptoms. Recent gradual dosing regimens and half-dosing regimens have limited the occurrence of these symptoms. Since it has poor absorption, alendronate must be taken on an empty stomach with a glass of water. Alendronate is equally as effective as estrogen in maintaining bone mass and decreasing fracture risk (72,73). However, unlike estrogen, the second generation of bisphosphonates maintains its efficacy after the treatment is withdrawn (74). The use of these drugs is advocated in situations where the use of estrogens is contraindicated, such as among patients with breast cancer and thrombophlebitis. In the setting of osteoporosis, one contraindication to the use of bisphosphonates is the presence of an acute fracture. Theoretically, the effect of bisphosphonates on remodeling may have an adverse impact on fracture healing.

Newer generations of bisphosphonates are rapidly becoming available which may be more potent and better tolerated than alendronate. Risedronate was evaluated in a study of 2,458 women (75). Over the 3-year course of the trial, patients taking risedronate had a 40% reduction in the incidence of new vertebral and nonvertebral fractures. Bone mineral density was increased 4.3% in the spine and 2.8% in the proximal femur. The incidence of adverse effects was equal to the placebo group. In a phase II trial, a single intravenous 4 mg dose of zoledronic acid increased bone mineral density and decreased markers of bone turnover for 1 year (76). Whether this treatment can significantly reduce fracture rates remains to be seen.

Calcitonin can down-regulate osteoclast function and has been used successfully in the treatment of Paget disease. In the osteoporotic, postmenopausal patient, calcitonin can increase total body calcium and lumbar bone mineral density (77,78). It has also been shown to decrease the spinal fracture rate by about 33% (79). The maximal effect of calcitonin is seen within the first 6 months of therapy and the elevations in bone mineral density persist over time (80). Calcitonin is indicated for female osteoporotic patients who have a high bone turnover rate on biopsy, are unable to take estrogen, are premenopausal with osteoporosis, and have persistent bone loss on estrogen, as well as for male patients with osteoporosis. Calcitonin is also very effective for use in the patient who has sustained an acute compression fracture, because calcitonin has a strong, short-term analgesic effect (81). Previously, calcitonin was administered subcutaneously, but there are bothersome side effects associated with this route of administration. The intranasal form is better tolerated. If therapy is to be initiated, 200 units should be given daily for a 6-month period.

The aforementioned therapies treat osteoporosis by preventing bone resorption; fluoride differs from these therapies because it can actually stimulate bone formation. Communities with fluorinated drinking water have a lower incidence of insufficiency fractures (82). With fluoride therapy, bone mass can be increased in the spine 4% to 5% per year (83). Initial studies evaluating treatment of osteoporosis with fluoride revealed concerns with the use of fluoride. These studies indicated that although fluoride therapy may increase bone density, it may also make the bone more fragile and more susceptible to fractures (84). These early investigations used high doses of fluoride, and did not give adequate calcium supplementation. Continuing work reveals that the rate of bone mass augmentation is important in stimulation of bone generation with the fluoride and should not outpace the ability of the body to mineralize that newly formed bone (85). It now appears that the susceptibility to bony fragility occurs when the bone is not given adequate time to mineralize. Pak et al. (83) have developed a cyclic, low-dose, slow-release fluoride form that may allow the bone to regenerate in a controlled fashion that does not jeopardize the mechanical stability of the bone. Their studies reveal a significantly decreased fracture rate with the use of this form of fluoride. This form awaits U.S. Food & Drug Administration approval. Should fluoride therapy be instituted, it must be done with low doses and supplemented with vitamin D and calcium to ensure adequate mineralization.

CONCLUSION

The spine surgeon may be the first clinician to detect the osteopenic patient. The patient may present in the office with a simple insufficiency fracture or with decreased bone density on routine spine radiographs. When osteopenia is discovered, the clinician should take the necessary steps to identify the underlying cause. Once a diagnosis is established with a proper history, physical examination and laboratory data; bone densitometry is useful to assess the patient's fracture risk, and to set a baseline for long-term follow-up. The most effective intervention to combat osteopenia is prevention. Patient education on proper diet, impact exercises, and avoidance of substances that promote bone loss is the cornerstone to prevention. Once osteopenia is established, there are medical therapies that can halt or retard the bone decay. In the future, new and exciting biologic technologies like gene therapy may allow us to rebuild the lost bone mass and ultimately prevent the occurrence of debilitating insufficiency fractures.

REFERENCES

1. Buckwalter JA, Cooper RR. Bone structure and function. In: Instructional course lectures, the American Academy of Orthopaedic Surgeons. Park Ridge, IL: The American Academy of Orthopaedic Surgeons, 1987;36:27–48.
2. Singh I. The architecture of cancellous bone. J Anat 1978;127: 305–310.
3. Recker RR. Embryology, anatomy, and microstructure of bone. In: Coe FL, Favus MJ, eds. Disorders of bone and mineral metabolism. New York: Raven Press, 1992,219–240.
4. Peck WA, Woods W. The cells of bone. In: Riggs BL, Melton LJ III, eds. Osteoporosis: etiology, diagnosis and management. New York: Raven Press, 1988:1–44.
5. Buckwalter JA, Glimcher MJ, Cooper RR, et al. Bone biology: part 1: structure, blood supply, cells matrix and mineralization. J Bone Joint Surg 1995;77-A:1256–1275.
6. Raisz LG, Kream BE. Regulation of bone formation. N Engl J Med 1983;309:29–35.
7. Russell RG, Bunning RA, Hughes DE, et al. Humoral and local factors affecting bone formation and resorption. In: Stephenson JC, ed. New techniques in metabolic bone disease. London: Butterworth, 1990:1–20.
8. Helfrich MH, Mieremet RH, Thesingh CW. Osteoclast formation in vitro from progenitor cells present in the adult mouse circulation. J Bone Miner Res 1989;4:325–334.
9. Ibbotson KJ, Roodman GD, McManus LM, et al. Identification and characterization of osteoclast-like cells and their progenitors in cultures of feline marrow mononuclear cells. J Cell Biol 1984;99: 471–480.
10. Vaes G. Cellular biology and biochemical mechanism of bone resorption. A review of recent developments on the formation, activation, and mode of action of osteoclasts. Clin Orthop 1988;231:239–271.
11. Herring GM. Methods for the study of glycoproteins of bone using bacterial collagenase. Determination of bone sialoprotein and chondroitin sulfate. Calcif Tissue Res 1977;24:29–36.
12. Triffit JT. The organic matrix of bone tissue In: Urist MR, ed. Fundamental and clinical bone physiology. Philadelphia: Lippincott, 1980:45–82.
13. Eastell R, Riggs BL. Calcium homeostasis and osteoporosis. Endocrinol Metab Clin North Am 1987;16:829–842.
14. Bell NH. Vitamin D-endocrine system. J Clin Invest 1985;76:1–6.
15. DeLuca HF. Metabolism and mechanisms of action of vitamin D. In: Peck WA, ed. Bone and mineral research. Amsterdam: Excerpta Medica, 1982:7–73.
16. Stern PH. The D vitamins and bone. Pharmacol Rev 1980;32:47–80.
17. Rosenblatt M. Pre-proparathyroid, proparathyroid hormone and parathyroid hormone. The biologic role of hormone structure. Clin Orthop 1982;170:270–276.
18. Hirsch PF, Munson PL. Thyrocalcitonin. Physiol Rev 1969;49: 548–622.
19. Martin TJ, Robinson CJ, MacIntyre I. The mode of action of thyrocalcitonin. Lancet 1966;1:900–902.
20. American Academy of Orthopaedic Surgeons. A position statement: prevention of hip fractures. Rosemont, IL: The American Academy of Orthopaedic Surgeons, 1993.
21. National Institutes of Health Consensus Development Conference. Statement on osteoporosis. JAMA 1984;252:799–802.
22. Lane JM, Riley EH, Wirganowicz PZ. Osteoporosis: diagnosis and treatment. J Bone Joint Surg 1996;78-A:618–632.
23. Kiel DP, Felson DT, Anderson JJ, et al. Hip fracture and the use of estrogens in postmenopausal women. The Framingham study. N Engl J Med 1987;317:1169–1174.
24. Poor G, Jacobsen SJ, Melton LJ III, et al. Mortality following hip fracture. Facts Res Gerontol 1994;7:91–109.
25. Melton LJ III, Chrischilles EA, Cooper C, et al. How many women have osteoporosis? J Bone Miner Res 1992;7:1005–1010.
26. Ray NF, Chan JK, Thamer M, et al. Medical expenditures for the treatment of osteoporotic fractures in the United States in 1995: report from the National Osteoporosis Foundation. J Bone Miner Res 1997;12: 24–35.
27. Melton LJ III. Epidemiology of spinal osteoporosis. Spine 1997;22: 2S–11S.
28. Cummings SR, Rubin SM, Black D. The future of hip fractures in the United States. Numbers, costs, and potential effects of postmenopausal estrogen. Clin Orthop 1990;252:163–166.
29. Schneider EL, Guralnik JM. The aging of America. Impact on health care costs. JAMA 1990;263:2335–2350.
30. Riggs BL, Melton LJ III. Evidence of two distinct syndromes of involutional osteoporosis. Am J Med 1983;75:899–901.
31. World Health Organization. Assessment of fracture risk and its application to screening for postmenopausal osteoporosis. Report of a World Health Organization Study Group. World Health Organ Tech Rep Ser 1994;843:1–129.
32. Kaplan FS. Prevention and management of osteoporosis. CIBA Clin Symp 1995;47:1–32.
33. Kanis JA, Melton LJ III, Christiansen C, et al. Perspective: the diagnosis of osteoporosis. J Bone Miner Res 1994;9:1137–1141.
34. Finsen V, Anda S. Accuracy of visually estimated bone mineralization in routine radiographs of the lower extremity. Skeletal Radiol 1988;17: 270–275.
35. Mayo-Smith W, Rosenthal DI. Radiographic appearance of osteopenia. Radiol Clin North Am 1991;29:37–47.
36. Glaser DL, Kaplan FS. Osteoporosis: definition and clinical presentation. Spine 1997;22:12S–16S.
37. Cohn SH, Abeisamis C, Yasumura S, et al. Comparative skeletal mass and radial bone mineral content in black and white women. Metabolism 1977;26:171–178.
38. Bikle DD, Genant HK, Cann C, et al. Bone disease in alcohol abuse. Ann Intern Med 1985;103:42–48.
39. Daniell HW. Osteoporosis of the slender smoker: vertebral compression fracture and loss of metacarpal cortex in relation to postmenopausal cigarette smoking and lack of obesity. Arch Intern Med 1976; 136:298–304.
40. Flawn LB. Amenorrhea, anorexia, and osteoporosis—the female triad. Curr Opin Orthop 1994;5:16–20.
41. Lane JM, Bernstein J. Metabolic bone disorders of the spine. In: Herkowitz HN, Garfin SR, Balderston RA, et al., eds. The spine, 4th ed. Philadelphia: WB Saunders, 1999:1259–1280.
42. Mankin HJ. Metabolic bone disease. In Jackson DW, ed. Instructional course lectures 44. Rosemont, IL: American Academy of Orthopaedic Surgeons, 1994:3–29.
43. Bostrom MPG, Boskey A, Kaufman JK, et al. Form and function of bone. In Buckwalter JA, Einhorn TA, Simon SR, eds. Orthopaedic basic science, 2nd ed. Rosemont, IL: American Academy of Orthopaedic Surgeons, 2000:320–369.
44. Price CP, Thompson PW. The role of biochemical tests in the screening and monitoring of osteoporosis. Ann Clin Biochem 1995;32:244–260.
45. Sanchez CP, Salusky IB. Biochemical markers in metabolic bone disease. Curr Opin Orthop 1994;5:66–72.
46. Grisso JA, Kelsey JL, Strom BL, et al. Risk factors for falls as a cause of hip fracture in women. The Northeast Hip Fracture Study Group. N Engl J Med 1991;324:1326–1331.
47. Cummings AR, Nevitt MC. A hypothesis: the causes of hip fractures. J Gerontol 1989;44:M107–M111.
48. Cummings AR, Nevitt MC, Browner WS, et al. Risk factors for hip fracture in white women. The Study of Osteoporotic Fractures Research Group. N Engl J Med 1995;332:767–773.

49. Matkovic V, Fontana D, Tominac C, et al. Factors that influence peak bone mass formation: a study of calcium balance and the inheritance of bone mass in adolescent females. Am J Clin Nutr 1990;52:878–888.
50. Hahn TJ. Steroid and drug-induced osteopenia. In: Favus MJ, ed. Primer on the metabolic bone diseases and disorders of mineral metabolism, 2nd ed. New York: Raven Press, 1993:250–255.
51. Meunier PH. Is steroid-induced osteoporosis preventable? N Engl J Med 1993;328:1781–1782.
52. Drinkwater BL, Grimston SK, Raab-Cullen DM, et al. ACSM position stand on osteoporosis and exercise. American College of Sports Medicine. Med Sci Sports Exerc 1995;27:745–750.
53. Madsen OR, Schaadt, O, Bliddal H, et al. Relationship between quadriceps strength and bone mineral density of the proximal tibia and distal forearm in women. J Bone Miner Res 1993;8:1439–1444.
54. Doty SB, Dicarlo EF. Pathophysiology of immobilization osteoporosis. Curr Opin Orthop 1995;6:45–49.
55. National Institutes of Health. Optimal calcium intake. NIH Consensus Statement 1994;12:1–31.
56. Chapuy MC, Arlot ME, Duboeuf F, et al. Vitamin D3 and calcium to prevent hip fractures in the elderly woman. N Engl J Med 1992;327:1637–1642.
57. Ettinger B, Genant HK, Cann CE. Long-term estrogen replacement therapy prevents bone loss and fractures. Ann Intern Med 1985;102:319–324.
58. Riis B, Thomsen K, Christiansen C. Does calcium supplementation prevent postmenopausal bone loss? A double-blind, controlled clinical study. N Engl J Med 1987;316:173–177.
59. Eriksen EF, Colvard DS, Berg NJ, et al. Evidence of estrogen receptors in normal human osteoblast-like cells. Science 1988;241:84–86.
60. Girasole G, Jilka RL, Passeri G, et al. 17 beta-estradiol inhibits interleukin-6 production by bone marrow-derived stromal cells and osteoblasts in vitro: a potential mechanism for the antiosteoporotic effect of estrogens. J Clin Invest 1992;89:883–891.
61. Pacifici R, Rifas L, McCracken R, et al. Ovarian steroid treatment blocks a postmenopausal increase in blood monocyte interleukin 1 release. Proc Nat Acad Sci 1989;86:2398–2402.
62. Horsman A, Gallagher JC, Simpson M, et al. Prospective trial of estrogen and calcium in postmenopausal women. BMJ 1977;2:789–792.
63. Hutchinson TA, Polansky SM, Feinstein AR, et al. Postmenopausal estrogens protect against fractures of hip and distal radius: a case control study. Lancet 1979;2:705–709.
64. Matthews KA, Meilahn F, Kuller LH, et al. Menopause and risk factors for coronary heart disease. N Engl J Med 1989;321:641.
65. Lane JM. Osteoporosis: medical prevention and treatment. Spine 1997;22:32S–37S.
66. Colditz GA, Egan KM, Stampfer MJ. Hormone replacement therapy and risk of breast cancer: results of epidemiologic studies. Am J Obstet Gynecol 1993;168:1473–1480.
67. Bergkvist L, Adami H, Persson I, et al. The risk of breast cancer after estrogen and estrogen-progestin replacement. N Engl J Med 1989;321:293–297.
68. Love R, Mazess RB, Barden HS, et al. Effects of tamoxifen on bone mineral density in postmenopausal women with breast cancer. N Engl J Med 1992;326:852–856.
69. Fisher B, Constantino JP, Wickerham DL, et al. Tamoxifen for prevention of breast cancer: report of the National Surgical Adjuvant Breast and Bowel Project P-1 Study. J Natl Cancer Inst 1998;90:1371–1388.
70. Ettinger B, Black DM, Mitlak BH, et al. Reduction of vertebral fracture risk in postmenopausal women with osteoporosis treated with raloxifene. Results from a 3 year randomized clinical trial. JAMA 1999;282:637–645.
71. Storm T, Steiniche T, Thamsborg G, et al. Changes in bone histomorphometry after long-term treatment with intermittent, cyclic etidronate for post-menopausal osteoporosis. J Bone Miner Res 1993;8:199–208.
72. Black DM, Cummings SR, Karpf DB, et al. Randomised trial of alendronate on risk of fracture in women with existing vertebral fractures. Lancet 1996;348:1535–1541.
73. Cummings SR, Black DM, Thompson DE, et al. Effect of alendronate on risk of fracture in women with low bone density but without vertebral fractures. Results from the Fracture Intervention Trial. JAMA 1998;280:2077–2082.
74. Rossini M, Gatti D, Zamberlan N, et al. Long-term effects of a treatment course with oral alendronate on postmenopausal osteoporosis. J Bone Miner Res 1994;9:1833–1837.
75. Harris ST, Watts NB, Genant HK, et al. Effects of risedronate treatment on vertebral and nonvertebral fractures in women with postmenopausal osteoporosis. JAMA 1999;282:1344–1352.
76. Reid IR, Brown JP, Burckhardt P, et al. Intravenous soledronic acid in postmenopausal women with low bone mineral density. N Engl J Med 2002;346:653–661.
77. Gruber HE, Ivey JL, Baylink DJ. Long-term calcitonin therapy in postmenopausal osteoporosis. Metabolism 1984;33:295–303.
78. Reginster JY, Denis D, Deroisy R, et al. Long-term (3 years) prevention of trabecular postmenopausal bone loss with low-dose intermittent nasal salmon calcitonin. J Bone Miner Res 1994;9:69–72.
79. Chesnut CH, Silverman S, Andriano K, et al. A randomized trial of nasal spray salmon calcitonin in postmenopausal women with established osteoporosis: The Prevent Recurrence of Osteoporotic Fractures Study. Am J Med 2000;109:267–276.
80. Reginster JY, Meurmans L, Deroisy R, et al. A 5-year controlled randomized study of prevention of postmenopausal trabecular bone loss with nasal salmon calcitonin and calcium. Eur J Clin Invest 1994;24:565–569.
81. Gennari C, Agnusdei D, Camporeale A. Use of calcitonin in the treatment of bone pain associated with osteoporosis. Calcif Tissue Int 1991;49:9S–13S.
82. Simonen O, Laitinen O. Does fluoridation of drinking water prevent bone fragility and osteoporosis? Lancet 1985;2:432–434.
83. Pak CY, Sakhaee K, Adams-Huet B, et al. Treatment of postmenopausal osteoporosis with slow-release sodium fluoride. Final report of a randomized controlled trial. Ann Intern Med 1995;123:401–408.
84. Riggs BL, Hodgson SF, O'Fallon WM, et al. Effect of fluoride treatment on the fracture rate in postmenopausal women with osteoporosis. N Engl J Med 1990;322:802–809.
85. Riggs BL, O'Fallon WM, Lane A, et al. Clinical trial of fluoride therapy in postmenopausal osteoporotic women: extended observations and additional analysis. J Bone Miner Res 1994;96:265–275.

CHAPTER 72

Surgical Options and Indications: Kyphoplasty and Vertebroplasty

Christopher M. Bono, Christopher P. Kauffman, and Steven R. Garfin

Osteoporosis is an increasingly recognized cause of fractures in the lumbar spine in the postmenopausal and older adult population (1–6). Women are more commonly affected (7), though men are also subject to the sequelae of progressive bone loss (8,9). Histologically, osteoporotic bone is normal, with a decreased amount of bone per volumetric unit caused by an imbalance between bone production and resorption (10). In contrast to osteomalacia, mineralization is unaltered. Though newer pharmacologic agents offer a promising future for the treatment and prevention of osteoporosis, they will have minimal impact on vast numbers of individuals with already advanced disease (11).

Decreased bone mineral density is related to skeletal weakening. Although all bones are affected, some regions are at greater fracture risk. The spine is the most commonly affected area, followed by the distal radius and proximal femur (7). Osteoporotic vertebral compression fractures (VCFs) are most common in the upper lumbar and lower thoracic spine (9,12). While injuries of the wrist and hip are clinically apparent, osteoporotic spine fractures are frequently asymptomatic. Often, however, they can be a troubling source of back pain, and potentiate medical morbidity and mortality. Multiple, consecutive VCFs are common in untreated individuals, leading to numerous levels of vertebral body (VB) height loss. This can lead to progressive anterior column shortening, resulting in thoracolumbar kyphosis, which can lead to functional disability, pulmonary compromise, and eating disorders, such as early satiety, in an older adult population that is likely to have many concomitant comorbidities (1,3–5).

VB augmentation has been developed to help treat osteoporotic VCFs. Currently available techniques are vertebroplasty and kyphoplasty. Vertebroplasty was first introduced in the mid- 1980s and involves direct injection of polymethylmethacrylate (PMMA) cement into the VB

(13). Cement fills the interstices of the cancellous bone under high pressure and hardens during final curing. It restores near normal stiffness and surpasses normal vertebral strength (14,15). Clinical reports of long-standing pain relief have demonstrated its effectiveness in treating symptomatic VCFs (16–19). Despite these positive attributes, vertebroplasty lacks the ability to restore VB height to a compressed segment.

Sagittal deformity (i.e., kyphosis) related to osteoporotic VCFs can lead to functional and respiratory impairment, as well biomechanically predispose the spine to further fractures (1,3). Thus, interest in minimally invasive methods of fracture reduction and stabilization has arisen. Kyphoplasty was developed in the early 1990s to fulfill these demands. Still in its infancy, it involves percutaneous insertion of an inflatable bone tamp into the VB to restore height (20,21). Cement is then injected under low pressure into the cavity created by the tamp; higher pressures are required for vertebroplasty. Preliminary clinical data indicate consistent restoration of vertebral height in addition to durable pain relief in over 90% of cases with low complication rates (20,21).

Both kyphoplasty and vertebroplasty are effective treatments of painful osteoporotic VCFs, with the former giving the added benefit of fracture reduction and deformity correction. Successful use of these techniques in the lumbar spine relies on a clear understanding of their indications, applications, complications, and outcomes.

INDICATIONS

Kyphoplasty

Pain Relief

Kyphoplasty is indicated for progressive or intractable pain associated with an osteoporotic VCF. Clinical data suggest more than 90% pain relief (20,21). The mode of relief remains speculative, though most believe it is fracture stabilization. Some hold that bony denervation from the heat produced during cement curing might contribute, though this remains conjectural.

Successful use of kyphoplasty requires that the practitioner first determine if the symptoms are genuinely originating from the VCF. The reliability of subjective reporting alone is limited, as complaints of chronic back pain might be related to other causes. Objective evidence that the vertebrae in question are the cause of pain must be sought. This is suggested by point tenderness on percussion of the spine that correlates with the fractured level on plain radiographs. If pain and tenderness are more generalized, this determination is difficult based on plain films alone, and other advanced imaging methods can be helpful. Magnetic resonance imaging (MRI) and bone scintigraphy can be used to gauge the acuteness of the injury (22,23). A positive signal on bone scan has been correlated with good pain relief after vertebral augmentation (22). It is likely that MRI is of similar use, though this remains to be demonstrated in a clinical study.

Pulmonary Function

VCFs have significant negative effects on pulmonary function (1,24). By measuring forced expiratory volume and resting vital capacities, Schlaich et al. (1) reported a strong correlation between the severity of kyphosis and decreases in lung capacity. Kado et al. (24) reported higher mortality rates secondary to pulmonary complications in patients with kyphotic VCFs versus those without deformity. It is not presently known if the converse relationship is true (i.e., if correction of the deformity reverses or prevents these effects). However, it is reasonable to assume that kyphoplasty may favorably affect pulmonary function of correctable osteoporotic kyphosis. Further study of the specific effects of kyphoplasty on postcorrection pulmonary function is warranted.

Deformity

Kyphoplasty is a relatively new technique. As a deformity correcting procedure, its indications must adhere to basic principles. Surgeons may be tempted to perform kyphoplasty on any, and every, VCF. Consideration of spinal balance and deformity progression is a more prudent measure. Though initial reports suggest its relative safety, further investigation is required to more clearly demonstrate a positive balance between the potential benefits of kyphosis correction versus procedural complications.

For both metabolic and mechanical reasons, the risk of subsequent VCFs increases with each additional injury. Realignment may help reduce the incidence of further fractures. Acute fractures (less than 3 months old) are more easily reduced than chronic ones (21). Although correction in VCFs one year or more after fracture have been obtained, this is difficult to predict. Severe, rigid deformities from multiple healed fractures that compromise function or quality of life might be better addressed by other surgical methods, if necessary. If detected radiographically, progressive collapse, even if not severely painful, is also an indication for kyphoplasty.

Vertebroplasty

The indications for vertebroplasty are limited to the treatment of pain associated with VCFs. Numerous series have documented high rates (90% to 95%) of pain relief in patients after vertebroplasty (16–19). Though it has been suggested that some vertebral height restoration can be obtained by positioning in the prone position with early fractures, this has not been substantiated in a clinical series. Fracture reduction cannot be considered an indication for this procedure. It is unlikely that vertebroplasty would have a direct impact on pulmonary function, as the deformities will be "fixed", although restoration of ambulation and mobility have positive effects on overall health. Kyphotic deformity related to osteoporotic VCFs cannot be considered an indication for vertebroplasty at this time.

CONTRAINDICATIONS

The contraindications for both kyphoplasty and vertebroplasty are similar. They are contraindicated in stable, healed, nonpainful fractures. They are also not indicated in the presence of infection. Associated medical problems can make the procedures dangerous. Coagulopathy can lead to epidural hematoma with VB cannulation, especially if the pedicle borders or posterior VB have been breached. At this time, a burst fracture pattern with retropulsed fragments is a relative contraindication to kyphoplasty or vertebroplasty, though some surgeons have used kyphoplasty in selected cases. In some situations such as vertebral plana, these procedures may not be technically possible because of inability to cannulate the VB due to severe vertebral compression. At present, it is also not used for traumatic, nonosteoporotic fractures in young individuals.

BIOMECHANICS AND BASIC SCIENCE

Osteoporotic VCFs are the result of alterations of the bone's mechanical or structural properties. Strength is diminished by decreases in quantity, while bone quality is unaffected. The proportion of mineral to bone matrix is physiologic, as a histologic sample would appear normal. The extent of osteoporosis can be assessed by measuring bone mineral density. Substantially low bone mineral density is associated with a predisposition to VCF with low-energy mechanisms.

VBs bear the majority of the axial compressive forces sustained by the spine. Flexion movements increase these forces. If they exceed the bone's capacity to resist them, fracture results. In its first stage, fractures involve the anterior aspect of the VB (i.e., anterior column). Flexion-compression fractures usually do not involve the posterior VB wall. With additional force, fracture lines can propagate into the middle column, creating a burst fracture. Alternatively, osteoporotic burst fractures can occur from pure axial loading, which might occur from a fall from height or other higher energy mechanism. These often fracture the posterior wall, and perhaps the posterior elements.

After VCF, the bone is weakened and compressed. Treatment can be directed at one or both of these problems. Medical management of osteoporosis addresses bone weakness by changing the metabolic balance of bone deposition and resorption. Agents such as alendronate, estrogen, and calcitonin have proven clinical efficacy in this manner (11). Though they are systemic treatments that affect the entire skeleton, they have limited effects on fracture risk in advanced cases.

Vertebroplasty and kyphoplasty address the bone fragility problem, but in a much more direct way than medical treatments. By injecting cement into the bone, mechanical properties are restored. Stiffness is defined as the slope of a force versus displacement curve and represents the elasticity of bone prior to permanent deformation. Strength is a reflection of the force required to permanently deform a specimen (25). Studies done in vitro have demonstrated that both stiffness and strength are affected with osteoporosis (14,15,25). As osteopenic bone is severely compromised, the mechanical properties of the augmented VCF are virtually entirely that of the bone cement. Thus, choice of bone filler (cement) affects the biomechanical effects of kyphoplasty and vertebroplasty.

Not all bone cements are equal. Different substances cause different changes in strength and stiffness. Orthocomp (Orthovita, Malvern, PA) has demonstrated significantly stronger and stiffer vertebrae than Simplex P (Howmedica, Rutherford, NJ) after in vitro vertebroplasty of human cadaveric osteopenic lumbar spinal segments (15). While Simplex P resulted in less stiffness than prefractured specimens, Orthocomp restored initial stiffness values. Similarly, other commonly used materials, such as cranioplastic cement (CMW, Blackpool, England) have demonstrated greater strength but lower stiffness than intact specimens (14). Other variables, such as the cement powder/monomer ratio and addition of media (e.g., barium) to increase the cement radiopacity, can alter material properties. The long-term clinical implications of these variables on augmentation durability remain to be seen (26). Additionally, it is not known how much strength is needed to support the osteoporotic bone and spinal column.

The volume of cement injected can influence mechanical properties after vertebral augmentation. In addition to cement viscosity, the method of injection can be a factor. In most cases a bilateral approach is recommended with kyphoplasty, while in some cases only unilateral injection might be possible. Bilateral injection maximizes cement delivery. Data from in vitro studies indicate significantly greater strength with bipedicular injection of 10 mL (5 mL on each side) versus unipedicular injection of 6 mL of cement in the lumbar spine (25). Interestingly, both methods resulted in restoration of initial stiffness.

Restoration of near normal levels of strength and stiffness is thought to be preferable. This procedure has limited use, however, because it is not clear what "normal" is in the osteoporotic spine. Osteoporotic VBs are weaker and more brittle than healthy specimens. In recent biomechanical studies cement augmentation resulted in strength greater than that of the prefractured state, while initial stiffness values were not exceeded. This is probably optimal. If augmentation had only restored, but not exceeded, the prefractured strength, it would have a similar risk of fracture as other osteoporotic vertebrae. However, if stiffer, it might act like a walnut in a column of banana slices, thereby increasing the chance of an adjacent segment fracture with slight compression.

Sagittal Balance

Kyphoplasty is a tool to treat pain and deformity through fracture reduction. As such, its indications should be subject to the same rigors as other methods of open surgical treatment. This relies on an understanding of the fundamental biomechanical principles of deformity correction.

The vertebral column is naturally contoured in the sagittal plane, while normally straight in the coronal plane. Sagittal contour is achieved by a combination of cervical and lumbar lordosis with intervening thoracic kyphosis. These curvatures are radiographically measured statically and represent the spine in a standing weight-bearing state. The thoracic spine normally has an average of 30° of kyphosis, with an approximate range of 20° to 40° (27). The apex of normal thoracic curvature is at T6 or T7. Thoracic kyphosis is produced primarily from anterior wedging of the VBs. Anterior and posterior disc heights are normally equal. The rib cage is an integral component in the stability of the thoracic spine providing an additional restraint to axial motion through costovertebral junctions. The lumbar spine is in lordosis, which is primarily produced by discs that are taller anteriorly than posteriorly. Average lumbar lordosis is approximately 50°, with values ranging from 30° to 80°.

Cervical, thoracic, and lumbar curvatures must be considered in concert. Together, they attempt to achieve vertebral balance. Sagittal balance can be assessed on a full-length lateral radiograph by dropping a vertical plumb line from the base of the occiput. Balance is realized if that line intersects the seventh cervical VB cranially and lies within 1 cm of the sacral promontory caudally. Mechanically, this ensures that the weight borne by the resting spine is acting to maintain its position within space. Relatively hyperkyphotic segments can be balanced by compensatory hyperlordosis in other segments. This carries the weight-bearing line back to its balanced position at the sacral promontory, which is centered over the hips.

Though compensation is common in other sagittal deformities, osteoporosis is usually characterized by uncompensated thoracic and lumbar kyphosis secondary to VCFs in both regions. These sagittal deformities can progress to a point at which the weight-bearing line can no longer return to its balanced position. This results in a self-propagating sagittal imbalance. To illustrate this, one can compare the hyperkyphotic spine to the Tower of Pisa. Balance is maintained if the center of mass lies within the boundaries of the base. Thus, the weight of the tower (or spine) functions to maintain its current position. However, if the tower leans over so much that the center of mass lies outside its base, the weight of the tower will cause it to fall. Corrective measures in deformity treatment attempt to restore the weight-bearing line or center of mass of the body to the anatomic base, which is the sacral promontory.

By increasing VB height at one or more levels, kyphoplasty can achieve this goal. Claims of vertebroplasty's ability to restore some vertebral height are unsupported in clinical trials, though some *in vitro* data suggest that as much as 28% can be regained with high-pressure injection (28). Laboratory investigations have demonstrated an average of 96% height restoration after kyphoplasty (28). Clinically, less height is gained if the procedure is performed more than 3 months after the fracture occurs (assuming the fracture correlates with pain onset). In an ongoing multicenter study, anterior and midline vertebral height was restored to within 99% and 92% of predicted dimensions, respectively, if performed less than 3 months after fracture occurrence (21).

Planning and Preoperative Assessment

History

Focus is initially on the disease course. Patients should be asked about prior workup, including results of bone densitometry (if performed), medications, and any surgery for extremity fractures. Careful evaluation by a primary care physician is helpful, as most patients have one or more comorbidities. Differential diagnoses must not be overlooked. Fevers and other constitutional symptoms can suggest infection or malignancy. A multidisciplinary approach is important, including internists, endocrinologists, and a spine surgeon.

Duration and location of pain are important factors in treatment decision making. Pain that follows an incident of low-energy trauma, such as a twist, exuberant cough, lifting a grocery bag, or opening a door suggests a VCF. The pain might be sharp and localized to one level, or dull and radiating to a number of levels. If the pain is resolving and the fracture is healing uneventfully, vertebral augmentation may not be indicated. Painless, progressive collapse, however, might be considered for reduction with kyphoplasty. A history of frequent falls may be an indicator of decompensated sagittal balance. This represents the patient's inability to overcome the forward shift of the center of gravity. Questions concerning intestinal bloating and appetite suppression are important, as this can occur with severe kyphosis from decreased abdominal volume.

Physical Examination

If the pain has not restricted the patient to a chair, initial examination should include observing the patient walking. Severe kyphotic deformities can lead to spinal imbalance. Some patients begin to trip because of forward shift of the center of gravity, and may eventually require a walker to safely ambulate. Some are in wheelchairs because of the pain with activity. Limb-length inequalities and scoliotic deformities can alter coronal balance, which may influence decisions regarding correction. Assessment of the symmetry of chest wall expansion with inspiration can be used as a rough estimate of pulmonary function. Minimal chest expansion can also broaden the differential diagnosis to include other conditions causing spinal deformities, such as ankylosing spondylitis. Complete neurologic examination, including normal and pathologic reflexes, is requisite.

Each spinous process is then systematically percussed for tenderness, symmetry, and step-off. Optimally, percussion at a single level will be painful with nontender adjacent segments. This strongly suggests an acute fracture at that level as the major source of pain. More often, numerous levels are painful, making determination of the most symptomatic segments challenging.

Plain Radiography

High-quality anteroposterior (AP) and lateral plain radiographs are first-line imaging modalities. Taping a radiopaque marker, such as a paper clip, to the point of maximal tenderness prior to taking radiographs can help identify symptomatic fractured regions. Sites of VB compression are visualized and Cobb angles measured. The anterior vertebral height is measured and compared to the posterior vertebral height to determine the percent of height loss. If the vertebra is uniformly compressed, height measurements are compared to those of adjacent vertebrae. Though a useful preoperative tool, plain films are limited in their ability to differentiate fracture age. Furthermore, fractures through the middle column (i.e., burst types) are difficult to detect because of the washed-out appearance of the osteopenic bone. For these reasons, advanced imaging modalities are strongly recommended.

Advanced Imaging

Treating physicians should obtain an MRI before deciding to perform kyphoplasty or vertebroplasty. MRI provides coronal, sagittal, and axial views of the vertebra, disc, spinal canal, and neural elements. Retropulsion is easily detected, as are epidural hematomas. Neoplasms and infections are better differentiated from VCFs with MRI than plain films. Spinal cord pathology including tumors and syringes can be visualized. Perhaps the greatest use of MRI before kyphoplasty is the ability to detect bone edema within the VB. This is an indication of the acuteness of the fracture. It must be noted, however, that increased signal intensity on T2-weighted images (i.e., edema) can remain for up to 2 years following an injury, even in clinically healed fractures. T2 images are better than T1 images in detecting bone edema, while STIR (short-time inversion recovery) images are best to differentiate malignant from benign osteoporotic fractures.

Computed tomography (CT) is useful to evaluate the bone. This study is often more helpful than MRI to differentiate tumors and infections from osteoporotic fractures. It also shows bone "quality" and defects. Another advantage of CT scan is that it is fast and readily obtainable. Often patients may not tolerate lying in the supine position for the extended period necessary with an MRI. They have decreased tolerance secondary to pain, CHF, and kyphotic deformity. In these individuals, CT may be necessary in place of MRI.

Bone scans can also be helpful in preoperative planning. By comparing the uptake at fractured versus adjacent nonfractured vertebrae, bone scans have proven highly predictive of pain relief after vertebral augmentation (22). Drawbacks include high radiation exposure and poor bony detail. For individuals in whom MRI is contraindicated, a CT combined with bone scan is a reasonable alternative to MRI.

SURGICAL TECHNIQUE: KYPHOPLASTY

General and local anesthesia both have been used with success. General anesthesia may be more appropriate for patients undergoing multiple levels of kyphoplasty, though local anesthetic with sedation is suitable for one or two segment procedures. If general anesthesia is chosen, the patient is induced and intubated in the supine position and then logrolled prone onto a radiolucent table. Patients should be positioned on transverse rolls across the chest and thighs/iliac crests, to extend the spine and help reduce the fracture.

Adequate visualization with an image intensifier (C-arm) should be done before the procedure is initiated. The pedicle and VB should be seen clearly on posteroanterior (PA), lateral, and *en face* views. The pedicle can be viewed *en face* by angling the beam 10° toward the midline. This approximates the posterolateral to anteromedial direction of the pedicle producing an end-on appearance. Cannulation with a spinal needle should appear as a perfectly centered ring in the *en face* view. If the surgeon is confident in visualization of these landmarks, the procedure may proceed. The patient is prepped and draped in the usual sterile fashion.

Approaches

There are three different methods of gaining access to the VB: transpedicular, extrapedicular, and posterolateral approaches. The extrapedicular approach is useful only in the thoracic spine and will not be discussed in this chapter, while the posterolateral approach is useful in the lumbar spine. The transpedicular technique is preferred and may be used at any level.

Transpedicular Approach

This is the preferred approach for the L1 to L5 level (Fig. 72-1). It requires a pedicle diameter of at least 4 to 5 mm. Some lumbar vertebrae are too small to safely accept the kyphoplasty instruments. Preoperative measurements on axial MRI or CT images are helpful in making this determination ahead of time. Both pedicles can be instrumented using the transpedicular approach. This approach endangers the spinal cord medially and the

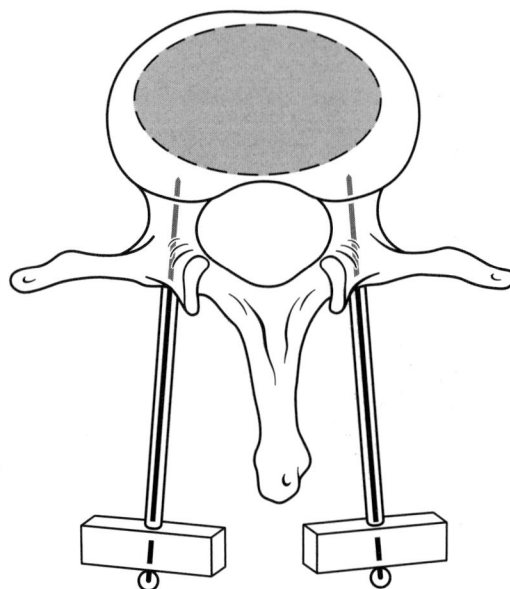

FIG. 72-1. The path of the instruments using the transpedicular approach.

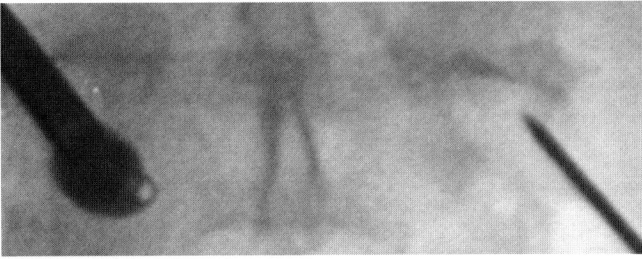

FIG. 72-2. The tip of the guidewire can be used to localize the point of insertion for the Jamshidi needle. In this case, the contralateral balloon tamp has already been placed. The guidewire tip lies directly over the center of the pedicle.

nerve root superiorly and inferiorly if the pedicle is missed or its cortex violated.

The spinous processes are palpated in the midline and the correct level of surgery is marked. This is confirmed on orthogonal views. In the PA view, the skin is marked just lateral to the lateral border of the pedicle. A spinal needle (Jamshidi needle) or guide pin is then introduced through a 1 cm longitudinal incision, angling approximately 10° toward the midline (Fig. 72-2). Needle location is then checked on a lateral to ensure proper orientation toward the pedicle center. Optimal radiographic appearance is the needle tip within the confines of the pedicle at all times. The C-arm is then moved to the *en face* or lateral position, and the needle is advanced under visual and tactile guidance.

The needle is inserted until the resistance of bone is felt. This may be difficult to discern because of the decreased bone density. With confirmation on all radiographic views, the needle is advanced to the posterior cortex of the VB. Once the needle is within the VB on the lateral view, it will appear slightly medial to the pedicle on the PA view (Fig. 72-3). As a general rule, the tip

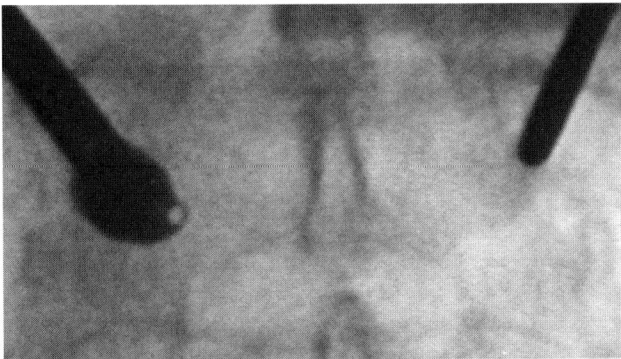

FIG. 72-3. After marking the proper insertion site, the Jamshidi needle is then percutaneously inserted into the skin. It is advanced through the soft tissues to lie on top of the bone. By localizing on anteroposterior and lateral views, the needle is inserted into the pedicle. It is angled slightly medial, to match the orientation of the pedicle. Although the needle tip is entirely contained within the pedicle, once it has passed the pedicle-body junction it may appear just medial to the pedicle.

should not cross the midline on the PA view at any point during insertion. If it does cross over to the contralateral side, careful investigation with a high quality *en face* view must confirm containment within the pedicle. Repositioning of the instrument should be considered if proper location cannot be ascertained.

The needle can be cranially or caudally directed through the pedicle, targeting toward a particular region of the VB. With compression of the superior end plate, the tool is directed toward the inferior half. Conversely, the needle is directed toward the superior half of the VB with compression fractures of the inferior end plate. This allows a greater amount of cancellous bone to be compressed beneath the fractured end plate. Cranial/caudal orientation is judged on the lateral view. If the vertebra is uniformly compressed the tool is advanced toward the mid-body.

Posterolateral Approach

This technique is useful for kyphoplasty of the L2 to L4 vertebrae. It enters the VB through its posterolateral cortex, anterior to the transverse process (Fig. 72-4). The pedicle is not cannulated at any time. The skin entry point is different than the transpedicular approach. It lies 8 to 10 cm lateral to the midline, similar to that for a discogram. The needle is directed approximately 45° toward the midline. The *en face* view is not useful with this approach. Instead, the lateral view is more critical. The needle should lie anterior to the transverse process and neural foramen, thus avoiding injury to the exiting nerve root. Because this method can only be performed unilaterally, the needle must cross the midline to ensure adequate augmentation of the contralateral aspect of the VB.

Bone Tamp Insertion

The center stylet is removed from the Jamshidi needle after confirmation of the position. A flexible guide pin is then inserted through the needle bore. The starting device (Jamshidi) is carefully removed with a twisting motion, maintaining the guidewire position within the vertebra. A centering stylet is passed over the guide pin to dilate the channel, followed by an outer cannula, which serves as the working channel. The guide pin and centering stylet can then be removed. A finger-held twist drill bit is introduced and advanced slowly to the anterior cortex of the VB. As the bone is soft, this must be performed under radiographic guidance to avoid penetration of the cortex. These steps are repeated on the opposite pedicle.

The drill bit is then removed while holding the working channel in position and the balloon tamp is inserted through the cannula. Different balloon sizes are available. The appropriate size can be determined on preoperative radiographs or MRI. In general, lumbar vertebrae can accommodate a large (20 to 25 mm) tamp.

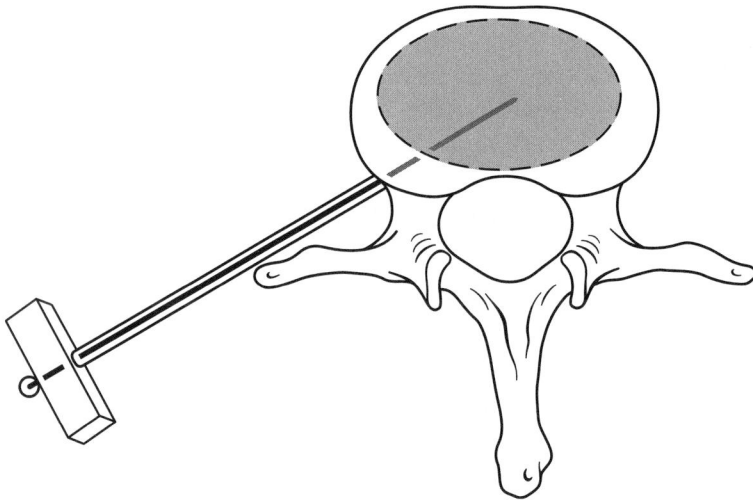

FIG. 72-4. The path of the instruments using the posterolateral approach.

The balloon tamp has several important features that should be noted. Instead of being a concentrically formed sphere, the balloon is narrowed at its midpoint. This effectively creates anterior and posterior tamps that can more uniformly fill the space within the compressed vertebra. This enables "en masse" reduction of the fractured end plate. In addition, radiopaque markers located on both sides of the balloon make its ends visible on fluoroscopy. This facilitates positioning of the bone tamp, which should be centered within the VB. The tamp is then inflated under controlled pressure, using a digital manometer, with a radiopaque dye (Fig. 72-5). Pressures should initially be low and then gradually increase as the balloon meets the resistance of the cancellous bone. Pressures can intermittently drop and rise again, representing "giving" of the end plates and, hopefully, reduction. Sudden and persistent drop in pressure suggests rupture of the balloon and warrants inspection of the device before

proceeding further. Volumes are also monitored to estimate the approximate quantity of cement needed to fill the bone void. Fracture reduction is judged on the lateral C-arm view. Up to 99% of predicted height can be restored if performed within 2 to 3 months of the onset of the fracture. However, this may vary and is not always related to fracture acuteness.

Cement Composition

The suggested formula for bone cement used during kyphoplasty includes PMMA, barium sulfate, and antibiotic powder. For consistency during each use, it is suggested that the surgeon use the same formula so as to minimize differences in curing time and consistency of cement. The following formula has been used successfully in practice: PMMA powder 40 cc, liquid monomer 10 cc, barium sulfate 6 g and antibiotic powder. Antibiotics that are heat stabile include cefazolin (1 g), vancomycin (1 g), and tobramycin (1.2 g).

Cement Delivery

The balloon tamp is deflated and removed while the working cannula is held in place. Several 3 cc syringes filled with a medium viscosity cement mixture of PMMA, barium, and antibiotic powder are prepared. These are used to fill several bone filler devices. In particularly unstable fractures, a contralateral tamp can remain inflated to maintain reduction while cement is injected ipsilaterally. Once the cement thickens to the desired consistency, the bone filler tubes are placed through the working cannula into the cavity in the VB. A stylet is then used to gently push the cement until the cavity created is filled (Fig. 72-6A,B). All steps at this point are followed fluoroscopically. Cement is injected under low pressure until one of the following occurs: cement has filled the anterior two-thirds of the VB, cement

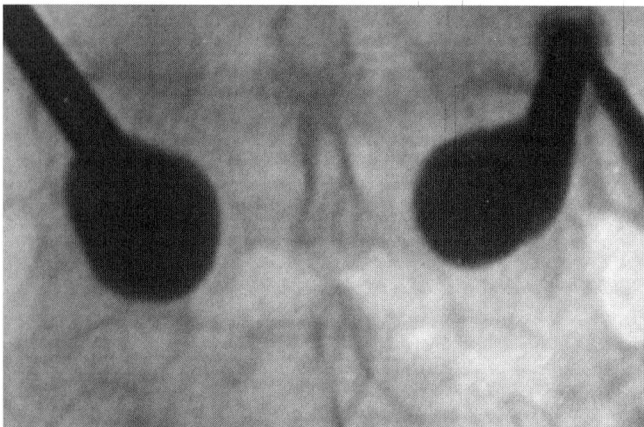

FIG. 72-5. The balloon tamps are inserted and inflated. On the anteroposterior view, the surgeon must be aware of lateral breakout of the tamp through the wall of the vertebral body. This intraoperative radiograph shows excellent orientation of two tamps being inflated simultaneously.

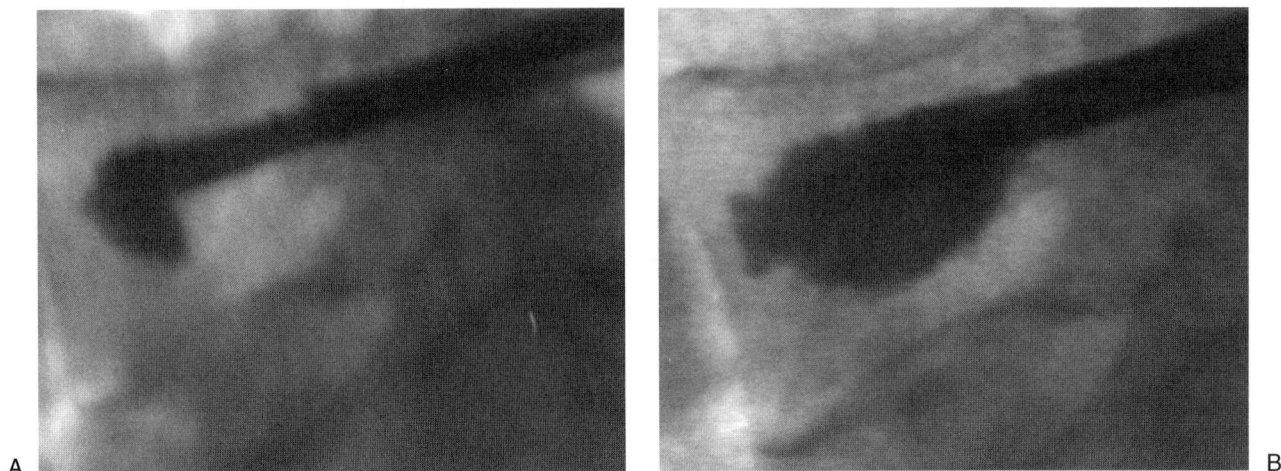

FIG. 72-6. A, B: The cement is then pushed into the vertebral body under low pressure. In these lateral radiographs, it can be seen that the body is filled anterior to posterior. This is facilitated by creation of the bone void, which allows the surgeon essentially to "pour" the cement into the vertebra.

begins leaking through the VB, or it starts to fill the posterior aspect of the body or pedicle. Cement leakage through the vertebra may occur with mixtures that are too fluid. In this case, injection can be temporarily stopped, allowing the peripheral cement to begin to cure. Then, injection is resumed into the vertebra, which has sealed off its leaks. The process is repeated on the contralateral side. Typically, 2 to 6 mL of cement can be injected on each side.

During injection, possible cement extrusion should be monitored on image intensification. In most cases cement extrusion has little clinical sequelae. Cement curing can take from 5 to 10 minutes and is affected by mixture proportion, room temperature, and product brand. Once the cement is hardened, the cannula and bone filler device are twisted to dissociate it from the surrounding PMMA and carefully removed. Final radiographs are used to confirm cement placement, fracture reduction, and restoration of alignment. The patient should remain in the prone position for 10 minutes to ensure final hardening in the reduced position.

SURGICAL TECHNIQUE: VERTEBROPLASTY

The setup and approach for vertebroplasty are similar to those for kyphoplasty. General or local anesthesia may be used. The techniques for cannulation of the VB are also similar. Vertebrograms can be performed before cement placement by injection of radiopaque dye through the working cannula. This gives an estimation of the path of least resistance, and thus, the most likely path of the cement. If enhancement of a nearby vessel occurs, the needle is moved to another position and retested. Mathis et al. (29) described three approaches: transpedicular, parapedicular (akin to extrapedicular), and posterolateral. The authors warn, however, of higher incidence of

cement leakage using posterolateral approaches in the lumbar spine. Leakage is probably more frequent with vertebroplasty than kyphoplasty because of the less viscous cement consistency required. In our experience, the posterolateral approach for kyphoplasty does not appear to be associated with a greater incidence of cement leakage.

Cement delivery is through a syringe filled with 2 to 3 mL of liquid PMMA cement attached to the cannulation needle. As with kyphoplasty, VB fill is monitored radiographically using the C-arm. Once cement has reached the posterior aspect of the VB, injection is stopped. The syringe is then removed, and the stylet is replaced into the needle to avoid leaving a "tail" of cement. Vertebroplasty can be performed unilaterally or bilaterally. Deramond et al. (30) recommend performing a unilateral vertebroplasty first. If adequate fill of more than 50% of the VB is achieved, this may be adequate. However, if less than 50% VB fill occurs, than contralateral augmentation is recommended. Biomechanical studies comparing unilateral versus bilateral cement injections have indicated comparable restoration of strength and stiffness with both methods (25).

POSTOPERATIVE CARE

Kyphoplasty or vertebroplasty can be performed as a same day procedure. Blood loss is minimal, and pain relief is often apparent within 24 hours. If general anesthesia is used, an overnight stay might be considered in these often older adult patients. Narcotic pain medication is usually not necessary for more than 2 days postoperatively, after which pain can be managed with extrastrength acetaminophen or nonsteroidal antiinflammatory drugs (NSAIDs). Bracing is usually not recommended. In most cases, some avoidance of heavy

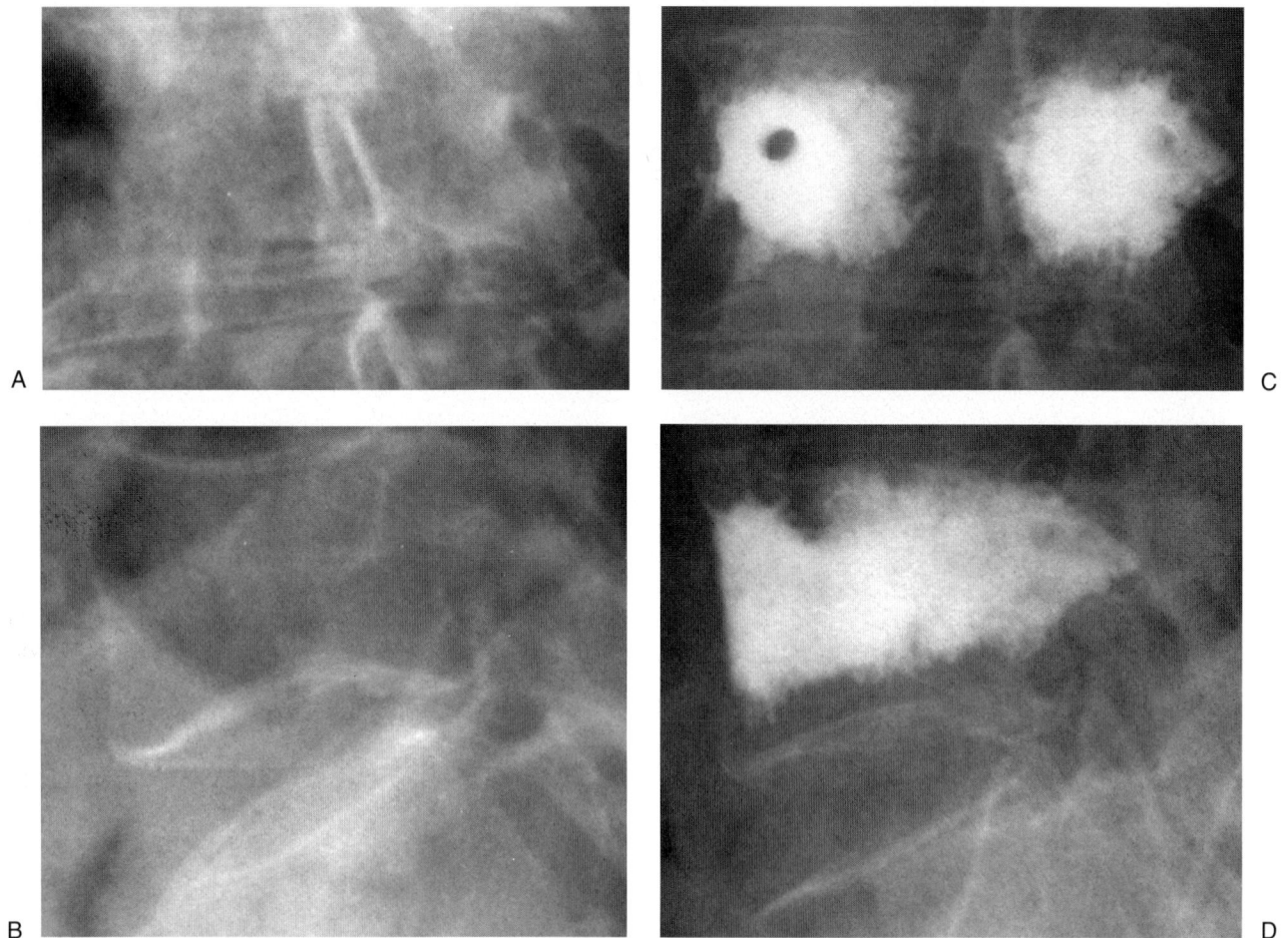

FIG. 72-7. A–D: Preoperative and postoperative radiographs after an L5 kyphoplasty. Note on the postoperative lateral view that cement was inserted until it reached the posterior border of the vertebral body. A small amount of cement entered the pedicle. This is a benign event and should not be considered extravasation. No extravasation into the spinal canal is seen. The small concentric holes noted on the anteroposterior view are the voids where the working cannulae were in place. This can be avoided by pulling the cannulae back to the pedicle-body junction during cement curing.

lifting for a few weeks is helpful for pain control and to avoid further fracture in patients who were forced to lead a sedentary lifestyle because of the pain. Follow-up radiographs should be obtained 1 month postprocedure, and repeated as indicated by the clinical picture (Fig. 72-7A–D). Radiographic follow-up may be considered for 1 year because of the propensity for subsequent fractures.

PROBLEMS AND COMPLICATIONS

The complication rate after kyphoplasty is very low. In a recent multicenter study clinical complications occurred in 1.2% of patients and 0.7% of fractures (20,21). The most common technical complication is cement leakage. This may occur in up to 8.6% of cases. These are infrequently associated with clinical sequelae. However, in both vertebroplasty and kyphoplasty neurologic deficit has been observed secondary to cement extrusion into the canal or neural foramina (21,31).

The most common clinical complication of vertebral augmentation is transient pyrexia (30). This is most likely from a mild systemic reaction to the cement. From available data, it appears to be more frequent after vertebroplasty than kyphoplasty. This may be related to the pressure of injection. As with joint arthroplasty, cement injection can also lead to mild intraoperative hypotension, though this has not been reported after kyphoplasty. Anticoagulation, if used by the patient, should be delayed for at least 4 days to avoid epidural hematoma formation.

Outcomes

Kyphoplasty

The senior author has had the opportunity to take part in evaluating an ongoing collection of kyphoplasty cases performed for osteoporotic VCFs. Early detailed evaluation of over 375 procedures has been reported. The results are extremely encouraging. At up to 18 months' follow-up, over 90% of patients reported symptomatic relief and functional improvement. Anterior and midline vertebral height was restored to within 99% and 92% of predicted dimensions, respectively. These results were highly consistent between centers and technicians. Only four clinical complications occurred. In one case, transient pyrexia was associated with a brief episode of intraoperative hypoxia after cement injection. We believe this was related to the cement being in too liquid a state. The patient's blood pressure quickly rebounded with no further complications. In another case an epidural hematoma developed after heparin anticoagulation had been initiated just 8 hours after the procedure. Anticoagulant administration should be delayed for 4 days. Two patients sustained neurologic complications. One developed an anterior cord syndrome after a thoracic vertebra had been augmented through an extrapedicular approach. In reexamining the preoperative MRI, there was an unrecognized fracture at the junction of the pedicle and VB, as the body was below the pedicle. The other neurologic complication was a case in which paraplegia resulted after cement extrusion into the spinal canal. This was secondary to improper needle placement with violation of the pedicle wall, and was not related to the inflatable bone tamp itself. The patient had paraparesis of the lower extremities, which responded somewhat to emergent laminectomy and decompression of the spinal cord. Deficits are most likely related to mechanical compression of the neural structures as experimental data has demonstrated little chance of thermal damage with cement hardening. All three major complications occurred within the first 100 fractures treated. These led to technique modifications. None have occurred since then.

Vertebroplasty

Numerous clinical reports of the results of vertebroplasty have been published. Barr et al. (17) retrospectively documented 95% marked or moderate pain relief in 38 patients treated for osteoporotic compression fractures. In contrast, only 50% of cases treated for metastatic lesions had substantial relief. The only neurologic complication was a case of T3 radiculitis that resolved with oral steroids.

In a similar retrospective analysis, Grados et al. (16) reported pain relief in 24 of 25 patients 1 month after the procedure. The authors used a percutaneous technique under general or local anesthesia. Unfortunately, they did not report immediate postprocedural pain relief, limiting the distinction between vertebroplasty's effects and eventual fracture healing. Two cases of transitory radiculitis treated with NSAIDs resolved. Seven cases of cement leakage into the disc space were noted on postoperative radiographs. Asymptomatic cement embolism to the lungs occurred in one patient. After an average of 48

months' follow-up, 34 new vertebral fractures occurred in 13 patients. The risk of fracture adjacent to a previously augmented level was higher than at other sites.

Heini et al. (18) performed percutaneous vertebroplasty under local anesthesia and sedation in 17 patients with 45 fractures. All patients reported significant pain relief at 1 day, 12 weeks, and 1 year after the procedure. Two patients sustained an additional fracture. The authors' rate of cement extrusion was high, with five cases of leakage into the paravertebral muscles, two cases into the spinal canal, and one case into a segmental spinal vein. However, no clinical complications were related to cement extrusion.

In response to a case of permanent nerve root deficit related to cement extrusion into the spinal canal, Wenger and Markwalder (19) performed open vertebroplasty in nine patients with osteoporotic compression fractures. Posterior cement leakage was removed under direct visualization in four cases. Interestingly, one fracture extended into the posterior VB cortex, but no PMMA leakage occurred. Internal fixation with pedicle screws was used to reinforce correction of a patient with multiple adjacent fractures. Pain relief was reported in all patients. One patient developed subsequent fractures that necessitated augmentation.

Other reported complications from vertebroplasty are transitory fever, temporary worsening of fracture pain, infection, and rib fracture (32–36). Spinal cord compression has been documented as well (31).

FUTURE DEVELOPMENTS

Kyphoplasty and vertebroplasty have been used primarily for osteoporotic lumbar VCFs in older adult or postmenopausal individuals. However, the future indications for these techniques may not be so limited. Techniques of sealing off the posterior part of the VB may facilitate augmentation of burst fractures with minimal retropulsion. Also, it is probable that the indications can be expanded to include compression fractures in younger nonosteoporotic adults, particularly if other bioresorbable fillers are introduced. Further investigation is warranted to study the *in vitro* effects of bone tamp inflation on retropulsed bone fragments. Concern has been raised about the balloon pushing the fragments posteriorly. However, with height reduction, ligamentotaxis may in fact reduce these fragments. As vertebroplasty has been successfully used in patients with destructive neoplastic processes (37,38), kyphoplasty may find its place in the treatment of collapsed, kyphotic metastatic lesions in the spine (39). Clinical trials in selected patients are an important next step to explore these options. With the advantages of minimal invasiveness, it is likely that kyphoplasty and vertebroplasty might have substantial benefits over larger open surgical stabilization procedures.

Currently, PMMA cement has been the only material used for vertebral augmentation. Although PMMA is biocompatible, it is not resorbable. Several biologic bone cements have recently been developed and demonstrated their usefulness in extremity fractures. It would be attractive to use such materials in the augmentation of VBs. However, the biomechanical, biochemical, and clinical effects of alternative bone cements in osteoporotic VCF remains to be elucidated. An optimal material would be both osteoinductive and osteoconductive, as well as restore strength and stiffness to near normal values (40). Additionally, the balloon tamp itself should be biocompatible and resorbable. This would further enhance safety by allowing the balloon itself to be left in, as a barrier to cement leakage.

REFERENCES

1. Schlaich C, Minne HW, Bruckner T, et al. Reduced pulmonary function in patients with spinal osteoporotic fractures. Osteoporos Int 1998;8:261–267.
2. Robb-Nicholson C. By the way, doctor. I'm interested in having vertebroplasty, the treatment for vertebral fractures mentioned in your August issue. When I called Medicare to see if the procedure is covered, I was told "Only if the FDA has approved it"; but when I checked with the FDA, I found that no one had applied for approval. Why is this? Is there some way to get vertebroplasty? Harv Womens Health Watch 1999;7:8.
3. Leech JA, Dulberg C, Kellie S, et al. Relationship of lung function to severity of osteoporosis in women. Am Rev Respir Dis 1990;141:68–71.
4. Lyles KW, Gold DT, Shipp KM, et al. Association of osteoporotic vertebral compression fractures with impaired functional status. Am J Med 1993;94:595–601.
5. Leidig-Bruckner G, Minne HW, Schlaich C, et al. Clinical grading of spinal osteoporosis: quality of life components and spinal deformity in women with chronic low back pain and women with vertebral osteoporosis. J Bone Miner Res 1997;12:663–675.
6. Tamayo-Orozco J, Arzac-Palumbo P, Peon-Vidales H, et al. Vertebral fractures associated with osteoporosis: patient management. Am J Med 1997;103:44S–48S; discussion 48S–50S.
7. Wasnich RD. Epidemiology of osteoporosis. In: Favus M. Primer on the metabolic bone diseases and disorders of mineral metabolism, 4th ed. Philadelphia: Lippincott Williams & Wilkins, 1999:257–259.
8. Baillie SP, Davison CE, Johnson FJ, et al. Pathogenesis of vertebral crush fractures in men. Age Ageing 1992;21:139–141.
9. Biyani A, Ebraheim NA, Lu J. Thoracic spine fractures in patients older than 50 years. Clin Orthop 1996;328:190–193.
10. Eastell R. Pathogenesis of postmenopausal osteoporosis. In: Favus M. Primer on the metabolic bone diseases and disorders of mineral metabolism, 4th edition. Philadelphia: Lippincott Williams & Wilkins, 1999:260–262.
11. Watts NB. Pharmacology of agents to treat osteoporosis. In: Favus MJ. Primer on the metabolic bone diseases and disorders of mineral metabolism, 4th edition. Philadelphia: Lippincott Williams & Wilkins, 1999:278–283.
12. Schneider PL, Dzenis PE, Kahanovitz N. Spinal trauma. In: Zuckerman JD. Compressive care of orthopaedic injuries in the elderly. Baltimore: Urban and Schwarzenberg, 1990.
13. Galibert P, Deramond H, Rosat P, et al. Note preliminaire sur le traitement des angiomes vertebraux par vertebroplastie acrylique percutanee. Neurochirurg 1984;233:166–168.
14. Belkoff SM, Maroney M, Fenton DC, et al. An in vitro biomechanical evaluation of bone cements used in percutaneous vertebroplasty. Bone 1999;25:23S–26S.
15. Belkoff SM, Mathis JM, Erbe EM, et al. Biomechanical evaluation of a new bone cement for use in vertebroplasty. Spine 2000;25:1061–1064.
16. Grados F, Depriester C, Cayrolle G, et al. Long-term observations of vertebral osteoporotic fractures treated by percutaneous vertebroplasty. Rheumatology (Oxf) 2000;39:1410–1414.
17. Barr JD, Barr MS, Lemley TJ, et al. Percutaneous vertebroplasty for pain relief and spinal stabilization. Spine 2000;25:923–928.
18. Heini PF, Walchli B, Berlemann U. Percutaneous transpedicular vertebroplasty with PMMA: operative technique and early results. A prospective study for the treatment of osteoporotic compression fractures. Eur Spine J 2000;9:445–450.
19. Wenger M, Markwalder TM. Surgically controlled, transpedicular methyl methacrylate vertebroplasty with fluoroscopic guidance. Acta Neurochir 1999;141:625–631.
20. Garfin SR, Yuan HA, Reiley MA. New technologies in spine: kyphoplasty and vertebroplasty for the treatment of painful osteoporotic compression fractures. Spine 2001;26:1511–1515.
21. Garfin SR, Yuan H, Lieberman IH. Early outcomes in the minimally-invasive reductions and fixation of compression fractures. Proceedings of the North American Spine Society, 2000;184–185.
22. Maynard AS, Jensen ME, Schweickert PA, et al. Value of bone scan imaging in predicting pain relief from percutaneous vertebroplasty in osteoporotic vertebral fractures. AJNR Am J Neuroradiol 2000;21:1807–1812.
23. Do HM. Magnetic resonance imaging in the evaluation of patients for percutaneous vertebroplasty. Top Magn Reson Imaging 2000;11:235–244.
24. Kado DM, Browner WS, Palermo L, et al. Vertebral fractures and mortality in older women: a prospective study. Study of Osteoporotic Fractures Research Group. Arch Intern Med 1999;159:1215–1220.
25. Tohmeh AG, Mathis JM, Fenton DC, et al. Biomechanical efficacy of unipedicular versus bipedicular vertebroplasty for the management of osteoporotic compression fractures. Spine 1999;24:1772–1776.
26. Jasper LE, Deramond H, Mathis JM, et al. The effect of monomer-to-powder ratio on the material properties of cranioplastic. Bone 1999;25:27S–29S.
27. White A, Panjabi M. Clinical biomechanics of the spine. Philadelphia: Lippincott-Raven, 1990.
28. Belkoff SM, Mathis JM, Fenton DC, et al. An ex vivo biomechanical evaluation of an inflatable bone tamp used in the treatment of compression fracture. Spine 2001;26:151–156.
29. Mathis JM, Barr JD, Belkoff SM, et al. Percutaneous vertebroplasty: a developing standard of care for vertebral compression fractures. AJNR Am J Neuroradiol 2001;22:373–381.
30. Deramond H, Depriester C, Galibert P, et al. Percutaneous vertebroplasty with polymethylmethacrylate. Technique, indications, and results. Radiol Clin North Am 1998;36:533–546.
31. Harrington KD. Major neurological complications following percutaneous vertebroplasty with polymethylmethacrylate: a case report. J Bone Joint Surg 2001;83A:1070–1073.
32. Cortet B, Cotten A, Boutry N, et al. Percutaneous vertebroplasty in patients with osteolytic metastases or multiple myeloma. Rev Rheum (English ed.) 1997;64:177–183.
33. Cortet B, Cotten A, Boutry N, et al. Percutaneous vertebroplasty in the treatment of osteoporotic vertebral compression fractures: an open prospective study. J Rheumatol 1999;26:2222–2228.
34. Cyteval C, Sarrabere MP, Roux JO, et al. Acute osteoporotic vertebral collapse: open study on percutaneous injection of acrylic surgical cement in 20 patients. AJR Am J Roentgenol 1999;173:1685–1690.
35. Chiras J, Sola-Martinez MT, Weill A, et al. [Percutaneous vertebroplasty]. Rev Med Interne 1995;16:854–859.
36. Jensen ME, Dion JE. Percutaneous vertebroplasty in the treatment of osteoporotic compression fractures. Neuroimaging Clin N Am 2000;10:547–568.
37. Weill A, Chiras J, Simon JM, et al. Spinal metastases: indications for and results of percutaneous injection of acrylic surgical cement. Radiology 1996;199:241–247.
38. Murphy KJ, Deramond H. Percutaneous vertebroplasty in benign and malignant disease. Neuroimaging Clin North Am 2000;10:535–545.
39. Dudeney S, Lieberman IH, Reinhart MK, and Hussein M. Kyphoplasty in the treatment of osteolytic vertebral compression fractures as a result of multiple myeloma. J Clin Oncol 2002;20:2382–2387.
40. Cunin G, Boissonnet H, Petite H, et al. Experimental vertebroplasty using osteoconductive granular material. Spine 2000;25:1070–1076.

CHAPTER 73

Osteopenia: Vertebrectomy and Fusion

Manabu Ito and Kiyoshi Kaneda

Primary management aims in thoracolumbar osteoporotic-fragile vertebral fractures should be alleviation of pain, early ambulation, preservation of the physiologic spinal balance with stability, and prevention of late neurologic complications. There has been a consensus that low-energy osteoporotic compression fractures in the thoracic and lumbar spine generally cause only localized pain and kyphosis without significant neurologic complications; therefore, urgent surgery is rarely indicated. Conservative treatment has been chosen for thoracolumbar compression fractures to relieve back pain. Usually these fractures can be treated successfully with a corset or hyperextension brace. Early ambulation and avoidance of prolonged bed rest are important. Late onset of vertebral collapse can occur in patients treated conservatively; therefore, clinical and radiographic follow-up is mandatory. In this chapter, the pathology and surgical management of osteoporotic and posttraumatic vertebral collapse with increasing kyphosis with or without neurologic complications are described.

LATE NEUROLOGIC COMPROMISE AFTER OSTEOPOROTIC FRACTURES

Gradually increasing kyphosis and late complications of the spinal cord or cauda equina can occur in some patients with an osteoporotic-fragile fracture of the thoraco-lumbar spine treated conservatively (Fig. 73-1). Taneichi et al.

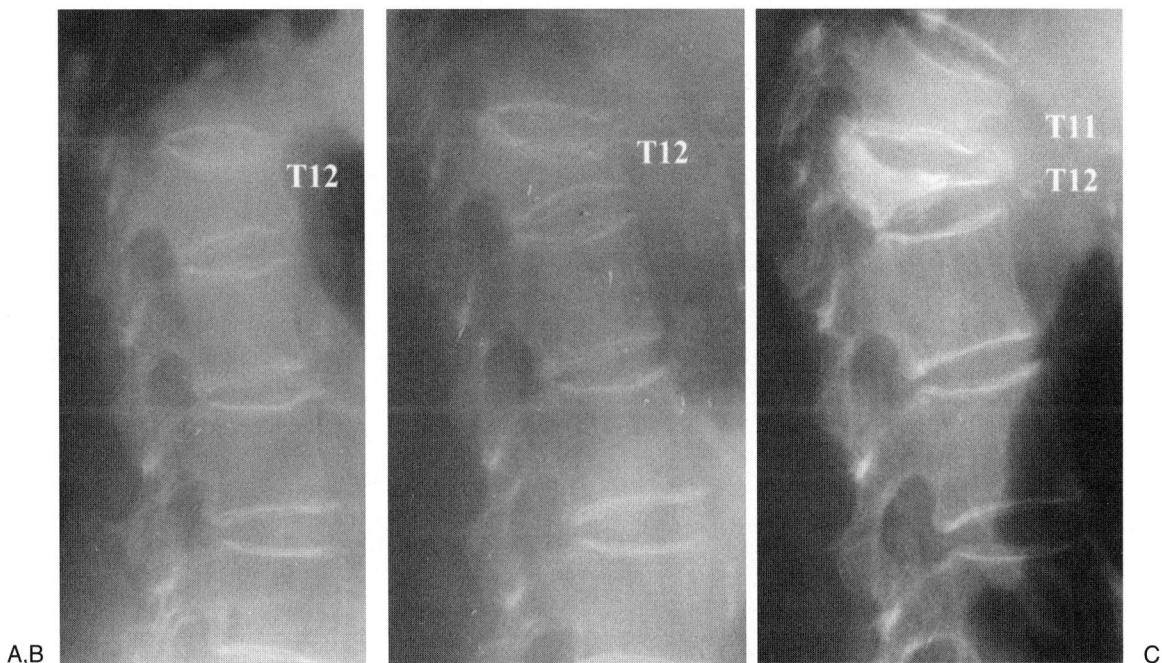

FIG. 73-1. A: This 88-year-old woman had a T12 compression fracture when she stumbled and fell. **B:** One month later, the fractured vertebral body of T12 collapsed and its vertebral body height decreased. **C:** Three months later, the T12 vertebral body completely collapsed and neurologic deficits occurred.

683

reported that 36.6% of patients with osteoporotic vertebral fractures showed progressive collapse of the fractured vertebrae, 13.9% showed pseudarthrosis at the fracture, and 3.5% showed neurologic deficits (1). This devastating neurologic compromise is brought about by anterior impingement of the neural tissues in the anterior spinal canal with the retropulsed bony mass of the collapsed vertebra(e) (2–8).

PATHOLOGIC FEATURES OF OSTEOPOROTIC AND POSTTRAUMATIC VERTEBRAL COLLAPSE

The cause of the delayed posttraumatic vertebral collapse and the mechanism of the late neurologic sequela have not been clarified completely, but it seems to be the secondary bone ischemia associated with nonhealing fractures of the vertebral trabeculae. Histology of the collapsed vertebral bodies shows massive fibrous tissues or necrotic tissues inside the collapsed vertebral bodies with minimal new bone formation (Fig. 73-2). Massive fibrous tissue of the fractured fragile trabeculae bring about disturbance of blood supply in the vertebral body, resulting in bone ischemia or pseudarthrosis, which eventually leads to vertebral collapse and neurologic compromise (9–11).

RECONSTRUCTIVE SURGERY OF OSTEOPOROTIC AND POSTTRAUMATIC VERTEBRAL COLLAPSE

Patient Demographics

Between January 1987 and December 1996, 101 patients (23 men and 78 women) with osteoporotic or posttraumatic vertebral collapse of the thoracic and lumbar spines were treated surgically in our department. The average age at surgery was 68 years (range, 43 to 89 years).

Indications for surgery were devastating neurologic compromise or increasingly unstable kyphosis at the fracture site. Eighty-four (83%) of the 101 patients suffered late devastating neurologic deficits, and the other 17 (17%) had severe back pain with increasing thoracolumbar kyphosis. The intervals between neurologic compromise and fracture were 3 months in 43%, 3 to 6 months in 22%, 6 to 12 months in 9%, and more than 1 year in 13%; the interval was unknown in 13%. The neurologic symptoms in 84 patients were: lesion of the spinal cord in 51 patients, the conus medullaris with the cauda equina in 10, the cauda equina in 22, and the nerve roots in one. The causes of injuries were: a fall while walking in 43 patients, a fall from a chair onto the floor in 24, lifting a

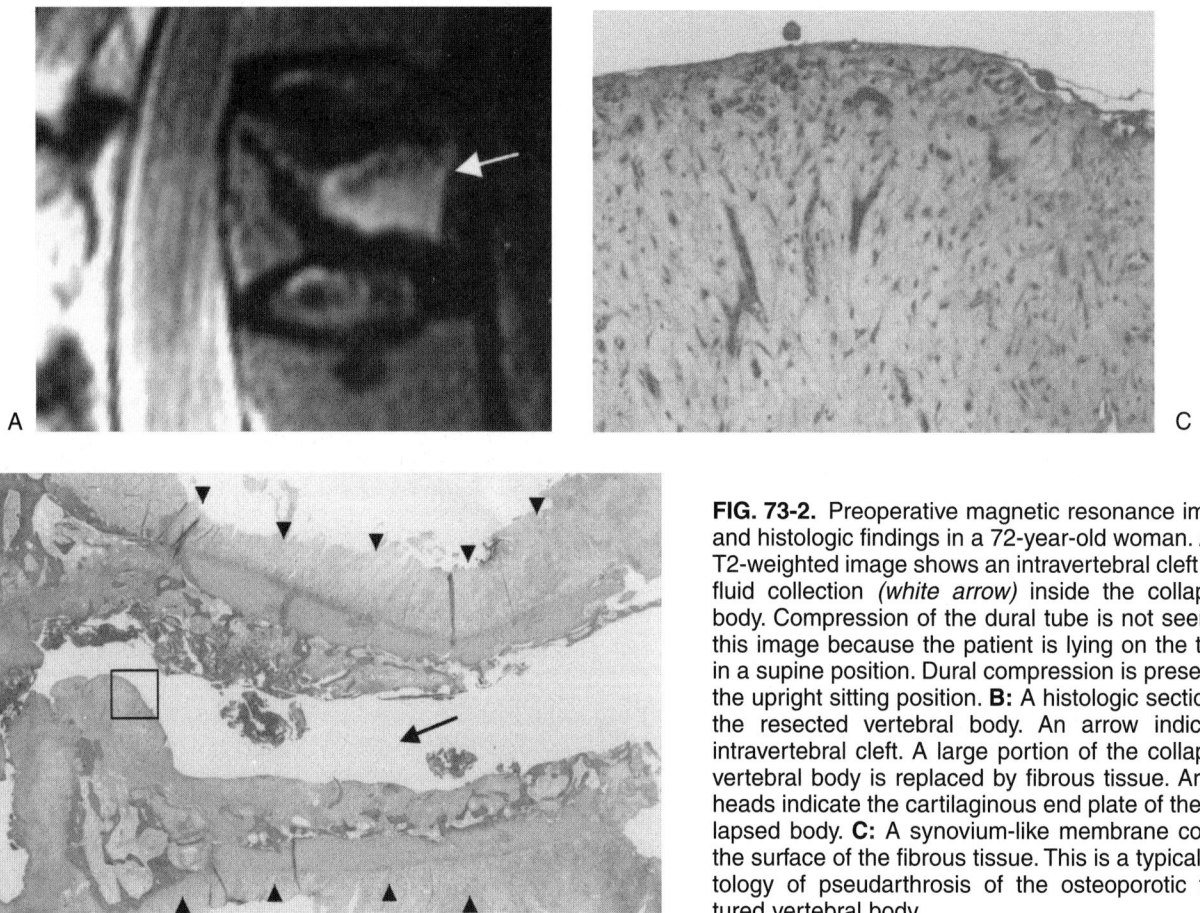

FIG. 73-2. Preoperative magnetic resonance image and histologic findings in a 72-year-old woman. **A:** A T2-weighted image shows an intravertebral cleft with fluid collection *(white arrow)* inside the collapsed body. Compression of the dural tube is not seen on this image because the patient is lying on the table in a supine position. Dural compression is present in the upright sitting position. **B:** A histologic section of the resected vertebral body. An arrow indicates intravertebral cleft. A large portion of the collapsed vertebral body is replaced by fibrous tissue. Arrowheads indicate the cartilaginous end plate of the collapsed body. **C:** A synovium-like membrane covers the surface of the fibrous tissue. This is a typical histology of pseudarthrosis of the osteoporotic fractured vertebral body.

heavy weight in 11, and no history of trauma in 23. The energy of trauma was thought to be low. Such low-energy trauma would not have resulted in compression fracture of the thoraco-lumbar spine in bone of normal quality and strength. The levels of collapsed vertebra(e) were: 28% at T12, , 33% at L1, 14% at L2, 5% at L3, 5% at T12 and L1, 2% at L1-2, 2% at T11-12, and 11% at other levels. Eighty of the 101 patients (79%) had osteoporotic posttraumatic vertebral collapse at the thoracolumbar junction of T12 and L1. The initial treatment was bracing with or without bed rest and prescription of nonsteroidal anti-inflammatory drugs in 75% of patients. The other 25% did not receive any treatment.

Surgical Procedures

The procedures used in the treatment of osteoporotic and posttraumatic vertebral collapse of the thoracolumbar spine were anterior spinal canal decompression by resection of the collapsed vertebra(e), correction of kyphosis, and reconstruction of anterior column support using a vertebral spacer and anterior instrumentation (Kaneda-SR, Depuy Acromed Corp., Cleveland, OH) (12–14). Surgical exposure of the thoracolumbar spine was via the extrapleural and retroperitoneal approach from the left side. Because osteoporotic and posttraumatic vertebral collapse usually occur below T11, exposure of the surgical portion of the thoracolumbar spine was achieved without thoracotomy (Fig. 73-3A). The resection was conducted using sharp osteotomes, chisels, curettes, and Kerrison rongeurs. The posterior longitudinal ligament was left intact during anterior spinal canal decompression to reduce bleeding from the epidural vein.

Following anterior spinal canal decompression by resection of the retropulsed bony mass compressing the neural tissue, application of Kaneda-SR anterior instrumentation was started. At first, the vertebral staples were placed properly and fixed with screws, as shown in figure 73-3.

Within 3 to 5 days after surgery, patients were encouraged to start walking with Thoraco-Lumbar Spinal Orthosis (TLSO). The brace was worn for about 6 months.

Surgical Results

Operating time was 228 minutes, blood loss was 588 mL, and postoperative follow-up period was 68 months on the average (range, 3 to 147 months). Preoperatively, 84 (83%) of the 101 patients suffered from devastating neurologic damage resulting from late posttraumatic vertebral collapse. Eighty-two of 84 patients showed remarkable neurologic recovery. Of 59 patients with preoperative bladder-bowel disturbance, complete or incomplete recovery occurred in 44 patients. Two patients who did not show any neurologic recovery in motor function in the lower extremities or the bladder-bowel function had satisfactory pain relief with correction of increasing kyphosis. These two patients kept their paralytic status with increasing kyphosis for over 1 year without spinal canal decompression.

In terms of radiographic evaluation, stable fusion was obtained in 77 (76%) of 101 patients treated by a single anterior surgery. Twenty-two patients (22%) required posterior reinforcement after anterior surgery because of their low bone mineral density (BMD) and severe kyphosis owing to vertebral collapse at multiple levels. Solid fusion

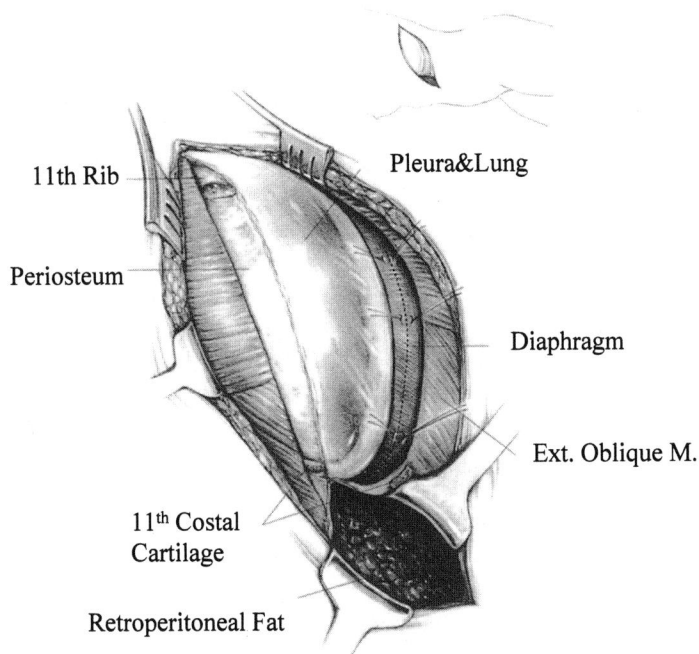

FIG. 73-3. Surgical procedures. **A:** The extrapleural retroperitoneal approach. The tenth or eleventh rib usually is resected for the extrapleural retroperitoneal approach. Retroperitoneal fat tissue can be seen after splitting the costal cartilage. Abdominal muscles are divided after separating the retroperitoneal fat and peritoneal contents from the anterior abdominal muscles.

(continued on next page)

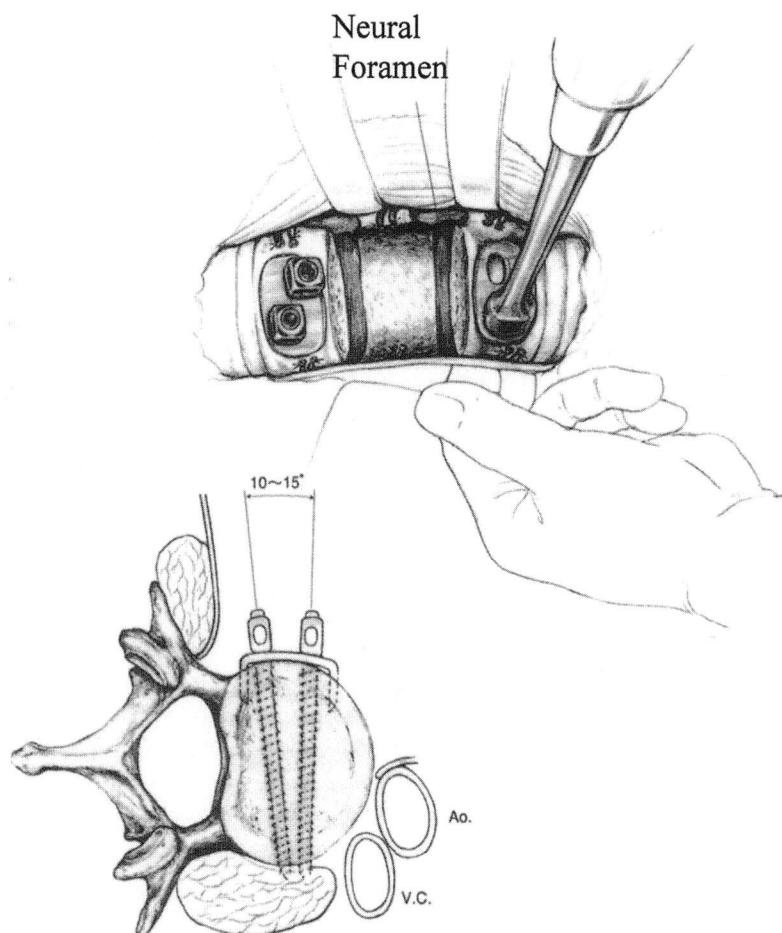

FIG. 73-3. (*Continued*) **B:** Placement of vertebral plates and screws. A vertebral plate is properly placed at the lateral aspect of vertebral body. The spikes of a plate must be placed parallel to the intervertebral space not penetrating into the disc spaces. Posterior vertebral screws must be inserted 10° to 15° anteriorly not to penetrate into the spinal canal. The screw tips must penetrate to the opposite cortex to achieve bicortical screw purchase. The screw tip is blunt to avoid additional tissue damage.

was not obtained in two patients who had postoperative deep infection. Correction of kyphotic deformity was from 33.2° preoperatively to 16.6° postoperatively and 20.2° at the survey. Overall, patients with single-level vertebral collapse with more than 0.7 g/cm² in BMD can be successfully treated by single anterior procedure consisting of corpectomy, decompression, and reconstruction.

Subsequent compression fractures at levels other than the reconstructed site occurred in 37 patients during follow-up. There was no fracture at the fused vertebrae where the vertebral staple and screws were inserted. It was not necessary to repair the subsequent compression fractures at adjacent vertebral bodies except in two

patients with severe collagen diseases treated with long-term steroid administration.

Complications were pseudarthrosis in two patients who had deep infection after surgery, dislodgement of the hooks of posterior instrumentation in one, temporary dementia in three, superficial infection in two, and urinary tract infection in one. There were no major complications including neurologic, respiratory, and circulatory complications. Death during follow-up occurred in 17 patients. Two died of pneumonia within 1 year postoperatively. Of the remaining 15 patients, four died within 1 to 2 years, six in 2 to 5 years, and five in over 5 years. The deaths had no relation to the spinal surgery.

FIG. 73-4. Case 1 represents a 74-year-old woman. The osteoporotic vertebral L1 collapse is shown. **A:** Myelogram under forward flexion. Arrows indicate that the intravertebral cleft closes. **B:** Myelogram under backward flexion. Arrows indicate that the cleft opens. **C, D:** X-ray films at 4 years postoperative.

Vertebral Spacer &
Autogenous Rib Graft

C

D

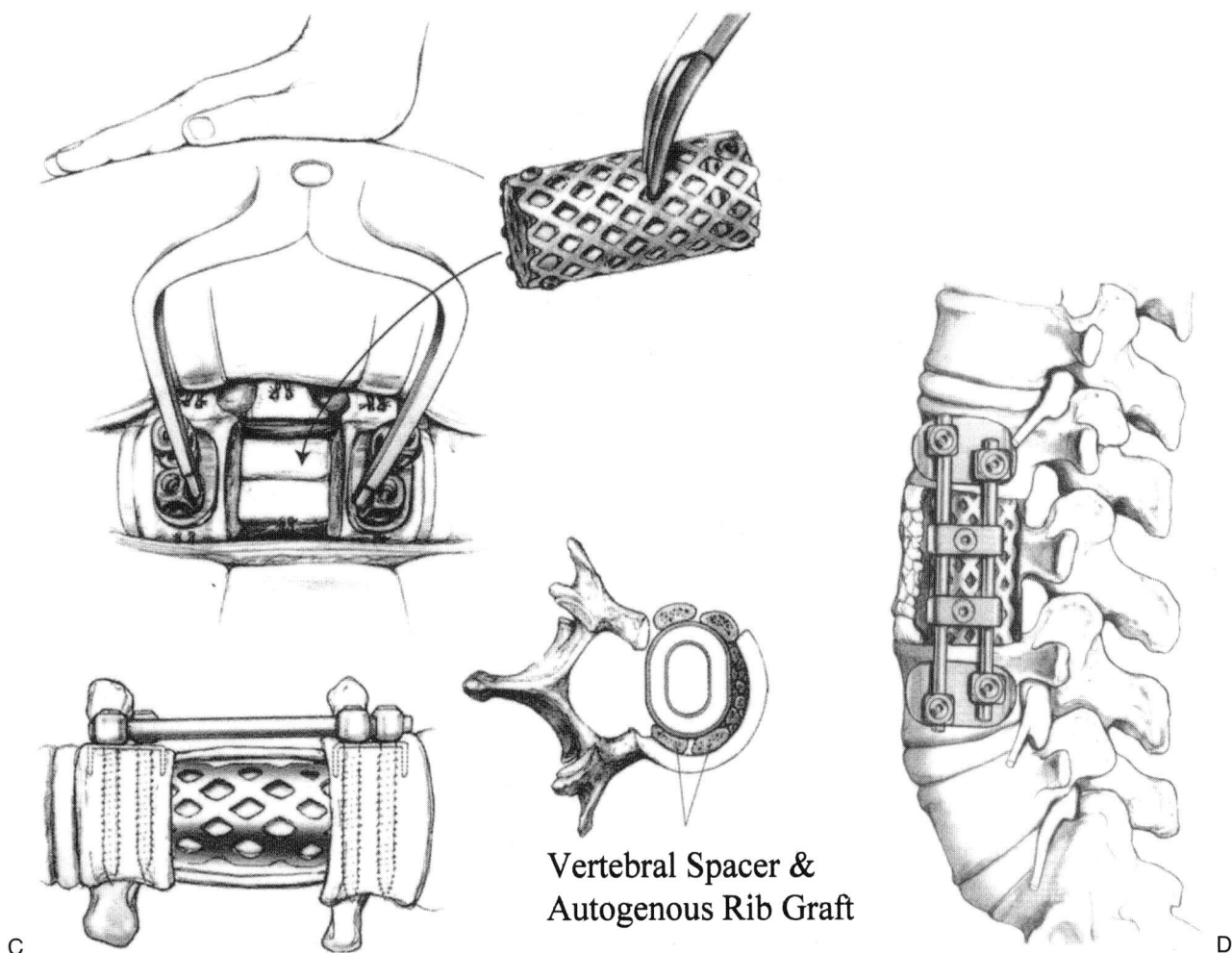

FIG. 73-3. (*Continued*) **C:** Placement of vertebral spacer. An autogenous rib graft and vertebral spacer of proper length are inserted after correcting the regional kyphotic deformity using a spreader. An autogenous rib graft at both sides of the vertebral spacer and a chip bone graft taken from the rib or healthy part of the vertebral body must be added. **D:** Completion of the Kaneda-SR system. Kaneda-SR instrumentation is completed by applying properly sized two-rod couplers.

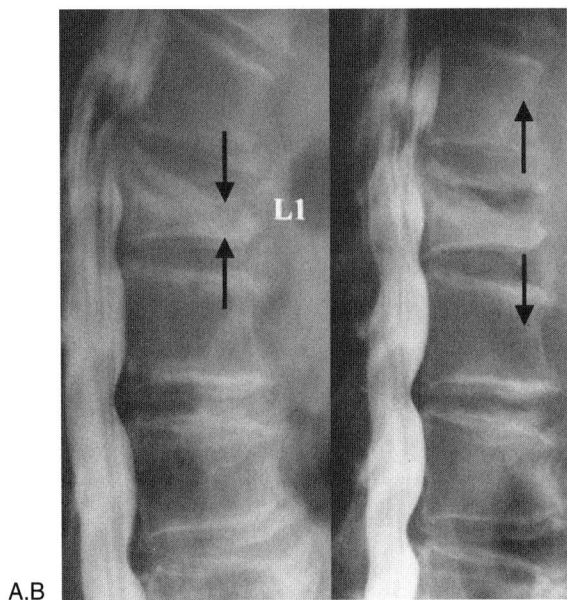

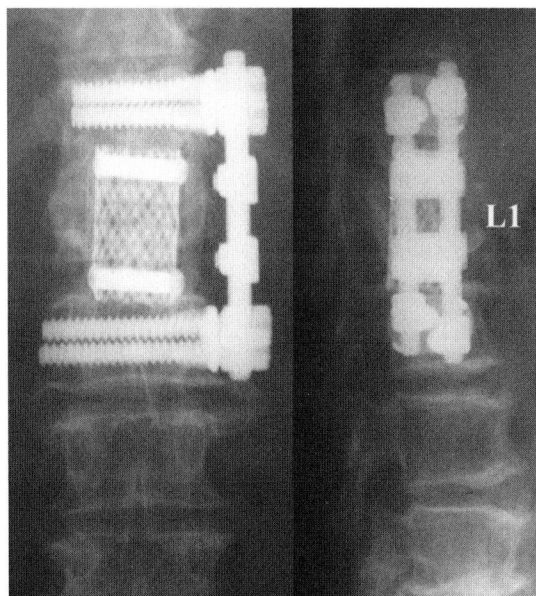

A,B

C,D

CASE REPORT

A 74-year-old woman suffered an L1 osteoporotic compression fracture when she stumbled and fell. She was treated conservatively with TLSO and nonsteroidal anti-inflammatory drugs by her physician (Fig. 73-4). Six months later, she suffered from a walking disturbance caused by motor weakness in the lower extremities and severe back pain. A functional lateral radiograph showed an intravertebral cleft inside the L1, which opened under backward flexion and closed under forward flexion (Fig. 73-4). Dural tube was compressed by the posterior wall of the collapsed vertebral body. Anterior spinal decompression at L1 and stabilization from T12 to L2 using Kaneda-SR, a titanium mesh cage, and an autogenous rib graft were conducted. Four years after surgery, bony fusion was complete and sagittal alignment of the thoracolumbar spine was acceptable (Fig. 73-4).

DISCUSSION

In our series, vertebral collapse after osteoporotic compression fracture of the thoracic and lumbar spine occurred in 41% within 3 months and 63% within 6 months. Eleven percent occurred at more than 1 year after fracture. The levels of vertebral collapse were concentrated at the T12 and L1 levels; therefore, osteoporotic compression fractures, especially at T12 and L1, should be followed-up carefully for at least 1 year after the initial fracture. Moreover, 23% of the patients in our series could not recognize the incidence of trauma in the past. If senile patients show neurologic deficits without cause, doctors should consider this pathology as a possible cause of neurologic impairment.

Causes of late vertebral collapse after osteoporotic compression fracture are unknown. From surgical findings, the collapsed vertebra was ischemic and fragile, and the resection of the collapsed vertebra could be conducted easily because of reduced bleeding owing to avascular necrosis of the collapsed body. Histologic study of the resected collapsed vertebra revealed massive necrotic or fibrous tissue, which might be the result of secondary bone ischemia. The normal fracture healing process of the osteoporotic trabeculae might be disturbed because of the fragility of the osteoporotic bone. As a result, osteoporotic fractured trabeculae led to massive scar formation, which would have disturbed the blood circulation in the vertebral body.

There were several reports of posterior reconstruction with instrumentation for treatment of this disease (15). Posterior reconstruction procedures have the following disadvantages: (a) indirect neural decompression; (b) destruction of intact posterior elements; (c) difficulty in reconstruction of anterior column support; and (d) prolonged levels of instrumentation. The pathology of the devastating neural damage and progressively unstable

kyphosis is located in the anterior pillar of the spinal column. The neural lesion is brought about by impingement of the neural tissue in the spinal canal by the retropulsed bony mass. Therefore, anterior spinal canal decompression by resection of the retropulsed bony fragment and the reconstruction of the stable anterior column support are the most reasonable choices. This concept is supported in our series and satisfactory results have been gained without severe complications even in very elderly patients.

Recently, vertebroplasty or kyphoplasty have been used by surgeons for the treatment of osteoporotic compression fractures (16). These procedures also have been performed for patients with progressive osteoporotic vertebral collapse of vertebral bodies. From the histologic point of view, cement injection to the collapsed vertebral bodies containing large fibrous or necrotic tissue may interfere with the healing process of the fractured bodies. Even though bioactive materials are injected, it is difficult to obtain biologic union by this technique because the collapsed vertebral bodies are filled with fibrous tissue and are severely ischemic. The efficacy of this new procedure awaits conformation by long-term follow-up studies.

In conclusion, late devastating neurologic complications can be brought about by osteoporotic and posttraumatic vertebral collapse of the thoracolumbar spine. The cause of this pathology is ischemic necrosis or pseudarthrosis of fractured vertebral bodies caused by secondary circulatory disturbance resulting from the formation of fibrous tissue around the fractured trabeculae. The principle of treatment should be anterior spinal canal decompression and reconstruction of the anterior spinal column using anterior instrumentation and a vertebral spacer.

REFERENCES

1. Taneichi H, Kaneda K, Oguma T, et al. Risk factor analysis for osteoporotic vertebral collapse and pseudarthrosis. Clin Orthop Surg 2002;37:437–442.
2. Arciero RA, Leung KYK, Pierce JH. Spontaneous unstable burst fracture of the thoracolumbar spine in osteoporosis. Spine 1989;14:114–117.
3. Golimbu C, Firooznia H, Rafii M. The intravertebral vacuum sign. Spine 1986;11:1040–1043.
4. Kaneda K, Asano S, Hashimoto T, et al. The treatment of osteoporotic-posttraumatic vertebral collapse using the Kaneda device and a bioactive ceramic vertebral prosthesis. Spine 1992;17:S295–S303.
5. Kaneda K, Ito M. Osteoporotic thoracic and lumbar fractures. With emphasis on osteoporotic-posttraumatic vertebral collapse. In: Obrant C, ed. Management of fractures in severely osteoporotic bone. Orthopaedic and pharmacological strategies. Sweden: Springer-Verlag, 2000:214–227.
6. Kaplan PA, Orton DF, Asleson RT: et al. Osteoporosis with vertebral compression fractures retropulsed fragments, and neurologic compromise. Radiology 1987;165:533–535.
7. Maruo S, Takekawa F, Nakano K. Paraplegia caused by vertebral compression fractures in senile osteoporosis. Z Orthop 1987;3:125–320.
8. Salomon C, Chopin D, Benoist M. Spinal cord compression; an exceptional complication of spinal osteoporosis. Spine 1988;13:222–224.
9. Lafforgue P, Chagnaud C, Daumer-Legre V. The intravertebral vacuum

phenomenon ("vertebral osteonecrosis") migration of intradiscal gas in a fractured vertebral body? Spine 1997;22:1885–1891.

10. Ito M, Kaneda K, Abumi K, et al. Influence of osteoporosis on healing process of vertebral fracture: a histological study. 69th Annual Meeting Proceedings of AAOS, Dallas, 2002.

11. Ryan P, Fogelman I. Osteoporotic vertebral fractures: diagnosis with radiography and bone scintigraphy. Radiology 1994;190:669–672.

12. Kaneda K. Anterior approach and Kaneda instrumentation for lesions of the thoracic and lumbar spine. In: Bridwell KH, Dewald RL, eds. Textbook of spinal surgery. Philadelphia, Lippincott, 1991: 959–990.

13. Ito M. Surgery for osteoporotic posttraumatic vertebral collapse: anterior decompression and stabilization. Spine Spinal Cord 2002;15: 89–96.

14. Yamamuro T. Reconstruction of the lumbar vertebrae of sheep with ceramic prosthesis. J Bone Joint Surg 1990;72B:889–893.

15. Shikata J, Yamamuro T, Iida H., et al. Surgical treatment for paraplegia resulting from vertebral fractures in senile osteoporosis. Spine 1990;15:485–489.

16. Lieberman I, Dudney S, Reinhardt MK, et al. Initial outcome and efficacy of kyphoplasty in the treatment of painful osteoporotic vertebral compression fractures. Spine 2001;26:1631–1638.

CHAPTER 74

Inflammatory Spondyloarthropathies

Philippe Goupille and David Borenstein

The inflammatory spondyloarthropathies (IS) are a cluster of interrelated chronic inflammatory rheumatic diseases including ankylosing spondylitis (AS), enteropathic arthritis (ulcerative colitis and Crohn disease), psoriatic arthritis (PA), and reactive arthritis (ReA) (postenteric and post-venereal arthritis) (Fig. 74-1). These disorders constitute a homogeneous group of inflammatory arthritides characterized by axial (sacroiliac and spinal joints) and peripheral enthesopathies, associated with peripheral arthritis and extraarticular (ocular, mucocutaneous, and genital) abnormalities. These disorders share a familial aggregation and a strong association with the HLA B27 antigen (1–4).

These shared characteristics of IS facilitate the use of international diagnostic validated criteria for inflammatory arthropathies (Table 74-1) (5) and group the pathogeneses of these disorders with the interaction between a predisposing immunogenetic predisposition and various environmental triggers (microorganisms).

COMMON CHARACTERISTICS OF IS

IS have common epidemiologic and pathologic characteristics. These are discussed in the following sections.

Age of Onset

The age of onset of IS is often at the end of the growth period (i.e., between 16 and 30 years) (6,7). Detailed study of chronic juvenile arthritis has recently shown that true IS can occur in children. These forms of childhood onset occur more frequently in certain regions: 10% to 15% of cases occur before the age of 15 years in Europe, whereas the rate is 30% in North African countries. Onset of certain forms occasionally occurs much later (after 50 years).

Male Predominance

There is a predominance of IS in men but the disease is not rare in women. The sex ratio depends on the type

of IS (Table 74-2). The forms in women, which have until recently probably been confused with other types of inflammatory rheumatism, have become more frequent.

Poorly Recognized Prevalence of Spondyloarthropathies (Table 74-2)

The prevalence reports depend on several factors such as the population studied, the diagnostic criteria used, and the study method (7). The prevalence of IS is in proportion to that of HLA B27 in all races. In black and Asian populations, where the prevalence of HLA B27 is lower than 2%, AS is much rarer than in Caucasian populations.

The prevalence of all types of IS is estimated at 0.5% of the overall population, but three tendencies warrant comment:

1. The prevalence of AS is increasing, especially because of greater awareness of childhood and female forms and undifferentiated forms.
2. The prevalence of PA also appears to be increasing because this condition is now better known.
3. The prevalence of true ReA is decreasing in Western countries, probably because of changes in ecologic bacteria and perhaps due to more frequent use of antibiotics.

Entheses: Main Sites of Inflammatory Involvement

Entheses are formed from bony elements parallel to the collagen of the tendon, which is anchored in the bone. Between the bone and the tendon is a cartilaginous area, the function of which is to absorb constraints in traction.

Onset of inflammation in IS is typically at the level of the entheses. After an initial inflammatory phase (osteitis), which is expressed as limited erosions of the bone, there is a cicatricial process consisting of bone proliferation and periosteal apposition forming entheso-

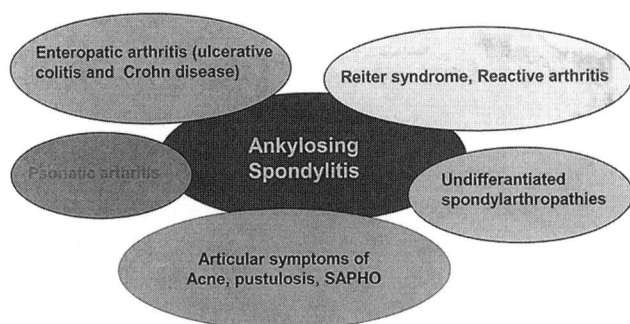

FIG. 74-1. Inflammatory spondyloarthropathies.

phytes. In developed forms the bone proliferation results in true bone fusion responsible for the ankylosing evolution of IS. This evolution explains the chronology of the osteitis-periostosis-hyperostosis triad which is characteristic of IS enthesopathies.

Explanation of the Radiographic Features Related to Enthesopathy

All the osteoarticular structures, which are components of entheses, may be involved.

The *sacroiliac joints* have only one very limited area of synovium because they are mainly composed of fibrous attachments. Sacroiliitis is therefore considered to be a sacroiliac enthesopathy, thus explaining the frequently observed ankylosis (Fig. 74-2).

The intervertebral disc consists of a fibrous annulus, which is a true enthesis surrounding the nucleus pulposus. The annulus is inserted into the periphery of the vertebral body and around the nucleus pulposus. The initial lesions are peripheral enthesopathies expressed as erosions of the anterior edge of the vertebra (Romanus sign), with vertebral "squaring" (Fig. 74-3). Subsequent development is then marked by the appearance of an enthesophyte known as a syndesmophyte. When there is enthesopathy of the central fibers of the annulus the lesions

TABLE 74-1. *European Spondyloarthropathy Study Group (ESSG) criteria*

Main criteria	Criteria

• Inflammatory spinal pain	Inflammatory spinal pain
	• History or present symptoms of spinal pain in back, dorsal or cervical region, with at least 4 of the following:
	    onset before age 45
	    insidious onset
	    improved by exercise
	    associated with morning stiffness
	    at least 3 mo duration

• Synovitis	Synovitis • Past or present asymmetric arthritis or arthritis predominantly in the lower limbs
Secondary criteria	
• Family history	Family history • Presence in first-degree or second-degree relatives of any of the following: ankylosing spondylitis, psoriasis, acute uveitis, reactive arthritis, and inflammatory bowel disease
• Psoriasis	Psoriasis • Past or present psoriasis diagnosed by a physician
• Inflammatory bowel disease	Inflammatory bowel disease • Past or present Crohn disease or ulcerative colitis diagnosed by a physician and confirmed by radiographic examination or endoscopy
• Alternative buttock pain	Alternative buttock pain • Past or present pain alternating between the right and left gluteal regions
• Enthesopathy	Enthesopathy • Past or present spontaneous pain or tenderness at examination of the site of the insertion of the Achilles tendon or plantar fascia
• Acute diarrhea	Acute diarrhea • Episode of diarrhea occurring within 1 mo before arthritis
• Urethritis	Urethritis • Nongonococcal urethritis or cervicitis occurring within 1 mo before arthritis
• Sacroiliitis	Sacroiliitis • Bilateral grade 2–4 or unilateral grade 3–4, according to the following radiographic grading system: 0 = normal, 1 = possible, 2 = minimal, 3 = moderate, 4 = ankylosis

From Dougados M, van der Linden S, Juhlin R, et al. The European Spondylarthropathy Study Group preliminary criteria for the classification of spondylarthropathy. Arthritis Rheum 1991;34:1218–1227, with permission.

TABLE 74-2. *Prevalence, association with HLA B27 and sex ratios of the different types of spondyloarthropathies*

Spondyloarthropathies	Prevalence (Caucasian population)[a]	Association HLA B27	Relative risk[b]	Sex ratio men:women
Ankylosing spondylitis	0.2%–0.5%	90%–95%	90	2–3:1
Reactive arthritis	0.1%	60%–80%	35	2–6:1 for genitourinary origin 1:1 for gastrointestinal origin
Psoriatic arthritis	0.1%	40%–70%	10	1:1
Enteropathic arthritis	0.01%	30%–60%	10	1:1

[a]Prevalence of HLA B27 is 7%–10% in Caucasian population.
[b]The relative risk estimates the probability of occurrence of spondyloarthropathy in HLA B27 carriers in Caucasian population.

seen radiographically can look like "pseudoptotic" spondylodiscitis. In certain advanced forms the bone fusion of the vertebral structures gives the typical "bamboo" appearance (Fig. 74-4).

All the other peripheral entheses can be involved. The most characteristic localizations are the calcaneum, the clavicular joints (acromiocostoclavicular and sternocostoclavicular), the symphysis pubis, and the distal interphalangeal joints. The example of the distal interphalangeal joints is very particular because the last phalanx is a complex enthesis system, characterized by a network of conjunctive tissue linking the last phalanx to the nail and the skin. Its characteristic involvement in PA may be expressed as true distal osteitis (sometimes without arthritis) associated with psoriatic onychosis and known as psoriatic onychopachydermoperiostitis (8–10).

Polymorphonuclear Neutrophils at the Origin of Inflammation in IS

The inflammatory synovial infiltrate in most inflammatory arthropathies, as in ReA, is made up of macrophages and lymphocytes. However, polymorphonuclear neutrophils (PMNs) predominate in the articular infiltrate (enthesis and synovium) in IS. This excess of PMNs is also present at the extra-articular sites such as cutaneous lesions in psoriasis and digestive lesions in enteropathies. These findings do not exclude the possi-

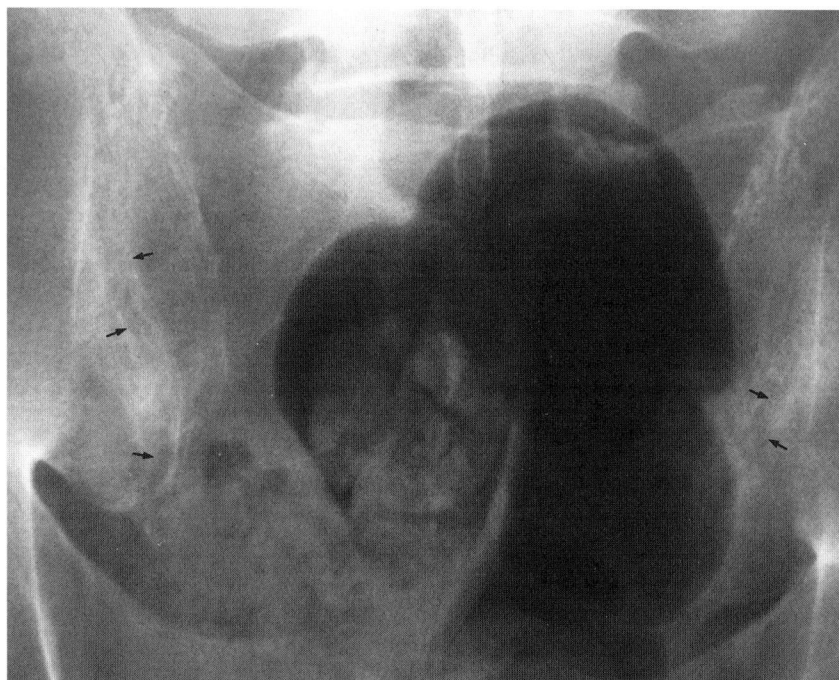

FIG. 74-2. A 45-year-old man with 10 years of inflammatory bowel disease and 5 years of low back stiffness and pain. Anteroposterior roentgenographic view of the pelvis reveals bilateral erosions and joint space widening *(black arrows)*.

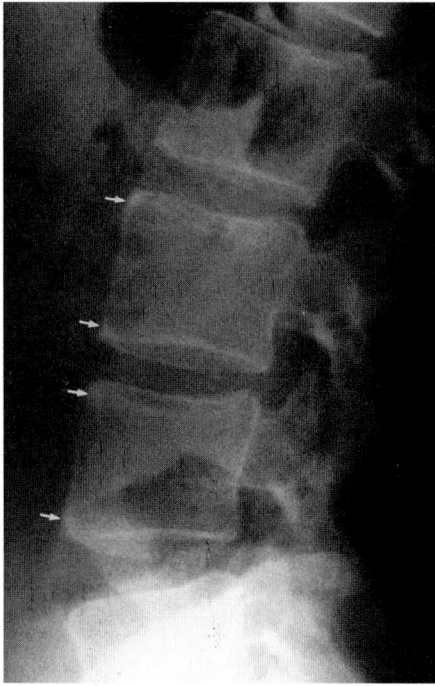

FIG. 74-3. Same patient as shown in Figure 74-1. A lateral roentgenographic view of the lumbar spine with squaring of the vertebral bodies *(white arrows).*

bility that the initial lesion might be lymphocytic, as demonstrated in the experimental models of IS (11,12).

Effectiveness of Nonsteroidal Antiinflammatory Drugs (NSAIDs)

The beneficial effects of NSAIDs can be dramatic, and this is a significant diagnostic criterion, but in certain forms of IS, NSAIDs may be only moderately or hardly effective, without changing the diagnosis.

Pathophysiology: Example of ReA

ReA is characterized by the interaction between a genetic predisposition and arthritogenic microorganisms (13–15).

Animal models of IS have contributed significantly to the existing understanding of the pathogenesis of IS. B27 transgenic rats, created by introducing copies of HLA B27 genes and β-2 microglobulin into the murine genome, develop a condition close to IS, with peripheral arthritis, colitis, genital inflammation, and skin and ungual abnormalities (11,12). It is interesting to note that if the newborn rats are raised in a germ-free environment they develop only a combination of the skin and genital signs, without arthritis or colitis. These findings confirm the need for an interaction between genetic predisposition and microorganisms to explain the occurrence of articular signs.

Role of Arthritogenic Microorganisms in ReA

ReA is defined as aseptic arthritis developing in the weeks following an extra-articular infection (genitourinary or gastrointestinal). This generally accepted concept enlarges the more restrictive concept of Fiessinger-Leroy-Reiter syndrome, of which the typical oculourethrosynovial form has become rare. The classic arthritogenic bacteria are urogenital in 50% of cases of ReA, and gastrointestinal in 50%. The percentages vary according to region. Other bacteria have been causally linked, but without certainty (Table 74-3).

The risks of ReA evaluated by clinical experience show that 0.5% to 3% of the general population and 10% to 20% of HLA B27 patients develop ReA after nongonococcal urethritis (mainly *Chlamydia trachomatis* and *Ureaplasma urealyticum*). Similar figures have been recorded after gastrointestinal infections with arthritogenic enterobacteria.

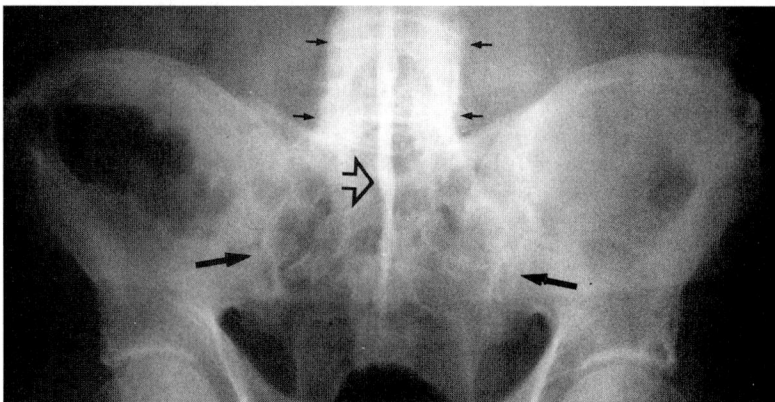

FIG. 74-4. A 55-year-old patient with ankylosing spondylitis with bilateral sacroiliitis *(large black arrows),* bamboo spine (syndesmophytes) *(small black arrows),* and interspinous ligament calcification *(open black arrow).*

TABLE 74-3. *Arthritogenic bacteria implicated in reactive arthritis*

	Urogenitary tract	Gastrointestinal tract	Other
Definite role	*Chlamydia trachomatis* *Ureaplasma urealyticum*	*Shigella flexneri* *Salmonella enteritidis* *Salmonella typhimurium* *Yersinia enterolitica* *Yersinia pseudotuberculosis* *Campylobacter jejuni*	
Possible role	*Neisseria gonorrhoeae*	*Shigella sonnei* *Clostridium difficile* *Leptospira icterohaemorrhagiae* *Escherichia coli* *Giardia lamblia* *Cryptosporidia* *Entamoeba histolytica* *Taenia saginata*	*Chlamydia pneumoniae* *Chlamydia psittaci* *Mycobacterium bovis* *Borrelia burgdorferi* *Streptococcus* *Staphylococcus aureus* *Propionibacterium acnes*

An important step in recent years has been the discovery of bacterial genomes (DNA and sometimes RNA) of Chlamydia in synovial samples from ReA using polymerase chain reaction (16–19). These results reinforce older studies that had already shown the existence of cytoplasmic inclusions of bacterial appearance (20).

However, for the moment questions remain unanswered, including:

- How do these bacteria persist in the articular cavity and escape from the immune system of the host?
- How can these bacteria cause arthritis?

An analysis of the microbiologic and immunologic data suggests the existence of two forms of ReA.

ReA of Chronic Infectious Arthritis Type

Certain forms of ReA could represent authentic chronic infectious arthritis caused by slow-growing organisms which are very difficult to cultivate and hence impossible to identify by the usual microbiologic methods. This hypothesis would appear to hold for Chlamydia, Mycoplasma, and Borrelia although not for enterobacteria. These microbes have an attenuated virulence, unlike those responsible for septic arthritis. Such forms of ReA are thus related to a "slow" intrasynovial infection, a condition also called "slow infectious arthritis" or "infectious ReA" (21).

ReA of Infection-Triggered Aseptic Arthritis Type

Some forms of ReA are probably aseptic and, if so, it is the persistence of bacterial antigens that could explain the appearance of an inflammatory reaction in the synovium. This hypothesis applies above all to enterobacteria (Yersinia, Salmonella, etc.). This type of arthritis, triggered by bacterial antigens in the absence of any viable intra-articular microbe, may be called "infection-triggered ReA."

What is the Role of HLA B27?

HLA B27 is certainly involved in the pathogenesis of IS because the prevalence of IS is proportional to that of HLA B27 for all ethnic groups and all forms of IS are associated, to varying degrees, with HLA B27.

HLA B27 is thus a genetic factor predisposing to IS, but those are only triggered by environmental factors, most commonly bacterial. With this hypothesis, HLA B27 may have different roles (22–24), including:

- HLA B27 may serve as a presentation molecule for bacterial arthritogenic peptides (traditional theory currently highly disputed).
- HLA B27 has molecular similarities to certain bacterial proteins (*Yersinia pseudotuberculosis* and *Shigella sonnei*). Because of these similarities, HLA B27 might become a target "by homology" for the host immune system.
- All bacteria do not have the same arthritogenic potential. As an example, certain strains of *Shigella flexneri* contain a plasmid with a gene coding for a peptide sequence homologous to the HLA B27 molecule, which could confer particular arthritogenic properties (25).
- Moreover, in some genetically predisposed individuals, HLA B27 would appear to lack the capacity to eliminate infected macrophages normally, thus facilitating the intra-articular persistence of the microbe.
- Arthritogenic bacteria like Yersinia or Salmonella are capable of modulating the function and structure of HLA B27 molecules. Affected HLA B27 molecules expressed specifically by infected cells might then serve as targets for the host immune system.

Despite these arguments it is possible that IS are not directly related to HLA B27, because 10% to 50% of IS are not HLA B27–related. The prevalence of AS is 1% to 3% in the B27 Caucasian population, but it is 20% if B27 subjects are related to a patient with AS. These figures suggest a familial predisposition independent of HLA B27.

Typical Evolution of Spondyloarthropathies

The evolution of IS has three characteristics:

1. Frequent spontaneous remissions occur in all types of IS, even in AS. This outcome is particularly characteristic of ReA, in which the first outbreak is usually followed after 1 to 6 months by complete remission. However, the condition recurs in nearly 60% of patients in 2 years, often in the same way.
2. All cases of IS can evolve toward a pattern of chronic AS. For example, 10% to 15% of patients develop an axial pattern 10 years after onset, similar to AS. The percentage reaches 25% to 40% after 15 years.
3. Transition from one form to another or the simultaneous occurrence of more than one IS is possible in the same patient. For example, the course of apparently primary AS may include episodes of ReA and, a few years later, the occurrence of true PA. These interrelationships with the different forms of IS illustrate the validity of this concept.

SPONDYLOARTHROPATHIES: DIAGNOSTIC PROCESS

A three-stage diagnostic process requires competent knowledge of the clinical characteristics and physiopathology of IS:

1. Evoke the diagnosis of IS by investigating a characteristic sign or symptom
2. Confirm the diagnosis of IS by eliminating other types of inflammatory arthritides and by investigating with other diagnostic procedures (Table 74-1)
3. Characterize the type of IS (Fig. 74-1).

Aims of the Clinical Interview

Aims of the clinical interview are:

- to investigate any familial aspect of IS as far as parents and grandparents
- to investigate any personal history of enthesopathy or articular involvement
- to investigate any recent or previous extra-articular condition such as psoriasis, acne, pustulosis, enteropathy, genitourinary or gastrointestinal infection, or ocular involvement. In some cases the presence of signs in parents and grandparents may also suggest the diagnosis.

Clinical Examination

Pelvic/Spinal Syndrome

Pelvic and spinal symptoms are mainly explained by axial enthesopathy which may involve the pelvis, spine, and anterior chest wall. Inflammatory back pain is mainly lumbar and dorsolumbar. The inflammatory nature is not always easy to confirm but it is probable if at least four of the following five characteristics are present:

- onset before the age of 40 years
- insidious onset
- evolution for over 3 months
- morning stiffness
- stiffness improved by exercise.

One feature of such back pain is that it can be easily controlled by NSAIDs. The other symptoms (limited mobility, deformation) occur later and do not contribute to early diagnosis.

Pain in the buttocks is a manifestation of sacroiliitis. This is usually bilateral but initially may be unilateral. The inflammatory pain occurs in the upper part of the thigh(s) and may radiate to the knees and occasionally to the calves. Clinical examination is difficult because few maneuvers are specific, especially when the patient has back pain. Pain reproduced on direct palpation is one of the best clinical signs.

Anterior (sternocostoclavicular and chondrosternal) and posterior thoracic pain (costovertebral) are very specific. Anterior lesions can be manifested by a true inflammatory tumefaction of the anterior chest wall.

Peripheral Enthesopathy

Retrocalcaneal and subcalcaneal inflammatory talalgia always suggests the diagnosis of IS in young patients. The inflammatory nature of this condition is usually expressed by pain on walking when arising from bed.

Other types of enthesopathy involving the anterior tibial tuberosity, the greater trochanter, and the pubic bone are expressed by characteristic inflammatory pain which should not be confused with microtraumatic tendinopathy.

Peripheral Articular Syndrome

The typical pattern is of oligoarthritis of the lower limbs, particular involving the knees and ankles. This oligoarthritis can occur in all types of IS, but it is very characteristic of ReA. It can occasionally be monoarticular or polyarticular. The polyarticular forms must not be confused with rheumatoid arthritis. Attention should be paid to two particular areas:

- Coxofemoral involvement (coxitis) is a sign of severity of IS. It is quite frequent in IS (20% to 40% of cases), especially in AS, and occurs approximately in the first 5 years in the course of the disease.
- "Sausage-shaped" toes and fingers (dactylitis) are characterized by an inflammatory erythematous, violaceous tumefaction that occurs particularly in ReA and PA. This very specific feature is generally rare, occurring in only 5% to 10% of cases of ReA secondary to *Chlamydia trachomatis*.

These peripheral forms are related to synovitis, which is often nonspecific. Sometimes the histologic features are more characteristic, with intense vascular hyperplasia and perivascular inflammation, but without significant necrosis or synovial hyperplasia. In practice, synovial histology is not of diagnostic value.

Extra-articular Manifestations

General Symptoms

Asthenia, weight loss, and fever are rare but may occur in acute ReA, particularly in forms following dysentery.

Uveitis

Uveitis is the most common extra-articular sign and takes the form of anterior uveitis expressed as red and painful eyes. The prevalence varies according to the form of IS. In AS it occurs in 30% of cases and may be an initial symptom in 2% to 5% of patients. The condition usually recovers without sequelae.

Other Extra-articular Manifestations

Various other extra-articular manifestations can occur, characteristic of each form of IS, sometimes successively and sometimes simultaneously in the same patient.

Cutaneous psoriasis, which occurs in PA, is often minimal and typically involves the scalp and body folds. Ungual involvement is very specific. Sometimes such lesions are only discovered on questioning, thus making definitive diagnosis difficult.

The gastrointestinal lesions of Crohn disease and ulcerative colitis often precede articular involvement. Occasionally the gastrointestinal involvement may be preceded, or sometimes revealed, by features of IS. In such cases the gastrointestinal signs are only detected on questioning. In practice, in the absence of any gastrointestinal signs, systematic gastrointestinal investigations (endoscopy) are not necessary, but it is interesting that systematic colonoscopies have shown inflammatory ileal lesions in more than 50% of cases of AS and ReA.

There are two types of extra-articular signs in ReA:

1. Signs of genitourinary (urethritis, prostatitis, salpingitis, cervicitis) or gastrointestinal infection (gastroenteritis) that precede onset of articular manifestations by 4 to 6 weeks. This entry route may pass unnoticed in more than half of cases, especially when it is an infection of the female genitalia.
2. Certain oculocutaneomucosal signs may mark the onset of ReA. These include: (a) common conjunctivitis, often bilateral; (b) mucosal lesions such as balanitis (20% of cases), which may be accompanied by macules or erosions on the scrotum, disappearing without sequelae; (c) lesions of the oral mucosa such as painless erythematous plaques; (d) papules or pustules, most often palmoplantar, which form hyperkeratosis which is sometimes difficult to differentiate from psoriasis (keratodermia blennorrhagica).

Other Visceral Complications of Spondyloarthropathies

Cardiac symptoms occur (valvular disease, myocarditis, and occasionally pericarditis), especially in AS and ReA. These conditions are rare (fewer than 5% of patients). Pulmonary involvement (upper lobe fibrosis) occurs almost exclusively with AS. Amyloid renal involvement occurs in 0.5% to 1% of cases of AS. Immunoglobulin A (IgA) nephropathy has sometimes been reported in AS. Neurologic involvement related to atlanto-axial subluxation occurs in 1% to 2% of cases. Aseptic arachnoiditis has also been reported, sometimes complicated by cauda equina syndrome characterized by an enlargement of the dural sac. Osteoporosis has been reported in advanced forms of AS, sometimes revealed by vertebral fractures.

VALUE OF DIAGNOSTIC METHODS

Value of Standard Blood Tests

Inflammatory syndrome is found in 60% to 80% of patients but the erythrocyte sedimentation rate (ESR) is often lower than 50 mm in the first hour, and cross-reacting protein (CRP) lower than 60 mg/L. A more intense inflammatory syndrome is more frequently observed in certain peripheral forms, particular in ReA of gastrointestinal or enteropathic origin, and in certain types of PA. On the other hand inflammatory syndrome may be very slight or absent in purely axial forms. When elevated ESR and CRP are present, the biologic signs overall indicate progression of IS.

Is Immunologic Monitoring Necessary?

Immunologic monitoring is of limited value but investigation of autoantibodies makes it possible to eliminate certain entities included in the differential diagnosis. In particular, it eliminates autoimmune diseases associated with peripheral articular signs (antinuclear antibodies), and particularly early RA (rheumatoid factors and anti-keratin). The only antibodies found in IS are rheumatoid factors, which are found in 5% to 10% of cases of AS and ReA and in 10% to 20% of cases of PA.

Is It Necessary to Biopsy the Synovium?

The synovial fluid and membrane do not contribute to the diagnosis of IS. However, the analysis of synovial fluid may eliminate infectious or microcrystalline arthritis.

Does an Infectious Workup Have Practical Implications?

Such a workup is only justified in ReA and undifferentiated IS. It has been demonstrated that there is *Chlamydia trachomatis* or *Ureaplasma urealyticum* infection in almost 30% of cases of undifferentiated oligoarthritis. In such cases there is a pathogenic value of identifying bacterial agents and there are therapeutic implications.

Investigation of genitourinary infection is justified, although extra-articular bacteria are rare once the articular symptoms have appeared. We currently recommend investigating the DNA of *Chlamydia trachomatis* in the first urine samples of the day in men and women and on cervical smears. This technique is more specific (about 100%) and more sensitive (about 80%) than classic methods. It also avoids the trauma of obtaining a urethral sample.

Stool samples are usually valueless in postdysentery forms because there are no pathogenetic bacteria in stools when the articular signs appear.

The practical value of routine bacteriologic studies of intra-articular samples has not been demonstrated.

Serologic investigations only occasionally provide diagnostic certainty because the presence of antibodies may simply be serologic cicatrization of a previous infection. In practice, only serologic studies are of value for *Chlamydia trachomatis*.

Value of Investigating HLA B27

Investigation of HLA B27 is only justified in early or atypical forms of IS. Discovery of HLA B27 must always be interpreted with caution in this context because 7% to 10% of the Caucasian population has at least one HLA B27 allele.

Value of Ophthalmologic Examination

Systematic examination for uveitis is warranted in childhood forms of IS with HLA B27.

Value of Radiographic Examination

Radiographic examination of typical sites can be performed (sacroiliac, dorsolumbar, and calcaneal articulations), even when there is no pain, because in some cases onset of lesions can be asymptomatic (26). Certain pitfalls can be avoided:

Enthesopathy should not be confused with growth-related epiphysitis in childhood forms. It should be noted that sacroiliac X-rays cannot be interpreted in children and adolescents because of physiologic pseudo-enlargement and irregularity. In adults, sacroiliitis can be confused with sacroiliac osteoarthri-

TABLE 74-4. *Differential diagnoses of spondyloarthropathies according to clinical or radiographic type of pelvic/spinal involvement*

Unilateral sacroiliac involvement	Infectious sacroiliitis • pyogenic infection • tuberculosis • brucellosis Paget disease Tumor
Bilateral sacroiliac involvement	Osteitis condensans ilii Sacroiliac osteoarthritis Variant of normal "pseudoerosion"
Spinal involvement	Scheuerman disease Diffuse idiopathic skeletal hyperostosis Infectious or microcrystalline (chondrocalcinosis) spondylodiscitis

tis or osteitis condensans ilii. Axial involvement must be distinguished from benign degenerative lesions (osteophytes) or from diffuse idiopathic skeletal hyperostosis (DISH) (Table 74-4).

Computed tomography scan is particularly valuable for the exploration of sacroiliac joints (axial slices) and thoracic and spinal involvement (cervicooccipital region). Scanning of the sacroiliac joint is warranted only if standard X-ray is not sufficiently clear or if there are doubts about the diagnosis (27).

Bone scintigraphy with technetium 99-labeled bisphosphonates is of limited value for early sacroiliitis because tracer uptake is usually bilateral and weak. Scintigraphy might be of greater value in the detection of peripheral enthesopathy. It can possibly be used in early atypical forms without objective radiographic evidence, or to investigate osteoarticular complications (fractures, fissures).

Magnetic resonance imaging currently has no practical value, but it might in the future facilitate the early diagnosis of axial and peripheral enthesopathies and make possible more precise exploration of neurologic complications (28,29).

PRACTICAL MONITORING OF CASES OF SPONDYLOARTHROPATHY

The routine aims in monitoring IS are to evaluate the evolution of the disease subjectively and objectively and to investigate extra-articular complications, particularly uveitis.

Evaluation of Symptoms

Symptoms can be evaluated by overall estimation of the pain, stiffness, and asthenia. Various indices have been validated but one of the easiest to use is the Bath Ankylosing Spondylitis Disease Activity Index (BAS-

TABLE 74-5. *The Bath Ankylosing Spondylitis Disease Activity Index (BASDAI)*

Please place a marker[a] on each line below to indicate your answer to each question, relating to *the past week.*
1. How would you describe the overall level of fatigue/tiredness you have experienced?
2. How would you describe the overall level of ankylosing spondylitis neck, back, or hip pain you have had?
3. How would you describe the overall level of pain/swelling in joints other than neck, back, or hip you have had?
4. How would you describe the overall level of discomfort you have had from any areas tender to touch or pressure?
5. How would you describe the overall level of morning stiffness you have had from the time you wake up?
6. How long does your morning stiffness last from the time you wake up?

---

[a]The patient places a marker on a 10 cm horizontal visual analog scale (VAS) for each question. Each VAS is scored from 0 to 10. The mean of the two scores relating to morning stiffness is taken, providing an aggregate score. The resulting 0–50 score for the overall index is converted to a 0–10 scale. The final BASDAI score has a range of 0–10.

From Garrett S, Jenkinson T, Kennedy G, et al. A new approach to defining disease status in ankylosing spondylitis: The Bath Ankylosing Spondylitis Disease Activity Index (BASDAI). *J Rheumatol* 1994;21:2286–2291, with permission.

DAI) (Table 74-5) that provides a practical and rapid estimate of a patient's functional abilities (30).

Objective Evaluation of Osteoarticular Involvement

This is based on study of mobility by various simple measurements that assess spinal damage (Schober test, fingertips-floor and occiput-wall distances) and thoracic involvement (chest expansion). Loss of height (due to kyphosis) and number of enthesopathies and sites of arthritis may also be included.

Blood Tests

Blood tests are of lesser value in the surveillance of IS because there is no absolute correlation between clinical evolution and increased levels of inflammatory proteins.

Investigation of Extra-articular Complications

The only extra-articular complication that must be systematically sought is uveitis. It is also necessary to be aware of the risk of valvular disorders.

SPECIFIC CLINICAL FEATURES

ReA

ReA is mainly manifested by peripheral articular signs (oligoarthritis of the lower limbs), sometimes associated

with extra-articular signs. "Sausage-shaped" fingers or toes are characteristic signs but do not always occur. In 10% to 30% of cases, the evolution of the disease occurs in an axial form on average 6 years after onset. Axial involvement is comparable to that of other forms of IS, although it is often less severe, more diffuse (cervical), and of asymmetric onset (unilateral sacroiliitis).

Psoriatic Arthritis (See Chapter 75)

Articular Manifestations of Inflammatory Enteropathy (Crohn Disease, Ulcerative Colitis)

In 10% to 30% of patients, the complications of these forms of enteropathy are peripheral arthritis usually involving the lower limbs (enteropathic rheumatism). These forms of arthritis usually develop in parallel with the gastrointestinal condition. The chronic forms, which are occasionally destructive (coxitis), sometimes occur with Crohn disease. In 5% to 15% of cases, such enteropathy is associated with axial involvement, which in more than one-third of cases may precede the onset of gastrointestinal symptoms, sometimes by several years. This form of IS, which evolves independently of the gastrointestinal disorder, often appears to be less severe and more often asymmetric (unilateral sacroiliitis).

Undifferentiated Spondyloarthropathies

Certain forms are characterized by oligoarthritis and enthesopathy of the lower limbs and are difficult to classify in the absence of axial symptoms and specific extra-articular manifestations. It is the clinical and immunogenetic characteristics (HLA B27 and history of familial IS) that place them in the nosologic group of IS.

OTHER FORMS OF SPONDYLOARTHROPATHIES

SAPHO Concept

The acronym SAPHO stands for synovitis, acne, pustulosis, hyperostosis, and osteitis. Certain dermatologic conditions (acne conglobata and fulminans, Verneuil disease, palmoplantar pustulosis) may have osteoarticular complications in the form of oligoarthritis or hyperostosis (usually sternocostoclavicular) or osteitis (31). Recurrent isolated multifocal osteitis and primary hyperostosis (Köhler disease) probably also belong to the SAPHO syndrome. Study of this group of conditions has shown that in 30% of cases there is sacroiliitis (unilateral in 50% of cases) and an association with HLA B27 in 20% to 35% of cases. It has been reported that inflammatory enteropathy occurs during the course of the disease. All of the characteristics indicate that SAPHO is a form of IS.

THERAPEUTIC PRINCIPLES

The treatment of IS is based mainly on drugs, particularly NSAIDs, and rehabilitation.

NSAIDs

NSAIDs are the basic treatment of IS. Several NSAIDs have been reported to be similarly effective for pain and joint mobility. It is impossible in practice to predict the most effective and best tolerated NSAID for an individual patient. It is necessary therefore to try a succession of NSAIDs, while explaining this to the patient. The initial dose prescribed is often the maximum, which will then be adapted to the course of the disease. NSAID treatment must be long term, as long as pain and stiffness persist. The prolonged treatment is of symptomatic value but it can also prevent bony ankylosis.

Analgesics

Analgesics are of value when NSAIDs are ineffective or not tolerated. All class I and II analgesics (World Health Organization classification) can be used effectively in combination with NSAIDs.

Disease Modifying Anti-Rheumatic Drugs (DMARDs)

Many of the DMARDs used in RA have also been used in IS. Among these are antipaladin drugs, gold salts, D-penicillamine, levamisole, sulfasalazine, methotrexate, and azathioprine. However, the efficacy is only demonstrated for peripheral IS.

Antitumor Necrosis α-Therapy (See Chapter 76)

Rehabilitation, Physiotherapy, and Rules Regarding Healthy Lifestyle

Functional rehabilitation is essential in the treatment of IS, although few studies have evaluated the real value of such measures. However, the success of rehabilitation depends largely on the motivation of the patient and the physiotherapist.

During painful phases it is necessary to use analgesics and to avoid deformation by rest and passive techniques such as positioning, analgesic physiotherapy, muscle-relaxing massage. Enthesopathy can be improved by cryotherapy and ionization. Wearing heel cushions is particularly valuable for talalgia. Corsets are prescribed in severe forms for posture and stabilization. Molded plastic antikyphosis corsets are sometimes used but they are often poorly tolerated.

TABLE 74-6. *Healthy lifestyle advice for patients with spondyloarthropathies*

Recommended	Not recommended
Firm mattress, low pillow	Carrying heavy loads
Alternating prone and supine lying positions	Lying on side
Sports activities (i.e., swimming)	Martial sports
Low-pain movement of affected joints	Prolonged sitting or standing
Positions and exercises several times a day	Excess body weight
	Smoking
Exercises at home	

The following exercises should be performed several times a day:
  stretching of all muscles of lower limbs
  spine stretching
  improvement of lordosis and spine mobility
  stretching of anterior chest wall and pectoral muscles
  breathing exercises.

During pain-free phases it is necessary to reestablish mobility and good axial and peripheral musculature using medical gymnastics and appropriate activities. Sports that encourage appropriate postures and balanced stretching of the spine are beneficial. Swimming, water games, and cross-country skiing are recommended. Running on soft ground, with appropriate shoes, can be recommended because maintained effort improves breathing capacity by developing mobility of the rib cage, and is beneficial for reducing the risk of osteoporosis.

Rehabilitation must be combined with healthy lifestyle, thus necessitating education and motivation of the patient (Table 74-6).

Local Treatment

Local treatment is particularly valuable in localized and resistant forms of arthritis.

Local Corticosteroids

The main indication for local treatment with corticosteroids is in peripheral arthritis, particularly the large joints (hips, knees, ankles). Intraarticular injection of the sacroiliac joints performed with radiographic visualization can be very beneficial (32). Enthesopathies sometimes benefit from topical corticosteroids, but injection of corticosteroids in contact with the tendon must be avoided because of the risk of secondary rupture (especially of patellar and Achilles tendons).

Synoviorthosis

Isotopic and osmic acid synoviorthosis are particularly valuable in involvement of large joints. They are much longer acting than corticosteroids and such treatment, which may be repeated, often makes it possible to delay prosthetic surgery.

Surgery

Early surgical synovectomy has not been shown to be particularly valuable, as in RA. It involves mainly surgical replacement (prosthesis) of the hip and knee. Corrective spinal surgery is the exception. It can only be envisaged where there is disabling kyphosis to improve walking or vision (inability to raise head).

Treatment and Prevention of Extra-articular Complications

The main complication is uveitis, which requires urgent treatment with topical corticosteroids that are readily absorbed by the cornea. This is combined with collyrium to dilate the pupil and avoid the development of synechiae. When the uveitis is generalized and resistant to topical treatment, subconjunctival injections and sometimes short courses of systemic corticosteroids can be used.

Other complications (neurologic, cardiac, etc.) occasionally warrant surgical treatment.

SPECIFIC THERAPEUTIC PRINCIPLES

ReA

Should Antibiotics Be Prescribed?

Altogether, clinical and experimental data exist to indicate that if antibacterial treatment of ReA can be started very early during the pathogenetic process, the disease can be prevented or the prognosis improved. In fully developed ReA, the value of antibacterial agents is less certain. All available evidence indicates that short-term conventional antibacterial treatment has no effect on the prognosis and final outcome of ReA, whereas prolonged (3-month) treatment with tetracycline shortens the duration of arthritis when triggered by *Chlamydia trachomatis*. Such treatment however has not proved effective in enteroarthritis (33,34). Several studies have in fact shown that cyclins, macrolides, and possibly quinolones can reduce the period of evolution of postvenereal ReA and the frequency of recurrence.

There is no ideal mode of therapy (type of antibiotic, dose, duration of treatment) and there is no consensus to date, but the principle of 3 months' antibiotic treatment with a cyclin or macrolide is accepted, especially during the first attack of postvenereal ReA. On the other hand, no study has yet to demonstrate the value of antibiotic treatment in postdysentery ReA.

Psoriatic Arthritis (See Chapter 75)

Inflammatory Enteropathies

How Should Peripheral Involvement of Crohn Disease and Ulcerative Colitis Be Treated?

Treatment of gastrointestinal diseases (corticosteroids, azathioprine, methotrexate) is often effective in peripheral arthritis. Topical or systemic corticosteroids can be used.

Can NSAIDs Be Used for Axial Forms?

Axial forms often pose complex treatment problems. NSAIDs sometimes exacerbate inflammatory episodes of enterocolitis. In practice, NSAIDs should be avoided during the active phase of enterocolitis. If the gastrointestinal disease is not actively progressing, courses of NSAIDs can be given, particularly to treat axial inflammatory signs that do not usually respond to other treatments (sulfasalazine, corticosteroids).

Which DMARDs Should Be Used?

Sulfasalazine can be beneficial in peripheral articular involvement, whereas mesalamine, which is the salicylic part of sulfasalazine and widely used today in gastrointestinal diseases, does not appear to be effective. Low doses of methotrexate can be valuable in peripheral forms.

CONCLUSION

Clinical and epidemiologic studies have shown that the seronegative types of IS can be classified as a distinct group of diseases.

However, many questions remain unresolved concerning the exact nature of the genetic haplotypes, the host's response, and the interaction between genetic factors and the suspected infectious agents.

REFERENCES

1. Stafford L, Youssef PP. Spondyloarthropathies: an overview. Intern Med J 2002;32:40–46.
2. Benoist M. Inflammatory spondyloarthropathies. In: Wiesel SW, Weinstein JN, Herkowitz HN, et al., eds. The lumbar spine, 2nd ed. Philadelphia: WB Saunders, 1996:797–811.
3. Calin A. Terminology, introduction, diagnostic criteria, and overview. In: Calin A, Taurog JD, eds. The spondylarthritides. Oxford: Oxford University Press, 1998:1–15.
4. Schumacher HR, Bardin T. The spondyloarthropathies: classification and diagnosis. Do we need new terminologies? Baillieres Clin Rheumatol 1998;12:551–565.
5. Dougados M, van der Linden S, Juhlin R, et al. The European Spondyloarthropathy Study Group preliminary criteria for the classification of spondyloarthropathy. Arthritis Rheum 1991;34:1218–1227.
6. Kennedy LG, Will R, Calin A. Sex ratio in the spondyloarthropathies

and its relationship to phenotypic expression, mode of inheritance and age at onset. J Rheumatol 1993;20:1900–1904.

7. Silman AJ. Ankylosing spondylitis and spondyloarthropathies. In: Silman AJ, Hochberg MC, eds. Epidemiology of the rheumatic diseases. Oxford: Oxford University Press, 2001:100–111.

8. Fournié B, Viraben R, Durroux R, et al. L'onycho-pachydermo-périostite psoriasique du gros orteil. Rev Rhum 1989;56:579–582.

9. Goupille P, Laulan J, Védère V et al. Psoriatic onycho-periostitis. Report of three cases. Scand J Rheumatol 1995;24:53–54.

10. Goupille P, Védère V, Roulot B, et al. Incidence of osteoperiostitis of the great toe in psoriatic arthritis. J Rheumatol 1996;23:1553–6.

11. Taurog JD. Animal models of the spondyloarthropathies. In: Calin A, Taurog JD, eds. The spondylarthritides. Oxford: Oxford University Press, 1988:223–237.

12. Taurog JD, Maika SD, Satumtira, et al. Inflammatory disease in HLA-B27 transgenic rats. Immunol Rev 1999;169:209–223.

13. Kuipers JG, Köhler L, Zeidler H. Reactive or infectious arthritis. Ann Rheum Dis 1999;58 :661–664.

14. Sieper J, Braun J. Pathogenesis of spondyloarthropathies: persistent bacterial antigen, auto-immunity or both? Arthritis Rheum 1995;38:1547–1554.

15. Sieper J, Kingsley J. Recent advances in the pathogenesis of reactive arthritis. Immunol Today 1996;17:160–162.

16. Bas S, Griffais R, Kvien TK, et al. Amplification of plasmid and chromosome Chlamydia DNA in synovial fluid of patients with arthritis and undifferentiated seronegative oligoarthritis. Arthritis Rheum 1995;38:1005–1013.

17. Li F, Bulbul R, Schumacher HR Jr, et al. Molecular detection of bacterial DNA in venereal associated arthritis. Arthritis Rheum 1996;39:950–958.

18. Rahman MU, Cheema MA, Schumacher HR, et al. Molecular evidence for the presence of Chlamydia in the synovium of patients with Reiter's syndrome. Arthritis Rheum 1992;35:521–529.

19. Hammer M, Nettelnbrecker E, Hopf S, et al. Chlamydial rRNA in the joints of patients with Chlamydia-induced arthritis and undifferentiated arthritis. Clin Exp Rheumatol 1992;10:63–66.

20. Schumacher HR, Magge S, Cherian PC, et al. Light and electron microscopic studies on the synovial membrane in Reiter's syndrome: immunocytochemical identification of chlamydial antigen in patients with early disease. Arthritis Rheum 1988;31:937–946.

21. Rook GAW, Stanford JL. Slow bacterial infections or autoimmunity? Immunol Today 1992;12:160–164.

22. Colbert RA, Prahalad S. Predisposing factors in the spondyloarthropathies: new insights into the role of HLA-B27. Curr Rheumatol Rep 2001;3:404–411.

23. Allen RL, Bowness P, McMichael A. The role of HLA-B27 in spondyloarthritis. Immunogenetics 1999;50:220–227.

24. Reveille JD, Ball EJ, Khan MA. HLA-B27 and genetic predisposing factors in spondyloarthropathies. Curr Opin Rheumatol 2001;13:265–272.

25. Ringrose JH. HLA B27 associated spondyloarthropathy, an autoimmune disease based on cross-reactivity between bacteria and HLA B27? Ann Rheum Dis 1999;58:598–610.

26. Braun J, Bollow M, Sieper J. Radiologic diagnosis and pathology of the spondyloarthropathies. Rheum Dis North Am 1998;24:697–735.

27. Yu W, Feng F, Dion E, et al. Comparison of radiography, computed tomography and magnetic resonance imaging in the detection of sacroiliitis accompanying ankylosing spondylitis. Skeletal Radiol 1998;27:311–320.

28. Bollow M, Braun J, Hamm B, et al. Early sacroiliitis in patients with spondyloarthropathy: evaluation with dynamic gadolinium-enhanced MR imaging. Radiology 1995;194:529–536.

29. Oostveen J, Prevo R, den Boer J, et al. Early detection of sacroiliitis on magnetic resonance imaging and subsequent development of sacroiliitis on plain radiography. A prospective, longitudinal study. J Rheumatol 1999;26:1953–1958.

30. Garrett S, Jenkinson T, Kennedy G, et al. A new approach to defining disease status in ankylosing spondylitis: the Bath Ankylosing Spondylitis Disease Activity Index (BASDAI). J Rheumatol 1994;21:2286–2291.

31. Kahn MF, Chamot AM. SAPHO syndrome. Rheum Dis Clin North Am 1992;18:225–246.

32. Maugars Y, Mathis C, Berthelot JM. Assessment of the efficacy of sacroiliac corticosteroid injections in spondyloarthropathies: a double-blind study. Br J Rheumatol 1996;35:767–770.

33. Leirisalo-Repo M. Are antibiotics of any use in reactive arthritis? APMIS 1993;101:575–581.

34. Toivanen A. Bacteria-triggered reactive arthritis: implications for antibacterial treatment. Drugs 2001;61:343–351.

CHAPTER 75

Psoriatic Arthritis

Philippe Goupille and David Borenstein

Psoriatic arthritis (PA) has common features with rheumatoid arthritis (RA) and ankylosing spondylitis (AS) and belongs in the spondyloarthropathy group. The variety of its clinical and radiologic manifestations warrants special emphasis.

HISTORICAL REVIEW

The first case of PA was reported by Alibert in 1818; the first report on its clinical and radiologic features was performed by Bourdillon in 1888. Subsequently, numerous clinical and epidemiologic studies have proved the validity of this disorder as a separate entity (1–5).

EPIDEMIOLOGY

The prevalence of inflammatory arthritis in patients with cutaneous psoriasis is about 5% to 7% and increases to 32% to 42% for the axial involvement (6,7); radiologic abnormalities of the sacroiliac joint have been reported in 43% of patients with cutaneous psoriasis (6,8). On the other hand, the prevalence of cutaneous psoriasis in patients with inflammatory arthritis is about 4% (9).

Epidemiology of Psoriasis

The prevalence of cutaneous psoriasis in the white population is about 1% to 3% (9), and lower in black Africans, black Americans, and Asians. The sex ratio is 1:1 (9) and the mean age of occurrence is 27 years.

Epidemiology of Psoriatic Arthritis

Prevalence

Commonly cited prevalence figures for the general population are 1 to 2 per 1,000 (10), but the lack of diagnostic criteria leads to an underestimation.

Role of Age and Sex

The age of occurrence is 30 to 50 years (11,12). The sex ratio is 1:1 (13,14), but varies according to clinical presentation. There is a predominance of men in axial (13,15) and distal interphalangeal joint involvement (12) and of women in the polyarticular forms (11).

Links with Cutaneous Psoriasis

Psoriasis precedes the arthritis in 64% to 87% of patients; the skin disease appears after the joint manifestations in about 6% to 18%; and skin and articular disease occur simultaneously in 8% to 30%.

GENETICS AND HLA

Psoriasis

Psoriasis is associated with HLA-B13, B17, CW6, and DR7 in the white population (16).

Psoriatic Arthritis

Family and epidemiologic studies have confirmed the genetic characteristic of PA. Moll and Wright have shown the presence of PA in 8.3% of first-degree parents of patients with PA (3). The link with HLA-B13, B17, CW6, and DR7 is present but weaker than in psoriasis (17). HLA-B27 is present in 18% to 30% of patients, especially in axial involvement (35% to 64%) (18,19). The association between HLA-B27 and radiologic sacroiliac involvement has been confirmed (18,20), especially in case of bilateral involvement (HLA-B27 in 22% of unilateral sacroiliitis and 85% of bilateral sacroiliitis). On the contrary, axial involvement without sacroiliitis is not associated with HLA-B27 (19). The association HLA-B38 and HLA-B39 is debated. HLA-B38 is present in

702

17% to 35% of cases compared with 4% to 6% of psoriasis in the white population (21).

PATHOGENESIS

Psoriasis is a multifactorial condition of hereditary and environmental pathogenesis. It is characterized by wide polymorphism of the cutaneous lesions and the presence of extracutaneous lesions, particularly articular.

The relationship between cutaneous psoriasis and articular lesions depends on the following factors.

- An epidemiologic link
- The existence of common trigger factors, particularly environmental and psychological factors
- The existence of common genetic factors
- The existence of similar elementary cutaneous and synovial membrane lesions characterized by a lymphocyte T infiltrate and excessive angiogenesis

Despite these shared factors, the following arguments suggest that the pathogenesis of skin lesions might be different from those of the articular lesions.

- The cutaneous and articular lesions begin simultaneously in only 15% of cases.
- There is no correlation between the severity and activity of the skin lesions and the severity of articular involvement.
- The articular involvement, which is particularly polymorphic, appears to be related to a particular genetic predisposition.
- Although the inflammatory cutaneous and synovial infiltrates are similar, it has been demonstrated that cutaneous and synovial lymphoid populations are different.

Genetic Factors

As in cutaneous psoriasis, the familial forms and genomic associations suggest the role of genetic factors.

Environmental Factors

Several environmental, microbial, mechanical, physical, drug, and psychosocial factors can cause cutaneous psoriasis. The same is the case for articular involvement, for which various trigger factors have been studied (22).

Infectious Factors

Streptococci

Vasey et al. demonstrated the more frequent existence of antiexotoxin streptococcal antibodies in PA than in cutaneous psoriasis (23). Ribosomal RNA of group A streptococci has been detected in the peripheral blood and synovium in patients with PA (24).

Viruses

Viruses (e.g., Epstein-Barr virus and cytomegalovirus) may act as trigger or maintaining factors, particularly in psoriatic synovitis. Human immunodeficiency virus and hepatitis C virus also may have triggering roles.

Toxic Factors

In contrast to skin lesions, it appears that toxins and drugs are not trigger or exacerbating factors in PA.

Mechanical Factors

Several reports have demonstrated the occurrence of posttraumatic PA defined by precise criteria (25,26). In a study of 700 patients, Punzi et al. reported posttraumatic arthritis in 8% of patients with PA compared to only 1.6% and 2% in RA and AS, respectively, in almost all cases involving peripheral forms of PA (26). The causal mechanisms might have been psychological or physical, by analogy with the reports on cutaneous lesions.

Immunopathology

Psoriatic lesions are characterized by lymphoid infiltrates, cutaneous and articular deposits of immunoglobulins, and neoangiogenesis, thus suggesting immunologic mechanisms.

Cutaneously, three hypotheses make it possible to establish a schematic relationship between specific abnormalities of keratinocytes in psoriasis and the lymphoid infiltrates (27).

1. Lymphocyte theory: The abnormalities of lymphocytes may cause abnormal proliferation and differentiation of keratinocytes.
2. Keratinocyte theory: The psoriatic keratinocytes may be abnormal and produce cytokines able to activate T lymphocytes.
3. Fibroblast theory: The dermal fibroblasts may be abnormal and trigger keratinocyte proliferation.

Psoriatic Synovitis

Psoriatic synovitis is not specific. Nevertheless, certain features appear to distinguish it from that of RA (i.e., less marked proliferation of synoviocytes and lymphoplasmacytic infiltrate, and presence of neoangiogenesis characterized by numerous vessels with thickened walls infiltrated by inflammatory cells).

This type of synovitis also is characterized by the early expression of various synovial membrane enzymes, metalloproteinase, cysteine proteases, and cathepsins, which must have a significant role in the occurrence of osteoarticular destruction.

Although predominantly lymphocytic, this type of synovitis can be distinguished from inflammatory cutaneous infiltrate for the following reasons.

- Injection of T lymphocytes from psoriasis plaques into severe combined immunodeficiency disease (SCID) mice does not cause arthritis.
- The infiltrate is mainly composed of CD4 T lymphocytes, which appear to be in greater quantities than in cutaneous lesions.
- Synovial T lymphocytes express fewer cutaneous lymphocyte antigen than lymphocytes of cutaneous tropism.

Psoriatic Enthesitis

The initial feature in most cases of PA is enthesitis; an experimental model in HLA B27 transgenic rats supports this (28). In fact, such rats developed spondyloarthropathy associated with skin and ungual lesions resembling psoriasis. Nevertheless, it has been difficult to establish the relationship between skin and enthesitis lesions, except for distal involvement, which sometimes is expressed as psoriatic onycho-pachydermo-periostitis. In this case there appears to be a direct relationship between cutaneo-ungual lesions and enthesitis.

Immunohistochemical analysis of psoriatic enthesitis appears to be characterized by the accumulation of monocytes and macrophages but few lymphocytes. These findings are not compatible with the widely developed lymphoid theory on the pathogenesis of cutaneous and synovial membrane lesions. In forms that mainly involve enthesitis, synovial membrane involvement might be "contiguous" synovitis related to release of various proinflammatory cytokines by enthesitis.

CLINICAL PRESENTATION AND DIAGNOSIS

Are there specific clinical features of PA that make it possible to differentiate it from other forms of inflammatory arthropathies? Compared to RA, PA has been reported to be equally distributed in both sexes, articular involvement is asymmetrical, there is an absence of subcutaneous nodules, frequent axial and distal interphalangeal involvement, a better prognosis, specific radiographic abnormalities, and absence of rheumatoid factor. It also has been demonstrated that among the group of patients with seronegative polyarthritis, those with psoriasis mostly have distal interphalangeal involvement, which is mainly erosive. Psoriatic arthritis includes more peripheral involvement, asymmetric sacroiliitis,

TABLE 75-1. *Clinical forms of psoriatic arthritis*

Involvement predominantly of distal interphalangeal joints
Mutilating arthritis
Symmetric seronegative polyarthritis
Asymmetric oligoarthritis or monoarthritis
Axial involvement (spondylitis and sacroiliitis)

and absence of masculine predominance than AS. Although spinal involvement in AS appears to progress from the lumbar spine to the cervical spine radiologically, the distribution appears more random in PA (29).

However, there are no criteria such as have been defined for lupus or RA. The usually accepted and used classification is that of Moll and Wright, which was established in 1973 (29) (Table 75-1). These clinical forms frequently overlap; reports of their respective proportions vary widely in the literature.

Clinical Forms

Symmetric or asymmetric involvement of one or more distal interphalangeal joints, with concomitant ungual psoriasis, occurs in 25% to 60% of patients with PA, in isolation or with other manifestations (2,6,12). Its course is benign generally.

Arthritis mutilans contributes fewer than 10% of cases. Onset is often abrupt, with constitutional symptoms and severely inflammatory arthritis in multiple joints. Severely deformed flail hand can result from this form of PA.

Symmetric polyarthritis similar to RA occurs in about 25% of cases. This form is slightly more common among women. Tests for rheumatoid factor are negative 85% to 90% of the time (11).

Asymmetric oligoarthritis or monoarthritis occurs in about 70% of cases. Exacerbations lasting several months occur, often separated by prolonged remissions. The asymmetric oligoarticular nature of this arthritis can result in involvement of all three joints of a single digit. Sausage digits (dactylitis) can develop as a result of concomitant arthritis of the distal and proximal interphalangeal joints and flexor tenosynovitis.

Psoriatic axial involvement often is accompanied with other forms of PA. The symptoms are similar to those of AS but may be less severe. The sacroiliac joints are involved in 30% to 50% of cases (1,12,20,30). Extraarticular involvement (lungs, heart, and eyes) seems less common than in RA. In addition, other patterns occur.

Enthesopathy (inflammatory disorder of the tendon–bone junction) can affect the sacroiliac joints, pubic symphyses, intervertebral joints, anterior chest wall, calcaneus, and ends of the digits. Peripheral enthesopathy manifesting as heel pain and Achilles tendinitis can be the first manifestations; and coexistence of psoriatic skin lesions should prompt a search for further evidence of PA.

TABLE 75-2. *Diagnostic criteria for psoriatic arthritis*

Primary criterion
  Psoriasis (cutaneous or ungueal) associated with pain
    and articular swelling limited mobility of at least one
    joint for more than 6 weeks
Secondary criteria
  Pain and swelling limited movement of at least one joint
    for more than 6 weeks identified by physician
  Inflammatory symptoms of distal interphalangeal joints,
    with the exclusion of Heberden nodules
  "Sausage-shaped" fingers or toes
  Asymmetric arthritis of hands and feet
  Absence of subcutaneous nodules
  Absence of rheumatoid factor
  Inflammatory synovial fluid. Absence of infection and
    sodium urate or calcium pyrophosphate crystals.
  Synovial biopsy revealing synovial hypertrophy, with
    infiltration predominantly of mononuclear cells and no
    granuloma or tumor
  Erosive damage to small joints revealed on radiography
    of peripheral joints, without obvious osteoporosis or
    erosive osteoarthritis.
  Axial radiography of skeleton revealing one or more of
    the following: sacroiliitis, syndesmophytes, or
    paravertebral ossification

Definite: Primary criterion and six secondary criteria.
Probable: Primary criterion and four secondary criteria.
Possible: Primary criterion and two secondary criteria.

Distinctive clinical patterns result from involvement of the foot in PA. The disease can affect the calcaneus and forefoot, particularly the great toe. Bauer toe is characterized by distal interphalangeal arthritis with psoriasis of the same toe or toenail. In psoriatic onychopachydermoperiostitis of the great toe, there is ungual psoriasis, thickening of the distal soft tissues, and osteoperiostitis of the distal phalanx without involvement of the interphalangeal joint (31,32).

TABLE 75-3. *Differential diagnosis of psoriatic arthritis and ankylosing spondylitis*

	Psoriatic arthritis	Ankylosing spondylitis
Gender	Men = women	Men > women
Distribution	Axial and peripheral	Axial
DIP involvement	5% Of patients	Absent
Syndesmophytes	Asymmetric, random distribution	Symmetric, usually with caudocranial progression
Sacroiliitis	Often asymmetric	Usually symmetric
HLA B27	40%–50%	80%–90%

DIP, distal interphalangeal; HLA, human leukocyte antigen.

TABLE 75-4. *Differential diagnosis of psoriatic arthritis and rheumatoid arthritis*

	Psoriatic arthritis	Rheumatoid arthritis
Gender	Men = women	Women > men
Distribution	Asymmetric	Symmetric
DIP involvement	Usual	Rare
Syndesmophytes	Usual	Absent
Sacroiliitis	Usual	Rare
Rheumatoid factor	Rare	Usually present

DIP, distal interphalangeal.

Extraarticular involvement is less frequent than in AS. Ocular and cardiac involvement are the most frequently reported.

Positive and Differential Diagnosis

The coexistence of skin lesions is a feature of PA. The rheumatologist must be aware of the specificity of articular conditions, but he must also systematically investigate the presence or history of psoriasis in all patients with osteoarticular disorders (axial or peripheral) and check the typical areas affected (e.g., elbows, knees, scalp, nails, and buttocks). The diagnostic criteria proposed by Wright and Moll in 1976 (10), and modified by Bennet in 1979 (Table 75-2) may be used, although the experience of the clinician is fundamental for this very unusual condition.

From the dermatologic point of view, the conditions likely to cause confusion are seborrheic dermatitis and mucosal infections. From the rheumatologic point of view, the main conditions to be eliminated are AS and RA (Tables 75-3 and 75-4). Microcrystalline disorders, particularly gout, sometimes are evoked in the setting of dactylitis, and erosive osteoarthritis of interphalangeal joints can cause diagnostic difficulty.

DIAGNOSTIC METHODS AND OUTCOME MEASURES

Imaging

Incidence

The incidence of radiographic evidence is difficult to define because of the variations in the populations studied and the methods used.

Typical Features

Certain typical features indicate the diagnosis (Table 75-5).

The overall asymmetric nature of the radiographic lesions has been demonstrated mainly in the fingers and toes. The following lesions appear to be indicative of PA.

TABLE 75-5. *Radiologic features of psoriatic arthritis*

Synovial, cartilaginous involvement and entheses
Most commonly asymmetric distribution
Interphalangeal joint involvement of fingers and toes
Sacroiliitis and spondylitis with paravertebral ossifications
Coexistence of erosions and bone proliferation
Bony ankylosis
Resorption of phalangeal tufts

- Pseudoenlargement of the articular space in fingers and toes, owing to erosion affecting the ends of the bones and progressively extending to the centre of the joint
- The classic "pencil-in-cup" deformity, associated with progressive thinning of the heads of metacarpal or metatarsal bones or the phalanges, and cupula-shaped hollowing of the bases of phalanges
- Bony ankylosis of the interphalangeal joints of the fingers and toes. The diagnosis is more obvious when osteolysis is followed by bony ankylosis or the coexistence of osteolysis of one joint and ankylosis of another.
- Resorption of phalangeal tufts, often associated with damage to the distal interphalangeal joint
- Periostosis of the calcaneum; tibial and peroneal, and femoral and trochanteric diaphyses; and lateral faces of the phalanges of the fingers

Sites of Involvement

Peripheral Skeleton

Hands

Predominance of PA in distal interphalangeal joints has been confirmed. Both erosive arthritis without osteophytes and pseudoenlargement features have been reported. Metacarpal-phalangeal, radiocarpal, and carpal joint involvement are less frequent than in RA.

Feet

The forefoot is a frequent site of PA and involvement of the big toe is very characteristic. This can take the form of simple osteoperiostitis of the phalanx (bone proliferation of the base, often associated with resorption of the tuft) without changes to the articular space, a very indicative and often early sign (32,33).

Calcaneum

Involvement of the calcaneum is more frequent in case of sacroiliitis. There may also be vague irregular posterior or plantar enthesopathy or postero-superior erosion.

Axial Skeleton

Involvement of the sacroiliac joint is the most common sign (Fig. 75-1). It is sometimes isolated, without spine involvement, or there is damage to the cervical spine while sparing the dorsolumbar spine. It is most often bilateral, but unilateral forms are more frequent than in AS (34). The joint may have a vague appearance in the early stages because of erosion and sclerosis usually predominating on the iliac side; later there is development into pseudoenlargement, pinching, and finally true fusion of the joint.

Spine involvement frequently is associated with sacroiliac involvement. This is characterized by the occurrence of syndesmophytes, two types of which have been described: (a) the classical features of vertical pointed ends, situated in contact with the disk perimeter, as seen in AS; and (b) more crude, irregular ossification further from the disk perimeter (and able to be confused with diffuse idiopathic skeletal hyperostosis [DISH]). Such syndesmophytes are more often asymmetrical and unilateral than in AS (29,34) and may appear at any level, and even affect only the cervical spine in contrast to AS in which progression is caudocranial (29). Involvement of the posterior dorsolumbar interapophyseal joints is rare, as are the features of osteitis, erosive Romanus spondylitis (squaring), "bamboo"-shaped spine, and symphysis pubis (29,34).

Involvement of the cervical spine, which is frequent and sometimes isolated, involves ossification of the anterior longitudinal ligament, arthritis of the posterior interapophyseal joints (particularly C3-C4, C4-C5, and C5-C6), syndesmophytes, and atlanto-axial subluxation (34,35). Finally, anterior chest wall involvement can occur, particularly of the manubriosternal and sternoclavicular joints.

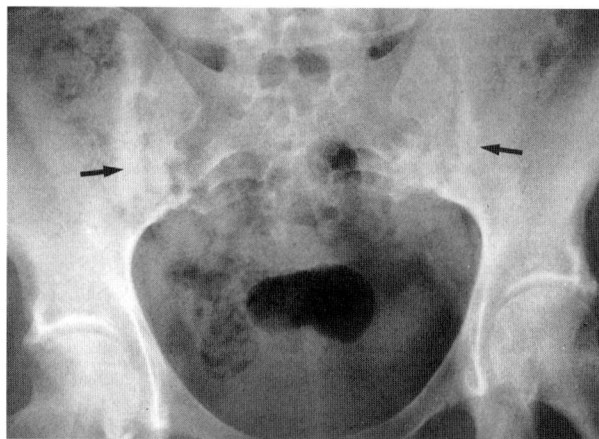

FIG. 75-1. A 38-year-old woman who had psoriasis for 8 years and back pain for 4 years. Antero-posterior roentgenograph of the sacroiliac joints revealing bilateral erosions and reactive sclerosis *(black arrows)*.

TABLE 75-6. *Radiologic features differentiating psoriatic arthritis (PA) from ankylosing spondylitis (AS)*

	Psoriatic arthritis	Ankylosing spondylitis
Asymmetric involvement of sacroiliac joint	++	+
Crude, asymmetric syndesmophytes	++	+
Resorption of phalangeal tufts	++	−
Osteitis	Rare	++
Vertebral "squaring"	Rare	++
Predominantly peripheral involvement	Distal (hands, feet)	Proximal (shoulders, hips)

Differential Diagnosis

These characteristic features of PA lesions visualized by radiography make it possible to differentiate RA (a frequent problem in polyarticular forms), AS (in axial forms), and DISH (axial forms with crude, irregular, and asymmetric paravertebral ossifications) (Tables 75-6, 75-7, and 75-8).

Laboratory Tests

Erythrocyte sedimentation rate (ESR), C reactive protein (CRP), and fibrinogen levels usually are raised (36), but can be normal, particularly in axial forms. Rheumatoid factor is present in about 10% of cases. Low levels of antinuclear antibodies may be detected, but the prevalence is not greater than 6% to 7%. Hyperuricemia, which is caused by increased cutaneous cell turnover, is present in less than 10% of patients with PA. The synovial fluid usually is inflammatory, but without any specific characteristics.

TABLE 75-7. *Radiologic features differentiating psoriatic arthritis from rheumatoid arthritis*

	Psoriatic arthritis	Rheumatoid arthritis
Areas involved	Synovial joints Symphyses Entheses	Synovial joints − −
Distal interphalangeal joints	++	−
Anterior chest wall	+	Rare
Asymmetric involvement	++	Rare
Bone proliferation	++	−
Resorption of phalangeal tufts	++	−
Articular ankylosis	Fingers, toes	Carpus
Spine and sacroiliac involvement	++	Rare

TABLE 75-8. *Radiologic features differentiating psoriatic arthritis from DISH*

	Psoriatic arthritis	DISH
Posterior interapophyseal joints	Erosion, sclerosis ankylosis	Degeneration
Sacroiliac joint	Erosion, sclerosis ankylosis	Osteophytes
Peripheral involvement	Erosion	Nonerosion

DISH, diffuse idiopathic skeletal hyperostosis.

OUTCOME AND NATURAL HISTORY

Psoriatic arthritis is classically considered relatively benign, or at least compared to RA (7,11,14,37,38). However, this is debatable and the different clinical forms of the condition must be taken into account.

Severity of Psoriatic Arthritis

In view of the favorable outcome of oligoarticular forms, the rarity of deformations, and the lesser degree of severity of lesions seen radiologically (7,11,37), PA is considered a condition that is never fatal and rarely affects functional outcome. In fact, polyarticular, symmetric, and progressively destructive and deforming forms that are responsible for significant dysfunction are not rare.

Kammer et al. confirmed the preponderance of oligoarticular forms of favorable outcome, but reported many cases of symmetric, progressively destructive, and deforming polyarticular forms (14). In a series of 220 patients, the majority of whom had polyarticular forms, Gladman et al. were much more guarded in their prognosis (13): 50% had an asymmetric condition, 16% had deformations, and 11% had marked dysfunction.

Outcome of Psoriatic Arthritis

More than 50% of patients had oligoarticular forms of unpredictable outcome (exacerbations lasting from a few weeks to a few months, interspersed with prolonged remissions) with no sequelae (11). However, there have been few longitudinal studies (11,38–40). Of these, the series reported by Gladman et al. on a majority of polyarticular forms demonstrated that, deformations and articular damage increased even when the inflammatory condition improved (40).

Prognostic Factors

Although poorly understood, these include gender, age at onset, sites of involvement, and genetic factors. The extent of the cutaneous involvement does not influence the articular prognosis (13). As in RA, recognizing these factors is essential for the most effective therapy, and certain forms of PA probably have been underestimated and insufficiently treated.

NOSOLOGY

Place within the Spondyloarthropathy Group

There is no doubt that PA belongs in the spondyloarthropathy group in view of its clinical signs (peripheral and axial involvement, enthesopathy, and extraarticular signs), radiographic evidence (sacroiliitis), and genetic background. However, it is an individual entity within this group, with variable manifestations and the current criteria used for the diagnosis of spondyloarthropathies are sometimes inadequate. For example, in a series of 205 patients with psoriasis, 75 (36%) patients with PA were diagnosed by clinicians (41). Only 49 patients (24%) met the criteria of spondyloarthropathy according to the European Spondyloarthropathy Study Group (42), with sensitivity of criteria at 65% and specificity 99% to 100%.

TREATMENT

The therapeutic principles are the same as for other inflammatory spondyloarthropathies, apart from certain points. Treatments for PA are influenced by: (a) its usually benign nature; (b) the variable course of the disease and uncertain prognosis making uncontrolled trials unreliable; and (c) the existence of associated dermatosis influences the choice and modalities of treatment (requires specific treatment). Few disease modifying anti-rheumatic drugs (DMARDs) have been evaluated; they are used based on their effectiveness in RA.

Why Is There a Dearth of Data on Disease Modifying Anti-rheumatic Drugs for Psoriatic Arthritis?

Several factors may be involved. Psoriatic arthritis is widely believed to be uncommon; therefore, the market represented by this disease holds little appeal. In addition, PA was long considered a benign disease that required only nonspecific symptomatic treatments.

Because PA shares clinical and radiologic features with RA and AS, DMARDs used in these two disorders are commonly used in PA, and no pressing need for formal validation of this practice is perceived.

What Specific Methodologic Obstacles Are Raised by Psoriatic Arthritis Evaluations?

There is no consensus about the diagnostic criteria. Thus, the criteria used for patient inclusion vary across therapeutic trials, making comparisons difficult.

Psoriatic arthritis covers a broad clinical spectrum. Most patients have a combination of these clinical patterns (e.g., oligoarthritis or axial involvement + enthesopathy, polyarthritis + distal interphalangeal arthritis, or oligoarthritis + axial involvement). Yet, reports of therapeutic trials, particularly the earliest ones, often provide little detail on the clinical features.

The therapeutic trials published to date included patients with various forms of PA. In the overwhelming majority of cases, different treatments are used for peripheral and axial forms, and few drugs have been found effective in axial forms. Yet many of the patents included in therapeutic trials had both peripheral and axial manifestations. This decreases the likelihood of finding clear evidence of efficacy. A more rational approach is to conduct separate studies of axial disease (which is similar to AS) and polyarthritis.

There are no specific criteria for evaluating disease activity. A number of tools that evaluate disease activity and functional impairment are available for investigating the efficacy of treatments for RA (disease activity score: American College of Rheumatology [ACR], 20, 50, and 70; health assessment questionnaire [HAQ]). In contrast, no specific tools have been developed for PA. The indices developed by Calin et al. for evaluating spondyloarthropathies (Bath Ankylosing Spondylitis Disease Activity Index and Bath Ankylosing Spondylitis Functional Index) are often used for axial forms of PA (43,44) and tools for evaluating RA in peripheral forms.

The course of PA usually is erratic. A fluctuating course with unpredictable but sometimes prolonged remissions is widely believed to be the rule. Thus, open-label studies of DMARDs can provide useful information on safety but are clearly inadequate for establishing efficacy.

The concomitant skin disease influences the choice of treatment. For instance, antimalarials and, to a lesser extent, gold, can cause exacerbations in the skin lesions or other severe adverse events. Extensive skin involvement may prompt treatment with methotrexate or cyclosporine, which improves the rheumatic manifestations.

Which Disease Modifying Anti-rheumatic Drugs Are Appropriate?

Six of the DMARDs used in RA and evaluated in polyarticular forms of PA deserve discussion: sulfasalazine, methotrexate, gold, antimalarials, cyclosporine, and azathioprine.

Sulfasalazine

Five randomized placebo-controlled studies have been published (45—49). The daily dosage was 2 to 3 g. Overall, sulfasalazine was significantly more effective than the placebo. Efficacy seemed greater with the 3 g per day dosage. Safety was satisfactory.

Methotrexate

The earliest studies used high dosages (30 to 50 mg/wk) and found incontrovertible evidence of efficacy at the expense of major side effects. When low-dose methotrexate was found effective in RA, open-label studies of low doses (15 mg/wk) were conducted in PA. The effects were favorable. The results were inconclusive in a prospective, randomized, placebo-controlled, double-blind trial of methotrexate, 7.5 to 15 mg per week, given to 37 patients for 12 weeks (50). However, this may be ascribable to the short treatment duration or small sample size.

Gold

Most studies used oral gold and found no evidence of efficacy. In contrast, efficacy has been reported in studies of intramuscular gold, including one conducted comparatively with oral gold and a placebo (51). Although controversial, the risk of skin lesion exacerbation deserves consideration.

Antimalarials

No controlled studies are available, and open-label studies provide little evidence of efficacy. However, they do show that the risk of skin lesion exacerbation is small (52,53). This adverse event has been reported mainly with chloroquine. Nevertheless, careful monitoring of the skin lesions is in order even with hydroxychloroquine.

Cyclosporine

Open-label studies and controlled but methodologically flawed studies suggest efficacy. Treatment-limiting side effects (e.g., arterial hypertension and serum creatinine elevation) can occur as with RA.

Azathioprine

Open-label studies in small numbers of patients suggest efficacy. In sum, only sulfasalazine has been evaluated in well-designed controlled studies; strong evidence of efficacy was found. However, available data strongly suggest that methotrexate and other drugs may be effective as well. No studies specifically designed to evaluate structural effects have been published. Combinations of DMARDs have not been evaluated.

What Can Be Expected of Anti-Tumor Necrosis Factor-α Agents?

Anti-tumor necrosis factor -α agents (i.e., infliximab and etanercept) were introduced recently for the treatment of RA. Several open-label studies and few controlled studies have been conducted in PA.

Etanercept

The results suggest dramatic improvements in the skin and joint abnormalities (54–56). An open-label study in

10 patients showed dramatic efficacy on the joint and skin involvement (57).

A randomized, placebo-controlled, double-blind trial of etanercept (25 mg twice a week) was conducted in 60 patients with PA. Efficacy was remarkable: The response rate (Psoriatic Arthritis Response Criteria, PSARC) was 87% with etanercept and 23% with the placebo. Corresponding figures were 73% versus 13% for the ACR 20, 50% versus 3% for the ACR 50, 75% versus 5% for the painful joint score, 72% versus 19% for the swollen joint score, and 83% versus 3% for the HAQ score. All of these differences were statistically significant (58). In each group, 19 patients with psoriasis were evaluable; a 75% or greater improvement in the psoriasis area and severity index (PASI) occurred in 26% of the etanercept patients versus 0% of the placebo patients. The mean PASI improvements in these two groups were 46.2% and 8.7%, respectively. No serious adverse events were recorded.

An open-label extension of the treatment period to 24 weeks confirmed these findings: Response rates were 82% for the PSARC, 74% for the ACR 20, 56% for the ACR 50, and 30% for the ACR 70, and the mean improvement in the PASI was 62% (59). Nine months into etanercept therapy, 28% of patients had no painful joints and 42% had no swollen joints. No serious adverse events occurred.

A large multicenter, randomized study has compared etanercept (n = 101; 25 mg ¥ 2/week subcutaneously) with placebo (n = 104) during 24 weeks (60). A statistically significant improvement of ACR 20, 50, and 70 scores (p < .001 in favor of etanercept), HAQ (p < .0001) and PASI (47% versus 0% in favor of etanercept) was observed.

Infliximab

A single-center, open-label pilot study evaluated 21 patients with spondylarthropathies, including nine with PA. The dosage was 5 mg/kg as an infusion at baseline and after 2 and 6 weeks. Rapid and dramatic improvements occurred in the axial and peripheral manifestations after the first infusion; these effects persisted throughout the 12-week study period. Similar improvements occurred in the skin lesions (61).

The same group has conducted a 12-week, randomized, placebo-controlled, double-blind trial (62). Forty patients with active spondyloarthropathies, including 18 with PA, were randomly assigned to receive an intravenous loading dose (weeks 0, 2, and 6) of 5 mg/kg infliximab or placebo. The primary end points were the improvements in patient and physician global assessments of disease activity on a 100-mm visual analog scale. Both primary end points improved significantly in the infliximab group compared with the baseline value, with no improvement in the placebo group. As early as week 2 and sustained up to week 12, there was a highly statistically significant difference between the values for these two end points in the infliximab versus the placebo group. In most of the other assessments of disease activity (laboratory measures and assessments of specific peripheral or axial disease), significant improvements were observed in the infliximab group compared with the baseline value and placebo. Moreover, preliminary studies indicate that infliximab is effective and safe in cutaneous psoriasis (63).

In the future, anti—TNF-α agents probably will have a place of choice in the therapeutic armamentarium for severe PA. However, several issues remain unsettled. We do not yet know whether anti—TNF-α agents are more likely to be effective in axial or peripheral forms of PA or whether they should be reserved for severe erosive polyarticular disease unresponsive to other DMARDs. Studies are needed to determine whether anti—TNF-α agents should be started immediately in patients with severe disease or only after failure of other DMARDs. Additional work will have to evaluate whether the dosage and frequency of infusions used in RA are appropriate for PA and whether the treatment should be stopped after a few infusions.

Local Treatment

Local treatment (e.g., intra-articular injection of corticosteroids, synoviorthosis, ergotherapy, physiotherapy, splints, and surgery) is as important as in RA.

Topical Treatment of Dermatosis

Topical treatment of dermatosis should be combined systematically, especially in preparation for surgery.

Indications

Nonsteroidal antiinflammatory drugs (NSAIDs) and local treatments should be used in monoarticular and oligoarticular forms. Patients who fail to improve with these treatments can receive the drugs used in polyarticular forms (sulfasalazine, 2 to 3 g/d; methotrexate, 7.5 to 15 mg/d, and gold). Evaluation of the need for DMARDs in polyarticular disease relies heavily on the clinician's experience. The risk-benefit ratio of anti—TNF-α agents remains to be determined. Immunosuppressant therapy (e.g., azathioprine and anti—TNF-α agents) is in order in arthritis mutilans. In axial forms, NSAIDs and probably sulfasalazine should be used. Axial disease may be an indication for anti—TNF-α therapy.

Methotrexate or cyclosporine may be the best choice in patients with extensive skin disease. Extreme caution is in order regarding the use of systemic glucocorticoids, antimalarials, and gold.

REFERENCES

1. Avila R, Pugh DG, Slocomb CH, et al. Psoriatic arthritis: a roentgenologic study. Radiology 1960;75:691–702.
2. Baker H, Golding DN, Thompson M. Psoriasis and arthritis. Ann Intern Med 1963;58:909–925.
3. Moll JMH, Wright V. Familial occurrence of psoriatic arthritis. Ann Rheum Dis 1973;32:181–201.
4. Wright V. Psoriasis and arthritis. Ann Rheum Dis 1956;15:348–356.
5. Wright V, Moll JMH. Psoriatic arthritis. Bull Rheum Dis 1971;21:627–632.
6. Green L, Meyers OL, Gordon W, et al. Arthritis in psoriasis. Ann Rheum Dis 1981;40:366–369.
7. Scarpa R, Oriente P, Pucino A, et al. Psoriatic arthritis in psoriatic patients. Br J Rheumatol 1984;23:246–250.
8. Moller P, Vinje O. Arthropathy and sacroiliitis in severe psoriasis. Scand J Rheumatol 1980;9:113–117.
9. Fraber EM, Nall ML. The natural history of psoriasis in 5600 patients. Dermatologica 1974;148:1–18.
10. Wright V, Moll JMH. Psoriatic arthritis. In: Wright V, Moll JMH, eds. Seronegative polyarthritis. Amsterdam: North-Holland, 1976:169–235.
11. Roberts MET, Wright V, Hill AGS, et al. Psoriatic arthritis: follow-up study. Ann Rheum Dis 1976;35:206–212.
12. Wright V. Rheumatism and psoriasis. A reevaluation. Am J Med 1959;27:454–462.
13. Gladman DD, Shuckett R, Russell ML, et al. Psoriatic arthritis. An analysis of 220 patients. Q J Med 1987;238:127–141.
14. Kammer GM, Soter NA, Gibson DJ, et al. Psoriatic arthritis: a clinical, immunologic and HLA study of 100 patients. Semin Arthritis Rheum 1979;9:75–97.
15. Lambert JR, Wright V. Psoriatic spondylitis: a clinical and radiological description of the spine in psoriatic arthritis. Q J Med 1977;46:411–425.
16. Murray C, Mann DL, Gerber LN, et al. Histocompatibility of allo-antigens in psoriasis and psoriatic arthritis: evidence for the influence of multiple genes in the major histocompatibility complex. J Clin Invest 1980;66:670–675.
17. Woodrow JC. Genetic aspects of the spondyloarthropathies. Clin Rheum Dis 1985;11:1–24.
18. Eastmond CJ, Woodrow JC. The HLA system and the arthropathies associated with psoriasis. Ann Rheum Dis 1977;36:112–120.
19. Lambert JR, Wright V, Rajah SM, et al. Histocompatibility antigens in psoriatic arthritis. Ann Rheum Dis 1976;35:526–530.
20. Gladman DD, Anhorn KA, Schachter RK, et al. HLA antigens in psoriatic arthritis. J Rheumatol 1986;13:586–592.
21. Arnett FC, Bias WB. HLA-BW38 and BW39 in psoriatic arthritis: relationships and implications for peripheral and axial involvement. Arthritis Rheum 1980;23:649–650.
22. Scarpa R, Mathieu A. Psoriatic arthritis: evolving concepts. Curr Opin Rheumatol 2000;12:274–280.
23. Vasey FB, Deitz C, Fenske NA, et al. Possible involvement of group A streptococci in the pathogenesis of psoriatic arthritis. J Rheumatol 1982;9:719–722.
24. Wang Q, Vasey FB, Mahfood JP, et al. V2 regions of 16S ribosomal RNA used as a molecular marker for the species identification of streptococci in peripheral blood and synovial fluid from patients with psoriatic arthritis. Arthritis Rheum 1999;42:2055–2059.
25. Punzi L, Pianon M, Rizzi E, et al. Prévalence du rhumatisme psoriasique post-traumatique. Presse Med 1997;26:420.
26. Sandorfi N, Freundlich B. Psoriatic and seronegative inflammatory arthropathy associated with a traumatic onset: 4 cases and a review of literature. J Rheumatol 1997;24:187–192.
27. Ortonne JP. Recent developments in the understanding of the pathogenesis of psoriasis. Br J Dermatol 1999;140(suppl):1–7.
28. Taurog JD. Animal models of the spondylarthropathies. In: Calin A, Taurog JD, eds. The spondylarthritides. Oxford, UK: Oxford University Press, 1988:223–237.
29. Moll JMH, Wright V. Psoriatic arthritis. Semin Arthritis Rheum 1973;3:55–78.
30. Scarpa R, Oriente P, Pucino A, et al. The clinical spectrum of psoriatic spondylitis. Br J Rheumatol 1988;27:133–137.
31. Fournié B, Viraben R, Durroux R, et al. L'onycho-pachydermo-périostite psoriasique du gros orteil. Rev Rheum 1989;56:579–582.
32. Goupille P, Laulan J, Védère V, et al. Psoriatic onycho-periostitis. Report of three cases. Scand J Rheumatol 1995;24:53–54.
33. Goupille P, Védère V, Roulot B, et al. Incidence of osteoperiostitis of the great toe in psoriatic arthritis. J Rheumatol 1996;23:1553–1556.
34. Killebrew K, Gold RH, Sholkoff SD. Psoriatic spondylitis. Radiology 1973;108:9–16.

35. Jeannou J, Goupille P, Avimadje MA, et al. Cervical spine involvement in psoriatic arthritis. Rev Rhum 1999;66:695–700.

36. Laurent MR, Panayi GS, Sheperd P. Circulating immune complexes, serum immuno-globulins and acute phase protein in psoriasis and arthritis. Ann Rheum Dis 1981;40:66–69.

37. Coulton BL, Thomson K, Symmons DP, et al. Outcome in patients hospitalized for psoriatic arthritis. Clin Rheumatol 1989;8:261–265.

38. Scarpa R, Pucino A, Iocco M, et al. The management of 138 psoriatic arthritis patients. Acta Dermatol Venereol 1989;146:199–200.

39. Brubacher B, Gladman DD, Buskila D, et al. Follow-up in psoriatic arthritis: relationship to disease characteristics. J Rheumatol 1992;19: 917–920.

40. Gladman DD, Stafford-Brady F, Chang CH, et al. Longitudinal study of clinical and radiological progression in psoriatic arthritis. J Rheumatol 1990;17:809–812.

41. Salvarini C, Lo Scocco G, Macchioni P, et al. Prevalence of psoriatic arthritis in Italian psoriatic patients. J Rheumatol 1995;22:1499–1503.

42. Dougados M, van der Linden S, Juhlin R, et al. The European Spondyloarthropathy Study Group preliminary criteria for the classification of spondyloarthropathy. Arthritis Rheum 1991;34:1218–12227.

43. Garrett S, Jenkinson T, Kennedy LG, et al. A new approach to defining disease status in ankylosing spondylitis: the Bath Ankylosing Spondylitis Disease Activity Index. J Rheumatol 1994;21:2286–2291.

44. Calin A, Garrett S, Whitelock H, et al. A new approach to defining functional ability in ankylosing spondylitis: the development of the Bath Ankylosing Spondylitis Functional Index. J Rheumatol 1994;21: 2281–2285.

45. Clegg DO, Reda DJ, Mejias E, et al. Comparison of Sulfasalazine and placebo for the treatment of psoriatic arthritis and cutaneous psoriasis. Arthritis Rheum 1996;39:2013–2020.

46. Combe B, Goupille P, Kuntz JL, et al. Sulfasalazine in psoriatic arthritis: a randomized, multicentre, placebo-controlled study. Br J Rheumatol 1996;35:664–668.

47. Farr M, Kiras GD, Waterhouse L, et al. Sulphasalazine in psoriatic arthritis: a double-blind placebo-controlled study. Br J Rheumatol 1990;29:46–49.

48. Fraser SM, Hopkins R, Hunter JA, et al. Sulphasalazine in the management of psoriatic arthritis. Br J Rheumatol 1990;32:923–925.

49. Gupta AK, Grober JS, Hamilton TA, et al. Sulfasalazine therapy for psoriatic arthritis: a double-blind, placebo controlled trial. J Rheumatol 1995;22:894–898.

50. Wilkens RF, Williams HJ, Ward JR, et al. Randomized, double-blind, placebo controlled trial of low-dose pulse methotrexate in psoriatic arthritis. Arthritis Rheum 1984;27:376–381.

51. Palit J, Hill J, Capell HA, et al. A multicentre double-blind comparison of auranofin, intramuscular gold thiomalate and placebo in patients with psoriatic arthritis. Br J Rheumatol 1990;29:280–283.

52. Kammer GM, Soter NA, Gibson DJ, et al. Psoriatic arthritis: a clinical, immunologic and HLA study of 100 patients. Semin Arthritis Rheum 1979;9:75–97.

53. Gladman DD, Blake R, Brubacher B, et al. Chloroquine therapy in psoriatic arthritis. J Rheumatol 1992;19:1724–1726.

54. Mease PJ. Cytokine blockers in psoriatic arthritis. Ann Rheum Dis 2001;60(suppl 3):37—40.

55. Mease PJ. Etanercept: a new era in the treatment of psoriatic arthritis. Am J Manage Care 2002;8(suppl 6):S181–S193.

56. Mease PJ. Tumour necrosis factor (TNF) in psoriatic arthritis: pathophysiology and treatment with TNF inhibitors. Ann Rheum Dis 2002;61:298–304.

57. Yazici Y, Erkan D, Lockshin MD. A preliminary study of etanercept in the treatment of severe, resistant psoriatic arthritis. Clin Exp Rheumatol 2000;18:732–734.

58. Mease PJ, Goffe BS, Metz J, et al. Etanercept in the treatment of psoriatic arthritis and psoriasis: a randomised trial. Lancet 2000;356:385–390.

59. Mease PJ, Goffe BS, Metz J, et al. Enbrel (Etanercept) in patients with psoriatic arthritis and psoriasis. Arthritis Rheum 2000;43(suppl 9): S403.

60. Mease PJ, Kivitz A, Burch F, et al. Improvement in disease activity in patients with psoriatic arthritis receiving etanercept (Enbrel): results of a phase 3 multicenter clinical trial. Arthritis Rheum 2001;44(suppl 9):S226.

61. Van Den Bosch F, Kruithof E, Baeten, et al. Effects of loading dose regimen of three infusions of chimeric monoclonal antibody to tumour necrosis factor alpha (infliximab) in spondyloarthropathy: an open pilot study. Ann Rheum Dis 2000;59:428–433.

62. Van Den Bosch F, Kruithof E, Baeten, et al. Randomized double-blind comparison of chimeric monoclonal antibody to tumor necrosis factor alpha (infliximab) versus placebo in active spondylarthropathy. Arthritis Rheum 2002;46:755–765.

63. Chaudhari U, Romano P, Mulcahy LD, et al. Efficacy and safety of infliximab monotherapy for plaque-type psoriasis: a randomised trial. Lancet 2001;357:1842–1847.

CHAPTER 76

Ankylosing Spondylitis

Federico Balagué and Jean Dudler

Historically, ankylosing spondylitis (AS) was first explicitly described at the end of the 19th century by Bechterew, von Strümpel, and Pierre Marie (1). In the early 1950s, Forestier, Rotes-Querol, and Scandinavian authors made further major contributions to its description (2). Nowadays, AS is considered the prototype of a group of different but closely interrelated disorders called seronegative spondyloarthropathies (3,4). Originally considered variants of rheumatoid arthritis, their characterized inflammatory involvement of axial skeleton, entheses, and their strong genetic association with the presence of the histocompatibility human leukocyte antigen (HLA)-B27 has clearly separated them as a different entity (3,4). The other diseases of this group have been described in detail in the previous chapters by Goupille and Borenstein, and this chapter concentrates uniquely on AS.

Epidemiologic figures vary widely in the literature (5). Ankylosing spondylitis is the second most common inflammatory arthritis, after rheumatoid arthritis, and commonly cited prevalence figures for the general population are 1 to 3 per 1,000 (5), with values increasing to 1% when considering the white adult population (6–8). Contrary to rheumatoid arthritis, where a fairly constant worldwide prevalence is recognized (9), AS shows strong racial differences, with extreme values ranging from almost nonexistent in African-Americans to 63 per 1,000 in specific American-Indian tribes (5). These data are consistent with the strong association of HLA-B27 and AS on one hand (8,10,11), and the observed racial variations in the prevalence of B27 on the other (10,11). Prevalence figures as low as .01%, and even .0065% (11), have been reported in Japan for AS where only 1% of the population is HLA-B27+ (6). On the opposite, in the Haida First Nation people and Bella Indians where over 50% of the population harbor the HLA-B27 antigen, the prevalence of AS is as high as 6% (5).

In Europe, Finland shows one of the highest prevalence of HLA-B27 with 14% (12), as compared to the usually reported 4% to 8% for the white population (5). In that country, the reported prevalence between 1980 and 1990 was .15% (95% confidence interval [CI]: .08% to .27%) and the annual incidence of AS requiring medication 6.9 (95% CI: 6.0 to 7.8) per 100,000 adults (13). A comparable study was repeated in 1995 with a similar incidence for AS of 6.3 (4.9 to 7.9) per 100,000 (12). Finally, a familial aggregation has been reported in different countries (14).

ETIOLOGY AND PATHOGENESIS

Ankylosing spondylitis is inflammatory rheumatism of unknown origin, generally thought to have an autoimmune pathogenesis. It now appears that AS represents a complex polygenetic disease influenced by various environmental factors. A complete review of this extensive field of research is not within the scope of this chapter, and the reader should refer to recent reviews for further reading.

Role of HLA-B27 and Other Genetic Factors

Despite considerable efforts since the initial description in 1973 of the strong association between HLA-B27 and AS (15,16), the links between this susceptibility gene and the observed clinical manifestations remain enigmatic (17,18).

Up to date, as much as 23 subtypes of HLA-B27 have been recognized and this number continues to increase (17,19). Some subtypes (e.g., B2706 and B2709) are not associated with AS (6), whereas variations in the respective distribution of subtypes across the world complicates epidemiologic studies, comparison among populations, and determination of their role in disease susceptibility (6,19,20). Furthermore, it appears that the risk associated with a high susceptibility subtype could be strongly influenced by the genetic background; that is, B2705 does not appear as a significant risk factor in West Africans (21).

The dominant paradigm that HLA-B27 favors a cross-reactive immune response because its antigenic structure mimics bacterial epitopes has been challenged (17,18).

There is also no compelling evidence for an arthritogenic peptide that could be uniquely presented by HLA-B27 molecules (17,18). There is growing evidence to suggest that the role of HLA-B27 is not explained by its physiologic function as an antigen-presenting protein, but rather by peculiarities of this molecule (17,18). HLA-B27 has been shown to increase the intracellular survival rate of bacteria and enhance the proinflammatory response to gram-negative infection (22,23). It also demonstrates an unusual tendency to misfold, with potential effects on the intracellular signaling (24–26). Finally, an apparently unique property to form homodimer could link HLA-B27 to autoimmunity (18,25,27,28).

Transgenic animal models have underlined the role of HLA-B27 in AS pathogenesis (29,30). However, they have not completely unraveled the mechanisms. Transgenic rats harboring multiple copies of the human HLA-B27 antigen develop a spontaneous inflammatory disease mimicking several features of human spondyloarthropathies (29,30). This observation could be interpreted as strong evidence for a role of HLA-B27 as a presenting-antigen molecule in the pathogenesis of AS, but it could also work through the nonphysiologic role of HLA-B27 on proinflammatory response, intracellular signaling, or bacterial survival. Furthermore, transgenic mice expressing functional HLA-B27 on their cell surface usually remain healthy, whereas they develop disease in the absence of mouse β2-microglobulin, which prevents surface expression of mature HLA-B27 molecules. This argues for a nonphysiologic role of HLA-B27 in the pathogenesis of AS (17,31).

Even if HLA-B27 is the strongest susceptibility factor, AS is a polygenetic disease (HLA-B27, B60, and HLA-A9); the exact number of genes involved is unknown (32). It appears that HLA-B27 contributes only 16% to 50% of the total genetic risk (19). This concept helps us to understand the known familial aggregation unexplained solely by HLA-B27 status. Models have been developed that suggest that a five-locus model best fits the observed data (33). Interestingly, this is in accordance to a genome-wide scan that identified four regions of interest on chromosomes 2, 10, 16, and 19 in addition to chromosome 6, which carries the HLA complex (34). However, the details of this polygenetic disease probably are more complex. Additional regions of interest have demonstrated a potential role in conferring disease susceptibility, such as cytochrome P-450, latent membrane protein 2 (LMP2), tumor necrosis factor (TNF) promoter region, or interleukin-1 receptor antagonist (17). To complicate the matter even further, possible non-B27 protective factors have been postulated (21).

Role of Infection and Other Environmental Factors

The importance of infection as a causative factor in reactive arthritis is well established, but the role of spe-

cific infections in the pathogenesis of AS is not as clear (35). A high fecal carriage of *Klebsiella pneumoniae* in patients with active disease, the presence of raised anti-Klebsiella antibodies, and possible molecular mimicry between HLA-B27 and bacterial antigens have led to the hypothesis that AS is a reactive arthritis to this specific bacteria (35). Despite numerous studies, such a role has not been demonstrated conclusively (35). However, animal models have underlined the importance of infection, because both transgenic rats and mice housed under specific pathogen- or germ-free conditions did not develop the disease (29,30).

Other strong arguments for the importance of environmental factor are twin studies, where the concordance rate for AS was 50% in monozygotic twins and 20% in dizygotic twins (36).

There is also a strong epidemiologic relationship between gut inflammation and the spondyloarthropathies, particularly Crohn disease, ulcerative colitis, and reactive arthritis (37). Ankylosing spondylitis patients without any known bowel disease also present with endoscopic lesions and histologic signs of gut inflammation at ileocolonoscopy (38). Finally, transgenic rats present with gut lesions reminiscent of inflammatory bowel disease (IBD) (29). However, the pathogenic relationship between gut and arthritis remains enigmatic (39), perhaps related to some increase small bowel permeability, as demonstrated in AS patients and their first-degree relatives (38). This could favor invasion, persistence, or transport of bacterial antigens as causative factors (39).

Others Factors

Others factors have been implicated as pathogenic or as risk factors for AS. Trauma (40), androgens (41), and even low birth order (42) have been reported, but no pathogenic mechanisms have been demonstrated.

CLINICAL PRESENTATION AND DIAGNOSIS

Ankylosing spondylitis classically presents as inflammatory rheumatism of the young male with characteristic axial involvement of the sacroiliac and spine joints and a unique propensity to affect entheses and adjacent soft tissue in the spine and peripheral skeleton. Hips and shoulders are involved more often than other peripheral joints, and various extraskeletal manifestations have been reported that underline the systemic nature of the disease (7,8,10,43).

Ankylosing spondylitis is usually a chronic, progressive disease with fluctuating activity (44), but it has been estimated that 1.5% to 10% of cases are totally asymptomatic and are diagnosed incidentally when a radiograph is taken for another reason (45,46).

Typically, AS begins in young adults. Age at time of diagnosis ranges from 6 to 61, with a mean age usually in the third decade (8,47–52). In two studies—one from Finland (12) and the other from Belgium (53)—AS was diagnosed at a mean age of 39.6 (10.3) and 32 years, respectively. Onset is uncommon after age 50, with only 6% of patients in a German study experiencing onset after age 40 (54). However, late-onset AS is a now well-recognized entity; the diagnosis of AS should not be discarded solely because of age (54).

Ankylosing spondylitis is regarded historically as a male disease. A male to female ratio up to 10:1 was reported in a recent review paper (7), whereas more conservative figures ranging from 2:1 to 3:1 (55) appear closer to reality (pooled data from the reviewed literature including more than 4,500 patients where males represented roughly three fourths of the cases). This discrepancy could result in part from ethnic variations: Male to female ratios as high as 16:1 have been reported in Asian countries (49).

Diagnosis and Classification Criteria

In a majority of cases, AS is diagnosed or at least suspected on clinical elements, particularly patient symptoms, family history, and physical findings (55). For a diagnosis of AS, a history of getting out of bed at night was shown to have a sensitivity of 65% and a specificity of 79%. The most sensitive items were morning stiffness (95%) and age less than 35 years (92%), whereas the most specific was relief by exercise (88%) (56). However, it has been reported in juveniles that pain usually is not relieved and sometimes is even aggravated by exercise (57). It is also important to keep in mind that the reproducibility of history-taking is not perfect, even for symptoms such as having to get out of bed at night (56).

The most commonly used set of criteria for classification is the Modified New York Criteria of 1984, where definite AS is defined by a unilateral sacroiliitis of grade 3 or 4 or bilateral grade 2 to 4, and any clinical criterion comprising low back pain of at least 3 months' duration improved by exercise and not relieved by rest, limitation of lumbar spine in sagittal and frontal planes, and chest expansion decreased relative to normal values for age and sex (55). Two more sets of criteria—the Amor criteria and those developed by the European Spondyloarthropathy Study Group (ESSG)—were published for spondyloarthropathies but actually used for AS (58). There are no validated diagnostic criteria for AS (55); the reader should keep in mind the difference between diagnostic and classification criteria (55,59). If the classification criteria of the ESSG sometimes have been used to aid diagnosis (59), their sensitivity in early cases is 66% compared to 94% in clinically definite AS, and they should not be used to establish a diagnosis of AS in individual patients (55).

The diagnosis of late-stage AS is not difficult but it can be challenging in the early stage. The delay between the first symptoms and the actual diagnosis ranges from 0 to 29 years, with a mean from 5 to 10 years (50,60). In a cohort, only two thirds of AS cases (50% of men and 85% of women) had been initially diagnosed when the medical records were reexamined within a research project (61). On the other hand, five pain characteristics considered typical of inflammatory disorders (back pain ≥ 3 months, morning stiffness, age of onset < 40 years, insidious onset of pain, and back pain improved by exercise) identify 10% to 15% of patients in primary care or other settings (55,62). This is much more than the prevalence of AS and represents a very high false-positive rate (55,62).

Finally, diagnosis is complicated by atypical presentations such as inflammatory back pain without radiographic sacroiliitis, inflammatory chest wall pain without sacroiliitis, juvenile onset (including tarsal enthesitis), late onset AS, acute anterior uveitis (with or without arthritis), and aortic regurgitation or complete heart block (with or without arthritis), which should be recognized as AS (55).

Axial Involvement

Axial involvement is the hallmark of AS and affects virtually 100% of patients at some time. It is the first manifestation in about three fourths of the cases and it is the cornerstone of diagnosis (see the preceding section on diagnosis and a later section on radiology). It encompasses not only the sacroiliac joints and spine itself, but also the thoracic cage and pelvis. This section focuses on little known or unrecognized aspects of this type of manifestation.

Among the uncommon localizations, AS has been reported to involve a transitional lumbosacral joint (63) and symphysis pubis (64). Pascual et al. (cited by Le) reported that up to 82% of AS patients with thoracic pain have an involvement of costovertebral joints with erosive lesions (65). Finally, a study including 50 patients with AS reported the following figures for the involvement of the anterior thoracic wall: interclavicular ligament and sterno-costo-clavicular joint (20%), manubriosternal symphysis (32%), and chondrocostal and costoxyphoidal ligaments (4%) (66).

Erosive spondylodiscitis (i.e., destructive changes at the discovertebral junction excluding lesions that may relate to cartilaginous nodes) were found in 8% of cases in a study including 147 patients with AS. The same number of cases had single-level as multilevel involvement, with a maximum number of six levels. Only 17% of the cases were symptomatic, and it seems that patients with this type of lesion have an earlier onset of AS (67). In 50 AS patients, 22% of the cervical and lumbar zygapophyseal joints were ankylosed on standard radiographs when evaluated by means of a new score. The authors conclude that ankylosis of the posterior joints may precede the syndesmophytes (53).

Geusens et al., in a cross-sectional study to decipher the etiology of hyperkyphosis, compared 38 AS patients with hyperkyphosis with 12 patients without such deformity. The lumbar spine did not contribute to the deformity, but thoracic disc wedging did. The sum of deformities of the thoracic vertebrae and discs explained 43% of the variance of the age-adjusted occiput-to-wall distance. There was no significant difference between genders and between patients aged more or less than 45 years (68).

An occult vertebral fracture, which may occur even with minor traumatic events, is one of the feared complications of AS. Mitra et al. compared 66 men with mild AS with 39 healthy controls. Despite the fact that the latter were roughly 15 years older, the AS patients had significantly more vertebral fractures (16.7% versus 2.6%) and significantly lower bone mineral density (BMD), both in the lumbar spine and femoral neck. However, there was no correlation between BMD and vertebral fractures in these patients (69). Kauppi et al. reported on one case and highlighted the fact that pain, neurologic symptoms, modification of the kyphosis, and increased mobility appearing after an accident should raise the suspicion of a fracture (70). Because the majority of such fractures occur at the cervico-thoracic junction, it is extremely difficult to obtain good-quality images (70). In a review of 21 cases, vertebral fractures were identified on a delayed basis and secondary neurologic deficits were described in three patients. Multiple non-contiguous fractures were found in several patients, and the diagnostic value of a specific MRI protocol was highlighted (71).

Other extensive studies with bone biopsy—like the one by Lee et al. comparing seven early patients with AS (mean duration 2 years and normal mobility) to seven late patients with AS (mean duration 27 years and limited spinal mobility) at baseline and at 15 months follow-up—confirmed the low BMD in AS but failed to demonstrate consistent change in bone turnover to explain it. It appeared that men with AS have both trabecular and cortical bone deficit that may result from genetic factors, inflammation, medication, or decreased mobility (72), whereas alteration in vitamin D metabolism and increased bone resorption–related high disease activity was suggested in another study by Lange et al. (73).

Peripheral Joint Involvement

Hips and shoulders are involved at some stage of the disease in about one third of patients (more commonly in patients with juvenile-onset AS); this should be regarded ultimately as a type of axial involvement (43). Hip disease usually is symmetric and insidious, and can result in severe disability (74). Shoulder symptoms and loss of mobility also are common in patients with AS and, in a survey including 1,515 subjects, the prevalence of severe or very severe pain and severe or very severe stiffness were 15.2% and 13.8%, respectively. Despite the high frequency and correlation with higher pain and arthritis

impact measurement scales (AIMS) scores, shoulder symptoms were rarely disabling (75).

True peripheral joint involvement is infrequent in AS; when present, it is usually regarded as asymmetric, transient, and rarely erosive and with a tendency to resolve without deformity (43).

A special case should be made for the temporomandibular joint. In one study, involvement of the temporomandibular joint was found in almost 50% of 65 patients aged 33 (±11). Condylar erosions and flattening, and sclerosis, as well as temporal flattening were significantly increased compared with controls (76), as were condylar erosions associated with longer duration of AS, neck complaints, and atlantoaxial subluxation (76). Magnetic resonance imaging (MRI) has been reported to show a high prevalence of temporomandibular degenerative changes or disc displacement which were, however, not specific for a diagnosis of AS (77). Temporomandibular joint involvement does not seem to be correlated with AS severity or peripheral joint involvement (77).

Entheses

Inflammation at the sites of attachment of a tendon or enthesitis can be a major disabling problem in some patients and is a hallmark of AS and the spondyloarthropathies (78,79). The entheses of the lower limbs are more frequently involved; heel enthesitis is the most common (79). Traditional methods of imaging, including plain film radiography and xeroradiography, have been supplanted by ultrasound and MRI, which demonstrated soft-tissue and bone edema and inflammation much before the classical erosions and bone proliferation seen in more advanced cases (79).

Extra-articular Manifestations

Various extra-articular manifestations have been associated with AS. Some can be considered as plain complications, often in late-stage disease, whereas others are more strongly disease-associated with shared pathogenesis.

Neurologic

Cauda equina syndrome (CES) is described as a rare complication of AS that manifests late in the course of the disease (46,80,81). Ahn et al. recently reviewed 52 papers on CES that included 86 patients (82). These patients had a mean age of 58.5 ± 2 years, with an average of 32 years of AS history. A slow onset of neurologic deficit was reported by 98% of patients. Motor deficit was found in 62%, whereas sensory deficit, reflex deficit, and bladder dysfunction were much more common (96%, 93%, and 95%, respectively). Of note, the clinical picture was initially misdiagnosed as prostatic hyperplasia and prostatectomy was performed in almost one third of males. Sciatica was the initial symptom in 22% of cases (82). Finally, only 40% of the patients treated surgically had some form of neurologic improvement, whereas steroids had no effect at all (82).

The hallmark of CES in AS is the presence of dorsal dura diverticula associated with a widened thecal sac and scalloped erosions of the posterior vertebral arch. This syndrome has been attributed to arachnoiditis and chronic inflammation (46,80–82), even though other hypotheses (arteritis, demyelination, fibrosis, etc.) have been raised (46). A published case report describes the coexistence of AS and spinal arteriovenous malformation with vasculitic changes (83).

Other neurologic manifestations of AS include isolated nerve root, cervical myelopathy, and possible combinations of nerve root and spinal cord compression in case of fractures (80). They have been attributed to instability (owing to subluxation or fracture), inflammation (arachnoiditis or single root lesions), or compression (ossified intraspinal ligaments, granulation tissue, or foraminal stenosis) (46).

One case of bilateral optic neuritis in a woman suffering from AS has been published, suggesting the possible connection between AS and multiple sclerosis (84). Dolan and Gibson published two cases of AS with spastic paraparesis because of undetermined intrinsic spinal cord lesions where the neurologic symptoms had been attributed to associated multiple sclerosis but were indeed a complication of AS (85).

Gastrointestinal

There is a clear association between IBD and the spondyloarthropathies (37). Cohorts of IBD develop inflammatory rheumatism that can be labeled as AS or enteropathic arthritis. The reader is referred to Chapter 74 by Goupille and Borenstein.

However, it is important to realize that AS patients without any known bowel disease present endoscopic lesions in 29.2% of cases and histologic signs of gut inflammation in 58.3% (acute inflammation in 8.3% acute and chronic inflammation in 50%) at ileocolonoscopy (38). This confirms previous studies where prevalence of inflammatory gut lesions observed by ileocolonoscopy ranged from 29% to 67% when looking only at the subgroup of AS patients (37).

Finally, a possible association may exist with celiac disease. Kallikorm et al. screened 18 patients with AS by means of different serologic tests (antigliadin and antireticulin antibodies—both IgA and IgG—and antiendomysium IgA) and discovered one case of celiac disease, corresponding to a prevalence of 5.5% as compared with an incidence of .37:1,000 live births in the same country (86).

Renal

In a cross-sectional study including 40 AS patients, 35% presented one or more renal abnormalities. The most common sign was microscopic hematuria followed by microalbuminuria, and reduced creatinine clearance. No case of proximal tubular impairment was found by means of the urinary excretion of retinol-binding protein (87).

In an extensive review of the literature, the overall prevalence of clinically relevant renal involvement in AS has been estimated to be around 10% with the following distribution: 62% of amyloidosis; 30% of IgA nephropathy; 5% of mesangioproliferative glomerulonephritis; and 1% each of membranous nephropathy, focal segmental glomerulonephritis, and focal proliferative glomerulonephritis (88). The figure for amyloidosis is in agreement with other studies. Histologic evidence of secondary amyloidosis was found in one of 15 (6.2%) specimens obtained during joint replacement procedures in AS patients without any clinical evidence of amyloidosis (aged 30, average disease duration 8.2 years) (89), whereas a systematic search for amyloidosis by subcutaneous abdominal fat aspiration in 137 patients yielded a positive test in 7% of the cases. These patients were significantly older, had longer duration of AS, and more peripheral erosive arthritis than the rest of AS patients (90). A more conservative estimate is around 3% for the prevalence of clinically recognizable secondary amyloidosis in live AS patients (89).

Pulmonary

Figures for pulmonary involvement range from 0% to 30% (91). In two papers from the same group, including 26 patients (women 23%; mean age 44.8 years; mean duration of AS 18.5 years, and 12% never smokers), six were symptomatic (23%) with mainly cough or dyspnea, whereas only two (8%) had basal crepitations on chest examination. However, pulmonary functions were abnormal in 11 patients (42%) with a restrictive pattern in eight and obstructive in three. Plain chest radiographs showed abnormalities in only 15%, whereas high-resolution CT was abnormal in 69%. The most common abnormalities on CT were interstitial lung disease, bronchial wall thickening and bronchiectasias, paraseptal emphysema, mediastinal lymphadenopathy, tracheal dilatation, and apical fibrosis unexplained by a history of smoking alone and suggesting a possible association between AS and interstitial lung disease (91,92). Others have reported similar findings. In a highly selected group of patients, where patients with histories of smoking or exposure to inhaled gases as well as patients with abnormal chest radiographs were excluded, prevalence of abnormalities was 71% for thin-section CT and 57% for pulmonary function tests, all with a restrictive pattern. The main types of lesions were interlobular septal thickening, linear septal thickening,

thickening of bronchial walls and pleural thickening (21 patients, mean age 43 ± 12, mean duration of AS 13 ± 7.5 years) (93).

Finally, a small study showed that smoking was associated with a poor outcome in terms of mobility and functional index in AS patients (60).

Cardiac

Several types of valve disease, arrhythmias, myocardial diseases, and pericarditis have been found in association with HLA-B27, most of them in patients with AS (94). A longitudinal study with a mean follow-up of 39 months found abnormalities of the aortic root and valves on transesophageal echocardiography in 82% of AS patients and 27% of controls ($p < .001$). These findings were unrelated to clinical features of AS. Twenty-four percent of patients developed new or other aortic root or valve abnormalities during follow-up, whereas another 12% demonstrated progression to a more severe regurgitation. However, the abnormalities detected at baseline also resolved in 20% (95).

Jimenez-Balderas et al. performed a two-dimensional echo Doppler study in cardiopulmonary asymptomatic patients with AS. They compared 20 cases with juvenile-onset AS, 31 with adult-onset AS, and 20 healthy males. Several abnormalities were found significantly more often among AS patients and some differences between juvenile- and adult-onset reported. Cardiomyopathy, increased aortic root diameter, and abnormal aortic ring reflectance were more frequent among patients with adult-onset despite a higher frequency of HLA-B27 among juveniles (90% versus 51%) but no difference in terms of increased mitral valve gradient was found between both subgroups of AS (96).

Ocular

Uveitis is the main type of eye involvement and the most common extra-articular manifestation (97). According to an extensive review, the likelihood of anterior uveitis in AS patients ranges from 20% to 30%. Conversely, the likelihood of AS in patients with uveitis is 15% for any uveitis, 30% to 50% for acute anterior uveitis with figures raising up to 84% to 90% for HLA-B27+ patients with acute anterior uveitis. The clinical patterns of uveitis most frequently associated with AS are the unilateral acute anterior recurrent uveitis and the unilateral acute anterior nonrecurrent uveitis (97).

Psychological

Different psychological aspects have been studied in AS patients. Günther et al. assessed 76 AS male patients and 16 healthy controls for their stress coping mechanisms. Patients were divided into four groups according to the duration of AS and overall patients differed from controls only in a few aspects. They used more cognitive coping and actionable strategies and less resignation and self-accusation, which led the authors to conclude that AS patients probably use the best coping mechanisms and that they conform with the notion of "healthy ill people" (98). Psychological well-being, as assessed by SCL-90-R, was found to be correlated with pain but neither with function nor spinal mobility measures (99).

Other studies have focused on sleep disturbances, which appear to be a significant problem for AS patients. A cross-sectional comparison of 70 AS patients and 3,558 controls demonstrated several differences between groups at all stages (i.e., pre-sleep, sleep, and wakefulness) (100). A previous study, including 11 patients and 11 controls, had already shown that sleep was different in AS patients and controls. Moreover, quality of sleep was correlated with lumbar flexibility, pain, and psychomotor performance (101). However, the same authors also stated in another study that the precise nature of the relationship among fatigue, disease activity, function, and sleep disturbance remained unclear (102).

In a study by Ward evaluating 175 patients with the Medical Outcomes Study Short Form 36 Health Survey (SF-36) among other tools, it appeared that mental health role limitations caused by emotional problems and social functioning were less affected than the rest of the subscales of the questionnaire (52). Nevertheless, it is also important to recognize that self-reported health status appeared more strongly related to personality traits than the degree of disability in a study that included 144 patients (103).

Finally, in a survey including 175 patients self-evaluated for the presence and importance of problems in 23 aspects of quality of life, the main concerns of patients were pain, stiffness, fatigue, and sleep problems. Less educated patients had lower quality of life. Moreover, women reported significantly more problems with fatigue, coping with illness, job performance, and self-care tasks. Pain and role limitations owing to physical problems are also more likely in women (52).

Various

Ankylosing spondylitis patients could be predisposed to lymphoid malignancies. In a subgroup of 1,137 HLA-typed patients selected from a Chinese marrow donor registry of 18,774 volunteer, ankylosing spondylitis was found in four of the 16 HLA-B27+ patients with lymphoid malignancies (three cases of acute lymphoblastic leukemia and one of Hodgkin lymphoma) (104).

In a study of 22 female patients with AS and 22 matched controls, enlarged thyroid volume, lower basal free T3, T4 and total T3, normal levels of TSH and total T4, and increased reverse-T3 were significantly more frequent in the AS group. This "low-T3 syndrome" was correlated to parameters of acute inflammatory activity (105).

Focal sialadenitis was found in 58% of AS patients and secondary Sjögren syndrome in 26%, figures quite similar to that concerning rheumatoid arthritis and other inflammatory diseases (106).

The prevalence of type A vitiligo was found to be 4.6% in a cohort of patients with AS ($n = 43$) versus 1.06% in a group of 468 control patients suffering from different rheumatic disorders excepted spondyloarthropathies (107).

Finally, AS patients could present with severe muscle wasting. There is no compelling evidence for an association of AS with inflammatory muscle disease, even if modest raised blood levels of muscle enzymes occasionally have been observed. Until proved otherwise, one should first exclude a neurologic complication, severe disuse, or malabsorption when a patient presents with such a clinical picture (43).

Of interest, despite AS being an inflammatory disease, it has been shown that some meteorologic variables have significant influence on the patient's quality of life as evaluated by the questionnaire (108).

Functional Capacity and Outcome

Different studies on this topic have been published; however, they are mainly cross-sectional (48,50,99, 109–111). A systematic review was published that summarized the information available up to 2001 (112). Despite the generalized opinion that most AS patients retain full work ability, it appears overall that AS has a substantial impact in terms of work disability (3% to 50%) and sick leave (12 to 46 days per patient per year) (112), but with large differences among countries (113).

Of course, life cannot be reduced to work capacity. According to Ward, mortality, quality of life, and physiologic or anatomic impairment are the major components of health outcomes (114). To evaluate health-related quality of life in AS, one should take into account several components: symptoms, physical functioning, role functioning, social interactions, psychological functioning, adverse effects of treatment, and both direct and indirect financial costs (114).

Juvenile Ankylosing Spondylitis

Juvenile ankylosing spondylitis (JAS) deserves a few comments. The definition is that of an ankylosing spondylitis occurring in individuals less than 16 years of age (57,115). However, no specific diagnostic criteria are available (116). The main characteristics of JAS are a male to female ratio of 7:1, mean onset age greater than 10 years, common enthesitis, HLA-B27+ in 90%, and no ANA or rheumatoid factor (115). The female to male ratio seems to increase as the age of onset decreases (117).

We have not found precise epidemiologic data, but rather indirect estimates. Lee et al. reported figures of prevalence of 10% to 15% for AS that start during childhood, with 29.2% of their patients originally diagnosed with juvenile chronic arthritis (late-onset pauciarticular type) (38). Much higher figures have been cited in selected referred rheumatic pediatric populations (57, 115,118).

Onset of JAS may be so acute that it mimics a septic disorder, or it may be much more subtle (115). Arthritis is often very episodic with long remission. The usual picture is that of an older boy with asymmetric oligoarthritis predominant in the lower limbs, often with enthesitis. Night pain and morning stiffness are characteristic. Hip joint arthritis at onset is common, and early onset is recognized as a risk factor for hip involvement (43). Multifactorial (e.g., synovitis, enthesitis, tenosynovitis, and bursitis) midfoot pain and tenderness also are frequent (115). One caveat is that evidence of arthritis of the sacroiliac joints and spine does not develop until 5 to 10 years after onset (57).

Constitutional symptoms such as high-grade fever, weight loss, muscle weakness and atrophy, fatigue, lymph node enlargement, leukocytosis, and anemia are present in 5% to 10% of patients (57). The usefulness of different imaging methods seems rather limited and they are not indicated routinely in this age group (115,116). Of note, in one study, not a single case presented with solely axial symptoms, and clinical signs in the absence of symptoms were extraordinarily rare (119).

INVESTIGATIONS AND OUTCOME MEASURES

Imaging

The main radiologic features of AS are: sacroiliitis, vertebral squaring, vertebral osteopenia, spondylitis anterior (Romanus lesion), shiny corner (marginal vertebral sclerosis), spondylodiscitis (Anderson lesion), joint capsule and ligament ossification, syndesmophytes, bamboo spine, and vertebral fractures (7,120).

Ankylosis of the sacroiliac joints can take years, but can also occur rapidly in approximately 20% of patients with very severe early disease (120). Sacroiliitis is central to diagnosis, and an agreement between pelvic antero-posterior (AP) views and sacroiliac joint incidences was found in 94% of cases. Therefore, the former should be preferred because they are cheaper, less irradiating, and also bring some information about the hip joints (121). A comparison of radiography, computed tomography (CT) scan, and MRI was performed in nine healthy volunteers and 24 patients with AS (mean age, 21.7 years). Magnetic resonance imaging showed the cartilage of all the sacroiliac joints of the volunteers to be normal, and both imaging techniques performed better than radiographs. Although only one patient was normal in each imaging technique, 11 sacroiliac joints were graded 0 in AP radiographs and 16 in oblique views (122). Moreover, CT was superior to MRI to identify sclerosis; on the other hand, MRI was able to reveal early cartilage changes and bone marrow edema (122). Two other recent studies have highlighted the usefulness of MRI, with or without enhancement, to detect early sacroiliitis (123,124) or Romanus lesions (125). Interestingly, a limited MRI examination used by McNally et al. to screen 1,042 cases suffering from LBP without radiculopathy and unresponsive to conservative treatment for more than 6 weeks demonstrated seven cases of AS, among other pathologies, even though the diagnostic criteria used were not reported (126).

The contribution of pathologic radiographs of the spine, irrespective of sacroiliac changes, to the diagnosis of AS is not clear (120). Early lesions of the spine in AS occur where the disc, anterior ligament, and edge of the vertebral body meet (120), and bone formation seems to parallel ongoing inflammation (120). As stated, it had been advocated that zygapophyseal joint ankylosis precede the syndesmophytes (53). The problem of occult fractures has been highlighted before and one should be aware that anterior atlantoaxial subluxation can occur in later stages of AS (120). Bone single photon emission computed tomography, evaluated in 28 patients, demonstrated abnormalities in the vertebral body and facet joints of 15 and 16 patients, respectively. Of note, multiple sites of uptake were common, but only three patients had elevated sacroiliac scores (127). Another technique, the ^{99m}Tc human IgG scintigraphy did not demonstrate usefulness (128).

The clinico-radiologic correlation appears poor in a study including 19 patients with AS. Actually, the frequency of symptoms at different specific localizations was only 20% to 25% of the prevalence of radiologic signs. Moreover, radiologic manifestations of enthesitis at the ischiatic tuberosity were present in 95% of patients, whereas none reported clinical symptoms (129).

The main validated scoring methods for reading standard radiographs in AS has been the object of multiple studies (44,130–133) and was highlighted in reviews (134). Spoorenberg et al. compared the existing methods of scoring; that is, the New York method and the Stoke Ankylosing Spondylitis Spine Score (SASSS) for the sacroiliac joints, the Larsen method for the hip joints, the Bath Ankylosing Spondylitis Radiology Index (BASRI) for AP and lateral views of the cervical and lumbar spine, and the SASSS for the lateral anterior and posterior aspects of the cervical and lumbar spine. Reliability and sensitivity to change over 1 year using the same radiograph techniques were evaluated for all methods. Only the SASSS (spine) and BASRI index reached good reliability. Moreover, observers agreed that no change occurred over 1 year in up to 89% of cases (133). Actually, only half of patients develop severe disease after 45 years, and 25% never develop cervical involvement.

There was a lack of correlation between the individual radiologic score and duration of disease. It appears that patients with hip involvement had more severe axial disease (130). It also appears from data obtained on the BASRI score that the AP view supplies more information than the lateral view (44).

A comparison of radiologic changes and mobility measures showed significant correlations among several variables, sometimes concerning different sections of the spine (e.g., cervical mobility was correlated with sacroiliac radiography) (135). An important drawback of radiographs is that, in contrast to the clinical status, radiographs cannot improve and sequential films are considered almost useless (10).

Laboratory Tests

Most laboratory tests are of limited value in AS. Levels of erythrocyte sedimentation rate (ESR) and C-reactive protein (CRP) are normal or only slighted increased in many patients with "active" AS, not allowing for further improvement (134). Neither is superior to the other in assessing disease activity (136). In their review, van den Hoogen et al. reported that raised ESR had sensitivity of .69 and specificity of .68 for diagnostic accuracy (56). Nevertheless, the latest recommendation promotes the use of ESR. Even if its predictive value and discriminative power remain to be defined by longitudinal studies (134). In a 6-week study including 443 patients, CRP was found to be increased at baseline in 39% of cases. Moreover, a reduction of CRP at follow-up occurred in 28% of cases in the placebo arm of the study (137).

Other tests, such as plasma viscosity and interleukin-6, have been used; however, laboratory tests are not very useful overall, and their correlation with the degree of impairment is minimal (10).

The strong association between HLA-B27 and AS has been discussed. A positive HL-B27 status has no real value in diagnosis. It will not make the diagnosis in a patient who failed clinical criteria. At best, AS is very unlikely with a negative result; an alternate diagnosis should be considered.

Outcome Measures

Traditionally, clinicians have relied heavily on physical measurement as measures of the efficacy of management. Viitanen et al. compared nine measurements of the cervical spine mobility either by means of a tape or an inclinometer; the results were correlated with radiologic changes of the whole spine. The authors concluded that cervical extension and lateral flexion as well as cervical rotation and occiput- or tragus-wall distance could be recommended as long-term outcomes measures (138). A method of assessment of the thoracolumbar rotation by means of a tape (the Pavelka method) has been shown to be a valid and reliable method in AS patients (139). The same group compared 17 repeated tests and correlated them with radiologic findings. They concluded that a modified Schober test, thoracolumbar flexion, lateral flexion, and rotation, chest expansion (after careful standardization), cervical rotation, and extension or lateral flexion could be used to assess disease progression (140). The sensitivity to change of different spinal, shoulder, and hip measurements also was tested in a 3-week inpatient course of intensive physiotherapy. Finger to floor distance, thoracolumbar rotation (Pavelka method), and thoracolumbar lateral flexion were the most sensitive, with effect sizes ranging between .32 and .43 (141). Finally, clinical and radiologic measures including dynamic radiographs were compared in 22 cases of AS with predominant involvement of the spine. The reproducibility of the clinical measures was reported to be excellent, whereas the correlation coefficients between radiologic and clinical measures ranged from .81 to .17 (142).

However, physical measurements represent only one of the different aspects or domains of the clinical evaluation. It includes taking a clinical history, physical examination, perception of the functional capacity and reported quality of life, as well as radiologic and laboratory data. Several tools have been developed specifically for AS, and core sets have been proposed for various tasks: daily clinical record keeping, evaluation of disease-modifying drugs, and evaluation of symptomatic treatments (134). This is an intense field of research still in progress (143,144). For example, a recent paper pooling five randomized controlled trials (RCTs), including more than 1,000 patients overall, proposed the use of "patient global assessment, pain, function, and inflammation" to define response to treatment or partial remission (145).

These instruments also can be used in sets defined to perform patient evaluation following the World Health Organization's recommendations (146). The group from the Royal National Hospital for Rheumatic Diseases (Bath, UK) has defined several sets of measurements that constitute different indexes: Bath Ankylosing Spondylitis Functional Index (BASFI), Bath Ankylosing Spondylitis Metrology Index (BASMI), Bath Ankylosing Spondylitis Disease Activity Index (BASDAI), Bath Ankylosing Spondylitis Psychological Index (BAS-PSYCH), and Bath Ankylosing Spondylitis Global status (BAS-G) (10,147–149). If these indexes are used widely in drug studies, they also may be used to evaluate impairment (BASDAI, BASMI, BAS-PSYCH, and radiographs), disability (BASFI and BAS-G), and handicap (cost, employment, and quality of life) according to Calin (10).

Numerous instruments to evaluate function are available and widely used in clinical research. They all have strengths and limitations, which should be kept in mind when evaluating an article. A recent study using data from a placebo-controlled RCT compared the most commonly used questionnaires for self-assessment of

patients' functional capacity: the BASFI, the Dougados Functional Index (DFI), and the specific version for AS of the Health Assessment Questionnaire (HAQ-S), and concluded that the BASFI performed better to identify either improvement or deterioration (51). In another study, the DFI and HAQ-S were compared with two more generic instruments—the Health Assessment Questionnaire (HAQ) and the Arthritis Impact Measurement Scales-2 (AIMS2)—with regard to construct validity and sensitivity to change. This was a longitudinal study with a 2-year follow-up of 216 patients. The authors concluded that HAQ-S performed similarly to the HAQ but better than the AIMS-2 and the functional index (150). AIMS2 has been described as a multidimensional but not AS-specific tool. On the other hand, BASFI, DFI, and HAQ-S are AS-specific; however, several important dimensions are missing (151). For this reason, the AS Arthritis Impact Measurement Scales 2 (AS-AIMS2), a new questionnaire based on AIMS2 and HAQ-S, has been developed and validated (151). In another study the scores of BASFI and DFI showed a Spearman correlation coefficient of .89 (152). With these indexes, 12% to 30% of patients were misclassified for disease activity. Finally, the authors could not make a definite choice even though the BASFI showed a slightly higher specificity (152).

Detailed review of all the available instruments is beyond the purpose of this chapter. Some information on the instruments used for radiologic and laboratory domains have been discussed in previous sections.

TREATMENT

Major short-term objectives of AS treatment are primarily pain relief and decrease stiffness. This should allow for long-term prevention of ankylosis, hyperkyphosis, and late-stage complications such as chest wall involvement with restrictive pulmonary failure (78,153). Finally, one could add control of inflammation, which should prevent complications such as secondary amyloidosis. It is not known if these measures prevent other long-term manifestations or complications, such as aortic insufficiency or pulmonary fibrosis.

Probably more than in most diseases, patient education and active participation in the treatment are crucial. Drug therapy is important and efficient, and the availability of biologic agents will probably radically change our approach to AS during the coming decades; however, self-management and physiotherapy remain a cornerstone in the management of AS at this time.

Monitoring the evolution of an AS patient and evaluating the efficacy of treatment is a laborious but important task. As stated, multiple domains should be considered for a thorough clinical evaluation. Core sets have been proposed to help us (143,144), but their validity in daily clinical practice for treatment guidance is unknown. Furthermore, a working knowledge of the clinically relevant differences among instruments is still missing (78,134, 154).

Physiotherapy

Even if controlled studies are rare, physiotherapy has demonstrated its importance through the years and is widely prescribed. Probably it should be used in a classical form, administered by a physical therapist, or more importantly as a self-exercise, alone or within a group of AS patients (153,155).

Significant benefits have been demonstrated in an RCT for home physiotherapy on a short-term basis of 4 months (156); manipulative therapy also can be helpful (153). Hydrotherapy appears also particularly valuable and is widely prescribed, even if no rigorous demonstration of its efficacy is available (153,155). Before prescription, one also should be aware that if aquatic therapy has great advantages, it also has contraindications and specific requirements (157).

Even if classically it has been associated with drug therapy, physiotherapy per se has some efficacy for symptomatic relief and could be sufficient alone (153). Finally, it is essential to insist on the importance of the lifelong regular practice of exercise (153). Sports also can be advocated, but the choice should be adapted to the type of involvement, cardiovascular status, and intrinsic risk of traumatism (158).

Drugs

Analgesic

Pure analgesics often are considered of limited value by doctors in the management of AS; however, they are widely used by patients. In one study, almost one third of patients take analgesics; this percentage increases with severity of disease (159). The use of narcotic analgesics is not uncommon because the patients' main concern is symptom relief (160). To our knowledge, there is no RCT on their efficacy in AS, but we are unaware of any demonstration that an antiinflammatory effect is necessary in AS.

Nonsteroidal Antiinflammatory Drugs

Nonsteroidal antiinflammatory drugs (NSAIDs) have been and are still extensively used in AS to provide symptomatic relief; more than 80% of the patients use them (160). The overall objective is to provide sufficient relief to allow the patient to realize free movements and regular exercise programs essential for the prevention of ankylosis (78,153,155). There is no convincing evidence to support the traditional assertion that phenylbutazone and indomethacin are the best NSAIDs for AS (even having possible effects on the calcification of syndesmophytes).

It seems that all NSAIDs are equally efficient at equivalent dosis (78,153,155). It is more local preferences and conventions, rather than prospective RCT studies, that appear to dictate the use of various NSAIDs.

It is important to stress that the efficacy of an NSAID usually can be assessed within 48 hours; one should change to another drug in case of inefficacy (78). New COX-2 specific NSAIDs appear equally effective as regular NSAIDs. Celecoxib has proved to be as efficient at relieving pain in AS as ketoprofen in a 6-week RCT (161). There is no reason to believe that the benefits from COX-2 specific inhibition with reduction in serious gastrointestinal adverse events observed in large osteoarthritis studies should not apply to AS patients (162,163).

Finally, it is important to remember that there is no evidence in the literature that prolonged antiinflammatory treatment improves radiologic or functional outcomes. Usage of NSAIDs should be restricted to painful periods of disease activity, because they do not have any disease-modifying properties per se (155).

Systemic Corticosteroids

Systemic oral corticosteroids have little use in AS (78,155). Some rare patients do benefit from intravenously pulsed methylprednisolone for severe flare; however, the improvement usually is limited in time (78). Dosage of 1 g did not appear more effective than 375 mg (78).

Disease-modifying Antirheumatic Drugs and Biologic Agents

Disease-modifying antirheumatic drugs (DMARDs) are classically prescribed for severe disease resisting or insufficiently controlled by NSAIDs; however, they have no disease-modifying effect in AS. Most of the classical DMARDs used for rheumatoid arthritis have been tried in AS and proved to be either totally inefficient or efficient only in a few cases (78,153,155). They can be prescribed in severe cases resistant to other treatment, so long as one recognizes the limitations and risks of this treatment, has a clear definition of the potential benefit, and is ready to interrupt the treatment if it does not achieve the goal.

Sulfasalazine is the DMARD most used by patients and recommended by rheumatologists for AS (159). Various studies have evaluated sulfasalazine in AS, both in patients with axial and peripheral joint involvement (164,165). A meta-analysis confirmed safety and some effectiveness in the short-term treatment of AS (166). However, efficacy is mainly limited to peripheral disease (164,165). These trials indicated that there is no clinically relevant beneficial effect, except for concomitant arthritis, which represents less than 25% of patients with AS (167). Of interest, sulfasalazine has demonstrated a potential for prevention of anterior uveitis (168).

Methotrexate (mtx) is the second most recommended DMARD for AS (159), although no RCT has proved its efficacy in AS. Efficacy was evaluated in two open-label studies (169,170). An Italian study treated 17 sulfasalazine-resistant or -intolerant AS patients with 7.5 to 10 mg oral mtx per week in association with indomethacin over 3 years. Unexpectedly, they showed significant improvement in axial disease as evaluated by the visual analog scale (VAS) for night pain, well-being and physical measurements, and absence of spine or sacroiliac joint disease progression on radiographs; however, they failed to demonstrate any decrease in the number of swollen or tender joints (170). On the other hand, the axial measures were not significantly different in 34 long-standing active AS patients who failed to improve on NSAIDs and were treated with intramuscular mtx 12.5 mg per week for 1 year in a prospective study, despite the fact that 53% were considered responders with clinical improvement, reduction of more than 50% in the dosage of NSAIDs, and 25% in ESR. Also, 16 out of 26 patients with peripheral involvement had significant improvement (169). Finally, a recent 1-year RCT with 51 AS patients compared treatment with oral mtx 7.5 mg per week and naproxen with naproxen alone. This study failed to demonstrate any superiority of the association, but dosage of mtx was very low for the actual standard; possibly, a higher dosage would show some efficacy (171).

Anti–tumor necrosis-a (anti–TNF-α) therapy has raised enormous hope in the treatment of AS and other spondyloarthropathies (172,173). In a 3-month open study, Brandt et al. demonstrated a more than 50% improvement in nine out of 11 AS patients for disease activity, as measured with the BASDAI, function, and pain scores. Disease was considered severe, with a mean duration of 5 years, and the patients received three perfusions of infliximab, an anti–TNF-α chimeric antibody at a dose of 5 mg/kg of weight at weeks 0, 2, and 6, a protocol similar to the one used for Crohn disease (174). These data have been confirmed in a multicenter German RCT of 70 patients with AS where 53% had significant (50%) short-term improvement in BASDAI and spinal pain on a VAS scale (175). Two randomized, double-blind studies comparing anti-TNF therapy to placebo have been published recently (176,177). In the first study, infliximab brought significant short-term (12-week) benefits in spondyloarthropathies as assessed on patient and physician global activity scales. Nineteen patients out of 40 had AS, and it should be noted that six out of 10 only had axial involvement in the placebo group, whereas six out of nine had axial and peripheral involvement in the treatment group. Treatment significantly improved primary end points and decreased CRP and ESR, but it failed to demonstrate improvement in axial involvement (176). The second study used twice-weekly subcutaneous injection of etanercept, a soluble Ig fusion receptor, in 40 AS patients. Again, there was a significant improvement in the global assessment, BASFI, ESR, and CRP, but not in measures assessing spinal involvement with the exception of chest expansion (177). At this time, it seems that anti–TNF-α therapy is efficient in the short term, particularly when assessing functional capacity or quality of life. This type of treatment appears less efficient using clinical and radiologic measures, but this could be a problem of study design, in particular with short-term studies, or sensitivity of the methods. Recent studies have hinted that MRI could be a good surrogate outcome parameter in this regard (174,178,179). Moreover, it should be remembered that if biologic agents bring us to the next dimension in the treatment of AS, they also can have severe adverse effects (e.g., tuberculosis) (175,176,180), regardless of price.

Finally, and as stated, most DMARDs have been used with little success, but one can always find an anecdotal dramatic response in a severe case of refractory AS. This hold true for thalidomide (181), anti-CD4, anti-interleukin-6 (182), azathioprine (183), and others (155). The authors do not recommend the utilization of such treatments.

Others

Pamidronate, an antiresorptive bisphosphonate, has demonstrated good efficiency in NSAID-refractory AS in two small open studies (184,185) and one 6-month RCT (186). At a dose of 60 mg intravenously monthly, pamidronate induced significant decrease in activity index (BASDAI) and improvement in function (BASFI). Interestingly, there was no significant amelioration of inflammatory parameters; the mechanisms of this beneficial effect remain enigmatic. Reduced bone marrow edema in affected joints after pamidronate has been described by the same group, which could explain some of the observed effects (185).

Finally, despite the sad experiment with induced leukemia after external spine radiotherapy (153), systemic treatment with radioisotopes has regained interest in Germany (187), but awaits the strict demonstration of its efficacy and lack of long-term adverse effects.

Local Treatment

The limited therapeutic response to systemic therapy and the restricted involvement of enthesis and peripheral arthritis make them good candidates for local treatment. Physical therapy and orthoses such as shoe insoles can be helpful, even if rigorous demonstration of their efficacy is still lacking. The same holds true for local injection of corticosteroids; one should be aware of the risk of rupture when the injection is done near the Achilles tendon. Local intra-articular corticosteroids certainly are helpful in the management of peripheral arthritis and refractory sacroiliac joint pain (188–190). Radioactive synovectomy has been advocated in chronic synovitis (153) despite the absence of evidence for its efficiency (191). Finally, external local radiotherapy remains indicated in rare, refractory cases of enthesitis (192).

Surgery

The surgical treatment of AS is the subject of Chapter 77 by Simmons, Simmons, and Zhengo.

REFERENCES

1. Russell AS. Ankylosing spondylitis: history. In: Klippel JH, Dieppe PA, eds. Rheumatology, 2nd ed. London: Mosby, 1998:6.14.1–6.14.2.
2. Benoist M. Inflammatory spondyloarthropathies. In: Wiesel SW, Weinstein JN, Herkowitz HN, et al., eds. The lumbar spine, 2nd ed. Philadelphia: WB Saunders, 1996:797–811.
3. Calin A. Terminology, introduction, diagnostic criteria, and overview. In: Calin A, Taurog JD, eds. The spondylarthritides. Oxford, UK: Oxford University Press, 1998:1–15.
4. Schumacher HR, Bardin T. The spondyloarthropathies: classification and diagnosis. Do we need new terminologies? Baillieres Clin Rheumatol 1998;12:551–565.
5. Silman AJ. Ankylosing spondylitis and spondyloarthropathies. In: Silman AJ, Hochberg MC, eds. Epidemiology of the rheumatic diseases. Oxford, UK: Oxford University Press, 2001:100–111.
6. Feltkamp T, Mardjuadi A, Huang F, et al. Spondyloarthropathies in eastern Asia. Curr Opin Rheumatol 2001;13:285–290.
7. El-Khoury GY, Kathol MH, Brandser EA. Seronegative spondyloarthropathies. Radiol Clin North Am 1996;34:343–357.
8. Sampaio-Barros PD, Bertolo MB, Kraemer MH, et al. Primary ankylosing spondylitis: patterns of disease in a Brazilian population of 147 patients. J Rheumatol 2001;28:560–565.
9. Silman AJ. Rheumatoid arthritis. In: Silman AJ, Hochberg MC, eds. Epidemiology of the rheumatic diseases. Oxford, UK: Oxford University Press, 2001:31–71.
10. Calin A. The individual with ankylosing spondylitis: defining disease status and the impact of the illness. Br J Rheumatol 1995;34:663–672.
11. Hukuda S, Minami M, Saito T, et al. Spondyloarthropathies in Japan: nationwide questionnaire survey performed by the Japan Ankylosing Spondylitis Society. J Rheumatol 2001;28:554–559.
12. Kaipiainen-Seppanen O, Aho K. Incidence of chronic inflammatory joint diseases in Finland in 1995. J Rheumatol 2000;27:94–100.
13. Kaipiainen-Seppanen O, Aho K, Heliovaara M. Incidence and prevalence of ankylosing spondylitis in Finland. J Rheumatol 1997;24:496–499.
14. Liu Y, Li J, Chen B, et al. Familial aggregation of ankylosing spondylitis in Southern China. J Rheumatol 2001;28:550–553.
15. Brewerton DA, Hart FD, Nicholls A, et al. Ankylosing spondylitis and HL-A 27. Lancet 1973;1:904–907.
16. Schlosstein L, Terasaki PI, Bluestone R, et al. High association of an HL-A antigen, W27, with ankylosing spondylitis. N Engl J Med 1973;288:704–706.
17. Colbert RA, Prahalad S. Predisposing factors in the spondyloarthropathies: new insights into the role of HLA-B27. Curr Rheumatol Rep 2001;3:404–411.
18. Allen RL, Bowness P, McMichael A. The role of HLA-B27 in spondyloarthritis. Immunogenetics 1999;50:220–227.
19. Reveille JD, Ball EJ, Khan MA. HLA-B27 and genetic predisposing factors in spondyloarthropathies. Curr Opin Rheumatol 2001;13:265–272.
20. Mardjuadi A, Nasution AR, Kunmartini S, et al. Clinical features of spondyloarthropathy in Chinese and native Indonesians. Clin Rheumatol 1999;18:442–445.
21. Brown MA, Jepson A, Young A, et al. Ankylosing spondylitis in West Africans—evidence for a non-HLA-B27 protective effect. Ann Rheum Dis 1997;56:68–70.
22. Virtala M, Kirveskari J, Granfors K. HLA-B27 modulates the survival of Salmonella enteritidis in transfected L cells, possibly by impaired nitric oxide production. Infect Immunol 1997;65:4236–4242.
23. Laitio P, Virtala M, Salmi M, et al. HLA-B27 modulates intracellular survival of Salmonella enteritidis in human monocytic cells. Eur J Immunol 1997;27:1331–1338.
24. Colbert RA. HLA-B27 misfolding: a solution to the spondyloarthropathy conundrum? Mol Med Today 2000;6:224–230.
25. Dangoria NS, DeLay ML, Kingsbury DJ, et al. HLA-B27 misfolding is associated with aberrant intermolecular disulfide bond formation (dimerization) in the endoplasmic reticulum. J Biol Chem 2002; 277: 23459–23468.
26. Mear JP, Schreiber KL, Munz C, et al. Misfolding of HLA-B27 as a result of its B pocket suggests a novel mechanism for its role in susceptibility to spondyloarthropathies. J Immunol 1999;163:6665–6670.
27. Allen RL, O'Callaghan CA, McMichael AJ, et al. Cutting edge: HLA-B27 can form a novel beta 2-microglobulin-free heavy chain homodimer structure. J Immunol 1999;162:5045–5048.
28. Edwards JC, Bowness P, Archer JR. Jekyll and Hyde: the transformation of HLA-B27. Immunol Today 2000;21:256–260.
29. Taurog JD. Animal models of the spondyloarthropathies. In: Calin A, Taurog JD, eds. The spondylarthritides. Oxford, UK: Oxford University Press, 1998:223–237.
30. Taurog JD, Maika SD, Satumtira N, et al. Inflammatory disease in HLA-B27 transgenic rats. Immunol Rev 1999;169:209–223.
31. Khare SD, Luthra HS, David CS. Animal models of human leukocyte antigen B27-linked arthritides. Rheum Dis Clin North Am 1998; 24:883–894, xi–xii.
32. van der Linden S, van der Heijde D. Clinical aspects, outcome assessment, and management of ankylosing spondylitis and postenteric reactive arthritis. Curr Opin Rheumatol 2000;12:263–268.
33. Brown MA, Laval SH, Brophy S, et al. Recurrence risk modelling of the genetic susceptibility to ankylosing spondylitis. Ann Rheum Dis 2000;59:883–886.
34. Brown MA, Pile KD, Kennedy LG, et al. A genome-wide screen for susceptibility loci in ankylosing spondylitis. Arthritis Rheum 1998; 41:588–595.
35. Uksila J, Toivanen P, Granfors K. Enteric infections and arthritis: bacteriological aspects. In: Calin A, Taurog JD, eds. The spondylarthritides. Oxford, UK: Oxford University Press, 1998:167–177.
36. Jarvinen P. Occurrence of ankylosing spondylitis in a nationwide series of twins. Arthritis Rheum 1995;38:381–383.
37. Mielants H, Veys EM. The bowel and spondylarthritis: a clinical approach. In: Calin A, Taurog JD, eds. The spondylarthritides. Oxford, UK: Oxford University Press, 1998:129–157.
38. Lee YH, Ji JD, Kim JS, et al. Ileocolonoscopic and histologic studies of Korean patients with ankylosing spondylitis. Scand J Rheumatol 1997;26:473–476.
39. Böcker U, Sartor RB. Mechanisms of arthritis associated with chronic intestinal inflammation. In: Calin A, Taurog JD, eds. The spondylarthritides. Oxford, UK: Oxford University Press, 1998:207–222.
40. Jun JB, Kim TH, Jung SS, et al. Seronegative spondyloarthropathy initiated by physical trauma. Clin Rheumatol 2000;19:348–351.
41. Giltay EJ, van Schaardenburg D, Gooren LJ, et al. Androgens and ankylosing spondylitis: a role in the pathogenesis? Ann NY Acad Sci 1999;876:340–364.
42. Baudoin P, van der Horst-Bruinsma IE, Dekker-Saeys AJ, et al. Increased risk of developing ankylosing spondylitis among first-born children. Arthritis Rheum 2000;43:2818–2822.
43. Kahn MA. Ankylosing spondylitis: clinical features. In: Klippel JH, Dieppe PA, eds. Rheumatology, 2nd ed. London: Mosby, 1998:6.16.1–6.16.19.
44. MacKay K, Mack C, Brophy S, et al. The Bath Ankylosing Spondylitis Radiology Index (BASRI): a new, validated approach to disease assessment. Arthritis Rheum 1998;41:2263–2270.
45. Mader R. Atypical clinical presentation of ankylosing spondylitis. Semin Arthritis Rheum 1999;29:191–196.
46. Tyrrell PN, Davies AM, Evans N. Neurological disturbances in ankylosing spondylitis. Ann Rheum Dis 1994;53:714–717.
47. Boyer GS, Templin DW, Bowler A, et al. Spondyloarthropathy in the community: clinical syndromes and disease manifestations in Alaskan Eskimo populations. J Rheumatol 1999;26:1537–1544.
48. Gran JT, Skomsvoll JF. The outcome of ankylosing spondylitis: a study of 100 patients. Br J Rheumatol 1997;36:766–771.

49. Koh WH, Boey ML. Ankylosing spondylitis in Singapore: a study of 150 patients and a local update. Ann Acad Med Singapore 1998; 27:3–6.
50. Roussou E, Kennedy LG, Garrett S, et al. Socioeconomic status in ankylosing spondylitis: relationship between occupation and disease activity. J Rheumatol 1997;24:908–911.
51. Ruof J, Sangha O, Stucki G. Comparative responsiveness of 3 functional indices in ankylosing spondylitis. J Rheumatol 1999;26: 1959–1963.
52. Ward MM. Health-related quality of life in ankylosing spondylitis: a survey of 175 patients. Arthritis Care Res 1999;12:247–255.
53. de Vlam K, Mielants H, Veys EM. Involvement of the zygapophyseal joint in ankylosing spondylitis: relation to the bridging syndesmophyte. J Rheumatol 1999;26:1738–1745.
54. Olivieri I, Salvarani C, Cantini F, et al. Ankylosing spondylitis and undifferentiated spondyloarthropathies: a clinical review and description of a disease subset with older age at onset. Curr Opin Rheumatol 2001;13:280–284.
55. van der Linden S, van der Heijde D. Ankylosing spondylitis. Clinical features. Rheum Dis Clin North Am 1998;24:663–676.
56. van den Hoogen HM, Koes BW, van Eijk JT, et al. On the accuracy of history, physical examination, and erythrocyte sedimentation rate in diagnosing low back pain in general practice. A criteria-based review of the literature. Spine 1995;20:318–327.
57. Burgos-Vargas R, Pacheco-Tena C, Vazquez-Mellado J. Juvenile-onset spondyloarthropathies. Rheum Dis Clin North Am 1997;23: 569–598.
58. Dougados M. Diagnostic features of ankylosing spondylitis. Br J Rheumatol 1995;34:301–303.
59. Muñoz Gomariz E, Cisnal del Mazo A, Pérez Guijo V, et al. The potential of ESSG spondyloarthropathy classification criteria as a diagnostic aid in rheumatological practice. J Rheumatol 2002;29: 326–330.
60. Averns HL, Oxtoby J, Taylor HG, et al. Smoking and outcome in ankylosing spondylitis. Scand J Rheumatol 1996;25:138–142.
61. Boyer GS, Templin DW, Bowler A, et al. A comparison of patients with spondyloarthropathy seen in specialty clinics with those identified in a community-wide epidemiologic study. Has the classic case misled us? Arch Intern Med 1997;157:2111–2117.
62. Underwood MR, Dawes P. Inflammatory back pain in primary care. Br J Rheumatol 1995;34:1074–1077.
63. Padula A, Barozzi L, Ciancio G, et al. Involvement of transitional lumbosacral joints in spondyloarthritis. Clin Exp Rheumatol 1999;17: 636–637.
64. Jajic Z, Jajic I, Grazio S. Radiological changes of the symphysis in ankylosing spondylitis. Acta Radiol 2000;41:307–309.
65. Le T, Biundo J, Aprill C, et al. Costovertebral joint erosion in ankylosing spondylitis. Am J Phys Med Rehabil 2001;80:62–64.
66. Fournie B, Boutes A, Dromer C, et al. Prospective study of anterior chest wall involvement in ankylosing spondylitis and psoriatic arthritis. Rev Rhum (Engl Ed) 1997;64:22–25.
67. Kabasakal Y, Garrett SL, Calin A. The epidemiology of spondylodiscitis in ankylosing spondylitis—a controlled study. Br J Rheumatol 1996;35:660–663.
68. Geusens P, Vosse D, van der Heijde D, et al. High prevalence of thoracic vertebral deformities and discal wedging in ankylosing spondylitis patients with hyperkyphosis. J Rheumatol 2001;28:1856–1861.
69. Mitra D, Elvins DM, Speden DJ, et al. The prevalence of vertebral fractures in mild ankylosing spondylitis and their relationship to bone mineral density. Rheumatology 2000;39:85–89.
70. Kauppi M, Belt EA, Soini I."Bamboo spine" starts to bend—something is wrong. Clin Exp Rheumatol 2000;18:513–514.
71. Finkelstein JA, Chapman JR, Mirza S. Occult vertebral fractures in ankylosing spondylitis. Spinal Cord 1999;37:444–447.
72. Lee YS, Schlotzhauer T, Ott SM, et al. Skeletal status of men with early and late ankylosing spondylitis. Am J Med 1997;103:233–241.
73. Lange U, Jung O, Teichmann J, et al. Relationship between disease activity and serum levels of vitamin D metabolites and parathyroid hormone in ankylosing spondylitis. Osteoporos Int 2001;12: 1031–1035.
74. Sochart DH, Porter ML. Long-term results of total hip replacement in young patients who had ankylosing spondylitis. Eighteen to thirty-year results with survivorship analysis. J Bone Joint Surg (Am) 1997;79-A:1181–1189.
75. Will R, Kennedy G, Elswood J, et al. Ankylosing spondylitis and the shoulder: commonly involved but infrequently disabling. J Rheumatol 2000;27:177–182.
76. Ramos-Remus C, Major P, Gomez-Vargas A, et al. Temporomandibular joint osseous morphology in a consecutive sample of ankylosing spondylitis patients. Ann Rheum Dis 1997;56:103–107.
77. Major P, Ramos-Remus C, Suarez-Almazor ME, et al. Magnetic resonance imaging and clinical assessment of temporomandibular joint pathology in ankylosing spondylitis. J Rheumatol 1999;26:616–621.
78. Koehler L, Kuipers JG, Zeidler H. Managing seronegative spondarthritides. Rheumatology 2000;39:360–368.
79. Olivieri I, Barozzi L, Padula A. Enthesopathy: clinical manifestations, imaging and treatment. Baillieres Clin Rheumatol 1998;12:665–681.
80. Bilgen IG, Yunten N, Ustun EE, et al. Adhesive arachnoiditis causing cauda equina syndrome in ankylosing spondylitis: CT and MRI demonstration of dural calcification and a dorsal dural diverticulum. Neuroradiology 1999;41:508–511.
81. Ginsburg WW, Cohen MD, Miller GM, et al. Posterior vertebral body erosion by arachnoid diverticula in cauda equina syndrome: an unusual manifestation of ankylosing spondylitis. J Rheumatol 1997; 24:1417–1420.
82. Ahn NU, Ahn UM, Nallamshetty L, et al. Cauda equina syndrome in ankylosing spondylitis (the CES-AS syndrome): meta-analysis of outcomes after medical and surgical treatments. J Spinal Disord 2001;14: 427–433.
83. Chen JY, Ho HH, Wu YJ, et al. Coexistence of spinal arteriovenous malformation and ankylosing spondylitis—are they related? Clin Rheumatol 1994;13:533–536.
84. Kang S, Lee E, Baek H, et al. Bilateral optic neuritis in ankylosing spondylitis. Clin Exp Rheumatol 1999;17:635–636.
85. Dolan AL, Gibson T. Intrinsic spinal cord lesions in 2 patients with ankylosing spondylitis. J Rheumatol 1994;21:1160–1161.
86. Kallikorm R, Uibo O, Uibo R. Coeliac disease in spondyloarthropathy: usefulness of serological screening. Clin Rheumatol 2000;19:118–122.
87. Vilar MJ, Cury SE, Ferraz MB, et al. Renal abnormalities in ankylosing spondylitis. Scand J Rheumatol 1997;26:19–23.
88. Strobel ES, Fritschka E. Renal diseases in ankylosing spondylitis: review of the literature illustrated by case reports. Clin Rheumatol 1998;17:524–530.
89. Escalante A, Weaver WJ, Beardmore TD. An estimate of the prevalence of reactive systemic amyloidosis in ankylosing spondylitis. J Rheumatol 1995;22:2192–2193.
90. Gratacos J, Orellana C, Sanmarti R, et al. Secondary amyloidosis in ankylosing spondylitis. A systematic survey of 137 patients using abdominal fat aspiration. J Rheumatol 1997;24:912–915.
91. Fenlon HM, Casserly I, Sant SM, et al. Plain radiographs and thoracic high-resolution CT in patients with ankylosing spondylitis. AJR Am J Roentgenol 1997;168:1067–1072.
92. Casserly IP, Fenlon HM, Breatnach E, et al. Lung findings on high-resolution computed tomography in idiopathic ankylosing spondylitis—correlation with clinical findings, pulmonary function testing and plain radiography. Br J Rheumatol 1997;36:677–682.
93. Turetschek K, Ebner W, Fleischmann D, et al. Early pulmonary involvement in ankylosing spondylitis: assessment with thin-section CT. Clin Radiol 2000;55:632–636.
94. Bergfeldt L. HLA-B27-associated cardiac disease. Ann Intern Med 1997;127:621–629.
95. Roldan CA, Chavez J, Wiest PW, et al. Aortic root disease and valve disease associated with ankylosing spondylitis. J Am Coll Cardiol 1998;32:1397–1404.
96. Jimenez-Balderas FJ, Garcia-Rubi D, Perez-Hinojosa S, et al. Two-dimensional echo Doppler findings in juvenile and adult onset ankylosing spondylitis with long-term disease. Angiology 2001;52:543–548.
97. Banares A, Hernandez-Garcia C, Fernandez-Gutierrez B, et al. Eye involvement in the spondyloarthropathies. Rheum Dis Clin North Am 1998;24:771–784.
98. Gunther V, Mur E, Traweger C, et al. Stress coping of patients with ankylosing spondylitis. J Psychosom Res 1994;38:419–427.
99. Dalyan M, Guner A, Tuncer S, et al. Disability in ankylosing spondylitis. Disabil Rehabil 1999;21:74–79.
100. Hultgren S, Broman JE, Gudbjornsson B, et al. Sleep disturbances in outpatients with ankylosing spondylitis: a questionnaire study with gender implications. Scand J Rheumatol 2000;29:365–369.
101. Jamieson AH, Alford CA, Bird HA, et al. The effect of sleep and noc-

turnal movement on stiffness, pain, and psychomotor performance in ankylosing spondylitis. Clin Exp Rheumatol 1995;13:73–78.

102. Jones SD, Koh WH, Steiner A, et al. Fatigue in ankylosing spondylitis: its prevalence and relationship to disease activity, sleep, and other factors. J Rheumatol 1996;23:487–490.

103. Hidding A, de Witte L, van der Linden S. Determinants of self-reported health status in ankylosing spondylitis. J Rheumatol 1994; 21:275–278.

104. Au WY, Hawkins BR, Cheng N, et al. Risk of haematological malignancies in HLA-B27 carriers. Br J Haematol 2001;115:320–322.

105. Lange U, Boss B, Teichmann J, et al. Thyroid disorders in female patients with ankylosing spondylitis. Eur J Med Res 1999;4: 468–474.

106. Helenius LM, Hietanen JH, Helenius I, et al. Focal sialadenitis in patients with ankylosing spondylitis and spondyloarthropathy: a comparison with patients with rheumatoid arthritis or mixed connective tissue disease. Ann Rheum Dis 2001;60:744–749.

107. Padula A, Ciancio G, La Civita L, et al. Association between vitiligo and spondyloarthritis. J Rheumatol 2001;28:313–314.

108. Challier B, Urlacher F, Vancon G, et al. Is quality of life affected by season and weather conditions in ankylosing spondylitis? Clin Exp Rheumatol 2001;19:277–281.

109. Barlow JH, Wright CC, Williams B, et al. Work disability among people with ankylosing spondylitis. Arthritis Rheum 2001;45:424–429.

110. Boonen A, Chorus A, Miedema H, et al. Withdrawal from labour force due to work disability in patients with ankylosing spondylitis. Ann Rheum Dis 2001;60:1033–1039.

111. Boonen A, Chorus A, Miedema H, et al. Employment, work disability, and work days lost in patients with ankylosing spondylitis: a cross sectional study of Dutch patients. Ann Rheum Dis 2001;60:353–358.

112. Boonen A, de Vet H, van der Heijde D, et al. Work status and its determinants among patients with ankylosing spondylitis. A systematic literature review. J Rheumatol 2001;28:1056–1062.

113. Boonen A, van Der Heijde D, Landewe R, et al. Work status and productivity costs due to ankylosing spondylitis: comparison of three European countries. Ann Rheum Dis 2002;61:429–437.

114. Ward MM. Quality of life in patients with ankylosing spondylitis. Rheum Dis Clin North Am 1998;24:815–827.

115. Cabral DA, Malleson PN, Petty RE. Spondyloarthropathies of childhood. Pediatr Clin North Am 1995;42:1051–1070.

116. Azouz EM, Duffy CM. Juvenile spondyloarthropathies: clinical manifestations and medical imaging. Skeletal Radiol 1995;24:399–408.

117. Gomez KS, Raza K, Jones SD, et al. Juvenile onset ankylosing spondylitis—more girls than we thought? J Rheumatol 1997;24: 735–737.

118. Prieur AM. Spondyloarthropathies in childhood. Baillieres Clin Rheumatol 1998;12:287–307.

119. Burgos-Vargas R, Vazquez-Mellado J. The early clinical recognition of juvenile-onset ankylosing spondylitis and its differentiation from juvenile rheumatoid arthritis. Arthritis Rheum 1995;38:835–844.

120. Braun J, Bollow M, Sieper J. Radiologic diagnosis and pathology of the spondyloarthropathies. Rheum Dis Clin North Am 1998;24: 697–735.

121. Battistone MJ, Manaster BJ, Reda DJ, et al. Radiographic diagnosis of sacroiliitis—are sacroiliac views really better? J Rheumatol 1998; 25:2395–2401.

122. Yu W, Feng F, Dion E, et al. Comparison of radiography, computed tomography and magnetic resonance imaging in the detection of sacroiliitis accompanying ankylosing spondylitis. Skeletal Radiol 1998;27:311–320.

123. Bollow M, Braun J, Hamm B, et al. Early sacroiliitis in patients with spondyloarthropathy: evaluation with dynamic gadolinium-enhanced MR imaging. Radiology 1995;194:529–536.

124. Oostveen J, Prevo R, den Boer J, et al. Early detection of sacroiliitis on magnetic resonance imaging and subsequent development of sacroiliitis on plain radiography. A prospective, longitudinal study. J Rheumatol 1999;26:1953–1958.

125. Jevtic V, Kos-Golja M, Rozman B, et al. Marginal erosive discovertebral "Romanus" lesions in ankylosing spondylitis demonstrated by contrast enhanced Gd-DTPA magnetic resonance imaging. Skeletal Radiol 2000;29:27–33.

126. McNally EG, Wilson DJ, Ostlere SJ. Limited magnetic resonance imaging in low back pain instead of plain radiographs: experience with first 1000 cases. Clin Radiol 2001;56:922–925.

127. Ryan PJ, Gibson T, Fogelman I. Spinal bone SPECT in chronic symptomatic ankylosing spondylitis. Clin Nucl Med 1997;22:821–824.

128. de Vlam K, Van de Wiele C, Mielants H, et al. Is 99mTc human immunoglobulin G scintigraphy (HIG-scan) useful for the detection of spinal inflammation in ankylosing spondylitis? Clin Exp Rheumatol 2000;18:379–382.

129. Secundini R, Scheines EJ, Gusis SE, et al. Clinico-radiological correlation of enthesitis in seronegative spondyloarthropathies (SNSA). Clin Rheumatol 1997;16:129–132.

130. Calin A, Mackay K, Santos H, et al. A new dimension to outcome: application of the Bath Ankylosing Spondylitis Radiology Index. J Rheumatol 1999;26:988–992.

131. Dawes PT. Stoke Ankylosing Spondylitis Spine Score. J Rheumatol 1999;26:993–996.

132. MacKay K, Brophy S, Mack C, et al. The development and validation of a radiographic grading system for the hip in ankylosing spondylitis: the bath ankylosing spondylitis radiology hip index. J Rheumatol 2000;27:2866–2872.

133. Spoorenberg A, de Vlam K, van der Heijde D, et al. Radiological scoring methods in ankylosing spondylitis: reliability and sensitivity to change over one year. J Rheumatol 1999;26:997–1002.

134. van der Heijde DM, van der Linden S. Measures of outcome in ankylosing spondylitis and other spondyloarthritides. Baillieres Clin Rheumatol 1998;12:683–693.

135. Viitanen JV, Kokko ML, Lehtinen K, et al. Correlation between mobility restrictions and radiologic changes in ankylosing spondylitis. Spine 1995;20:492–496.

136. Spoorenberg A, van der Heijde D, de Klerk E, et al. Relative value of erythrocyte sedimentation rate and C-reactive protein in assessment of disease activity in ankylosing spondylitis. J Rheumatol 1999;26: 980–984.

137. Dougados M, Gueguen A, Nakache JP, et al. Clinical relevance of C-reactive protein in axial involvement of ankylosing spondylitis. J Rheumatol 1999;26:971–974.

138. Viitanen JV, Kokko ML, Heikkila S, et al. Neck mobility assessment in ankylosing spondylitis: a clinical study of nine measurements including new tape methods for cervical rotation and lateral flexion. Br J Rheumatol 1998;37:377–381.

139. Viitanen JV, Kokko ML, Heikkila S, et al. Assessment of thoracolumbar rotation in ankylosing spondylitis: a simple tape method. Clin Rheumatol 1999;18:152–157.

140. Viitanen JV, Heikkila S, Kokko ML, et al. Clinical assessment of spinal mobility measurements in ankylosing spondylitis: a compact set for follow-up and trials? Clin Rheumatol 2000;19:131–137.

141. Heikkila S, Viitanen JV, Kautiainen H, et al. Sensitivity to change of mobility tests; effect of short term intensive physiotherapy and exercise on spinal, hip, and shoulder measurements in spondyloarthropathy. J Rheumatol 2000;27:1251–1256.

142. Rahali-Khachlouf H, Poiraudeau S, Fermanian J, et al. Validité et reproductibilité des mesures cliniques rachidiennes dans la spondylarthrite ankylosante. Ann Readapt Med Phys 2001;44:205–212.

143. van der Heijde D, Calin A, Dougados M, et al. Selection of instruments in the core set for DC-ART, SMARD, physical therapy, and clinical record keeping in ankylosing spondylitis. Progress report of the ASAS Working Group. Assessments in ankylosing spondylitis. J Rheumatol 1999;26:951–954.

144. van der Heijde D, van der Linden S, Bellamy N, et al. Which domains should be included in a core set for endpoints in ankylosing spondylitis? Introduction to the ankylosing spondylitis module of OMERACT IV. J Rheumatol 1999;26:945–947.

145. Anderson JJ, Baron G, van der Heijde D, et al. Ankylosing spondylitis assessment group preliminary definition of short-term improvement in ankylosing spondylitis. Arthritis Rheum 2001;44: 1876–1886.

146. Classification internationale du fonctionnement, du handicap et de la santé: CIF. Genève: Organisation mondiale de la Santé; 2001.

147. Calin A, Nakache JP, Gueguen A, et al. Defining disease activity in ankylosing spondylitis: is a combination of variables (Bath Ankylosing Spondylitis Disease Activity Index): an appropriate instrument? Rheumatology 1999;38:878–882.

148. Jenkinson TR, Mallorie PA, Whitelock HC, et al. Defining spinal mobility in ankylosing spondylitis (AS). The Bath AS Metrology Index. J Rheumatol 1994;21:1694–1698.

149. Kennedy LG, Jenkinson TR, Mallorie PA, et al. Ankylosing spondyli-

tis: the correlation between a new metrology score and radiology. Br J Rheumatol 1995;34:767–770.

150. Ward MM, Kuzis S. Validity and sensitivity to change of spondylitis-specific measures of functional disability. J Rheumatol 1999;26:121–127.

151. Guillemin F, Challier B, Urlacher F, et al. Quality of life in ankylosing spondylitis: validation of the ankylosing spondylitis Arthritis Impact Measurement Scales 2, a modified Arthritis Impact Measurement Scales Questionnaire. Arthritis Care Res 1999;12:157–162.

152. Spoorenberg A, van der Heijde D, de Klerk E, et al. A comparative study of the usefulness of the Bath Ankylosing Spondylitis Functional Index and the Dougados Functional Index in the assessment of ankylosing spondylitis. J Rheumatol 1999;26:961–965.

153. Haslock I. Ankylosing spondylitis: management. In: Klippel JH, Dieppe PA, eds. Rheumatology, 2nd ed. London: Mosby, 1998:6.19.1–6.19.10.

154. Ward MM. Response criteria and criteria for clinically important improvement: separate and equal? Arthritis Rheum 2001;44:1728–1729.

155. Dougados M, Revel M, Khan MA. Spondyloarthropathy treatment: progress in medical treatment, physical therapy and rehabilitation. Baillieres Clin Rheumatol 1998;12:717–736.

156. Kraag G, Stokes B, Groh J, et al. The effects of comprehensive home physiotherapy and supervision on patients with ankylosing spondylitis—a randomized controlled trial. J Rheumatol 1990;17:228–233.

157. McNeal RL. Aquatic therapy for patients with rheumatic disease. Rheum Dis Clin North Am 1990;16:915–929.

158. Dudler J. Sports et rhumatismes inflammatoires. Méd et Hyg 1998;56:586–592.

159. Pal B. Use of simple analgesics in the treatment of ankylosing spondylitis. Br J Rheumatol 1987;26:207–209.

160. Ward MM, Kuzis S. Treatments used by patients with ankylosing spondylitis. Comparison with the treatment preferences of rheumatologists. J Clin Rheumatol 1999;5:1–8.

161. Dougados M, Behier JM, Jolchine I, et al. Efficacy of celecoxib, a cyclooxygenase 2-specific inhibitor, in the treatment of ankylosing spondylitis: a six-week controlled study with comparison against placebo and against a conventional nonsteroidal antiinflammatory drug. Arthritis Rheum 2001;44:180–185.

162. Silverstein FE, Faich G, Goldstein JL, et al. Gastrointestinal toxicity with celecoxib vs nonsteroidal anti-inflammatory drugs for osteoarthritis and rheumatoid arthritis: the CLASS study: a randomized controlled trial. Celecoxib Long-term Arthritis Safety Study. JAMA 2000;284:1247–1255.

163. Bombardier C, Laine L, Reicin A, et al. Comparison of upper gastrointestinal toxicity of rofecoxib and naproxen in patients with rheumatoid arthritis. VIGOR Study Group. N Engl J Med 2000;343:1520–1528.

164. Clegg DO, Reda DJ, Weisman MH, et al. Comparison of sulfasalazine and placebo in the treatment of ankylosing spondylitis. A Department of Veterans Affairs Cooperative Study. Arthritis Rheum 1996;39:2004–2012.

165. Clegg DO, Reda DJ, Abdellatif M. Comparison of sulfasalazine and placebo for the treatment of axial and peripheral articular manifestations of the seronegative spondyloarthropathies: a Department of Veterans Affairs cooperative study. Arthritis Rheum 1999;42:2325–2329.

166. Ferraz MB, Tugwell P, Goldsmith CH, et al. Meta-analysis of sulfasalazine in ankylosing spondylitis. J Rheumatol 1990;17:1482–1486.

167. Kirwan J, Edwards A, Huitfeldt B, et al. The course of established ankylosing spondylitis and the effects of sulphasalazine over 3 years. Br J Rheumatol 1993;32:729–733.

168. Benitez-Del Castillo JM, Garcia-Sanchez J, Iradier T, et al. Sulfasalazine in the prevention of anterior uveitis associated with ankylosing spondylitis. Eye 2000;14:340–343.

169. Sampaio-Barros PD, Costallat LT, Bertolo MB, et al. Methotrexate in the treatment of ankylosing spondylitis. Scand J Rheumatol 2000;29:160–162.

170. Biasi D, Carletto A, Caramaschi P, et al. Efficacy of methotrexate in the treatment of ankylosing spondylitis: a three-year open study. Clin Rheumatol 2000;19:114–117.

171. Altan L, Bingol U, Karakoc Y, et al. Clinical investigation of methotrexate in the treatment of ankylosing spondylitis. Scand J Rheumatol 2001;30:255–259.

172. Braun J, Sieper J. Anti-TNF-alpha: a new dimension in the pharmacotherapy of the spondyloarthropathies? Ann Rheum Dis 2000;59:404–407.

173. Sieper J, Braun J. New treatment options in ankylosing spondylitis: a role for anti-TNF-alpha therapy. Ann Rheum Dis 2001;60(iii):58–61.

174. Brandt J, Haibel H, Cornely D, et al. Successful treatment of active ankylosing spondylitis with the anti-tumor necrosis factor alpha monoclonal antibody infliximab. Arthritis Rheum 2000;43:1346–1352.

175. Braun J, Brandt J, Listing J, et al. Treatment of active ankylosing spondylitis with infliximab: a randomised controlled multicentre trial. Lancet 2002;359:1187–1193.

176. Van Den Bosch F, Kruithof E, Baeten D, et al. Randomized double-blind comparison of chimeric monoclonal antibody to tumor necrosis factor alpha (infliximab) versus placebo in active spondyloarthropathy. Arthritis Rheum 2002;46:755–765.

177. Gorman JD, Sack KE, Davis JC. Treatment of ankylosing spondylitis by inhibition of tumor necrosis factor alpha. N Engl J Med 2002;346:1349–1356.

178. Stone M, Salonen D, Lax M, et al. Clinical and imaging correlates of response to treatment with infliximab in patients with ankylosing spondylitis. J Rheumatol 2001;28:1605–1614.

179. Braun J, de Keyser F, Brandt J, et al. New treatment options in spondyloarthropathies: increasing evidence for significant efficacy of anti-tumor necrosis factor therapy. Curr Opin Rheumatol 2001;13:245–249.

180. Keane J, Gershon S, Wise RP, et al. Tuberculosis associated with infliximab, a tumor necrosis factor alpha-neutralizing agent. N Engl J Med 2001;345:1098–1104.

181. Breban M, Gombert B, Amor B, et al. Efficacy of thalidomide in the treatment of refractory ankylosing spondylitis. Arthritis Rheum 1999;42:580–581.

182. Wendling D, Racadot E, Toussirot E, et al. Combination therapy of anti-CD4 and anti-IL6 monoclonal antibodies in a case of severe spondyloarthropathy. Br J Rheumatol 1996;35:1330.

183. Durez P, Horsmans Y. Dramatic response after an intravenous loading dose of azathioprine in one case of severe and refractory ankylosing spondylitis. Rheumatology 2000;39:182–184.

184. Maksymowych WP, Jhangri GS, Leclercq S, et al. An open study of pamidronate in the treatment of refractory ankylosing spondylitis. J Rheumatol 1998;25:714–717.

185. Maksymowych WP, Lambert R, Jhangri GS, et al. Clinical and radiological amelioration of refractory peripheral spondyloarthritis by pulse intravenous pamidronate therapy. J Rheumatol 2001;28:144–155.

186. Maksymowych WP, Jhangri GS, Fitzgerald AA, et al. A six-month randomized, controlled, double-blind, dose-response comparison of intravenous pamidronate (60 mg versus 10 mg) in the treatment of nonsteroidal antiinflammatory drug-refractory ankylosing spondylitis. Arthritis Rheum 2002;46:766–773.

187. Braun J, Lemmel EM, Manger B, et al. [Therapy of ankylosing spondylitis (AS) with radium chloride (224SpondylAT)]. Z Rheumatol 2001;60:74–83.

188. Maugars Y, Mathis C, Vilon P, et al. Corticosteroid injection of the sacroiliac joint in patients with seronegative spondyloarthropathy. Arthritis Rheum 1992;35:564–568.

189. Gunaydin I, Pereira PL, Daikeler T, et al. Magnetic resonance imaging guided corticosteroid injection of the sacroiliac joints in patients with therapy resistant spondyloarthropathy: a pilot study. J Rheumatol 2000;27:424–428.

190. Maugars Y, Mathis C, Berthelot JM, et al. Assessment of the efficacy of sacroiliac corticosteroid injections in spondyloarthropathies: a double-blind study. Br J Rheumatol 1996;35:767–770.

191. O'Duffy EK, Clunie GP, Lui D, et al. Double blind glucocorticoid controlled trial of samarium-153 particulate hydroxyapatite radiation synovectomy for chronic knee synovitis. Ann Rheum Dis 1999;58:554–558.

192. Zvaifler NJ, Seagren SL. Local radiotherapy for painful heels with spondyloarthropathies. In: Klippel JH, Dieppe PA, eds. Rheumatology, 2nd ed. London: Mosby, 1998:6.20.7–6.20.8.

CHAPTER 77

Ankylosing Spondylitis: Operative Treatment

Edward H. Simmons, Edward D. Simmons, and Yinggang Zheng

It is well recognized that severe flexion deformities of the spine may occur in patients with ankylosing spondylitis. Despite emphasis on early recognition and current advances in medical treatment, patients are still seen with advanced kyphotic deformities of the trunk who are very severely disabled and who present a major challenge for definitive surgical correction of their deformity (1–4).

Lumbar osteotomy is the first type of surgical correction for kyphotic deformity of spine in ankylosing spondylitis, reported by Smith-Petersen et al. in 1945 (5). The initial procedure as reported by Smith-Petersen et al. was done under general anesthesia with the patient lying prone. This was further reported by LaChapelle, Herbert, Nunziata, Wilson and Turkell, Law, and others (6–13). To avoid difficulties with the use of the prone position for patients with kyphotic deformity, Adams recommended that surgery be done with patients on their sides. He used a three-point rack to manipulate the spine for correction (14).

Some have recommended a two-stage or double-exposure procedure with division of the longitudinal ligament anteriorly. In our experience this is not required, and correction can be consistently done from the posterior approach alone. It should be appreciated that gastric dilatation and abdominal ileus is a major and consistent complication of lumbar osteotomy. When the spine is extended with the costal margin moving away from the pelvis, the superior mesenteric artery is stretched over the third part of the duodenum, producing a functional block to the outlet of the stomach and predisposing to gastric dilatation. If this hazard is not anticipated, patients may vomit a large amount. With a stiff rigid neck in the supine position, there is a major risk of aspiration, which could prove fatal. It is necessary to have a nasogastric tube in position postoperatively with suction drainage until intestinal motility is established and the patient is passing gas.

Early workers recognized the risk of general anesthesia in the performance of lumbar osteotomy (15,16). A review of the results of all reported cases of lumbar osteotomy under general anesthesia prior to 1969 indicated that the

mortality was 8% to 10% and that neurologic deficit of some degree, including paraplegia, had an incidence of 30%. In analyzing the causes of death, two thirds appeared related to the use of general anesthesia. As a result, we routinely carried out correction on the lumbar spine under local anesthesia beginning in 1969, which was found to be a safe, reliable, and practical procedure (1,17–21).

With improvement in anesthesia (particularly the ability to carry out fiberoptic intubation with the patient awake) and the development of spinal cord monitoring, the risks of surgery under general anesthesia have markedly decreased. General anesthesia is a reasonably safe option if the patient's general health is good, if he or she has had previous surgery under general anesthesia without complication, and if reasonable neck mobility remains. Our current technique is for the patient to be intubated while awake. With the endotracheal tube in position the patient is able to stand and place himself or herself on an adjusted Tower table with the hips and knees flexed and supports adjusted for the pelvis, chest, and head. These are adjusted until the patient is comfortable, avoiding any strain on the neck or elsewhere. When comfortable, the patient gives an OK signal with the hand, and general anesthesia is commenced. Spinal cord monitoring is done throughout the procedure. It is important to have valid preoperative tracings for comparison with the findings during surgery. The use of general anesthesia makes the resection easier to perform and allows easier undercutting of the pedicles above and below, with a more thorough decompression of the nerve roots. When the hips are extended to produce anterior osteoclasis with extension of the lumbar spine, the knees should be kept flexed to avoid any sciatic nerve tension that would alter the evoked spinal responses if posterior tibial nerve stimulation is used at the ankles (Fig. 77-1).

The initial recommendation of Smith-Petersen et al. (5) was to carry out a posterior wedge resection of the mid-lumbar spine in a V-fashion, with fracturing of the anterior longitudinal ligament. A midline resection was car-

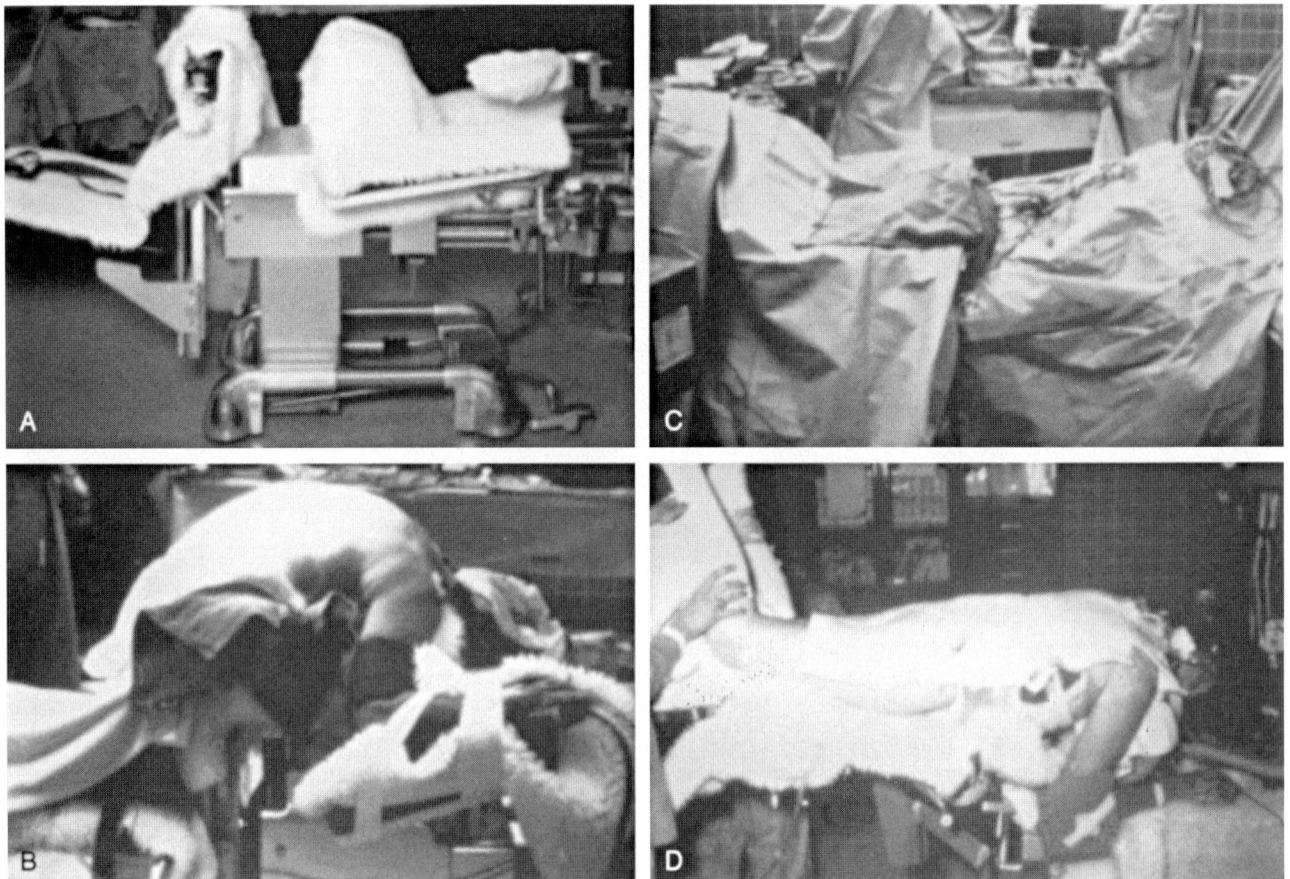

FIG. 77-1. A: Side view of a Tower table prepared for lumbar osteotomy under general anesthesia. The patient is intubated while awake and positioned on the table awake. Adjustments are made so that head is supported in a comfortable position with the eyeballs free of pressure. The chest and pelvis are supported with the abdomen free. The knees bear part of the patient's weight, with the hips and knees flexed. When the patient is comfortable, general anesthesia is begun. **B:** Lateral view of a patient with lumbar flexion deformity in position on a Tower table with knees flexed at 90 degrees. **C:** Operative view showing correction of the flexion deformity after lumbar resection-extension osteotomy. The hips are extended with the spine fracturing anteriorly and the resected defect closing posteriorly. The knees are kept flexed to avoid stretching of the sciatic nerves and interference with spinal cord monitoring. The resected defect closes, allowing Luque instrumentation with Wisconsin buttons, and grafting. **D:** Postoperative view with application of posterior shell to support the patient when turned supine. (From Simmons EH. Ankylosing spondylitis: surgical considerations. In: Herkowitz HN, Garfin SR, Balderston RA, et al, eds. Rothman-Simeone: the spine, 4th ed. Philadelphia: WB Saunders, 1999:1303–1356, with permission.)

ried upward and outward through the superior facet of the vertebrae above and the inferior facet of the vertebrae below in an oblique fashion. The obliquity of the osteotomy was to allow locking of the vertebrae following correction in an effort to prevent displacement. This technique is the basis for our current procedure.

INDICATIONS FOR LUMBAR OSTEOTOMY

Lumbar osteotomy is commonly done for surgical correction of lumbar hypolordosis or kyphosis giving rise to a fixed flexion deformity. The indications are variable and depend on the extent of the deformity, the degree of functional embarrassment, the age and general condition of the patient, the feasibility of correction, and above all else, the earnest desire of the patient to accept the risks and rehabilitation measures required for correction.

The contraindications include patients who are not suitable candidates for medical reasons and where the severity of the deformity does not warrant the procedure. Severe osteopenia is also a relative contraindication.

ASSESSMENT OF SPINAL FLEXION DEFORMITY

In assessing patients for possible surgical correction, it is important to recognize the primary site of the deformity and accurately measure the angle of deformity.

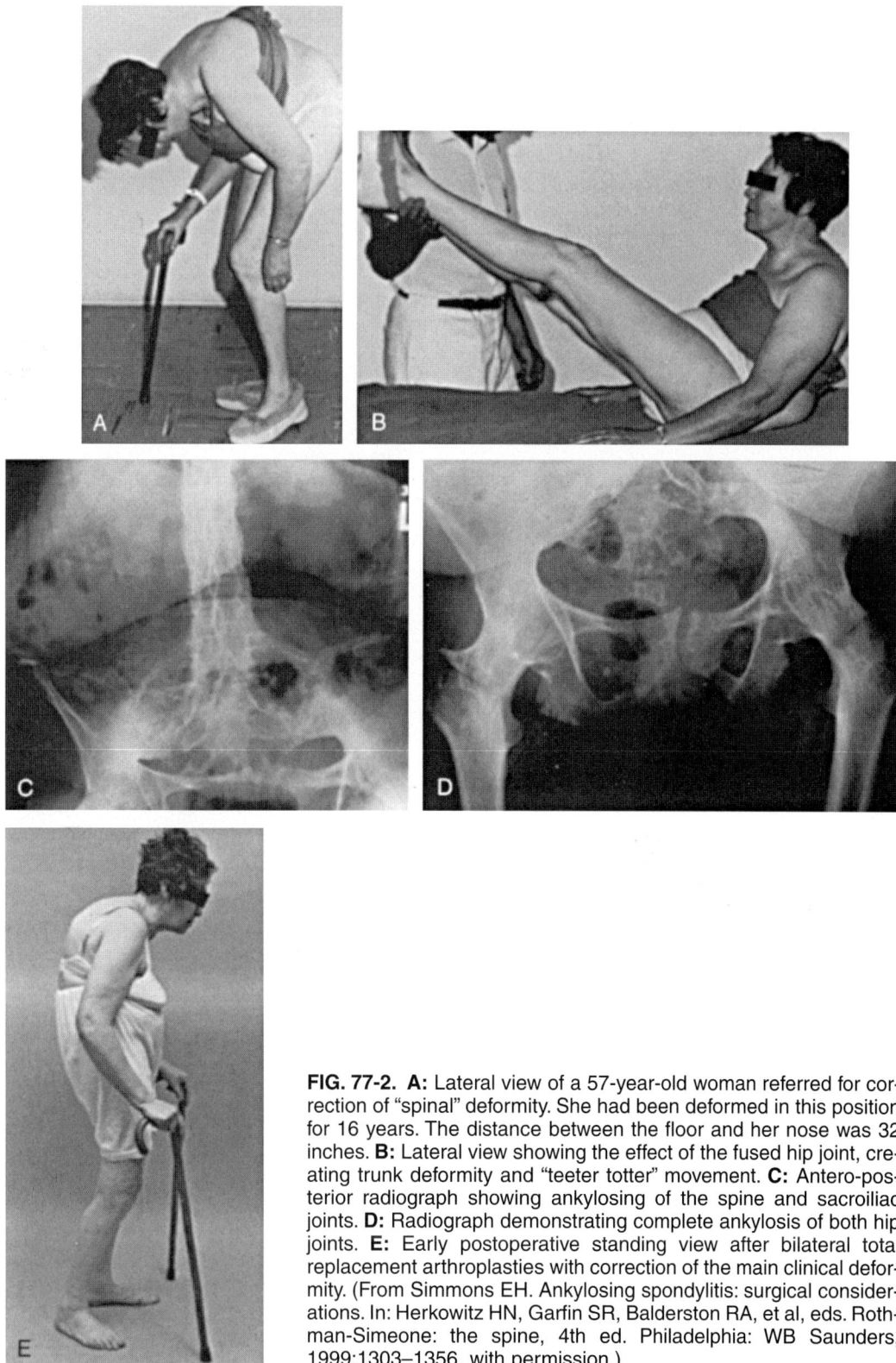

FIG. 77-2. **A:** Lateral view of a 57-year-old woman referred for correction of "spinal" deformity. She had been deformed in this position for 16 years. The distance between the floor and her nose was 32 inches. **B:** Lateral view showing the effect of the fused hip joint, creating trunk deformity and "teeter totter" movement. **C:** Antero-posterior radiograph showing ankylosing of the spine and sacroiliac joints. **D:** Radiograph demonstrating complete ankylosis of both hip joints. **E:** Early postoperative standing view after bilateral total replacement arthroplasties with correction of the main clinical deformity. (From Simmons EH. Ankylosing spondylitis: surgical considerations. In: Herkowitz HN, Garfin SR, Balderston RA, et al, eds. Rothman-Simeone: the spine, 4th ed. Philadelphia: WB Saunders, 1999:1303–1356, with permission.)

The surgeon may attempt to improve spinal alignment and patient function by operating at a level somewhat distant from the area of primary deformity; however, if any major correction is to be attempted, the correction must be done at the site of the main deformity. If this is not done, disturbance of balance could occur and the ability to walk and stand upright could be impaired. Patients who present with apparent spinal deformity may have the main deformity in their hip joints rather than their spine. The main deformity may be in the lumbar, thoracic, or even cervical spine (4).

Figure 77-2A shows a 57-year-old woman who was referred for correction of her "spinal" deformity. Once a woman of normal height, she was flexed so much that the distance from her nose to the floor was only 32 inches. She had been held rigidly in this position for 16 years. Her knees were held inflexibly together in adduction, and she wore a protective pad on her right knee as a result of impingement of one knee against the other. The spine and hip joints were both solidly ankylosed so that she could be moved up and down in a "teeter totter" fashion by lifting up on her extremities or pushing down on her head (Fig. 77-2, B—D). It was evident also that her main flexion deformity was at the fused hip joints, and if her lower limbs were placed below her, in line with her trunk, the main deformity would be corrected. She was not treated by spinal osteotomy, but by bilateral total hip replacement arthroplasties mobilizing the hips and correcting the hip

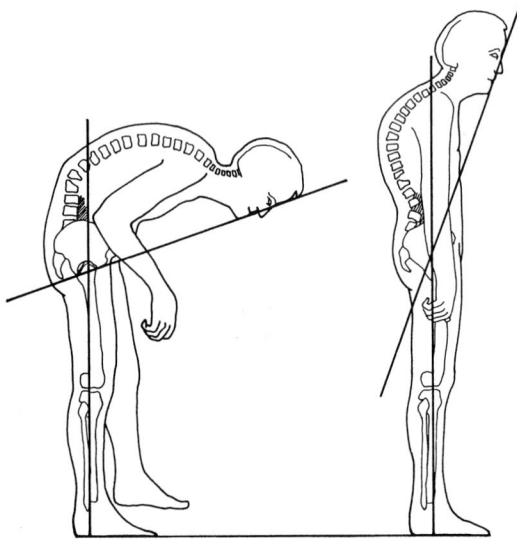

FIG. 77-3. Technique for measuring the degree of flexion deformity of the spine in ankylosing spondylitis. The chin-brow to vertical angle is measured from the brow to the chin to the vertical, with the patient standing with the hips and knees extended and the neck in its fixed or neutral position. (From Simmons EH. Surgery of the spine in ankylosing spondylitis and rheumatoid arthritis. In: Chapman MW, ed. Operative orthopaedics, vol. 3. Philadelphia: JB Lippincott, 1988:2077–2114, with permission.)

flexion deformities, placing the lower limbs in more normal alignment below the trunk. After this she was able to stand and look ahead (Fig. 77-2E). As far as she was concerned, her main problem had been relieved. She continued to progress well, walking with aids, and was able to look after her own home.

Accurate assessment and measurement of lumbar flexion deformity are required in planning surgical treatment and evaluating its results. The most effective and consistent measure of trunk flexion deformity is the chin-brow to vertical angle. This is a measure of the angle from a line extending from the chin to the brow measured to the vertical, when the patient stands with the hips and knees extended and the neck in its neutral or fixed position. Based on this, the size of the wedge in lumbar spine to be removed posteriorly is determined (Fig. 77-3).

The patient is admitted prior to the proposed surgery for careful medical assessment, including pulmonary function tests and electrocardiography. A physiotherapy program of deep breathing and extremity exercises is given, to be used postoperatively. Psychological preparation includes preoperative visits by the anesthetist as well as the surgeon, to explain the whole procedure to the patient and gain his or her confidence (21).

TECHNIQUES

Patients who have primarily a lumbar kyphotic deformity with loss of lumbar lordosis are selected. The deformity is determined by clinical and radiologic assessment. The angle of lumbar spine correction that is required is indicated by measurement of the chin-brow to vertical angle. This angle is transposed to a lateral radiograph of the lumbar spine, with the apex of the angle at the posterior longitudinal ligament of the L3-4 disc space (Fig. 77-4).

The osteotomy is done at the L3-4 level, which is the normal center of lumbar lordosis. This is also below the conus medullaris and the spinal canal volume is fairly reasonable at this level. It is at or below the bifurcation of the aorta. A preoperative computed tomography scan should be done to evaluate the spinal canal preoperatively. A midline exposure is made and the proposed osteotomy site is confirmed radiographically, because operative localization is difficult owing to the fused confluent nature of the posterior elements of the spine. The posterior elements are removed in a V-fashion to accomplish the realignment of the spine. Following resection of the angle and closure posteriorly, an opening wedge of the same amount is created anteriorly, which results in correction of the patient's deformity. It is essential that full correction be obtained and that the weight-bearing line of gravity be shifted posterior to the osteotomy site, so that gravity will tend to maintain and even increase correction as well as stimulate bone formation across the osteotomy site at the resected fused posterior masses of the spine (Fig. 77-5).

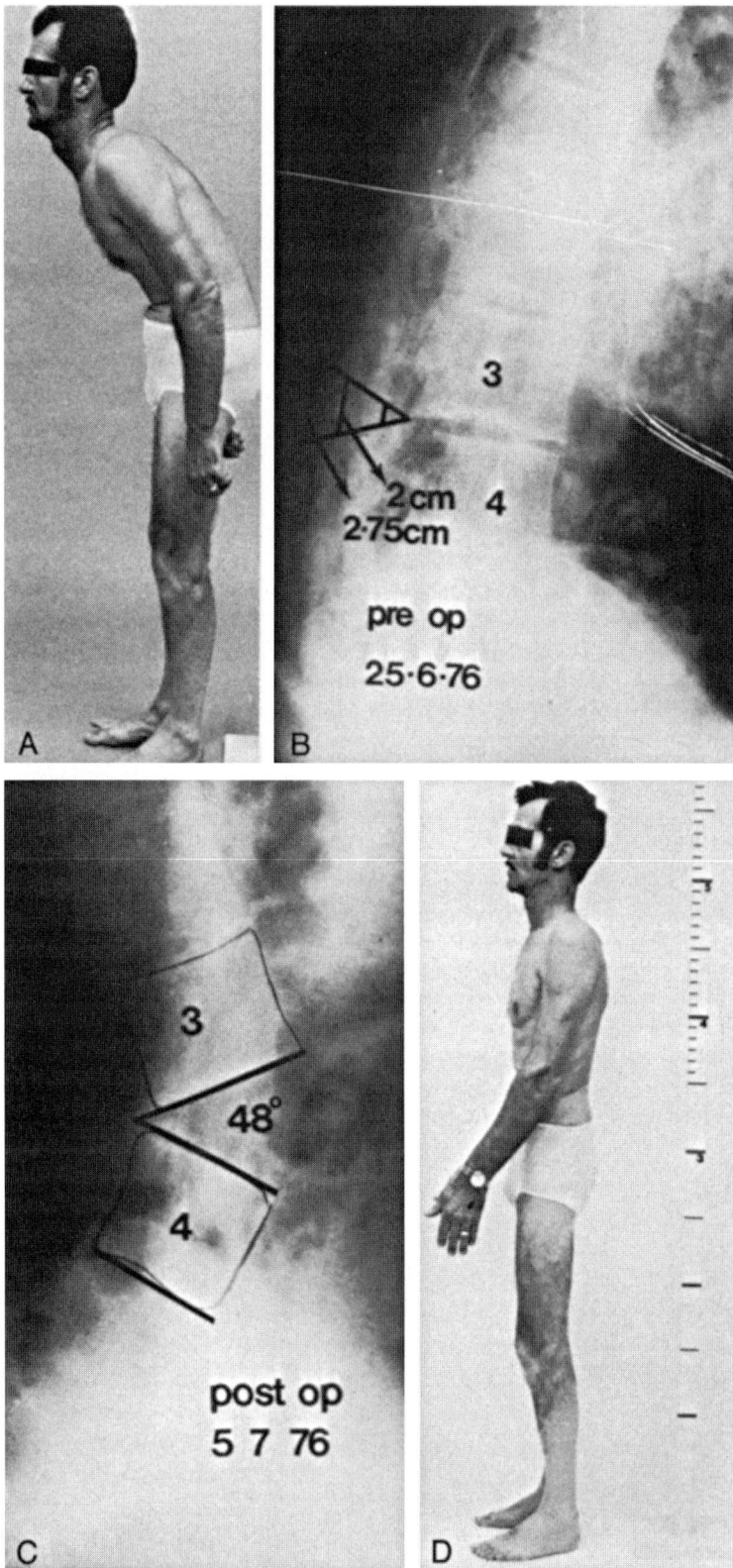

FIG. 77-4. A: Lateral view of a patient standing with hips and knees extended. This patient still had mobility of his cervical spine and was compensating with the neck hyperextended. When the neck was in the neutral or comfortable position, he had a chin-brow to vertical angle of 45 degrees. B: Lateral radiograph of lumbar spine showing the chin-brow to vertical angle superimposed with the apex at the L3-4 disc space. The amount of bone to be resected is indicated at each depth posteriorly. C: Postoperative lateral radiograph showing the angle of correction obtained after closure of the resected defect posteriorly with an opening osteoclasis at L3-4 of 48 degrees. The weight-bearing line has been shifted posterior to the osteotomy site. D: Postoperative standing lateral radiograph showing complete correction of the deformity following removal of a calculated wedge of bone based on preoperative assessment. (From Simmons EH. Surgery of the spine in ankylosing spondylitis and rheumatoid arthritis. In: Chapman MW, ed. Operative orthopaedics, vol. 3. Philadelphia: JB Lippincott, 1988:2077–2114, with permission.)

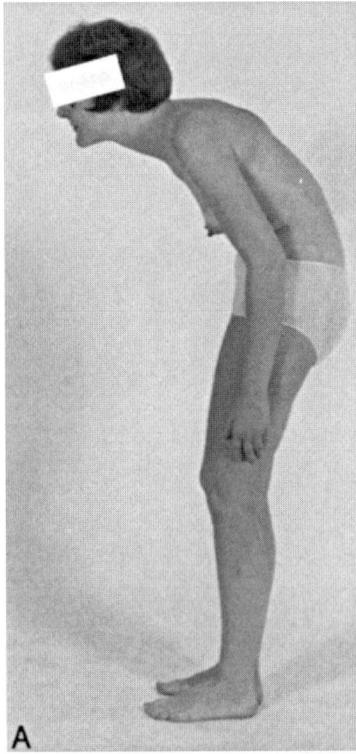

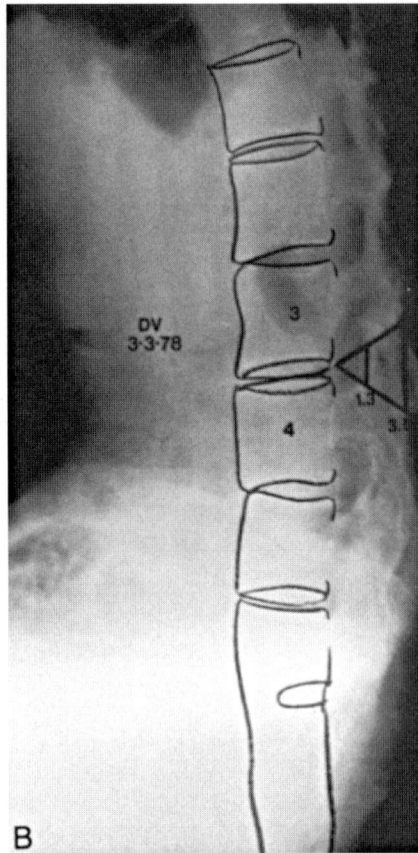

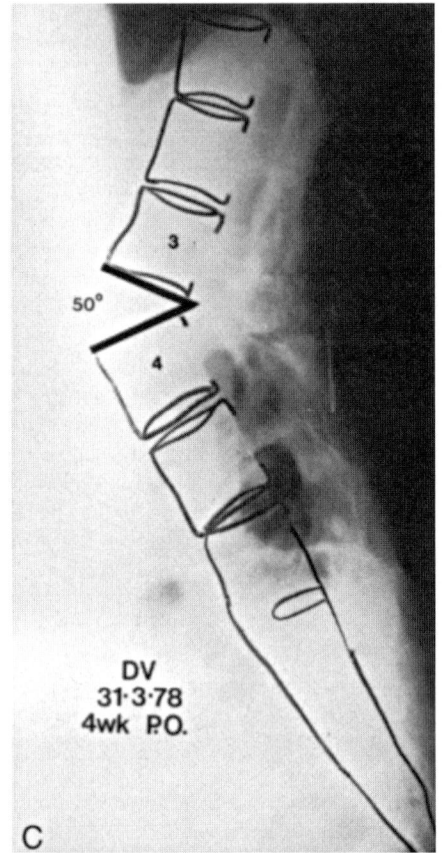

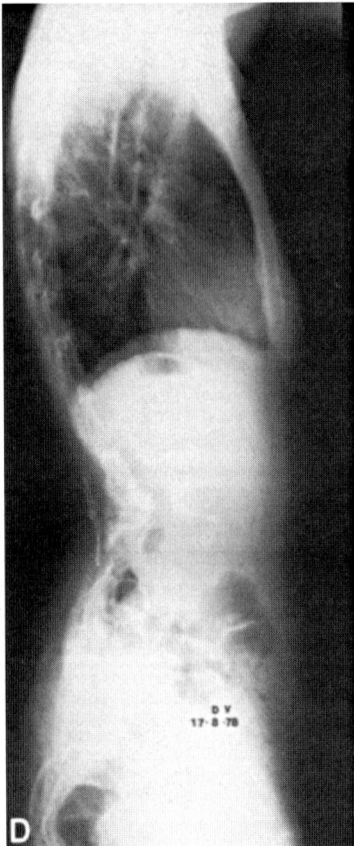

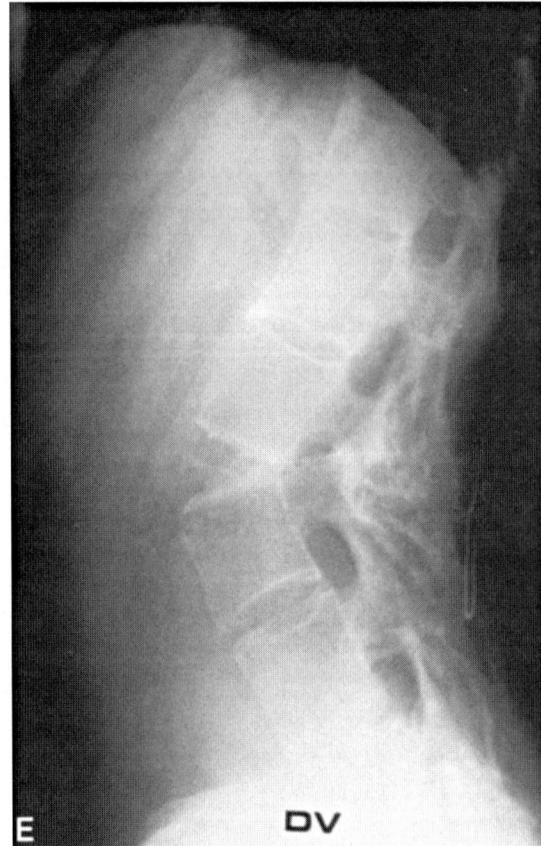

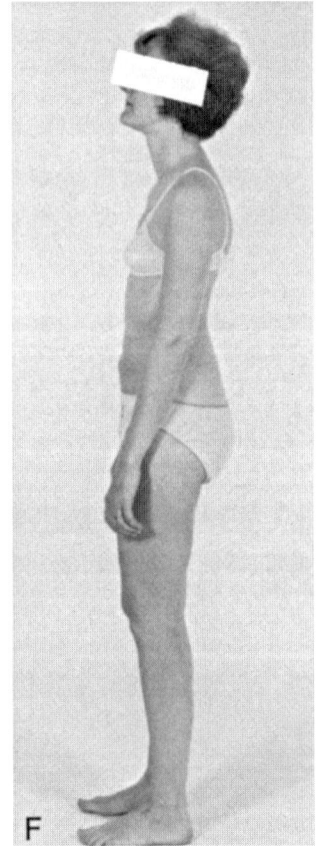

The reasons for greater vascular safety of osteotomies done at L3-4 or L4-5 are the increased mobility of the aortic bifurcation and iliac arteries related to lower limb motion, the segmental vessels of L5 arise from the internal iliac arteries, and that the segmental vessels of L5 and L4 are smaller vessels than higher-segmental arteries. The reasons for greater vascular risk of osteotomies at higher levels are that the aorta becomes less mobile proximally; the renal arteries arise at L2-3, adding to fixation of the aorta; and the segmental vessels increase in size proximally.

EARLIER TECHNIQUE

Initially the operation was done under local anesthesia. This avoided pulmonary complications and mortality related to it. It provided the best intraoperative monitoring of neurologic, vascular, and other vital functions (4,17,20,22). The results of the first 64 cases done under local anesthesia were reported by Wills in 1985 (21). Stabilization of the osteotomy when performed under local anesthesia initially was based on a V-shaped locking osteotomy with plaster shells and a turning frame for 6 to 8 weeks. Later, wire-loop fixation was applied (Fig. 77-5). A Luque rectangle was then used with Drummond buttons and wires; Cotrel–Dubousset instrumentation also was used, all possible under local anesthesia. Regardless of whether or not internal fixation and the type of fixation used, the most important factor in the successful maintenance of correction is to correct the deformity completely, shifting the weight-bearing line posterior to the osteotomy site so that gravity will maintain and tend to increase correction with stimulation of bone formation through the weight-bearing lines of the fusion masses posterolaterally. Postoperative management used well-molded posterior and anterior plaster body shells extending from head to knee in which the patient could be firmly strapped for turning onto a CircOlectric bed, later a Stryker turning frame, and finally a Roto-Rest bed (23–25).

CURRENT TECHNIQUE

Our current technique of fiberoptic intubation with the patient awake is described in the preceding. The patient is placed in the prone position on an adjusted Andrews table while awake. The patient must be carefully positioned on the operating table in a flexed knee-chest position. Careful positioning is also necessary because these patients have fixed ankylosed spines and undue pressure in any one particular area must be avoided. The thoracic chest support often must be elevated considerably to accommodate the patient on the operating table. Anesthesia is commenced when the patient is comfortable. Routine monitoring of vital signs and spinal cord monitoring are carried out throughout the procedure. A wake-up test also can be used if necessary. Pulse oximetry, CO_2 analyzer, and systemic blood gases are used to monitor the patient. A Doppler apparatus is fixed to the patient's chest to detect any possible air embolisms.

Be certain of the L3-4 level at which you are preparing to perform the osteotomy because the landmarks are obscured. Radiographic confirmation is necessary.

At this point pedicle screws are inserted in L1, L2, (L3), L5, and S1. The pedicle screws are inserted in a standard fashion, using anatomic and image-guided techniques as required. It is not usually possible to have screws in L4 because they will impinge on the L3 screws following extension correction of the spine.

I then carry out the resection. The interspinous ligaments usually are ossified and at the beginning, the osteotomy can be started with large bone cutters to trim away the intervening bone and spinous processes in a V-shaped fashion. The laminae can be thinned out with Leksell rongeurs and the bony fragments maintained for autogenous bone graft. A high-powered burr also can be used; however, if this is used exclusively, there will be less bone available for the bone grafting.

When the spinal canal is opened, the dura is carefully stripped from the bone with a seeker and protected with cottonoid patties. In many long-standing cases, the dura is quite atrophic, similar to that of long-standing spinal

FIG. 77-5. A: Standing lateral view of a female patient with gross kyphosis confined to the lumbar spine. She has no flexion deformity of the neck or thoracic spine. **B:** Lateral view of the lumbar spine showing complete loss of lumbar lordosis with kyphosis beyond the neutral. The sacrum is in a straight line with the lumbar spine. Resection-extension osteotomy of the mid-lumbar spine is ideal for this type of deformity. The amount to be resected has been indicated on the lateral radiograph with the apex at the L3-4 disc space. **C:** Postoperative lateral radiograph showing an anterior opening wedge correction of 50 degrees (following closing wedge osteotomy posteriorly). A normal lordosis has been established. **D:** Standing lateral 3-foot radiograph of the spine 6 months after surgery showing normal lordosis. The weight-bearing line is posterior to the osteotomy site. **E:** Lateral radiograph of the lumbar spine 3½ years after surgery showing solid fusion posteriorly in the weight-bearing line. Bone is slow to form anteriorly away from the area of weight bearing. **F:** Postoperative lateral view of the patient showing complete correction of deformity with the establishment of a normal lordosis and normal chin-brow to vertical angle. (From Simmons EH. Surgery of the spine in ankylosing spondylitis and rheumatoid arthritis. In: Chapman MW, ed. Operative orthopaedics, vol. 3. Philadelphia: JB Lippincott, 1988:2077–2114, with permission.)

stenosis. In rare instances, it may be adherent to the laminae, making its separation difficult. The entire L4 lamina is removed along with a portion of the L3 and L5 laminae with undercutting of the laminae to bevel them so that there is no impingement on closure of the osteotomy site. The cauda equina must be decompressed well laterally out to the level of the pedicles. The entire superior L4 facet is removed and the L3-4 neuroforamina widely exposed laterally and undercut with a medium-angle Kerrison rongeur, again so as to prevent any impingement on closure of the osteotomy site.

The precise amount of bone removed posteriorly is calculated to arrive at the amount of correction desired. On closure of the osteotomy with osteoclasis of the spine anteriorly, the lateral masses should meet with good bone surface contact. The pedicles also must be undercut, removing the superior edge of the L4 pedicle and inferior edge of the L3 pedicle again to allow adequate room for the nerve root during the extension correction of the spine.

The osteoclasis is carried out by extending the foot-end of the table, bringing the hips and thighs up into an extended position. On doing so, pressure also can be applied manually by pushing downward at the L3-4 site, causing a fulcrum for the osteoclasis to occur. An audible and palpable osteoclasis of the spinal column often is present and the lateral masses then come together in apposition. The lower extremities and hips are now kept in an extended position, preferably with the knees flexed, to avoid any tension on the sciatic nerve roots. Rods are then cut and contoured to the appropriate length and shape for each side of the spine and then fitted into the pedicle screws and secured. Posterolateral and posterior bone grafting is done using the removed morselized bone, which is usually quite generous.

A well-molded posterior plaster shell is applied extending from head to knee. The patient is strapped into the shell and transferred in the shell to a Roto-Rest bed. It is important to recognize that this is an essential part of the procedure. A modification of this technique has been provided by Simmons. Good orthotists can make a rigid plastic shell (Crystaplex) rather than plaster. It should be emphasized that this must be rigid and not flexible so that it will give the patient rigid support. Two shells allow approximation to take up any slack caused by weight loss of the patient and provide rigid mobilization for turning activities. This has worked very effectively. However, recognize that the principle is the same.

The rigid thoracic kyphosis is more prominent than the pelvis after extension osteotomy, and if the patient is lying on a flat surface, gravity tends to push to the thorax forward and allow the pelvis and lower lumbar spine to come posteriorly. If the trap door of the bed is removed for a bowel movement, the spine is unsupported. A well-contoured padded rigid posterior plaster shell provides a contoured well-fitted surface on which the rigid trunk can

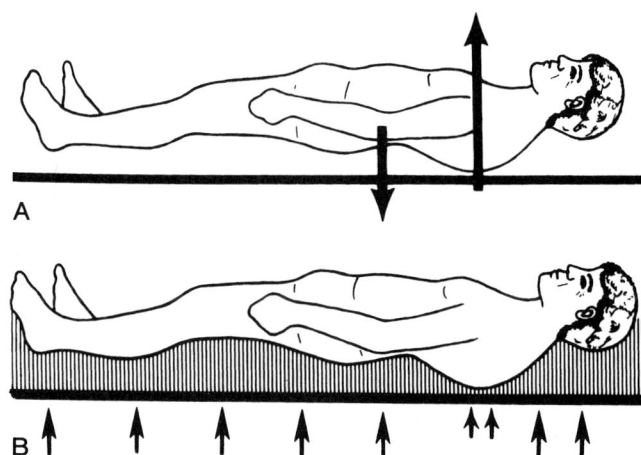

FIG. 77-6. A: Lateral diagrammatic view showing the contour of the corrected spine when lying supine unsupported. The posteriorly projecting thoracic hump bears most of the weight, with less support on the lumbar spine and the spine below the osteotomy. As a result the rigid thoracic hump tends to be displaced forward and the lumbar spine posteriorly. B: With the patient supine in a well-molded, rigid shell equal support is created throughout the spine, with elimination of any uneven contact forces that would tend toward displacement. (From Simmons EH. Surgery of the spine in ankylosing spondylitis and rheumatoid arthritis. In: Chapman MW, ed. Operative orthopaedics, vol. 3. Philadelphia: JB Lippincott, 1988:2077–2114, with permission.)

lie, protecting the osteotomy site (Fig. 77-6). A nasogastric suction tube is placed before the patient leaves the operating room. It is maintained until the patient is passing gas, with normal gastric function.

The advantages of the current technique are that it allows easier and more liberal decompression. It provides more rigid internal fixation with less risk of displacement, easier and more rapid mobilization, and probably greater comfort for the patient. Its disadvantages are increased operative time, the altered anatomy for screw insertion into the pedicles, and the potential risks of bone screws. At this time it appears that the advantages outweigh the disadvantages; to date it has provided excellent results (Fig. 77-7).

RESULTS AND COMPLICATIONS

One of the concerns that have been raised about extension osteotomy of the lumbar spine is the possibility of injury to the major vessels, particularly the abdominal aorta (14,26,27). All the reported cases of major vascular injury associated with resection-extension osteotomy of the lumbar spine for ankylosing spondylitis have been reviewed, and we documented the level at which the osteotomy was performed in each case. It is noted that in all cases with injury to the abdominal aorta the osteotomy was done at T12-L1, L1-2, or L2-3. There is no reported case of aortic injury with osteotomy performed at L3-4 or

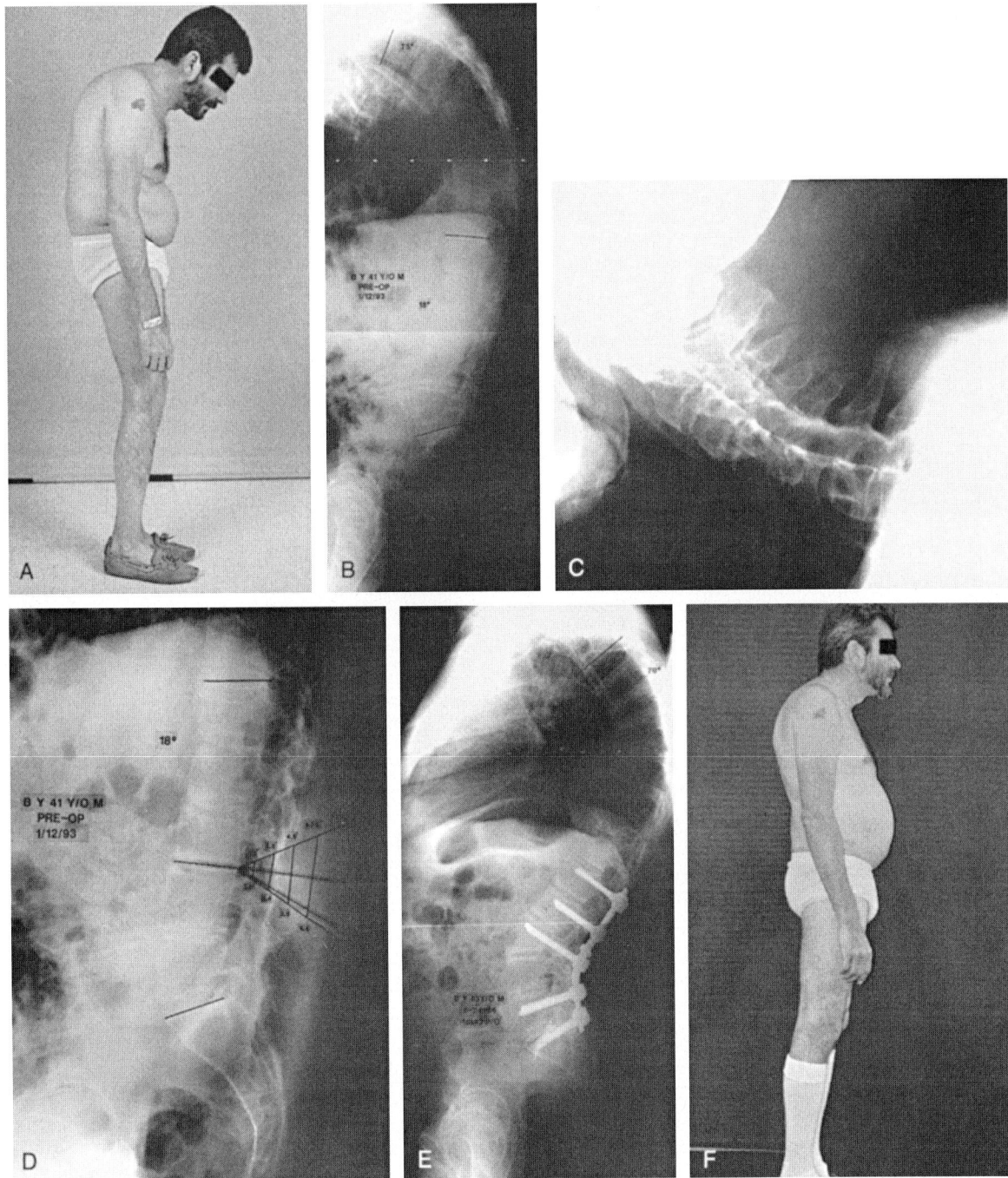

FIG. 77-7. A: Lateral view of a 41-year-old man with a 21-year history of ankylosing spondylitis. He had suffered with a major kyphotic deformity for 10 years, which prevented him from working for 5 to 6 years. His chin-brow to vertical angle measured 55 degrees. **B:** Lateral standing 3-foot film of the spine showing increased thoracic kyphosis measuring 75 degrees but decreased lumbar lordosis measuring 18 degrees. His weight-bearing line is well anterior to the mid-lumbar spine. **C:** Lateral standing radiograph of the cervical spine showing a compensatory increase in cervical lordosis with ossification from C2 distally. **D:** Preoperative lateral radiograph of the lumbar spine showing planned resection-osteotomy at L3-4 of 50 to 55 degrees. **E:** Lateral standing 3-foot radiograph 16 months postoperatively showing healed osteotomy with lumbar lordosis measuring 74 degrees. Thoracic kyphosis was corrected slightly to 70 degrees. The spine is in balance. The main weight-bearing line is posterior to the osteotomy site. **F:** Standing lateral view of the patient 16 months postoperatively. He has returned to a normal lifestyle. His correction prompted an uninformed observer to state that his wife was living with "different man." (From Simmons EH. Ankylosing spondylitis: surgical considerations. In: Herkowitz HN, Garfin SR, Balderston RA, et al, eds. Rothman-Simeone: the spine, 4th ed. Philadelphia: WB Saunders, 1999:1303–1356, with permission.)

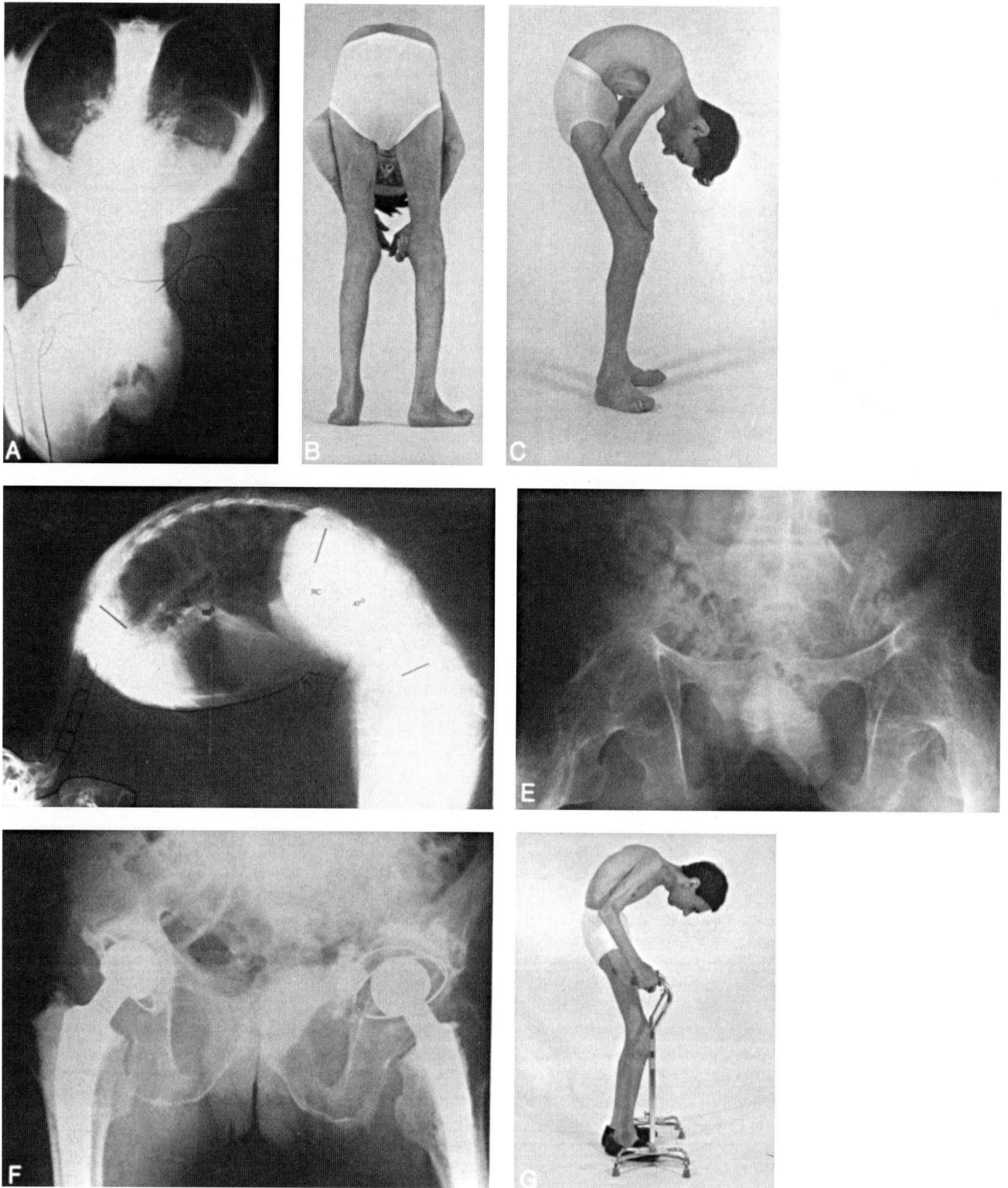

FIG. 77-8. A: Standing anteroposterior radiograph of spine of a patient with severe combined deformity. The anteroposterior film of the chest resembles a computed tomography axial view. **B:** Posterior standing view of patient. The patient could only see and moved about by walking backward. **C:** Standing lateral view showing chin-brow to vertical angle of 134 degrees. Assessment reveals combined deformities of thoracic kyphosis, gross lumbar flexion deformity, and hip flexion deformity. **D:** Standing lateral radiograph showing thoracic kyphosis of 68 degrees, complete loss of normal lordosis and 47 degrees of lumbar kyphosis, with hip flexion deformities. **E:** Antero-posterior radiograph showing fused hip joints. **F:** Postoperative view following bilateral total hip replacement arthroplasties. **G:** Standing lateral view of patient following bilateral hip arthroplasties. The deformity is improved but the patient can now see neither backward nor forward for walking.

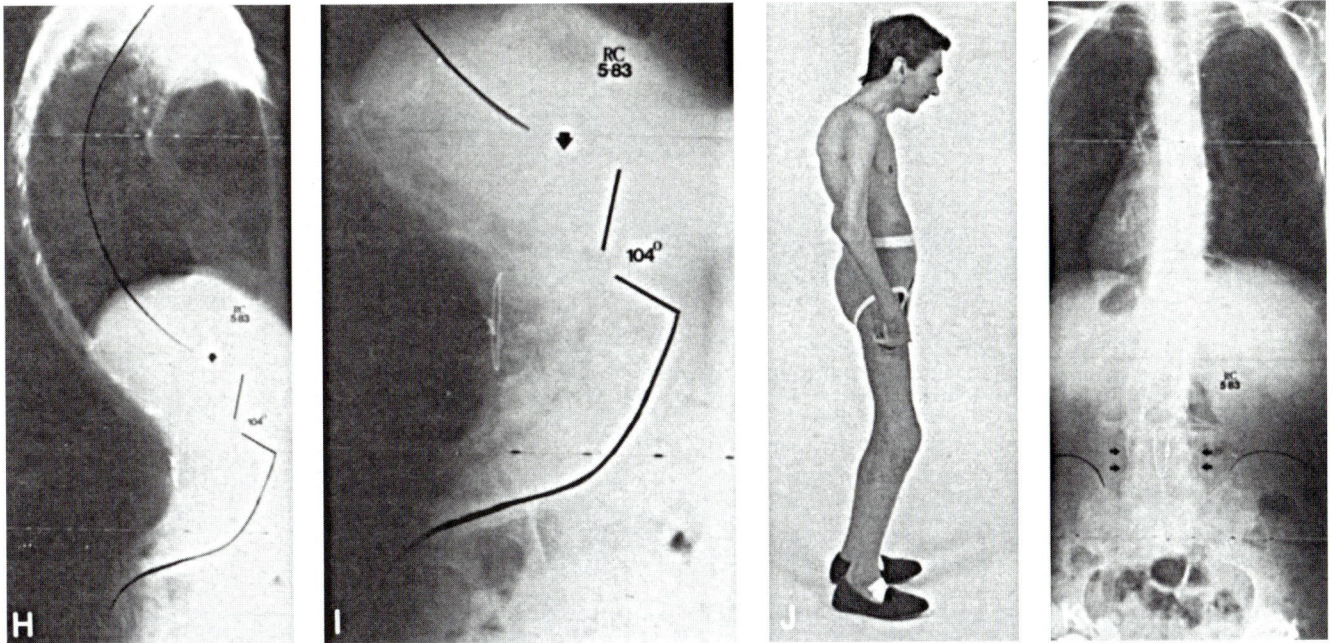

FIG. 77-8. (*Continued*) **H:** Standing lateral radiograph of spine following resection-extension osteotomy of 104 degrees done under local anesthesia. The weight-bearing line has been shifted posterior to the osteotomy site. **I:** Lateral radiograph of the lumbar spine showing osteotomy with weight-bearing line posteriorly. Patient had associated spondylodiscitis (*arrow*), which has gone on to healing. **J:** Postoperative standing lateral view of patient showing correction of major deformities. He still has some flexion deformity of the knees and neck, but is able to stand, look ahead, and walk ahead in a normal fashion. (From Simmons EH. Surgery of the spine in ankylosing spondylitis and rheumatoid arthritis. In: Chapman MW, ed. Operative orthopaedics, vol. 3. Philadelphia: JB Lippincott, 1988:2077–2114, with permission.)

L4-5. One hundred sixteen consecutive lumbar osteotomies performed by us also were reviewed. Of these, 113 were done at L3-4, two at L4-5, and only one at L2-3. There was no incidence of major arterial injury. The presence of previous radiation or atheromatous change did not result in major vessel injury. The extent of correction also was not a factor. Correction ranged from 40 to 140 degrees, with an overall average of 58 degrees (Fig. 77-8).

The only vascular injury we encountered was an inferior vena cava thrombosis extending above the renal veins. This occurred in a markedly obese male who had undergone previous extension osteotomy at L2-3 but still had major deformity. The thrombosis was likely related to the weight of his corpulent abdomen resting on his stretched vena cava after extension correction. The patient did well in the early postoperative interval, but 4 to 5 days postoperatively gradually increasing edema developed, which became massive and extended up to the mid-chest, with his scrotum "the size of a football." There was no change in arterial pulses or evidence of arterial insufficiency. Routine Doppler studies of his lower extremities did not reveal the diagnosis initially, which was established by nuclear venography. With the increased intraspinal venous pressure, neurologic deficit developed based on venous stasis of the conus, as described by Aboulker et al. (28). The neurologic deficit was maximal when the edema was greatest. Most patients with this disease are relatively thin, which is likely the reason that this has not been encountered in other cases. There was no change in arterial pulses or evidence of arterial insufficiency.

Regular potential complications can occur with any spinal procedure. Major neurologic problems are relatively infrequent; however, obviously it can be a major problem when they occur. Potential complications specific to this procedure include intestinal obstruction, problems related to instrumentation owing to osteopenia, and difficulty with surface landmarks in terms of inserting the instrumentation. Removal of too little or too much bone posteriorly can result in too little or too great a correction. Careful preoperative planning is necessary to determine the amount of correction desired and the appropriate amount of bone removed in accordance with this. Other possible complications, such as intraspinal hematoma, loss of fixation and correction, and other difficulties inherent to spinal surgery may occur. However, when the procedure is carefully planned and executed, the results are most gratifying both to the patient and the surgeon.

REFERENCES

1. Simmons ED, Simmons EH. Ankylosing spondylitis. In: Farcy JPC, ed. Complex spinal deformities. Philadelphia: Hanley & Belfus, 1994: 589–603.
2. Simmons EH. Arthritic spinal deformity: ankylosing spondylitis. In: White AH, Schofferman JA, eds. Spine care. St. Louis: Mosby, 1995: 1652–1719.
3. Simmons EH. Ankylosing spondylitis: surgical considerations. In: Herkowitz HN, Garfin SR, Balderston RA, et al, eds. Rothman-Simeone: the spine, 4th ed. Philadelphia: WB Saunders, 1999: 1303–1356.
4. Simmons EH. Ankylosing spondylitis: surgical considerations. In: Rothman RH, Simeone FA, eds. Rothman-Simeone: the spine, 3rd ed. Philadelphia: WB Saunders, 1992:1447–1511.
5. Smith-Petersen MN, Larson CB, Aufranc OE. Osteotomy of the spine for correction of flexion deformity in rheumatoid arthritis. J Bone Joint Surg 1945;27:1.
6. Herbert JJ. Vertebral osteotomy for kyphosis, especially in Marie-Strumpell arthritis: a report on 50 cases. J Bone Joint Surg 1959; 41A:291.
7. Herbert JJ. Vertebral osteotomy, technique, indications and results. J Bone Joint Surg 1948;30A:680.
8. LaChapelle EH. Osteotomy of the lumbar spine for correction of kyphosis in a case of ankylosing spondylarthritis. J Bone Joint Surg 1959;28A:270.
9. Law WA. Lumbar spinal osteotomy. J Bone Joint Surg 1959;41B:270.
10. Law WA. Osteotomy of the spine. J Bone Joint Surg 1962;44A:1199.
11. Law WA. Osteotomy of the spine. Clin Orthop 1969;66:70.
12. Nunziata A. Osteotomia de la columna: operacio de Smith-Petersen. Prensa Med Argent 1948;35:1536.
13. Wilson MJ, Turkell JH. Multiple spinal wedge osteotomy: its use in the case of Marie-Strumpell spondylitis. Am J Surg 1949;77:777.
14. Adams JC. Technique, dangers, and safeguards in osteotomy of the spine. J Bone Joint Surg 1952;34B:226–232.
15. Emneus H. Wedge osteotomy of spine in ankylosing spondylitis. Acta Orthop Scand 1968,39:321–336.
16. Kallio KE. Osteotomy of the spine in ankylosing spondylitis. Ann Chir Gynaecol 1963;52:615.
17. Simmons EH. Kyphotic deformity of the spine in ankylosing spondylitis. Clin Orthop 1977;128:65.
18. Simmons EH. Surgery of rheumatoid arthritis. Philadelphia: JB Lippincott, 1971:100–104.
19. Simmons EH. Surgery of rheumatoid arthritis. In: Cruess RL, Mitchell NS, eds. Surgery of the spine in rheumatoid arthritis and ankylosing spondylitis. Philadelphia: JB Lippincott, 1971:93–110.
20. Simmons EH. Surgery of the spine in ankylosing spondylitis and rheumatoid arthritis. In: Chapman MW, ed. Operative orthopaedics, vol. 3. Philadelphia: JB Lippincott, 1988:2077–2114.
21. Wills DG. Anesthetic management of posterior lumbar osteotomy. Can Anesth Soc J 1985;83:248–257.
22. Simmons EH. Surgery of the spine in rheumatoid arthritis and ankylosing spondylitis. In: Evarts CM, ed. Surgery of the musculoskeletal system, vol. 2. New York: Churchill Livingstone, 1983:85.
23. McKenzie KG, Dewar FP. Scoliosis with paraplegia. J Bone Joint Surg 1949;31B:162.
24. McMaster PE. Osteotomy of the spine for fixed flexion deformity. Pacific Med Surg 1965;73:314.
25. Mason C, Cozen L, Adelstein L. Surgical correction of flexion deformity of the cervical spine. Calif Med 1953;79:244.
26. Lichtblau PO, Wilson PD. Possible mechanism of aortic rupture in orthopaedic correction of rheumatoid spondylitis. J Bone Joint Surg 1956;38A:123–127.
27. Weatherley C, Jaffray D, Terry A. Vascular complications associated with osteotomy in ankylosing spondylitis: a report of two cases. Spine 1988;13:43–46.
28. Aboulker J, Aubin ML, Leriche H, et al. L'hypertension veineuse intrarachidienne par anomalies multiples du systeme cave. Acta Radiol Suppl 1975;347:395–401.

CHAPTER 78

Pyogenic and Fungal Lumbar Spine Infections

Matthew J. Geck and Frank J. Eismont

Vertebral osteomyelitis is an infection of the spine that can include the disc, bony elements, the epidural space, as well as adjacent structures. In the preantibiotic era, spine infections had uniformly high morbidity and mortality (1). Even today, paralysis and death can still be sequelae, especially in the immunocompromised patient. Diagnosis is often delayed even with current clinical vigilance and diagnostic testing. With adequate clinical suspicion, radiographic work-up, and biopsy and cultures to establish the offending organism, the vast majority of spine infections can be successfully treated with 6 or more weeks of the appropriate antibiotic. However, even with appropriate conservative therapy, there are patients who may need surgical treatment for a clinically significant abscess, open biopsy, severe deformity, neurologic deficit, and failure of conservative treatment with continued chronic infection.

PYOGENIC INFECTIONS

Incidence

Originally thought to be a rare entity, Kulowski (1) in 1936 described 102 cases, of which 60 were from his own institution, comprising approximately 4% of all the patients with musculoskeletal osteomyelitis at his home institution in the reviewed time. Nagel et al. (2) found the incidence at Yale Medical Center to be 8% of all osteomyelitis. In a review of 178 cases in the literature (3), 52% of the patients were older than age 50 (52%). Younger patients often had a history of intravenous (IV) drug use (4).

Pathogenesis

Spine infections most often are caused by hematogenous spread from another source. Risk factors include urinary tract infections or instrumentation, soft-tissue infections, respiratory tract infections, IV catheter infections, and IV drug abuse (3,4). Direct inoculation from surgical intervention also has been reported (3). However, it is notable that a source cannot be identified in 37% of cases. Other less common sources are salmonellosis (5), infectious endocarditis (6), otitis media (7), dental infections (8), surgery (9), and discograms (10,11).

Diabetes mellitus also has been thought to be a risk factor for vertebral osteomyelitis. In one review of patients with infections, patients with diabetes had twice the incidence versus historical controls (3). This may result from immunocompromise or diabetic-related vascular disease and peripheral neuropathy with associated soft-tissue ulcers and bladder dysfunction, both of which can lead to systemic bacteremia.

Human immunodeficiency virus (HIV) also has been associated with spine infections. In a review of patients with HIV from 1994 to 2000, Weinstein et al. (12) found that the incidence of spine infections in patients with HIV was 0.095% (17/17,717). This is higher than the incidence in the general population, but much less than originally suspected. The CD4 count in patients with pyogenic infections averaged 339.6, and the organism identified was *Staphylococcus aureus*. These patients responded to conservative treatment with IV antibiotics for 6 to 12 weeks. Six patients with spinal tuberculosis had a mean CD4 count of 57. One patient died and the others were treated with antituberculous medications. Three patients with epidural abscesses had a mean CD4 count of 21. Two of the patients had *Nocardia* as the organism and both died; the third patient had Group A streptococcus. Thus, patients with HIV have a higher incidence of spinal infection than the general population, and the organism and type of infection vary with the degree of immunocompromise. Identification of the organism is essential for the success of treatment of this complex patient population.

Bacteriology

Hematogenous vertebral osteomyelitis is usually a single-organism infection (13). *Staphylococcus aureus* is the most common isolate and accounts for more than 50% of isolates in most series. Gram-negative infections can be seen in elderly men who have a history of urinary tract infection, as well as in IV drug abusers. Intravenous drug users on the West Coast of the United States have a significant incidence of *Pseudomonas,* as well as the more common *Staphylococcus aureus* (4). In patients with chronic low-grade infections, thought must be given to coagulase negative *Staphylococcus, Diphtheroids, Propionibacter,* or unusual gram-negative organisms (14). Owing to their slow growing time, suspect cultures should be held for 10 days before they are discarded as negative. If a low grade pathogen grows in culture, it should not be regarded as a contaminant.

Pathophysiology

Infection by hematogenous routes typically begins in the vertebral metaphysis (15). There is a significant paravertebral venous plexus (16) as well as a rich arterial anastomosis of end arterioles within the metaphyseal region of the vertebral body (17). Both routes may play a role. Once established in the metaphysis, the infection may spread through the vasculature at the intervertebral disc periphery or more commonly rupture through the end plate into the disc and then infect the adjacent vertebral end plate and body. The disc is avascular, and once infected is rapidly broken down by bacterial enzymes and proteolytic enzymes from inflammatory cells. Untreated pyogenic infections often progress to abscess formation, into either the spinal canal as epidural abscesses (18) or the adjacent soft-tissue structures. Very often this develops into a psoas abscess in the lumbar spine.

Clinical Presentation

The clinical presentation of vertebral osteomyelitis is dependent on the virulence of the organism involved, as well as various patient factors such as immunocompromise, age, general health, and nutrition. Fulminant presentation with subsequent high mortality is relatively uncommon today with antibiotics, diagnostic imaging, biopsy, and surgical care. However, this presentation is still often seen in the severely immunocompromised patient with a virulent organism. Very often these patients present with some degree of paralysis.

The most common complaint is localized spine pain, which occurs in about 90% of patients (3). This can be associated with tenderness and muscle spasm. Fever, defined as a temperature of greater than 100°, was present only 50% of the time. Symptom duration varied widely, with 20% less than 3 weeks, 30% 3 weeks to 3

months, and 50% with symptoms of more than 3 months' duration on presentation. The lumbar spine is the most common location of the infection (48%), followed by the thoracic spine (35%), cervical spine (6.5%), and thoracolumbar and lumbosacral junctions account for the rest. Noncontiguous infection occurs in 4% to 5% of patients (11).

Occult infections with low virulence organisms are even more difficult to properly diagnose (14). In one series of nine patients with chronic low-grade back pain (14), fever was present in only four patients, the sedimentation rate was normal in seven, and the white blood cell count (WBC) was normal in six. The average duration of symptoms was 9.5 months in this group before a diagnosis was made. The diagnosis was made by biopsy. Theses cases demonstrate that a normal erythrocyte sedimentation rate (ESR) and a normal WBC do not rule out infection. Only by combining clinical suspicion with history, evaluation of risk factors, and radiographic findings, as well as laboratory work-up and biopsy, can the proper diagnosis be made.

Eismont and colleagues (11) evaluated patients with vertebral osteomyelitis with paralysis, and compared them with a group of patients who were evaluated and treated in the same period in the same city, but who did not have paralysis. Factors predisposing to paralysis were older age, more cephalad level of infection, diabetes mellitus, rheumatoid arthritis, and steroid use. Youth seemed protective; the younger IV drug abusers were spared paralysis. Microbiologically, *Staphylococcus aureus* was the causative organism in the vast majority of the patients with severe paralysis.

Vertebral osteomyelitis in infants is different from pediatric discitis. In a report of four patients (19), infants 2 to 13 weeks old were treated for vertebral osteomyelitis. All four had severe dissolution of the vertebral bodies, with end plates of the adjacent vertebrae being normal or near normal, suggesting that the origin of the infection was in the vertebrae rather than the discs. The patients were uniformly systemically ill and had no neurologic deficits, and three of the four patients had septicemia from *Staphylococcus aureus*. Three patients who had short courses of antibiotics (2 weeks or less) relapsed, necessitating longer courses. The late radiographic appearance of these patients was similar to congenital kyphosis, and we recommended early bracing with posterior fusion if progression occurred.

The presence of a tumor does not eliminate the possibility of infection. Eismont and colleagues (20) reported three cases of metastatic tumors to the spine with an infection existing concurrently, with no clinical evidence to suggest infection. This was attributed to vascularity of the tumor, seeding of the necrotic portion of the tumor, and immunosuppression. Biopsy and culture should be performed in known metastatic disease if there is anything atypical on presentation (e.g., leukocytosis, fever, sepsis, or atypical radiographic appearance). All biopsies should be sent for both culture and pathology.

Intravenous drug abusers are a subset of patients who often develop vertebral osteomyelitis. In a case report and review of the literature, Sapico and Montgomerie (4) reviewed 67 IV drug users who had vertebral osteomyelitis and noted that these patients tended to be younger (89% were 20 to 49 years old) than pyogenic infections from other sources (52% > 50) (3). One other major difference is that gram-negative rods comprised 82.5% of isolates, with *Pseudomonas* species most common followed by *Serratia, Klebsiella,* and *Enterobacter.* No patient had a permanent paralysis.

Diagnosis

Laboratory Studies

The initial work-up of vertebral osteomyelitis includes a complete blood count, differential, and other general laboratory studies. However, ESR is the only laboratory test of diagnostic value other than biopsy and culture. In two reviews of the literature (3,4) the ESR was elevated about 90% of the time in patients with biopsy-confirmed vertebral osteomyelitis on initial presentation. However, the ESR is not sensitive and only moderately specific; low-grade infections can have normal values (14).

The ESR is useful in assessing the response to treatment (4,21). In one series, the sedimentation rate was down to two thirds the presentation value at the time of successful completion of the parenteral therapy, and in most of these patients it fell to half (3). In another series, it fell to normal after the disease was fully treated (21).

For the biopsy and culture, it is important to hold the specimen a full 10 days, to allow low-grade infections to grow out in the culture media (14).

Imaging Evaluation

Plain radiographs are negative early in the disease process, with characteristic changes not evident for 2 to 4 weeks (11,22). Narrowing of the disc space is evident in 74% of patient at presentation (3), and as the disease progresses, there are additional destructive changes evident on both sides of the disc space with erosion of the end plates (Fig. 78-1). In late stages, there is destruction of the vertebral bodies on either side of the infected disc. Gas in the disc space may be indicative of a gas-forming organism (23). In a blinded study, plain radiographs were found to have a sensitivity of 82%, specificity of 57%, and accuracy of 73% (24).

Even with treatment, radiographic findings continue to lag up to 3 months behind the clinical picture (15). Patients often develop reactive bone formation, sclerosis, and progressive disc space narrowing. Spontaneous fusion may occur in up to 50% of patients, usually in those with the most severe degrees of destruction. This fusion may take up to 5 years to consolidate (25,26).

Computed tomography (CT) scans are the best for demonstrating bony detail and erosion. Lytic areas, paraspinous soft-tissue masses, local tissue swelling, and gas formation all can be evident. Significant prevertebral soft-tissue swelling can help differentiate an infection from a tumor, because tumors usually demonstrate little or no prevertebral soft-tissue swelling (27). Computed tomography can be a valuable adjunct for biopsy localization, and myelography combined with post-myelography CT can be useful to evaluate neural compression in indicated cases.

Radionuclide studies are a useful adjunct in patients in whom magnetic resonance imaging (MRI) is contraindicated or a multifocal process is in the differential. These changes are thought to be present earlier than radiographic presentation with an animal model study of technetium scanning showing 71% positive results in 15 days and a near absolute true-positive rate over time (28). In a blinded study of 23 patients suspected of having vertebral osteomyelitis, [99m]technetium HDP bone scanning was found to have 90% sensitivity and 78% specificity (24). Combined with gallium-67 scanning, there was a sensitivity of 90%, specificity of 100%, and accuracy of 94%. The accuracy was not superior to MRI (24). False-negative rates have been reported for technetium scanning in infants and elderly people because of regional ischemia to the area (29). There can be a very high false-negative rate of radionuclide scanning in low-grade infections (14). Single photon emission computed tomography scanning and [111]indium leukocyte imaging are other radionuclide modalities that can be helpful.

Magnetic resonance imaging is considered the ideal imaging study for infections. It has multiplanar imaging capability, visualization of all compartments in and around the spine, and provides direct imaging of the disc, spinal cord, and nerve roots. Its exquisite sensitivity to changes in water content in structures makes it ideal for evaluating the vascular and edema characteristics in and around a spine infection (30). Increased water is demonstrated on MR images by areas of low signal on T1-weighted images and high signal on T2-weighted images. The addition of gadolinium-diethylenetriamine penta-acetic acid (Gd-DTPA) IV contrast enables MR imaging to detect active viable inflammatory tissue such as infected discs (31). Currently we recommend gadolinium contrast when MRI is being done for any patient for whom infection is in the differential diagnosis. In a blinded study of 37 patients, MRI was found to have a sensitivity of 96%, a specificity of 92%, and an accuracy of 94%, making it at least as accurate as combined technetium and gallium scanning.

The characteristic findings on MRI of a disc space infection are decreased signal of the vertebral bodies and the intervertebral disc on T1-weighted imaging, and sig-

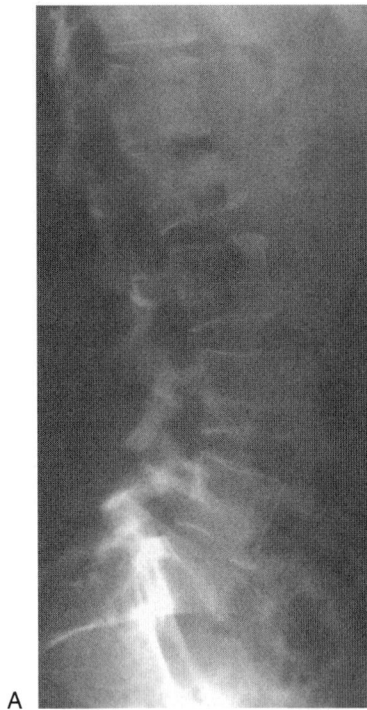

A

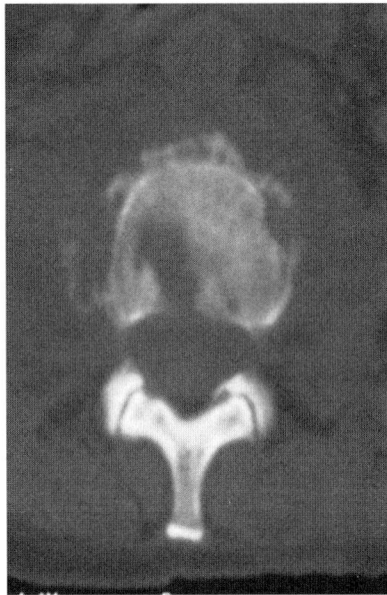

B

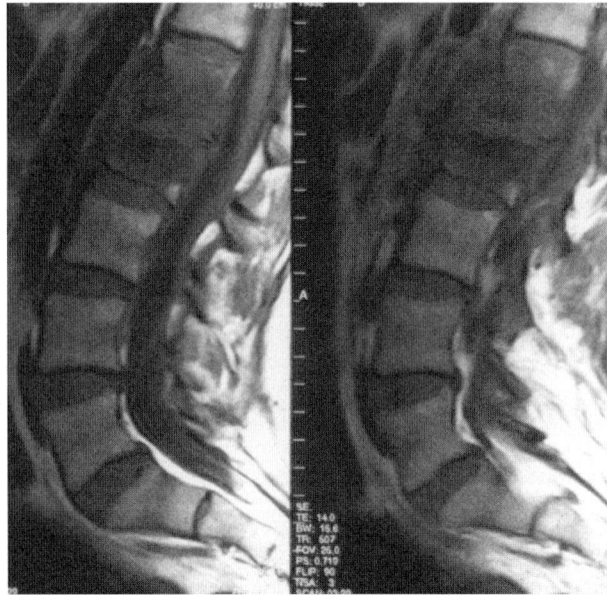

C

FIG. 78-1. This 55-year-old woman with chronic liver disease from alcohol abuse presented with complaints of 8 weeks of low back pain. **A:** Plain radiographs showed narrowing of the disc space with erosion of the end plates on both sides of the L1-2 disc space. **B:** Computed tomography scan showed end plate erosion, sclerosis, and some prevertebral soft-tissue swelling. **C:** T1-weighted magnetic resonance imaging shows decreased signal of the vertebral bodies and the intervertebral disc. **D:** T2-weighted imaging shows loss of the internuclear cleft.

nal intensity of the same bodies and disc on T2-weighted imaging with loss of the intranuclear disc cleft. Gadolinium contrast results in enhancement of both the adjacent vertebral bodies and the involved disc on T1-weighted imaging, with any sequestered abscesses spared from the enhancement (30,31).

Disadvantages of MRI include access, artifact from spinal instrumentation, poor resolution in patients who move during the scan, and contraindications such as pacemakers, aneurysm clips, metallic fragments in the eye or spinal cord, and severe claustrophobia.

Biopsy Techniques

Despite the excellent characteristics of the current imaging studies, especially MRI, definitive diagnosis and treatment require either microscopic or bacteriologic confirmation by biopsy. The only case in which biopsy can be avoided is in the patient with clear radiographic and clinical signs of spondylitis and positive blood cultures (15). However, blood cultures are positive in only 25% of patients with vertebral osteomyelitis (3).

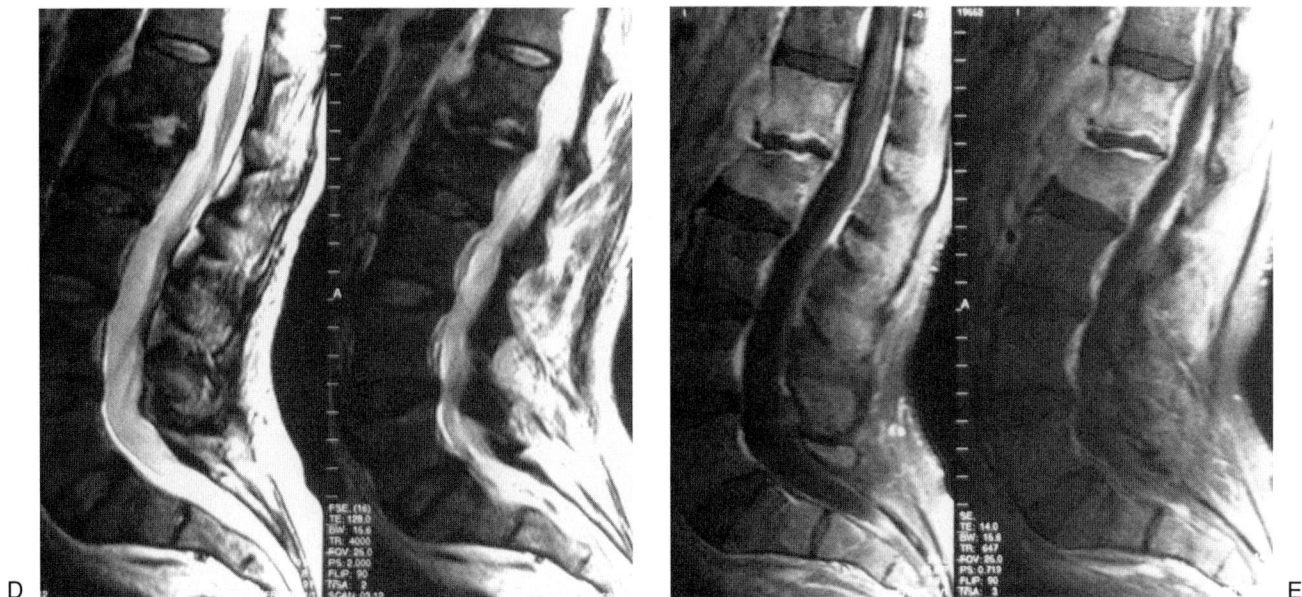

FIG. 78-1. (*Continued*). **D:** T2-weighted imaging shows loss of the internuclear cleft. **E:** Addition of gadolinium contrast to a fat/saturation image again showed the increased uptake in the adjoining vertebral bodies. Computed tomography–guided biopsy grew a pan-sensitive *Staphylococcus aureus* that was treated conservatively with a 6-week course of antibiotics. The sedimentation rate dropped to half. Clinical follow-up showed no recurrence of infection.

Percutaneous closed biopsy techniques are safe (32) and their use is widespread. Fluoroscopic or CT guidance is routine. Craig needle biopsy instrumentation is preferred because of the larger sample size and bone coring capacity (15). Diagnostic yield varies but was 70% in a review of the literature (3). Needle biopsy is possible in all areas of the spine, but open biopsy may be preferable in the cervical spine and occasionally in the thoracic spine for reasons of safety, access, and risk of paralysis. Even after a negative first closed biopsy, it is recommended that a second closed biopsy be obtained. This second biopsy often is positive when the first was negative. This is advisable only if it is medically safe to continue to withhold antibiotics.

Indications for open biopsy include failed or nondiagnostic initial closed biopsy, unsafe closed biopsy, or need for concurrent surgical treatment and débridement. Similarly, an open biopsy is recommended if the first closed biopsy is negative and antibiotics can no longer be withheld. The advantage of an open biopsy is primarily that this allows a larger sample and has a lower false-negative rate. In one compilation of the literature, open biopsy had a false-negative rate of 14% compared with 30% for closed biopsies (3). Failure of closed biopsy often results from empiric treatment with antibiotics without a full or proper work-up.

Nonoperative Management

Historically, mortality has ranged from 25% to 70% for pyogenic infections of the spine (1,33). In one early series

of 102 cases, mortality was 25%, with an increase in mortality to 50% with the additional onset of central nervous system involvement such as neural compression, meningitis, subdural purulence, or infarction of the cord (1). However, morbidity and mortality can be controlled, mortality of the disease reduced to less than 5%, and residual neurologic deficits reduced to less than 7% with modern management, including full medical work-up, modern antibiotics, reversal of metabolic defects and hypoxia, improved control of systemic illnesses such as diabetes mellitus, and source and alternate foci control (3). One key issue is the withholding of antibiotics until an organism is identified. If the patient has severe sepsis, maximal broad-spectrum antibiotic therapy should be instituted once an adequate biopsy has been performed. If there is vertebral osteomyelitis but a negative open biopsy, then a full course of this broad-spectrum therapy must be given for 6 to 8 weeks.

Antibiotic choice for spine infections is paramount. The antibiotic must be specific for the organism diagnosed, and the least toxic agent should be used. Some studies show that bone penetration for normal and osteomyelitic bone is equal to serum concentration for such large molecules as cephalosporins. However, for disc tissue and abscesses, penetration may be more class dependent (34–39). Vancomycin, teicoplanin, gentamicin, tobramycin, and clindamycin penetrate the nucleus pulposus with adequate concentrations (34,35,39). Cephalosporins and penicillins are less reliable with regard to penetration (35,37,39) and are even lower with increased serum binding (38). In general, antibiotics with a positive charge and smaller size have a better chance of penetrating the intervertebral disc (40).

At least 6 weeks of IV antibiotic therapy has been the mainstay of conservative treatment of spine infections (11). Four weeks of IV therapy followed by 2 weeks of an appropriate oral antibiotic may be sufficient as well (25,41). However, with regimens of less than 4 weeks, the relapse rate goes up to 25% (3).

Progress of therapy should be monitored with clinical signs, physical examination, and laboratory data. Patients with signs of sepsis, continued unrelenting pain, or laboratory values that remain elevated warrant further evaluation of the progress of treatment. The sedimentation rate should be a useful guide; in one review of the literature it decreased to two thirds of the presentation value in all patients and to less than one half the presentation value in over one half of the patients at the completion of 6 weeks of therapy (3). At final follow-up, patients with successful therapy should have a normalized sedimentation rate (21). Appropriate antibiotic therapy was noted to relieve severe pain within a few days. Bracing is recommended to control pain and prevent progression of deformity, which may otherwise be a sequela of infection (25).

Operative Management

Most pyogenic spine infections can be managed nonoperatively with an adequate trial of specific IV antibiotics that target the causative organism. Indications for operative management include multiple negative closed biopsies; location of infection that precludes a safe closed biopsy; clinically significant abscess with spiking temperatures and a septic clinical picture; severe deformity (Fig. 78-2), body destruction, or failure of conservative management with elevated sedimentation rate; radiographic progression; and continued severe pain. The final indication is neurologic deficit with neural compression.

Historically, the decompressive operation of choice was laminectomy; however, early on it was thought to be deleterious to neural recovery in infection, prompting Seddon to state, "The operation may be of some value in certain rare forms of paraplegia, but as a routine procedure it is to be condemned." This was chiefly because of approaching an anterior disease from a posterior approach and removing the one part of the spine that is usually still intact in case of spine infection. Seddon noted a transient improvement of the clinical picture, probably because of posterior cord displacement. However, residual pressure of the anterior infection compressing the spinal cord combined with increasing instability often leads to later neurologic deterioration (42). Problems with postoperative instability and deformity have plagued the modern series of this approach to a pyogenic spine infection (11,43), especially in the cervical and thoracic spine.

Posterior laminectomy with *in situ* fusion following a thorough débridement of the disc infection, however, is a reasonable option below the level of the conus medullaris. This is with the prerequisite that there is minimal anterior body destruction and collapse and that adequate decompression can be obtained using this approach. This is effective in the lordotic lumbar spine so long as the facets are preserved. The *in situ* transverse process fusion is added to prevent unstable spondylolisthesis and foraminal narrowing that may occur with collapse. This approach is often best in patents who are medically ill and in those high-risk patients in whom a small procedure is ideal.

The majority of the time infections should be approached anteriorly. The anterior approach provides

FIG. 78-2. This 29-year-old intravenous (IV) drug user presented with complaints of axial low back pain. **A:** Initial plain radiographs showed disc space height loss with mild end plate erosion. **B:** Magnetic resonance imaging confirmed the diagnosis with gadolinium uptake in the adjoining vertebral bodies and an obvious L2-3 disc space infection. Computed tomography–guided biopsy confirmed infection of the disc space with *Staphylococcus aureus* sensitive to fluoroquinolones. The patient was discharged with a 30-day supply of medication despite leaving against medical advice. She lost the medications and never followed up in the clinic. She presented 2 months later, again complaining of severe low back pain with no neurologic symptoms, a normal examination, and normal urologic function. **C:** Plain films taken at that time show severe osteomyelitis of the L2 and L3 vertebral bodies with erosion and marked kyphosis. **D:** Magnetic resonance imaging confirmed compression of the neural elements and spread of the infection. She was brought to the operating room for urgent initial anterior débridement with subtotal carpectomies of L2 and L3, decompression of the infection out of the spinal canal, and placement of a structural autogenous iliac crest bone graft. Intraoperative cultures grew out *Staphylococcus aureus* yet again. Postoperatively she was placed on IV vancomycin. **E,F:** She was brought back a few days later for pedicle screw instrumentation and osteotomy to correct the kyphosis and stabilize the anterior graft. **G:** Computed tomography scan confirmed that the graft was in a good position. The patient was kept in the hospital for a full course of IV vancomycin, her sedimentation rate normalized, and she was discharged on Bactrim.

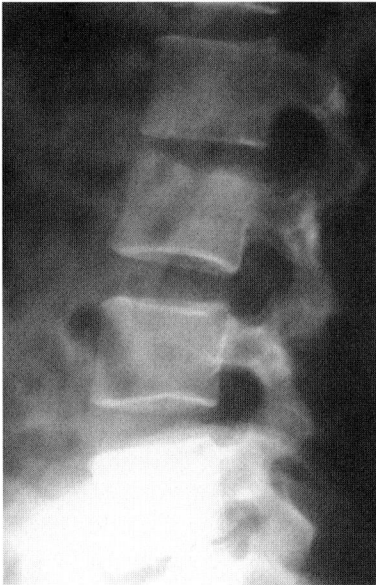

A

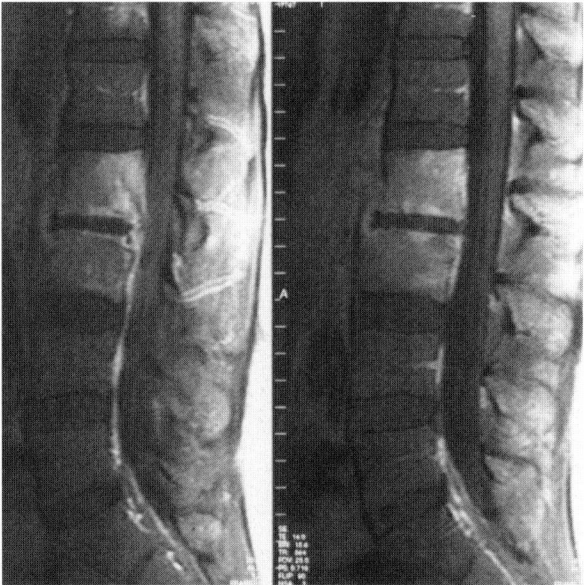

B

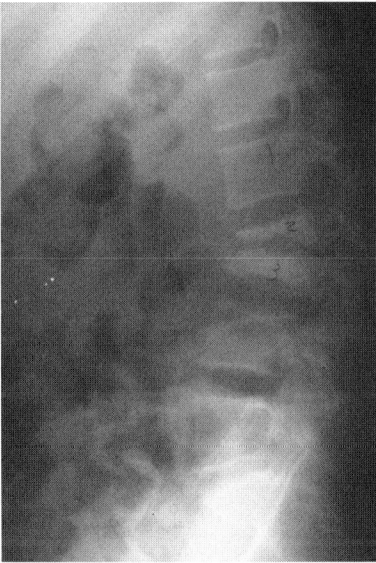

C

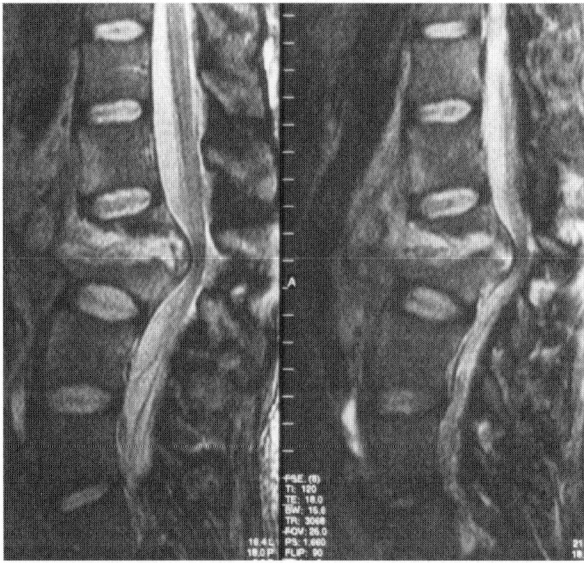

D

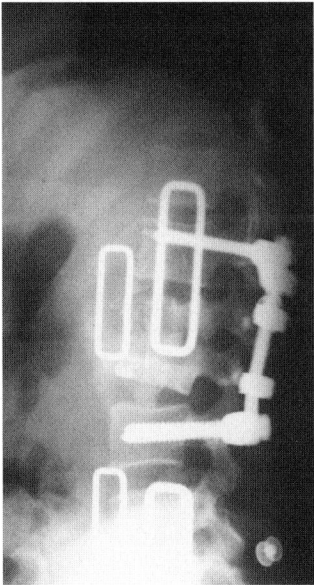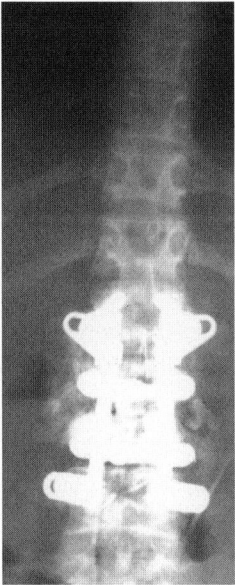

E,F

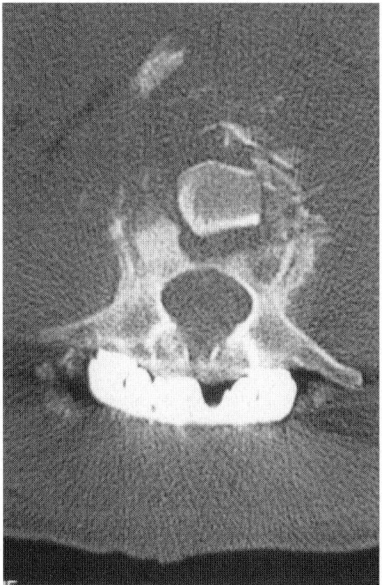

G

direct access to the infection without neural retraction; the disc space can be grafted acutely with a very high fusion rate (96%) in order to prevent collapse (44). The anterior graft heals rapidly, which facilitates rehabilitation (3,11,45,46).

In terms of technique for the anterior approach, great care must be taken with the anterior vascular structures, especially in the lower lumbar spine because these may be adherent and friable from the adjoining infection. The surgeon can check for abscess extension on the contralateral aspect of the affected vertebral bodies and explore the psoas muscle. Reconstruction with autograft iliac bone is the gold standard (44,46); however, a rib is suitable if there is no kyphosis and minimal body destruction, although it lacks the structural integrity of tricortical iliac grafts.

The use of autograft has been established as the gold standard in the literature for spine infections (44,47,48) treated with a single-stage procedure. Posterior instrumentation has been noted to be an adjunct that can be safely used (49). Single-stage anterior instrumentation has been associated with persistent infection as well as instrumentation failure from poor fixation (49). The use of cages has been advocated as well as an anterior graft in conjunction with posterior instrumentation (49) despite evidence in their series of a high rate of persistent infection in patients with anterior instrumentation or cages. In addition, cages have been associated with persistent infection requiring explantation and revision two body carpectomies with a long antero-posterior reconstruction in at least one instance (50). In the cervical spine, anterior instrumentation combined with autogenous iliac bone grafting has been very successful in treating infection.

Surgery for Paralysis

Eismont and colleagues (11) evaluated patients with vertebral osteomyelitis with paralysis and compared them with a group of patients who did not have paralysis but who were evaluated and treated in the same period in the same city. Factors predisposing to paralysis were older age, more cephalad level, diabetes mellitus, and rheumatoid arthritis with concurrent steroid use. Youth seemed protective, with the younger IV drug abusers being spared paralysis. Microbiologically, *Staphylococcus aureus* was the causative organism in the vast majority of the patients with severe paralysis.

Patients with cervical or thoracic infections had better neurologic recovery with surgery than patients treated nonoperatively. Patients treated with a laminectomy either worsened or failed to improve neurologically. Patients treated with anterior decompressions and fusions tended to improve neurologically. However, at the root level in the lumbar spine, patients had similar rates of recovery with operative and nonoperative treatment. Similarly, there was no difference in neurologic recovery in the lumbar spine between patients treated with anterior and posterior operations, except for one patient in whom paralysis failed to improve following a wide laminectomy and subsequent spondylolisthesis (11).

Prognosis

The prognosis is good in the era of modern antibiotics, with mortality less than 5% (15). There is increased morbidity and mortality in patients with systemic diseases such as diabetes and rheumatoid arthritis (15,22). In terms of deformity, there is a risk of progression (25), especially in patients with significant kyphosis on presentation (51). Paralysis is a significant source of morbidity (11), but with proper treatment, less than 7% of patients have a permanent neurologic deficit (3).

EPIDURAL ABSCESS

Spinal epidural abscess is a clinical entity that requires rapid diagnosis and treatment with appropriate antibiotics and usually surgery to minimize the significant morbidity and especially the paralysis that often occurs because of this type of infection. The incidence of epidural abscess is .2 to 1.2 cases per 10,000 hospital admissions (18). It generally is a disease of adults (52), with an equal male to female ratio, and may a higher incidence associated with invasive procedures, IV drug abuse, and elderly patients (52). Other risk factors are diabetes mellitus, trauma, and alcoholism (53).

The source of infection can be identified in 70% to 80% of cases (18,52). The route of infection can be hematogenous (Fig. 78-3), contiguous, or by inoculation (as in a procedure or surgery). Hematogenous infection can come from skin and soft-tissue infections, respiratory tract infections, and urinary tract infections (52). Most commonly, a bacteremia seeds the epidural space, which contains fatty tissue and a rich venous plexus (18). The most common location for a spinal epidural abscess is in the posterior spinal canal (79%). The majority of the anterior epidural abscesses are from direct spread from an anterior osteomyelitis. Fourteen percent of these epidural abscesses occur in the cervical spine, 51% in the thoracic spine, and 35% in the lumbar spine. The epidural infection leads to a mass effect from the granulation tissue or pus, which produces neural element compression and paralysis. In severe paralysis owing to infection, there can be secondary subarachnoid vascular injury and thrombosis (18).

The range of organisms mirrors vertebral osteomyelitis, with *Staphylococcus aureus* responsible for

62% of the infections. Aerobic gram-negative rods are isolated in 18%, aerobic streptococci in 8%, coagulase-negative staphylococcus in 2%, anaerobes in 2%, and no organism isolated in 6% (52). A large proportion can have positive blood culture (69%) (52).

The clinical course can be acute or chronic. For an acute epidural abscess the clinical picture has been described in four phases (54): spinal ache, root pain, weakness including bowel and bladder dysfunction, and paralysis. The spinal ache usually is localized to the level of the affected spine and can bring the patient to the physician quickly. In the next few days, the patient can then get root pains radiating from the localized painful area. Fever and leukocytosis usually are present, as is an elevated sedimentation rate (18). Signs and symptoms of neurologic involvement are consistent with the level of the spine infection. Chronic infection differs in that these events occur over weeks or months, and the signs and symptoms of concurrent sepsis usually are absent. However, rapid neurologic deterioration can still be a hallmark of a chronic epidural abscess despite the initially slow course and can be the presenting feature in chronic epidural abscess (18). The differential diagnosis includes meningitis, spinal subdural abscess, acute transverse myelitis, disc herniation, vascular lesion, and tumors in the spinal canal.

Diagnosis begins with a detailed clinical history and physical examination. The majority of acute epidural abscess patients present with septicemia, with a mean peripheral WBC of about 16,000 (18,53). Chronic infections can have a normal peripheral WBC (18). The sedimentation rate is almost always elevated above 25 mm (89%), whether the infection is acute or chronic (52). Radiographs are usually normal unless there is evidence of a contributing or concurrent disc space infection. Myelography, now combined with CT, was once the diagnostic imaging modality of choice to document the neural compression. If pus was aspirated in the epidural space before the intradural space was entered, a diagnosis was established with gram stain and culture. However, this test carried the risk of converting the epidural abscess into an intradural infection, and is no longer recommended (53). Radionuclide studies are not appropriate because they are nonspecific with a false-negative rate for epidural abscess, and are time-consuming (54). Magnetic resonance imaging is the study of choice with gadolinium contrast, allowing the differentiation of the epidural abscess from adjacent compressed thecal sac that previously was not possible with noncontrast MRI (30,31).

The presence of an epidural abscess is generally regarded as a surgical emergency, especially in the presence of any neurologic deficit. Even if the patient initially has intact motor strength, the presence of root symptoms or early urine retention is a sign of possible impending neurologic collapse (Fig. 78-3). The goals of treatment are to preserve neurologic function, eliminate infection, relieve pain, diagnose the pathogen, and stabilize the spine if necessary.

The surgical approach is dictated by abscess location and extent. Because epidural abscesses are generally posterior and can range over many levels, surgical drainage generally is performed with a laminectomy. Care is taken to preserve the facet joints for postoperative stability (18,54). In cases with an anterior abscess with concurrent vertebral osteomyelitis, anterior decompression and grafting usually are indicated for complete débridement and may require supplemental posterior laminectomy to decompress proximal and distal abscess extensions. The wounds may be closed over drains or be packed open in instances of severe tissue necrosis (52).

Antibiotic therapy should be started once an adequate spine culture has been performed and gram stain obtained. Broad-spectrum antibiotics should be administered until identification and sensitivities are available. Most authors recommend 3 to 4 weeks of parenteral therapy (18), with therapy extending to 6 to 8 weeks in the presence of a concurrent vertebral osteomyelitis.

There are small series documenting the treatment of epidural abscesses with antibiotics alone (52,55,56). The majority of these patients were neurologically intact with no signs of sepsis. However, numerous other references report neurologic progression and even cord infarction under these same circumstances (18,52–54,57). Combined surgical decompression with appropriate antibiotic treatment remains the standard of care. Indications for initial nonoperative management include poor surgical candidates, diffuse involvement of the spinal canal, no neurologic deficit, and complete neurologic deficit for more than 3 days (55,56). Patients deteriorating neurologically should undergo surgical decompression.

With the advent of the modern antibiotic era and the facility in diagnosing spinal epidural abscess with MRI, the mortality of spinal epidural abscess has dropped from nearly universal at the turn of the 20th century, to 34% from 1954 to 1960, to 15% from 1991 to 1997 in one review of the literature (53). In regard to paralysis, Currier (58) noted in another review of the literature that 38% had full recovery, 29% had some weakness, 21% had paralysis, and 12% died. Neurologic recovery is directly related to the time and severity of the paralysis (52–54). Recovery is observed in most patients presenting with minimal paralysis or significant paresis of less than 36 hours (54). No recovery has been observed with complete paralysis of more than 36 to 48 hours (54,59). Acute onset with paralysis within 12 hours carries a poor prognosis because cord infarction may be the mechanism of paralysis as opposed to simply mechanical compression (57).

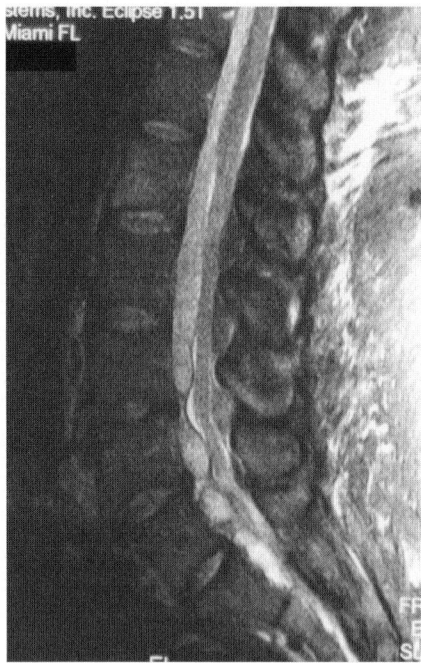

A

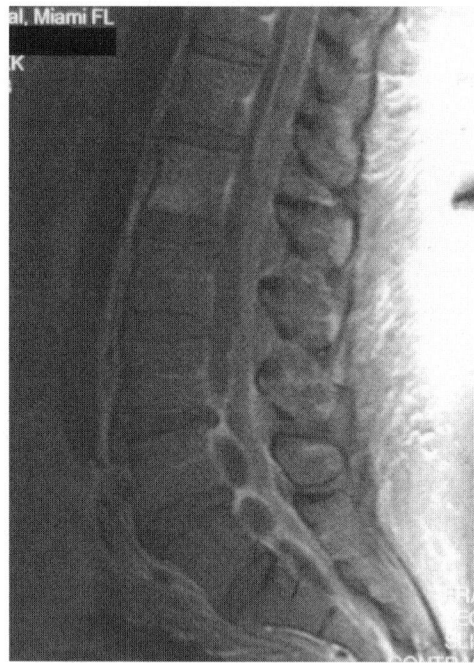

B

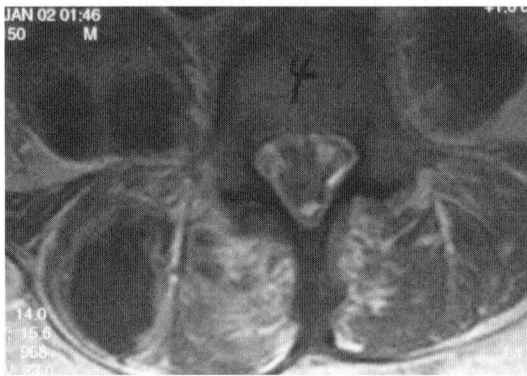

C

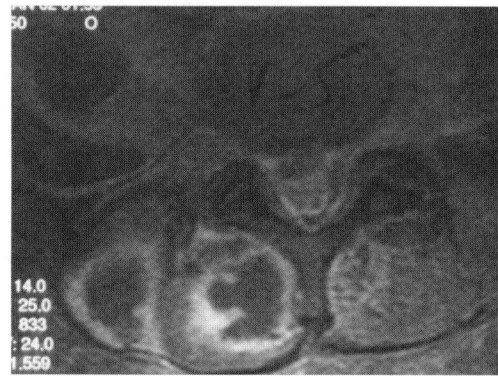

D

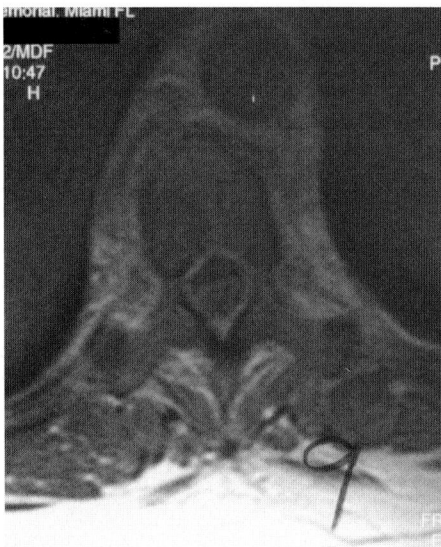

E

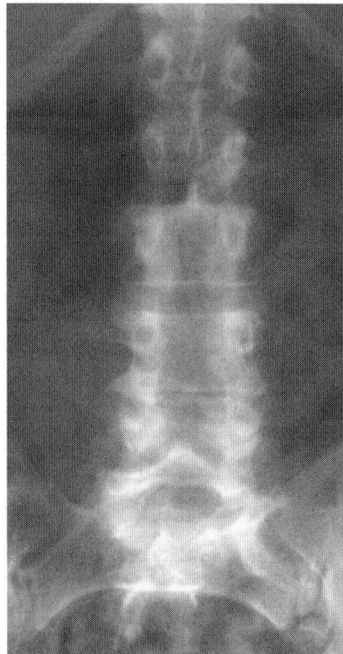

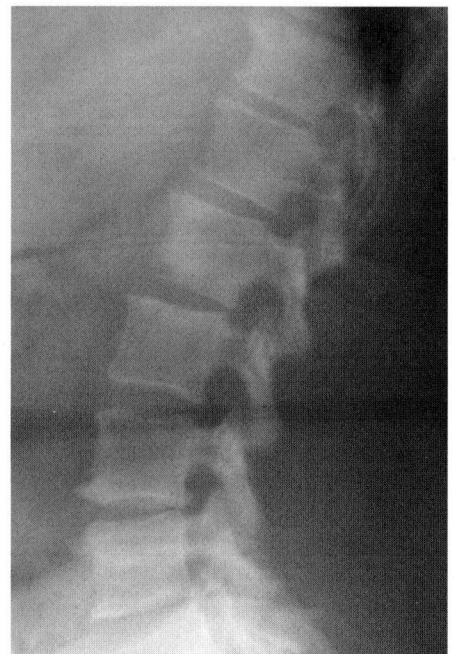

F,G

FUNGAL INFECTIONS

Fungal infections of the spine are relatively uncommon and are typically seen in immunocompromised patients. However, these infections must be considered in the differential diagnosis of infectious spondylitis. A delay in diagnosis occurs frequently because the infectious course often is indolent. The principles of diagnosis and treatment remain the same as for pyogenic infections (Fig. 78-4). Diagnosis rests primarily on obtaining a good biopsy and a positive tissue specimen culture. Biopsies must be evaluated with fungal stains as well as cultures, because the latter may be negative or take weeks to months to become positive. The differential diagnosis should include pyogenic and tuberculous infections, metastatic disease, axial neuroarthropathy, and spinal sarcoidosis (15). Spinal infections caused by aspergillosis, candidiasis, cryptococcus, blastomycosis, and coccidioidomycosis have been reported in both immunocompetent and immunocompromised patients (Table 78-1) (15,58,60).

In one series of 11 patients with fungal spine infections with long-term follow-up (61), the source of the fungal spondylitis was hematogenous seeding from sepsis in four, postoperative spondylitis in three, local extension from an adjacent fungal infection in two, direct traumatic implantation in one, and unknown in one. All of the patients except two had risk factors consistent with immunosuppression or chronic medical illness.

At the time of clinical presentation (61), 10 of the 11 patients had severe unremitting pain localized to the level of the infection and nine patients had some degree of paralysis. The clinical presentation was characterized by a long delay between the onset of symptoms and administration of an antifungal agent (Table 78-2), the delay ranging from 7 to 365 days (average 99 days) in 10 patients; the outlying eleventh patient had a draining sinus for 9 years. Only one patient had a fever of more than 101°F. The sedimentation rate was elevated in 10 patients, and the WBC was elevated in only three patients, and greater than 20,000 cells/mm^2 in only one. Radiographic presentation showed peridiscal erosions and decreased disc space height in 10 patients. In the eleventh, the most chronic patient, there was diffuse vertebral involvement.

Tissue obtained by closed or open biopsy revealed the diagnosis in all 11 patients (61). Half of the closed biopsies were negative, whereas all of the open biopsies were positive. The organism was identified with a positive fungal culture, KOH (potassium hydroxide) slide preparation, or Gomori methenamine silver stain. Seven of the 11 patients had *Candida* alone, and one patient had *Aspergillus* alone. Two of the patients had mixed infections with a fungus plus other fungi or bacteria. Ten of the 11 patients were treated with amphotericin B, and the remaining patient had a resistant organism treated with IV miconazole and oral ketoconazole.

Ten of the 11 patients were treated with surgical débridement of the spine to obtain the biopsy, débride the spine and drain abscesses, decompress the neural elements, and treat a failure of conservative treatment.

FIG. 78-3. A 34-year-old African-American woman was transferred to the medical service with the primary complaint of worsening axial low back pain. She had a long history of type 2 diabetes, and a recent history significant for a right large toe osteomyelitis that had been treated with débridement 2 weeks earlier. A Hickman catheter had been placed for long-term intravenous antibiotics, but was removed after spiking fevers and a line culture positive for methicillin-resistant *Staphylococcus aureus* (MRSA) confirmed a diagnosis of line sepsis. On initial consult, her plain films were negative for any obvious disc space erosions. She was neurologically normal, with no long tract signs, and normal perirectal sensation, rectal tone, and volition. **A–D:** Urgent magnetic resonance imaging revealed a massive epidural abscess with large psoas and paraspinous muscle abscesses. Reexamination revealed a stable, intact motor examination, with normal strength, mildly decreased distal vibratory sensation, a stocking glove distribution in both feet, and a normal sensory and volitional rectal examination. Postvoid residual, however, was 300 cc of urine. **E:** She had evidence of abscess tracking up to the mid thoracic spine but no clinical symptoms or signs of myelopathy She was taken to the operating room for decompressive laminectomies of L2-4, and decompression and drainage of the psoas abscess through an intertransverse approach, and the paraspinous abscesses as well. Gross pus in the canal was encountered largely centered at L3-4, the level of the psoas and paraspinous abscesses. Gram stain showed gram-positive cocci in clusters, and intraoperative cultures grew methicillin-resistant *Staphylococcus aureus*. Above L2 there was no residual mass effect and instead of purulence, just some granulation tissue. She was treated with vancomycin and rifampin for 8 weeks, and afterward with Bactrim. **F,G:** Postoperative radiographs showed no instability. She had no postoperative neurologic deficit and recovered normal urodynamics.

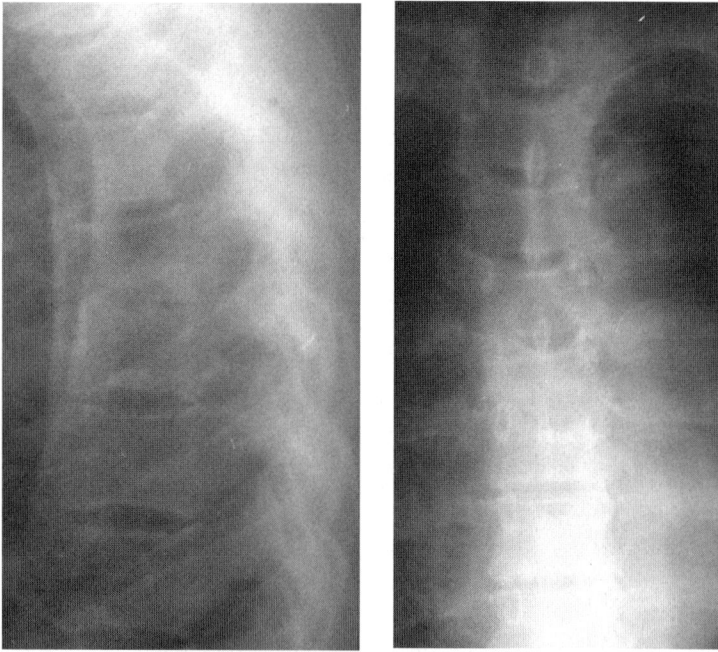

A,B

FIG. 78-4. A 68-year-old woman presented to the emergency room complaining of mid-thoracic back pain for 8 months with slow worsening. She was neurologically normal, had a negative travel history of any significance, and had lived in the same city for 20 years. **A,B:** The work-up revealed a sedimentation rate of 80, and plain films with some end plate erosions at T5-6. Computed tomography (CT) scan confirmed significant prevertebral soft tissue mass at T5-6 **(C)** as well as at T8 **(D). E:** Magnetic resonance imaging (MRI) confirmed the pattern of disc space infection at T5-6 on T1-weighted images with some intrusion into the canal. **F:** Gadolinium-enhanced images showed the extent of the anterior infection and vertebral body edema. **G:** T2-weighted images showed the infection with a large thoracic spinal canal and no cord compression.

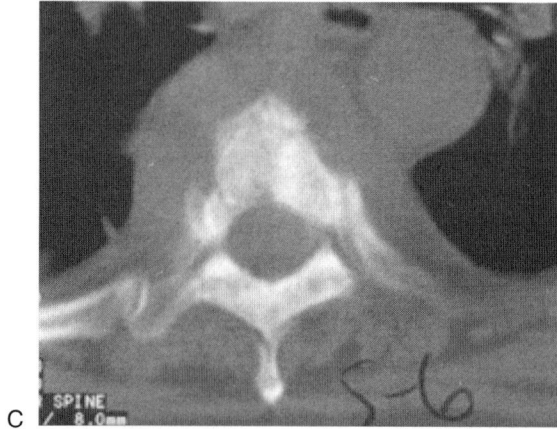

C

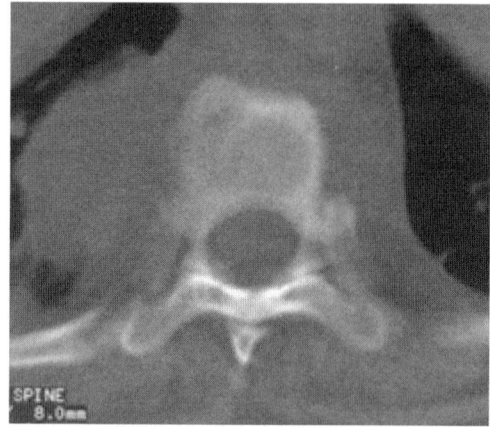

D

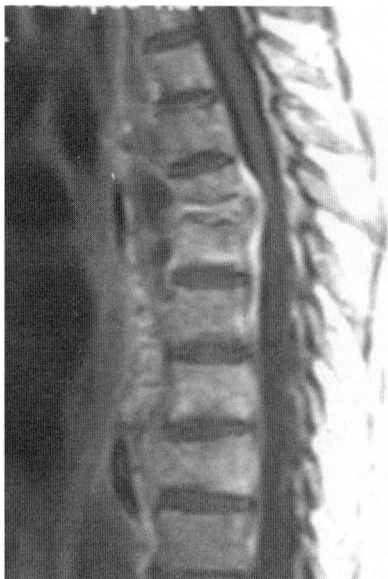

E,F

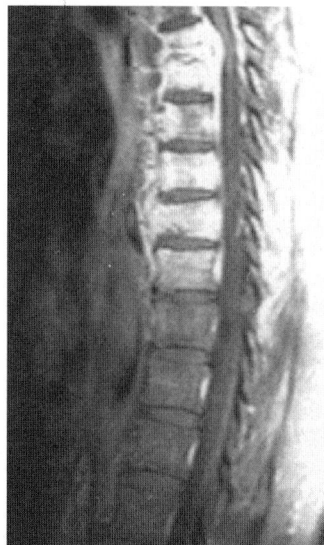

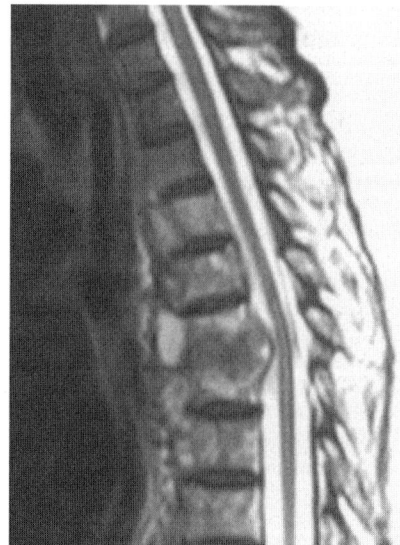

G

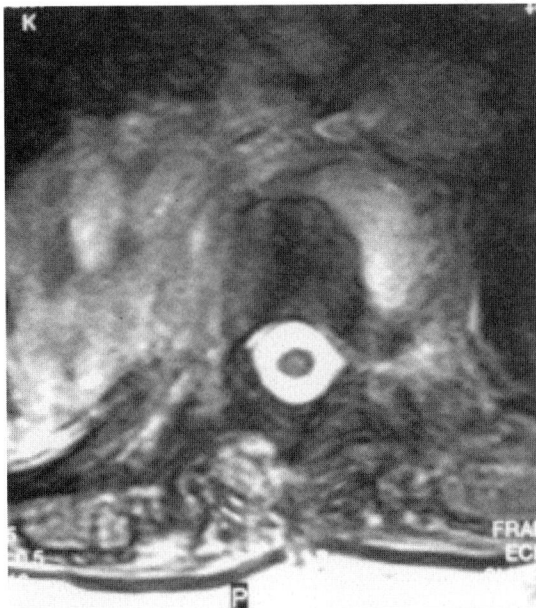
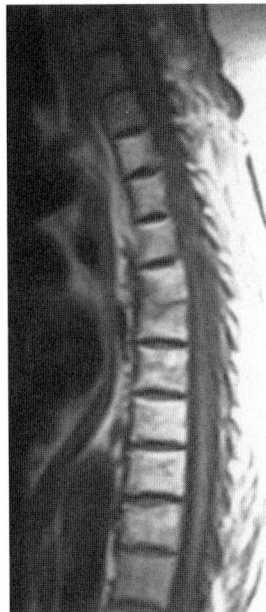

H,I

J

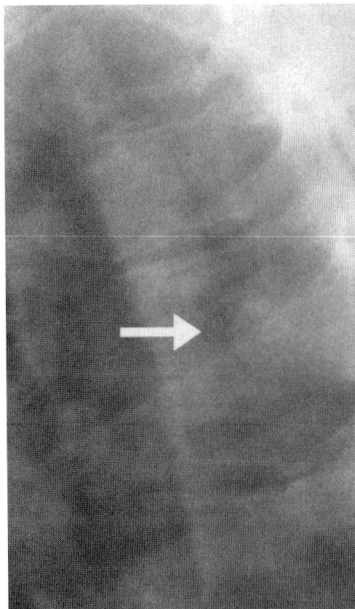
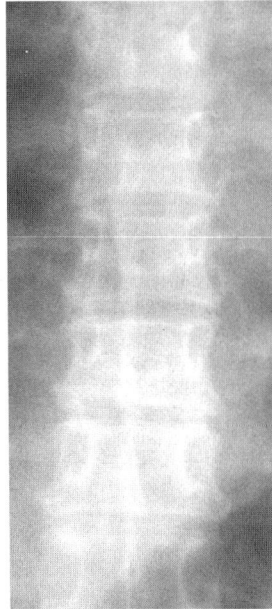

K,L

FIG. 78-4. (*Continued*). **H:** Other images confirmed the large soft-tissue abscess. Computed tomography–guided biopsy was negative on conventional cultures twice at the 10-day mark, and she was monitored with frequent neurologic examinations while in the hospital. Because she felt well, she left against medical advice, upon which her fungal cultures grew out *Blastomyces dermatitidis.* She was readmitted, and was adamantly against any surgery on discussion of alternatives and their risks and benefits. She was started on *amphotericin B,* to which she had significant renal toxicity. A trial of AmBisome resulted in neutropenia. Itraconazole was started and well tolerated. Her sedimentation rate normalized over the course of 1 month, and after 4 months of conservative treatment, itraconazole was discontinued. At 6 months, MRI scans confirmed resolution of the infection as well as the prevertebral abscesses **(I,J),** and plain films showed spontaneous fusion of T5-6 (**K,** *arrow;* **L,** *top*) with no deformity.

Two patients died, one of disseminated aspergillus infection, and one of a massive upper gastrointestinal hemorrhage. The authors concluded that even when neural decompression was not needed, the results were better with an anterior surgical approach. Once treatment was completed, only four of the nine survivors were neurologically normal. Four of these nine patients had persistent mechanical spine pain, and two were functionally disabled from the pain. However, once full medical and surgical treatment was completed, no patient had a recurrence of the infection with an average of 6.3 years of follow-up.

TABLE 78-1. *Fungal pathogens with a propensity for spine and musculoskeletal involvement and their characteristics*

Fungal pathogen	Endemic area/ecosystem	Host	Mode of infection	Non-MSK sites	Dissemination
Coccidiomycosis	Soil, desert ecosystem Arid southwestern United States San Juaquin Valley fever	Travel, endemic exposure	Airborne spore Skin abrasions	Pulmonary Cutaneous Osseous Prostatic Central nervous system	Hematogenous
Blastomycosis	Warm moist soil rich in organic debris Mississippi and Ohio river valleys Great Lakes, St. Lawrence River	Endemic exposure	Spore inhalation	Lung, skin	Hematogenous
Cryptococcus	Throughout the world Pigeon feces and soil	AIDS	Inhalation of fungal form	Lung/central nervous system	Hematogenous
Candidiasis	Normal skin commensals Gastrointestinal tract, sputum, skin Urine of catheterized patients	Immuno-compromised Vascular access IVDA Burns	Endogenous	Blood Endocarditis Meningitis Fungemia	Hematogenous
Aspergillus	Dead plant and animal matter Threshing areas and mills	Immuno-compromised Farm workers	Inhalation of conidia	Pulmonary	Direct extension

IVDA, intravenous drug abuse; MSK, musculoskeletal.

TABLE 78-2. *Antifungal agents and their characteristics*

Agent	Mechanism	Route	Side effects	Indication	Pathogens
Amphotericin B	Plasma membrane permeability, cell death	IV	Bone marrow dysfunction Liver and renal toxicity	Life-threatening disease Central nervous system involvement Medically ill	Blastomycosis Coccidiomycosis
Flucytosine	Inhibits DNA synthesis	IV		With amphotericin B	Aspergillosis Candida Cryptococcus Blastomycosis Coccidiomycosis
Ketoconazole Fluconazole Itraconazole	Block the biosynthesis of fungal lipids in the cell membranes	PO		HIV Good central nervous system penetration	
Ambisome	Liposomal formulation of amphotericin B	IV	Similar amphotericin B	Fail amphotericin B Not tolerating amphotericin B	Aspergillosis Candidiasis Cryptococcal

CONCLUSION

Diagnosis and treatment of spine infections begins with clinical suspicion, meticulous history and physical, as well as appropriate laboratory work-up. Imaging, especially MRI, can enhance clinical suspicion and guide treatment decisions. However, biopsy and culture are the key elements needed to guide antibiotic choice and the success of conservative treatment. Even with appropriate conservative therapy, there are patients who may need surgical treatment for a clinically significant abscess, open biopsy, severe deformity, neurologic deficit, or failure of conservative treatment with continued chronic infection.

REFERENCES

 1. Kulowski J. Pyogenic osteomyelitis of the spine. An analysis and discussion of 102 cases. JBJS 1936;18:147.
 2. Nagel DA, Albright JA, Keggi KJ, et al. Closer look at spinal lesions: open biopsy of vertebral lesions. JAMA 1965;191:103.
 3. Sapico FL, Montgomerie JZ. Pyogenic vertebral osteomyelitis: report of nine cases and review of the literature. Rev Infect Dis 1979;1:754–776.
 4. Sapico FL, Montgomerie JZ. Vertebral osteomyelitis in intravenous drug abusers: report of three cases and review of the literature. Rev Infect Dis 1980;2:196–206.
 5. Santos EM, Sapico FL. Vertebral osteomyelitis due to salmonellae: report of two cases and review. Clin Infect Dis 1998;27:287–295.
 6. Sapico FL, Liquete JA, Sarma RJ. Bone and joint infections in patients with infective endocarditis: review of a 4-year experience. Clin Infect Dis 1996;22:783–787.
 7. Bonfiglio M, Lange TA, Kim YM. Pyogenic vertebral osteomyelitis. Disk space infections. Clin Orthop Rel Res 1973;96:234–247.
 8. Pinckney LE, Currarino G, Highgenboten CL. Osteomyelitis of the cervical spine following dental extraction. Radiology 1980;135:335–337.
 9. Rawlings CE, III, Wilkins RH, Gallis HA, et al. Postoperative intervertebral disc space infection. Neurosurgery 1983;13:371–376.
10. Bernard TN Jr. Lumbar discography followed by computed tomography. Refining the diagnosis of low-back pain. Spine 1990;15:690–707.
11. Eismont FJ, Bohlman HH, Soni PL, et al. Pyogenic and fungal vertebral osteomyelitis with paralysis. J Bone Joint Surg Am 1983;65:19–29.
12. Weinstein M, Lebwohl NH, Brown MD, et al. Infections of the spine in patients with HIV. North American Spine Society, Seattle, October 31–November 3, 2001:18–19.
13. Sapico FL. Microbiology and antimicrobial therapy of spinal infections. Orthop Clin North Am 1996;27:9–13.
14. Schofferman L, Schofferman J, Zucherman J, et al. Occult infections causing persistent low-back pain. Spine 1989;14:417–419.
15. Slucky AVEF. Spinal infections. In: Bridwell KJDR, ed. The textbook of spinal surgery, 2nd ed. Philadelphia: Lippincott-Raven, 1997:2141–2183.
16. Batson OV. The function of the vertebral veins and their role in the spread of metastasis. Ann Surg 1940;112:138.
17. Wiley AMTJ. The vascular anatomy of the spine and its relationship to pyogenic vertebral osteomyelitis. J Bone Joint Surg (Br) 1959;41:796.
18. Baker AS. Spinal epidural abscess. N Engl J Med 1975;293:463–468.
19. Eismont FJ, Bohlman HH, Soni PL, et al. Vertebral osteomyelitis in infants. J Bone Joint Surg (Br) 1982;64:32–35.
20. Eismont FJ, Green BA, Brown MD, et al. Coexistent infection and tumor of the spine. A report of three cases. J Bone Joint Surg (Am) 1987;69:452–458.
21. Digby JM, Kersley JB. Pyogenic non-tuberculous spinal infection: an analysis of thirty cases. J Bone Joint Surg (Br) 1979;61:47–55.
22. Garcia AGS. Hematogenous pyogenic vertebral osteomyelitis. J Bone Joint Surg (Am) 1960;42A:429–436.
23. Charles RW, Mody GM, Govender S. Pyogenic infection of the lumbar vertebral spine due to gas-forming organisms. A case report. Spine 1989;14:541–543.
24. Modic MT, Feiglin DH, Piraino DW, et al. Vertebral osteomyelitis: assessment using MR. Radiology 1985;157:157–166.

25. Frederickson B, Yuan H, Olans R. Management and outcome of pyogenic vertebral osteomyelitis. Clin Orthop 1978;160–167.
26. King DM, Mayo KM. Infective lesions of the vertebral column. Clin Orthop 1973;96:248–253.
27. Van Lom KJ, Kellerhouse LE, Pathria MN, et al. Infection versus tumor in the spine: criteria for distinction with CT. Radiology 1988;166:851–855.
28. Szypryt EP, Hardy JG, Hinton CE, et al. A comparison between magnetic resonance imaging and scintigraphic bone imaging in the diagnosis of disc space infection in an animal model. Spine 1988;13:1042–1048.
29. Schlaeffer F, Mikolich DJ, Mates SM. Technetium Tc 99m diphosphonate bone scan. False-normal findings in elderly patients with hematogenous vertebral osteomyelitis. Arch Intern Med 1987;147:2024–2026.
30. Post MJ, Quencer RM, Montalvo BM, et al. Spinal infection: evaluation with MR imaging and intraoperative US. Radiology 1988;169:765–771.
31. Post MJ, Sze G, Quencer RM, et al. Gadolinium-enhanced MR in spinal infection. J Comput Assist Tomogr 1990;14:721–729.
32. Ottolenghi CE. Aspiration biopsy of the spine: technique for the thoracic spine and results of 28 biopsies in this region and overall results of 1050 biopsies of other spinal segments. J Bone Joint Surg (Am) 1969;51:1531.
33. Goldman AB, Freiberger RH. Localized infectious and neuropathic diseases. Semin Roentgenol 1979;14:19–32.
34. Currier BL, Banovac K, Eismont FJ. Gentamicin penetration into normal rabbit nucleus pulposus. Spine 1994;19:2614–2618.
35. Eismont FJ, Wiesel SW, Brighton CT, et al. Antibiotic penetration into rabbit nucleus pulposus. Spine 1987;12:254–256.
36. Fraser RD, Osti OL, Vernon-Roberts B. Iatrogenic discitis: the role of intravenous antibiotics in prevention and treatment. An experimental study. Spine 1989;14:1025–1032.
37. Gibson MJ, Karpinski MR, Slack RC, et al. The penetration of antibiotics into the normal intervertebral disc. J Bone Joint Surg (Br) 61987;9:784–786.
38. Guerrero IC, MacGregor RR. Comparative penetration of various cephalosporins into inflammatory exudate. Antimicrob Agents Chemother 1979;15:712–715.
39. Scuderi GJ, Greenberg SS, Banovac K, et al. Penetration of glycopeptide antibiotics in nucleus pulposus. Spine 1993;18:2039–2042.
40. Riley LH, III, Banovac K, Martinez OV, et al. Tissue distribution of antibiotics in the intervertebral disc. Spine 1994;19:2619–2625.
41. Sapico FL, Montgomerie JZ. Vertebral osteomyelitis. Infect Dis Clin North Am 1990;4:539–550.
42. Seddon HJ. Pott's paraplegia. Br J Surg 1935;22:769–771.
43. Kemp HBS. Laminectomy in paraplegia due to infective spondylosis. Br J Surg 1974;61:66–72.
44. McGuire RA, Eismont FJ. The fate of autogenous bone graft in surgically treated pyogenic vertebral osteomyelitis. J Spinal Disord 1994;7:206–215.
45. Bohlman HH, Eismont FJ. Surgical techniques of anterior decompression and fusion for spinal cord injuries. Clin Orthop 1981;57–67.
46. Hodgson AR. Anterior spine fusion for the treatment of tuberculosis of the spine. The operative findings and results of treatment in the first on hundred cases. J Bone Joint Surg (Am) 1960;42:295.
47. Cahill DW, Love LC, Rechtine GR. Pyogenic osteomyelitis of the spine in the elderly. J Neurosurg 1991;74:878–886.
48. Przybylski GJ, Sharan AD. Single-stage autogenous bone grafting and internal fixation in the surgical management of pyogenic discitis and vertebral osteomyelitis. J Neurosurg 2001;94:1–7.
49. Hee HT, Majd ME, Holt RT, et al. Better treatment of vertebral osteomyelitis using posterior stabilization and titanium mesh cages. J Spinal Disord Tech 2002;15:149–156.
50. Polly D. Corpectomy cage explants. 2002. Personal communication.
51. Rajasekaran S, Shanmugasundaram TK. Prediction of the angle of gibbus deformity in tuberculosis of the spine. J Bone Joint Surg (Am) 1987;69:503–509.
52. Danner RL, Hartman BJ. Update on spinal epidural abscess: 35 cases and review of the literature. Rev Infect Dis 1987;9:265–274.
53. Reihsaus E, Waldbaur H, Seeling W. Spinal epidural abscess: a meta-analysis of 915 patients. Neurosurg Rev 2000;23:175–204.
54. Heusner AP. Nontuberculous spinal epidural infections. N Engl J Med 1948;239:845–854.
55. Leys D, Lesoin F, Viaud C, et al. Decreased morbidity from acute bac-

terial spinal epidural abscesses using computed tomography and non-surgical treatment in selected patients. Ann Neurol 1985;17:350–355.

56. Mampalam TJ, Rosegay H, Andrews BT, et al. Nonoperative treatment of spinal epidural infections. J Neurosurg 1989;71:208–210.

57. Koppel BS, Tuchman AJ, Mangiardi JR, et al. Epidural spinal infection in intravenous drug abusers. Arch Neurol 1988;45:1331–1337.

58. Currier BL, Eismont FJ. Infections of the spine. In: Herkowitz HN, ed. The spine, 4th ed. Philadelphia: WB Saunders, 1999:1207–1259.

59. Hakin RN, Burt AA, Cook JB. Acute spinal epidural abscess. Paraplegia 1979;17:330–336.

60. Govender TS. Fungal infections of the spine. In Weinstein SL, ed. The pediatric spine, 2nd ed. Philadelphia: Lippincott Williams & Wilkins, 2001:649–657.

61. Frazier DD, Campbell DR, Garvey TA, et al. Fungal infections of the spine. Report of eleven patients with long-term follow-up. J Bone Joint Surg (Am) 2001;83-A:560–565.

CHAPTER 79

Tuberculosis

S. Rajasekaran

Tuberculosis is rampant in many parts of the world: In the year 1993 alone, more than 3 million tuberculosis-related deaths were reported (1). Roughly 3% to 4% of all tuberculous infections involve the skeletal system and more than 50% of those involve the spine. Even by a conservative estimate, there are about 3 million patients with active spinal tuberculosis in the world today (2). The eradication of the disease appears remote because of the poor economic and social standards of the developing world, increasing global travel, the emergence of multi–drug-resistant strains, and the increasing incidence of patients coinfected with tuberculosis and acquired immunodeficiency syndrome (AIDS).

PATHOLOGY

Mycobacterium tuberculosis, characterized by its acid-fast staining properties, is the organism commonly responsible for human infections. The spinal infection is always a secondary lesion by hematogenous spread from a pulmonary (Gans focus), gastrointestinal, or genitourinary lesion, but an active primary source is detected in less than 10% of patients. Apart from arterial channels, the spread also can occur through the Batson plexus of veins; this accounts for the increased involvement of the lumbar spine (Fig. 79-1). Skip lesions with multilevel involvement are possible and are detected in about 5% of patients with plain radiography and in 15% of patients when magnetic resonance imaging (MRI) is used.

Anterior lesions affecting the vertebral body account for 85% to 90% of the lesions (2). Many types of body involvement are seen—paradiscal, central, complete, and anterior lesions. The paradiscal variety is the most common, especially in adolescents and young adults (Fig. 79-2). Here the infection spreads through the epi-

physeal arteries, which branch to supply the paradiscal region of adjacent vertebrae. The initial picture is loss of definition of the paradiscal margins of consecutive vertebrae with narrowing of disc space; there is further destruction of the vertebral bodies with progress of the disease. Complete destruction of one or more vertebrae is commonly found in children below the age of 10 years and is predisposed by poor nutritional status (3). Here the anterior column deficit is extensive; such children are prone to buckling collapse of the spine, leading to late progress in deformity and late paraplegia. The central type of lesion is more common in children. There can be collapse of the body without any change in the disc spaces, which simulates a radiologic picture of Calves disease. Anterior lesions are frequent in the thoracic region and the infection can quickly spread beneath the anterior longitudinal ligament to many consecutive levels.

Posterior lesions affecting the pedicle, laminae, and spinous process constitute 10% to 15% of lesions; however, they are important because they are associated with late diagnosis and a higher incidence of neurologic deficit (4). Computed tomography (CT) and MRI studies must be used for an early diagnosis whenever there is a suspicion. Rarely the disease starts at the posterior margin of the body with profuse granulation tissue. The patient presents with neurologic deficit without any radiologic abnormality and the clinical picture mimics a spinal cord tumor (spinal tumor syndrome). Irregular destruction of the vertebral bodies can lead to scoliosis and may cause confusion with hemivertebrae in healed cases. Destruction of more than two vertebral bodies leads to facetal dislocation during the period of collapse in children and can precipitate complete translocation of the spine, resulting in a complex deformity (Fig. 79-3).

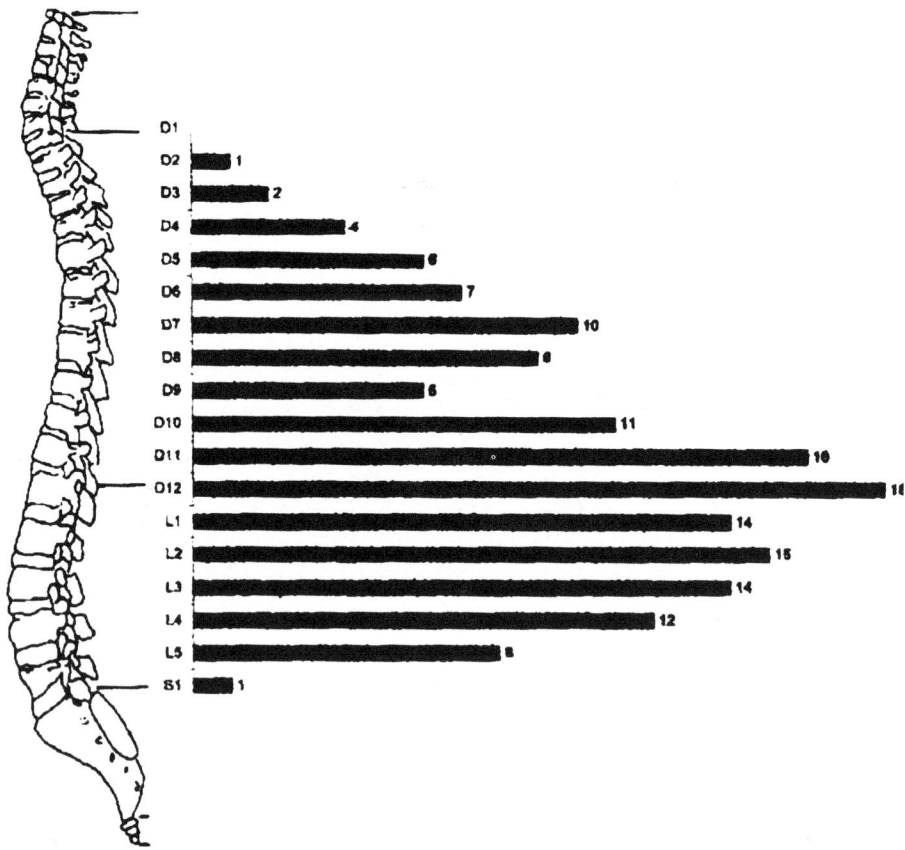

FIG. 79-1. The thoracolumbar and lumbar regions are most commonly affected in spinal tuberculosis. The larger mass of bone, increased range of movements in the region, spread by Batson plexus of veins and the proximity to cisterna chyli are quoted as reasons.

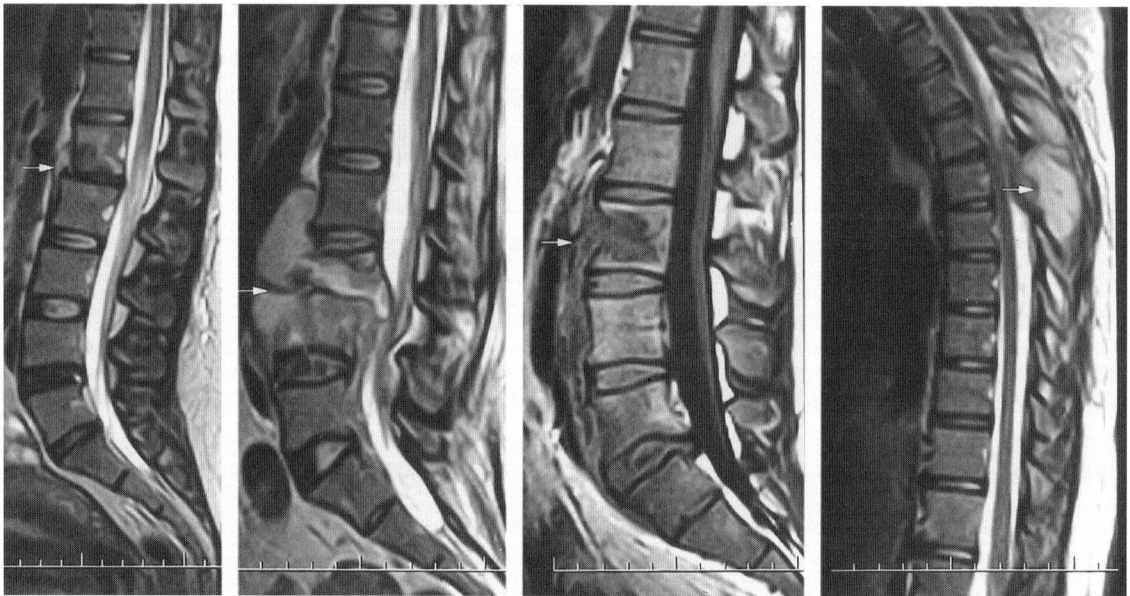

A–D

FIG. 79-2. The various types of lesions seen commonly in spinal tuberculosis. **A:** Paradiscal lesions with destruction of the discs and involvement of the adjacent vertebral bodies is the most common lesion. **B:** With progression of the disease and especially in children, entire vertebral bodies are destroyed with the formation of caseous material and abscess. **C:** Body lesions without the involvement of discs are relatively rare. **D:** Posterior lesions without involvement of the anterior column are also rare and are more easily identified in computed tomography and magnetic resonance imaging scans.

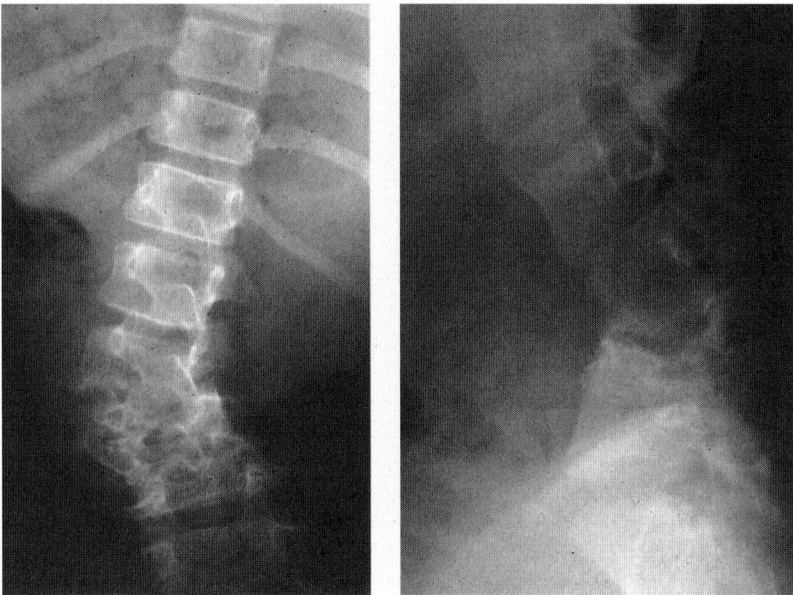

FIG. 79-3. In patients with destruction of two or more vertebral bodies, the facetal joints dislocate to allow the normal vertebral bodies to come into contact and consolidate anteriorly. The disruption of the posterior arch in the presence of anterior column deficit leads to global instability and the spine often heals with varying degrees of scoliosis, kyphosis, and rotation.

A,B

THE NATURAL HISTORY OF THE DISEASE

Untreated spinal tuberculosis has a vicious clinical course of progressive destruction of vertebral bodies with potential for persistent sinuses, abscess, and early- or late-onset neurologic deficit (Pott paraplegia). Effective chemotherapy can arrest the progress at any stage with healing and consolidation of the focus. In minimal disease, the disc is destroyed early and the cancellous bone of the adjacent vertebrae consolidates with bony fusion, which is the hallmark of healing in spinal tuberculosis. In severe disease with extensive destruction of the anterior column, facet joints frequently give way and destabilize the spine. The superior healthy vertebra then rotates and descends so that its anterior surface comes into contact with the superior surface of the inferior healthy vertebra. The deformity often increases to more than 60° and in children can progress during the period of growth even after cure of the disease.

The progress of deformity depends on the age at the time of involvement, the level of lesion, and the severity of disease. The deformity progresses in two distinct phases: phase I, or the active phase, which includes changes in the first 18 months during the period of active disease. Changes that occur after the disease is cured are termed phase II, or healed phase, changes (5).

Adults have a lesser deformity at presentation, a lesser increase during phase I, and virtually no change after cure of the disease. The progression of deformity usually is less than 30° and is restricted to the first 12 to 18 months when consolidation of the focus is complete (3). In contrast, children have a higher deformity at presentation, a greater tendency for collapse during the active phase, and continued progression until growth is complete. Children are more susceptible to deformity because

of the increased severity of destruction at presentation (3,6,7), increased flexibility of the spine (8), a relative destruction of the growth plates anteriorly interfering with future growth (9,10), and the suppressive effect of the mechanical forces of kyphosis on the growth of the anterior half of the fusion mass and adjacent normal vertebrae (11).

Distinct types of progress are seen in children during the growth phase that determine the extent of the final deformity (5). Unlike other spinal deformities, which usually deteriorate with growth, there is both a beneficial or worsening effect during the period of growth spurt (Figs. 79-4 and 79-5).

Type 1 Progression

There is continued progress through the entire period of growth; this is noticed in 44% of children (Fig. 79-6). The increase could occur continuously after phase I (type 1A) or a lag period of 3 to 6 years after the disease is cured (type 1B). Type IB progression is important because the lag period may result in the progression being missed. It is common practice to follow-up children only for 2 to 3 years after the disease is cured; therefore, the late increase in deformity can be missed.

Type II Progression

Type II progression shows beneficial effects during growth with a decrease in deformity after healing (Fig. 79-7). This can occur immediately after phase 1 (type II a) or a period of 3 to 6 years (type IIb). Children with type II progression have the best outcome because they have lesser increase during phase I and greater improvement during phase II.

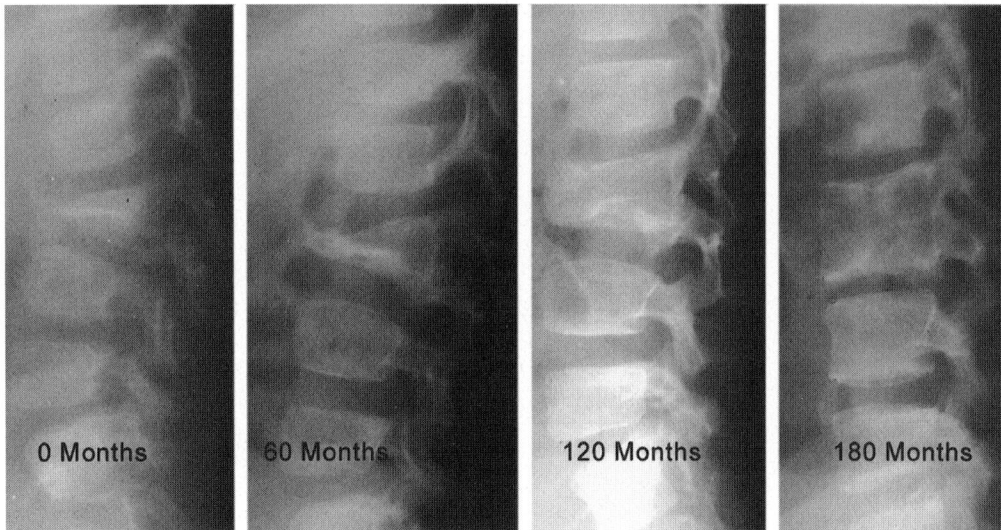

FIG. 79-4. Lateral radiographs of the lumbar spine of a 4-year-old child with severe destruction of L2 and L3 at the start of treatment. Follow-up shows excellent improvement with growth at 60, 120, and 180 months. The fusion mass of L2 and L3 begins to show increased anterior growth. By 15 years the fusion mass almost resembles a normal vertebra except for the attachments of the pedicles of two levels. (Reproduced with permission from Rajasekaran S. The natural history of post tubercular kyphosis in children. J Bone Joint Surg (Br) 2001;83.B:954–962.)

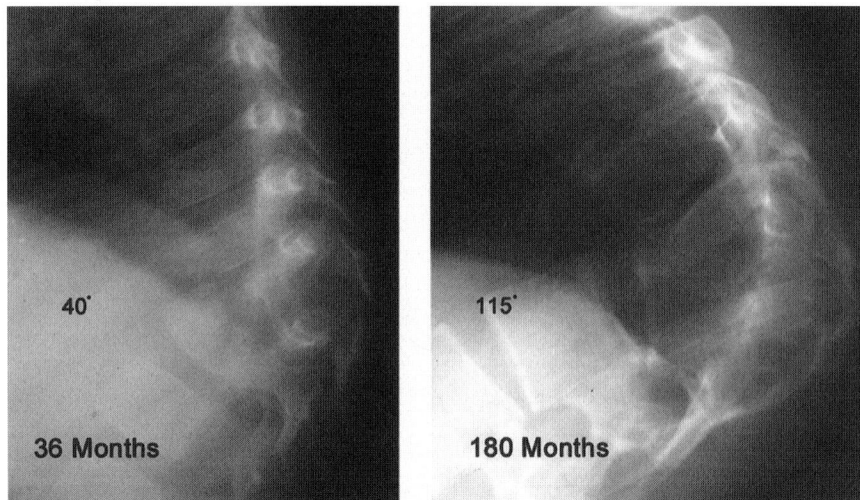

FIG. 79-5. Radiographs showing extensive thoracic lesions in a 3-year-old girl with a deformity of 40° at 3-year follow-up. The disease was completely cured, but the deformity progressed to 115° at 15 years follow-up. (From Rajasekaran S. The natural history of post tubercular kyphosis in children. J Bone Joint Surg (Br) 2001;83.B:954–962, with permission.)

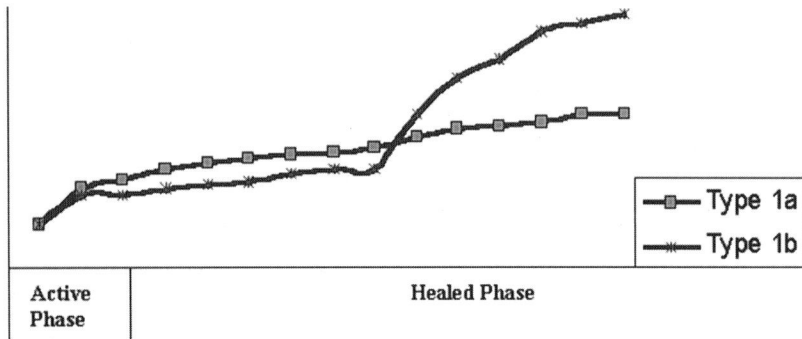

FIG. 79-6. Graph showing that type 1 progression showed deterioration in the deformity even after healing of the disease. In type 1a progression, this deterioration continued throughout growth, whereas in type 1b progression there was a lag period of a few years before the deterioration started. The progression was more severe in type 1b. (From Rajasekaran S. The natural history of post tubercular kyphosis in children. J Bone Joint Surg (Br) 2001;83.B:954–962, with permission.)

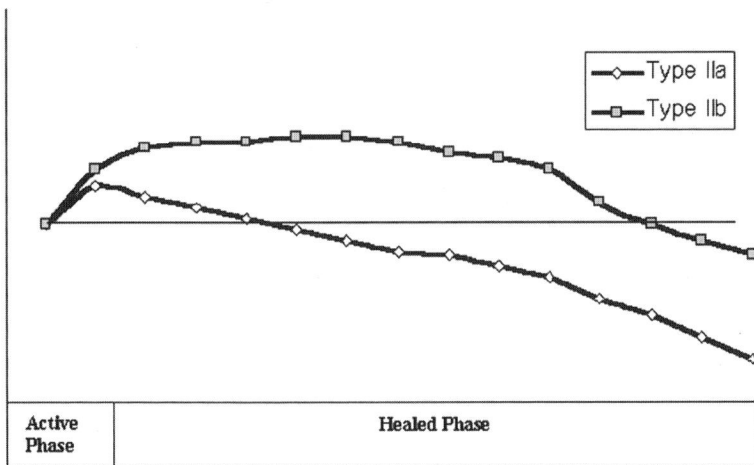

FIG. 79-7. Graph showing that in children with type 2 progression a decrease in deformity occurred during the healed phase. In type 2a the improvement started soon after healing of the disease and in type 2b after a lag period of a few years. (From Rajasekaran S. The natural history of post tubercular kyphosis in children. J Bone Joint Surg (Br) 2001;83.B:954–962, with permission.)

Type III Progression

Children who have minimal disease or lower lumbar lesions without loss of lordosis do not have any major change in deformity during phases I and II (Fig. 79-8).

Facetal dislocation leading to spinal instability determines the course of the disease. The failure of the posterior arch and the instability that follows is identifiable by the following instability signs, termed "spine at risk" radiologic signs (Fig. 79-9)(5).

Separation of the Facet Joints

With progressive kyphosis, the facet joint at the apex of the curve is subluxed followed by frank dislocation. In patients with severe involvement, there is separation at more than one level, with wide distraction of the spinous processes at the corresponding levels.

Retropulsion of the Diseased Vertebral Segments

With progressive destruction, the remnants of the destroyed vertebral bodies are retropulsed. This is assessed by drawing two lines along the posterior surface of the normal vertebrae above and below the level of the lesion. Retropulsion is confirmed when the diseased segments are seen to lie posterior to the drawn lines.

Lateral Translation of the Vertebral Column

Translation is confirmed when the line drawn form the center of a pedicle of the lower vertebrae does not intersect the pedicle of the upper vertebrae in an antero-posterior (AP) radiograph.

Toppling Sign

The separation of the facet joint allows the superior normal vertebral segment to tilt or topple, so that the anterior surface of the vertebra comes into contact with the superior surface of the vertebra below the level of the lesion. A line drawn along the anterior surface of the inferior vertebra intersects the superior first normal vertebra above the middle of its anterior surface.

Each of these signs is given a score of 1, with a maximum possible instability score of 4. Of all the variables, an instability score of more than 2 is the most significant factor in determining an increase of more than 30° or a final deformity of more than 60° (5). The radiologic signs of instability are found to be particularly useful because

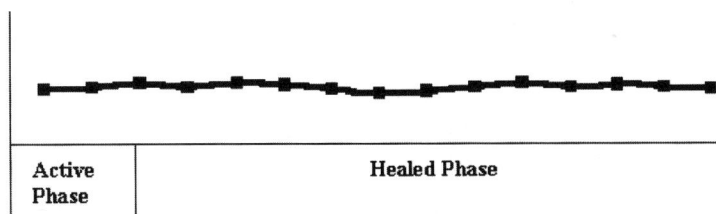

FIG. 79-8. Graph showing type 3 progression had only a minimal increase during the active phase and little change during the healed phase. This was found in children with only minimal destruction or lesions of the lower lumbar region. (From Rajasekaran S. The natural history of post tubercular kyphosis in children. J Bone Joint Surg (Br) 2001;83.B:954–962, with permission.)

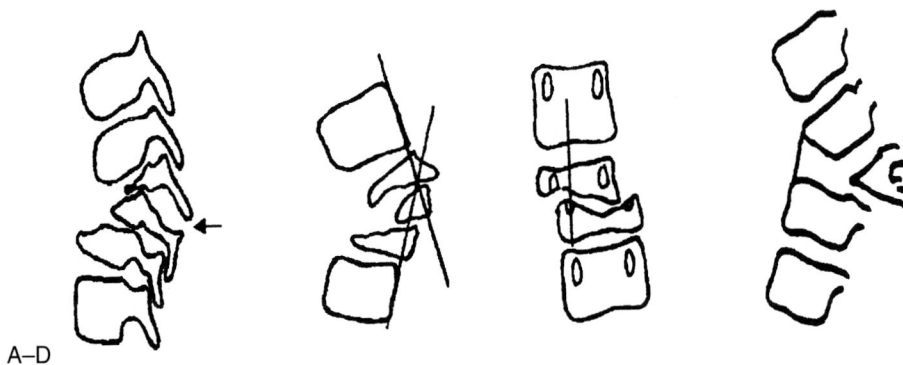

FIG. 79-9. Spine at risk radiologic signs in children. **A:** Separation of the facet joint. The facet joint dislocates at the level of the apex of the curve, causing instability and loss of alignment. In severe case the separation can occur at two levels. **B:** Posterior retropulsion. This is identified by drawing two lines along the posterior surface of the first upper and lower normal vertebrae. The diseased segments are found to be posterior to the intersection of the lines. **C:** Lateral translation. This is confirmed when a vertical line drawn through the middle of the pedicle of the first lower normal vertebra does not touch the pedicle of the first upper normal vertebra. **D:** Toppling sign. In the initial stages of collapse, a line drawn along the anterior surface of the first lower normal vertebra intersects the inferior surface of the first upper normal vertebra. Tilt or toppling occurs when the line intersects higher than the middle of the anterior surface of the first normal upper vertebra. (From Rajasekaran S. The natural history of post tubercular kyphosis in children. J Bone Joint Surg (Br) 2001;83.B:954–962, with permission.)

they appear early during the active stage of the disease itself when surgical intervention is easier and can be performed with fewer complications.

CLINICAL FEATURES

Pain in the region of involvement with paraspinal muscle spasm and restriction of movements is the usual mode of presentation. Weight loss, loss of appetite, malaise, and evening temperature elevation are present in most patients, but may be absent in patients with good nutrition and health (2). Patients with extensive involvement and instability have a guarded gait and frequently exhibit reluctance to alter the position or ambulate. Deformities are present in most patients; the spinous process becomes prominent, producing a knuckle deformity when one vertebra is destroyed. A gibbus deformity of varying degree develops when many vertebrae are destroyed (Fig. 79-10). In lower lumbar lesions, lordosis protects the spine from an external kyphotic deformity and the severe collapse is manifested as foreshortening of the trunk (6).

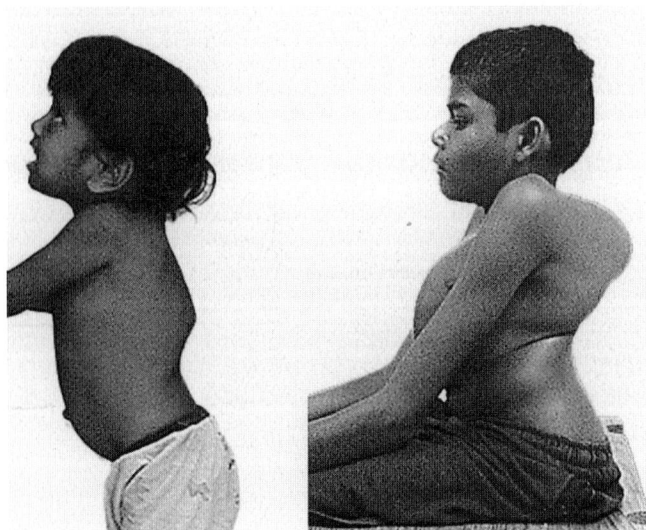

FIG. 79-10. A 4-year-old child with a healed tuberculosis and a prominent kyphotic deformity of the dorsolumbar region **(A)**. These lesions require early intervention; otherwise, they progress to severe deformities with risk for late-onset neurologic deficit, as seen in **(B)**.

COLD ABSCESS

Abscess is a common feature of spinal tuberculosis. Its clinical or radiologic identification greatly helps in the diagnosis of spinal tuberculosis. The abscess, composed of caseous material, serous exudates, and bone debris, spreads in various directions along the lines of least resistance and often presents subcutaneously. Absence of signs of inflammation at the site of presentation has led to the term cold abscess. In lumbar lesions, the abscess enters the psoas sheath and gravitates to form a psoas mass. It may then track down to the Petit triangle or may appear below the inguinal ligament or medial aspect of the thigh. It also can follow the great vessels into the pelvis, gluteal region, or posterior aspect of the thigh. Lesions of the sacrum and coccyx form abscess that track along the sciatic nerve to present in the posterior aspect of the thigh or popliteal region.

NEUROLOGIC INVOLVEMENT

The incidence of a significant neurologic deficit in spinal tuberculosis is less than 3%, although some form of mild involvement can be present in up to 30% of patients (2,12). Compromise of the spinal canal with compression of the spinal cord by abscess, granulation tissue, and sequestrated bone or disc material is the usual cause of paraplegia (Fig. 79-11A). The neurologic involvement caused by such compression usually progresses insidiously, but precipitous paraplegia can occur

because of infective vasculitis compromising the blood supply to the cord or a pathologic dislocation of severely destroyed vertebrae (Table 79-1). Other rare causes are spinal tumor syndrome and progressive fibrosis around the cord at the region of deformity apex.

The incidence of neurologic deficit is more common in thoracic and thoracolumbar lesions and is rare in lesions below the second lumbar vertebrae. The capacious spinal canal in the lower lumbar level and the fact that the spinal cord ends at the lower border of the first lumbar vertebra account for the lower incidence of neurologic deficit in lumbosacral lesions. When the involvement is at the cord level the disease passes through characteristic stages (Table 79-2). Lumbar lesions mainly produces radiculopathy and a full-blown cauda equina syndrome only rarely results. Magnetic resonance imaging has replaced myelography and is superior in accurately demonstrating the extent and cause of cord compression. It also shows the presence or absence of primary change in the cord and helps to prognosticate the outcome of treatment and recovery.

Paraplegia was initially divided into early and late onset, depending on its occurrence within or after 2 years of onset of the disease. This differentiation is less useful than the classification paraplegia of active disease (occurring however late) and paraplegia of healed disease. The prognosis is more favorable in paraplegia in active disease because the pathology is inflammation, and conservative treatment with adequate chemotherapy may be sufficient. Good recovery with chemotherapy is seen

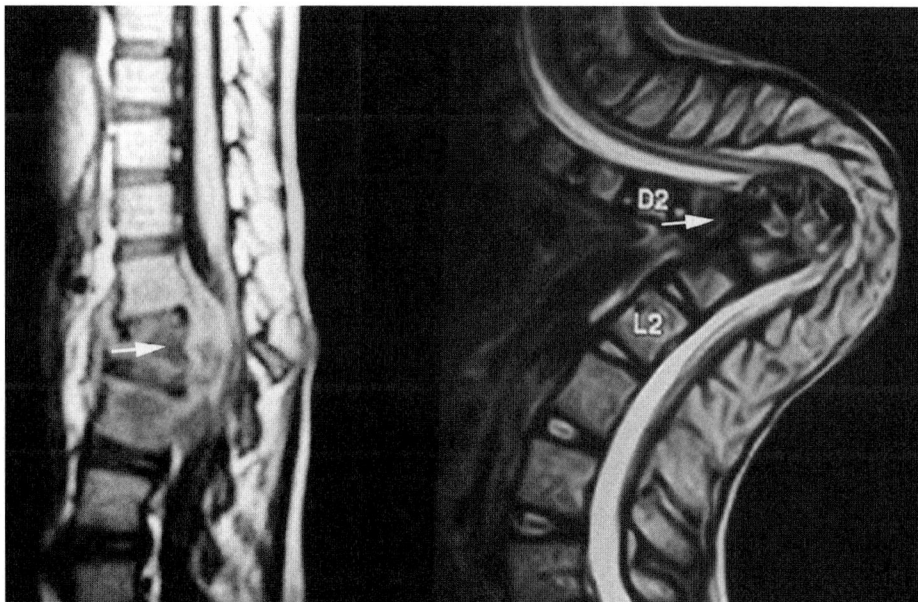

FIG. 79-11. A: An active lumbar lesion with neurologic deficit owing to compression of the dural sac by abscess, granulation tissue, retropulsed bone debris, and disc material. B: In contrast, the cause for neurologic deficit in healed disease is caused by stretching the cord over the apex of the bony deformity (internal gibbus).

TABLE 79-1. *Causes of neurologic deficit in active and healed disease*

Paraplegia of active disease (occurring however late)
  Compressive pathology caused by
    Inflammatory edema
    Granulation tissue
    Caseous tissue and abscess
    Sequestrated bone and disc material
  Infective vasculitis
  Spinal tumor syndrome
  Pathologic dislocation of the spine
  Direct infiltration of the cord
Paraplegia of healed disease
  Stretching of the cord over the apex during progressive
    deformity (internal gibbous)
  Progressive extradural fibrosis

in the presence of active disease with an inflammatory cause of compression, incomplete involvement, short duration of deficit, minimal kyphotic deformity, younger age, and good nutritional status. When surgical decompression is indicated, surgery must be done at the earliest possible moment. Decompression done after 1 year rarely produces good results.

In paraplegia of healed disease, the pathology is mechanical compression; surgical decompression is mandatory (Fig. 79-11B). The prognosis is less favorable and surgery is fraught with complications (13).

RADIOLOGY FINDINGS

Plain Radiography

Radiographic appearance changes depend on the type of body lesion, severity of involvement, and stage of the disease. Osteoporosis of the vertebral body with haziness of margins of the adjacent vertebrae and narrowing of disc space are the initial findings in paradiscal lesions (Fig. 79-12A). Progressive destruction of the vertebral bodies are noted in advanced lesions, leading to gross kyphosis (Fig. 79-12B). Posterior spinal disease can be missed easily and AP radiographs are more useful in early

TABLE 79-2. *Stages of Potts paraplegia*

Patient has no symptoms; physician detects plantar
  extensor response or ankle clonus
    ↓
Patient has incoordination but can walk with support
    ↓
Paraparesis severe enough to confine the patient to bed
    ↓
Paraplegia in extension with variable level of sensory
  blunting
    ↓
Paraplegia in flexion with sphincter involvement
    ↓
Flaccid paraplegia

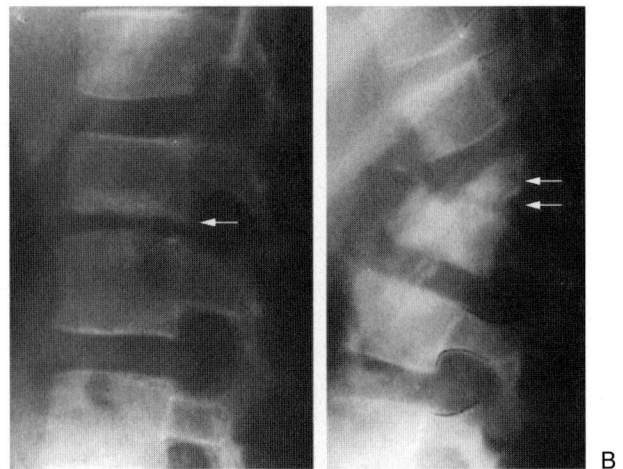

FIG. 79-12. A: Reduction of disc space with irregularity of the vertebral margins is the earliest radiologic sign. B: With progression of the disease, complete destruction of the vertebral bodies occur leading to a kyphotic deformity.

diagnosis than lateral radiographs (Fig. 79-13, A–C). Cold abscesses are seen as fusiform paravertebral shadows in the dorsal lesion and a bulge of the lateral margins of the psoas shadow in the lumbar lesions. After the start of chemotherapy, radiologic changes of healing usually

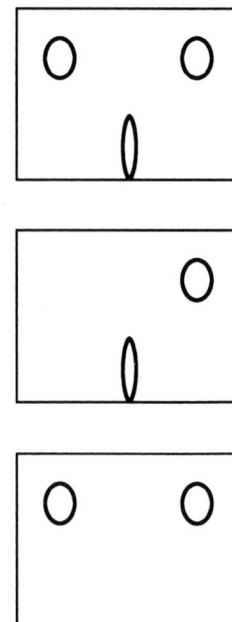

FIG. 79-13. A: In the antero-posterior radiographs, a normal vertebra has two pedicles and a spinous process resembling the eyes and the beak of an owl. A lesion of the spinous process gives rise to a loss of the beak, and a destructive lesion of the pedicle gives the appearance of a "winking" owl sign. B: Destruction of a pedicle as shown in the figure leads to loss of a pedicle, resulting in the "winking owl" sign. C: A lesion of the spinous process leads to the loss of the beak, resulting in a "beakless" owl sign.

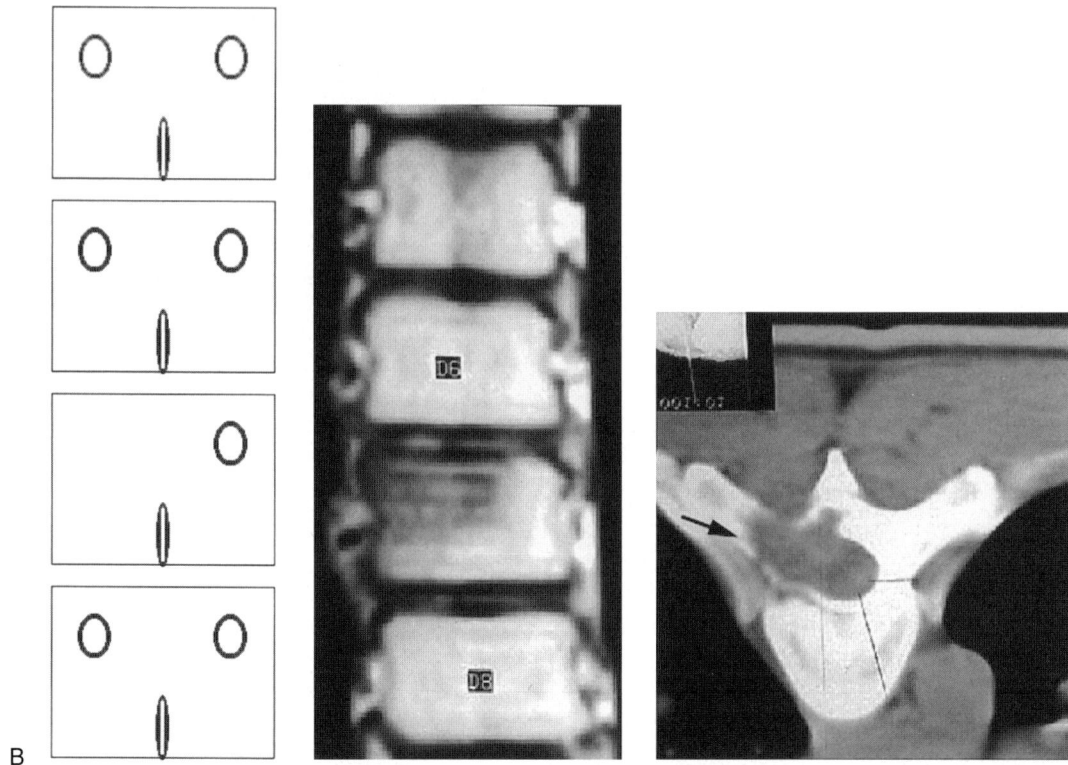

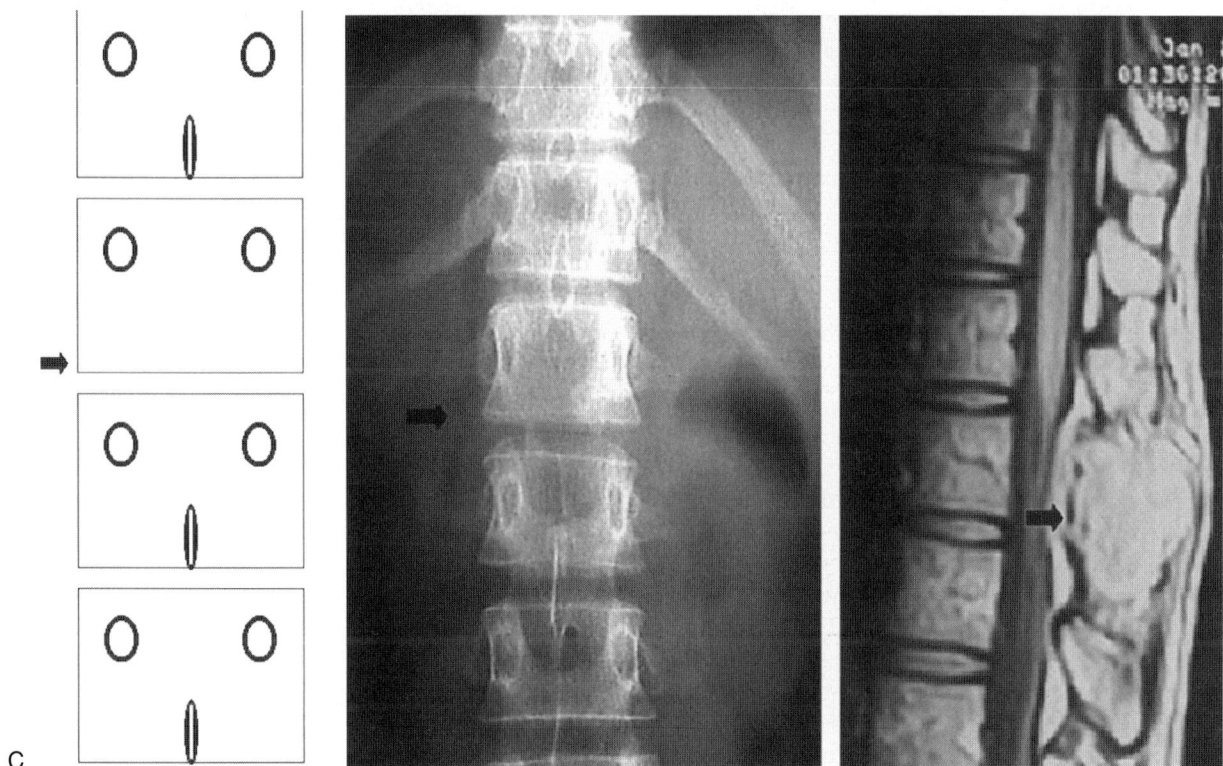

FIG. 79-13. (*Continued*). **B:** Destruction of a pedicle as shown in the figure leads to loss of a pedicle, resulting in the "winking owl" sign. **C:** A lesion of the spinous process leads to the loss of the beak, resulting in a "beakless" owl sign.

lag by 6 to 8 weeks after clinical improvement is noticed. Decrease in osteoporosis and sclerosis of the margins of the destroyed vertebra are the first signs of good response to treatment.

Computed tomography scans are useful in assessing the extent of bony destruction and the early diagnosis of lesions not easily visualized by plain radiography, such as those involving the craniovertebral and cervicodorsal junction, sacroiliac joint, sacrum, and posterior spinal disease.

Magnetic resonance imaging is superior in defining the extent of soft-tissue mass in both the sagittal and coronal planes and clearly differentiates the nature and extent of compression of the spinal cord (Fig. 79-11 A,B). Magnetic resonance imaging is of special use in the evaluation of the cause of compression in patients with neurologic deficit and in pure intramedullary and isolated extradural disease. Although MRI can strongly suggest tuberculosis, it is important to remember that there are no specific findings that can conclusively differentiate tuberculosis from other spinal infections or neoplasm. Gadolinium enhancement helps to accurately delineate the abscess wall from the compressed dura and localize portions of paraspinal masses most likely to yield a positive percutaneous biopsy. It is also well to remember that MRI often shows an exaggerated picture of the involvement because of signal intensity changes related to marrow edema and assessment of the extent of vertebral destruction is more accurately done by assessment from plain radiographs.

Radioisotope scans that are useful in pyogenic osteomyelitis are negative in one third of patients with tuberculosis. Gallium scans also are negative in the majority of patients, and their diagnostic value in tuberculosis is limited.

DIAGNOSIS

A typical clinical picture of insidious onset of pain in the region of involvement, paraspinal muscle spasm with restriction of spinal movements, low-grade constitutional symptoms, and a typical radiologic picture of paradiscal type of involvement of adjacent vertebrae is considered sufficient evidence clinically tò start specific antituberculous therapy in most endemic areas. Relative lymphocytosis with elevated erythrocyte sedimentation rate and a positive enzyme-linked immunosorbent assay (ELISA) test may contribute to the diagnosis, but is normal in many patients with good nutrition. The work-up must include a thorough clinical examination and tests to rule out extraskeletal involvement, which may be present in 15% of patients. In parts of the world where the incidence of tuberculosis is rare and whenever the diagnosis is in doubt, histologic confirmation by a CT-guided biopsy should be the procedure of choice. The material obtained by a thin needle routinely used for fine-needle aspiration

cytology (FNAC) is usually insufficient and the use of a thicker needle (e.g., the Jamshidi needle) is recommended. Aspiration of a paravertebral abscess also helps to establish a diagnosis, but the yield for culture from the pus is low.

Tuberculous infections have to be differentiated from pyogenic discitis and brucellosis. Pyogenic discitis has a more precipitous presentation with severe pain, high fever, and profound clinical symptoms. The organism can be isolated either by a blood culture or from needle aspiration material. Brucellosis also is common in geographic regions where tuberculosis is endemic. Undulating fever, less vertebral destruction, new bone formation (even in the active stage of the disease), marked sclerosis, and a positive serologic test for brucella antigen help to clinch the diagnosis.

Central types of lesions and pedicle involvement have to be differentiated from secondaries and myeloma in elderly patients and lymphoma and eosinophilic granuloma in young patients. The presence of paravertebral mass in MRI and a rim enhancement sign in CT scan point toward a tuberculous infection.

TREATMENT

Modern antituberculosis drugs have made disease cure highly possible because of their ability to achieve adequate therapeutic concentration in caseous tissues and abscesses, and excellent results have been reported by conservative therapy alone (2,7,14–16). On the other hand, surgery has become safer, and has better outcomes when performed under chemotherapeutic cover, which has prompted new surgical approaches and procedures (17,18). The reasons advocated for surgery were earlier recovery owing to débridement of the disease focus, feasibility for correction of deformity, fusion with bone grafts, and the possibility of obtaining tissues for histologic confirmation. The conflicting claims prompted the international multicenter trials at the Medical Research Council, Great Britain. Their conclusions now form the basis of treatment in patients without neurologic deficit (Table 79-3) (7,14–18). Favorable status, defined as no residual neurologic impairment, sinuses, clinically evident abscess, or impairment of physical activities owing to the spinal lesion, and with radiologic quiescent disease was achieved equally by radical surgery and chemotherapy at 3 years; this was maintained at 10 years. The major advantage was that equal results could be achieved by chemotherapy in places were there was a dearth of surgical expertise, adequate anesthetic facilities, and a high postoperative standard. Also, perioperative mortality of about 4%, reported even in the hands of the originators of the surgery, could be avoided. The study in Madras, India, further proved that these results could be achieved even with short-course (9-month) chemotherapy (7,16). Ninety-eight percent of patients with chemotherapy

TABLE 79-3. *Conclusions of Medical Research Council trials*

Ambulant outpatient chemotherapy treatment is highly successful.

Daily addition of streptomycin is not necessary.

No extra benefit from rest in hospital.

No benefit from plaster jacket for first few months.

Débridement alone offers no advantage over ambulant chemotherapy.

Ambulant chemotherapy equals radical surgery in achieving of favorable status.

Radical surgery achieves favorable status quickly and has decreased tendency for progress in deformity.

Short-course chemotherapy with daily isoniazid and rifampicin for 9 months achieved higher rate (98%) of favorable status than radical surgery (88%) at 5 years.

Favorable status: No residual neurologic impairment, sinuses, clinically evident abscess, or impairment of physical activities owing to the spinal lesion and with radiologically quiscent disease.

Inclusion criteria: Patients with clinical and radiologic evidence of tuberculosis involving any vertebra from the first dorsal to the first sacrum and without neurologic involvement.

Exclusion criteria: Presence of severe extraspinal disease, tuberculous or nontuberculous or with a previous history of antituberculous chemotherapy or surgical intervention.

Bony fusion and the severity of deformity were not considered in the criteria for favorable status.

---

achieved a favorable status, compared with only 88% with radical surgery. The rate of occurrence of bony union and the extent of deformity was identical in both groups. Achievement of solid bony fusion was considered as a desirable end of treatment because it was firm evidence for cure of the disease. Also, the chance for the further progress of the deformity was minimal. However, the increased risk for disease recurrence in the absence of bony union has not been borne out in long-term follow-up. The absence of bony union has been found to be a risk factor for increased deformity in children but not adults (7).

TABLE 79-4. *Indications for surgery in patients without neurologic deficit (middle path regimen)*

Failure of clinical improvement after 6 to 10 weeks of treatment

Recurrence of disease

Primary drug resistance or history of irregular chemotherapy

To prevent deformity (Table 79-5)

Rare indications

To establish diagnosis (needed only when computed tomography-guided biopsy is inconclusive)

Patients with persistent sinuses and abscess

Tuberculosis of cervical spine with paravertebral abscess causing difficulty in deglutition and respiration

Source: Adapted from Tuli SM. Results of treatment of spinal tuberculosis by "Middle Path" regimen. J Bone Joint Surg 1975;57-B(1):13–23, with permission.

TABLE 79-5. *Risk factors for severe increase in deformity*

Patients less than 10 years of age and with "spine at risk" radiologic signs

An initial kyphotic angle of >30 degrees

Vertebral body loss of >1.5

Involvement of more than three vertebral bodies

Computed tomography scan showing involvement of both anterior and posterior structures

Children who have partial or no fusion during adolescent growth spurt

---

The main shortcoming of the Medical Research Council (MRC) trials has been the exclusion of deformity severity as an assessment criterion for favorable status. Fifteen percent of patients treated by chemotherapy alone may end up with an unacceptable degree of deformity, and about 3% may have a deformity in excess of 60° (2,5,7,9,10). These patients would benefit from surgery, where the deformity can be corrected and solid anterior bony fusion can be achieved. It is appropriate to advocate surgery selectively to this group, because the expertise and infrastructure required for it are not freely available where tuberculosis is endemic. In patients without neurologic deficit, Tuli has proposed the "middle path" regimen, which takes advantage of the efficacy of modern antituberculous drugs and offers surgery only to the most needy (Table 79-4) (21). Here ambulant chemotherapy is advocated in all patients and surgery is advocated selectively when there is recurrence of disease, possibility of severe deformity, or onset of neurologic deficit (Table 79-5). This protocol not only helps to prevent unnecessary surgery in most patients with spinal tuberculosis, but also offers the benefits of the surgery when needed. We have followed this principle as a routine in our clinical practice; in patients without neurologic deficit, fewer than 15% require surgery.

ANTITUBERCULOUS CHEMOTHERAPY

It is imperative that the chemotherapy regimen consists of combination chemotherapy and lasts an adequate duration of time, so that cure is established and emergence of resistant strains is prevented. Two phases of chemotherapy are ideal in skeletal tuberculosis to increase the success rate and prevent the emergence of drug-resistant strains: an intensive phase, consisting of chemotherapy with three or four drugs, followed by a continuation phase consisting two drugs.

The current recommendation for the treatment of adults, with or without HIV infection, is 300 mg of isoniazid (INH) per day, 600 mg of rifampicin per day, and 20 to 30 mg/kg of body weight per day of pyrazinamide. In this intensive phase, which is carried on for 2 months, ethambutol (or streptomycin for children, who are too young to be monitored for visual acuity) should be included when: (a) the severity of the lesion is extensive and there are complicating factors such as neurologic involvement; (b) the patient population has a high primary resistance to INH; and (c) there is a suspicion of drug resistance. After the 2-month intensive phase with either the three- or four-drug regimen, a continuation phase with INH and rifampicin can be continued for 9 to 12 months.

SURGERY FOR SPINAL TUBERCULOSIS

Although chemotherapy forms the mainstay of treatment, a surgical procedure may be indicated in the following situations:

1. To obtain material for establishing diagnosis in doubtful situations
2. To drain an abscess cavity around the spine or pelvis
3. To radically débride the entire focus and perform an anterior arthrodesis with bone grafts.
4. In addition to anterior arthrodesis, to also perform a posterior fusion with or without instrumentation, either primarily or as a second stage to obtain global fusion

Computed tomography–guided biopsy and percutaneous transpedicular biopsy procedures have made indications for open biopsy rare. Similarly, abscesses (however large) clear adequately with chemotherapy; surgical intervention is required only in rare circumstances. Other than retropharyngeal abscesses, which can present as clinical emergencies with dysphagia and dyspnea, even large abscesses in other regions usually are asymptomatic and rarely require intervention. When indicated, drainage

TABLE 79-6. *Factors leading to poor outcome after surgery*

Poor nutritional status
Surgery performed without chemotherapeutic cover
Vertebral body loss of >2
Junctional lesions (cervicothoracic and thoracolumbar)
Marked preoperative kyphosis
Use of grafts spanning more than two disc spaces
Spinal instability with radiological "spine at risk" signs

must be performed under the cover of antituberculous drugs and the wound must be carefully closed in layers.

Surgical procedures for obtaining disease clearance must involve complete débridement of focus and reconstruction of anterior defect with suitable bone grafts, with protection of the grafts by instrumentation whenever necessary. Débridement of the disease focus alone without addition of bone grafts gives poor results and does not add an advantage to the chemotherapy regimen. In performing a radical surgery procedure, it is important not to remove the entire bones that have been affected and to limit the débridement when the margins of the healthy bones are reached. Plain radiographs allow a better judgment of the extent of involvement than MRI. Magnetic resonance imaging studies show an exaggerated picture of bone involvement because of signal intensity changes in the marrow and may unnecessarily lead to a overly extensive débridement. Excessive removal of bone increases the deficit of the anterior column, and this leads to a high incidence of graft failure (7,20). Four types of

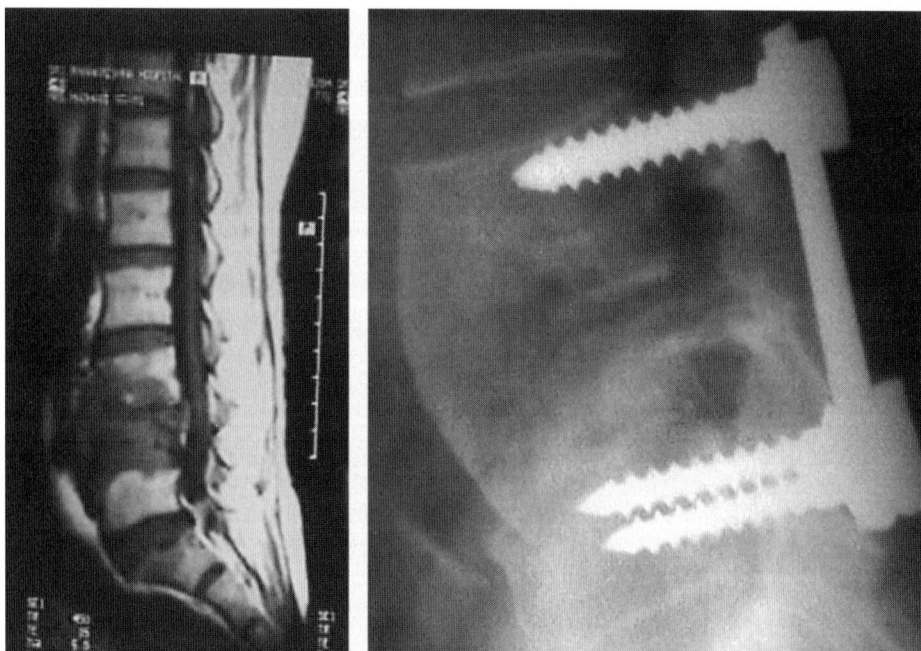

FIG. 79-14. Lumbar lesion in an adult with complete destruction of the fourth lumbar and partial involvement of the adjacent vertebrae. Fusion has been achieved with good incorporation of the tricortical iliac graft with posterior instrumentation performed in a single stage.

graft failures have been observed when the graft length exceeds two disc spaces: dislodgement, fracture, absorption, and subsidence, of which graft dislodgement is the most common (Table 79-6). Complications related to grafts are more common in the dorsal and dorsolumbar regions, and patients with one or more unfavorable factors benefit from additional posterior instrumentation and fusion, either as a single or second stage following anterior fusion (Fig. 79-14).

Spinal implants can be used safely in the presence of active tuberculous infections (21,22). Persistence of biomaterial-centered infections is caused by preferential bacterial colonization of the inert surfaces and production of a biofilm (glycocalyx), which protects them from the host defenses and chemotherapeutic agents. *Mycobacterium tuberculosis* is less adhesive and produces less biofilm than other bacteria; implants and titanium cages can be used safely to achieve good results (23).

TREATMENT IN PRESENCE OF NEUROLOGIC DEFICIT

All patients with neurologic complications warrant a thorough clinical and radiologic evaluation; the presence or absence of active infection influences patient management.

Paraplegia of active disease is caused by compression by inflammatory material and most patients respond to conservative therapy with rest and antituberculous drugs. Conservative regimen can be used confidently, especially in less privileged countries where adequate facilities for radical surgical treatment may not be available (24,25). Surgical decompression has been advocated because it may provide an earlier and higher rate of recovery, quick improvement in general condition, the reduction of deformity, and anterior spine fusion (26). Tuli has advocated a policy of selective surgical management where patients are treated with chemotherapy, bed rest, and surgery performed only for specific indications (2). Only less than 20% require surgical intervention; the remaining show good improvement with chemotherapy alone.

Surgical technique in the presence of active disease must involve complete decompression of the dura in the entire region of apex of the kyphosis and include bone-grafting procedures to prevent a collapse. Laminectomy as an isolated procedure has no role except in a rare patient in whom the lesion is confined to posterior structures and in patients with spinal tumor syndrome. The posterior approach is not an ideal route to decompress a lesion that lies anteriorly; laminectomy can completely destabilize the spine, resulting in rapid deterioration. Costotransversectomy is useful and safer in patients with very severe kyphosis and in centers where there is a lack of expertise to perform radical surgery. Paraplegia in healed disease is a much more difficult therapeutic problem and requires decompression of the spinal cord that is stretched over the internal gibbus. Anterior decompression with removal of the internal gibbus is the treatment of choice, but it is a technically difficult surgery and the outcome is less satisfactory in comparison to those obtained in paraplegia with active disease (13).

REFERENCES

1. Satyasri S. Global epidemiology of tuberculosis. In: Sathya Sri S, ed. Textbook of pulmonary and extra-pulmonary tuberculosis. Madras, India: Interprint, 1993:13–18.
2. Tuli SM. Tuberculosis of the skeletal system. New Delhi, India: Jaypee Brothers Medical Publications, 1991.
3. Rajasekaran S. A longitudinal study on the progress of deformity in children with spinal tuberculosis. PhD thesis. The Tamil Nadu Medical University, Chennai, India, 1999.
4. Kumar KA. Clinical study and classification of posterior spinal tuberculosis. Int Orthop 1985;9:147–152.
5. Rajasekaran S. The natural history of post tubercular kyphosis in children. J Bone Joint Surg (Br) 2001;83.B:954–962.
6. Rajasekaran S, Dheenadayalan J, Shetty DK, et al. Tuberculosis lesions of the lumbosacral region. A 15 year follow-up of patients treated by ambulant chemotherapy. Spine 1998;23(10):1163–1167.
7. Parthasarathy R, Sriram K, Santha T, et al. Short course chemotherapy for tuberculosis of the spine: a comparison between ambulant treatment and radical surgery: ten year report. J Bone Joint Surg (Br) 1999; 81(3):464–471.
8. Leventhal HR. Birth injuries of the spinal cord. J Pediatr 1960;56: 557–563.
9. Moon MS, Lee MK. The changes of the kyphosis of the tuberculous spine in children following ambulant treatment. J Korean Orthop Assoc 1971;6:189–195.
10. Tuli SM. Severe kyphotic deformity in tuberculosis of the Spine. Int Orthop (SICOT) 1995;19:327–331.
11. White A, Panjabi M, Thomas CL, et al. The clinical bio-mechanics of Kyphotic deformity. Clin Orthop 1977;128:8–17.
12. Moon MS. Spine update: tuberculosis of the spine, controversies and a new challenge. Spine 1997;22(15):1791–1797.
13. Hsu LCS, Cheng CC, Leong JCY. Pott's paraplegia of late onset: the causes of compression and results after anterior decompression. J Bone Joint Surg 1988;70B:534–538.
14. Medical Research Council Working Party on Tuberculosis of the Spine. A 10-year assessment of controlled trials of inpatient and outpatient treatment and a plaster of Paris jackets for tuberculosis of the spine in children on standard chemotherapy. Studies in Masan and Pusan, Korea. J Bone Joint Surg 1985;67B:103–110.
15. Medical Research Council Working Party on Tuberculosis of the Spine. Controlled trial of short course regimens of chemotherapy in the ambulatory treatment of spinal tuberculosis. J Bone Joint Surg 1993;75-B:240–248.
16. Indian Council of Medical Research/British Medical Research Council. A controlled trial of short course regimen of chemotherapy in patients receiving ambulatory treatment or undergoing radical surgery for tuberculosis of the spine. Ind J Tuberculosis 1989;36: 1–21.
17. Medical Research Council Working Party on Tuberculosis of the Spine. A controlled trial of anterior spinal fusion and débridement in the surgical management of tuberculosis of the spine in patients on standard chemotherapy. Br J Surg 1974;61:853–866.
18. Medical Research Council. A 5 year assessment of controlled trials of ambulatory treatment, débridement and anterior spinal fusion in the management of tuberculosis of the spine. Studies in Bulawayo (Rhodesia) and in Hong Kong. VI Report. J Bone Joint Surg 1978;60B: 163–177.
19. Tuli SM. Results of treatment of spinal tuberculosis by 'middle-path' regimen. J Bone Joint Surg 1975;57-B(1):13–23.
20. Rajasekaran S, Soundarapandian S. Progression of kyphosis in tuberculosis of the spine treated by anterior arthrodesis. J Bone Joint Surg 1989;71-A:1314–1323.
21. Oga M, Arizona T, Takasita M, et al. Evaluation of the risk of instrumentation as a foreign body in spinal tuberculosis. Clinical and biological study. Spine 1993;18(13):1890–1894.

22. Gristina AG, Costerton JW. Bacterial adherence to biomaterials and tissue. The significance of its role in clinical sepsis. J Bone Joint Surg (Am) 1985;67(2):264–273.
23. Louw JA. Spinal tuberculosis with neurological deficit. J Bone Joint Surg 1990;72B:686–693.
24. Rajeshwari R, Balasubramanian R, Venkatesan P, et al. Short course chemotherapy in the treatment of Pott's paraplegia. Int J Tuberculosis Lung Dis 1997;1:152–158.
25. Jain AK, Kumar S, Tuli SM. Tuberculosis of the spine. Spinal Cord 1999;37(5):362–369.
26. Hodgson AR, Skinsnes OK, Leong CY. The pathogenesis of Pott's paraplegia. J Bone Joint Surg 1967;49A:1147–1156.

CHAPTER 80

Postoperative Lumbar Spine Infections

Eric C. Chamberlin and Edward N. Hanley Jr.

Despite continuing advances in medicine and surgery, there remains a quantifiable risk of infection in lumbar spine surgery. Since the advent of antibiotics and the use of aseptic technique, there have been continuing improvements in the prevention of perioperative infection. However, coincident with improvement in prophylaxis came increases in surgical complexity and operative times, which may have served to mitigate the positive effects of these improvements. Postsurgical infection, although relatively infrequent, can be a major cause of morbidity in the patient undergoing lumbar spine surgery.

INCIDENCE

Multiple studies have addressed the incidence of infection after spine surgery, with reported values between 0% and 11.3% depending on the study and procedure performed (1–16). Reported infection rates are approximately 2% in uninstrumented fusions and 7% for instrumented spinal fusions. As might be expected, the lowest incidence of infection has been reported in isolated disc excision surgery at less than 1%. Weinstein et al. published a .86% incidence of infection in simple discectomy procedures in their 9-year experience with 2,391 spinal operations (2).

The incidence of infection tends to increase as the complexity of the procedure and operative time increase. Massie et al. found a 1.3% incidence of infection in 376 noninstrumented spine fusions and 6.6% in 258 instrumented fusions (3). Multiple other studies have supported their conclusions. Spinal fusion without instrumentation has a reported risk of .4% to 5% (2,3). Instrumented fusions increase the incidence to .06 to 11.9%, depending on the study (1–10,12–16). Many risk factors have been identified that increase the incidence of infection.

ETIOLOGY: PATIENT AND SURGICAL FACTORS

Patient

Multiple risk factors have been established that tend to increase the potential for infection in spine surgery patients. Factors such as diabetes mellitus, obesity, malnutrition, smoking, previous or ongoing metachronous infection, rheumatoid arthritis, and iatrogenic or other states of immunodeficiency all have been implicated as predisposing to infection (2,4,11,12,17–22).

Diabetes is associated with an increased incidence of infective complications with many types of surgery. Wimmer et al. reported an increased incidence of infection in patients with diabetes in a retrospective review of 850 spine surgery cases (11). This may result from the cardiovascular, peripheral vascular, renal, and immune effects of the disease as well as the altered glucose metabolism.

Obesity has been shown to increase the incidence of postoperative complications including infection (11). Karduan found that the complication rate correlated with obesity in a study of patients undergoing discectomy (23). However, other articles call obesity into doubt as an independent risk factor. Andreshak found in a prospective study of 159 patients, 55 of whom were obese, no difference in infection rates between groups. The discrepancy in the literature in part may result from differing definitions of obesity. In general, the preponderance of the literature suggests a connection between infection and obesity in those patients with morbid obesity (23,24).

The nutritional state of the patient has been shown to be crucial to the ability to heal wounds and resist infection (19,21). Klein found a strong correlation between nutrition and postoperative infection with 10 of 13 malnourished patients in a group of 114 becoming infected. Nutrition is important in both the presurgical and postsurgical period because of the catabolic state caused by the surgery and the usual poor caloric intake associated with the perioperative period. Several markers of nutritional fitness have been suggested for use in patient evaluation. Total lymphocyte count of less than 1,500, albumin of less than 3.4, and weight loss of more than 10 pounds are all useful markers of malnutrition and can be used both preoperatively and postoperatively to monitor and optimize patient caloric intake (25).

Smoking has been shown to increase the incidence of infection as well as decrease fusion rates (26,27). Thalgott found 90% of patients with wound infection following spine fusion to be smokers. These patients also showed an increases incidence of myonecrosis within the infected wound (27).

Surgery

Efforts to control the surgical factors that contribute to the incidence of infection have been continuously studied and implemented since the time of Lister. Although clouds of carbolic acid have given way to monitored air exchange, the operative environment, operative team, and patients themselves are common sources of the offending organisms. The incidence of infection increases with longer duration operations and increased operating room traffic (2,11). Both of these factors provide opportunities for wound contamination. They also allow a greater likelihood of shedding of organisms both from the patient and staff (28).

Increasing the number of operative personnel and traffic in the room significantly increases the bacterial colony counts in the operating room (29,30). Efforts should be made to eliminate excess traffic in the room, as often is done in arthroplasty procedures. Laminar flow with an air exchange rate of at least 25 times an hour has been shown to reduce colony counts in the operating room (31).

Studies have shown that over time, the skin recolonizes after surgical preparation. The source of the recolonization appears to be the hair follicles. Some have advocated re-prepping patients periodically during long cases. Zdeblick et al. reported povidone-iodine scrub and paint inferior to paint alone in decreasing bacterial counts. There were no infections in either group in their study. Night before surgery showers with hexachlorophene also decreased bacterial colony counts (32). Others have stressed the importance of shaving the patient in the immediate preoperative period. Shaving the night before surgery has been implicated in an increased incidence of infection (29).

As stated, there is an increased incidence of infection in instrumented fusions versus noninstrumented fusions. The reason for this association is most likely multifactorial. Length of procedure has been shown to be an independent influence on infection, and in general is increased with instrumentation placement. The other

important consideration is the implant itself. Instrumentation is a good medium for bacterial adherence, decreasing the host's ability to clear colonized bacteria and prevent infection. Chang stated that instrumentation acts as a nidus for bacteria, which secrete a glycocalyx. The glycocalyx serves to allow more effective colonization and protects the bacteria from the effects of antibiotics (33).

Another key advance in the decreased incidence of infection is the use of preoperative antibiotics. Although there is no universal standard regimen, studies suggest that antibiotics dosed one half to 2 hours before skin incision decrease the incidence of infection (34). The most common antibiotic used is a first-generation cephalosporin such as cephalexin. Cephalexin is excellent against gram-positive organisms and has good activity against *Escherichia coli* and *Proteus* species. Cephalexin also has the longest half-life of the first-generation cephalosporins in serum and bone. The one area that may have decreased concentrations of cephalexin is the nucleus pulposus, whose high concentration of positively charged glycosaminoglycans repels the positively charged cefazolin (35).

Boscardin tested the efficacy of cefazolin for prophylaxis of postoperative discitis. In 40 patients, serum and intradiscal samples were taken at intervals. They found that cefazolin does enter the disc and is at optimum level 15 to 80 minutes following a 2-gram dose (36).

Because of the relative frequency of gram-negative infections reported with lumbar spine surgery, some authors recommend adding gentamicin or another gram-negative effective antibiotic. Gentamicin also is negatively charged and may have better penetration of the nucleus pulposus for reasons stated previously (35). Dimick, in a review of antimicrobial prophylaxis, concluded that cefazolin should be dosed within 30 minutes of incision, redosed for blood loss greater than 1,500 cc or for duration of greater than 4 hours, and not given for more than 24 hours postoperatively. Dimick suggested the need for randomized controlled trials before adding other agents such as gentamicin to the standard prophylaxis (35).

Microbiology

Most studies show a preponderance of gram-positive (primarily staphylococcus skin flora) organisms in spine surgery perioperative infections (2,9,35). However, Massie et al. found a significant number of gram-negative and -positive organisms in their study population. Enterobacter, serratia, pseudomonas, Acinetobacter, bacteroides, and clostridium represented the gram-negative organisms. Other gram-positive organisms were enterococcus faecalis, strep viridans and epidermidis, diphtheroids, propionibacter, Peptococcus, and Peptostreptococcus. A large number of the infections were polymicrobial, which may have been due to the postoperative regimen of body casts and long hospital stays (3).

Rechtine reported in a study of 12 infections associated with instrumented fusions for spine fractures, nine deep, and three superficial infections. Two were gram-positive only infections. Both of these were superficial infections. Three were gram-negative only infections and seven were multiple organisms. All of the deep infections were either gram-negative or multiple organisms (4).

Brook and Frazier found a large number of different organisms on aspiration of spine wound infections. They found 36% aerobic, 16% anaerobic, and 48% mixed flora. Predominant aerobes included *E. coli* and proteus species; anaerobes included Bacteroides, and Peptostreptococcus. They found increased bacteroides and *E. coli* infections in incontinent patients (37).

The reason for the relatively high incidence of polymicrobial and gram-negative infections reported in lumbar spine surgery is not known. Perry found a high incidence of gram-negative aerobic bacilli in patients undergoing procedures to the sacrum and in those with urinary incontinence (12). Some possible explanations include the common use of only a first-generation cephalosporin for prophylaxis, and the proximity of the incision to the perineum.

Diagnostic Work-up

Presentation

Superficial infections (located beneath the dermis and subcutaneous tissues and above the fascia) present most often with tenderness and local erythema, drainage, and fluctuance. Deep infections (deep to the fascia) often are more difficult to diagnose because of a lack of findings typical of infection. Patients may experience a deep back or radicular-type pain and malaise, and usually are febrile (3). Weinstein noted only 14 of 46 patients had pyrexia at presentation for infection (2). A high index of suspicion must be maintained, especially in patients with unexplained fevers. Because of the effects of pus under pressure and often a delay in diagnosis, these infections are characterized by a greater degree of tissue necrosis, and patients are more likely to be systemically affected.

Blood laboratory studies are the first step in the workup of patient suspected of having a postoperative infection. The white blood cell count may or may not be elevated early in the infection. A left shift in the differential is often present. The primary markers of infection are the erythrocyte sedimentation rate (ESR) and C-reactive protein (CRP). Studies have clearly delineated the timing of rise and fall of these blood markers (38–40). Thelander found that the CRP peaks at 2- to days following spine surgery and returns to normal at 5 to 14 days. The ESR peaks at 5 to 7 days and returns to normal at around 21 to 42 days (39). A peak outside of these parameters is suggestive of infection. Meyer found that with serial testing to day 5 following disc surgery, CRP was the most sensitive and specific marker (Table 80-1).

TABLE 80-1. *Comparison of c-reactive protein (CRP), erythrocyte sedimentation rate (ESR), and complete blood count (CBC) as markers of infection*

	Sensitivity	Specificity
CRP	100%	95.8%
ESR	78.1%	38.1%
CBC	21.4%	76.8%

Adapted from Meyer B, Schaller K, Rohde V, et al. The C-reactive protein for detection of early infections after lumbar microdiscectomy. *Acta Neurochirurgica* 1995;136(3–4):145–150, with permission.

Sterile aspiration is advocated in patients with suspected deep infection (febrile, increased WBC with shift and a benign-appearing wound). Vigilant and aggressive monitoring of the postoperative spine patient can prevent unnecessary delay in diagnosis of infection.

The principal imaging diagnostic tool for postoperative infection of the lumbar spine is MRI. Magnetic resonance imaging finds fluid collections and bone and tissue edema as increased signal intensity on T2-weighted images. Because of the ability of MRI to precisely localize an abscess, it may be superior to aspiration for the evaluation of the patient suspected of having a postoperative abscess (41).

Treatment

The primary treatment for a postoperative wound infection in the lumbar spine is surgical drainage of purulent material and complete débridement of all necrotic and grossly infected tissues (42). The débridement should progress systematically from superficial to deep by lay-

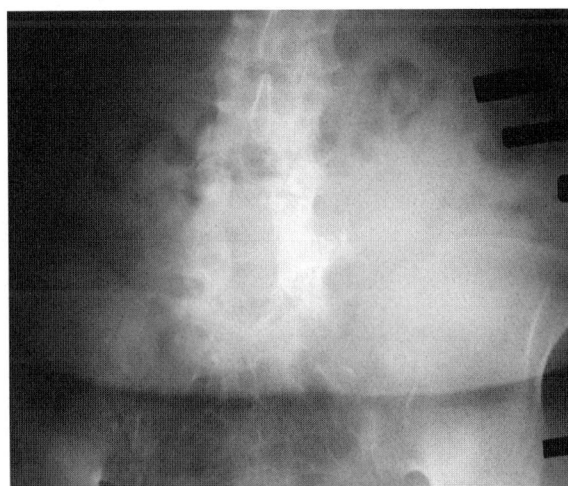

FIG. 80-1. Antero-posterior radiographs of a 54-year-old woman with back pain and neurogenic claudication. She had previously undergone decompressive surgery at L4-5 and L5-S1 and suffered from chronic renal failure caused by glomerulosclerosis.

Broad-spectrum antibiotics should be started once intraoperative cultures have been obtained. The antibiotic coverage is then narrowed according to the culture and sensitivity results.

In general, wounds can be closed over closed suction drainage (31). Dernbach treated 10 patients with postoperative deep infections with I&D, antibiotics, and closure over large suction drains; all healed (43). However, in some cases the loss of soft tissue or the severity of infection may dictate leaving the wound open and either packing it open or placing a wound vacuum (Figs. 80-1 through 80-4). Weinstein obtained primary closure in

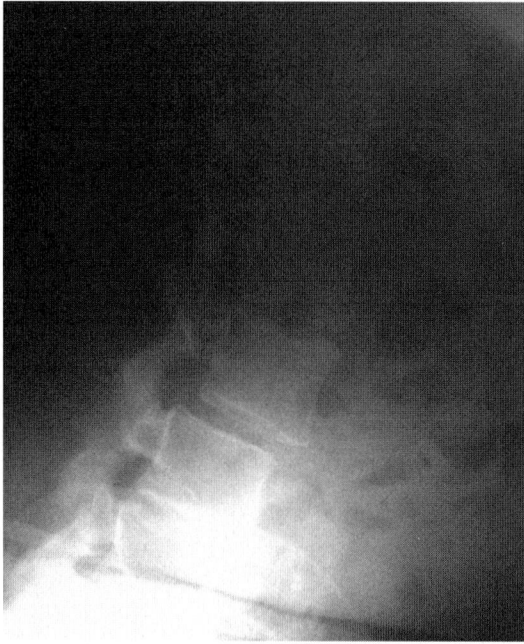

FIG. 80-2. Lateral radiographs of a 54-year-old woman with back pain and neurogenic claudication. She had previously undergone decompressive surgery at L4-5 and L5-S1 and suffered from chronic renal failure caused by glomerulosclerosis.

ers. A sequential progression of the débridement helps to avoid infecting potentially unaffected lower levels (3,31).

The literature is inconclusive as to the optimal treatment of infected implants. Bone graft may be left in place if not grossly contaminated and, in general, removal of implants that would lead to an unstable spine may be delayed until fusion has occurred (2). Often more than one operation may be necessary to eradicate the infection. The instrumentation should be removed in a late infection in which fusion has occurred.

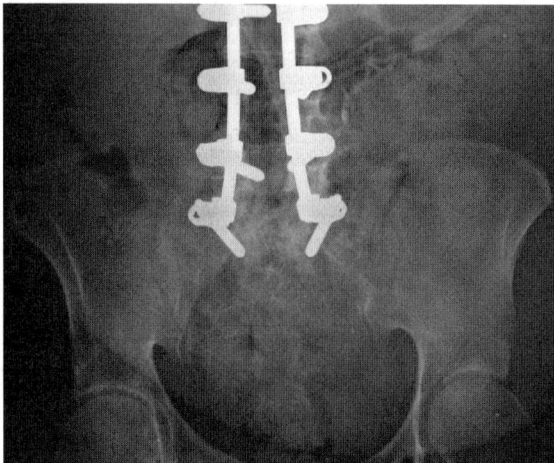

FIG. 80-3. Antero-posterior lumbar spine following repeat decompression and instrumented fusion surgery.

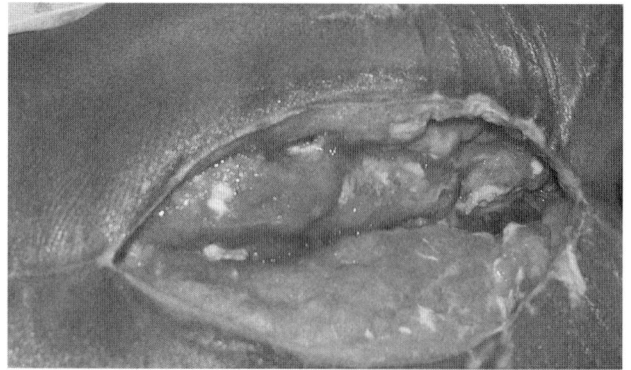

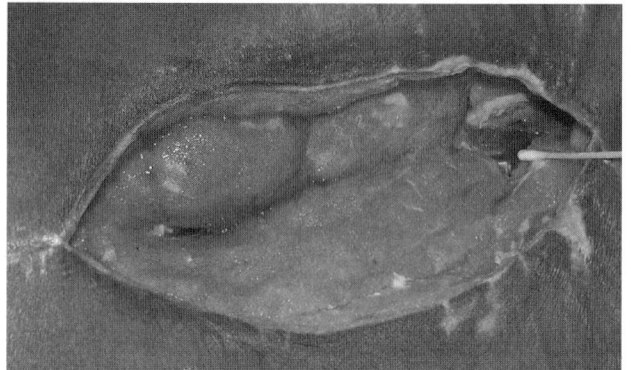

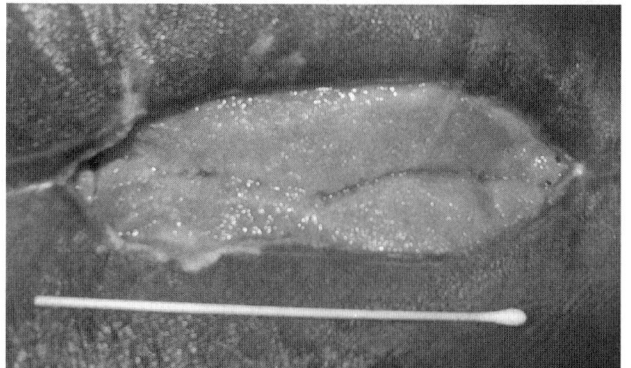

FIG. 80-4. A: Deep wound infection after débridement at beginning of subatmospheric wound vacuum dressing treatment. **B:** After 4 days. **C:** After 22 days.

only seven of 22 infections; all others underwent delayed closure (2).

Multiple studies have shown the efficacy of vacuum wound coverage (44–46). Argenta noted that subatmospheric pressure treatment removes chronic edema, leading to increased localized blood flow and resulting in an increased rate of granulation tissue formation (44). Fortunately, the muscle and soft-tissue envelope is substantial around back wounds, allowing many options for local flap coverage of defects (47–49).

OUTCOMES AND SEQUELAE OF LUMBAR SPINE INFECTIONS

Postoperative lumbar spine infections are an infrequent, but important, source of morbidity and mortality. These infections also have further ramifications for the health care system. Capen et al. estimate that an infection increases the cost of treatment more than four times. The average cost of a postoperative infection of the lumbar spine in their study was over $100,000. Five of 11 patients with infections went on to pseudarthrosis, and only 20% returned to work (50).

Weiss et al. studied the incidence of pseudarthrosis after postoperative wound infection in the lumbar spine. After successful débridement, 62.1% had successful arthrodesis. They found that female sex, allograft use, and extension of the fusion to the sacrum increase the rate of pseudarthrosis following postoperative infection of the lumbar spine (51).

In a direct comparison of 11 patients with low back fusion complicated by infection versus 15 patients with fusion and without infection, Calderone found a clear difference in fusion rates, but uniformly poor return rates and poor ratings of quality of life. These results are tempered by the fact that these were workers' compensation cases, but still suggest poor outcomes with infection and reinforce the finding of decreased fusion rates found in other studies (52).

CONCLUSION

Postoperative lumbar spine infections are detrimental to the patient as well as the medical system as a whole. A quantifiable incidence of infection remains despite advances in technique and prophylaxis. In order to decrease the morbidity associated with these complications, a high degree of suspicion must be maintained by the spine surgeon during the postoperative period. Prompt diagnosis followed by meticulous and aggressive débridement as well as appropriate antibiotics are essential to eradicate the infection and prevent further damage. The infection and soft-tissue wound can in most cases be controlled; despite this, there remains an increase in the rate of pseudarthrosis and functional impairment.

REFERENCES

1. Sponseller PD, LaPorte DM, Hungerford MW, et al. Deep wound infections after neuromuscular scoliosis surgery: a multicenter study of risk factors and treatment outcomes. Spine 2000;25(19):2461–2466.
2. Weinstein MA, McCabe JP, Cammissa FP Jr. Postoperative spinal wound infection: a review of 2,391 consecutive index procedures. J Spinal Disord 2000;13(5):422–426.
3. Massie JB, Heller JG, Abitbol JJ, et al. Postoperative posterior spinal wound infections. Clin Orthop Rel Res 1992;284:99–108.
4. Rechtine GR, Bono PL, Cahill D, et al. Postoperative wound infection after instrumentation of thoracic and lumbar fractures. J Orthop Trauma 2001;15(8):566–569.
5. Eck KR, Bridwell KH, Ungacta FF, et al. Complications and results of long adult deformity fusions down to L4, L5 and the sacrum. Spine 2001;26(9):E182–E191.
6. Capen DA, Calderone RR, Green A. Perioperative risk factors for wound infections after lower back fusions. Orthop Clin North Am 1996;27(1):83–86.
7. Hee HT, Castro FP Jr, Mafd ME, et al. Anterior/posterior lumbar fusion versus transforaminal lumbar interbody fusion: analysis of complications and predictive factors. J Spinal Disord 2001;14(6):533–540.
8. Aydinli U, Karaeminogullari O, Tiskaya K. Postoperative deep wound infections in instrumented spinal surgery. Acta Orthop Belg 1999;65 (2):182–187.
9. Wimmer C, Nogler M, Frischhut B. Influence of antibiotics on infection in spinal surgery: a prospective study of 110 patients. J Spinal Disord 1998;11(6):498–500.
10. Hodges SD, Humphrey SC, Eck JC, et al. Low postoperative infection rates with instrumented fusions. South Med J 1998;91(12):1132–1136.
11. Wimmer C, Gluch H, Franzreb M, et al. Predisposing factors for infection in spine surgery. J Spinal Disord 1998;11(2):124–128.
12. Perry JW, Montgomery JZ, Swank S, et al. Wound infections following spinal fusion with posterior segmental spinal instrumentation. Clin Infect Dis 1997;24(4):558–561.
13. Abbey DM, Turner DM, Warson JS, et al. Treatment of postoperative wound infections following spinal fusion with instrumentation. J Spinal Disord 1995;8(4):278–283.
14. West JL III, Ogilvie JW, Bradford DS. Complications of the variable screw plate pedicle screw fixation. Spine 1991;16(5):576–579.
15. Esses SI, Sachs BL, Dreyzin V. Complications associated with the technique of pedicle screw fixation. A selected survey of ABS members. Spine 1993;18(15):2238–2239.
16. Dave SH, Meyers DL. Complications of lumbar spinal fusion with transpedicular instrumentation. Spine 17(6 Suppl):S184–189.
17. Andreshak TG, An HS, Hall J, et al. Lumbar spine surgery in the obese patient. J Spinal Disord 1997;10(5):376–379.
18. Viola RW, King HA, Adler SM, et al. Delayed infection after elective spinal instrumentation and fusion. A retrospective review of eight cases. Spine 1997;22(20):2450–2451.
19. Klein JD, Hey LA, Klein BB, et al. Perioperative nutrition and postoperative complications in patients undergoing spinal surgery. Spine 1996;22(21):2676–2682.
20. Swank SM, Lonstein JE, Moe JH, et al. Surgical treatment of adult scoliosis. J Bone Joint Surg 1981;63AS:268.
21. Klein JD, Garfin SR. Nutritional status in the patient with spinal infections. Orthop Clin North Am 1996;27(1):33–36.
22. Heary RF, Hunt CD, Krieger AJ, et al. HIV status does not affect microbiologic spectrum or neurologic outcome in spinal infections. Surg Neurol 1994;42(5):417–423.
23. Karduan JW, White LR, Shaffer WO. Acute complications in patients with surgical treatment of lumbar herniated disc. J Spinal Disord 1990;3(1):30–38.
24. Cronquist AB, Jakob K, Lai L, et al. Relationship between skin microbacterial counts and surgical site infection after neurosurgery. Clin Infect Dis 2001;33(8):1302–1308.
25. Jensen JE, Jensen TG, Jensen JE. Nutrition in orthopedic surgery. J Bone Joint Surg 1982;84(A):1263–1272.
26. Porter SE, Hanley EN. The musculoskeletal effects of smoking. J AAOS 2001;9(1):9–17.
27. Thalgott JS, Colter HB, Sasso RC, et al. Postoperative infections in spinal implants. Classification and analysis—a multicenter study. Spine 1991;16(8):981–984.

28. Ritter MA. Surgical wound environment. Clin Orthop 1984;190:11–13.

29. Cruse PJ, Foord R. A five year prospective study of 23,649 surgical wounds. Arch Surg 1973;107:206–209.

30. Bethune DW, Blowers R, Parker M, et al. Dispersal of staphylococcus aureus by patients and operating room staff. Lancet 1976;40:480–483.

31. Heller JG, Levine MJ. Postoperative infections of the spine. Semin Spine Surg 1996;8(2):105–114.

32. Zdeblick TA, Lederman MM, Jacobs MR, et al. Preoperative use of povidone-iodine. A prospective, randomized study. Clin Orthop Rel Res 1986;(213):211–215.

33. Chang CC, Merritt K. Infection at the site of implanted materials with and without preadhered bacteria. J Orthop Res 1994;12:526–531.

34. Classen DC, Evans RS, Pestotnik SL, et al. The timing of prophylactic antibiotics and the risk of surgical-wound infection. N Engl J Med 1992;326:281–286.

35. Dimick JB, Lipsett PA, Kostuik JP. Spine update: antimicrobial prophylaxis in spine surgery: basic principles and recent advances. Spine 2000;25(19):2544–2548.

36. Boscardin JB, Ringus JC, Feingold DJ, et al. Human intradiscal levels with cefazolin. Spine 1992;17(6 Suppl):S145–148.

37. Brook I, Frazier EH. Aerobic and anaerobic microbiology of surgical-site infection following spinal fusion. J Clin Microbiol 1999;37(3):841–843.

38. Meyer B, Schaller K, Rohde V, et al. The C-reactive protein for detection of early infections after lumbar microdiscectomy. Acta Neurochirurg 1995;136(3–4):145–150.

39. Thelander U, Larrson S. Quantitation of C-reactive protein levels and erythrocyte sedimentation rate after spinal surgery. Spine 1992;17(4):400–404.

40. Jonsson B, Soderholm R, Stromqvist B. Erythrocyte sedimentation rate after lumbar spine surgery. Spine 1991;16(9):1049–1050.

41. Rothman SL. The diagnosis of infections of the spine by modern imaging techniques. Orthop Clin North Am 1996;27(1):15–31.

42. Rubayi S. Wound management in spinal infection. Orthop Clin North Am 1996;27(1):137–153.

43. Dernbach PD, Gomez H, Hahn J. Primary closure of infected spinal wounds. Neurosurgery 1990;26(4):707–709.

44. Argenta LC, Morykwas MJ. Vacuum-assisted closure: a new method for wound control and treatment: clinical experience. Ann Plastic Surg 1997;38(6):563–576.

45. Morykwas MJ, Argenta LC, Shelton-Brown EI, et al. Vacuum-assisted closure: a new method for wound control and treatment: animal studies and basic foundation. Ann Plastic Surg 1997;38(6):553–562.

46. Philbeck TE, Whittington KT, Millsap MH, et al. The clinical and cost effectiveness of externally applied negative pressure wound therapy in the treatment of wounds in home healthcare medicare patients. Ostomy/Wound Manage 1999;45(11):41–50.

47. Hochberg J, Ardenghy M, Yuen J, et al. Muscle and musculocutaneous flap coverage of exposed spinal fusion devices. Plastic Reconstruct Surg 1998;102(2):385–389.

48. Wendt JR, Gardner VO, White JI. Treatment of complex postoperative lumbosacral wounds in nonparalyzed patients. Plastic Reconstruct Surg 1997;10(6):482–487.

49. Ramasastry SS. Muscle and musculocutaneous flap coverage of exposed spinal fusion devices. Plastic Reconstruct Surg 1998;102(2):390–392.

50. Calderone RR, Garfin DE, Capen DA, et al. Cost of medical care for postoperative spinal infections. Orthop Clin North Am 1996;27(1):171–182.

51. Weiss LE, Vaccaro AR, Scuderi G, et al. Pseudarthrosis after postoperative wound infection in the lumbar spine. J Spinal Disord 1997;10(6):482–487.

52. Calderone RR, Thomas JC Jr, Haye W, et al. Outcome assessment in spinal infections. Orthop Clin North Am 1996;27(1):201–205.

CHAPTER 81

Primary Spine Tumors

Edward D. Simmons and Yinggang Zheng

Spine tumors are clinically classified into three categories: primary benign tumor, primary malignant tumor, and metastatic tumor. The treatment of spine neoplasm represents a challenge to spine care professionals. Surgery plays a major role in the selected patients with spinal tumors. To avoid disastrous complications, the existing and potential neurologic involvement must be considered. Besides the histologic nature of tumors, the anatomic complexity of spinal structure and failure to obtain en block resection of the involved spinal segment make the surgical treatment much more difficult. Fortunately, the incidence of new cases of primary malignant bone tumor is low compared with other tumors. In the United States, approximately 2,000 malignant bone tumors out of 7,000 new sarcomas are diagnosed each year. Four percent to 20% of bone tumors are spinal tumors, constituting 80 to 400 tumors (1–3).

Metastatic tumors are both the most frequent tumor of bone and the spinal column, regardless of origin of primary tumor. Cancer is the second leading cause of death in the United States, accounting for 21% of all deaths in 1981 and 25% in 1985 (4,5). Breast cancer alone strikes approximately one in nine women worldwide. There are more than one million women in the United States presently living with metastases of breast cancer (4). Each year 494,000 patients die of cancer. It is estimated that 24,700 new cases of metastatic spinal cord diseases will be diagnosed per year (3,6). It has been demonstrated that 30% to 70% of patients who die from cancer have evidence of vertebral metastases that are visible on careful postmortem examination (7,8). This number could reach 85% in women with breast cancer (9–11); however, only less than 10% of patients with spinal instability require surgical treatment, accounting for approximately 18,000 new cases yearly (12–15). Patient survival after diagnosis of malignant neoplasm has improved dramatically over the past decade concomitant with advances in chemotherapy, immunotherapy, hormonal manipulation, radiotherapy, surgical intervention, or a combination of these modalities (4,5,14,16).

SPINE TUMORS CLASSIFICATION

In addition to metastatic diseases to the spine, primary spine tumors are from different tissues of origin. There is no universally accepted classification of primary spine tumors. Schimidek and Schiller proposed the classification summarized in Table 81-1 (17).

AGE

Age is an important factor when considering a differential diagnosis of bone tumors. A specific tumor has a peak incidence in a range of age (18,19). Dahlin, in a series of 8,542 bone tumors, reported 60% of benign spinal tumors occurred in the second or third decades of life (20). Tumors of the sacrum in children are more likely to be malignant (21). Benign (e.g., osteoid osteoma, osteoblastoma, and eosinophilic granuloma) and malignant tumors (e.g., osteosarcoma and Ewing sarcoma) are commonly seen in the 10- to 30-year-old age group; whereas multiple myeloma, chordoma, and chondrosarcoma are common in the 40- to 60-year-old age group. For patients aged between these two periods, other neoplasms are commonly diagnosed. They include giant cell tumor, enchondroma, lymphoma, and fibrosarcoma. There are more metastatic diseases in patients more than 60 years old. However, suspicion of metastatic tumors for spinal lesion following malignant tumor should be aroused for patients of any age (18,19,22,23).

LOCATION

The location of neoplasm lesion within the vertebra is significantly correlated with the type of tumor, symptoms, neurologic deficit, and the choice of surgical regimens.

TABLE 81-1. *Classification of primary tumors of the osseous spine*

Tissue of origin	Benign tumors	Malignant tumors
Fibrous tissue	Fibroma	Fibrosarcoma
	Fibrous dysplasia	Malignant fibrous histiocytoma
Cartilage	Chondroblastoma	Chondrosarcoma
	Osteochondroma	
	Enchondroma	
	Chondromyxoid fibroma	
Bone	Osteoid osteoma	Osteosarcoma
	Osteoblastoma	Osteosarcoma associated with Paget disease and previous radiation
Hematopoietic elements		Multiple myeloma, Solitary plasmacytoma Lymphoma
Fate cell	Lipoma	Liposarcoma
Vascular system	Hemangioma	Angiosarcoma
Blood vessels		Hemangiopericytoma
Lymphatics	Lymphangioma	Lymphangiosarcoma
Nerve	Schwannoma (neurilemmoma)	Malignant nerve sheath tumor
	Neurofibromatosis	
	Pigmented nerve sheath tumors	
	Ganglioneuroma	
Notochord		Chordoma
Unknown	Eosinophilic granuloma	Giant cell tumor
	Aneurysmal bone cyst	Ewing sarcoma

Source: Adapted from Schimidek HH, Schiller AL. Premalignant lesions of the osseous spine and classification of primary tumors. In: Sundaresan N, Schmidek HH, Schiller AL, et al., eds. Tumors of the spine: diagnosis and clinical management. Philadelphia: WB Saunders, 1990:3–5, with permission.

Spine tumors occur more commonly in the thoracic, lumbar, and sacral areas than in the cervical area, and are more prevalent in the vertebral body than in posterior elements. Giant cell tumors, aneurysmal bone cysts, and eosinophilic granulomas occur more frequently in the thoracic spine than the lumbar vertebral bodies (24).

Among benign tumors, eosinophilic granuloma and hemangioma have a tendency to occur in the anterior vertebral body rather than the posterior elements, whereas osteoid osteomas and osteoblastomas almost always involve the posterior elements of the vertebra. However, aneurysmal bone cysts and giant cell tumors may affect either the vertebral body or posterior elements. Of malignant neoplasms, multiple myeloma, solitary plasmacytoma, lymphoma, chondrosarcoma, chordoma, Ewing sarcoma, and metastases are more commonly seen in the anterior column, but osteosarcomas occur either anteriorly or posteriorly (25,26).

The majority of metastases affect the vertebral body, compared with only 14% of metastases involved in posterior elements. The common portion of vertebra initially affected is the pedicle (18,27). Seventy-five percent of vertebral metastases originate from carcinoma of the breast, prostate, kidney, thyroid, or lymphoma and myeloma. Carcinomas originating from different organs spread to different spine areas because of the anatomic character of the venous system. Carcinomas of the breast or lung most commonly metastasize to the thoracic spine, whereas prostatic carcinomas usually affect the lumbar spine, sacrum, and pelvis (28,29).

Location of a neoplasm within the vertebra is also related to symptoms and neurologic deficits. Neoplasm in the cervical and lumbar levels often causes radicular pain, whereas in the thoracic area it causes more cord compression because of the smaller vertebral canal. Lesions within vertebral bodies grow posteriorly and encroach on the anterior column of the spinal cord, causing motor function loss first. Conversely, lesions from posterior elements encroach on the spinal cord, causing sensory function loss as the initial neurologic deficit.

PRIMARY AND METASTATIC TUMORS

Clinical Presentation

Patients with spinal tumors commonly present with pain, spinal deformity, and neurologic deficit; and uncommonly with a palpable local mass as well. Systemic symptoms may be present in malignant lesions.

Back pain is the most common symptom (24). It may result from neurologic or mechanical compression, or the tumor itself. Pain caused by tumor is sometimes confused with pain from minimal trauma or degenerative low back pain. Pain with stiffness is often persistent, gradually worsening, and unrelieved by rest. Night pain is another symptom of certain skeletal neoplasms (e.g., osteoid osteoma and osteoblastoma) in that pain can be relieved by aspirin. If the tumor is involved in neural structures, there is radicular pain with or without numbness, mimicking the radiculopathy of lumbar intervertebral disc herniation (30). If this happens in teenagers, suspicion of neoplasm should be aroused.

Pain with metastatic disease usually is more severe. Most metastatic tumors to the thoracic or lumbar spine involve the anterior and middle columns. Following expansion of the tumor, pathologic fracture of vertebral body can occur and cause severe acute pain similar to that seen in traumatic vertebral compression fractures. However, the former usually results from minimal or no obvious trauma. Approximately 85% of metastases causing spinal instability and neurologic compromise arise anteriorly from the vertebral body (31–33). Spinal nerve and cord compression owing to pathologic fracture or invasion of neoplasm results in local pain, radicular pain along the affected nerve roots, and myelopathy (34). In addition, it should be kept in mind that metastases frequently are asymptomatic initially. Tumors themselves often are discovered incidentally (35).

Spinal deformity such as scoliosis is also commonly seen in certain spinal tumor patients (36,37), and may be caused by primary benign tumor, malignant tumor, or metastatic disease. Benign tumors such as osteoid osteoma or osteoblastoma are often associated with scoliosis, typically presenting with paraspinal muscle spasm and stiffness. Different from adolescent idiopathic scoliosis, this type of scoliosis presents with pain, rapid progression of curve, and rigidity. Structurally, there is absence of both vertebral rotation and wedging, which usually are present in adolescent idiopathic scoliosis (25). Deformity in patients with a malignant tumor, such as spinal neuroblastoma, may result from the involvement of the spine or spinal cord (38). The etiology of spinal deformity in patients with neuroblastoma may have intrinsic causes such as involvement of the axial skeleton with the tumor or neurologic deficits from spinal nerve or cord compression (38,39). The extrinsic causes may be the treatment itself and the sequelae of asymmetric irradiation of the spine, especially in children; soft-tissue fibrosis and contracture; laminectomy; and paraplegia secondary to epidural spread of tumor. Destruction of vertebral body in metastatic tumor results in compression fracture, associated with deformity and paraspinal muscular spasm, but the kyphosis is seldom dramatic enough to warrant much notice or be the presenting complaint (24).

Benign or malignant lesions or the neurologic compromise of the spinal cord or nerve root may occur after the progression of a spinal tumor. Malignant tumors present more neurologic deficits than benign tumors because of their invasive nature. Major causes of neurologic deficits are the direct encroachment of a tumor on spinal nerve roots or the spinal cord, or pathologic fracture secondary to destruction of vertebral body. When the nerve root is compressed, the patient presents with local back pain, radicular pain, and paresthesias that are commonly seen in lesions involving the cervical and lumbar spine. When such symptoms are persistent, thorough investigation for spinal neoplasm should be considered. Furthermore, spinal cord compromise results in more severe clinical symptoms and signs. Depending on the level of the lesion, patients may present with increasing extremity weakness, sensory disturbance, and sphincter dysfunction of bowel and bladder. Compression of the neoplasm may occur on the cervical or thoracic spinal cord, conus, and cauda equina causing varied neurologic deficits. A mixed neurologic picture may occur, particularly when metastatic lesions are present at multiple levels (40). Compression on the cervical spinal cord can cause quadriplegia, whereas neoplasm of the thoracolumbar spine can result in leg weakness, spasticity, difficult ambulation, sensory loss along the affected dermatomes, or paraplegia below the level of the lesion (41).

Although spinal tumor seldom presents with a mass as the initial finding, a local palpable mass or systemic symptoms for patients with spine tumor may be present. Tumor mass in the cranial or caudal regions of the spine is more likely to be found than in the thoracic or lumbar areas. Sacral tumors, such as chondrosarcoma or chordoma, following the growth of an anterior mass, may cause bowel or bladder symptoms and be palpable on rectal examination (24,25). Systemic symptoms usually are present in malignant lesions, especially with round cell tumors such as lymphoma and myeloma, Ewing sarcoma, and metastatic diseases. With the progression of lesions, patients present with weight loss, fever, fatigue, and general deterioration.

Imaging Studies

A correct diagnosis of spinal tumor depends on the teamwork of clinician, radiologist, and pathologist. Diagnosis of spinal tumor includes plain radiograph, bone scan, computed tomography (CT), magnetic resonance imaging (MRI), angiography, and biopsy. Other modalities may include single photon emission computed tomography (SPECT) bone scanning (42), positron emission tomography (PET) scan, or laboratory work-up.

Plain Radiograph

Roentgenology is the primary investigation for patients with suspicious spinal neoplasms. Antero-posterior (AP) and lateral radiographs are most commonly used. An open mouth AP view is necessary to evaluate the odontoid. The upper thoracic levels are difficult to see on the lateral view; therefore, an augmented tomography is helpful in highly suspicious cases. Specific radiographic appearance is often suggestive of different neoplasms.

Benign and malignant tumors have different radiographic characteristics. The major radiographic appearance of neoplasm in the vertebra is osteoblastic or sclerotic, osteolytic, or mixed. The location of lesion within the vertebra, presence of calcification, and extent of mass are the important clues for diagnosis (41). According to the progression of tumor showing on radiograph, slow-growing and expanding tumors are often benign and have a better prognosis, whereas aggressive lesions usually are malignant with deterioration of general condition in a short time. As commonly seen, benign tumors, osteoid osteomas, and osteoblastomas are frequently seen as sclerotic lesions in the posterior elements of the spine, with a central lytic area surrounded by reactive bone (26,43). These sclerotic lesions in the pedicles differ from the osteolytic changes of metastases (43). Certain metastases, such as prostate and breast cancer, can also show osteoblastic changes within vertebral bodies.

Lytic destruction of pedicle, contour changes of the vertebral body, sparing of the intervertebral disc, and soft-tissue invasion are the characteristics of primary malignant tumors and metastatic disease. The "winkle owl" sign seen on an AP radiograph for a destroyed pedicle is the most classic early sign of vertebral involvement, usually by malignant lesions, although the vertebral body typically is affected first. Thirty percent to 50% of the

vertebral body must be destroyed before osteolytic changes can be recognized radiographically. In contrast, minimum lysis of pedicular bone can be involved early; the pedicle can be seen well in cross section on an AP radiograph (29,44–46). Destruction of cortex and bone trabeculae by tumor results in contour change of the vertebral body, with localized kyphosis (Fig. 81-1). A pathologic compression fracture, which could happen in multiple levels, needs to be differentiated from an osteoporotic compression fracture. Bowing or "fish mouthing" at multiple end plates is suggestive of diffuse osteopenia, which may be secondary to multiple myeloma (40). Usually there is no lytic change of pedicle in osteoporotic vertebra. The intervertebral disc is usually preserved in patients with neoplasms, which is different from pyogenic infection in that the disc is frequently destroyed along with the adjacent vertebral body (13). Furthermore, the soft-tissue shadow on a radiograph from extension of a vertebral body lesion is also an important sign of malignancy.

Bone Scan

Bone scans, using technetium-99m (^{99m}Tc) labeled phosphate compounds, are widely used in the initial diagnosis and follow-up of bone tumors. Technetium scans

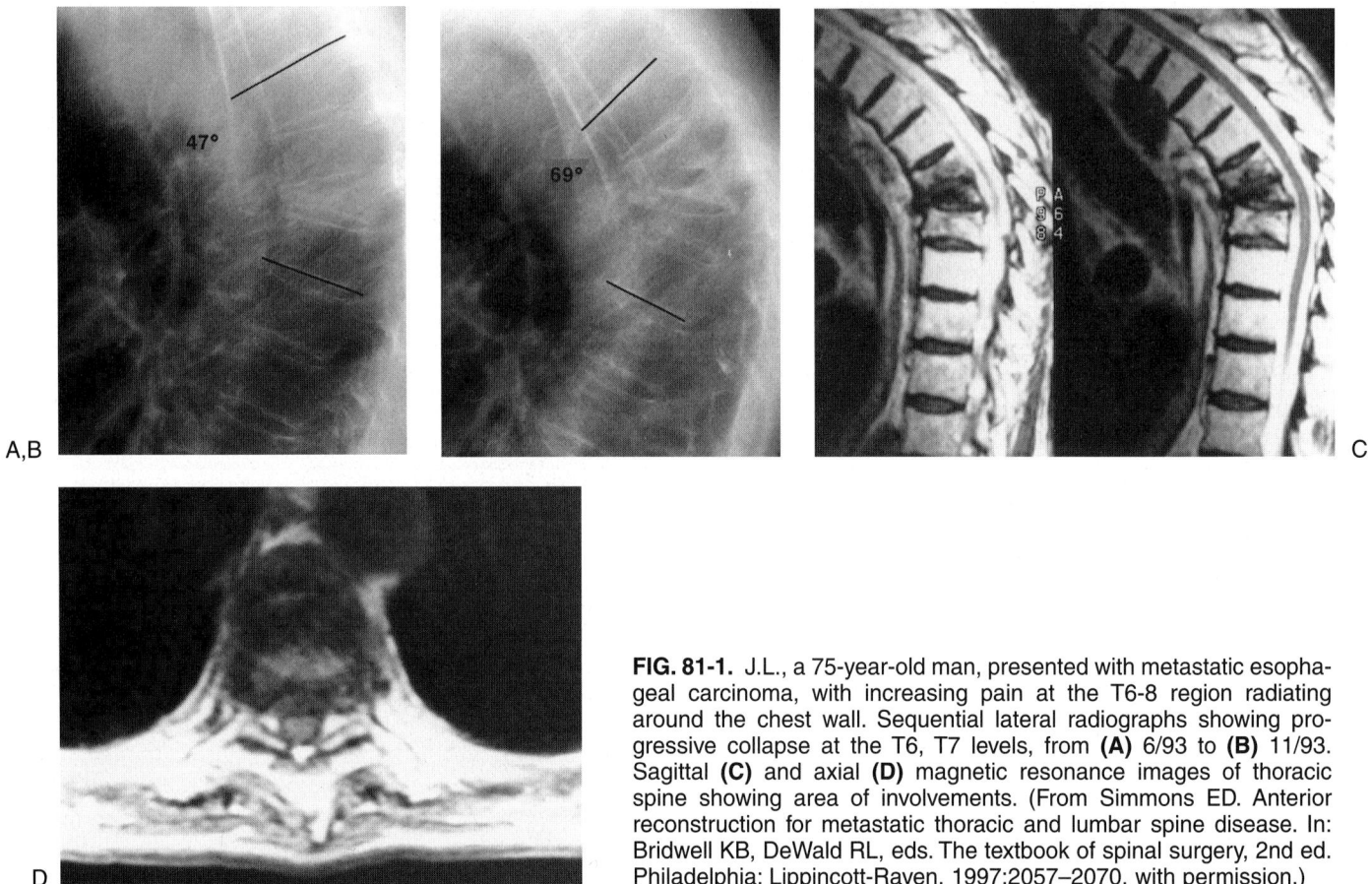

FIG. 81-1. J.L., a 75-year-old man, presented with metastatic esophageal carcinoma, with increasing pain at the T6-8 region radiating around the chest wall. Sequential lateral radiographs showing progressive collapse at the T6, T7 levels, from (A) 6/93 to (B) 11/93. Sagittal (C) and axial (D) magnetic resonance images of thoracic spine showing area of involvements. (From Simmons ED. Anterior reconstruction for metastatic thoracic and lumbar spine disease. In: Bridwell KB, DeWald RL, eds. The textbook of spinal surgery, 2nd ed. Philadelphia: Lippincott-Raven, 1997;2057–2070, with permission.)

are extremely sensitive to any area of increased osteoid reaction of the host to destructive processes within bone, and can detect lesions as small as 2 mm (19). They can detect as little as a 5% to 15% alteration in local bone turnover; whereas a minimum size of 1 cm and a 50% decrease in bone density are required for plain radiographs to detect a lytic lesion, and a 30% increase in bone density is required to detect sclerotic lesions. Radionuclide bone imaging is thus 50% to 80% more sensitive in detecting early skeletal metastases (47,48), and may predate radiographic changes of osteolytic or osteoblastic disease by 2 to 18 months (40–51). Total body scans can demonstrate all of the skeletal lesions, thus they are usually used: (a) as screening tests, (b) to determine whether a lesion is solitary or multifocal in expression, and (c) the local extent (47,48,52).

A high-quality radiograph should be obtained of any region where there is increased radionuclide uptake. Patients with a single or few areas of increased uptake and normal radiographs should have CT scans of these areas (10,53). Using this technique, the false-positive incidence is extremely small. Processes of new bone formation (e.g., fracture healing, infection, inflammation, and degenerative arthritis) may produce "hot spots"— focal areas of increased isotope uptake—whereas neoplastic processes that produce intense bone destruction without concomitant new bone deposition (e.g., solitary plasmacytoma, multiple myeloma, or lung carcinoma) may produce "cold spots," or negative bone scans (47). Because the uptake of a bone-seeking radionuclide is nonspecific, a bone scan cannot be used to differentiate between benign and malignant lesions. However, when a scan is strongly positive in multiple skeletal sites, metastatic disease should be suspected, even if the primary lesion is unknown (41).

Computed Tomography and Myelography

Once the area of disease is identified by plain radiographs or bone scan, further imaging with either CT or MRI should be undertaken to fully define the extent and nature of the lesion (25,54). Computed tomography, with its excellent resolution of bone anatomy, has been used to delineate small areas of bone destruction and the nature of fragments within the canal in pathologic fracture (55). Tumor margins in bone can be clearly seen with CT, because MRI gives relatively poor images on cortical bone. Computed tomography also can help to identify soft-tissue features of lesions that are not apparent on plain radiographs (56). The emergence of spiral CT allows quick performance of thin axial sections (1 to 1.5 mm), and improved computer software allows rapid reformatting into the appropriate plane (57).

Myelography is frequently applied in the past to find out spinal canal compression. Magnetic resonance imaging is now more widely used for this purpose because it is noninvasive. The combination of CT and myelography (myelo-CT) delineates the intrathecal structure on axial view; therefore, any encroachment on the spinal cord can be demonstrated. Myelography or myelo-CT now is used for the imaging study of patients with recurrent disease, especially those with stainless steel implants, because MRI cannot be applied owing to the artifact from this implant.

Magnetic Resonance Imaging

Magnetic resonance imaging has the advantage of producing excellent imaging in soft tissues and the axial skeleton. With its superior soft-tissue and tumor contrast, MRI can delineate the local extent of the tumor and involvement of surrounding soft tissues. Axial, sagittal, and coronal planes can be obtained without exposure to ionizing radiation (47,58). Magnetic resonance imaging is also recommended for determining the level and extent of suspected single or multiple neoplasm lesions, without the risk or invasiveness of myelography (40). It also helps in accurate local staging of tumor and obtaining adequate safety margins for surgery. For spinal canal encroachment, MRI clearly demonstrates ventral versus posterior compression. Intramedullary lesions also can be demonstrated clearly.

Unlike plain radiograph or CT, MRI provides valuable information in detecting vertebral bone marrow infiltration by tumors. Variations in MRI signal intensity depend on cellularity. Neoplasm lesions replace the normal marrow elements with higher cellularity, which results in a decreased signal on the T1-weighted images and a slightly higher signal on T2-weighted images. The benign cavernous hemangioma is the only lesion that shows increased signal relative to normal marrow on T1-weighted sequences and variable signal relative to normal marrow on T2-weighted or gradient echo sequences (58). Magnetic resonance imaging is more sensitive than a radionuclide bone scan in the detection of spinal metastases (59), and can detect metastatic lesions larger than 3 mm in size (60). The sensitivity of MRI in the detection of bone metastases is 90%, compared with the 49% sensitivity of CT (Fig. 81-1) (61).

Gadolinium-enhanced MRI provides additional information for detection of metastases. A study suggests that subarachnoid metastatic tumors enhance prominently and can be detected relatively easily against the background of nonenhanced normal nerve tissue and spinal fluid. Contrast scan also helps to distinguish disc disease from epidural tumor and select biopsy sites (62).

Magnetic resonance imaging also has used for monitoring response to chemotherapy, and for detecting postoperative tumor recurrence. Postcontrast MRI studies are helpful for evaluating the presence or absence of tumor necrosis during chemotherapy. Dynamic MRI after intravenous bolus administration of gadolinium-diethylenetriamine pentaacetic acid or other paramagnetic contrast media is particularly useful for assessing response to chemotherapy. Diffusion-weighted MRI is a new technique that is potentially capable of detecting and quantitating the amount of tumor necrosis after chemotherapy or radiation therapy (63).

Magnetic resonance imaging is also applied for the differential diagnosis among tumor, infection, and fracture. For a malignant lesion, MRI shows homogeneous and diffuse vertebral signal abnormality, a convex vertebral border, pedicle involvement, and sparing of the intervertebral disc (64). For pyogenic osteomyelitis, there is decreased signal on T1-weighted images and increased signal on T2-weighted images in the vertebra, with the erosion of end plates, intervertebral disc, and adjacent vertebra. Because of the marrow changes from fracture hematoma and edema, it is sometimes difficult to differentiate osteoporotic fracture from malignant compression fracture by MRI.

Compared with CT, MRI has less signal artifact of titanium implant; however, MRI does have disadvantages. In certain tumors (e.g., osteoid osteoma, osteoblastoma, or eosinophilic granuloma), the MRI signal of the inflammatory response in the soft tissue surrounding the tumor simulates soft-tissue involvement, giving the impression of a more aggressive tumor than actually exists (25,55, 65,66).

Angiography

Spinal angiography can be applied for some tumors with rich vascular structure, such as aneurysmal bone cyst, hemangiosarcoma, and metastatic renal cell. Angiography can identify the exact location and anatomic configuration of the lesion, and the vascularity of all feeding and draining vessels. Angiography with selective embolization can also be used for such lesions to reduce intraoperative blood loss (23).

Biopsy

The establishment of a definite diagnosis for spinal neoplasm lesion is of the utmost importance for the treatment, either surgical or nonoperative, and the prediction of prognosis. Because surgery is still the major treatment for excisable tumors, a pathologic diagnosis is essential for surgical planning. There are two major forms of biopsy for obtaining a sample of a suspected tumor lesion: percutaneous needle biopsy and open biopsy. The open biopsy consists of excisional and incisional biopsy.

Percutaneous needle biopsy has advantages compared with open biopsy. Needle biopsy, including bone marrow biopsy, is a simple, safe, and fast technique. Needle biopsy may save the patient from an open surgical procedure, especially when the final treatment is not surgical. It has fewer complications and morbidity, with a reported successful diagnosis in 75% to 95% of cases (67,68). The indications for needle biopsy include the following conditions: (1) confirmation of suspected round cell tumors (e.g., myeloma and lymphoma); (2) primary tumors that require reconstructive surgery; (3) eosinophilic granuloma for which aggressive surgery usually is not warranted; (4) known or suspected metastatic diseases before initiating radiotherapy or chemotherapy (69).

Fluoroscopic or CT guidance is necessary to localize the lesion and avoid neurologic and vascular complications. Computed tomographic guidance provides a great margin of safety for surrounding structures (24,69).

Obviously the limitation of needle biopsy is the small tissue sample, which sometimes makes it difficult to formulate a definite pathologic diagnosis. Large needles are recommended when performing a biopsy on osteoblastic lesions. Several specimens should be obtained because the success in obtaining positive results has been shown to be as low as 20% to 25% (70). Hemorrhage is always a concern for this procedure, especially when obtaining a sample from a suspected vascular lesion, for instance, hemangioma or aneurysmal bone cyst (67,69). When high risk for hemorrhage exists, needle biopsy should not be applied; switch to another diagnostic regimen.

A careful consideration is needed in selecting an approach for biopsy. When approaching an open biopsy, the potential need for a definitive surgical procedure must be considered. To avoid spreading tumor by contamination, the biopsy tract or incision should be placed so that it may be excised with the tumor during the definitive procedure (19). Using the most direct route to the lesion, biopsies of lesions affecting the posterior elements can be easily done with a straight posterior approach. Biopsies of lesions involving the vertebral body can be performed either from a transpedicular approach or after a costotransversectomy. Transpedicular biopsy is used for intraosseous lesions of the thoracic and especially the lumbar spine. A costotransversectomy approach is preferred in the presence of involvement of a vertebral body with an extended soft-tissue mass (41). Because of the potential morbidity involved with thoracotomies and retroperitoneal approaches, they should be reserved for definitive surgical intervention (40). An incisional biopsy should be the last step in the staging of the patient, performed just before the definitive surgical resection. Both procedures may be performed under the same anesthetic if the frozen section provides a clear diagnosis (19).

Intraoperatively, a frozen section should be obtained to confirm adequate material sampling. Adequate specimens should be obtained from the soft-tissue component accompanying lytic areas and blastic lesions, with an adequate amount of specimen allowing for pathologic diagnosis, including special stains and immunohistochemical studies. Whenever a bone biopsy is performed, blood is aspirated for cytologic analysis, and a sample is cultured to rule out infection (40).

BENIGN PRIMARY SPINE TUMORS

Osteoid Osteoma and Osteoblastoma

Osteoid osteoma and osteoblastoma of the spine are rare. Histologically, the two lesions are from the same osteoblastic origin, characterized by a rich fibrovascular stroma and abundant osteoblasts. The difference between these two lesions is their respective sizes and differing biologic behavior (71–74). An osteoblastic lesion less than 1.5 cm in size is arbitrarily defined as osteoid osteoma; one larger than that is named an osteoblastoma (75,76). Osteoid osteoma represents about 3% of primary bone tumors and 20% of reported cases in the vertebral column (20,72), whereas osteoblastoma is 1% and 41%, respectively (72,77,78).

Patients usually present in the second or third decade, with osteoid osteoma in a younger age group. The male to female ratio is 2:1 (79). These two benign lesions show a distinct propensity for spinal involvement, usually in the posterior elements. Besides being larger in size in comparison with osteoid osteoma, osteoblastoma grows more extensively and often forms extraskeletal soft tissue. The clinical manifestations include back pain and spinal scoliosis. The pain is typically persistent and presents at night in half of the patients. In the majority, weight-bearing activities aggravate the pain. Aspirin classically provides dramatic relief of pain in 30% to 73% of the patients with osteoid osteoma, but lack of a response to aspirin does not rule out the diagnosis (19,80). Scoliosis can occur in 60% to 77% of patients, with the tumor situated in the concave side of the apex (73,81,82). The neurologic deficit is seen more often in patients with osteoblastoma than in patients with osteoid osteoma (83).

Radiographically, osteotic osteoma presents as an isolated radiolucent area, surrounded by a zone of reactive sclerosis. Because of its small size, osteoid osteoma is easily obscured by the overlapping shadows of the vertebral column, whereas osteoblastoma is more apparent by its larger size in expansion of the cortical bone. Osteoblastoma has a thin rim of reactive bone between the lesion and the surrounding soft tissue; this rim separates the lesion from the rest of medullary bone. The involvement of the vertebral body is usually from the extension of tumor in the pedicle and has a limited extent (Fig. 81-2).

The radionuclide bone scan is the most sensitive and reliable screening technique of finding these two types of neoplasms (19,74). It is useful in the detection of small vertebral lesions and can usually localize the lesion to a specific level. The appearance of an osteoblastoma is a typical hot spot (84). Computed tomography scan is the best imaging procedure for defining the location of the lesion and the exact extent of the osseous involvement, and is helpful for surgical planning. For patients with neurologic deficits, MRI help in the evaluation of spinal cord and nerve compression (Fig. 81-2).

The treatment for either of these lesions is wide surgical excision of the entire lesion, with radical curettage of the surrounding normal vertebral bone (36).

Osteochondroma

Osteochondromas are the most common primary benign bone tumors, representing approximately 12% of all bone tumors. Most of these tumors occur in the long bones and in teenagers, and only 3% of these lesions are in the spine (20,85,86). Posterior elements, especially the spinous processes, are the common sites for these lesions (85).

Osteochondromas usually are asymptomatic. When lesions grow large, they cause impingement of nearby structures and precipitate symptoms. The symptoms vary greatly, from a painful bursa over the lesion to different neurologic deficits. Some authors report neurologic compromise .5% to 1% of the time (87), whereas others show myelopathy occurring in up to 47% of cases (88–92). A growing osteochondroma with pain after puberty should always raise the suspicion of sarcomatous transformation.

The distinguishing feature of an osteochondroma on plain radiograph is the continuity of the cortex and marrow between the normal bone and tumor, with trabeculae coursing from the tumor into the normal bone (93). Unfortunately, this characteristic does not always show on plain radiographs (88). Differential diagnosis needs further investigation by bone scan, CT, and MRI. Wide surgical excision is the choice when surgery is indicated.

Aneurysmal Bone Cyst

Aneurysmal bone cysts (ABCs) are rare lesions, constituting only 1% of biopsied primary bone tumors. Eleven percent to 20% of these lesions are located in the spine (94,95). The etiology of aneurysmal bone cysts remains unclear, but may result from the alternation of bone hemodynamics by vascular anomaly (96).

Aneurysmal bone cysts are primarily seen in patients younger than 20 years of age (94,97). When involving the spine, these lesions are more commonly in the lumbar spine, and are seen more in the posterior elements of vertebrae than in the vertebral body. In a reported series, 60% of lesions were located in the posterior elements and 40% in the vertebral body (95). Not limited to one single level, many aneurysmal bone cysts affect adjacent vertebra. Back pain is the most common symptom. Neurologic deficits may also occur with variable presentations.

On plain films the lesion shows an expansile, osteolytic cavity with periosteal new bone formation. The cortex of the cavity is eggshell-thin, making the lesion bubbly in appearance. Computed tomography and MRI can further detail the features of these lesions. Magnetic resonance imaging with gadolinium can demonstrate the multiple septations within these lesions and is used for differentiation with other cystic or fluid-filled lesions (98). A bone

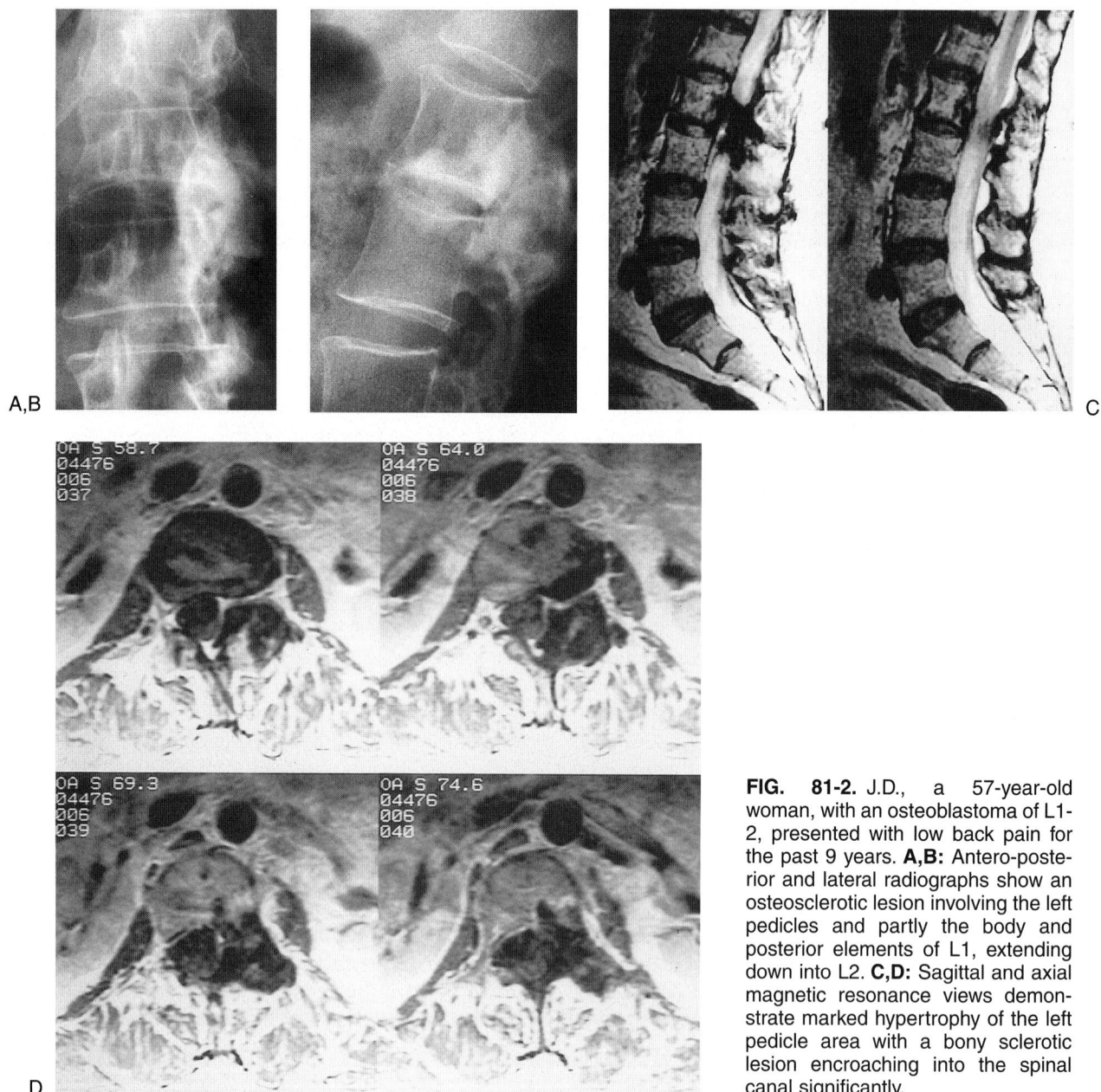

FIG. 81-2. J.D., a 57-year-old woman, with an osteoblastoma of L1-2, presented with low back pain for the past 9 years. **A,B:** Antero-posterior and lateral radiographs show an osteosclerotic lesion involving the left pedicles and partly the body and posterior elements of L1, extending down into L2. **C,D:** Sagittal and axial magnetic resonance views demonstrate marked hypertrophy of the left pedicle area with a bony sclerotic lesion encroaching into the spinal canal significantly.

scan usually shows increased uptake in the area of the tumor (99). Angiography provides useful information for the suspected lesions, because it can demonstrate the vascular blood-filled spaces caused by the arteriovenous shunting (96).

Management of these lesions includes embolization, surgical curettage or excision, and low-dose radiation.

Giant Cell Tumor

Giant cell tumors (GCTs) appear as lytic lesions and are eccentrically located in the epiphysis. These lesions are histologically benign, but their clinical behavior is

sometimes unpredictable and capricious (100). Most patients are young adults with a large age range. Turcotte and coauthors reported a group of 186 Canadian patients with a mean age of 36 years (range, 14 to 72 years) (101). Giant cell tumors are slow growing and locally aggressive and have a tendency to recur locally (102,103).

Giant cell tumors are characterized by their typical location in the epiphysis of long bone (101). In the spine, they are more commonly seen in the vertebral body than the posterior elements. They are also most common in the sacrum (104,105). Patients present with local pain or a painless, slowly enlarging mass in the sacrum. Most giant cell tumors are benign but occasionally have malignant behavior with pulmonary metastases in 3% of patients (106–108). Mononuclear round cells and randomly scattered osteoclast-type giant cells are the pathologic features of these lesions. The histologic grading system (grades I, II, and III), however, has not proved useful for prognosis (109).

The lesions are radiographically expansile, lytic, septate, and lack calcification. The lesions are somewhat soap bubble in appearance. Usually the lesions are limited by a rim that appears faint on plain radiograph but is well defined on CT. There is no periosteal reaction. The radiographic hallmark of these lesions is that they abut the subchondral bone plate of the adjacent joint. In the sacrum, these tumors have a tendency to occur proximally and eccentrically. This is in contradistinction to chordoma, which is more likely to be central and distal in the sacrum (103). In the vertebra, large areas of tumor are solid, accompanying blood-filled cystlike spaces that should be distinguished from aneurysmal bone cyst (109). Positive isotope scan helps with the diagnosis.

Giant cell tumor has potential to recur after treatment such as curettage or incomplete resection. The great majority of recurrences appear within 2 to 3 years (110–112), with a range of 25% to 50% (76,109, 113,114). Wide marginal resection is necessary for these lesions. To enhance surgical procedures, adjuvant measures such as liquid nitrogen, acrylic cement, and local delivered chemotherapy are applied. Reconstruction is usually done following the aggressive surgery.

Eosinophilic Granuloma

Eosinophilic granuloma is a benign tumor-like condition that produces focal bone destruction (115). The histologic features of these lesions are sheets of histiocytes and inflammatory cells, particularly eosinophils. A defect of the immune system is considered as the major cause of this condition. Eosinophilic granulomas represent less than 1% of all tumor-like conditions of bone (116); 7% to 20% of these lesions are located in the spine (117,118). Eosinophilic granulomas are seen commonly in the first or second decades of life, with a peak incidence under the age of 10 years. Males are more like to have this lesion than females, with a ratio of more than two to one (86).

Lesions may occur in solitary or multiple bone forms, with or without system involvement (93). Lesions of the skull are most commonly seen. Tumors are more often in the thoracic spine followed by the lumbar and then the cervical spine (119).

Back pain and stiffness are the major complaints of this lesion. Neurologic deficit is rare. System involvement termed as histocytosis X manifests as triad of syndromes: eosinophilic granuloma, acute form of Letterer-Siwe disease, and chronic form of Hand-Schüller-Christian disease (119,120).

Vertebra plana is the typical characteristic of this lesion on plain radiograph. A lesion appears as a solitary central lytic lesion on the vertebra. The adjacent discs are usually preserved and soft-tissue mass is rare. When the vertebral body collapses and settles, radiographs demonstrate the "coin-on-end" appearance: flattened discs of dense cortical bone retained between the two intact intervertebral discs (121,122). Bone scans usually show cold images (118). Magnetic resonance imaging may show a "flare" reaction with extensive high signal areas on T2-weighted images in the surrounding bone marrow and soft tissue. Biopsy is necessary to differentiate among other malignant lesions (123–125).

Because many lesions are self-limiting and can heal spontaneously without treatment, the prognosis for recovery is excellent. Vertebral height can reconstitute spontaneously with time, even though sometime it is partial or with residual deformity (119). Aggressive surgery is only reserved for those with significant instability and neurologic compromise (123–125).

Hemangioma

Hemangiomas are the most common benign lesions with a vascular origin. Tumors consist of thin-walled capillaries that are engorged with red blood cells. There are cavernous, capillary, or mixed types. The majority of these tumors in the spine are of the cavernous or mixed types. They can occur at any age but most commonly are found after the age of 40 (83). These tumors show no significant gender predominance (86). The vertebra of thoracolumbar or lumbar spine is most commonly involved.

Most spinal hemangiomas are asymptomatic and are found as incidental findings; therefore, they are of less clinical importance. Patients may present with pain and kyphosis or scoliosis following compression fracture. Neurologic symptoms are rare but can occur following spinal cord compression or nerve root encroachment.

The typical appearance of these lesions on plain radiograph is prominent vertical striations of thickened trabeculae within vertebral body, which can be best seen on the lateral view. The number of bone trabeculae is decreased owing to replacement by the sinusoid. This appearance is called "celery stalk" or "honeycomb" (93). At least one third of the vertebral body must be involved for the classic findings to be recognizable on plain radiograph. A significant characteristic is that compression fracture due to vertebral hemangioma is rare and can often heal with time if it happens. The cortex and disc space are usually intact on plain film, but the affected cortex, if any, can be demonstrated on the axial view of CT scan. The thickened trabeculae showed on CT are in a "polka dot" pattern (126).

Most hemangiomas do not warrant special treatment. Clinical observation is adequate. For symptomatic lesions, radiotherapy is usually the first choice because this tumor is radiosensitive and frequently responds well. Surgery is rare indicated with these lesions and may be necessary for some cases with spinal cord compression. Caution about severe hemorrhage should be taken when operating on these lesions. Preoperative angiography with selective embolization helps control bleeding from these vascular lesions during surgery (127–130).

MALIGNANT PRIMARY SPINE TUMORS

Multiple Myeloma

Multiple myeloma is the most common primary malignant tumor either in all of the skeleton or the spinal column (25). It originates from plasm cells of marrow. This lesion is usually seen in the older age group, from 50 to 75 years, with a mean of 62 years (131,132). The hematopoietic marrow in the vertebral bodies, ribs, pelvic bone, and skull is usually affected, representing the systemic nature of this lesion. Because of the widespread bone marrow involvement, patients usually present with normocytic and normochromic anemia. Such patients are susceptible to infection of any kind (33). The expansion of the spinal lesion can cause pain and fracture of the vertebral body.

The typical characteristics of this lesion on radiograph are punched-out lytic lesions within the bones without bone reaction. Radiographs of vertebral bodies may demonstrate osteopenia, wedging, and compression fracture. Bone scan has proved to be of little value in assessing patients with myeloma. The lack of bone reaction to the tumor lysis accounts for this poor result (133). Serum protein electrophoresis shows reversal of the albumin to globulin ratio. Bone marrow biopsy is the definitive means for making diagnosis (Fig. 81-3) (41).

Surgery is rarely indicated for multiple myeloma. The primary treatment for multiple myeloma is chemotherapy. Radiation therapy can be used for localized painful lesions. Surgical intervention is reserved for the treatment of disease complications, such as neurologic

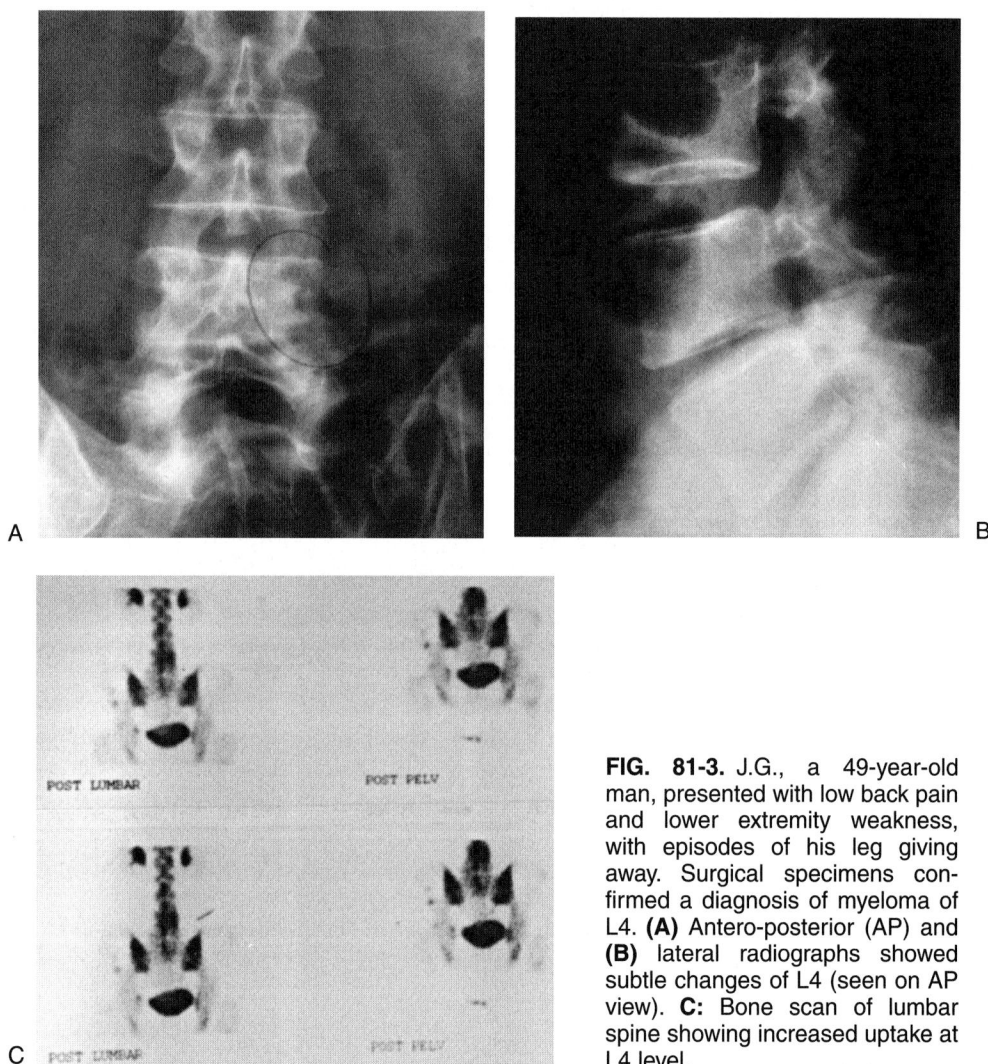

FIG. 81-3. J.G., a 49-year-old man, presented with low back pain and lower extremity weakness, with episodes of his leg giving away. Surgical specimens confirmed a diagnosis of myeloma of L4. (A) Antero-posterior (AP) and (B) lateral radiographs showed subtle changes of L4 (seen on AP view). C: Bone scan of lumbar spine showing increased uptake at L4 level.

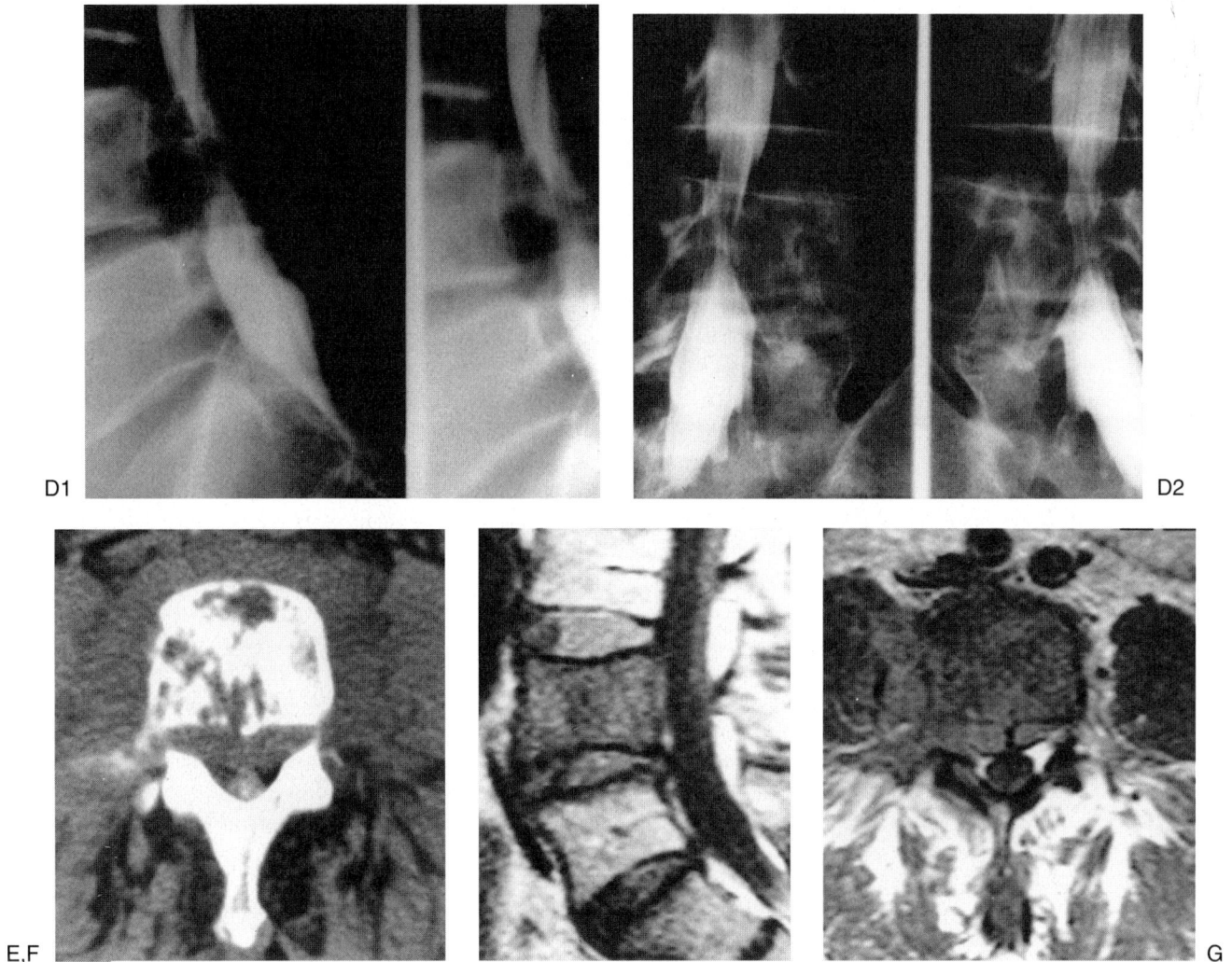

FIG. 81-3. (*Continued*). **D:** Myelograph showing involvement of spinal canal with thecal sac compression and permeative involvement of vertebral body. **E:** Computed tomography scan studies showing involvement of spinal canal with thecal sac compression and permeative involvement of vertebral body. **F:** Sagittal and **(G)** axial magnetic resonance images of lumbar spine showing involvement of L4 vertebral body and spinal canal. (From Simmons ED. Anterior reconstruction for metastatic thoracic and lumbar spine disease. In: Bridwell KB, DeWald RL, eds. The textbook of spinal surgery. Philadelphia: Lippincott-Raven, 2nd ed. 1997:2057–2070, with permission.)

deficits owing to spinal cord compression by pathologic fracture. The prognosis for survival of multiple myeloma patients involving spine, despite all recent advances, still remains poor. Median survival ranges from 11.5 to 32 months (131,134).

Solitary Plasmacytoma

Solitary plasmacytoma, like multiple myeloma, is also a plasm cell neoplasm. However, these lesions are rare with only 3% of all plasma cell neoplasms (135). Because of the significant different natural history of multiple myeloma and solitary plasmacytoma, these two lesions are considered as two manifestations in a continuum of B-cell lymphoproliferative diseases (19). Spinal lesions,

most in the thoracic spine, constitute 25% to 50% cases (136,137). Overall, men have a higher incidence than women (138).

Clinical manifestations of solitary plasmacytoma may present with back pain and neurologic deficit. Initial radiographs of spine demonstrate a lytic lesion within vertebra, usually first seen in the pedicle then extended to the anterior vertebral body. Vertebral plana and collapse can occur following the progression of lesion. Fifty percent of these lesions may develop to systemic disease and multiple myeloma (139). Like multiple myeloma, bone scan has little value for the diagnosis because of lack of sclerotic bone reaction, whereas bone marrow aspiration and serum and urine protein electrophoresis are necessary. Computed tomography can identify the lesion that can be not seen on plain radiograph. Magnetic resonance imaging provides useful information for evaluating the location and extent of the lesion.

Radiotherapy is the major treatment for this tumor because of its radiosensitivity (41). Patients with solitary plasmacytoma may have prolonged survival compared with multiple myeloma. It was reported that 5-year survival rates range from 35% to 70% (136,140). Mclain and Weinstein reported that the 5-year disease-free survival in 84 cases of spinal lesions was approximately 60%, with a median survival of 92 months (141).

Lymphoma

Primary bone lymphoma is an uncommon malignancy. It accounts for less than 5% of the primary bone tumors and 5% of the extranodal non-Hodgkin lymphoma (142,143). It has the same histologic features of other lymphomas arising from the lymphoid and soft tissue. Hodgkin disease rarely presents with bony lesions. Non-Hodgkin lymphoma may occur as a solitary lesion of bone or, more commonly, as systemic disease with associated bony lesions in 20% of patients (143–145). In spine, vertebral body is more commonly involved than posterior elements. Patients are usually in the middle age of life, with a range of 18 to 69 years (146).

Lymphoma has a destructive nature and can cause collapse of the vertebral body with extraosseous extension of the lesion to the paravertebral area and into the spinal canal. The symptoms and signs vary from localized back pain to a partial or complete neurologic deficit (147). The tumor on radiographs is a lytic lesion with an ill-defined margin that gradually expands and breaks through the cortex (147); however, these radiographic features are inclusive and variable. Percutaneous or open biopsy is desirable to clarify the diagnosis (146).

The treatment of choice traditionally is a combination of chemotherapy and radiation therapy. Radiation therapy may be unnecessary for children. Surgery usually is appropriate for patients with neurologic deficits by spinal cord compression owing to pathologic fractures.

Osteosarcoma

Osteosarcoma is the second most common malignant primary bone tumor after myeloma, constituting 20% of all primary malignant tumors of bone (143,148,149). It usually occurs in the metaphyses of extremity long bones. The peak age of onset is in the second decade. The estimated incidence of this tumor in the United States is approximately 1.7 cases per million per year, representing about 500 to 600 new cases annually (150,151). Primary osteosarcomas of the spine are extremely rare, constituting only 3% of all primary osteosarcomas and 5% primary malignant tumors of the spine (1,152,153). Primary osteosarcomas in the spine tend to occur in patients in an older age group than does the same tumor in the extremities (152).

Osteosarcoma of spine commonly occurs at the vertebral body. Back pain from the affected vertebra area is the main symptom. Most patients also have variable sensory or motor deficits (152,154). Malignant features on radiographs include osteoblastic and osteolytic changes, cortical destruction, and soft-tissue calcification. The radiographic hallmarks of osteosarcoma in the extremities—Codman triangle of reactive bone and "sunburst" appearance—are not present in spinal lesions. The level of serum alkaline phosphatase is usually elevated in these patients and can be used for differentiation. Computed tomography, MRI, and bone scan are helpful for identifying the extent of tumor and diagnosis. For case with suspected osteosarcoma, biopsy is necessary before initiating chemotherapy (152).

Prognosis for patients with osteosarcoma has traditionally been poor. Before early 1970s, amputation was the primary treatment of osteosarcoma of long bones, with a poor 5-year survival rate of 20% (143,148,150,155–157). During the last 15 to 20 years, since the use of adjuvant and neoadjuvant chemotherapy by eradicating micrometastasis, the survival rate has been improved dramatically, to 50% to 70% (158–161). Like the lesions in the long bones, the survival of patients with osteosarcoma of the spine is also poor, with a median survival of 6 to 10 months (152,162). To improve the prognosis, chemotherapy followed by aggressive surgical excision of lesion is proposed. Anterior and posterior wide excision or complete spondylectomy has been applied in addition to chemotherapy. Postoperative radiotherapy to the primary site in conjunction with postoperative chemotherapy is used to improve the survival rate.

Chondrosarcoma

Chondrosarcoma is the third most common primary malignant tumor of the bone next to multiple myeloma and osteogenic sarcoma (147). About 4% to 8% of chondrosarcomas occur in the spine (20,163). The basic neoplastic tissue is cartilage without osteoid, formed directly by sarcomatous stroma (143,164). It may occur as a primary lesion or secondary to a preexisting benign tumor. The average of age for chondrosarcomas is 40 years, with a broad range (163,165–168).

Clinically, chondrosarcomas is most common in long bones and pelvis, but it is not unusual for the spine column to be affected, especially the lumbar and sacral region (147). Local discomfort or pain and a slow-growing mass are common manifestations. Lumbar or sacral lesions may result in a large pelvic or intraabdominal mass. Chondrosarcomas are histologically divided into low, intermediate, and high grades. Low-grade tumors seldom metastasize, whereas high-grade lesions have early metastases to the lungs and other areas of the body.

Bony destruction and a growing lobulated mass with calcific mottling are the common signs of chondrosarcomas on radiographs. Computed tomography can clearly demonstrate the location, cortical destruction, and extent of the tumor. Bone scans are positive in most chondrosarcomas (169). Biopsy is usually necessary for final diagnosis.

Radiotherapy and chemotherapy have little value for the treatment of chondrosarcoma. Wide surgical resection is the treatment of choice (164), but this is frequently restrained by spinal structures. The most important factors for patient survival are augmented chromosomal content and tumor size. Kreicbergs et al. found that chondrosarcoma with normal DNA content were associated with a significantly higher 10-year survival rate than those with abnormal chromosome content, 81% versus 21% (170,171).

Chordoma

Chordomas are rare primary malignant tumors of the axial skeleton, arising from the remnants of embryonic notochord (172,173). These lesions constitute 1% to 4% of primary malignant bone tumors (20,143), yielding an annual incidence of approximately 25 afflicted persons in the United States (173,174). A little more than half of the tumors occur in the sacrum, 35% at the base of skull, and 15% in the spine vertebrae and other areas (20,173,175, 176–179). Although chordomas have been reported in all age groups, they are commonly seen in the fifth through seventh decades of life (104,180–182). Males are more affected than females, with a ratio of 2:1 (20).

Chordomas are slow-growing masses. The symptoms vary from months to several years before patients see the physician. The symptoms and signs of the tumor are related to the location and are usually nonspecific. Pain is the frequent symptom of tumor in the sacral coccygeal region. Most of these tumors extend anterior to the sacrum; therefore, the tumor can grow to a large size before being diagnosed because of the relatively large space available for expansion within the posterior pelvis. Rectal and bladder dysfunction can occur in 20% to 40% of patients and are late features (41,173). A careful rectal examination either with finger or proctoscope is necessary for diagnosis. A firm and fixed presacral mass can be palpated on rectal examination. Neurologic deficits of these tumors at the base of skull, cervical, thoracic, and lumbar regions of spine column are relevant to their location. Although this tumor is aggressive locally, it also can metastasize to other distant sites of the body, such as lymph nodes, lung, liver, and other intraabdominal viscera. Metastases can be discovered as early as 1 year and as late as 10 years after diagnosis of primary tumor, with variable incidence from 5% to 40% (177,179,183).

The characterized radiographic finding in sacral chordomas is a lytic lesion involving several segments of the sacrum associated with an expansile ballooning soft-tissue mass anterior to it (180,181). Peripheral calcification can be seen in 40% to 80% of tumors (184–186). Tumors involving the true vertebrae usually originate in a single vertebral body and are lytic with surrounding reactive sclerosis (181). Computed tomography can disclose the extent of tumor mass and calcification. Heterogeneous signals and internal septations on T2-weighted MRI are predominant features (186). Bone scans are rarely positive for these lesions. Biopsy can be done for diagnosis.

Although chordomas are considered low-grade malignant lesions and are slow to metastasize, their proximity to the spinal cord and cauda equina and the extent of tumor at time of initial presentation make them extremely difficult to treat effectively (187). Wide surgical resection with adjuvant radiotherapy has been recommended for the treatment of chordoma. Chemotherapy has not proved even modestly effective (104,188). In sacrococcygeal chordomas, the level of lesion significantly affects the mode of treatment. The removal of the S1 vertebra impairs the stability of the pelvic girdle. There is a significant difference in surgical treatment between lesions involving the third sacral segment distally and those involving the more proximal portion of the sacrum. Distal chordoma can be excised posteriorly (104,188). Sphincter control of bowel and bladder is directly related to the number of preserved nerve roots. If the most caudad nerve root preserved is the first sacral nerve, no control can be expected, and the patient may be unable to walk without orthotic assistance. If both second sacral nerve roots are spared, 50% of patients regain at least partial bowel and bladder control. If one third of the sacral nerve root is preserved, most patients regain sphincter control. Stener and Gunterberg have described surgical techniques for high radical sacrectomy, either above or through the anterior foramina of the S1 nerve root. They believe that it is possible to sacrifice all sacral nerve roots unilaterally without significant disturbance of bowel or bladder function (189).

Because the tumor in the vertebral column is usually located at the vertebral body, an anterior approach or a combination of anterior and posterior procedures is carried out to excise the lesion and reconstruct the stability of spine column. Because the recurrence rate and ultimate failure rate are much higher for these tumors, adjuvant proton-beam therapy has been used both for palliation of recurrent tumors and for otherwise inoperable lesions (173,190).

The reported survival rates have been poor in the past. The surgical treatment of spine chordoma is less satisfactory than that of sacrococcygeal lesion. Sundaresan reported the disease-free survival rate is less than 10% (173). However, aggressive excision with adjuvant radiotherapy achieves the best results with a disease-free survival of more than 5 years for 50% to 77% of patients (104,186,191).

Ewing Sarcoma

Ewing sarcoma of bone was first described in 1921 by James Ewing (192). It accounts for approximately 6% of all malignant primary bone tumors (20). Ewing sarcomas are the second most common primary malignant tumors of bone in childhood and adolescence, with an annual incidence rate in whites of 3 per 1 million children less than 15 years of age. The average age of patients is 15 years, with a range from the first to the fourth decade of life (193,194).

Ewing sarcoma of the spine is rare, representing only about .5% of all primary malignant tumors of bone, and 8% to 10% of all Ewing sarcoma (20,195,196). Primary sites are sacral and vertebra. Pain and neurologic deficits are the most common presenting features. Metastases may occur in patients at the time of diagnosis, commonly involving the lungs or other locations in the spinal column. Many patients have low-grade fever, anemia, leukocytosis, and elevated erythrocyte sedimentation rate.

Plain radiographs reveal a lytic destruction lesion, often with peripheral sclerosis and a soft-tissue mass. Computed tomography and MRI are needed to further identify the location and extent of tumor. Bone scan is used to rule out other metastases. An accurate diagnosis is made by pathology. Showing histopathologically as small blue round cell tumors, Ewing sarcomas show a typical chromosomal rearrangement in more than 95% of cases (197).

Because of the obvious limitations in excising the tumor and achieving adequate margins, standard treatment for local control of the primary lesion, historically, has been chemotherapy and radiation. The overall 5-year survival rate in the past is low, approximately 20% (195,198). Great strides have been made in the diagnosis and treatment of patients with Ewing sarcoma. Currently, surgical resection has become a more effective option in the multidisciplinary treatment of patients with this disease. The response to induction chemotherapy is a strong prognostic factor (199,200). Cotterill and coauthors, by analyzing 975 patients, also found that metastases at diagnosis, primary site, and age are the prognostic factors (201). With the advent of modern chemotherapy, the long-term survival has improved to approximately 50% to 70% (194,197,202).

REFERENCES

1. Dreghorn C, Newman R, Hardy G, et al. Primary tumors of the axial skeleton: experience of Leeds Regional Bone Tumor Registry. Spine 1990;15:137–140.
2. Hart RA, Boriani S, Biagini R, et al. A system for surgical staging and management of spine tumors: a clinical outcome study of giant cell tumors of the spine. Spine 1997;22:1773–1778.
3. Silverberg E. Cancer statistics, 1985. CA Cancer J Clin 1985;35:19–35.
4. Harrington KD. Orthopaedic management of extremity and pelvic lesions. Clin Orthop 1995;312:136–147.
5. Seidman H, Mushinski MH, Gelb SK. Probabilities of eventually developing or dying of cancer, United States, 1985. CA Cancer J Clin 1985;35:36–56.
6. Silverberg E, Lubera JA. Cancer statistics, 1989. CA Cancer J Clin 1989;39:3–20.
7. Jaffe WL. Tumors and tumorous conditions of the bones and joints. Philadelphia: Lea & Febiger, 1958.
8. Thompson JE, Keiller VH. Multiple skeletal metastases from cancer of the breast. Surg Gynecol Obstet 1924;38:367–375.
9. Galasko CSB. Diagnosis of skeletal metastases and assessment of response to treatment. Clin Orthop 1995;312:64–75.
10. Galasko CSB. Incidence and distribution of skeletal metastases. In: Galasko CSB, ed. Skeletal metastases. London: Butterworth, 1986:14–21.
11. Weinstein JN, Collalto P, Lehmann TR. Long-term follow-up of non-operative treated thoracolumbar spine fractures. J Orthop Trauma 1988;3:152–159.
12. Barron KD, Hirano A, Araki S. Experience with metastatic neoplasms involving the spinal cord. Neurology 1959;9:91.
13. Black P. Spinal metastasis: current status and recommended guideline for management. Neurosurgery 1979;5:726–746.
14. Harrington KD. The use of methylmethacrylate for vertebral body replacement and anterior stabilization of pathological fracture-dislocations of the spine due to metastatic malignant disease. J Bone Joint Surg 1981;63A:36–46.
15. Young RF, Post EM, King GA. Treatment of spinal epidural metastases. Randomized prospective comparison of laminectomy and radiotherapy. J Neurosurg 1980;53:741–748.
16. Sundaresan N, Galicich JH, Bains MB, et al. Vertebral body resection in the treatment of cancer involving the spine. Cancer 1984;53:1393–1396.
17. Schimidek HH, Schiller AL. Premalignant lesions of the osseous spine and classification of primary tumors. In: Sundaresan N, Schmidek HH, Schiller AL, et al, eds. Tumors of the spine: diagnosis and clinical management. Philadelphia: WB Saunders, 1990:3–5.
18. Tillotston CL, Rosenthal DI. Radiology of spine tumors: general considerations. In: Sundaresan N, Schmidek HH, Schiller AL, et al, eds. Tumors of the spine: diagnosis and clinical management. Philadelphia: WB Saunders, 1990:34–45.
19. Weinstein JN, McLain RF. Tumors of the spine. In: Rothman RH, Simeone FA, eds. The spine, 3rd ed. Philadelphia: WB Saunders, 1992:1279–1318.
20. Dahlin DC, Unni KU, eds. Bone tumors, general aspects and data on 8542 cases, 4th ed. Springfield, IL: Charles C Thomas, 1986.
21. Kozlowski K, Barylak A, Campbell J, et al. Primary sacral bone tumors in children (report of 16 cases with a short literature review). Australas Radiol 1990;34:142–149.
22. Weinstein JN, McLain RF. Primary tumors of the spine. Spine 1987;12:843–851.
23. Weinstein JN. Spinal tumors. In: Weinstein JN, Wiesel SW, eds. The lumbar spine, 2nd ed. Philadelphia: WB Saunders, 1996:917–944.
24. Enneking WF. Spine. In: Enneking WF, ed. Musculoskeletal tumor surgery. New York: Churchill Livingstone, 1983:303–354.
25. Gelb DE, Bridwell KH. Benign tumors of the spine. In: Bridwell KH, DeWald RL, eds. The textbook of spinal surgery, 2nd ed. Philadelphia: Lippincott-Raven, 1997:1959–1981.
26. Meislin RJ, Neuwirth MG, Bloom ND. Tumors of the thoracolumbar spine. In: Lewis MM, ed. Musculoskeletal oncology: a multidisciplinary approach. Philadelphia: WB Saunders, 1992:227–241.
27. Willis RA. Secondary tumors of bones. In: The spread of tumors in the human body, 3rd ed. London: Butterworth, 1973:229.
28. Harrington KD. Anterior decompression and stabilization of the spine as a treatment for vertebral collapse and spinal cord compression from metastatic malignancy. Clin Orthop 1988;233:177–197.
29. Harrington KD. Metastatic disease of the spine. J Bone Joint Surg 1986;68A:1110–1115.
30. Sinar EJ, Maurice-Williams RS. Spinal extradural tumours mimicking a lumbar disc protrusion. J R Coll Surg Edinburgh 1987;32:179–180.
31. Constans JP, de Devitis E, Conzelli R, et al. Spinal metastases with neurological manifestations. Review of 600 cases. J Neurosurg 1983;59:111–118.
32. Dunn RC Jr, Kelly WA, Wohns RNW, et al. Spinal epidural neoplasis: a 15-year review of the results of surgical therapy. J Neurosurg 1980;52:47–51.

33. Fielding JW, Pyle RN Jr, Fietti VG Jr. Anterior cervical vertebral body resection and bone grafting for benign and malignant tumors. A survey under the auspices of the Cervical Spine Research Society. J Bone Joint Surg 1979;61A:251–253.

34. Griffin JB. Benign osteoblastoma of the thoracic spine. J Bone Joint Surg 1978;60A:833–835.

35. Schaberg JC, Gainor BJ. A profile of metastatic carcinoma of the spine. Spine 1985;10:19–20.

36. Akbarnia BA, Rooholamini SA. Scoliosis caused by benign osteoblastoma of the thoracic and lumbar spine. J Bone Joint Surg 1981;63A:1146–1155.

37. Pettine KA, Klassen RA. Osteoid-osteoma and osteoblastoma of the spine. J Bone Joint Surg 1986;68A:354–361.

38. Mayfield JK. Neuroblastoma and spinal deformity. In: Akbarnia BA, ed. Spine: state of the art reviews. Philadelphia: Hanley & Belfus, 1988:351–362.

39. Galasko CS, Norris HE, Crank S. Spinal instability secondary to metastatic cancer. J Bone Joint Surg 2000;82A:570–594.

40. Asdourian PL. Metastatic disease of the spine. In: Bridwell KH, DeWald RL, eds. The textbook of spinal surgery, 2nd ed. Philadelphia: Lippincott-Raven, 1997:2007–2050.

41. Levine AM, Crandall DG. Treatment of primary malignant tumors of the spine and sacrum. In: Bridwell KH, DeWald RL, eds. The textbook of spinal surgery, 2nd ed. Philadelphia: Lippincott-Raven, 1997:1938–2006.

42. Gates GF. SPECT bone scanning of the spine. Semin Nucl Med 1998;28:78–94.

43. Sweriduk ST, DeLuca SA. The sclerotic pedicle. Am Fam Physician 1987;35:161–162.

44. Brice J, McKissock W. Surgical treatment of malignant extradural spinal tumors. BMJ 1965;1:1341.

45. Jacobson JG, Poppel MH, Shapiro JH, et al. The vertebral pedicle sign. AJR Am Roentgenol 1958;80:817.

46. Livingston KE, Perrin RG. The neurosurgical management of spinal metastases causing cord and cauda equina compression. J Neurosurg 1978;49:839–843.

47. MacDonald DR. Clinical manifestations. In: Sundaresan N, Schmidek HH, Schiller AL, et al, eds. Tumors of the spine: diagnosis and clinical management. Philadelphia: WB Saunders, 1990:6–21.

48. Rosenthall L, Lisbona R. Skeletal imaging. Norwalk, CT: Appleton-Century-Crofts, 1984.

49. Galasko CS, Doyle FH. The detection of skeletal metastases from mammary cancer. A regional comparison between radiology and scintigraphy. Clin Radiol 1972;23:295–297.

50. Joo KG, Parthasarathy KL, Bakshi SP, et al. Bone scintigrams: their clinical usefulness in patients with breast carcinoma. Oncology 1979;36:94–98.

51. Roberts JG, Gravelle IH, Baum M, et al. Evaluation of radiography and isotopic scintigraphy for detecting skeletal metastases in breast cancer. Lancet 1976;1(7953):237–239.

53. Mehta RC, Wilson MA, Perlman SB. False-negative bone scan in extensive metastatic disease: CT and MR findings. Case report. J Comput Assist Tomogr 1989;13:717–719.

54. Body JJ. Metastatic bone disease: clinical and therapeutic aspects. Bone 1992;13:S57–S62.

55. Crim JR, Mirra JM, Eckardt JJ, et al. Widespread inflammatory response to osteoblastoma: the flare phenomenon. Radiology 1990;177:835–836.

56. Brown KT, Kattapuram SV, Rosenthal DI. Computed tomography analysis of bone tumors: Patterns of cortical destruction and soft tissue extension. Skel Radiol 1986;15:448–451.

57. Kaiser JA, Holland BA. Imaging of the cervical spine. Spine 1998;23:2701–2712.

58. Witte RJ, Miller GM. Spine. In: Berquist TH, ed. MRI of the musculoskeletal system, 4th ed. Philadelphia: Lippincott Williams & Wilkins, 2001:143–194.

59. Avrahami E, Tadmor R, Dally O, et al. Early MR demonstration of spinal metastases in patients with normal radiographs and CT and radionuclide bone scans. J Comput Assist Tomogr 1989;13:598–602.

60. Petren-Mallmin M, Nordstrom B, Andreasson I, et al. MR imaging with histopathological correlation in vertebral metastases of breast cancer. Acta Radiol 1992;33:213–220.

61. Algra PR, Bloem JL, Tissing H, et al. Detection of vertebral metas-

tases: comparison between MR imaging and bone scintigraphy. Radiographics 1991;11:219–232.

62. Sundaresan N, Krol G, Digiacinto GV. Metastatic tumors of the spine. In: Sundaresan N, Schmidek HH, Schiller AL, et al, eds. Tumors of the spine: diagnosis and clinical management. Philadelphia: WB Saunders, 1990:279–304.

63. Lang P, Johnston JO, Arenal-Romero F, et al. Advances in MR imaging of pediatric musculoskeletal neoplasms. Magn Reson Imaging Clin North Am 1998;6:579–604.

64. Moulopoulos LA, Yoshimitsu K, Johnson DA, et al. MR prediction of benign and malignant vertebral compression fractures. JMRI 1996;6:667–674.

65. Beltran J, Aparisi F, Bonmati LM, et al. Eosinophilic granuloma: MRI manifestations. Skeletal Radiol 1993;22:157–161

66. Woods ER, Martel W, Mandell SH, et al. Reactive soft-tissue mass associated with osteoid osteoma: correlation of MR imaging features with pathologic findings. Radiology 1993;186:221–225.

67. Mink J. Percutaneous bone biopsy in the patient with known or suspected osseous metastases. Radiology 1986;161:191–194.

68. Tehranzadeh J, Freiberger RH, Ghelman B. Closed skeletal needle biopsy: review of 120 cases. AJR Am J Roentgenol 1983;140:113–115.

69. Kattapuram SV, Rosenthal DI. Percutaneous needle biopsy of the spine. In: Sundaresan N, Schmidek HH, Schiller AL, et al, eds. Tumors of the spine: diagnosis and clinical management. Philadelphia: WB Saunders, 1990:46–51.

70. Boland PJ, Lane JM, Sundaresan N. Metastatic disease of the spine. Clin Orthop 1982;169:95–102.

71. Byers PD. Solitary benign osteoblastic lesions of bone. Osteoid osteoma and benign osteoblastoma. Cancer 1968;22:43–57.

72. Jackson RP, Reckling FW, Mantz FA. Osteoid osteoma and osteoblastoma: similar histologic lesions with different natural histories. Clin Orthop 1977;128:303–313.

73. Kirwan EOG, Hutton PAN, Pozo JL, et al. Osteoid osteoma and benign osteoblastoma of the spine. J Bone Joint Surg 1984;66B:21–26.

74. Sypert GW. Osteoid osteoma and osteoblastoma of the spine. In: Sundaresan N, Schmidek HH, Schiller AL, et al, eds. Tumors of the spine: diagnosis and clinical management. Philadelphia: WB Saunders, 1990:117–125.

75. McLeod RA, Dahlin DC, Beabout JW. The spectrum of osteoblastoma. Am J Roentgenol 1976;126:321–325.

76. Unni KK. Dahlin's bone tumors. General aspects and data on 11,087 cases, 5th ed. Philadelphia: Lippincott-Raven, 1996.

77. Lichtenstein L, Sawyer WR. Benign osteoblastoma: further observations and report of twenty additional cases. J Bone Joint Surg 1964;46A:755–765.

78. Marsh BW, Bonfiglio M, Brady LP, et al. Benign osteoblastoma: range of manifestations. J Bone Joint Surg 1975;57A:1–9.

79. Cohen MD, Harrington TM, Ginsberg WW. Osteoid osteoma: 95 cases and a review of the literature. Semin Arthritis Rheum 1983;12:265–281.

80. Healey JH, Ghelman B. Osteoid osteoma and osteoblastoma: current concepts and recent advances. Clin Orthop 1986;204:76–85.

81. Nemoto O, Moser RP, Van Dam BE, et al. Osteoblastoma of the spine. A review of 75 cases. Spine 1990;15:1272–1280.

82. Ozaki T, Liljenqvist U, Hillmann A, et al. Osteoid osteotome and osteoblastoma of the spine: experiences with 22 patients. Clin Orthop 2002;397:394–402.

83. Boriani S, Capanna R, Donati D, et al. Osteoblastoma of the spine. Clin Orthop 1992;278:37–45.

84. Janin Y, Epstein JA, Carras R, et al. Osteoid osteomas and osteoblastomas of the spine. Neurosurgery 1981;8:31–38.

85. Novick GS, Pavlov H, Bullough PG. Osteochondroma of cervical spine: case reports. Skeletal Radiol 1982;8:13–15.

86. Schajowicz F. Tumors and tumor like lesions of bone and joints. New York: Springer-Verlag, 1981.

87. Malat J, Virapongse C, Levine A. Solitary osteochondroma of the spine. Spine 1986;11:625–628.

88. Albrecht S, Crutchfield JS, SeGall GK. On spinal osteochondromas. J Neurosurg 1992;77:247–252.

89. Gottlieb A, Severi P, Ruelle A, et al. Exostosis as a cause of spinal cord compression. Surg Neurol 1986;26:581.

90. Kak VK, Prabhakar S, Khosla VK, et al. Solitary osteochondroma of

spine causing spinal cord compression. Clin Neurol Neurosurg 1985; 87:135–138.

91. Marchand EP, Villemure JG, Rubin J, et al. Solitary osteochondroma of the thoracic spine presenting as spinal cord compression. A case report. Spine 1986;11:1033–1035.

92. Prasad A, Renjen PN, Prasad ML, et al. Solitary spinal osteochondroma causing neural syndromes. Paraplegia 1992;30:678–680.

93. Merenda JT. Other primary benign tumors and tumor-like lesions of the spine. In: Akbarnia BA, ed. Spine: state of the art reviews. Philadelphia: Hanley & Belfus, 1988:275–287.

94. Capanna R, Albisinni U, Picci P, et al. Aneurysmal bone cyst of the spine. J Bone Joint Surg 1985;67A:527–531.

95. Hay MC, Paterson D, Taylor TKF. Aneurysmal bone cysts of the spine. J Bone Joint Surg 1978;60B:406–411.

96. Wu KK. Diagnosis and treatment of benign and malignant monostotic tumors of the spine. Detroit: National Production Corporation, 1985.

97. Worlock P, Clifford P. Aneurysmal bone cyst of the sacrum. J Roy Coll Surg Edinb 1985;30:196–199.

98. Caro PA, Mandell GA, Stanton RP. Aneurysmal bone cyst of the spine in children. MRI imaging at 0.5 tesla. Pediatr Radiol 1991;21:114–116.

99. Akbarnia BA. Aneurysmal bone cysts of the spine. In: Akbarnia BA, ed. Spine: state of the art reviews. Philadelphia: Hanley & Belfus, 1988:265–274.

100. Campanacci M. Giant cell tumor. In: Gaggi A, ed. Bone and soft-tissue tumors. Bologna: Springer-Verlag 1990:117–153.

101. Turcotte RE, Wunder JS, Isler MH, et al. Giant cell of long bone: a Canadian sarcoma group study. Clin Orthop 2002;397:248–258.

102. Campanacci M, Baldini N, Boriani S, et al. Giant cell tumor of bone. J Bone Joint Surg 1987;69A: 106–113

103. Turcotte RE, Sim FH, Unni KK. Giant cell tumor of the sacrum. Clin Orthop 1993;291:215–221.

104. Samson IR, Springfield DS, Suit HD, et al. Operative treatment of sacrococcygeal chordoma. A review of 21 cases. J Bone Joint Surg 1993;75A:1476–1484.

105. Walker DR, Rankin RN, Anderson C, et al. Giant-cell tumour of the sacrum in a child. Can J Surg 1988;31:47–49.

106. Bertolini F, Present D, Enneking WF. Giant cell tumor of bone with pulmonary metastases. J Bone Joint Surg 1985;67A:890–900.

107. Rock MG, Sim FH, Unni KK, et al. Secondary malignant giant cell tumor of bone: clinicopathological assessment of nineteen patients. J Bone Joint Surg 1986;68A:1073–1079.

108. Siebenrock KA, Unni KK, Rock MG. Giant-cell tumor of bone metastasizing to the lung: a long-term follow-up. J Bone Joint Surg 1998;80B:43–47.

109. Campanacci M, Boriani S, Giunti A. Giant cell tumors of the spine. In: Sundaresan N, Schmidek HH, Schiller AL, et al, eds. Tumors of the spine: diagnosis and clinical management. Philadelphia: WB Saunders, 1990:163–172.

110. Campanacci M, Giunti A, Olmi R. Giant-cell tumor of bone. A study of 209 cases with long-term follow up in 130. Ital J Orthop Traumatol 1975;1:249.

111. Persson BM, Wouters HW. Curettage and acrylic cementation in surgery of giant cell tumors of bone. Clin Orthop 1976;120:125–133.

112. Pritchard DJ. The surgical management of giant cell tumors of bone. Orthop Surg 1980;1:2.

113. Dahlin DC, Cupps R, Johnson EW. Giant cell tumor: a study of 195 cases. Cancer 1980;25:1061–1070.

114. Trieb K, Bitzan P, Dominkus M, et al. Giant cell tumor of long bone. J Bone Joint Surg 2000;82A:1360–1361.

115. Ippolito E, Farsetti, Tudisco C. Vertebra plana. J Bone Joint Surg 1984;66A:1364–1368.

116. Makley JT, Carter JR. Eosinophilic granuloma of bone. Clin Orthop 1986;204:37–44.

117. Silberstein MJ, Sundaram M, Akbarnia B, et al. Eosinophilic granuloma of the spine. Orthopedics 1985;8:264,267–274.

118. Villas C, Martinez-Peric R, Barrios RH, et al. Eosinophilic granuloma of the spine with and without vertebra plana: long-term follow-up of six cases. J Spinal Disord 1993;6:260–268.

119. Nesbit ME, Kieffer S, D'Angio GJ. Reconstruction of vertebral height in histiocytosis X: a long term follow-up. J Bone joint Surg 1969;51A:1360–1368.

120. Fowles JV, Bobechko WP. Solitary eosinophilic granuloma of bone. J Bone Joint Surg 1970;52B:238–243.

121. Compere EL, Johnson WE, Coventry MB. Vertebra plana (Calve's disease) due to eosinophilic granuloma. J Bone Joint Surg 1954; 36A:969–980.

122. Sherk HH, Nicholson JT, Nixon JE. Vertebra plana and eosinophilic granuloma of the cervical spine in children. Spine 1978;3:116–121.

123. Dickinson LD, Farhat SM. Eosinophilic granuloma of the cervical spine. A case report and review of the literature. Surg Neurol 1991;35:57–63.

124. Kornberg M. Erythrocyte sedimentation rate following lumbar discectomy. Spine 1986;11:766–767.

125. Ruff SJ, Taylor TKF, Nicholson OR. Eosinophilic granuloma of the spine. J Bone Joint Surg 1984;66B:780.

126. Mirra JM. Bone tumors: diagnosis and treatment. Philadelphia: JB Lippincott, 1980.

127. Baker ND, Klein MJ, Greenspan A. Symptomatic vertebral hemangiomas: a report of four cases. Skeletal Radiol 1986;15:458–463.

128. Bartels RH, Grotenhui JA, Van Der Spek JA. Symptomatic vertebral hemangiomas. J Neurosurg Sci 1991;35:187–192

129. Nguyen JP, Djindjian M, Gaston A, et al. Vertebral hemangiomas presenting with neurologic symptoms. Surg Neurol 1987;27:391–397.

130. Smith TP, Koci T, Mehringer CM, et al. Transarterial embolization of vertebral hemangioma. J Vasc Interv Radiol 1993;4:681–685.

131. Kapadia S. Multiple myeloma: a clinicopathologic study of 62 consecutively autopsied cases. Medicine (Baltimore) 1980;59:380–392.

132. Kyle RA. Multiple myeloma: review of 869 cases. Mayo Clin Proc 1975;50:29.

133. Goodman MA. Plasma cell tumors. Clin Orthop 1986;204:86–92.

134. Durie B. Multiple myeloma: what's new. CA Cancer J Clin 2001;51: 263,271–272.

135. Corwin J, Lindberg RD. Solitary plasmacytoma of bone vs. extramedullary plasmacytoma and their relationship to multiple myeloma. Cancer 1979;43:1007–1013.

136. Bataille R, Sany J. Solitary myeloma: clinical and prognostic features of a review of 114 cases. Cancer 1981;48:845–851.

137. Wiltshaw E. The natural history of extramedullary plasmacytoma and its relation to solitary myeloma of bone in myelomatosis. Medicine (Baltimore) 1976;55:217–238.

138. Quowling MA, Harwood AR, Bergsal DE. Comparison of extramedullary plasmacytoma with solitary and multiple plasma cell tumors of bone. J Clin Oncol 1983;1:255.

139. Bacci G, Savini R, Calderoni P, et al. Solitary plasmacytoma of the vertebral column. A report of 15 cases. Tumori 1982;68:271–271.

140. Bergsagel DE. Plasma cell myeloma: biology and treatment. Annu Rev Med 1991;42:167–168.

141. McLain RF, Weinstein JN. Solitary plasmacytomas of the spine: a review of 84 cases. J Spinal Disord 1989;2:69–74.

142. Baar J, Burkies Rl, Gospodarowicz M. Primary non-Hodgkin's lymphoma of bone. Semin Oncol 1999;26:270–275.

143. Huvos AG. Bone tumors: diagnosis, treatment, and prognosis. Philadelphia: WB Saunders, 1979.

144. Ostrowsky ML, Unni KK, Banks PM, et al. Malignant lymphoma of bone. Cancer 1986;58:2646–2655.

145. Vassalo J, Roessner A, Vollmer E, et al. Malignant lymphoma with primary bone manifestation. Pathol Res Pract 1987;182:381–389.

146. Camargo OPD, Machado TMDS, Croci AT, et al. Primary bone lymphoma in 24 patients treated between 1955 and 1999. Clin Orthop 2002;397:271–280.

147. Aprin H. Primary malignant tumors of the spine. In: Akbarnia BA, ed. Spine: state of the art reviews. Philadelphia: Hanley & Belfus, 1988: 289–299.

148. Dahlin DC, Coventry MB. Osteosarcoma: a study of 600 cases. J Bone Joint Surg 1967;49A:101–110.

149. Lane JM. malignant bone tumors. In: Alfonson AE, Cardner E, eds. The practice of cancer surgery. New York: Appleton-Century-Crofts, 1982:307–324.

150. Goorin AM, Abelson HT, Frei III, E. Osteosarcoma: fifteen years later. N Engl J Med 1985;313:1637–1643.

151. Lane JM, Hurson B, Boland PJ, et al. Osteogenic sarcoma. Clin Orthop 1986;204:93–110.

152. Shives TC, Dahlin DC, Sim FH, et al. Osteosarcoma of the spine. J Bone Joint Surg 1986;68A:660–668.

153. Talac R, Yaszemski MJ, Currier BL, et al. Relationship between surgical margins and local recurrence in sarcomas of the spine. Clin Orthop 2002;397:127–132.

154. Sundaresan N, Rosen G, Huvos AG, et al. Combined treatment of osteosarcoma of the spine. Neurosurgery 1988;23:714–719.

155. Carter SK. The dilemma of adjuvant chemotherapy of osteogenic sarcoma. Cancer Clin Trials 1980;3:29–36.
156. Marcove RC, Mike V, Hajek JV, et al. Osteogenic sarcoma under the age of twenty-one. A review of one hundred and forty-five operative cases. J Bone Joint Surg 1970;52A:411–423.
157. McKenna RJ, Schwin CP, Soong KY, et al. Sarcomata of osteogenic series (osteosarcoma, fibrosarcoma, chondrosarcoma, parosteal osteogenic sarcoma, and sarcomata arising in abnormal bone). An analysis of 552 cases. J Bone Joint Surg 1966;48A:1–26.
158. Goorin AM, Andersen JW. Experience with multiagent chemotherapy for osteosarcoma. Improved outcome. Clin Orthop 1991;270:22–28.
159. Jaffe N, Frei E III, Traggis D, et al. Adjuvant methotrexate and citrovorum factor treatment of osteogenic sarcoma. N Engl J Med 1974;291:994–997.
160. Link MP, Goorin AM, Miser AN, et al. The effect of adjuvant chemotherapy on relapse-free survival in patients with osteosarcoma of the extremity. N Engl J Med 1986;314:1600–1606.
161. Rosen G, Caparros B, Huvos AG, et al. Preoperative chemotherapy for osteogenic sarcoma: selection of postoperative adjuvant chemotherapy based on the response of the primary tumor to preoperative chemotherapy. Cancer 1982;49:1221–1230.
162. Barwick KW, Huvos AG, Smith J. Primary osteosarcoma of the vertebral column: a clinicopathologic correlation of ten patients. Cancer 1980;46:595–604.
163. Henderson ED, Dahlin DC. Chondrosarcoma of bone: a study of 288 cases. J Bone Joint Surg 1963;45A:1450–1458.
164. Healey JH, Lane JM. Chondrosarcoma. Clin Orthop 1986;204:119–129.
165. Campanacci M, Guernelli N, Leonessa D. Chondrosarcoma: a study of 133 cases, 80 with long-term follow-up. Ital J Orthop Traumatol 1975;1:387.
166. Kilpatrick SE, Inwards CY, Fletcher CD, et al. Myxoid chondrosarcoma (chordoid sarcoma) of bone: a report of two cases and review of the literature. Cancer 1997;79:1903–1910.
167. Marcove RC. Chondrosarcoma: diagnosis and treatment. Orthop Clin North Am 1977;8:811–820.
168. Pritchard DJ, Lunke RJ, Taylor WF, et al. Chondrosarcoma. A clinicopathologic and statistical analysis. Cancer 1980;45:149–157.
169. Hudson TM. Radionuclide bone scanning of medullary chondrosarcoma. AJR Am J Roentgenol 1982;139:1071–1076.
170. Kreicbergs A, Boquist L, Borssen B, et al. Prognostic factors in chondrosarcoma: a comparative study of cellular DNA content and clinicopathologic features. Cancer 1982;50:577–583
171. Kreicbergs A, Zetterberg A, Soderberg G. The prognostic significance of nuclear DNA content in chondrosarcoma. Anal Quant Cytol 1980;2:271–279.
172. Dahlin DC, Unni KK. Chordoma. Arch Pathol Lab Med 1994;118:596–597.
173. Sundaresan N. Chordomas. Clin Orthop 1986;204:135–142.
174. Fechner RE, Mills SE. Tumors of the bones and joints. In: Rosai J, Sobin L, eds. Atlas of tumor pathology, 3rd ed. Washington, DC: Armed Forces Institute of Pathology, 1993:239–244.
175. Gladstone HB, Bailet JW, Rowland JP. Chordoma of the oropharynx: an unusual presentation and review of the literature. Otolaryngol Head Neck Surg 1998;118:104–107.
176. Kendall BE. Cranial chordomas. Br J Radiol 1977;50:687–698.
177. Mindell ER. Chordoma. J Bone Joint Surg 1981;63A:501–505.
178. Penzin KH, Pushiparaj M. Non-epithelial tumors of the nasal cavity, paranasal sinuses, and nasopharynx chordoma. Cancer 1986;57:784–796.
179. Sundaresan N. Huvos AG, Krol G, et al. Spinal chordomas: results of surgical treatment. Arch Surg 1987;122:1478–1482.
180. Higinbotham NL, Philips RF, Farr HW, et al. Chordoma: thirty-five year study at Memorial Hospital. Cancer 1967;20:1841–1850.
181. Sundaresan N, Galicich JH, Chu FC, et al. Spinal chordomas. J Neurosurg 1979;50:312–319.
182. Wold LE, Laws ER. Cranial chordomas in children and young adults. J Neurosurg 1983;59:1043–1047.
183. Chamber PW, Schwinn CP. Chordoma: a clinicopathologic study of metastases. Am J Clin Pathol 1979;72:765–776.
184. Krol G, Sundaresan N, Deck MDF. Computed tomography of axial chordomas. J Comput Asst Tomogr 1983;7:286–289.
185. Smith J, Ludwig RL, Marcove RC. Clinical radiologic features of chordoma. Skeletal Radiol 1987;16:37–44.
186. Soo MY. Chordoma: Review of clinicoradiological features and factors affecting survival. Australas Radiol 2001;45:427–434.
187. Azzarelli A. Quagliuolo V, Cerasoli S, et al. Chordoma: natural history and treatment results in 33 cases. J Surg Oncol 1988;37:185–191.
188. Kaiser TE, Pritchard DJ, Unni KK. Clinicopathologic study of sacrococcygeal chordoma. Cancer 1984;54:2574–2578.
189. Stener B, Gunterberg B. High amputation of the sacrum for extirpation of tumors. Principles and technique. Spine 1978;3:351–366.
190. Colli B, Al-Mefty O. Chordomas of the craniocervical junction: follow-up review and prognostic factors. J Neurosurg 2001;95:933–943.
191. Crockard HA, Steel T, Plowman N, et al. A multidisciplinary team approach to skull base chordomas. J Neurosurg 2001;95:175–183.
192. Ewing J. Diffuse endothelioma of bone. Proc NY Pathol Soc 1921;21:17–22.
193. Dunst J, Ahrens S, Paulussen M, et al. Prognostic impact of tumor perfusion in MR-imaging studies in Ewing tumors. Strahlenther Onkol 2001;177:153–159.
194. Paulussen M, Frohlich B, Jurgens H. Ewing tumour: incidence, prognosis and treatment options. Paediatr Drugs 2001;3:899–913.
195. Bradway JK, Pritchard DJ. Ewing's tumor of the spine. In: Sundaresan N, Schmidek HH, Schiller AL, et al, eds. Tumors of the spine: diagnosis and clinical management. Philadelphia: WB Saunders, 1990:235–239.
196. Venkateswaran L, Rodriguez-Galindo C, Merchant TE, et al. Primary Ewing tumor of the vertebrae: clinical characteristics, prognostic factors, and outcome. Med Pediatr Oncol 2001;37:30–35.
197. Paulussen M, Ahrens S, Dunst J, et al. Localized Ewing tumor of bone: final results of the cooperative Ewing's Sarcoma Study CESS 86. J Clin Oncol 2001;19:1818–1829.
198. Rosen G, Caparros B, Nirenberg A, et al. Ewing's sarcoma: ten-year experience with adjuvant chemotherapy. Cancer 1981;47:2204–2213.
199. Marcus RB Jr, Berrey BH, Graham-Pole J, et al. The treatment of Ewing's sarcoma of bone at the University of Florida: 1969 to 1998. Clin Orthop 2002;397: 290–297.
200. Oberlin O, Patte C, Demeocq F, et al. The response to initial chemotherapy as prognostic factor in localized Ewing's sarcoma. Eur J Cancer Clin Oncol 1985;21:463–467.
201. Cotterill SJ, Ahrens S, Paulussen M, et al. Prognostic factors in Ewing's tumor of bone: analysis of 975 patients from the European Intergroup Cooperative Ewing's Sarcoma Study Group. J Clin Oncol 2000;18:3108–3114.
202. Weber KL, Sim FH. Ewing's sarcoma: presentation and management. J Orthop Sci 2001;6:366–371.

CHAPTER 82

Metastatic Spine Tumors

Stanley D. Gertzbein

One million new cases of cancer are diagnosed every year in this country (1). Metastases occur in approximately two thirds of patients, with the skeleton being the most common site for metastatic tumors, after the lung and liver (2). A metastasis of the spine is defined as a malignancy whose cells have been transferred from the primary site of the tumor to the spinal column with continued unchecked growth. The spine is the most common site of spread (3), one third of which are symptomatic (4). Up to 5% of patients are diagnosed with symptomatic spinal cord lesions (2,5).

The highest incidence of metastases in the spine is in the lumbar region, followed by the thoracic and cervical levels (6). Most associated spinal *cord* lesions, however, are located in the thoracic spine, related to the smaller spinal canal size, vascular supply (7), and predisposition of the thoracic spine to kyphotic deformity (8).

ETIOLOGY, SPREAD, AND GROWTH

Secondary spread of metastatic disease to the skeleton occurs from the following organs in order of frequency: breast, prostate, lung, and kidney. These organs make up approximately 80% of all secondary spread to the spine (4). Of the epidural metastases, the order of frequency is breast, lung, prostate, and kidney (6).

Metastatic lesions are commonly spread by the arterial side of the circulation, particularly from the lung and prostate (9). However, the venous route through Batson plexus may be a source of contamination by tumor cells in the pelvis and abdomen from retrograde spread. The lack of venous valves allows backflow into the vessels of the vertebrae with increased pressure in the abdomen (10). A combination of both of these routes may also be operative (11). Tumors may also spread to the spinal column directly, such as in the mediastinum from lung and from retroperitoneal structures, including the pancreas.

Metastatic lesions enlarge through biochemical and mechanical factors. Osteoclast activating factor (12), col-

lagenase (13), and prostaglandin (14,15) release result in the breakdown of ground substance and collagen, allowing tumor cells to grow and expand. As the mass of the tumor increases, there may be direct pressure on the bony trabeculae, resulting in ischemia and subsequent resorption of bone.

INSTABILITY

Spinal stability relies on the intact spine. As proposed by Denis (16), there are three structural components of the spine, the anterior, middle, and posterior columns. With tumor spread throughout these columns, there is an

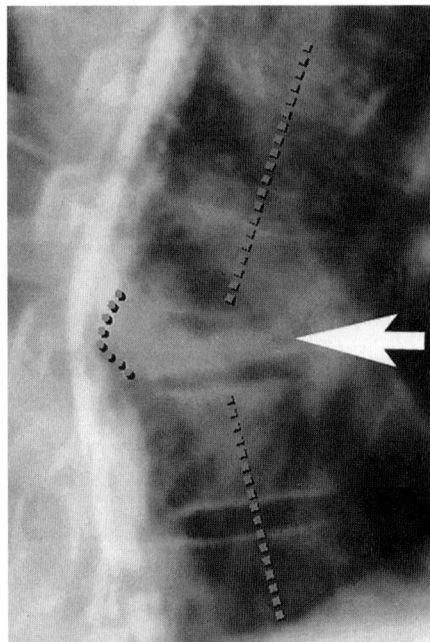

FIG. 82-1. Spinal instability. This lateral radiograph demonstrates collapse of a metastatic lesion resulting in a pathologic fracture *(white arrow)* with moderate angulation *(dotted lines).*

increase in the degree of instability. The middle column accounts for approximately 60% of the axial strength (17) so that when this component is compromised, the spine is at risk for collapse with the potential to create a pathologic fracture. Along with flexion forces, a kyphotic deformity may result with further loss of vertebral height. The fulcrum of the spine in each motion segment, located in the middle column, may migrate posteriorly toward the posterior elements as the forces act on the weakened structures with the result that deformity occurs (Fig. 82-1). In some cases, however, there can be an even collapse of the spine, which does not result in kyphosis, although the expansion of tumor and bone into the spinal canal may result in compromise to the spinal canal and neurologic impairment.

CLINICAL FEATURES

History

Most patients complain of fatigue, malaise, and weight loss because of their underlying disease. Although many metastatic lesions to the spine are asymptomatic, a significant proportion of patients complain of pain because of involvement of the bony elements by tumor tissue. As the tumor replaces bone, the trabeculae weaken, resulting in microfractures or full pathologic fractures, deformity, and instability. Posterior element involvement leading to instability may be a source of pain as well. Pain is the most common presentation in up to 96% of patients, resulting from these sequelae (18). The deposition of peridural tumor in the spinal canal causes compression of the neural elements, and this may also result in pain (Fig. 82-2) (6,19).

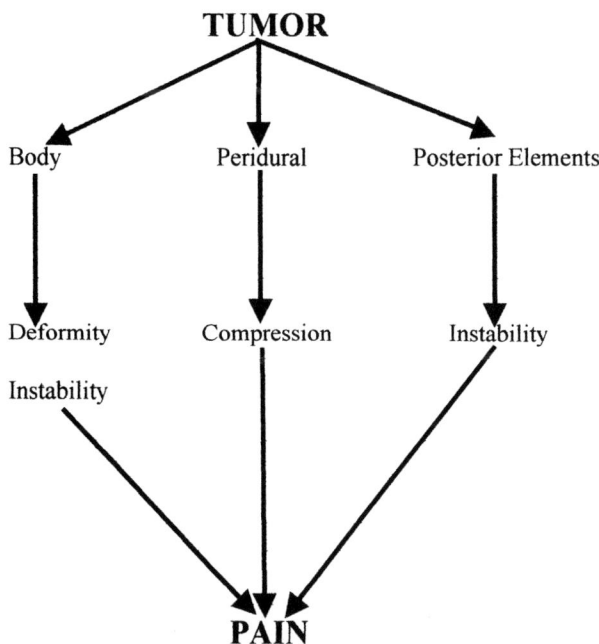

FIG. 82-2. Mechanisms of pain with spinal metastasis.

Neurologic symptoms include weakness, numbness, and paresthesias of the limbs and, with spinal cord involvement, spasms, and bowel and bladder complaints. Neurologic compromise is most common in the thoracic spine, with approximately 70% of all neurologic deficits found in this region, and 15% each in the cervical and lumbar spine (6).

Physical Examination

Although there may be no deformity, the most common observation of malalignment on inspection is that of kyphosis, where there has been collapse from a pathologic fracture. Local tenderness is often present. Neurologic examination may be normal early but with neural compromise the physical examination elicits features associated with upper motor or lower motor neuron findings, depending on the involvement of the spinal cord, the cauda equina, or the nerve roots. A rectal examination is essential in all neurologically compromised patients to identify bowel or bladder dysfunction.

INVESTIGATION OF SPINAL METASTASES

Laboratory Evaluation

Blood work includes a complete blood count, including a sedimentation rate, electrolytes, blood urea nitrogen, calcium, phosphorus, alkaline phosphatase, serum proteins, and protein electrophoresis. This blood profile may be helpful in determining the extent of systemic involvement but does not identify the primary tumor. The immunologic status can be determined from some of these studies as well. Prostatic-specific antigen is useful for identifying prostatic tumor, and carcinoembryonic antigen may be useful in monitoring the progress of tumor therapy (20).

Plain Radiographs

It has been estimated that up to 70% of bone mass loss must be present to visualize an osteolytic lesion on normal X-rays (21). Often, a missing pedicle is the first radiographic finding (Fig. 82-3) (22). Destruction of the vertebral body with or without collapse and the presence of prevertebral soft-tissue findings are late signs of involvement. Although most lesions are osteolytic, several are known to be osteosclerotic. The prostate is the most frequently identified osteosclerotic lesion, but a small proportion of the following lesions are also associated with osteoblastic findings on plain radiographs: breast, bladder, thyroid, and gastrointestinal tumors.

Magnetic Resonance Imaging

Magnetic resonance imaging (MRI) is very useful in not only determining the extent of the lesion within the

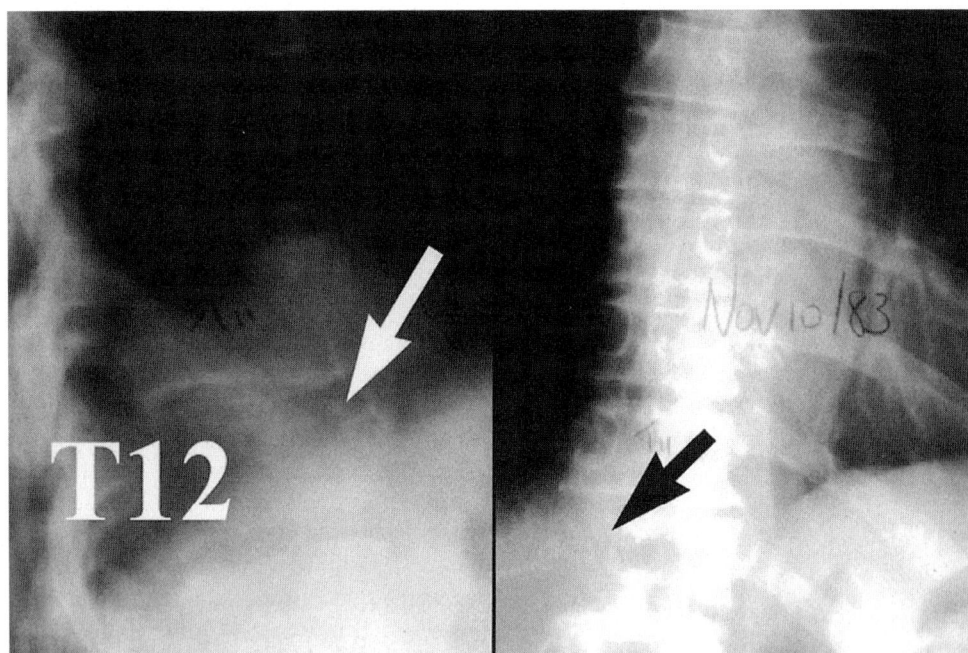

FIG. 82-3. Antero-posterior (AP) and lateral radiograph of the thoracic spine. The lateral projection demonstrates a pathologic fracture of T12 *(white arrow)*. On the AP projection the pedicle is absent because of destruction by the tumor, which is often an early sign of involvement.

spinal canal and its relationship to the spinal cord and cauda equina, but also in helping to differentiate osteoporotic fractures from pathologic fractures caused by tumors of the spine. The distinction is best evaluated on T2-weighted images, where high intensity is seen with

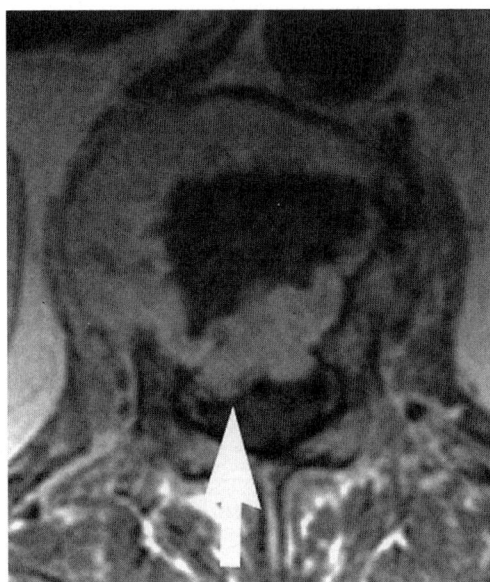

FIG. 82-4. Magnetic resonance image. T2-weighted image of a secondary metastasis to the lumbar spine with hyperintensity of the tumor *(white arrow)* clearly identifying the significant encroachment of the lesion into the spinal canal.

tumors as opposed to normal intensity with osteoporotic fractures (Fig. 82-4). Lesions as small as 3 mm can be detected (23). The use of contrast agents when studying T1-weighted images also assists in interpreting metastases, especially when suppressing the fatty component in the marrow (24). Contrast material injected at the time of MRI scanning also may be helpful in following the effectiveness of chemotherapy or radiation over time (25).

Computed Tomography Myelogram

Although a computed tomography myelogram (myelo-CT) is useful in some cases to define the extent of a block when tumor tissue is present within the spinal canal, the MRI, for the most part, has superseded the use of this study. The CT scan alone, however, provides excellent detail by defining the extent of osseous involvement of the metastasis (Fig. 82-5). This can be helpful in planning the type of surgery.

Bone Scan

Bone scans usually are not helpful in assessing the specific lesion because most secondary tumors demonstrate increased uptake. However, rapid proliferation of some tumors, such as lung, kidney, and myeloproliferative disorders, may not be positive (26). The bone scan, however, is useful in identifying the extent of spread within the spine and other parts of the skeleton and may detect a more accessible lesion to perform a biopsy.

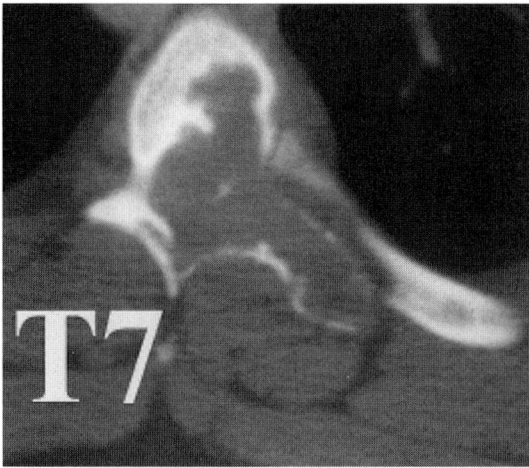

FIG. 82-5. Computed tomography scan accurately identifies the extent of bony involvement at T7, indicating lateral infiltration of the vertebral body. This lesion could readily be addressed surgically from a postero-lateral approach.

Biopsy

Prior to initiating treatment, a biopsy should be performed in all lesions where possible when the diagnosis is deemed necessary. Biopsy can be performed under CT-guided assistance. The entry point of the needle in the skin is 6 to 7 mm lateral to the midline at an angle of about 35°. The success rate in obtaining a tumor specimen is as high as 75% to 95% (27), with an accuracy rate as high as 95% (28,29). The complication rate is low (5), but includes neurologic complications, hemopneumothorax, and excessive bleeding (30,31).

MANAGEMENT OF METASTATIC TUMORS OF THE SPINE

A team approach is essential in treating patients with metastatic disease. This includes the orthopedic surgeon, neurosurgeon, oncologist or radiotherapist, radiologist, and pathologist.

Variables in determining the type of treatment include the type of tumor and the response of the tumor to nonoperative measures. If the tumor is sensitive to chemotherapy or radiotherapy, nonsurgical treatment may be the treatment of choice, especially if the lesions are stable biomechanically and neurologically (32). In cases where there are multiple tumors and widespread involvement of the vertebrae, palliative measures are more appropriate (33). Finally, with patients whose medical status is poor and cannot undergo the trauma of surgery, a less aggressive approach is indicated.

NONOPERATIVE TREATMENT

Chemotherapy

The use of chemotherapeutic drugs will likely have been initiated according to the protocol of the particular primary tumor before the discovery of the spinal lesion. The various regimens are supervised by the oncologist and are beyond the scope of this chapter.

Steroids have been used to reduce edema and inflammation associated with spinal cord compression. This should be considered as an adjunct to management because significant cord compression requires surgical intervention (20), although some protocols have shown a positive effect in combination with radiotherapy (34).

Radiotherapy

Radiation therapy is an effective modality in the treatment of spinal metastases, especially where a painful radiosensitive tumor such as prostate and breast (35) can be treated before there is a major neurologic deficit and before the bony architecture has been significantly destroyed. Although it usually does not return a patient to ambulatory status (33), it is effective in pain control in many instances, especially with multiple site involvement. The dose of radiotherapy to the spinal cord should not exceed 5,000 cGy in 25 fractions over a 5-week period to avoid radiation myelopathy (33,33a). If surgery is performed, adjunctive radiotherapy should be given well before the date of surgery or at least 21 days after the surgery to avoid problems with healing of the soft tissues (36) as well as fusion (37).

External Orthoses

Braces in the thoracolumbar spine are useful during and after treatment for healing and pain control. The halo-vest is similarly effective for patients with cervical lesions (38), but care must be taken in its use because of the concern for skin breakdown in a neurologically or nutritionally compromised patient.

SURGERY

Before performing surgery, several factors require evaluation, including life expectancy. Life expectancy should be evaluated in terms of the prognosis of the primary tumor. It is clear that some tumors have a short survival time irrespective of spread to the spine, such as gastric carcinoma. Other primary lesions have a longer prognosis, including prostate and breast (39). Surgery, therefore, for the most part, should be directed at prevention of local progression and complications such as neurologic sequelae, deformity, and pain. The exception is a solitary metastasis where total spondylectomy is considered for possible cure (40).

The nutritional (41) and immunologic status (42) of the patient as well as the pulmonary status, especially for anterior surgery (20) must be assessed. If these factors are favorable, or if they can be improved, then surgery can be considered. The goals of surgery include: (a)

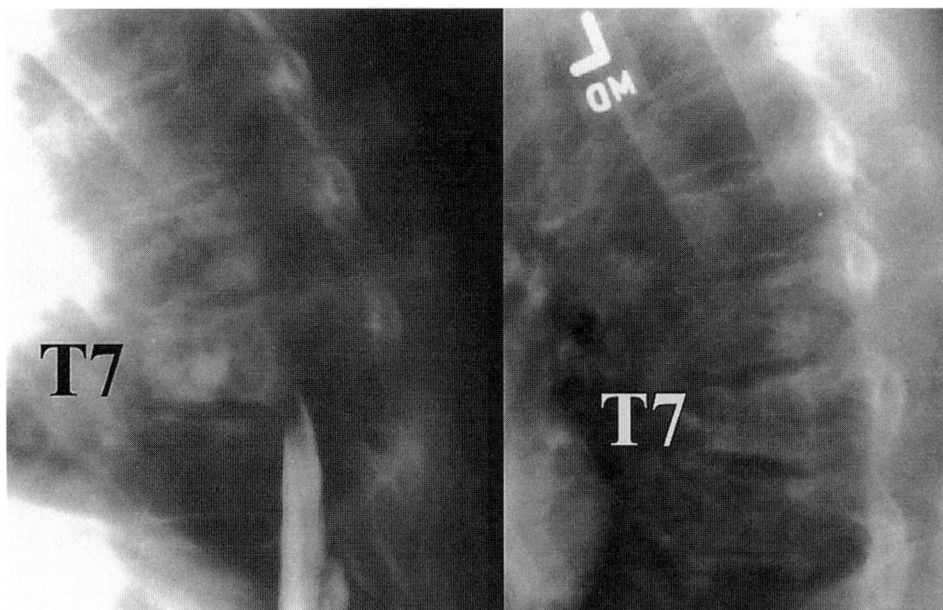

FIG. 82-6. Nonoperative treatment, antero-posterior and lateral radiographs. This breast metastasis at T7 was associated with a major block to the spinal canal, but with only a minor neurologic deficit. The patient was treated with radiation therapy and bracing with relief of the neurologic deficit. One and a half years later the vertebrae maintained its integrity and no neurologic sequelae were seen.

decompression of the neural tissues, (b) prevention of neural injury by stabilization of the unstable spinal column, or (c) pain control. Those patients with no or mild neural deficit and minimal erosion of bone without collapse of the spine and demonstrate good alignment who are chemosensitive or radiosensitive can be treated with these therapies along with a brace and analgesics, as mentioned in the preceding (Fig. 82-6). The remaining patients require surgery. The principles of surgery include tumor reduction, decompression of the neurologic tissues, and stabilization of the spine. There is some controversy as to whether prophylactic surgery is indicated in patients with less than 50% involvement of the vertebral body (43–45). Patients who progress to greater than 50% often collapse (43,44). It is also known that a significant number of patients with spinal metastases go on to neurologic compromise (2,5). For these reasons, cases with greater than 50% vertebral body collapse, especially where there is imminent involvement of the spinal cord, should be stabilized after clearing of the tumor. When pain is the primary indication for surgery, a good response can be expected from the surgery but the life expectancy remains unaltered (46).

STAGING AND CLASSIFICATION OF METASTATIC LESIONS

Recent interest in more aggressive surgery for metastatic disease has been spurred on, in part, by improvements in surgical technology. It is now feasible to perform a total

excision of a vertebra and stabilize the segment (40,47–50), depending on the extent of bony involvement (Fig. 82-7).

Scoring systems have been devised that address the important aspects of tumor surgery and include classifications that describe the extent of instability (51), the neurologic involvement along with instability (52), prognostic factors to determine if surgery should be performed (53), and factors that determine the type of surgery to be performed (54,55), specifically whether en bloc surgery is feasible over major excision, palliative surgery, or no surgery. Caution must be exercised in attempting to precisely determine tumor containment because spread can extend beyond tissues commonly held to be natural barriers, such as the posterior longitudinal ligament (46).

In a recent paper on surgical strategy for spinal metastasis (55), an attempt was made to determine the type of surgery necessary based on three prognostic factors: grade of malignancy, visceral metastases, and bony metastases (Fig. 82-8). Points are awarded according to the aggressiveness of the primary tumor and the extent of visceral and bony spread. A low score leads to total excision surgery, whereas a high score does not merit surgery.

The results indicated that the en bloc patients had a survival of 38 months, whereas the intralesional excision patients survived 22 months. The palliative surgery patients lived 10 months and those without surgical treatment died at 5 months. Satisfactory pain control occurred in 80% of patients and neurologic improvement in 74%. These results suggest that an ordered approach to surgical intervention has merit, although the outcomes are not

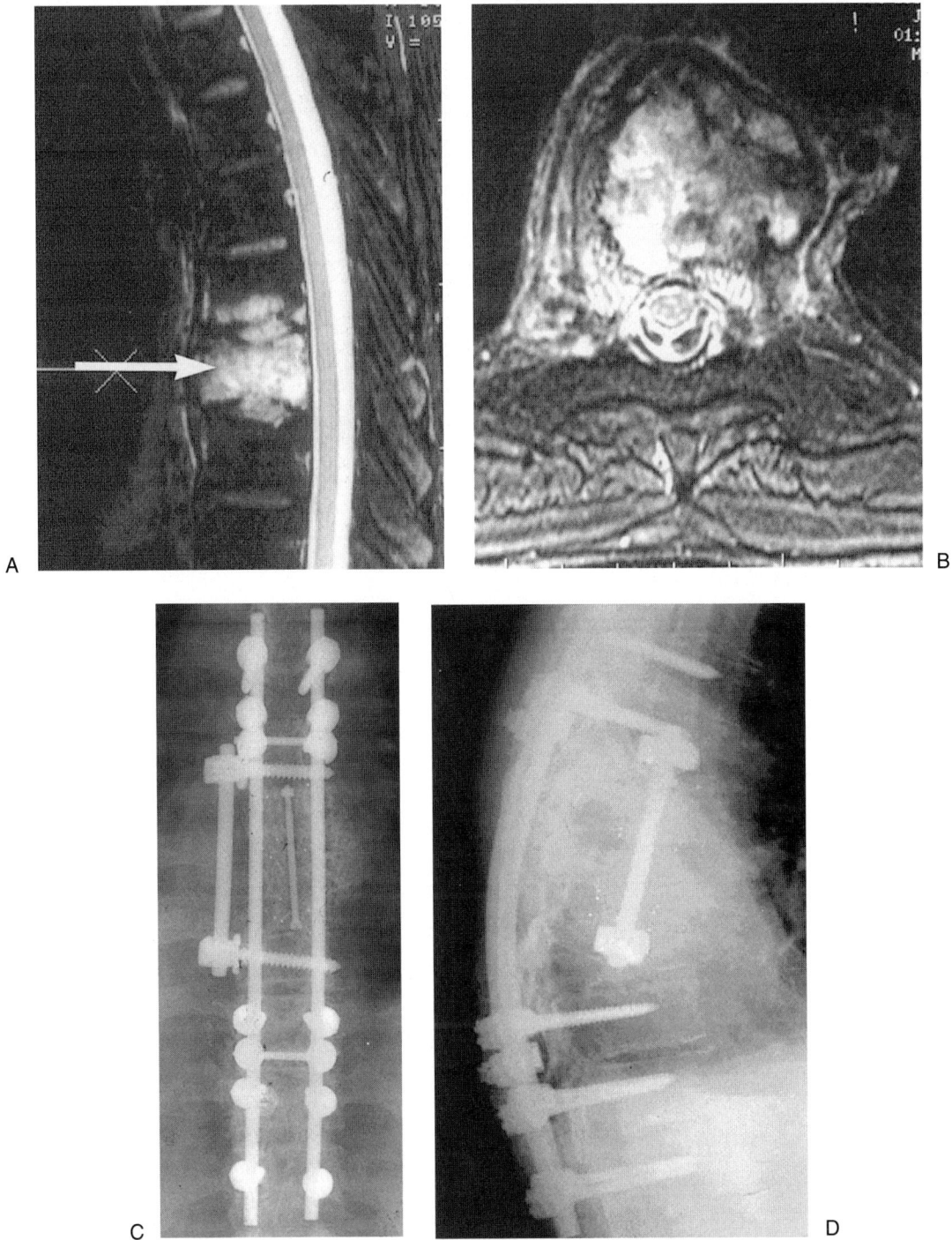

FIG. 82-7. Vertebrectomy. **A:** Lateral magnetic resonance image of the thoracic spine demonstrating increased intensity of metastasis in T8 with spread into the inferior aspect of T7 and the T8-9 disc. **B:** Computed tomography scan of T8 demonstrating containment of the tumor within the bone without involvement of the spinal canal. **C,D:** Antero-posterior and lateral radiograph postoperatively following complete vertebrectomy of T7 and T8, anterior fixation with methyl methacrylate and rod fixation, and posterior pedicle screw and rod instrumentation. (From Dr. Rex Marco, with permission.)

that much different than earlier surgical series (56–58). Long-term survival is obviously related to the aggressiveness of the primary tumor, but if local extirpation is effective, then local recurrence should not be an issue in the long-term survivors.

As an adjunct to surgery, the use of preoperative embolization of metastatic spinal tumors has been shown to be effective not only in allowing for more extensive removal of the tumor, but also in reducing the intraoperative bleeding significantly with less intraoperative complications (59).

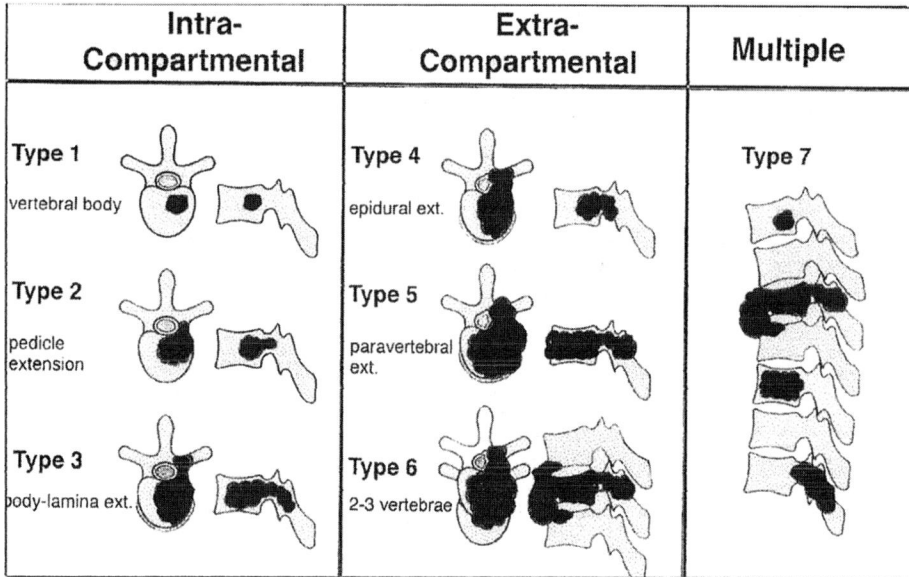

FIG. 82-8. Classification of the involvement of metastatic tumors grouped into intracompartmental, extracompartmental, and multiple lesions. (From Tomita K, Kowahara N, Kobayashi T, et al. Surgical strategy for spinal metastases. Spine 2001;26(3): 298–306, with permission.)

THE ANTERIOR APPROACH TO THE SPINE

When there is a need to reduce the tumor size and decompress the neurologic tissues, the most direct approach is anteriorly because the most common site is in the verte-bral body, although a posterolateral approach may be performed in some instances (Fig. 82-5) (60,61). Stabilization of the spine also can be performed anteriorly when decompression anteriorly is required (62,63). Methyl methacrylate is a useful material as an anterior spacer (51,58,64,65),

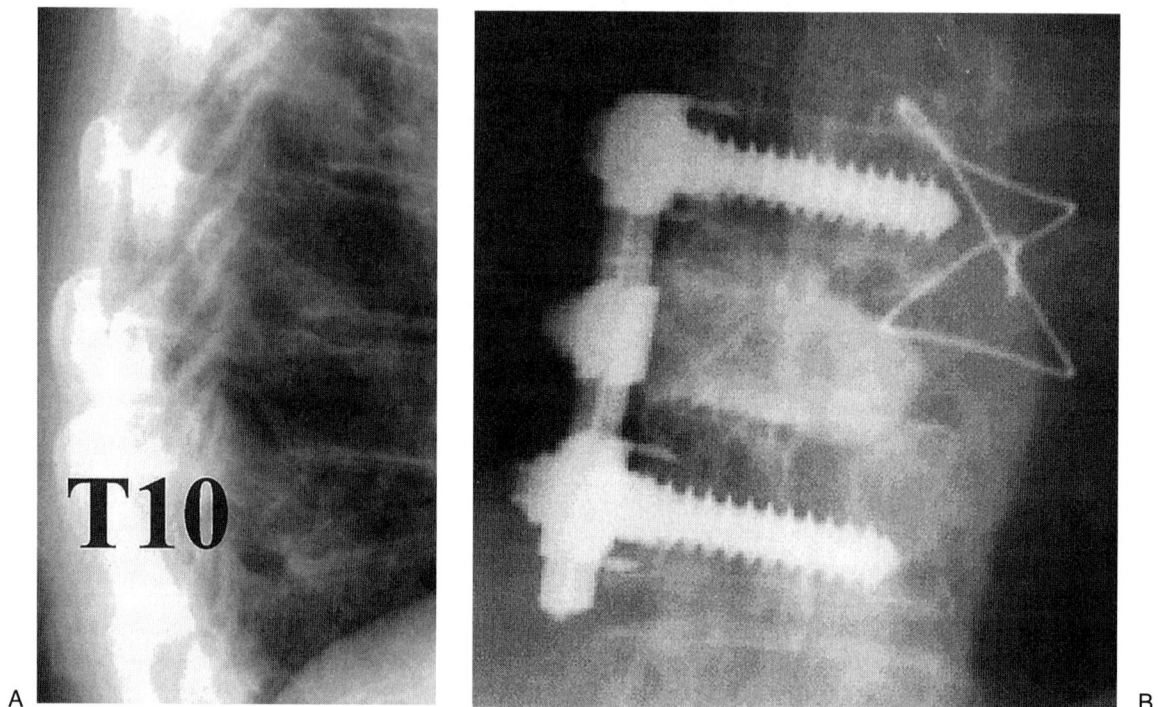

FIG. 82-9. Anterior approach. **A:** Lateral radiograph of the thoracic spine demonstrating a pathologic fracture of T10 secondary to lung carcinoma. **B:** Antero-posterior projection following anterior corpectomy and decompression of the tumor with methyl methacrylate and rib strut grafting along with anterior instrumentation T9 to T11.

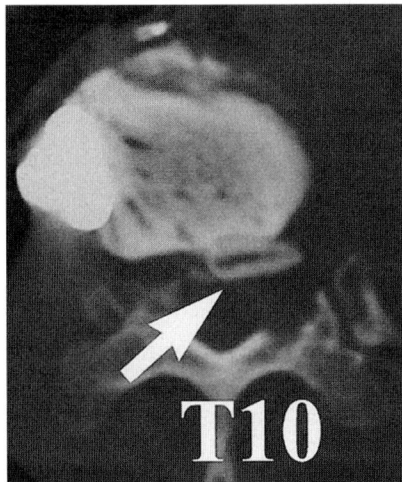

FIG. 82-9. (*Continued*). **C:** Computed tomography scan outlining the presence of methyl methacrylate and rib strut grafts. There is a complete decompression of the spinal canal *(white arrow).*

especially in patients with a shorter estimated time of survival. The use of mesh cages is also effective when filled with cement or allograft. Anterior iliac strut grafts combined with internal fixation is an option in patients with a longer survival time (Fig. 82-9). Prosthetic devices also have been described but are not widely used (66–69).

THE POSTERIOR APPROACH TO THE SPINE

Laminectomy alone is not effective in improving neurologic function (70–72). Furthermore, attempting to remove tumor tissue from the anterior spinal canal from the posterior approach, especially at the thoracic and cervical levels, has a high risk of neurologic deterioration (73) and often destabilizes the level, leading to deformity with the potential for additional neurologic impairment. Nevertheless, the posterior approach is more accessible, less hazardous, and effective in the correction of deformity if combined with instrumentation (Fig. 82-10). Seg-

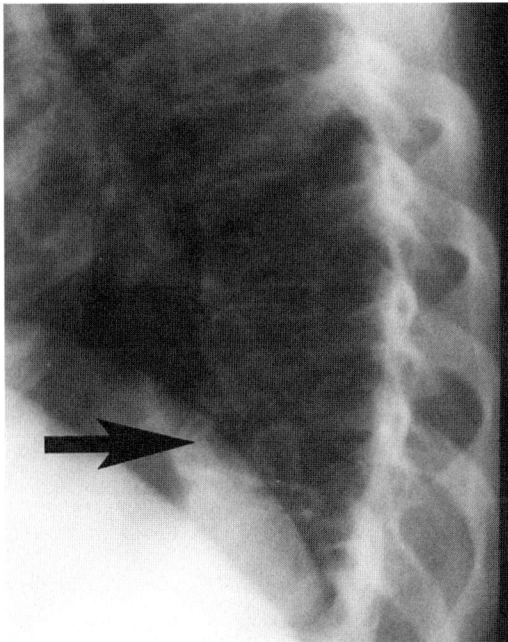

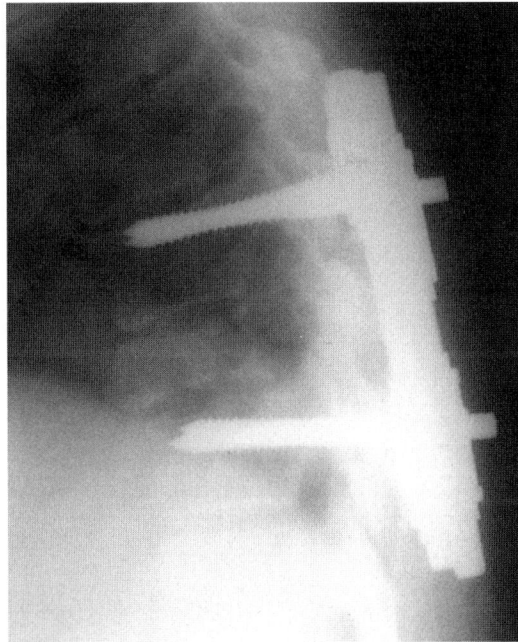

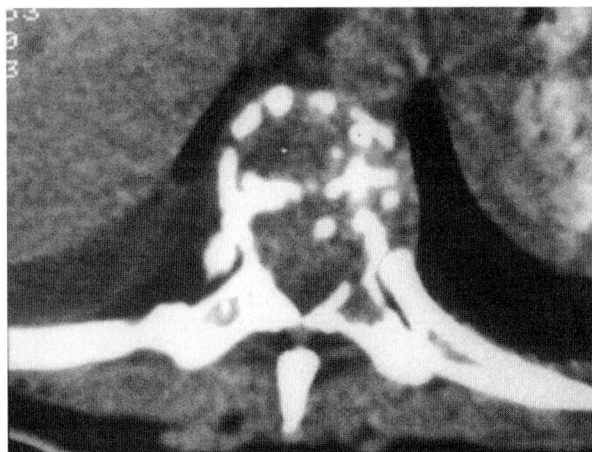

FIG. 82-10. Posterior surgery. **A:** Lateral radiographs of a breast carcinoma at T9. The patient had quite significant pain from this pathologic fracture and tumor. **B:** Computed tomography scan demonstrating significant involvement of the vertebral body and encroachment on the spinal canal although the she was neurologically intact. **C:** Lateral postoperative radiographs demonstrating fixation of the lesion and bone grafting followed by radiation therapy with good pain relief and no neurologic deterioration.

mental fixation using pedicle screws is often the treatment of choice, although sublaminar wiring may be used as well, particularly if there is multiple segment involvement in an osteoporotic spine (74). For posterior or lateral pathology, particularly at the lower lumbar region, a posterolateral approach often is sufficient.

COMBINED APPROACH

The combined approach is required for those cases where there is major involvement of the spinal columns both anteriorly and posteriorly. Anterior grafting or spacers along with posterior instrumentation, with either pedicle screw fixation or segmental fixation, is often required to be performed in two stages under one anesthetic or a few days apart. Alternatively, the anterior and posterior procedures can be effectively accomplished through a posterior approach (65,75). If complete vertebrectomy is feasible in an isolated lesion of the vertebra, then stabilization using an anterior bone strut combined with anterior and posterior stabilization is necessary following the vertebrectomy (Fig. 82-7) (40,57,61,76).

RESULTS OF SURGERY

In most studies, pain relief is significant, as high as 92% (77,51,61). Neurologic deficits following surgery improve by about 80%, especially with anterior surgery (Table 82-1) (56–58,72,76,78–85). Ambulation has been reported to be as high as 93% (86), particularly with anterior surgery.

TABLE 82-1. *Maintenance and recovery of neurologic function after spinal decompression*

Investigator	n	Percent improvement
Anterior decompression		
Sundaresan (59)	110	82
Siegal (67)	75	80
Fidler (60)	17	73
Harrington (35)	77	84
Kostuik (62)	70	73
Manabe (61)	28	82
Total	427	79
Posterior decompression		
Wright (63)	86	35
White (64)	226	38
Hall (65)	123	39
Gilbert (45)	65	45
Nather (66)	42	13
Siegal (50)	25	39
Sherman (68)	149	27
Kostuik (47)	30	33
Total	746	33

Source: Adapted from Weinstein JN, Spine Tumors. In: Wiesel SW, Weinstein JN, Herkowitz H, et al., eds. The lumbar spine, 2nd ed. New York: Lippincott Williams & Wilkins, 1996, p. 932.

COMPLICATIONS

Surgical complications tend to be higher than in other conditions in the spine but with improving surgical and anesthesia techniques, the incidence of major problems should decrease as was observed in a recent review where 75% of patients had no complications (87).

Mortality for the anterior approach or the posterior approach with instrumentation is as high as 8% (88–90). Worsening of neurologic function may occur in up to 5% of patients undergoing an anterior approach and up to 25% for patients treated by laminectomy alone (20). Wound healing can also be a significant problem because of malnutrition and concurrent radiotherapy (91), as high as 32% in one series. Failure of fixation with resulting deformity or recurrence of deformity is less common with the use of pedicle screw fixation and anterior reconstruction techniques, dropping from as high as 79%, to 0% to 4% (60,61,68,92).

INNOVATIVE AND NEWER TECHNIQUES

Investigative tools are becoming more sophisticated and include performing MRIs with contrast measuring blood perfusion time-intensity curves to distinguish osteoporotic fractures from pathologic fractures secondary to metastases (93). Another imaging study, single photon emission computed tomography has been found useful in distinguishing benign disease from metastases (94). Percutaneous ablation of certain metastatic tumors of the spine is currently performed for unresectable lesions for pain control (95) and endoscopic surgery for removal of metastases at the cervico-thoracic junction (96). These innovative techniques are examples of some of the future directions that will be pursued as technological breakthroughs continue.

SUMMARY

Although many metastatic lesions can be treated nonoperatively with bracing, analgesics, chemotherapy, or radiotherapy, those cases with instability and loss of vertebral height as well as deformity; those cases in which there is significant neurologic deficit will require operative intervention. The approach should be tailored to fit the lesion employing the anterior approach for decompression surgery and anterior stabilization, whereas the posterior approach with instrumentation should be reserved for patients with minimal neurologic involvement but in whom instability and deformity are of concern. With newer procedures such as bone conductive spacers, combined anterior and posterior surgery techniques and vertebrectomy surgical outcomes will continue to improve with less risk and complications.

REFERENCES

1. Silverberg E, Lubera J. Cancer statistics, 1987. CA, Cancer J Clin 1987;37(1):2–16.
2. Boland PJ, Lane JM, Sundaresan N. Metastatic disease of the spine. Clin Orthop 1982;169:95-102.
3. Berrettoni BA, Carter JR. Mechanisms of cancer metastasis to bone. J Bone Joint Surg 1986;68A(2):308–320.
4. Schaberg JC, Gainor BJ. A profile of metastatic carcinoma of the spine. Spine 1985;10:(11):19–20.
5. Barron KD, Hirano A, Araki S, et al. Experiences with metastatic neoplasms involving the spinal cord. Neurology 1959;9:91–98.
6. Brihaye J, Ectors P, Lemont M, et al. The management of spinal epidural metastases. Adv Tech Stand Neurosurg 1988;16:121–130.
7. Nottebaert M, von Hochstetter AR, Exner GU, et al. Metastatic carcinoma of the spine: a study of 92 cases. Int Orthop 1987;7(4):345–357.
8. Urist MR, Gurvey MS, Fareed DO. Long-term observations of aged women with pathological osteoporosis. In: Barzel US, ed. Osteoporosis. New York: Grune and Stratton, 1970.
9. Coman DR, Delong RP, McCutcheon J. Studies on the mechanisms of metastases: the distribution of tumors in various organs in relation to the distribution of arterial emboli. Cancer Res 1951;11:648–658.
10. Batson OV. The role of the vertebral veins in the metastatic process. Am Int Med 1942;16:38–45.
11. Yuh, WTC, Quets JP, Lee HG, et al. Anatomic distribution of metastases in the vertebral body and modes of hematogenous spread. Spine 1996;21(19):2243–2250.
12. Galasko CSB. The development of skeletal metastases. In: Weiss L, Gilbert AJ, eds. Bone metastases. Boston: GA Hall Medical, 1981.
13. Powles TJ, Dowset MD, Eastey GC, et al. Breast cancer osteolysis, bone metastases and the anti-osteolytic effect of aspirin. Lancet 1978;1:608-1610.
14. Galasko CSB, Bennett A. Relationship of bone destruction in skeletal metastases to osteoclast activation and prostaglandins. Nature 1976;263(5577):508–516.
15. Greaves M, Ibbotson K, Athens D, et al. Prostaglandins as mediators of bone resorption in renal and breast tumors. Clin Sci 1980;58(3):201–205.
16. Denis F. The three-column spine and its significance in the classification of acute thoracolumbar spinal injuries. Spine 1983;8(8):817–831.
17. Haher TR, Tozzi JM, Lospinuso MS, et al. The contribution of the three columns of the spine to spinal stability: biomechanical model. Paraplegia 1989;27:432–441.
18. Onimus M, Papin P, Gangloff S. Results of surgical treatment of spinal thoracic and lumbar metastases. Eur Spine J 1966;5(6):407–411.
19. Applegren L, Nordborg C, Sjoberg M, et al. Spinal epidural metastasis: implications for spinal analgesia to treat "refractory" cancer pain. J Pain Symptom Manage 1997;13(13):25–42.
20. Asdourian PL. Metastatic disease of the spine. In: Bridwell KH, DeWald RL, eds. The textbook of spinal surgery, 2nd ed. Philadelphia: Lippincott-Raven, 1997.
21. Edelsyn GA, Gillespie PJ, Gribbell FS. The radiological demonstration of osseous metastases. Experimental observation. Clin Radiol 1967;18(2):158–167.
22. Jacobson JG, Poppel MH, Shapiro JH, et al. The vertebral pedicle sign. AJR Am J Roentgenol 1958;80:817–821.
23. Petren-Mallmin M, Nordstrom B, Andreasson I, et al. MR imaging with histopathological correlation in vertebral metastases of breast cancer. Acta Radiol 1992;33(3):213–223.
24. Smoker WRK, Godersky JC, Knutzon RK, et al. The role of MR imaging in evaluating metastatic spinal disease. AJR Am J Roentgenol 1987;149(6):1241–1252.
25. Sugimura K, Kajitani A, Okizuka R, et al. Assessing response to therapy of spinal metastases with gadolinium-enhanced MR imaging. J Magn Reson Imaging 1991;1(4):481–490.
26. Galasko CSB. Skeletal metastases. Clin Orthop 1986;210:18–221.
27. Tehranzadeh J, Freiberger RH, Ghelman B. Closed skeletal needle biopsy: review of 120 cases. AJR Am J Roentgenol 1983;140(1):113–117.
28. Mink J. Percutaneous biopsy in the patient with known or suspected osseous metastases. Radiology 1986;161(1):191–199.
29. Schiff D, O'Neill BP, Sumar BP. Spinal epidural metastases as the initial manifestation of malignancy: Clinical features and diagnostic approach. Neurology 1997;49(2):452–456.
30. Fyfe IS, Henry APS, Mulholland RC. Closed vertebral biopsy. J Bone Joint Surg 1983;65B(2):140–145.
31. Jacobsson H. Percutaneous bone biopsy with a simple punch instrument. Acta Radiol Diagn 1982;23(4):415–419.
32. Rau S, Badani K, Schildhauer T, et al. Metastatic malignancy of the cervical spine. A non-operative history. Spine 1992;17(10 supp):S407–S410.
33. Tomita T, Galicich JH, Sundaresan N. Therapy for spinal epidural metastases with complete block. Acta Radiol Oncol 1983;22(2):135–145.
33a. Cramer S, Southard MF, Mansfield CM. Radiation effects and tolerance of the central nervous system. Front Radiat Ther Oncol 1972;6:332–339.
34. Greenberg HS, Kim JH, Posner JB. Epidural spinal cord compression for metastases: for results with a new treatment protocol. Ann Neurol 1980;8(4):361–366.
35. Bruckmann JE, Bloomer WD. Management of spinal cord compression. Semin Oncol 1978;5:135–140.
36. Vanderbrouck C, Sancho F, LeFur R, et al. Results of a randomized clinical trial of preoperative irradiation versus postoperative in the treatment of tumors of the hypopharynx. Cancer 1997;39:1445–1449.
37. Bouchard JA, Anuradha K, Bensusan JS, et al. Effects of irradiation on post-spinal fusions. Spine 1994;19(16):1836–1841.
38. Danzig LA, Resnick D, Akeson WH. The treatment of cervical spine metastases from prostate with the halo-cast. Spine 1980;5:395–398.
39. Tatsui H, Onomura T, Morishita S, et al. Survival rates of patients with metastatic spinal cancer after scintigraphic detection of abnormal radioactive accumulation. Spine 1996;18:2143–2148.
40. Tomita K, Kawalahara M, Baba H, et al. Total en bloc spondylectomy for solitary spinal metastases. Int Orthop 1994;18:291–298.
41. DeWys, WD. Anorexia as a general effect of cancer. Cancer 1979;43(5 suppl):2013–2020.
42. DeWald RL, Bridwell KH, Prodromas C, et al. Reconstructive spinal surgery as palliation for metastatic malignancies of the spine. Spine 1985;10(1):21–26.
43. Findlay GFC. The role of vertebral body collapse in the management of malignant spinal cord compression. J Neurol Neurosurg Psychiatry 1987;50:151–154.
44. Ominus M, Sehraub S, Bertin D, et al. Surgical treatment of vertebral metastases. Spine 1986;11(9):883–896.
45. Solini A, Paschero B, Orsini G, et al. The surgical treatment of metastatic tumors of the lumbar spine. Ital J Orthop Traumatol 1985;11(4):427–439.
46. Chataigner H, Onimous M. Surgery in spinal metastasis with spinal cord compression: Indications and strategy related to risk of recurrence. Eur Spine J 2000;9(6):523–527.
47. Fujita T, Ueda Y, Kawahara N. Local spread of metastatic vertebral tumors. Spine 1997;22:1905–1912.
48. Magerl F, Coscia MF. Total posterior vertebrectomy of the thoracic or lumbar spine. Clin Orthop 1988;232:62–69.
49. Stener B. Complete removal of vertebrae for extirpation of tumors. Clin Orthop 1989;245:72–82.
50. Sundaresan N, DiGiacinto GV, Krol G, et al. Spondylectomy for malignant tumors of the spine. J Clin Oncol 1989;14:85–91.
51. Kostuik JP, Errico TJ, Gleason TF, et al. Spinal stabilization of vertebral column tumors. Spine 1988;13(3):250–256.
52. Harrington KD. Metastatic disease of the spine. J Bone Joint Surg 1986;68A:1110–1115.
53. Tokuhashi Y, Matsuzaki H, Toriyami S, et al. Scoring system for the pre-operative evaluation of metastatic spine tumor prognosis. Spine 1990;15:1110–1113.
54. Weinstein JN. Spine neoplasms. In: Weinstein SL, ed. The pediatric spine: principles and practice. New York: Raven Press, 1994:887–916.
55. Tomita K, Kowahara N, Kobayashi T, et al. Surgical strategy for spinal metastases. Spine 2001;26(3):298–306.
56. Siegal T, Siegal T. Surgical decompression of anterior and posterior malignant epidural tumors compressing the spinal cord: a prospective study. Neurosurgery 1985;17(3):424–430.
57. Fidler MW. Pathological fractures of the cervical spine. J Bone Joint Surg 1985;67B:352–357.
58. Harrington KD. Anterior decompression and stabilization of the spine as a treatment for vertebral collapse and spinal cord compression from metastatic malignancy. Clin Orthop 1988;233:177–194.
59. Hess T, Kramann B, Schmidt E, et al. Use of pre-operative vascular

embolization in spinal metastasis resection. Arch Orthop Trauma Surg 1997;116(5):279–282.

60. Bauer HC. Posterior decompression and stabilization for spinal metastases. Analysis of 67 consecutive patients. J Bone Joint Surg 1998;79(4):514–522.

61. Bilsky MH, Boland P, Lis E, et al. Single stage posterolateral transpedicular approach for spondylectomy, epidural decompression and circumferential fusion of spinal metastases. Spine 2000;25(17):2240–2249.

62. Gokaslan ZL, York JE, Walsh GL, et al. Transthoracic vertebrectomy for metastatic spinal tumors. J Neursurg 1998;89(4):599–609.

63. Chen LH, Chen WJ, Niu CH, et al. Anterior reconstructive spinal surgery with Zielke instrumentation for metastatic malignancies of the spine. Arch Orthop Trauma Surg 2000;120(1–2):27–31.

64. Yen D, Kuriachar V, Yach J, et al. Long term outcome of anterior decompression and spinal fixation after placement of the Wellesley Wedge for thoracic and lumbar spinal metastases. J Neurosurg 2002;96(1 suppl):6–9.

65. Cahill DW, Kumar R. Palliative subtotal vertebrectomy with anterior and posterior reconstruction via a single posterior approach. J Neuro Surg 1999;(1 suppl):42–47.

66. Ono K, Tada K. Prosthesis of the cervical vertebra. J Neurosurg 1975;42(5):42–49.

67. Solini A, Orsini G, Broggi S. Metal cementless prosthesis for vertebral body replacement of metastatic malignant disease of the cervical spine J Spinal Disord 1989;2(4):254–260.

68. Hosono N, Yonenohu K, Fuji T, et al. Vertebral body replacement with a ceramic prosthesis for metastatic spinal tumors. Spine 1995;20(22):2454–2462.

69. Kaneda K, Takeda N. Reconstruction with a ceramic vertebral prosthesis and Kaneda device following subtotal or total vertebrectomy in metastatic thoracic and lumbar spine. In: Bridwell KH, DeWald RI, eds. The textbook of spinal surgery, 2nd ed. Philadelphia: Lippincott-Raven, 1999:2071–2087.

70. Nicholls PJ, Jarecky TW. The value of posterior decompression by laminotomy for malignant tumors of the spine. Clin Orthop 1985;201:210–213.

71. Constans JP, DeVitus E, Donzelli R, et al. Spinal metastases with neurological manifestations. Review of 600 cases. J Neurosurg 1983;59:111–118.

72. Gilbert RW, Kim JH, Posner JB. Epidural spinal cord compression from metastatic tumor: diagnosis and treatment. Ann Neurol 1978;3:40–51.

73. Martin NS, Williamson J. The role of surgery in the treatment of malignant tumors of the spine. J Bone Joint Surg 1970;52B:227–237.

74. Ghogawala Z, Mansfield FL, Borges LF. Spinal radiation before surgical decompression adversely affects outcomes of surgery for symptomatic metastatic spinal cord compression. Spine 2001;26(7):818–824.

75. Akeyson EW, McCucheon IE. Single stage posterior vertebrectomy and replacement combined with posterior instrumentation for spinal metastases. J Neurosurg 1996;85(2):211–220.

76. Sundaresan N, Steinberger AA, Moore F, et al. Indications and results of combined anterior-posterior approaches for spine tumor surgery. J Neurosurg 1996;85(3):438–446.

77. Hammerberg KW. Surgical treatment of metastatic spine disease. Spine 1992;17(10):1148–1153.

78. Menabi S, Tateishi A, Abe M, et al. Surgical treatment of metastatic tumors of the spine. Spine 1989;14:41–47.

79. Kostuik JP. Anterior spinal cord decompression for lesions of the thoracic and lumbar spine: techniques, new methods of anterior fixation results. Spine 1983;8:513–531.

80. Wright RL. Malignant tumors in the spinal extradural space: results of surgical treatment. Ann Surg 1963;157:227–231.

81. White AA III, Panjabi MM. Clinical biomechanics of the spine. Philadelphia: JB Lippincott, 1978.

82. Hall AJ, MacKay NN. The results of laminectomy of the cord or cauda equina by extradural malignant tumour. J Bone Joint Surg 1973;55B:497–505.

83. Nather A, Bose K. The results of decompression of the cord or cauda equina compression from metastatic extradural tumors. Clin Orthop 1982;169:103–108.

84. Siegal T, Tiqva P, Seigal T. Vertebral body resection for epidural compression by decompression by malignant tumors. J Bone Joint Surg 1985;67A:375–382.

85. Sherman MS, Waddell JP. Laminectomy for metastatic epidural spinal cord tumors. Clin Orthop 1986;207:55–63.

86. Weigel B, Maghsudi M, Neumann C, et al. Surgical management of symptomatic spinal metastases. Post-operative outcome and quality of life. Spine 1999;24(21):2240–2246.

87. Wise JJ, Fischgrund JS, Herkowitz HN, et al. Complications, survival rates, and risk factors of surgery for metastatic disease of the spine. Spine 1999;24(18):1943–1951.

88. McAffe PC, Zdeblick T. The thoracic and lumbar spine: Surgical treatment via the anterior approach. J Spinal Disord 1989;2(3):145–157.

89. O'Neil J, Gardner V, Armstrong G. Treatment of tumours of the thoracic and lumbar spine. Clin Orthop 1986;227:103–114.

90. Perrin RG, McBroom RJ. Anterior versus posterior decompression for symptomatic spinal metastases. Can J Neurol Sci 1987;14(1):75–83.

91. McPhee IB, Williams, RP, Swanson, CE. Factors influencing wound healing after surgery for metastatic disease of the spine. Spine 1998;23(6):726–733.

92. Hussein AA, El-Karef E, Hafez M. Resconstructive surgery in spinal tumors. Eur J Surg Oncol, 2001;27(2):196–199.

93. Chen WT, Shih TT, Chen RC, et al. Blood perfusion of vertebral lesions evaluated with gadolinium-enhanced dynamic MRI: in comparison with compression fracture and metastasis. J Magn Reson Imaging 2002;15(3):308–314.

94. Savelli G, Grasselli G, Maccauro M, et al. The role of bone SPET study in diagnosis of single vertebral metastases. Anticancer Res 2000;20(2B):1115–1120.

95. Gronemeyer DH, Schirp S, Gevargez A. Image-guided radiofrequency ablation of spinal tumors: preliminary experience with an expandable array electrode. Cancer 2002;8(1):33–39.

96. Le Huec JC, Lesprit E, Guibaud JP, et al. Minimally invasive endoscopic approach to the cervico-thoracic junction for vertebral metastases: report of 2 cases. Eur Spinal J 2001;10(5):421–426.

CHAPTER 83

Lumbar Spine Tumors: Posterior Approach

K. Anthony Kim, Babak Kateb, Peter Dyck, Srinath Samudrala

Spinal cord tumors account for approximately 15% of central nervous system tumors (1). Metastatic tumors aside, common tumors of the spine can be divided by location into extramedullary (two-thirds of cases) and intramedullary types. Intramedullary tumors include astrocytoma, ependymoma, hemangioblastoma, lymphoma, and primitive neuroectodermal tumors, among others. Aside from drop metastasis, hemangioblastoma of the conus and nerve roots, and ependymomas of the filum terminale, the surgeon is rarely faced with intramedullary tumors in the lumbar spine. Extramedullary tumors of the lumbar region include nerve sheath tumors such as neurofibromas and schwannomas (40%), meningiomas (40%), filum ependymoma (15%), and dermoid and epidermoid tumors, among others (2–7). Tumors in the lumbar spine are discussed in detail in Chapters 81 and 82. In this chapter, we will focus on posterior approaches to these intradural and extradural tumors of the lumbar spine.

INDICATIONS

As in any spine surgery, decompression of neural elements, correction of orthopedic deformity, and stabilization of acute or glacial instability are the main goals of the posterior approach (8). Posterior surgery is simple, does not require specialized approach surgeons, and allows for three-column stabilization with transpedicular instrumentation in most cases. However, historically, the posterior approach has been limited in terms of total tumor resection simply due to the proclivity of tumors in the anterior column.

Tumor surgery challenges the spine surgeon to develop minimally invasive methods of neural decompression without worsening the existing deformity and instability brought on by the pathologic process. In the past, limitations of three-column stabilization from anterior surgery alone have necessitated two-stage operations. The 360° operations are particularly significant in tumor surgery in

that excision of tumor naturally worsens a pathologic deformity and contributes to the instability of the spine. The anterior column is supported with graft or caging, and supplementation with posterior instrumentation is considered. To compound the issue, extensive tumor involvement of multiple posterior spinal levels may be an impediment for posterior fusion and instrumentation. The least invasive and least destructive operation is often ideal. The patient is often weakened from chemotherapy and may have had radiosurgery, thus being a suboptimal candidate for bony fusion. Anterior transperitoneal or retroperitoneal approaches are not tolerated in some patients, and the surgeon may consider transpedicular approaches to the vertebral column instead. To summarize, in the era of improved instrumentation, innovative fusion material with minimally invasive interventional drug and cement delivery systems and image-guidance, the posterior approach may well afford simple circumferential decompression and stabilization in patients who are unable to undergo long or multiple spine surgeries or cannot tolerate anterior decompression. Although tumor localization in the spine is predominantly in the anterior column, more posterior-directed tumor surgeries go beyond the simple palliative decompression and stabilization in preference for aggressive decompression and *en bloc* spondylectomy (9–11).

The posterior approach is a well-established method for decompression of neural elements involved by intradural tumors, neural foraminal, and spinal bony tumors that mainly involve the posterior column. A translaminar approach with preservation of the facets is sufficient for exposure to ependymomas, hemangioblastomas, and dermoid or epidermoid tumors involving the cauda equina and conus medullaris.

A simple laminectomy can be extended with facetectomy and a transpedicular approach to access the posterior vertebral column with decompression of the ipsilateral anterior extradural space and associated nerve root. *En bloc* tumor resections or limited posterior debulking can be accomplished by experienced surgeons from the posterior approach alone for metastatic tumor. Hemilaminectomy with facetectomy allows visualization of the neural foramen and the exiting nerve root in the case of a nerve sheath tumor. Posterior fusion and instrumentation follows in the standard manner. Fluoroscopic-, endoscopic-, or navigation-guided delivery of cement, methylmethacrylate, or fusion protein substances (e.g., bone morphogenic protein) may replace the need for some anterior instrumentation surgeries in the future (12–23).

PREOPERATIVE ASSESSMENT

Minimizing Blood Loss—Erythropoietin and Preoperative Embolization

Patients with malignant tumors frequently present with malnutrition, anorexia, and anemia. Certain patients have already undergone radiation to the tumor bed or chemotherapy. They are in a state of iatrogenic immunocompromise, leukopenia, coagulopathy, and anemia. Preoperative autologous blood donation of 3 units of whole blood may not be possible in these patients. Cell-saver is not optimal in patients with tumor. Lee et al. studied the minimal effective dosage of recombinant human erythropoietin for posterior decompression and instrumentation of the lumbar spine. In a prospective randomized clinical trial of n = 45, 50 units per kilogram of recombinant human erythropoietin facilitated the build-up of a patient preoperative hematocrit and enabled preoperative autologous blood donation (24).

The goal of preoperative embolization is for reduction of blood loss in patients undergoing surgery for hypervascular spinal tumors (25,26). Prabhu et al. evaluated 51 patients with magnetic resonance (MR) imaging and angiography. MR imaging had a supportive role in predicting the vascularity of a majority of the tumors studied, and arterial embolization was precluded in patients who shared a vascular pedicle between a radiculomedullary artery and the tumor ($p = .02$) (27).

The main predictor of successful preoperative embolization to minimize operative blood loss is not imaging but the tumor pathology itself. Tumors frequently benefiting from preoperative embolization include renal cell carcinoma (11,27,28), aneurysmal bone cyst (29), chordoma (30), hemangiopericytomas (31), multiple myeloma (11), bony sarcoma (11), neuroectodermal tumors, pheochromocytomas, and hepatocellular carcinoma (11).

Computer-Assisted Navigation

A disadvantage of traditional tumor surgery is that the extension of the tumor is not accurately determinable intraoperatively. The surgeon is often limited in the extent of neural decompression and hemilaminectomy due to concern for overall spinal stability and unknown extension of tumor into the canal, conus medullaris, and soft tissue structures. Additionally, tumor involvement of the posterior column may impede intraoperative identification of essential anatomy. Tumor margins are often difficult to appreciate intraoperatively and the extent of resection becomes clear only in a delayed fashion with postoperative imaging (32). Posterior instrumentation for stabilization is complicated when landmarks become unclear secondary to tumor erosion, iatrogenic debulking or prior surgery (33–36). Prior application of bone cement, in particular, renders the re-do open surgery extremely difficult (34). Addressing the frustrations of the aforementioned points, navigation with computer-assistance versus intraoperative real-time imaging may allow for improved resection of tumor and safer application of instrumentation (10).

Computer-assisted tomography or MR navigation has received mixed reviews, namely for its cumbersome preoperative planning and intraoperative real-time inaccuracies compared to preoperative imaging. Accuracy of computer-assisted navigation depends on (a) how mobile the spine segments are in relation to the other, (b) the number of registration points available, and (c) size of the target desired, be it pedicle or tumor (37,38). The presence of a fusion mass impedes conventional intraoperative assessment but can aid computer-assisted navigation by limiting local motion (33,34). Austin et al. studied seven embalmed cadaveric spines. The posterior elements of four spines were covered with bone cement. Pedicle screw placement by standard laminoforaminotomy alone resulted in an overall pedicle breach rate of 21.43% in the spines with fusion mass compared to pedicle breach rates of 6% to 10% using standard fluoroscopy. No pedicle breaches were noted in the navigation-guided pedicle insertions in the spines with fusion masses (34). The multifaceted morphology of the posterior column renders itself to increased navigational accuracy compared to the anterior column.

Buchowski et al. studied 26 pedicle and 8 lateral mass screws in human cadavers using two registration techniques. The trajectory accuracy was 2.5 1.0 mm and 2 degrees from T12 to L5. In this study, only the posterior column could be accurately registered, and there was a discrepancy of accuracy at the cervicothoracic and thoracolumbar junction (39). The use of virtual fluoroscopy offers several advantages over conventional fluoroscopy as well. While maintaining a mean trajectory difference of $2.7° \pm 0.6°$ and a mean probe tip error of less than 1 mm, virtual fluoroscopic navigation marries the benefits of real-time fluoroscopy with those of computer-assistance (35,40).

Clearly, there are limitations that override the benefits with the current computer-assisted navigation systems. Still in its infancy, the future navigation systems will facilitate midlumbar posterior tumor resection and fusion surgeries. Caution with computer-assistance is advocated in the highly unstable spine and at junctions of the spine.

Real-Time Navigation

Intraoperative computed tomography (CT) holds great promise for tumor resection and instrumentation with greater accuracy than current intraoperative fluoroscopy alone (35,41). Holly and Foley evaluated the use of isocentric, three-dimensional, C-arm fluoroscopic-guided percutaneous placement of thoracic and lumbar pedicle screws in three cadaveric specimens. They had no pedicle breaches in the lumbar spine and an 8% breach rate of the thoracic spine confirmed by CT (42). Experience at our institution comparing thin-slice CT with the same device confirms that the isocentric three-dimensional C-arm has more of an increased sensitivity to pedicle breaches than conventional CT (in submission).

Real-time intraoperative CT and MR imaging facilitate complete tumor resection, particularly if the tumor is contrast-enhancing. Whereas a low Tesla intraoperative magnet may be suboptimal for low-enhancing tumors such as low-grade gliomas, gadolinium-enhanced MR imaging is the study for choice during resection of a dumbbell schwannoma at the neural foramen. Though still experimental, phosphorus MR spectroscopic analysis of spinal tumors may replace gadolinium dependence in the future (43). Intraoperative imaging eliminates the anterior dural space blind spot when the transpedicular approach is used for extradural circumferential tumor resection such as in anterior meningiomas and metastases. Intraoperative navigation facilitates the delivery of chemotherapy or bone substitution agents to the anterior column in the case of pathologic fracture from a posterior approach, be it transpedicular or percutaneous (12–23).

An example of the fusion properties of osteogenic protein 1 (OP-1) is seen in the work of Grauer et al. These researchers performed single-level, intertransverse process lumbar fusion in rabbits and assessed for fusion by biomechanics and palpation at 5 weeks postoperatively. Experimental arms were divided into those who underwent carrier-alone fusion and carrier-plus–OP-1 fusion. Whereas only five of eight rabbits in the carrier-alone arm evidenced fusion, all eight rabbits in the carrier-plus–OP-1 group demonstrated stable fusion. There was statistically significant loss of multidirectional movement, including flexion, in the carrier-plus–OP-1 group compared to the carrier-alone group. Although fusion rates of OP-1 determined by manual palpation were not significant from autograft fusion rates, biomechanical testing demonstrated OP-1 fusion to be more stable than the time-matched autograft fusion (17). Quicker and stronger fusion through a minimally invasive corridor is precisely the goal in tumor debulking and reconstructive surgery.

Disadvantages of the intraoperative MR imaging for the spine includes a severe limitation in instrumentation and tools that are MR-compatible, the current lack of availability of high Tesla systems, the price of open MR imaging and its continued need for maintenance, and the restriction of the open MR imaging space (44).

In an ever-growing market of navigational and intraoperative imaging techniques, the patient with difficult anatomy, especially re-do spine cases, will benefit from image guidance.

Neurophysiologic Monitoring

The goal of intraoperative nerve root monitoring on the lumbosacral spine is to minimize risk to the cauda equina during intradural tumor resection (e.g., ependymoma) and to reduce risk of misplaced pedicle screws. Nerve root injury has been reported to occur in as many as 11% to 15% of operations (45). The goal of intraoperative somatosensory evoked potentials (SEPs), spontaneous electromyographic (EMG) activity, and compound muscle action potential monitoring are to allow for early warning of injury to the cauda equina, spinal cord, and individual nerve roots so that the surgeon is able to correct the issue immediately. Balzer et al. studied 44 patients who underwent lumbosacral spinal decompression and instrumentation for degeneration, trauma, and tumor. Baseline peroneal and tibial SEPs were taken. Quadriceps and biceps femoris, gastrocnemius, and anterior tibialis muscle groups were recorded for spontaneous EMG. Intraoperative pedicle, pedicle screw, and nerve root stimulation were recorded during instrumentation. Most helpful was EMG recording that became aberrant in cases and required decompression of nerve root or redirection of instrumentation. Simultaneous SEP recordings were "falsely negative" as expected (45). In a separate study, Heyde et al. used intraoperative EMG stimulation of 334 implanted pedicle screws which led to corrected redirection of 3.9% of screws (46).

In the setting of lumbosacral tumor resection, EMG monitoring coupled with nerve root stimulation provides ideal monitoring during surgery. Nerve root monitoring and bladder sphincter monitoring is frequently helpful when débriding a conus myxopapillary ependymoma or tethered cord with dermoid tumor. Nerve root monitoring can provide an early warning of pedicle breach during instrumentation, although its sensitivity and specificity are yet to be clarified (47).

THE POSTERIOR APPROACH

Standard Laminectomy Approach to Intradural Lesion

The patient is brought to the operating room and intubated in the supine position. EMG and SEP monitoring, including placement of a bladder sphincter monitor around the Foley catheter, occurs during this period. Arte-

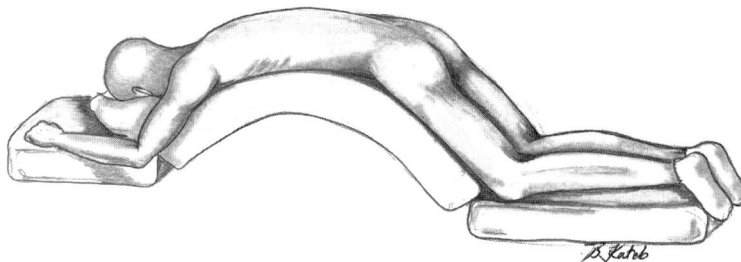

FIG. 83-1. Illustration of the prone position for the posterior approach to the spine. The patient is on a radiolucent table. Ideally, the patient is intubated with gel-foam protection of the face, gel-rolls on the chest and the iliac crest pressure points, gel-pads on the knees, and pillows around the ankles. The arms are placed at right angles to minimize retraction of the brachial plexus. The abdomen is freed of pressure to minimize intraoperative bleeding. Electromyographic and somatosensory evoked potential recording devices are placed. A fluoroscopic C-arm is placed under or over the abdomen and included in the sterile field for real-time navigation as needed.

rial line access and central access, if needed, are established. The patient is then placed on a radiolucent table in the prone position with adequate gel protection of the head and gel-rolls on the chest and iliac pressure points. The arms are placed at right angles to arrest retraction of the brachial plexus. The knees are padded and the leg and feet elevated with appropriate pillows. Leg squeezers are placed for deep venous thrombosis prophylaxis. The abdomen is noted to be free of pressure as increased intra-abdominal pressure will aggravate intraoperative bleeding. Navigation equipment is placed in the appropriate positions, including real-time fluoroscopy as needed. A preoperative pelvic X-ray may be taken to ascertain the absence of tumor involvement of the pelvis in case autograft from the iliac crest is required (Fig. 83-1).

The sterile field is draped to include the medial 10 cm of bilateral iliac crest and extended superiorly as needed for the surgical approach. Frequently, an X-ray is taken with a spinal needle to mark the correct levels of surgery prior to complete field preparation and drape. In the case of sacral chordomas, extensive field draping may be needed in case of muscle flap or plastic reconstructive surgery to follow the tumor debulking.

A standard midline incision is placed and extended down to the supraspinous ligament. The erector spinae muscle is dissected away from the spinous process and laminae. Care is taken not to disrupt the interspinous and intraspinous ligaments during the subperiosteal dissection that is performed with Cobb retractors and monopolar electrocautery. Care is also taken to expose only the levels and structures needed, as additional ligamentous/muscle disruption may add to future glacial instability of the spine.

The spinous process and interspinous ligaments of the involved levels are removed with a double-action rongeur or spinous process cutter (Fig. 83-2). The inferior portion of the superior lamina is drilled down to a thin "eggshell" using a high-speed drill. The remaining lamina is removed with Kerrison rongeurs keeping above the ligamentum flavum as the ligamentum flavum at this level

will reduce the risk of inadvertent tearing of the dura. Laminectomy is carried out superiorly and inferiorly once the dura is visualized using the combination of high-speed drilling and Kerrison rongeur technique. Ligamentum flavum is removed with the rongeur to expose the extradural space and dura. Laminectomy is carried out to the laminar-facet border laterally and care is taken not to disrupt the facet joints.

Alternatively, laminectomy may be performed using a 3- to 5-mm burr high-speed drill to drill out troughs or gutters on both sides of the facet-laminar border (Fig. 83-3). At this laminofacet junction, the outer cortical lamina

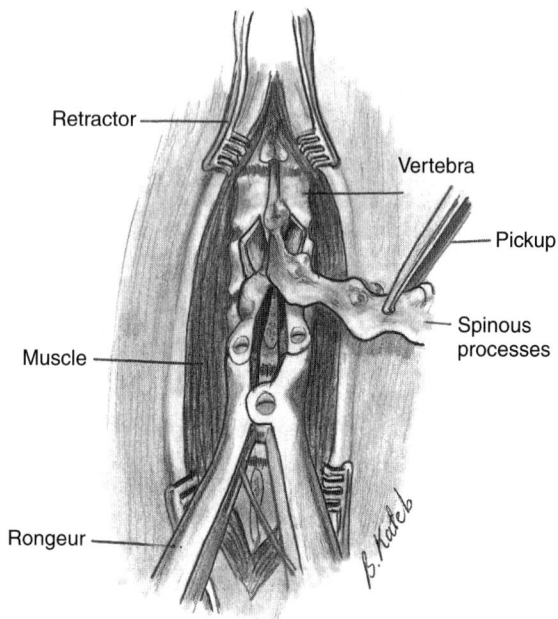

FIG. 83-2. Illustration of a standard approach to lumbar laminectomy. The spinous processes of the involved levels are removed with a spinous process cutter or double-action rongeurs. Care is taken not to remove supraspinous, interspinous ligaments of uninvolved levels to minimize injury to the posterior tension band.

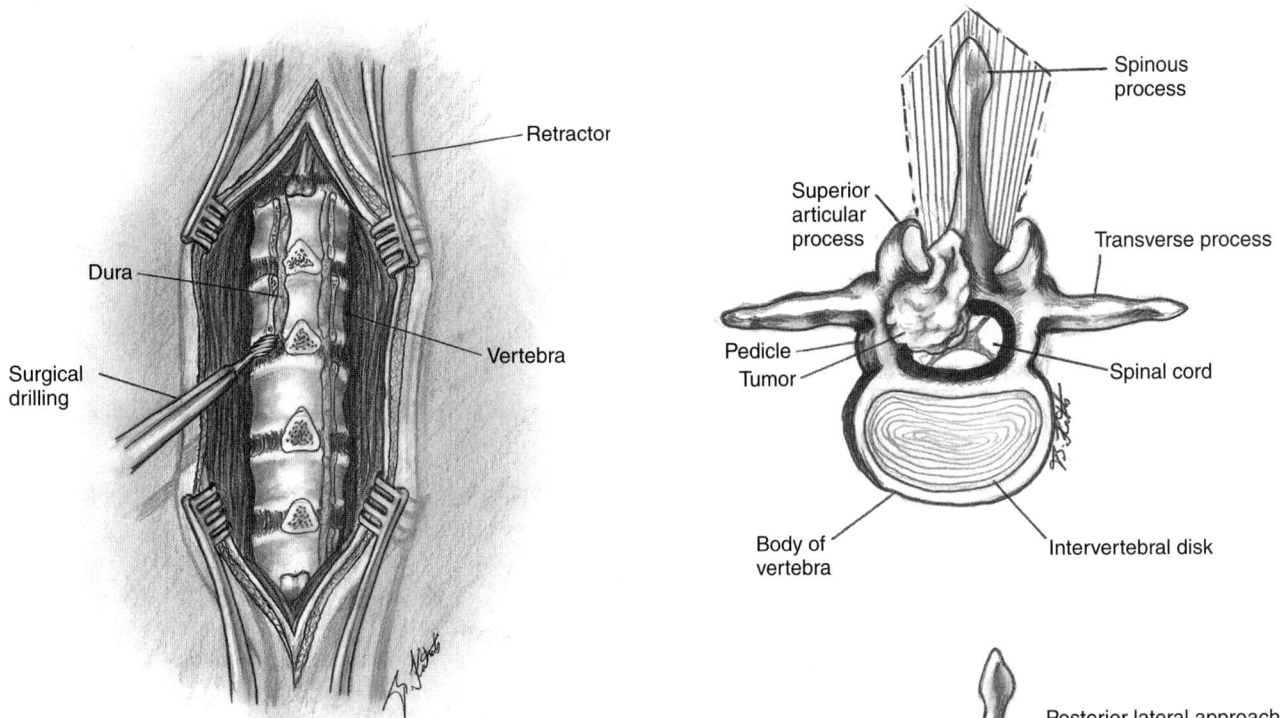

FIG. 83-3. Illustration of laminectomy of the lumbar spine. The spinous processes have been removed along with the associated interspinous ligaments. A high-speed drill is used to decorticate the facet-laminar junction while taking great care not to violate the facets. Once the troughs are drilled down to a thin 9eggshell,9 they may be removed with Kerrison rongeurs.

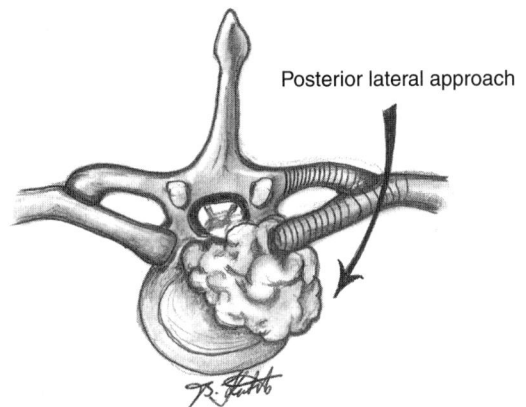

FIG. 83-4. Illustration of the spine postlaminectomy. The ligamentum flavum is removed and the borders of the lamina are smoothed out with the Kerrison rongeur. Once again, the facets are preserved. The dura is exposed.

is drilled down, leaving a thin rim of bone to the point where Kerrison rongeurs may be used to remove the inner cortex, thereby separating the lamina from the facet complex. The spinous process along with the associated interspinous ligament is removed with a spinous process cutter or double-action rongeur. Essentially, the lamina is de-roofed from the epidural space (Fig. 83-4). In children, the laminectomy may be performed *en bloc* along with the intact spinous process and replaced after surgery with small, absorbable bio-implant material. This laminoplasty method with bone cement, however, is most common in approaches to cervical intramedullary tumors with concern for progressive kyphosis secondary to denervation muscle atrophy in the posterior neck.

Epidural bleeding is arrested with bipolar technique and the use of gel-foam powder. Any remaining ligamentum flavum and epidural fat is removed carefully with Kerrison rongeurs.

The microscope is introduced at this time and the dura is sharply divided at the midline. In the case of a myxopapillary ependymoma, great care is taken to visualize from the conus to the end of the dural sac. Each sleeve of the dura is then gently retracted with several 4-0 stitches to provide optimal visualization of the intradural con-

tents. Dural tears are repaired with 5-0 and 6-0 nonabsorbable stitches and fibrin glue. Short long cottonoids provide for protection of nerve root elements during the debulking of the tumor in question. Standard microneurosurgical technique is followed at this time for tumor debulking. In the case of ependymoma, gentle suction may be sufficient to debulk the tumor from around the nerve roots (Fig. 83-5). The filum terminale can be differentiated from the rest of the nerve roots by intraoperative nerve root stimulation and by the presence of the artery of the filum terminale.

In the case of meningioma, the dura may need to be resected, in which case, bovine pericardium or other dura substitutes are used to perform a duraplasty with a 4-0 nylon stitch. Fibrin glue is placed over the duraplasty edges.

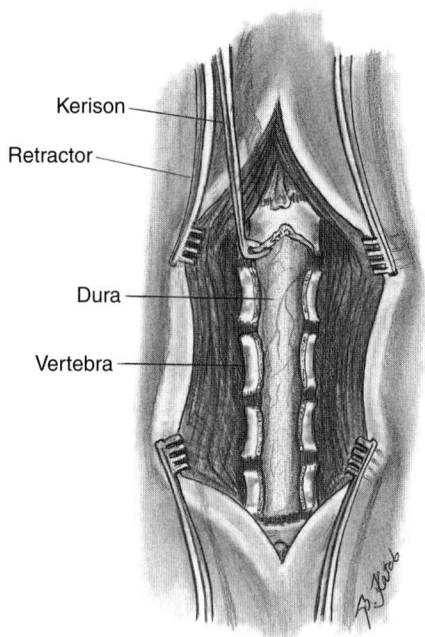

FIG. 83-5. Illustration of an intradural neurofibroma of the cauda equina. Often, several neurofibromas may exist in the intradural space regardless of preoperative magnetic resonance imaging findings. Note the dura has been divided and tacked up with 4-0 nylon. Nerve root monitoring and microscope-guided dissection is recommended for this portion of the surgery.

The dura is closed in running non-interlocking fashion with 4-0 nonabsorbable nylon. An intradural lumbar drain is usually not necessary. Valsalva maneuver will detect any unnoticed dural tears. The wound is irrigated and closed in standard fashion.

Approach to Nerve Sheath Tumors

Prior to approaching a nerve sheath tumor, exact knowledge of the tumor's pathology is helpful. Discussion is held as to what the patient may want done if the tumor is not a benign one or cannot be eggshelled out. In malignant nerve sheath tumors or extensive neurofibromas, the nerve root may need to be excised. Grafting of the nerve root with sural nerve is an option as well.

The combination of hemilaminectomy with limited facet resection may be sufficient for exposure to the lateral recess and neural foramen. A similar approach is used for paramedian microdiscectomy. However, the facet may need to be excised to afford better visualization of the nerve root's path. Discussing with the patient the possibility of unilateral transpedicular screw insertion with rod placement is recommended prior to surgery in the case of a large neural foraminal tumor.

The dissection is carried out with exposure of the transverse process superiorly and, if needed, inferiorly. The surgical window is centered with the neural foramen medially and the pedicles and transverse processes as the superior and inferior margins. In the case of a schwannoma, the tumor can be debulked from the core outward with a combination of bipolar and suction technique, or "shelled out" with sharp dissectors. Retraction of the nerve root is best minimized and we prefer the debulking from the core outward. Depending on the degree of injury to the bony elements by approach and by the tumor, the surgeon decides on the extent of stabilization instrumentation.

The Posterolateral Transpedicular Approach

The transpedicular approach is a powerful tool for the treatment of lumbar spine tumors. Aggressive tumor debulking versus limited decompressive laminectomy is often debated and depends to an extent on the patient's life expectancy and comorbid condition. The posterolateral transpedicular approach addresses the controversy of aggressive debulking versus limited laminectomy in that the added debulking can be accomplished in the same procedure without excessively prolonged surgical time or morbidity.

Posterior approach vertebrectomy was first demonstrated as early as 1922 by MacLennan, who performed an apical resection from a posterior-only approach with postoperative casting for severe scoliosis. Since then, posterior approaches to the vertebral column have become increasingly more popular (48,49). Posterior approaches with aggressive decompression and stabilization are now feasible with spondylectomy *en bloc* tumor resection (9,50) or with the transpedicular posterolateral approach (11,51–53). Some variations of the *en bloc* and transpedicular techniques are addressed subsequently.

Through a bi-transpedicular approach with fine threadwire saws, *en bloc* vertebrectomy was achieved in 14 patients with malignant or benign vertebral tumors by Abe et al. In this study, nerve roots had to be sacrificed in 7 cases with marginal surgical margin achieved in 10 cases. All 14 cases experienced pain relief and ambulation in the immediate postoperative period, with recurrence of tumor in 3 cases at mean 3-year follow-up (9). Bilsky et al. reported a promising 15-month follow-up in 25 patients who underwent a single-stage posterolateral transpedicular approach for spondylectomy, epidural decompression, and circumferential fusion for spinal metastasis. Twelve of these patients had either circumferential or 270° epidural spinal cord compression. Fifteen patients had cerebrospinal fluid (CSF) space obliteration with cord compression. All patients underwent prone position laminofacetectomy with transpedicular excision of tumor. Spine reconstruction is initiated through fluoroscopy-guided placement of methylmethacrylate mixed with tobramycin followed by segmental instrumentation using pedicle screws or hooks as needed. Two patients had progression of neurologic deterioration. Disadvantages of these approaches include the possible need to sacrifice the nerve root, the need for dura and nerve root retraction (similar to microdiscectomy), the increased risk to nerve root and dura injury through the use of the osteotome or high-speed drill close to the dura, the need for posterior stabilization instrumentation, and the need for some sort of anterior stabilization from the posterior approach (e.g., the methylmethacrylate injection discussed previously) (11). The transpedicular approach has a blind spot roughly at the junction of the lateral recess and anterior dural space. Navigation promises to eliminate this blind spot in the future.

Posterolateral approach to decompression of nerve root and neural elements of the symptomatic side can be stabilized using a single diagonal fusion cage at the surgical bed and supplemented with transpedicular screw and rod instrumentation. A prospective 2-year analysis of 27 patients with degenerative spine disorders who underwent unilateral posterolateral interbody fusion (PLIF) using one diagonal fusion cage PLIF demonstrated radiographic fusion in 25 patients at 1 year (54). Fusion rates will likely be less in patients with malignant tumors, especially those patients undergoing radiation therapy. Novel alternatives, such as the titanium alloy screws connected by elastic synthetic compounds, remain to be better tested prior to standard use (55).

Technique

Depending on the location of the tumor, either a bilateral transpedicular or a unilateral transpedicular approach is considered. In the thoracic spine, a bilateral approach is frequently necessary for posterior vertebral column resection (56) but a unilateral approach may be sufficient in the lumbar spine (11). The transpedicular approach for removal of a unilateral versus bilateral pedicle and posterior vertebral column mass is a destabilizing procedure. Above and below segment instrumentation is recommended with anterior column grafting.

A standard laminectomy is performed over the area of tumor involvement and over the segmental areas that are to be instrumented. The facets of all areas to be fused are removed with double-action rongeurs, and, with the high-speed drill, insertion sites for pedicle screws are prepared with decortication. Decortication is continued at the transverse process and surrounding laminar areas. Discectomy may be performed using sharp dissection of the disc followed by pituitary rongeurs to remove the disc and to prepare the end plate with curettage in the standard fashion for interbody fusion. Pedicle screws are then inserted in all pedicles except for the pedicles that are to be subtracted for the approach. The pedicle that is to be drilled down is identified and the nerve roots beneath it and above it are visualized clearly. For visualization purposes, hemostasis is meticulous with gel-foam powder and microscope- or loupe-resolution is recommended. Using a 3-mm high-speed drill, the center of the pedicle

is drilled down at the angle similar to pedicle screw placement, and the pedicle is eggshelled to the level of the posterior vertebral body (Fig. 83-6). The outer edges ("shells") of the pedicle are removed with small rongeurs. A trough is then created in the posterior vertebral body using the high-speed drill followed by thin osteotomes. At this point, the pedicle will have been removed, exposing a one-inch gap between the two nerve roots. With small osteotomes, the end plate is prepared along with further resection of the posterior body. Real-time fluoroscopy is used to delineate the depth of resection and the nerve roots are carefully spared. The corridor is limited by the dura medially, the nerve roots superiorly and inferiorly, and the anterior longitudinal ligament ventrally. The lateral borders are protected by the fasciae of the psoas and quadratus lumborum muscles. This fascia continues as the transversalis fascia of the abdomen. It is worthwhile to remember that the lumbar plexus resides within the psoas muscle and the psoas muscle and fascia are preserved as much as possible as they hug the vertebral body.

The removal of the pedicle and facet joint enable a 30° corridor of visualization compared to a simple laminectomy (Fig. 83-7A,B). With bilateral pedicle take down, the visualization of the posterior body is almost complete, except for a small piece directly anterior to the dural sac. Down-going Epstein curettes are used to stomp down any small bony or tumor elements compressing the anterior dura. Depending on the extent of the posterior

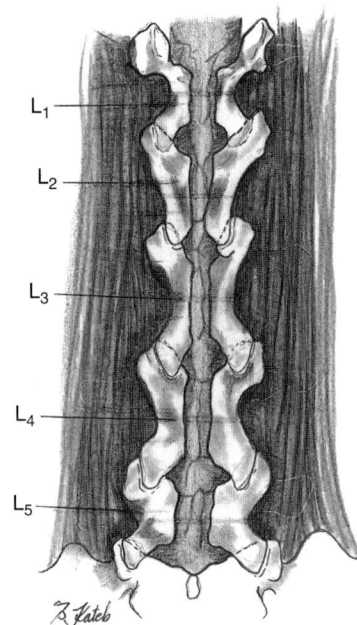

FIG. 83-6. Illustration of a pedicle finder (in this case, curved) inside the pedicle and the posterior vertebral column. In pedicle-subtraction technique, the 1 cm area around the pedicle finder is roughly the bone subtraction desired for access to the posterior vertebral column.

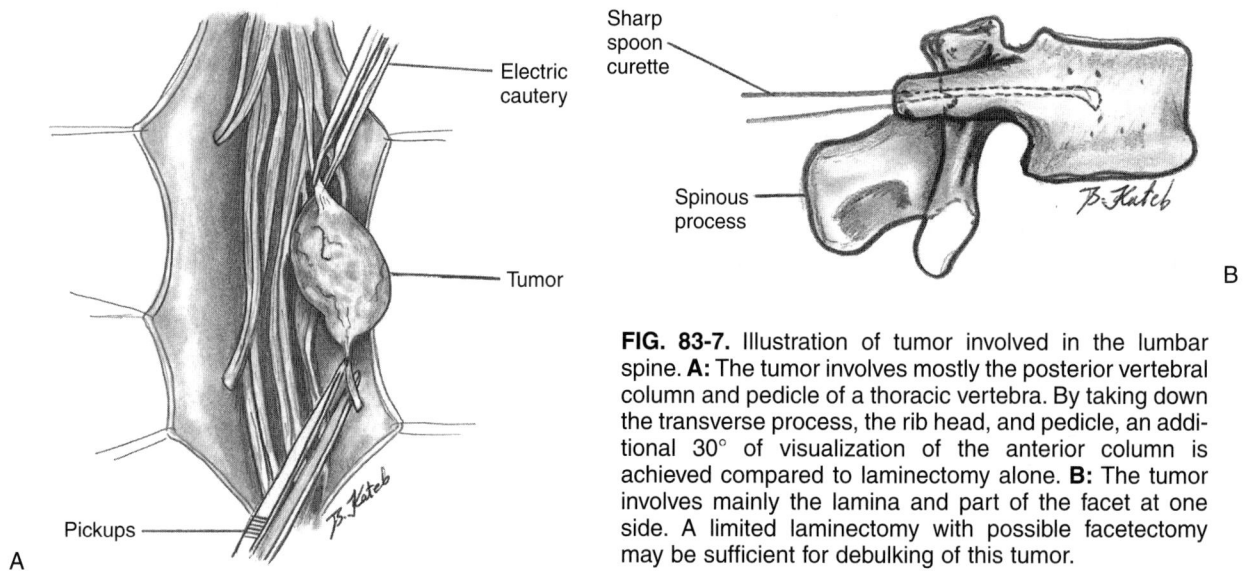

Electric
cautery

Tumor

Pickups

A

Sharp
spoon
curette

Spinous
process

B

FIG. 83-7. Illustration of tumor involved in the lumbar spine. **A:** The tumor involves mostly the posterior vertebral column and pedicle of a thoracic vertebra. By taking down the transverse process, the rib head, and pedicle, an additional 30° of visualization of the anterior column is achieved compared to laminectomy alone. **B:** The tumor involves mainly the lamina and part of the facet at one side. A limited laminectomy with possible facetectomy may be sufficient for debulking of this tumor.

column resection, methylmethacrylate may be used or stackable cages may be placed one on top of the other to complete the anterior column stabilization. Rods are placed in the pedicle screws and placed in compression. The remaining areas are prepared for fusion with decortication. Bone graft is placed in the standard manner, followed by closure.

COMPLICATIONS

The most common complications following posterior lumbar surgery are wound infections, CSF leak, nerve root injury, and destabilization of the spine. Infections and failed surgery are discussed elsewhere (Chapters 80 and 91, respectively). Wound infections are exceptionally high in patients who are on steroids postirradiation for malignant tumors. Patients should be weaned off steroids as soon as possible. Optimal glucose control and nutrition are important. A patient with spinal headaches in the postoperative period may benefit from 48 hours of flat bed rest. Should there be a CSF leak from the wound, organism-directed antibiotics and placement of a lumbar drain for 3 to 4 days while the leak heals is recommended. The drain is set to remove 10 cc an hour and is clamped on the last day while the patient is mobilized and assessed for CSF leak. Blood or fibrin patch are alternatives to treatment of CSF leak.

REFERENCES

1. Sloof JL, Kernohan JW, MacCarthy CS. Primary intramedullary tumors of the spinal cord and filum terminale. Philadelphia: WB Saunders, 1964.
2. McCormick PC. The lateral extracavitary approach to the thoracic and lumbar spine. In: Holtman RRN, McCormick PC, Farcy JPC, eds. Spinal instability. New York: Springer-Verlag, 1993:335–348.
3. McCormick PC. Anatomic principles of intradural surgery. Clin Neurosurg 1994;41:204–223.
4. McCormick PC, Post KD, Stein BM. Intradural extramedullary tumors in adults. Neurosurg Clin North Am 1990;1:591–608.
5. McCormick PC, Torres R, Post KD, et al. Intramedullary ependymoma of the spinal cord. J Neurosurg 1990;72:523–533.
6. McCormick PC, Stein BM. Intramedullary tumors in adults. Neurosurg Clin North Am 1990;1:609–630.
7. McCormick PC, Stein BM. Miscellaneous intradural pathology. Neurosurg Clin North Am 1990;1:687–700.
8. White AA, Panjabi MM. Clinical biomechanics of the spine, 2nd ed. Philadelphia: Lippincott, 1990:30–342.
9. Abe E, Kobayashi T, Murai H, et al. Total spondylectomy for primary malignant, aggressive benign, and solitary metastatic bone tumors of the thoracolumbar spine. J Spinal Disord 2001;14 (3):237–146.
10. Arand M, Hartwig E, Kinzl L, et al. Spinal navigation in tumor surgery of the thoracic spine: first clinical results. Clin Orthop Rel Res 2002;1 (399):211–218.
11. Bilsky MH, Boland P, Lis E, et al. Single-stage posterolateral transpedicle approach for spondylectomy, epidural decompression, and circumferential fusion of spinal metastases. Spine 2000;25(17): 2240–2250.
12. Blattert TR, Delling G, Dalal PS, et al. Successful transpedicular lumbar interbody fusion by means of a composite of osteogenic protein-1 (rhBMP 7) and hydroxyapatite carrier: a comparison with autograft and hydroxyapatite in the sheep spine. Spine 2002 27(23):2697–2705.
13. Boden SD, Martin GJ, Horton WC, et al. Laparoscopic anterior spinal arthrodesis with rhBMP-2 in a titanium interbody threaded cage. J Spinal Disord 1998;11:95–101.
14. Boden SD, Martin GJ, Morone M, et al. The use of coralline hydroxyapatite with bone marrow, autogenous bone graft, or osteoinductive bone protein extract for posterolateral lumbar spine fusion. Spine 1999; 24:320—327.
15. Cook SD, Dalton JE, Tan EH, et al. In vivo evaluation of recombinant human osteogenic protein (rhOP-1) implants as a bone graft substitute for spinal fusions. Spine 1994;19:1655–1663.
16. Cunningham BW, Kanayama M, Parker LM, et al. Osteogenic protein versus autologous interbody arthrodesis in the sheep thoracic spine: a comparative endoscopic study using the Bagby and Kuslich interbody fusion device. Spine 1999;24:509–518.
17. Grauer JN, Patel TC, Erulkar JS, et al. Evaluation of OP-1 as a graft substitute for intertransverse process lumbar fusion. Spine 26;2001(2): 237–133.
18. Hect BP, Fishgrund JS, Herkowitz HN, et al. The use of recombinant human bone morphogenic protein 2 (rh BMP-2) to promote spinal fusion in a nonhuman primate anterior interbody fusion model. Spine 1999;24:629–636.

19. Helm GA, Sheehan JM, Sheehan JP, et al. Utilization of type I collagen gel, demineralized bone matrix, and bone morphogenic protein-2 to enhance autologous bone lumbar spinal fusion. J Neurosurg 1997;86: 93–100.
20. Magin MN, Delling G. Improved lumbar vertebral interbody fusion using rhOP-1: a comparison of autogenous bone graft, bovine hydroxyapatite (Bio-Oss), and bMP-7 (RhOP-1) in sheep. Spine 2001;26: 469–478.
21. Minamide A, Kawakami M, Hashizume H, et al. Evaluation of carriers of bone morphogenic protein for spinal fusion. Spine 2001;26: 933–939.
22. Minamide A, Tamaki T, Kawakami M, et al. Experimental spinal fusion using sintered bovine bone coated with type I collagen and recombinant human bone morphogenetic protein-2. Spine 1999;24:1863–1872.
23. Sandhu HS, Kanim LEA, Toth JM, et al. Experimental spinal fusion with recombinant human bone morphogenetic protein-2 without decortication of osseous elements. Spine 1997;22:1171–1180.
24. Lee JH, Lee SH, Oh JH. Minimal effective dosage of recombinant human erythropoietin in spinal surgery. Clin Orthop Rel Res 2003;412: 71–76.
25. Chiras J, Cognard C, Rose M, et al. Percutaneous injection of an alcoholic embolizing emulsion as an alternative preoperative embolization for spine tumor. AJNR 1993;14(5):1113–1117.
26. Shi H, Jin Z, Suh DC, et al. Preoperative transarterial embolization of hypervascular vertebral tumor with permanent particles. Chinese Med J 2002;115(11):1683–1686.
27. Prabhu VC, Bilsky MH, Jambhekar K, et al. Results of preoperative embolization for metastatic spinal neoplasms. J Neurosurg 2003;98[2 Suppl]:156–164.
28. Jackson RJ, Loh SC, Gokaslan ZL. Metastatic renal cell carcinoma of the spine: surgical treatment and results. J Neurosurg 2001;94[1 Suppl]:18–24.
29. Dekeuwer P, Odent T, Cadillac C, et al. Aneurysmal bone cyst of the spine in children: a 9 year follow-up of 7 cases and review of the literature. Revue de Chirurgie Orthopedique et Reparatrice de 1 Appareil Moteur 2003;89 (2):97–106.
30. Winant D, Bertal A, Hennequin L, et al. Imaging of cervical and thoracic chordoma. J Radiologie 1992;73(3):169–174.
31. Muraszko KM, Antunes JL, Hilal SK, et al. Hemangiopericytoma of the spine. Neurosurgery 1982;10(4):473–479.
32. Bauer HC. Posterior decompression and stabilization for spinal metastasis. Analysis of sixty-seven consecutive patients. J Bone Joint Surg 1997;79A:514–522.
33. Amiot L, Lang K, Putzier M, et al. Comparative results between conventional and computer-assisted pedicle screw installation in the thoracic, lumbar, sacral spine. Spine 2000;25:606–614.
34. Austin MS, Vaccaro AR, Brislin B, et al. Image-guided spine surgery: a cadaveric study comparing conventional open laminoforaminotomy and two image-guided techniques for pedicle screw placement in postero-lateral fusion and nonfusion models. Spine 2002;27(22):2503–2508.
35. Foley KT, Simon DA, Rampersaud YR. Virtual fluoroscopy: computer-assisted fluoroscopic navigation. Spine 2001;26:347–351.
36. Glossop ND, Hu RW, Randle JA. Computer-aided pedicle screw placement using frameless stereotaxis. Spine 1996;21:2026–2034.
37. Laine T, Schlenzka D, Makitalo K, et al. Improved accuracy of pedicle screw insertion with computer-assisted surgery. Spine 1997;22: 1254–1258.
38. Rampersaud YR, Simon DA, Foley KT. Accuracy requirements for image-guided spinal pedicle screw placement. Spine 2001;26: 352–359.
39. Buchowski JM, Helm PA, Huckell CB, et al. Evaluation of registration methods used in frameless stereotactic surgery for the lumbar and cervical regions of the spine. Am J Orthop 2003;32(2):90–97, discussion 97.
40. Foley KT, Smith MM. Image-guided spine surgery. Neurosurg Clin North Am 1996;7:171–186.
41. Ebmeier K, Giest K, Kalff R. Intraoperative computerized tomography for improved accuracy of spinal navigation in pedicle screw placement of the thoracic spine. Acta Neurochir [Suppl] 2003;85:105–113.
42. Holly LT, Foley KT. Three dimensional fluoroscopy-guided percutaneous thoracolumbar pedicle screw placement. Technical note. J Neurosurg 2003;99[3 Suppl]:324–329.
43. Sijens PE, Van Den Bent MJ, Ouderk M. Phosphorus-31 chemical shift imaging of metastatic tumors located in the spinal region. Invest Radiol 1997;32(6):344–350.
44. Verheyden P, Katscher S, Schulz T, et al. Open MR imaging in spine surgery: experimental investigations and first clinical experience. Eur Spine J 1999;8(5):346–353.
45. Balzer JR, Rose R, Welch WC, et al. Simultaneous somatosensory evoked potential and electromyographic recordings during lumbosacral decompression and instrumentation. Neurosurgery 1998;42(6): 1318–1324.
46. Heyde CE, Bohm H, el-Saghir H, et al. First experience of intraoperative nerve root monitoring with the INS-1 device on the lumbosacral spine. Zeitschrift fur Orthopadie und Ihre Grenzgebiete 2003;141(1): 79–85.
47. Weiss DS. Spinal cord and nerve root monitoring during surgical treatment of lumbar stenosis. Clin Orthop Rel Res 2001;1(384):82–100.
48. Heinig CF, Boyd BM. One stage vertebrectomy or egg-shell procedure. Orthop Trans 1985;9:130.
49. Murray DB, Brigham CD, Kiebzak GM, et al. Transpedicular decompression and pedicle subtraction osteotomy (eggshell procedure): a retrospective review of 59 patients. Spine 2002;27(21):2338–2345.
50. Boriani S, Biagini R, DeFure F, et al. Resection surgery in the treatment of vertebral tumors. Chir Organi Mov 1998;1–2:53–64.
51. Bridwell K, Jenny A, Sault T, et al. Posterior segmental spinal instrumentation with posterolateral decompression and debulking for metastatic thoracic and lumbar spine disease: limitation and technique. Spine 1998;13:1383–1394.
52. Cahill DW, Kumar R. Palliative subtotal vertebrectomy with anterior and posterior reconstruction via single posterior approach. J Neurosurg (Spine 1) 1999;90:42–47.
53. Gambardella G, Gervasio O, Zaccone C. Approaches and surgical results in the treatment of ventral thoracic meningiomas. Review of our experience with a postero-lateral combined transpedicular-transarticular approach. Acta Neurochir 2003;145(5):385–392.
54. Zhao J, Hou T, Wang X, et al. Posterior lumbar interbody fusion using one diagonal fusion cage with transpedicular screw/rod fixation. Eur Spine J 12 2003;(2):173–177.
55. Stoll TM, Dubois G, Schwarzenbach O. The dynamic neutralization system for the spine: a multi-center study of a novel fusion system. Eur Spine J 2002;11[Suppl 2]:S170–178.
56. Suk SI, Kim JH, Kim WJ, et al. Posterior vertebral column resection for severe spinal deformities. Spine 2002;27(21):2374–2382.

CHAPTER 84

Anterior Procedures

Mark A. Knaub, Douglas S. Won, and Harry N. Herkowitz

Neoplastic lesions of the spine may arise from local lesions arising from within the spinal column or surrounding structures or from spread of distant malignancies through hematogenous or lymphatic routes. Local involvement of the spine may result from primary tumors of bone, lesions originating from the neural elements or their coverings, or by direct extension of tumors arising in the paraspinal soft tissues. Metastatic disease to the spine may occur with nearly any solid tumor of the body, with osseous malignancies of the appendicular skeleton, and with lymphoreticular malignancies such as lymphoma and multiple myeloma. The likely diagnosis for any given lesion depends greatly on patient characteristics as well as the location and radiographic appearance of the lesion on imaging studies. Given this information, a physician should be able to generate a reasonable differential diagnosis which will assist in the formulation of a plan for further evaluation and for eventual treatment.

Advances in systemic treatment modalities have increased the life expectancy of patients with malignancies. As a result, the surgical treatment of spinal tumors in these patients has become more common in an attempt to improve their quality of life. The goals of such surgical procedures are to improve the patient's quality of life and to minimize the morbidity and mortality associated with the surgery. Indications for surgical intervention vary depending upon the general health of the patient, the tumor type, and previous treatment rendered. General surgical indications include: (a) an isolated primary or solitary metastatic lesion or a solitary relapse in which the goal of treatment is to cure the patient; (b) pathologic fracture producing neurologic deficit or pain; (c) neurologic deficit arising from direct expansion of the tumor; (d) a tumor that is resistant to the radiation therapy; and (e) segmental instability secondary to bony destruction (1–6). These recommendations assume that the patient is medically stable enough to tolerate an invasive, lengthy surgical procedure and that the expected survival is measured in months or years, not weeks.

Specific goals of surgical intervention in a patient with a spinal tumor are to decompress the neural elements, to provide stability in the setting of preexisting instability or impending pathologic or iatrogenic instability, to decrease or alleviate pain, and in some circumstances to completely excise the tumor. Surgical approaches can be divided into those that provide access to the thecal sac anteriorly (vertebrectomy), posteriorly (laminectomy), laterally (costotransversectomy or posterolateral approach), and combined anterior and posterior access. The choice of surgical approach depends upon the location and extent of neural element compromise, the number of vertebral levels involved, the exact region of the spine affected, the presence of or potential development of spinal instability, and the patient's general medical condition.

The focus of this chapter will be on the anterior approach to tumors in the lumbar spine. Posterior procedures and combined anterior and posterior procedures are covered in detail in other chapters in this book. A brief discussion on the specific surgical indications for an anterior approach will be followed by a description of surgical techniques. A section dealing with the use of anterior instrumentation and various graft options is included to highlight these controversial topics. Finally, complications and results of anterior approaches for lumbar spine tumors are discussed.

PATIENT EVALUATION

Both primary and malignant tumors can be found in all age groups and at all levels throughout the spine. Metastatic lesions account for a vast majority of all spinal neoplasms and are found more frequently in the thoracic and thoracolumbar spine. These metastatic foci are found most frequently in the vertebral body (7). The etiology of this phenomenon is believed to be related to the vascular supply of the spine, namely the vertebral venous system or the Batson plexus (8). Primary spinal tumors are most commonly found in the thoracic and sacral regions (9).

Primary lesions arising from the posterior elements of the vertebral body are more likely to be benign while those originating in the vertebral body are likely malignant.

The most common presenting complaint of patients with spinal cord neoplasms is pain. More than 75% of all patients diagnosed with a spinal tumor present with back pain, radicular pain, or a combination of both. Fewer than 10% of patients present with isolated motor weakness. Of those who present with back pain, about 50% are also found to have weakness on exam. Pain at night is a common presenting symptom. It is frequently continuous and unrelenting in character. There tends not to be an association with activity as there is with mechanical back pain. When radicular symptoms are present they too tend to be progressive and unrelenting in nature. They are typically not relieved by recumbency or rest as is typical with a disc herniation. Structural deformities may also be associated with spinal neoplasms. Osteoid osteoma and osteoblastoma have been associated with painful scoliosis. The onset and progression of the deformity may be rapid in this situation (10). Deformities associated with neoplasms are usually flexible and easily correctible if treated early but may become rigid and structural if neglected (11).

An algorithmic approach should be used when evaluating a patient with a spinal tumor. A sample algorithm is presented in Figure 84-1. The urgency of this evaluation depends largely on the neurologic status of the patient. After a thorough history and physical examination, initial imaging should consist of high-quality plain radiographs. Lateral and anteroposterior images of the symptomatic segment are many times sufficient to identify the characteristics of the lesion such as tumor growth and bony destruction. Computed tomography (CT) may be used when suspicion is high and initial radiographs are negative or equivocal. Assessing the amount of actual bony destruction is also best accomplished with CT scans and may be enhanced with the addition of sagittal, coronal, or three-dimensional reconstructions. Bone scans may also be used to evaluate the patient in whom suspicion is high and initial radiographs are normal. Nuclear imaging is also helpful in identifying any skip lesions within the spine and sites of distant metastasis. Magnetic resonance imaging (MRI) has replaced myelography as the "gold standard" for evaluation of epidural metastasis and neural compromise. MRI is noninvasive, safe, and readily available at nearly all centers. It provides greater contrast for soft-tissue evaluation and allows for direct evaluation of the neural structures. Direct tumor extension into the spinal canal and the paravertebral soft tissues can be visualized. Multiplanar images produced by MRI are of superior quality when compared to reconstructions obtained with CT scanning. Identification of multilevel involvement is also possible secondary to the ease of imaging the entire spinal column as well as the sensitivity of MRI at detection of spinal tumors.

Additional evaluation of these patients should include laboratory analysis of blood and urine. Further imaging

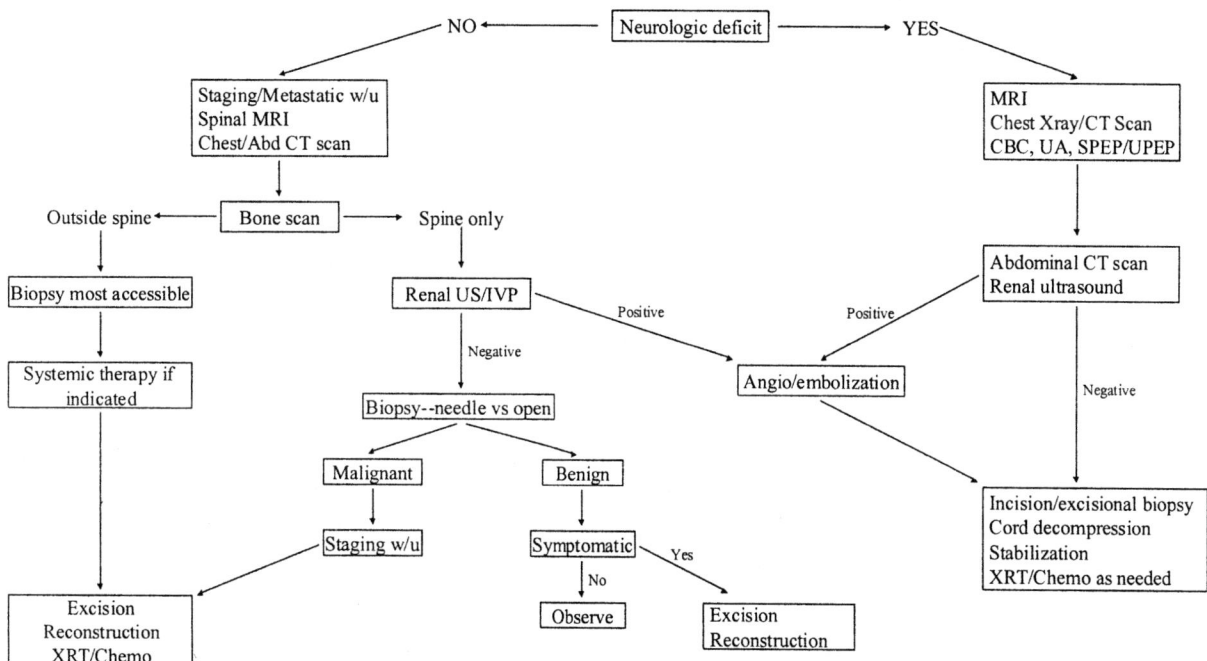

FIG. 84-1. An algorithm for the evaluation and management of a patient with a suspected spinal column neoplasm.

of the chest, abdomen, pelvis, and skeletal system should be performed to assess for other foci of disease or for a primary lesion when one is suspected. The exact nature of the neoplasm must be determined prior to the formulation of a treatment plan. A vertebral body lesion in an older patient with a history of malignancy is likely to be metastatic disease. Tumors in younger patients or those with no known history of malignancy may require a tissue specimen for diagnosis and subsequent treatment. A discussion pertaining to the method of obtaining a tissue sample for pathologic diagnosis is beyond the scope of this chapter. If an incisional biopsy is performed, strict adherence to the principles of oncologic surgery is a necessity.

SURGICAL INDICATIONS FOR THE ANTERIOR APPROACH

A multidisciplinary effort during the evaluation process will allow for a more global understanding of the ramifications of the patient's disease. The decision to proceed with surgical intervention in these patients should be made only after thorough evaluation of the patient's life expectancy, medical condition, and quality of life before and after any proposed surgical treatment.

When the diagnosis of a primary neoplasm of bone has been made or is suspected from the evaluation, the vertebral body can be divided into four anatomic zones for surgical planning. Tumor extension is designated as intraosseous, extraosseous, and distant tumor spread (12). A graph illustration of this anatomic staging system can be seen in Figure 84-2. Surgical planning not only requires attention to the bony involvement of the vertebral body but also the involvement or extension of the tumor into the surrounding vital structures. Involvement of the spinal cord, aorta, or vena cava likely renders the tumor unresectable.

Obtaining the widest surgical margin possible is essential in malignant and most aggressive benign tumors. The location of the lesion within the vertebral body as well as the extent of soft tissue extension determines the feasibility of wide surgical excision. Wide excision of B-type lesions in the lumbosacral regions may render the patient with a significant neurologic deficit. Lesions in zone I are best approached posteriorly. Lesions in zone II must be approached posterolaterally (13). Lesions in zone IV often require combined anterior and posterior surgical approaches. These scenarios are discussed in detail in other chapters in this text.

Lesions in zone III should be approached anteriorly. Tumors confined to a single vertebral body (type A) can be adequately resected throughout the lumbar spine. Careful scrutiny of type B lesions must be performed preoperatively to assess for invasion into vital surrounding soft-tissue structures. Segmental instability created by removal of large portions of a vertebral body should be addressed with structural bone grafting. The addition of anterior instrumentation may afford sufficient stability to avoid a posterior instrumented fusion. Lesions that require the resection of the fifth lumbar vertebral body are not amenable to an anterior approach alone. While difficult, resection of the vertebral body is feasible, but the addition of instrumentation is nearly impossible secondary to the fact that caudal fixation must be obtained in the anterior portion of the sacrum. Fixation methods available currently are not suited for placement into the anterior sacrum and any instrumentation in this region is dangerous secondary to the proximity to the great vessels. A more thorough discussion on the use of structural grafts and anterior instrumentation in the lumbar spine is included later in this chapter.

Metastatic lesions occurring in the spine are most often found within the vertebral body. As a result, most epidural compression stemming from metastatic tumors

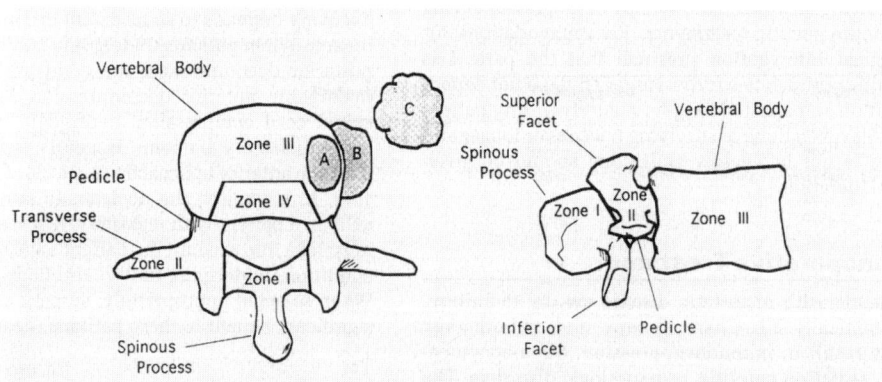

FIG. 84-2. An anatomic staging system for spinal tumors. The location of the tumor within the body is described relative to zones I through IV. Extension of the tumor is described as intraosseous (A), extraosseous (B), or distant metastatic disease (C). (From McClain R. Spinal neoplasms. In: An HS, ed. Principles and techniques of spine surgery. Philadelphia: Lippincott Williams & Wilkins, 1998, with permission.)

develops ventral to the thecal sac. Early studies failed to take this fact into consideration when they reported the poor neurologic results when posterior decompression alone was used to treat neurologic deterioration. These studies reported no advantage of laminectomy over radiation therapy alone. As a result, many physicians have been taught that surgical intervention should be used only as a last resort. With recent advances in the understanding of the metastatic disease process and in surgical techniques for canal decompression and the stabilization of spinal instability, surgical intervention has become an accepted treatment modality in the care of patients with metastatic spinal disease.

The overall goals of treatment of patients with symptomatic spinal metastasis are to provide pain relief, to stabilize or prevent neurologic deterioration, to maintain a maximal quality of life, and to prevent the complications of the metastatic disease process. Various treatment modalities are available to treat symptomatic spinal metastasis including hormonal manipulation, chemotherapy, radiation therapy, steroids, and surgical intervention. In patients with acute neurologic deterioration only steroids and surgical decompression have been shown to be effective in stabilizing or reversing neurologic deterioration. An in-depth discussion on the nonoperative treatment of symptomatic spinal metastasis is beyond the scope of this chapter.

Prior to recommending surgical intervention, one must thoroughly evaluate the entire patient. The nutritional, immunologic, and pulmonary status must be considered as should the life expectancy. Patients with bone marrow suppression from systemic chemotherapy or radiation are susceptible to wound sepsis and the profound consequences that accompany it (14,15). No consensus exists as to the required life expectancy to warrant surgical intervention. Some investigators suggest that a predicted survival of 6 months be required to justify surgical intervention while others use a predicted survival of 3 months (16–21). Because of the difficulty in accurate prediction of survivability, the decision to operate on a patient should include consideration of the patient's quality of life, which can be greatly enhanced by timely surgical intervention.

At present, the indications for operative intervention in the treatment of metastatic spinal disease include progressive neurologic deficit before, during, or after radiation therapy (17,18,20,22–31); intractable pain unresponsive to conservative treatment (18,29,31,32); need for histologic diagnosis (25, 33); radioresistant tumors (23–27); and spinal instability or vertebral collapse, with or without neurologic deficit (14,23,34,35). Entering into surgery with well thought out goals will provide an environment for surgical success. Preservation or improvement in neurologic function, alleviation or lessening of the patient's pain, and stabilization of the patient's spine so that the patient can be mobilized are the main objectives of all surgical intervention for symptomatic metastatic spinal disease. Attainment of these goals will require decompression of the neural elements in conjunction with debulking or removal of the tumor mass, correction of any preexisting spinal deformity, and stabilization of the spine.

ANTERIOR SURGICAL APPROACH TO THE LUMBAR SPINE

Standard surgical approaches to the lumbar spine are used in the treatment of tumors of the lumbar spine. The assistance of a general or vascular surgeon is usually recommended for the actual surgical approach. Exposure to the midportion of the lumbar spine is accomplished through a standard retroperitoneal approach. The retroperitoneal space may be accessed either through a standard oblique flank incision or a longitudinal incision made at the lateral border of the rectus sheath. The traditional oblique flank incision allows for a wider exposure and should be used in most situations. In lesions confined to the vertebral body, the left side is used by most surgeons because of the location of the abdominal aorta. Tumors with extension into the paraspinal soft tissues should be approached from the side of the soft-tissue involvement. Approaching the lumbar spine from the right side places the inferior vena cava at greater risk for injury from excessive retraction and misdirected surgical instruments.

An anterior-only approach for lesions arising from the upper lumbar spine (particularly L1) necessitates the exposure of the T12 vertebral body for placement of instrumentation. Detachment of at least the crus of the diaphragm or possibly the entire hemi-diaphragm will be necessary to work at the level of the body of T12. Therefore, a combined thoracoabdominal approach may be used. The 10th or 11th rib is exposed and removed and can be used for bone graft purposes. A transpleural exposure of the lower thoracic spine is then combined with a retroperitoneal approach to the upper lumbar spine after the diaphragm has been released approximately 1 cm from its insertion on the body wall. Some surgeons prefer to avoid violation of the thoracic cavity during the surgical approach to the upper lumbar spine. To accomplish this, the 12th rib is exposed and removed from its bed, taking care to stay extrapleural. The retroperitoneal space is entered in a standard fashion. Because of the small size of the 12th rib it cannot be used for structural grafting.

Access to the anterior portion of the lower lumbar spine is more difficult because of the bifurcation of the great vessels. Exposure down to the midportion of the L5 vertebral body can be accomplished with a standard retroperitoneal approach in which the anterior portion of the flank incision is curved parallel to the lateral border of the rectus sheath. Mobilization of the great vessels adjacent to the lower lumbar spine is difficult because of the tethering effect of the iliolumbar veins. These vessels are especially prone to injury and will bleed profusely if injured. Ligation of the iliolumbar veins is often required for adequate mobilization of the great vessels.

Lesions arising in the L5 vertebral body are best approached directly anterior. A skin incision oriented longitudinally in the midline or just off the midline is used to gain access to the peritoneal cavity for a transperitoneal approach or the retroperitoneum for a retroperitoneal approach. The bifurcation of the aorta anterior to the L4 vertebral body allows for direct anterior access to the lumbosacral junction in the window between the common iliac vessels. Because of the variability in vascular anatomy, preoperative imaging studies such as a CT scan or MRI should be used to determine the exact level of bifurcation prior to proceeding with surgical incision.

Once the anterior portion of the lumbar spine has been exposed and the great vessels retracted, the segmental vessels adjacent to the involved vertebral body as well as the bodies cranial and caudal to it should be ligated. Identification of the involved body is straightforward if a large soft-tissue mass is present or if extensive bony destruction has occurred. In situations where identification of the level of involvement is difficult or impossible, a localizing radiograph should be obtained. The removal of the diseased vertebral body is begun by performing complete discectomies at the adjacent levels. This allows for preparation of the adjacent vertebral end plates and identification of the exact location of the posterior longitudinal ligament and the spinal canal. The diseased vertebral body is removed with a combination of large osteotomes, Leksell rongeurs, and pituitary rongeurs. The anterior portion of the vertebral body is removed first. This creates a cavity into which the material close to the canal can be pulled anteriorly. The addition of distraction will assist in visualization of the posterior vertebral cortex and is especially useful if vertebral collapse and kyphosis are present. This can be accomplished with a large vertebral spreader or distractor. If the posterior cortex is intact, a high-speed burr may be used to thin the bone. Small curettes can then be used to pull the posterior cortex anteriorly, thereby avoiding any posteriorly directed force toward the canal. In situations in which the posterior cortex of the body has been compromised, great care must be exercised to avoid pushing tumor or bone fragments posteriorly into the canal. Penfield dissectors and small curettes may be used to free tumor found in the epidural space from the thecal sac. Care must be taken to avoid injury to the dura. Epidural venous bleeding can be controlled with the use of Gelfoam soaked in thrombin.

After complete decompression of the neural elements and removal of the diseased vertebral body, stabilization must be performed. There are many different choices for both grafting material as well as instrumentation. The details of these are discussed in the next section of this chapter.

RECONSTRUCTION OF THE ANTERIOR LUMBAR SPINE: GRAFTING AND INSTRUMENTATION OPTIONS

Decompression of the neural elements and removal of the pathologic tissue fulfill only two of the goals of the surgical treatment of spinal tumors. Correction of preexisting deformity and preventing future deformity by stabilization of the spine are also paramount to the success of surgical intervention. Tumor removal and decompression of the neural elements results in further destabilization of the already compromised anterior column. Many choices for anterior reconstruction of the lumbar spine exist. The method chosen must be able to withstand the physiologic loads imparted on it and must be able to remain functional for the remainder of the patient's life expectancy.

The defect created by decompression and tumor removal can be reconstructed by both biologic and nonbiologic struts. Examples of biologic struts include vascularized and nonvascularized autogenous rib grafts and various allograft struts including fibula, tibia, femur, and humerus. Autogenous nonvascularized rib grafts have been used in anterior reconstruction following resection of metastatic disease in the thoracic spine (36). Concerns about the lack of strength and small cross-sectional area limit their use in anterior lumbar reconstruction. Vascularized rib grafts have been used with success in reconstruction of kyphotic deformities but the limited life expectancy of patients with metastatic disease precludes their use in this situation. The use of fibular strut allografts for anterior column reconstruction has been described (37,38), although late collapse and recurrent deformity have been reported when they were used in metastatic disease (39). Structural rigidity combined with a small cross-sectional diameter predisposes fibular grafts to subsidence into the adjacent vertebral bodies. Concerns over subsidence into the adjacent end plates really preclude their use in this situation although some surgeons have placed two fibula grafts, "double stacking" them side-by-side in the defect. Fibular autografts may also be considered, but the relatively high complication rates from the donor site likely outweigh the benefits of using autograft in this patient population.

Allografts such as tibia, humerus, and femur have larger surface contact area and are composed of cortical bone. Therefore, they are less prone to subside into the adjacent end plates and result in kyphosis. The cortical bone that comprises these grafts allows for sufficient strength for these grafts to withstand the normal physiologic loads they will encounter. An example of anterior reconstruction with an allograft femoral strut combined with anterior instrumentation is shown in Figure 84-3. In patients with long life expectancies, the cylindric geometry of these allografts allows for placement of additional bone graft material in the center of the graft. Filling the

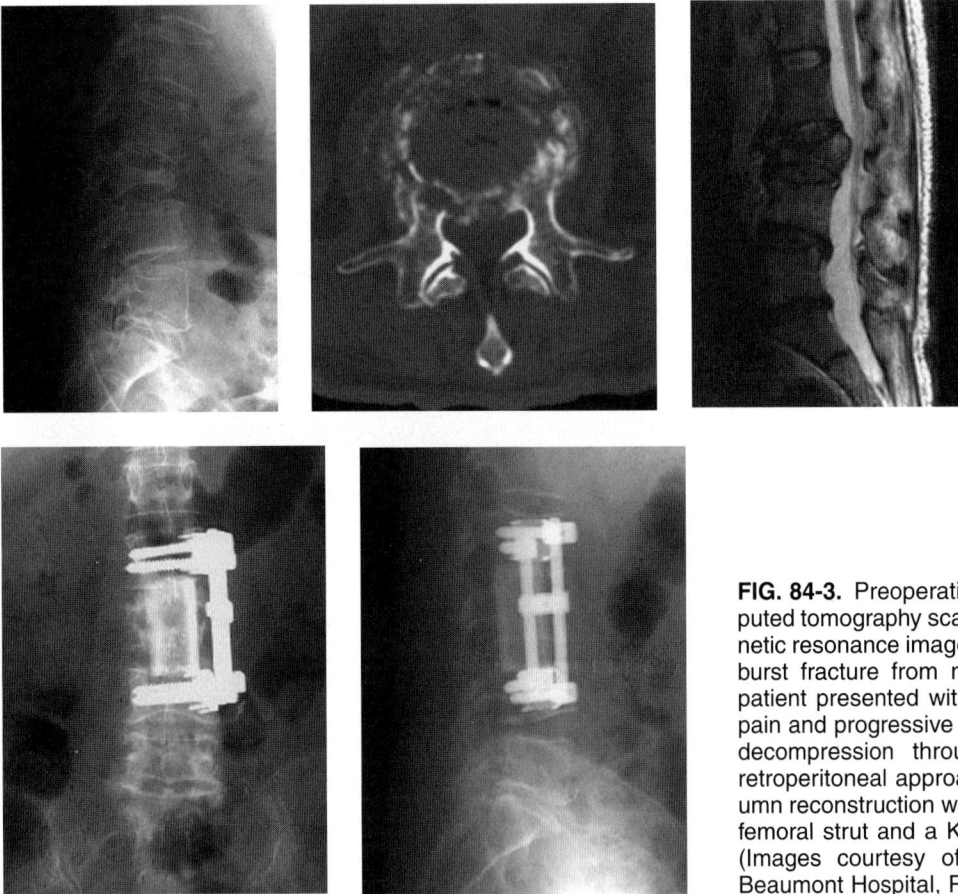

FIG. 84-3. Preoperative lateral radiograph, axial computed tomography scan, and sagittal T2-weighted magnetic resonance image of a patient with a pathologic L3 burst fracture from metastatic adenocarcinoma. The patient presented with an acute increase in low back pain and progressive neurologic deterioration. Anterior decompression through an oblique flank incision, retroperitoneal approach was performed. Anterior column reconstruction was accomplished with an allograft femoral strut and a Kaneda dual rod/screw construct. (Images courtesy of Eeric Truumees, MD, William Beaumont Hospital, Royal Oak, MI.)

center of an allograft with cancellous autograft from the iliac crest many increase fusion rates and decrease time to solid arthrodesis. The use of both bone graft substitutes, including bone morphogenetic proteins may also have beneficial effects on time to arthrodesis and pseudoarthrosis rates.

Various nonbiological struts may also be used for reconstruction of anterior defects created by decompression and tumor removal. Titanium mesh cages (40–42), carbon fiber implants (43), ceramic vertebral body replacements (44,45), and methylmethacrylate (46–48) have been described for anterior column reconstruction following corpectomy. When methylmethacrylate is used alone, it merely functions as an internal splint and will fail in time. Therefore, the role of methylmethacrylate without bone grafting is limited to patients with short life expectancy (48). If polymethylmethacrylate (PMMA) is used, reinforcing it with wires or wire mesh will improve its strength and decrease its bending flexibility. The addition of Steinmann pins to the construct will also increase the bending resistance and can be used to anchor the cement spacer to the adjacent vertebrae. These Steinmann pins are placed though the intact vertebral bodies, spanning the defect, prior to placing liquid cement into the defect (27). Great care must be exercised to avoid thermal

injury to the nearby dural sac and adjacent great vessels. Placement of a sheet of Gelfoam adjacent to the dura and the use of more "doughy" cement, in addition to constant cool saline irrigation, can be helpful in avoiding this complication (6).

Metallic and carbon fiber cage devices initially function as internal splints as well. The long-term function of these implants relies on the development of a solid arthrodesis. Like the long bone allografts mentioned previously, these devices are typically filled with bone graft. The choice of grafting material depends somewhat on the life expectancy of the patient and the preference of the surgeon. Choices for packing of these grafts include autograft cancellous iliac crest, rib autograft, allograft cancellous bone, and various bone graft substitutes/expanders. In the future, the use of bone morphogenetic proteins may eliminate the need for autograft harvest, decrease the time to union, and decrease the rate of pseudoarthrosis and hardware failure.

Anterior strut grafts function to maintain correction of any preexisting deformity by distributing load across the end plates of the adjacent vertebral bodies. Release of distractive forces used for graft insertion results in compression across the strut graft. Despite these compressive forces and the interference fit between the graft and the adjacent end plate, these struts alone do not provide enough stability to allow for mobilization of the patient and are frequently used in combination with anterior instrumentation. Grafts placed anteriorly without additional support are likely to displace and may do so into the spinal canal with devastating consequences. The addition of anterior instrumentation alone or in combination with posterior instrumentation and fusion will provide adequate stability to protect against graft displacement when the patient is mobilized. Concerns about excessive torque and lateral bending moments in the lumbar spine have resulted in some surgeons advocating the addition of posterior instrumentation and fusion when anterior lumbar vertebrectomy and fusion are performed after tumor resection (49). Combined anterior and posterior procedures are covered elsewhere in this text.

Anterior instrumentation for the thoracic and lumbar spine comes in many forms. Many screw/plate devices and screw/rod devices are available for anterior column reconstruction and stabilization. The use of many of these devices in the lower lumbar spine is difficult because they are not "low profile." Any hardware placed outside of the confines of the bony spinal column will be adjacent to the great vessels as they descend in the retroperitoneum. Erosion of the implant into the vessel could result in pseudoaneurysm formation or catastrophic bleeding. Screw and rod constructs such as the Kaneda device or the Xia anterior system, are high-profile devices that protrude laterally from the bony spinal column. Their insertion in the lower lumbar spine is challenging secondary to the difficulty in mobilization of the psoas muscle in this area. The close proximity of the vessels to these implants in the lower lumbar spine typically precludes their use. These screw/rod constructs can be used safely in the thoracolumbar and upper lumbar spine. The details of the precise surgical technique for these devices are beyond the scope of this chapter.

Plate/screw devices are also available for anterior reconstruction of the lumbar spine. These devices are lower profile than the screw/rod constructs but they still extend beyond the confines of the vertebral body, therefore, the potential exists for damage to the surrounding soft-tissue structures. Loosening and back-out of the screws can also result in damage to the adjacent structures. These devices are available in many different sizes and may be precontoured to fit the spine (contoured anterior spinal plates, or CASP plates). Multiple-hole designs allow for variable placement of the screws in the intact, adjacent vertebral bodies and the intervening allograft strut. Slots have been added to some systems to allow for the transmission of dynamic compressive forces across the allograft. Locking screws have also been designed to allow these plates to function as fixed angle devices. Hook and distraction rod devices, such as the Knodt distraction rod/hook system and the Rezaian distraction device, do not extend beyond the confines of the verte-

bral bodies, therefore the risk of vascular injury is low. Unfortunately, the stability provided by these devices, even when they are combined with cement augmentation, is insufficient without posterior stabilization.

The existing clinical literature does not support the superiority of one specific structural graft or instrumentation system for reconstruction of the anterior lumbar spine following corpectomy for neoplastic disease. Clinical studies evaluating the use of various anterior instrumentation systems for the treatment of burst fractures have documented varied rates of implant failure and pseudoarthrosis (50–53). Biomechanical studies have been performed in an attempt to determine the optimum construct for anterior spinal reconstruction. Lee et al. used a calf lumbar spine corpectomy model to study the effect of different anterior grafts on the stability of different anterior reconstruction constructs (54). They found that the use of a titanium mesh cage (Harms cage) increased the torsional rigidity when combined with either anterior or posterior instrumentation. They compared the mesh cage to a block of PMMA or a calf tricortical iliac crest graft also combined with anterior or posterior instrumentation. No differences in stability were found in flexion/extension or in lateral bending. The authors hypothesized that improved friction at the graft/bone interface from the serrated edges of the cage resulted in a more rigid construct in torsion.

Biomechanical studies aimed at evaluating anterior instrumentation systems have also been published. Zdeblick et al. reported that the Kaneda anterior rod/screw construct provided greater stability than earlier systems such as the CASP and the Kostuik-Harrington devices (55). In a study by An et al., the Kaneda device, anterior TSRH system, the Z-plate, and the University anterior plating system were all found to restore stability in all loading modes when combined with an interbody graft (56). Lim et al. also evaluated the Kaneda device and the University anterior plating system in an unstable calf spine model. These devices, when combined with an anterior graft, restored the stability of the spine to at least that of the intact state (57). Kotani (57a) used a synthetic spine testing model to evaluate the static and fatigue properties of 12 anterior thoracolumbar instrumentation systems. The instrumentation systems were applied according to manufacturer's recommendations to two synthetic cylinders that were standardized to represent vertebral bodies. Compressive loading was applied which resulted in lateral bending forces on the implants. The bending strength and fatigue properties are illustrated in Figures 84-4A and 84-4B, respectively.

The authors also included a description of the failure modes for each device. This "worst-case scenario" testing did not include the addition of a strut between the simulated vertebral elements. However, the addition of a biomechanical strut would improve both the bending strength and the fatigue properties of these devices. This study clearly demonstrates the *in vitro* superiority of some of the

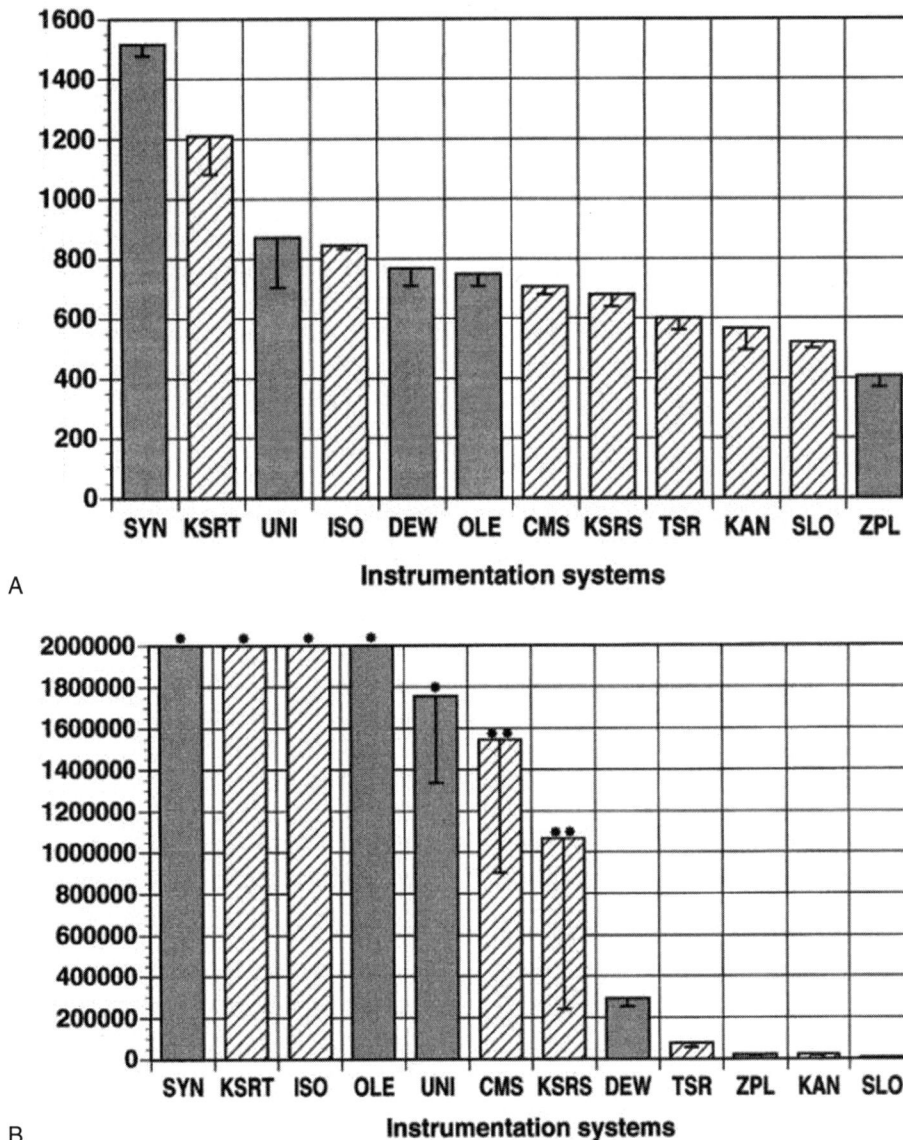

FIG. 84-4. A: Bending strength *(N)* and **(B)** failure cycles (at 500 N) of 12 different anterior instrumentation systems. *SYN,* Synthes thoracolumbar locking plate; *KSRT,* Kaneda SR titanium; *UNI,* University plate titanium system, ISO, anterior ISOLA; *DEW,* Dewald-LDI; *OLE,* Olerud plate; *CMS,* Cross Medical Synergy; *KSRS,* Kaneda SR stainless steel; *TSR,* TSRH system; *KAN,* Kaneda device; *SLO,* Slot-Zielke device; *ZPL,* Z-plate. [From Kotani Y, Cunningham B, Parker L, Kanayama M, et al. Static and fatigue biomechanical properties of anterior thoracolumbar instrumentation systems: a synthetic testing model. Spine 1999;24(14):1406, with permission.]

anterior instrumentation systems. Despite this, the authors are careful to point out that most of these devices have been used with reasonable success in clinical situations. This suggests that perhaps strict attention to surgical technique and careful patient selection are the keys to success when performing anterior-only reconstruction after resection of a tumor in the thoracolumbar or lumbar spine.

RESULTS

The anterior approach to the thoracolumbar and lumbar spine has been used successfully to address spinal cord compression and instability caused by lesions such as neoplasm, fracture, infection, and deformity. Many studies have documented significant neurologic improvement in patients who underwent anterior decompression. The results of these studies must be carefully evaluated secondary to the variability among studies including surgical indications, timing of operations, methods of defining patient function, definition of surgical complications, and length of follow-up. In addition, extrapolation of these data to the lumbar spine is also difficult because these studies combined surgical treatment of the tumors involving the cervical, thoracic, and lumbar spines.

The vast majority of malignant primary spine tumors and metastatic lesions of the spine occur in the vertebral body. When neurologic compromise does occur it is most likely related to compression of the neural elements from ventral pathology. Retropulsed fragments of bone from a pathologic fracture, direct extension of tumor, epidural metastasis ventral to the thecal sac, and draping of the neural elements over a kyphotic segment created by a fracture can account for compression of the neural structures. Initial studies that documented the results of the surgical treatment of neurologic deterioration in the setting of spinal tumors found that surgical decompression, in the form of a posterior decompression, had no benefit when compared to radiation therapy alone. These studies failed to take into account the fact that neural compression occurs ventrally and therefore, is not directly addressed by posterior decompression.

Several studies have been published that compare anterior and posterior approaches for the treatment of metastatic or primary lesions of the anterior column. Kostuik et al. reviewed 100 consecutive patients with tumors involving the anterior column (2). Metastatic lesions comprised 71% of the patients in this study. The stated indications for the surgical intervention included spinal instability, impending pathologic fracture, and rapid progression of neurologic deficits. Decompression and reconstruction of the thoracic and lumbar spine were performed through anterior, posterior, or combined anterior and posterior approaches. In the group of patients with metastatic disease, 30 of the 41 (73%) patients who underwent an anterior decompression achieved significant neurologic recovery, compared with only 16 (40%) patients who were decompressed with a posterior approach. Siegal compared the neurologic status of patients with primary and metastatic tumors of the spine that underwent anterior decompression versus posterior decompression (24). Eighty percent of patients treated with anterior decompression retained or regained the ability to walk postoperatively, compared to only 40% of those treated with a laminectomy. In addition, 5 of 25 patients who underwent laminectomy experienced neurologic deterioration. In comparison, 12 of 13 patients treated with anterior decompression regained at least one grade in neurological function. McLain performed a review of the literature and reported on 427 cases of anterior decompression. He found that 78% of patients that were decompressed anteriorly had a significant improvement in neurologic function and that a satisfactory outcome was obtained in 80% of the patients. Weinstein reviewed 746 cases of posterior decompression found in the published literature (58). He compared the neurologic and functional outcomes of these patients to those reported by McLain (59). Only 33% of patients that underwent posterior decompression showed neurologic improvement postoperatively. Weinstein also found that only 37% of these patients had satisfactory clinical out-

comes. While these two literature reviews combine studies with great variability, they highlight the fact that patients with neurologic decline secondary to metastatic spinal lesions benefit from anterior decompression of their spinal canal.

A strong correlation has been repeatedly reported between preoperative neurologic status and postoperative outcome, regardless of the surgical approach for decompression. Most studies have found that 60% to 95% of the patients who had the ability to ambulate at the time of diagnosis retained the ability to ambulate postoperatively. Conversely, only 35% to 65% of the patients with paraparesis regained the ability to ambulate after decompression. Those patients with complete paraplegia have less than 30% likelihood of regaining the ability to ambulate (1,2,30,60–64). The rate of progression of neurologic deficit is also an important prognostic factor. Harrington reported that if the neurologic deficit progresses rapidly, in less than 24 hours, the prognosis for neurologic recovery is poor, irrespective of the treatment rendered (3). Slow onset and progression of the neurologic deficit tended to have a much more favorable prognosis.

A review of 36 patients with metastatic disease of thoracic and lumbar spine treated with anterior corpectomy and stabilization was published by Kaneda (65). A majority of these patients presented with pain as their main complaint. Following surgery, only 1 of 36 patients required occasional narcotic pain medication. Nearly 60% of the patients were pain-free while 20% reported only minimal pain. Of the 27 patients with preoperative neurologic deficit, 19 (70.4%) patients improved at least one Frankel grade postoperatively. Of the 14 patients who were bedridden before surgery, 11 became ambulatory and 2 were able to transfer from a bed to a chair. Local recurrence occurred in 5 patients who underwent subtotal corpectomy and 3 patients who underwent total corpectomy. Recurrence occurred at an average of 16 months (7 to 28 months), and all 8 patients had radioresistant tumors.

Harrington also reported on 52 patients with spinal instability secondary to metastatic lesions of the spine (20). These patients underwent anterior decompression and stabilization with methylmethacrylate in situ. Of 52 patients, 26 had a metastasis to the cervical spine, 18 to the thoracic spine, 4 to the thoracolumbar spine, and 4 to the lumbar spine. Preoperatively, 40 of the 52 patients had a major neurologic deficit that required spinal cord or nerve root decompression. Of these, 40% had complete neurologic recovery following anterior decompression and stabilization. Twenty-five percent showed significant improvement while five patients remained unchanged. Only one patient deteriorated neurologically after an anterior decompression and stabilization.

Despite the variability in patient characteristics found in published reports on the surgical treatment of primary spine tumors and metastatic lesions of the spine, three major themes have emerged:

1. The presence of a preoperative neurologic deficit correlates with poorer outcomes regardless of the treatment rendered.
2. Rapidly progressive neurologic deterioration is predictive of less likely return of neurologic function after decompression.
3. Because of the anatomic location of most malignant primary and metastatic tumors in the spine, compression of the neural elements occurs ventrally in the vertebral body.

Accordingly, decompression through an anterior approach results in a greater chance of neurologic recovery, greater pain relief, and better clinical outcomes.

COMPLICATIONS

Complications related to the surgical treatment of spinal tumors are common. Adverse events such as infection, recurrent instability, recurrence of disease, vascular injury, pseudoarthrosis, and medically related complications have been reported in approximately 25% of cases. The occurrence of a new neurologic deficit following anterior decompression for spinal tumors is approximately 2% to 4% (20,24,66). The development of complications in this patient population can be devastating. They may result in multiple return trips to the operating room and prolonged hospitalizations, which negatively affect the quality of life of these patients. As with any procedure, prevention of the complication is the best treatment.

McAfee et al. retrospectively analyzed 24 patients who had major complications after undergoing stabilization with methylmethacrylate. Initial instability was related to metastatic tumor in 9 patients and to a traumatic condition in 15 patients (67). Postoperative neurologic deficit occurred in 11 patients. The authors thought that the recovery of the neurologic function was hindered by cement in 6 of these patients. The most common complication in this group of patients was loosening and loss of fixation. Hardware failure occurred in 12 of 15 of the trauma patients and in 8 of 9 patients with neoplasm. A deep wound infection developed in 6 patients. Based on the findings of this review, the authors recommended combined anterior and posterior procedures for the reconstruction of instability in the setting of tumor. The use of methylmethacrylate alone, without bone grafting, will fail because a solid, bony fusion will not occur. This technique should be reserved for patients with a limited life expectancy. In patients whose long-term prognosis is good, biologic (autograft or allograft) struts should be used to allow for eventual union across the fused segments.

The use of radiation therapy for the treatment of spinal tumors has also been shown to affect complication rates. McLain et al. reported that patients undergoing preoper-

ative radiation therapy accounted for 42% of all complications (68). This group also suffered 70% of the major complications in this study. Wise et al. also reported higher complication rates (40%) in those patients treated with radiation therapy preoperatively (15). In McLain's study, 36% of patients developed transient neurologic deficits in the postoperative period (68). Wound infection and vascular injuries also occurred in 18% of patients. Clinically significant pseudoarthrosis developed in two patients while progression of renal cell carcinoma led to late instability in another two patients. Failure of fixation occurred in four patients and was attributed to inadequate reconstruction of the anterior column that was compromised from tumor involvement.

Wise et al. (15) retrospectively reviewed 80 patients who underwent surgical treatment for metastatic disease of the spine. Mean survival time after the diagnosis of spinal metastasis was 26 months, while mean survival time after surgery was 15.9 months. Twenty (25%) of 80 patients had 35 complications. The authors found a relationship between the Harrington classification and complication rates. Increased rates of complications occurred in those patients with greater neurologic deficits, lower Frankel grades before and after surgery, and those who were treated with radiation preoperatively.

Patients with spine tumors are more likely to be immunosuppressed secondary to their primary disease as well as the treatment of that disease. These patients may also be malnourished because of the systemic effects of their malignancy and its treatment. Both immunosuppression and poor nutritional status have been associated with higher rates of postoperative complications (69–73). The urgency with which many of these patients present many times precludes the optimization of nutritional parameters prior to operative intervention. If elective decompression and stabilization is planned, laboratory studies such as albumin, serum transferrin, and total lymphocyte count may be used to guide preoperative nutritional supplementation. Optimization of the nutritional status of the patient may help to prevent postoperative complications that could negatively affect the patient's quality of life.

REFERENCES

1. Manabe S, et al. Surgical treatment of metastatic tumors of the spine. Spine 1989;14:41–57.
2. Kostuik JP, et al. Spinal stabilization of vertebral column tumors. Spine 1988;13:250–256.
3. Harrington KD, Metastatic disease of the spine, current concepts. J Bone Joint Surg Am 1986;68A:1110–1115.
4. Fraser RD, Paterson DC, Simpson DA. Orthopaedic aspects of spinal tumors in children. J Bone Joint Surg Br 1977;59B:143–151.
5. Flatley TJ, Anderson MN, Anast GT. Spinal instability due to malignant disease. Treatment by segmental spinal stabilization. J Bone Joint Surg Am 1984;66A:47–52.
6. Dolin MG. Acute massive dural compression secondary to methyl methacrylate replacement of a tumorous lumbar vertebral body. Spine 1989;14(1):108–110.

7. Brihaye J, et al. The management of spinal epidural metastases. Adv Tech Stand Neurosurg 1988;16:121–176.
8. Harada M, et al. Role of the vertebral venous system in metastatic spread of cancer cells to the bone. Adv Exp Med Biol 1992;324:83–92.
9. Weinstein JN, McLain RF. Primary tumors of the spine. Spine 1987; 12(9):843–851.
10. Keim HA, Reina EG. Osteoid-osteoma as a cause of scoliosis. J Bone Joint Surg Am 1975;57(2):159–163.
11. Pettine KA, Klassen RA. Osteoid-osteoma and osteoblastoma of the spine. J Bone Joint Surg Am 1986;68(3):354–361.
12. Weinstein JN. Surgical approach to spine tumors. Orthopedics, 1989;12(6):897–905.
13. Lesoin F, et al. Posterolateral approach to tumours of the dorsolumbar spine. Acta Neurochir (Wien) 1986;81(1–2):40–44.
14. DeWald RL, et al. Reconstructive spinal surgery as palliation for metastatic malignancies of the spine. Spine 1985;10(1):21–26.
15. Wise JJ, et al. Complication, survival rates, and risk factors of surgery for metastatic disease of the spine. Spine 1999;24(18):1943–1951.
16. Phillips E, Levine AM. Metastatic lesions of the upper cervical spine. Spine 1989;14(10):1071–1077.
17. O'Neil J, Gardner V, Armstrong G. Treatment of tumors of the thoracic and lumbar spinal column. Clin Orthop 1988;227:103–112.
18. Lee CK, Rosa R, Fernand R. Surgical treatment of tumors of the spine. Spine 1986;11(3):201–208.
19. Hammerberg KW. Surgical treatment of metastatic spine disease. Spine 1992;17(10):1148–1153.
20. Harrington KD. Anterior cord decompression and spinal stabilization for patients with metastatic lesions of the spine. J Neurosurg 1984;61 (1):107–117.
21. Cybulski GR, et al. Luque rod stabilization for metastatic disease of the spine. Surg Neurol 1987;28(4):277–283.
22. Dunn RC Jr, et al. Spinal epidural neoplasia. A 15-year review of the results of surgical therapy. J Neurosurg 1980;52(1):47–51.
23. Onimus M, et al. Surgical treatment of vertebral metastasis. Spine 1986;11(9):883–891.
24. Siegal T. Surgical decompression of anterior and posterior malignant epidural tumors compressing the spinal cord: a prospective study. Neurosurgery 1985;17(3):424–432.
25. Siegal T, Tiqva P. Vertebral body resection for epidural compression by malignant tumors. Results of forty-seven consecutive operative procedures. J Bone Joint Surg Am 1985;67(3):375–382.
26. Tomita T, Galicich JH, Sundaresan N. Radiation therapy for spinal epidural metastases with complete block. Acta Radiol Oncol 1983;22(2):135–143.
27. Sundaresan N, et al. Treatment of neoplastic epidural cord compression by vertebral body resection and stabilization. J Neurosurg 1985;63(5): 676–684.
28. Sundaresan N, Galicich JH, Lane JM. Harrington rod stabilization for pathological fractures of the spine. J Neurosurg 1984;60(2):282–286.
29. Kleinman WB, Kiernan HA, Michelsen MJ. Metastatic cancer of the spinal column. Clin Orthop 1978(136):166–172.
30. Harrington KD. Anterior decompression and stabilization of the spine as a treatment for vertebral collapse and spinal cord compression from metastatic malignancy. Clin Orthop 1988(233):177–197.
31. Cusick JF, et al. Distraction rod stabilization in the treatment of metastatic carcinoma. J Neurosurg 1983;59(5):861–866.
32. Ramsey RG, Zacharias CE. MR imaging of the spine after radiation therapy: easily recognizable effect. Am J Roentgenol 1985;144:1131–1135.
33. Edelson RN, Deck MD, Posner JB. Intramedullary spinal cord metastases. Clinical and radiographic findings in nine cases. Neurology 1972;22(12):1222–1231.
34. Solini A, et al. The surgical treatment of metastatic tumours of the lumbar spine. Ital J Orthop Traumatol 1985;11(4):427–442.
35. Findlay GF. Adverse effects of the management of malignant spinal cord compression. J Neurol Neurosurg Psychiatry 1984;47(8): 761–768.
36. Shirakusa T, et al. Anterior rib strut grafting for the treatment of malignant lesions in the thoracic spine. Arch Orthop Trauma Surg 1989;108 (5):268–272.
37. Graziano GP, Sidhu KS. Salvage reconstruction in acute and late sequelae from pyogenic thoracolumbar infection. J Spinal Disord 1993;6(3):199–207.
38. Pun WK, et al. Tuberculosis of the lumbosacral junction. Long-term follow-up of 26 cases. J Bone Joint Surg Br 1990;72(4):675–678.
39. Lord CF, Herndon JH. Spinal cord compression secondary to kyphosis associated with radiation therapy for metastatic disease. Clin Orthop 1986(210):120–127.
40. Akamaru T, et al. Healing of autologous bone in a titanium mesh cage used in anterior column reconstruction after total spondylectomy. Spine 2002;27(13):E329–E333.
41. Nishida J, et al. Leiomyosarcoma of the lumbar spine: case report. Spine 2002;27(2):E42–E46.
42. Lowery L, Harms J. Titanium surgical mesh for vertebral defect replacement and intervertebral spacers. In: Thalgott JS, ed. The manual of internal fixation of the spine. Philadelphia: Lippincott-Raven, 1996:127–146.
43. Boriani S, et al. The use of the carbon-fiber reinforced modular implant for the reconstruction of the anterior column of the spine. A clinical and experimental study conducted on 42 cases. Chir Organi Mov 2000; 85(4):309–335.
44. Kaneda K, et al. The treatment of osteoporotic-posttraumatic vertebral collapse using the Kaneda device and a bioactive ceramic vertebral prosthesis. Spine 1992;17[8 Suppl]:S295–S303.
45. Matsui H, Tatezaki S, Tsuji H. Ceramic vertebral body replacement for metastatic spine tumors. J Spinal Disord 1994;7(3):248–254.
46. Panjabi MM, et al. Biomechanical study of cervical spine stabilization with methylmethacrylate. Spine 1985;10(3):198–203.
47. White AAI, Panjabi MM. Surgical constructs employing methylmethacrylate. In: White AA, Panjabi MM, eds. Clinical biomechanics of the spine. Philadelphia: JB Lippincott Co, 1978:423–431.
48. Clark CR, Keggi KJ, Panjabi MM. Methylmethacrylate stabilization of the cervical spine. J Bone Joint Surg Am 1984;66(1):40–46.
49. Harrington KD. Metastatic tumors of the spine: diagnosis and treatment. J Am Acad Ortho Surg 1993;1(2):76–86.
50. Kaneda K, et al. Anterior decompression and stabilization with the Kaneda device for thoracolumbar burst fractures associated with neurological deficits. J Bone Joint Surg Am 1997;79(1):69–83.
51. Ghanayem, AJ, Zdeblick TA. Anterior instrumentation in the management of thoracolumbar burst fractures. Clin Orthop 1997;335:89–100.
52. Esses SI, Botsford DJ, Kostuik JP. Evaluation of surgical treatment for burst fractures. Spine 1990;15(7):667–673.
53. Been HD, Anterior decompression and stabilization of thoracolumbar burst fractures by the use of the Slot-Zielke device. Spine 1991;16(1): 70–77.
54. Lee SW, et al. Biomechanical effect of anterior grafting devices on the rotational stability of spinal constructs. J Spinal Disord 2000;13(2): 150–155.
55. Zdeblick TA, et al. Anterior spinal fixators. A biomechanical in vitro study. Spine 1993;18(4):513–517.
56. An HS, et al. Biomechanical evaluation of anterior thoracolumbar spinal instrumentation. Spine 1995;20(18):1979–1983.
57. Lim TH, et al. Biomechanical evaluation of anterior and posterior fixations in an unstable calf spine model. Spine 1997;22(3):261–266.
57a. Kotani Y, et al. Static and fatigue biomechanical properties of anterior thoracolumbar instrumentation systems. A synthetic testing model. Spine 1999;24:1406–1413.
58. Weinstein JN. Differential diagnosis and surgical treatment of primary benign and malignant neoplasms. In: Frymoyer JW, ed. The adult spine: principles and practice. New York: Raven Press, 1991:829–860.
59. McLain RF, Weinstein JN. Tumors of the spine. Semin Spine Surg 1990;2:157–180.
60. Black P. Spinal metastasis: current status and recommended guidelines for management. Neurosurgery 1979;5(6):726–746.
61. Fidler MW. Pathological fractures of the cervical spine. Palliative surgical treatment. J Bone Joint Surg Br 1985;67(3):352–357.
62. Hall AJ, Mackay NN. The results of laminectomy for compression of the cord or cauda equina by extradural malignant tumour. J Bone Joint Surg Br 1973;55(3):497–505.
63. Harrington KD. Metastatic disease of the spine. In: Harrington KD, ed. Orthopaedic management of metastatic bone disease. St. Louis: Mosby, 1988:309–383.
64. Nather A, Bose K. The results of decompression of cord or cauda equina compression from metastatic extradural tumors. Clin Orthop 1982;169:103–108.
65. Kaneda K, Takeda N. Reconstruction with a ceramic vertebral prosthesis and Kaneda device following subtotal or total vertebrectomy in metastatic thoracic and lumbar spine. In: Bridwell KH, DeWald, RL, eds. The textbook of spinal surgery, Vol 2, 2nd ed. Philadelphia: Lippincott-Raven, 1997:2071–2088.

66. Sundaresan N, et al. Vertebral body resection in the treatment of cancer involving the spine. Cancer 1984;53(6):1393–1396.
67. McAfee PC, et al. Failure of stabilization of the spine with methylmethacrylate. A retrospective analysis of twenty-four cases. J Bone Joint Surg Am 1986;68(8):1145–1157.
68. McLain RF, Kabins M, Weinstein JN. VSP stabilization of lumbar neoplasms: technical considerations and complications. J Spinal Disord 1991;4(3):359–365.
69. Hill GL, et al. Malnutrition in surgical patients. An unrecognised problem. Lancet 1977;1(8013):689–692.
70. DeWys WD. Anorexia as a general effect of cancer. Cancer 1979;43[5 Suppl]:2013–2019.
71. Dick J, Boachie-Adjei O, Wilson M. One-stage versus two-stage anterior and posterior spinal reconstruction in adults. Comparison of outcomes including nutritional status, complications rates, hospital costs, and other factors. Spine 1992;17[8 Suppl]:S310–S316.
72. Lenke LG, et al. Prospective analysis of nutritional status normalization after spinal reconstructive surgery. Spine 1995;20(12):1359–1367.
73. Smith TK. Prevention of complications in orthopedic surgery secondary to nutritional depletion. Clin Orthop 1987;222:91–97.

CHAPTER 85

Combined Anterior-Posterior Procedures

Osamu Shirado, Naoki Takeda, Akio Minami, and Kiyoshi Kaneda

The survival time of patients with malignant tumors has been increasing, not only because of the advances of adjunctive treatments such as chemotherapy and radiotherapy, but also because of advances in surgical treatments. Thus, raising the quality of life (QOL), as well as lengthening life expectancy, has become another important concern for clinicians who treat patients with malignant tumors.

The surgical treatment of primary malignant and metastatic spine tumors has progressed with the development of surgical techniques and spinal instrumentations. Laminectomy proved to have no advantage over conventional radiation therapy in 1970s (1). Following this evidence, simultaneous laminectomy and stabilization with spinal instrumentation provided better results than laminectomy alone (2). The technique of posterolateral decompression or costotransversectomy (3) in thoracic lesions has also provided much better surgical results for metastatic spinal disease (4). However, the main goals of those surgical procedures were to relieve and prevent deteriorating paralysis, thus those procedures were palliative treatments. As a result, local recurrences inevitably arose if the patients survived for a long enough time after surgery (4,5).

In the modern era, when patients with cancer may experience medium- or long-term survival, we now see patients with spinal metastases who will require more radical and aggressive surgery to decrease the rate of local recurrence. Accordingly, total spondylectomy through combined anterior-posterior procedure or posterior procedure alone is needed and indicated for patients with primary malignant or metastatic spinal tumors who are expected to have a long-term survival (6–9).

Total spondylectomy can be performed using two approaches: the anterior-posterior combined approach (6,7,10) or the posterior approach alone (8,9,11). Our preferred and recommended method is the combined approach. On the other hand, one of the most popular posterior approaches is known as total *en bloc* spondylec-

tomy, or TES (8,9). From the oncologic standpoint, either approach results in intralesional resection if the tumor has invaded both pedicles. No matter how *en bloc* resection of the involved vertebra with tumors is performed, it is impossible to curatively resect the tumor with a wide margin in such cases. Contamination by the remaining tumor cells is almost inevitable when dissecting the posterior and anterior elements of the vertebra at the pedicle during surgery. However, this procedure is currently recommended as the most aggressive treatment and is likely to have the most successful outcome in patients with primary malignant or metastatic spinal tumors. In this chapter, the surgical indications and techniques for the combined anterior-posterior procedure for resecting spine tumors are described.

INDICATIONS FOR THE COMBINED ANTERIOR-POSTERIOR PROCEDURE (TABLE 85-1)

A number of different surgical approaches are available to spine surgeons. The surgical approaches for spinal tumors, however, can be divided into three main procedures: anterior, posterior, and the combined anterior-posterior approach. Spine surgeons must consider several factors before determining the most appropriate approach for each case. The most suitable choice of approach for patients with spinal tumors depends upon (a) the patient's life expectancy, (b) the number of vertebrae involved, (c) the location and extent of neural impingement, (d) the presence and degree of spinal instability, and (e) the patient's general medical condition (12). The most appropriate surgical approach is determined only after considering the following factors: the efficacy of adjunctive therapy such as radiotherapy, tumor biology including the grade of malignancy, the extent of tumor, the degree of spinal instability, vertebral involvement, and life expectancy. More basic factors should be taken into account as well such as the patient's immunologic, nutritional, and psychosocial condition.

824

TABLE 85.1. *Indications for the combined anterior and posterior procedure for spinal tumors*

Anticipated life expectancy longer than 6 months
Three-column involvement of the tumor
High-grade instability such as the three-column instability
Involvement of contiguous vertebral bodies
Solitary metastases
Destructive benign tumor such as giant cell tumor

After considering all of the above, indications for combined anterior and posterior procedures in primary malignant and metastatic spinal tumors are as follows (6,7,10): (a) three-column tumor involvement of the spine, (b) high-grade instability such as the three-column instability, (c) involvement of contiguous vertebral bodies, (d) the presence of solitary metastases, (e) anticipated life expectancy longer than 6 months, and (f) destructive benign tumor such as a giant cell tumor. Solitary metastasis limited to the vertebral body may also be an indication for this combined procedure, as TES can be performed more safely using this approach.

From the prognostic point of view, it is very important to predict the patient's life expectancy as exactly as possible. Some prognostic scoring systems are advocated to evaluate the life expectancy in patients with spine tumors, especially metastatic tumors. Tokuhashi et al. (13) proposed an assessment system for the prognosis of metastatic spine tumors. They employed six parameters: (a) the patient's general condition, (b) the number of extraspinal bone metastases, (c) the number of metastases in the vertebral body, (d) the presence of metastases to major internal organs, (e) the primary site of the cancer, and (f) the severity of spinal cord palsy. Each parameter ranged from 0 to 2 points, for a possible total score of 12 points. The more the points the patient receives the better the prognosis. The authors pointed out that the total score is likely to be well correlated with the prognosis in each patient. An excisional operation should be performed on those cases scoring 9 points or above. Tomita et al. (9) proposed a prognostic score using three prognostic factors: grade of malignancy, the presence of both visceral metastases, and bone metastases. Based on the scoring system, they suggested a surgical strategy for spinal metastases. As a result, they recommended that all patients with solitary tumors have the potential for long-term survival, thus justifying a more aggressive strategy.

SHORT REVIEW OF THE LITERATURE ON THE SURGICAL APPROACHES FOR SPINAL TUMORS

Kaneda and Takeda (6) recommended the anterior procedures for corpectomy when (a) the metastasis is confined to one, or two to three contiguous vertebrae, (b) a metastatic lesion is confined to the vertebral body of a radioresistant tumor, (c) there is anterior instability (i.e., a vertebral collapse is more than 50% likely), (d) there is epidural expansion in the anterior spinal canal and the main mass is confined to the vertebral body, or (e) the anticipated life expectancy is longer than 6 months.

Simultaneous corpectomy with posterior-element resection of the vertebra (i.e., total spondylectomy) is indicated in solitary metastases to the spine in radioresistant tumors such as those encountered in renal, thyroid, and breast cancers (9,10). There are two types of surgical approaches for total spondylectomy: posterior approach alone and a combined anterior and posterior approach. In 1971, Stener (14,15) removed three vertebrae in a patient with a chondrosarcoma of the spine using the posterior approach alone. He recommended complete spondylectomy of the thoracic and lumbar vertebrae down to the third lumbar vertebra using the posterior approach alone. For complete removal of the fourth lumbar vertebra, however, he advised using both an anterior and posterior approach. There were two reasons for this recommendation: one was the close relationship between the lower lumbar spine and several large vessels; the other was the hindrance caused by the iliac wings when exposing the L5 vertebral body from behind.

Roy-Camille (11) performed a thoracic one-stage total vertebrectomy through a simple posterior approach. However, he pointed out that the psoas and iliac muscle insertions on the vertebral body, as well as the vascular lumbar pedicles, make the posterior-only approach to the lumbar vertebra impossible. A two-stage operation should be recommended in such a case. Magerl and Coscia (16) reported a posterior vertebrectomy of the thoracic and lumbar spine. However, it would be contraindicated to attempt a total vertebrectomy using the posterior procedure alone in a situation of extension of the tumor into the soft tissues surrounding the vertebral body. More recently, Tomita et al. (8) reported a TES that resected the involved vertebra in two major blocs using the posterior approach alone. This technique is the most appropriate surgical procedure for primary vertebral malignancy.

Conversely, Sundaresan et al. (17) recommended that spondylectomy should be carried out as a two-stage operation with stage 1 the posterior phase and stage 2 the anterior phase. They recommended a staged operation in order to minimize the possibility of neurologic deficits resulting from ischemic damage to the nerve tissues. Fidler (18) reported a radical resection of the spine from a posterior approach (the first stage), and then an anterior and posterior combination (the second stage). He concluded that a purely posterior approach was not feasible in some cases, because of lung involvement, extensive adhesions after a previous operation, paravertebral hematoma, and the difficulty of mobilizing and delivering a large tumor through the posterior approach alone. A combined approach enabled radical resection of all the involved tissues allowing direct visualization, and also permitted the unhindered access to, and control of, the blood supply to the tumor.

PREOPERATIVE MANAGEMENT

Adjunctive treatment such as radiotherapy and chemotherapy is carefully considered and planned during the preoperative period. Preoperative radiotherapy is often very effective for some radiosensitive malignant tumors such as prostatic and lymphoreticular tumors. In such tumors excellent clinical results can sometimes be obtained by irradiation alone in many patients.

The effectiveness of spine surgery in treating tumor cases is sometimes compromised by excessive bleeding. Metastatic renal cell and thyroid carcinomas can be highly vascular, increasing patients' morbidity and mortality. Angiography with selective embolization of the segmental vessels in the involved vertebra, including the vertebrae above and below, can be an effective way to manage such lesions, and may be safely carried out up to 24 hours prior to surgery. The use of this technique can decrease intraoperative blood loss and perioperative morbidity and mortality. It may also be helpful to identify the origin of the Adamkiewicz artery. We recommend this procedure one day before surgery. Thoracolumbosacral orthosis (TLSO) for postoperative external support should be manufactured preoperatively.

SURGICAL TECHNIQUES IN THE COMBINED ANTERIOR-POSTERIOR PROCEDURE

The posterior procedure precedes the anterior one. The combined procedure is usually performed under the same anesthesia.

Step 1: Posterior Procedure

Resection of the posterior elements (including the spinous process, laminae, articular processes, transverse processes, and the pedicles) is performed first. Patients are positioned prone on the Hall frame in a comfortable fashion without pressure on the thorax or abdomen. The skin is suitably prepared, and is infiltrated only into subcutaneous tissues with a 1:500,000 epinephrine solution. A midline skin incision is made over at least two spinal segments, above and below the involved segment, followed by subperiosteal exposure. Dissection should be extended laterally along the ribs with the thoracic spine and the transverse processes in the lumbar spine. Wide resection is needed to make the total spondylectomy feasible. The ribs of the involved vertebra should then be dissected 3 to 4 cm from the midline. The periosteum should be carefully removed from the ribs to avoid opening the pleura. This posterior procedure should be performed extrapleurally and retroperitoneally.

Both costotransverse ligaments are divided, and both rib heads should be carefully removed. Both superior articular facets of the involved vertebra are then exposed by removing the proximal lower laminae and inferior articular processes of the adjacent cranial vertebra. A threadwire saw, or T-saw (a flexible, multifilament device, 0.54 mm in diameter, designed and developed by Tomita), is used to perform *en bloc* resection of the posterior element (8,9). The T-saw is inserted into the epidural space beneath the lamina through a T-saw guide, and is pulled out of the neural foramen (Fig. 85-1A). The T-saw guide should be introduced along the medial cortex of the pedicle so that the spinal cord and the nerve root are not damaged. Both ends of the T-saw are pulled around the pedicle of the involved vertebra with a sawing motion. This maneuver is performed in a lateral direction with the help of a T-saw manipulator and guide (Fig. 85-1B, C).

Thus, both pedicles of the involved vertebra are cut off using the T-saw. Finally, after incising the interspinous ligament, the facet capsules, and ligament flavum, posterior elements of the involved vertebra can be removed *en bloc* (Fig. 85-1D). To maintain spinal stability after resection of the vertebral body for the next step, a temporary spine fixation is performed with a unilateral posterior instrument such as the pedicle screw system (Fig. 85-1E, F). Otherwise, the spine could be completely temporarily destabilized and at even greater risk of neurologic compromise.

The segmental arteries, which lie inferior-lateral to the pedicle, should be identified and tightly, bilaterally ligated. The pleura are pushed aside from the lateral aspect of the body. The segmental arteries and the aorta are carefully dissected from the vertebral body using the fingers. A curved spatula or malleable retractor is inserted to protect and displace the anterior structures. The discs above and below the pathology are carefully identified, and resected posterolaterally from both sides. Great effort should especially be paid to resecting the contralateral sides of the disc from which the anterior approach is performed. With the dura visible, the posterior longitudinal ligament can then be carefully cut with a knife. Following these procedures, the final posterior instrumentation is adjusted, and the spinal deformity or lesion should be corrected appropriately.

Step 2: Anterior Procedure

The involved spine can be approached from either the right or left side, depending upon the location of the pathology. If there is no special consideration regarding the pathology, then our preferred approach to the thoracolumbar and lumbar spine is from the left side. The aorta is located on the left and anterior to the spinal column at this level, and is much easier and safer to manipulate than

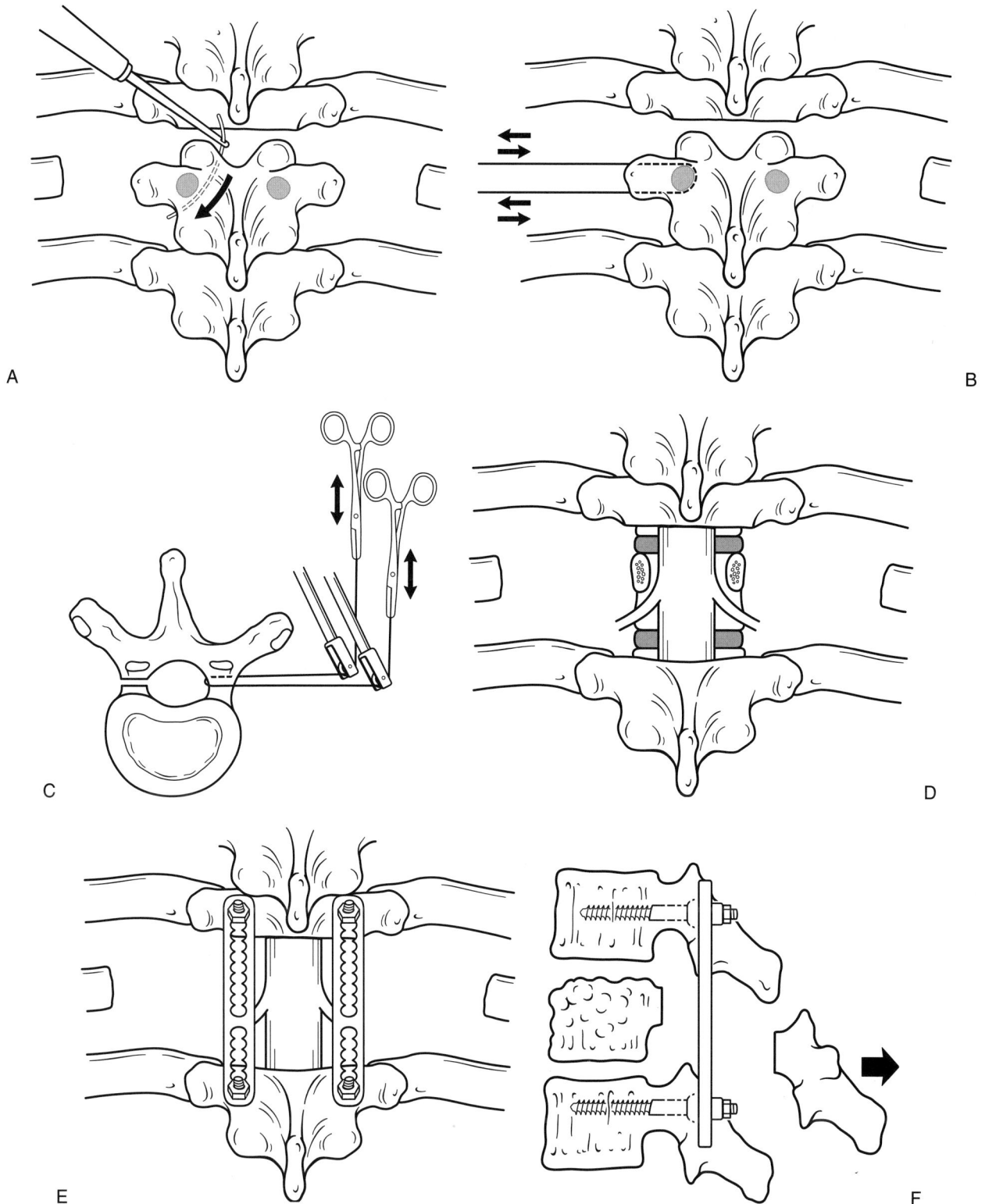

FIG. 85-1. A: After widely exposing the posterior element and resecting the proximal ribs of the involved vertebra, the threadwire saw (T-saw) is introduced into the epidural space under the lamina through a T-saw guide, and is pulled out of the neural foramen. **B,C:** Both ends of the T-saw are pulled around the pedicle of the involved vertebra in a sawing motion. This procedure is carried out in a lateral direction with the T-saw manipulator. **D:** After the resection of the whole posterior element of the involved verte-bra, the dural tube, costal nerve, and posterolateral aspect of the anterior element can be directly visu-alized. **E,F:** To preserve the stability after resection of the vertebral body, the spine is temporally fixed with posterior instrumentation.

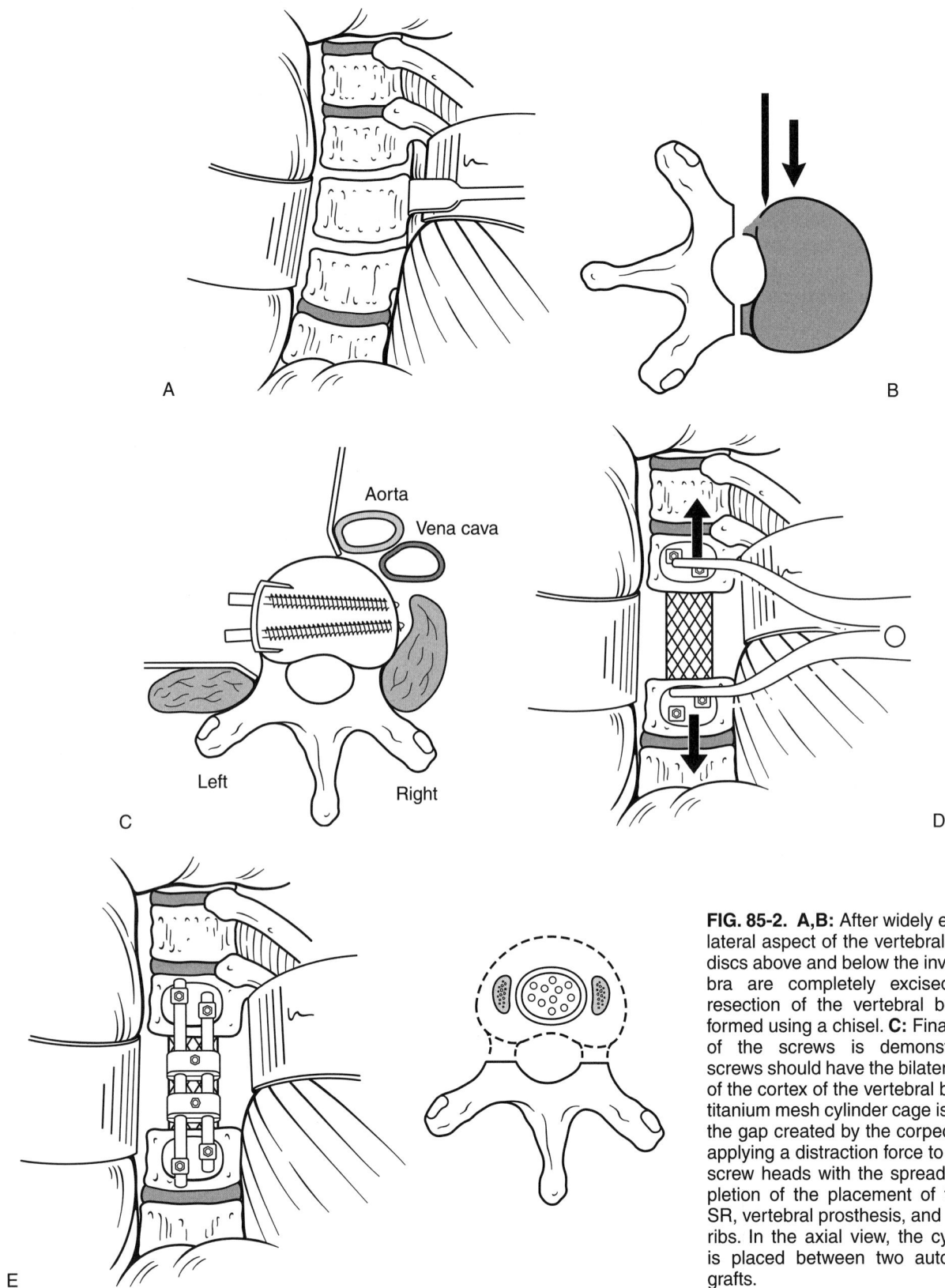

FIG. 85-2. A,B: After widely exposing the lateral aspect of the vertebral bodies, the discs above and below the involved vertebra are completely excised. *En bloc* resection of the vertebral body is performed using a chisel. C: Final placement of the screws is demonstrated. The screws should have the bilateral purchase of the cortex of the vertebral body. D: The titanium mesh cylinder cage is placed into the gap created by the corpectomy, while applying a distraction force to the anterior screw heads with the spreader. E: Completion of the placement of the Kaneda SR, vertebral prosthesis, and autogenous ribs. In the axial view, the cylinder cage is placed between two autogenous rib grafts.

the vena cava. The left-sided approach can usually be performed up to the level of T9 or T10. The thoracic vertebrae above T9 or T10 are approached from the right side, because the aorta at this level is located on the left side of the thoracic spines (6,7).

The thoracolumbar spines (T10-L2) are usually exposed using an extrapleural and retroperitoneal approach by the resection of the 10th or 11th rib. Even for the thoracic spines above the 10th vertebra, surgeons should make every effort to expose the spines extrapleurally. However, thoracotomy is usually needed for the exposure at this level. At the lumbar spine below L2, a retroperitoneal exposure is usually performed.

After exposure of the anterior spine, the involved vertebral body can be carefully dissected from the surrounding organs and soft tissues. The segmental vessels on the three vertebrae, including those above and below the involved vertebrae, are then tightly ligated and cut. The lateral aspect of the vertebral bodies must be adequately exposed for total or subtotal corpectomy, and appropriate application of the anterior spinal instrumentation, such as the Kaneda SR, should be performed. For lesions involving the lumbar spine, the psoas major muscle must be sufficiently retracted posteriorly. After exposing the lateral aspect of the vertebral bodies, the discs above and below the involved vertebra should be completely excised, including the anterior longitudinal ligament. *En bloc* resection of the vertebral body is then easily carried out because the pedicles, posterior longitudinal ligament, and contralateral side of the disc have already been resected in step 1 (Fig. 85-2A, B).

After the resection of the involved vertebra, the anterior spinal instrumentation was applied to secure the unstable vertebra created by the total spondylectomy. The Kaneda SR is our preferred anterior instrumentation, and has proved to be safe and biomechanically rigid enough to reconstruct unstable spines produced by a variety of pathologies such as tumor, trauma, spinal deformity, and degenerative spondylosis (19). First, the spinal plates marked with the letters A (anterior), P (posterior), and C/R (caudal and rostral) are placed on the lateral aspect of the vertebral body. Second, the appropriate screw size is measured with the specially designed vertebral-width gauge. Then, the spinal screws are inserted into the vertebral bodies through the plate holes. The screw tips must penetrate the opposite vertebral cortex by approximately 2 to 3 mm. Screws with blunt tips can alternatively be used if the risk to the major vessels is anticipated due to the presence of these sharp screw tips (Fig. 85-2C).

Third, kyphotic deformity can be corrected by applying a distraction force to the anterior screw heads with the distractive spreader. A vertebral prosthesis such as an allograft and titanium mesh cylinder cage can be tapped into the gap created by the corpectomy (Fig. 85-2D). The resected autogenous rib taken earlier may be added as a strut-graft material if a secure and rigid bony fusion is required. Fourth, the vertebral prosthesis is securely fixed by applying an appropriate compressive force using the compressor or other compressing device. Then, two rods may be inserted into the screw head holes, and the vertebral prosthesis firmly kept in place by applying the compressive force. Finally, the set screws can be used to fix the rods into the screw head holes that are then firmly tightened, and two rod couplers can then be added between the rods (Fig. 85-2E) (6,7).

POSTOPERATIVE MANAGEMENT

If the patient is in a stable medical condition after the surgery, he or she can be ambulatory with the TLSO within a week after the operation. The TLSO is usually worn for 12 to 16 weeks. However, it depends upon several factors such as life expectancy, spinal stability, and QOL. Postoperative adjuvant radiotherapy can be attempted when a subtotal spondylectomy instead of a total spondylectomy is performed.

CONCLUSIONS

As patients with a primary malignant or metastatic tumor may now be expected to live longer, the chance of local recurrence increases. Thus, the life span of cancer patients depends upon how the local recurrence can be controlled. Missenard et al. (5) investigated local tumor recurrence in 58 patients who survived 1 year or more. They highlighted the following results. First, the sensitivity of the primary cancer to adjuvant treatment and correct timing of the critical postoperative radiation therapy seemed to significantly reduce local tumor recurrence. Second, complete excision of the tumor should be indicated when the patient has a tumor that is insensitive to the adjuvant treatment (either radiotherapy or chemotherapy), and when the patient's life expectancy reaches 1 year or more.

Investigators pointed out that the local recurrence rate after corpectomy or total vertebrectomy was 22% (6) and 32% (20), respectively. This rate seems to diminish if *en bloc* total vertebrectomy is performed. As a result, *en bloc* total vertebrectomy should be recommended if the patient has a solitary spinal metastasis from a radioresistant tumor such as that from a renal, thyroid, or breast cancer (Figs. 85-3, 85-4). Combined anterior and posterior procedures described in this chapter are a powerful tool for surgeons who are willing to manage patients in need of a total spondylectomy.

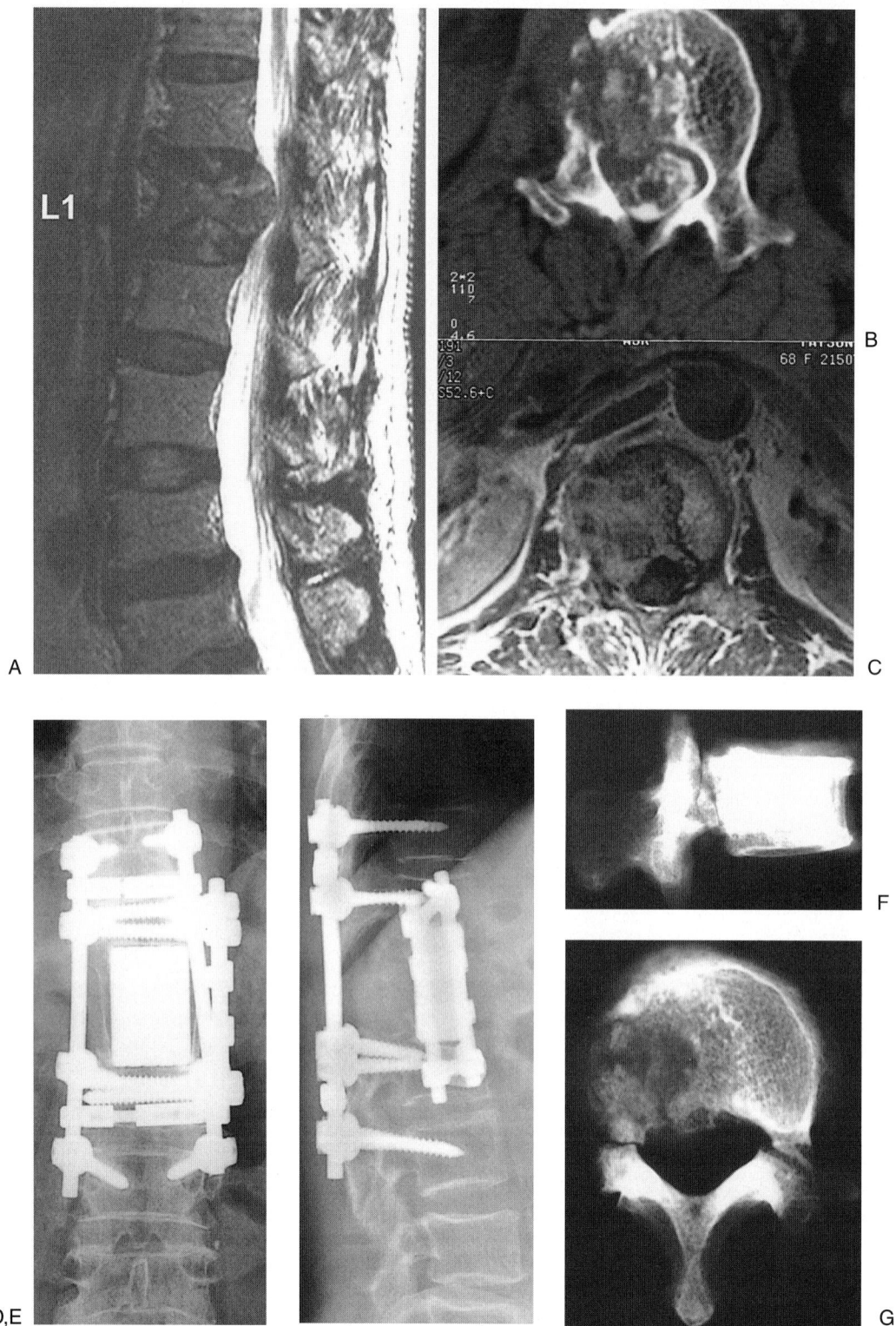

FIG. 85-3. Case 1: Metastatic thyroid carcinoma at L1 with intractable low back pain and paraparesis in a 68-year-old woman. After tumor embolization, total en bloc vertebrectomy was performed with the anterior and posterior combined procedure. **A:** A T2-weighted sagittal magnetic resonance (MR) image demonstrated marked collapse of L1 vertebral body and spinal cord compression at L1. **B,C:** A computed tomography-myelograph and a gadolinium-enhanced axial MR image showed the tumor involving the vertebral body and the right pedicle. **D,E:** Plain X-rays 4 years after the operation. En bloc total spondylectomy of L1 was performed through the combined approach. First, the posterior element of L1 was resected, followed by reconstruction with a pedicle screw system from T11 to L3. Second, the vertebral body was resected en bloc, followed by reconstruction with an A-W glass ceramic vertebral prosthesis and the Kaneda SR system. The patient is still ambulatory with no evidence of disease, and solid biologic bony fusion has been obtained. The A-W glass ceramic spacer has now been taken off the market due to the manufacturer's circumstances. **F,G:** Plain radiographs demonstrated the L1 vertebra resected in the en bloc fashion. The vertebra was dissected only at the pedicles with no destruction of the other part.

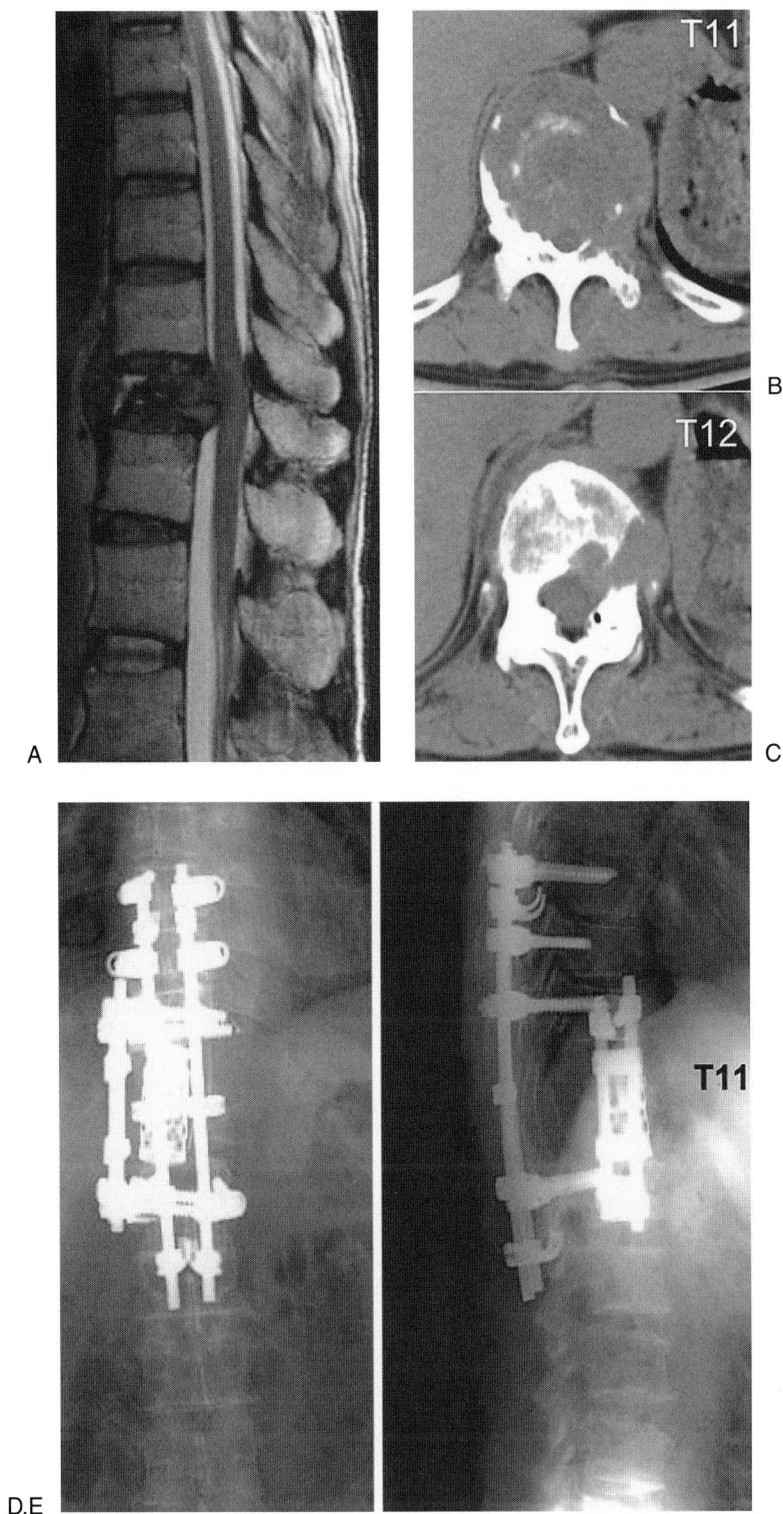

A

B

C

D,E

FIG. 85-4. Case 2: Metastatic renal cell carcinoma at T11 and T12 with severe back pain and paraparesis in a 52-year-old man. After tumor embolization, total vertebrectomy was performed with the combined procedure. **A–C:** A sagittal T1- and T2-weighted magnetic resonance (MR) image **(A)** demonstrated collapse of T11 vertebral body and spinal cord compression at T11. The tumor extended into the spinal canal as well as into the paravertebral area. The MRI and computed tomography films also showed that the tumor invaded to the superoposterior portion of T12 vertebral body. **D,E:** The plain X-P films after the surgery. The spine was firmly stabilized, both anteriorly and posteriorly, and the neurologic deficits completely recovered.

REFERENCES

1. Gilbert RW, Kim JH, Posner JB. Epidural spinal cord compression from metastatic tumor: diagnosis and treatment. Ann Neurol 1978;3: 40–51.
2. Sherman RMP, Waddell JP. Laminectomy for metastatic epidural spinal cord tumors. Clin Orthop 1986;207:55–63.
3. Cybulski GR, Stone JL, Opesanmi O. Spinal cord decompression via a modified costotransversectomy approach combined with posterior instrumentation for management of metastatic neoplasms of the thoracic spine. Surg Neurol 1991;35:280–285.
4. Bridwell KH, Jenny AB, Saul T, et al. Posterior segmental spinal instrumentation (PSSI) with posterolateral decompression and debulking for metastatic thoracic and lumbar spine disease. Spine 1988;13: 1383–1394.
5. Missenard G, Lapresle P, Cote D. Local control after surgical treatment of spinal metastatic disease. Eur Spine J 1996;5:45–50.
6. Kaneda K, Takeda N. Reconstruction with a ceramic vertebral prosthe-

sis and Kaneda device following subtotal or total vertebrectomy in metastatic thoracic and lumbar spine. In: Bridwell KH, DeWald RL, eds. The textbook of spinal surgery. Philadelphia: Lippincott-Raven, 1996:2071–2087.

7. Kaneda K. Anterior fixation. In: Bradford DS, ed. Master technique in orthopaedic surgery. The spine. Philadelphia: Lippincott-Raven, 1997: 471–486.

8. Tomita K, Kawahara N, Baba H, et al. Total en bloc spondylectomy. Spine 1997;22:324–333.

9. Tomita, K, Kawahara, N, Kobayahi, T, et al. Surgical strategy for spinal metastases. Spine 2001;26(3):298–306.

10. Sundaresan N, Steinberger AA, Moore F, et al. Indications and results of combined anterior-posterior approaches for spine tumor surgery. J Neurosurg 1996;85:438–446.

11. Roy-Camille R, Mazel C, Saillant G, et al. Treatment of malignant tumors of the spine with posterior instrumentation. In: Sundaresan N, Schmidek HH, Schiller AL, eds. Tumors of the spine. Philadelphia: WB Saunders, 1990:473–487.

12. Asdourian PL. Metastatic disease of the spine. In: Bridwell KH, DeWald RL, eds. The textbook of spinal surgery, 2nd edition. Philadelphia: Lippincott-Raven, 1996:2007–2050.

13. Tokuhashi, Y, Matsuzaki, H, Toriyama, S, et al. Scoring system for the preoperative evaluation of metastatic spine tumor prognosis. Spine 1990;15(11):1110–1113.

14. Stener B. Technique of complete spondylectomy in the thoracic and lumbar spine. In: Sundaresan N, Schmidek HH, Schiller AL, et al., eds. Tumors of the spine. Philadelphia: WB Saunders, 1990:432–437.

15. Stener B. Technique of complete spondylectomy in the thoracic and lumbar spine. In: Sundaresan N, Schmidek HH, Schiller AL, et al., eds. Tumors of the spine. Philadelphia: WB Saunders, 1990:432–437.

16. Magerl F, Coscia M. Total posterior vertebrectomy of the thoracic or lumbar spine. Clin Orthop 1988;232:62–69.

17. Sundaresan N, DiGiacinto GV, Krol G, et al. Complete spondylectomy for malignant tumors. In Sundaresan N, Schmidek HH, Schiller AL, et al., eds. Tumors of the spine. Philadelphia: WB Saunders, 1990:438–445.

18. Fidler MW. Radical resection of vertebral body tumours. J Bone Joint Surg [Br] 1994;76-B(5):765–772.

19. Zdeblick TA, Shirado O, McAfee PC, et al. Anterior spinal fixation after lumbar corpectomy. A study in dogs. J Bone Joint Surg 1991;73-A:527–534.

20. Sundaresan N, Rothman A, Manhart K, et al. Surgery for solitary metastases of the spine. Spine 2002;27(16):1802–1806.

CHAPTER 86

Prognosis and Results of Surgery for Primary and Metastatic Tumors

Jonathan N. Grauer and Alan S. Hilibrand

Previous chapters have described the incidence and work-up of primary and metastatic tumors of the spine. Surgical indications and techniques also have been presented. This chapter reviews the prognosis and results of operative treatment for spinal tumors. In general, surgical intervention has been shown to improve outcomes with regard to longevity and quality of life for most benign (1–3) and all malignant (4–8) primary spinal tumors. On the other hand, the role of surgery for metastatic spinal disease is more controversial (9–11).

For most spinal tumors, the extent of resection has been correlated with lower rates of recurrence and improved survivorship (7,8,12). However, the unique anatomy and function of the spine often limit the ability to perform even a wide excision of some tumors. The surgeon must find a balance between attaining adequate surgical margins and preserving vital neurovascular structures.

The potential for postsurgical instability is also an important issue. For example, decompressive laminectomy can be complicated by progressive kyphosis (13). Although the most rigid stabilization can be achieved through a posterior approach, posterior instrumentation can only stabilize the posterior column. Because many surgeons now approach lesions from the column of primary involvement, which is often anterior (9,14,15), there has been a greater emphasis on anterior resections and anterior or circumferential reconstructions. This is discussed in later sections.

Adjuvant therapies have been evolving in parallel with surgical techniques for the treatment of spinal tumors. Radiation can provide local cytotoxicity and reduce neural compression by shrinking tumor mass. However, this effect is limited in field, raises concern for inducing sarcomatous changes, and can compromise future surgical approaches within the radiation field. Chemotherapy affords more systemic cytotoxicity, which can be both beneficial and limiting. Finally, as reviewed in this chapter, evolution in surgical techniques has led to improvements in prognosis and results of surgery for tumors of the spine. Because it is difficult to generalize about prognosis of spinal tumor surgery, primary benign, primary malignant, and metastatic tumors are discussed separately, and the results of surgery for individual tumor types are reviewed.

PRIMARY TUMORS

Primary tumors of the spine are relatively uncommon, especially in comparison with metastatic disease. As such, most studies are small and retrospective, with larger series including patients from multiple medical centers or over prolonged periods of time. As a result, there is great variability in surgical techniques and adjuvant therapies within and between study populations. Furthermore, published studies often report outcomes in different forms and with varying lengths of follow up. In this chapter, an emphasis is placed on larger series. Comparable data and outcome measures are presented where available.

Benign

The six most common benign tumors of the spine that present for treatment are: osteoblastomas, osteoid osteomas, osteochondromas, giant cell tumors, aneurysmal bone cysts, and hemangiomas in order of decreasing frequency. This is as noted in a retrospective review of 31 such tumors by Weinstein and McLain (7). Outcomes were usually good with relatively low long-term morbidity and mortality. The overall recurrence rate was 21%, and the overall 5-year survival rate was 86%.

Osteoblastomas and osteoid osteomas are both benign osteoblastic lesions, of which 36% and 10% occur in the

Spine respectively (16). Surgical excision can afford immediate pain relief and facilitate early patient mobilization (3). Recurrence rates for osteoblastomas and osteoid osteomas have been found to be 0% to 10% and 9%, respectively (17,18). Such recurrences have been related to incomplete excisions. In cases of osteoblastoma with poorly defined margins, adjuvant radiation can improve results (17). Alternative treatments, such as high-frequency radiowave ablation, have been tried recently for osteoid osteomas with minimal morbidity and good initial success (19).

Osteochondromas are osteocartilaginous exostoses, of which 1% to 4% occur in the spine as solitary lesions or as manifestations of familial osteochondromatosis (1). In most cases, surgery is indicated only if there is neurologic compromise or secondary scoliosis (2,20). Approximately 90% of patients have been reported to have relief of symptoms (1,2). Recurrences are rare but have been reported (21,22).

Giant cell tumors are locally aggressive lesions of large multinucleated cells, of which 1.8% to 9.3% occur in the spine (23). Because of the locally aggressive nature of giant cell tumors, they do not share the same favorable prognosis as other benign lesions (7). For this reason, radical resection is recommended, if possible (24). Radiation has been found to improve results for patients with incomplete excisions or local recurrences (23). Nevertheless, recurrence rates of 22% to 42% have been reported (23,25), and half of the recurrences reported in the series by Weinstein and McLain were giant cell tumors (7).

Aneurysmal bone cysts are highly vascular lesions of unknown origin, of which 10% to 30% occur in the spine (26,27). With early excision with or without bone grafting or embolization, recurrences have been reported in the 2% to 19% range (12,26,27). Selective arterial embolization has been associated with superior clinical results because of decreased operative bleeding. In fact, some studies have suggested that embolization alone may be sufficient treatment (26); however, others additionally recommend routine curettage and bone grafting (12,27). Radiation has not been found to decrease the rate of recurrence (28).

Hemangiomas often are noted incidentally or never detected. Surgical decompression or excision is considered for those with neurologic symptoms, or when the structural integrity of a vertebra is compromised. Similar to aneurysmal bone cysts, embolization offers a means to minimize surgical bleeding (29,30). Recurrence was noted in 27% of patients in one surgical series (29). Postoperative radiation thus was recommended to minimize recurrence if subtotal tumor resection is performed. Vertebroplasty (31) or ethanol injections (32) may provide an alternative means of treatment for these tumors, although long-term results of these treatments have not yet been reported.

Malignant

The six most common primary malignant tumors of the spine are: solitary plasmacytomas, chordomas, chondrosarcomas, lymphomas, Ewing sarcomas, and osteosarcomas, in order of decreasing frequency. This is as noted in a retrospective review of 51 such tumors by Weinstein and McLain (7). Overall 5-year survival rates correlated with tumor type and extent of initial surgical excision (Table 86-1). Survival was greatest for patients with chondrosarcomas and solitary plasmacytomas and was shortest for those with osteosarcomas and primary lymphomas. The overall local recurrence rate was 21%, and metastatic disease developed in 27% of these patients.

Solitary plasmacytomas are treated to prevent local progression and dissemination to multiple myeloma. Although initial treatment often consists of radiation, partial resection or curettage is recommended for progressive neurologic symptoms or cord compression. The role of chemotherapy is controversial (33). The prognosis for plasmacytoma is much better than of multiple myeloma. Five- and 10-year survival rates have been found to be 86% to 100% and 85%, respectively (34,35). Disease-free survival at 5 and 10 years has been found to be 40-% to 60% and 0%, respectively (33,35). Recurrence is correlated with the appearance or increase of the M light-chain component (35).

Chordomas are low-grade, locally invasive tumors that are slow to metastasize. The 5-year survival rate for these tumors has been reported to be 58% to 86% (5,36). Achieving tumor-free margins has been shown to be important for preventing local recurrence and improving survival (5,36). Additionally, more proximal lumbosacral

TABLE 86.1. *5-Year survival rates for primary malignant tumors of the spine*

Primary bone malignancy	5-Year survival rate	References
Solitary plasmacytoma	86%–100%	Meis et al. (34), Delauche-Cavallier et al. (35)
Chordoma	58%–86%	Cheng et al. (36), Ozaki et al. (5)
Chondrosarcoma	55%–72%	Bergh et al. (4), Shives et al. (38), York et al. (8)
Ewing sarcoma	33%	Grubb et al. (13)
Lymphoma	22%–24%	DiMarco et al. (41), Salvati et al. (40)
Osteosarcoma	4%–10%	Barwick et al. (48), Shives et al. (6)

location and initial radiation have been correlated with longer survival (36). Metastases develop in 5% to 40% of patients studied (5), and preservation of the mid-sacral roots has been found to be important for maintaining bowel and bladder function.

Chondrosarcomas are malignant cartilage producing tumors. Approximately 9% of these lesions are in the axial skeleton (Fig. 86-1) (37). Five- and 10-year surgical survival rates have ranged from 40% to 72% (4,8,38). Lower histologic grade (4), wider tumor resection (4,8,37), and younger age (4) have been associated with improved survival. Neither radiation nor chemotherapy has been found to be beneficial (8).

Although some consider an epidural lymphoma primary to the spine only if the original foci are in the spine (38,40), others report all lymphomas presenting with spinal cord compression within this group, irrespective of the presence of other previously undetected neoplastic foci (41,42). Traditionally, these tumors have been treated with decompressive laminectomy and radiation with poor clinical outcomes; one such study reported six of 12 dead within 6 months and the remaining six dead within 4 years (39). With adjuvant chemotherapy and improved surgical techniques, outcomes have improved; 5-year survivals of 22% to 40% are now reported (40–42). Neurologic status was found to be an independent prognostic

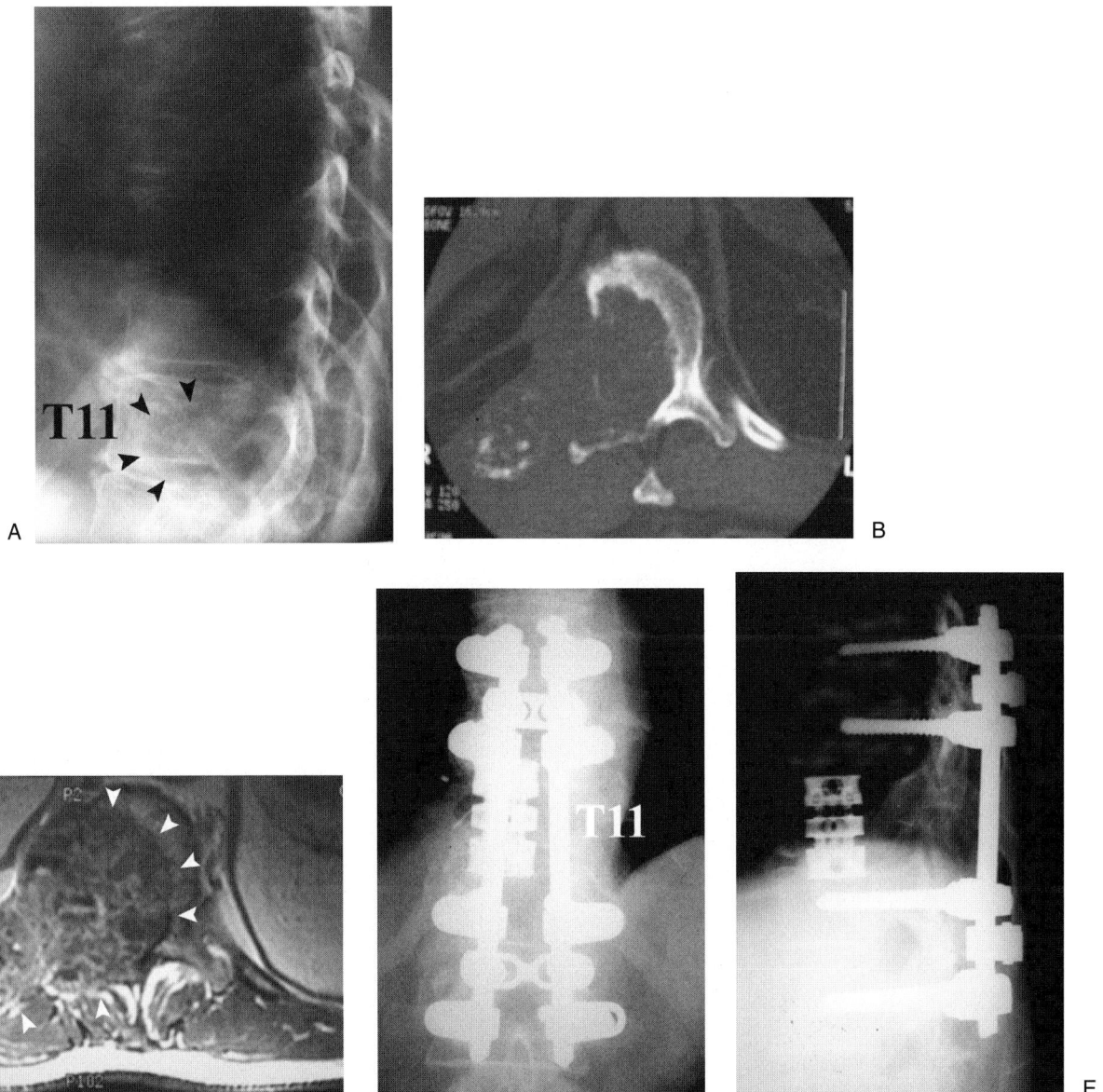

FIG. 86-1. Case example of a 54-year-old man with a chondrosarcoma arising from the right T11 costovertebral junction. Preoperative plain film **(A)**, computed tomography **(B)**, and magnetic resonance imaging **(C)** demonstrate the lesion. Postoperative plain films **(D,E)** show the anterior and posterior reconstruction after resection was performed.

factor for this group of patients (40,42), but tumor histology was not (42).

Ewing sarcomas are malignant tumors of unknown cell origin, of which only 4% to 7% are found in the spinal column (43,44). Early work suggested that spinal involvement was a poor prognostic feature, with 6% survival compared with overall 16% survival (43). With newer regimens of chemotherapy and radiation tailored to this disease process, survival rates of primary spinal Ewing have improved (45). A recent review of 36 cases found the 5-year survival rate to be 33% (13). It has been suggested that sacrococcygeal tumors may have a worse prognosis that those elsewhere in the axial skeleton (46).

Osteosarcomas are malignant osteoid producing tumors, of which 1.5% to 3% occur in the spine (6,47). Reported outcomes have been poor. With or without decompressive laminectomy, attempted excision, radiation, or chemotherapy, all but one patient died of the disease in two series (5-year survival rates of 4% to 10%) (6,48). Furthermore, the mean length of survival was only 6 to 10 months for those who did not survive 5 years.

In summary, primary malignant tumors of the spine pose a significant surgical challenge. Aggressive surgical excision with appropriate adjuvant therapy provides the best chance of preventing local recurrences and distant metastases. However, regardless of the treatment regimen, long-term outcomes are not good for most subtypes.

METASTATIC TUMORS

The surgical indications for metastatic disease of the spine are less well defined than those for primary tumors.

The risks of significant morbidity in chronically ill patients with limited life spans must be weighed against the potential for pain relief, restoration of quality of life, and prolongation of survival. A clear understanding between surgeons and patients of the variables affecting prognosis and results of surgery aids in the decision-making process.

General indications for surgical management include progressive neurologic deficit, intractable pain, spinal instability, radio-resistant tumors, and the need for histologic diagnosis (Fig. 86-2) (11,49). Radiation with or without chemotherapy is the mainstay of treatment for metastatic disease. Surgery is an adjunct to these primary modalities. Goals of surgery include decompression of neural structures, with debulking the tumor mass, correction of deformity, and stabilization for the relief of pain.

Historically, most resections were done from posterior approaches, despite the fact that the majority of metastatic lesions occur anteriorly, in the vertebral body. Consequently, the results of such procedures were disappointing (50,51), and some authors found no significant difference in outcome between those undergoing decompressive laminectomy and radiation and those receiving radiation alone (52). However, adjuvant stabilization did improve results (53).

Anterior decompression and stabilization has been found to provide significantly better results for patients with anterior disease isolated to one or two continuous segments (Fig. 86-1) (9,14,15,49). In a review of the literature, Weinstein found the average percentage of patients with satisfactory outcome to be 37% after posterior decompression and 80% after anterior decompres-

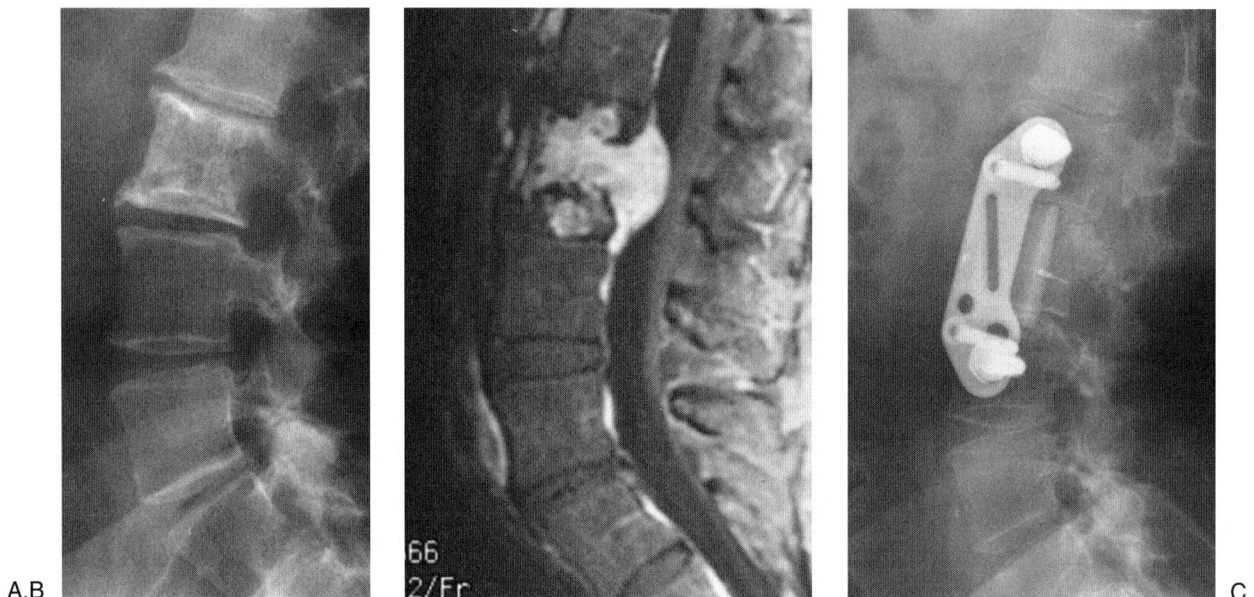

FIG. 86-2. Case example of a 61-year-old woman with metastatic disease of L3. Preoperative plain film **(A)**, preoperative magnetic resonance imaging **(B)**, and postoperative laterals **(C)** show anterior column reconstruction with femoral allograft and an anterior plate.

sion (15). Patients with more than two segments of continuous disease pose a much greater challenge. If anterior collapse or neural element compression exists, an anterior decompression and posterior stabilization is indicated. A posterior approach may be considered if there is extensive disease over many levels (54), although such extensive disease suggests a poor prognosis and may militate against any significant benefit from operative treatment.

Pretreatment neurologic status, duration of neurologic compromise, and rate of neurologic decline have been identified as prognostic factors in treatment (55,56). For this reason, some have recommended early surgical intervention for spinal metastases once neurologic manifestations are recognized. Significant neurologic improvements have been described after anterior decompression and reconstruction of metastatic tumors. Among patients with neurologic deficits undergoing operative treatment, Harrington described complete recovery in 42% and significant improvement in an additional 26% (9). Kostuik et al. found a significant neurologic return in 40% of posterior decompressions and 71% in anterior decompressions (14). Siegal and Siegal found a 31% increase in patients' ability to walk from pre-decompressive to postdecompressive laminectomy and a 52% increase with anterior decompression (49).

Tumor type also has been found to affect outcome (11,55,56). The most common primary tumors metastatic to bone are tumors of breast and prostate (84%), thyroid (50%), lung (44%), and kidney (37%) (15). As expected, the more aggressive the primary tumor, the worse the long-term prognosis. Wise et al. found postoperative survival rates were the longest for myeloma and soft-tissue sarcomas and the shortest for adenocarcinoma of unknown primary origin and prostate cancer (11).

The decompression site can be reconstructed with autograft, allograft, or methyl methacrylate. The advantage of autograft or allograft is the potential for incorporation and biologic fusion, which can provide long-term stability. However, fusion is often compromised in the tumor patient by local factors such as abnormal tumor biology, local radiation effects, and chemotherapeutics. Some authors have recommended the use of methylmethacrylate if expected survival is limited (generally less than 1 year) (9,14). However, care must be exercised in placing methyl methacrylate in proximity to the neural elements to avoid injury from the exothermic curing process.

Perioperative complications can significantly limit the potential benefits of surgical treatment in this patient population and dramatically alter the postoperative course. The most common complication is postoperative wound infection (11). This can result from impaired wound healing, which is seen in the setting of prior radiation treatment (11), and chronic malnutrition (57,58), both of which are common in this population. These variables also lead to relative states of immunosuppression by limiting vascular ingrowth and thus further predisposing to local infections.

In summary, surgery for metastatic disease of the spine is indicated for correction of deformity, preservation of neurologic function, and control of intractable pain. Mean survival time after surgery for metastatic disease is only about 11 to 16 months (10,11,14), although this is primarily related to the natural history of the underlying primary tumor. Nevertheless, as surgical techniques and adjuvant therapy regimens are refined, surgical goals are becoming more attainable and outcomes are improving.

CONCLUSIONS

Neoplastic lesions of the spine pose a significant clinical problem. Most are found in older patients and are the result of metastatic disease. Although the follow-up of such patients treated surgically is limited, the results reviewed in this chapter provide some indication of the relative benefits of surgery for the different tumor subtypes. Adequate tumor resection, appropriate stabilization, and targeted adjuvant therapy are important considerations in all such patients. The past 20 years have seen tremendous strides in the surgical management of all types of spinal tumors—primary and metastatic. In particular, an increased appreciation of the need for direct decompression of the tumor via an anterior approach, followed by anterior column reconstruction and (often) posterior stabilization has extended the benefits of surgery to many more cancer patients. However, more large multicenter studies are needed to prove the efficacy of these more extensive surgical procedures in improving patient quality of the life and survivorship.

REFERENCES

1. Albrecht S, Crutchfield S, SeGall GK. On spinal osteochondromas. J Neurosurg 1992;77:247–252.
2. Fiumara E, Scarabino T, Guglielmi G, et al. Osteochondroma of the L-5 vertebra: a rare case of sciatic pain. J Neurosurg 1999;91(Suppl 2):219–222.
3. Kirwan EO, Hutton PAN, Pozo JL, et al. Osteoid osteoma and benign osteoblastoma of the spine: clinical presentation and treatment. J Bone Joint Surg 1984;66B:21-26.
4. Bergh P, Gunterberg B, Meis-Kindblom JM, et al. Prognostic factors and outcome of pelvic, sacral, and spinal chondrosarcomas: a center-based study of 69 cases. Cancer 2001;91:1201–1212.
5. Ozaki T, Hillmann A, Winkelmann W. Surgical treatment of sacrococcygeal chordoma. J Surg Oncol 1997;64:274–279.
6. Shives TC, Dahlin DC, Sim FH, et al. Osteosarcoma of the spine. J Bone Joint Surg 1986;68A:660–668.
7. Weinstein JN, McLain RF. Primary tumors of the spine. Spine 1987;12:843–851.
8. York JE, Berk RH, Fuller GN, et al. Chondrosarcoma of the spine: 1954–1997. J Neurosurg 1999;90:73–78.
9. Harrington KD. Anterior decompression and stabilization of the spine as a treatment for vertebral collapse and spinal cord compression from metastatic malignancy. Clin Orthop 1988;233:177–197.
10. O'Neil J, Gardner V, Armstrong G. Treatment of tumors of the thoracic and lumbar spinal column. Clin Orthop 1988;227:103–112.
11. Wise JJ, Fishgrund JS, Herkowitz HN, et al. Complication, survival

rates, and risk factors of surgery for metastatic disease of the spine. Spine 1999;24:1943–1951.

12. deKleuver M, vanderHeul RO, Veraart BE. Aneurysmal bone cyst of the spine: 31 cases and the importance of the surgical approach. J Pediatr Orthop 1998;B7:286–292.

13. Grubb MR, Currier BL, Prichard DJ, et al. Primary Ewing's sarcoma of the spine. Spine 1994;19:309–313.

14. Kostuik JP, Errico TJ, Gleason TF, et al. Spinal stabilization of vertebral column tumors. Spine 1988;13:250–256.

15. Weinstein JN. Spinal tumors. In: Weisel SW, Weinstein JD, Herkowitz H, et al, eds. The lumbar spine, 2nd ed. Philadelphia: WB Saunders, 1990:917–944.

16. Jackson RP, Reckling FW, Mantz FA. Osteoid osteoma and osteoblastoma: similar histologic lesions with different natural histories. Clin Orthop 1977;128:303–313.

17. Boriani S, Capanna R, Donati D, et al. Osteoblastoma of the spine. Clin Orthop 1992;278:37–45.

18. Raskas DS, Graziano GP, Herzenberg JE, et al. Osteoid osteoma and osteoblastoma of the spine. J Spinal Disord 1992;5:204–211.

19. Osti OL, Sebben R. High-frequency radio-wave ablation of osteoid osteoma in the lumbar spine. Eur Spine J 1998;7:422–425.

20. Mexia MJ, Nunez EI, Garriga CS, et al. Osteochondroma of the thoracic spine and scoliosis. Spine 2001;26:1082–1085.

21. Bell MS. Benign cartilaginous tumours of the spine: a report of one case together with a review of the literature. Brt J Surg 1971;58:707–711.

22. Yablon JS. Osteochondroma of the vertebral column (Letter). Neurosurgery 1990;27:659–660.

23. Sanjay BKS, Sim FH, Unni KK, et al. Giant-cell tumors of the spine. J Bone Joint Surg 1993;75B:148–154.

24. Shikata J, Yamamuro T, Shimizu K, et al. Surgical treatment of giant-cell tumors of the spine. Clin Orthop 1992;278:29–36.

25. Savini R, Gherlinzoni F, Morandi M, et al. Surgical treatment of giant-cell tumor of the spine:the experience at the Istituto Orthopedico Rizzoli. J Bone Joint Surg 1983;65A:1283–1289.

26. Boriani S, DeLure F, Campanacci L, et al. Aneurysmal bone cyst of the mobile spine: report on 41 cases. Spine 2001;26:27–35.

27. Papagelopoulos PJ, Currier BL, Shaughnessy WJ, et al. Aneurysmal bone cyst of the spine: management and outcome. Spine 1998;23:621–628.

28. Capanna R, Albisinni U, Picci P, et al. Aneurysmal bone cyst of the spine. J Bone Joint Surg 1985;67A:527–531.

29. Fox MW, Onofrio BM. The natural history and management of symptomatic and asymptomatic hemangiomas. J Neurosurg 1993;78:36–45.

30. Nguyen JP, Djindjian M, Gaston A, et al. Vertebral hemangiomas presenting with neurologic symptoms. Surg Neurol, 1987;27:391–397.

31. Cotton A, Boutry N, Cortet B, et al. Percutaneous vertebroplasty: state of the art. Radiographics 1998;18:311–320.

32. Doppman JL, Oldfield EH, Heiss JD. Symptomatic vertebral hemangiomas: treatment by means of direct intralesional injection of ethanol. Radiology 2000;214:341–348.

33. McLain RF, Weinstein JN. Solitary plasmacytomas of the spine: a review of 84 cases. J Spinal Disord 1989;2:69–74.

34. Meis JM, Butler JJ, Osborne BM, et al. Solitary plasmacytoma of the bone and extramedullary plasmacytoma. A clinicopathologic and immunohistological study. Cancer 1987;59:1475–1485.

35. Delauche-Cavallier MC, Laredo JD, Wybier M, et al. Solitary plasmacytoma of the spine: long-term clinical course. Cancer 1988;61:1707–1714.

36. Cheng EY, Ozerdemoglu RA, Transfeldt EE, et al. Lumbosacral chordoma: prognostic factors and treatment. Spine 1999;24:1639–1645.

37. Prichard DJ, Lunke RJ, Taylor WF, et al. Chondrosarcoma: a clinicopathologic and statistical analysis. Cancer 1980;45:149–157.

38. Shives TC, McLeod RA, Unni KK, et al. Chondrosarcoma of the spine. J Bone Joint Surg 1989;71A:1158–1165.

39. Rao TV, Narayanaswamy KS, Shankar SK, et al. "Primary" spinal epidural lymphomas: a clinico-pathological study. Acta Neurochirurgica 1982;62:307–317.

40. Salvati M, Cervoni L, Artico M, et al. Primary spinal epidural non-Hodgkin's lymphomas: a clinical study. Surg Neurol 1996;46:339–344.

41. DiMarco A, Campostrini F, Garusi GF. Non-Hodgkin lymphomas presenting with spinal epidural involvement. Acta Oncol 1989;28:485–488.

42. Eeles RA, O'Brien P, Horowich A, et al. Non-Hodgkin's lymphoma presenting with extradural spinal cord compression: functional outcome and survival. Br J Cancer 1991;63:126–129.

43. Prichard DJ, Dahlin DC, Dauphine RT, et al. Ewing's sarcoma: a clinicopathological and statistical analysis of patients surviving five years of longer. J Bone Joint Surg 1975;57A:10–16.

44. Whitehouse GH, Griffiths GJ. Roentgenologic aspects of spinal involvement by primary and metastatic Ewing's tumor. J Can Assoc Radiol 1976;27:290–297.

45. Sharafuddin MJA, Haddad FS, Hitchon PW, et al. Treatment options in primary Ewing's sarcoma of the spine: report of seven cases and review of the literature. Neurosurgery 1992;30:610–619.

46. Pilepich MV, Vietti TJ, Nesbit TJ, et al. Ewing's sarcoma of the vertebral column. Int J Radiat Oncol Biol Phys 1981;7:27–31.

47. Dahlin DC, Coventry MB. Osteogenic sarcoma. A study of six hundred cases. J Bone Joint Surg 1967;49A:101–110.

48. Barwick KW, Huvos AG, Smith J. Primary osteogenic sarcoma of the vertebral column: a clinicopathologic correlation of ten patients. Cancer 1980;46:595–604.

49. Siegal T, Siegal T. Surgical decompression of anterior and posterior malignant epidural tumors compressing the spinal cord: a prospective study. Neurosurgery 1985;17:424–431.

50. Hall AJ, MacKay NNS. The results of laminectomy for compression of the cord or cauda equina by extradural malignant tumour. J Bone Joint Surg 1973;55B:497–505.

51. Nicholls PJ, Jarecky TW. The value of posterior decompression by laminectomy for malignant tumors of the spine. Clin Orthop 1985;201:210–213.

52. Gilbert RW, Kim JH, Posner JB. Epidural spinal cord compression from metastatic tumor: diagnosis and treatment. Ann Neurol 1978;3:40–51.

53. Sherman RM, Waddell JP. Laminectomy for metastatic epidural spinal cord tumors. Clin Orthop 1986;207:55–63.

54. Riley LH, Frassica DA, Kostuik JP, Frassica FJ. Metastatic disease to the spine: diagnosis and treatment. Instructional Course Lectures 2000;49:471–477.

55. Constans JP, DeDivitiis E, Donzelli R, et al. Spinal metastases with neurologic manifestations. Review of 600 cases. J Neurosurg 1983;59:111–118.

56. Nather A, Bose K. The results of decompression of cord or cauda equina compression from metastatic extradural tumors. Clin Orthop 1982;169:103–108.

57. Dick J, Boachie-Adjei O, Wilson M. One stage versus two stage anterior and posterior spinal reconstruction in adults: comparison of outcomes including nutritional status, complication rates, hospital cost and other factors. Spine 1992;17(Suppl):S310–S316.

58. Klein JD, Hey LA, Yu CS, et al. Perioperative nutrition and postoperative complications in patients undergoing spinal surgery. Spine 1996;21:2676–2682.

CHAPTER 87

Determining Reasons for Failed Surgery

Christopher S. Raffo and Sam W. Wiesel

Surgery on the lumbar spine is not always successful. An estimated 300,000 new laminectomies are performed yearly in the United States and 45,000 of these patients will continue to be disabled (1). The patient who has undergone multiple surgeries with continued or worsening pain and disability is of increasing concern. As lumbar surgeries continue to grow, the problem will continue to expand. With this expansion comes an ever-growing cost of treating these patients, an obvious concern in the era of rigid cost containment. The complexity of a multiply operated patient necessitates a methodical, precise, and cost-efficient evaluation.

It seems obvious, but is worth restating, that the best chance for an excellent outcome from spine surgery is appropriate indications for that surgery. Conversely, surgery with inaccurate or inappropriate indications must be avoided due to its dismal chance for good outcome (2,3). Precise correlation of physical symptoms and findings with the diagnostic imaging studies is essential, owing to the high incidence of clinically false-positive myelograms, discograms, computed tomograms (CT), and magnetic resonance imaging (MRI) (4–6). Exploration of the spine is unacceptable, without well-defined and correctable pathology that matches the data gathered from advanced imaging. Also, due to increasing complexity with each revision operation, the first surgical procedure has the greatest chance for success.

The first decision point in the evaluation of *failed back surgery syndrome (FBSS)*, the term describing the complex problem of the multiply operated and failed spine, is to separate mechanical from nonmechanical pathology. Mechanical pathology includes herniated discs, segmental instability, and spinal stenosis. These conditions often respond favorably to surgical treatment, because they cause direct compression of the neural elements. Nonmechanical causes of lumbar spine pain include scar, discitis, psychosocial conditions, and general medical problems. Nonmechanical conditions will not improve with surgery and, in fact, will probably further deteriorate.

Differentiating between the two is the critical first step in selecting surgical candidates.

The keystone in establishing a good outcome when treating lumbar spine pathology is obtaining an accurate diagnosis. While this seems intuitive, failure to accomplish this primary goal will lead to a treatment course fraught with difficulty.

EVALUATION

An organized approach to the evaluation of a patient who has undergone multiple low back operations is required to simplify the evaluation and to prevent missing significant details. The history can be quite detailed and complex. Many patients have a desire to relate their entire history of back problems, and it is best to let them do so. After deciphering these often complex stories, three historical points must be gathered.

1. The number of previous spine surgeries correlates with the outcome for future surgeries. The chance for a successful result is dramatically reduced with additional operations. Historically, a second procedure for a given problem has only a 50% success rate and further procedures often worsen the patient's condition (7–9)

2. The length of the pain-free interval must be clearly understood. If the patient awoke from a previous operation with the exact pain that brought him or her to surgery, it is likely that the nerve root was not decompressed completely or the improper nerve root was decompressed. However, if the interval from surgery to the present complaint is 6 months or more, the new pain may be the result of a recurrent disc herniation at the same or different level. If the pain-free interval is only 1 to 6 months, and the new symptoms gradually progressed, scar tissue is suspected (7,10). Both epidural fibrosis and arachnoiditis can cause this pain pattern.

3. The patient's pain pattern must be recorded. If leg pain predominates, a herniated disc or spinal stenosis is likely the diagnosis. Scar tissue may also result predomi-

nantly in leg pain. Back pain, however, is suggestive of infection, instability, tumor, or possibly scar tissue. Having both back and leg pain is suggestive of spinal stenosis or scar tissue.

After a thorough and detailed history, the physical exam is the next most important aspect of evaluation. Objective neurologic findings and the presence of a tension sign, such as the sitting straight-leg raise, must be sought. A dependable presurgical exam is very helpful, as it allows comparison with the current postoperative exam. If the neurologic exam is unchanged from before the surgery, and no tension sign is present, then mechanical compression is unlikely. If a new neurologic deficit is present and a tension sign also is present, then compression on the neural elements is possible. The tension sign is not pathognomonic for neural compression; however, it can also be caused by epidural or perineural fibrosis.

Special attention should be paid to inorganic physical findings. Red flags include nonanatomic pain distributions or distraction signs. Waddell et al. showed that presence of three or more nonorganic signs predicts a poor outcome from repeat lumbar surgery (8). Also, it is essential to identify litigation or secondary gain issues that may influence treatment and outcomes. Multiple authors have shown that unresolved litigation or compensation is a significant risk for poor outcome. While formal testing, such as the Minnesota Multiphasic Personality Inventory, can be useful, it should not replace the surgeon's attempt to identify well-motivated and adjusted patients (11). These patients are most likely to benefit from surgery.

DIAGNOSIS

Arriving at the correct diagnosis is the primary goal in the evaluation of the patient with the multiply operated back. The lesions most commonly responsible for FBSS include persistent or recurrent disc herniation (12% to 16%), lateral (58%) or central (7% to 14%) stenosis, arachnoiditis (6% to 16%), epidural fibrosis (6% to 8%), and instability (less than 5%) (10,12). To standardize and simplify the approach to treatment of this complex problem, an algorithm has been developed. The aim of the algorithm is to assist by organizing diagnostic criteria, helping identify the correct diagnostic category, and directing treatment principles (Fig. 87-1; Table 87-1).

An important step in the algorithm is identifying nonorthopedic causes for back pain. Important diagnoses to consider are pancreatitis, diabetes, and abdominal aneurysm. All can mimic FBSS and will potentially respond to disease-specific therapy. A general medical evaluation, by an internist or equivalent physician, should be routinely obtained and appropriate treatment initiated. In addition, any psychosocial abnormality should be identified. These include alcoholism, drug dependency,

anxiety, or depression. A psychiatric evaluation is necessary in these cases. Again, it is worth restating that patients with unresolved litigation or compensation issues do not respond to further surgery (13).

Of course, patients with psychiatric disorders may have legitimate orthopedic pathology. It is wise to address the psychiatric diagnoses before proceeding with any further surgery. Hopefully, treatment of the psychiatric condition will eliminate or significantly reduce the somatic back symptoms and disability.

The remaining patients, after eliminating those with medical or psychiatric diagnoses and those motivated by secondary gain, will have either back or leg pain. The goal is to identify which patients have specific mechanical problems that may respond to further surgery from those with symptoms resulting from scar tissue or inflammation.

Mechanical Lesions

Herniated Intervertebral Disc

If the pain of FBSS is from a herniated disc, three possibilities exist. The prior decompression may have been inadequate. This may occur when the correct level was insufficiently decompressed, an incorrect level is decompressed, or disc material is left behind. Typically leg pain predominates and mimics the original symptoms. The pain pattern is identical because the nerve root remains mechanically compressed. The neurologic findings, tension signs, and radiographic pattern will be unchanged from the preoperative findings. The key historical point is the absence of a pain-free interval: the patient awoke in the recovery room with the same pain he or she had preoperatively. Patients in this category will benefit from a proper and complete decompression.

A recurrent herniation may also occur at the previous level, despite an adequate decompression at the index procedure. Typically, the patient awoke in the recovery room pain-free and remained so for at least 6 months. The recurrent disc then irritates and compresses the original nerve root, causing the identical symptoms. If contrast-enhanced CT or gadolinium-enhanced MRI demonstrates herniated disc material, then further decompression is warranted.

Lastly, a different disc may herniate at a new level, causing a different constellation of symptoms. The pain-free interval is typically greater than 6 months, but can be shorter. Leg pain usually predominates, in an anatomic pattern consistent with mechanical compression of a different nerve root. The tension sign should be positive. Again, if contrast-enhanced CT or gadolinium- enhanced MRI demonstrates a disc at a level consistent with the symptoms then the patient will benefit from another decompression.

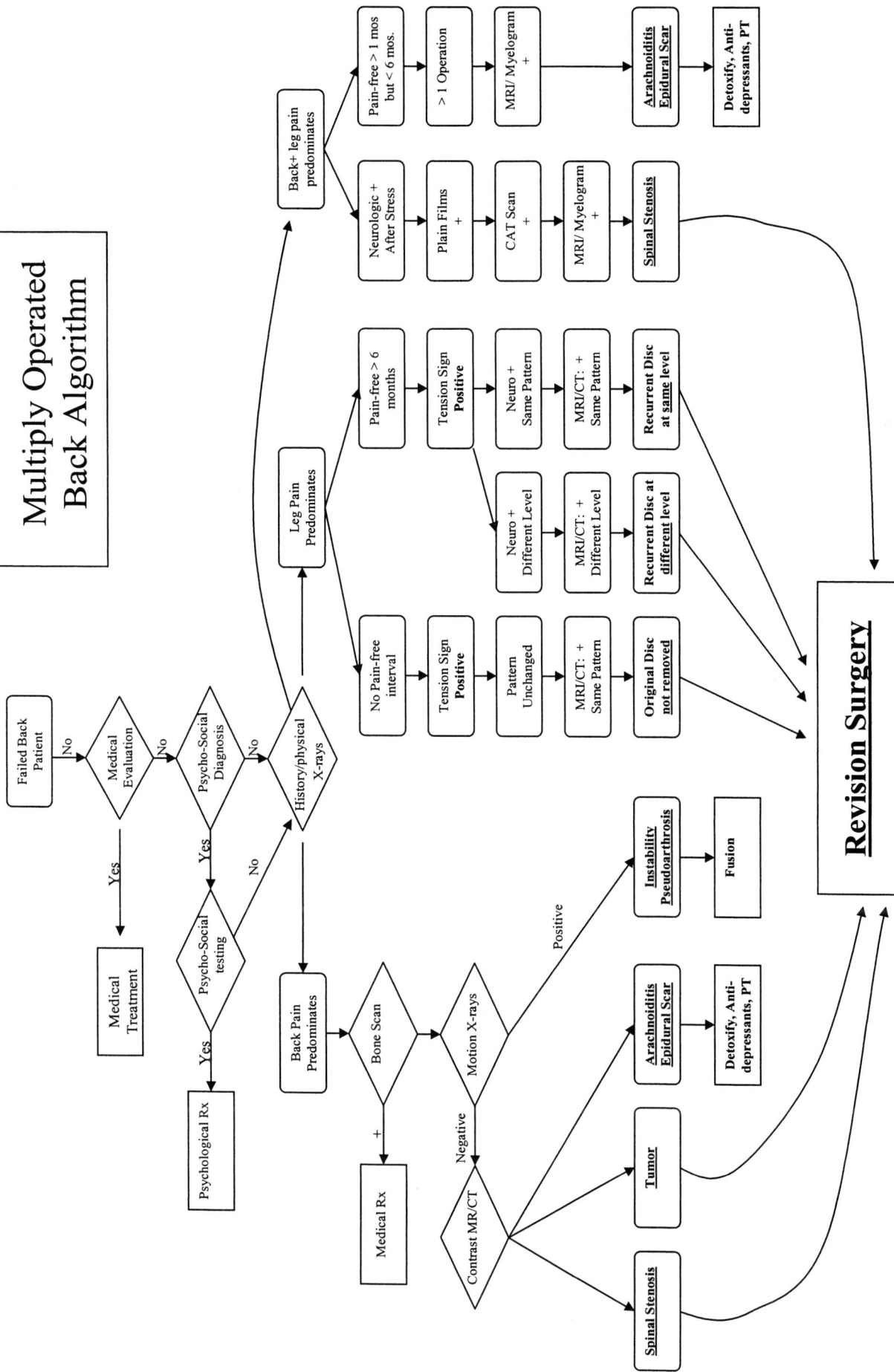

FIG. 87-1. An algorithm for evaluating patients with failed lumbar spine surgery. (Modified from Boden SD, Wiesel SW, Laws ER Jr, et al. The aging spine. Philadelphia: WB Saunders, 1991, with permission.)

TABLE 87.1. *Table format of algorithm for treatment of failed back surgery syndrome: differential diagnosis of the multiply operated back*

History and physical radiographs	Original disc not removed	Recurrent disc at same level	Recurrent disc at different level	Spinal Instability	Spinal Stenosis	Arachnoiditis	Epidural Scar Tissue
No. of previous operations						>1	
Pain-free interval	None	>6 months	>6 months			>1 month but <6 months	>1 month gradual onset
Predominant pain (leg vs. back)	Leg pain	Leg pain	Leg pain	Back pain	Back and leg pain	Back and leg pain	Back and/or leg pain
Tension sign	+	+	+			May be positive	May be positive
Neurologic exam	+ same pattern	+ same pattern	+ different level		+ after stress		
Plain X-rays	+ if wrong level				+		
Lateral motion X-rays				+			
Metrizamide myelogram	+ but unchanged	+ same level	+ different level		+	+	+
CT scan	+	+	+		+		+
MRI	+	+	+		+		+

Lumbar Instability

Segmental instability is a poorly understood cause of persistent back pain in the FBSS patient. Instability, the abnormal motion between two vertebrae, results from the inability of the spinal motion segments to bear normal physiologic loads. While deformity or neurologic deficits are potential complications of instability, pain is the most frequent finding (14). The cause in the FBSS patient may be related to the underlying disease, or it may be iatrogenic. The common iatrogenic causes are excessive facet resection during surgery or pseudoarthrosis (15).

The pain felt from segmental instability may be episodic. Particular activities, such as rising from a chair or straightening after forward bending, may provoke symptoms. Less commonly, instability can produce dynamic stenosis creating leg pain. The physical exam is often normal, although a characteristic reversal of normal spinal rhythm may be noted on return from forward bending (16).

The key to diagnosis may be the weight-bearing, lateral flexion, and extension radiographs. Relative sagittal translation of 12% or angulation of 11° is considered positive. At L5-S1, a more modest 25% translation or 19° angulation is considered a positive test (17). Progressive scoliosis or listhesis on subsequent radiographs is also indicative of instability.

Radiographic evidence of motion should be interpreted cautiously since not all patients with abnormal motion will be symptomatic. In the absence of another identifiable mechanical cause for pain, patients with both pain and abnormal motion may benefit from fusion of the affected levels (18). Additionally, exploration of a pseudoarthrosis may be indicated if abnormal motion can be documented. However, without documented motion or a thorough exclusion of other potential causes for the symptoms, surgery for pseudoarthrosis has a low probability of success (19).

Spinal Stenosis

In all patients, including patient who has experienced multiple back surgeries, lumbar spinal stenosis may produce back and leg pain. The pain may result from progression of an inherent degenerative spinal disorder, a previous incomplete decompression, or by overgrowth of a fusion mass.

The pain-free interval will vary depending on the circumstances. If the previous surgery failed to completely decompress a stenotic canal, there may be no pain-free interval. Alternatively, the patient may be free of symptoms for months to years before the canal becomes sufficiently stenotic to produce symptoms.

In general, the history and physical should be similar to any patient with lumbar spinal stenosis. Back and leg pain are typically present, and leg pain often is exacerbated by exercise, although this is not essential to the diagnosis. The neurologic exam is typically normal, unless neurogenic claudication can be produced during an exercise stress test. Tension signs are generally absent (20,21). It is crucial to differentiate true neurogenic claudication from pain produced by vascular insufficiency.

Plain radiographic findings suggestive of stenosis are facet hypertrophy and degeneration, decreased interpedicular distance, decreased sagittal canal diameter, and degenerated disc spaces. Spondylolisthesis is commonly associated with central and lateral stenosis. While it occurs most commonly at the L4-L5 level, it can occur at the previous operative level. MRI clearly shows thecal sac narrowing and, following gadolinium injection, can differentiate between compression caused by epidural scar and by hypertrophied normal soft-tissue structures. Postmyelographic CT provides excellent visualization of bony encroachment on the neural elements centrally, as well as in the lateral recesses and foramina. However, CT cannot reliably differentiate scar from hypertrophied soft tissue (22).

If direct evidence of bony encroachment or mechanical pressure from hypertrophied soft tissue can be found on advanced imaging, then the patient will potentially respond well to decompression of the neural elements. Good results can be expected from surgery in at least 70% of properly selected patients. However, if gadolinium-enhanced MRI shows substantial scar tissue is present, the degree of pain relief that may be anticipated is less certain. Perhaps related to this fact, patients who have undergone previous laminectomy and fusion respond less well to repeated surgical decompression (23).

Nonmechanical Spinal Lesions

Scar tissue and discitis are nonmechanical sources of recurrent pain in the FBSS patient. Although the location and pathology of these entities differ, they are discussed in common because neither improves with further surgery. Postoperative scar formation in the spine is divided into two main types based on anatomic location. Scar tissue that forms within the dura is referred to as *arachnoiditis*. Scar tissue that forms outside the dura is appropriately termed *epidural fibrosis*.

Arachnoiditis

Arachnoiditis is strictly defined as inflammation of the pia-arachnoid membrane surrounding the spinal cord or cauda equina (12). The extent of scarring may vary from person to person. At its most severe, the subarachnoid space may be obliterated and the flow of cerebrospinal fluid or contrast agents obstructed. While the precise cause is uncertain, previous lumbar spine surgery, intraoperative dural tears, and the injection of oil-based contrast agents are precipitating factors (24). Postoperative infection may also play a role in the pathogenesis of arachnoiditis (25,26).

There is no consistent clinical presentation for arachnoiditis. A typical patient complains of back and leg pain that developed after a brief pain-free interval, between 1 and 6 months. A history of multiple back surgeries is also common. The physical exam is generally not helpful, with any neurologic deficits being attributed to previous pathology or surgery. CT myelography and MRI may confirm the diagnosis.

At present there is no effective treatment for arachnoiditis. Surgery has proved ineffective at relieving pain or reducing scar formation. Combined with much needed encouragement, various nonoperative therapies can be employed (3,12,26,27). The administration of epidural steroids, transcutaneous electrical nerve stimulation, spinal cord stimulation, operant conditioning, bracing and patient education have all been tried, with varying success. None of these therapies cures the condition, but all may provide some relief to some patients for varying periods. Patients should be detoxified of all narcotics, started on amitriptyline hydrochloride (Elavil; Zeneca Pharmaceuticals, Wilmington, DE), and encouraged to be as active as possible. Treating these patients remains a significant challenge, requiring devotion and patience by both the physician and patient, to achieve optimal results.

Epidural Fibrosis

Formation of scar outside the dura, on the cauda equina or directly on the nerve roots, is unfortunately relatively common (28). The epidural scar tissue acts as a constrictive force on the neural elements and may cause postoperative pain. However, while most postsurgical patients have epidural scar formation to some extent, only an unpredictable few are symptomatic.

Patients with epidural scarring may present with symptoms at any time, from several months to more than a year after surgery. The onset is insidious and patients often report back or leg pain. New neurologic deficits are unexpected but a tension sign may be present due to constriction and scarring around the nerve root. The condition is best differentiated from a recurrent herniated disc with a gadolinium-enhanced MRI.

As with arachnoiditis, there is no definitive treatment for epidural scar formation. Prevention may be the best strategy. In the past, a free fat interpositional graft was used after laminectomy (29). A study comparing the use of Gelfoam (Upjohn; Kalamazoo, MI), interposed free fat, and placebo showed no statistical difference in relieving or exacerbating epidural fibrosis (30). Adcon-L (Gliatech, Inc.; Cleveland, OH), a recently introduced biodegradable gel matrix that was approved by the U.S. Food and Drug Administration for use after single-level laminectomy or laminotomy, reduces epidural scar formation in experimental studies. While its use is attractive in preventing scarring, its clinical efficacy is not entirely proven. Although Adcon-L is now available for patients thought to be high risk for scarring, its routine use should be avoided until further studies show a distinct benefit in outcomes (31).

Once epidural fibrosis has formed, surgical treatment is not beneficial. More scar, in fact, would form from repeated surgical exploration. The treatment program described for arachnoiditis should also be employed for epidural fibrosis.

Discitis

Discitis is an uncommon but debilitating complication of lumbar spine surgery. The pathogenesis, although not completely understood, is thought to be direct inoculation of the avascular disc space (32). Severe back pain, usually about one month after surgery, is the usual presentation. Signs on physical exam that may corroborate the diagnosis are fever, presence of a tension sign, and possibly a superficial abscess.

If discitis is suspected, plain radiographs, blood cultures, an erythrocyte sedimentation rate (ESR), and a C-reactive protein (CRP) should be obtained. CRP is more specific than ESR, especially in the early phases of infection. Also, it normalizes more quickly than the ESR, and in other orthopedic infections is commonly used as a marker of response to treatment. The classic plain radiographic findings of disc space narrowing and end-plate erosion may not be present early in the disease. Contrast-enhanced MRI confirms the diagnosis.

The treatment of discitis is controversial (32). Most commonly, the patient is restricted to short-term bed rest and immobilization with a brace or corset. If the patient has progressive pain despite immobilization or has constitutional symptoms, a needle aspiration is recommended. If an organism can be isolated by aspiration, appropriate intravenous antibiotics are administered, usually for 6 weeks. Open disc space biopsy is unnecessary if the patient improves with treatment outlined above. With improvement of symptoms, and normalization of the ESR and CRP, the patient may ambulate as tolerated.

Instrumentation

The use of instrumentation as an adjunct to lumbar spinal fusion has become enormously popular in the last 10 years, almost exclusively in the form of pedicle-screw–based implants. This complicates the approach to the FBSS patient. It is our anecdotal experience that more patients are undergoing lumbar spine fusion without objective indications, resulting in a high failure rate. The presence of the implant itself raises several technical considerations relating to possible revision surgery, including the significance of screw breakage, implant loosening, infection, and aberrant screw placement. Finally, because of adverse publicity surrounding the use of these devices, their presence raises legal implications that at times further cloud a complicated clinical picture.

Pedicle screw instrumentation systems are inert orthopedic implants with an exceedingly low incidence of true allergy. Mechanical failure of the implant does not always represent an indication for removal or revision. The most dramatic mode of failure is breakage of the screw, typically at the shank-thread junction, which has been reported at a rate of 0.5% to 2.5% (33,34). Screw failure was historically quite common, even early in the postoperative period. With advancements in material science and manufacturing, implant failure is now far less common. Furthermore, a broken screw has questionable clinical significance and does not eliminate the possibility of a successful fusion. However, a study by Lonstein et al. reported a correlation between screw breakage and pseudoarthrosis. In this study, 12 of 19 patients who had a fractured screw had a pseudoarthrosis (33). The authors recommended that all symptomatic patients with broken pedicle screws have the implants removed.

Other mechanisms of failure of these systems include screw loosening in the pedicle and vertebral body. This is a more common long-term finding, typically noted as a small zone of lucency above the screw on routine radiographs. Again, no correlation between loosening and symptoms has been reported. Therefore, asymptomatic loosening, in the absence of pseudoarthrosis with instability, warrants observation.

Finally, the risk of infection appears to be increased with the use of these bulky implants and has been reported as high as 5% (35). Although infection in the perioperative period is more readily diagnosed, late developing infection has been reported and may represent a source of recurrent back pain after a pain-free interval. The patient with worsening pain several months or even years after an otherwise successful fusion may be manifesting late infection and should be evaluated accordingly. CT scanning, looking for a fluid collection around the implant, and aspiration of the wound may aid in this diagnosis.

SURGICAL TECHNIQUES IN THE MULTIPLY OPERATED SPINE

Operating on the previously operated lumbar spine can be a considerable technical challenge. The actual technique of a repeated laminectomy is different than the initial procedure. There is certainly increased morbidity, with increased risk of damage to the dura and neural elements. The specific technique for repeated laminectomy and repair of a dural tear are presented in the following sections.

Repeated Decompression

The goal of decompression in the multiply operated back patient is identical to the goal for any spinal decompression: to safely and completely free the neural elements, without causing excessive hemorrhage. Unfortunately, after prior decompression, the anatomic features are no longer normal, and the presence of scar tissue may complicate exposure and ease of decompression. Thus, several technical aspects of performing a repeated laminectomy are different from those for a primary procedure.

The first difference involves the operative approach. Stripping the paraspinal muscles away with impunity is not possible, because no lamina or ligamentum flavum is present to protect the neural elements at the previously operated sites. This means that the approach begins at a new anatomic level, which is normal and protected. This allows the surgeon to find the correct depth of the cauda equina (neural elements).

The surgeon may also be tempted, after the depth of the neural elements is determined, to remove the extradural scar tissue directly from the dura. Technically, this is difficult, and there is a great deal of hemorrhage and a high possibility of injury to the dura. Even if the scar tissue is successfully removed, there is no good way to prevent its reformation. Therefore, it is recommended that, in most cases, that extradural scar tissue should be left intact. Only tissue that is covering the area of pathologic change should be removed. Otherwise, the operative plane should be developed by elevating the scar (and dura) away from the bone at the lateral margin of the old laminectomy.

Finally, the nerve roots must be visualized laterally and any mechanical pressure on them removed. This is accomplished by extension of the laminectomy from the new level down to the lateral gutters, leaving the central scar tissue intact. Each nerve root is then identified and any bony encroachment or herniated disc material at that level can be easily removed. It is essential not only to visualize the nerve root to the dorsal root ganglion and to enlarge the foramen, but also to ensure that the root is mobile.

Routine fusion in a multiply operated back patient is not necessary. If there are preoperative signs of instability on the lateral, weight-bearing flexion and extension radiographs, a fusion is indicated. Also, widening the laminectomy so that bilaterally 50% of the facet joints are destroyed at any one level, or the pars interarticularis is thinned, potentially destabilizes the spine. A bilateral, lateral fusion is recommended in these circumstances. The preoperative patient counseling and the surgical planning should reflect this possibility.

The integrity of a previous fusion mass should be checked during all revision surgeries, for the possibility of a pseudoarthrosis. A pseudoarthrosis can be extremely difficult to detect, even by direct visualization during revision surgical procedures. Unless there are objective signs on flexion-extension radiographs of instability with horizontal translation, a nonunited fusion mass can be easily missed. After identifying the fusion mass laterally, use an osteotome to shave off the outer surface. In a solid fusion, the bone is contiguous throughout. If a defect were identified, the area should be decorticated and new bone graft added. However, even determining if a known pseudoarthrosis is responsible for a patient's symptoms can be particularly challenging. As stated previously, many pseudoarthroses are not symptomatic. Thus, caution should be used when deciding to treat an *apparently* painful pseudoarthrosis with revision surgery and fusion.

Repair of Dural Tears

The rate of dural injury or tear is definitely increased in the patient who has undergone multiple back operations. The surgeon must be skilled in handling this complication. Although each dural tear is unique, certain basic principles always should be applied.

A dural tear usually occurs as the surgeon is gaining visualization of the spinal canal. This can result when a bone-biting instrument inadvertently pinches a small fold of the dura. Alternatively, removal of the adherent dura from the undersurface of bone can initiate a tear. When a tear does occur, the wound usually fills quickly with cerebrospinal fluid (CSF), obscuring the extent of the damage. The surgeon's first impulse is to try to see the tear by using suction in the approximate area of the problem. This is a mistake because individual nerve roots may be drawn into the suction tip, causing extensive neurologic damage. Suction should only be applied through a Cottonoid patty (Codman & Shurtleff, Inc.; Raynham, MA) so that no damage is done to the neural elements. After the tear is visualized, the surgeon places a piece of absorbable gelatin sponge (Gelfoam) over the injury site—with a large Cottonoid covering the entire area—and obtains adequate exposure of the tear. The patient's head should be tilted down to decrease the flow of CSF in the wound.

After adequate exposure is obtained, the surgeon's attention can be focused on repairing the tear. The goal is a watertight closure. If this cannot be accomplished, a CSF fistula potentially may form, raising the risk of meningitis or of forming a subarachnoid cyst. A subarachnoid cyst can exert mechanical pressure on the neural elements.

The operative field should be dry, with meticulous hemostasis. Magnification loupes and adequate lighting facilitate the repair. The technique used to close the dura depends on the size and location of the tear. For simple lacerations, 4-0 silk sutures on a tapered, one-half circle needle are used. A running locking suture (Fig. 87-2A) or simple sutures incorporating a free fat graft (Fig. 87-2B) give a watertight closure. If a large tear is present, a graft from the lumbar fascia is obtained and sutured in place with interrupted dural silk sutures (Fig. 87-2C). If the defect is in an inaccessible area, a small tissue plug of muscle or fat is introduced through a second midline durotomy and pulled against a tear from the inside of the dura.

To test the repair, place the patient in the reverse Trendelenburg position and perform the Valsalva maneuver. This maneuver increases intrathecal pressure and stresses

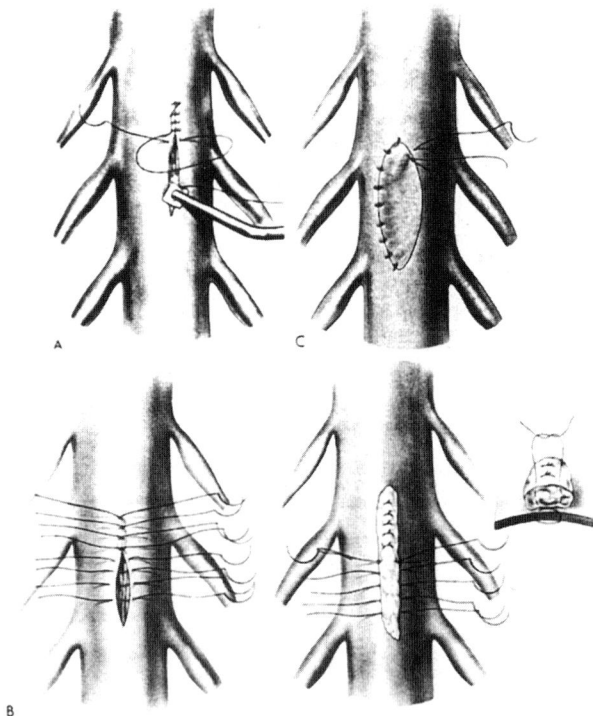

FIG. 87-2. Treatment of dural repair. (From Eismont FJ, Wiesel SW, Rothman RH. Treatment of dural tears associated with spinal surgery. J Bone Joint Surg 1981;63A: 1132–1137, with permission.)

the watertight closure. The fascia is then closed with a heavy nonabsorbable suture to create another watertight barrier to the egress of CSF. Drains should not be used, as drains promote fistula formation. Postoperatively, the patient should be kept flat, on strict bed rest, for at least 3 days. The repair should heal by this time.

Diagnosing a CSF leak in the postoperative period can be challenging. Clear drainage emanating from either the drain site or the wound should raise suspicion for a dural leak. No helpful, noninvasive diagnostic techniques exist at present. The best diagnostic test is a myelogram performed with water-soluble contrast medium; this is recommended if a dural leak is seriously suspected. After the postoperative CSF leak is identified, the patient should be returned quickly to the operating room for dural repair to prevent infection in the CSF.

Closed subarachnoid drainage is a nonoperative alternative treatment for dural leaks (36). A subarachnoid shunt can be placed percutaneously into the lumbar canal, which results in the resolution of some CSF leaks. If a shunt is not quickly successful, the patient should be returned to the operating room for an open dural repair.

Prevention of dural tears is best achieved by excellent visualization and meticulous technique during exposure. Complete hemostasis should always be maintained. If there is any question about the presence of dura in the jaws of a bone-biting instrument, a Cottonoid patty

should be placed between the dura and the bony structures to prevent dural injury. This is an easy and safe preventive measure.

CONCLUSION

The incidence of FBSS will likely continue to rise with the high rate of lumbar spine surgery in our society. Prevention of FBSS is unquestionably more beneficial to the patient, as out treatment of this condition is limited. Properly selecting candidates for lumbar spine surgery will lead to a high rate of success. Unfortunately, many patients with FBSS were inappropriately selected for their original surgery and further surgery only worsens the patient's condition. When considering revision surgery in these patients, a clear-cut diagnosis of nerve root compression or instability should be present. Consider exhausting nonoperative measures before operating.

The evaluation of patients with FBSS is a critical step in their treatment. The cause of the patient's symptoms must be accurately localized and identified, and a thorough investigation of the patient's psychosocial and general medical status is needed. Critical historical points are the number of previous operations, predominance of back or leg pain, and the duration of the pain-free interval. Neurologic deficits and tension signs are sought on physical exam. All imaging studies available should be thoroughly reviewed to corroborate the history and physical findings. When all the information is integrated, the physician can usually identify patients with correctable mechanical problems from those with epidural fibrosis, arachnoiditis, and discitis.

Physicians involved in the treatment of FBSS should realize there is little likelihood the patient will return to a pain-free state. Some level of permanent pain or disability generally remains. These patients should be counseled and encouraged to resume as functional a role as possible in society.

REFERENCES

1. Spengler DM, Freeman DW. Patient selection for lumbar discectomy: An objective approach. Spine 1979;4:129.
2. Laurie JD. Clinical problem solving: a pain in the back. N Engl J Med 2000;343:723–726.
3. Rothman RH, Simeone FA. The spine, 2nd ed. Philadelphia: WB Saunders, 1982.
4. Boden SD, Davis DO, Dma TS, et al. Abnormal magnetic-resonance scans of the lumbar spine in asymptomatic subjects. A prospective investigation. J Bone Joint Surg Am 1990;72:403–408.
5. Holt EP. The question of lumbar discography. J Bone Joint Surg Am 1968;50:720–726.
6. Wiesel SW, Bell GR, Feffer HL, et al. A study of computer assisted tomography. Part I. The incidence of positive CAT scans in an asymptomatic group of patients. Spine 1984;9:549–551.
7. Finnegan WJ, Tenline JM, Marvel JP, et al. Results of surgical intervention in the symptomatic multiply-operated back patient. J Bone Joint Surg Am 1979;61:1077.
8. Waddell G, Kummell EG, Lotto WN, et al. Failed lumbar disc surgery and repeat surgery following industrial injuries. J Bone Joint Surg Am 1979;61:201.

9. Loupasis GA, Stanos K. Seven to twenty year outcome of lumbar discectomy. Spine 1999;24:2313–2317.
10. Fritsch EW. The failed back surgery syndrome: reasons, intraoperative findings and long-term results. A report of 182 operative treatments. Spine 1996;21:626–633.
11. Southwick SM, White AA. Current concepts review: the use of psychological tests in the evaluation of low back pain. J Bone Joint Surg Am 1983;65:560–565.
12. Burton CV. Lumbosacral arachnoiditis. Spine 1978;3:24–30.
13. Waring EM, Weisz GM, Bailey SI. Predictive factors in the treatment of low back pain by surgical intervention. Adv Pain Res Ther 1979; 1:939–942.
14. White AA, Panjabi MM, Posner I, et al. Spinal stability: evaluation and treatment. In: AAOS Instructional Course Lectures. St. Louis: Mosby, 1981:30:457.
15. Hazlett JW, Kinnard P. Lumbar apophyseal process excision and instability. Spine 1982;7:171–174.
16. Paris SV. Physical signs of instability. Spine 1985;10:277–279.
17. Boden SD, Wiesel SW. Lumbosacral motion in normal individuals: have we been measuring instability properly? Spine 1990;12:571–576.
18. Byrd SE, Cohn ML, Biggens SL, et al. The radiographic evaluation of the symptomatic postoperative lumbar spine patient. Spine 1985;10: 652–661.
19. Lauerman WC, Bradford DS, Ogilvie JW, et al. Results of lumbar pseudarthrosis repair. J Spinal Disord 1992;5:149–157.
20. Spengler DM. Degenerative stenosis of the lumbar spine. Current concepts review. J Bone Joint Surg Am 1987;69:305–308.
21. Hall S, Onofrio BM, et al. Lumbar spinal stenosis: clinical features, diagnostic procedures, and results of treatment in 68 patients. Ann Intern Med 1985;103:271–275.
22. Bolender NF, Schonstrom NSR, Spengler DM. Role of computed tomography and myelography in the diagnosis of central spinal stenosis. J Bone Joint Surg Am 1985;67:240–246.
23. Nasca RJ. Surgical management of lumbar spinal stenosis. Spine 1987;12:809–816.
24. Quiles M, Marchisello PJ, Tsairis P. Lumbar adhesive arachnoiditis: etiologic and pathologic aspects. Spine 1978;3:45–50.
25. Epstein BS. The spine. Philadelphia: Lea & Febiger, 1962.
26. Coventry MG, Staufer RN. The multiply operated back. In: American Academy of Orthopaedic Surgeons: symposium on the spine. St. Louis: CV Mosby, 1969:132–142.
27. Mooney V. Innovative approaches to chronic back disability. Instructional course lecture. The 1974 Annual Meeting of the American Academy of Orthopaedic Surgeons; January 1974; Dallas, TX.
28. LaRocca H, Macnab I. The laminectomy membrane: studies in its evolution, characteristics, effects and prophylaxis in dogs. J Bone Joint Surg Br 1974;56:545–550.
29. Lahde 5, Puranen J. Disk space hypodensity in CT: the first radiological signs of postoperative diskitis. Eur J Radiol 1985;5:190–192.
30. Hinton JL Jar, Wreck DJ. Inhibition of epidural scar formation after lumbar laminectomy in the rat. Spine 1995;20:564–570.
31. Fischgrund JS. Use of Adcon-L for epidural scar prevention. J Am Acad Orthop Surg 2000;8:339–343.
32. Dall BE, Rowe DE, Odette WG, et al. Postoperative discitis: diagnosis and management. Clin Orthop 1987;224:138–148.
33. Lonstein JE, Denis F, Perra JH, et al. Complications associated with pedicle screws. J Bone Joint Surg 1999;81A:1519–1528.
34. Steffe AD, Brantigan JW. The variable screw placement spinal fixation system: report of a prospective study of 250 patients enrolled in FDA clinical trials. Spine 1993;18:1160–1172.
35. Masferrer R, Gomez CH, Karahalios DG, et al. Efficacy of pedicle screw fixation and the treatment of spinal instability and failed back surgery. A five year review. J Neurosurg 1988;89:371–377.
36. Kitchel SR, Eismont FJ, Green DA. Closed subarachnoid drainage for management of cerebral spinal fluid leakage after an operation of the spine. J Bone Joint Surg 1989;71A:984–987.

CHAPTER 88

Failed Back Surgery Syndrome

Nonoperative Interventional Management Options

Richard Derby and Connor O'Neill

Failed back surgery syndrome (FBSS) is not a diagnosis but a label describing the patient who continues to experience chronic pain following one or more spinal surgeries. Unfortunately, FBSS often connotes psychological pain exaggeration and a centralized self-sustaining pain process in which further diagnostic tests are inappropriate and treatment options directed at a specific structural cause are useless. Although some patients with chronic pain do develop psychological and behavioral problems, in its extreme this condition should be labeled *chronic pain syndrome,* not FBSS. Here FBSS is considered an outmoded phrase for describing patients with persistent intermittent or constant spinal pain following one or more spinal surgeries. Although these patients have an increased likelihood of problematic pain sources such as fibrosis, neuropathic nerve roots, and segmental instability, the diagnostic work-up and treatment options are similar to those of patients without prior surgery.

With more physicians and societies devoted to pain management and musculoskeletal spine and sport medicine, diagnosis and nonoperative treatment algorithms are evolving to include not only pastoral care modalities (e.g., functional restoration, behavioral modification, and psychological counseling), but also algorithms including aggressive pharmacologic pain management and interventional procedures for identifying and treating specific sources of pain. The proliferation of interventional procedures characterizing many nonoperative spine practices has been controversial. Although detractors argue that many of these procedures are dubious, risky, scientifically unproved, and do not lead to long-term functional improvement, they are ubiquitous. Even more procedures are being investigated in both pilot and randomized studies. Some, such as epidural injections have stood the test of time, but others, such as pulsed radiofrequency treatments are recent concepts that may or may not be in common use in 3 to 5 years. In this chapter, we survey the most common procedures currently in use (1–3).

Most of these interventional procedures are directed at specific peripheral sources of pain originating within the posterior, middle, or anterior columns. However, there is continued doubt that one can identify specific pain sources in chronic low back pain. It has been estimated that using clinical and radiologic data, the source of low back pain can be accurately determined in only 15% to 20% of patients (4) with the exception of imaging (5). Contrary to this view, many spine specialists believe pain sources can be identified using pain reproduction and relief following precise localized and spinal injection techniques (International Spinal Injection Society [ISIS] standards) (6). Based on Schwarzer's studies using precision diagnostic injection as the criterion standard for diagnosis, Bogduk postulated that a definite diagnosis could be made in 70% to 80% of patients (7). Although arriving at a different percentage prevalence of specific pain sources, Manchikanti (3) was able to identify the z-joint, sacroiliac (SI) joint, or disc as the primary source of pain in 68% of patients.

POSTERIOR COLUMN

The prevalence of specific posterior column pain generators in postsurgical patients is unknown. However, the effects of spinal surgery could increase the likelihood of chronic pain originating from z-joints, SI joints, and muscles or ligaments. Such effects may include increased segmental motion above or below a spinal fusion or increased or abnormal segmental motion owing to partial removal the intervertebral disc.

Facet Blocks

Attempts to identify a clinical "facet syndrome" have largely been fruitless. Revel (8) has suggested that patients with facet pathology can be reliably identified by clinical criteria. Pain relief following placebo-controlled medial branch blocks is the current standard for diagnosing z-joint pain (9). Using this standard, the prevalence of z-joint pain in younger injured workers with chronic low back pain is approximately 15% and approximately 40% in older rheumatologic patients (10,11). A more recent study found a 40% incidence of facet-related pain in a series of 120 consecutive patients (12).

Relief following local anesthetic denervation does not, however, determine the cause. If pain is caused by inflammation, then injection of corticosteroid into the joint might be expected to give short-term pain relief; if the cause of inflammation is an acute episode, then relief might last until another event causes s pain to return. However, in the postsurgical patient persistent z-joint pain is probably more often caused by mechanical strain of facet capsules secondary to abnormal segmental motion, rather than inflammation. Randomized placebo-controlled z-joint treatment trials with chronic low back pain have not shown a significant difference in pain relief between corticosteroid injection and placebo (13,14).

Medial Branch Neurotomy

Because of the poor long-term results following corticosteroid z-joint injections (15), medial branch blocks have become the standard for diagnosis and treatment of z-joint–related pain. Blocking the medial branches at two consecutive levels temporarily denervates the joints. If pain is caused by the z-joints, pain relief should follow. Studies (16) have shown that lumbar medial branch blocks were target-specific and a valid test of z-joint pain. Carefully diagnosed with controlled diagnostic medial branch blocks, Dreyfuss et al. also showed that 60% of patients obtained at least 90% pain relief at 12 months, and 87% obtained at least 60% relief following radiofrequency medial branch neurotomy (17). In a randomized placebo-controlled study, van Kleef et al. showed that lumbar medical branch neurotomy was not a placebo (18).

However, medial branches do regenerate. In clinical practice the average patient may expect an average of 50% decrease in pain between 6 and 12 months, but the procedure can be repeated with a success rate of approximately 75% (19). In the case of a specific z-joint injury, the purpose of repeat neurotomies is to provide partial pain relief while the injury heals. However, lasting resolution of pain may depend on gradual stabilization of the spinal segment, which may take many years. Over time some patients develop different sources of pain and become unresponsive to further denervation.

Restorative Injection Therapy of Failed Back Surgery

The medial branches innervate both facet capsules and interspinous ligaments. If pain is caused by chronic ligamentous strain arising from increased or abnormal motion, medial branch neurotomies do not treat the underlying problem. Although there is no evidence to show that multifidus muscle denervation following medial branch neurotomy increases instability, nonsurgical treatments directed at increasing the strength of the ligamentous structures are more appealing.

For many years practitioners of orthopedic medicine have advocated injecting injured connective tissues with of proliferative agents (20–22). Theoretically, tissue proliferation could afford increased motion, segment stability, and reduced pain. Although remaining a contentious form of treatment, data showing connective tissue proliferation in animal models has provided some support for this approach (23). In addition, some clinical data have suggested that injection treatments may be of benefit to some FBSS patients. For example, Gedney treated patients with massive degeneration of intervertebral discs by injecting ligaments in the lumbar area and sacroiliac ligament with sclerosing solution (20,21), and Klein et al. (24) successfully treated a group of patients with low back pain, including patients with unsuccessful lumbar fusion.

Despite the continued widespread use of proliferative injections, controlled perspective outcome studies of prolotherapy are few and have not permitted a definitive evaluation. Although Klein et al. (25) showed significantly better results in patients treated by proliferative solution than patients injected with placebo, Dechow (26) failed to show significant differences between patients treated with proliferative solutions and those treated with lidocaine. However, it is significant to note that successful case studies required a period of treatment longer than 6 months and repetition of injections. In the Klein study, treatment included six injections with 1-week intervals between treatments and an exercise program, whereas in the Dechow study patients received only three injections and neither exercise treatment nor manipulations. Follow-up in both studies was 6 months. It is significant that successful case studies required a period of treatment longer than 6 months and injections were repeated. Manipulation and special exercises also were important.

Intramuscular Botulinum Toxin Injections

Muscle overreactivity resulting in spasms is frequently observed in various pathologic conditions associated with pain (27). It is not clear whether spasm itself causes pain, or is simply a component of a more complex pathologic process. Electromyographic studies have shown that electrical activity of paraspinal muscle is higher in patients with low back pain (28). Although the role of chronic muscle spasm in chronic back pain is unclear, many physicians believe that overactive paraspinal muscles contribute to chronic spinal pain; this belief has led to the investigation and use of botulinum toxin.

Botulinum toxin's therapeutic efficacy has been established in randomized controlled studies for the treatment of spasticity and dystonia, and there has been an increasing empiric use of botulinum toxin for the diagnosis and treatment of chronic spinal pain.

Intramuscular injection of botulinum toxin causes localized muscle paralysis by inhibiting acetylcholine release from neuromuscular junctions. In a randomized double-blind study pain relief following intramuscular injection of 40 units of botulinum toxin A at each of the five lumbar paravertebral levels was measured relative to placebo (29). At 8 weeks, nine of 15 patients (60%) in the botulinum toxin group and two of 16 (12.5%) of the normal saline group had pain relief exceeding 50% as measured by Visual Analogue Scale (VAS) score. Several possible mechanisms of pain relief using this method were proposed, and include spasm relief mediated via nocioreceptors, and neuronal innervation of nociceptors or spinal cord neurons.

Middle Column

Although not the most common sources of spinal pain, recurrent disc herniation, stenosis, instability, and fibrosis are commonly sited structural sources of early or late recurrence of nociceptive pain following lumbar spinal surgery (30). However, even with direct surgical inspection it may be impossible to determine the primary source of axial pain. Many patients may have an undetermined degree of neuropathic symptoms unlikely to resolve following repeated surgical intervention. Many physicians continue to view FBSS as a syndrome characterized by neuropathic pain exacerbated by psychosocial factors (31).

Epidural Injections

Nociceptive pain unresponsive to oral antiinflammatories and aggravated by inflammatory dural sensitization caused by disc herniations and stenosis is often treated with epidural injections of anesthetic and corticosteroids.

The effectiveness of epidural injections has been evaluated in numerous studies with mixed results (32–34). Performed by nonspecialists without the use of fluoroscopic imaging on patients with an unclear diagnosis current data does not support the application of blind translaminar injections (13). However, the efficacy of transforaminal epidural injections using fluoroscopic verification of targeting is more convincing.

Because of attenuation of the epidural space, postlaminectomy transforaminal injection offers a more selective and reliable method of targeting injectant to the anterior epidural space (35,36). In a randomized study in

patients presenting with lumbosacral radicular pain secondary to herniated disc, Lutze et al. compared the transforaminal injection of local anesthetic and corticosteroid versus trigger point injection (37) and showed an 84% success rate for transforaminal injections versus a 48% success rate for trigger point injections at an average follow-up time of 1.4 years. Subsequent work showed a 50% or greater reduction in pain at an average of 80 weeks following injections (38). In a randomized controlled study of 55 patients requesting surgery for radicular pain, Reiw found that 20 of 28 patients randomized to undergo fluoroscopically guided transforaminal injections with bupivacaine and betamethasone decided not to have an operation at follow-up (13 to 29 months). Among patients receiving betamethasone alone, only nine of 27 decided against surgery. In a prospective evaluation of 30 patients with pain secondary to a foraminal or extraforaminal herniation, Weiner (39) found that 22 of the 28 patients available for long-term follow-up showed sustained relief from their symptoms following transforaminal injection of local anesthetic and corticosteroids.

In a recent randomized controlled trial comparing the effectiveness of transforaminal local anesthetic and corticosteroid injections against a placebo injection of normal saline, Karppinen (40) showed both cost and short-term pain effectiveness for contained lumbar disc protrusions. These benefits were not obtained with disc extrusions.

The efficacy of treating spinal stenosis with transforaminal injections remains understudied. Using computed tomography (CT)–guided transforaminal injections in patients with spinal stenosis showed 72% short- and 28% long-term success rates compared with patients with disc herniations of the lumbar spine, who showed 95% short-term and 69% extended-term success rates.

Although epidural steroid injections are frequently effective for treating middle column inflammation at unoperated levels, the results when treating recurrent herniations and spinal stenosis at operated levels are less predictable. Because the nerve root obtains as much as 50% of its nutrition through cerebral spinal fluid within the dural cuff (41), postsurgical fibrosis may cause nerve root ischemia and neuropathic pain. If this process were responsible for a substantial portion of postoperative pain, epidural steroid injections would not be of significant benefit. However, treatment failure could be of prognostic value by suggesting the presence of irreversible processes unlikely to benefit from further surgery.

Derby et al. retrospectively studied a group of patients undergoing primary and repeat lumbar spinal surgery for extremity pain and determined that greater than 50% relief of extremity pain for more than 1 week following selective epidural block with local anesthetic and corticosteroids correlated with 50% or greater relief of leg pain at 1 year postsurgery. All patients had temporary relief of leg pain for the duration of the local anesthetic. When duration of leg pain was less than 1 year, both steroid responders and nonresponders had good outcomes. However, when the duration of leg pain exceeded 1 year, patients unresponsive to corticosteroids (two of 13 patients, or 15%) showed a favorable outcome compared with 11 of 13 patients (85%) who responded to corticosteroids. Derby concluded that in patients with leg pain greater than 1 year in duration, not responding to corticosteroids injection, the probability of resolution following surgery was low. The chance of resolution in patients with previous surgery and no significant structural abnormalities was even less likely (42).

Although not specifically addressing the number of injections to perform in situations where the pathology is at an operated level, ISIS guidelines suggest that a series of injections should be limited to no more than four injections at intervals of 7 to 14 days within a 6-month period. Failure to obtain at least 40% relief of pain after any injection is sufficient reason to stop the series unless there is a strong desire to avoid surgery, absence of a surgical lesion, or the patient experienced relief followed by an acute exacerbation of symptoms. The American Academy of Pain Medicine (AAPM) has similar guidelines.

Lysis of Adhesions

Whether fibrosis is a source of pain remains controversial (43–45). Because fibrosis is often seen in patients with and without continued spinal pain following surgery, some have concluded that continued pain is more psychological than physiologic (46,47–50). Traction on neural structures via fibrous adhesions could theoretically lead to pain; however, coexisting processes (e.g., sensitization because of inflammation, nerve damage, or segmental instability) must be present for pain to be symptomatic.

Surgical neurolysis of adhesions has generally shown poor long-term results (51), although some studies have shown pain relief for 3 to 6 months (52). This apparent short-term surgical relief has prompted the study and use of various percutaneous neurolysis methods.

Although perhaps the simplest method of treating epidural adhesions is the epidural injection of hyaluronidase, local anesthetic and corticosteroid, when Devulder (53) compared the results of transforaminal injection of hyaluronidase, and local anesthetic and a combination of hyaluronidase, local anesthetic, and Depo-Medrol in a randomized study of 60 patients with FBSS owing to fibrosis there was no difference in outcome between the groups at 6 months, although all groups did show a decrease in pain at 1 month. Interestingly only the two groups without corticosteroid showed a statistically significant decreased efficacy at 3 and 6 months.

Another common neurolysis method is the forceful injection of fluid into the caudal epidural space. Using this approach, several randomized comparative studies have investigated the efficacy of providing pain relief in postoperative patients with back and leg pains without an obvious structural source other than epidural fibrosis. Using fluoroscopic and contrast-verified injections, both Revel (54) and Meadeb (55) compared the efficacy of forced saline injection with or without added corticosteroids versus low-volume corticosteroid alone. Revel showed a 6-month success rate of 45% and 29% for leg pain and back pain, respectively. At 18 months postinjection, there was a statistically significant improvement in patients in back (31%) and leg (39%) compared with the group treated with steroids alone. Meadeb did not follow enough cases to reach statistical significance. However, a modest 15% decrease was seen in 47% of the forceful injection group patients at 1 month following three injections administered at 1-month intervals. No complications were reported.

A more aggressive approach involves fluoroscopically guiding an epidural catheter to the site of fibrosis and using both injected fluid pressure and mechanical disruption by the catheter to lyse adhesions. Racz and Holubec (56) reported the first use of epidural hypertonic saline to facilitate lysis. Originally, Racz followed a 3-day in-hospital protocol using repeat treatments and included, in addition to normal saline and corticosteroids the injection of a hypertonic (10%) saline solution, which presumably decreased edema and attenuated small pain fiber activity. In a randomized comparative study to determine if hyaluronidase or hypertonic saline increased outcome, the Racz group found a 25% or more reduction in VAS scores in 83% of the patients at 1 month, and approximately 50% of the patients at 3, 6, 9, and 12 months. However, there was no difference in the groups, although the groups receiving hypertonic saline with or without hyaluronidase required slightly fewer treatments. More recently, Manchikanti found that a single day protocol using reduced volumes of both normal saline and 10% NaCl achieved similar 50% number of patients who achieved "significant" relief of pain at a 1-year follow-up (57). The use of a catheter directed through the intervertebral foramen also has been advocated as an alternative or perhaps more reliable method of catheter placement when one wants to lysis adhesions within the neural foramen (58).

One recent neurolysis method combines use of fluoroscopy with direct visualization via a fiberoptic endoscope directed through the caudal canal. This approach may facilitate disruption of neural adhesions using injected fluid or the endoscope itself (59). Manchikanti recommends endoscopic neurolysis if neurolysis by catheter technique is ineffective (60).

In addition to pain presumed to be secondary to epidural fibrosis, in a small retrospective study Manchikanti reviewed the charts of 18/239 patients with moderate to severe spinal stenosis who underwent a lysis protocol of 1 to 10 sessions. A 50% or greater reduction in pain for an average of 10.7 weeks was found (61). Seventeen percent and 11% of patients maintained relief at 1 and 2 years, respectively.

Epidural injection of corticosteroids and hyaluronidase is relatively safe (62–64). However, use of hypertonic saline may significantly increase the risk of complications if the solution inadvertently enters the subarachnoid space. Most reported complications, however, have resulted from pressure following injections of relatively large volumes of fluid.

Thermal Treatment

In theory, treatment of nociceptive pain by reducing or modifying small fiber input through dorsal root ganglions or dorsal horns is attractive. Surgical interruptions (dorsal root entry zone [DREZ] lesions), however, have not shown an acceptable long term success rate (65).

Since the early 1980s Sluijter has pioneered percutaneous treatment procedures directed at the dorsal root ganglion (DRG) (66). One approach involves a 67°C "cool burn" applied by a radiofrequency (RF) needle positioned close to the DRG after the pain source has been identified via local anesthetic relief. Data suggest that RF heating of the dorsal root ganglion is more effective than placebo in chronic cervicobrachialgia (67,68). Use of this technique for lumbosacral pain, however, is limited. In a retrospective analysis of 279 patients undergoing RF treatment of the DRG, 59% of patients reported satisfactory pain relief at 2 months postprocedure, with a mean duration of 3.7 years (69). Wright reported successful treatment of low back pain via RF directed at the L2 DRG (70). The concept that cooler temperatures permit selective destruction of small fibers has recently been questioned (71).

Although this technique continues to be practiced, it is worth noting that procedures that reduce input into the dorsal horns in neuropathies afford abnormal synaptic connections. In many cases in which chronic extremity pain following surgical intervention, central, neuropathic, and nociceptive pain are present in variable degrees. As Sluijter points out, "when for reasons we do not fully understand the dorsal horn may become permanently altered in its capacity to respond to normal peripheral input, pain centralization and therefore neuroablative procedures are doomed to failure and have the potential of creating additional neuropathic pain." (72).

Pulsed Radiofrequency Treatment

When radiofrequency treatment does not depend on neuroablation, but derives its effect from exposure of the DRG to electrical fields created by the RF probe, some problems associated with thermal injury may be eliminated. One approach involves use of a pulsed field. Slappendel et al. (73) found that pulsed RF treatment of the cervical DRG at 40°C and 67°C showed an equal 3

month significant reduction in pain in approximately 50% of both groups. This approaches again the idea of Sluijter, who in his own preliminary studies feels that he can achieve a similar favorable outcome. His preliminary results, theory, experimental data, treatment guidelines, and techniques are presented in his latest book (72).

Because of its low potential for adverse outcome and promotion by medical device manufactures, use of this technique is widespread. However, published outcome studies are lacking. Anecdotally, pain management physicians appear divided on the benefits of this technique.

Spinal Cord Stimulation

As discussed elsewhere in this volume, neuropathic extremity pain refractory to oral medication is commonly treated with a spinal cord stimulator. In the United States, FBSS is the most common reason for application of spinal cord stimulation therapy (74). The analgesic efficacy ranges from 52% to 72%. A recent analysis of the national Italian register of implantable systems found that 81% of the patients reported a positive assessment for pain control, with a reduction in drug needs reported by 71% of positive responders (75). Some consider spinal cord stimulation a first-choice treatment in FBSS caused by lumbosacral fibrosis (76).

ANTERIOR COLUMN

The primary structure in the anterior column responsible for continued or recurrent pain after lumbar surgery is the intervertebral disc. In the unoperated spine, the prevalence of pain owing to an internally disrupted disc is at least 39% (77). The prevalence of failed surgery because of continued pain from an intervertebral disc is unknown. Nevertheless, it is known that the surgical failure rate (unrelated to recurrent herniations) is significantly higher when discectomies alone are performed for smaller disc protrusions (78) and significantly higher when posterior reconstructive surgeries without anterior fusions are performed in patients with a low-pressure positive discography (79).

Because of nerve ingrowth in the degenerative, injured, or postoperative disc, continued pain from remaining disc tissue may be responsible for ongoing symptoms (80,81). Although the existence of discogenic pain is now well accepted, use of discography for identifying a painful disc remains controversial because of recent studies showing pain provocation during disc injection in asymptomatic subjects. If one excludes patients with somatization, applying more precise criteria for determining a positive level and use of a manometric grading scale (described by Derby et al. and recently adapted by the International Association for the Study of Pain and International Spinal Injection Society), the specificity of lumbar discography becomes 80% to 100% (82). In previously operated discs, however, the false-positive rate may be higher (83).

A more rational stepwise approach to patients with axial and referred extremity pain owing to an internally disrupted disc is evolving. Of particular interest are patients with lesser degrees of internal disruption, maintained disc heights, and pain provocation during discography at pressures less than 15 psi above opening pressure. Consistent with our current understanding of peripheral sensitization, there may be significant chemical sensitization causing increased pain response relative to the degree of structural pathology (79). Identifying these patients before surgical intervention and offering less invasive treatment options is a focus of current clinical investigations. Whether newer microinvasive techniques will be successful in previously operated discs or discs above or below spinal fusions is uncertain.

Intradiscal Injections

A logical first step might be use of intradiscal corticosteroid injections either during discography or as a series. Although many discographers inject corticosteroid into painful discs at the time of discography, and others consider intradiscal steroid injection a treatment option, the outcome is often unrewarding (84). Outcome studies on the use of intradiscal corticosteroids have, however, included a heterogeneous mixture of disc pathologies. Injected agents may benefit patients with chemically sensitized discs (85).

There is a growing interest in intradiscal solutions that could promote healing of an injured annulus. Animal studies suggest growth factors may modulate repair of the nucleus and transition zone. A single injection of tumor growth factor-β has been shown to induce 3 weeks of proteoglycan synthesis and healing of full-thickness cartilage lesions, indicating that continuous exposure to growth factors may not be necessary for healing to occur. Intradiscal injection of a solution of glucosamine, chondroitin sulfate, and hypertonic dextrose is currently being studied. When injected into a disrupted intervertebral disc, these agents could upregulate the biosynthesis of proteoglycans directly and indirectly through the release of endogenous growth factors. In a recent study, a group of 30 patients with chronic low back pain, including five patients with previous lumbar surgery and positive manometric controlled discograms, underwent a series of one to three injections at 2-month intervals. The investigators found 25 of the 30 patients achieved a 50% average decrease in pain and disability scores (24,86). Pain reduction has been postulated to occur because of improvement in the intradiscal chemical environment.

Thermal Treatment

If pain following disc injury arises in part from ingrowth and the subsequent sensitization of nociceptive fibers within annular fissures, pain reduction may occur by reducing or eliminating nociceptive input by destroying pain sensitive fibers with heat. Percutaneous intradiscal heating treatment was first introduced in 1993 by Sluijter (87) using a standard radiofrequency needle inserted into the center of the disc and heated 90 seconds at 70°. Although this original did not survive a randomized controlled study, better methods have been developed. Currently available methods involve either a resistive thermal coil threaded circumferentially around the annulus (Oratec SpineCath) or an ionic heating catheter threaded across the posterior annulus (Tyco-Radionics Disc Trode). Outcome data on the former method has shown an approximate 60% success rate in selected patients (88–91). Patients best suited are those with maintained disc heights and more limited degrees of disruption with a chemically sensitized outer annulus. Although animal and human data suggest annular temperatures above 45°C are required to destroy nociceptive fibers, the mechanism of pain relief is unclear. A combination of processes including thermal fiber destruction, collagen modification, and perhaps even biochemical modification of the inflammatory process may be involved

Coblation

Other alternative microinvasive intradiscal treatment techniques are emerging. One technique is the use of a microinvasive decompressive procedure using coblation technology. In this approach energy capable of breaking chemical bonds in tissue is generated via a highly focused plasma field. Using this technique an approximate 10% volumetric reduction in nuclear tissue is observed. The resulting decrease in intradiscal pressure is thought to be responsible for pain reduction. Because this is a new method, relatively few outcome studies have been completed. In one study using this method, nucleoplasty gave an overall 79% success rate with a 67% success rate in a group of patients with previous surgery (92). Similar to other decompressive techniques, the procedure is designed to treat patients with extremity pain owing to smaller disc protrusions. There is a growing trend to perform both nuclear decompression and a heating treatment in the same session (Fig. 88-1) (3).

Central Pain

Neuropathic pain is caused by the hyperexcitability of neurons in the peripheral and central nervous system (93). The experience of chronic constant pain may have a primary or secondary component of sympathetic neuropathic pain. That is why even when the primary source of the pain is exterminated, particularly after spine surgery, patients can continue to perceive pain owing to the continued excitation of neurons that are responsible for pain sensation. The mechanism by which this occurs is not fully understood. The normal neurologic pathway in

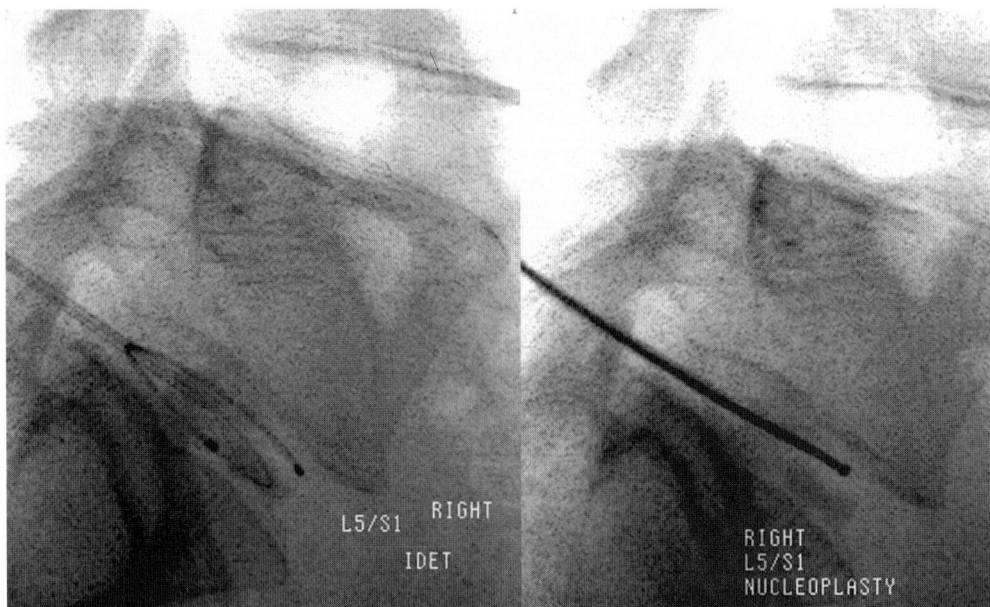

FIG. 88-1. Nucleoplasty intradiscal electrothermal therapy (IDET) combined procedure. Patient with painful internally disrupted disc successfully treated with combined nucleoplasty/IDET. Figure shows nucleoplasty needle and electrode in L5-S disc. Following nucleoplasty, IDET catheter is passed through introducer needle and heated using 85° protocol.

response to and injury travels along the A-δ and C fibers through peripheral nerves to enter the spinal cord through the dorsal root and synapse on the dorsal horn with interneurons carrying the impulses to ascending tracts, the anterior horn, and intermediolateral cell column, where the painful message is relayed to the sympathetic nerve cell bodies. A sympathetic reflex is activated by efferent sympathetic impulses sent out of the spinal cord through the ventral roots to a ramus communicans albus and then into the sympathetic chain to synapse in a sympathetic ganglion. The postganglionic sympathetic fiber leaves the ganglia, where it travels with the peripheral nerve producing vasoconstriction. If this sympathetic reflex arc does not shut down but continues to function and accelerate, a sympathetic hyperdynamic state ensues. This results in increased vasoconstriction and tissue ischemia, causing more pain and thus increasing the barrage of afferent pain impulses traveling in the spinal cord and reactivating the sympathetic reflex. Hypothetically, repeated sympathetic blocks could be used to treat pain perpetuated or enhanced by this overactive sympathetic state (94). Prospective controlled study has not, however, confirmed effectiveness of this treatment in patients with failed back surgery syndrome (95).

Another cause of neuropathic pain after spine surgery may be direct injury during the procedure, scar tissue, damage to small peripheral nerves of the soft tissues and skin with retraction instruments, insertion of venous catheters, or superficial skin irritants.

Several classes of medications have been shown to be effective in the treatment of neuropathic pain by dampen-

ing the threshold to excitation in the postganglionic sympathetic neurons. Tricyclic antidepressants act as balanced inhibitors of reuptake of both cartooning and noradrenaline at the sympathetic junction that act to suppress pain transmission, resulting in the prolongation of serotonin activity at the receptor (96). It was shown (97) that tricyclic antidepressants via L-tryptophan were effective in the treatment of postoperative pain.

Calcium channel blockers reduce nerve conductibility and excitability (98). Neurolytics such as Gabapentin (Neurontin) act by blocking Ca^+ voltage-dependent channels in the neuron membrane, and thus reducing excitability (99). It is effective in the treatment of intractable neuropathic pain (100) or is used as an adjuvant treatment (101,102). Case studies have demonstrated gabapentin to be effective in the treatment of failed back surgery syndrome caused by epidural fibrosis (103).

Other classes of medications currently being used as adjuvant therapies include N-methyl-D-aspartate (NMDA) inhibitors, α-blockers, and topical anesthetics.

Large groups of medications act as opioid receptor agonists. Analgesic opioids have been used for pain alleviation for ages, and remain to this day the most controversial solution. Cases of iatrogenic addiction owing to the use of opioid analgesics date back the 19th century. Physicians hesitate to prescribe them for fear of their potential addictive qualities. The use of opioids for patients suffering from malignant terminal cancer pain has found wide-ranging acceptance in medical practice. However, in patients suffering with profound pain from nonmalignant sources such as failed back surgery syndrome where long-term survival is expected, physicians hesitate, assuming the potential for addition is high. However, the rate of addiction is 0.8% with the use of long-acting medication formulations now on the market (104). The medical literature is fraught with contradictory reports showing the abuse rate in this same population as high as 24% (105). Schofferman (106) found no psychological, psychophysiologic, or clinical characteristics predicting the probability of addiction. This same study demonstrated that opioid analgesics could provide significant improvement in quality of life for patients suffering with chronic low back pain following failed back surgery who had no other treatment alternatives.

Although most patients exposed to opioid analgesics for an extended period develop some degree of physical dependence (107), psychologically their dependence differs from that in drug-addicted individuals seeking euphoria (108). Drug addicts use drugs purely for the euphoric effects despite it destroying their normal life, causing them to withdraw from family and society as well as endangering their health. In contrast, patients suffering from chronic pain take opioid medications in order to restore normal life, relations, and participation with family, and to return to work (109). Another problem that is mostly associated with short-acting analgesics is the development of tolerance to opioids. This occurs because of the upregulation of opioid receptors on the cell membrane, requiring higher doses of the drug to create the same perceived analgesic effect (110). It has been shown in patients without chronic pain who received methadone for opioid dependence that the analgesic effect for both methadone and morphine was diminished. Higher doses were necessary to reach the same analgesic effect (111,112). Studies have shown that chronic pain patients who are being managed on long-acting opioid preparations are able to maintain stable analgesic doses for years (106). It was suggested that chronic pain itself could activate analgesic tolerance (110). Some adjuvant medications can inhibit cellular mechanisms responsible for analgesic tolerance. Namely is has been shown that NMDA blocks opioid receptors, restoring opioid analgesic capacity to both reduce not only tolerance but also allows for dose reduction (113).

Common adverse side effects of oral opioid administration include constipation, sedation, cognitive impairment, pruritus, nausea, and vomiting (114). Usually these complications take place at the beginning of treatment and resolve in a few weeks.

However, in a selected group of patients these adverse reactions do not diminish in time even in the face of adequate pain control. They find that the adverse side effects from the opioids cause even greater levels of disability and diminished functional status. For these select patients alternative methods of administration of the medications via indwelling epidural catheters are now possible. By delivering the opioid medication directly into the epidural space a fraction of the per oral dose can be used to obtain the same degree of pain control without the medication's systemic adverse side effects.

Implantable self-infusion pump systems are being used in selected cases for the treatment of severe chronic pain in patients with failed back surgery (115). It has been shown that intrathecal morphine pumps are effective in the management of failed back syndrome in more than 60% of patients who had been unresponsive to oral therapy who had been suffering for 5 years or longer (116). Despite the high cost of surgical pump implantation, in long-term prospective studies (11 months and longer) intrathecal morphine therapy is more cost effective than traditional oral opiate therapy (117). Even though this system of opioid delivery solves many of the problems associated with oral administration, some of the same adverse side effects are still possible and do occur with the implantable systems, such as nausea, pruritus, constipation, and urinary retention. These symptoms usually can be controlled with antiemetics, antihistamines, and stool softeners with stimulants (116). In patients where these adverse effects become intolerable and resistant to medical management or in the case of drug tolerance or pump failure, these systems eventually are removed (117).

Physicians should consider long-term opioids as the last option in the treatment of failed back surgery (109,116,118). Psychological evaluation of a patient's potential for addiction is highly recommended before considering the use long term opioid management of chronic failed back syndrome (106). In the case of intrathecal pump placement a 3-day trial in an inpatient setting of intermittent intrathecal opioid administration through a temporary catheter allows for the adjustment of individual dosing with proper analgesic response and diminished adverse side effects (116).

SUMMARY

This chapter discusses interventional procedures commonly used for the treatment of chronic spinal pain. Many of these procedures are controversial and lack definitive evidence-based medical support. On the other hand, there is a growing use of these procedures both as supplementary optional methods of pain control and as methods to help confirm that a specific structure is a source of pain.

Although the treatment ideally should be directed at the source of pain, in many cases of FBSS either the source of pain is elusive or there are multiple pain sources. In these cases, the more "benign" and least invasive procedures should be tried first. Several different procedures can be performed in the same session (Fig. 88-2).

Interventional procedures used to treat painful posterior column structures include percutaneous medial

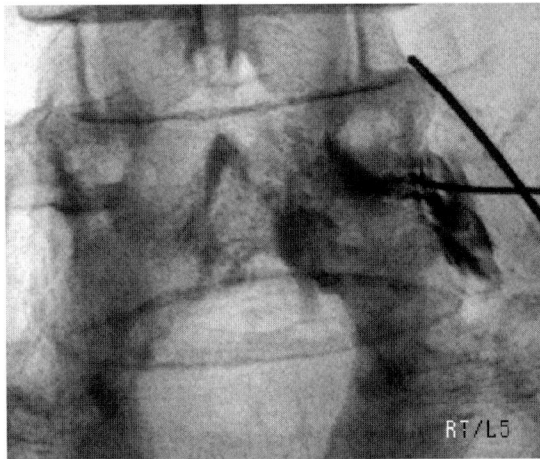

FIG. 88-2. Combined neurotomy and transforaminal epidural block. The patient 4 years post L4-S1 intertransverse fusion with continued unilateral low back and leg pain. Back pain is reduced by more than 50% following L2 and L3 (shown above) medial branch neurotomies performed at 6- to 12-month intervals. The patient's leg pain, which is secondary to L4 foraminal stenosis, is reduced following transforaminal epidural injections. The patient continues to work and does not want another surgery.

branch neurotomies to denervate the z-joints and intramuscular botulinum toxin injections to temporarily paralyze the paravertebral muscles. Both procedures are relatively benign, have an approximate duration of action of 6 and 3 months, respectively, and can be repeated. In those patients thought to have increased or abnormal segmental movement, a series of three to six injections of hypertonic solutions into the posterior compartment ligaments at 1- to 4-week intervals might be of benefit in increasing stability by promoting a proliferation of connective tissue.

In the middle column, transforaminal epidural blocks may help reduce inflammation and edema secondary to recurrent disc protrusions and spinal stenosis and thereby provide short-term pain reduction. Repeat sessions to mechanically lysis epidural adhesions using a fluoroscopically directed epidural catheter with or without direct visualization may help reduce pain in selected patients but is only weakly validated by a few authors. Pulsed radiofrequency treatments of the dorsal root ganglion is newly proposed and relatively benign method that theoretically reduces pain by exposing the dorsal root ganglion to an electrical field rather than radiofrequency-generated heat, but outcome studies are yet to be published. In contrast, "cool burns" of the dorsal root ganglion, although effective for some patients, carry a significant potential to amplify neuropathic pain and should be undertaken with caution.

Continued discogenic pain at the same or adjacent levels of surgery is a common source of early or late recurrence of anterior column pain. Surgical removal of the entire disc with interbody fusion is the definitive treatment option. Newer less invasive treatment options, including intradiscal heating, nucleoplasty, or both, may be considered when either the patient does not want another surgery or the number of adjacent painful levels would require excessive surgery. However, these procedures are more likely to be successful before surgical intervention and when the painful disc has limited annular disruption and a preserved disc height.

Pharmacologic management is the first step in treating central neuropathic pain. When medications are either ineffective or cause unacceptable side effects, implantable systems are available. Spinal cord stimulation is commonly performed to reduce neuropathic extremity pain, but reduction in axial pain is more difficult to achieve. Intrathecal implantable drug delivery systems are a last resort.

ACKNOWLEDGMENTS

We are very grateful to Janine Talty for her valuable suggestions for improving the chapter. We also thank Marina Kurgansky and Todd Bellicci, who worked on the text and prepared the manuscript for submission.

REFERENCES

1. Manchikanti L, Singh V, Cyrus E, et al. Interventional techniques in the management of chronic pain: Part 1. Pain Phys 2000;3(1):7–42.
2. Bogduk N. Practise guidelines and protocols: lumbar medial branch blocks. International Spinal Injection Society, 9th Annual Scientific Meeting. Orlando, FL, 2002.
3. Derby R. Lumbar algorithm with treatment guidelines. International Spinal Injection Society, 9th Annual Scientific Meeting. Orlando, FL, 2002.
4. Nachemson A. Advances in low-back pain. Clin Orthop 1985;200:266–278.
5. Nachemson A, Vingard E. Assessment of patients with neck and back pain: a best-evidence synthesis. In: Nachemson A, Johnsson E, eds. Neck and back pain: the scientific evidence of causes, diagnosis, and treatment. Philadelphia: Lippincott Williams & Wilkins, 2000:189–235.
6. Standards for the performance of seine injection procedures. http://www.spinalinjection.com/ISIS1/standard/stand1.htm
7. Bogduk N. Musculoskeletal pain: toward precision diagnosis. Progress in pain research and management. In: Jensen TS, Turner JA, Wiesenfeld-Hallin Z, eds. Proceeding of the 8th World Congress on Pain. Seattle: IASP Press, 1997:507–525.
8. Revel M, Poiraudeau S, Auleley GR, et al. Capacity of the clinical picture to characterize low back pain relieved by facet joint anesthesia. Proposed criteria to identify patients with painful facet joints. Spine 1998;23(18):1972–1976; discussion 1977.
9. Lord SM, Barnsley L, Bogduk N. The utility of comparative local anesthetic blocks versus placebo-controlled blocks for the diagnosis of cervical zygapophysial joint pain. Clin J Pain 1995;11(3):208–213.
10. Schwarzer AC, Aprill CN, Derby R, et al. Clinical features of patients with pain stemming from the lumbar zygapophysial joints. Is the lumbar facet syndrome a clinical entity? Spine 1994;19(10):1132–1137.
11. Schwarzer AC, Wang SC, Bogduk N, et al. Prevalence and clinical features of lumbar zygapophysial joint pain: a study in an Australian population with chronic low back pain. Ann Rheum Dis 1995;54(2):100–106.
12. Manchikanti L, Singh V, Pampati V, et al. Evaluation of the relative contributions of various structures in chronic low back pain. Pain Phys 2001;4(4):308–316.

13. Carette S, Marcoux S, Truchon R, et al. A controlled trial of corticosteroid injections into facet joints for chronic low back pain. N Engl J Med 1991;325:1002–1007.
14. Lilius G, Laasonen E, Myllynen P, et al. Lumbar facet join syndrome. A randomized clinical trial. J Bone Joint Surg (Br) 1989;71:681–684.
15. Carette S, Leclaire R, Marcoux S, et al. Epidural corticosteroid injections for sciatica due to herniated nucleus pulposus. N Engl J Med 1997;336(23):1634–1640.
16. Dreyfuss P, Schwarzer A, Lau P, et al. Specificity of lumbar median branch and L5 dorsal ramus blocks: a computed tomographic study. Spine 1997;22:895–902.
17. Dreyfus P, Halbrook B, Pauza K, et al. Efficacy and validity of radiofrequency neurotomy for chronic lumbar zygapophysial joint pain. Spine 2000;25:1270–1277.
18. van Kleef M, Barendse GA, Kessels A, et al. Randomized trial of radiofrequency lumbar facet denervation for chronic low back pain. Spine 1999;24(18):1937–1942.
19. Derby R. A prospective evaluation of medial branch neurotomy for zygapophyseal joint pain. North American Spine Society, 10th Annual Conference. Washington, DC, 1995.
20. Gedney E. Use of sclerosing solution may change therapy in vertebral disc problem. The osteopathic profession. 1952;19:11–13, 34–41.
21. Gedney E. Conservative management of recurring symptoms in postlaminectomy cases. The osteopathic profession. 1955;22:22–25, 45.
22. Barbor R. A treatment for chronic low back pain. IVth International Congress of Physical Medicine. Paris, 1964.
23. Schultz LW. A treatment for sublaxation of the temporomandibular joint. JAMA 1937;109(13):1032–1035.
24. Klein RG, Eek B, O'Neill C, et al. Biochemical injection treatment for discogenic low back pain: a pilot study. Spine J 2003;3:220–226.
25. Klein RG, Eek BC, DeLong WB, et al. A randomized double-blind trial of dextrose-glycerin-phenol injections for chronic, low back pain. J Spinal Disord 1993;6(1):23–33.
26. Dechow E, Davies RK, Carr AJ, et al. A randomized, double-blind, placebo-controlled trial of sclerosing injections in patients with chronic low back pain. Rheumatology 1999;38:1255–1259.
27. Ward AB. A summary of spasticity management: a treatment algorithm. Eur J Neurol 2002;9(1 Suppl):48–52.
28. Nowen A, Bush C. The relationship between paraspinal EMG and chronic low back pain. Pain 1984;20:109–123.
29. Foster L, Clapp L, Erickson M, et al. Botulinum toxin A and chronic low back pain: a randomized, double-blind study. Neurology 2001;56(10):1290–1293.
30. Jonsson B, Stromqvist B. Repeat decompression of lumbar nerve roots. A prospective two-year evaluation. J Bone Joint Surg Br 1993;75(6):894–897.
31. Loeser J, Bigos S, Fordyce W, et al. Low back pain. In: Bonica J, ed. The management of pain. Philadelphia: Lea & Febiger, 1990:1148–1183.
32. Serrao JM, Marks RL, Morley SJ, et al. Intrathecal midazolam for the treatment of chronic mechanical low back pain: a controlled comparison with epidural steroid in a pilot study. Pain 1992;48(1):5–12.
33. Papagelopoulos PJ, Petrou HG, Triantafyllidis PG, et al. Treatment of lumbosacral radicular pain with epidural steroid injections. Orthopedics 2001;24(2):145–149.
34. Abouleish E, Vega S, Blendinger I, et al. Long-term follow-up of epidural blood patch. Anesth Analg 1975;54(4):459–463.
35. Andrade S, Eckman E. Distribution of radiographic contrast media in the epidural space of normal human volunteers using a midline trans ligamentum flavum vs a selective epidural nerve canal injection technique. Int Spine Injection Soc Newsl 1992;1(4):6–8.
36. Andrade S, Eckman E, Yates G. The value of preliminary interlaminar epidurography during the performance of interlaminar epidural injections. Int Spine Injection Soc Newsl 1993;1(6):28–31.
37. Lutze M, Stendel R, Vesper J, et al. Periradicular therapy in lumbar radicular syndromes: methodology and results. Acta Neurochir 1997;139(8):719–724.
38. Lutz G, Vad V, Wisneski R. Fluoroscopic transforaminal lumbar epidural steroids: an outcome study. Arch Phys Med Rehabil 1998;79(11):1362–1366.
39. Weiner B, Fraser RD. Foraminal injection for lateral lumbar disc herniation. J Bone Joint Surg (Br) 1997;79(5):804–807.
40. Karppinen J, Ohinmaa A, Malmivaara A, et al. Cost effectiveness of periradicular infiltration for sciatica: subgroup analysis of a randomized controlled trial. Spine 2001;26(23):2587–2595.
41. Rydevik B, Holm S, Brown M, et al. Diffusion from the cerebrospinal fluid as a nutritional pathway for spinal nerve roots. Acta Physiol Scand 1990;138(2):247–248.
42. Derby R, Kine G, Saal J, et al. Response to steroid and duration of radicular pain as predictors of surgical outcome. Spine 1992;17(6S):S176–S183.
43. Annertz M, Jonsson B, Stromqvist B, et al. No relationship between epidural fibrosis and sciatica in the lumbar postdiscectomy syndrome. A study with contrast-enhanced magnetic resonance imaging in symptomatic and asymptomatic patients. Spine 1995;20(4):449–453.
44. Grane P, Tullberg T, Rydberg J, et al. Postoperative lumbar MR imaging with contrast enhancement. Comparison between symptomatic and asymptomatic patients. Acta Radiol 1996;37(3):366–372.
45. Cervellini PCD, Volpin L, Bernardi L, et al. Computed tomography of epidural fibrosis after discectomy: a comparison between symptomatic and asymptomatic patients. Neurosurgery 1988;23(6):710–713.
46. Coskun EST, Topuz O, Zencir M, et al. Relationships between epidural fibrosis, pain, disability, and psychological factors after lumbar disc surgery. Eur Spine J 2000;9(3):218–223.
47. Schofferman J, Anderson D, Hines R, et al. Childhood psychological trauma and chronic refractory low-back pain. Clin J Pain 1993;9(4):260–265.
48. Love AW, Peck CL. The MMPI and psychological factors in chronic low back pain: a review. Pain 1987;28(1):1–12.
49. Connally GH, Sanders SH. Predicting low back pain patients' response to lumbar sympathetic nerve blocks and interdisciplinary rehabilitation: the role of pretreatment overt pain behavior and cognitive coping strategies. Pain 1991;44(2):139–146.
50. Fordyce WE. Psychological factors in the failed back. Int Disabil Stud 1988;10(1):29–31.
51. Daniel JN, Polly DW Jr, Van Dam BE. A study of the efficacy of nonoperative treatment of presumed traumatic spondylolysis in a young patient population. Mil Med 1995;160(11):553–555.
52. Heavner J, Racz G, Raj P. Percutaneous epidural neuroplasty: prospective evaluation of 0.9% NaCl versus 10% NaCl with or without hyaluronidase. Reg Anesth Pain Manag 1999;24(3):202–207.
53. Devulder J, Deene M, De Laat M, et al. Nerve root sleeve injections in patients with failed back surgery syndrome: a comparison of three solutions. Clin J Pain 1999;15(2):132–135.
54. Revel M, Auleley G, Alaoui S, et al. Forceful epidural injections for the treatment of lumbosciatic pain with post-operative lumbar spinal fibrosis. Rev Rhum Engl Ed 1996;63(4):270–277.
55. Meadeb JRS, Duquesnoy B, Kuntz JL, et al. Forceful sacrococcygeal injections in the treatment of postdiscectomy sciatica. A controlled study versus glucocorticoid injections. Joint Bone Spine 2001;68(1):43–49.
56. Racz GB, Holubec JT. Lysis of adhesions in the epidural space. In: Racz GB, ed. Techniques of neurolysis. Boston: Kluwer Academic, 1989:57–72.
57. Manchikanti L, Pakanati R, Bakhit C, et al. Role of adhesiolysis and hypertonic saline neurolysis in management of low back pain. Evaluation of modification of Racz protocol. Pain Digest 1999;9:91–96.
58. Hammer M, Doleys DM, Chung OY. Transforaminal ventral epidural adhesiolysis. Pain Phys 2001;4(3):273–279.
59. Richardson J, McGurgan S, Cheema, et al. Spinal endoscopy in chronic low back pain with radiculopathy. A prospective case series. Anaesthesia 2001;56(5):454–460.
60. Manchikanti L, Bakhit C. Percutaneous lysis of epidural adhesions. Pain Phys 2000;3(1):46–64.
61. Manchikanti L, Pampati V, Fellows M, et al. Effectiveness of percutaneous adhesiolysis with hypertonic saline neurolysis in refractory spinal stenosis. Pain Phys 2001;4(4):366–373.
62. Riew K, Yin Y, Gilula L, et al. The effect of nerve-root injections on the need for operative treatment of lumbar radicular pain. A prospective, randomized, controlled, double-blind study. J Bone Joint Surg Am 2000;82-A(11):1589–1593.
63. Bush K, Hillier S. A controlled study of caudal epidural injections of triamcinolone plus procaine for the management of intractable sciatica. Spine 1991;16(5):572–575.
64. Schmid G, Vetter S, Gottmann D, et al. CT-guided epidural/perineural injections in painful disorders of the lumbar spine: short- and extended-term results. Cardiovasc Intervent Radiol 1999;22(6):493–498.

65. Wetzel F, Phillips F, Aprill C, et al. Extradural sensory rhizotomy in the management of chronic lumbar radiculopathy: a minimum 2-year follow-up study. Spine 1997;22(19):2283–2291; discussion 2291–2292.

66. Sluijter ME, Mehta M. Treatment of chronic back and neck pain by percutaneous thermal lesions. In: Lipton S, Miles J, eds. Persistent pain, modern methods of treatment. London, Toronto, Sydney: Academic Press, 1981:141–179.

67. Geurts JW, van Wijk RM, Stolker RJ, et al. Efficacy of radiofrequency procedures for the treatment of spinal pain: a systematic review of randomized clinical trials. Reg Anesthesiol Pain Med 2001;26(5): 394–400.

68. van Kleef M, Liem L, Lousberg R, et al. Radiofrequency lesion adjacent to the dorsal root ganglion for cervicobrachial pain: a prospective double blind randomized study. Neurosurgery 1996;38(6): 1127–1131; discussion 1131–1132.

69. van Wijk RM, Geurts JW, Wynne HJ. Long-lasting analgesic effect of radiofrequency treatment of the lumbosacral dorsal root ganglion. J Neurosurg 2001;94(2 Suppl):227–231.

70. Wright RE, Howell A. Medial brunch neurotomy for lumbar facet denervation in clinical practice. International Spine Injection Society 5th Annual Meeting. Denver, 1997.

71. de Louw AJ, Vles HS, Freling G, et al. The morphological effects of a radio frequency lesion adjacent to the dorsal root ganglion (RF-DRG)—an experimental study in the goat. Eur J Pain 2001;5(2): 169–174.

72. Sluijter M. Radiofrequency part 1: the lumbosacral region. Amsterdam: Spinhex & Industrie, 2001.

73. Slappendel R, Crul BJ, Braak GJ, et al. The efficacy of radiofrequency lesioning of the cervical spinal dorsal root ganglion in a double blinded randomized study: no difference between 40 degrees C and 67 degrees C treatments. Pain 1997;73(2):159–163.

74. North R, Roark G. Spinal cord stimulation for chronic pain. Neurosurg Clin North Am 1995;6:45–61.

75. Soldati E. National Italian register of implantable systems for spinal cord stimulation (SCS): analysis of preliminary data. Neuromodulation 2002;5(1):5–15.

76. Fiume D, Sherkat S, Callovini G, et al. Treatment of the failed back surgery syndrome due to lumbo-sacral epidural fibrosis. Acta Neurochir Suppl (Wien) 1995;64:116–118.

77. Schwarzer AC, Bogduk N. In response: letters. Spine 1996;21: 776–777.

78. Keskimäki I, Seitsalo S, Österman H, et al. Reoperations after lumbar disc surgery: a population-based study of regional and interspecialty variations, point of view. Spine 2000;25:1500–1508.

79. Derby R, Howard M, Grant J, et al. The ability of pressure controlled discography to predict surgical and non-surgical outcomes. Spine 1999;24(4):364–371.

80. Freemont AJ, et al. Nerve ingrowth into diseased intervertebral disc in chronic back pain. Lancet 1997;350(9072):178–181.

81. Coppes MH, Marani E, Thomeer RTWM, et al. Innervation of "painful" lumbar discs. Spine 1997;22:2342–2349.

82. Bogduk N, April C, Derby R. Discography. In: White A, Schofferman A, eds. Spine care. Diagnosis and conservative treatment. St. Louis: Mosby, 1995:219–236.

83. Carragee EJ, Chen Y, Tanner CM, et al. Provocative discography in patients after limited lumbar discectomy. Spine 2000;25:3065–3071.

84. Simmons ED, Simmons EH. Spinal stenosis with scoliosis. Spine 1992;17(6 Suppl):S117–1120.

85. Schellhas K. Epidurography and therapeutic epidural anesthetic and steroid injections. Int Spine Injection Soc Newsl 1992;1(4):3.

86. Mooney V, Klein RG. Intradiscal proliferant therapy. In: Corbin T, et al, eds. Advanced spine surgical technologies. St. Louis: Quality Medical Publishing, in press.

87. van Kleef M, Spaans F, Dingemans W, et al. Effects and side effects of a percutaneous thermal lesion of the dorsal root ganglion in patients with cervical pain syndrome. Pain 1993;52(1):49–53.

88. Derby R, Eek B, Ryan DP. Intradiscal electrothermal annuloplasty. Sci Newsl Int Spinal Injection Soc 1998;3(1).

89. Shadid E, Kazala K, O'Neill C, et al. An independent assessment of the one to two year clinical outcomes of intradiscal electrothermal anuloplasty (IDET) for discogenic low back pain. ISIS 9th Annual Scientific Meeting. Orlando, FL, 2002.

90. Mayer HM. Discogenic low back pain and degenerative lumbar spinal stenosis: how appropriate is surgical treatment? Schmerz 2001;15(6): 484–491.

91. Saal JA, Saal JS. Intradiscal electrothermal treatment for chronic discogenic low back pain: a prospective outcome study with minimum 1-year follow-up. Spine 2000;25(20):2622–2627.

92. Sharps LS, Issac Z. Percutaneous disc decompression using nucleoplasty. Pain Phys 2002;5(2):121–126.

93. Sindrup SH, Jensen TS. Efficacy of pharmacological treatments of neuropathic pain: an update and effect related to mechanism of drug action. Pain 1999;83(3):389–400.

94. Aldrete JA. Extended epidural catheter infusion with analgesic for patients with noncancer pain at their homes. Reg Anesth 1997;22:35–42.

95. Fredman B, Zohar E, Nun MB, et al. The effect of repeated epidural sympathetic nerve block on "failed back surgery syndrome" associated chronic low back pain. J Clin Anesthesiol 1999;11(1):46–51.

96. Gyermek L. Pharmacology of serotonin as related to anesthesia. J Clin Anesthesiol 1996;8(5):402–425.

97. Ceccherelli F, Diani MM, Altafini L, et al. Postoperative pain treated by intravenous L-tryptophan: a double-blind study versus placebo in cholecystectomized patients. Pain 1991;47(2):163–172.

98. Tremont-Lukats IW, Megeff C, Backonja MM. Anticonvulsants for neuropathic pain syndromes: mechanisms of action and place in therapy. Drugs 2000;60:1029–1052.

99. Field MJ, Hughes J, Singh L. Further evidence for the role of the alpha(2)delta subunit of voltage dependent calcium channels in models of neuropathic pain. Br J Pharmacol 2000;131(2):282–286.

100. Rosner H, Rubin L, Kestenbaum A. Gabapentin adjunctive therapy in neuropathic pain states. Clin J Pain 1996;12(1):56–58.

101. Hays H, Woodroffe MA. Using gabapentin to treat neuropathic pain. Can Fam Phys 1999;45:2109–21112.

102. Eckhardt K, Ammon S, Hofmann U. et al. Gabapentin enhances the analgesic effect of morphine in healthy volunteers. Anesthesiol Analges 2000;91(1):185–191.

103. Braverman DL, Slipman CW, Lenrow DA. Using gabapentin to treat failed back surgery syndrome caused by epidural fibrosis: a report of 2 cases. Arch Phys Med Rehabil 2001;82:691–693.

104. Passik SD, Whitcomb LA, Dodd S, et al. Pain outcomes in long-term treatment with opioids: preliminary results with a newly developed physician checklist. Annual Meeting of the American Association of Pain Management. San Francisco, 2002.

105. Manchikanti L, Pampati V, Damron KS, et al. Prevalence of opioid abuse in interventional pain medicine practice settings: a randomized clinical evaluation. Pain Phys 2001;4(4):358–365.

106. Schofferman J. Long-term opioid analgesic therapy for severe refractory lumbar spine pain. Clin J Pain 1999;15(2):136–140.

107. Fishbain DA, Rosomoff HI, Rosomoff RS. Drug abuse, dependence and addiction in chronic pain patients. Clin J Pain 1992;(8):77–85.

108. Foley KM. Controversies in cancer pain. Medical perspectives. Cancer 1989;63(11 Suppl):2257–2265.

109. Neuburger O, Aels A, Boggan J, et al. The painful dilemma: the use of narcotics for the treatment of chronic pain. http://mojo.calyx. net/schaffer/asap/dilemma.html, 1990.

110. South SM, Smith MT. Analgesic tolerance to opioids. Pain Clin Updates 2001;9(5):1–4.

111. Doverty M, Somogyi AA, White JM, et al. Methadone maintenance patients are cross-tolerant to the antinociceptive effects of morphine. Pain 2001;93(2):155–163.

112. Doverty M, White JM, Somogyi AA, et al. Hyperalgesic responses in methadone maintenance patients. Pain 2001;90(1–2):91–96.

113. Mao J. NMDA and opioid receptors: their interactions in antinociception, tolerance and neuroplasticity. Brain Res Brain Res Rev 1999;30 (3):289–304.

114. Portenoy R. Opioid therapy for nonmalignant pain. In: Fields HL, Liebeskind JC, eds. Pharmacological approach to the treatment of chronic pain: new concept and critical issues. Seattle: IASP Press, 1994.

115. Sjoberg M, Appelgren L, Einarsson S, et al. Long-term intrathecal morphine and bupivacaine in "refractory" cancer pain. I. Results from the first series of 52 patients. Acta Anaesthesiol Scand 1991;35(1):30–43.

116. Angel IF, Gould HJ Jr, Carey ME. Intrathecal morphine pump as a treatment option in chronic pain of nonmalignant origin. Surg Neurol 1998;49(1):92–98; discussion 98–99.

117. de Lissovoy G, Brown RE, Halpern M, et al. Cost-effectiveness of long-term intrathecal morphine therapy for pain associated with failed back surgery syndrome. Clin Ther 1997;19(1):96–112; discussion 84–85.

118. Harvey SC, O'Neil MG, Pope CA, et al. Continuous intrathecal meperidine via an implantable infusion pump for chronic, nonmalignant pain. Ann Pharmacother 1997;31(11):1306–1308.

CHAPTER 89

Psychological Approaches to the Management of Failed Surgery and Revision Surgery

Robert J. Gatchel and Chris J. Main

^Today, low back pain (LBP) is a pervasive medical problem in industrialized countries. In addition to the pain and emotional suffering that LBP patients experience, LBP presents enormous costs to society. Such costs include lost earnings, decreased productivity, and increased health care utilization expenses in disability benefits. For example, studies have calculated the annual cost of chronic LBP in the United States alone to be between $20 and $60 billion when measures such as lost productivity and social disability insurance benefits were calculated, along with treatment costs (1). Gevirtz et al. (2) have indicated that 80% of Americans suffer back pain at some point in their lives, and about 18% develop chronic LBP disability. Indeed, chronic LBP is the chief cause of disability in people under age 45. Moreover, following an initial episode of LBP, relapses are reported to be 30% to 70% of patients sampled (3).

Thus, as is apparent, the costs of LBP can be viewed in terms of costs to the individual and society. As far as the individual is concerned, costs include both pain-associated suffering and limitations. Suffering can range from mild discomfort to associated distress triggering suicidal ideation, and (rarely) suicide. Pain-associated limitations can include impact on activities of daily living, personal relationships, and work. Most LBP resolves spontaneously or with early focused interventions such as manipulation. Most such treatment, or indeed the passage of time, is successful, although recurrences are to be expected. In the presence of red flags (4), early surgery should be considered; but unless there are clear and equivocal surgical indications, surgery is usually considered only after failed conservative treatment. The problem then may become chronic, and carry with it the psychosocial "baggage" characteristic of the chronic pain patient. Of course, sometimes surgery is successful, but sometimes it is not so, and the costs of failed low back

surgery is considerable to both the individual patient and society as a whole.

Spine surgery is the next line of medical care when conservative treatment for LBP fails. Of course, whenever surgery is performed, there is always the possibility of complications or failure. Fortunately, necessary spine surgery is often successful when performed by an experienced spine surgeon. However, spine surgery has become a controversial area because of the high cost, frequent use, and some research suggesting limited effectiveness. For example, earlier studies focused attention on the complications and perceived poor outcomes of spine fusion surgery, particularly in the lumbar region (5,6). Discectomy, which is usually performed earlier than fusion after symptom onset, is often viewed to be less invasive or controversial. However, although short-term pain relief and improvement in vocational status appear to be supported, reoperations are often common, with rates as high as 17% to 20% reported in early studies (7,8). Nevertheless, more recent studies have suggested that spine surgery is cost effective, and it can lead to significant improvement in lifestyle. For example, Atlas et al. (9) conducted a 4-year follow-up study of patients with lumbar spinal stenosis and found that those treated surgically (primarily with a decompression laminectomy) had significantly less back and leg pain and greater satisfaction than those treated nonsurgically. Moreover, Malter et al. (10) reported that quality of life for patients with herniated lumbar discs, operated on with discectomy, were significantly greater than that of patients treated conservatively for up to 5 years. In addition, the cost effectiveness of the discectomy was found in this study to be significantly greater than that for such procedures as coronary artery bypass grafting for single-artery disease, and greater than medical therapy for moderate hypertension.

PREVALENCE OF LOW BACK SURGERY

There are wide differences in surgery rates for LBP among countries. It has been estimated by Waddell (11), derived from data by Cherkin et al. (12), that surgical rates in Europe and Australia (in comparison with the United States) are between one third and two thirds (although there is a fivefold difference between the United Kingdom and the United States). This is seen most clearly in a direct comparison of rates of spinal fusion (13). The reasons for this are not entirely clear, because presumably there are not major differences in surgically remediable pathology. The fact that there are even greater differences in back surgery rates *within* the United States suggests that differences are probably influenced also by a range of factors such as access to surgery (in terms of third-party coverage), differences in selection for surgery, and willingness to undergo surgery. A clear majority of patients appear to be satisfied with surgery (14). Early studies (15,16) estimated a success rate for surgery of 65% to 75%; even though later studies have been somewhat optimistic, they estimated an average failure rate of only 15% (17) and 10% (18). Given that approximately 192,000 patients with chronic intractable back pain undergo spinal fusion each year (19), there are still a significant number of surgical failures, with a reoperation rate of 10% for discectomy (15), and 23% for spinal fusion (16). Surgical enthusiasts argue that improvements in surgical technique (including instrumentation) permit a wider range of surgical options and, indeed, surgical rates are increasing; but this increase in surgical intervention does not appear to have been matched by a corresponding improvement in surgical outcome (20).

Poor surgical outcome is costly not only to the individual and his or her family, but also to society. In all studies of LBP, 10% to 15% of patients account for 80% to 90% of the total health care consumption and costs for spinal disorders, and the 1% to 2% who undergo surgery are the most expensive group (21). Furthermore, a recent comparison of societal costs of LBP in various countries has shown that *indirect* costs, in terms of sickness benefits and lost productivity, were considerably greater than *direct* health care costs (22). Clearly it is important, therefore, to consider the determinants of poor surgical outcome. In attempting to address this problem, it is necessary to appraise the evidence concerning the predictors of surgical outcome in general and of poor surgical outcome in particular.

CONSEQUENCES OF FAILED SURGERY

Of course, spine surgery is certainly not a panacea for all patients. In a comprehensive review of all lumbar discectomies conducted up to the time of their publication, Hoffman et al. (15) reported that the mean success rate

was 67%. Likewise, in reviewing all research on spinal fusion, Turner et al. (16) reported a successful clinical outcome obtained in 65% to 75% of patients, with success rates lower the more levels fused, and generally the more invasive the procedure. Subsequently, Franklin et al. (23) reported that 68% of workers compensation patients who underwent lumbar fusion, were work disabled and 23% required additional lumbar spine surgery 2 years postfusion. These results, therefore, highlight the fact that spine surgical success is not guaranteed. It should also be kept in mind that the way one determines surgical success or failure can be quite variable. We discuss this issue later in this chapter. Nevertheless, spinal surgeons are quite aware of the consequences of FBSS.

Oaklander and North (24) define FBSS as persistent or recurrent chronic pain after one or more surgical procedures on the lumbosacral spine. Unfortunately, as noted, this syndrome is much more common than desired. The surgeon many times becomes "wedded" to these failed back surgery patients. Some of the frustrations and demands subsequently encountered by the surgeon include the following:

- The patient may make increasing demands on the surgeon for pain relief. The surgeon, in turn, feels a strong sense of responsibility to provide relief when the surgery has been ineffective.
- The patient may become increasingly angry with the surgeon because of the failed surgery and, perhaps, litigious.
- Pain medication use by the patient often escalates, thus increasing chances of dependence or addiction. Patients often overuse medication and demand refills before the designated time.
- In an attempt to provide relief, the surgeon may order additional conservative treatments that have little chance of success, thereby increasing length and cost of the case. Moreover, patients may decide to additionally undergo increasingly invasive surgery, with subsequent opportunities for infection, instrumentation failure, or other iatrogenic complications. Unfortunately, the probability of successful outcome significantly decreases with each spine surgery.
- The probability of reducing pain and returning the patient back to work decreases as length of disability increases. Because failed back surgery lengthens the period of disability, these patients are less likely to ever recover. Thus, the total cost of the initial injury dramatically increases because of direct treatment and surgeries plus resultant disability income benefits.
- Finally, there may be financial incentives to remain disabled that far outweigh incentives for recovery.

Thus, the spine surgeon is often faced with a conundrum. The surgeon feels obligated to the patient but, at the same time, becomes frustrated and the target of the patient's distress. The intervention subsequently proposed often becomes more invasive, but the outcomes are less satisfactory. For example, a failed simple laminectomy or discectomy is frequently followed by a much more extensive fusion (perhaps with instrumentation), leading to greater opportunity for failure. Indeed, many studies concur with the conclusion made by Waddell (25) that the probability of a successful spine surgery outcome leading to pain relief decreases significantly with each successive procedure. For example, in an early study, Pheasant et al. (26) reported that patients who had multiple surgeries had a lower probability of obtaining a good outcome than did patients who only had a single surgery. North et al. (27) also suggest that the long-term success rate in reoperated patients is approximately one third. The only solution to this conundrum is better methods to prescreen patients before surgery in order to eliminate those who have a poor probability of success.

HOW DOES ONE DETERMINE SURGICAL SUCCESS OR FAILURE?

It should be kept in mind that when one talks about surgical outcome, its assessment is not a straightforward matter. Of course, the most straightforward fashion to determine surgical success is the determination of whether the identified pathology was corrected. Unfortunately, however, patients frequently fail to experience or report any symptomatic improvement despite excellent surgical correction because of the biopsychosocial nature of pain. Therefore, a determination of surgical success requires the evaluation of major areas in which the back pain patient's life is affected, such as activities of daily living and socioeconomic outcomes such as return to work and decrease in health care use. In the past, the great majority of studies on spine surgery have used some variation of the criteria proposed by Stauffer and Coventry (28) to assess outcome. These criteria evaluate outcome in terms of reduced pain sensation, job impairment, use of narcotic medications, and improvement in functional activity. For example, Trief et al. (29) evaluated the percent of patients reporting improvement in back and leg pain, the percent working, and functional disability status using the Dallas Back Pain Questionnaire. More recently, Klekamp et al. (30) have suggested a modification of the original Stauffer and Coventry (28) outcome criteria, which is somewhat more comprehensive in nature. These criteria are listed in Table 89-1.

As can be seen, these criteria appear to capture the major life areas affected by chronic pain. However, there are many gray areas in terms of ratings. For example, what is the precise definition of "infrequent" use of analgesics? Moreover, under the good outcome category, what if a patient meets three of the four criteria? Thus, as can be seen, there may not be any definitive and totally objective criteria that are generic enough to capture success or failure in all patients. In appreciation of the difficulties involved in defining success or failure, it should be kept in mind that, whenever evaluating spine surgical outcome results, no totally accepted criteria are consistently used across all studies.

Problems in Evaluation of Outcome

The nature of pain, chronic pain in particular, is complex. Surgery is directed primarily at the correction or remediation of some sort of surgical lesion. According to Waddell (11), much current orthopedic practice derives from the discovery of the "ruptured disc" as a cause for sciatica by Mixter and Barr (31), and apparently the first surgeons made the diagnosis on hard neurologic signs; although, their successors came to rely much more on symptoms, and the diagnosis of discogenic back pain became established. It was argued further that, if sciatica was caused by disc prolapse, then LBP might be caused by disc degeneration. Surgery such as lumbar fusion was offered for LBP, and outcome was evaluated in terms of the technical success of the procedure, such as stabilizing the spine and avoidance of complications. It was assumed that surgical intervention would improve (if not abolish) pain, restore function, and facilitate return to work. It became clear that, in a number of patients, not only did surgical success not guarantee improvement in pain, function, and work compromise, but also that evaluation of success simply in terms of surgical parameters was inadequate as a single outcome measure.

Evaluation of success or failure is made difficult also because there are various stake holders. Prior to the advent of managed care and outcome-related funding, outcome was evaluated primarily by the success of the surgery in correction (or amelioration) of structural abnormality, and the avoidance of complications thereafter. Outcome was determined primarily, therefore, by the surgeon's appraisal of the technical success of the operation. However, the move to patient-centered out-

TABLE 89.1. *Criteria for spine surgery outcome*

	Pain relief	Employment	Activities	Analgesics
Good	Most (76%–100%)	No limits	No limits	Infrequently
Fair	Partial (26%–75%)	Lighter work	Limited	Occasionally
Poor	Little to none	Disabled	Greatly limited	Frequently

Source: Adapted from Klekamp J, McCarty E, Spengler D. Results of elective lumbar discectomy for patients involved in the workers' compensation system. J Spin Disord 1998;11:277–282, with permission.

come in terms of pain and function complicated the picture, because technical success was not always accompanied by commensurate improvement in pain and function. The advent of managed care and outcome-related health care funding has led to the incorporation of economic and occupational outcomes (e.g., change in benefit status or rate of return to work), thus complicating the picture still further. The issue is of more than academic importance. Rates of success or failure of surgery can only be accurately compared where there are a clear assessment of indication of surgery, a clear description of the surgical intervention, and comparable outcome measures.

Types of Outcome Assessment

There are two principal types of outcome appraisal: clinical appraisal of the individual and aggregated data on efficacy of treatment (usually for audit or research purposes). The principal domains are shown in Table 89-2.

Implicit in the surgical view of intervention is the assumption that correction of the physical abnormality will produce a commensurate improvement in pain and function. There are undoubtedly many patients in whom global improvement is achieved; however, in a significant minority of patients there is a residual degree of pain or pain-associated incapacity despite surgical "success." The lack of a direct correspondence between physical impairment and pain severity requires a broadening of the discogenic model of pain. Indeed, there is a similar dis-

cordance among pain, functional disability, and work loss (11). Explaining outcome necessitates an understanding of its determinants and, as far as functional disability and work are concerned, a broader model of illness is required than the narrow pathology-based model. The biopsychosocial model of LBP disability (32), drawing inspiration from Loeser's earlier pain model (33), and its several later derivatives (25,34), offers a different way of understanding pain-associated disability. If indeed pain-associated disability is multifactorial, then so perhaps are the determinants of disability and (conversely) the obstacles to successful recovery. A wider perspective on outcome is needed.

Outcome Assessment

The need for a variety of outcome measures has been increasingly recognized. According to Bombardier (35): "Clinical success in the treatment of spinal disorders has traditionally been measured in terms of morbidity, physiologic changes (e.g., nerve conduction) or improvement in physical findings (e.g. weakness). More recently, outcome measures have been introduced that take into account the patients' self-report of their physical function and health" (p. 3,097). She points out that the use of outcome measures is relatively new, and that "several areas still remain controversial such as the need for and choice of utility measures, which concept of satisfaction should be used, or how to measure reduced work-productivity" (p. 3,098). She offers a set of key questions to ask about an outcome measure, as presented in Table 89-3.

TABLE 89.2. *Outcome evaluation: examples of important domains*

Posttreatment clinical domains
  Surgical: technical success
  Surgical: absence of complications
  Pain
  Self-rated interference
    Self-reported disability
    Clinical appraisal
    Behavioral observation
  Psychological
    Beliefs and fears
    Emotional responses
    Coping strategies
  Patient satisfaction
Maintenance and follow-up
  Relapse
  Length of follow-up
Occupational domains
  Time to return to work
  Work performance
  Further sick leave
Cost-effectiveness
  Costs of treatment
    Further health care use
  Disability/benefit saving
    Reduction in presenteeism
    Reduction in absenteeism

TABLE 89.3. *Key questions to ask about an outcome measure*

Content, population/setting, purpose
  Which outcomes do you want to measure?
  Which population will you be studying and in what setting?
  What is the purpose of your study: to describe, or predict or to measure change?
Content validity
  What domains and items are included? Are there important omissions or inappropriate conclusions?
Face validity
  Is each question phrased in a suitable way?
  Are the response categories appropriate?
  Is there an overall score summarizing across questions? How is it calculated?
Feasibility
  Is it easy to understand?
  Is it easy to use (i.e., clear instruction manual)?
  Is it acceptable?
  What format is available (self-administered, telephone, interviewer-administered)?
  How long does it take to administer?

Source: Adapted from Bombardier C. Spine Focus Issue Introduction. Outcome assessments in the evaluation and treatment of spinal disorders. Spine 2000;25:3097–3099, with permission.

Implications of the Need for Broad-Based Outcomes

Consideration of outcomes from a wide range of perspectives has a number of implications for clinical practice in general, and the evaluation of surgery in particular. There are important implications for clinical decision making. As has been stated, a majority of patients appear to be satisfied with surgery. Nonetheless, there is a significant minority dissatisfied to a greater or lesser extent, and outcome of surgery is coming under increasing scrutiny (36). It used to be argued that surgical intervention is designed to correct a physical abnormality, and that all that can reasonably be asked from a surgical intervention is correction of that abnormality. Outcome assessment was confined to evaluation of technical success (e.g., in stability of fusion or whether or not complications such as instability or infection resulted). Outcome evaluation in terms of physical signs seems to be relatively straightforward, at least from the conceptual point of view. However, most patients seek treatment as a consequence of painful symptoms or pain-associated limitations in function and, unfortunately, technical surgical success guarantees neither cure of pain, complete restoration of function, work retention, nor return to work, even in the treatment of sciatica, which usually is considered to be a better bet for surgery for low back pain (37). Such considerations have important implications for clinical decision making, and require reconsideration of the nature of pain-associated disability and outcome of treatment. Of the many factors that have been examined, psychological factors appear to be particularly important.

Influence of Psychosocial Factors on Outcome

A number of studies have demonstrated a relationship between psychosocial factors and outcome of surgery. The influence of preexisting or coexisting psychological vulnerability was investigated in a number of early studies (38–40). More recently, in a series of related Scandinavian papers, Graver et al. demonstrated a positive relationship between preoperative psychological distress after lumbar disc surgery, both at 1- and 7-year follow-up (41,42). The precise psychological mechanisms, however, are not entirely clear. Psychological variables influence postoperative anxiety and physical complaints (43). The results concerning postoperative functional disability are inconsistent. Some studies (29,44) have found a positive association between psychological factors and functional disability at outcome, whereas others (18) have failed to demonstrate an association. This may be a consequence of differences in patient selection, whether in terms of screening out patients with positive psychological features, or in terms of better physical indications for surgery (45). A clear association has been found between psychological factors and return to work (29,46). In one of the few predictive studies attempting to disentangle the vari-

ous sorts of psychological factors on return to work after surgery, Schade et al. (46) found that return to work 2 years after surgery was influenced not by clinical findings, such as magnetic resonance imaging (MRI)–identified abnormalities, but by depression and psychosocial aspects of work. This finding is consistent with recent primary care perspectives on secondary prevention of back pain disability, in which early attention to the psychosocial aspects of pain-associated disability is recommended (47). More recent consideration of obstacles to recovery, with differentiation of these yellow flags, focuses on patients' beliefs about pain, disability and treatment, and occupationally focused blue and black flags (48). The blue flags have their origin in the stress literature. They are perceived features of work that generally are associated with higher rates of symptoms, ill health, and work loss (49), which, in the context of injury, may delay recovery or constitute a major obstacle to it. They are characterized by features such as high demand or low control, unhelpful management style, poor social support from colleagues, perceived time pressure, and lack of job satisfaction. Individual workers may differ in their perception of the same working environment. According to Bigos et al. (50), perception may be more important than the objective characteristics because, "Once an individual is off work, perception about symptoms, about the safety of return to work, and about impact of return to work on one's personal life can affect recovery even in the most well-meaning worker" (50). It should be emphasized that blue flags incorporate not only issues related to the perception of job characteristics such as job demand, but also perception of social interactions (whether with management or fellow workers). Black flags are *not* a matter of perception, and affect all workers equally. They include both nationally established policy concerning conditions of employment and sickness policy, and working conditions specific to a particular organization.

Because psychosocial factors seem to have such a powerful influence on outcome, appraisal of such features needs to become an integral aspect of patient evaluation. Many clinics now undertake some sort of presurgical screening or psychological evaluation prior to surgery.

PRESURGICAL SCREENING

Presurgical psychological evaluation is carried out for a number of reasons, illustrated in Table 89-4.

TABLE 89.4. *Purposes of presurgical psychological evaluation*

Identifying contraindications; consider legitimacy and ethics of this
For prior psychological intervention
For conjoint psychological therapy
To flag for postsurgical psychological management

Identification of Contraindications to Surgery

The costs of surgical failure are considerable, both in terms of financial cost and human suffering. Factors such as distress, unrealistic expectations of outcome, and maladaptive coping strategies are all associated with poor outcome, and a case could be made for simply denying surgery to any patients demonstrating such features. Certainly, such a strategy would improve overall surgical success rates. However, there are two major ethical concerns. First, although adverse psychological factors have been demonstrated among groups of patients, the strength of the relationships with outcome is not sufficiently strong to enable accurate prediction in the individual case. Second, denial of surgery in the presence of good *surgical* indications is regarded by some as an abrogation of clinical responsibility. It might reasonably be argued that surgery is a necessary but not sufficient intervention to produce satisfactory outcome in such patients.

Prior Psychological Intervention

Coping with surgery requires a certain degree of resilience and, in some patients, a degree of prior psychological preparation may be necessary, with therapy focused on emotional support, the establishment of appropriate and realistic expectations, and the development of effective coping strategies both before and after surgery. Block et al. (44) have presented methods for providing the following.

Conjoint Psychological Therapy

The opportunity for conjoint psychological therapy clearly is limited, but additional emotional support immediately before surgery or at the time of postsurgical recovery in patients who demonstrate high levels of anxiety about surgery itself or the anticipated sequelae is important.

Flag for Postsurgical Psychological Management

Patients with a nervous disposition, or poor pain coping skills and low pain tolerance prior to surgery, may not be psychologically oriented for postsurgical management and rehabilitation. Furthermore, it could be argued that *all* failed surgery patients should be considered for psychologically oriented pain management, if not individualized psychological therapy.

Nature of Screening Tools

Psychological screening, for whatever purpose, usually has involved administration of a self-report questionnaire, ranging from full-scale personality inventories (51) to fairly simple measures of distress (52). Recently, however, Block et al. (44) developed a specific screening tool, the Psychological Screening Scorecard (PPS), incorporating interview-based assessment of medical and psychological risk factors derived from the Minnesota Multiphasic Personality Inventory (MMPI) and the Coping Strategies Questionnaire (53). The instrument is imaginative and potentially useful, but requires further methodologic development, because the cutoffs for decision making are still not completely quantitative, and the actual sensitivity and specificity in terms of different sorts of outcomes (for whatever purpose) needs to be demonstrated. However, screening does not constitute a comprehensive clinical assessment, and should not be confused with such.

RISK FACTORS AND OBSTACLES TO RECOVERY

Main (48) has recommended a conceptual shift from *risks* to *obstacles to recovery*. It is possible to take a narrow or a broad view of obstacles to recovery. It may be helpful to base prevention not on risk as such, but to refocus attention on obstacles to recovery, which can be considered either in terms of contraindications to surgery, potential targets for adjunctive psychologically oriented pain management (54), or a functional rehabilitation approach (55). Because surgery is directed first and foremost at correction of physical abnormality, it is perhaps not surprising that good surgical outcome is associated with better surgical indications (45). However, according to Mayer et al. (55): "poor surgical outcomes may result from outmoded postoperative methods, rather than failures of patient selection or surgical technique"; and, according to Polatin et al. (56), "surgery may correct the anatomic dysfunction, but subsequent recovery and return to productivity will be governed by non-surgical factors." Again, Block et al. (44) reviewed the importance of postsurgical rehabilitation in producing good clinical outcomes.

SOME PRELIMINARY CONCLUSIONS

In designing a successful clinical intervention in the context of failed surgery, we need to be mindful of lessons learned about the nature of pain-associated disability in terms of its development and prevention. The advent of third-party professional practice audits requires a broader perspective on outcomes. In the case of the failed surgery patient, consideration of further treatment needs to incorporate a biopsychosocial rather than a biomedical perspective. The need for a systems approach, involving all key stake holders, is now recognized, particularly in connection with intended occupational outcomes. However, even good clinical outcome does not guarantee return to work. Comprehensive pain management programs and functional restoration programs include an occupational component. However, certain aspects of work can only be tackled in the actual work place. Successful occupation outcomes may require specific work place interventions, such as phased return to work or transient work adaptations.

In patients who have already failed surgery, iatrogenic misunderstanding and distress may be particularly important features in their overall clinical presentation. Therefore, if the patient is considered to require both surgery and pain management, it is necessary to establish a clinically led systems approach involving all key stake holders in planning the scheduling of different treatment components, and in enlisting the patient's full understanding and cooperation.

CONCLUDING REFLECTIONS (KEY POINTS)

1. Outcome of surgery is dependent both on the nature of the physical indications for surgery and the patient's psychological reaction to pain and pain-associated limitation in function. This is true for first-time surgery and probably even more so for repeat surgery.
2. Outcome can be considered from a number of perspectives.
3. There may be a lack of concordance between different sorts of outcomes and among different stake holders.
4. Patients with poor outcome of surgery are likely to require psychologically oriented pain management. Consideration may have to be given to presurgical preparatory pain management as well as psychologically oriented postsurgical rehabilitation.
5. Arguably, surgery represents the most powerful example of the "bio" part of biopsychosocial intervention. Achieving optimal outcome requires not only clear surgical indications, but also addressing the psychosocial aspects of the patient's pain and pain-associated disability, both at the time of initial assessment and in the entire treatment that may be necessary to achieve satisfactory outcome.
6. Although such methodologic considerations are a critical component in research design, often a more pragmatic approach to outcome has been adopted, and the issue of choosing outcomes becomes the prime focus of concern. A focus group of spinal researchers (57) recommended five key domains for outcome assessment in spinal disorders:
   • Back-specific function
   • Generic health status
   • Pain
   • Work disability
   • Satisfaction (back-specific)

ACKNOWLEDGMENT

This work was supported in part by grant numbers 2K02-MH1107, 2R01-MH46452, and 2R01-DE010713 from the National Institutes of Health.

REFERENCES

1. Gatchel RJ, Mayer TG. Occupational musculoskeletal disorders: introduction and overview of the problem. In: Mayer TG, Gatchel RJ, Polatin PB, eds. Occupational musculoskeletal disorders: function, outcomes, and evidence. Philadelphia: Lippincott Williams & Wilkins, 2000:3–8.
2. Gevirtz RN, Hubbard DR, Harpin RE. Psychophysiologic treatment of chronic lower back pain. Prof Psychol Res Pract 1996;27:561–566.
3. Garofalo JP, Polatin PB. An epidemic in industrialized countries. In: Gatchel RJ, Turk DC, eds. Psychosocial factors in pain: critical perspectives. New York: Guilford, 1999.
4. AHCPR. Acute low back pain problems in adults. Clinical practice guidelines No. 14. Rockville, MD: United States Department of Health and Human Services, Agency for Health Care Policy and Research, 1994.
5. Deyo R, Cherkin D, Loeser J, et al. Morbidity and mortality in association with operations on the lumbar spine: the influence of age, diagnosis, and procedure. J Bone Joint Surg (Am) 1992;74:536–543.
6. Deyo RA, Ciol M, Cherkin D, et al. Lumbar spinal fusion: a cohort study of complications, reoperations, and resource use in the Medicare population. Spine 1993;18:1463–1470.
7. Abramovitz J, Neff S. Lumbar disc surgery: results of the prospective lumbar discectomy study of the joint section on disorders of the spine and peripheral nerves of the American Association of Neurological Surgeons and the Congress of Neurological Surgeons. Neurosurgery 1991;29:301-308.
8. Dvorak J, Gauchat MH, Valach L. The outcome of surgery for lumbar disc herniation: I. A 4-17 years' follow-up with emphasis on somatic aspects. Spine 1988;13:1418–1422.
9. Atlas SJ, Keller RB, Robson D, et al. Surgical and non-surgical management of lumbar spinal stenosis. Spine 2000;25:556–562.
10. Malter AD, Larson EB, Urban N, et al. Cost-effectiveness of lumbar discectomy for the treatment of herniated intervertebral disc. Spine 1996;21:1048–1055.
11. Waddell G. The back pain revolution. Edinburgh: Churchill Livingstone, 1998.
12. Cherkin DC, Deyo RA, Loeser JD, et al. An international comparison of back surgery rates. Spine 1994;19:1201–1206.
13. Waddell G. Low back pain: a 20th century health care enigma. Spine 1996;21:2820–2825.
14. Ljunggren AE. Natural history and clinical role of the herniated disc. In: Wiesel SW, Weinstein JN, Herkowitz H, et al., eds. The lumbar spine, 2nd ed., Volume 1. Philadelphia: W.B. Saunders, 1996:102–131.
15. Hoffman RM, Wheeler KJ, Deyo RA. Surgery for herniated lumbar discs: a literature synthesis. J Gen Int Med 1993;8:487–496.
16. Turner J, Ersek M, Herron L, et al. Patient outcomes after lumbar spinal fusions. JAMA 1992;268:907–911.
17. Gill K, Frymoyer JW. Management of treatment failures after decompressive surgery. Surgical alternatives and results. In: Frymoyer JW, ed. The adult spine: principles and practice, 2nd ed. Philadelphia: Lippincott-Raven, 1997.
18. Tandon V, Campbell F, Ross ERS. Posterior lumbar interbody fusion: association between disability and psychological disturbance in non compensation patients. Spine 1999;24:1833–1838.
19. Owings MF, Kosak LJ. Ambulatory and inpatient procedures in the United States, 1996. Vital Health Stat 13. 1998;139:1–119.
20. Haider TT, Kishino ND, Gray TP, et al. Functional restoration: comparison of surgical and nonsurgical spine patients. J Occup Rehabil 1998;8:247–253.
21. Waddell G, Gibson JNA, Grant I. Surgical treatment of lumbar disc prolapse and degenerative lumbar disc disease. Cochrane Review, 2000.
22. Norlund AI, Waddell G. Cost of back pain in some OECD countries. In: Nachemson A, Jonsson E, eds. Neck pain and back pain: the scientific evidence of causes, diagnosis and treatment. Philadelphia: Lippincott Williams & Wilkins, 2000:421–425.

23. Franklin G, Haug J, Heyer N, et al. Outcome of lumbar fusion in Washington state worker's compensation. Spine 1994;17:1897–1904.

24. Oaklander AL, North RB. Failed back surgery syndrome. In: Loeser JD, Butler SH, Chapman CR, et al, eds. Bonica's management of pain. Philadelphia: Lippincott Williams & Wilkins, 2001.

25. Waddell G. A new clinical model for the treatment of low-back pain. Spine 1987;12:632–644.

26. Pheasant HC, Gelbert D, Goldfarb J, et al. The MMPI as a predictor of outcome in low back surgery. Spine 1979;4:78–84.

27. North RB, Campbell JN, James CS, et al. Failed back surgery syndrome: 5-year follow-up in 102 patients undergoing repeated operation. Neurosurgery 1991;28:685–691.

28. Stauffer R, Coventry M. Posterolateral lumbar spine fusions: analysis of Mayo Clinic series. J Bone Joint Surg (Am) 1972;54:1195–1204.

29. Trief PM, Grant W, Fredrickson B. A prospective study of psychological predictors of lumbar surgery outcome. Spine 2000;25:2616–2621.

30. Klekamp J, McCarty E, Spengler D. Results of elective lumbar discectomy for patients involved in the workers' compensation system. J Spinal Disord 1998;11:277–282.

31. Mixter WJ, Barr JS. Rupture of the intervertebral disc with involvement of the spinal canal. N Engl J Med 1934;211:210–215.

32. Waddell G, Bircher M, Finlayson D, et al. Symptoms and signs: physical disease or illness behavior? BMJ 1984;289:739–741.

33. Loeser JD. Perspectives on pain. In: Turner P, ed. Clinical pharmacy and therapeutics. London: Macmillan, 1980:313–316.

34. Main CJ, Waddell G. A comparison of cognitive measures in low back pain: statistical structure and clinical validity at initial assessment. Pain 1991;56:287–298.

35. Bombardier C. Spine focus issue introduction: outcome assessments in the evaluation of treatment of spinal disorders. Spine 2000;25:3097–3099.

36. Mayer TG, Prescott M, Gatchel RJ. Objective outcomes evaluation: m and evidence. In: Mayer TG, Gatchel RG, Polatin PB, eds. Occupational musculoskeletal disorders: function, outcomes, and evidence. Philadelphia: Lippincott Williams & Wilkins, 2000.

37. Atlas S, Deyo R, Keller R, et al. The Maine lumbar spine study: Part II. One-year outcomes of surgical and nonsurgical management of sciatica. Spine 1996;21:1777–1786.

38. Davis RA. A long-term outcome analysis of 984 surgically treated herniated lumbar discs. J Neurosurg 1994;80:415–421.

39. Dvorak J, Valach L, Fuhrimann P, et al. The outcome of surgery for lumbar disc herniation. II. A 4-17 year follow-up with emphasis on psychosocial aspects. Spine 1988;13:1423–1427.

40. Sorensen LV. Pre-operative psychological testing with the MMPI at first operation for prolapsed lumbar disc. Five-year follow-up. Danish Med Bull 1992;39:186–190.

41. Graver V, Llungren AE, Malt UF, et al. Can psychological traits predict the outcome of lumbar disc surgery when anamnestic and physiological risk factors are controlled for? Results of a prospective cohort study. J Psychosom Res 1995;39:338–349.

42. Graver V, Haaland AK, Magnaes B, et al. Seven-year clinical follow-up after lumbar disc surgery: results and predictors of outcome. Br J Neurosurg 1999;2:178–184.

43. de Groot KI, Boeke S, van den Berge HJ, et al. The influence of psychological variables on postoperative anxiety and physical complaints in patients undergoing lumbar surgery. Pain 1997;69:19–25.

44. Block A, Gatchel RJ, Deardoff W, Guyer R. The psychology of spine surgery. Washington, D.C.: American Psychological Association Press, 2003.

45. Waddell G, Morris EW, Paola MP, et al. A concept of illness tested as an improved basis for surgical decisions in low back disorders. Spine 1986;11:712–719.

46. Schade V, Semmner N, Main CJ, et al. The impact of clinical, morphological, psychosocial and work-related factors on the outcome of lumbar discectomy. Pain 1999;80:239–249.

47. Kendall NAS, Linton SJ, Main CJ. Guide to assessing psychosocial yellow flags in acute low back pain: risk factors for long-term disability and work loss. In: Accident Rehabilitation and Compensation Insurance Corporation of New Zealand and the National Health Committee, 1997.

48. Main CJ. Concepts of treatment and prevention in musculoskeletal disorders. In: Linton SJ, ed. New avenues for the prevention of chronic musculoskeletal pain and disability. Amsterdam: Elsevier, 2002.

49. Bongers P, de Winter C, Kompier MAJ, et al. Psychosocial factors at work and musculoskeletal disease. Scand J Work Environ Health 1993;19:297–309.

50. Bigos SJ, Battie MC, Nordin M, et al. Industrial low back pain. In: Weinstein J, Wiesel S, eds. The lumbar spine. Philadelphia: WB Saunders, 1990:846–859.

51. Butcher JN, Dahlstrom WG, Graham JR, et al. MMPI-2: Manual for the administration and scoring. Minneapolis: University of Minnesota Press, 1989.

52. Main CJ, Wood PLR, Hollis S, et al. The distress assessment method: a simple patient classification to identify distress and evaluate risk of poor outcome. Spine 1992;17:42–50.

53. Rosenstiel A, Keefe F. The use of coping strategies in low back pain patients: Relationship to patient characteristics and current adjustment. Pain 1983;17:33–40.

54. Main CJ, Spanswick CC. Pain management: an interdisciplinary approach. Edinburgh: Churchill-Livingstone, 2000.

55. Mayer TG, Gatchel RJ. Functional restoration for spinal disorders: the sports medicine approach. Philadelphia: Lea & Febiger, 1988.

56. Polatin P, Rainville J, Haider T, et al. Post operative treatment: outpatient medical rehabilitation. In: Mayer TG, Gatchel RJ, Polatin P, eds. Occupational musculoskeletal disorders: function, outcomes and evidence. Philadelphia: Lippincott Williams & Wilkins, 2000.

57. Bombardier C. Outcome assessments in the evaluation of treatment of spinal disorders. Spine 2000;25:3100–3103.

CHAPTER 90

Surgical Treatment of Symptomatic Recurrent Disc Herniation

Ragnar Johnsson

The crucial watershed for surgical treatment of recurrent disc herniation (DH) is the extent of clinical symptoms, as it is for first-time disc herniation. The combination of the relatively high frequency of asymptomatic lumbar disc herniations of various degree in adults (1), and the potentially confounding effect of a prior disc herniation episode with surgical treatment warrant increased attention to the interpretation of clinical symptoms and signs and spine morphology on imagery. The risk for symptomatic recurrent DH has been estimated to be 5% to 10% after first time discectomy in the lower lumbar spine (2–4), the majority on the same side of the disc (ipsilateral recurrent DH) and the minority on the opposite side (contralateral recurrent DH). In ipsilateral recurrent DH epidural or periradicular fibrosis after the primary discectomy can confound the clinical and imaging evaluation, which normally is not the case for recurrent DH on the nonoperated contralateral side. However, the primary discectomy might have weakened the annulus in general, which could be a predisposing factor for recurrent DH on both sides of the disc.

This chapter proposes guidelines for surgical treatment of symptomatic ipsilateral or contralateral recurrent DH at a previously operated disc level based on basic clinical evaluation, preoperative imaging studies, surgical principles, known surgical results, and functional outcome.

DIAGNOSTIC PROCEDURES

Clinical Evaluation

Ipsilateral Radiating Leg Pain

The clinical symptoms and signs can indicate to a certain degree whether radiating leg pain is caused by an ipsilateral recurrent DH or another cause as epidural or periradicular fibrosis after the primary discectomy, disc herniation at another disc level, spinal stenosis, or any other cause. A pain-free period of at least several months after the prior discectomy, severely reduced walking capacity, present radicular pain distribution consistent with the previously operated disc level, radiating leg pain on cough, and straight leg raising test positive at less than 30° increase the likelihood for true symptomatic ipsilateral recurrent DH (5). If there has been no substantial pain-free period of at least some months, the case should be regarded as a failure of the prior discectomy rather than a possible recurrent DH (6).

Contralateral Radiating Leg Pain

Because normally no surgery has been performed on the contralateral side of the disc, the clinical picture of a contralateral recurrent DH resembles symptomatic first-time disc herniation.

Imaging Studies

Magnetic resonance imaging (MRI) is the imaging method of choice to study recurrent DH (7). By comparing T1-weighted images of the previously operated disc level before and after intravenous injection of the contrast medium gadolinium, which enhances vascularized soft-tissue structures, including postoperative scar formations, a recurrent DH with or without sequester and neural structures often can be distinguished from postoperative epidural or periradicular fibrosis (Figs. 90-1 to 90-4). Further, conventional T1- and T2-weighted images yield good information on disc herniation at another disc level, spinal stenosis, or any other lumbar cause that might explain the radiating leg pain.

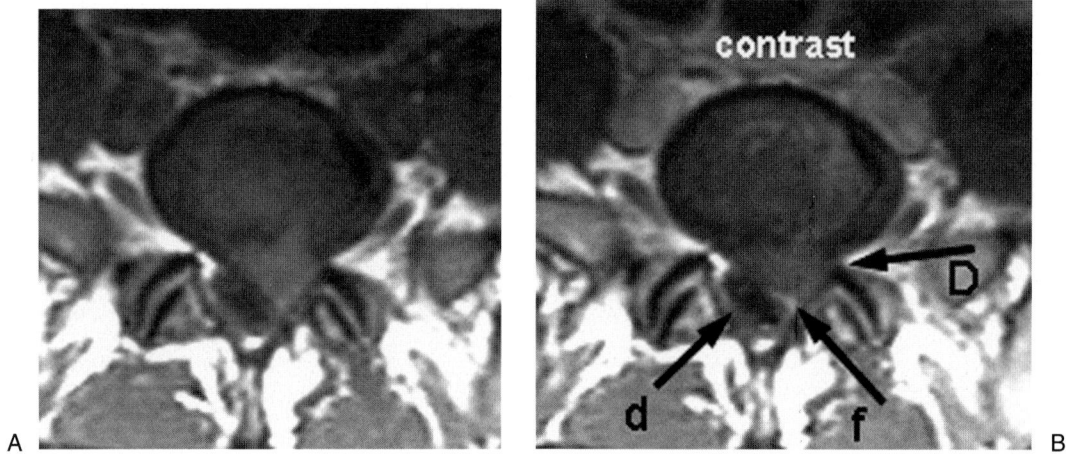

FIG. 90-1. T1-weighted axial magnetic resonance images without **(A)** and with **(B)** contrast. With contrast, minimal epidural or periradicular fibrosis *(f)* is distinguished between dura *(d)* and recurrent disc herniation or sequester *(D)*.

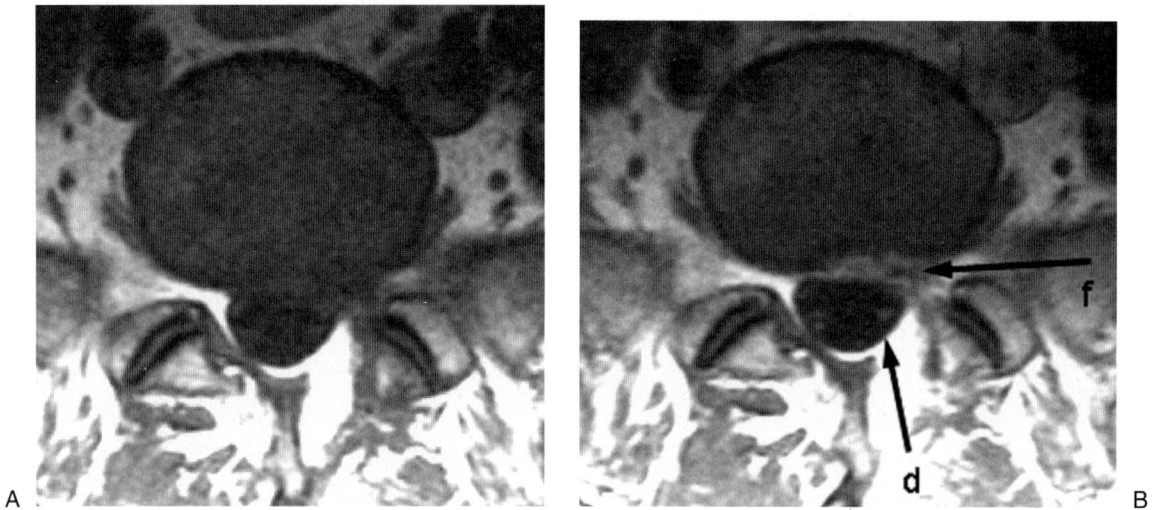

FIG. 90-2. T1-weighted axial magnetic resonance images without **(A)** and with **(B)** contrast. With contrast, epidural or periradicular fibrosis *(f)* is distinguished from dura *(d)* but no recurrent disc herniation is present.

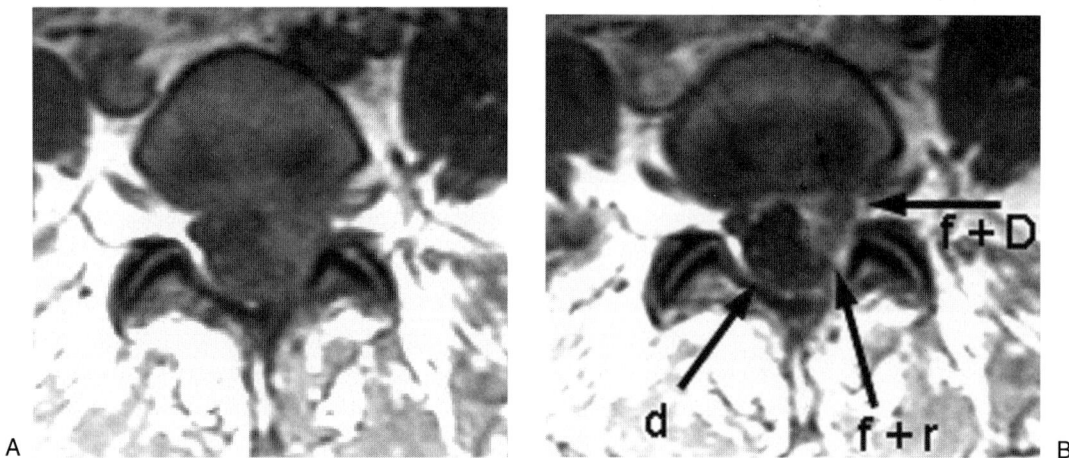

FIG. 90-3. T1-weighted axial magnetic resonance images without **(A)** and with **(B)** contrast. With contrast, epidural or periradicular fibrosis *(f)* is distinguished from dura *(d)*, S1 nerve root *(r)*, and disc sequester *(D)*.

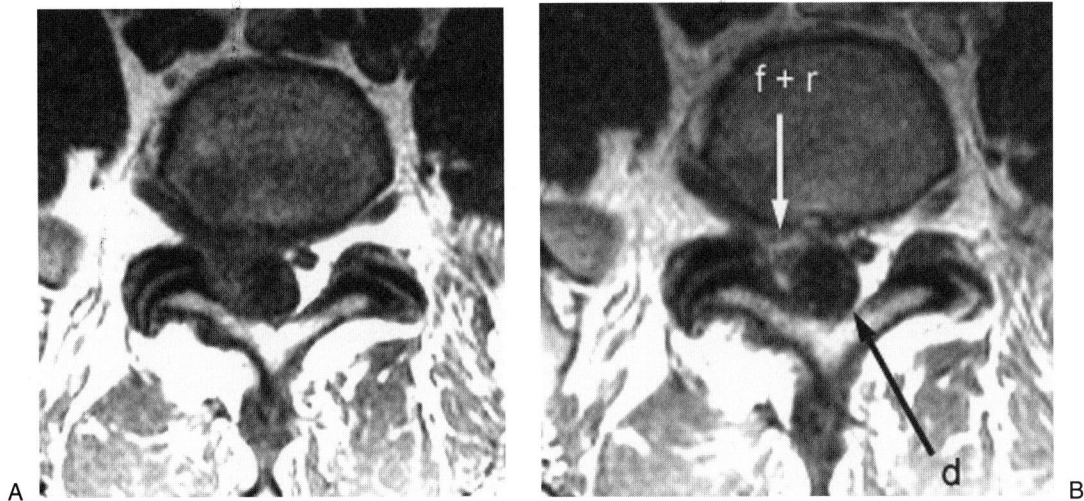

FIG. 90-4. T1-weighted axial magnetic resonance images without **(A)** and with **(B)** contrast. With contrast, epidural or periradicular fibrosis *(f)* is distinguished from dura *(d)* and S1 nerve root *(r)*, but no recurrent disc herniation is present.

RATIONALES FOR SURGERY

Our knowledge of the natural history and effectiveness of nonoperative treatment of symptomatic recurrent DH is limited (6). Because the intraspinal morphology has been altered with various degrees of epidural or periradicular fibrosis on the side of the primary discectomy and postoperative alteration of the disc tissue has occurred, it is rational to assume a somewhat worse or at best the same course of events as for primary disc herniation. It is also rational to assume that ipsilateral recurrent DH with epidural or periradicular fibrosis, which might trigger radicular pain by itself and limit the mobility of the affected nerve root, behaves less like primary disc herniation than does contralateral recurrent DH without fibrosis. Thus, the rationale for surgery of both types of recurrent DH are similar to primary disc herniation; that is, absolute indication for early discectomy in the rare cases with cauda equina syndrome and relative indication for discectomy in declining order in cases with progressive and severe pain and neurologic deterioration, intractable radicular pain, and long-standing disturbing radicular pain not responding to a trial of adequate nonoperative treatment. Epidural or periradicular fibrosis by itself, however, is not an indication for surgery, because excision of fibrosis and neurolysis without concomitant recurrent DH or any other nerve root compromise does not yield substantial long-lasting pain relief (8).

It has been argued that the occurrence of a symptomatic recurrent DH is a sign of a more severe disc pathology, which should be addressed with combined discectomy and fusion to treat and prevent both radicular leg pain and discogenic back pain. To date, no data support this addition of a fusion to the surgical strategy as a solution for the vast majority of patients with symptomatic recurrent DH (2,3,8,9). In the few cases with symptomatic recurrent DH and pronounced disc degeneration with intractable presumably discogenic back pain; however, combined discectomy and fusion ought to be considered. This surgical combination also might be contemplated in the rare case of multiple symptomatic recurrent DH at the same disc level, preferably as combined extensive discectomy and interbody fusion.

SURGICAL TECHNIQUE

A somewhat wider surgical exposure in ipsilateral recurrent DH than at the primary discectomy is usually needed to clear postoperative extraspinal fibrosis. The prior laminotomy or partial laminectomy is increased as much as needed in a facet joint–saving fashion to get a proper exposure of the transition zones between postoperative epidural or periradicular fibrosis, dura, nerve root, and herniated disc material. Magnification of the visual field should be used to optimize this soft-tissue distinction and thereby decrease the risk for damage of the dura or nerve root. The choice of operating microscope or magnification glasses is up to the surgeon, but the microscope improves the educational facility and illumination of the deep surgical field. Enough epidural or periradicular fibrosis is cleared to facilitate the identification and excision of the herniated disc material without compromising the dura or the nerve root. Concomitant lateral stenosis of the nerve root is removed. To decrease the risk for new postoperative fibrosis, the neural structures can be covered with an anti-adhesion barrier gel (10) or a free fat autograft (11), although the effect of both methods on future radicular symptoms is questioned (11,12). The surgical technique for contralateral recurrent DH is similar to primary discectomy.

SURGICAL COMPLICATIONS

Intraoperative undue handling of the intraspinal soft-tissue structures can easily cause a dural tear and associated leakage of cerebrospinal fluid (CSF). The standard treatment of a dural tear is to suture the defect and then cover the suture line with a fibrin sealant. To ensure proper early healing of the dural defect preventing leakage of CSF with associated postural cerebral symptoms, pseudocyst or fistula, postoperative bed rest in a strict horizontal position minimizing the intradural pressure for 2 days is advised. A systemic prophylactic antibiotic is given to prevent postoperative meningitis. A superficial nerve root lesion is left unattended and superficial epineural sutures are used to approach the nerve root endings in the rare case of complete nerve root lesion. The use of an anti-adhesion barrier gel might induce late symptomatic dural defects according to recent reports (13,14). A too-large free fat autograft can be pressed into the spinal canal and cause a cauda equina syndrome. These risks of an anti-adhesion barrier gel and a free fat autograft, and the questioned effect of both methods on future radicular symptoms (11,12) should be kept in mind when reflecting on covering the neural structures with either gel or fat.

POSTOPERATIVE MANAGEMENT

The aim of the patient is to attain the normal level of physical and functional activities as quickly as possible. It has been shown that immediately after primary discectomy all activity restrictions can be lifted as soon as the specific domestic, recreational, and occupational activities can be tolerated by the patient without increasing the risk for complications (15). This also probably can be the guiding principle after discectomy of recurrent DH. The rehabilitation process can be further enhanced by adding specific physical exercises 1 month postoperatively to strengthen back and abdominal muscles (16–18).

RESULTS AND FUNCTIONAL OUTCOME

There is a general expectation of worse results after repeat surgery at a previously operated level in the lumbar spine. The chance for a satisfactory result after discectomy of a recurrent DH is good, however, providing that high-quality pain relief also has been obtained after surgery of the primary disc herniation. The scientific documentation on the results of discectomy in recurrent DH, both ipsilateral and contralateral, implies similar improvement of radicular leg pain, back pain, and functional outcome during the first years postoperatively as after primary discectomy (2,3,8,9). Documentation on long-term results is still lacking. The risk for another recurrent DH at the same level is unknown and there are no specific preventive measures except combined extensive discectomy and interbody fusion. However, this is not a fruitful surgical option for the vast majority of patients with symptomatic recurrent DH (2,3,8,9).

REFERENCES

1. Jensen M, Brant-Zawadzki MN, Obuchowski N, et al. Magnetic resonance imaging of the lumbar spine in people without back pain. N Engl J Med 1994;331:69–73.
2. Cinotti G, Roysam GS, Eisenstein SM, et al. Ipsilateral recurrent lumbar disc herniation. A prospective, controlled study. J Bone Joint Surg 1998;80-B:825–832.
3. Cinotti G, Gumina S, Giannicola G, et al. Contralateral recurrent lumbar disc herniation. Results of discectomy compared with those in primary herniation. Spine 1999;24:800–806.
4. Yorimitsu E, Chiba K, Toyama Y, et al. Long-term outcomes of standard discectomy for lumbar disc herniation. A follow-up study of more than 10 years. Spine 2001;26:652–657.
5. Jönsson B, Strömqvist B. Clinical characteristics of recurrent sciatica after lumbar discectomy. Spine 1996;21:500–505.
6. Postacchini F. Management of herniation of the lumbar disc. J Bone Joint Surg 1999;81-B:567–576.
7. Runge VM, Muroff LR, Jinkins JR. Central nervous system: review of clinical use of contrast media. Topics MRI 2001;12:231–263.
8. Jönsson B, Strömqvist B. Repeat decompression of lumbar nerve roots. A prospective two-year evaluation. J Bone Joint Surg 1993;75-B:894–897.
9. Suk K-S, Lee H-M, Moon S-H, et al. Recurrent lumbar disc herniation. Results of operative management. Spine 2001;26:672–676.
10. Tribolet N, Porchet F, Lutz T, et al. Clinical assessment of a novel anti-adhesion barrier gel: Prospective, randomized, multicenter, clinical trial of ADCON-L to inhibit postoperative peridural fibrosis and related symptoms after lumbar discectomy. Am J Orthop 1998;27:111–120.
11. Toftgaard Jensen T, Asmussen K, Berg-Hansen E-M, et al. First-time operation for lumbar disc herniation with or without free fat transplantation. Prospective triple-blind randomized study with reference to clinical factors and enhanced computed tomographic scan 1 year after operation. Spine 1996;21:1072–1076.
12. Richter HP, Kast E, Tomczak R, et al. Results of applying ADCON-L gel after lumbar discectomy: the German ADCON-L study. J Neurosurg 2001;95(2 Suppl):179–189.
13. Hieb LD, Stevens DL. Spontaneous postoperative cerebrospinal fluid leaks following application of anti-adhesion barrier gel. Spine 2001;26:748–751.
14. Le AN, Rogers DE, Dawson EG, et al. Unrecognized durotomy after lumbar discectomy. A report of four cases associated with the use of ADCON-L. Spine 2001;26:115–118
15. Carragee EJ, Han MY, Yang B, et al. Activity restrictions after posterior lumbar discectomy. Spine 1999;24:2346–2351.
16. Danielsen JM, Johnsen R, Kibsgaard, SK et al. Early aggressive exercise for postoperative rehabilitation after discectomy. Spine 2000;25:1015–1020.
17. Dolan P, Greenfield K, Nelson RJ, et al. Can exercise therapy improve the outcome of microdiscectomy? Spine 2000;25:1523–1532.
18. Kjellby-Wendt G, Styf J. Early active training after lumbar discectomy. A prospective, randomized, and controlled study. Spine 1998;21:2345–2351.

CHAPTER 91

Management of Failed Lumbar Surgery: Recurrent Stenosis

Jayesh Trivedi and Stephen Eisenstein

Lumbar spinal stenosis is a disabling syndrome affecting older patients. Surgical decompression forms the mainstay of operative treatment. However, the beneficial results of surgical decompression may deteriorate with time, resulting in recurrence of symptoms or development of new symptoms. The purpose of this chapter is to discuss the causes of poor results after surgical decompression for lumbar stenosis and offer management options.

Lumbar stenosis is caused by constriction in the dimensions of the spinal canal or intervertebral foramen. Degenerative stenosis, the most common form, is characterized pathologically by degenerative hypertrophy of the facet joints and vertebral body margins, thickening of the ligamentum flavum, and narrowing of the intervertebral discs (1). The combined effect of these changes is a narrowing of the spinal canal and reduction in the space available to the cauda and exiting nerve roots. Clinically it is characterized by lower limb pain and paraesthesias, varying degree of back pain, and a limitation of walking distance in the presence of good peripheral circulation. The lower limb pain is relieved by stooping or sitting, which increases the spinal canal capacity. This constellation of symptoms constitutes neurogenic claudication (Table 91-1).

Anatomically, the stenosis is classified as "central" when the compression affects mainly the thecal sac, or "lateral" when it affects the nerve roots in the nerve root canals (Figs. 91-1, 91-2) (2). Etiologically, Arnoldi et al. classified stenosis into congenital or developmental, acquired (including degenerative, iatrogenic, and posttraumatic), or combined varieties (3).

The incidence of degenerative lumbar stenosis is 1.7% to 8% (4,5). Symptoms usually develop after the fifth decade of life. The initial management is symptomatic, consisting of analgesics including nonsteroidal antiinflammatory drugs (NSAIDs), epidural injections, physical therapy, and lifestyle modification. Johnsson et al. studied the natural history of 32 patients with lumbar stenosis who did not undergo surgical decompression (6). Seventy percent of the patients were symptomatically unchanged at follow-up. In the remainder, half were better and the other half were worse. At 1 year, the Maine Lumbar Spine Study reported that the patients treated nonoperatively were symptomatically stable, although there was no clinical improvement (7). Other authors have reported a similar success rate with aggressive nonoperative treatment (8,9,10)

TABLE 91.1. *Comparison between vascular and spinal claudication*

Signs and symptoms	Vascular	Neurogenic
Claudication distance	Fixed	Variable
Relief on cessation of walking	Immediate	Lingering symptoms
Effect of posture on pain relief	Standing relieves pain	Flexion of spine and sitting relieves pain
Back pain	Infrequent	Frequent
Walking up hill	Painful	Not painful
Bicycle riding	Painful	Not painful
Peripheral pulses	Absent	Present

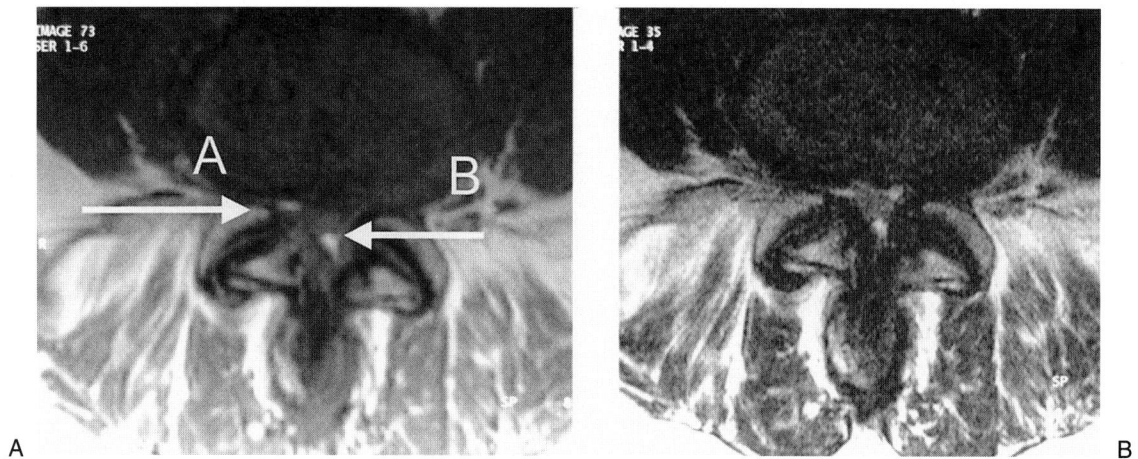

FIG. 91-1. Magnetic resonance imaging scan axial cuts showing central and lateral stenosis. **A:** Lateral recess. **B:** Central canal.

SURGERY AND ITS OUTCOME

Surgery for patients with lumbar stenosis is that of decompression with or without concomitant fusion. A variety of techniques to decompress the spine have been reported in literature. These include laminectomy, laminotomies (11,12), and distraction laminoplasty (13). Successful outcomes from surgical decompression have varied from 57% to 95% (14–18), depending on the duration of the follow-up. In most studies the outcome deteriorated with the length of follow-up. Jonsson et al. prospectively studied 140 patients treated surgically, and reported an average improvement of 82% in leg pain and 71% in back pain at 3 years (19). Herron et al. reported satisfactory results in 67% patients at 2 years after surgery that deteriorated to 52% at 5-year follow-up (20). Katz et al., reporting on 88 consecutive patients undergoing laminectomy, found that the initial 89% relief of pain deteriorated to 57% at 4 years after surgery (15). At 7 to

10 years follow-up after surgery, they found that 23% of patients had received repeat surgery, with 33% complaining of severe back or buttock pain. Postacchini reported a 67% satisfactory result in 64 patients followed up to 8.2 years after surgery (21). Meta-analysis has shown a similar outcome in patients with a long-term follow-up (22). Thus, the initial good results after surgery may deteriorate with time but this does not necessarily mean a failure of the initial index procedure.

FAILED SURGERY FOR STENOSIS

The incidence of unsatisfactory results after surgery for lumbar stenosis is not known. The incidence of failed lumbar surgery syndrome is reported to be 15% to 40% (22–24). The rate of repeat operation in lumbar stenosis has been reported to be 5% to 13% in some studies (13,25). Failed lumbar stenosis surgery may pose a prob-

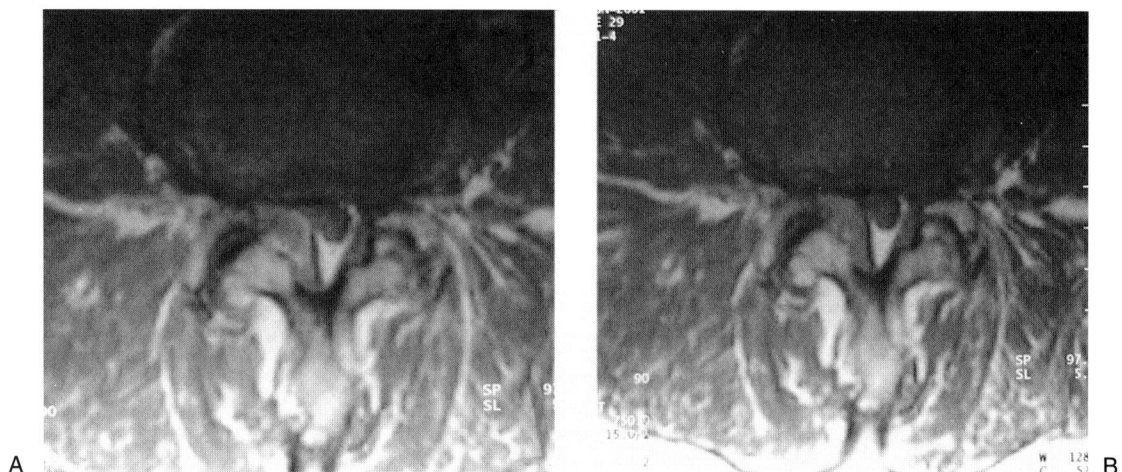

FIG. 91-2. Magnetic resonance imaging scan axial cuts demonstrating facet hypertrophy and lateral stenosis.

lem in diagnostic evaluation and management for the spinal surgeon. Furthermore, the likelihood of obtaining a successful outcome after repeat surgery in this situation may be limited. Unsatisfactory results after surgery for lumbar stenosis may result from: (a) wrong diagnosis, (b) presence of comorbidity, (c) inadequate decompression, (d) recurrent stenosis either at the same level or previously noninvolved levels, or (e) new or increased back pain resulting from iatrogenic mechanical instability owing to surgery or spondylosis, and spondylolisthesis present before surgery and not addressed at surgery.

WRONG DIAGNOSIS

Distinguishing spinal claudication from vascular claudication is important (Table 91-1). The age for spinal claudication is also an age when peripheral arterial disease is common.

Clinical examination in these patients should include palpation for the presence of pulses in the dorsalis pedis and posterior tibial arteries. A Doppler study in a clinic setting is indicated if the latter are not felt. Absent pulses represent an indication for referral to the vascular surgeon for further investigations to rule out peripheral vessel pathology.

Confirmation of diagnosis with appropriate imaging is essential in patients presenting with symptoms typical of spinal claudication. The authors' preference is for all patients to undergo a magnetic resonance imaging (MRI) scan. Magnetic resonance imaging is reported to have 75% to 85% accuracy in diagnosing stenosis (26). A myelography-computed tomography (myelo-CT) is the investigation of choice if the MRI scan is inconclusive or for patients who can not undergo an MRI.

The use of nerve root sheath injections may be diagnostic and even therapeutic in patients with symptoms predominantly suggestive of a lateral stenosis. These may be combined with electrophysiologic studies of nerve conduction. In patients who have had previous surgery in the lumbar area, the use of contrast-enhanced MRI is essential to estimate the extent of postoperative fibrosis. This involves the intravenous administration of gadolinium (Gd-DPTA). T1-weighted images obtained immediately after the administration of Gd-DPTA demonstrate increased signal intensity in perithecal fibrosis.

COMORBID FACTORS

Katz et al., reporting on the long-term results of patients undergoing decompression for lumbar stenosis, found that an unsatisfactory long-term outcome is associated with the presence of comorbid medical conditions and laminectomy confined to a single level (15). Preexisting cardiovascular disease, rheumatoid or osteoarthritis, and chronic pulmonary disease were found to influence the long-term results following decompression. The effect of these factors was found to be additive.

Oldridge et al. reported on 34,148 patients with average age of 71 years and undergoing lumbar surgery; they found the mortality rate to be 0.5% (27). They reported that patients older than 80 years had increased mortality. Smith and Hanigan reported that patients with three or more comorbidities had a higher rate of complications when undergoing lumbar surgery (28). Benz et al., in a retrospective review of 68 patients older than 70 years and undergoing decompression, found that serious complications occurred in 12% with an early mortality of 1.4% (29). They were unable to show a significant relationship between comorbidities and postoperative complications.

It is likely that the presence of comorbidities may affect the patient's perception or tolerance to pain and thus influence outcome after decompression.

Recurrent Stenosis

Postacchini reviewed 40 patients treated surgically for lumbar stenosis and found varying degrees of bony regrowth of the resected posterior arches in 35 of the 40 patients (30). These patients were evaluated at an average of 8.6 years after operation. Two types of bony regrowth were identified. There was either a gradual regrowth of the laminae and the articular surfaces resected at surgery or a coalescence of islets of bone tissue within a fibrous sheet filling the laminectomy defect. Complete resection of the inferior articular processes was found to be preventive against this regrowth. Furthermore, the wider the initial decompression, the less likelihood there was of this regrowth. Patients with degenerative spondylolisthesis were more likely to have regrowth if they had not been fused at the time of the index operation. The clinical outcome was found to be satisfactory in patients with little or no bony regrowth. In patients with moderate or marked bony regrowth, the proportion of satisfactory results was 55% and 40%, respectively. There are other reports of bony regrowth after surgery (31,32). We have not encountered bony regrowth so far in our practice.

Stenosis at previously uninvolved levels may also contribute to recurrence of symptoms. Katz et al., in a longterm review of surgically treated patients with stenosis, found that a single level laminectomy was associated with poor results (15). Degenerative changes and stenosis can occur throughout the lumbar spine so that previously uninvolved levels may become stenotic with time.

Inadequate Decompression

Inadequate decompression is probably the most common cause of failed surgery in spinal stenosis and persisting symptoms after surgery. Scrutiny of preoperative imaging to ascertain where the compression is, and knowledge of spinal anatomy at decompression is important. Degenerative lumbar stenosis is usually circumferential and multifactorial in terms of structures that intrude into the space intended for neural anatomy. Therefore, decompression should deal with bone, joint (facet), ligamentum flavum, and disc at all relevant levels if subsequent failure is to be avoided. The surgical technique should address the central canal and lateral recesses. Decompression of the latter should as a rule involve undercutting of the medial aspects of the hypertrophic superior facets of the caudad vertebra. The adequacy of decompression may be assessed by the free passage of a probe along the path of the nerve.

Stenosis and Low Back Pain

Mechanical low back pain may coexist with stenosis in some patients. It may also be iatrogenic after surgery for spinal stenosis.

Degenerative spondylolisthesis is a radiographic finding often associated with stenosis. It is commonly seen at the L4-5 level and tends to be more common in women. Satomi et al. reported on 41 patients treated surgically with decompression (33). Twenty-seven patients had anterior interbody fusion, whereas 14 patients had decompression alone. The fusion group had 93% good to excellent results as opposed to 72% in the nonfused group. Nasca also reported a better outcome in patients who had concomitant fusion and decompression compared to decompression alone (34). Herkowitz and Kurz published a controlled prospective study of patients with stenosis and degenerative spondylolisthesis who were randomized to either decompression alone or decompression with *in situ* intertransverse fusion (35). A better outcome was reported in the group that underwent concomitant fusion. Other authors have reported similar findings (36,37).

Iatrogenic radiographic instability may result from a radical decompression in which more than 50% of each facet joint has been sacrificed. In this situation flexion-extension lateral radiographs of the patient may detect segmental instability. If these radiographs demonstrate either a 4-mm translational movement or greater than 10° angulation between vertebrae, "instability" is present and fusion may be indicated (38).

We (39) recommend concomitant fusion in the presence of the following: significant low back pain, spondylolisthesis, and radical decompression. Relative contraindications to fusion include age more than 75 years and the presence of comorbidities, including diabetes or cardiopulmonary disease. Our preference is for intertransverse fusion with pedicular screw fixation, the latter depending on adequate bone quality.

MANAGEMENT

Nonoperative Treatment

Not all patients with recurrence of symptoms after surgical decompression for stenosis require a repeat opera-

tion. In a retrospective review of 317 patients, Herno et al. found that patients undergoing repeat surgery were less likely to have a successful outcome following surgery (40). In their study excellent to good results were obtained in 67% of the singly operated patients as opposed to 46% in the repeat surgery group. Coexisting disease and surgery within 18 months after the index procedure was associated with poor outcome after repeat surgery. Echeverria and Lockwood in a comparative study of 17 patients undergoing surgery with 10 patients who had undergone previous spinal surgery found excellent to good outcomes in 76% in the former and 50% in the latter group (41). Although other studies have disputed a poorer outcome in revision spinal surgery, it is clear that the outcome in revision surgery is still controversial. Furthermore, there may be no correlation between postoperative radiological findings and the patients' symptoms. This has been shown to be the case by Herno, Finnegan and other authors (40,42,43). Nonsteroidal antiinflammatory drugs, activity modification, use of mobility aids such as trolleys or wheelchairs and epidural steroids are all reasonable options for patients who have failed to have a satisfactory result from previous surgery.

Surgery: Indications and Technique

Failure to respond to nonoperative treatment, inadequate decompression demonstrable on radiologic imaging, spinal "instability" with intractable back pain not addressed at initial surgery are all indications for further surgery. The patient should be fit to undergo further spinal surgery. The presence of advanced cardiopulmonary disease forms a contraindication for revision surgery. Previously listed causes for recurrence of symptoms should be diligently addressed at repeat surgery to ensure a satisfactory outcome. The technique of surgery is tailored to the patient but concomitant fusion is considered for those demonstrating instability or where radical decompression is deemed necessary.

Repeat decompression surgery presents a daunting prospect, with every expectation of dural injury, neural injury, and unsatisfactory symptom response. Many patients present an anesthetic challenge at the first surgery, by virtue of the intercurrent afflictions of advanced years on all systems. Apart from the difficulties of revision surgery, patients may be disqualified from revision surgery because it presents too great a risk to life.

The fact remains that careful technique can produce a gratifying result in those rare instances where revision decompression is deemed appropriate and possible (44). The surgery can be much simplified by the routine application of one of the commercial polysaccharide pastes to all exposed dural surfaces at the completion of the original operation. These products are expensive but useful in leaving a plane of cleavage between dura and surrounding bone, annulus, and ligament. The authors have a small but gratifying experience of revision surgery in these circumstances, and use such a product routinely in decompression surgery in the lumbar spine.

Once the dorsal aspects of the relevant segments have been exposed, careful further dissection reveals the junction between the residual lateral or laminar bone margin, and the scar of previous dissection. A sharp elevator separates the scar from bone and usually allows re-entry into the spinal canal without mishap. Careful probing in directions away from the scar ensures a plane between bone and unscarred dura.

A margin of the bony surround is then removed, allowing a leisurely approach from fresh anatomy back toward the previous battleground. Postoperative scar densely adherent to dura is left in place: Too much striving for its removal is unnecessary and dangerous. The elements most likely responsible for persistent or recurrent neural symptoms are new facet joint osteophytes, stenosis of entry to the nerve root foramen, or a new disc prolapse. With patience, care, and persistence, these areas can be reached eventually without major injury, and the intruding tissue excised. All levels demonstrated to be stenotic on imaging should be addressed.

Where recurrence of stenosis is found to be the development of spondylolisthesis since the original surgery, the options are distinctly unattractive. Ideally, revision decompression should be accompanied by fusion, in order to halt further vertebral shift. The difficulty then is that most patients have bone too soft and weak to hold fixation implants. Bone grafting has to be protected by old-fashioned external bracing of some kind for an extended period, probably beyond the tolerance and capability of many elderly patients.

The ancient recommendation that the need for revision surgery is better prevented than that revision surgery is skillfully executed sounds insufferably sanctimonious. It remains true, however, that stenosis surgery over several segments is tedious, tiring, and somewhat frightening, if performed with thoroughness and attending to all elements circumferentially, centrally, and laterally.

SUMMARY

Management of failed surgery involves a thorough attempt to establish the cause for failure in the index procedure and addressing this at repeat surgery. Development of stenosis at previously unaffected levels may also account for a recurrence of symptoms. The presence of comorbid factors plays an important role in influencing surgical outcome. The technique of revision surgery is tailored to the individual patient, but a satisfactory outcome can be obtained with proper preoperative evaluation and meticulous surgical technique.

REFERENCES

1. Hilibrand AS, Rand N. Degenerative lumbar stenosis: diagnosis and management. J Am Acad Orthop Surg 1999;7:239–249.
2. Kirkaldy-Willis WH, Wedge JH, Yong-Hing K, et al. Pathology and pathogenesis of lumbar spondylosis and stenosis. Spine 1978;3:319–328.
3. Arnoldi CC, Brodsky AE, Cauchoix J, et al. Lumbar spinal stenosis and nerve root entrapment syndromes: definition and classification. Clin Orthop 1976;115:4–5.
4. Roberson GH, Llewellyn HJ, Taveras JM. The narrow lumbar spinal canal syndrome. Radiology 1973;107:89–97.
5. De Villiers PD, Booysen EL. Fibrous spinal stenosis: a report on 850 myelograms with a water-soluble contrast medium. Clin Orthop 1976;115:140–144.
6. Johnsson KE, Rosen I, Uden A. The natural course of lumbar spinal stenosis. Clin Orthop 1992;279:82–86.
7. Atlas SJ, Deyo RA, Keller RB. The Maine Lumbar Spinal Study, Part III: 1 year outcomes of surgical and nonsurgical management of lumbar spinal stenosis. Spine 1996;21:1787–1795.
8. Dilke TW, Burry HC, Grahame R. Extradural corticosteroid injection in the management of lumbar nerve root compression. BMJ 1973;2:635–637.
9. Hoogmartens M, Morelle P. Epidural injection in the treatment of spinal stenosis. Acta Orthop Belg. 1987;53:409–411.
10. Aryanpur J, Ducker T. Multilevel lumbar laminotomies: an alternative to laminectomy in the treatment of lumbar stenosis. Neurosurgery 1990;26:429–432.
11. Getty CJM, Johnson JR, Kirwan E, et al. Partial undercutting facetectomy for bony entrapment of the lumbar nerve root. J Bone Joint Surg Br 1981;63:330–335.
12. O'Leary PF, McCance SE. Distraction laminoplasty for decompression of lumbar spinal stenosis. Clin Orthop 2001;(384):26—34.
13. Getty CJM. Lumbar spinal stenosis. The clinical spectrum and results of operation. J Bone Joint Surg (Br) 1980;62:481–485.
14. Herkowitz HN, Garfin SR. Decompressive surgery for spinal stenosis. Sem Spine Surg 1989;1:163–167.
15. Katz JN, Lipson SJ, Larson MG, et al. The outcome of decompressive laminectomy for degenerative lumbar stenosis. J Bone Joint Surg Am 1991;73(6):809–816.
16. Spengler DM. Degenerative stenosis of the lumbar spine. J Bone Joint Surg Am 1987;69:305–308.
17. Herno A, Airaksinen O, Saari T. Long term results of surgical treatment of lumbar spinal stenosis. Spine 1993;18:1471–1474.
18. Airaksinen O, Herno A, Turunen V, et al. Surgical outcome of 438 patients treated surgically for lumbar spinal stenosis. Spine 1997;22:2278–2282.
19. Jonsson B, Stromquist B. Decompression for lateral stenosis. Results and impact on sick leave and working conditions. Spine 1994;19:2381–2386.
20. Herron LD, Mangelsdorf C. Lumbar spinal stenosis. J Spinal Disord 1991;4:426–433.
21. Postacchini F, Cinotti G, Gumina S. Long term results of surgery in lumbar stenosis. 8 year review of 64 patients. Acta Orthop Scand 1993;64(Suppl 251):78–80.
22. Turner JA, Ersek M, Herron L, et al. Surgery for lumbar spinal stenosis: attempted meta-analysis of the literature. Spine 1992;17:1–8.
23. Wiesel SW. The multiply operated lumbar spine. Instr Course Lect 1985;34:68–77.
24. Biondi J, Greenberg BJ. Redecompression and fusion in failed back pain syndrome patients. J Spinal Disord 1990;3:362–369.
25. Paine KWE. Results of decompression for lumbar spinal stenosis. Clin Orthop 1976;115:96–100.
26. Bischoff RJ, Rodriguez RP, Gupta K, et al. A comparison of computed tomography-myelography, magnetic resonance imaging and myelography in the diagnosis of herniated nucleus pulposus and spinal stenosis. J. Spinal Disord 1993;6:289–295.
27. Oldridge NB, Yuan Z, Stoll JE, et al. Lumbar spine surgery and mortality among medicare beneficiaries. Am J Public Health 1994;84(8):1292–1298.
28. Smith EB, Hanigan WC. Surgical results and complications in elderly patients with benign lesions of the spinal canal. J Am Geriatr Soc 1992;40(9):867–870.
29. Benz RJ, Ibrahim ZG, Afshar P, et al. Predicting complications in

elderly patients undergoing lumbar decompression. Clin Orthop 2001;384:116–121.

30. Postacchini F, Cinotti G. Bone regrowth after surgical decompression for lumbar spinal stenosis. J Bone Joint Surg Br 1992;74:862–869.
31. Brodsky AE. Post-laminectomy and post fusion stenosis of the lumbar spine. Clin Orthop 1976;115:130–139.
32. Verbiest H. Results of surgical treatment of idiopathic developmental stenosis of the lumbar vertebral canal: a review of twenty-seven years' experience. J Bone Joint Surg (Br) 1977;59:181–188.
33. Satomi K, Hirabayashi K, Toyama Y, et al. A clinical study of degenerative spondylolisthesis. Radiographic analysis and choice of treatment. Spine 1992;17:1329–1336.
34. Nasca RJ. Rationale for spinal fusion in lumbar spinal stenosis. Spine 1989;14:451–454.
35. Herkowitz HN, Kurz LT. Degenerative lumbar spondylolisthesis with spinal stenosis. A prospective study comparing decompression with decompression and intertransverse process arthrodesis. J Bone Joint Surg (Am) 1991;73:802–808.
36. Yone K, Sakou T, Kawauchi Y, et al. Indication of fusion for lumbar spinal stenosis in elderly patients and its significance. Spine 1996;21:242–248.
37. Yone K, Sakou T. Usefulness of Posner's definition of spinal instability for selection of surgical treatment for lumbar spinal stenosis. J Spinal Disord 1999;12:40–44.
38. Booth RE Jr, Spivak J. The surgery of spinal stenosis. Inst Course Lect 1994;43:441–449.
39. Eisenstein S. Fusion for spinal stenosis: a personal view. J Bone Joint Surg (Br) 2002;84:9–10.
40. Herno A, Airaksinen O, Saari T, et al. Surgical results of lumbar spinal stenosis:A comparison of patients with or without previous back surgery. Spine 1995;20(8):964–969.
41. Echeverria T, Lockwood RC. Lumbar spinal stenosis, experience at a community hospital. NY J Med 1979;79:872–873.
42. Finnegan WJ, Fenlin JM, Marvel JP, et al. Results of surgical intervention in the symptomatic multiply-operated back patient. J Bone Joint Surg (Am) 1979;61:1077–1082.
43. Kim SS, Michelsen CB. Revision surgery for failed back surgery syndrome. Spine 1992;17:957–960.
44. Hansraj KK, O'Leary PF, Cammisa FP Jr, et al. Decompression, fusion, and instrumentation surgery for complex lumbar spinal stenosis. Clin Orthop 2001;384:18–25.

CHAPTER 92

Failed Surgery and Revision Surgery: Failed Instrumentation

Frank M. Phillips

The role of spinal instrumentation is to obtain and maintain spinal alignment and stabilize the spine until fusion occurs. Failure of instrumentation is typically the result of a surgeon applying the instrumentation in a situation where the deforming forces exceed the ability of the instrumentation to stabilize the spine. To reduce the likelihood of failure, the surgeon must understand the capabilities of the instrumentation as well as the biomechanical environment across which the instrumentation is applied.

Posterior instrumentation comprising pedicle screws attached to a longitudinal plate or rod is frequently applied in the lumbar spine. Hooks, wires, or cables are alternate posterior techniques for achieving spinal fixation that are less frequently used in the lumbar spine. Anterior instrumentation includes threaded intradiscal devices, vertical cages, or struts and rod or plate-screw constructs. Failure of instrumentation most frequently involves loosening or less commonly breakage of the implant, implying failure of fusion and often associated with a loss of correction of spinal deformity.

When instrumentation fails by implant breakage or screw pullout, plain radiographs usually confirm the diagnosis. In some instances, subtle instrumentation failure, such as screw loosening, may be less obvious on radiographs. Lucencies visualized around the screws should raise concern for ongoing spinal motion, implying failure of fusion. Failure of fusion is difficult to identify radiographically and additional studies such as computed tomography (CT) scans or bone scans may be helpful in the work-up of these patients (1,2). Computed tomography scans are also helpful for assessing the architecture of the pedicle if revision fixation is being considered. The quality of bone, as well as the pedicle diameter and screw length within the vertebral body, can be determined from CT scans.

Instrumentation failure in and of itself may not cause symptoms, and identifying failed instrumentation should prompt a diligent search for the source of the patient's symptoms. Instrumentation failure may alert the physician to a pseudarthrosis that may be the source of the patient's symptoms. Failure of instrumentation may also lead to the development of spinal deformity that requires further surgery. Even in the presence of failed instrumentation, unless a well-defined source of the patient's symptoms is identified, surgery directed toward revising or removing the instrumentation is unlikely to provide relief of symptoms (3).

POSTERIOR INSTRUMENTATION FAILURE

Posterior constructs secured to the spine via screws placed through the pedicle and into the vertebral body have been popularized over the last decade. Pedicle screw instrumentation allows for segmental control of all three columns of the spine from a posterior approach. The rigidity achieved with these implants may reduce the number of fixation points necessary for stability, thereby reducing the number of levels that are fused. Early pedicle screw fixation systems used an unconstrained linkage of the screws to the rod or plate spanning the involved levels. These systems had high failure rates in terms of implant loosening, breakage, and pseudarthrosis (4) and have been superseded by systems with rigid, constrained connections between the screws and the longitudinal rod or plate. Pedicle screw systems have been shown to provide significant stabilization to the treated motion segment and improve lumbar fusion rates (5–7).

It is uncommon for contemporary pedicle screw systems to fail by breakage or screw-connector disengagement (8,9). These implants are extremely strong and rigid and are more likely to fail by loss of fixation of the screws to the spine. Posterior instrumentation failures typically occur when the implant is placed in an environment in which the bending loads produced by forces acting eccentrically to the implant's neutral axis exceed the load-bearing capabilities of the implant.

Posterior instrumentation failure may occur:

1. When pseudarthrosis develops, subjecting the instrumentation to continuing bending moments until fatigue failure of the device occurs
2. With anterior column deficiencies, such as might occur with vertebral body tumors or unstable vertebral fractures
3. With spinal deformities, such as advanced spondylolisthesis or kyphosis
4. When the bony anchorage of the screw to the spine is insufficient often because of osteoporosis, and screw loosening or pullout occurs (10)

Pseudarthrosis

Instrumentation failure often heralds the presence of a pseudarthrosis (3,4,11). If the pseudarthrosis is thought to be symptomatic, revision arthrodesis may be considered. In general, repeat arthrodesis should be performed in the anatomic location where the most favorable environment for fusion exists. If an initial postero-lateral instrumented fusion was attempted, success of repeat postero-lateral arthrodesis may be compromised by the devascularized and scarred "fusion bed." This should prompt the surgeon to consider performing an interbody arthrodesis. Advantages of the interbody technique for arthrodesis include the large surface area available for achieving fusion and the favorable biomechanical environment for fusion (12–14). Autograft bone remains the gold standard for achieving lumbar fusion. The detailed treatment of pseudarthrosis is discussed elsewhere in this volume.

Anterior Column Deficiencies

Anterior spinal column deficiencies may occur with vertebral body destruction caused by tumor, infection, or trauma (Figs. 92-1 to 92-5). Approximately 80% of the spinal load is transmitted through the anterior column so that deficiencies of this column place large bending stresses on posterior instrumentation constructs (15). McLain et al. (16) reported a 60% rate of instrumentation failure when comminuted vertebral body thoracolumbar fractures were treated with posterior pedicle-based instrumentation extended to the level above and below the fractured level. Furthermore, *in situ* contouring of the rods predisposed to failure. Similarly, Kramer et al. (17) reported that four of 11 patients with thoracolumbar fractures treated with short-segment transpedicular instrumentation had breakage or disengagement of the caudal screw. The kyphosis across the operated levels increased

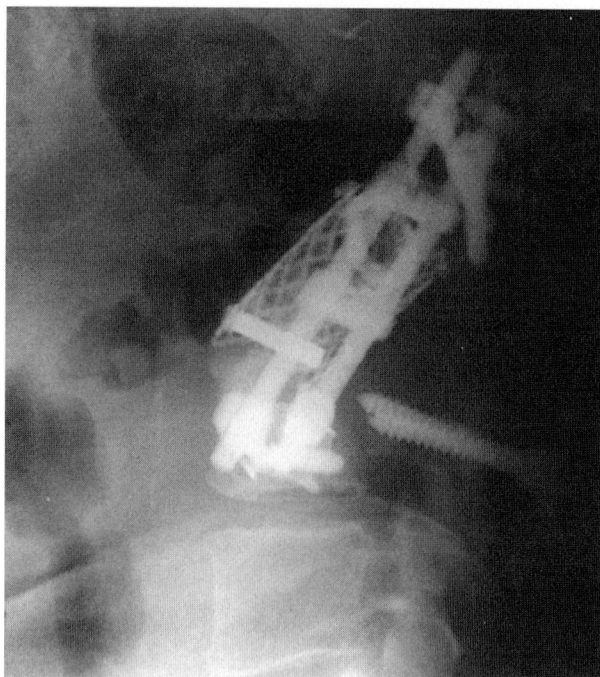

FIG. 92-1. A 60 year-old man with metastatic renal carcinoma to L3 that was treated by anterior decompression and instrumented L2-4 antero-posterior fusion. Radiograph 5 years after initial surgery, when the patient presented with destruction of the L2 vertebral body by tumor, resulting in loss of fixation of the posterior instrumentation and anterior Kaneda device breakage with cage migration, leading to gross spinal instability.

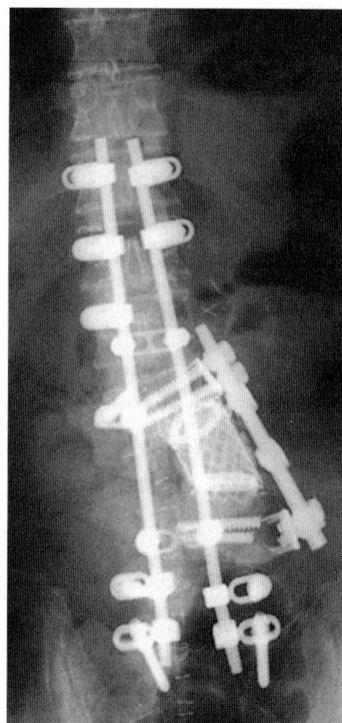

FIG. 92-2. The patient was treated with initial posterior stabilization to restore stability and spinal alignment. The antero-posterior radiograph is shown.

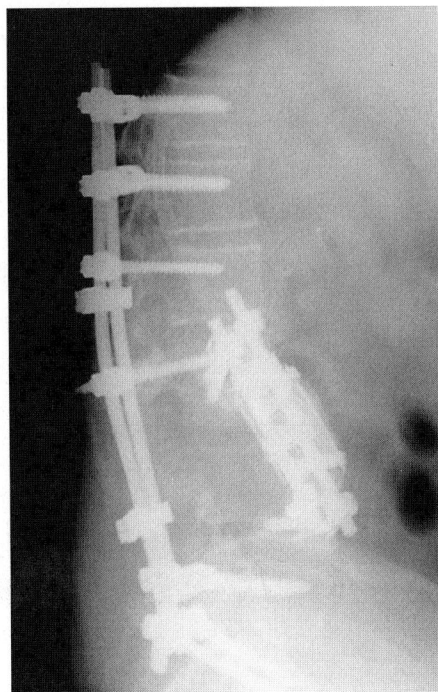

FIG. 92-3. The patient was treated with initial posterior stabilization to restore stability and spinal alignment. The lateral radiograph is shown.

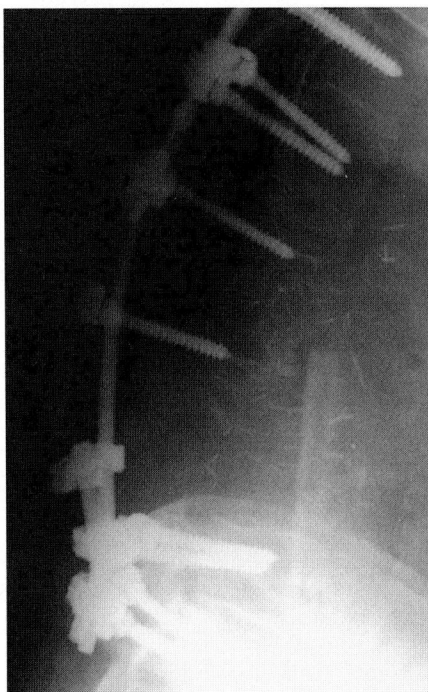

FIG. 92-5. One year later, the patient presented with further anterior column destruction as a result of tumor growth, resulting in fibular dislodgement and posterior instrumentation failure with rod breakage.

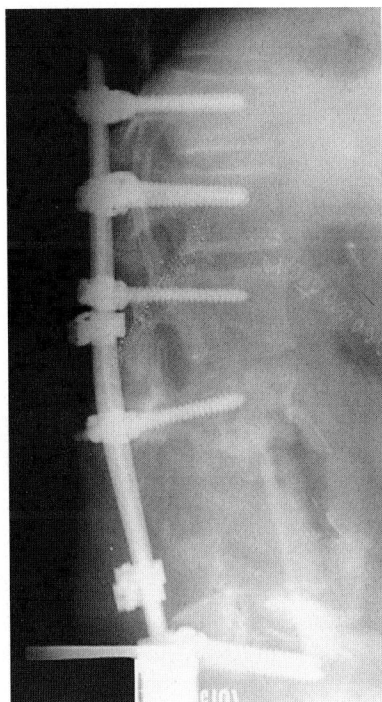

FIG. 92-4. The patient then underwent anterior instrumentation removal and placement of a fibular strut graft spanning L1 to L4. (Extensive scarring and resulting inability to safely mobilize vessels prevented a more extensive anterior reconstruction.)

by 12.9° postoperatively. Posterior instrumentation may be inadequate in situations in which the anterior column is deficient, and supplemental anterior column support is advisable.

When posterior instrumentation fails in the face of anterior column deficiency, reconstructive strategies should include restoring anterior structural support. This is typically accomplished with placement of a strut or cage to reinforce the anterior column. If interbody support is required, this can be accomplished through either an anterior or posterior approach to the disc space. If vertebral body re-enforcement or replacement is required, a separate anterior approach to the lumbar spine usually is required. In addition to the anterior column reconstruction, revision of the failed posterior instrumentation to enhance stability typically is required. This may be accomplished by using wider-diameter or longer pedicle screws or obtaining additional points of fixation to the spine by incorporating additional levels in the instrumentation construct. The choice to extend the instrumented fusion to improve stability of the construct must be balanced against the increased morbidity associated with the additional level surgery.

Deformity

Angular and translational deformities of the lumbar spine are frequently addressed with posterior instrumented arthrodesis. With advanced degrees of spondylolisthesis or kyphosis, posterior instrumentation may be inadequate to immobilize the involved motion segment and fusion may be less likely. Furthermore, if reduction of the deformity is attempted, large forces are placed on posterior instrumentation that can lead to instrumentation failure or recurrence of the deformity.

With advanced degrees of spondylolisthesis, posterior instrumentation may fail by implant breakage or pullout of the screws. In these situations, revision surgery usually includes the addition of anterior column support as well as posterior implant revision that may require including additional levels in the construct. When lumbosacral arthrodesis is performed, the sacrum is typically the least secure point of fixation of the construct (18). If instrumentation placed into the sacrum has failed, the surgeon might consider improving distal fixation by placing multiple sacral screws such as medial and laterally directed screws at S1, supplemental S2 pedicle screws, placing screws or rods into the ileum, or adding interbody structural support (19,20).

Osteoporosis

As larger reconstructive spine surgeries are performed on older patients, the ability of the osteoporotic spine to support spinal implants must be considered. Posterior instrumentation failure has been shown to correlate with bone mineral density (BMD) (21–23). In the osteoporotic spine the weak link in the instrumentation construct is the implant–bone interface, and the majority of instrumentation failures involve screw loosening and pullout that may lead to failure of fusion or the development of recurrent or *de novo* deformity

At the time of pedicle screw insertion, the surgeon may recognize the poor screw purchase in osteoporotic bone. This is usually a result of the surgeon noticing the low insertion torque required to advance the screw. Insertion torque has been correlated with BMD and screw pullout, and may predict early screw failure (18,24,25). If poor screw purchase is recognized intraoperatively, the surgeon should attempt to salvage the situation rather than relying on inadequate fixation to achieve the goals of instrumentation.

The surgeon may consider increasing the length or diameter of the pedicle screw placed in an attempt to improve the screw purchase in bone. Increasing screw length does increase screw pullout strength, although this effect may be less pronounced in osteoporotic bone (26,27). The inability to accurately gage the anterior vertebral body cortex intraoperatively may affect the surgeon's ability to safely place longer screws, because screws extending beyond the anterior vertebral body may predispose to vascular injury. At the sacrum, bicortical purchase may be safely accomplished with medially directed pedicle screws with a low risk of vascular injury. Increasing screw diameter also increases pullout strength

(27–30); however, the dimensions of the pedicle being cannulated limit the screw diameter.

Another strategy to improve reliability of the pedicle screw construct in osteoporotic bone is to increase the number of points of fixation to the spine by including additional levels in the construct. This approach must be weighed against the added immediate morbidity of the additional level surgery as well as the potential long-term consequences of a fusion spanning additional levels. The bone–screw interface also may be improved by injecting bone cement (polymethylmethacrylate) into the pedicle. A twofold to threefold increase in screw pullout has been demonstrated with the use of bone cement injected into the vertebral body through a cannulated pedicle (22,26). Other cements, such as hydroxyapatite cement, calcium phosphate, and carbonated apatite, also have been shown to enhance the screw–bone interface and increase pedicle screw pullout strength (30–32). Possible risks of these techniques include cement extravasation outside of the vertebra, with potential for leakage into the spinal canal or neural foramina. The surgeon also may augment the pedicle screw construct with offset sublaminar hooks that are well suited for use in the osteoporotic spine by relying on the relatively sparred cortical laminar bone for fixation (21,33).

Revision surgery after instrumentation failure in elderly osteoporotic patients is often a large undertaking with significant risks. Nonsurgical treatment may be attempted, and bracing may be helpful if early instrumentation failure is suspected. Failure of posterior instrumentation in the osteoporotic spine usually occurs as the result of loss of fixation of the screws, with screw toggling, loosening, and eventual pullout. In osteoporotic bone, this often results in a relatively large void around the screw that precludes reusing the same pedicle for revision screw fixation. If revision surgery is considered, the previously mentioned strategies for enhancing posterior fixation should be considered. In addition, strong consideration should be given to anterior column structural support and fusion as part of the revision strategy. The anterior vertebral end plates provide a wide surface area that is advantageous for promoting fusion and also for load bearing of structural struts (13,14). Anterior column support also helps to reduce flexion-bending moments on the posteriorly placed instrumentation reducing risks of instrumentation failure.

ANTERIOR INSTRUMENTATION FAILURE

Anterior approaches to the lumbar spine may be preferred in patients with neurologic deficit resulting from anterior pathologies, for anterior release with deformity, and to allow for short segment fixation. Anterior arthrodesis allows for reconstruction of both the anterior and middle spinal columns as well as for placement of bone graft under compression, which provides a favorable mechanical environment for fusion (13,14).

Anterior plate and rod-screw fixation is frequently used for anterior column reconstruction at the thoracolumbar junction and in the upper lumbar spine. These implants are customarily applied to the lateral aspect of the vertebral body and may be less suited for use in the lower lumbar spine because of the vascular anatomy (iliac artery and vein) and because the pelvis may prevent achieving an appropriate trajectory for screw placement. Anterior instrumentation is designed to be load sharing and is typically used in combination with a longitudinally oriented bone graft, strut, or cage to re-enforce the deficient anterior column. The use of anterior instrumentation may allow for fusion of fewer mobile segments than might be required with posterior fixation.

Anterior construct failure typically occurs with implant loosening or with subsidence of the strut or cage into the cancellous bone of the adjacent vertebral body, both of which may lead to failure of fusion and recurrence of deformity. Intravertebral screws may loosen if fixation is poor, as is common in osteoporotic bone. Fixation can be improved by obtaining bicortical purchase of the vertebral body with wide diameter screws (34). Care also must be taken not to penetrate an unfused disc space with the screws. The risk of construct failure as a result of settling of the longitudinal strut or cage into the adjacent vertebral bodies may be reduced by maintaining the integrity of the vertebral end plates during their preparation (35). In addition, small-diameter struts or cages should be avoided, because these tend to cut into the vertebral end plates and piston into the vertebral body. If the surgeon is concerned about the stability of the anterior reconstruction, the construct should be supplemented with posterior instrumentation.

If anterior instrumentation fails with implant loosening or settling of the construct, salvage with posterior instrumentation and fusion to stabilize the involved motion segments may be adequate. However, if the anterior device has lost its structural integrity or has migrated toward adjacent vascular or visceral structures, anterior device removal or revision will be required in addition to the posterior surgery. If the anterior strut has telescoped into the adjacent vertebral body or screw failure has created voids in the vertebral body, additional levels often need to be incorporated in any revision construct so as to obtain fixation to healthy bone. A repeat anterior approach to the previously operated spine may be extremely difficult because of the adherent vessels in close proximity to the spine. If the vascular anatomy precludes safely revising the anterior instrumentation, the surgeon might consider removing the failed anterior construct and then placing a strut only anteriorly, and supplementing this with posterior instrumentation.

INTERBODY DEVICE FAILURE

Interbody devices may be placed by anterior, posterior, or lateral approaches to the disc (36–40) and include both impacted implants that rest on the vertebral end plates, and threaded implants whose threads engage the vertebral end plates. Biomechanical studies have shown that interbody devices significantly stabilize the motion segment in all directions except for extension (13,41). Annular tension achieved by disc space distraction is thought to be important for the stability of these devices.

Although early studies reported high clinical and radiographic success with interbody devices used without posterior fixation, it became apparent that with widespread use these results were not necessarily reproduced (14,37,38). Many cases of so-called "failed interbody devices" actually represent failures of patient selection by the surgeon rather than any failure of the device. In addition, poor surgical technique in applying these devices is a common reason for failure (38). Undersized devices may lead to inadequate motion segment stability and ultimately failure of fusion. To achieve successful results with an interbody device, the surgeon must understand both the biomechanics of the device and of the treated motion segment. Situations in which a "stand-alone" interbody device may not be ideal and supplemental posterior fixation should be considered include: (a) interbody device insertion through a posterior approach that necessitates significant bony resection, (b) multilevel constructs, (c) significant instability (e.g., advanced degrees of spondylolisthesis), (d) loss of posterior stabilizers such as may occur with wide laminectomy, (e) poor fixation of the interbody device in osteoporotic bone, and (f) tall disc without a stabilization response.

The more common "implant failures" with the use of an interbody device include failure of fusion, device loosening and migration, and malpositioned devices. Immediate radiographic imaging and work-up is prudent if a patient presents with neurologic symptoms after interbody arthrodesis surgery. If the interbody device is identified as causing neural compression, it should be removed and, where possible, revised. If the revised interbody construct does not restore stability, posterior instrumentation should be added. Alternatively, if a patient presents with back pain after interbody surgery, a prolonged period of observation and conservative treatment is in order before considering further surgical solutions.

Removal or revision of an interbody device is technically challenging with risks of neural or vascular injury with a posterior or anterior approach to the disc space, respectively. If the goal of revision surgery is to address a pseudarthrosis after a previously placed stand-alone interbody implant, often this can be accomplished by performing a postero-lateral instrumented arthrodesis without the need for interbody implant revision. Unless the interbody device is malpositioned and causing symptoms or is posing a risk to neurovascular or visceral structures, the risks of device removal likely outweigh the potential advantages of device revision. When interbody implant revision surgery is necessary, the decision as to the optimal surgical approach must take into account the added morbidity of a new approach to the spine and weigh this against the difficulties of repeat surgery through the previous surgical field. In general, if interbody device revision is performed in the early postoperative period, this usually can be accomplished through the same surgical approach to the disc as was used for device insertion.

If late interbody device removal is required, the approach to the disc space depends on the location of the implant within the disc space, the extent of access required for device extraction, and local vascular and neural anatomy. After late interbody device removal, it is unlikely that adequate stabilization will be achieved with placement of another (larger) interbody device alone, and adding posterior instrumentation is advisable. If interbody device removal requires extensive bony resection or if peri-implant bone deficiency has developed as a result of settling of a nonintegrated implant, a more extensive anterior column reconstruction is required. In this situation, the reconstruction usually includes an anterior strut with supplemental posterior stabilization to ensure stability and prevent settling and subsidence.

CONCLUSION

When confronted with a patient with failed instrumentation the surgeon should determine the likely reason for failure of the instrumentation. The surgeon must also elucidate the source of the patient's symptoms and any relationship of these to the finding of failed instrumentation. If revision surgery is contemplated, the surgery should be primarily directed to the likely symptom generator. If revision reconstruction of the spine is undertaken, any implants applied must be able to withstand the forces acting across the instrumented spinal segments. Revision surgery often involves posterior instrumentation as well as establishing anterior column support.

REFERENCES

1. Brodsky AE, Kovalsky ES, Khalil MA. A correlation of radiologic assessment of lumbar spine fusions with surgical explorations. Spine 1991;16:261–265.
2. Slizofski WJ, Collier BD, Flatley TJ, et al. Painful pseudarthrosis following lumbar spinal fusion: detection by combined SPECT and planar bone scintigraphy. Skeletal Radiol 1987;16:136–141.
3. Hume M, Capen DA, Nelson RW, et al. Outcome after Wiltse pedicle screw removal. J Spinal Disord 1996;9:121–124.
4. Wetzel FT, Brustein M, Phillips FM, et al. Hardware failure in an unconstrained lumbar pedicle screw system. A 2-year follow-up study. Spine 1999;24:1138–1143.
5. Fischgrund JS, Mackay M, Herkowitz HN, et al. Degenerative lumbar spondylolisthesis with spinal stenosis; a prospective, randomized study comparing decompressive laminectomy and arthrodesis with and without spinal instrumentation. Spine 1997;22:2807–2812.
6. Yuan HA, Garfin SR, Dickman CA, et al. A historical cohort study of pedicle screw fixation in thoracic, lumbar and sacral spinal fusions. Spine 1994;19:2279–2296.
7. Zdeblick TA. A prospective, randomized study of lumbar fusion: preliminary results. Spine 1993;18:983–991.
8. Bailey S, Blumenthal S, Gill K. Complications of the Wiltse pedicle screw fixation system. Spine 1994;18:1867–1871.
9. Bailey SJ, Barttolozzi P, Bertagnoli R, et al. The BMW spinal fixator system. A preliminary report of a 2-year prospective, international multicenter study in a range of indications requiring surgical intervention for bone grafting and pedicle screw fixation. Spine 1996;21:2006–2015.
10. Sidhu KS, Herkowitz HN. Spinal instrumentation in the management of degenerative disorders of the spine. Clin Orthop 1977;335:39–53.
11. Lonstein JE, Dennis F, Perra JH, et al. Complications associated with pedicle screws. J Bone Joint Surg 1999;81:1519–1528.
12. Chen D, Fay LA, Lok J, et al. Increasing neuroforaminal volume by anterior interbody distraction in degenerative lumbar spine. Spine 1995;20:74–79.
13. Lund T, Oxland TR, Jost B, et al. Interbody cage stabilisation in the lumbar spine. Biomechanical evaluation of cage design, posterior instrumentation and bone density. J Bone Joint Surg 1998;80-B:351–359.
14. McAfee PC. Interbody fusion cages in reconstructive operations of the spine. J Bone Joint Surg 1999;81-A:859–880.
15. Haher TR, O'Brien M, Dryer JW, et al. The role of lumbar facet joints in spinal stability. Identification of alternate paths of loading. Spine 1994;19:2667–2670.
16. McLain RF, Sparling E, Benson DR. Early failure of short-segment pedicle instrumentation for thoracolumbar fractures. A preliminary report. J Bone Joint Surg 1993;75A:162–167.
17. Kramer DL, Rodgers WB, Mansfield FL. Transpedicular instrumentation and short-segment fusion of thoracolumbar fractures: a prospective study using a single instrumentation system. J Orthop Trauma 1995;9:499–506.
18. Lu WW, Zhu Q, Holmes AD, et al. Loosening of sacral screw fixation under in vitro fatigue loading. J Orthop Res 2000;18:808–814.
19. Kuklo TR, Bridwell KH, Lewis SJ, et al. Minimum 2-year analysis of sacropelvic fixation and L5-S1 fusion using S1 and iliac screws. Spine 2001;26:1976–1983.
20. Jackson RP. Intrasacral fixation with C-D. In: Brown CW, ed. Spinal instrumentation technique. Rosemont, IL: Scoliosis Research Society, 1994.
21. Coe JD, Warden KE, Herzig MA, et al. Influence of bone mineral density on the fixation of thoracolumbar implants. A comparative study of transpedicular screws, laminar hooks and spinous process wires. Spine 1990;15:902–907.
22. Soshi S, Shiba R, Kondo H, et al. An experimental study on transpedicular screw fixation in relation to osteoporosis of the lumbar spine. Spine 1991;16:1335–1341.
23. Yamagata M, Kitahara H, Minami S, et al. Mechanical stability of the pedicle screw fixation systems for the lumbar spine. Spine 1992;7(suppl 3):51–54.
24. Okuyama K, Sato K, Abe E, et al. Stability of transpedicle screwing for the osteoporotic spine. An in vitro study of the mechanical stability. Spine 1993;18:2240–2245.
25. Zdeblick TA, Kunz DN, Cooke ME, et al. Pedicle screw pullout strength. Correlation with insertional torque. Spine 1993;18:1673–1676.
26. Zindrick MR, Wiltse LL, Widell EH, et al. A biomechanical study of intrapedicular screw fixation in the lumbosacral spine. Clin Orthop 1986;203:99–112.
27. Polly DW, Orchowski JR, Ellenbogen RG. Revision pedicle screws. Bigger, longer shims. What is best? Spine 1998;23:1374–1379.
28. Brantley AG, Mayfield JK, Koeneman JB, et al. The effect of pedicle screw fit: an in vitro study. Spine 1994;19:1752–1758.
29. McLain RF, McKinley TO, Yerby SA, et al. The effect of bone quality on pedicle screw loading in axial instability. A synthetic model. Spine 1997;22:1454–1460.
30. Yerby SA, Toh E, McLain RF. Revision of failed screws by using hydroxyapatite cement. A biomechanical analysis. Spine 1998;23:1657–1661.
31. Moore DC, Maitra RS, Farjo LA, et al. Restoration of pedicle screw fixation with an in situ setting calcium phosphate cement. Spine 1997;22:1696–1705.
32. Lotz JC, Hu SS, Chiu DF, et al. Carbonated apatite cement augmentation of pedicle screw fixation in the lumbar spine. Spine 1997;22:2716–2723.
33. Chiba M, McLain RF, Yerby SA, et al. Short-segment pedicle instru-

mentation. Biomechanical analysis of supplemental hook fixation. Spine 1996;21:288–294.

34. Spiegel DA, Cunningham BW, Oda I, et al. Anterior vertebral screw strain with and without solid interspace support. Spine 2000;25: 2755–2761.

35. McBroom RJ, Hayes WC, Edwards WT, et al. Prediction of vertebral body compressive fracture using quantitative computed tomography. J Bone Joint Surg 1985;67:1206–1214.

36. Brantigan JW, Steffee AD, Lewis ML, et al. Lumbar interbody fusion using the Brantigan I/F cage for posterior lumbar interbody fusion and variable pedicle screw placement system. Spine 2000;25:1437–1446.

37. Kuslich SD, Ulstrom CL, Griffith DL, et al. The Bagby and Kuslich method of lumbar interbody fusion. History, techniques and 2-year fol-low-up results of a United States prospective, multicenter trial. Spine 1998;23:1267–1278.

38. McAfee PC, Cunningham BW, Lee GA, et al. Revision strategies for sal-vaging or improving failed cylindrical cages. Spine 1999;24:2174–2183.

39. McAfee PC, Regan JR, Zdeblick T, et al. The incidence of complica-tions in endoscopic anterior thoracolumbar spinal reconstructive surgery. A prospective multicenter study comprising the first 100 con-secutive cases. Spine 1995;20:1624–1632.

40. Phillips FM, Cunningham B. Intertransverse lumbar interbody fusion. Spine 2002;27:E37–41.

41. Oxland TR, Hoffer Z, Nydegger T, et al. A comparative biomechanical investigation of anterior lumbar interbody cages: Central and bilateral approaches. J Bone Joint Surg 200;82A:383–393.

CHAPTER 93

Management of Failed Surgery: Adjacent Segment to Fusion

Thomas S. Whitecloud III and Paul Pagano

Adjacent segment degeneration describes disc degeneration above or below previously fused spinal segments, also called *transitional syndrome*. The reported incidence of transition zone degeneration by radiographic criteria is approximately 25% to 40%. Not all such patients are symptomatic. Some may benefit from further surgery if nonoperative management has failed (1–4).

The pathophysiology of transitional syndrome merits discussion. One generally accepted hypothesis is that fusion of a spinal segment causes hypermobility, and therefore increased stress, at adjacent mobile segments. However, is transitional syndrome simply a natural progression of disc deterioration? In other words, would the observed radiographic changes and symptoms have occurred if no surgery had been performed? Several *in vitro* biomechanical studies have been published that indicate increased stress and alteration of motion segment biomechanics (5–12).

Panjabi, using an *in vitro* sheep model, showed alteration in spinal segment function above and below a disc injury. The injury was to the annulus either with or without nuclear removal. These asymmetric injuries altered the kinematics of the functional spinal units above and below the traumatized disc segment. Similar changes could lead to a degenerative cascade in an *in vivo* situation (13).

Is adjacent segment degeneration accelerated by spinal fusion? In another *in vitro* study, the effects of instrumentation on adjacent segment intradiscal pressures were reported by Weinhoffer et al. Transducers placed into the disc above a stabilized motion segment showed a greater than normal increase in pressure with flexion. This change in pressure increased with increasing motion (12).

Does the type of fusion (antero-posterior, instrumented, or circumferential) accelerate this disease process? Lee compared stability and adjacent segment effects of posterior, posterolateral, and anterior lumbosacral fusions in a cadaver model. All types of fusion produced increased stress on the adjacent spinal segment, with the facet joints above the stabilized segment demonstrating the highest amount of stress (9).

Several other publications indicate that stabilizing a motion segment does adversely affect the biomechanics of the segment above (5–12). These *in vitro* studies indicate there are mechanical changes above a simulated fusion. They cannot account for functioning muscle mass, bone density, and so on, or take into account load transfers to other adjacent segments of the spine (7).

The patient with transitional syndrome experiences low back pain. In most instances, a cascade of events has already occurred, initiated by disc deterioration, followed by any combination of facet arthrosis, degenerative spondylolisthesis, retrolisthesis, acquired spondylolisthesis, or associated osteoporosis (Fig. 93-1) (2,7,14–17). Several clinical studies discuss the incidence of this problem (1–4). Few address optimum surgical treatment (1,14,16–18).

Lehmann et al. (2) evaluated 62 patients who had undergone lumbar fusion at L3 or lower. The median follow-up was 33 years. Thirty-three of these patients had follow-up roentgenographic studies. The incidence of segmental instability above the previous fusions was 45%. Although approximately 50% of the patients had lower back symptoms, none were considered surgical candidates.

Forty-two patients, each having undergone a posterolateral fusion of the lumbar spine approximately 20 years earlier, were evaluated thoroughly by Hambly et al. (14) A variety of degenerative changes in the transitional zone above the fused segments were found. The intervertebral disc space two levels above the fusion developed abnormalities as frequently as the disc space immediately

A

B

A

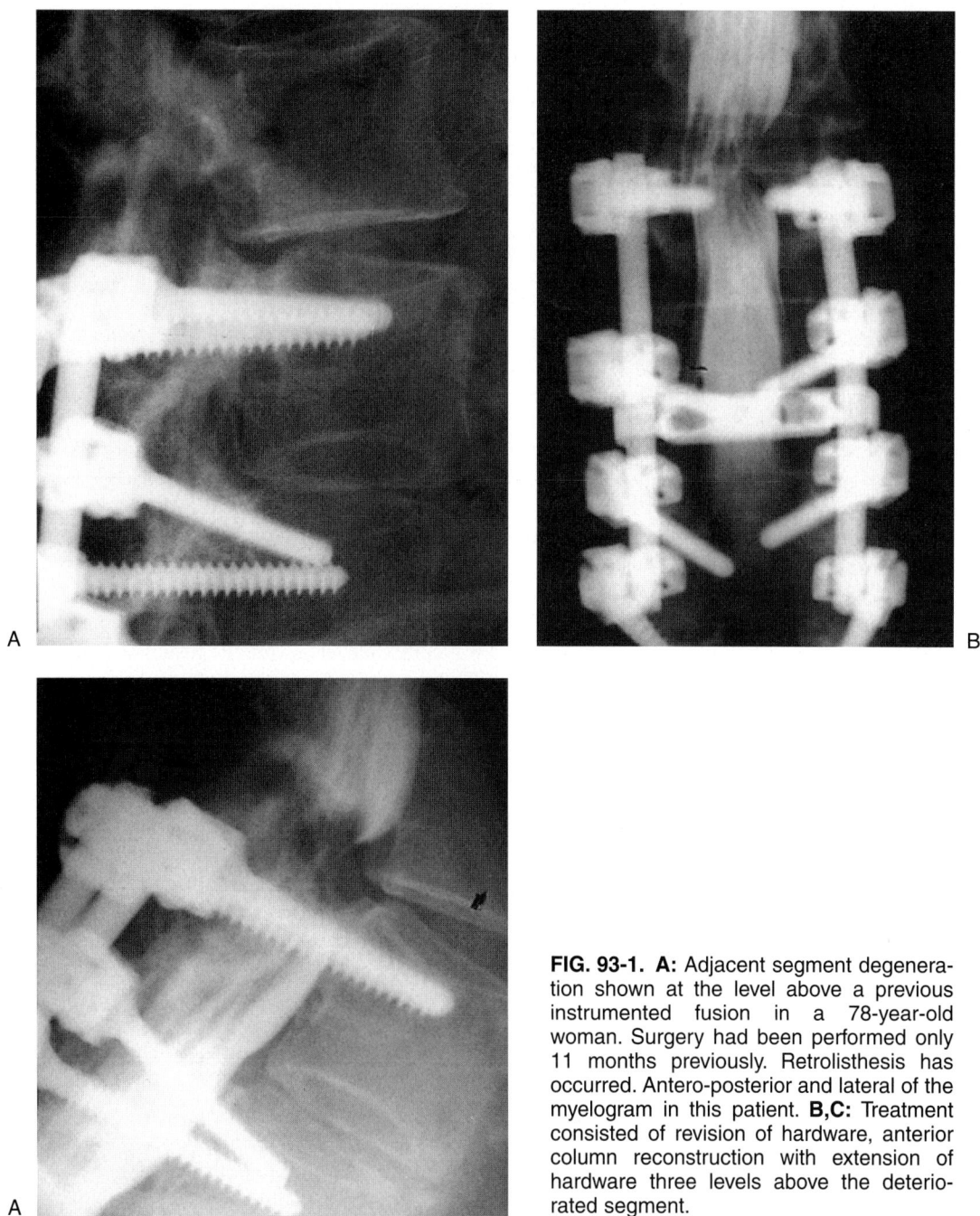

FIG. 93-1. A: Adjacent segment degeneration shown at the level above a previous instrumented fusion in a 78-year-old woman. Surgery had been performed only 11 months previously. Retrolisthesis has occurred. Antero-posterior and lateral of the myelogram in this patient. **B,C:** Treatment consisted of revision of hardware, anterior column reconstruction with extension of hardware three levels above the deteriorated segment.

above the fusion. This finding was also noted by Penta (3). Despite the abnormalities noted in roentgenographic evaluation, 76% of the patients studied reported good to excellent results. No surgery was recommended.

Possible accelerated degeneration of adjacent segments *in vivo* was reported by Rahm (4). Forty-nine patients who had undergone an instrumented lumbar fusion were evaluated. Twenty-five of these patients also had received a posterior lumbar interbody fusion. The time of follow-up varied, but minimally was 2 years. The average was 5.1 years. Thirty-five percent of the patients showed

degenerative changes above the fused segment per X-ray evaluation. A logistic regression model demonstrated that older patients who underwent circumferential fusion with instrumentation were more likely to have deterioration with time. Eight of these patients underwent further surgery. Four of these had poor results, two had insufficient follow-up to be reported, and two were classified as good. A trend to have a pseudoarthrosis in the segments below was noted in the patients who did not show transitional zone changes. I did not feel, because of the variables involved, that there was an increased incidence of adjacent segment degeneration when compared to post-operative fusion alone.

Aota suggested in 1995 that age is the most significant predictor for developing adjacent segment deterioration in instrumented fusion. Patients over the age of 55 had an incidence of 37%, whereas the incidence of patients under this age was 12%. Posterior translation was the most common finding. The average follow-up time was 39 months. The number of patients evaluated was 65. Overall, the incidence of postfusion instability was 24.6%. Older patients appear to be more susceptible, and failure to correct sagittal and coronal balance accelerates the process (1).

Hypolordosis across the instrumented segments may accelerate adjacent segment degeneration by causing compensatory hyperlordosis in the adjacent mobile segments. Biomechanically, a significant load increase in the adjacent hyperlordotic segments has been described (11).

Spinal surgeons recognize adjacent segment degeneration as a cause of failed back syndrome. However, surgical management of patients with adjacent segment degeneration, if unresponsive to nonoperative management, has not been precisely defined. The literature provides few guidelines as to optimal operative intervention for this diagnosis. Generally, surgical treatment when required is usually decompression, decompression with fusion with or without instrumentation, or additionally with anterior column reconstruction.

In 1994, I presented a small series of patients undergoing surgery for adjacent segment degeneration (17). There were 14 patients in this series, and 12 had undergone more than one previous lumbar procedure. Average time from the first fusion to the adjacent segment degeneration requiring surgery was 11.5 years. All these patients were stenotic with instability either primarily or secondarily following decompression. All had extension of their fusion, five without instrumentation, and nine with pedicle fixation. Without instrumentation, only one patient obtained arthrodesis, resulting in an unacceptable 80% pseudoarthrosis rate for the patient series. Because of this, pedicle instrumentation was used primarily in the next nine patients. Three of the five patients who had not been instrumented, subsequently were revised with pedicle fixation. With instrumentation use, primarily or for revision, the pseudoarthrosis rate was 17%. The authors concluded that pedicle instrumentation is generally needed for stabilization of adjacent segment degeneration. However, the clinical results in this series were not outstanding. The authors felt that this reflected chronicity of patients' symptoms and the salvage nature of the procedure. Because there continued to be a greater than 15% pseudoarthrosis rate using instrumentation, I have been adding anterior column reconstruction with titanium surgical mesh for this condition since 1994.

Other authors subsequently recommended that pedicle fixation be used for adjacent segment degeneration. Chen et al. reported on 39 patients who had undergone decompression and instrumented fusion for degenerative spondylolisthesis with stenosis, who then developed lumbar instability with stenosis (18). All underwent a decompression and instrumented fusion at the adjacent segment. The average interval from the index procedure to the second operation was 5.2 years. Follow-up after the second procedure was 62 months. The rate of arthrodesis was 37 of 39 patients, or 95%. Clinical results were satisfactory in 77% of the patients. Five patients subsequently developed a segmental breakdown above the second fused area. These patients had poor results. Pedicle fixation provided immediate segmental stability, and we felt its use contributed to the exceptional rate of fusion and patient satisfaction.

Schlegal (16) reported on 58 patients who had undergone a fusion procedure for a variety of conditions. Their symptom-free period averaged 13 years from the time of their first surgery. A return of symptoms led to operative intervention at adjacent segments. Thirty-seven patients were then followed for at least 2 years. It was noted that segmental deterioration was as likely to occur in the segment two levels above the fusion as at the one at the level adjacent to the fusion. Diagnosis leading to further surgery was spinal stenosis, disc prolapse, or instability with olisthesis. Of the 37 patients with 2-year follow-up, 23 were decompressed without fusion, and 14 decompressed and fused. Three of those patients decompressed without fusion were subsequently stabilized, two of them underwent fusion revision, and two had hardware removal. At 2 years, nine patients were rated as excellent, 17 as good, eight as fair, and two as poor. We concluded that adjacent segment deterioration may simply represent a natural progression of a disease process, and fusion is often necessary if an adjacent segment requires decompression.

The series with the longest patient follow-up following adjacent segment surgery was reported on in 2000 (15). Bohlman performed decompression for spinal stenosis at symptomatic adjacent segments in 39 patients who had undergone lumbar fusion. The patients had been asymptomatic for approximately 7 years following their first procedure. Twenty-six were followed for an average of 5 years. Of the 26 patients, 22 then underwent extension of their posterolateral fusion following decompression. The four patients who were not fused appeared early in the series when we did not appreciate that decompression could destabilize the adjacent segment. Fifteen patients reported satisfactory results, six were neutral about the operative procedure, and five were dissatisfied. Overall, the surgery performed was most effective in relieving leg discomfort in most patients; most patients continued to have some back discomfort. Of the 26 patients studied, six had further lumbar surgery during the follow-up period. Two fusions were revised with instrumentation. One patient had a herniated disc above the fused segment and three required further decompression for stenosis above the adjacent segment surgery. Five of these six requiring further surgery had poor results. Again, this may reflect the salvage nature of the subsequent procedures in patients with failed back syndrome.

We feel that both surgeon and patient should have realistic expectations about surgery for adjacent segment degeneration. Older individuals are more prone to the condition, possibly because of osteoporosis. Certainly, coronal or sagittal malalignment in the older person

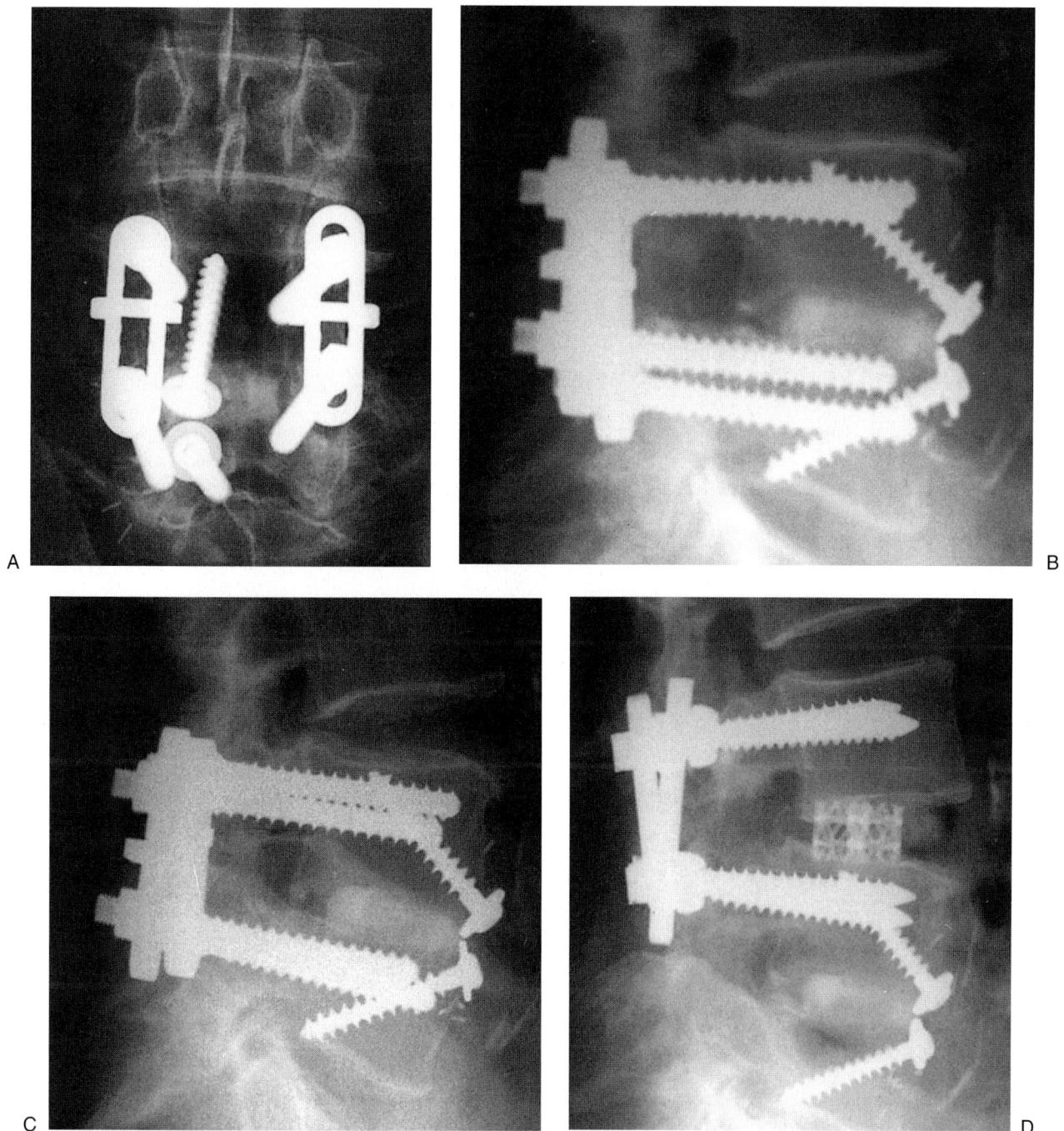

FIG. 93-2. A,B: Antero-posterior and lateral of circumferential fusion performed in a 42-year-old man. Symptoms were relieved for approximately 5 years until the patient began developing back pain and symptoms of spinal stenosis. **C:** Further deterioration of the segment immediately above the spinal arthrodesis. **D:** Lateral X-ray following circumferential reconstruction by a unilateral transforaminal approach. Autogenous bone was placed in the anterior disc space followed by two titanium surgical mesh cages packed with bone. The patient's symptoms have been improved by the operative intervention.

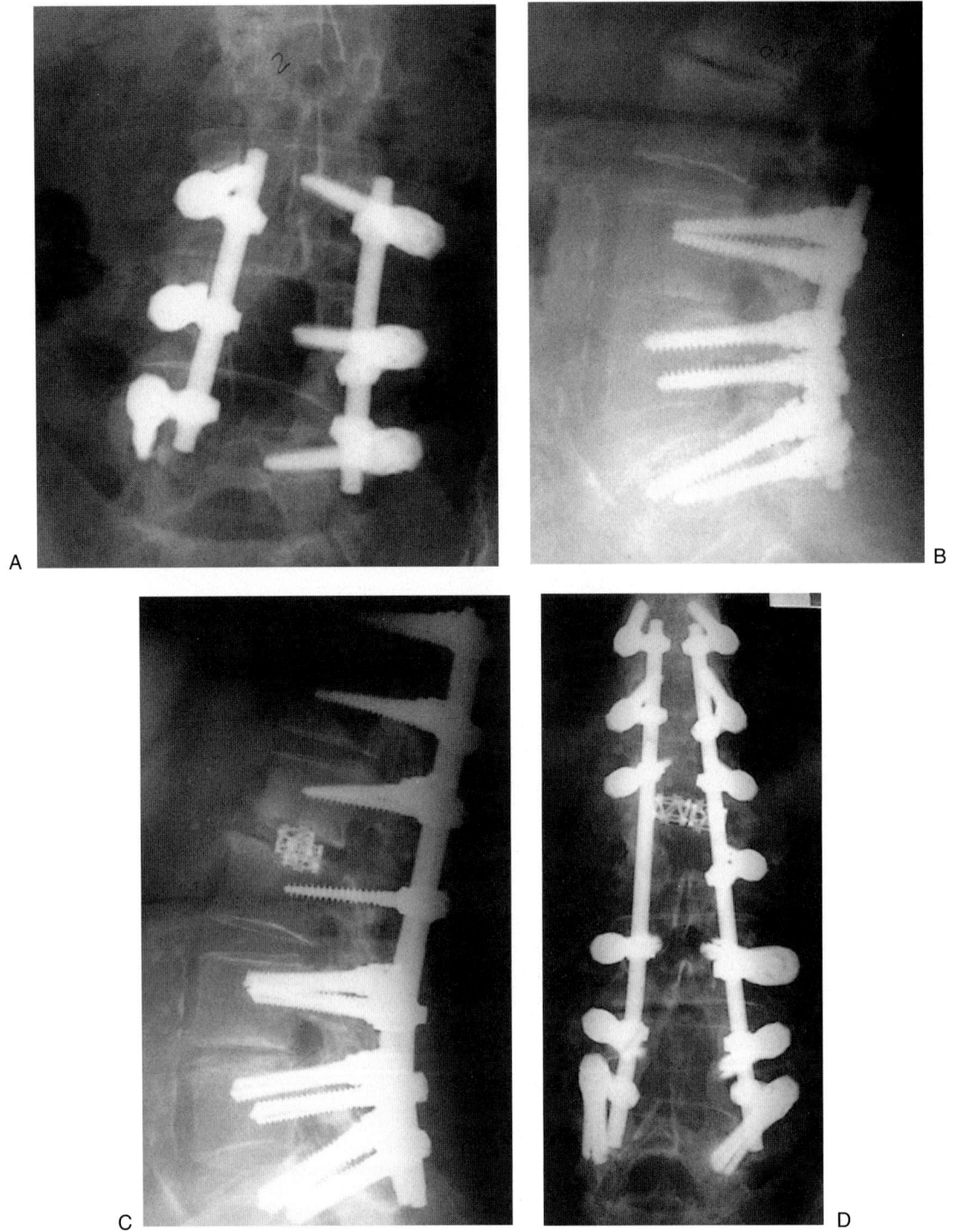

FIG. 93-3. A,B: Antero-posterior and lateral X-ray of a 67-year-old woman who had previously undergone a decompression and stabilization for spinal stenosis. **C,D:** Within 2 years, the segment above the adjacent segment had deteriorated with retrolisthesis with return of symptoms. Antero-posterior and lateral X-ray of reconstruction performed in this patient. At the time of surgery, it was found that the lower fusion was not solid. The patient was osteoporotic and she was revised with expandable screws in the previous fusion mass. A transforaminal approach was made to insert titanium surgical mesh at the collapsed L1-2 inner space. Because of the osteoporosis, the segmental instrumentation was carried three levels above the area of concern. L1-2 was also decompressed. The patient's symptoms have been relieved by the procedure.

rapidly leads to adjacent segment degeneration. Surgery for back pain only, without instability, should be avoided.

The pathology that often leads to surgical intervention is segmental instability and spinal stenosis. This condition requires decompression of neural elements followed by stabilization. Decompression alone simply destabilizes the motion segment to a greater degree than it was before operative intervention. Stabilization without instrumentation results in an unacceptable pseudoarthrosis rate. With instrumentation, the anterior column is often deficient and reconstruction should be considered. Reduction also should be attempted if possible.

In the patient younger than 55 who presents with adjacent segment degeneration and a previous fusion of one or two levels, decompression and extension of the fusion over the involved segment generally is sufficient. With a degenerative slip at the involved segment, a circumferential fusion should be considered (Fig. 93-2).

The most challenging patients are often older with a longer original construct, associated sagittal or coronal imbalance, and osteoporosis. These patients require correction of their spinal imbalance, decompression of the involved segments, with selective anterior column reconstruction. A longer pedicle screw construct should extend above the area of pathology (Fig. 93-3).

Adjacent segment degeneration is a common cause of failed back syndrome. Nonoperative management should be used whenever possible. If both the patient and surgeon recognize that operative intervention will likely not be as successful as the index procedure, surgery can be considered. Careful preoperative planning is required. It must be realized that continued progression at the next adjacent segment is possible after further extension of a previous fusion.

REFERENCES

1. Aota Y, Kumano K, Hirabayashi S. Postfusion instability at the adjacent segments after rigid pedicle screw fixation for degenerative lumbar spinal disorders. J Spinal Disord 1995;8(6):464–473.
2. Lehmann TR, Spratt KF, Tozzi JE, et al. Long-term follow-up of lower lumbar fusion patients. Spine 1987;12(2):97–104.
3. Penta M, Sandhu A, Fraser RD. Magnetic resonance imaging assessment of disc degeneration 10 years after anterior lumbar interbody fusion. Spine 1995;20(6):743–747.
4. Rahm MD, Hall BB. Adjacent-segment degeneration after lumbar fusion with instrumentation: a retrospective study. J Spinal Disord 1996;9(5):392–400.
5. Axelsson P, Johnsson R, Strömqvist B. The spondylolytic vertebra and its adjacent segment. Spine 1997;22(4):414–417.
6. Dekutoski MB, Schendel MJ, Ogilvie JW, et al. Comparison of in vivo and in vitro adjacent segment motion after lumbar fusion. Spine 1994;19(15):1745–1751.
7. Eck JC, Humphreys SC, Hodges SD. Adjacent-segment degeneration after lumbar fusion: a review of clinical, biomechanical, and radiologic studies. Am J Orthop 1999;28(6):336–340.
8. Ha K-Y, Schendel MJ, Lewis JL, et al. Effect of immobilization and configuration on lumbar adjacent-segment biomechanics. J Spinal Disord 1993;6(2):99–105.
9. Lee CK, Langrana NA. Lumbosacral spinal fusion: a biomechanical study. Spine 1984;9(6):574–581.
10. Olsewski JM, Schendel MJ, Wallace LJ, et al. Magnetic resonance imaging and biological changes in injured intervertebral discs under normal and increased mechanical demands. Spine 1996;21(17):1945–1951.
11. Umehara S, Zindrick MR, Patwardhan AG, et al. The biomechanical effect of postoperative hypolordosis in instrumented lumbar fusion on instrumented and adjacent spinal segments. Spine 2000;25(13):1617–1624.
12. Weinhoffer SL, Guyer RD, Herbert M, et al. Intradiscal pressure measurements above an instrumented fusion. A cadaveric study. Spine 1995;20(5):526–531.
13. Panjabi MM, Krag MH, Chung TQ. Effects of disc injury on mechanical behavior of the human spine. Spine, 1984;9(7):707–713.
14. Hambly MF, Wiltse LL, Raghavan N, et al. The transition zone above a lumbosacral fusion. Spine 1998;23(16):1785–1792.
15. Phillips FM, Carlson GD, Bohlman HH, et al. Results of surgery for spinal stenosis adjacent to previous lumbar fusion. J Spinal Disord 2000;13(5):432–437.
16. Schlegel JD, Smith JA, Schleusener RL. Lumbar motion segment pathology adjacent to thoracolumbar, lumbar, and lumbosacral fusions. Spine 1996;21(8):970–981.
17. Whitecloud TS III, Davis JM, Olive PM. Operative treatment of the degenerated segment adjacent to a lumbar fusion. Spine 1994;19(5):531–536.
18. Chen W-J, Lai P-L, Niu C-C, et al. Surgical treatment of adjacent instability after lumbar spine fusion. Spine 2001;26:E519–E524.

CHAPTER 94

Lumbar Pseudoarthrosis

S. Govender

Lumbar arthrodesis has been well established for the treatment of infections, deformity, and trauma (1–8). The introduction of spinal instrumentation, advances in imaging and refinement of surgical techniques have led to the expansion of surgical indications for lumbar spine fusion in patients with instability, back pain owing to mechanical degeneration of the intervertebral disc, and neurologic deficit (9–20). Stauffer and Coventry defined radiographic fusion as "a pattern of continuous trabeculae traversing the grafted region and the adjacent vertebral bodies with no evidence of motion when the patient was bending" (21). The diagnosis of pseudarthrosis cannot be confirmed with certainty until a year after surgery, although it may be suspected within 6 months of the primary procedure (22). A pseudarthrosis rate of more than 30% has been reported when lumbar spine fusion of three or more levels was undertaken (23–28). Patients with documented asymptomatic pseudarthrosis have been observed to develop symptoms when followed for longer periods of time (29,30).

INCIDENCE OF LUMBAR PSEUDOARTHROSIS

Steinman and Herkowitz reported that the incidence of lumbar pseudarthrosis ranged from 0% to 68% and depended on the technique of fusion, indications for fusion, and the methods used to detect pseudarthrosis (31). A pseudarthrosis of 20% after posterior spinal fusion and 10% following posterolateral fusion was reported by Cleveland et al. (26). In their series failure of fusion was identified on plain radiographs in 11% of the patients; this increased to 21% when flexion-extension radiographs were used to detect pseudarthrosis. McNabb and Dall found that following two-segment intertransverse fusions (L4-S1), the pseudarthrosis was lower (7%) when compared with anterior interbody (30%) and posterior (17%) fusions (32). The reasons for the low incidence of pseudarthrosis following intertransverse fusions were

attributed to an extensive uninterrupted vascular graft bed extending from the zygo-apophysial joints, the lateral aspects of the superior articular facets to the transverse process.

Brodsky et al. found that posterolateral fusions without instrumentation led to 31.5% rate of pseudarthrosis and only 13% pseudarthrosis with instrumentation (33). Similar results were reported by Zdeblick, who reported pseudarthrosis in 5% of patients with instrumentation compared with 35% without instrumentation (20). Following posterolateral fusion for degenerative spondylolisthesis Fischgrund et al. reported 18% pseudarthrosis in instrumented fusions and 55% for uninstrumented fusions (10).

CAUSES OF LUMBAR PSEUDOARTHROSIS

De Palma and Rothman stated that lumbar pseudarthrosis was iatrogenic after inadequate surgical technique and failure to immobilize the spine with appropriate instrumentation or external immobilization (27). Fusion masses that are subjected to increased shear or tensile stresses and abnormal motion following inadequate immobilization develop a higher incidence of pseudarthrosis. Thorough decortication of the transverse processes and end plate preparation are essential in promoting vascular ingrowth (26,34–36). A pseudarthrosis will develop if these local factors are inadequate.

Pseudarthrosis also has been reported in patients who have undergone multiple operations, in those who are nutritionally depleted as a result of chronic granulomatous disease, steroid use, diabetes, osteoporosis, drug abuse, smoking, peripheral vascular disease, following postoperative wound infection, workers' compensation cases, and pending litigation (8,37–48). Corticosteroids decrease the synthesis of major components of bone matrix necessary for bone healing (37,47,49). Nonsteroidal antiinflammatory drugs (NSAIDs) suppress the

890

inflammatory response and may inhibit bone repair. Deguchi et al. reported lower fusion rates in patients who were on NSAIDS for the first 3 months after surgery and have concluded that NSAIDs inhibited osteoclastic bone resorption in the trabecular area (50). Multiple spinal operations result in increased scar tissue, which in turn result in poor functional outcomes. It has been suggested that individuals undergoing multiple operations are in poor physical condition at surgery, thus impeding rehabilitation efforts and early return to work (51,52). Failure to restore sagittal plane balance and inadequate bone graft surface area after multiple operations predisposes to recurrent deformity and pseudarthrosis (43).

Pseudarthrosis in smokers after spinal fusion has been noted to be three to four times higher than in nonsmokers (37,39,46,47,49). Studies also have shown the influence of smoking on bone mineral loss, especially in postmenopausal women who smoke (38,47). Tobacco smoke extracts have been reported to induce calcitonin resistance and interfere with osteoblastic formation. Deguchi et al. showed a significantly higher rate of pseudarthrosis in patients who continued to smoke after surgery (50). Brown et al. noted significantly lower blood gas levels in smokers as a result of increased carbon monoxide levels and reported a pseudarthrosis of 40% in smokers and 8% in nonsmokers following posterolateral lumbar fusion (39). In smokers, Carpenter et al. found a negative linear association between the outcome scores and the number of pack years (25). Cessation of smoking prior to the operation positively affected the outcome including return to full-time work.

Lower fusion rates have been reported in patients with a postoperative hematocrit of less than 30%, shoulder pain, headaches, educational level of less than 12 years, sciatica, and a family member who had back surgery (47). Narcotic use and neurologic deficit increased the incidence of pseudarthrosis. Between 75% and 100% of the patients with failure outcomes reported severe pain, were out of work, used narcotics on a regular or addictive basis, and could not walk several blocks (53).

Pseudarthrosis may occur following postoperative wound infections (8,37,48). Keller and Pappas postulated that the lack of spinal stability following early removal of instrumentation in the management of sepsis, in addition to septic involvement of the graft, played a major role in the development of a pseudarthrosis (44). The modification of the inflammatory response resulting from the degradation of the bacteria as well as the host enzymatic lysosomal activity are thought to play a role in the diminution of differentiation and activity of osteoprogenitor cells (44). They recommended that it was essential not to remove spinal instrumentation after postoperative infection because it provides the necessary stability to allow for the eradication of infection and improve the potential for fusion.

CLASSIFICATION OF LUMBAR PSEUDOARTHROSIS

Heggeness and Esses classified pseudarthrosis of the lumbar spine following surgical exploration (54). The most common form of pseudarthrosis in their series was a horizontal or transverse defect within the remodeled bone fusion. The shingle type is a defect in the fusion mass that passes obliquely through the sagittal plane and may create an onion skin impression of the fusion mass. A complex pseudarthrosis results from defects in the fusion mass at multiple levels; a different type of pseudarthrosis may be noted on each side. The atrophic variety reveals resorption of the graft and is associated with an intact facet joint in 89.5% of cases. They postulated that in atrophic pseudarthrosis an intact facet joint may provide stress shielding to bone graft placed in the intertransverse area. Sixty-one percent of patients fused with metal ware developed atrophic pseudarthrosis, whereas only 38% without instrumentation developed an atrophic pseudarthrosis. Transverse, shingle, and complex pseudarthrosis are caused by excessive movement of the affected levels despite adequate stress stimulation. Asymptomatic pseudarthrosis (shingle, transverse, and complex) may provide sufficient stability to a previously painful lumbar spine despite the absence of a solid fusion.

CORRELATION BETWEEN LUMBAR PSEUDOARTHROSIS AND FUNCTIONAL OUTCOME

The correlation between bony fusion and clinical outcome is controversial. Achieving a successful fusion does not necessarily lead to improvement of preoperative pain or disability (22,25,53,55). De Palma and Rothman studied 448 patients who had lumbar intertransverse spinal fusions (27). Thirty-nine (9%) patients developed pseudarthrosis, which was demonstrated on flexion and extension views. They compared these patients to 39 patients who had a solid fusion and found no difference in the ability to return to work or activity levels. The authors noted that the back pain and sciatica improved in patients with a solid fusion, but the difference was not marked when compared to the pseudarthrosis group. Similar results were reported by Bragg and Watkins and Bosworth, who reported 43% of lumbar pseudarthrosis being asymptomatic (23,24). O'Beirne et al. reviewed 81 patients following posterior spinal fusion for low back pain and 74% were satisfied with the outcome, although 34% had a pseudarthrosis (56). There was no clear relationship between the integrity of the fusion and clinical success.

Greenough et al. and Flynn and Hoque found no correlation between anterior interbody lumbar fusion and clinical outcome (11,13). The association between fusion and clinical outcome in compensation and litigation patients was intriguing. Greenough et al. found that the noncompensation patients mobilized more actively inducing axial stresses that promoted union (13). Penta and Fraser reported that the clinical outcome using the low back outcome score was not affected by the presence of radiologic fusion at a minimum 10-year follow-up (57). Greenough et al. reviewed the results of posterolateral lumbar arthrodesis with instrumentation in 135 patients and compared these outcomes with outcomes reported by Penta and Fraser, who performed anterior interbody arthrodesis in 108 patients (13,57). Overall there was a twofold difference in the low back outcome scores, with anterior interbody arthrodesis yielding better results regardless of the patient's workers' compensation status.

Lauerman et al. noted a significantly improved functional outcome in patients in whom a solid fusion was obtained and in those who had undergone only one prior surgery on the lumbar spine (55). Deguchi et al. found a strong positive correlation between radiologic fusion and clinical success following posterolateral fusion for isthmic spondylolisthesis in adults (50). In multiple-operated symptomatic back patients several studies have reported an increased number of poor results in patients who underwent repair of pseudarthrosis and good results in those who had mechanical decompression, although the differences were not statistically significant (7,22,31,52,55,58).

When comparing these series, one should take into account that patient demographic variables and the clinical and radiographic assessment may have been different with regard to known risk factors. The clinical outcomes should be evaluated with a reproducible method of scoring the outcome to facilitate elucidation of the role of confounding factors, such as compensation status and preoperative psychological disturbance.

DIAGNOSIS

The physical findings generally are nonspecific and include tenderness and restriction of motion. Objective neurologic deficit may be present depending on the initial diagnosis. The development of new neurologic symptoms and objective signs more likely are indicative new pathologic changes on a surgical complication (22,59).

The ability to diagnose pseudarthrosis is important if one accepts the premise that the presence of a pseudarthrosis is potentially the cause of pain, deformity, and instability. No highly specific or sensitive noninvasive method has been developed to detect pseudarthrosis. Plain radiography is certainly the most widely used in many centers and reported in scientific articles, although they judge the structural integrity and not the functional integrity (9,33,60). Rigid internal fixation is unlikely to

be of benefit in judging the functional integrity of the fusion mass unless there is obvious loosening, displacement, or breakage of the metal ware (61). The associated findings with late symptomatic pseudarthrosis (i.e., pain, loss of correction, and failure of instrumentation) do not pose a diagnostic challenge. Surgical exploration is the most accurate means of detecting pseudarthrosis in a symptomatic patient but this is not always practical and cost effective (9,14,33,54,60,62). Therefore, the detection of pseudarthrosis rests to a great extent on the surgeon's ability to interpret the antero-posterior, lateral, and oblique radiographs to assess fusion. A continuous trabecular pattern transversing the grafted segments denotes a solid fusion. Flexion-extension radiographs that demonstrate gross motion may be insensitive when subtle motion, muscle guarding, or both are present, and following transpedicular fixation (14,61,63). Blumenthal and Gill found that the overall agreement between radiographic assessment of fusion and actual surgical results was 69% in patients stabilized with rigid internal fixation (60). Preoperatively the assessment of fusion from anteroposterior and lateral radiographs was undertaken by two spinal surgeons and two musculoskeletal radiologists. Intraoperatively the fusion was explored bilaterally to determine the presence or absence of fusion. In addition a mechanical stress test of the motion segment was performed with a Kocher clamp and observations were recorded. The authors concluded that plain radiographs can predict the presence or absence of pseudarthrosis in approximately two thirds of patients.

Rothman and Glenn found reformatted computed tomography (CT) scan very useful in the evaluation of patients with pseudarthrosis although CT scan does not provide a measure of motion but only the integrity of the fusion (64). Lang et al. reported that three-dimensional (3D) sagittal planar and coronal reformations were more reliable than any other imaging method to detect instability following spinal fusion (62). The understanding and interpretation of 3D-reformatted image is essential in the diagnosis of pseudarthrosis. In the assessment of fusion integrity with 3D the cleft in the fusion may be obscured from view by overlying unattached shards of bone that blend with the underlying bone into one solid-appearing fusion mass. Clefts less than 1 mm were generally not detected in 3D surface cuts. Undulations in the fusion mass may produce fictitious clefts in the 3D image of a solid fusion. However, the amount and position of previously grafted bone can be determined. Larsen et al. performed a prospective study comparing plain radiographs, flexion-extension views, CT scanning and bone scintigraphy with operative findings in the assessment of pseudarthrosis in pedicle screw fusion (61). The combination of the results of plain radiography, CT, and bone scintigraphy did not predict pseudarthrosis or fusion at a statistically significant level. Similarly, Brodsky et al.

noted a poor correlation of the preoperative radiologic assessment (plain X-rays, bending films, tomography, and CT scan) of pseudarthrosis with surgical exploration (33). Albert et al. analyzed the efficacy of single photon emission computed tomography (SPECT) in pseudarthrosis and found that it was sensitive in only 50% and specific in 58% when comparing the results of the blind readings with surgical exploration (53). In the instrumented fusions the sensitivity (.42) and specificity (.56) was lower, which may result from the SPECT scan interpretation. Single photon emission computed tomography scanning may be more useful in diagnosing pseudarthrosis in the noninstrumented spine (65). Bohnsack et al. evaluated planar bone scintigraphic scan (^{99m}Tc) to detect bone union after posterior spinal fusion in cases clinically and radiologically suggestive of pseudarthrosis (66). The sensitivity and positive predictive value of bone scintigraphy were low to detect pseudarthrosis after spinal fusion. Pape et al. found that surgical exploration confirmed the adequacy of roentgen stereophotogrammetric analysis (RSA) as a reliable *in vivo* method to evaluate lumbosacral stability after anteroposterior fusion (16). Roentgen stereophotogrammetric analysis was used to study vertebral motions after posterolateral fusion with transpedicular fixation and proved to be able to differentiate between patients with and without fusion (14,63).

Interbody fusion cage devices that provide axial load-bearing capability in the anterior column interfere with surgeons' ability to interpret the status of the fusion. Anterior fusion (extra cage) was noted in 81% of patients with interbody cage by independent observers following the use of structural titanium mesh cages (67–69).

TREATMENT

Pseudarthrosis has been identified as one of the causes of failure following lumbar spine surgery (10,23–25, 29,37,42,51,53). The patient with a failure after lumbar spine surgery may present with evidence of one or more of these entities and the contribution of each to the patients' pain pattern as well as the likely response of a given pathology to surgical treatment need to be determined. Nonoperative care should be attempted initially in the majority of patients with symptomatic pseudarthrosis because of a high failure rate at surgical attempts to repair pseudarthrosis (7). If symptoms persist despite prolonged rehabilitation a meticulous selection of patients is essential in achieving acceptable results. The timing of revision fusion should not be considered before 1 year to allow fusion to consolidate unless there is progressive instability or increasing neurologic deficit and pain (70). A thorough clinical evaluation should localize the anatomic source of pain. The evaluation of pseudarthrosis repair in patients who initially had no indication for fusion must be carefully taken into consideration before surgery. The

rationale for previous surgical treatment must be reviewed, including review of all imaging studies. The technical details of the prior procedure should be evaluated. It is also possible that a new pathologic condition has risen since the last procedure and is responsible for the patient's current symptoms (25,53,55).

Low back pain is uniquely personal and invariably has a physical basis (58). The psychological ramifications are universal and usually become more important after failed or multiple surgery and should be given due consideration before any decision is taken to operate. Social factors may contribute to disability and the social consequences of disability are unavoidable. The presence of compensation undoubtedly alters these psychological and social aspects (25,53,55). Depression; conversion mechanisms; and economic, legal, and work-related factors can affect a patient's response to treatment. These extenuating factors, which are frequently overlooked, must be evaluated before considering further surgery. The clinician should refer patients with identifiable psychological stress to trained professionals and community resources including counselors and self-help groups. Patients in whom clear operative indications are lacking, may benefit from programs incorporating cognitive therapy with physical, vocational training, and disability management (25,41,42,51,53,57). In addition prior to surgery other factors to be excluded include infection, adjacent segment degeneration, and inadequate rehabilitation or incorrect diagnosis.

Waddell et al. analyzed the results of repeat back surgery for degenerative disc disease in 103 Workmen's Compensation Board patients (7,58). The authors found that the results were better when the preceding operation provided pain relief for greater than 6 months, when sciatica was worse than back pain and when a recurrent disc herniation was noted. Pseudarthrosis, previous infection, scarring, and adverse psychological factors precluded a good result. They recommended rigorous patient selection, including a psychological assessment prior to repeat surgery.

Although efforts are made to ensure a solid fusion is achieved, a partially failed fusion or pseudarthrosis is not detrimental. Pseudarthrosis may well be desirable because patients whose fusions develop pseudarthrosis might be less susceptible to subsequent adjacent-segment degeneration (71). Attempted repair of a pseudarthrosis is based on a doubtful rationale because there appears to be no correlation between the presence of a pseudarthrosis and persisting back pain. Operative repair of a pseudarthrosis is a salvage procedure in a patient who has already had at least one previous attempt at spinal arthrodesis (25). The use of bone growth factors (bone morphogenetic proteins, basic fibroblast growth factor) may be helpful in preventing nonunions, particularly in conditions of impaired vascularization, such as smoking, diabetes, spinal instability, and insufficient bone graft (38,72,73). However, there are few reports on the functional outcome in these patients. In a multicenter pilot study 14 patients underwent anterior interbody fusion at L5-S1 with titanium fusion cages. Eleven patients had fusion cages filled with rhBMP-2/carrier and three controls had autogenous iliac graft filled in the cages. At 6 months and 1 year 100% of patients with rhBMP-2 had solid fusion and only two patients with autograft had fused (72).

Repair of a pseudarthrosis is challenging in terms of the technical difficulties, approach, and selection of patients. It is frequently difficult to decide which patients require a combined procedure versus either an anterior or posterior operation alone for symptomatic pseudarthrosis (53). Most techniques of pseudarthrosis repair have reported on posterior fusion without instrumentation, posterior fusion, with instrumentation or anterior fusion alone (21,26,51,55,59). The poor vascularity and scar tissue following revision posterior surgery and loss of sagittal alignment of the lumbar spine have been suggested as reasons for low success rates of pseudarthrosis repair (6,7,55,74). Anterior interbody fusion may be more appropriate in patients who had multiple posterior operations resulting in inadequate bone stock for fusion or insertion of posterior instrumentation. In addition the graft is placed closer to the center of vertebral motion, theoretically achieving greater stiffness when fusion has occurred. The intervertebral height may be restored and a smaller volume of bone graft may be used compared with that required for posterior techniques (36,42). An anterior interbody fusion with tricortical iliac crest autograft and more recently femoral ring allografts packed with autograft have been recommended (34,35,75,76). The increased vascularity of the vertebral body, superior biomechanical environment, and large surface area of contact offer an optimal environment for a fusion. Structural iliac crest grafts have several limitations (i.e., donor site morbidity, limited amount of graft available for multiple-level fusion, and graft subsidence). Femoral ring allografts take a longer time to incorporate but there is less graft subsidence and loss of correction when compared with iliac crest grafts. In addition, femoral ring allografts can be used at multiple levels without subjecting the patient to significant donor site morbidity. Thorough preparation of the vertebral end plate is essential to promote fusion. Cohen et al. obtained a 100% anterior fusion rate with femoral ring allografts and anterior instrumentation (35). The Bridwell-Lenke grading scale (34) was used to evaluate the anterior fusion; they noted no difference in the return to work between patients involved in litigation and those not involved in litigation. In addition, they found no significant difference in the fusion rate or long-term functional outcome when using iliac crest allograft and femoral cortical allografts. However, graft site morbidity was not evaluated in their study. Interbody fusion cages have been approved only for limited investigational applications in humans because the long-term

effects are not yet known (68,74). The most reliable radiographic indication of fusion is the sentinel sign or the presence of bridging bone anterior to the fusion cage. High rates of fusion (greater than 90%) following anterior interbody arthrodesis have been reported with the BAK and Ray cages at 2-year follow-up. The 5-year functional outcomes are currently in progress (67–69).

Several studies have reported that despite a solid fusion the functional results have not been uniformly satisfactory (25,28,43,51,57,77–79). Kozak and O'Brien obtained 85% fusion rate for repair of pseudarthrosis but only 30% of their patients had good clinical results (77). Similarly, Kostuik et al. reported 91% fusion rate but only 43% of patients returned to work (6). Others have noted that a successful fusion was important in predicting a satisfactory outcome (21,37,55). Kim and Michelsen reported 81% of patients who had a successful fusion following pseudarthrosis repair had a satisfactory outcome, whereas 95% who had a poor functional outcome did not achieve a fusion (52).

Albert et al. achieved 90% fusion rate following repair of pseudarthrosis with a combined anterior and posterior approach (53). The advantages of the circumferential fusion include elimination of all potential sources of pain both anteriorly and posteriorly as well as maximization of stability with resulting increase in the rate of fusion (18,19,25). This hypothesis is supported by reports of back pain that persisted despite solid posterior fusion but was subsequently relieved after the addition of anterior discectomy and interbody arthrodesis (80). A functional failure of 31% was noted despite a successful fusion. The authors identified functional failures in those patients using two or more doses of narcotic medication per day prior to surgery and those with abnormal neurologic findings, compensation, or legal claims were at more than twice the risk for functional failure after pseudarthrosis repair (53). The association of perineural fibrosis emphasizes the difficulty in obtaining a good functional outcome in patients who had multiple surgery and nerve root injury.

CONCLUSION

Prevention of pseudarthrosis is the most successful treatment that entails appropriate patient selection, meticulous surgical technique, and well-managed postoperative rehabilitation. Clearly, not every patient with pseudarthrosis after lumbar spine fusion requires repeat surgery. Nonoperative treatment is an option in patients who had multiple attempts at fusion and have associated risk factors. Successful pseudarthrosis repair leads to a successful surgical result if the rationale for the original procedure was sound. It is equally important to exclude other potential pathologic conditions responsible for the pain. The expectations of revision surgery must be explained to the patient.

REFERENCES

1. Albee F H. Transplantation of a portion of the tibia into the spine for Pott disease. A preliminary report. JAMA 1991;57:885–886.
2. Cummine JL, Lonstein JE, Moe JH, et al. Reconstructive surgery in the adult for failed scoliosis fusion. J Bone Joint Surg 1979;61A:1151–1161.
3. Hibbs RA. An operation for progressive spinal deformities. NY Med J 1911;93:1013–1016.
4. Hodgson AR, Stock FE. Anterior spine fusion for the treatment of tuberculosis of the spine. J Bone Joint Surg 1960;42B:295–310.
5. Kaneda K, Abumi K, Fujiya M. Burst fractures with neurologic deficits of the thoraco-lumbar spine. Results of anterior decompression and stabilization with anterior instrumentation. Spine 1984;9:788–795.
6. Kostuik JP, Maurais GR, Richardson WJ, et al. Combined single stage anterior and posterior osteotomy for correction of iatrogenic lumbar kyphosis. Spine 1988;13:257–266.
7. Lauerman WC, Bradford DS, Transfeldt EE, et al. Management of pseudarthrosis of the spine for idiopathic scoliosis. J Bone Joint Surg 1991;73A:222–236.
8. Weinstein MA, McCabe JP, Cammisa FB. Postoperative spinal wound infection: a review of 2,391 consecutive index procedure. J Spinal Disord 2000;13:422–426.
9. Albert TJ, Pinto S, Smith MD, et al. Accuracy of SPECT scanning in diagnosing pseudarthrosis: a prospective study. J Spinal Disord 1998;13:197–199.
10. Fischgrund JS, Mackay M, Herkowitz HN, et al. Degenerative lumbar spondylolisthesis with spinal stenosis: a prospective, randomized study comparing decompressive laminectomy and arthrodesis with and without spinal instrumentation. Spine 1997;22:2807–2812.
11. Flynn JC, Hoque A. Anterior fusion of the lumbar spine: end result study with long-term followup. J Bone Joint Surg 1979;61(A):1143–1150.
12. Fujimaki A, Crock HV, Bedbrook GM. The results of 150 anterior lumbar interbody fusion operations performed by two surgeons in Australia. Clin Orthop Rel Res 1982;165:164–167.
13. Greenough CG, Peterson MD, Hadlow S, et al. Instrumented posterolateral lumbar fusion. Results and comparison with anterior interbody fusion. Spine 1998;23:479–486.
14. Johnsson R, Axelsson P, Gunnarsson G, et al. Stability of lumbar fusion with transpedicular fixation determined by roentgen stereophotogrammetric analysis. Spine 1999;24:687–690.
15. Kozak JA, Heilman AE, O'Brien JP. Anterior lumbar fusion options. Clin Orthop Rel Res 1994;300:45–51.
16. Pape D, Fritsch E, Kelm J, et al. Lumbosacral stability of consolidated anteroposterior fusion after instrumentation removal determined by Roentgen stereophotogrammetric analysis and direct surgical exploration. Spine 2002;27:269–274.
17. Stauffer RN, Coventry MB. Posterolateral lumbar sine fusion. J Bone Joint Surg 1972;54A:1195–1204.
18. Stewart G, Sachs BL. Patients outcome after reoperation on the lumbar spine. J Bone Joint Surg 1996;78A:706–711.
19. Thalgott J, La Rocca H, Gardner V, et al. Reconstruction of failed lumbar surgery with narrow AO DCP plates for spinal arthrodesis. Spine 1991;16:170–175.
20. Zdeblick TA. A prospective, randomized study of lumbar fusion: preliminary results. Spine 1993;18:983–991.
21. Stauffer RN, Coventry MB. Anterior interbody lumbar spine fusion. J Bone Joint Surg 1972;54A:756–768.
22. Larsen JM, Capen DA. Pseudarthrosis of the lumbar spine. J Am Ac Orthop Surg 1997;5:153–162.
23. Bosworth DM. Technique of spinal fusion: pseudarthrosis and method of repair. Instructional Course Lectures 1948;5:295–313.
24. Bragg C, Watkins MB. Lumbosacral fusion results with early ambulation. Surg Gynecol Obstet 1956;102:604–610.
25. Carpenter CT, Dietz JW, Leung KYK, et al. Repair of pseudarthrosis of the lumbar spine. J Bone Joint Surg 1996;78A:712–720.
26. Cleveland M, Bosworth DM, Thompson FR. Pseudarthrosis in the lumbosacral spine. J Bone Joint Surg 1948;30A:302–312.
27. DePalma AF, Rothman RH. The nature of pseudarthrosis. Clin Orthop 1968;59:113–118.
28. Rothman RH, Booth R. Failures of the spinal fusion. Orthop Clin North Am 1975;6:299-304.
29. Frymoyer JW, Matteri RE, Hanley EN, et al. Failed lumbar disc surgery requiring second operation: a long-term follow-up study. Spine 1978;3:7–11.
30. Frymoyer JW, Hanley EN, Howe J, et al. A comparison of radiographic findings in fusion and nonfusion patients 10 or more years following lumbar disc surgery. Spine 1979;4:435–440.
32. McNabb I, Dall D. The blood supply of the lumbar spine and its application to the technique of intertransverse lumbar fusion. J Bone Joint Surg 1991;53B:628–638.
33. Brodsky AE, Kovalsky ES, Khalil MA. Correlation of radiologic assessment of lumbar spine fusions with surgical exploration. Spine 1991;16(6 suppl):S261–S265.
34. Bridwell KH, Lenke LG, McEnery KW, et al. Anterior fresh frozen allografts in the thoracic and lumbar spine. Spine 1995;20:1410–1418.
35. Cohen D B, Chotivichit A, Fujita T, et al. Pseudarthrosis repair autogenous iliac crest versus femoral ring allograft. Clin Orthop Rel Res 2000;371:46–55.
36. Fraser RD. Interbody, posterior and combined fusions. Spine 1995;20:167S–177S.
37. Bernard TN. Repeat lumbar surgery. Factors influencing outcome. Spine 1993;18:2196–2200.
38. Boden SD, Sumner DR. Biologic factors affecting spinal fusion and bone regeneration. Spine 1995;20(24 suppl):102S–112S.
39. Brown CW, Orme TJ, Richardson HD. The rate of pseudarthrosis (surgical non-union) in patients who are smokers and patients who are non smokers. A comparison study. Spine 1986;11:942–943.
40. DeBerard MS, Masters KS, Colledge AL, et al. Outcomes of posterolateral lumbar fusion in Utah patients receiving worker's compensation. Spine 2001;26:738–747.
41. Greenough CG, Fraser RD. Assessment of outcomes in low-back pain. Spine 1992;17:36-41.
42. Hanley EN, David SM. Current concepts review. Lumbar arthrodesis for the treatment of low back pain. J Bone Joint Surg 1999;81A:716–730.
43. Hinkley BS, Jarenko ME. Effect of 360-degree lumbar fusion in a workers' compensation population. Spine 1997;22:312–323.
44. Keller RB, Pappas AM. Infection after spinal fusion using internal fixation instrumentation. Orthop Clin North Am 1972;3:99–111.
45. Mandelaum BR, Tolo VT, McAfee PC, et al. Nutritional deficiencies after staged anterior and posterior spinal reconstructive surgery. Clin Orthop Rel Res 1988;234:5–11.
46. Silcox DH, Daftari T, Boden SD, et al. The effect of nicotine on spinal fusion. Spine 1995;20:1549–1553.
47. Snider RK, Krumwiede NK, Snider LJ, et al. Factors affecting lumbar spinal fusion. J Spinal Disord 1999;12:107–114.
48. Theiss SM, Lonstein JE, Winter RB. Wound infections in reconstructive spine surgery. Orthop Clin North Am 1996;27:105–110.
49. Turner JA, Ersek M, Herron L, et al. Patient outcomes after lumbar spinal fusion. JAMA 1992;268:907–911.
50. Deguchi M, Rapoff A, Zdeblick TA. Posterolateral fusion for isthmic spondylolisthesis in adults. Analysis of fusion rate and clinical results. J Spinal Disord 1998;11:459–464.
51. Finnegan WJ, Fenlin JM, Marvel JP, et al. Results of surgical intervention in symptomatic multiply-operated back patient: analysis of sixty-seven cases followed for three to seven years. J Bone Joint Surg 1979;61A:1077–1082.
52. Kim SS, Michelsen CB. Revision surgery for failed back surgery syndrome. Spine 1992;17:957–960.
53. Albert T J, Pinto M, Denis F. Management of symptomatic lumbar pseudarthrosis with anteroposterior fusion. Spine 2000;25:123–130.
54. Heggeness MH, Esses SL. Classification of pseudarthroses of the lumbar spine. Spine 1991;16(85):5449–5454.
55. Lauerman WC, Bradford DS, Ogilvie JW, et al. Results of lumbar pseudarthrosis repair. J Spinal Disord 1992;5:149–157.
56. O'Beirne J, O'Neill D, Gallagher J, et al. Spinal fusion for back pain. A clinical and radiological review. J Spinal Disord 1992;5:32–38.
57. Penta M, Sandhu A, Fraser RD. A long term assessment of adjacent disc degenerations following anterior lumbar interbody fusions. Spine 1995;20:743–747.
58. Waddell G, Kummel EG, Lotto WN, et al. Failed lumbar disc surgery and repeat 78. Surgery following industrial injuries. J Bone Joint Surg 1979;61A:201–207.
59. Watkins MB. Posterolateral fusion in pseudarthrosis and posterior element defect of the lumbosacral spine. Clin Orthop Rel Res 1964;35:80–95.

60. Blumenthal SL, Gill K. Can lumbar spine radiographs accurately determine fusion in post operative patients? Correlation of routine radiographs with a second surgical look at lumbar fusions. Spine 1993;18: 1186–1189.
61. Larsen JM, Rimoldi RL, Capen DA, et al. Assessment of pseudarthrosis in pedicle screw fusion:A prospective study comparing plain radiographs, flexion-extension radiographs, CT scanning and bone scintigraphy with operative findings. J Spinal Disord 1996;9:117–120.
62. Lang T, Genant HK, Chafetz N, et al. Three dimensional computer tomography and multiplane reformation in the assessment of pseudarthrosis in posterior lumbar fusion patients. Spine 1988;13:69–75.
63. Johnsson R, Selvik G, Strompvist B, et al. Mobility of the lower lumbar spine after posterolateral fusion determined by roentgen stereophotogrammetric analysis. Spine 1990;15:347–350.
64. Rothman SL, Glenn WV. CT evaluation of interbody fusion. Clin Orthop Rel Res 1985;193:47–56.
65. Slizofsky WJ, Collier BD, Flatley TJ, et al. Painful pseudarthrosis following lumbar spinal fusion: detection by combined SPECT and plainer bone scintigraphy skeletal radiology. Skeletal Radiol 1987;16: 36–41.
66. Bohnsack M, Gosse F, Ruhmann O, et al. The value of scintigraphy in the diagnosis of pseudarthrosis after spinal fusion surgery. J Spinal Disord 1999;12:482–484.
67. Kuslich SD, Ulstrom CL, Griffith SL, et al. The Bagby and Kuslich method of lumbar interbody fusion. History techniques and 2 year follow-up results of a United States prospective multicenter trial. Spine 1998;23:1267–1279.
68. McAfee PC. Current concepts review. Interbody fusion cages in reconstructive operations on the spine. J Bone Joint Surg 1999;81A: 859–880.
69. Ray CD. Threaded fusion cages for lumbar interbody fusions. An economic comparison with 360 fusions. Spine 1997;22:681–685.
70. Salvini R, Di Silvestre M, Gargiulo G. Late paraparesis due to pseudarthrosis after posterior spinal fusion. J Spinal Disord 1990; 3:427–432.
71. Muggleton JM, Kondracki M. Allen R. Spinal fusion for lumbar instability: does it have a scientific basis. J Spinal Disord 2000;13:200–204.
71. Steinmann JC, Herkowitz HN. Pseudarthrosis of the spine. Clin Orthop 1992;284:80–90.
72. Boden SD, Zdeblick TA, Sandhu HS, et al. The use of rhBMP-2 in interbody fusion cages. Definitive evidence of osteoconduction in humans: a preliminary report. Spine 2000;25:376–381.
73. Ludwig SC, Kowalski JM, Boden SD. Osteoinductive bone graft substitutes. Eur Spinal J 2000;(9 Suppl 1)S119–125.
74. Lehman TR, Spratt KF, Tozzi JE, et al. Long term follow-up of lower lumbar fusion patients. Spine 1987;12:97–104.
75. Butterman GR, Glazer PA, Bradford DS. The use of bone allografts in the spine. Clin Orthop 1996;324:75–85.
76. Kumar A, Kozak JA, Doherty BJ, et al. Interspace distraction and graft subsidence after anterior lumbar fusion with femoral strut allograft. Spine 1993;18:2393–2400.
77. Kozak JA, O'Brien JP. Simultaneous combined anterior and posterior fusion: an independent analysis of treatment for disabled low back pain patient. Spine 1990;15:322–328.
78. O'Brien JP, Dawson MH, Heard CW, et al. Simultaneous combined anterior and posterior fusion:A surgical solution for failed spinal surgery with brief review of the first 150 patients. Clin Orthop Rel Res 1986;203:191–195.
79. O'Brien JP, Holte BC. Simultaneous combined anterior/posterior fusion. A review of its concept in 10 years of refinement of the technique: a solution for the patient with severe back and leg pain. Eur Spine J 1992;1:2–6.
80. Weatherly CR, Prickett CF, O'Brien JP. Discogenic pain persisting despite solid posterior fusion. J Bone Joint Surg 1986;68B:142–143.

CHAPTER 95

Management of Failed Surgery

Posttraumatic Spinal Deformity

Jeff S. Silber and Alexander R. Vaccaro

Each year in the United States there are more than 1 million acute injuries to the spine, with approximately 50,000 of these resulting in fractures to the bony spinal column (1). Although there are 7,000 to 10,000 new cases of spinal cord injury each year, for the most part, the majority of spinal injuries are minor and without long-term consequence (2). The majority of spinal injuries often only involve the paraspinal soft tissues and do not require surgical stabilization or even prolonged orthotic immobilization.

The vast majority of unstable spinal injuries are recognized early and managed appropriately, either nonoperatively or operatively. In rare cases requiring surgery, the operative management may have been inadequate, either in alleviating neural compression or in achieving adequate spinal stability. In clinical scenarios in which inadequate biomechanical stability is achieved, continued unrelenting exposure to physiologic stresses may result in a gradual posttraumatic deformity, further impeding the functional and emotional recovery of the trauma patient.

The management of failed surgery for traumatic injuries of the thoracolumbar spine leading to posttraumatic deformity can be extremely challenging. Various clinical situations may be responsible for a failed surgical posttraumatic deformity. These include:

1. Inadequate selection of fusion levels
2. Inadequate placement of instrumentation
3. Pseudoarthrosis or nonunion
4. Junctional breakdown above or below the fusion segment. The development of a Charcot or neuropathic spinal deformity may be considered under this category
5. Implant failure

A careful history and examination of all initial presurgical imaging studies is necessary to determine the appropriate classification of the initial injury and to determine if the index procedure was biomechanically sufficient as a treatment alternative. During the consultant's evaluation, up to date imaging studies are obtained to get an understanding of the patient's global balance. Dynamic plain radiographs are also obtained to evaluate for any objective evidence of instability.

SYMPTOMS

Pain

Usually the first and most common symptom after a failed surgical procedure for thoracolumbar trauma is increasing pain. This may be secondary to iatrogenic spinal imbalance in the coronal or sagittal plane, failed instrumentation leading to a progressive deformity, or the result of a symptomatic pseudoarthrosis. Typically, patients initially complain of a constant aching discomfort most commonly located in the apical segment of the deformity. The complaints of pain are exacerbated with activity such as bending, walking, lifting, and twisting but also can be aggravated with prolonged sitting or standing (3). This pain is caused by spinal column imbalance and resultant abnormal forces placed on the soft-tissue structures, leading to gradual soft-tissue fatigue and pain. Furthermore, pain also may be a consequence of premature degenerative changes associated with the spinal deformity.

Neurologic Dysfunction

A minority of patients with a failed surgical procedure leading to posttraumatic spinal deformity may manifest symptoms of neurologic deterioration (Fig. 95-1).

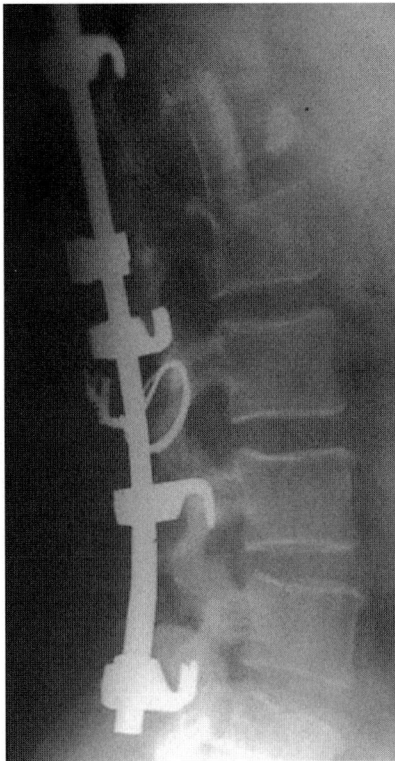

FIG. 95-1. Lateral radiograph after an anterior decompression and strut grafting followed by posterior segmental instrumentation. The neural elements were decompressed and the sagittal alignment re-established, resulting in functional improvement and decreased pain.

Recently, it has been reported that patients developing a posttraumatic kyphosis of less than 15° or canal stenosis of less than 25% had a 50% less likely chance of developing a hydromelia (spinal cord cyst) than patients developing a greater deformity (4). Neurologic dysfunction without spinal cord cystic degeneration has been shown to result from progressive kyphosis, stenosis, instability, arachnoiditis, and cord tethering (4). It is important not to underestimate the potential for progressive myelopathy in the setting of a static long-term kyphotic deformity, which may manifest neurologically only with activity. In this setting, patients may present with no obvious pathologic findings on physical examination but give a clear history of lower extremity weakness, incoordination, and loss of balance with ambulation. This is attributed the active tethering of the scarred neural elements (spinal cord) over the prominent vertebral fracture fragment or deformity during ambulation.

Neurologic worsening following initial neural improvement or plateauing may result from the development of an intracord or intramedullary cyst or cavity known as either a posttraumatic syringomyelia or progressive posttraumatic cystic myelopathy. Because of the wide availability of advanced imaging studies such as magnetic resonance imaging, these processes can be rec-

ognized and diagnosed early in patients with complaints of neural deterioration. The prevalence of this abnormality has been reported to be 3.2% to 40% (3,5). There are many causes of intracord or intramedullary cyst or cavity development. These include spinal cord tethering, microcystic cord degeneration, arachnoiditis, and spinal column instability resulting in spinal cord compression. The pathoanatomy of posttraumatic syringomyelia consists of a confluent cyst within the spinal cord parenchyma. When the presence of numerous microcysts exists in the absence of a large cyst, it is referred to as posttraumatic myelomalacic myelopathy (6). Surgical intervention for this syndrome consists of cyst shunting or fenestration and releasing any existing tether. Unfortunately, shunting of the cyst alone has resulted in disappointing long-term improvement with shunt revisions frequently needed (7).

CAUSES OF FAILED SURGERY

Pseudoarthrosis (Bone Union Failure)

A postoperative pseudoarthrosis or nonunion may result in a progressive spinal deformity. This may occur in the presence of a previously well-performed spinal reconstructive procedure, but is more common in the setting of inadequate fusion level selection or inadequate instrumentation. The concomitant use of nicotine products or pharmacologic agents that retard osteoblast function may also contribute to bony nonhealing. Patients with a symptomatic nonunion often present with increasing pain, with or without activity localized to the operative site. Pain intensity usually heightens approximately 6 to 9 months after the index procedure and may plateau or worsen gradually, depending on the integrity of the spinal instrumentation. Patients or their relatives may also notice a change in the patient's posture over time. Radiographic examination may reveal evidence of instrumentation loosening or failure, and bone nonhealing. It is imperative to exclude the possibility of an occult deep infection when a symptomatic nonunion is identified. Fortunately, the vast majority of nonhealed spinal fusions are asymptomatic and do not result in a progressive spinal deformity.

Instrumentation Failure

As mentioned, implant loosening or failure may result in a pseudoarthrosis and deformity progression. This is the most common reported complication resulting in a posttraumatic deformity. In some series, it has been reported in up to 16% of patients following a posterior instrumented stand-alone fusion procedure. Often, a mistake in judgment in selecting appropriate fusion levels or the extent of stabilization, or an error in technique is the etiologic factor for posterior-only instrumentation failure. Instrumentation failure in this setting eventually results from excessive forces at the implant bone junction leading to migration, displacement, or breakage. Revision stabilization often is required when early failure of instrumentation occurs.

Inadequate Biomechanical Stability

This cause of surgical failure is closely related to the causes of instrumentation failure. Postsurgical deformity progression may occur in the setting of inadequate restoration of spinal stability. This is commonly encountered following anterior or posterior-alone procedures in which significant incompetence exists in the nonsurgically treated spinal columns. Additionally, fusion procedures of inadequate length may not adequately stabilize a three-column spinal injury leading to a gradual spinal deformity. Keene reported on 106 patients who underwent operative stabilization for unstable thoracolumbar fractures. Sixteen patients (15%) eventually required additional surgery for chronic instability and deformity progression 4 months to 16 years after the index procedure. The authors reported on several risk factors responsible for the posttraumatic deformity progression. These included the presence of a laminectomy or a short fusion segment (Fig. 95-2). The authors found that long-term adequate spinal alignment without significant progres-

sion of deformity was observed when at least five levels or more were incorporated posteriorly into the fusion segment (Fig. 95-3). They also reported the same observations when a posterior laminectomy was not performed at the initial surgery (8).

Charcot Spine

Charcot spine is a rare neuropathic spinal deformity, which often leads to a significant posttraumatic deformity in active young patients with a complete spinal cord injury. The pathophysiology of a neuropathic spine involves abnormal motion between vertebrae, resulting in cartilage and ligament breakdown, end plate fracture, and failure of subchondral bone ultimately leading to vertebral collapse. The end stage of this destructive process is a massive pseudoarthrosis. Although this process is initiated in the environment of insensate vertebral segments, patients commonly complain of worsening back pain, increased lower extremity spasticity, palpable and audible crepitans with increased motion at the Charcot segment, and a progressive gibbus formation with loss of sitting balance. If pronounced, decubitus ulcers may develop over the acute kyphotic segment (9,10). In the early stages, radiographic examination demonstrates hypertrophic bone formation. This is seen in vertebral seg-

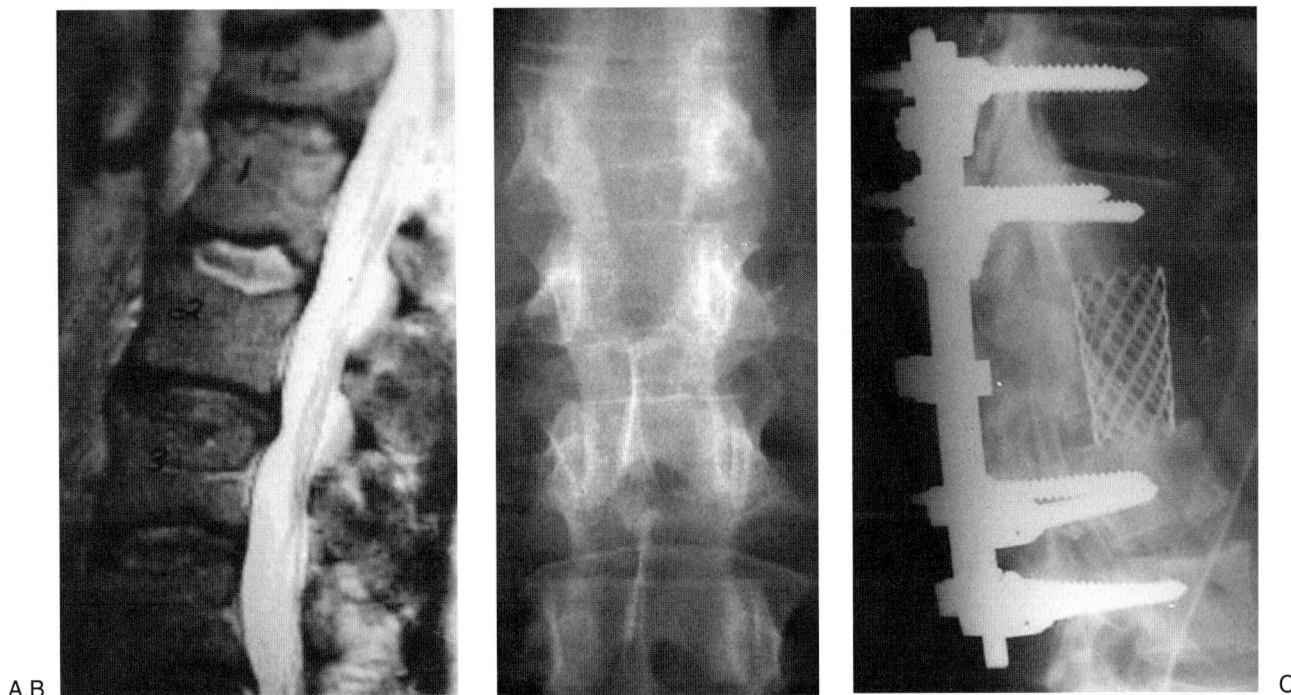

A,B

C

FIG. 95-2. A: Sagittal magnetic resonance image 12 months after a T12 burst fracture managed with a posterior decompressive procedure alone. A focal kyphotic deformity developed, producing increased pain and neural dysfunction. **B:** Antero-posterior radiograph revealing the decompressive laminectomy defect. **C:** Postoperative lateral radiograph of an anterior T12 corpectomy and strut grafting followed by a posterior stabilization procedure. Note the improvement in sagittal spinal alignment.

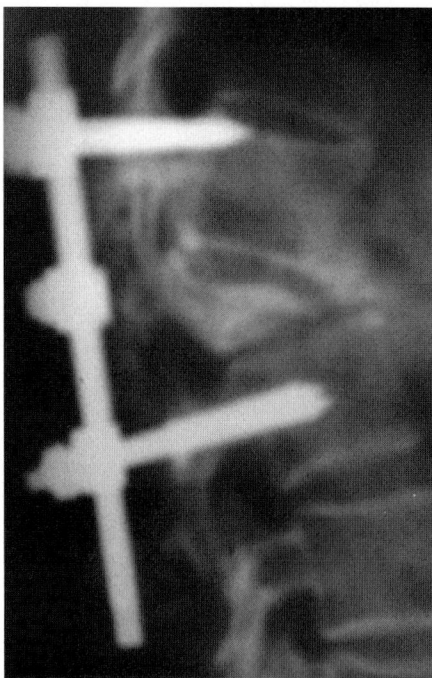

FIG. 95-3. Lateral radiograph showing a failed short-segment posterior instrumented fusion in the management of an L1 burst fracture. The patient developed an increased kyphotic deformity with posterior skin breakdown.

ments adjacent to and below the level of the spinal cord lesion. This hypertrophic bone formation also may develop immediately below a previous fusion segment (9,11). Further progression of the process results in fragmentation of the intervertebral disc space and end plates. The final stage of this process is massive hypertrophic periosteal bone formation and a giant pseudoarthrosis, resulting in an audible and palpable crepitans with spinal motion (11). In order to prevent the development of a rapid spinal deformity with this disorder, early detection through physical and radiographic evaluation is necessary (12,13).

SURGICAL CONSIDERATIONS

The combination of all imaging data along with a history defining the impact of the present deformity on the functional status of the patient determines if revision surgical intervention is necessary. Revision surgical intervention may be considered if:

1. The spinal deformity is progressive.
2. There is a static or progressive neurologic deficit.
3. The deformity is considered responsible for unrelenting back pain or functional disability recalcitrant to conservative management.

Various surgical options can be employed to treat a failed surgery resulting in a posttraumatic spinal defor-

mity. These include a posterior- or anterior-only approach or any variation of a combined anterior and posterior procedure. It has been shown that in most cases of failed surgery resulting in a posttraumatic deformity, a posterior-only revision approach is often inadequate for optimal deformity correction and stabilization.

The long-term outcome following surgical management of failed surgery leading to posttraumatic deformity has been satisfactory. The earlier intervention is provided to the patient, the better the overall outcome. There is an increased risk of operative complications seen in this difficult group of patients, including wound breakdown or infection, neurologic worsening, or fusion nonhealing. The most feared complication, neurologic worsening, is often the consequence of the existing kyphotic spinal deformity resulting in the draping, scarring, or tethering of the neural elements over the posterior aspect of the anterior vertebral elements. Often the patient in this setting has a baseline neurologic deficit; any neural manipulation, especially a subtle tension force, may result in progressive neural dysfunction.

OPERATIVE APPROACHES

Many surgical strategies are available in the setting of a radiographically identified spinal deformity following failed surgery. The goal of surgical intervention includes relief of symptomatic neurologic compression, correction of spinal malalignment and spinal stabilization, and hopefully, the alleviation of pain. The surgical approach may be a posterior- or anterior-only approach or any variation of a combined anterior and posterior procedure. It has been shown that in the management of a late posttraumatic thoracolumbar kyphotic deformity, a posterior stabilization procedure alone, unless an adequate posterior column shortening osteotomy is performed, is often insufficient to achieve both optimal spinal alignment correction and long-term stabilization. An obvious biomechanical disadvantage exists in a posterior-only fusion in the presence of an existing kyphotic deformity owing to the considerable tension placed on the posterior instrumentation and bone graft. These stresses often exist regardless of the adequacy of sagittal plane correction and result from the large bending moments challenging the corrective forces needed to obtain adequate spinal alignment provided by the instrumentation. This assumes an osteotomy was not used to obtain the desired sagittal correction. To improve on the biomechanical integrity of a posterior-only revision procedure, a sagittal plane osteotomy often is required to balance the C7 vertebral body over the sacral elements. Recently, the posterior transforaminal interbody approach has gained increased popularity in reconstructing the anterior lumbosacral column when significant deformity is not present. This technique has the advantage of allowing for anterior graft placement without excessive retraction of the neural elements. Polly et al. have reported the usefulness of the bilateral transforaminal approach. They report on the biomechanical advantage of anterior structural graft placement that functions as a pivot point of rotation followed by posterior compressive forces. The combination of anterior strut grafting and posterior compressive force helps to restore sagittal (lumbar lordosis) alignment. This approach allows for an indirect circumferential fusion and is extremely useful, especially in patients where an anterior approach is undesirable (14).

An alternative revision strategy that has proved to provide long-term stability involves either an initial anterior release or decompressive procedure and grafting followed by a posterior segmental stabilization procedure. This strategy provides a favorable biomechanical environment, allowing significant manipulation and restoration of spinal alignment. Furthermore, improved fusion success is seen when anterior column reconstruction is accomplished. An anterior-alone approach has been shown to provide good long-term stability in the setting of a native fracture and correctable sagittal plane deformity with a stable posterior spinal column (15). This is rarely the clinical situation in the setting of a failed surgical procedure resulting in a posttraumatic spinal deformity.

When a fixed lumbar kyphotic deformity (flat back) is present, the surgeon may select one of several surgical strategies. These include a combined anterior and posterior approach or a posterior-alone approach involving a pedicle subtraction, eggshell, or Smith-Peterson osteotomy. As much as 35° of focal sagittal plane correction may be achieved with a closing wedge osteotomy (14).

Kostuik et al. reported on 54 patients managed with a combined anterior opening wedge osteotomy and instrumentation followed by a posterior closing extension osteotomy with instrumentation for a fixed iatrogenic flat back deformity. The average increase in lumbar lordosis went from a preoperative measurement of 21.5° to 49° postoperatively. They also reported significant postoperative pain reduction in over 90% of the patients (16). The back-front-back procedure popularized by Shufflebarger consists of an initial posterior release with removal of existing instrumentation, the performance of necessary osteotomies and facetectomies, followed by an anterior release and reconstruction. Posterior placement of instrumention is then performed to restore the posterior spinal element tension band (17).

OSTEOTOMY TECHNIQUES

Two commonly performed posterior extension osteotomy techniques used in the correction of flat back (kyphotic) deformities include the Smith-Peterson osteotomy and the pedicle subtraction osteotomy (PSO) (18). The Smith-Peterson osteotomy removes a predetermined V-shaped wedge of bone from the posterior elements in

order to rebalance sagittal alignment (18,19). The amount of bone resected is determined preoperatively and is determined by the degree of sagittal deformity present. With a Smith-Peterson osteotomy, approximately 1° of sagittal correction is usually achieved for each millimeter of bone resected. If 20-mm of bone is resected, this will achieve 20° of sagittal plane correction. It is usually easy to close an osteotomy defect that is up to 15 mm in height without additionally releasing the anterior intervertebral disc. If needed, multilevel osteotomies can be performed or a thorough release of the anterior annulus and removal of the disc may be performed to achieve greater sagittal plane correction. All posterior bone removed is kept for subsequent grafting. A V-shaped osteotomy is created often beginning superiorly below the L2 or L3 pedicle. This is well above the iliac vessel bifurcation and below the rib cage. A symmetric amount of bone is removed from both sides leading to the removal of the pars interarticularis bilaterally. A V-shaped osteotomy is chosen so as to prevent the possibility of rotation once the osteotomy is closed. In the presence of a coronal plane deformity, the symmetry of posterior bone removal may be adjusted depending on the degree of coronal alignment correction necessary. The decompression exposes the pedicles above and below the level of bone resection. The remaining lamina is undercut in order to avoid dural impingement when the osteoclasis is performed. Once the osteotomy is completed, the hips are gradually extended as the surgeon applies an anterior to posterior force to close down the osteotomy site (Fig. 95-4) (18,19).

A pedicle subtraction osteotomy involves the posterior removal of the pedicles at the desired level followed by the planned decancellation of the vertebral body up to, but not involving, the anterior vertebral cortex. The bone anterior to the pedicles may be removed in a V-shaped fashion with the base of the triangle being the posterior vertebral cortex, or the entire vertebrae may be decancellized. Using this technique at one level, usually at L2 or L3, often achieves 30° to 35° of sagittal correction. A variation of this technique involves the removal of the pedicles bilaterally along with the superior vertebral body in a posterior inferior to anterior superior direction including removal of the cephalad intervertebral disc. Fluoroscopic guidance may be used with this technique. The outer margins of the pedicles may be removed last as the pedicles are cannulized in order to protect the neural elements medially and inferiorly at the pedicle level. Once the pedicles are cannulated, curettes are inserted through the pedicle on one side to perform the decancellation as pituitary rongeurs aid in the removal of loose bone through the opposite pedicle (Fig. 95-5). The anterior vertebral body cortex is left intact to act as a fulcrum for subsequent osteoclasis. Once adequate bone is removed within the vertebral body, the posterior vertebral body cortex is tamped into the vacant vertebral body cavity. The pedicles then are removed and the osteotomy is

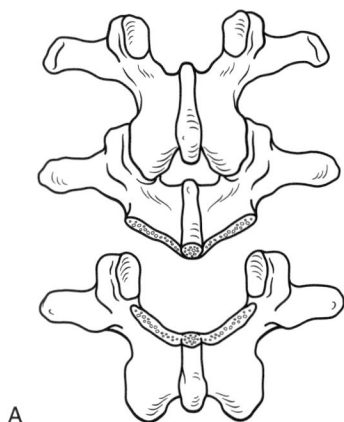

A

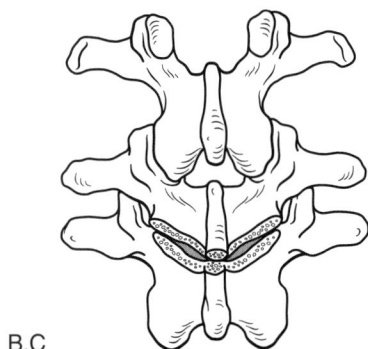

B,C

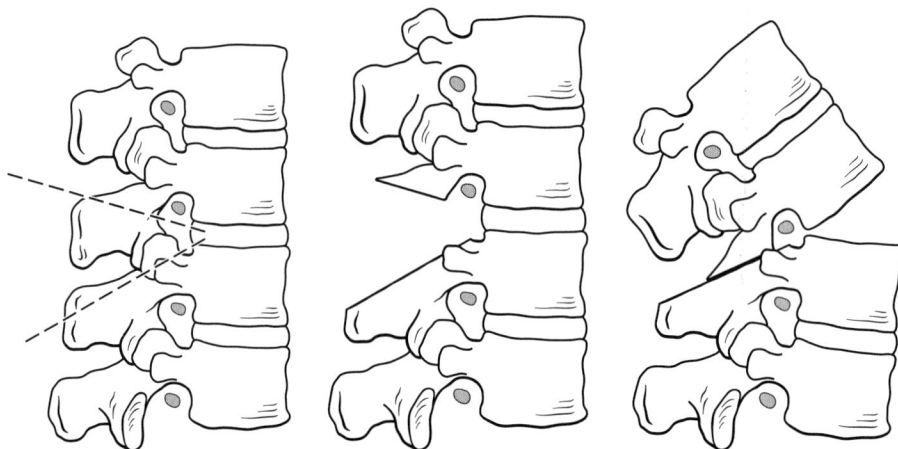

D,E

FIG. 95-4. An illustration of the Smith-Peterson V-shaped osteotomy after bony resection **(A)**, and osteoclasis and closing of the osteotomy site **(B).** An illustration showing the desired preoperative osteotomy defect **(C)**, bony osteotomy resection **(D)**, and reduction of the extension osteotomy **(E).**

complete. Extension of the hips along with anterior directed force applied at the osteotomy site closes down the created posterior defect. All neural structures are carefully inspected during the osteotomy reduction (Fig. 95-6). Before the completion of the osteotomy, a temporary rod is placed on one side and locked so as to prevent

inadvertent premature catastrophic translation at the working site. This rod is allowed to glide though the spinal anchors when the reduction force is subsequently applied. An intraoperative lateral radiograph or fluoroscopic views then are obtained to assess the adequacy of the reduction.

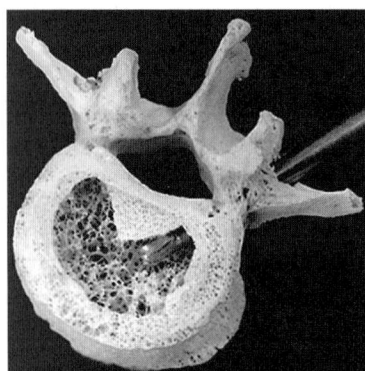

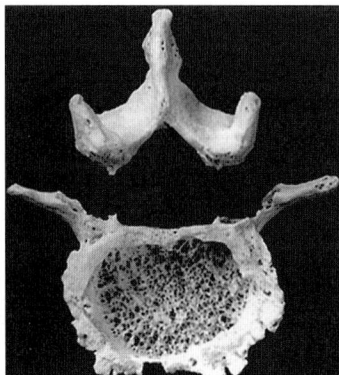

A,B

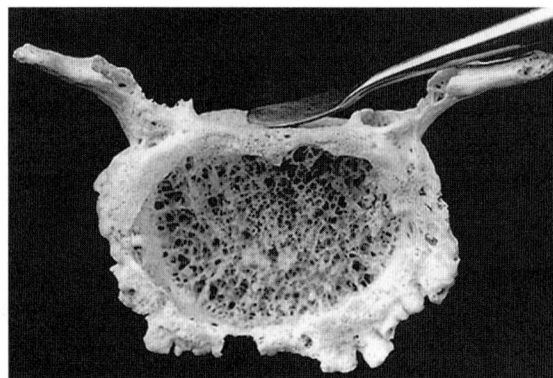

C

FIG. 95-5. Cadaveric specimen demonstrating bipedicular cannulation **(A)**, following completion of the decancellation and tamping of the posterior vertebral body cortex into the void created after adequate removal of the cancellous portion of the vertebral body **(B).**

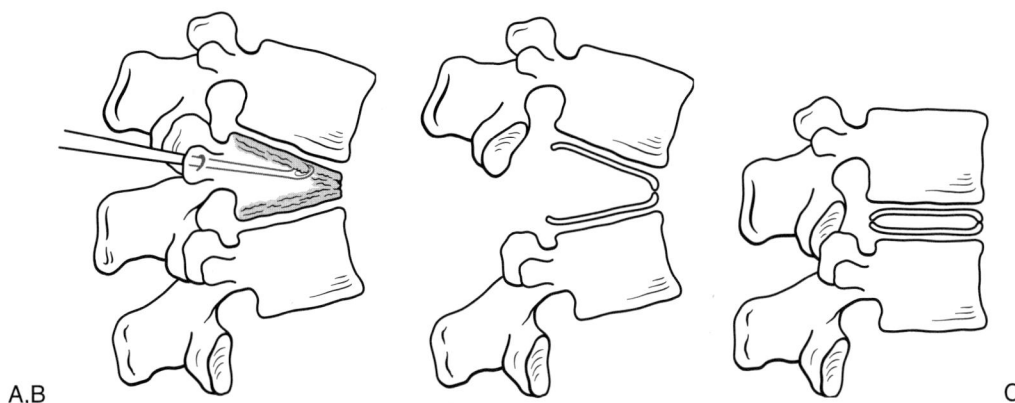

FIG. 95-6. Illustrations demonstrating removal of the cancellous portion of the vertebral body **(A)**, after osteotomy completion **(B)**, and osteotomy osteoclasis **(C)**.

COMPLICATIONS

The potential for neurologic injury in the surgical management of a failed surgery resulting in posttraumatic spinal deformity is significantly increased over the index procedure because of the complexity of the deformity, the anterior draping of the neural elements over the anterior vertebral elements, and the presence of neural scarring. The incidence is significantly higher in the surgical management of failed spinal surgery and posttraumatic deformity. The presence of preexisting spinal cord injury with associated spinal cord tethering, vascular ischemia, and scarring also sensitize the neural elements to the potential for stretch injury from manipulation. New onset or progressive neurologic injury is reported to be approximately 1% following all spinal surgery. Intraoperative spinal monitoring should be used during deformity correction as an aid to detect early changes in neurologic function during surgical manipulation and hardware placement (1). If any neurologic changes are noted during spinal manipulation or hardware placement, the decision of releasing the correction or removal of hardware must be seriously considered.

SUMMARY

The long-term outcomes following the surgical management of postoperative deformity or posttraumatic instability are influenced by many factors. These include patient age and medical status, the type or mechanism of initial injury, the time period between the initial injury and surgical deformity correction, the quality and availability of bone stock for hardware placement, and most important, the experience of the surgical team. Trauma to the spinal cord and column is a devastating injury that may be fraught with many complications, including posttraumatic deformity. Certainly the best treatment is prevention of initial spinal deformity through adherence to biomechanical principles and close follow-up with early intervention if needed. Once failure of the index proce-

dure presents itself, treatment of the posttraumatic deformity follows basic principles consisting of neural decompression and re-establishment of the integrity of the compromised spinal columns. This may involve an anterior, posterior, or combined surgical approach. Great care must be given when manipulating the sagittal profile of the spinal column so as not to over-lengthen the neural elements, which is poorly tolerated, especially in the setting of a pre-existing spinal cord injury. The surgical management of posttraumatic deformity is a challenging problem. The treating physician must pay strict attention to the biomechanics of the entire spinal column and be cognizant of the response of the neural elements to any form of manipulation. Hopefully, this will allow a successful surgical and functional outcome.

REFERENCES
1. Connelly PJ, Abitbol JJ, Martin RJ, et al. Spine: trauma. In: Garfin SR, Vaccaro AR, eds. Orthopaedic knowledge update: spine. Rosemont, IL: American Academy of Orthopedic Surgeons, 1997:197–217.
2. National Spinal Cord Injury Statistical Center. Spinal cord injury facts and figures at a glance. Birmingham: University of Alabama, 1999.
3. Malcolm BW, Bradford DS, Winter RB, et al. Posttraumatic kyphosis. A review of forty-eight surgically treated patients. J Bone Joint Surg 1981;63A:891–899.
4. Abel R, Gerner HJ, Smit C, et al. Residual deformity of the spinal canal in patients with traumatic paraplegia and secondary changes of the spinal cord. Spinal Cord 1999;37:14–19.
5. Curati WL, Kingsley DPE, Moseley IF. MRI in chronic spinal trauma. Neuroradiology 1992;35:30–35.
6. Lee TT, Alameda GJ, Gromelski EB, et al. Outcome after surgical treatment of progressive posttraumatic cystic myelopathy. J Neurosurg 2000;92:149–154.
7. Batzdorf U, Klekamp J, Johnson JP. A critical appraisal of syrinx cavity shunting procedures. J Neurosurg 1998;89:382–388.
8. Keene JS, Lash EG, Kling TF Jr. Undetected posttraumatic instability of "stable" thoracolumbar fractures. J Orthop Trauma 1988;2:202–211.
9. Bolesta MJ, Bohlman HH. Late sequelae of thoracolumbar fractures and fracture-dislocations: Surgical treatment. In: Frymoyer JW, ed. The adult spine: principles and practice, 2nd ed. Philadelphia: Lippincott-Raven, 1997:1513–1533.
10. Standaert C, Cardenas DD, Anderson P. Charcot spine as a late complication of traumatic spinal cord injury. Arch Phys Med Rehabil 1997; 2:221–225.
11. McBride GG, Greenberg D. Treatment of Charcot spinal arthropathy following traumatic paraplegia. J Spinal Disord 1991;2:212–220.

12. Brown CW, Jones B, Donaldson DH, et al. Neuropathic (Charcot) arthropathy of the spine after traumatic spinal paraplegia. Spine 1992;6:S103-8.
13. Sobel JW, Bohlman HH, Freehafer AA. Charcot's arthropathy of the spine following spinal cord injury. J Bone Joint Surg 1985;67A:771–776.
14. Polly DW Jr, Klemme WR, Shawen S. Management options for the treatment of posttraumatic thoracic kyphosis. Semin Spine Surg 2000; 12:110–116.
15. Roberson JR, Whitesides TE Jr. Surgical reconstruction of late post-traumatic thoracolumbar kyphosis. Spine 1985;10:307–312.
16. Kostuik JP, Gilles RM, Richardson WJ, et al. Combined single stage anterior and posterior osteotomy for correction of iatrogenic lumbar kyphosis. Spine 1988;13:257–266.
17. Shufflebarger HL, Clark CE. Thoracolumbar osteotomy for postsurgical sagittal imbalance. Spine 1992;17:S287–S290.
18. Simmons EH. Kyphotic deformity of the spine in ankylosing spondylitis. Clin Orthop 1977;128:65–77.
19. Smith-Peterson MN, Larson CB, Aufranc OE. Osteotomy of the spine for correction of flexion deformity in rheumatoid arthritis. J Bone Joint Surg 1945;27:1–11.

CHAPTER 96

Management of the Failed Back Patient

Spinal Cord Stimulation

Donna D. Ohnmeiss and Ralph F. Rashbaum

Spinal cord stimulation (SCS) has been used for decades in the treatment of chronic, intractable pain. The concept of stimulation for decreasing pain may initially appear paradoxic. The exact mechanism by which SCS provides relief is not fully understood. However, it is thought to be rooted in the gate control theory of Melzack and Wall (1). They theorized that one could modulate pain by stimulating low-threshold, large-diameter, afferent A-δ fibers responsible for inhibiting impulses from the small unmyelinated C-fibers associated with pain sensation. Therefore, SCS is thought to produce a pain-relieving effect by stimulating the inhibition of pain signals. It does not directly address the source of the pain. The first article on spinal cord stimulation for pain control was published by Shealy in 1967 (2). Since that time it has been used to treat a broad range of painful conditions, including angina, spinal cord injury, ischemic limb pain, peripheral vascular disease, failed back syndrome, tumors, phantom limb pain, and brachial plexus injuries. Since the early days of SCS there have been continual developments of the stimulators including the leads, batteries, transmitters, and programming units. Dual lead systems are now available as well. The literature related to SCS is difficult to synthesize because of the wide variety of devices used, differences in study methodology, variation in surgical technique, and the fact that many studies deal with mixed diagnostic groups. In the past, some have viewed SCS as a treatment of last resort. It was thought to be applicable to patients in whom no clear pathology related to their ongoing pain complaints could be identified, or for patients whose pain was related to problems such as arachnoiditis that was not likely to respond to other treatments. Added to the fact that many SCS patients have concomitant health problems or failed surgery at least once, this created a very difficult popula-

tion of patients to treat. With time, indications for SCS have been better defined in failed back surgery (FBSS) patients; at the same time the role of SCS has expanded. In this chapter, we review the literature on SCS primarily for the treatment of FBSS. The discussion of complications focuses primarily on recent literature because this better reflects the problems encountered with modern stimulation systems.

PREOPERATIVE PLANNING AND EVALUATION

Patient Education

As part of screening candidates for SCS, prospective recipients need to be evaluated to determine that they can understand the operation of the external programming unit. At our facility, a nurse educator spends time with each patient, and preferably a family member, explaining the trial procedure, implant procedure, and basic operation of the device. After the implant procedure, patients receive more detailed education about the operation of the programming device they will use.

Realistic Expectations

It is imperative that realistic exceptions be set by the patient, family, insurer, and physician before the surgery. Spinal cord stimulation for FBSS, like any other treatment for this condition, is not likely to yield complete pain relief. Realistic goals must be discussed. Typically these are reduced pain and increased function. For some patients, return to work is realistic, for many it is not. Another issue to address is fluctuations in pain. This can be related to weather, increased activity, and psychological factors, particularly those related to increased stress and depression. There are technical reasons for failure of SCS. The most obvious of these is getting the correct lead placement. Only if the leads are positioned to achieve coverage of the symptomatic areas can a good result be achieved. At some point, many SCS patients require repositioning of their leads to regain optimal coverage in the areas needed. Rarely is there a device failure. One difficulty we have observed with SCS patients is changing expectations. One problem is the degree of pain relief, and the other item is pain location. Some patients initially report great satisfaction and good pain relief. With time the pain relief is the same, but they are less satisfied because they want more. Many times before surgery patients indicate that pain in one particular region is the primary problem they want to address. Postoperatively, with this pain under control, they return with different complaints, or more likely want relief of pain that was present but was not their primary concern at the time of SCS implantation.

Role of the Psychologist

Teaming with a psychologist in the treatment of SCS and FBSS patients is essential. The psychologist can provide comprehensive preoperative screening. The screening typically consists of an interview and formal psychological testing including the MMPI (Minnesota Multiphasic Personality Inventory). Based on the results, some patients who are at risk of having a poor outcome can be identified and SCS not undertaken. The psychologist also can provide treatment strategies for improving coping skills, relaxation, and stress reduction. He or she also may play a role in determining if the patient has realistic expectations or in setting these. At our facility, the psychologist who performs the patient screening is in the operating room during the SCS trial to keep the patient relaxed and at ease during the procedure.

SURGICAL PROCEDURE

There are several variations in surgical procedures for SCS implantation. Presented here is an overview of the procedure that has been used in our facility for several years and has been described in detail elsewhere (3). The procedure is performed under local anesthesia and the patient is only lightly sedated. The psychologist who performed the preoperative evaluation and screening is in the operating room to help keep the patient distracted and relaxed. It is essential that the patient be awake during the placement and testing of the leads in order to provide feedback concerning which areas are being stimulated. After preparing the operative area in the usual sterile manner, imaging is used to identify the spinal levels. At the T12 or L1 level the skin is anesthetized and a stab wound is made midline or slightly off-midline depending on the location of the patient's symptoms. A Touchy needle is progressed caudally into the epidural space. A lead is introduced and progressed into the thoracic region. Imaging is used to check the position of the lead. Trial stimulation is initiated after the lead in introduced. Various stimulation settings are used, with the patient providing feedback for each concerning how well coverage is being achieved in the target symptomatic regions. Also, any stimulation in undesirable regions, such as into the chest or abdomen, is noted. The lead may be repositioned to gain optimal coverage. If coverage of all target symptomatic regions cannot be achieved with one lead, a second lead can be introduced and the trial continued. After satisfactory coverage is achieved with no undesirable stimulation, the trial is over. The extension wires to the leads are brought through the skin at a location away from the implant site. These wires are connected to an external screening unit that powers the leads. The patient then uses the device for a period of several days to determine the degree of pain relief during daily activities. Typically, the system is implanted if the patient achieves 50% or greater pain relief during this trial period. Spinal cord stimulation had an advantage over many procedures in that it can be undertaken in steps and is reversible. That is, if the patient fails the trial period, there is no procedure to implant the battery or internal receiver. The percutaneously placed leads are easily removed.

It should be noted that there are two primarily types of SCS systems. One is totally implantable, including the battery. The other has a receiver that is implanted and is powered by a radiofrequency transmitter that is powered by a common 9-volt battery worn externally. With either system, the patient has a programming unit that can be used to turn the device on and off and to change the intensity of the stimulation.

REPORTED RESULTS

In one of the older studies involving FBSS patients that was published in 1975, Long and Erickson reported that 29% of patients had a good result (4). They noted that they changed their patient selection criteria based on their experience. Initially they had used SCS in some patients with poor psychological profiles. They also noted that another reason for some patients having poor results was that coverage was not achieved in their symptomatic areas. This is related to the fact that the system was implanted while the patient was anesthetized. During SCS it is important that the patient be awake and be able to provide feedback concerning coverage of the stimulation with regard to the painful body regions. This is the only way to optimize the lead placement for pain relief. Although the overall results were not impressive, the authors noted that some patients had remarkable pain relief from the SCS.

Racz et al. reported on their experience with SCS in a group of 26 patients with chronic pain following multiple prior spine interventions (5). The follow-up was 21.2 months. The results were encouraging with 68% of patients having good to excellent pain relief, 84% reduced or eliminated narcotic use, and 72% with lifestyle improvement. In the early 1990s the results of two studies, each with 23 patients, were published (6,7). Both studies reported good or good to excellent results in 74% of patients. The study by LeDoux and Langford also noted a reduction in narcotics use (7).

North et al. reported the long-term follow-up, averaging 7.1 years, in a group of 171 patients (8). With regard to results, 52% of patients reported 50% or greater pain relief and 60% indicated that they would undergo the procedure again for the same result. Although this study had the strength of involving a large number of patients and a long follow-up, in did include a mix of stimulator types used over the long period needed to accumulate such a large number of patients.

In 1996, two prospective studies on SCS were published (9,10). Burchiel et al. reported a 1-year follow-up on 70 patients enrolled in a multicenter study (9). They found that 56% of patients had 50% or greater pain relief. They noted there was no significant change in medication use. In a prospective study involving a group of 40 FBSS patients who underwent SCS for primary complaints of the lower extremity, both functional testing and questionnaires were used to assess outcome at various time periods up to 24 months (10). There was a significant improvement in pain as assessed by Visual Analogue Scales (VAS). However, 50% or greater pain relief was noted in 53% of patients at 6 months and in only 26% of patients at the longer follow-up periods. At 12- and 24-month follow-up, at least 65.6% of patients had reduced or eliminated narcotic use. Bilateral isometric extremity function was assessed. Significant functional improvement was noted at 6 weeks and remained improved throughout the 24-month study period. A worse case analysis was performed in which a negative response was assigned for any patients lost to follow-up. With this method, 70% of patients indicated that the procedure had helped them and they would recommend it to someone with similar problems.

North et al. collected follow-up data on a group of 45 patients who underwent SCS for FBSS (11). The mean follow-up was 5 years. Success was defined as 50% or greater pain relief and the patient indicated that he or she would undergo the procedure again for the same result. At a mean follow-up of 2 years, 53% of patients had a successful result. At the mean follow-up of 5 years, 47% of patients were classified as a success. At both follow-up periods, another 7% of patients experienced 50% or greater pain relief, but would not undergo the procedure again. At follow-up the majority of patients were not taking analgesics. Before SCS, 74% of patients were taking narcotic medication. After SCS this figure reduced to 12%, and one half of these patients were using a reduced dosage.

In 1995, Turner et al. published the results of a review on the use of SCS for FBSS (12). They found that when synthesizing the data from the various studies, 59% of patients experienced 50% or greater pain relief and 75% received 50% or greater relief of leg pain.

For many years SCS was used in FBSS patients with no other operative option. Patients with diagnoses such as symptomatic pseudoarthrosis, recurrent disc herniation, and so on, were not generally considered for SCS. North et al. reported the results of a prospective randomized study comparing SCS to conventional reoperation (13). Patients had what was described as "surgically remediable disease." The study excluded patients with neural compression, primary complaints of back pain, and those with significant psychological problems. At 6 months follow-up, patients were allowed to decide if they wanted to cross over to receive the unassigned treatment. Twenty-seven patients reached the 6-month follow-up. Two of 12 patients (17%) in the SCS group chose to cross over to traditional reoperation. Among the 15 patients who underwent reoperation after being assigned to that group, 10 patients (67%) opted to cross over and undergo SCS. These studies supports that SCS may be a viable treatment alternative in patients who may otherwise undergo much more invasive surgery.

Arachnoiditis

Arachnoiditis is difficult to treat. A few studies have focused on the use of SCS for its treatment and have reported favorable results (14–17). In 1982, Siegfried et al. reported on a series of 191 patients with this condition who underwent a trial for SCS (17). Eighty-nine patients passed the trial stimulation and progressed to implantation of the system. At 1-year follow-up, 71% of patients had a successful outcome. This figure decreased to 61% at 4- to 8-year follow-up. However, considering the difficult population being addressed and the long follow-up duration, these results are quite good. The authors noted that the results were decreased among patients with significant psychological problems. A year later another study dealing with SCS specifically for the treatment of arachnoiditis was published (14). Their study involved 38 patients with a mean of 3.5 previous surgeries. The mean follow-up was 38.5 months. There was a 60% improvement in pain, and 40% of patients substantially reduced their use of pain medication. In 1995 Fiume et al. reported on a group of 36 patients who underwent SCS for pain related to arachnoiditis (15). They reported that 56% of patients had 50% or greater pain relief a mean of 55 months after the SCS surgery. They noted that the results were better in female patients and those who had primarily radicular, rather than axial pain.

Probst reported good results from SCS for pain related to epi-/intradural fibrosis in a group of 112 patients with a mean follow-up of 54 months (16). He reported that patients in whom the electrodes were implanted epidurally had a better outcome than did patients in whom the electrodes were placed endodurally (67% versus 45%). Analgesic use was reduced or eliminated in 40% of patients.

Case Report

Presented here is a case report of a 36-year-old man who had worked in his family's iron-working business since a young age. He first underwent a discectomy at age 16. In his twenties, he reinjured his back and eventually underwent a series of lumbar surgeries including a repeat discectomy combined with a Harrington rod fusion from L3-4 to the sacrum. The rods were later removed and this was followed by an infection requiring débridement. He was able to work only sporadically during these years because of pain. Upon presentation to our clinic the patient reported back pain rated as 10 of 10 in intensity and equally severe leg pain. He was obese at 5'8" tall and 250 pounds. The patient was also a two-pack-a-day smoker. He had been disabled from work for the previous 3 years. As seen in Figure 96-1, the patient had severe arachnoiditis. The patient underwent SCS implantation. He reported being significantly improved at his 2-week postoperative follow-up office appointment. At his most recent office visit, approximately 4 years after SCS implantation, his ambulation improved and he had lost more than 40 pounds. With regard to activity, the patient reported that he had been able to go on a vacation with his family and that he had returned to full-time employment in the iron-working business. The patient is still using some analgesic medication. There was one reoperation to replace his depleted battery.

Low Back Pain

Among FBSS patients, SCS was traditionally indicated for patients with primary complaints of leg pain. With the development of dual lead systems, the indications for SCS expanded to include patients with primary complaints of back pain as well. There have been two studies published recently that dealt specifically with patients having primarily complaints of low back pain. Ohnmeiss and Rashbaum published the results in a group of 41 patients, 38 of whom were diagnosed with FBSS (3). The length of follow-up ranged from 5.5 to 19 months. A negative response to a patient follow-up questionnaire was assigned for the four patients who had the device removed. Also, a worst-case analysis was performed in which a negative response was assigned for patients lost to follow-up or who elected not to respond to a question. At follow-up (the number in parentheses is the worst-case analysis figure), patient responses to questionnaires indicates that 79% (72%) of patients would recommend the treatment, 70% (58%) were satisfied, 76% (69%) would do it again, and 60% considered themselves improved.

Barolat et al. reported on a group of 41 patients in whom SCS was used to treat chronic back pain (18). The authors reported excellent results at 1 year, with 88% of

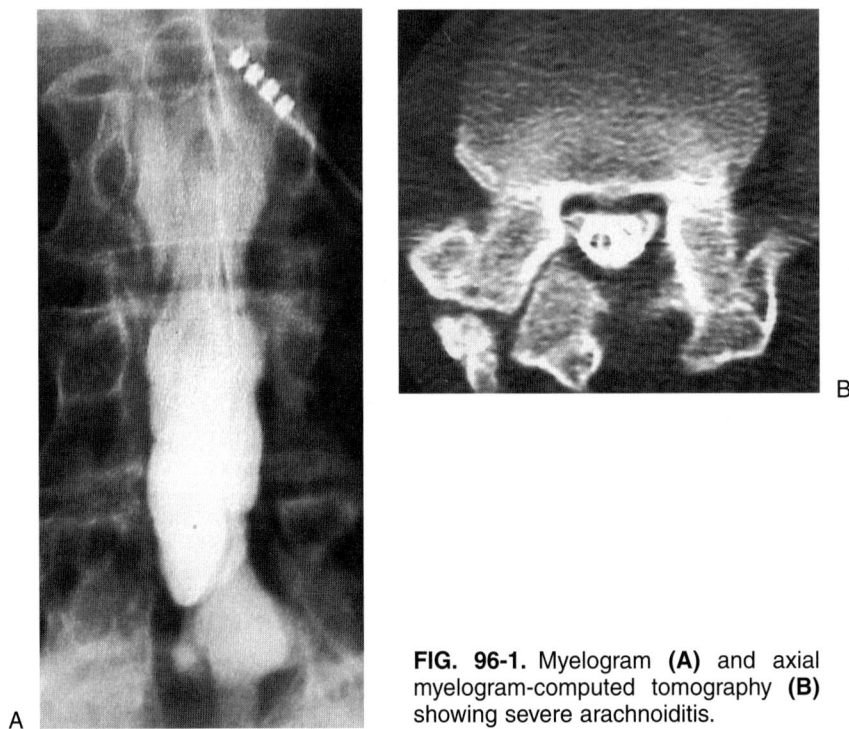

FIG. 96-1. Myelogram **(A)** and axial myelogram-computed tomography **(B)** showing severe arachnoiditis.

patients having excellent relief of leg pain, 69% excellent relief of back pain, and 88% satisfaction with their outcome. However, results of this study must be read with caution. The 12-month follow-up included only 17 of the original 41 patients. Patients in whom the device was removed, who were lost to follow-up, or who were removed from the study for unexplained reasons, were not included in the 12-month data. It is likely that at least some of these patients had a poor outcome that was not reflected in the reported results.

Factors Related to Outcome

Burchiel et al. investigated possible prognostic factors for SCS treatment outcome in a group of primarily FBSS patients (19). They found that the best prognostic factors with regard to change in the VAS scales were patient age and the depression score on the MMPI. Factors not related to outcome were gender, educational level, pain location, compensation, pain duration, Oswestry scores, Beck Depression Inventory, McGill Pain Questionnaire, Sickness Impact Profile, and the other scales of the MMPI. However, the stepwise linear regression analysis that was used to generate the predictive equation included the depression scale, age, and the McGill Pain Questionnaire. The analysis revealed that 54% of variation in the preoperative to postoperative VAS could be explained by these three variables. One significant drawback to this study was the inclusion of only 34 patients with a 3-month follow-up. With so few patients, prognostic factors are difficult to evaluate. However, this study indicates that more work involving a larger number of patients is warranted.

COMPLICATIONS

This review of complications is limited to newer SCS devices and to those studies dealing specifically with FBSS or back pain patients. Complications of SCS are not infrequent, but fortunately they are generally not serious. North et al. reported on complications in a series of patients with a mean 7.1-year follow-up (8). Clinical data were available for 171 patients, and 298 patients were available for analysis of device-related problems. They reported no cases of spinal cord injury, bacterial meningitis, or life-threatening infection. There was a 5% rate of wound infections. These were all treated successfully by removal of the SCS system and a course of antibiotics. After the infection was addressed, the SCS unit was reimplanted. The authors reported that electrode and lead assembly failed because of fatigue fracture of the conductors or insulation failure occurred in 7% of cases. The radiofrequency receiver failed in 5% of systems. The authors did not provide the number of patients who underwent reoperation for revision of migrated leads.

In the review of SCS literature, Turner reported that across multiple studies, on average 42% of patients had a complication, ranging from 20% to 75% (12). Infection occurred in 5% of patients, and what was termed a biological complication other than infection was reported in 9% of patients. Thirty percent of patients had a stimulator complication, ranging from 0% to 75% in the various studies. Problems with the electrodes were noted in 24% of patients, problems with the lead wires occurred in 7%, and 2% of patients had a problem with the pulse generator. The authors noted that although the complication rate was rather high at 42%, the complications were minor and few if any resulted in permanent neurologic damage or death. It should be noted that the review included studies dating back to the 1970s and included a variety of devices.

In more recent studies, the most frequently occurring complication related to SCS is migration of the lead(s) requiring reoperation (3,7,10). This has been reported in up to 43% of patients in various studies (7). Lead migration typically presents as patients who have done well suddenly report that they no longer have coverage in their painful regions. One can take radiographs to compare the current location of the leads to that seen on earlier radiographs. One can try reprogramming the leads to restore coverage. If this does not adequately address the problem, the patient is scheduled for a procedure to reposition the leads. Hopefully, with new developments in the technology, an anchoring system is incorporated into the design that reduces the problem with lead migration, without increasing the risk of injury to the dura or nerve roots.

Several studies have reported that about 10% of patients have the SCS system removed because it has ceased to provide them relief (3,10,19,20). Another study reported a greater rate of removal, at 26% of patients (7). Another problem noted early in a series of patients was the need to relocate the stimulator to a more comfortable position after initially placing it under the patient's belt line (10). In another study the authors reported a 17% incidence of patients reported pain at the receiver implant site (7). A few other miscellaneous complications have been reported, including unpleasant sensations at the lead or generator (5.7%), shorting-out (2.8%), muscle spasm (1.4%), urinary hesitancy (1.4%), and lead fracture (1.4%) (9).

POSTOPERATIVE REHABILITATION

Spinal cord stimulation patients are typically a group who have experienced pain for many months and in most cases several years. During that time, many have undergone and failed surgical intervention. Because of pain, they have significantly reduced their activity level and are typically deconditioned. These patients need to be encouraged to initiate an exercise program. The patients need to start slowly with activities and gently progress. They need to be aware that there may well be a flare up in pain particular related to increased activity. When this occurs, simply reduce activities for a brief time and then more gradually progress.

DISCUSSION

Patients who have failed to gain acceptable pain relief, or who report new severe pain following spine surgery represent a difficult to treat patient population. In patient with well-defined pain origins such as pseudoarthrosis, neural compression, recurrent disc herniation, adjacent segment breakdown, or instability, further traditional surgery may be indicated and many surgeons are comfortable addressing these problems. However, patients in whom pain is related to arachnoiditis, scarring around the nerve roots, or in whom the source of symptoms is not well defined represent a very difficult to treat population. In either group of FBSS patients, on must be acutely aware of the potential for psychological problems in this group of patients. This may be part of the reason for the initial failed surgery or may have developed after failing one or more surgeries.

In the early use of SCS, there was a tendency to use it in patients for whom no other treatment option was available. As discussed, some of the early reported results for SCS were likely compromised because patients were included who were poor psychological risks for an operative intervention. As with spine surgery in chronic pain patients in general, there has been a growing appreciation for the importance of psychological screening for SCS patients. Also, results of some of these earlier studies were compromised because the leads were placed with the patient anesthetized. Unless the patient is awake, there is no way to determine if the lead is positioned to provide optimal pain relief.

In recent years, several studies have indicated that the role of SCS is expanding in the treatment of FBSS patients. Traditionally, it was reserved for patients with primary complaints of lower extremity pain and for those who were not considered candidates for traditional spine surgery intervention. Advances in stimulator technology have now broadened the use for FBSS patients with primary complaints of low back pain rather than axial pain. Two recent studies have reported good results for this application (3,18). Based on the randomized study by North et al., it appears that SCS is a viable alternative to traditional reoperation in FBSS patients (13). More studies on this application are warranted. Spinal cord stimulation may provide a treatment to allow patients to avoid more invasive traditional intervention and may be a viable option for patients who are otherwise poor operative candidates owing to general health problems. However, as with other spine surgery procedures, one should not pursue using SCS simply because the surgeon feels obligated to do something.

Surgeons and patients must understand that the treatment of SCS patients is an ongoing process. The leads

may need to be repositioned, the system may need reprogramming, implanted batteries need to be replaced, there may be fluctuation in pain that needs attention, and pain medication needs to be refilled.

As with many spine surgery procedures, the reported results of SCS vary. Overall, the results of SCS have been good, particularly considering the population being treated. Several studies defined success as 50% or greater pain relief. This is a more stringent criterion than used in many studies dealing with other forms of operative intervention for back pain. In the study by Ohnmeiss et al. (10) based on the VAS, only 26% of patients met this rigid criterion at the 24-month follow-up. However, even in the worst-case analysis 70% of patients reported benefit from the procedure and would have it again for the same result. Also in that study, patients reduced narcotic use and significantly improved lower extremity function and maintained these improvements throughout the 24-month follow-up period.

As seen in this review of some of the SCS literature, the results generally have improved over time. This is likely because of improvements in the technology, better definition of selection criteria, and improved operative technique using fluoroscopic imaging to check lead placement and performing the procedure with the patient awake and able to provide feedback concerning pain relief with various lead placements and device settings. The development of SCS technology will continue. The primary problem with SCS systems is migration of the leads. Hopefully, new developments in the design of the leads will address this problem. Based on the literature, it appears that the role of SCS is increasing to include patients with primary complaints of back pain. Of importance, based of the work of North et al., SCS appears to have a role in a broad spectrum of FBSS patients. Further investigation is needed to confirm its efficacious role in FBSS rather than performing traditional surgery. Spinal cord stimulation can be an effective treatment for many patients with chronic pain. However, physicians using this treatment must be carefully trained in patient selection, operative technique, and dealing with the long-term treatment of these chronic pain patients.

REFERENCES

1. Melzack R, Wall PD. Pain mechanisms: a new theory. Science 1965; 150:971–979.
2. Shealy CN, Mortimer JT, Reswick JB. Electrical inhibition of pain by stimulation of the dorsal columns: preliminary clinical report. Anesth Analg 1967;46:489–491.
3. Ohnmeiss DD, Rashbaum RF. Patient satisfaction with spinal cord stimulation in the treatment of predominant complaints of chronic, intractable low back pain. Spine J 2001;1:358–363.
4. Long DM, Erickson DE. Stimulation of the posterior columns of the spinal cord for relief of intractable pain. Surg Neurol 1975;4:134–143.
5. Racz GB, McCarron RF, Talboys P. Percutaneous dorsal column stimulator for chronic pain control. Spine 1989;14:1–4.
6. Devulder J, de Colvenaer L, Rolly G, et al. Spinal cord stimulation in chronic pain therapy. Clin J Pain 1990;6:51–56.

7. LeDoux MS, Langford KH. Spinal cord stimulation for the failed back syndrome. Spine 1993;18:191–194.
8. North RB, Kidd DH, Zahurek M, et al. Spinal cord stimulation for chronic, intractable pain: Experience over two decades. Neurosurgery 1993;32:384–395.
9. Burchiel KJ, Anderson VC, Brown FD, et al. Prospective, multicenter study of spinal cord stimulation for relief of chronic back and leg pain. Spine 1996;21:2786–2794.
10. Ohnmeiss DD, Rashbaum RF, Bogdanffy GM. Prospective outcome evaluation of spinal cord stimulation in patients with intractable leg pain. Spine 1996;21:1344–1350.
11. North RB, Campbell JN, James CS, et al. Failed back surgery syndrome: 5-year follow-up in 102 patients undergoing repeated operation. Neurosurgery 1991;28:685–690.
12. Turner JA, Loeser JD, Bell KG. Spinal cord stimulation for chronic low back pain: a systematic literature synthesis. Neurosurgery 1995;37:1088–1096.
13. North RB, Kidd DH, Lee MS, et al. A prospective, randomized study of spinal cord stimulation versus reoperation for failed back surgery syndrome: initial results. Stereotact Funct Neurosurg 1994;62:267–272.
14. de la Porte C, Siegfried J. Lumbosacral spinal fibrosis (spinal arachnoiditis). Its diagnosis and treatment by spinal cord stimulation. Spine 1983;8:593–603.
15. Fiume D, Sherkat S, Callovini GM, et al. Treatment of the failed back surgery syndrome due to lumbo-sacral epidural fibrosis. Acta Neurochir Suppl (Wien) 1995;64:116–118.
16. Probst C. Spinal cord stimulation in 112 patients with epi-/intradural fibrosis following operation for lumbar disc herniation. Acta Neurochir (Wein) 1990;107:147–151.
17. Siegfried J, Lazorthes Y. Long-term follow-up of dorsal cord stimulation for chronic pain syndrome after multiple lumbar operations. Appl Neurophysiol 1982;45:201–204.
18. Barolat G, Oakley JC, Law JD, et al. Epidural spinal cord stimulation with a multiple electrode paddle lead is effective in treating intractable low back pain. Neuromodulation 2001;4:59–66.
19. Burchiel KJ, Anderson VC, Wilson BJ, et al. Prognostic factors of spinal cord stimulation for chronic back and leg pain. Neurosurgery 1995;36:1101–1111.
20. de la Porte C, Van de Kelft E. Spinal cord stimulation in failed back surgery syndrome. Pain 1993;52:55–61.

Subject Index

Page numbers followed by f indicate figures; page numbers followed by t indicate tables.

in outcomes assessment, 135–137
Asymptomatic disc herniation, 23–25, 24f–25f, 437–439, 438t
Asymptomatic disc prolapse
  natural history of, 437–438, 438t
Atenolol
  intraoperative hypotension induced by, 205
Athletes
  pars interarticularis fractures in, 579–583
    history and physical examination in, 580
    imaging in, 580–581
    nonoperative treatment of, 581, 582t, 583
    surgical treatment of, 583
  spondylolysis in, 567, 569, 591
Atrophy
  muscle
    in back pain, 430–431
Auriculotherapy
  defined, 160
Australia
  chemonucleolysis results in, 449
Autograft, 249f–250f, 249–251. See also Bone grafting
  advantages of, 249
  allograft combined with, 251–252
  allograft versus, 252
  alternatives to, 75
  ceramic bone graft substitutes versus, 257
  disadvantages of, 250
  in fusion
    in spondylolisthesis, 531, 531f
  indications for, 249
  in osteomyelitis, 746
  results with, 252
  sources of, 249, 249f–250f
  in tumor surgery, 837
Autoimmune reaction
  in nerve root pain
    theories of, 20
Autologous blood transfusion
  preoperative considerations in, 204
  in transpedicular instrumentation, 277
Autologous bone graft. See Autograft
Autologous growth factor
  autologous platelet concentrate and
    as bone graft substitute, 262
Autologous platelet concentrate
  as bone graft substitutes, 262
Axial compression
  compression fractures and, 88
  end plates in, 47, 63
  in spinal instrumentation, 63–64
    artificial disc in, 79, 79f
  testing of
    in disc degeneration, 36–38
Axial skeleton
  in ankylosing spondylitis, 714–715
  in psoriatic arthritis, 706, 706t
Azathioprine
  in psoriatic arthritis, 709

B

Back injury
  disc degeneration as sequela of, 301
Back pain. See also Low back pain
  classification of, 167–168, 168f
    epidemiology and, 4
  epidemiology and economics of, 3–9, 4t–6t, 6f
  in failed surgery
    evaluation of, 839–840
  genetics of, 103–104
  intermittent exacerbations in, 168, 168f
  issue of increasing incidence of, 7–8
  occupational risk factors for, 33–34

in osteosarcoma, 786
prevalence of, 3–4, 4t, 167
  historical, 7–8
  tumor-related, 776–777
Bacterial infection, 739–746, 742f–743f, 745f. See also Pyogenic infection
  in ankylosing spondylitis, 713
  in disc herniation
    asymptomatic, 438, 438t
    postoperative, 770–771
  in reactive arthritis, 693, 694t
Bacteroides
  in postoperative infection, 771
Bagby and Kuslich interbody fusion cage. See BAK interbody fusion device
BAK interbody fusion device, 286, 287f, 289
  complications of, 362–364
  construct testing in, 67–69, 68f, 68t
  Food and Drug Administration status of, 397
  results with, 334, 345, 347
BAK-Proximity cage
  complications of, 363
Ball exercises
  in spondylolysis, 581, 582t
Balloon cannula
  in endoscopic procedures, 240
Balloon insertion
  in kyphoplasty, 91, 677–678, 678f
Barbell cage
  axial compression force in, 63–64
Barium sulfate
  in kyphoplasty, 678
Bath Ankylosing Spondylitis Disease Activity Index, 697–698, 698t
Bath Ankylosing Spondylitis Radiology Index, 719
Beakless owl sign
  in tuberculosis, 763f
Behavioral treatment
  of low back pain, 172–173
Belgium
  recurrent back pain in, 168
  sciatica prevalence in, 7
Bending
  back pain from
    work-related, 180, 180t, 183
  in disc degeneration
    spinal kinematics and, 39–40
  in disc herniation, 403, 403f
  radiographs of
    in low back pain, 55
    in scoliosis, 609
Benign tumor, 781–784
  aneurysmal bone cyst as, 782, 834
  classification of, 776t
  eosinophilic granuloma as, 783
  giant cell tumor as, 782–783, 834
  hemangioma as, 783–784, 834
  location of, 776
  metastatic versus, 778
  osteoblastoma as, 781, 782f, 833–834
  osteochondroma as, 781, 834
  osteoid osteoma as, 781, 833–834
  results of treatment of, 833–834
Bias
  in back pain epidemiology, 3
Bioartificial disc
  in spinal instrumentation, 81–82
Biocoral
  as bone graft substitute, 256
Biofilm
  in tuberculosis surgery, 767
Biomechanical mode
  video-based, 189–190

Biomechanical testing
  of artificial discs, 387–389, 389t
  in disc degeneration, 36–40
    elastic behavior in, 36
    internal disc mechanics in, 37–39, 39f
    spinal kinematics in, 39–40
    viscoelastic behavior in, 36–37
  of spinal instrumentation, 59–70
    animal models in, 70–71
    axial compression force in, 63–64
    cage-related studies in, 67–70, 68f, 68t
    construct testing in, 64f, 64–70, 68f, 68t
    device-vertebra interface in, 60–63, 61f, 61t
    osteoligamentous cadaver models in, 65–67
    overview of, 59–60
    plastic vertebra models in, 64f, 64–65
Biomechanical tolerance
  pain and, 181–185, 184t
    adaptation and, 183
    facet joint limits and, 183
    functional spinal unit limits and, 182–183
    ligament limits and, 183
    pathways between tissue stimulation and, 181–182
    physiologic limits and, 184–185
    psychophysical limits and, 183–184, 184t
Biomechanics
  of disc degeneration, 31–42
    mechanical versus, 35
  testing of. See Biomechanical testing
Biomechanics logic
  in ergonomics, 180–181, 181f
Biopsy
  in fungal infection, 749
  fusion assessment with, 344
  in multiple myeloma, 784
  in osteomyelitis, 742–743
  in tuberculosis, 764
  in tumors, 780–781
    metastatic, 795
Biopsychosocial paradigm
  in proactive low back pain treatment, 169
Bisphosphonates
  in osteopenia prevention, 669
  in Paget disease, 656, 657t, 658f–659f, 659
Blastomyces
  infection with, 750f–751f, 752t
Bleeding
  in lumbosacral procedures, 229–231
  in microscopic discectomy, 459–460
  in posterior fusion, 327, 327f, 329–330
  surgical
    strategies to minimize, 205t, 205–206
Blindness
  from lumbar surgery, 226
  from scoliosis surgery, 624
B-Blockade
  intraoperative hypotension induced by, 205
Blood conservation
  preoperative and perioperative, 204–205
Blood loss
  in spinopelvic fixation, 646
  surgical field and, 205t, 205–206
  in transpedicular instrumentation, 281
  in tumor surgery, 804
Blood supply. See also Vasculature
  end plate, 47
Blood tests. See also specific tests
  in inflammatory spondyloarthropathies, 696, 698
  in metastatic tumors, 793
Blood transfusion
  preoperative considerations in, 204

in nerve root pain, 21–23, 22f
treatment of, 23

D

Dacron
in artificial discs, 387
Dahllite
bone graft substitutes and, 256
Dead bug exercise
in spondylolysis, 581, 582t
Débridement
in epidural abscess, 747
in fungal infection, 749
in postoperative infection, 771–772, 772f
in tuberculosis, 766
Decompression
complications of, 533
in epidural abscess, 747
in failed surgery
treatment of, 844–845
fusion and
in degenerative scoliosis, 271
in degenerative spinal stenosis, 271–272
in degenerative spondylolisthesis,
269–270, 270f, 528–533, 540–546
in osteomyelitis, 744
in scoliosis, 550
fusion and, 551–553, 552f, 554f
in spinal stenosis, 497–499, 498f, 504–505,
505f, 507, 550
in failed surgery, 872–874
fusion and, 551–553, 552f, 554f
in Paget disease, 656
in spondylolisthesis, 524–530, 587–588, 592
fusion and, 269–270, 528–533, 530f–531f,
540–546, 541f–544f
instrumentation and, 540–541
overview of, 524, 526–527
radiographic findings in, 524, 525f
results of, 525–526
slippage after, 526
technique of, 524–525, 526f
in tumor surgery, 803. *See also* specific
procedures
Decubitus position
for lumbar procedures, 222
Deep vein thrombosis prophylaxis
in degenerative spondylolisthesis, 544
Deformation
mechanical
in nerve root pain, 16
Deformity, 604–660. *See also* specific
deformities
in ankylosing spondylitis, 727
artificial disc contraindicated in, 385, 385t
bone cement fracture repair and, 94, 95f
in failed surgery, 897–903, 898f–900f,
902f–903f
instrumentation in, 879–880
in Paget disease, 647
posttraumatic
epidemiology of, 897
in failed surgery, 897–903, 898f–900f,
902f–903f
symptoms of, 897–898, 898f
treatment of, 900–903, 902f–903f
range of, 628
sagittal plane, 628–634, 629f–632f, 634f
scoliosis as. *See* Scoliosis
spinal fusion for, 59
spinopelvic fixation for, 636–646, 637f–646f.
See also Spinopelvic fixation
in spondylolisthesis, 598–599, 599f–601f,
602

surgical approach for, 218
in tuberculosis, 755, 757, 758f–760f,
759–760, 765, 765t
tumor-related, 777
in vertebral compression fracture
kyphoplasty in, 673
Degeneration
adjacent segment. *See* Adjacent segment
degeneration
instability from, 53–54, 54f
Degenerative disc disease. *See also* Disc
degeneration
disc replacement in, 334, 335f, 356–357,
357f–358f. *See also* Artificial disc
complications of, 369–370
end plates in, 46–49
epidemiology of
changing views of, 98
fusion in, 273, 317–322, 324–336, 338–341
cages in, 286–290, 287f, 289f, 342–350,
344f, 346f
complications of, 360–369
as gold standard, 352
minimally invasive, 352–358, 353f–355f–,
353t–354t, 357f–358f
gene therapy in, 107–111, 109f–111f
genetics of, 98, 101–103, 102f
nonoperative treatment of, 342–343
pain in, 342, 353
scoliosis and, 474f, 604–605, 606f, 611
spondylolisthesis and
direct pars repair in, 588
stability in, 338
translaminar screw fixation in, 294
Degenerative scoliosis, 604–605, 605f–606f, 614
fusion in, 270–271
spinopelvic fixation in, 636, 641–643, 646f
Degenerative spondylolisthesis
after spinal fusion, 516, 517f, 521
anatomic features of, 524, 525f
causes of, 514
classification of, 514, 565
clinical presentation of, 519–521, 520f
defined, 514, 535, 558
diagnosis of, 517–519, 518f
differential, 519
fusion in, 269–270, 270f, 353, 353f
imaging in, 517f, 517–518, 524, 525f–526f
ischemic, 518f
low back pain in, 489
lytic *versus*, 482, 485f, 485t
natural history of, 514–517, 515f–517f, 515t
overview of, 514, 524, 535
primary *versus* secondary, 514–515
progression of, 485f
stenosis and
imaging in, 472, 475f, 479, 482,
482f–488f, 485t, 487
prevalence of, 524
recurrent postoperative, 545–546
synovial cysts and
imaging of, 482, 486f–487f
treatment of
anterior fusion in, 535–539, 537t–538t
decompression in, 524–527, 525f–526f
decompression with instrumented fusion
in, 540–546
decompression with posterolateral fusion
in, 528–533
fusion in, 269–270, 270f, 353, 353f
nonoperative, 521–522
options in, 528, 535
surgical indications in, 528–529, 536,
540–541

Degenerative stenosis
defined, 465, 495
fusion in, 271–272
simple, 495
Demineralized bone matrix
as bone graft substitutes, 251, 260
Denervation
radiofrequency
facet joint, 307–311, 309f
Density
apparent
defined, 85
estimates of, 85–87
Depression
in low back pain
work retention and, 175
Developmental stenosis
defined, 495
Device-vertebra interface
in spinal instrumentation, 60–63, 61f, 61t
Diabetes
degenerative spondylolisthesis in, 516
osteomyelitis risk in, 739
in postoperative infection risk, 769
preoperative concerns in, 203
spinal stenosis treatment and, 497
Diabetic neuropathy
spondylolisthesis *versus*, 519
Diagonal transfixation
construct testing and, 66
Diaphragm
anatomy of, 214, 215f
Diathermy
in discectomy, 444
Diffuse idiopathic hyperostosis
psoriatic arthritis *versus*, 707t
Diffuse idiopathic skeletal hyperostosis
spondylolisthesis *versus*, 519
Diffusion
in disc solute transport, 47
Disability
in ankylosing spondylitis, 718
chronic back pain and, 8
comorbidity and, 171
defined, 8
in failed surgery, 861
pain *versus*, 8
performance and, 9
psychosocial factors in, 7, 170–171, 174–175
in sagittal place deformity, 628
specific *versus* nonspecific types in, 168
subjectivity of, 8
in Sweden, 6t, 6–7
in the United States, 5
Disc
anatomy of, 121–122
antibiotic penetration of, 206
artificial
in spinal instrumentation, 77–70, 78f–79f
bioartificial
in spinal instrumentation, 81–82
defined, 121
degeneration of. *See* Degenerative disc
disease; Disc degeneration
disorders of, 299–304. *See also* specific
disorders
degenerative, 300–303, 301t–303t,
302t–303t
nonoperative treatment of, 304, 304t
soft tissue, 299–300, 300t
disruption of
in disc herniation, 428–429
taxonomy for, 303, 303t
herniation of. *See* Disc herniation

osteoporotic
    prevalence of, 665

X

X-Stop distraction system
    in dynamic stabilization, 377, 377f

Y

Yang
    in acupuncture, 159
Yellow flags
    in low back pain evaluation, 170–171, 300,
        300t

Yin
    in acupuncture, 159

Z

Zietek cage
    in spinal instrumentation
        cyclic loading in, 70
Zoledronate
    in osteopenia prevention, 669
    in Paget disease, 657t
Zone classification
    in spinal stenosis, 465
Zone therapy

reflexology as, 158
Zoonosis
    Paget disease as possible,
        648
Z-plate
    in spinal instrumentation
        construct testing in, 65–66
    in tumor surgery, 818, 819f
Zygapophysial joint. *See also*
    Facet joint
    disc function and, 32, 32f
    innervation of, 121f,
        121–123